Donald School

Textbook of Ultrasound in Obstetrics & Gynecology

Donald School
Textbook of Ultrasound in Obstetrics & Gynecology

Fifth Edition

Editors

Asim Kurjak MD PhD
Professor
Department of Obstetrics and Gynecology
Medical School University of Zagreb
Zagreb, Croatia
Professor Emeritus
International University Sarajevo School of Science and Technology
Sarajevo, Bosnia and Herzegovina

Frank A Chervenak MD MMM
Chair, Obstetrics and Gynecology
Lenox Hill Hospital
Hugh RK Barber, MD Chair in Obstetrics and Gynecology
Associate Dean for International Medicine
Zucker School of Medicine at Hofstra/Northwell
New York, USA

JAYPEE

JAYPEE BROTHERS MEDICAL PUBLISHERS
The Health Sciences Publisher
New Delhi | London

Jaypee Brothers Medical Publishers (P) Ltd

Headquarters
Jaypee Brothers Medical Publishers (P) Ltd
EMCA House, 23/23-B
Ansari Road, Daryaganj
New Delhi 110 002, India
Landline: +91-11-23272143, +91-11-23272703
+91-11-23282021, +91-11-23245672
Email: jaypee@jaypeebrothers.com

Corporate Office
Jaypee Brothers Medical Publishers (P) Ltd
4838/24, Ansari Road, Daryaganj
New Delhi 110 002, India
Phone: +91-11-43574357
Fax: +91-11-43574314
Email: jaypee@jaypeebrothers.com

Overseas Office
JP Medical Ltd.
83, Victoria Street, London
SW1H 0HW (UK)
Phone: +44 20 3170 8910
Fax: +44 (0)20 3008 6180
Email: info@jpmedpub.com

Website: www.jaypeebrothers.com
Website: www.jaypeedigital.com

Inquiries for bulk sales may be solicited at: jaypee@jaypeebrothers.com

Donald School Textbook of Ultrasound in Obstetrics & Gynecology

First Edition: 2004
Second Edition: 2008
Third Edition: 2011
Fourth Edition: 2017

Fifth Edition: **2025**

ISBN: 978-93-5696-813-4

Printed at Sanat Printers

Dedicated to

Ian Donald

(Brilliant Visionary, Role Model,

Globalist, Teacher, and Friend)

Contributors

Agnieszka Nocun
Consultant
Gynecology and Oncology Clinic
University Hospital in Krakow
Krakow, Poland

Aida Salihagic Kadic
Professor of Physiology
and Neuroscience
Department of Physiology
Medical School University of Zagreb
Zagreb, Croatia

Ajlana Mulic-Lutvica
Senior Consultant
Department of Obstetrics and
Gynecology
Uppsala University Hospital
Uppsala, Sweden

Alaa Ebrashy
Professor
Department of Obstetrics and Gynecology
Consultant in Fetal Medicine
Cairo University
Cairo, Egypt

Aleksandar Ljubic
Professor
Pronatal Hospital
Belgrade, Serbia
Dubrovnik International University
Libertas, Dubrovnik, Croatia

Alessandra Giocolano
Specialist
Department of Obstetrics and Gynecology
III Obstetrics and Gynecology Unit
University Medical School of Bari
Bari, Italy

Alexandra Matias MD PhD
Full Professor
Department of Obstetrics and Gynecology
Faculty of Medicine University of Porto
Centro Hospitalar Universitário São João
Porto, Portugal

Anna Maroto
Associate Professor
Maternal-Fetal Medicine Department
Hospital Universitari de Girona
Dr Josep Trueta
Universitat de Girona
Girona, Spain

Antonella Cromi
Specialist
Department of Obstetrics and
Gynecology
University Medical School of Insubria
Varese, Italy

Aris J Antsaklis
Professor of Obstetrics and Gynecology
Department of Maternal and Fetal
Medicine
University of Athens
IASO Maternity Hospital
Athens, Greece

Ashok Khurana
Consultant in Reproductive Ultrasound
The Ultrasound Lab
New Delhi, India

Asim Kurjak
Professor
Department of Obstetrics and
Gynecology
Medical School University of Zagreb
Zagreb, Croatia
Professor Emeritus
International University
Sarajevo School of Science and
Technology
Sarajevo, Bosnia and Herzegovina

Autumn Broady
Specialist
Division of Maternal-Fetal Medicine
Department of Obstetrics, Gynecology
and Women's Health
John A Burns School of Medicine
University of Hawaii, Honolulu, USA

Berivoj Miskovic
Professor
Medical School University of Zagreb
Medifem Obs/Gyn Clinic with Day
Surgery
Zagreb, Croatia

Biserka Funduk Kurjak
Professor (Emeritus)
Department of Obstetrics and
Gynecology
Medical School University of Zagreb
Zagreb, Croatia

Carlota Rodó
Specialist
Fetal Medicine Department
Hospital Universitari Vall d'Hebron
Barcelona, Spain

Carmen Comas Gabriel
Chief of Obstetrics Services
Department of Obstetrics and
Gynecology
Hospital Germans Trias i Pujol
Badalona (Barcelona), Spain
Associated Professor in Obstetrics
and Gynecology
Autonomic University of Barcelona

Costin Berceanu
Professor
Department of Obstetrics and
Gynecology
The University of Medicine and
Pharmacy of Craiova
Emergency University Hospital
Craiova, Romania

Eberhard Merz
Professor
Centre for Ultrasound and Prenatal
Medicine
Frankfurt/Main Germany

Edoardo Di Naro
Associate Professor
I Obstetrics and Gynecology Unit
University Medical School of Bari
Bari, Italy

Elena Carreras
Chief
Department of Obstetrics and Gynecology
Hospital Universitari Vall d'Hebron, Barcelona
Professor
Universitat de Vic-Universitat Central de Catalunya
Associate Professor
Universitat Autònoma de Barcelona
Spain

Eva Meler Barrabés
I+D+i Obstetric Clinic
Department of Obstetrics, Gynecology and Reproductive Medicine
University Hospital Quirón Dexeus
Barcelona, Spain

Fernando Bonilla-Musoles
Professor
Department of Obstetrics and Gynecology
University of Valencia, School of Medicine
Valencia, Spain

Francesc Figueras
Specialist
Service of Fetal Medicine
Clinical Institute of Gynecology, Obstetrics and Neonatology
University of Barcelona
Barcelona, Spain

Francisco Bonilla Jr
Specialist
Department of Obstetrics and Gynecology
University of Valencia, School of Medicine
Valencia, Spain

Francisco Raga
Specialist
Department of Obstetrics and Gynecology
University of Valencia, School of Medicine
Valencia, Spain

Frank A Chervenak
Chair, Obstetrics and Gynecology
Lenox Hill Hospital
Hugh RK Barber, MD Chair in Obstetrics and Gynecology
Associate Dean for International Medicine
Zucker School of Medicine at Hofstra/Northwell
New York, USA

Frederico Rocha
Specialist
Division of Maternal-Fetal Medicine
Department of Obstetrics, Gynecology, and Women's Health
John A Burns School of Medicine
University of Hawaii
Honolulu, Hawaii, USA

Gabriella Minneci
Specialist
Department of Obstetrics and Gynecology
Maternal Fetal Medicine Unit
ARNAS Civico Hospital
Palermo, Italy

Geeta Sharma
Specialist in Maternal-Fetal Medicine
New York University School of Medicine
New York, USA

George A Partsinevelos
Specialist
1st Obstetrics-Gynecology Clinic
Medical School, University of Athens
Alexandra Hospital
Athens, Greece

Giovanni Centini
Foundation President
"Danilo Nannini" for Motherhood and Childhood
Santa Maria alle Scotte Hospital
Siena, Italy

Giuseppe Calì
Specialist
Department of Obstetrics and Gynecology
Maternal Fetal Medicine Unit
ARNAS Villa Sofia-Cervello Hospital
Casa di Cura Candela
Palermo, Italy

Grazia Volpe
Specialist
Prenatal Diagnosis and Fetal Surgery Unit
Department of Obstetrics and Gynecology
Medical School, University of Milan
Milan, Italy

Helena Dukić
Affiliate Lecturer
Academy of Music
University of Zagreb
Zagreb, Croatia

Ivica Zalud
Professor and Chair
Kosasa Endowed Chair
Department of Obstetrics, Gynecology and Women's Health
John A Burns School of Medicine
University of Hawaii
Honolulu, Hawaii, USA

Jaideep Malhotra
Professor
Managing Director
ART Rainbow IVF
Agra, Uttar Pradesh, India

Jiri Sonek
Specialist
Department of Obstetrics and Gynecology
Wright State University
President
Fetal Medicine Foundation of the USA
Dayton, Ohio, USA

Jon Hyett
Professor
Department of Obstetrics and Gynecology
Western Sydney University
Head of Maternal and Fetal Medicine
Liverpool Hospital
Sydney NSW Australia

José M Carrera
President
Matres Mundi
Barcelona, Spain

Juan Carlos Castillo
Specialist
Department of Obstetrics and Gynecology
University of Valencia, School of Medicine
Valencia, Spain

Juan Luis Alcázar
Professor
Department of Obstetrics and Gynecology
Hospital Quirónsalud Málaga
Málaga, Spain

Judith L Chervenak
Professor
Department of Obstetrics and Gynecology
New York University School of Medicine
New York, USA

Jure Knez
Specialist
Clinic for Gynecology and Perinatology
Maribor University Medical Centre
Maribor, Slovenia

Kazunori Baba
Professor
Center for Maternal, Fetal and Neonatal Medicine
Saitama Medical Center, Saitama Medical University
Saitama, Japan

Kazuo Maeda
Professor (Emeritus)
Department of Obstetrics and Gynecology
Tottori University Medical School
Yonago, Japan

Kohei Shiota
Professor
Department of Anatomy and Developmental Biology
Congenital Anomaly Research Center
Kyoto University Graduate School of Medicine
Kyoto, Japan

Lucia Rosignoli
Specialist
Prenatal Diagnosis Unit
University Hospital Meyer
Florence, Italy

Luigi Raio
Specialist
Department of Obstetrics and Gynecology
University of Bern
Bern, Switzerland

Maja Predojevic
Specialist
Department of Obstetrics and Gynecology
Medical School, University of Zagreb
Clinical Hospital "Sveti Duh"
Zagreb, Croatia

Marcin Wiechec
Consultant
Fetal Anomalies and Ultrasound
Coordinator, Interclinical Ultrasound Lab
Chair, Gynecology and Obstetrics
Jagiellonian University in Krakow
Krakow, Poland

Miguel Pereira-Macedo
Resident Physician
Centro Hospitalar Universitário Lisboa Norte
Lisbon, Portugal

Milan Stanojevic
Professor
Department of Obstetrics and Gynecology
Medical School University of Zagreb
Neonatal Unit
University Hospital Sveti Duh
Zagreb, Croatia

Mohamed Ahmed Mostafa AboEllail
Specialist
Department of Obstetrics and Gynecology
Faculty of Medicine
Sohag University
Sohag, Egypt

Narendra Malhotra
Professor
Managing Director
Global Rainbow Healthcare
(Ujala-Cygnus-Rainbow Hospital)
Director, ART Rainbow IVF
Director, FOGSI SMRITI Manyata CSE
Agra, Uttar Pradesh, India

Neharika Malhotra Bora
Director
Malhotra Nursing and Maternity Home (P) Ltd
Director, Rainbow IVF
Agra, Uttar Pradesh, India

(Late) Nuno Montenegro
Professor
Porto Medical Faculty of Medicine
Department of Obstetrics and Gynecology
Hospital of S João
Porto, Portugal

Oliver Vasilj
Specialist
University North Department
Medifem Ob-Gyn Clinic with Day Surgery
Zagreb, Croatia

Oscar Caballero
Specialist
Department of Obstetrics and Gynecology
University of Valencia, School of Medicine
Valencia, Spain

Panagiotis Antsaklis
Assistant Professor
1st Obstetrics-Gynecology Clinic
Medical School, University of Athens
Alexandra Hospital
Athens, Greece

Radu Vlădăreanu
Professor and Chairman
Department of Obstetrics and Gynecology
Carol Davila University of Medicine and Pharmacy
Elias University Hospital
Bucharest, Romania

Ritsuko K Pooh
Professor and Director
Fetal Diagnostic Center/
Fetal Brain Center
CRIFM Prenatal Medical Clinic
Osaka, Japan

Robin B Kalish
Specialist
Division of Maternal-Fetal Medicine
Department of Obstetrics and Gynecology
Weill Medical College of Cornell University
New York, USA

Sanja Kupesic Plavsic
Professor Emerita
Department of Obstetrics and Gynecology
Paul L Foster School of Medicine
Texas Tech University Health Sciences Center
El Paso, Texas, USA

Sonal Panchal
Ultrasound Consultant
Dr Nagori's Institute for Infertility and IVF
Ahmedabad, Gujarat, India

Sonila Pashaj
Specialist
Centre for Ultrasound and Prenatal Medicine
Frankfurt/Main, Germany

Stephen T Chasen
Specialist
Weill Medical College of Cornell University
New York, USA

Takahito Miyake
President
Department of Obstetrics and Gynecology
Miyake Clinic
Ofuku, Okayama, Japan
Clinical Professor
Department of Perinatology and Gynecology
Kagawa University Graduate School of Medicine
Miki, Kagawa, Japan

Tamara Illescas
Specialist
Department of Obstetrics and Gynecology
Hospital Universitario La Paz
Madrid, Spain

Tatjana Bozanovic
Specialist
School of Medicine
Belgrade University
Institute for Obstetrics and Gynecology
Clinical Center of Serbia
Belgrade, Serbia

Toshiyuki Hata
Special Adviser
Department of Obstetrics and Gynecology
Miyake Clinic
Ofuku, Okayama, Japan
Professor Emeritus
Department of Perinatology and Gynecology
Kagawa University Graduate School of Medicine
Miki, Kagawa, Japan

Tuangsit Wataganara
Associate Professor
Division of Maternal-Fetal Medicine
Department of Obstetrics and Gynecology
Faculty of Medicine
Siriraj Hospital
Bangkok, Thailand

Ulla Marton
Specialist
Department of Obstetrics and Gynecology
Polyclinic Dr Marton
Zagreb, Croatia

Ulrich Honemeyer
Consultant (Obstetrics, Gynecology and Fetal Medicine)
King's College Hospital, Dubai
NMC Royal Hospital
Sharjah, UAE

Veljko Vlaisavljevic
Professor
IVF Adria consulting d.o.o.
Maribor, Slovenia

Vincenzo D'Addario
Professor
Department of Obstetrics and Gynecology
Medical School University of Bari
Bari, Italy

Waldo Sepulveda
Professor
Director
FETALMED—Maternal-Fetal Diagnostic Center
University of Santiago de Chile (USACH)
Santiago, Chile

William Goh
Clinical Instructor
Department of Obstetrics, Gynecology and Women's Health
John A Burns School of Medicine
University of Hawai'i at Mānoa
Honolulu, Hawaii, USA

Yasunari Miyagi
Director
Department of Gynecology
Miyake Ofuku Clinic
Ofuku, Okayama, Japan
Representative
Medical Data Labo
Yamasaki, Okayama, Japan

Zoltán Papp
Professor
Semmelweis University
Maternity Private Clinic of Obstetrics and Gynecology
Budapest, Hungary

Zoltán Tóth
Professor
Department of Obstetrics and Gynecology
Debrecen University
Debrecen, Hungary

Preface to the Fifth Edition

The Ian Donald International School of Ultrasound bears testament to globalization in its most successful and worthwhile form. The school was founded in Dubrovnik in 1981. In the Preface of the First Edition in 2004, we were proud to announce that the school had grown to 8 branches. Since then, the growth has been meteoric and now consists of 129 branches in almost every corner of the globe. The reason for this success has been the tireless and selfless efforts of the world's leading authorities in ultrasound who are willing to dedicate their valuable time without reimbursement to teach sonologists and sonographers throughout the world. Our teachers put national, religious, political, and other parochial considerations aside as they strive to improve the care of all women and fetal patients. Politicians in the countries represented by our school have much to learn from the purity of spirit that exists throughout our international family. We believe that Ian Donald is smiling down from heaven at the school that bears his name.

In the educational efforts of the 129 branches of the Ian Donald School, there is clearly a need for a textbook to complement and supplement lectures and didactic sessions. The first, second, third, and fourth textbooks were successful in this endeavor, but with the explosion of knowledge, it was clear that an expanded and updated fifth edition would be invaluable. The current edition illustrates the latest developments Silhouette ultrasound and four-dimensional ultrasound which have been pioneered by our school. For the sake of simplicity, our book is divided into three sections. *Section 1* deals with a variety of topics that lay the foundation for the rest of the book. *Section 2* addresses the myriad subtopics in obstetric ultrasound that optimize the care of pregnant women and fetal patients. The last section addresses the essential role that ultrasound plays in many dimensions of clinical gynecology.

A special word of thanks to Jadranka, our tireless secretary, for her hundreds of dedicated hours of quality work.

We are grateful to many course Directors and Lecturers of the Ian Donald School who have enabled its growth and have selflessly contributed to this volume. In order to maximize the reach of this textbook by minimizing its price, all contributors have waived any honorarium or royalty. Their dedication to the dream of globalized quality ultrasound has enabled its reality.

Asim Kurjak
Frank A Chervenak

Preface to the First Edition

Ultrasound is the backbone of modern obstetrics and gynecology practice. For those of us old enough to remember the dark ages of clinical practice prior to ultrasound, this is not an overstatement. Younger physicians may find it hard to imagine the clinical realities of doctors who delivered undiagnosed twins presenting at delivery, who performed unnecessary surgeries for the clinical suspicion of a pelvic mass that was not present, and who consoled anguished parents when an anomalous infant was born unexpectedly. Recent technological breakthroughs in diagnostic ultrasound, including the advent of color Doppler, power Doppler, three-dimensional and four-dimensional imaging, have led ultrasound to surpass the expectations of Ian Donald, its visionary father.

The Ian Donald School was founded in 1981 and is devoted to international education and research cooperation concerning all aspects of diagnostic ultrasound. The first chapter was founded in Dubrovnik at that time and has now expanded to 7 additional national branches.

To facilitate the educational efforts of the Ian Donald School, we believed a textbook would be of value. The text is divided into three parts general aspects, obstetrics, and gynecology. All contributors are either present or former teachers in the 8 branches of the Ian Donald School. We believe this comprehensive text with state-of-the-art images will be of value for both new learners and experienced practitioners.

We are grateful to all of the teachers in the school and especially to all of the contributors to this textbook for their tireless efforts to enhance the quality of ultrasound practice throughout the world.

Asim Kurjak
Frank A Chervenak

Acknowledgments

The editors are indebted to the selfless members of the Ian Donald School who contribute their time and efforts without honorarium as do all contributors to this volume in the relentless pursuit of improving care of maternal, fetal, and neonatal patients throughout the world.

We are especially indebted to the indefatigable Jadranka Cerovec—the keystone of our Ian Donald educational efforts.

Contents

SECTION 1: General Aspects

SECTION 2: Obstetrics

SECTION 1

General Aspects

CHAPTER 1

Safety of Ultrasound in Obstetrics and Gynecology

Kazuo Maeda

INTRODUCTION

Although no adverse effects of ultrasound diagnosis have been reported, bioeffect and safety issues have been studied and discussed by various medical ultrasound organizations.[1-9] It is emphasized that, for safe use, ultrasonic examinations are only performed when medically indicated. Secondly, the users are responsible for safety and should recognize that biological tissues of developing embryos and fetuses may be damaged by intense ultrasound.[6] The main biological effect is the thermal effect due to the temperature rise induced by ultrasound absorption, because teratogenicity was reported in fetal animals exposed to high temperature.[2] Non-thermal effects of ultrasound are inertial cavitation and other mechanical effects. Diagnostic ultrasound users are requested to know the ultrasonic intensity of their devices, the mechanisms of ultrasound bioeffects and prudent use of their ultrasound devices. No hazardous thermal effects are expected when the temperature rise in exposed tissue is less than 1.5°C and local temperature is lower than 38.5°C,[1] the fetus was tolerable to 50 hours exposure up to 2°C rise,[5] while 5 minutes at 41°C can be hazardous to the tissue.[1] No hazardous thermal effects are expected in simple B-mode imaging devices because there is minimum heat production due to low ultrasound intensity. World Federation of Ultrasound in Medicine and Biology (WFUMB) concluded that the use of simple imaging equipment is not contraindicated on thermal grounds.[1] Simple transvaginal B-mode, simple three-dimensional (3D) and four-dimensional (4D) imaging are included in this category. The International Society of Ultrasound in Obstetrics and Gynecology (ISUOG) also stated the safe use of Doppler ultrasound.[7] More practical plans on the safe use of Doppler ultrasound from the user's view is discussed in this chapter. Direct subject heating with transvaginal transducer is avoided where the transducer is lower than 41°C.

Thermal index: 1.0 thermal index (TI) is the ultrasound power to rise the temperature of exposed tissue for one degree centigrade. Soft tissue TI (TIs) is lower than bone TI (TIb) and transcranial TI (Tic). TIb is used in the safety of ultrasound, where the TI less than 1.0 is safe. Mechanical effect of ultrasound is expressed by mechanical index (MI), where MI is rarefactional pressure (Megapascal, Pr) divided by the square root of ultrasound frequency (Megahertz, MHz). Obstetric diagnostic devices are set at ultrasonic intensity lower than 1.0 TI and lower than 1.0 MI. Output intensity of simple B mode equipment was regulated below SPTA 10 mW/cm^2 in 1980 by Japanese Industrial Standard (JIS), where the level was 1/24 of non-hazardous threshold of ultrasound, which is SPTA 240 mW/cm^2, and it was the results of our experimental study.[11] Ultrasound of Doppler flow velocity measurements, color and power Doppler mappings are set at the level lower than 1.0 TI and 1.0 MI.

Recent two studies[12,18] reported hazardous ultrasound effect, however, the effects are doubted, because the effects could not be expected because ultrasound intensity was lower than 240 mW/cm^2 but can be resulted by the heating with attached ultrasound probes. As the increase of hepatic apoptosis of animal fetus by Doppler ultrasound was reported,[19] ISUOG[21] regulated the use of Doppler ultrasound in early pregnancy.

DIAGNOSTIC ULTRASOUND DEVICES AND ULTRASOUND INTENSITY

Ultrasonic imaging devices and Doppler blood flow studies utilize pulsed wave (PW) ultrasound, while continuous wave (CW) ultrasound is applied in fetal functional tests **(Table 1)**.

TABLE 1: Diagnostic ultrasound.

Index	***Mortality/1,000 live births***
Pulsed wave (PW) for imaging and blood flow studies	Continuous wave (CW) for the functional tests
B-mode imaging, 3D/4D ultrasound, pulsed Doppler flow velocity wave, Color/power flow mapping	Fetal heart Doppler detector, fetal heart rate tracing, fetal movement record (actocardiogram), CW Doppler flow velocity wave
• High peak intensity and low temporal average intensity in simple B-mode and 3D/4D ultrasound • High peak and average intensities in pulsed Doppler flow velocity wave • High peak intensity and medium average intensity in color/power Doppler flow mapping	Low peak and average intensities

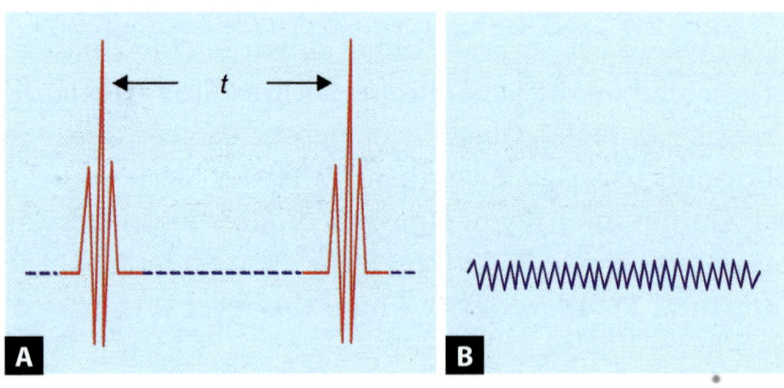

Figs. 1A and B: Two types of diagnostic ultrasound waves. (A) Pulse wave (PW) for the imaging and Doppler: 1/t is repetition frequency; (B) Continuous wave (CW) for fetal functional studies in fetal heart detector.

The ultrasound intensity differs between PW and CW devices **(Figs. 1A and B)**, i.e., temporal peak intensity is large in PW and weak in CW ultrasound, while temporal average intensities are nearly the same to temporal peak of CW.

NON-HAZARDOUS EXPOSURE TIME OF THE FETUS TO THE HEAT

The revised safety statement on diagnostic ultrasound of American Institute of Ultrasound in Medicine (AIUM)[5] published in 1998, is based on the NCRP report[2] in 1992, where inverse relation is found between hazardous temperature level and exposure time. They stated that the fetus tolerated 1 minutes at 6°C temperature rise (absolute temperature is 43°C). They showed the relation of the temperature rise above 37°C and the non-hazardous exposure time was 1,000 minutes if the temperature rise was 1°C.[2]

DIAGNOSTIC ULTRASOUND INSTRUMENTS AND ULTRASOUND INTENSITY

Ultrasonic imaging devices and Doppler blood flow studies utilize pulse wave (PW) ultrasound, while continuous wave (CW) ultrasound is applied in fetal functional tests **(Table 1)**. The ultrasound intensity differs between PW and CW machines **(Figs. 1A and B)**, i.e., temporal peak intensity is large in PW and weak in CW ultrasound, while temporal average intensity is almost identical in simple PW B-mode imaging device and CW machines **(Table 1)**. However, pulsed Doppler flow velocity measurement tends to use high peak and average intensity due to its long pulse and high repetition frequency **(Figs. 1A and B)**. The temporal average intensity of color and power Doppler flow mapping is lower than pulsed Doppler but tends to be higher than simple B-mode machine. Ultrasound intensity is usually represented by spatial peak (SP) temporal average (TA) intensity, i.e., by SPTA intensity, e.g., cultured cell growth curve was not injured, if ultrasound intensity was lower than SPTA 240 mW/cm^2 in our experiment.[11]

ULTRASOUND INTENSITY OF DOPPLER ULTRASOUND

The maximum intensity of adult Doppler ultrasound was 1–3 W/cm^2, which was as high as the ultrasonic physiotherapy with the tissue heating, where young patient's bone and pregnant women were contraindicated from the concern on ultrasound effect. The difference between therapeutic ultrasound and pulsed Doppler device was the exposure duration, which was shorter in Doppler ultrasound. Temperature rises not only at the sample volume but also in all tissues passed by the Doppler ultrasound beam. Ultrasound intensity is lower in color/power Doppler flow mapping than pulsed Doppler flow wave because of scanning ultrasound beam in the region of interest (ROI) of flow mapping. Ultrasound intensity of color Doppler is lower than pulsed Doppler and within the limit of nonhazard waves FDA intensity, which was 720 mW/cm^2. Thermal effect was discussed firstly in pulsed Doppler, where the safety was determined by ultrasound intensity and exposure duration, where thermal index and mechanical index <1.0 is safe in the use of Doppler ultrasound.

THE EFFECT OF DIRECT HEATING ON MAMMAL FETUSES

The presence of teratogenicity was reported by biologists in the direct exposure of mammal animal embryos and fetuses to experimental high temperature of 39–50°C in various mammals, avoiding the heating of pregnant small animals, to eliminate the influence of maternal animal reaction to the heat. The results were fetal animal head and neck anomalies,[2] where a discriminal line clearly separated hazardous and non-hazardous areas. Non-hazardous exposure time was as short as 1 minute in 43°C and infinite in physiological body temperature, 37°C. Ultrasound intensity is very low to be regulated in autocorrelation fetal heart rate meter, actocardiography and CW ultrasound Doppler devices.

THE ULTRASOUND INTENSITY OF NO BIOEFFECT

The effect of ultrasound exposure was studied using JTC-3 human amniotic cell origin cultured cell strain. Our experiments aimed the suppression of cultured cell growth curves with CW and PW ultrasound, in the study group of Japan, Ministry of Health and Welfare in 1973–1975, where the exposure experiment was performed avoiding the heat of ultrasound probe by inserting at 37°C stabilized water between the probe and exposure subjects.

The cultured cell growth curve was suppressed by exposure to PW ultrasound at 2 MHz SPTA 240 or more mW/cm^2, 3 μs pulse duration and 1 kHz repetition PW ultrasound, and 2 MHz, 1,000 or more mW/cm^2 CW ultrasound. No suppression was detected when the ultrasound intensity was lower than 240 mW/cm^2 in PW and 1,000 mW/cm^2 in CW.

Official bioeffect threshold to suppress the cultured cells was 240 mW/cm^2, where ultrasound intensity was determined by the manufacturer's data and furthermore by our steel-ball moving method. Exposure duration was 30–60 minutes.

The 1.0 TI intensity was determined deducting standard propagation attenuation and standard perfusion from the threshold intensity, and the 1.0 TI intensity was around SPTA 210 mW/cm^2.

The most important conclusion on the results of or experiments is "the ultrasound is totally safe, if its intensity is lower than SPTA 240 mW/cm^2 or lower than 1.0 TI", namely, the safety of diagnostic ultrasound was objectively established, where no ultrasound bioeffect was recognized when the intensity was lower than SPTA 240 mW/cm^2.

"ALARA" PRINCIPLE

The output intensity of commercial diagnostic ultrasound devices were regulated to be lower than 10 mW/cm^2 by the Japan Industrial Standard (JIS) in 1982, which was about 1/20 of 1.0 TI intensity, therefore, the ultrasound safety of diagnostic ultrasound device was established in Japan, while international ultrasound safety is kept when obstetrical setting is lower than 1.0 in TI and MI. However, Sande et al.[21] reported useful Doppler flow wave was obtained using 0.1 TI pulsed ultrasound, which was 1/10 of 1.0 TI, equal to about 20 mW/cm^2, and close to JIS regulation. The ultrasound intensity of Doppler actocardiogram, invented by the author, was only 1 mW/cm^2 in its TOITU commercial model.

ALARA (As Low AS Reasonably Achievable) principle, which is another principle of diagnostic ultrasound safety, that is further reduction of ultrasound intensity below 1.0 TI, getting sufficient clinical results even in Doppler study with the intensity lower than 1.0 TI.

Low TI will be determined correctly using TI measurement device provided by ISUOG.

ABSOLUTE TEMPERATURE OF THE TISSUE EXPOSED TO ULTRASOUND

Absolute tissue temperature is determined by the addition of temperature rise estimated by TI to 37°C, e.g., absolute temperature is 38°C, when TI is 1, and 39°C when TI is 2. TI is an useful value for various purposes.

THERMAL AND MECHANICAL SAFETIES OF DIAGNOSTIC ULTRASOUND BY USING THERMAL AND MECHANICAL INDICES

The thermal safety of ultrasound is shown by the thermal index, which is theoretically equal to temperature rise due to ultrasound absorption of the subject tissue.

Although electrical and structural safeties of diagnostic ultrasound devices are proved by the manufacturer, the device user is responsible to the ultrasound safety,[3] studying physics of medical ultrasound, mechanism of ultrasound images, ultrasound output intensity of user devices, thermal and mechanical indices, the threshold output intensity to develop bioeffect, how to reduce ultrasound device output intensity, non-medical use of ultrasonic imaging, regulation of ultrasound use in early pregnancy, etc., related diagnostic ultrasound safety. This is particularly important in obstetric application of ultrasound.

Thermal effect of ultrasound appears along with the temperature elevation due to the absorption of ultrasound by the tissue, where immature fetal tissues are sensitive to high temperature, and thermal teratogenicity or embryonal cell damage can be concerned in some occasions. Mechanical effect of ultrasound is cavitation, which is production and rupture of microbubbles in the liquid developing high temperature, strong pressure and free radical formation. Neonatal animal lung develops hemorrhage by the cavitation. Negative pressure of ultrasound pulse is related cavitation, while positive pressure, streaming and static wave were not discussed in the mechanical effect of ultrasound.

THERMAL SAFETY OF ULTRASOUND

As direct heating of animal fetus developed head and neck anomaly in biological experiment,[2] 1°C temperature rise was selected to set an objective index, which avoid excess exposure in clinical ultrasound, i.e., the thermal index was prepared. TI is set below 1.0 for the thermal safety of ultrasound devices. 1.0 TI produces 1°C temperature rise of subject tissue, which will be less than SPTA 240 mW/cm^2 which is the lowest intensity to suppress cultured cell growth. Any ultrasound device output is controlled to safe condition, if the output is less than 1.0 TI, preventing excess heating.

The thermal index, mechanical index, and other values related ultrasound safety are displayed on the monitor screen,[3] making the users to keep the safe ultrasound diagnosis. Obstetric setting should be confirmed before ultrasound imaging and Doppler studies in pregnancy to keep the safety of ultrasound. Although ISUOG safety statement[7] reported that there is no reason to withhold the use of scanners that have received FDA clearance, AIUM[5] stated that in the FDA regulatory limit at 720 mW/cm^2, the maximum temperature rise can exceed 2°C. As ultrasound intensity to suppress cultured cell-growth was 240 or more mW/cm^2 in our studies,[11] the FDA regulation intensity would not be accepted from the safety reasons.

Thermal Index to Prevent Thermal Effect of Ultrasound Exposure

Thermal index is a useful index to know the temperature rise by ultrasound exposure. Ultrasound intensity is estimated by the subject temperature rise due to ultrasound absorption under standard ultrasound attenuation and perfusion, where TI is 1.0, when the temperature rises 1°C above 37°C and absolute temperature is 38°C, while TI is 3.0 when temperature rises for 3°C and absolute temperature is 40°C, i.e., TI represents the ultrasound intensity to rise subject temperature for TI °C above 37°C. Since the subject temperature rises due to the absorption of ultrasound, TIs, soft tissue TI, is low and TIb of bone and TIc of cranium are higher than TIs. TIb is used to estimate ultrasound bioeffect, while TIs is applied embryo of no bone before 10 weeks of pregnancy, whereas bone TIb is applied in the fetus with bone.

No hazardous thermal effect is expected when the temperature rise of exposed tissue is less than 1.0°C and an ultrasound examination is safe when the TI is less than 1.0 in daily practice, particularly in the screening of pregnancy and research works. The output power is reduced until the TI is lower 1.0, if the displayed TI is 1.0 or more, though revised safety statement AIUM[5] stated that equal or less than 2°C temperature rise above 37°C was tolerated by the fetus for short time.

Other Thermal Issues

Caution should be paid for the temperature of the tissue exposed to Doppler ultrasound in febrile patients, where the basic temperature is higher than 37°C. If ultrasound TI is 2 in 38°C febrile patient, the temperature rise above physiologic condition is 3°C, the situation corresponds to TI 3 in nonfebrile normal temperature case, therefore, ultrasound study will be contraindicated until the recovery of febrile condition.

Thermal effect of transvaginal ultrasound was discussed, and the surface temperature of transvaginal probe was regulated to be lower than 41°C.

Analysis of Ultrasonic Fetal Brain Damage Reports

Ang et al.[12] reported the delay of neural cell migration after exposure to real time B-mode ultrasound for more than 30 minutes attaching ultrasound probe to the pregnant mice.

Ultrasound intensity maybe around SPTA 2 mW/cm^2. Ping et al.[17] exposed pregnant rats to 106 mW/cm^2 ultrasound for 60 minutes in total, and found the damage of learning and memory function and hippocampus in 2 month' infants.

They reported the damage was caused by ultrasound. However, the conclusion would be controversy, because their ultrasound intensity were lower than 240 mW/cm^2, by which no bioeffect of ultrasound was expected, and suggest the presence of the other cause.

There may be difference in the effects of two reports, if it is ultrasound effect, because ultrasound intensity was 50 times larger in Ping et al., but actually the effect was the same brain neuronal damage. The effects would be caused by the heat of ultrasound probe, because the probe suspectedly heated for 41 or more °C was attached pregnant small animal for 30–60 minutes, that may be enough to warm up small animal. Direct heating effect in NCRP report was head anomaly which suggested fetal brain neuronal damage by heating in their experiments. The experiments are recommended to repeat cutting off the heat of ultrasound probe, as we did in the exposure of cultured cells to detect ultrasound intensity to suppress the cultured ell growth curve. The recommendation is based on the experience in our study group in 1970s, namely, mouse fetuses did not develop anomaly by the ultrasound exposure to pregnant mice when animals were isolated from heated ultrasound probe by the 37°C thermostat water inserted between the probe and pregnant mice, while the fetuses developed head anomaly after the heating of pregnant mice with directly attached ultrasound probe at the abdomen of pregnant mice in a Japanese report in 1972.

MECHANICAL INDEX OF ULTRASOUND

Mechanical effect of ultrasound is prevented setting mechanical index lower than 1.0, even in Doppler ultrasound in obstetrical setting, because high MI ultrasound produced pulmonary hemorrhage of animal neonate. The MI is determined by rarefactional pressure (negative pressure) of the pulse wave (Megapascal)/ Square root of ultrasound frequency (Megahertz). Low MI prevents the development of cavitation, which is caused by the rupture of micro-bubbles produced by intense ultrasound, and characterized by high temperature, high pressure and free radical formation. There will be furthermore the microstreaming and blood cell stasis due to standing wave, of which bioeffects have not been reported.

SAFETY OF DIAGNOSTIC ULTRASOUND DEVICES

1. *Simple abdominal scan B-mode imaging device:* Simple B-mode imaging is not concerned for the thermal effect, because of its very low output intensity, e.g., the output of B-mode machine is regulated in Japan[10] to be lower than SPTA 10 mW/cm^2. In addition, either TI or MI should be lower than 1.0. Associated use of Doppler ultrasound should be controlled by the regulation listed in the chapter of Doppler Ultrasound, particularly the use in early pregnancy should be regulated by the opinion of ISUOG.[21]
2. *Transvaginal scan ultrasound:* Its use is the same as abdominal scan. Only difference is the regulation of transvaginal scan probe temperature, which should be lower than 41°C.
3. *Three-dimensional (3D) ultrasound:* As the 3D ultrasound image is obtained by multiple simple B-mode scan in a few seconds, it is as safe as simple B-mode, of which TI and MI are less than 1.0. It is regulated when Doppler ultrasound is associated.
4. *Four-dimensional (4D) ultrasound:* As the 4D ultrasound is the repetition of 3D ultrasound, basically 4D is as safe as simple B-mode ultrasound, however, fetal 4D image observation is recommended to be shorter than 30 minutes. Either TI or MI should be less than 1.0.
5. *Ultrasonic Doppler method:* Pulsed Doppler ultrasound is concerned in fetal study. Either TI or MI should be less than 1.0, as low as possible. Pulsed Doppler ultrasound beam should not pass fetal body in Doppler examination of maternal or umbilical cord blood flow. Doppler ultrasound is recommended to perform under as low intensity as 0.1 TI, which was successful in Sande's trial.[20]

Transient Increase of Hepatic Cell Apoptosis after Doppler Ultrasound Exposure

Pellicer et al.[19] reported transient increase of hepatic cell apoptosis index after 20 or more sec exposure to 140 mW/cm^2 pulsed Doppler ultrasound in fetal rat fetuses. ISUOG[21] responded with a regulation of pulsed Doppler ultrasound in 11–13 weeks of pregnancy as:

1. No pulsed Doppler ultrasound is studied in the routine ultrasound in 11–13 weeks of pregnancy.
2. Pulsed ultrasound is used only to confirm fetal aneuploidy in 11–13 weeks of pregnancy.
3. The ultrasound safety should be teached in obstetric ultrasound education.

Pellicer et al. used 140 mW/cm^2 Doppler ultrasound, which is lower than 240 mW/cm^2, it was the intensity of no ultrasound effect, and lower than 1.0 TI, therefore, the presence of any artifact is doubted but it has not been reported. ISUOG[21] declared a regulation on the use of Doppler ultrasound in 11–13 weeks of pregnancy.

Two kinds of apoptosis, extrinsic and intrinsic, are classified,[20] and intrinsic apoptosis will be physiologic, while it is difficult to define the apoptosis as intrinsic in Pellicer report. As Sande et al.[20] reported the success of clear pulsed Doppler flow record with 0.1 TI ultrasound, Pellicer's study will be recommended to repeat using 0.1 TI ultrasound, where the usage regulation will be cleared, if no apoptosis develops after the Doppler study with 0.1 TI ultrasound. In summary, ultrasound bioeffect will be hardly established by animal experiments due to possible presence of various artifacts.

NONMEDICAL USE OF DIAGNOSTIC ULTRASOUND

Although the use of diagnostic ultrasound should be limited for medical purposes and users are responsible to the safety of ultrasound, i.e., users must keep the knowledge on possible ultrasound bioeffect and use the ultrasound under the ALARA (as low as reasonably achievable) principle. Nonmedical ultrasound in entertainment or keepsake ultrasound, fetal portrait studios or prenatal boutiques which record intrauterine fetal 3D/4D ultrasound on DVD are recent problems concerning ultrasound safety. There are also ethical concerning and false reassuring problems in the topics.[13-16] WFUMB[13] disapproved the use of ultrasound for the sole purpose of providing souvenir images of the fetus. Because the safety of an ultrasound examination cannot be assured, the use of ultrasound without medical benefit should be avoided. Furthermore, ultrasound should be employed only by health professionals who are well trained and updated in ultrasound clinical usage and bioeffects. The use of ultrasound to provide keepsake images or video of the fetus may be acceptable if it is undertaken as part of normal clinical diagnostic ultrasound examination, provided that it does not increase exposure to the fetus. Ultrasound imaging for nonmedical reasons is not recommended unless carried out for education, training or demonstration purposes. Live scanning of pregnant models for equipment exhibition at ultrasound congresses is considered a nonmedical practice that should be prohibited since it provides no medical benefit and afford potential risk to the fetus. When using ultrasound for nonmedical reasons, the ultrasound equipments display should be used to ensure that TI <0.5 and MI <0.3.[13]

SAFE LEVEL OF ULTRASOUND INTENSITY

The safe obstetric ultrasound intensity level was reported to be one thermal index (1.0 TI) and one mechanical index (1.0 MI) in general opinions of medical ultrasound authorities. There can be possible biological hazardous effects in the ultrasound intensity above the levels.

In our detailed ultrasound radiation experiments insulating the heating of the transducer by 37°C stabilized water, the cultured fetal amniotic origin JTC-cell line floated in the culture medium held in ultrasound translucent container was exposed to quantitatively identified ultrasound for 30–60 minutes and the cell growth curve was compared to the sham of no radiation in the same temperature stabilized water.

The cell growth curve showed no difference to the sham below the SPTA 240 mW/cm^2 (SPTP 80 W/cm^2) of pulsed ultrasound, while the growth curve was suppressed after the exposure to the output intensity ultrasound above SPTA 240 mW/cm^2.[11] Since Japan Society of Ultrasonics in Medicine authorized the results, and Japan Industrial Standard (JIS)[10] regulated medical ultrasound output intensity at the level lower than SPTA 10 mW/cm^2, therefore the medical ultrasound safety was established in Japan.

Although the regulated intensity is low level, the standing wave in reflected ultrasound may increase the intensity, and deformed pulse ultrasound waves may further increase the intensity. The prudent JIS setting will contribute the safety of medical ultrasound even in its accidental increase, while possible increase of output intensity to get further clear fetal image in nonmedical entertainment will easily exceed the safe threshold intensity level. The risk should be prevented by the skillful medical staff with rich safety knowledge and prudent use of diagnostic ultrasound equipment.

In summary of opinions of ultrasound safety specialists, the non-medical use of diagnostic ultrasound for solely entertainment is not recommended or not permitted from the standpoint of diagnostic ultrasound safety.[13-16]

CONCLUSION

The strategies to keep the safety of each diagnostic ultrasound equipments depends on their system, because the thermal effect estimated by TI has been the main criteria in the safety. Simple B-mode, 3D and 4D ultrasound, fetal heart detector and fetal monitor, are not contraindicated due to thermal effect because of their low temporal average intensity. Pulsed Doppler machines are the main target in the safety due to the tendency of its high temporal average intensity. Non-hazardous exposure time of NCRP/AIUM criteria and the temperature rise estimated by TI are useful in retrospective criticism on the past examination. The principle of safe diagnostic ultrasound in daily practice is to keep the TI and MI below 1.0, where obstetrical setting is important. Research works and pregnancy screening strictly follow these principles of ultrasound safety. The ALARA principle should be remembered decreasing the intensity to 0.5–0.1 TI in necessary situations. As for the safe output intensity, the intensity level lower than 240 mW/cm^2 will be safe, because no ultrasound bioeffect was found at the intensity level in the experiment, while cultured cell growth was suppressed by the exposure to 240 or higher mW/cm^2 ultrasound.[11]

REFERENCES

1. Barnett S, Kossoff G. WFUMB Symposium on Safety and Standardisation in Medical Ultrasound. Issues and recommendations regarding thermal mechanisms for biological effects of ultrasound. Ultrasound Med Biol. 1992; 18(9):731-810.
2. National Council on Radiation Protection and measurements; Exposure Criteria for Medical Diagnostic Ultrasound: I. Criteria Based on Thermal Mechanisms. NCRP Report No.113; 1992.
3. American Institute of Ultrasound in Medicine/National Electrical Manufacturers Association; Standard for Real Time Display of Thermal and Mechanical Acoustic Output Indices on Diagnostic Ultrasound Equipment; 1992.
4. Barnett S, ter Haar GR, Ziskin MC, et al. Current status of research on biophysical effects of ultrasound. Ultrasound Med Biol. 1994;20:205-18.
5. AIUM Official Statement Changes; Revised statements; Clinical safety. AIUM Reporter. 1998;154:5-7.
6. Barnett S, Rott HD, ter Haar GR, et al. The sensitivity of biological tissue to ultrasound. Ultrasound Med Biol. 1997; 23(6):805-12.
7. ISUOG Bieffect and Safety Committee; Safety statement 2000 (reconfirmed 2002). Ultrasound Obstet Gynecol. 2002; 19:105.
8. Ide M. Japanese policy and status of standardization. Ultrasound Med Biol. 1986;12:705-08.
9. The Safety Group of the British Medical Ultrasound Society. Guidelines for the safe use of diagnostic ultrasound equipment. BMUS Bulletin. 2000;3:29-33.
10. Maeda K, Ide M. The limitation of the ultrasound intensity for diagnostic devices in the Japanese Industrial standards. IEEE Trans Ultrason Ferroelectr, Freq Control. 1986;33: 241-4.
11. Maeda K, Murao F, Tsuzaki T, et al. Experimental studies in the suppression of cultured cell growth curves after irradiation with CW and pulsed ultrasound. IEEE Trans Ultrason, Ferroelectrics, Freq control. 1986;33(2):186-93.
12. Ang SB Jr, Gluncic V, et al. Prenatal exposure to ultrasound waves impacts neuronal migration in mice. PNAS. 2006; 103(34):12909.
13. Barnett S, Abramowicz JS, Ziskin MC, et al. WFUMB symposium on safety of nonmedical use of ultrasound, Ultrasound Med Biol. 2010;36:1209-12.
14. Abramowicz JS. Nonmedical use of ultrasound: bioeffects and safety risk. Ultrasound Med Biol. 2010;36:1213-20.
15. Philips RA, Stratmeyer ME, Harris GR. Safety and US regulatory considerations in the nonmedical use of medical ultrasound devices. Ultrasound Med Biol. 2010;36: 1224-8.
16. Brezinka C. Nonmedical use of ultrasound in pregnancy: Ethical issue, patients' rights and potential misuse. Ultrasound Med Biol. 2010;35:1233-6.
17. Ping Li, et al. Prenatal exposure to ultrasound affects learning and memory in young rats. Ultrasound Med Biol. 2015;41:644-53.
18. Pellicer B, et al. Ultrasound bioeffects in rats: quantification of cellular damage in the fetal liver after pulsed Doppler imaging. Ultrasound in Obstet Gynecol. 2011;3:643-8.
19. Guicciardi ME, Malhi H, Molt JL, et al. Apoptosis and necrosis in the liver. Compr Physiol. 2013;10.1002/cphy.C10020.
20. Salvesen KA, Lees C, Abramowicz J, Brezinka C, ter Haar G, Maršál K. Opinion: Safe use of Doppler ultrasound during the 11 to 13+6week scan: is it possible? Ultrasound Obst Gynecol. 2011;37:625-8.
21. Sande RK, Matre K, Kiserad T, et al. Ultrasound safety in early pregnancy: reduced energy setting does not compromise obstetric Doppler measurements. Ultrasound Obstet Gynecol. 2012;39:438-43.

2

CHAPTER

Development of Three-dimensional Ultrasound

Kazunori Baba

INTRODUCTION

Short History of 3D Ultrasound

Szilard developed a mechanical three-dimensional (3D) display system to see a fetus three-dimensionally in 1974.[1] Brinkley and colleagues invented a 3D position sensor for a probe. They took many tomographic images of a stillborn baby underwater, traced its outline manually and showed its wire-framed 3D images in 1982.[2]

A modern 3D ultrasound system was first developed by Baba and colleagues in 1986 and a live fetus in utero was depicted three-dimensionally.[3,4] The system was comprised of an ultrasound scanner, position sensor and computer. An imaging technology, named surface rendering, was used for 3D image construction. This system was also applied to placental blood flows (by combining 3D ultrasound with color Doppler) and breast ducts and cysts (by using so-called inversion mode).[5]

A 3D probe and an ultrasound scanner, that displayed three orthogonal planes on a screen, were developed and became commercially available in 1989. In the early 1990s, clinical applications of the 3-orthogonal-plane display in obstetrics were reported.[6,7] Sohn reported translucent display by using volume rendering in 1991.[8] Since 1994, the number of reports on fetal 3D images has increased rapidly because a 3D ultrasound scanner, that could construct and display a 3D image as well as three orthogonal planes, became commercially available.

Two unique 3D ultrasound technologies were also developed. One was defocusing lens method[9,10] and the other was real time ultrasonic beam tracing.[11] In the former method, a fetal volume image was obtained only by using a probe with a defocusing lens. In the latter method, construction of a 3D image and 3D scanning were performed simultaneously and a complete 3D image could be obtained just when a 3D scanning was completed without any delay.

The first world congress on 3D ultrasound in obstetrics and gynecology was held in Mainz, Germany in 1997 and also the first English book on it was published in the same year.[12] Development of 3D ultrasound has been accelerated afterwards and all major manufacturers of ultrasound scanners now provide 3D ultrasound scanners.

WHAT CAN 3D ULTRASOUND DO?

Three-dimensional ultrasound handles 3D data, whereas conventional 2D ultrasound can take care of only 2D data **(Figs. 1A and B)**. Some functions that only 3D ultrasound can perform are:

- Display of a 3D image
- Display of an arbitrary section
- Measurement in 3D space (including volume measurement)
- Display of a 3D blood flow image
- Saving, copying and transmission of all information in 3D space
- Re-examination with a saved 3D data set, without the patient.

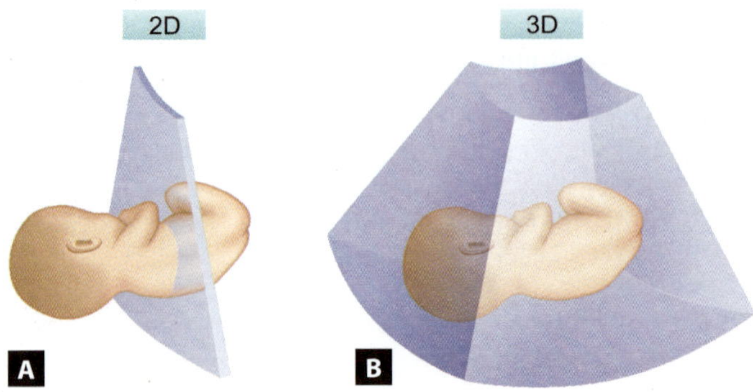

Figs. 1A and B: (A) Two-dimensional data for conventional 2D ultrasound; (B) 3D data for 3D ultrasound.[13]

TECHNICAL ASPECTS OF 3D ULTRASOUND

Various images are obtained through the following processes in 3D ultrasound **(Fig. 2)**:

- Acquisition of 3D data (3D scanning)
- Construction of a 3D data set
- Volume visualization.

Acquisition of 3D Data

Three-dimensional data is usually acquired as a large number of consecutive tomographic images through movements of an ultrasound transducer array (conventional 2D ultrasound probe). The most popular way is to use a 3D probe because of its easiness for scanning. A 3D probe has a built-in transducer array (2D ultrasound probe), which tilts in the 3D probe and 3D data are obtained automatically **(Fig. 2)**.

There are some other 3D scanning methods for wide scanning area **(Figs. 3A to C)**. Each tomographic image should be acquired with its positional information for construction of a 3D data set. Accurate positional information can be obtained through an electromagnetic position sensor, an electric gyroscope attached to the probe **(Fig. 4)** or a mechanical position sensor.

Ultrasound travels in a soft tissue at an average speed of 1,540 m/s. This speed limits 3D scanning speed. Parallel receiving technique is a method to overcome the limitation. In this technique, one broad ultrasonic beam is transmitted and its echoes are received as plural ultrasonic beams. In a 2D array probe **(Fig. 5)**, a high degree of parallel receiving (at least 1:16) is used and high-speed 3D scanning is possible.[17,18]

Construction of a 3D Data Set

A set of tomographic images obtained through 3D scanning must be constructed three-dimensionally into a 3D data set for further computer processing **(Fig. 6)**. This construction process involves interpolation and improvement of data quality by filtering.[15] A 3D data set is composed of a set of voxels (volume elements). Each voxel has a gray value (and color information in 3D color Doppler ultrasound).

For scanning of the heart, a gated technique (so called STIC: spatiotemporal image correlation) is applied[19,20] to avoid distortion of a 3D data set due to movement. Tomographic images are rearranged according to the phase of the cardiac cycle and a 3D data set is constructed

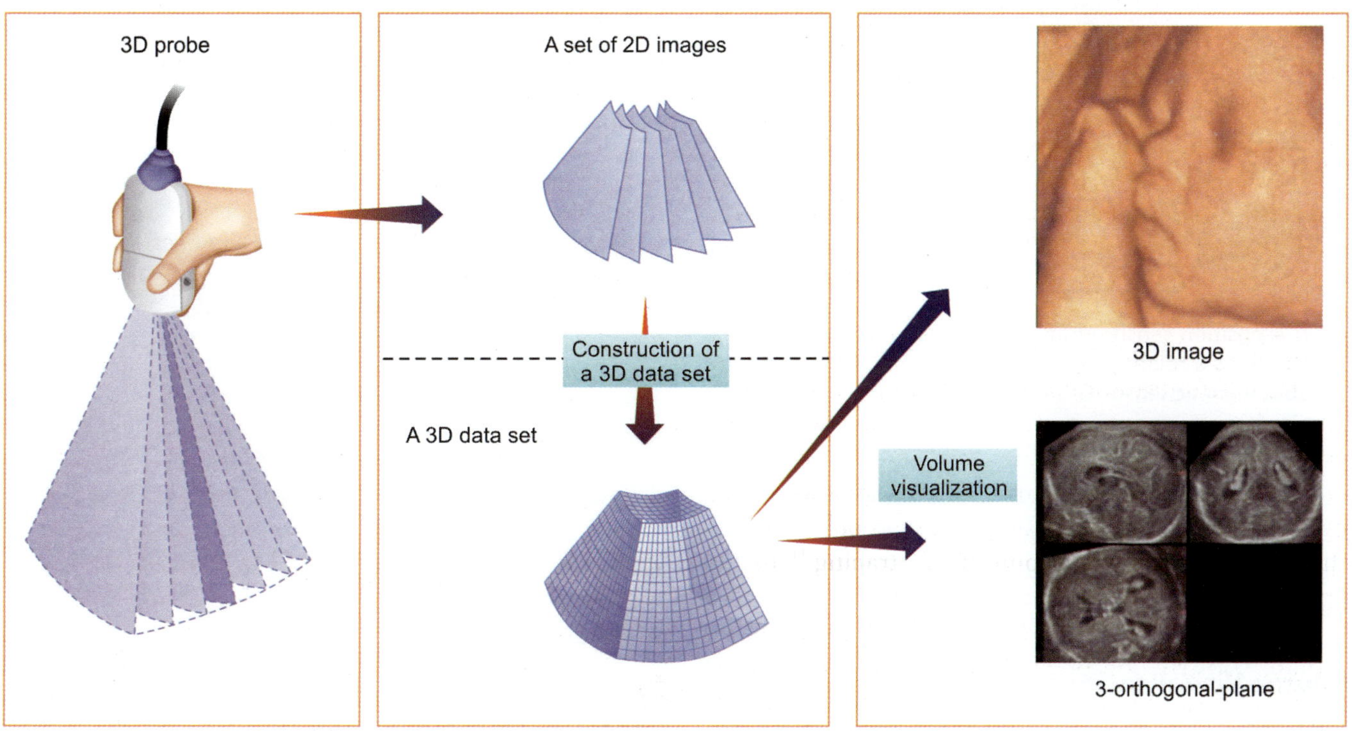

Fig. 2: Basic processes in 3D ultrasound.[14]

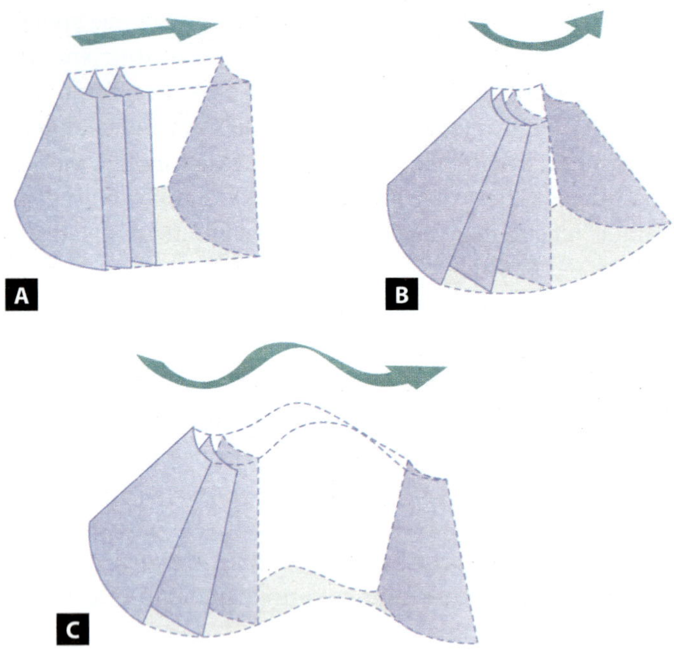

Figs. 3A to C: 3D scanning methods. (A) Parallel scanning; (B) Fan-like scanning; (C) Free surface scanning.[15]

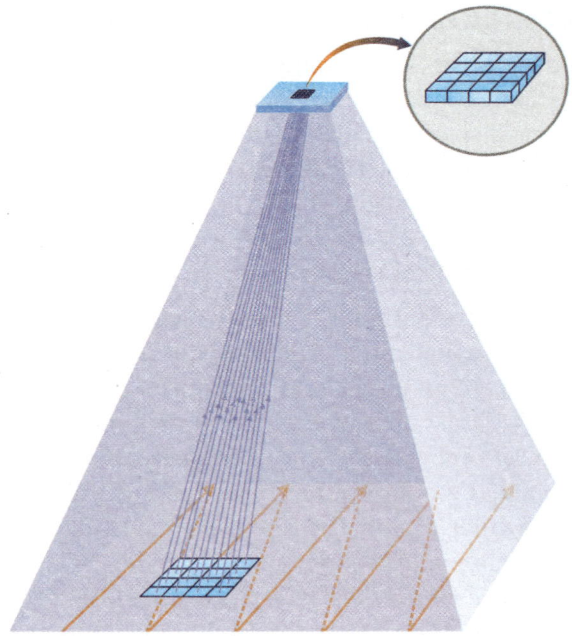

Fig. 5: 3D scanning by a 2D array probe. A large number of tiny transducers are arranged two-dimensionally and 3D scanning is performed electrically. High-speed 3D scanning is possible by 1:16 parallel receiving.[13]

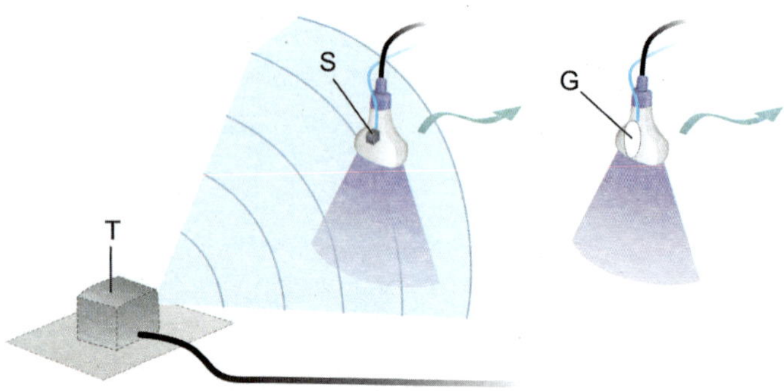

Fig. 4: A position sensor or an electric gyroscope attached to a probe detects a relative position of the probe. (T: transmitter; S: electromagnetic sensor; G: electric gyroscope).[16]

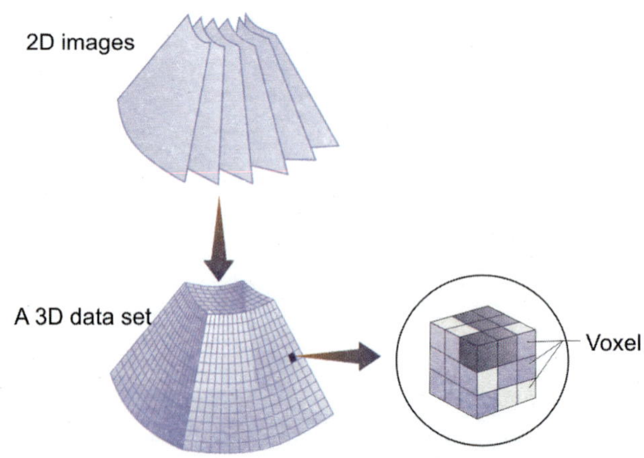

Fig. 6: Construction of a 3D data set.[16]

with only tomographic images at the same phase of the cardiac cycle **(Fig. 7)**. The heart can be seen beating three-dimensionally by constructing many 3D data sets in a single cardiac cycle.

Volume Visualization

A 3D data set is processed by a computer to be displayed on a 2D screen. This process is called volume visualization. These three methods are usually used for volume visualization in 3D ultrasound:

1. Section reconstruction
2. Volume rendering
3. Surface rendering.

Section Reconstruction

Three orthogonal planes are displayed on a screen immediately after 3D scanning in most of 3D ultrasound

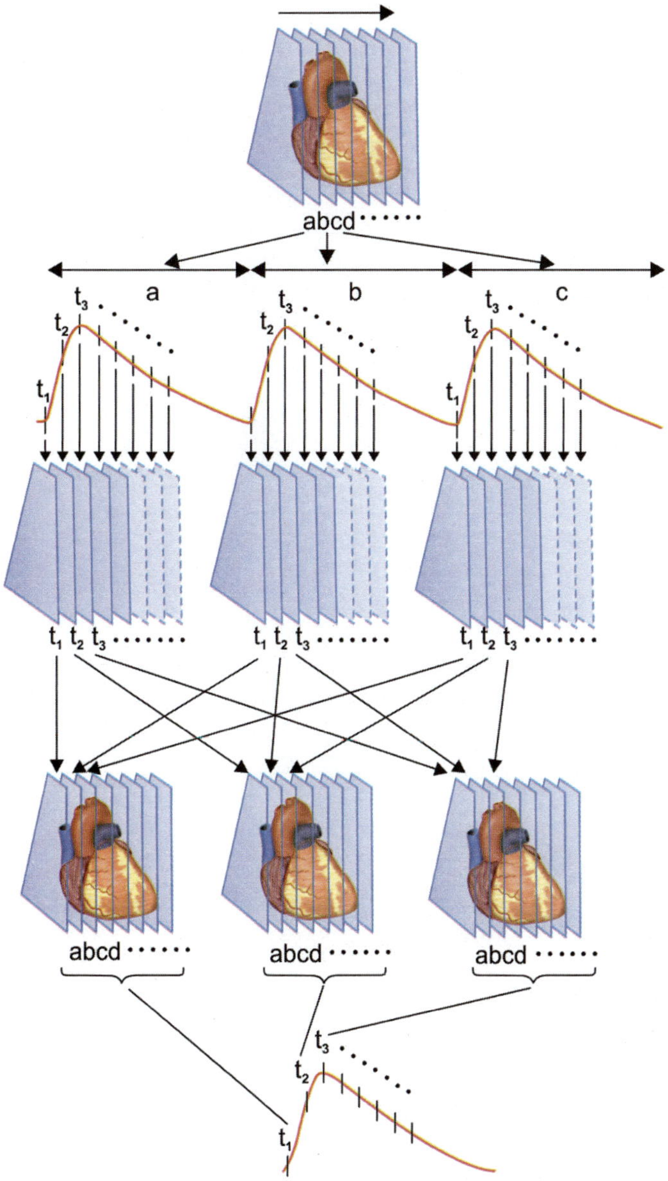

Fig. 7: A gated technique for 3D scanning of the fetal heart.[13]

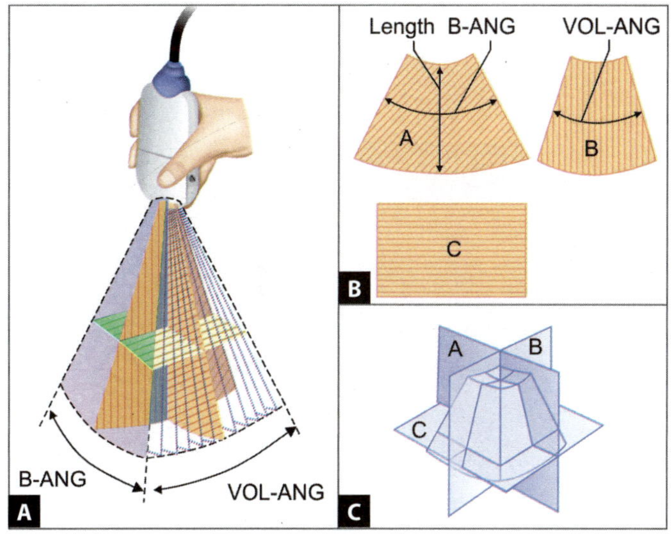

Figs. 8A to C: (A) Relation between a 3D probe; (B) Initial three orthogonal planes on the screen; (C) 3D data set.[14]

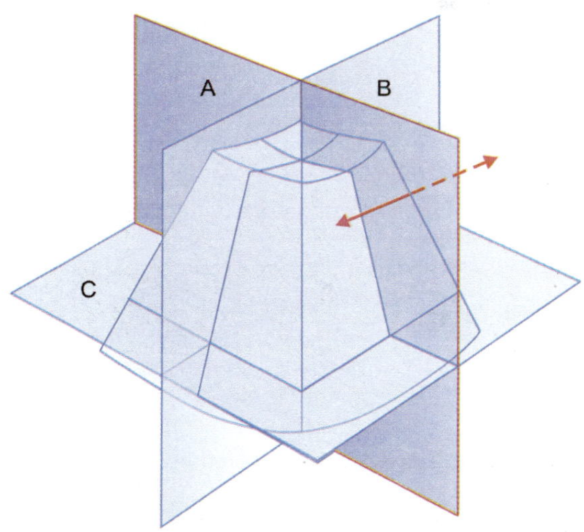

Fig. 9: Arbitrary section display by translating. Not only plane A but also B and C planes can be translated individually.[14]

scanners **(Figs. 8A to C)**. An arbitrary section can be selected and displayed through translation **(Fig. 9)** and rotation **(Figs. 10A and B)** of the 3D data set. This means that re-examination can be done after the patient has left, only if 3D data sets are saved.

Usually, 3-orthogonal-plane display **(Figs. 11A to C)** or parallel-plane display **(Fig. 12)** are used for better understanding of the position and orientation of each section in 3D space. These reconstructed sections, some of which cannot be obtained by conventional 2D ultrasound, are very useful for diagnosis in some cases. Three orthogonal sections may also be allocated three-dimensionally **(Figs. 13A to C)**.

Volume Rendering

Three-dimensional images are obtained by an algorithm called volume rendering. A smaller 3D data set for rendering (3D image generation) is extracted first from the original 3D data set to eliminate unnecessary parts around the object as much as possible **(Fig. 14)**. A 3D data set for rendering is projected directly on a projection plane **(Fig. 15)** in volume rendering. Rays are assumed

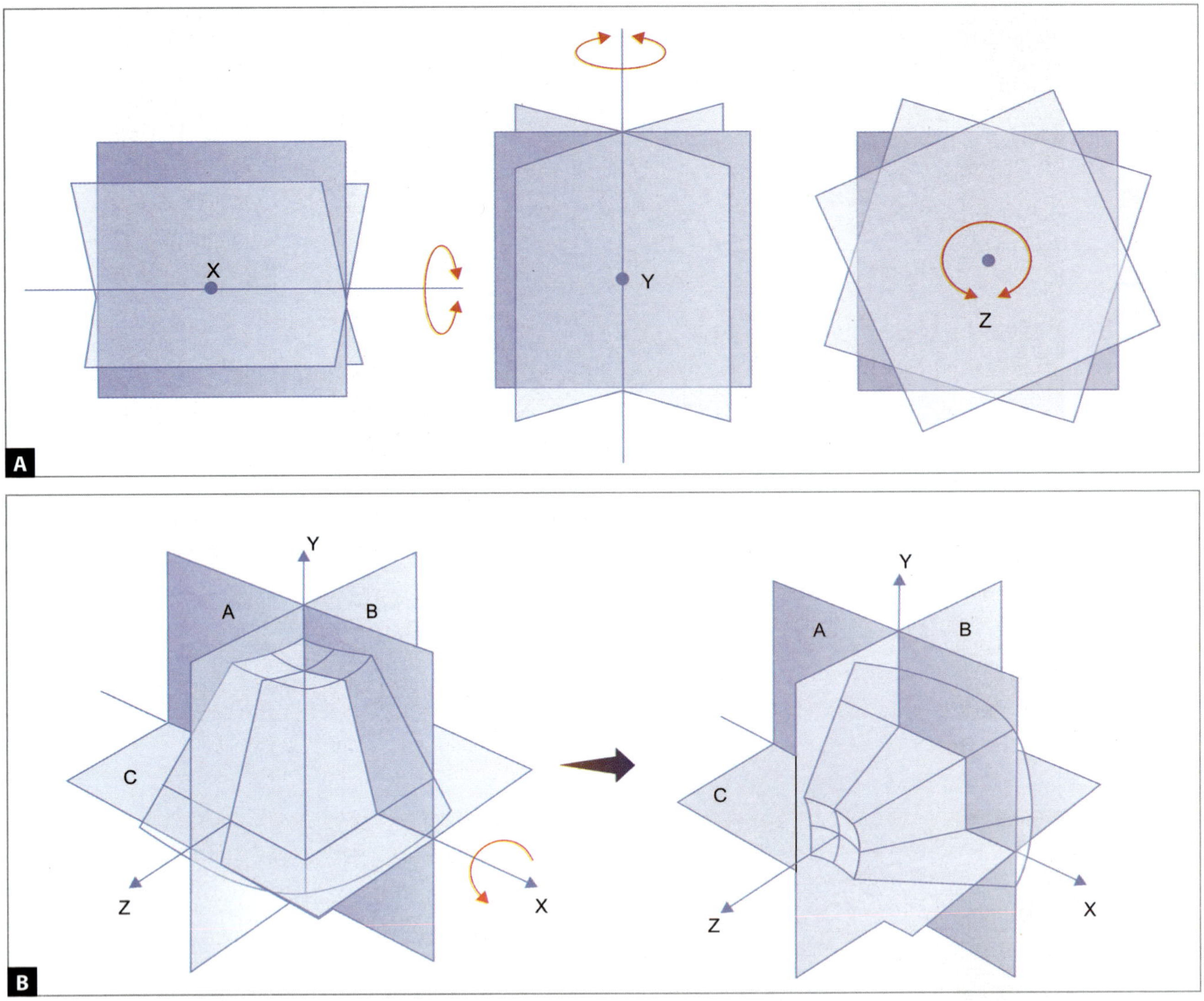

Figs. 10A and B: Arbitrary section display by rotating the 3D data set. One of 3 axes (X, Y, Z) is selected for rotation.[14]

from each pixel on the projection plane into the 3D data set. Brightness of each pixel is determined based on gray values of voxels on each corresponding ray. **Figure 16** illustrates how brightness is calculated through voxels in the original volume rendering.[21,22]

A fetal surface image **(Fig. 17)** is obtained through volume rendering. Boundaries of the object do not need to be outlined strictly in volume rendering because low level noises around the object become transparent and do not affect the final 3D image much. An inside view of the heart can also be depicted three-dimensionally by using a 3D data set constructed with a gated technique **(Figs. 18A and B)**.

Some other kinds of 3D images can be obtained by volume rendering. A fetal skeletal image is obtained when only the maximum gray values on each ray are displayed on the projection plane (maximum intensity projection) **(Fig. 19)**. A 3D image of cystic parts and blood vessels is obtained when only the minimum gray values on each ray are displayed on the projection plane (minimum intensity projection) **(Figs. 20A to D)**. However, a 3D image shows only silhouettes in this way. A surface rendered 3D image of cystic parts is obtained by inverting black and white and processing cystic parts as solid parts (so-called inversion mode).[5] **Figures 21A to C** show the difference between images by so-called minimum mode (minimum intensity projection) and by inversion mode.

Speckle noises are accumulated in volume rendering and a higher contrasted and clearer image than a sectional

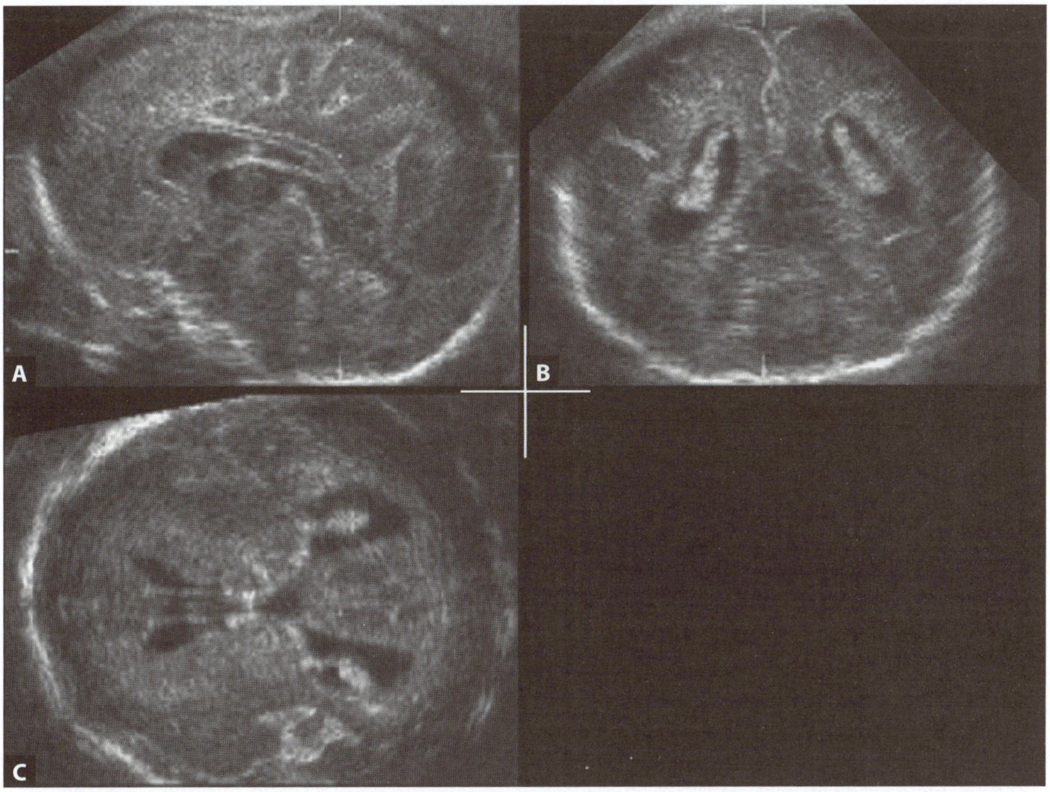

Figs. 11A to C: Three-orthogonal-plane display of a fetal head. (A) Midsagittal plane; (B) Coronal plane; (C) Axial plane are displayed on a screen simultaneously.

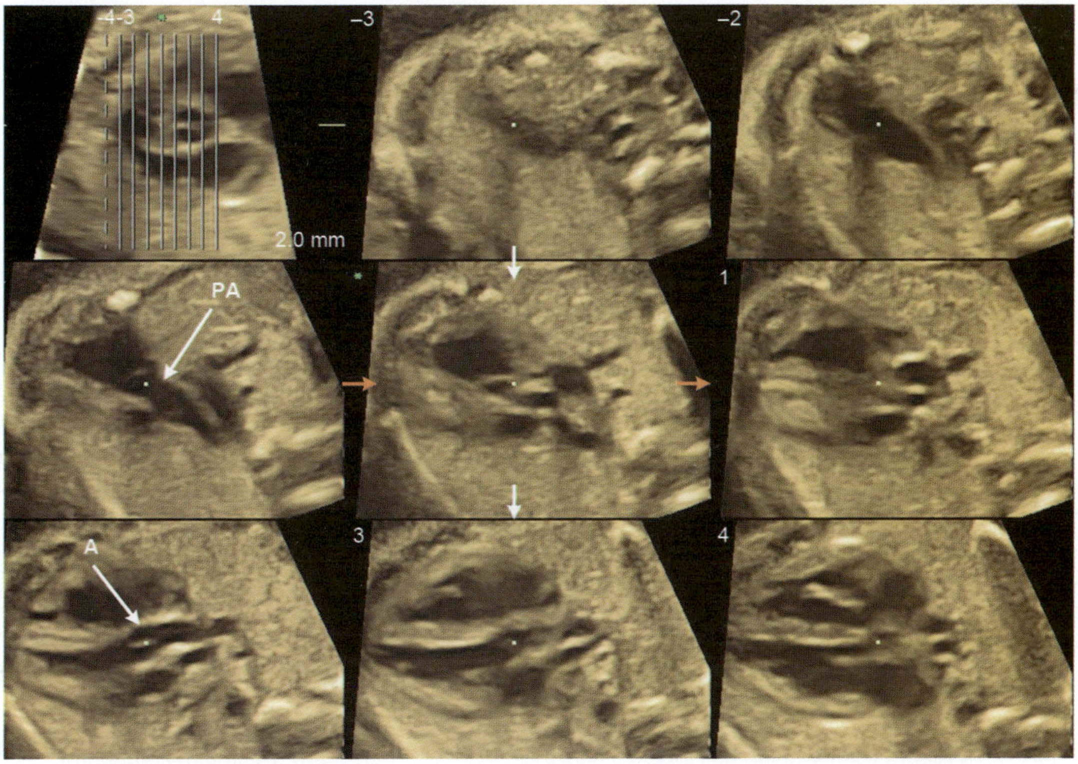

Fig. 12: Parallel-plane display of a fetal heart. Both pulmonary artery (PA) and aorta (A) are depicted on an image.

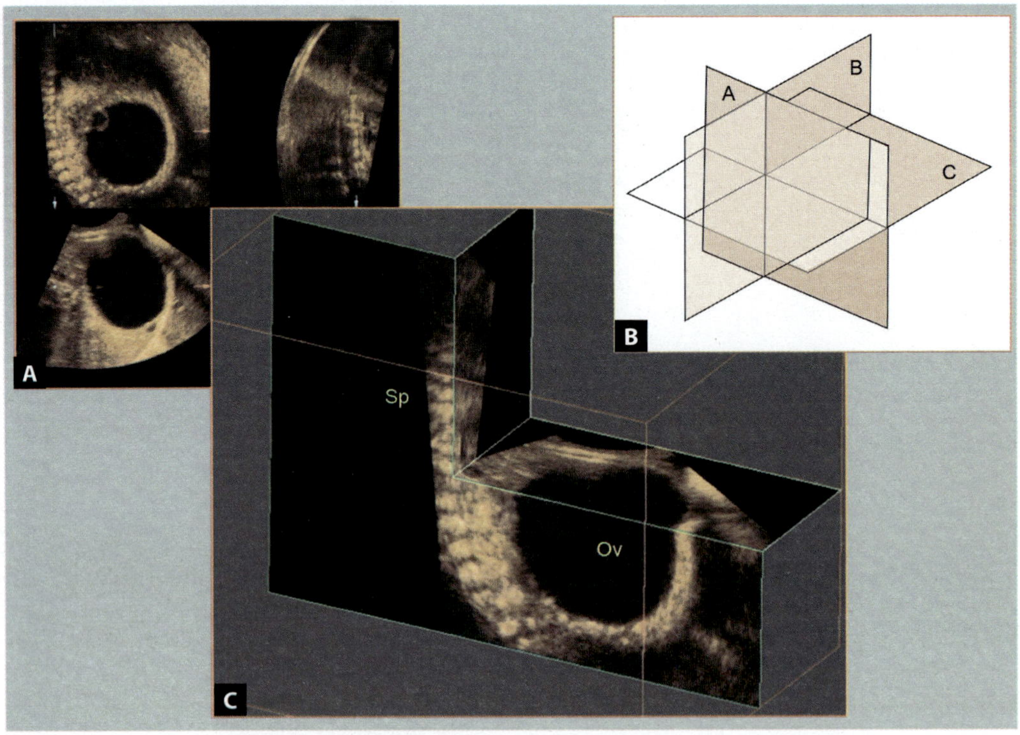

Figs. 13A to C: A fetal ovarian cyst at 36 weeks of gestation. (A) Three-orthogonal-plane display; (B) A display in which three orthogonal planes are allocated three-dimensionally; (C) As shown in the schema. (Sp: spine; Ov: ovarian cyst)

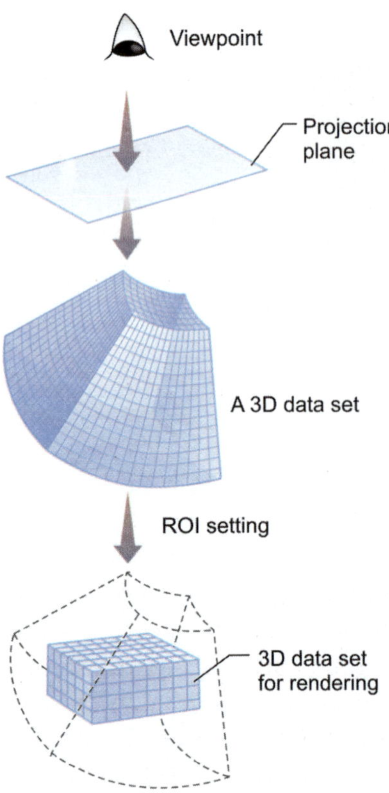

Fig. 14: Settings of a viewpoint and ROI (region of interest) for a 3D data set for rendering.[16]

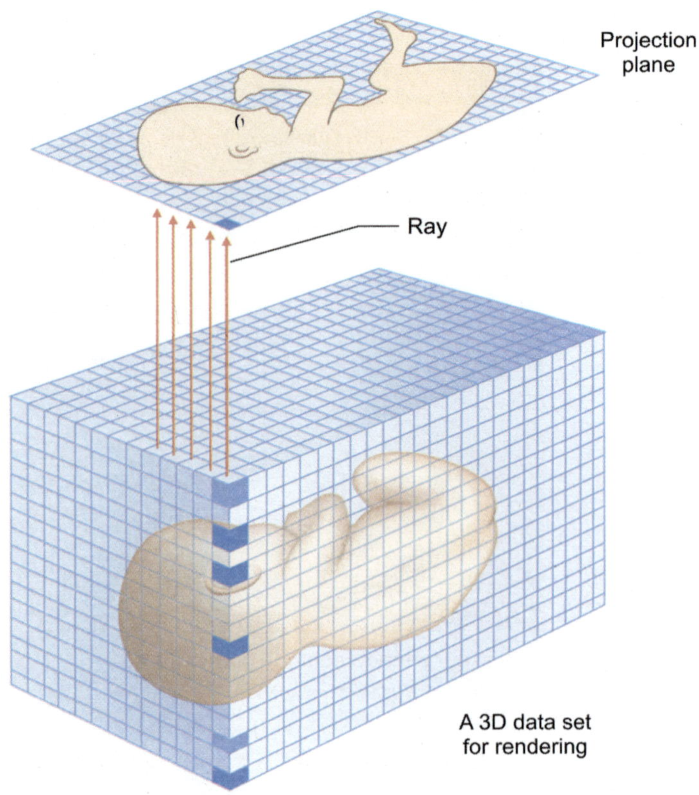

Fig. 15: Volume rendering.[16]

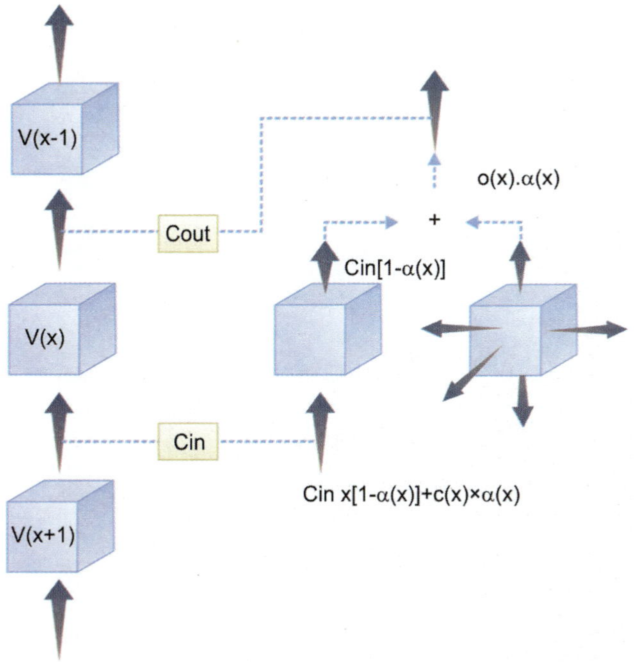

Fig. 16: The original method of calculation in volume rendering.[15]

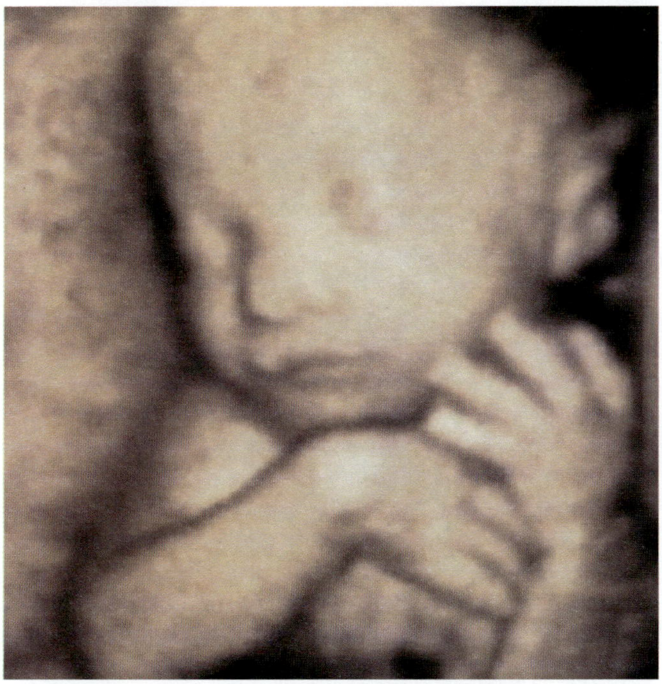

Fig. 17: A surface-rendered image of a fetus at 33 weeks of gestation by volume rendering.

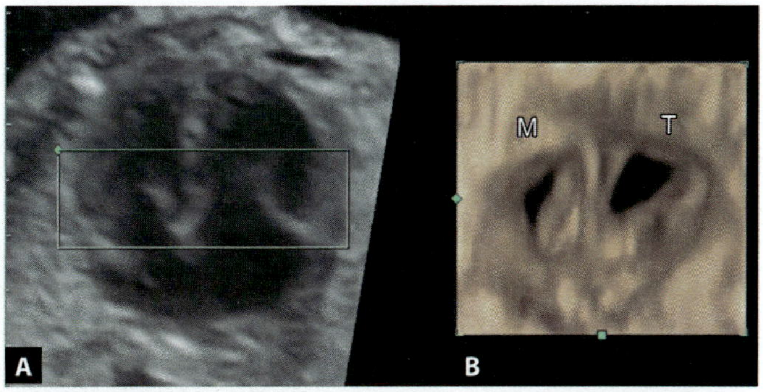

Figs. 18A and B: (A) A tomographic image for ROI setting; (B) A 3D image of openings of mitral (M) and tricuspid (T) valves. A normal fetus at 28 weeks of gestation.

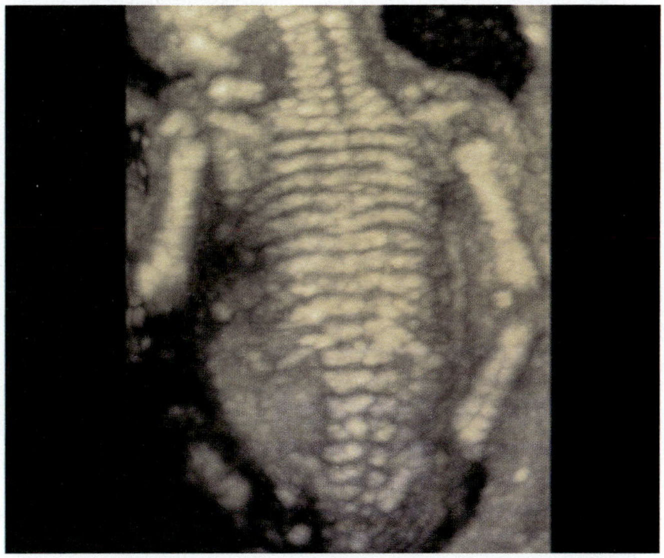

Fig. 19: A 3D image of the fetal skeleton by maximum intensity projection.

image can be obtained in some cases **(Figs. 22A and B)**. A 3D image of blood flows (blood vessels) is obtained by using color Doppler or power Doppler images instead of B-mode images **(Fig. 23)**. Volume rendering is a good rendering method for observation but not for volume measurement.

Surface Rendering

Three-dimensional surface images are also obtained by an algorithm called surface rendering. **Figure 24** illustrates the principle of surface rendering. The object is extracted from a 3D data set, transformed to a set of intermediate geometrical data and projected on a 2D plane. Intermediate geometrical data is composed of small cubes or small polygons **(Figs. 25A and B)**. A 3D image looks more three-dimensional by shading **(Figs. 26A and B)**.[15]

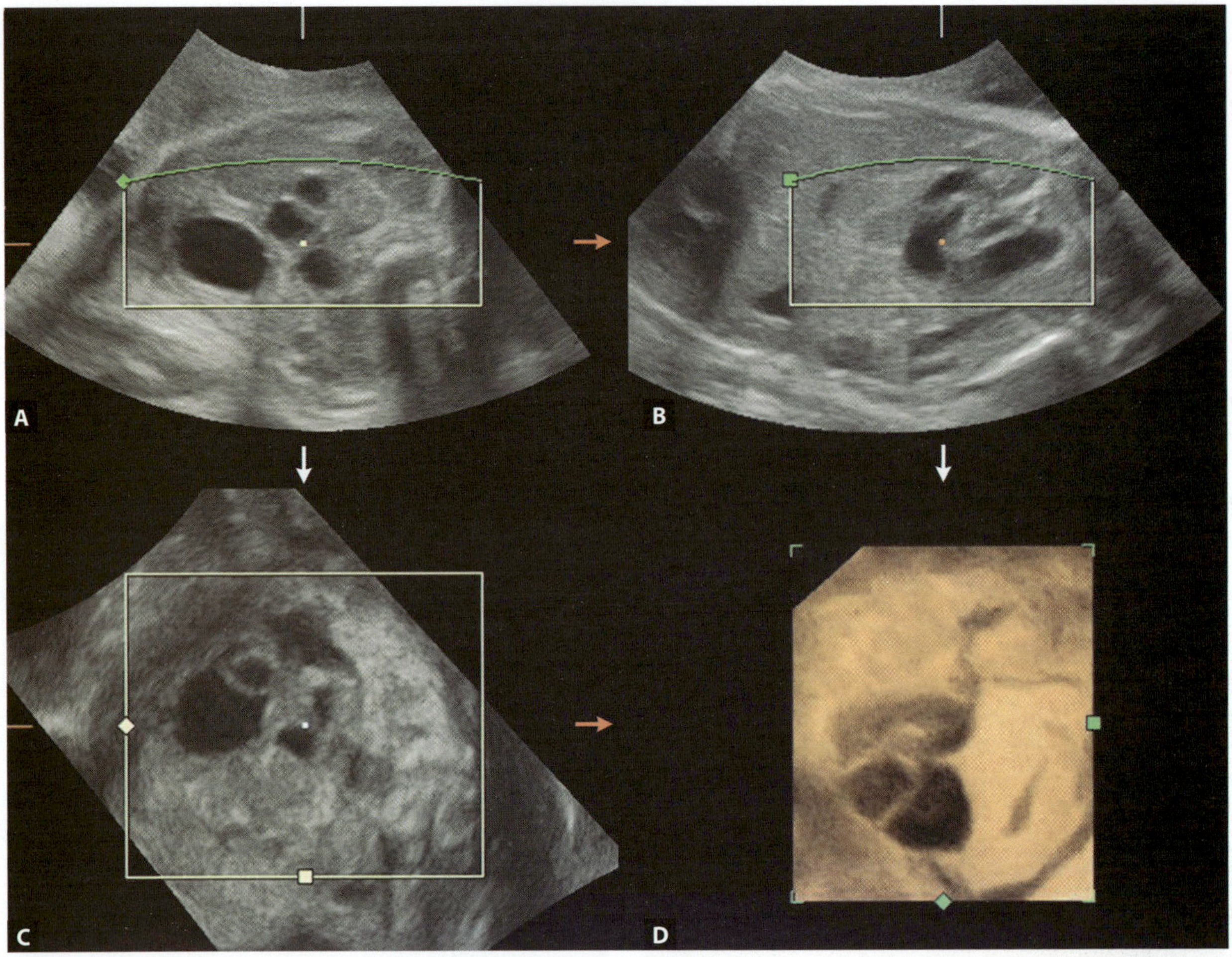

Figs. 20A to D: (A to C) Three orthogonal planes; (D) A 3D image of a hydroureter by minimum intensity projection.[14]

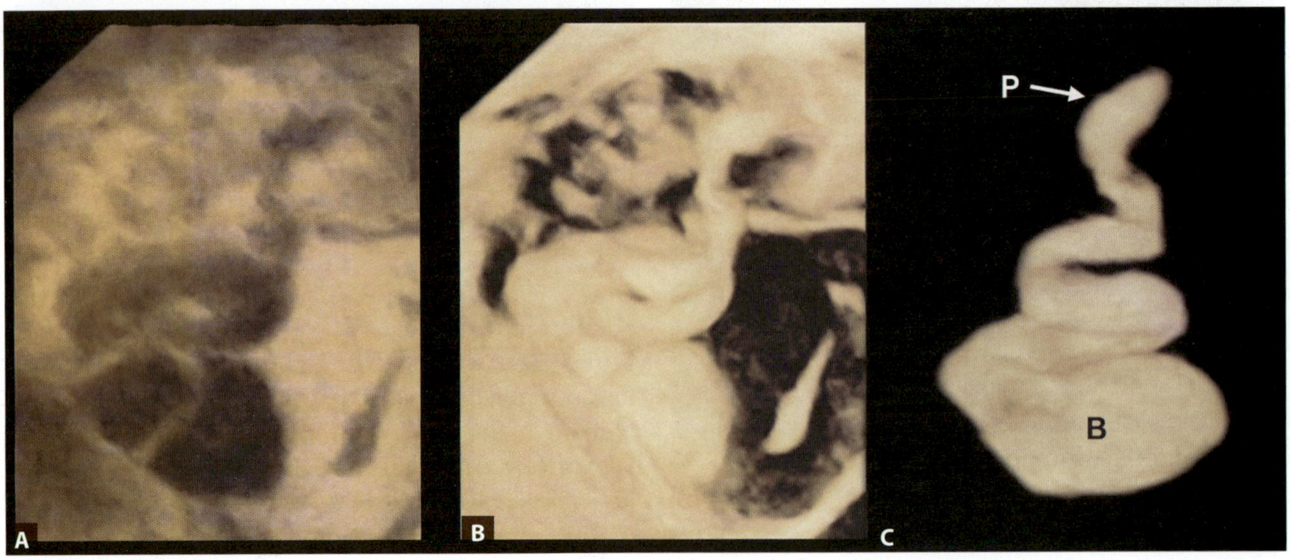

Figs. 21A to C: (A) A 3D image of a hydroureter by minimum intensity projection (same image in **Figure 20**); (B) A 3D surface image of the hydroureter by inversion mode; (C) A 3D surface image of the hydroureter by inversion mode after removal of surrounding unnecessary parts.[14] (P: pelvis; B: bladder)

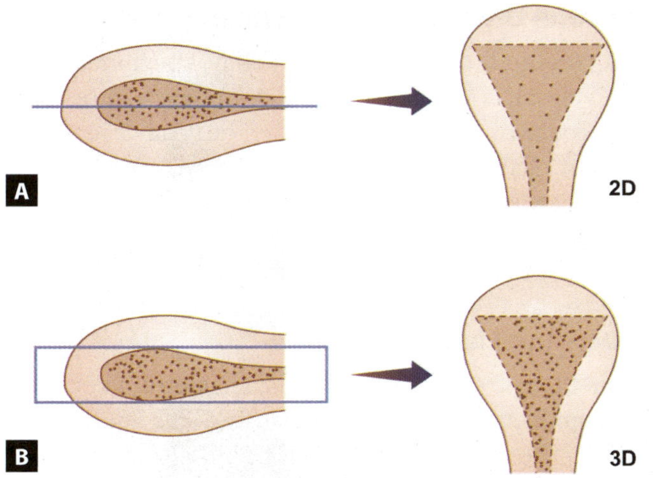

Figs. 22A and B: (A) A plane image of a coronal section of the uterus; (B) A 3D image (lower right). A higher contrasted image can be obtained by volume rendering.

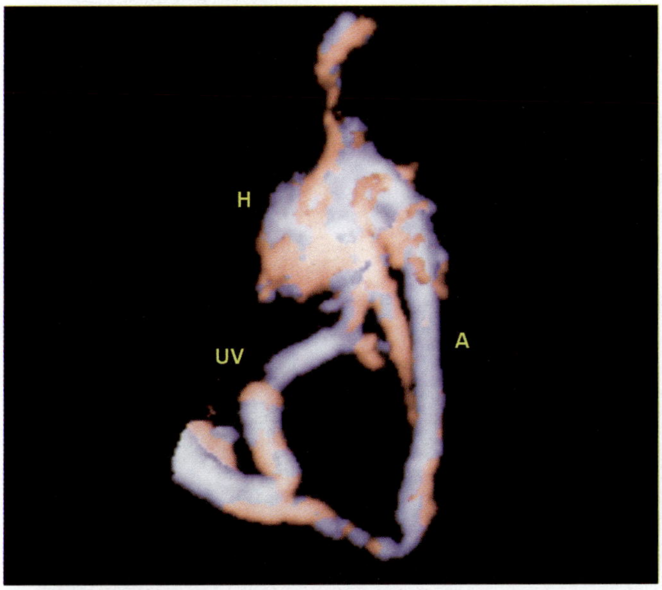

Fig. 23: A 3D image of fetal circulation. The heart (H), the aorta (A) and the umbilical vein (UV). A normal fetus at 19 weeks of gestation.

Extraction of the object may be performed by setting an appropriate threshold **(Fig. 27)**. But in most of the cases, extraction is done by manual tracing **(Figs. 28A and B)** because boundaries of the object should be outlined strictly in surface rendering. Thus, surface rendering is more troublesome than volume rendering. But once the object is extracted, not only 3D image is displayed but also its volume can be calculated **(Figs. 29A to E)**.

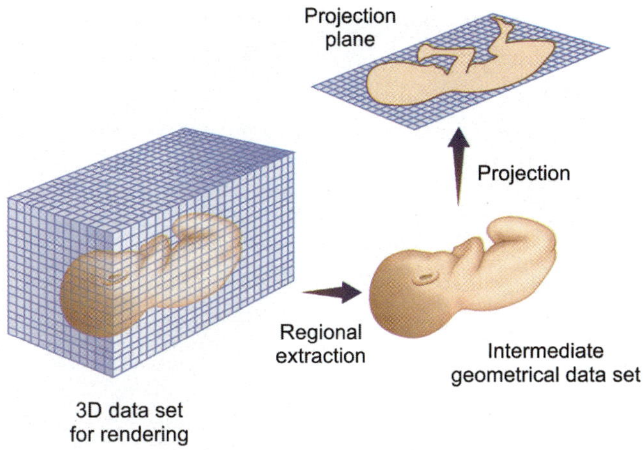

Fig. 24: Surface rendering.[16]

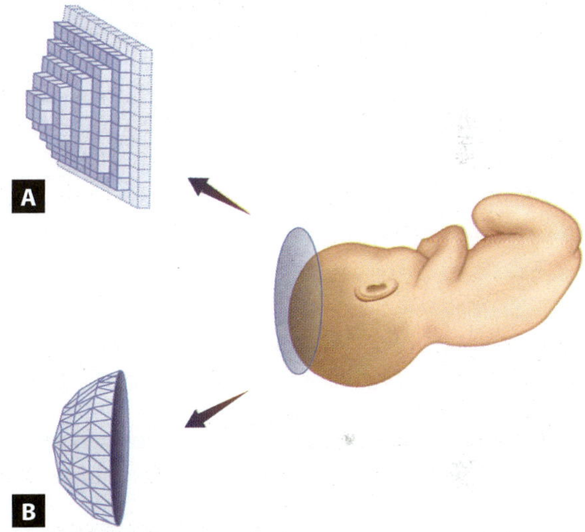

Figs. 25A and B: (A) Intermediate geometrical data set composed of small cubes; (B) Small polygons.[16]

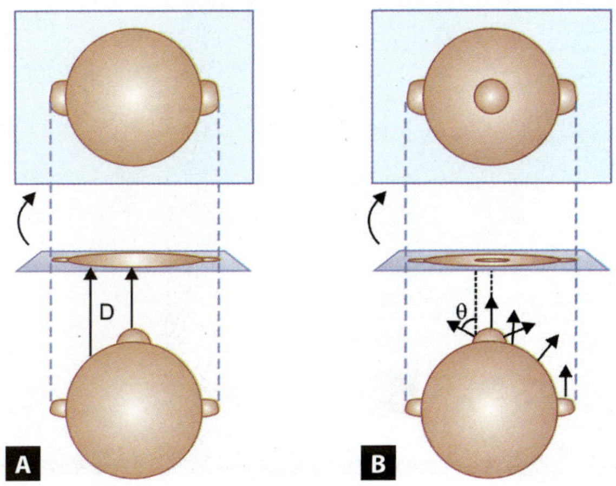

Figs. 26A and B: Shading makes a 3D image more realistic. (A) Depth-only shading; (B) Shading with the orientation of the object surface.[16] (D: depth; θ: angle of orientation)

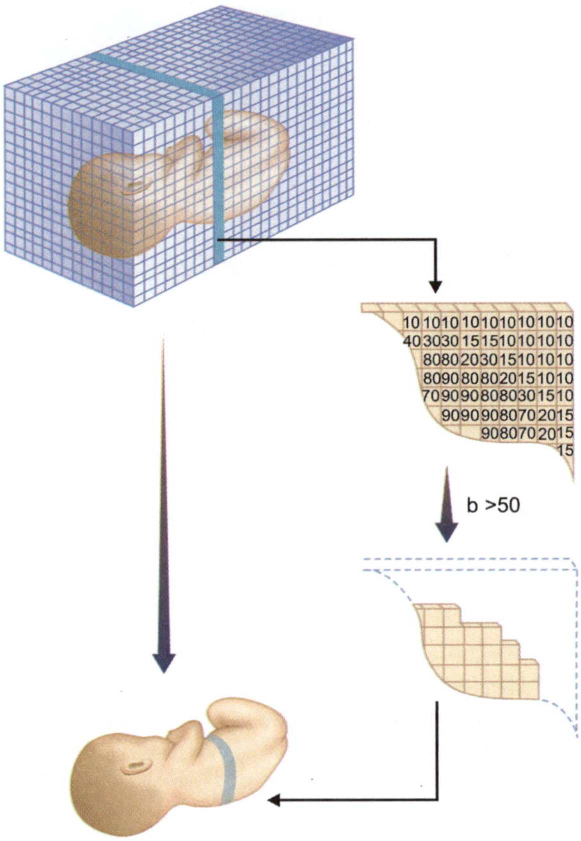

Fig. 27: Extraction of the object (segmentation) may be performed by setting a threshold properly.[16]

Real Time Ultrasonic Beam Tracing

In this method, each ultrasonic beam is regarded as a ray in volume rendering. Calculation for each ultrasonic beam is performed immediately after the beam is received **(Fig. 30)**. This means that 3D scanning and volume rendering are performed simultaneously. This method does not require construction of a 3D data set, but a 3D image is always displayed as seen from the probe.

Defocusing Lens Method

This method is referred to as volume imaging or thick slice 3D imaging. A thick slice by defocusing lens attached to

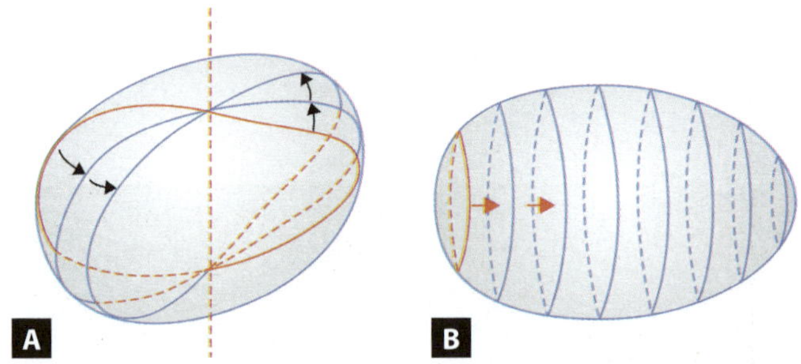

Figs. 28A and B: Manual extraction of the object (segmentation) is done on several sections). The sections are selected by (A) Rotating or; (B) Translating the 3D data set.[14]

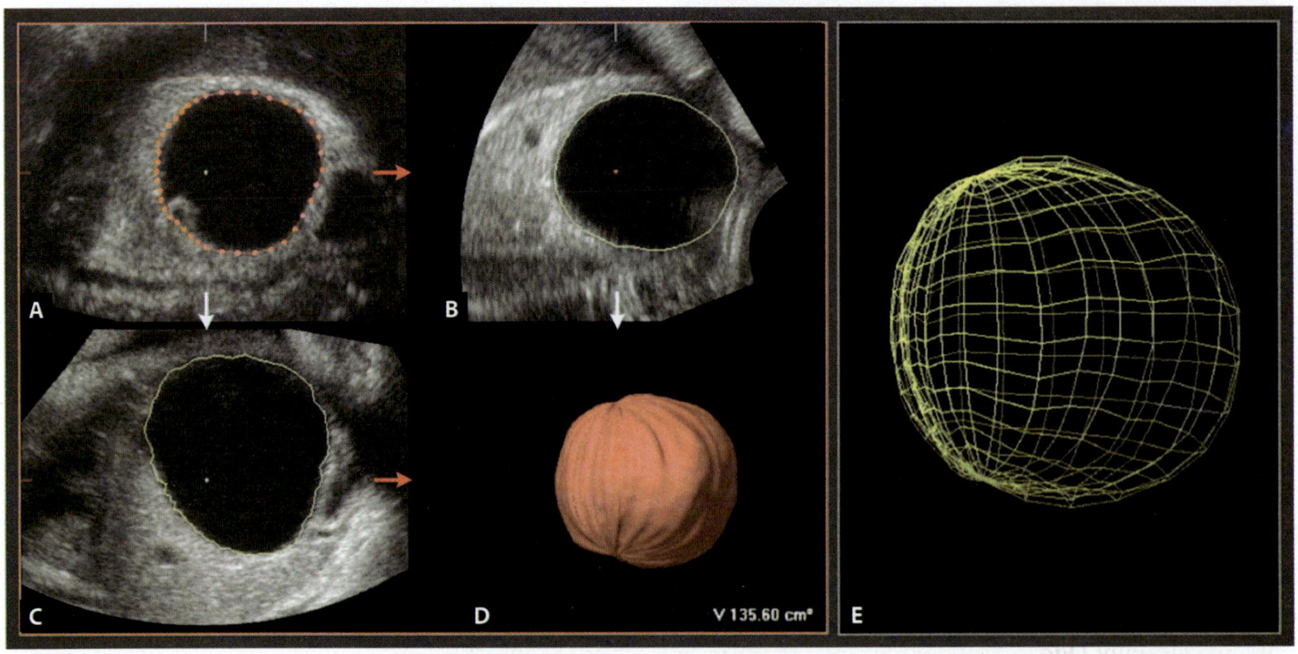

Figs. 29A to E: Surface rendering and measurement of the volume of a fetal ovarian cyst at 36 weeks of gestation. (A to C) The outlines of the cyst were traced manually on three orthogonal planes like "A" in **Figure 28**; (D) A 3D image by surface rendering is displayed; (E) The 3D image is based on a set of small polygons and the volume is calculated automatically with the polygon data.

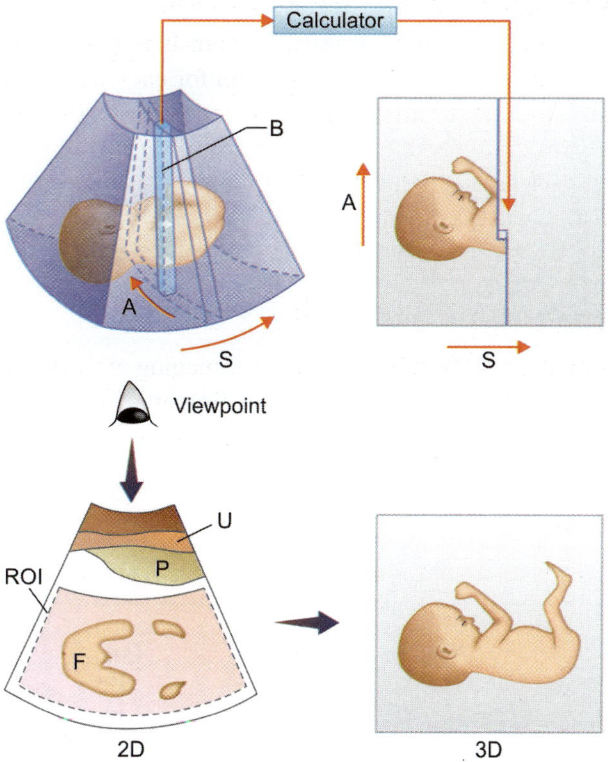

Fig. 30: 3D image generation by real time ultrasonic beam tracing.[16]

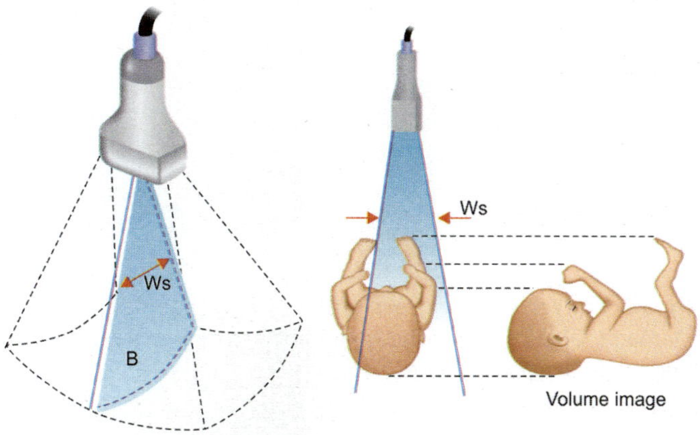

Fig. 31: Volume imaging. Slice width (Ws) is widened by a defocusing lens attached to the surface of a conventional probe.[16]

the surface of a conventional probe captures an object three-dimensionally **(Fig. 31)**. Real time observation is possible, but the clinical application of this method is very limited.

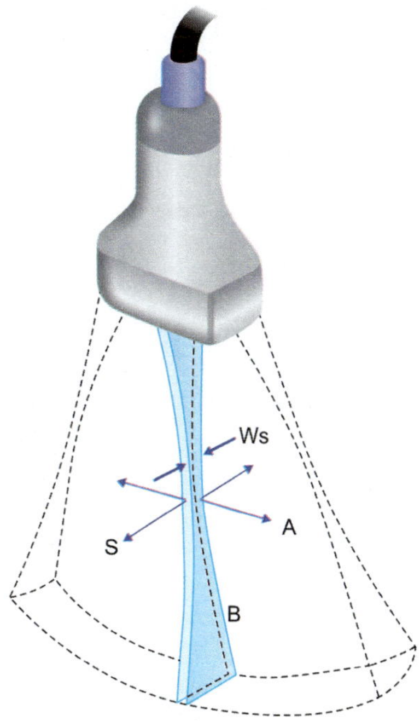

Fig. 32: Widths of an ultrasonic beam (B). The width (Ws) in the direction of slice width (S) is much wider than the width in the direction of transducer array (A).[16]

PRACTICAL TIPS

3D Scanning

The first point is to find a proper probe position and orientation for 3D scanning. For a fetal surface image, a position and orientation where a sufficient amount of amniotic fluid is seen over the fetus should be selected.

The second point is to consider the direction of 3D scanning. An ultrasonic beam is converged electrically in the direction of transducer array. In the direction perpendicular to the tomogram (the direction of slice width), only an acoustic lens is used for converging the beam **(Fig. 32)**. But convergence by an acoustic lens is not good enough and the object in the 3D data set tends to be expanded in the direction of slice width or in the direction of 3D scanning **(Fig. 33)**. Consequently, the width of the object on a 3D image **(Figs. 34A and B)** and resolution of a 3D image **(Figs. 35A and B)** varies on the direction of 3D scanning.

Region of Interest

Figure 36 illustrates the relation between three orthogonal planes and a 3D image. A 3D data set for rendering is extracted by setting a region of interest (ROI) on the three

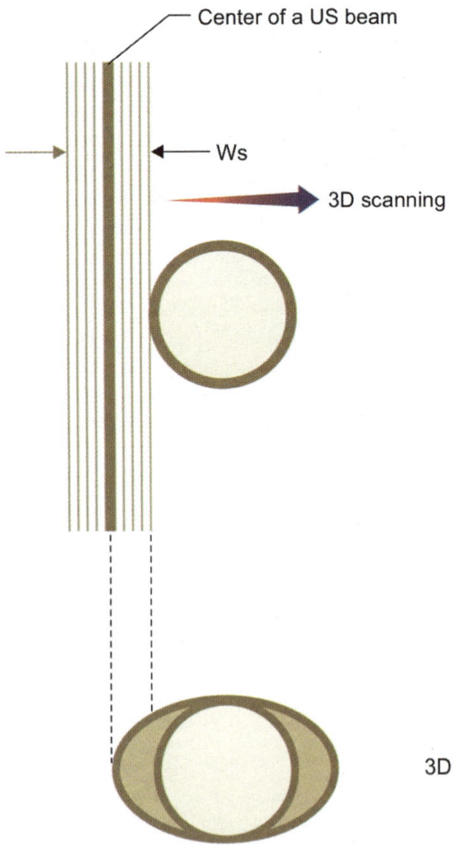

Fig. 33: Influence of slice width (Ws) on 3D data. The 3D data of the object is expanded in the direction of 3D scanning.[15]

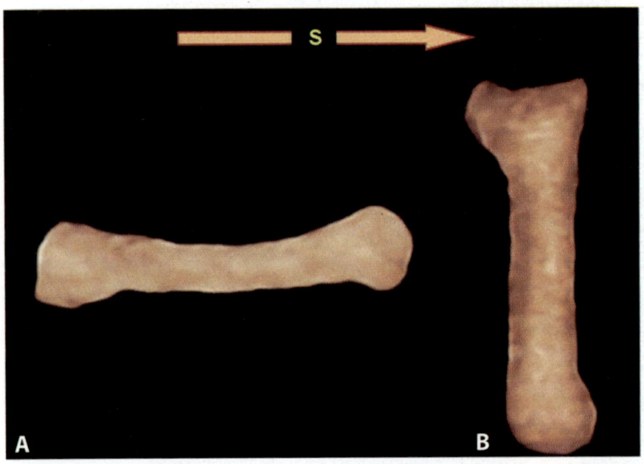

Figs. 34A and B: An example of influence of slice width on a 3D image. The same fetal femur was scanned in different directions. The femur looks thicker in B than in A. (S: direction of 3D scanning)

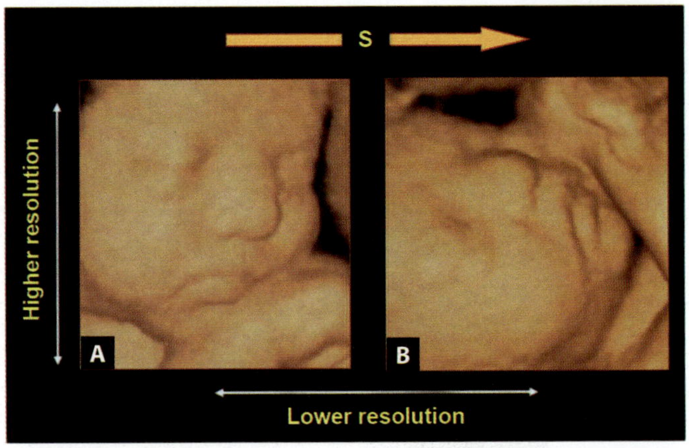

Figs. 35A and B: An example of influence of slice width on a 3D image. The same fetal face was scanned in different directions. A gap between eyelids is seen clearer in A than in B. (S: direction of 3D scanning)

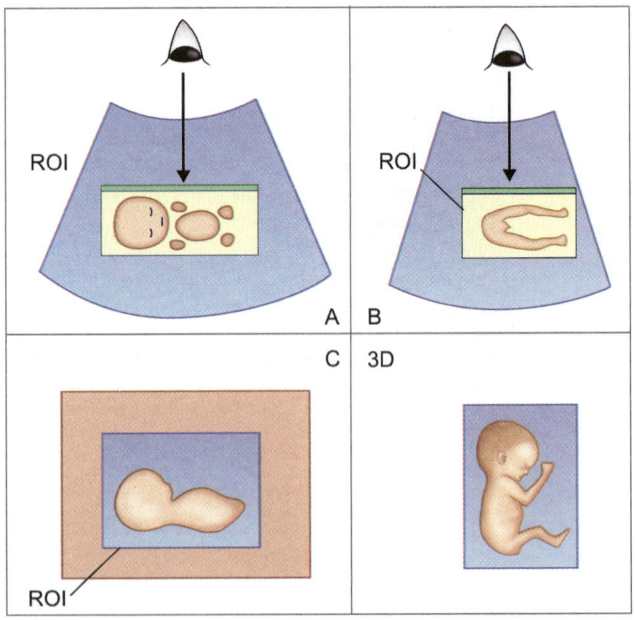

Fig. 36: The relation between three orthogonal planes and a 3D image. Objects under the green line are depicted on the 3D image.[14] (ROI: region of interest)

orthogonal planes. The point is to fit the ROI to the object as much as possible, by translating and rotating the original 3D data set and by selecting ROI size **(Figs. 37A and B)**.

Threshold

Setting the threshold properly is also very important to obtain a good 3D image. By doing so, unnecessary weak noises around the object can be removed **(Fig. 27)** and a clear 3D image can be obtained. When the threshold is too low, weak noises around the object hide it. When the threshold is too high, parts of the object get eliminated **(Figs. 38A to C)**.

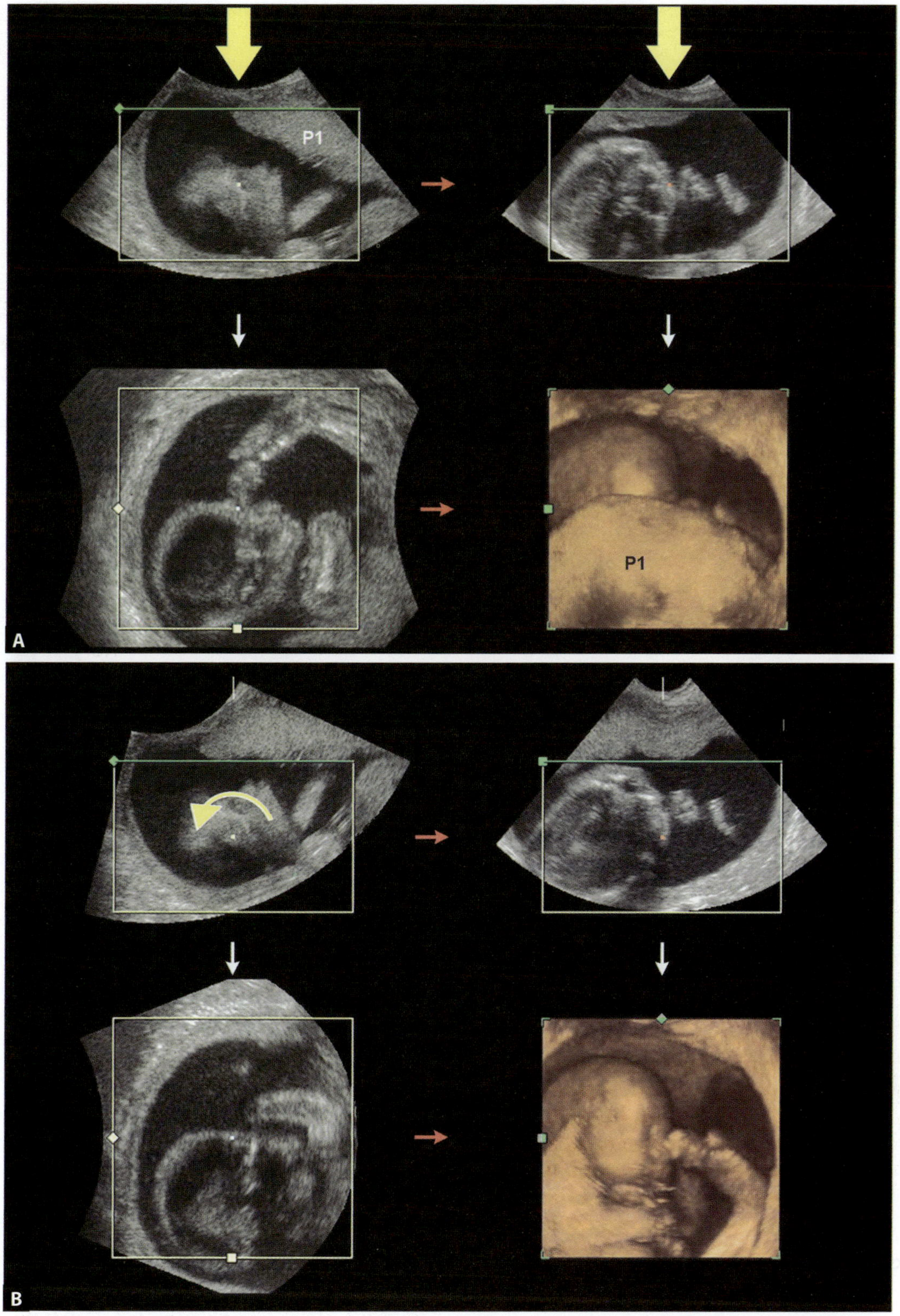

Figs. 37A and B: (A) The placenta (P1) hides a part of a fetus on the 3D image; (B) By rotating upper left plane counterclockwise around Z axis, hidden parts can be seen on the 3D image.

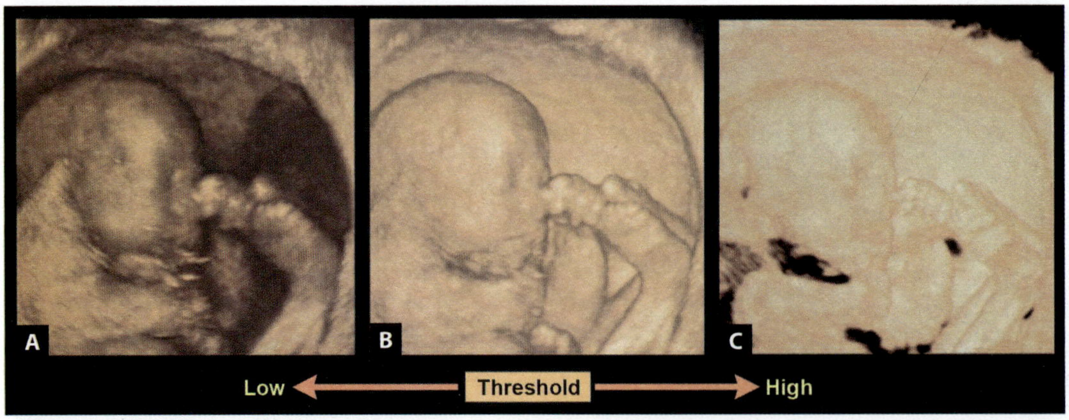

Figs. 38A to C: Three-dimensional images of the same fetus as in **Figure 37**. (A) Left leg cannot be seen with a low threshold; (B) It can be seen with increasing the threshold; (C) Parts of the fetus are also eliminated when the threshold is set too high.

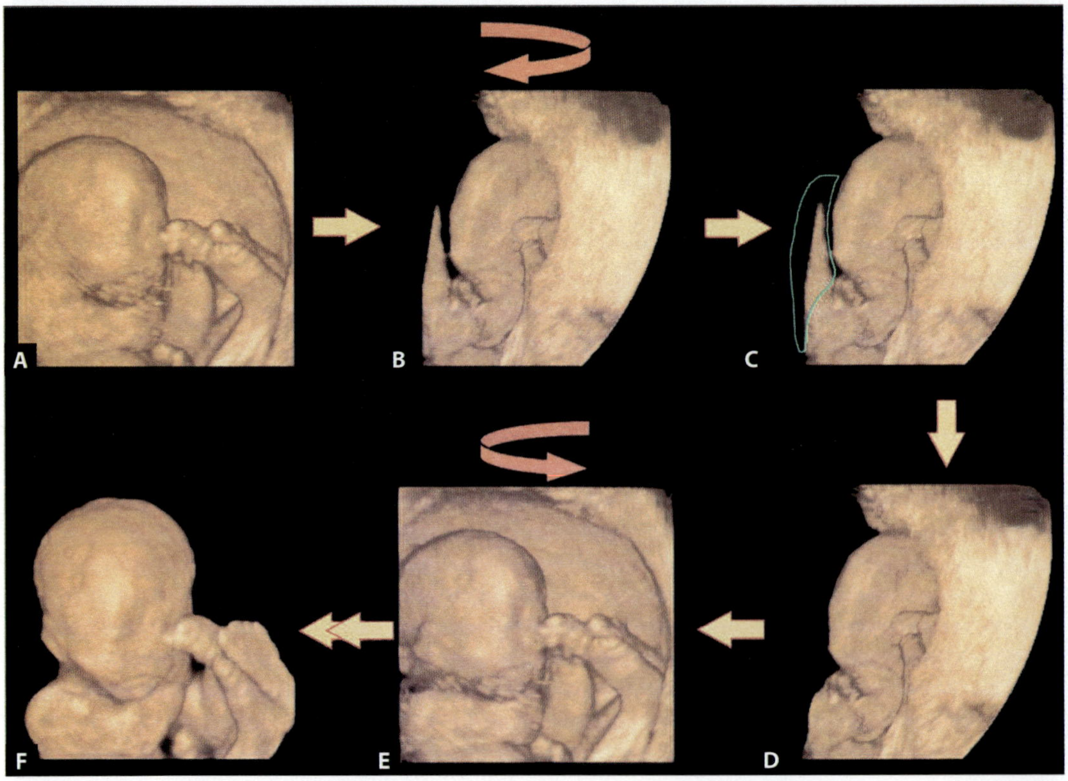

Figs. 39A to F: Removal of unfavorable parts around a fetus. (A) The fetus is partially covered by the uterine wall; (B to E) The uterine wall over the right shoulder is eliminated after rotating the 3D image and surrounding the uterine wall with green line. The remaining uterine wall and umbilical cord around the fetus can also be eliminated in the same manner; (F) A 3D image after removal of all unfavorable parts around the fetus.

Electrical Scalpel

Even when unfavorable images remain around a 3D image of the object after proper settings of ROI and threshold, unnecessary parts in the 3D data set can be removed in the computer and unfavorable images can be eliminated **(Figs. 39A to F)**. This function is called electrical scalpel or 3D cutting. Even a separated fetal bone can be displayed by this function **(Figs. 34A and B)**.

CONCLUSION

Three-dimensional ultrasound has many functions and possibilities that are not involved in conventional 2D ultrasound. Both volume rendering and surface rendering give a 3D image. Volume rendering provides various kinds of 3D images as well as a surface-rendered image. In surface rendering, the intermediate geometrical 3D data set can be easily used for volume measurement of the object as well as 3D image generation. Some considerations are required in 3D scanning, ROI setting, threshold setting and electrical scalpel to obtain a clearer 3D image.

REFERENCES

1. Szilard J. An improved three-dimensional display system. Ultrasonics. 1974;12(6):273-6.
2. Brinkley JF, McCallum WD, Muramatsu SK, et al. Fetal weight estimation from ultrasonic three-dimensional head and trunk reconstructions: evaluation in vitro. Am J Obstet Gynecol. 1982;144(6):715-21.
3. Baba K, Satoh K. Development of the system for ultrasonic fetal three-dimensional reconstruction. Acta Obst Gynaec Jpn. 1986;38:1385.
4. Woo J. A short history of the development of ultrasound in obstetrics and gynecology. [online]. Available from http://www.ob-ultrasound.net/history 3D. html [Accessed on July, 2016, 2011].
5. Baba K. Leaps of obstetrics and gynecology by ultrasonography - from transabdominal to transvaginal, from 2-dimensional to 3-dimensional - Osaka, Japan: Nagai Shoten; 1992.
6. Merz E, Macchiella D, Bahlmann F, et al. Fetale Fehlbildungsdiagnostik mit Hilfe der 3D-Sonographie. Ultraschall Klin Prax. 1991;6:147.
7. Kuo HC, Chang FM, Wu CH, et al. The primary application of three-dimensional ultrasonography in obstetrics. Am J Obstet Gynecol. 1992;166(3):880-6.
8. Sohn C, Stolz W, Nuber B, et al. Three-dimensional ultrasound diagnostics in gynaecology and obstetrics. Geburtshilfe Frauenheilkd. 1991;51:335-40.
9. Chiba Y, Yamazaki S, Takamizawa K, et al. Real-time three-dimensional effect using acoustic wide-angle lens for the view of fetuses. Jpn J Med Ultrasonics. 1993;20(suppl.1):611-2.
10. Kossoff G, Griffiths KA, Warren PS. Real-time quasi-three-dimensional viewing in sonography, with conventional gray-scale volume imaging. Ultrasound Obstet Gynecol. 1994;4(3):211-6.
11. Baba K, Okai T, Kozuma S. Real-time processable three-dimensional fetal ultrasound. Lancet. 1996;348(9037):1307.
12. Baba K, Jurkovic D (Eds). Three-dimensional Ultrasound in Obstetrics and Gynecology. Carnforth, UK: Parthenon Publishing; 1997.
13. Baba K. Introduction to three- and four-dimensional ultrasound. In: Kurjak A, Jackson D (Eds). An Atlas of Three- and Four-Dimensional Sonography in Obstetrics and Gynecology. New York, USA: Taylor and Francis; 2004. pp. 3-18.
14. Baba K. Basis of 3D ultrasound. In: Baba K (Ed). Ultrasound in Obstetrics and Gynecology. Tokyo, Japan: Tokyo Igaku Publishing; 2010. pp. 27-37.
15. Baba K, Okai T. Basis and principles of three-dimensional ultrasound. In: Baba K, Jurkovic D (Eds). Three-dimensional Ultrasound in Obstetrics and Gynecology. Carnforth, UK: Parthenon Publishing; 1997. pp. 1-19.
16. Baba K. Basis and principles of three-dimensional ultrasound. In: Takeuchi H, Baba K (Eds). Master three-dimensional ultrasound. Tokyo, Japan: Medical View; 2001. pp. 12-29.
17. Smith SW, Trahey GE, von Ramm OT. Two-dimensional array ultrasound transducers. Ultrason Imaging. 1992;14(3):213-33.
18. von Ramm OT, Smith SW, Carroll BA. Advanced real-time volumetric ultrasound scanning. J Ultrasound Med. 1995;14(suppl):S35.
19. Nelson TR, Pretorius DH, Hagan-Ansert S. Fetal heart assessment using three-dimensional ultrasound. J Ultrasound Med. 1995;14(suppl):S30.
20. Deng J, Gardener JE, Rodeck CH, et al. Fetal echocardiography in three and four dimensions. Ultrasound Med Biol. 1996;22:979-86.
21. Baba K, IO Y. Three-dimensional ultrasound in obstetrics and gynecology. Tokyo, Japan: Medical View; 2000.
22. Levoy M. Display of surfaces from volume data. IEEE Computer Graphics and Applications. 1988;8(3):29-37.

3

CHAPTER

Artifacts, Pitfalls and Normal Variants

Ivica Zalud, Frederico Rocha

INTRODUCTION

Artifacts in ultrasound are common problem in everyday clinical practice. Differentiating real findings and deceptive artifacts is very important. A good understanding of the physical principles of ultrasound waves, equipment and their interaction with anatomy being examined is essential in distinguishing reality, normal variants and artifacts.

What is the Problem?

- What gives the multiple appearance of an intrauterine contraceptive device?
  Answer: Reverberation.
- Why does an early single intrauterine pregnancy sometimes look like a twin gestation?
  Answer: Duplication artifact.
- Why is a large cyst-like structure occasionally seen in the pelvis when it does not exist?
  Answer: Mirror image artifact.
- Why does a simple cyst sometimes appear to contain a sludge-like layer?
  Answer: Slice thickness artifact.
- Why are dermoids, even large ones, sometimes not detectable sonographically?
  Answer: Shadowing (tip of the iceberg phenomenon).
- What does it all mean?
  Answer: In this chapter, these intriguing artifacts are described and explained. Advice on how to recognize and in some cases, how to minimize them is also given. On the other hand, the presence of artifacts can sometimes even be helpful in clinical practice and give additional information.

DEFINITION

Artifacts in ultrasound imaging occur as structures that are one of the following:

- Not real
- Missing
- Of improper brightness
- Of improper shape
- Of improper size.

Some artifacts are produced by improper equipment operation (e.g., improper transducer location and orientation information sent to the display) or settings (e.g., incorrect receiver compensation settings). Some are caused by improper scanning technique (e.g., allowing patient or organ movement during scanning). Other as inherent in the ultrasound diagnostic method and can occur even with proper equipment and technique.

MECHANISM

Artifacts are merely errors in presentation that result from the following assumptions:

Echoes come from interfaces that are:

- Directly in front of the transducer
- At a depth equal to half the time of flight of the sound pulse multiplied by a constant velocity (1,540 m/s).

In other words, if the pulse is reflected, refracted or otherwise affected in the body, the ultrasound machine has no way of knowing that. A blip that does not correspond to an actual interface at a corresponding point in the body may appear on the screen. The blip always appears on the screen at a point corresponding to the time since the production of the pulse and from the direction that the transducer was pointing.

CLASSIFICATION

Commonly encountered artifacts include:

- Reverberation and ring-down (comet tail)
- Shadowing
- Enhancement
- Mirror (multipath) artifacts
- Refraction and side lobes

- Curved and oblique reflector
- Propagation speed error
- Resolution
- Doppler artifacts
- Three-dimensional artifacts.

These artifacts are seen daily. Although some of these artifacts are more pronounced in the upper abdomen, chest or neck (the examples chosen are mainly those encountered in obstetric and gynecologic ultrasound examinations).

REVERBERATION

Reverberation results in reflectors that are not real, being placed on the image. They will be placed behind the second real reflector at separation intervals equal to the separation between the first and second real reflectors. Each subsequent reflection will be weaker than prior ones. This can occur from the anterior wall of the urinary bladder, especially in an obese person **(Fig. 1)**. The sound pulse is reflected back from the anterior wall of the bladder to the transducer face. As the transducer has to produce the true echo, it absorbs some of the pulse. However, some of that sound is reflected from the transducer-skin interface back into the body. It again hits the anterior bladder interface and is reflected back for a second time to the transducer. This produces a first reverberation artifact on the image. The ultrasound equipment assumes (incorrectly) that the signal has returned from a point in the body that is twice the distance from the transducer, as it is aware only of the time taken for the signal to return and not of the path actually travelled. This artifact is seen as a blip on the screen at twice the depth of the true echo. This is because the time taken for the first reverberation artifact is the same time taken for the pulse to travel the original distance and back. This same reverberation can occur a second and third time to give the second or third reverberation artifact. This is commonly known as "near-field" artifact, especially in obese patients. The echoes may be more diffuse and fuzzy if they bounce around in various directions in the subcutaneous fat before returning to the transducer.[1] Occasionally, care must be taken not to confuse this artifact for an anterior placenta.

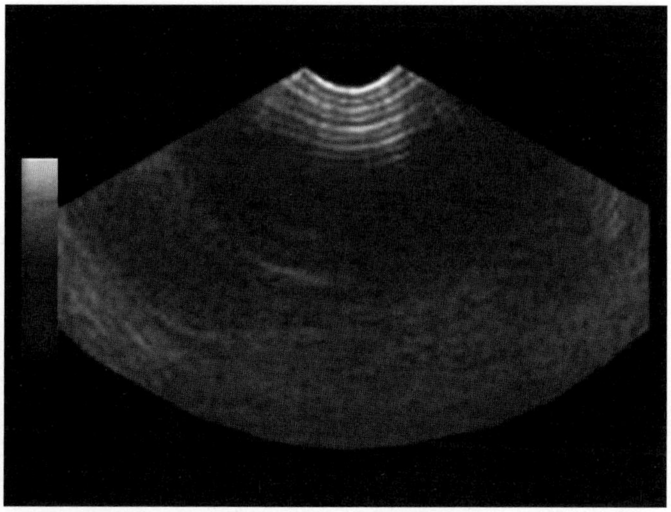

Fig. 1: Reverberation: Anterior wall of the urinary bladder in an obese person.

Ring-down is another type of reverberation artifact. It occurs when the sound hits a metallic structure, such as a metallic surgical clip or a group of small gas bubbles. In this situation, the sound bounces back and forth numerous times within the structure, each time sending some of the sound back to the transducer. This, therefore, appears on the screen as numerous tiny parallel echoes deep to the structure. This artifact has also been called a "comet tail". Certain situations are there, where there are only one or two reverberations deep to a structure. This can occur with intrauterine device (IUD) in the uterus.

Since reverberation artifacts are produced by sound bouncing back and forth within the body, it is virtually impossible to adjust the machine to get rid of them. Although one can turn down the near gain, the real echoes will be lost along with the artifactual ones. The presence of a ring-down artifact enables the identification of gas. When this is found in an abnormal, extraluminal location, it may indicate that the patient has an abscess. In other situations, a ring-down artifact indicates that there is gas and therefore, the "mass" seen deep to it is likely to be an artifact. When needle biopsies are done under ultrasound guidance, the needle also produces a ring-down artifact, which is particularly helpful in identifying the location of the needle on the image.

SHADOWING

Shadowing is the reduction in reflection amplitude from reflectors that lie behind a strongly reflecting or attenuating structure. Shadows in ultrasound may be due to reflection, absorption or refraction. The reflective or absorptive shadows are entirely analogous to the shadow cast by a tree in the sun. All of the light is reflected and/or absorbed by the tree trunk, so that there is a relative shadow on the tar side. With ultrasound, all of the sound beam must be blocked by a calcification to produce a shadow. There should be an echo from the near side of the structure as well. It is possible to produce an echo without a shadow if the structure only impinges on part of the sound beam without being large enough to block it completely. It is therefore possible to have small clumps of calcification that do not produce a shadow. One cannot change the size of the calcified structure. However, one can choose the correct transducer or the correct focal level to maximize the chance of identifying the shadow. The narrowest beam and narrowest portion of the beam are necessary to identify a shadow. If the focal depth of a transducer is adjusted either too close or too far, the echoes may be identified but not the shadows. If shadowing is not present, the calcified nature of a lesion or structure may be missed.

Air can also cause shadowing **(Figs. 2 and 3)**. Most of the time, this causes great interference on the ultrasound examination by obscuring the deeper structures. For this reason, patients have to be examined with a full bladder to displace the air-containing bowel from the pelvis. The shadow deep to gas is different from the shadow deep to a calcified structure. With the latter, although some of the sound is reflected, much of it is absorbed. With gas, the acoustic mismatch is so great that virtually all of the sound is reflected. This sound bounces around in the tissues between the transducer and the gas, and can cause numerous reverberations and other mirror image artifacts, which on the image appear deep to the echo from the gas interface. This has been called a "dirty" shadow as opposed to the "clean" shadow deep to bone or other calcified (sound-absorbing) structures. This distinction does not always hold true but most of the shadows due to gas are easily differentiated from shadows due to hard and/or calcified structures. As previously mentioned, the presence of ring-down is of further value in recognizing gas. Another type of shadowing is associated particularly with dermoid cysts. This is a peculiar situation in which there is a strong "dirty" shadow that is likely due to the inhomogeneous structures within a dermoid. These include hair, cartilage, fat and so on. This appearance of strong shadowing can cause a difficulty in diagnosing dermoids because they can look very similar to gas and stool in the bowel, in both transverse and longitudinal scans. This is the so-called tip of the iceberg sign.[2] The stool-filled rectum can mimic a dermoid or a dermoid can be overlooked by assuming that it is the rectum. When there is a clinical suspicion, a digital examination or water enema during ultrasound visualization may help differentiate between the two.

Another kind of shadow occurs at the edge of structures when the sound beam passes through an oblique interface. When the sound beam passes through a curved or oblique interface, some of the sound beam can be refracted away from the central line. This can result in a defocusing of the sound beam deep to the oblique interface and can be seen at the edge of the fetal skull, especially when the beam passes through the placenta. Occasionally, these can be at the edges of cysts in the ovaries. Refractive shadowing can also cause a drop-out of echoes deep to the bladder in the

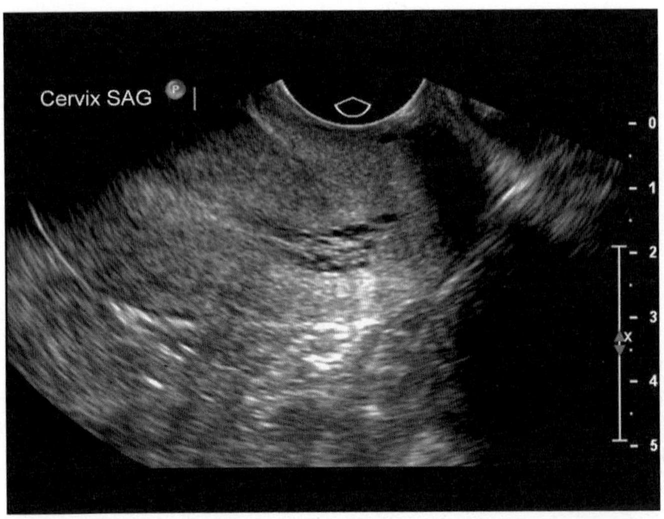

Fig. 2: Shadowing artifacts on transvaginal ultrasound caused by air in the condom. Portion of the cervix and cul-de-sac are "in the dark."

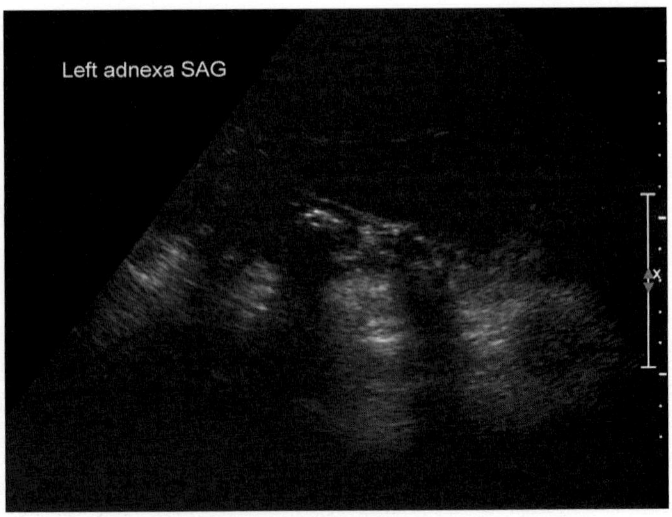

Fig. 3: Another example of shadowing caused by air in the bowels.

lower uterine segment or in the region of the cervix. This is especially true in patients with leiomyomas.

ENHANCEMENT

Enhancement is the opposite of shadowing. It is the increase in reflection amplitude from reflectors that lie behind a weakly attenuating structure **(Figs. 4 and 5)**. Shadowing and enhancement result in reflectors being placed on the image with amplitudes that are too low and too high, respectively. In this situation, the echoes returning from structures deep to cysts appear more intense than if the cyst were not interposed. There are two explanations for this phenomenon. One is that the fluid replaces normal soft tissue in the intervening space, decreasing its attenuation.[3] The time gain compensation (TGC) is set to expect tissue between the transducer and the deepest echoes. If there is fluid instead, especially if the fluid occupies only the central portion of the image, the echoes returning from deep to the fluid collection will be more intense than expected.[3] This appears as a posterior enhancement of the beam and this finding indicates that a lesion is truly cystic, even if there are internal echoes within the cyst. Occasionally, enhancement will be noted deep to a very small cystic structure, more than what can be explained by a lack of attenuation. The small cyst acting as a lens and refocusing the sound beam may cause this enhancement.[4] This is the opposite of refractive shadowing where the oblique interface defocusses the beam. Often the two co-exist.

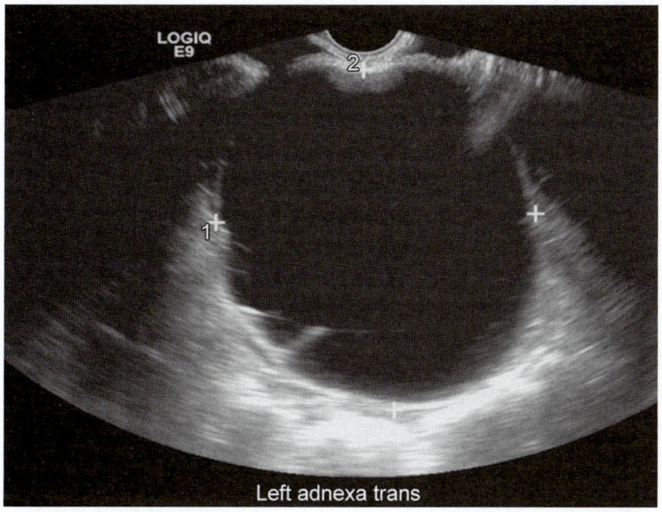

Fig. 4: Enhancement: The echoes returning from structures deep to the cyst appear more intense than if the ovarian cyst was not interposed.

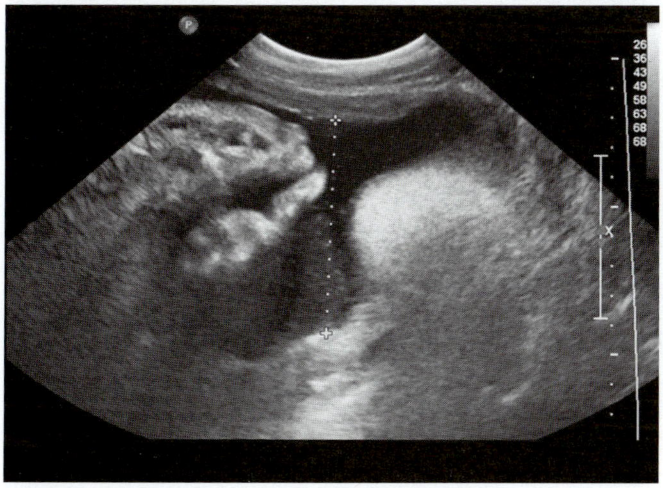

Fig. 5: Enhancement caused by amniotic fluid. Bright edges are clearly seen.

MIRROR ARTIFACTS

The term mirror or multipath artifact describes the situation in which the paths to and from a reflector are different. This artifact results in improper reflector image positioning. If separation is not sufficient, two reflectors are seen as one (missing-reflector artifact). Whereas reverberations and ring-downs are reflections that occur back and forth within the direction of the original sound beam, a mirror image artifact is one in which the sound beam is deflected away from the transducer. The reflected sound may hit a strong interface, be bounced back to the "mirror" and then back to the transducer. The machine will therefore receive an echo and display a blip on the screen in the direction that the transducer was pointing and at a distance corresponding to the time taken. However, this will be a phantom echo since there is no interface in that position. It can also cause significant trouble when it produces a mirror image of the bladder deep to the rectum or sigmoid colon. In this situation, the phantom can closely resemble a cyst, ovarian tumor or leiomyoma.[1] This kind of artifact can fool even the most experienced sonologists. Differentiating between a true lesion and a mirror image artifact can be difficult. However, the phantom cyst frequently has an unusual, somewhat triangular shape on the longitudinal scan. The back wall is often very ill defined, whereas true cystic lesions invariably have a good, clear posterior wall. It is important to realize that this artifact is seen on both transverse and longitudinal scans. One can have the patient partially empty the bladder. This will cause the phantom mass to become proportionately smaller. It is, however, important that the patient does not empty the bladder completely as real lesions can then be missed. Transvaginal scanning can be very useful in difficult cases.

REFRACTION (DUPLICATION) AND SIDE LOBES

This most interesting artifact occurs uniquely when the transducer is held in a transverse plane over the linea alba. The sound is refracted toward the midline when the transducer is pointing to the medial edge of the rectal muscle on either side. This makes small midline structures appear duplicated on the screen. This phenomenon can cause an erroneous appearance of early twins due to duplication of a single small gestational sac. In addition, intrauterine device can appear duplicated. One could similarly diagnose a bicornuate uterus erroneously. This artifact does not occur in a sagittal or transverse section once the transducer is moved to either side of the midline.[5,6] Not only is the beam not as narrow as anticipated, but also there is a phenomenon called "side lobes." Due to refraction, there are relatively strong beams of sound outside the main beam. If one of these "side lobes" strikes an interface and especially if that interface is concave toward the transducer, an echo is received by the transducer. Once again, the transducer and machine have no way of knowing that this came from outside the main beam and it will be displayed as though it were an interface directly in front of the transducer. These artifacts generally appear as curved lines that can be followed back to their origin. They are commonly seen in the bladder, coming off the concave surface anterior to the fundus of the uterus. Occasionally, they come from a loop of bowel that indents the bladder slightly. Refraction can cause a reflector to be improperly positioned on the display. A similar occurrence can be caused by reflections from side lobes. Refraction and propagation speed error can also cause a structure to be displayed with incorrect shape.

OTHER ARTIFACTS

A curved reflector can produce a reflection low in amplitude because some of the reflection is missed by the transducer. Oblique reflection can produce a reflection low in amplitude or the reflection may be completely missed by the transducer. Resolution also increases the apparent size of a reflector on a display. Propagation speed error occurs when the assumed value for propagation speed in the range equation is incorrect. Diagnostic instrumentation assumes a speed of 1,540 m/s. If the propagation speed that exists over a path traveled is greater than 1,540 m/s, the calculated distance to the reflector is too small and the display will place the reflector too close to the transducer. If the actual speed is less than 1,540 m/s, the reflector will be displayed too far from the transducer. The minimum displayed lateral and longitudinal dimensions will be the beam diameter and one-half the spatial pulse length, respectively.

DOPPLER ULTRASOUND ARTIFACTS

Aliasing

Aliasing is the most common artifact encountered in Doppler ultrasound.[7] There is an upper limit to Doppler shift that can be detected by pulsed instruments. If the Doppler shift frequency exceeds one half the pulse repetition frequency (normally in the 1–30 kHz range), aliasing occurs and improper Doppler shift information (improper direction and improper value) results. Higher pulse repetition frequencies permit higher Doppler shifts to be detected but also increase the chance of the range ambiguity artifact **(Figs. 6 and 7)**. Aliasing in a color flow system is exposed in a spatial two-dimensional plane in which the aliased flow is shown in reversed color surrounded by non-aliased flow **(Fig. 8)**. This pattern mimics the color flow appearance of separate streams in differing directions. The two patterns

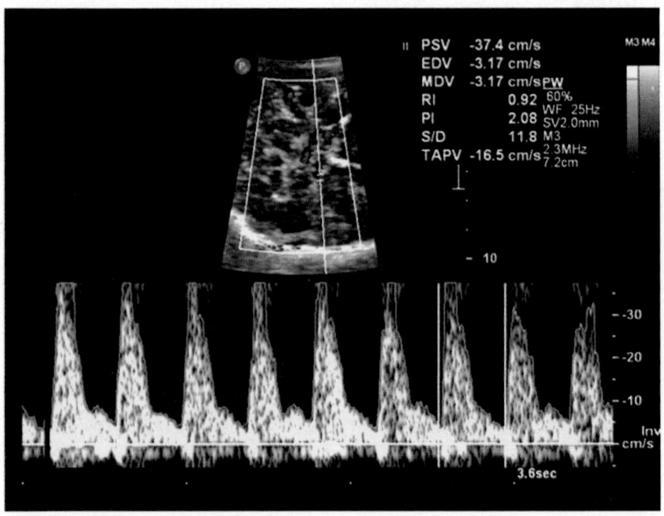

Fig. 6: Aliasing: Higher pulse repetition frequencies (PRF) permit higher Doppler shifts to be detected but also increase the chance of the range ambiguity artifact.

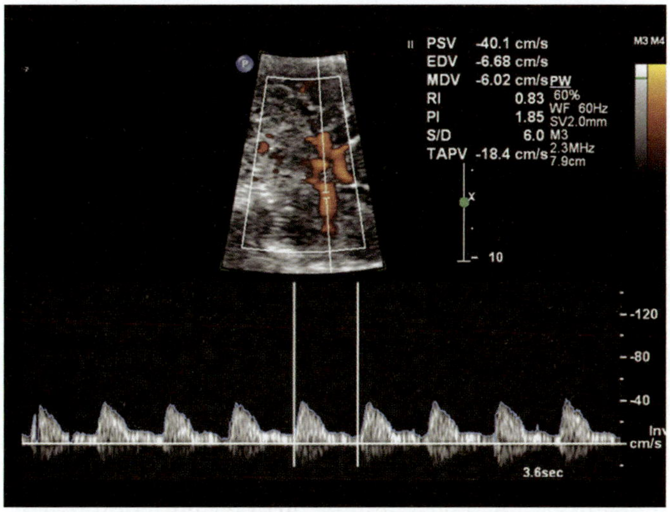

Fig. 7: Appropriate PRF setting to avoid aliasing in pulsed Doppler waveform analysis.

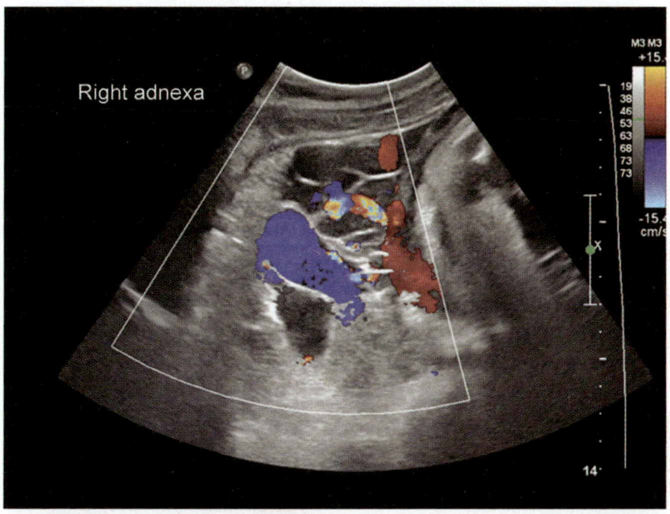

Fig. 8: Right complex, mostly cystic adnexal mass. Color Doppler aliasing shown in the middle of the mass (neovascularization) with normal red (uterine vein) and blue color (internal iliac vein) displayed on side.

are, however, clearly distinguishable. In an aliased flow, the higher velocity generates a higher Doppler shifted frequency that is depicted with greater brightness. The higher the frequency shifts, the brighter the color. The brightest level in the color calibration bar (the uppermost for the flow toward the transducer and lowermost for the flow away from the transducer) represents the Nyquist limit. As the velocity and therefore, the frequency shift exceeds this limit, the color wraps around the calibration bar and appears at the other end as the most luminous color of the opposite direction. For example, a flow toward the transducer with an increasing velocity is depicted with an increasingly bright red color changing to yellow. As the Nyquist limit is reached, the color flow shows brightest yellow in the color bar and as the limit exceeds, flow is shown in the brightest blue. Thus in an aliased flow, bright or pale color of one direction is juxtaposed against bright color of the opposite direction. In contrast, in genuine flow separation the distinct flow streams are depicted in the directionally appropriate colors that are separated by a dark margin. It should be noted that the hue that demarcates an aliased flow would depend on the choice of the color-mapping scheme.

Aliasing can be eliminated by increasing pulse repetition frequency, increasing Doppler angle (which decreases the Doppler shift for a given flow) or by baseline shifting. The latter is an electronic “cut and paste” technique that moves the misplaced aliasing peaks over to their proper location. It is a successful technique as long as there is no legitimate Doppler shifts in the region of the aliasing. If there are, they will get moved over to an inappropriate location along with the aliasing peaks. Other approaches to eliminating aliasing include changing to a lower frequency Doppler transducer or changing to a continuous-wave instrument. Aliasing occurs with the pulsed system because it is a sampling system.[8] If samples are taken often enough, the correct result is achieved. Sufficient sampling yields the correct result. Insufficient sampling yields an incorrect result.

Range Ambiguity

In an attempt to solve the aliasing problem by increasing pulse repetition frequency, the range ambiguity problem can be encountered.[9] This occurs when a pulse is emitted before all the echoes from the previous pulse have been received. When this happens, early echoes from the last pulse are simultaneously received with late echoes from the previous pulse. This causes difficulty with the ranging process. The instrument is unable to determine whether an echo is an early one (superficial) from the last pulse or a late one (deep) from the previous pulse. To avoid this difficulty, it simply assumes that all echoes are derived from the last pulse and that these echoes have originated from some depth. As long as all echoes are received before the next pulse is sent out, this will be true. However, with high pulse repetition frequencies, this may not be the case. Doppler flow information may, therefore, come from locations other than the assumed one (the gate location).

In effect, multiple gates or sample volumes are operating at different depths. Instruments often increase pulse repetition frequency (to avoid aliasing) into the range where range ambiguity occurs. Multiple sample gates are shown on the display to indicate this condition. Range ambiguity in color-flow Doppler, as in sonography, places echoes (color Doppler shifts in this case) that have come from deep locations after a subsequent pulse was emitted in shallow locations where they do not belong. In practice, however, most Doppler color flow devices prevent this problem by automatically reducing the depth when the pulse repetition frequency is increased to the threshold of range ambiguity.

Temporal Ambiguity

Temporal ambiguity occurs when Doppler color flow mapping fails to depict hemodynamic events with temporal accuracy. Specifically, such a situation arises when the frame rate for color flow is too slow relative to the circulatory dynamics. As discussed earlier, the basic unit of color flow depiction is a single frame which when completed shows the average mean frequency shifts color coded and superimposed on the gray scale tissue image. The flow dynamics are, therefore, summarized for the duration of one frame. As we have noted above, the frame rate is inversely proportional to the number of scan lines and the number of samples per scan line. The slower the frame rates the better the color image quality in terms of both spatial resolution and Doppler sensitivity. Herein lies the paradox as a slower rate means longer duration of a frame. As the frame duration increases, there is a progressive loss of the ability to recognize discrete hemodynamic events.

Angle of Insonation

Angle dependency of the Doppler shifted frequencies is also a critical factor in blood-flow analysis. In sector scanning, multiple scan lines spread out from the transducer in a fan-like manner. When the sector scanner is used to interrogate a circulatory system in which the direction of flow is across these scan lines in a color window, the angle of insonation between the flow axis and the ultrasound beam changes. The angle is smallest when the flow stream enters in the sector field and progressively rises to 90° as the flow approaches the center of the field. Concurrently, the Doppler shifted frequencies progressively decline and may become undetectable at the center of the color field. A sector scanner may also create apparently contradictory directional information in a vessel traversing across the color field. As the flow approaches the midline of the field, the flow is depicted in color encoding for flow toward the transducer which usually is red; as the flow moves away, it will be encoded blue. Thus, the same vessel will show bidirectional flow. This paradox actually highlights the basic concept of representation of flow directionality by any Doppler system.

Doppler Mirror Artifact

The mirror image artifact can also occur with Doppler systems. This means that an image of a vessel and a source of Doppler shifted echoes can be duplicated on the opposite side of a strong reflector (such as a bone). The duplicated vessel containing flow could be misinterpreted as an additional vessel. It will have a spectrum similar to that for the real vessel **(Fig. 9)**. A mirror image of a Doppler spectrum can appear on the opposite side of the baseline when, indeed, flow is unidirectional and should appear only on one side of the baseline.[10] This is an electronic duplication of the spectral information. It can occur when receiver gain is set too high (causing overloading in the receiver and cross talk between the two flow channels) or with low gain (where the receiver has difficulty determining the sign of the Doppler shift). It can also occur when Doppler angle is near 90°. Here the duplication is usually legitimate and this is because beams

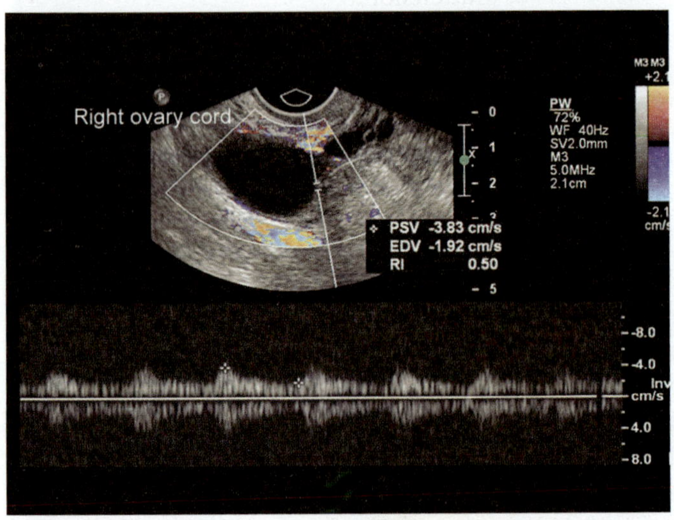

Fig. 9: Mirror effect: A mirror image of a Doppler spectrum appeared on the opposite side of the baseline when blood flow was unidirectional and should appear only on one side of the baseline.

are focused and not cylindrical in shape. Thus, portions of the beam can experience flow toward while other portions can experience flow away.

3D ULTRASOUND ARTIFACTS

Three-dimensional (3D) ultrasonography is a rapidly developing area with increased application in obstetrics and gynecology. Unfortunately, its technology is not only susceptible to artifacts, but the volume acquisition also can present unique artifacts. The images obtained are usually acquired by a series of 2D image planes that are rendered to a volume 3D image. Motion or vibration of the targeted organ during the acquisition of a volume introduces a motion artifact into the volume. The motion artifact affects the overall quality of a volume and is particularly relevant in obstetric imaging because of the movement of the fetus.[11] Shadowing from adjacent structures can reproduce, e.g., an apparent limb defect or cleft lip and palate **(Fig. 10)**.[12]

Technical aspects of imaging must be considered as this new technology is learned by practitioners in our field. Not only are there artifacts inherent to 2D imaging present in 3D ultrasound but additional artifacts specific to volume imaging have also emerged. Such acoustic artifacts as dropout and shadowing which are well known to the ultrasound community are present in 3D imaging, although more difficult to recognize due to different and unfamiliar displays. Color and power Doppler artifacts relating to gain and flash may also be confusing in rendered images. Three-dimensional volume sets are hampered by fetal movement, cardiac motion, as well as movement of adjacent structures. Acoustic shadowing and other artifacts look very different when displayed in 3D volumes and may be more difficult to recognize than on standard 2D due to lack of specific training of personnel. Acquiring data from multiple orientations may avoid artifacts of this type.

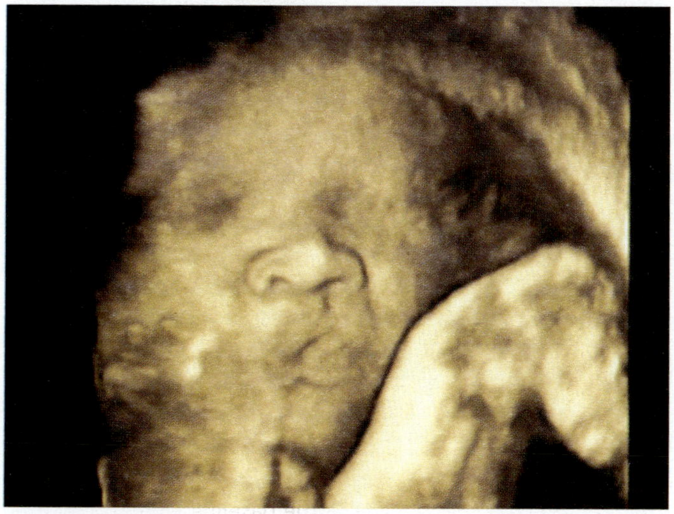

Fig. 10: 3D artifact: Shadowing from adjacent structures reproduced an apparent cleft lip and palate.

CONCLUSION

A prerequisite for optimal utilization of ultrasound in obstetrics and gynecology is an in-depth knowledge of the principles and limitations of this dynamic technique. It is important to appreciate that the appearance of Doppler images is influenced by the operational setting of the equipment that must be taken into account for any reliable interpretation. Only persons with sufficient training and education should perform diagnostic ultrasound. One of the major reasons for so many conflicting and controversial results in the ultrasound literature originates from technique complexity and rather limited education in physics and technique. With all artifacts, but especially with mirror image artifacts, it is important not to let a superficial knowledge cause trouble. Once the cause and nature of an artifact are understood, it is important not to misinterpret a real lesion as an artifact and miss the true pathology. This can happen, particularly with pelvic masses such as leiomyomas with poor through transmission in which the deep wall is not well seen. If there is also an artifact situated near where the deep wall would be, the actual mass might be dismissed as simply an artifact. One must pay attention at all times not only to identify artifacts, but also not to let them interfere with the identification of true lesions. While the more common artifacts seen on ultrasound images frequently are ignored and appreciated as such, it is certainly interesting to know why they occur. On the other hand, the usefulness of artifacts cannot be underestimated. Occasionally, the identification of an artifact may prevent the novice from making an important error in diagnosis or management. An appreciation and understanding of how to avoid artifacts can help even the more experienced practitioner decide whether a structure is real. It is also important not to ignore real pathology under the assumption that it is caused by an artifact.

REFERENCES

1. Laing FC, Brown DL, DiSalvo DN. Gynecologic ultrasound. Radiol Clin North Am. 2001;39(3):523-40.

2. Guttman PH. In search of the elusive benign cystic ovarian teratoma: application of the ultrasound "tip of the iceberg" sign. J Clin Ultrasound. 1977;5(6):403-6.
3. Filly RA, Sommer FG, Minton MJ. Characterization of biological fluids by ultrasonic computed tomography. Radiology. 1980;134(1):167-71.
4. Robinson DE, Wilson LS, Kossoff G. Shadowing and enhancement in ultrasonic echograms by reflection and refraction. J Clin Ultrasound. 1981;9(4):181-6.
5. Buttery B, Davison G. The ghost artifact. J Ultrasound Med. 1984;3(2):49-52.
6. Sauerbrei EE. The split image artifact in pelvic ultrasonography: the anatomy and physics. J Ultrasound Med. 1985;4(1):29-34.
7. Zalud I, Kurjak A, Maulik D, et al. Transvaginal Doppler: measurements and errors. In: Kurjak A, Kupesic S (Eds). An Atlas of transvaginal color Doppler. New York-London, Parthenon Publishing. 2000;255-62.
8. Mitchell DG. Color Doppler imaging: principles, limitations, and artifacts. Radiology. 1990;177(1):1-10.
9. Kremkau FW. Doppler color imaging: principles and instrumentation. Clin Diagn Ultrasound. 1992;27:7-60.
10. Burns PN. Principles of Doppler and color flow. Radiol Med. 1993;85(5 Suppl 1):3-16.
11. Nelson TR, Pretorius DH, Hull A, et al. Sources and impact of artifacts on clinical three-dimensional ultrasound imaging. Ultrasound Obstet Gynecol. 2000;16(4):374-83.
12. Hull AD, Pretorius DH, Lev-Toaff A, et al. Artifacts and the visualization of fetal distal extremities using three-dimensional ultrasound. Ultrasound Obstet Gynecol. 2000;16(4):341-4.

4

CHAPTER

Routine Use of Obstetric Ultrasound

Geeta Sharma, Stephen T Chasen, Frank A Chervenak

INTRODUCTION

Ultrasound examination of the fetus became integrated into prenatal care soon after its introduction in the late 1950s. The past four decades have seen further improvements in ultrasound technology and advances in its utility, as well as the promotion of respect for patient's autonomy and involvement in medical care. There is concomitant support for and opposition to the routine use of ultrasound in pregnancy. Questions remain regarding the benefits and harms of routine obstetric ultrasound. How often should a "routine" ultrasound be performed? When should the "routine" ultrasound be performed? Who should receive an ultrasound? Who should perform the ultrasound? How should the results be interpreted? Many of these questions do not have a clear answer. These answers gain importance as ultrasound burgeons with the dynamic field of obstetrics and gynecology research unveils a multitude of applications for this remarkable tool.

BASIC ULTRASOUND

The real-time obstetric ultrasound examination is usually performed with the pregnant patient in the supine position. A distended bladder aids in displacing bowel loops and can facilitate visualization with the transabdominal approach.[1] Sonogram gel is applied to the transabdominal or transvaginal transducer. The gel simulates a liquid interface that permits optimum travel of the sound waves.

Ultrasound consists of high frequency sound waves that encounter a tissue interface and are reflected, refracted, attenuated or absorbed. The mechanical vibration required for the most obstetric imaging ranges between 3–7 MHz (megahertz), million cycles per second. A transducer or ultrasound probe contains piezoelectric material and a crystal that together generate ultrasound waves. The crystal resonates when electrical current traverses the piezoelectric ceramic.[2]

The ultrasound beam is emitted radially and transmits through tissue as a longitudinal wave influenced by the velocity of the ultrasound between interacting particles and density of particles encountered. Therefore, ultrasound penetration is dependent on the tissue particles' elasticity and mass, which both contribute to the tissue's acoustic impedance. The velocity of ultrasound in soft tissue is relatively constant, except in adipose tissue where the speed is reduced by approximately 20%. In most of the soft tissues, changes in acoustic impedance are dependent on changes in tissue density. When the ultrasound beam contacts large differences in tissue interfaces, reflection of the beam can occur. Only 2–10% reflection occurs between soft tissues, permitting most of the ultrasound waves to travel deeper to distant structures. However, interfaces such as air-tissue or bone/calculus-tissue allow 100% and 67% reflection of the incident ultrasound beam, respectively, creating a distal acoustic shadow.[2]

After processing the reflected beams received by the transducer, an image is constructed and displayed on a monitor. Most obstetric ultrasound imaging uses the pulse-echo method that measures the time delay between the insonant beam to the echo reflected by the tissue back to the transducer. An image is recreated from these echoes and reflected waves. Real-time ultrasound relies on a continual sweep of pulsed waves. With rapid repetition, the transducer sweeps the area being scanned approximately 30 times in one second.[3]

Other ultrasound wave behaviors include refraction, attenuation and absorption. In addition to reflecting the insonant beam, tissue can refract or scatter the normally coherent waves. Ultrasound energy is lost by refraction, resulting in diminished energy returned to the transducer. Thus, the received signal is attenuated. Further attenuation can occur from the conversion of acoustic energy to thermal energy by tissues and energy is absorbed. A larger degree of absorption is seen with tissue containing larger molecules, greater viscosity and with higher frequency ultrasound. Although higher frequency ultrasound, with its shorter wavelengths, allows for greater resolution, its transabdominal use can be limited due to absorption. Conversely, endovaginal ultrasound minimizes both the distance between the transducer and the area being scanned and contact with tissue with high acoustic impedance, i.e., bone. The frequencies employed in diagnostic ultrasound do not generate significant thermal energy as is possible and often desired with therapeutic ultrasound.[2]

Ultrasound intensity is a temporal measure of energy (watts) exposure over a surface (cm^2). The special peak temporal average intensity represents the peak intensity. Devices for fetal heart auscultation use continuous wave ultrasound with a special peak temporal average intensity ranging between 0.6–80 mW/cm^2. The range for pulse echo imaging is between 1–200 mW/cm^2. The fetal dose depends on both intensity and exposure time, which are influenced by maternal habitus and operator skill.[4,5] It is prudent to minimize the number and duration of ultrasound examinations in order to keep the in utero exposure as low as reasonably achievable, i.e., the ALARA principle.[5]

SAFETY

Diagnostic ultrasound of the developing fetus has largely been considered safe without apparent deleterious effects. Greater image resolution and pulsed Doppler mode are possible with greater acoustic output. With this technological innovation, the fetal intensity may be increased up to eight fold. The potential teratogenicity of sound energy conversion to thermal energy and mechanical bioeffects of cavitation have not been proven or ascribed to diagnostic ultrasound.[6] These effects are associated with the higher intensities of continuous wave therapeutic ultrasound. Cavitation refers to the escape of dissolved gases in tissues due to localized low pressure created by very high intensity ultrasound.[2]

The American Institute of Ultrasound in Medicine (AIUM) 1998 conference on mechanical bioeffects encouraged continued research regarding ultrasound safety, especially in tissues with known gas bodies, i.e., lung and intestine. The conference did conclude "there is no known risk of lung or intestinal hemorrhage in the fluid-filled human fetal lung or intestine that is exposed to diagnostic ultrasound during a routine obstetrical examination."[7] In 2002, the AIUM stated "although there are no confirmed biological effects from ultrasound at the present time, the possibility exists that such biological effects may be identified in the future."[8]

In order to monitor the potential bioeffects, newer ultrasound equipment can display the acoustic output, measured by the thermal and mechanical indices. The thermal index measures the temperature absorption; a value below 1.0 is not considered concerning. The mechanical index measures the likelihood of cavitation by measuring the decompressive and compressive forces of ultrasound pulses. Some machines will display one index; the thermal index will be shown for Doppler imaging and the mechanical index for imaging.[5]

Long-term follow up of randomized controlled studies of routine versus selected ultrasound in Norway[9,10] and in Sweden[11,12] do not show a significant affect on subsequent childhood neurological development **(Fig. 1)**. In addition, a meta-analysis of childhood malignancies and birth weight showed, overall, no significant negative effects from antenatal ultrasound.[13] An association has been described between left-handedness in a retrospective cohort study

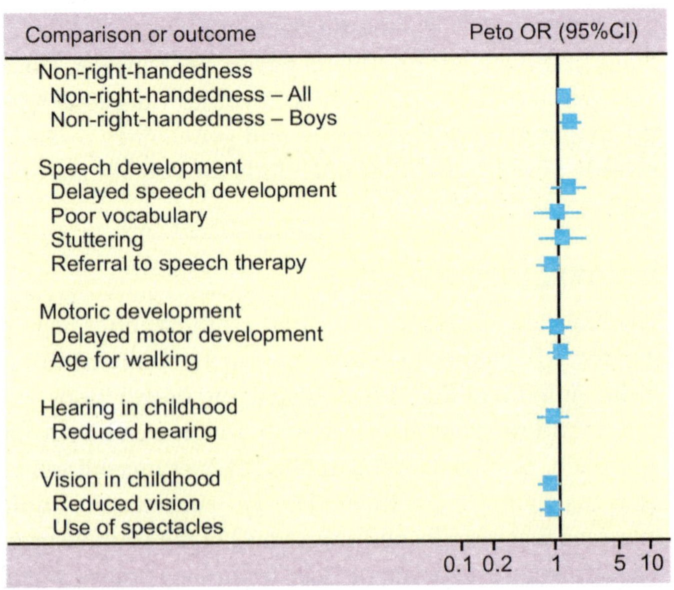

Fig. 1: Meta-analysis of Nordic and Swedish studies on routine ultrasound during pregnancy and childhood neurological development.

Note: Meta-analysis from ultrasound during pregnancy and birthweight, childhood malignancies and neurological development. Ultrasound in Med. and Biol. 1999;25(7):1028. Reproduced with permission.

of males enlisting in the military. Their exposure or nonexposure to ultrasound was assumed in accordance to local practices based on their place of birth.[14] However, follow-up in the aforementioned randomized controlled trials did not show an increase in non-right-handedness in children randomized to routine ultrasound when subgroup gender analysis was not performed and intention to treat maintained.[15] A provocative study from Yale School of Medicine showed a dose (duration of exposure) - response effect at 7.5 MHz in neuronal migration in mice exposed to ultrasound waves. As the gestational period and alignment of mice fetuses in the U-shaped mouse uterus differs greatly from human gestations, it is difficult to extrapolate this study to significant clinical effects in human fetuses.[16] In addition, the aforementioned long-term studies show that routine ultrasound does not have deleterious effects in humans.

GUIDELINES FOR THE USE OF OBSTETRIC ULTRASOUND

The 1984 National Institutes of Health (NIH) Consensus Development Conference on Diagnostic Ultrasound Imaging in Pregnancy called for studies to evaluate the efficacy of antenatal ultrasound and its affect on perinatal morbidity and mortality.[17,18] The consensus statement suggested 28 scenarios that may benefit from ultrasound evaluation **(Box 1)**. However, "this document is no longer viewed by NIH as guidance for current medical practice."[17] In 1993 and 1997, the AIUM and Royal College of Obstetricians and Gynecologists, respectively, set forth standards for the "antepartum obstetrical ultrasound examination" **(Box 2 and Fig. 2)**.[19] Further detail for performing the anatomical survey is found in **Table 1**.[20] The AIUM has also delineated guidelines for ultrasound accreditation to ensure proper technique and expertise.[21]

Responsible utilization of this technology obligates expert training in performance and interpretation of antenatal sonography to minimize false positive and false negative diagnoses.

Routine obstetric ultrasound has been implemented in the United Kingdom, Sweden (1976), Germany (1980), Denmark, Norway (1986), Iceland (1987), Austria (1988), Greece, France, Canada and Australia.[22-26] The rate of antenatal ultrasound performance in the United States by women with live births has steadily increased from 47.7% in 1989 to more than 67% in 2001. Since data was acquired from birth certificate information, this percentage is underestimated, as it does not include spontaneous fetal losses and abortions.[27] The American College of Obstetrics and Gynecology (ACOG) now recommends routine ultrasound for the general population as their 2007 Practice Bulletin supports first trimester nuchal translucency measurement as part of a combined first trimester risk assessment for fetal aneuploidy.[28]

RANDOMIZED CONTROLLED TRIALS OF ROUTINE ULTRASOUND

The wide acceptance of antenatal ultrasound by physicians and patients precludes the fulfillment of a study that adequately and accurately evaluates the impact of ultrasound on prenatal care and perinatal outcomes. In addition, in the setting of uncertainty where benefits outweigh potential risks, respect for a patient's autonomy obligates the physician to offer obstetric ultrasound where available.[29]

Antecedent ultrasound studies randomized patients to routine versus selective antenatal sonography, but were of insufficient power to detect a reduction in perinatal mortality or morbidity. An early prospective randomized trial of routine obstetric ultrasound was performed by Bennet et al. in London.[30] In this study, 1,062 women underwent routine ultrasound at 16 weeks menstrual age. The fetal biparietal diameter (BPD) was measured and dates corrected in 25% of the patients, mostly due to an overestimation from the last menstrual period. Patients were then randomized to one of two groups, using the last digit of the patients' hospital number. In the study group, the BPD information was shared with the clinician while it was withheld in the control group. However, the authors conceded BPD results were revealed, due to ethical obligations, in 30% (161/531) of the patients in the control group in which there was a high degree of clinical concern. Intention to treat analysis between the two groups did not show a difference in fetal outcome (birth weight centile, Apgar score at 1 minute and perinatal mortality) or rate of labor induction. Subgroup analysis demonstrated a significantly greater labor induction rate for suspected growth retardation in the revealed control group, 34.8% (56/161) than in either the concealed control group, 13.8% (51/370) or the study group, 19.6% (104/531). The study did not look at differences in neonatal morbidity; therefore, the clinical significance of the ultrasound information could not be completely assessed. The authors concluded that accurate dating information was critical in assessment

BOX 1: 1984 NIH indications for ultrasound assessment.
(No longer viewed by NIH as guidance for current medical practice)

1. **Estimation of gestational age for patients with uncertain clinical dates, or verification of dates for patients who are to undergo scheduled elective repeat cesarean delivery, indicated induction of labor, or other elective termination of pregnancy:** Ultrasonographic confirmation of dating permits proper timing of cesarean delivery or labor induction to avoid premature delivery.
2. **Evaluation of fetal growth** (e.g., when the patient has an identified etiology for uteroplacental insufficiency, such as severe preeclampsia, chronic hypertension, chronic renal disease, severe diabetes mellitus or for other medical complications of pregnancy where fetal malnutrition, i.e., IUGR or macrosomia, is suspected): Following fetal growth permits assessment of the impact of a complicating condition on the fetus and guides pregnancy management.
3. **Vaginal bleeding of undetermined etiology in pregnancy:** Ultrasound often allows determination of the source of bleeding and status of the fetus.
4. **Determination of fetal presentation:** When the presenting part cannot be adequately determined in labor for the fetal presentation is variable in late pregnancy. Accurate knowledge of presentation guides management of delivery.
5. **Suspected multiple gestation:** Based upon detection of more than one fetal heartbeat pattern, or fundal height larger than expected for dates, and/or prior use of fertility drugs. Pregnancy management may be altered in multiple gestations.
6. **Adjunct to amniocentesis:** Ultrasound permits guidance of the needle to avoid the placenta and fetus, to increase the chance of obtaining amniotic fluid, and to decrease the chance of fetal loss.
7. **Significant uterine size/dates discrepancy:** Ultrasound permits accurate dating and detection of such conditions as oligohydramnios and polyhydramnios, as well as multiple gestation, IUGR and anomalies.
8. **Pelvic mass detected clinically:** Ultrasound can detect the location and nature of the mass and aid in diagnosis.
9. **Suspected hydatidiform mole:** On the basis of clinical sign of hypertension, proteinuria and/or the presence of ovarian cysts felt on pelvic examination or failure to detect fetal heart tones with a Doppler ultrasound device after 12 weeks. Ultrasound permits accurate diagnosis and differentiation of this neoplasm from fetal death.
10. **Adjunct to cervical cerclage placement:** Ultrasound aids in timing and proper placement of the cerclage for patients with incompetent cervix.
11. **Suspected ectopic pregnancy:** When pregnancy occurs after tuboplasty or prior ectopic gestation. Ultrasound is a valuable diagnostic aid for this complication.
12. **Adjunct to special procedures,** such as fetoscopy, intrauterine transfusion, shunt placement, in vitro fertilization, embryo transfer or chorionic villi sampling. Ultrasound aids instrument guidance, which increases safety of these procedures.
13. **Suspected fetal death:** Rapid diagnosis enhances optimal management.
14. **Suspected uterine abnormality** (e.g., clinically significant leiomyomata, or congenital structural abnormalities, such as bicornuate uterus or uterus didelphys, etc.). Serial surveillance of fetal growth and state enhances fetal outcome.
15. **Intrauterine contraceptive device localization:** Ultrasound guidance facilitates removal, reducing chances of IUD-related complications.
16. **Ovarian follicle development surveillance:** This facilitates treatment of infertility.
17. **Biophysical evaluation for fetal well being** after 28 weeks of gestation. Assessment of amniotic fluid, fetal tone, body movements, breathing movements and heart rate patterns assists in the management of high-risk pregnancies.
18. **Observation of intrapartum events** (e.g., version/extraction of second twin, manual removal of placenta, etc.). These procedures may be done more safely with the visualization provided by ultrasound.
19. **Suspected polyhydramnios or oligohydramnios:** Confirmation of the diagnosis is permitted, as well as identification of the cause of the condition in certain pregnancies.
20. **Suspected abruptio placentae:** Confirmation of the diagnosis and extent assists in clinical management.
21. **Adjunct to external version from breech to vertex presentation:** The visualization provided by ultrasound facilitates performance of this procedure.
22. **Estimation of fetal weight and/or presentation in premature rupture of membranes and/or premature labor:** Information provided by ultrasound guides management decisions on timing and method of delivery.
23. **Abnormal serum alpha-fetoprotein value** for clinical gestational age when drawn. Ultrasound provides an accurate assessment of gestational age for the AFP comparison standard and indicates several conditions (e.g., twins, anencephaly) that may cause elevated AFP values.
24. **Follow-up observation of identified fetal anomaly:** Ultrasound assessment of progression of lack of change assists in clinical decision making.
25. **Follow-up evaluation of placenta location for identified placenta previa.**
26. **History of previous congenital anomaly:** Detection of recurrence may be permitted or psychological benefit to patients may result from reassurance of no recurrence.
27. **Serial evaluation of fetal growth in multiple gestation:** Ultrasound permits recognition of discordant growth, guiding patient management and timing of delivery.
28. **Evaluation of fetal condition in late registrants for prenatal care:** Accurate knowledge of gestational age assists in pregnancy management decisions for this group.

BOX 2: 1993 AIUM Standards reproduced from AIUM.

Equipment

These studies should be conducted with real-time equipment, using an abdominal and/or vaginal approach. A transducer of appropriate frequency should be used. Fetal ultrasound should be performed only when there is a valid medical reason. The lowest possible ultrasonic exposure setting should be used to gain the necessary diagnostic information.

Documentation

Adequate documentation of the study is essential for quality patient care. This should include a permanent record of the ultrasound images, incorporating whenever possible the measurement parameters and anatomical findings proposed [herein]. Images should be appropriately labeled with the examination date, patient identification, and, if appropriate, image orientation. A report of the ultrasound findings should be included in the patient's medical record. Retention of the ultrasound examination should be consistent both with clinical need and with relevant legal and local healthcare facility requirements.

Standards for First Trimester Sonography

1. The uterus and adnexa should be evaluated for the presence of a gestational sac. If a gestational sac is seen, its location should be documented. The presence or absence of an embryo should be noted and the crown-rump length recorded.
2. Presence or absence of cardiac activity should be reported.
3. Fetal number should be documented.
4. Evaluation of the uterus, adnexal structures and cul-de-sac should be performed.

Standards for Second and Third Trimester Sonography

1. Fetal life, number, presentation and activity should be documented.
2. An estimate of amniotic fluid volume (increased, decreased, normal) should be reported.
3. The placental location, appearance and its relationship to the internal cervical os should be recorded. The umbilical cord should be imaged.
4. Assessment of gestational age should be accomplished at the time of the initial scan using a combination of cranial measurement such as biparietal diameter or head circumference and limb measurement such as the femur length.
   A. The standard reference level for the measurement of the biparietal diameter is an axial image that includes the thalamus.
   B. Head circumference is measured at the same level as the biparietal diameter, around the outer perimeter of the calvarium.
5. Fetal weight should be estimated in the late second and in the third trimesters and requires the measurement of abdominal diameter of circumference.
   A. Abdominal circumference should be determined on a true transverse view, preferably at the level of the junction of the left and right portal veins.
   B. If previous fetal biometric studies have been performed, an estimate of the appropriateness of interval growth should be given.
6. Evaluation of the uterus (including the cervix) and adnexal structures should be performed.
7. The study should include, but not necessarily be limited to, assessment of the following fetal anatomy: cerebral ventricles, posterior fossa (including cerebellar hemispheres and cisterna magna), four-chamber view of the heart (including its position within the thorax), spine, stomach, kidneys, urinary bladder, fetal umbilical cord insertion site and intactness of the anterior abdominal wall. While not considered part of the minimum required examination, when fetal position permits, it is desirable to examine other areas of the anatomy.

The minimum standard for a "20 week" anomaly scan:

Gestational age can be established by measurement of biparietal diameter, head circumference and femur length. The inclusion of abdominal circumference would be optional.

Fetal Normality:

- Head shape + internal structures cavum pellucidum cerebellum ventricular size at atrium (<10 mm)
- Spine—longitudinal and transverse
- Abdominal shape and content at level of stomach
- Abdominal shape and content at level of kidneys and umbilicus
- Renal pelvis (< 5 mm AP measurement)
- Longitudinal axis—abdominal-thoracic appearance (diaphragm/bladder)
- Thorax at level of 4 chamber cardiac view
- Arms—three bones and hand (not counting fingers)
- Legs—three bones and foot (not counting toes)

Contd...

Contd...

The optimal standard for the "20 week" anomaly scan. If resources allow, the following could be added to the features listed above:
- Cardiac outflow tracts
- Face and lips

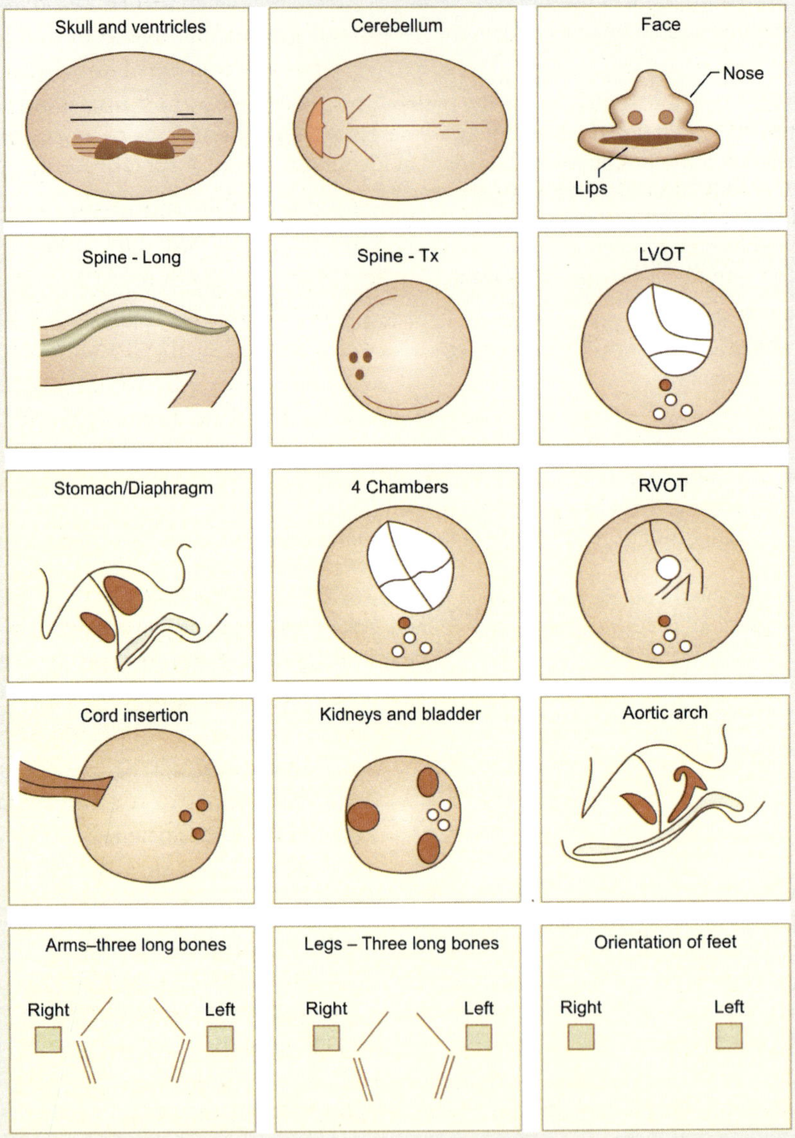

Fig. 2: Baseline examination views—20 weeks anomaly scan.

Reproduced with permission from: 2000: Routine Ultrasound Screening in Pregnancy—Protocol, Standards and Training Supplement to Ultrasound Screening for Fetal Abnormalities Report of the RCOG Working Party *http://www.rcog.org.uk/mainpages.asp?PageID=439*

for growth retardation and the ultrasound findings were of obstetric value in 25% of the patients. This study illustrates the difficulty of performing a randomized controlled trial of ultrasound utility, as concern surrounding the information generated from ultrasound obligated disclosure of the BPD in 15% of the population.

In another study designed to investigate early detection of growth restriction and perinatal outcome, Neilson et al.[31] in Glasgow, Scotland, conducted a practice-based randomized controlled trial between 1979–1981 of 877 (90%) low risk women without prior risk of growth restriction. All patients had gestational age confirmed by ultrasound prior to 24 weeks gestation and underwent crown-rump length and trunk area measurements at 34–36.5 weeks. Patients were randomized by hospital number to a study group or control group. The study group

TABLE 1: Fetal measurements and anatomic features visualized on the routine scan between 18 and 22 weeks.

1. Standard fetal measurements:
   - Biparietal diameter
   - Head circumference
   - Abdominal circumference
   - Femoral length
2. Fetal anatomic features and measurements:
   - *Brain*
     - Ventricular section—anterior and posterior horns of the cerebral ventricles; measurement: anterior and posterior ventricle-hemisphere ratio
     - Posterior fossa section—cerebellum, vermis, cisterna magna and nuchal skinfold; measurement: trans-cerebellar diameter, and nuchal skinfold
   - *Skull:* Shape
   - *Face:*
     - Orbits (and both lenses) measurement—interorbital, external orbital diameters
     - Nose, lips, palate and mandible
   - *Spine:* "Anterior" view of spinous processes down to tip of sacrum; clear view of skin margin throughout length of spine
   - *Chest*
     Heart: 4-chamber view, aortic root and arch, pulmonary artery and ductus
   - *Abdomen:*
     - Diaphragm
     - Cord insertion
     - Liver, stomach and intestines
     - Both kidneys for parenchyma and renal pelvis size
     - Bladder
     - Genitalia
   - *Limbs:*
     - Femur, tibia, fibula, foot and toes (both limbs)
     - Humerus, radius, ulna, hand and fingers (both limbs)
   - *Placenta:* Morphology and site
   - *Cord:* Number of vessels
   - *Amniotic Fluid:* Volume assessment

Reproduced with permission from Campbell S. The obstetric ultrasound examination. In: Chervenak FA, Isaacson GC, Campbell S (Eds). Ultrasound in Obstetrics and Gynecology. Boston: Little Brown; 1993. p. 188.

comprised of 433 patients whose results were shared with the obstetricians, while the results of 455 patients in the control group were concealed with the exception of breech presentation (nine cases) or placenta previa (one case). The control group information was made available by clinician request; no requests were made. The two-stage ultrasound approach was 94% sensitive and 90% specific for the detection of birth weight below the 5th percentile. There were no differences noted between the two groups. The groups were compared with respect to many parameters, including number of labor inductions overall and for suspicion of growth restriction, number of emergency cesarean sections, unfavorable Apgar scores, mean gestational age at delivery, mean birth weight and number of small-for-dates neonates.

Bakketeig et al.[32] investigated the use of a two-stage ultrasound regimen in patients randomly selected for ultrasound examination compared to a control group of patients that did not undergo antenatal ultrasound. This randomized controlled practice-based trial was conducted between 1979–1980 in Trondheim, Norway. A total of 1,009 patients were enrolled. The 510 women in the screened group underwent ultrasound examination at 18 weeks and 32 weeks gestation. When compared to the background rate of low birth weight, 4.2%, the rate in the study population, 3.9%, suggested that the study population was biased towards being more low risk and may not have accurately reflected the populace. A power analysis to assess perinatal mortality was not provided. There were no statistical differences between the screened and control groups, except for an unexplained greater number of antenatal admissions, mostly for pre-eclampsia, in the screened group. There was a trend towards earlier detection of twin gestations, fewer post-date inductions and fewer low birth weight neonates in the screened group.

With regards to routine ultrasound specifically after 24 weeks gestation, the 2009 Cochrane review,[33] a meta-analysis of eight trials, including a total of 27,024 women from unselected population, showed no difference in neonatal outcome but did show a trend towards a higher cesarean delivery rate in the screened group.

Another Norwegian trial was conducted from 1979–1980 in Ålesund. Eik-Nes et al. reported preliminary results in 1984 and subsequently published a complete analysis in 2000.[34] This prospective randomized trial involved 1,628 patients. Routine ultrasound screening at 18 and 32 weeks gestation was performed in the study group (n = 825) and ultrasound examinations were performed upon clinician request in 34% of the control group (n = 803). The screened group had significantly less post-term inductions, fewer neonates with five minutes Apgar scores below eight and fewer neonates that required positive pressure ventilation for more than one minute. Also, twins were detected earlier in the screened group, but there were no significant differences in twin outcome between the groups. The study lacked power to assess perinatal mortality (PNM), but did show a trend towards improved perinatal outcomes in the ultrasound screened group for both singleton and twin pregnancies.

In Copenhagen, Denmark, Secher et al.[35] recruited patients between 1980–1983 and studied a low-risk population that underwent ultrasound gestational age assessment before 22 weeks gestation and subsequently underwent third trimester screening for growth retardation. All patients were screened at 32 and 37 weeks gestation. An additional ultrasound was performed at 34 weeks if the estimated fetal weight was at or less than the 15th percentile at 32 weeks. There were 184 fetuses suspected to be at or less than the 15th percentile at one or more third trimester ultrasound examinations. These patients were randomized to a treatment (n = 96) or control (n = 88) group. The ultrasound results were withheld from the control group, but were revealed in 28 cases due to clinical concern. The treatment group was followed with weekly non-stress tests (NST) and serum estradiol and human placental lactogen. There were no differences between the two groups with respect to the number of neonates weighing <2,500 grams and maternal and neonatal complications. There were statistically more labor inductions in the treatment group, although the indications for induction were not detailed. There was suggestion of a marginal, not statistically significant, benefit of a reduced occurrence of neonatal hypoxia, measured by arterial cord pH <7.15, in the treatment group. The authors acknowledge that there was insufficient power in the study and was further weakened by the 32% of the control group whose results were revealed.

The first randomized controlled trial in the United States included enrolled patients from 1984–1986. Ewigman et al.[36] randomized 42% (915/2171) patients presenting for prenatal care to a study group that received an ultrasound at 10–12 weeks gestation or to a control group that received indicated ultrasonography; 23.9% of the control group underwent ultrasound scans. The strict inclusion and exclusion criteria of the study still did not ensure minimum control group exposure to ultrasound and the demographics of this study's population was not reflective of the general United States. Patient recruitment was practice-based, not population-based, with Caucasians representing over 90% of the patients. The power calculations permitted a 64% chance of detecting a 50% reduction in post-term inductions and a 70% chance of detecting a 50% reduction in adverse perinatal outcome. Adverse perinatal outcome was defined as perinatal death, neonatal intensive care unit (NICU) admission of or more days or Apgar score at 5 minutes less than 6. The groups did not differ in the number of post-term inductions, total inductions or adverse perinatal outcomes. Ultrasound was beneficial in both groups for adjustment of estimated date of confinement.

Waldenström et al.[37] in Stockholm, Sweden randomized 4,997 women without clinical indication for ultrasound into a screening group (n = 2482) and a control group (n = 2511). Patients were recruited between 1985–1987 from all local antenatal clinics. The screening group underwent an ultrasound at 15 weeks gestation. Subsequent ultrasound examinations were performed in either group at the request of the clinician. Excluding the initial screening ultrasound in the screening group, the 31.8% of unscreened group that underwent ultrasound, utilized more ultrasound examinations after 19 weeks than the screened group, 1,279 and 736, $P = 0.039$, respectively. Gestational age estimation by ultrasound prior to 19 weeks had been performed in 103 patients in the control group. Compared to the control group, the screening group had significantly fewer inductions for post-term pregnancy (9.1% versus 5.9% $P<0.0001$), greater average birth weight (3497 ± 557, 3521± 527 $P = 0.008$) and fewer low birth weight neonates (4% versus 2.5%, $P = 0.005$). There were 48 sets of twins between the two groups. All 24 sets of twins in the screening group were identified by 24 weeks and the 20 sets of twins in the control group were identified by 32 weeks. There were no significant differences in twin pregnancy outcomes, i.e., gestational age at delivery, birth weight, Apgar scores and perinatal death, between the two groups.

The largest European randomized controlled trial assessing routine versus selective antenatal ultrasound screening was also the first to compare systematically the detection of fetal abnormalities. The study took place in Helsinki, Finland and patients were recruited from 1986–1987. Saari-Kemppainen et al.[38] randomized 9,310 patients into a study group (n = 4691) that routinely underwent ultrasonography between 16–20 weeks and a control group (n = 4619) that selectively underwent ultrasonography. In the latter group, 77% of patients received an ultrasound during the course of the pregnancy, while most ultrasound examinations were performed prior to 20 weeks in the study group. The large number of controls exposed to ultrasound could account for the lack of significant difference in labor inductions and mean birth weights between the two groups. The study group utilized less antenatal care outpatient visits than the control group (2.3 versus 2.6, *P* <0.0001) and had improved detection of twins by 24 weeks (100% versus 76.3%). Most importantly, the perinatal mortality of singletons was reduced by 49.2% in the study group (4.6/1,000) as compared to the control group (9.0/1,000). This difference was attributed to the detection of severe fetal abnormalities and the participants' acceptance of pregnancy termination. The rate of fetal abnormality detection varied according to ultrasound site. The detection rate at the City Hospital was less than that of the University Hospital, 36.0% versus 76.9%. The overall perinatal mortality rate was reduced, but the small number of twins restricted further analysis between the two groups; though it appeared that the perinatal mortality rate for twins was less in the study group than in the control group, 27.8/1,000 versus 65.8/1,000. The reduction in overall perinatal mortality rate was impressive as Finland already exhibited one of the lowest perinatal mortality rates in the world confirming the impact of congenital malformations on perinatal mortality.

Geerts et al.[39] in South Africa, assessed the utility of a single screening ultrasound in a developing country. After randomization, 8% of patients were excluded; 909 patients remained with 457 in the routine ultrasound group and 452 in the selective ultrasound group. Patients were recruited from 1991–1992 and study patients received a screening ultrasound between 18–24 weeks gestation. As seen in other similar studies, ultrasound examinations were performed in 25% of the control group. Compared to the study group, the control group had a greater degree of suspected post-dates pregnancies (9 versus 38, *P* = 0.00002) and more ultrasounds (3 versus 23, *P* = 0.0001) and inductions (1 versus 14, *P* = 0.002) were performed for this indication. Five patients in the control group required confirmation of lung maturity by amniocentesis while no patients in the study group underwent fetal lung maturity testing, *P* = 0.03. There were no differences seen in adverse pregnancy outcomes (perinatal mortality, NICU admission or long-term morbidity) in singletons between the two groups. The routine group did have a greater proportion of low birth weight infants (*P* = 0.007, or 1.61; 95% CI 1.13-2.30), but the numbers were too small for statistical comparison of perinatal outcome. Similarly, as there were only a total of 6 sets of twins, perinatal outcomes for multiple gestations could not be compared. More major congenital anomalies were detected in the routine group (n = 8) than in the control group (n = 3). Within each group, there were two pregnancy terminations due to these fetal abnormalities. The authors concluded that the selective use of ultrasound did not increase adverse pregnancy outcomes and that the results did not support the additional cost accrued by routine ultrasound.

In response to the 1984 NIH Consensus Conference, the Routine Antenatal Diagnostic Imaging with Ultrasound (RADIUS)[40] trial was created as the largest prospective randomized controlled trial of routine versus selective antenatal ultrasound. The RADIUS trial was a practice-based study that attempted to evaluate the effect of two-stage routine ultrasound screening in a low-risk population on perinatal morbidity and mortality. Patients were recruited from 1987–1991 from 109 private practices in five Midwestern states and one New England state. A total of 55,744 patients registered for prenatal care in the participating clinics. Ignoring patients that were lost to follow-up, 61% (32,317/53,367) of screened registrants were deemed ineligible or were excluded. Another 26% were then lost to follow-up or declined screening. The remaining 15,530 patients, representing 28% of the original registrants, were randomized. The study group (n = 7,812) underwent sonography at 15–22 weeks and again at 31–35 weeks. Power calculations were performed but did not state the percent chance of detecting their primary goal of a 20% reduction in adverse perinatal outcomes (fetal or neonatal death or moderate or severe neonatal morbidity). Secondary outcome measures included the incidence neonates born small for gestational age or post-term and rate of labor induction in presumed post-term pregnancies. Multiple gestations were analyzed separately according to birth weight and rate of premature births.

The RADIUS trial did not demonstrate significant differences between the routine and selective screening groups with respect to maternal and perinatal morbidity and perinatal mortality.[40] However, there were significant differences in the detection of fetal anomalies and multiple gestation, use of tocolysis and diagnosis of post-date pregnancy.[41,42] Prior to 24 weeks gestation, 4.9% (8/163) of fetal anomalies in the control group were detected, as opposed to the three-fold increase in the detection of fetal anomalies, 16.6% (31/187), seen in the routine screening group. Subgroup analysis revealed a 35% (19/54) detection rate of fetal anomalies at the tertiary centers while nontertiary centers detected 13% (8/64). Twin pregnancies were detected by 24 weeks in 98.5% (67/68) of patients in the study group. The one missed patient was noncompliant with the screening regimen. Conversely, 37% (23/61) of twin pregnancies were detected by 24 weeks in the control group. Tocolysis was utilized by 3.4% (260/7617) patients in the study group versus 4.2% (318/7534) in the control group. The study group had significantly less pregnancies past 41 weeks and past 42 weeks than the control group, 19.1% versus 21.4%, *P* <0.001, 3.2%, 4.6%, *P* <0.001, respectively.

CRITIQUE OF RADIUS TRIAL

Although the magnitude of the RADIUS trial is impressive, there are four important points to consider regarding its conclusions.[43]

Applicability of Results

An extremely low-risk population was enrolled in the RADIUS trial. Selection bias commenced with enrollment in prenatal care and in private clinics. Most patients were whites (93%), English speaking (100%), had ideal body weight (90%), had received college level education (70%)[44] and were indifferent to pregnancy termination. The stringent exclusion criteria removed 60% of patients at initial enrollment and 45% of the remaining 40% of patients considered low risk subsequently underwent ultrasonography.[45] Therefore, the conclusions of the trial are applicable to less than 40% of low-risk private patients, who are deemed low risk after extensive scrutiny.[43]

Outcomes Emphasized

Although a power analysis was performed, the number of participants was insufficient to draw definitive conclusions on the lack of effect of a single technology, ultrasound, on perinatal morbidity and mortality. Therefore, the potential for improvement in perinatal morbidity and mortality cannot be dismissed. Published estimated power calculations show a minimum of 6,250 patients in each group to demonstrate a 50% decrease in perinatal mortality (from 10/1,000–5/1,000).[46] Ultrasound screening could possibly predict approximately half of the congenital malformations or intrauterine growth restriction cases that lead to fetal or neonatal demise. Thus, a more realistic reduction from 10 to 8 per 1,000 perinatal deaths would require 46,820 patients in each group.[47]

The RADIUS trial also ascribed therapeutic properties to ultrasound examination, which serves purely a diagnostic role. Romero asserted it is unreasonable to expect ultrasound to reduce the rate of prematurity and small for gestational age neonates without the combination of an effective treatment modality.[48]

There were significant findings in the RADIUS trial that deserve emphasis. Routine ultrasound examination led to an increased detection of fetal anomalies, earlier diagnosis of twin pregnancies, fewer cases of tocolysis and induction of labor for post-dates.[49] With larger numbers, the benefits of these significant findings may have translated into improved perinatal morbidity and mortality.

Ultrasound Quality

The non-uniform detection rate of fetal anomalies between tertiary and non-tertiary centers highlights a critical issue regarding the quality of the ultrasound examinations performed in the study. The detection rate prior to 24 weeks gestation of 16.6% was much lower than that seen in European studies. Romero compared the sensitivity of the RADIUS trial with a series of European trials for which a combined sensitivity was generated, 16.6% versus 50.9%, *P*<0.00001.[48] Proper and frequent ultrasound accreditation, training and auditing is required in any ultrasound setting to maximize the full potential of ultrasonography and to minimize harm.

Cost Analysis

According to the cost analysis proposed by the RADIUS trial, the additional 1.6 ultrasound scans at $200/scan would incur an increased cost of $500 million. However, DeVore illustrated that the cost per fetal anomaly detected in tertiary centers is 48% below the RADIUS trial's projected cost and also less than the cost of universal screening with maternal serum alpha-fetoprotein.[50] The RADIUS trial also did not address the financial cost of caring for infants with severe congenital anomalies.[49]

META-ANALYSES OF RANDOMIZED CONTROLLED TRIALS

Thacker summarized the first four randomized controlled trials of routine ultrasound in 1983.[30-32,34] The combined results did not show a significant difference in frequency of low Apgar score at one minute or in the rate of perinatal mortality between the pooled study and control groups. However, a significant reduction in labor induction for incorrectly presumed post-dates was seen.[46]

Bucher and Schmidt also analyzed four randomized control trials with a combined total of 15,935 pregnancies.[32,36-38] This meta-analysis demonstrated a significant reduction in perinatal mortality, largely due to the contribution of the Helsinki study. The Helsinki study achieved a reduction in perinatal mortality due to their reasonable early detection rate of fetal abnormalities that permitted the option of induced abortion.[51]

A Cochrane review in 2002 concluded, "routine ultrasound in early pregnancy appears to enable better gestational age assessment, earlier detection of multiple pregnancies and earlier detection of clinically unsuspected fetal malformation at a time when termination of pregnancy is possible. However, the benefits for other substantive outcomes (perinatal mortality) are less clear."[52] The use of routine ultrasound, overall, significantly improved detection of twin pregnancies by 20 and 24 weeks gestation, reduced the rate of post-term labor inductions and led to a greater proportion of pregnancy terminations. The meta-analysis did not show a difference in antenatal hospital admissions, Apgar score below 7 at 1 or 5 minutes, low birth weight or special care admissions for singletons or in perinatal mortality (twins and singletons). The follow-up studies of ultrasound safety also did not show a difference between routine and unscreened groups in school related oral reading, reading comprehension, spelling, arithmetic, overall performance, dyslexia, reduced vision, reduced hearing, spectacle use, non-right-handedness, left-handedness and ambidexterity.[52] The 2009 Cochrane review of routine ultrasound after 24 weeks gestation did not show a difference in neonatal outcome, but did not assess long-term outcomes of neurological development. The cesarean delivery rate was slightly higher in the group that received routine ultrasound after 24 weeks gestation, but trend was not significant.[33]

DIAGNOSTIC ABILITY OF ROUTINE ULTRASOUND

One of the pioneer programs integrating routine ultrasound in prenatal care began in Malmö, Sweden in 1973 in order to improve the diagnosis of twin pregnancies. A retrospective study of their screening program from 1973–1978 revealed most (94.4%) twin pregnancies were diagnosed by 19–20 weeks gestation. The benefit of early diagnosis of twins, compared to prior diagnosis by 27 weeks was seen in the reduction of premature births (from 33–10%) and perinatal mortality (from 6–0.6%).[53] In addition, placenta previa was better identified and greater accuracy of gestational age led to a reduction in post-term induction of labor from 8–2.6%. The authors estimated that the improved outcomes reduced the use of hospital care resources by 10%.[54]

Another early site for routine ultrasound, Barcelona, Spain, reported 22 years, 1970–1991, of ultrasound screening for fetal abnormalities in a mixed high and low-risk population. As expected, the improving skill and technology led to better detection rates of major fetal abnormalities in the second decade of examination, 19.75–96.4%; detection rates prior to 22 weeks increased from 8.63–84.8%. The specificity remained 99%. Overall, 59.4% (598/1,006) fetal anomalies were detected early in pregnancy. Termination of pregnancy procedures paralleled the increase in fetal anomaly detection and the perinatal mortality rate declined from 8.4/1,000 in 1981–1985 to 5.5/1,000 in 1986–1990. Although the population included many high-risk referrals, the majority of fetal abnormalities, 85–90%, were detected in low-risk patients.[25]

In Finland, Rosendahl and Kivinen[55] performed routine ultrasonography on 9,012 patients between 1980–1988. For the first two years, a routine scan was completed at 18 weeks, subsequently; a second scan was added at 34 weeks. The additional third trimester survey increased the sensitivity of major malformations to 63.8% from 41.7%. The sensitivity of structural anomaly detection prior to 24 weeks was 39.4%. Fetal abnormality detection correlated with clinical suspicion of an abnormality in only 25.8% of cases; therefore, the authors "emphasized the necessity for ultrasound examination of all pregnancies."[55]

In Belgium, Levi et al.[56] described a multicenter experience of ultrasonography performed in each trimester from 1984–1989. In this unselected population, a total of 16,361 fetuses were evaluated. Between 12–22 weeks, 62.1% (259/417) of fetal malformations were scanned with a 21% (59/259) sensitivity, 100% specificity and 100% positive predictive value. The sensitivity rose to a 40% (154/318) detection rate of abnormal fetuses with additional sonograms later in pregnancy. There were 66 false negative and 8 false positive cases. Anomaly detection was analyzed according to type, gestational age at detection, gestational age-based probability of detection and severity. Eighty-five percent of lethal anomalies were correctly diagnosed antenatally. The authors evaluated the appropriateness of ultrasound as a screening test and found it to be suitable in their population.

In a similar analysis, Gonçalves et al.[57] conducted a retrospective case-control study of congenital anomaly detection from 1987–1991. Participants were referred for indicated ultrasound examination. Infants and fetuses were selected based upon hospital discharge diagnoses.

The study and control groups each contained 287 women. There were 152 true positives for 287 cases, yielding an overall sensitivity of 53%. Congenital anomalies were also analyzed according to diagnostic category and gestational age at detection. Advanced gestational age, lethality of the anomaly and high-risk categorization of the pregnancy all increased sensitivity. From 20–23 weeks, the sensitivity was 59% while it reached 68% after 24 weeks. A high percentage, 89%, of lethal anomalies was detected. Sensitivity of detecting an anomaly was higher in high-risk patients as compared to low or unknown risk patients, 71%, 36%, 46%, respectively. Since the study did not have a reference population and many false-negative cases may have been omitted.[58]

In another retrospective trial, Chitty et al.[59] correctly identified 93 of 125 fetal anomalies in 8,342 fetuses prior to 24 weeks gestation for a sensitivity of 4%. The study was conducted between 1988–1989. All patients who registered early for prenatal care underwent ultrasonography prior to 24 weeks gestation. There were 14 trisomies that were not included in the calculation of sensitivity; their inclusion would reduce the sensitivity to 63%. The authors were able to demonstrate the utility of ultrasonography for antenatal fetal anomaly detection in a low-risk population. They also addressed problems encountered with routine ultrasonography in this population. These problems are:

- Technical problems such as maternal obesity, fetal position and multiple gestations hindered diagnosis of some structural anomalies.
- Uncertain outcomes of recognizable anomalies such as mild ventriculomegaly.
- Late presentation of some findings such as duodenal atresia.
- The abnormality may not be detectable, i.e., tracheo-esophageal fistula.
- Evolving data on minor markers such as choroids plexus cysts, mild pyelectasis.
- Late registration for prenatal care.

Shirley et al.[60] performed a combined retrospective and prospective study in an unselected pregnant population. The study evaluated 6,183 (96%) infants delivered from 1989–1990 who had been scanned in the second trimester. Of the 84 abnormal fetuses scanned prior to 22 weeks gestation, 51 had fetal anomalies detected yielding a sensitivity of 60.7%. The sensitivity for detecting lethal anomalies by 22 weeks gestation was 73% (41/56). There was one false-positive diagnosis of omphalocele that was a hemangioma at birth. The specificity was 99.98%. The authors supported a routine screening program that allowed patients the opportunity to adapt to or to consider termination of an abnormal fetus and acknowledged its potential to reduce perinatal mortality.

Papp et al.[61] prospectively studied two-stage routine sonography in 51,675 women between 1988–1990. Of the 63,794 patients offered screening, 81% participated. Sensitivity of maternal serum alpha fetoprotein (MSAFP) was compared with the sensitivity of ultrasound scanning at 18–24 weeks and at 28 weeks. Of the 496 severe anomalies detected, 317 were detected by ultrasonography between 18–20 weeks. The sensitivity of ultrasound screening of major fetal anomalies was 63.9% and significantly exceeded that of MSAFP screening. The efficiency of prenatal detection in this study supports the contention of perinatal mortality reduction by offering patients the option of pregnancy termination.

Luck[62] examined the impact of routine ultrasonography at 19 weeks gestation in an unselected population. All pregnant women from 1988–1991 were offered to participate and 96% (8,523/8,849) accepted. There were 160 fetal anomalies of which 140 were detected at 19 weeks gestation. According to Luck, the majority of anomalies occur in low-risk pregnancies and thus routine screening of pregnant women by trained and skilled ultrasonographers is advocated. Additional benefits of early anomaly detection included appropriate and timely tertiary care referrals and emotional preparation for parents with a fetal anomaly. A cost analysis demonstrated cost effectiveness of termination of pregnancy for lethal, crippling deformities detected with expert ultrasonography.

The Multicentric Eurofetus Study[63] investigated the sensitivity of fetal anomaly detection in a large unselected population involving 14 European countries. Routine ultrasound examination was performed between 18–22 weeks gestation from 1990–1993. Fetal abnormalities occurred in 3,686 fetuses, 44% of all these cases were detected prior to 24 weeks while 55% of severe anomalies were identified. The information from this study supports the use of routine ultrasound performance and enhances physician-patient discussion regarding pregnancy options, limitations of ultrasonography (i.e., a negative test cannot provide absolute assurance) and areas to focus on to improve detection.

Routine obstetric ultrasonography in low-risk patients was assessed by Skupski et al.[64] from 1990–1994. A retrospective review of 860 fetuses revealed a 1.2% (10/860) incidence of major anomalies. Considering only diagnoses identifiable by ultrasound, a 75% (3/4) sensitivity for major anomaly detection was reported. As the incidence of major fetal anomalies detectable sonographically was 0.5%, the authors analogize amniocentesis performance for a similar incidence of aneuploidy. With early prenatal diagnosis patients received nondirective counseling and 2 out of 3 patients with ultrasound detected major anomalies opted for pregnancy termination; thereby, availing themselves of autonomy enhancing facets of prenatal care.

Quisser-Luft et al.[65] performed a retrospective case control analysis of patients with and without antenatally detected fetal anomalies. Cases from 1990–1994 were reviewed and 298 malformed cases were identified from 20,248 livebirths, stillbirths and abortuses; 30.3% (95/298) were identified antenatally. As per standard policy in Germany, each patient underwent a minimal of three ultrasounds. Specific detection rates for anomalies detectable with ultrasound were described. The detection rates improved during the course of the study and with increasing gestational age with 38% sensitivity for ultrasound examinations prior to 24 weeks gestation and 50% after 24 weeks. Anamnestic data was collected for the 298 cases and high-risk criteria developed retrospectively to identify women with abnormal fetuses **(Table 2)**.[65] Retrospective application of the risk factors identified 22% (4,525/20,248) of the population as high risk of which 3.2% (145/4,525) newborns had detectable anomalies as opposed to 0.9% (142/15,723) in the remainder of the population. However, the absolute number of detectable anomalies between the two groups remained the same, i.e., scanning for indications would potentially miss the opportunity to detect half of the anomalies.

In a 6 year retrospective analysis of antenatal fetal anomaly detection with ultrasound, Boyd et al.[66] demonstrated an increase in sensitivity over time from 1991–1997. Cases (n = 725) were selected from an ongoing birth and malformations registry (n = 33,376) and matched with antenatal ultrasound data. In the first 3 years, 42% of fetal anomalies were detected versus 68% in the latter half. However, there was a concomitant twelve-fold increase in false-positive diagnoses largely attributed to the incorporation of soft markers in screening. This study emphasized the cautious use of soft markers as isolated anomalies and respect for autonomy enhancing practices of non-directive counseling and offering of abortion. An estimated 23% reduction in congenital malformations occurred due to pregnancy termination.

TABLE 2: High-risk characteristics identified from anamnestic data.

	Statistically significant increased odds ratios		
Risk factors	***OR***	***CI***	***P value***
Anamnestic risk factors:			
Sibling with malformation	4.6	1.3–16	0.02
Mother/father with malformation	4.1	1.3–13	0.01
Consanguinity	3.1	1.4–6.6	0.004
Neonatal death/stillbirth	1.9	1.1–3.6	0.001
Alcohol abuse (mother)	2.4	1.1–6.3	0.04
Maternal age >35	1.3	1.1–1.7	0.007
Drug exposure (first trimester)	1.2	1.1–1.3	0.008
Clinical signs:			
Polyhydramnios*	13.5	9.5–19.0	0.001
Oligohydramnios*	8.7	5.2–14.0	0.001
Premature labor•	4.7	3.8–4.9	0.001
Placental insufficiency*	1.9	1.1–2.7	0.01
Growth retardation*	1.8	1.3–2.6	0.001
Vaginal bleeding*	1.5	1.2–1.8	0.001
Pre-eclampsia*	1.3	1.1–1.6	0.003

*(<32 weeks)
•(<28 weeks)
Reproduced with permission from Queisser-Luft A, Stopfkuchen H, Stolz G, et al. Prenatal diagnosis of major malformations: quality control of routine ultrasound examinations based on a five-year study of 20,2248 newborn fetuses and infants. Prenat Diag. 1998;18:573.

Sprigg et al.[67] conducted a prospective trial from 1992–1994 comparing routine versus selective ultrasound practices for the detection of fetal anomalies. The detection of fetal malformations from the year prior to establishing routine ultrasound surveillance was compared with the new policy. The incidence of major anomalies remained the same between the two scanning regimens. However, the routine scan permitted ultrasound detection of 29 anomalies of which 17 were true positives. There were 11 severe anomalies and 7 patients opted for pregnancy termination that led to a significant estimated cost savings. Weighing the benefit burden calculus of screening, the authors found the use of routine screening justified.

A large difference in detection of fetal anomalies between women screened routinely versus based on indication was seen in the prospective trial conducted by VanDorsten et al., 47.6% versus 75.0%, $P = 0.001$.[68] From 1993–1996, 2,031 patients enrolled for prenatal care at a tertiary care center. The indicated scans were primarily performed at a maternal-fetal medicine unit whereas the screening ultrasounds took place in a primary care center.

TABLE 3: Comparison of sensitivity of fetal anomaly detection.

Reference	*Period*	*n*	*Gestational age (weeks)*	*Prevalence of anomalies*	*Sensitivity*	*Specificity*	*PPV*	*NPV*
Saari-Kamppainen[38]	1986–87	4,073	16–20	0.99%	40% (18/45)	99.8% (4,636/4,646)	64.3% (18/28)	99% (4,636/4,663)
Levi[56]	1984–89	16,072	12–20	1.61%	20.8% (54/259)	100% (15,972/15,972)	100% (54/54)	98.7% (15,972/16,177)
Rosendahl[55]	1980–88	9,012	<24	1.03%	39.8% (37/93)	*	*	*
Shirley[60]	1989–91	6,183	19	1.36%	60.7% (51/84)	99.9% (6,098/6,099)	98.1% (51/52)	99.5% (6,098/6,131)
Chitty[59]	1988–89	8,432	<24	1.48%	74.4% (93/125)	99.9% (8,305/8,307)	97.9% (93/95)	99.6% (8305/8337)
Luck[62]	1988–91	8,523	19	1.95%	84.3% (140/166)	99.9% (8,355/8,357)	98.6% (140/142)	99.7% (8,355/8,381)
Overall	**1980–91**	**52,295**	**<24**		**52.9%** (393/772)	**99.9%** (43,366/43,381)	**95.9%** (356/371)	**99.26%** (43,366/43,689)

Reproduced with permission from Romero R. Routine obstetric ultrasound. Ultrasound Obstet Gynecol. 1993;306.

There were 15 anomalous fetuses that were not detected antenatally, 73% (11/15) were in the screening group. These false-negative diagnoses included eight missed cardiac anomalies, five ventricular septal defects, one atrial septal defect, one valvular incompetence and one atrioventricular canal defect. Detection rates of specific anomalies were analyzed. VanDorsten supported routine ultrasound as a screening test as it potentially can improve patients' healthcare with respect to morbidity, mortality, disfigurement and anxiety. He acknowledged that more experience and better equipment promotes antenatal ultrasound and that "low risk for adverse perinatal outcome does not confer low risk for anomalies."[68]

Routine prenatal ultrasound prior to 22 weeks for the detection of congenital anomalies was strongly supported by the Euroscan study.[69] Included were 709,030 unselected pregnancies from 12 European countries. A total of 20 Congenital Malformation Registries participated from 1993 to 1996; 18 registries were population-based and 16 collaborated with the EUROCAT program. Congenital malformations existed in 8,126 cases and 44.3% (3,601/8,126) were detected with antenatal ultrasound screening. All categories of major congenital anomalies capable of prenatal detection were detected less frequently in countries without a routine antenatal ultrasound policy and in Eastern Europe. These findings suggest that operator experience, equipment and gestational age at examination are important factors affecting the sensitivity of congenital anomaly detection. From the results of this largely population based trial, the authors recommend single-stage routine ultrasound screening for fetal anomalies as the majority occur in pregnancies without ascertainable risks.[69,70]

A compilation of studies yielded a combined sensitivity of 50.9% for ultrasound detection of fetal anomalies before 24 weeks gestation **(Table 3)**.[48] In this analysis, Romero proposed if prenatal care should encompass detection of fetal anomalies, then routine ultrasound screening by experts can achieve this goal. Clementi also supported the use of routine ultrasound as the detection of congenital anomalies continues to improve concomitant with experience and advances in ultrasound technology. In addition, congenital malformations impact heavily on perinatal morbidity and mortality and their detection can be amendable to secondary and tertiary prevention.[70]

In order to maximize visualization of fetal anatomy and minimize follow-up ultrasound examinations, the ideal time to perform the second trimester ultrasound is between 20–22 weeks gestation. Schwärzler et al.[24] determined this optimum gestational age by randomizing 1,206 women who were available for follow up and had undergone normal first trimester ultrasonography. Three groups were established; group 1 was scanned between 18 weeks–18 weeks 6 days, group 2 was scanned between 20 weeks–20 weeks 6 days and group 3 was scanned between 22 weeks–22 weeks and 6 days. The anatomy scan was more likely to be completed and within a shorter time period between 20–22 weeks than at 18 weeks, 88–90% versus 76%, ($P = 0.001$).

FIRST TRIMESTER ULTRASONOGRAPHY

The benefits of antenatal ultrasound examination can proceed from assessment in the first trimester. Determination of risk assessment of aneuploidy in singleton and multiple gestations, fetal viability, accurate gestational age, multiple gestations, and chorionicity and amnionicity[71] and detection of fetal anomalies have been described with first trimester ultrasonography. Fetal nuchal translucency measurement has emerged as a valuable tool for aneuploidy screening and fetal nasal bone assessment is gaining importance.[72] Although the first trimester scan continually advances its ability to detect fetal anomalies, it does not currently substitute for the second trimester sonogram.[73,74]

Crowther et al.[75] demonstrated the utility of first trimester sonography performed at the first prenatal visit. There were 648 eligible patients randomized to ultrasound versus no ultrasound prior to routine screening at 18–20 weeks. Patients presented for prenatal care at mean gestational ages of 10.7±2.7 and 10.6±2.6 weeks, respectively. The study group who underwent early sonography had more accurate estimation of gestational age and expressed more positive feelings towards their pregnancy. There was a trend towards earlier detection of twins in the study group compared to the control group. Earlier diagnosis of twins and accurate gestational age determination are important factors in maternal biochemical screening.

Studies evaluating first trimester sonographic detection of structural anomalies demonstrate sensitivities similar to those reported for second trimester ultrasonography. Economides et al.[74] assessed first trimester fetal anomaly detection in 1,632 low-risk pregnancies. The incidence of anomalous fetuses was 1% (17/1,632) of which 64.7% (11/17) were detected in the first trimester. The routine second trimester ultrasound identified an additional three anomalous fetuses for a combined trimester sensitivity of 82.3% (14/17). The specificity at each screening ultrasound was greater than 99%. Analysis by the time of detection and specific anomaly revealed similar disparities in the detection rates of central nervous system and cardiac anomalies in first and second trimester ultrasound examinations in low-risk populations. However, with nuchal translucency screening, the first trimester ultrasound can potentially identify those fetuses at increased risk of cardiac anomalies.[76,77] Whitlow et al.[77] expanded the aforementioned study to include an additional 4,811 viable pregnancies (n = 6443). There were 92 abnormal fetuses yielding an incidence of 1.4% that included 63 fetuses with prenatally detected structural anomalies of which 43 were aneuploid. There were three false-positive initial diagnoses of exophthalmos that were cancelled upon subsequent rescanning. First trimester sensitivities for the detection of structural anomalies and chromosomal abnormalities were 59% (37/63) and 78% (31/40). Chromosomal abnormalities, except for three cases of Klinefelter's syndrome, were suspected by fetal structural anomalies and/or nuchal translucency greater than the 99th percentile for crown-rump length. Combining first and second trimester scans, increased the sensitivity for structural anomaly detection to 81% (51/63). The authors concluded that most structural and chromosomal abnormalities can be detected by fetal ultrasound examination between 11–14 weeks, ideally at 13 weeks, but should not replace second trimester ultrasound.

Carvalho et al.[78] evaluated 2,853 pregnancies with first trimester transabdominal and transvaginal ultrasound, median gestational age 12 weeks and 4 days. Patients enrolled in antenatal care at a tertiary referral center. There were a total of 130 fetal anomalies during the study period, 93 (71.5%) of which were detected with antenatal ultrasound. First trimester ultrasonography detected 29 out of 130 (22.3%) fetal anomalies representing 31.2% (29/93) of the prenatally detected fetal anomalies. Of the structural anomalies, 50.8% major anomalies (66/130) were noted and 78.8% (52/66) detected antenatally. The first trimester scan detected 37.8% (25/66) of all major anomalies.

With an increasing proportion of pregnant women of advanced maternal age, the incidence of trisomy 21 in the second trimester increased from 1/740 in 1974 to 1/504 in 1997.[73] Early detection of aneuploidy allows women to consider invasive diagnostic testing and termination of pregnancy in the first trimester or early second trimester. However, many of these aneuploid fetuses may result in spontaneous fetal demise. The advent of nuchal translucency screening in the first trimester has facilitated earlier detection of fetal aneuploidy. Nicolaides et al.[79] in 1992 described an association between increased first trimester nuchal translucency thickness and aneuploidy and introduced first trimester nuchal translucency screening for abnormal karyotypes. He reported a sensitivity of 64% for aneuploidy using a nuchal translucency cutoff of ≥3 mm. Snijders et al.[80] in 1998 reported a detection rate of 82%, false positive rate 8.3%, for trisomy 21 fetuses. This multicenter European trial involved 22 centers, 306 sonographers and 96,127 fetuses. Each fetus had a nuchal translucency measurement obtained from which a gestational age (by crown-rump length) related likelihood ratio was used to combine the maternal age and nuchal thickness-related risks to estimate an adjusted risk. Nuchal translucency measurements vary normally with gestational age and a single cutoff should not be used to adjust risk since it will lead to a lower sensitivity than if nuchal translucency is treated as a continuous variable. Studies using nuchal translucency screening as a continuous, not dichotomous, variable, demonstrate similar detection rates for trisomy 21 and other abnormal karyotypes as reported by the Fetal Medicine Foundation.[81-84] After the introduction of a nuchal translucency screening protocol, Zoppi et al.[85] compared the rate of declining an invasive diagnostic procedure in women of advanced maternal. Prior to the initiation of such a screening program, the incidence of declined invasive procedures was 22% and detection of aneuploidy by transabdominal chorionic villi sampling was 31.5%. However, 30% of women who underwent nuchal translucency screening declined invasive procedures, yet the fewer number of chorionic villi samples revealed a higher rate, 65%, of chromosomal abnormalities. Therefore, nuchal translucency screening in a high-risk population was able to influence a reduction in the number of invasive diagnostic procedures.[85,86] This reduction was also seen in the work of Chasen et al.[86]

Nuchal translucency screening for aneuploidy has been used successfully in unselected populations. Economides et al.[87] retrospectively investigated first trimester anatomy and nuchal translucency screening for detecting chromosomal abnormalities in 2,281 consecutive, unselected gravidas. Of the 16 chromosomal abnormalities, 44% (7/16) were diagnosed between 11–14 weeks due to a nuchal translucency measurement at or greater than the 99th percentile for gestational age. Of the eight cases of trisomy 21, 63% (5/8) were detected by nuchal translucency screening. The sensitivity of detection improved when combined with evaluation of first trimester anatomy. The combined sensitivities were 81% for all chromosome abnormalities and 75% for trisomy 21. Schwärzler et al.[88] investigated the applicability of nuchal translucency screening in an unselected population of 4,523 consecutive, viable fetuses. There were 230 patients (5.1%) that were screen-positive for fetal aneuploidy. Patients were screen-positive, if the nuchal translucency measurement translated to an adjusted risk greater than 1:270. Chromosomal abnormalities were found in 23 (0.51%) cases. The sensitivity of nuchal translucency screening for the detection of an abnormal karyotype was 78%, with a false-positive rate of 4.7%, specificity of 95.3%, positive and negative predictive values of 7.8% and 99.9%, respectively.

The First Trimester Maternal Serum Biochemistry and Ultrasound Fetal Nuchal Translucency Screening Study (BUN)[89] found this test to be efficacious. In this prospective observational trial, the detection rate of trisomy 21 in 7,668 patients based on maternal age and nuchal translucency measurement was 84.2% with a false positive rate of 12.0%. With the same sensitivity, the false positive rate was reduced to 9.4% with the advent of combined screening—the addition of first trimester maternal serum screening with pregnancy-associated plasma protein A (PAPP-A) and free β-human chorionic gonadotropin (fβ-hCG). The BUN trial also assessed the feasibility of widespread implementation of nuchal translucency screening. Quality sonographic images for assessment was possible with interventions such as diligent individual feedback and occasional equipment tuning.[89]

The credibility, greater sensitivity and acceptability[90,91] of first trimester combined (nuchal translucency measurement plus PAPP-A and fβ-hCG) screening has been supported by large international trials.[89,91-95] Large prospective trials assessing first and second trimester biochemical and sonographic screening for aneuploidy were completed in North America and in the United Kingdom. In North America, the FASTER[95] (First and Second Trimester Evaluation of Risk for aneuploidy) trial and in the United Kingdom, the SURUSS (Serum Urine and Ultrasound Screening Study) trial addressed comparisons between and among these screening modalities.[92]

ETHICAL DIMENSIONS

Controversy exists surrounding the practice of routine obstetric ultrasound with objections to its use, inadequately addressing the central ethical principles of beneficence and respect for autonomy.

Beneficence

Beneficence, the oldest principle of medical ethics dating back to Hippocrates, obligates physicians to seek greater good than harm for patients. Using sound clinical judgment, physicians should seek clinical treatments that engender a greater balance towards good. Health-related interests should be promoted and protected rather than harmed. Therefore, the concept of nonmaleficence is subordinate to beneficence in obstetric ethics as avoiding harm for one patient in the mother-fetus unit, may portend worse harm for the other.[43] A beneficence-based discussion regarding routine obstetric ultrasound centers on potential benefits and harms from application of this technique.[96] Arguments against ultrasound screening wrongly assume its benefits are diminutive with respect to its harms. The reported benefits include decreased postdatism, decreased labor induction and use of tocolytics and improved detection of multiple gestations.[52] Additional benefits of ultrasonography develop from continued research. In the case of multiple gestations, which are known to have an increased risk of anomalies, preventing the birth of an anomalous twin can be advantageous to decreased morbidity of the surviving co-twin. This tertiary prevention approach requires the early detection of multiple gestations, an accurate determination of chorionicity and a thorough evaluation of fetal anatomy.[49] The putative harms involve the theoretical risk of fetal damage from ultrasound exposure and false positive diagnoses yielding unnecessary interventions and maternal anxiety. No in vivo data exist to suggest that diagnostic two-dimensional ultrasound, performed adeptly and within reasonable time constraints is harmful.[6,21,52,97] It is the sonologist's integrity centered responsibility to ensure quality ultrasound performance. Expert quality ultrasonography can detect many lethal and disabling anomalies during a routine 18–20 week scan, even in low-risk pregnancies. Quality of ultrasound performance underlies the wide range of rates of detection of anomalies.[98] Poor quality ultrasound can lead to a higher incidence of false-positive and false-negative diagnoses. These circumstances can lead to more harm than good incurring additional interventions such as invasive diagnostic testing with chorionic villi sampling, amniocentesis, and cordocentesis and procedure-related fetal loss.[99] Minor ultrasound markers of aneuploidy may cause maternal anxiety, especially in low-risk populations.[99] However, one is unable to discern with certainty for an individual whether a specific minor marker occurs as a normal variant or as a sign of aneuploidy. Careful scrutiny to reduce false positive diagnoses is reasonable and achievable. In order to maximize the potential benefits of ultrasound and to minimize false positive prenatal diagnoses, serial and composite screening modalities have evolved.[91,100-102] First trimester serum analyte testing coupled with nuchal translucency screening can reach 90% sensitivity and 5% false-positive rate for aneuploidy detection.[91] As seen with the introduction of nuchal translucency screening, improved sensitivity for aneuploidy with decreasing frequency of false-positive diagnoses can reduce both the number of invasive prenatal testing procedures and resulting fetal losses.[85,86] Nuchal translucency measurement also offers patients the ability to decline invasive prenatal testing or to decide whether to undergo chorionic villi sampling versus amniocentesis. The former may have slightly higher miscarriage and mosaicism rates and does not permit simultaneous screening for neural tube defects with amniotic fluid α-fetoprotein determination.[103] Since beneficence-based clinical judgment supports routine obstetric ultrasound practice, when quality ultrasound is available, patients should not be denied access to its use just as their autonomy should not be disrespected.[43,104,105]

Autonomy

The physician's role of patient advocate is supported by beneficence and autonomy-based ethical principles. The physician's perspective on the patient's interests provides the basis for beneficence-based obligations owed to her; the patient's perspective on those interests provides the basis for autonomy-based obligations owed to her.[43] Respect for patient autonomy underlies medical, and therefore, obstetric ethics. Autonomy-based practice warrants careful discussion with patients regarding the use of antenatal ultrasound as well as relevant antenatal diagnostic and therapeutic alternatives and acknowledgment by the physician of the patient's preferences and values. Eliciting a patient's views is integral in respecting one's autonomy since these views may influence management, barring any compelling contstraints.[106] Chervenak et al.[29] stated "the standard of care demands that prenatal informed consent for sonogram be accepted as an indication for the prudent use of obstetric ultrasonography performed by qualified personnel." Implementing autonomy-based principles requires a three step process:

1. Adequate information transfer regarding the patient's condition and management.
2. Patient comprehension of the information.
3. Voluntary action by the patient to either accept or decline clinical management.[43]

Diagnostic and therapeutic alternatives should be discussed with the patient as a central component of prenatal care and autonomy enhancing practice. Non-disclosure of alternatives, such as not routinely offering obstetric ultrasound, impairs the patient's exercise of autonomy and may preclude options of diagnosis of severe anomalies and pregnancy termination.

The fetus, prior to viability, does not directly posses autonomy, unless proscribed by the mother. Therefore, autonomy-based obligations to the fetus must be balanced with maternal autonomy and beneficence principles and practices.[43] Autonomy-based obligation to the gravida seeking obstetric ultrasound is not diminished by controversy regarding lack of benefit or excess cost. Studies that did not show improvement in perinatal morbidity and mortality were limited by insufficient power[46-48,51] and exclusive definition of benefits. Beneficence-based clinical judgment would not condone ignoring outcomes that could reduce or prevent harm in a small but important subset of patients.[104] Regarding excessive cost, the argument to strip away autonomy due to financial concerns falls short of both cost-effective and cost-beneficial analysis. Cost-effectiveness of routine ultrasound was demonstrated by Devore[50] in California where the cost of anomaly detection with ultrasound was less than that detected by serum screening. Cost-benefit analysis incorporates long-term emotional and financial benefits that are often ignored in discussions of implementation costs across a population. The costs to an individual and to the society are harder to measure with regards to care of a child with severe malformation.

CONCLUSION

Routine first trimester ultrasound for nuchal translucency measurement in conjunction with maternal serum analyses is an effective tool for adjusting risk for aneuploidy.[27,89-95] Routine midtrimester ultrasound is an effective diagnostic tool. Establishment of accurate gestational age, detection of fetal anomalies and multiple gestations, and reduction in postdate pregnancies and labor inductions are proven benefits of routine ultrasound. The benefit burden calculus of routine antenatal ultrasonography support its use and fulfillment of ethical principles of beneficence and respect for patient's autonomy.

REFERENCES

1. Fleischer AC. Ultrasound in obstetrics and gynecology. In: Grainer and Allison's Diagnostic Radiology: A Textbook of Medical Imaging, 4th edition. Churchill Livingstone; 2001. pp. 2177-85.
2. Cosgrove DO. Ultrasound: general principles. In: Grainer and Allison's Diagnostic Radiology: A Textbook of Medical Imaging, 4th edition. Churchill Livingstone; 2001. pp. 43-57.
3. Woo J. Obstetric Ultrasound: A comprehensive guide. Available at www.ob-ultrasound.net. Accessed on February 2011.
4. NIH Consensus Conference. The use of diagnostic ultrasound imaging during pregnancy. JAMA. 1984;252(5):669-72.
5. American College of Obstetricians and Gynecologists. New Ultrasound Output Display Standard. ACOG Committee Opinion No. 180. Washington, DC: ACOG, 1996.
6. Reece EA, Assimakopoulos E, Zheng XZ. The safety of obstetric ultrasonography: concern for the fetus. Obstet Gynecol. 1990;76(1):139-46.
7. AIUM Bioeffects Report. Mechanical bioeffects from diagnostic ultrasound: AIUM consensus statements. J Ultrasound Med. 2002;29:73-6.
8. AIUM News Release: AIUM opposes use of ultrasound for entertainment. Laurel, MD: November 5, 2002.
9. Salvesen Kå, Bakketeig LS, Eik-Nes SH, et al. Routine ultrasonography in utero and school performance at 8-9 years. Lancet. 1992;339:85-9.
10. Salvesen Kå. Routine ultrasonography in utero and development in childhood – a randomized controlled follow-up study. Acta Obstet Gynecol Scand. 1995;74:166-7.
11. Kieler H, Haglund B, Waldenström U, et al. Routine ultrasound screening in pregnancy and the children's subsequent growth, vision and hearing. Br J Obstet and Gynaecol. 1997;104:1267-72.
12. Kieler H, Ahlesten G, Haglund H, et al. Routine ultrasound screening in pregnancy and the children's subsequent neurologic development. Obstet Gynecol. 1998;91 (5 Pt 1):750-6.
13. Salvesen Kå, Eik-Nes SH. Ultrasound during pregnancy and birthweight, childhood malignancies and neurological development. Ultrasound Med Biol. 1999;25(7):1025-31.
14. Kieler H, Cnattingius S, Halund B, et al. Sinistrality – a side-effect of prenatal sonography: a comparative study of young men. Epidemiology. 2001;12:618-23.
15. Salvesen Kå, Eik-Nes SH. Ultrasound during pregnancy and subsequent childhood non-right handedness: a meta-analysis. Ultrasound Obstet Gynecol. 1999;13:241-6.
16. Ang ES, Gluncic V, Duque A, et al. Prenatal exposure to ultrasound waves impacts neuronal migration in mice. Proc Natl Acad Sci USA. 2006;103(34):12903-10.
17. National Institute Health Consensus Development Conference Consensus Statement. 1984;5(1):17. Available at http://hstat.nlm.nih.gov/hq/Hquest/screen/HquestHome/s/45672 . Accessed on February, 2011.
18. Ultrasound Screening: Implications of the RADIUS Study [draft summary]. NIH Technol Assess Statement Online. 1993;12:1-5.

19. American Institute of Ultrasound In Medicine. Standards for Performance of the Antepartum Obstetrical Examination. J Ultrasound Med. 1996;29:185-7. Available at www.aium.org. Accessed on February 2011.
20. Campbell S. The obstetric ultrasound examination. In: Chervenak FA, Isaacson GC, Campbell S (Eds). Ultrasound in Obstetrics and Gynecology. Boston: Little Brown; 1993. pp. 187-98.
21. American Institute of Ultrasound in Medicine (2002). Standards and Guidelines for the Accreditation of Ultrasound Practices (online). Available at www.aium.org/consumer/statement_selected.asp?statement=27. Accessed February 2011.
22. Marinac-Dabic D, Krulewitch CJ, Moore RM. The safety of prenatal ultrasound exposure in human studies. Epidemiology. 2002;13:S19-22.
23. Anderson G. Routine prenatal ultrasound screening. In: Canadian Task Force on the Periodic Health Examination. Canadian Guide to Clinical Preventive Health Care. Ottawa: Health Canada; 1994. pp. 4-14.
24. Royal College of Obstetricians and Gynaecologists. Ultrasound Screening for Fetal Abnormalities Report of the RCOG Working Party. London, UK: RCOG; 1997.
25. Schwarzler R, Senat M-V, Holden D, et al. Feasibility of the second-trimester ultrasound examination in an unselected population at 18, 20 or 22 weeks of pregnancy: a randomized controlled trial. Ultrasound Obstet Gynecol. 1999;14(2):92-7.
26. Carrera JM, Torrents M, Mortera C, et al. Routine prenatal ultrasound screening for fetal abnormalities: 22 years' experience. Ultrasound Obstet Gynecol. 1995;5(3):174-9.
27. Martin JA, Hamilton BE, Ventura SJ, et al. Births: Final data for 2001. National vital statistics reports; Hyattsville, MD: National Center for Health Statistics. 2002; 51.
28. American College of Obstetricians and Gynecologists. Screening for fetal chromosomal abnormalities. ACOG Practice Bulletin No. 77. Washington, DC: ACOG; 2007.
29. Chervenak FA, McCullough LB, Chervenak JL. Prenatal informed consent for sonogram: an indication for obstetric sonography. Am J Obstet Gynecol. 1989;161(4):857-60.
30. Bennett MJ, Little G, Dewhurst J, et al. Predictive value of ultrasound measurement in early pregnancy: a randomized controlled trial. British J Obstet Gynaecol. 1982;89(5):338-41.
31. Neilson JP, Munjanja SP, Whitfield CR. Screening for small for dates fetuses: a controlled trial. Br Med J. 1984; 289(6453):1179-82.
32. Bakketeig LS, Eik-Nes SH, Jacobsen G, et al. Randomised controlled trial of ultrasonographic screening in pregnancy. Lancet. 1984;2(8396):207-11.
33. Bricker L, Neilson JP, Dowswell T. Routine ultrasound in late pregnancy (after 24 weeks' gestation). Cochrane Database of Systematic Reviews [1469-493X]. 2008;4: CD001451.
34. Eik-Nes SH, Salvesen Kå, Økland O. Routine ultrasound fetal examination in pregnancy: the 'ålesund' randomized controlled trial. Ultrasound Obstet Gynecol. 2000; 15(6):473-8.
35. Secher NJ, Kern Hansen P, Lenstrup C, et al. A randomized study of fetal abdominal diameter and fetal weight estimation for detection of light-for-gestation infants in low-risk pregnancies. Br J Obstet Gynaecol. 1987;94(2):105-9.
36. Ewigman B, LeFevre M, Hesser J. A randomized trial of routine prenatal ultrasound. Obstet Gynecol. 1990;76:189-94.
37. Waldenström U, Axelsson O, Nilsson S, et al. Effects of routine one-stage ultrasound screening in pregnancy: a randomized controlled trial. Lancet. 1988;2(8611):585-8.
38. Saari-Kemppainen A, Karjalainen O, Ylöstalo P, et al. Ultrasound screening and perinatal mortality: controlled trial of systemic one-stage screening in pregnancy. Lancet. 1990;336:387-91.
39. Geerts L, Brand E, Theron G. Routine obstetric ultrasound examinations in South Africa: cost and effect on perinatal outcome – a prospective randomized controlled trial. Br J Obstet Gynaecol. 1996;103(6):501-7.
40. Ewigman BG, Crane JP, Frigoletto FD, et al. Effect of prenatal ultrasound screening on perinatal outcome. RADIUS Study Group. N Engl J Med. 1993;329(12):821-7.
41. LeFevre ML, Bain RP, Ewigman BG, et al. A randomized trial of prenatal ultrasonographic screening: impact on maternal management and outcome. RADIUS (Routine Antenatal Diagnostic Imaging with Ultrasound) Study Group. Am J Obstet Gynecol. 1993;169(3):483-9.
42. Crane JP, LeFevre ML, Winborn RC, et al. A randomized trial of prenatal ultrasonographic screening: Impact on the detection, management, and outcome of anomalous fetuses. The RADIUS Study Group. Am J Obstet Gynecol. 1994; 171(2):392-9.
43. Skupski DW, Chervenak FA, McCullough LB. Is routine ultrasound screening for all patients? Clin Perinatol. 1994;21(4):707-22.
44. Berkowitz RL. Should every pregnant woman undergo ultrasonography? New Eng J Med. 1993;329(12):874-5.
45. Gunderson EW. Cost of routine ultrasonography. Am J Obstet Gynecol. 1994;171(2):581-2.
46. Thacker SB. Quality of controlled clinical trials. The case of imaging ultrasound in obstetrics: a review. Br J Obstet Gynaecol. 1985;92(5):437-44.
47. Lilford RJ, Chard T. The routine use of ultrasound. Br J Obstet Gynaecol. 1985;92:434-6.
48. Romero R. Routine obstetric ultrasound. Ultrasound Obstet Gynecol. 1993;3(5):303-7.
49. Chasen ST, Chervenak FA. What is the relationship between the universal use of ultrasound, the rate of detection of twins, and outcome differences? Clin Obstet Gynecol. 1998;41(1):66-77.
50. DeVore GR. The routine antenatal diagnostic imaging with ultrasound study: another perspective. Obstet Gynecol. 1994;84(4):622-6.

51. Bucher HC, Schmidt JG. Does routine ultrasound scanning improve outcome in pregnancy? Meta-analysis of various outcome measures. BMJ. 1993; 307(6895):13-7.
52. Neilson JP. Ultrasound for fetal assessment in early pregnancy (Cochrane Review). In: The Cochrane Library, Issue 4, 2002. Oxford: Update Software.
53. Grennert L, Persson PH, Gennser G. Benefits of ultrasonic screening of a pregnant population. Acta Obstet Gynecol Scand. 1978; Suppl 78: 5-14.
54. Persson PH, Kullander S. Long-term experience of general ultrasound screening in pregnancy. Am J Obstet Gynecol. 1983;146(8):942-7.
55. Rosendahl H, Kivinen S. Antenatal Detection of Congenital Malformations by Routine Ultrasonography. Obstet Gynecol. 1989;73(6):947-51.
56. Levi S, Hyjazi Y, Schaapst JP, et al. Sensitivity and specificity of routine antenatal screening for congenital anomalies by ultrasound: the Belgian multicentric study. Ultrasound Obstet Gynecol. 1991;1(2):102-10.
57. Gonçalves LF, Jeanty P, Piper JM. The accuracy of prenatal ultrasonography in detecting congenital anomalies. Am J Obstet Gynecol. 1994; 171(6):1606-12.
58. Boyle JG. The accuracy of prenatal ultrasonography in detecting congenital anomalies (letter). Am J Obstet Gynecol. 1995;173(2):667-8.
59. Chitty LS, Hung GH, Moore J, et al. Effectiveness of routine ultrasonography in detecting fetal structural abnormalities in a low risk population. BMJ. 1991;303(6811):1165-9.
60. Shirley IM, Bottomley F, Robinson VP, et al. Routine radiographer screening for fetal abnormalities by ultrasound in an unselected low risk population. Br J Radiol. 1992;65(775):564-9.
61. Papp Z, Tóth-Pál E, Papp C, et al. Impact of prenatal mid-trimester screening on the prevalence of fetal structural anomalies: a prospective epidemiological study. Ultrasound Obstet Gynecol. 1995;6(5):320-6.
62. Luck CA. Value of routine ultrasound scanning at 19 weeks: a four year study of 8849 deliveries. BMJ. 1992;304(6840): 1474-8.
63. Grandjean H, Larroque D, Levi S, et al. The performance of routine ultrasonographic screening of pregnancies in the Eurofetus Study. Am J Obstet Gynecol. 1999;181(2):446-54.
64. Skupski DW, Newman S, Edersheim T, et al. The impact of routine obstetric ultrasonographic screening in a low-risk population. Am J Obstet Gynecol. 1996;175(5):1142-5.
65. Queisser-Luft A, Stopfkuchen H, Stolz G, et al. Prenatal diagnosis of major malformations: quality control of routine ultrasound examinations based on a five-year study of 20,248 newborn fetuses and infants. Prenat Diag. 1998;18:567-76.
66. Boyd PA, Chamberlain P, Hicks NR. 6-year experience of prenatal diagnosis in an unselected population in Oxford, UK. Lancet. 1998;352(9140):1577-81.
67. Long G, Sprigg A. A comparative study of routine versus selective fetal anomaly ultrasound scanning. J Med Screen. 1998;5(1):6-10.
68. VanDorsten JP, Hulsey TC, Newman RB, et al. Fetal anomaly detection by second-trimester ultrasonography in a tertiary center. Am J Obstet Gynecol. 1996;178:742-9.
69. Stoll C, Tenconi R, Clementi M, et al. Detection of congenital anomalies by fetal ultrasonographic examination across Europe. Community Genet. 2001;4(4):225-32.
70. Clementi M, Stoll C. The Euroscan Study. Ultrasound Obstet Gynecol. 2001;18(4):297-300.
71. Sepulveda W, Odibo A, Sebire NJ, et al. The lambda sign at 10-14 weeks of gestation as a predictor of chorionicity in twin pregnancies. Ultrasound Obstet Gynecol. 1996;7(6):421-3.
72. Cicero S, Curcio P, Papageorghiou A, et al. Absence of nasal bone in fetuses with trisomy 21 at 11-14 weeks of gestation: an observational study. Lancet. 2001;358(9294):1665-7.
73. Souter VL, Nyberg DA. Sonographic screening for fetal aneuploidy: first trimester. J Ultrasound Med. 2001;20(7): 775-90.
74. Economides DL, Braithwaite JM. First trimester ultrasonographic diagnosis of fetal structural abnormalities in a low risk population. Br J Obstet Gynaecol. 1998;105(1):53-7.
75. Crowther CA, Kornman L, O'Callaghan S, et al. Is ultrasound assessment of gestational age at the first antenatal visit of value? A randomized clinical trial. Br J Obstet Gynaecol. 1999;106(12):1273-9.
76. Hyett JA, Perdu M, Sharland GK, et al. Using fetal nuchal translucency to screen for major congenital cardiac defects at 10-14 weeks of gestation: population based cohort study. BMJ. 1999;318(7176):81-5.
77. Whitlow BJ, Chatzipapas IK, Lazanakis ML, et al. The value of sonography in early pregnancy for the detection of fetal abnormalities in an unselected population. Br J Obstet Gynaecol. 1999;106(9):929-36.
78. Carvalho MHB, Brizot ML, Lopes LM. Detection of fetal structural abnormalities at the 11-14 weeks ultrasound scan. Prenat Diagn. 2002;22:1-4.
79. Nicolaides KH, Azar G, Byrne D, et al. Fetal nuchal translucency: ultrasound screening for chromosomal defects in first trimester of pregnancy. BMJ. 1992;304(6831): 867-9.
80. Snijders RJ, Noble P, Sebire N, et al. UK multicentre project on assessment of risk of trisomy 21 by maternal age and fetal nuchal-translucency thickness at 10-14 weeks of gestation. Fetal Medicine Foundation First Trimester Screening Group. Lancet. 1998;352(9125):343-6.
81. Fukada Y, Takizawa M, Amemiya A, et al. Detection of aneuploidy with fetal nuchal translucency and maternal serum markers in Japanese women. Acta Obstet Gynecol Scand. 2000;79(12):1124-5.
82. Acacio GL, Barini R, Pinto Junior W, et al. Nuchal translucency: an ultrasound marker for fetal chromosomal abnormalities. Sao Paulo Med J. 2001;119(1):19-23.

83. Comas C, Torrents M, Munoz A, et al. Measurement of nuchal translucency as a single strategy in trisomy 21 screening: should we use any other marker? Obstet Gynecol. 2002;100(4):648-54.
84. Sharma G, Chasen ST, Kalish RB, et al. Aneuploidy screening with nuchal translucency: performance in a single institution. Am J Obstet Gynecol. 2002;187 part 2:S177.
85. Zoppi MA, Ibba RM, Putzolu M, et al. Nuchal translucency and the acceptance of invasive prenatal chromosomal diagnosis in women aged 35 or older. Obstet Gynecol. 2001;97:916-20.
86. Chasen ST, McCullough LB, Chervenak FA. Is nuchal translucency screening associated with different rates of invasive testing in an older obstetric population? Am J Obstet Gynecol. 2004;190:769-4.
87. Economides DL, Whitlow BJ, Kadir R, et al. First trimester sonographic detection of chromosomal abnormalities in an unselected population. Br J Obstet Gynaecol. 1998;105(1):58-62.
88. Schwärzler P, Carvalho JS, Senat MV, et al. Screening for fetal aneuploidies and fetal cardiac abnormalities by nuchal translucency thickness measurement at 10-14 weeks of gestation as part of routine antenatal care in an unselected population. Br J Obstet Gynaecol. 1999;106(10):1029-34.
89. Snijders RJM, Thom EA, Zachary JM, et al. First trimester trisomy screening: nuchal translucency measurement training and quality assurance to correct and unify technique. Ultrasound Obstet Gynecol. 2002;19:353-9.
90. Sharma G, Gold HT, Chervenak FA, et al. Patient preference regarding first-trimester aneuploidy risk assessment. Am J Obstet Gynecol. 2005;193(4):1429-36.
91. Nicolaides KH, Chervenak FA, McCullough LB, et al. Evidence-based obstetric ethics and informed decision-making by pregnant women about invasive diagnosis after first-trimester assessment of risk for trisomy 21. Am J Obstet Gynecol. 2005;193(2):322-6.
92. Bindra R, Heath V, Liao A, et al. One-stop clinic for assessment of risk for trisomy 21 at 11-14 weeks: a prospective study of 15,030 pregnancies. Ultrasound Obstet Gynecol. 2002;20:219-25.
93. Wald NJ, Rodeck C, Hackshaw AK, et al. First and second trimester antenatal screening for Down's syndrome: the results of the Serum, Urine and Ultrasound Screening Study (SURUSS). Health Technol Assess. 2003;7(11):1-77.
94. Wapner R, Thom E, Simpson JL, et al. First-trimester screening for trisomies 21 and 18. N Engl J Med. 2003;349:1405-13.
95. Malone FD, Canick JA, Ball RH, et al. First- and Second-Trimester Evaluation of Risk (FASTER) Research Consortium. First-trimester or second-trimester screening, or both, for Down's syndrome. N Engl J Med. 2005;353(19):2001-11.
96. McCullough LB, Chervenak FA. Ethics in Obstetrics and Gynecology. New York, NY: Oxford University Press; 1994.
97. Salvesen, Kå. Ultrasound and left-handedness: a sinister association? Ultrasound Obstet Gynecol. 2002;19(3):217-21.
98. Chitty LS. Ultrasound screening for fetal abnormalities. Prenat Diag. 1995;15:1241-57.
99. Smith-Bindman R, Hosmer W, Feldstein V, et al. Second-trimester ultrasound to detect fetuses with Down syndrome. A meta-analysis. JAMA. 2001;285(8):1044-55.
100. Nyberg DA, Luthy DA, Resta RG, et al. Age-adjusted risk assessment for fetal Down's syndrome during the second trimester: description of the method and analysis of 142 cases. Ultrasound Obstet Gynecol. 1998;12(1):8-14.
101. Wald NJ, Watt HC, Hackshaw AK. Integrated screening for Down's syndrome based on tests performed during the first and second trimesters. New Engl J Med. 1999;341(7):461-7.
102. Spencer K. Accuracy of Down syndrome risks produced in a first-trimester screening program incorporating fetal nuchal translucency thickness and maternal serum biochemistry. Prenat Diag. 2002;22:244-6.
103. Chasen ST, Skupski DW, McCullough LB, et al. Prenatal informed consent for sonogram – the time for first-trimester nuchal translucency has come. J Ultrasound Med. 2001;20:1147-52.
104. Skupski DW, Chervenak FA, McCullough LB. A clinical and ethical evaluation of routine obstetric ultrasound. Curr Opin Obstet Gynecol. 1994;6(5):435-9.
105. Sharma G, McCullough LB, Chervenak FA. Ethical considerations of early (first vs second trimester) risk assessment disclosure for trisomy 21 and patient choice in screening versus diagnostic testing. Am J Med Genet Part C Semin Med Genet. 2007;145C(1):99-104.
106. Chervenak FA, McCullough LB, Ledger WJ. Advocacy for routine obstetric ultrasound. ACOG Clinical Review. 1996;1:1-4.

5

CHAPTER

Medicolegal Issues in Obstetric and Gynecologic Ultrasound

Frank A Chervenak, Judith L Chervenak

INTRODUCTION

Ultrasound has revolutionized the practice of obstetrics and gynecology in one generation more than any other innovation. However, practitioners should be aware of the medicolegal risks.

Obstetric ultrasound plays a vital and increasingly frequent role in legal actions, either as the focus in a case alleging wrongful birth in which an anomaly was not diagnosed, and the mother was deprived of a chance to terminate her pregnancy; or as a significant or contributing factor in a case alleging negligent obstetric care with resulting damage to the infant-plaintiff or mother.

This chapter will focus upon the general aspects of a medical negligence case as they relate to the performance of the obstetric ultrasound examination, summarize the recommendations of both the American College of Obstetrics and Gynecology (ACOG) and the American Institute of Ultrasound in Medicine (AIUM), regarding the performance of these examinations, and outline potential areas of negligence and discuss ways to avoid them.

MEDICAL NEGLIGENCE

In order to establish negligence, the plaintiff must show that there was:

- A duty recognized by the law.
- A breach of that duty, in that there was a failure on the part of the physician to meet what was considered to be the standard of care at the time the treatment was rendered.
- A causal relationship between the treatment and the resulting injury, and
- Actual loss or damage to the plaintiff.[1]

Obstetric ultrasound cases may include allegations of a failure on the part of the maternal-fetal medicine specialist performing the ultrasound to fully advise the obstetric patient regarding the medical aspects of her case, given his specialized training in the field of high-risk obstetrics. The maternal-fetal medicine specialist has a duty to the patient and should clearly define the extent of his role in the patient's care, whether he or she is comanaging a patient, rendering consultative services or only performing antenatal diagnoses.

Generally, damages are easily established, granting either or both the departure from the accepted standards of care and the causal connection between that breach and the damages as the major focus of the litigation. Standard of care is most commonly established by the testimony of an expert witness whose knowledge, training or experience qualifies him to testify as to the standard of care.[2] These experts are limited by the state of medical knowledge and standards of practice at the time of the alleged negligence.[2] While these standards were previously limited to local legal requirements, they have expanded to those practiced nationally, given the recent advances in communication and dissemination of medical information.

Although guidelines promulgated by various organizations do not establish the standard of care introduced at trial, the obstetric ultrasound practitioner should be aware of the recommendations of ACOG and the AIUM. These organizations have published recommendations regarding guidelines, instrumentation and safety, documentation, indications, examination content and quality control. They periodically issue clinical recommendations. These guidelines are designed to inform the practitioner so that he or she is aware of currently suggested practices in this ever evolving discipline.

GUIDELINES

ACOG's recent publications include a Practice Bulletin entitled *Ultrasonography in Pregnancy* issued in December of 2004[3] and a *Committee Opinion on Guidelines for*

Diagnostic Imaging During Pregnancy in September of 2004.[4] In 2003, the AIUM published a *Practice Guideline for the Performance of an Antepartum Obstetric Ultrasound Examination* in conjunction with ACOG and the American College of Radiology (ACR).[5] The AIUM guidelines were originally published in 1985 and are now in their fourth revision.

INSTRUMENTATION AND SAFETY

While acknowledging that manufacturers offer machines with 3D capability, the practice bulletin indicates that proof of a clear advantage over 2D imaging has not yet been demonstrated.[3] ACOG also recommends that practitioners should have a method of storing images and equipment should be serviced on a regular basis.[3]

The US Food and Drug Administration has arbitrarily limited energy exposure from ultrasonography to 94 mW/cm^2.[4] In the 2004 *Committee Opinion on Guidelines for Diagnostic Imaging During Pregnancy*, ACOG noted that there had been no documented reports of adverse fetal effects from diagnostic ultrasound procedures, including duplex Doppler imaging.[4] The AIUM concurs and emphasizes the "as low as reasonably achievable" (ALARA) principle, which means that the lowest possible ultrasonic exposure setting should be used to gain the necessary information.[5]

DOCUMENTATION

The AIUM has published a standard for documentation of an ultrasound exam which can be obtained from the AIUM's website, www.aium.org.[6] These guidelines recommend that a permanent record of both the images and the interpretation of the ultrasound be recorded in a retrievable format and should be kept in accordance with the relevant requirements of local legal and healthcare facilities. The AIUM suggests that the documentation include the patient's name and identifying numbers, such as a social security or medical record number, the date of ultrasound exam and image orientation on all recorded images. Additionally, the healthcare provider's name, type of ultrasound examination and identification of the sonographer/sonologist should be included on the accompanying report.[6]

A preliminary report of the findings may be provided, and a final report should be included in the patient's medical record. Within the final report, limitations of the examination should be noted, biometric data, including variations from normal size, should be accompanied by measurements and a final report should be completed, and transmitted to the patient's healthcare provider. Depending on the circumstances, the results may need to be directly conveyed to the patient's referring health care provider and documentation of this communication is recommended.[6]

ACOG has noted "Absence of visual image documentation eliminates the possibility of future review or clinical reintegration and weakens the defense against an allegation that an incomplete or inadequate study was performed."[3]

INDICATIONS

The AIUM has published indications for first and second obstetric ultrasound examinations, which are listed in **Tables 1 and 2**.[5] When there is no indication, ACOG has commented that, while it is reasonable to honor a patient's request for an ultrasound, based upon the limitations of the various studies analyzing the benefits of routine screening and their equivocal results, a physician is not obligated to perform an ultrasound in a low-risk patient without indications.[3] The authors have argued that all pregnant women should be offered a quality second trimester ultrasound examination in clinical settings where it is available.[7] Further, it has been argued that pregnant women should also be offered a quality first trimester ultrasound examination in clinical settings where it is available.[8] Currently, ACOG has recommended that all pregnant women, regardless of their age, should be offered screening for Down syndrome in a quality manner.[9]

TABLE 1: First trimester ultrasound examination.[5]

Indications: A sonographic examination can be of benefit in many circumstances in the first trimester of pregnancy, including, but not limited to, the following indications:

- To confirm the presence of an intrauterine pregnancy
- To evaluate a suspected ectopic pregnancy
- To define the cause of vaginal bleeding
- To evaluate pelvic pain
- To estimate gestational (menstrual*) age
- To diagnose or evaluate multiple gestations
- To confirm cardiac activity
- As an adjunct to chorionic villus sampling (CVS), embryo transfer, and localization and removal of an intrauterine device (IUD)
- To evaluate maternal pelvic masses and/or uterine abnormalities
- To evaluate suspected hydatidiform mole.

*For the purpose of this document, the terms "gestational age" and "menstrual age" are considered equivalent.

TABLE 2: Second and third trimester examination.[5]

Indications: Sonography can be of benefit in many situations in the second and third trimesters, including, but not limited to, the following circumstances:

- Estimation of gestational age
- Evaluation of fetal growth
- Vaginal bleeding
- Abdominal/pelvic pain
- Incompetent cervix
- Determination of fetal presentation
- Suspected multiple gestation
- Adjunct to amniocentesis
- Significant discrepancy between uterine size and clinical dates
- Pelvic mass
- Suspected hydatidiform mole
- Adjunct to cervical cerclage placement
- Suspected ectopic pregnancy
- Suspected fetal death
- Suspected uterine abnormality
- Evaluation of fetal well-being
- Suspected amniotic fluid abnormalities
- Suspected placental abruption
- Adjunct to external cephalic version
- Premature rupture of membranes and/or premature labor
- Abnormal biochemical markers
- Follow-up evaluation of a fetal anomaly
- Follow-up evaluation of placental location for suspected placenta previa
- History of previous congenital anomaly
- Evaluation of fetal condition in late registrants for prenatal care.

In certain clinical circumstances, a more detailed examination of fetal anatomy may be indicated.

(*Adapted from:* National Institutes of Health. Diagnostic Ultrasound Imaging in Pregnancy: Report of a Consensus. NIH Publication 84-667. Washington, DC: US Government Printing Office; 1984).

EXAMINATION CONTENT

The AIUM has published a practice guideline for the performance of an antepartum obstetric ultrasound examination in conjunction with ACOG and the American College of Radiology (ACR).[5] The components of a first trimester ultrasound examination and second and third trimester examinations are listed in **Tables 3 and 4**. The AIUM and ACOG use the terms "standard," "limited" and "specialized" to describe the types of obstetric ultrasound performed during the second and third trimesters. Standard and limited examinations are defined by their components and the components of a specialized exam are determined on a case-by-case basis.[3,5]

Standard examinations include an evaluation of fetal presentation, amniotic fluid volume, cardiac activity, placental position, biometry and an anatomic survey. An examination of the uterus and adnexa is also suggested if technically feasible.[3,5]

TABLE 3: Contents of first trimester ultrasound examination.[5]

- Scanning in the first trimester may be performed either transabdominally or transvaginally. If a transabdominal examination is not definitive, a transvaginal scan or transperineal scan should be performed whenever possible
- The uterus and adnexa should be evaluated for the presence of a gestational sac. If a gestational sac is seen, its location should be documented. The gestational sac should be evaluated for the presence or absence of a yolk sac or embryo and the crown-rump length should be recorded, when possible
- Presence or absence of cardiac activity should be reported
- Fetal number should be reported
- Evaluation of the uterus, adnexal structures, and cul-de-sac should be performed.

Limited exams are performed for a specific indication such as identification of fetal presentation, evaluation of fetal cardiac activity or amount of amniotic fluid and are appropriate when a standard examination has already been performed. In such cases, an anatomic survey is not necessary.

Specialized examinations include the biophysical profile, fetal Doppler studies, fetal echocardiography and those examinations that are done when it is necessary to evaluate a specific question or to evaluate a specific or suspected fetal anomaly or maternal biochemical screening test. These examinations should be performed by operators with specific experience in the relevant area.[3,5]

QUALITY CONTROL

Following the results of the Routine Antenatal Diagnostic Imaging with Ultrasound trial (RADIUS) published in 1993[10] and other studies which indicated that the detection of anomalies was dependent on the experience of the operator, the AIUM began to offer voluntary medical facility accreditation for ultrasound practices. This process reviews the qualifications of the facility's practitioners, the type of equipment and its maintenance, including the proper methods of antimicrobial cleaning and/or chemical sterilization and storing of transducers to prevent contamination between patients, and methods of reporting and storage.[11]

The acquisition and maintenance of such accreditation ensures compliance with current organizational standards, is recommended and is often required for reimbursement for obstetric ultrasound studies by various insurance companies. A recent study in which practices

TABLE 4: Contents of a standard second and third trimester obstetric ultrasound examination.[5]

- Fetal cardiac activity, number and presentation should be reported.
- A qualitative or semiquantitative estimate of amniotic fluid volume should be reported
- The placental location, appearance, and relationship to the internal cervical os should be recorded. The umbilical cord should be imaged and the number of vessels in the cord should be evaluated, when possible
- Gestational age assessment
- Fetal weight estimation
- Maternal anatomy. Evaluation of the uterus and adnexal structures should be performed
- Fetal anatomic survey
- The following areas of assessment represent the essential elements of a standard examination of fetal anatomy. A more detailed fetal anatomic examination may be necessary if an abnormality or suspected abnormality is found on the standard examination.
  - Head and neck:
    - Cerebellum
    - Choroid plexus
    - Cisterna magna
    - Lateral cerebral ventricles
    - Midline falx
    - Cavum septi pellucidi
  - Chest:
    - The basic cardiac examination includes a 4-chamber view of the fetal heart.
    - If technically feasible, an extended basic cardiac examination can also be attempted to evaluate both outflow tracts.
  - Abdomen:
    - Stomach (presence, size and sinus)
    - Kidneys
    - Bladder
    - Umbilical cord insertion site into the fetal abdomen
    - Umbilical cord vessel number
  - Spine: Cervical, thoracic, lumbar and sacral spine
  - Extremities: Legs and arms (presence or absence)
  - Gender: Medically indicated in low-risk pregnancies only for evaluation of multiple gestations.

that sought and received accreditation were re-evaluated three years later, found that these practices had improved compliance within accepted standards, and therefore concluded that this improvement would translate into an enhancement of the quality of practice.[11]

LITIGATION RELATED TO ULTRASOUND

Sanders had tracked litigation related to ultrasound. Since there is no reliable system of tabulating legal cases that are filed, many cases are dropped following the review of a competent expert, the majority of cases settle out of court and not all of those that do go to court are reported, this task has been made especially difficult. In 2003, Sanders published his latest series documenting the types of cases he reviewed that were filed between 1997–2002.[12]

TABLE 5: Nineteen possible ways to get sued for ultrasound.[13]

1.	Missing the sonographic finding.
2.	Misinterpretation of the sonographic finding.
3.	Failure to compare findings with previous ultrasound.
4.	Failure to properly communicate the sonographic report to the referring physician or the patient.
5.	Failure to personally examine the patient or take a proper history.
6.	Incorrect sonographic approach for a specific condition.
7.	Incomplete examination.
8.	Inadequate quality of films.
9.	Slip and fall injuries.
10.	Complications from puncture techniques under ultrasound control.
11.	Failure to obtain informed consent.
12.	Complications of ultrasound such as induced vaginal bleeding or abortion.
13.	Equipment complications (e.g., electric shocks).
14.	Failure to recommend additional sonographic or radiologic studies or biopsy.
15.	Failure to order a sonographic examination.
16.	Inclusion of sonologist in a shotgun suit.
17.	Loss of films, inadequate filing system, misplacement of films or reports.
18.	Abuse of patient by sonologist or sonographer (sexual, physical or mental).
19.	Miscellaneous anxiety produced by misdiagnosis, invasion of privacy, etc.

When categorizing suits by specialty, predictably those relating to obstetric ultrasound were the most common of all those involving ultrasound examinations, followed by gynecologic examinations. Suits relating to obstetric ultrasound can be expected to have large economic damages because damages are based upon the life-expectancy of the infant-plaintiff, thereby rewarding plaintiff's attorneys with large contingency fees. Sanders found that the missed fetal anomalies are now the most common reason for litigation, comprising over half of the cases in his most recent series.[13] **Table 5** documents Sander's tabulation of the possible ways to be sued when performing ultrasound.[13]

NONMEDICAL USE OF ULTRASONOGRAPHY

The AIUM has published the following "prudent use" statement, endorsed by ACOG.

"The AIUM advocates the responsible use of diagnostic ultrasound. The AIUM strongly discourages the non-medical use of ultrasound for psychosocial or entertainment purposes. The use of either two-dimensional or three-dimensional ultrasound only to view the fetus, obtain a picture of the fetus or determine the fetal gender without a medical indication is inappropriate and contrary to responsible medical practice. Although there are no confirmed biological effects on patients caused by exposures from present diagnostic ultrasound instruments, the possibility exists that such biological effects may be identified in the future. Thus, ultrasound should be used in a prudent manner to provide medical benefit to the patient."[14] This position has been ethically defended.[15]

CONCLUSION

Physicians who perform obstetric ultrasound can expect to be subjected to increasing legal risk. While knowledge of and comportment with the published recommendations and guidelines of ACOG and the AIUM does not offer complete protection from legal risk, they help to both avoid and to defend oneself. Failure to comply with such standards has the potential to make any subsequent legal case more difficult to defend.

REFERENCES

1. Prosser W, Keeton WP, Dobbs DB, et al. Prosser and Keeton on the Law of Torts, 5th edition. Minnesota: West Publishing Group; 1984, p.187.
2. Moore T, Gaier M. Medical Malpractice. New York Law Journal;2004:1.
3. Ultrasonography in Pregnancy. ACOG Practice Bulletin(58), 2004. www.acog.org.
4. Guidelines for Diagnostic Imaging During Pregnancy. ACOG Committee Opinion, 2004. 299. www.acog.org.
5. AIUM Practice Guideline for the performance of an antepartum obstetric ultrasound examination. J Ultrasound Med. 2003;22(10):1116-25.
6. American standard for documentation of an ultrasound examination. American Institute of Ultrasound in Medicine. J Ultrasound Med. 2002:21(10):1188-9.
7. Chervenak FA, McCullough LB, Chervenak JL. Prenatal informed consent for sonogram (PICS): an indication for obstetric ultrasound. Am J Obstet Gynecol. 1989;161: 857-60.
8. Chasen S, Skupski DW, McCullough LB, Chervenak FA. Prenatal consent for sonogram: the time for first trimester nuchal translucency has come. J Ultrasound Med. 2001; 20:1147-52.
9. Barclay L. Screening for fetal chromosomal abnormalities. Obstet Gynecol. 2007.
10. Ewigman BG, Crane JP, Frigoletto FD, et al. Effect of prenatal ultrasound screening on perinatal outcome. RADIUS Study Group. N Engl J Med. 1993; 329(12):821-7.
11. Abuhamad AZ, Benacerraf B, Woletz P, et al. The accreditation of ultrasound practices-impact on compliance with minimum performance guidelines. J Ultrasound Med. 2004:23(8):1023-9.
12. Sanders RC. Changing patterns of ultrasound-related litigation: a historical survey. J Ultrasound Med. 2003:22(10): 1009-15.
13. Sanders RC. The effect of the malpractice crisis on obstetrics and gynecologic ultrasound. In: Chervenak FA, Isaacson GC, Campbell S (Eds). Ultrasound in Obstetrics and Gynecology. Boston: Little Brown and Company; 1993. pp.263-76.
14. ACOG Committee Opinion, Non-medical Use of Obstetric Ultrasonography. 2004;297.
15. Chervenak FA, McCullough LB. An ethical critique of boutique fetal imaging: a case for the medicalization of fetal imaging. Am J Obstet Gynecol. 2005; 192(1):31-3.

SECTION 2

Obstetrics

6

CHAPTER

Fetal and Maternal Physiology and Ultrasound Diagnosis

Aida Salihagic Kadic, Maja Predojevic, Asim Kurjak

INTRODUCTION

Human life does not begin with birth. Normal development of the human being lasts 280 days before parturition. In prenatal growth and development, the placenta plays a key role. It has numerous functions essential for maintaining the pregnancy and promoting normal fetal development. During intrauterine period, the fetus gradually begins to perform many vital physiological functions. Furthermore, through 9 months of gestation, a repertoire of fetal functions and activities constantly expands. Development of modern imaging methods has revealed the existence of a full range of fetal movement patterns, even facial movements similar to emotional expressions in adults. Indeed, the world in utero is fascinating. Therefore, the birth is not the beginning, but only a new chapter in the story of human life.

PLACENTA

"The vessels join to the uterus like the roots of plants, and through them the embryo receives its nourishment."

—***Aristotle, De Generatione Animalium, Book II.***

DEVELOPMENT OF THE PLACENTA

The placenta is an organ that is indispensable for the transfer of nutrients and gases from the mother to the fetus and the removal of fetal waste products. Placenta can be defined as a fusion of fetal membranes with the uterine mucosa. The development of the placenta starts with the implantation, in the moment when the blastocyst begins the invasion of the endometrium, about the 6th day after conception.[1] Prior to implantation in the uterine lining, blastocyst consists of an external, single-layer, cellular component named the trophoblast and the inner cell mass, embryoblast. After the trophoblast has attached to the endometrial epithelium, rapid cellular proliferation occurs and the trophoblast differentiates into two layers consisting of the inner cytotrophoblast and an outer syncytiotrophoblast, a multinucleated mass without cellular boundaries. Syncytial trophoblast processes extend through the endometrial epithelium to invade the endometrial stroma. Stromal cells surrounding the implantation site become laden with lipids and glycogen, develop into polyhedral shape, and are referred to as decidual cells. These decidual cells degenerate in the region of the invading syncytiotrophoblast and provide nutrition to the developing embryo.[2] At day 7–8 after conception, the blastocyst has completely crossed the epithelium and is embedded within the endometrium. At day 8–9 postconception, the syncytiotrophoblast generates a number of fluid-filled spaces within its mass. These spaces flow together forming larger lacunae and are finally separated by parts of the syncytiotrophoblast (trabeculae) that cross the syncytial mass from the embryonic to the maternal side. The development of the lacunar system leads to the division of the placenta into several compartments. The embryonically oriented part of the trophoblast will become the chorionic plate, the lacunae will develop into the intervillous space **(Fig. 1)**, while the trabeculae will become the anchoring villi, with the growing branches developing into floating villi. Finally, the maternally oriented part of the trophoblast will develop into the basal plate.[3]

At day 12 after conception, the process of implantation is completed. The developing embryo with its surrounding extraembryonic tissues is totally embedded in the endometrium and the syncytiotrophoblast surrounds the whole surface of the conceptus. Mesenchymal cells derived from the embryo spread over the inner surface of the trophoblast, thus generating a new combination of trophoblast and mesoderm, termed chorion. Starting on day 12 postconception, proliferation

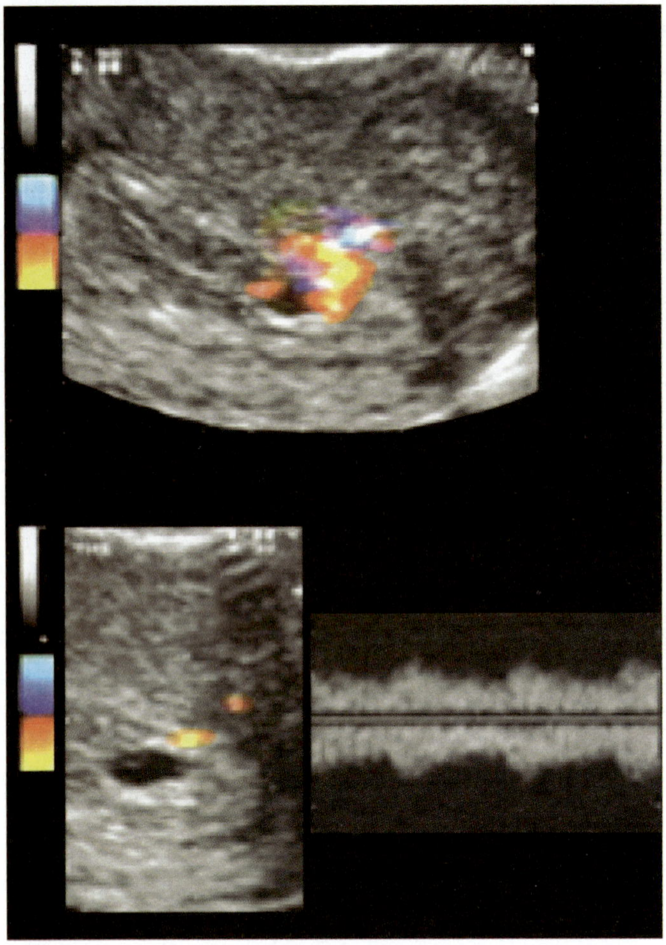

Fig. 1: Image recorded by 2D color Doppler sonography, showing intervillous blood flow.

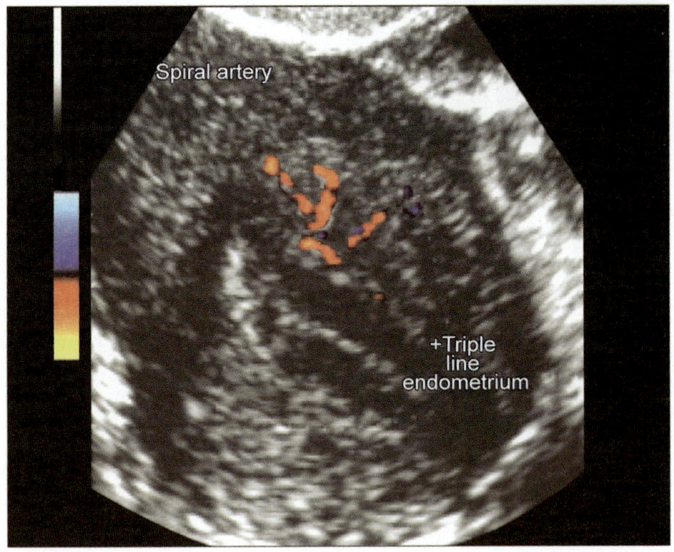

Fig. 2: Image recorded by 2D color Doppler sonography showing blood flow in spiral arteries.

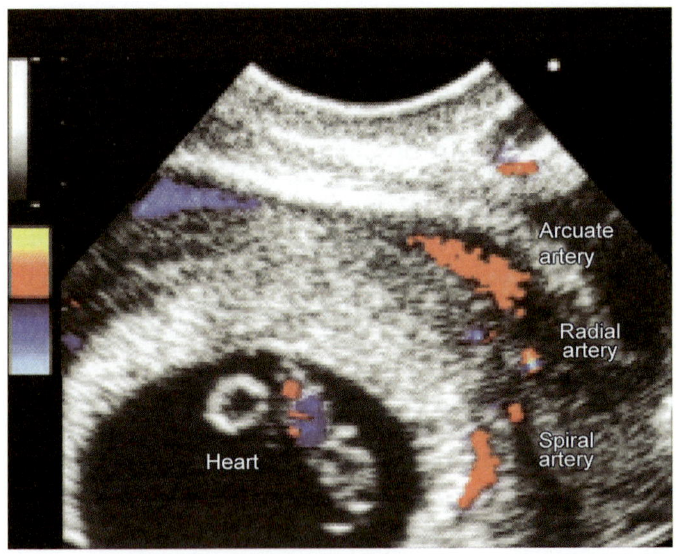

Fig. 3: Image recorded by 2D color Doppler sonography showing blood flow in part of uteroplacental circulation (arcuate, radial and spiral arteries). The terminal segments of spiral arteries will be remodelated by trophoblast cell invasion.

of cytotrophoblast pushes trophoblast cells to penetrate into the syncytial trabeculae, reaching the maternal side of the syncytiotrophoblast by day 14. Further proliferation of trophoblast cells inside the trabeculae (day 13) stretches the trabeculae resulting in the development of syncytial side branches filled with cytotrophoblast cells (primary villi). Shortly after, the mesenchymal cells from the extraembryonic mesoderm too follow the cytotrophoblast and penetrate the trabeculae and the primary villi, thus generating secondary villi. At this stage there is always a complete cytotrophoblast layer between the penetrating mesenchyme and syncytiotrophoblast. Around day 20–21, vascularization within the villous mesenchyme gives rise to the formation of the first placental vessels (tertiary villi). Only later, the connection to the fetal vessel system will be established. The villi are organized in villous trees that cluster together into a series of spherical units known as lobules or placentones. Each placentone originates from the chorionic plate by a thick villous trunk stemming from a trabecula. Continuous branching of the main trunk results in daughter villi mostly freely ending in the intervillous space.[3]

In normal pregnancies, decidual and myometrial segment of the spiral arteries **(Fig. 2)**, undergo changes to convert them into large vessels of low resistance **(Figs. 3 and 4)**. Two types of migratory cytotrophoblast

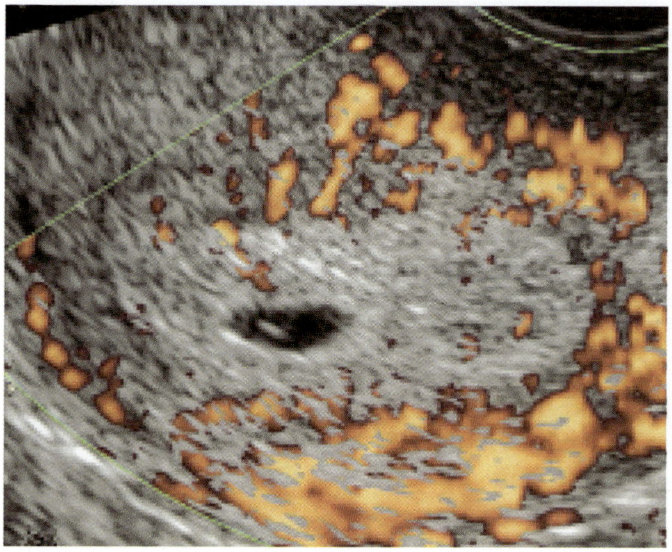

Fig. 4: Image recorded by 2D power Doppler sonography showing increased blood flow that surrounds the gestational sac as a direct consequence of the spiral arteries dilation.

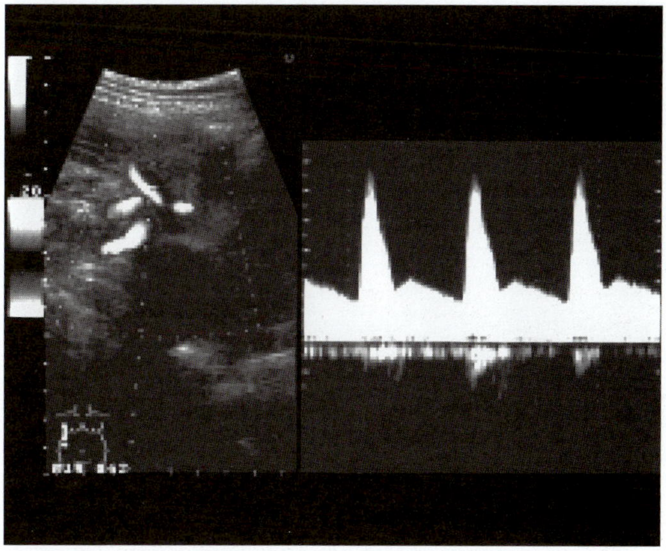

Fig. 5: Image recorded in the 30th week of gestation showing increased impedance to flow in the uterine artery with early diastolic notching.

cause this—endovascular and interstitial cytotrophoblast. Endovascular cytotrophoblast invades spiral arteries on the decidua and myometrium and replaces arterial endothelium, destroying muscle and elastic tissues in the tunica media. Interstitial cytotrophoblast destroys the ends of decidual blood vessels, promoting the flow of blood into the lacunae. The maternal arteries are opened up and functionally denervated so that they are completely dilated and unresponsive to circulatory pressor substances or autonomic neural control. Behind this, at uterine radial artery level, local prostacyclin maintains vasodilatation.[1] Free transfer of maternal blood to the intervillous space is established at the end of the first trimester of pregnancy.[3]

ABNORMAL PLACENTAL DEVELOPMENT AND ULTRASOUND

Trophoblast invasion is a key process during human placentation. Failure of trophoblast invasion and spiral artery transformation leads to reduced perfusion of the placenta and fetus, and inadequate fetal nutrition and oxygenation. This condition is called uteroplacental insufficiency because the metabolic demands of the fetus and placenta exceed the uteroplacental transport capacity. It is considered that there are two phases of trophoblast invasion. The first wave of trophoblastic invasion converts the decidual segments of the spiral arteries between 6–10 weeks of the pregnancy. The second wave converts the myometrial segments between 14–16 weeks of the pregnancy.[2] As a result of these physiological changes, the diameter of the spiral arteries increase from 15–20 mm to 300–500 mm, reducing impedance to flow and optimizing fetomaternal exchange in the intervillous space.[4] In pregnancies complicated by preeclampsia and intrauterine growth restriction (IUGR), trophoblast invasion is limited to the decidualized endometrium, which results in failure of the spiral arteries to become low-resistance vessels.[5] Using Doppler ultrasound, uteroplacental and fetal vessels conversion of the uterine spiral arteries and placental development may be assessed.

Successful trophoblast invasion results in loss of early diastolic notching in the uterine artery Doppler waveform by the end of the first trimester.[6,7] The failure to undergo physiological trophoblastic vascular changes is reflected by the high impedance to the blood flow at the level of the uterine arteries and with the characteristic waveform of early diastolic notching **(Fig. 5)**. In normal pregnancies, due to progressive maturation of the placenta, impedance to flow in the umbilical artery decreases and end-diastolic velocity establishes by the end of the first trimester. Doppler indices continue to fall towards term as umbilical blood flow resistance decreases[6-8] **(Fig. 6)**. In cases of placental insufficiency, because of inadequate ramification of villi and increased degradation due to degenerative processes, surface of the capillary network is reduced and blood flow resistance in the placenta is elevated. These conditions reflect in the abnormal umbilical

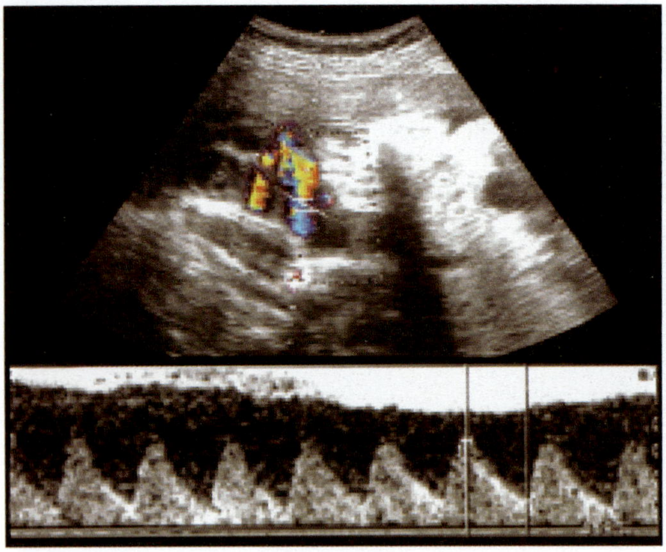

Fig. 6: Normal Doppler waveforms from the umbilical artery.

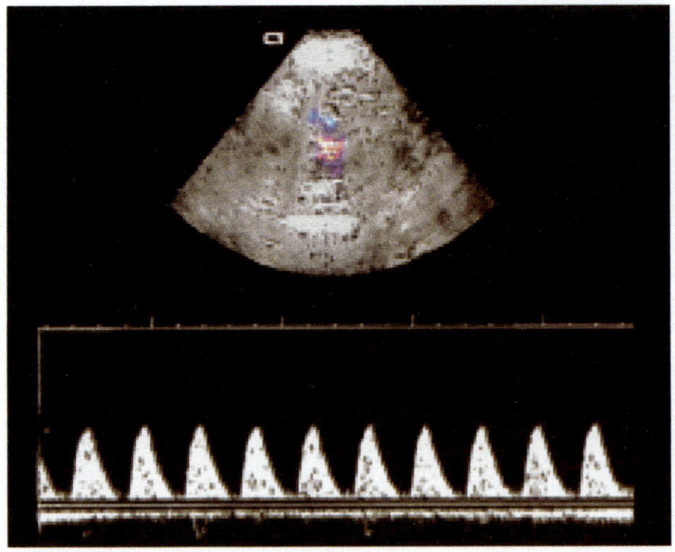

Fig. 7: Increased impedance to flow in the umbilical artery with an absent end-diastolic flow.

artery blood velocity waveforms. However, pathological studies have demonstrated that increased impedance in the umbilical arteries becomes evident only when at least 60% of the placental vascular bed is obliterated.[9] In pregnancies with reversed or absent end-diastolic flow in the umbilical artery, compared to those with normal flow, mean placental weight is reduced and the cross-sectional diameter of terminal villi is shorter.[10] Absent diastolic velocity or retrograde diastolic velocity in the umbilical artery indicate extremely increased placental vascular impedance **(Fig. 7)**.

Endangered by placental insufficiency, fetus activates compensatory mechanisms. Fetal response to placental dysfunction evolves from early compensatory reactions to late decompensation in multiple organ systems.[11] Fetal hypoxia activates a range of biophysical, cardiovascular, endocrine and metabolic responses. Fetal cardiovascular responses to hypoxia, which include modification of the heart rate, an increase in arterial blood pressure and redistribution of the cardiac output towards vital organs, are probably the most important adaptive reactions responsible for maintaining fetal homeostasis.[12] The redistribution of blood flow towards the fetal brain is known as the "brain-sparing effect" **(Figs. 8 and 9)**. Doppler assessment of the fetal cerebral and umbilicoplacental circulations can detect fetal blood flow redistribution towards the brain during hypoxia and quantify the degree of this redistribution using the C/U ratio.[12-14] In normal pregnancies, cerebral vascular resistance

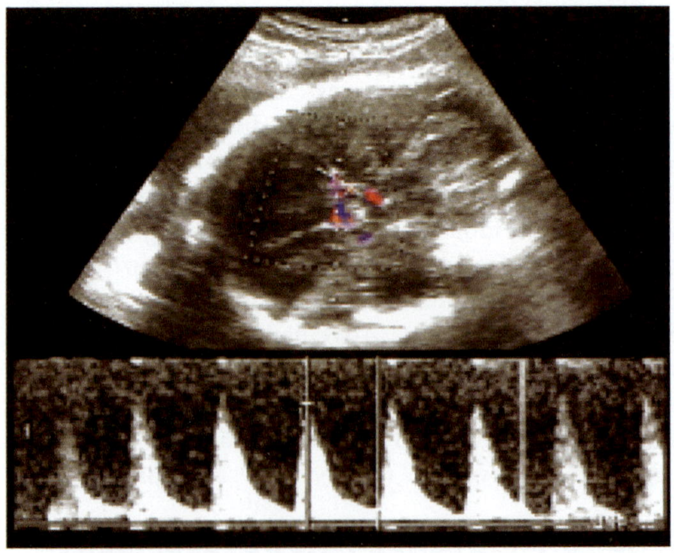

Fig. 8: Normal flow of the middle cerebral artery in the third trimester.

remains higher than placental vascular resistance. Therefore, the cerebroumbilical (C/U) ratio, expressed as the cerebral resistance index/the umbilical remains resistance index, remains higher than 1. This ratio becomes less than 1 in case of blood flow redistribution in favor of the fetal brain.[13] Previous experimental studies on animal models have shown that the C/U ratio decreases in proportion to fetal pO_2.[12,15]

Although, the brain-sparing effect attempts to compensate for the reduced oxygen delivery to the fetal brain, it has become clear that this phenomenon cannot

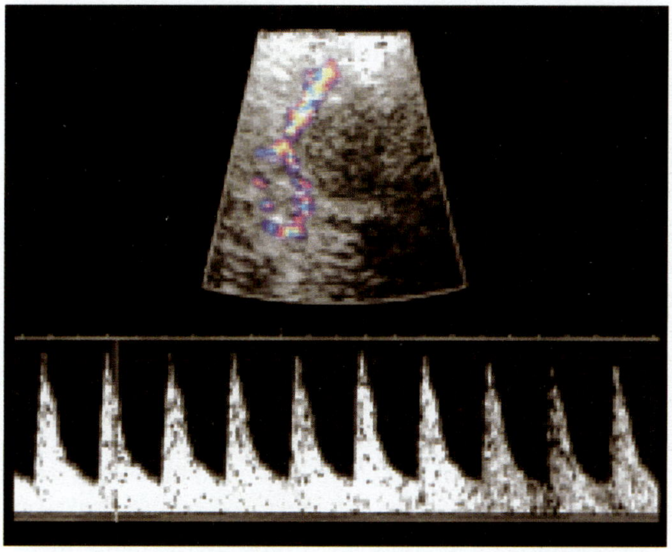

Fig. 9: Decreased impedance to flow in the middle cerebral artery ("brain-sparing effect").

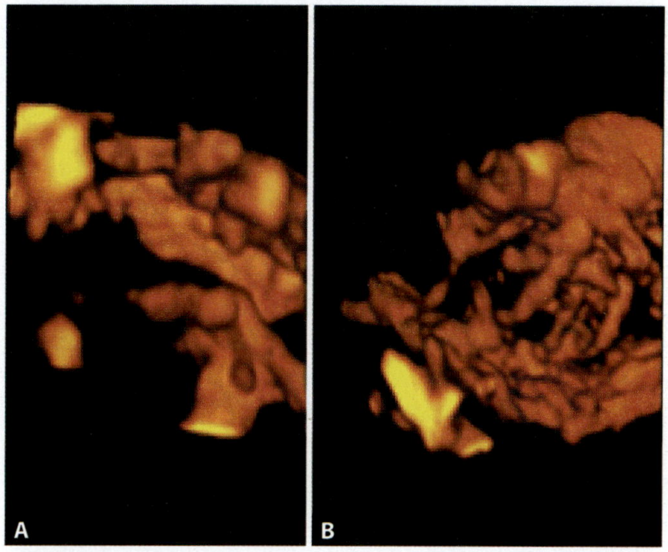

Figs. 10A and B: 3D power Doppler angiography of the placental vascular tree at the (A) 16th week of pregnancy and at the (B) 36th week of pregnancy.

always prevent the development of brain lesions.[15-17] Our studies have demonstrated the existence of several phases in the hemodynamic response of the fetal brain to chronic hypoxia. During the early phase of Doppler surveillance, cerebrovascular variability was still observed; this was followed by a loss of cerebrovascular variability and finally an increase in cerebrovascular resistance with a reduction in brain perfusion. Maximal redistribution of blood flow in favor of the fetal brain was reached 5–8 days prior to the onset of fetal heart rate abnormalities.[16,18]

FUNCTIONS OF THE PLACENTA

The placenta has multiple roles in fetal metabolism and growth. The major function of the placenta is to provide diffusion of nutrients and oxygen from the mother's blood into the fetus's blood and diffusion of excretory products from the fetus back into the mother.[19] The placenta also produces hormones that affect fetal growth. The placenta is usually fully formed and functional as a nutritive, respiratory, excretory and endocrine organ by the end of the third month of pregnancy. However, well before this time, oxygen and nutrients are diffusing from maternal to embryonic blood, and embryonic metabolic wastes are passing in the opposite direction.[20] Most of the early nutrition is due to trophoblastic digestion and absorption of nutrients from the endometrial deciduas. This is the only source of nutrients for the embryo during the first week after implantation. The embryo continues to obtain at least some of its nutrition in this way for another eight weeks, although the placenta also begins to provide nutrition after about the 16th day after fertilization (a little more than one week after implantation).[19] Molecules of low molecular weight such as blood gases, sodium, water, urea, fatty acids, nonconjugated steroids, pass through placental membrane by simple diffusional exchange between the circulations. Hexose sugars, conjugated steroids, amino acids, nucleotides, water-soluble vitamins, plasma proteins, cholesterol will not gain access to the fetal circulation unless either special transport mechanisms exist or the integrity of the barrier is breached.[21] In the early months of pregnancy, the placental membrane is still thick because the placenta is not fully developed. Therefore, its permeability is low. Further, the surface area is small because significant placental growth has not occurred yet. In later pregnancy, the permeability increases due to the thinning of the membrane diffusion layers and the multiple expansion of the surface area, giving way to a tremendous increase in placental diffusion **(Figs. 10A and B)**.[19] In addition to the placental thickness, the factors that will influence exchange between the mother and the fetus include the maternal and the fetal blood flow; the fetal and the maternal concentrations of the substances to be transported; and the types of transport mechanisms available. The exchange of more freely diffusible molecules such as O_2 is to a larger extent dependent on the blood flow than placental thickness.[21]

Fetal Growth and Metabolism

As soon as within the 1st month following the fertilization of the ovum, all the organs of the fetus have already begun to develop and in the next 2–3 months, the fine anatomic structures of the organs will be formed. After the 4th month, the organs of the fetus, including the majority of their substructures, are for the most part the same as those of the neonate. However, the development of the cells in the structures is still far from complete and will require the remaining 5 months of pregnancy to complete development.[19]

Normal fetal growth requires macronutrients—carbohydrates, lipids, proteins and micronutrients—vitamins and minerals. Also, other factors influence growth, like growth factors and hormones. The main ingredient of the fetal diet is carbohydrate. The fetus has a low capacity for gluconeogenesis, largely because the necessary enzymes, although present, are inactive due to a low fetal arterial pO_2. The fetus must therefore obtain its glucose from the maternal blood.[21] The growing fetus requires approximately 87 kcal/kg/per day.[22] About half of the calories needed for fetal growth and metabolism come from the mother's glucose, and the other half from her amino acids and placental lactate.[21] The fetus has a high ability of storing proteins and fats.[19] Protein accumulation occurs early in fetal development, to reach its maximum by week 35. Protein deposition precedes fat deposition.[21] Fetal fat content is low at 26 weeks. Fat acquisition starts sometime between the 26–32 weeks and continues intensively thereafter, being a result of glucose utilization rather than placental fatty acid uptake.[22] By term, about three times as much energy is stored as fats than as proteins. In addition, glucose is also stored as glycogen in the fetal liver. Glycogen is an important nutrient in the period immediately after birth, before nutrients from breast milk are used.[21]

Fetal metabolism shows some particularity in relation to calcium, phosphate, iron, and some vitamins. About 22.5 grams of calcium and 13.5 grams of phosphorus are accumulated in an average fetus during gestation. About one-half of these accumulate during the last four weeks of gestation, which is coincident with the period of rapid ossification of the fetal bones and with the period of rapid weight gain of the fetus. Iron accumulates in the fetus even more rapidly than calcium and phosphate. Most of the iron is in the form of hemoglobin, which begins to be formed as early as in the third week after fertilization of the ovum. Small amounts of iron are concentrated in the mother's uterine progestational endometrium even before implantation of the ovum. This iron is used to form the early red blood cells. About one-third of the iron in a fully developed fetus is normally stored in the liver. Interestingly, the fetus needs an equal intake of vitamins as the adult. The B vitamins, especially vitamin B_{12} and folic acid, are necessary for formation of red blood cells and the nervous tissue, as well as for the overall growth of the fetus. Vitamin C is necessary for appropriate formation of intercellular substances, especially the bone matrix and fibers of connective tissue. Vitamin D is needed for normal bone growth in the fetus. The mother needs it for adequate absorption of calcium from her gastrointestinal tract. If the mother has plenty of this vitamin in her body fluids, large quantities of the vitamin will be stored by the fetal liver to be used by the neonate for several months after birth. Vitamin E, although the mechanisms of its functions are not clear, is necessary for normal development of the early embryo. In its absence in laboratory animals, spontaneous abortion usually occurs at an early stage of pregnancy. Vitamin K is used by the fetal liver for formation of blood coagulation factors. Prenatal storage in the fetal liver of vitamin K derived from the mother is helpful in preventing fetal hemorrhage, particularly hemorrhage in the brain when the head is traumatized by squeezing through the birth canal.[19]

The fetus actively participates in endocrine regulation of its metabolism and growth by synthesis and secretion of hormones. For instance, the rate at which glucose is utilized by growing fetal tissues is probably determined largely by the actions of fetal insulin. The storage of glucose as fat is also regulated primarily by fetal insulin. Fetal adrenocorticotropic hormone (ACTH) and glucocorticoids stimulate the storage of glucose as glycogen.[21] Hormonal regulation of fetal growth differs from hormonal regulation of growth during postnatal life. Furthermore, fetal growth hormone (GH) has a small role in stimulating fetal growth. Although pituitary begins to produce and secrete GH during the 5th week of gestation, fetal GH does not significantly affect fetal growth, possibly due to the lack of functional GH receptors on fetal tissues.[23] Data have shown that pituitary aplasia and congenital hypopituitarism do not cause severe IUGR.[24,25] On the contrary, fetal insulin significantly stimulates fetal growth. It is a known fact that pancreatic agenesis is associated with severe growth restriction[26] and that fetal hyperinsulinemia leads to fetal mass overgrowth. It is believed that insulin-like growth factors (IGFs or somatomedins) produced by a large range of fetal cell types and particularly by the fetal liver, provide a major endocrine stimulus to fetal growth.[21] They have the potent effect of increasing all aspects of bone growth in postnatal life.[19] IGFs are present in human fetal tissue extracts after 12 weeks gestation.[22] IGF-1 has the most important role in stimulation of fetal growth.[21] Its levels in fetal and cord circulation directly correlate with the fetal length and mass.[27] Reduced plasma concentration of IGF-1 has been reported in intrauterine growth restriction (IUGR).[28] Furthermore, maternal starvation leads to a rapid decrease in fetal plasma IGF-1 concentration, which is generally associated with the cessation of intrauterine growth.[29] It is considered that glucose is the major regulator of fetal IGF-1 secretion.[30] Maternal IGF-1, IGF-2 and insulin do not cross the placenta, and do not have a direct effect on fetal growth, but may have an effect on placental function, thus altering the nutrient exchange between the placenta and the fetus.[31] It has been found that maternal plasma IGF-1 concentration correlates with fetal growth.[32] Production of fetal IGFs is stimulated by prolactin, insulin and human chorionic somatomammotropin (HCS).[33] In the fetus, HCS acts via lactogenic receptors to stimulate growth, regulate intermediary metabolism and stimulate the production of IGFs, insulin, adrenocorticotropic hormones and pulmonary surfactant.[23] Fetal thyroid hormones also stimulate growth, especially in the later stage of pregnancy, but their most significant role is the one they have in the central nervous system development.[21]

Additional factors that affect birth weight include parity (primiparous mothers have smaller babies than multiparous mothers), maternal size, multiple pregnancy.[21] Maternal nutrition is also of great significance for fetal growth and the adverse effects of severe malnutrition on fetal well-being and neonatal survival have been long known. Data have confirmed a great impact of maternal diet during pregnancy on fetal growth and development, as well as on postnatal development and health.[34-43] It is during intrauterine life that the diet has significant effect on the brain development. It has been known for some time that folic acid plays a protective role in neurodevelopmental processes. Periconceptional use of folic acid has been proven to significantly reduce the risk of neural tube birth defects.[34] Such birth defects can cause death or permanent physical disability. Periconceptional use of folic acid decreases the occurrence of anencephaly and spina bifida by at least 50%.[35] Hence, some countries (USA, Canada) have decided to fortify food with folic acid. A recent study on the prevalence of congenital abnormalities following folic acid fortification of grain in the United States found a modest, yet statistically significant decrease in prevalence of transposition of the great arteries, cleft palate, pyloric stenosis and omphalocele.[35] Yet, other studies provide no evidence of folate being an important factor in the prevention of birth defects other than neural tube defects.[36] Furthermore, a significant protective effect was seen with large doses of folic acid (approximately 6 mg/d) and iron (150–300 mg/d of ferrous sulfate) during the first gestational month against Down's syndrome.[37]

Numerous findings have shown a favorable impact of essential fatty acids on prenatal development.[38-40,42,43] Omega-3 and omega-6 fatty acids are necessary for human growth and development. Since, their endogenous synthesis is impossible, they need to be taken into the body through diet. The arachidonic (AA) and docosahexaenoic acids (DHA) are the key components of all membranes and are incorporated into the structural lipids of the developing brain. Fetal demand for essential fatty acids is at its peak during the third trimester of pregnancy.[21] A recent study has demonstrated that DHA supplemented during pregnancy plays a role in the maturation of the visual system and benefits infant visual acuity at four but not six months of age.[38] Also, results of a recent study indicate that DHA consumption in pregnancy significantly affects problem solving abilities at the age of nine months, but does not affect memory processes.[39] Additionally, children's mental processing scores at 4 years of age correlated significantly with maternal intake of DHA during pregnancy.[40] Seafood (especially sardine and tuna) is a rich source of omega-3 fatty acids. Essential fatty acids can be also found in linseed oil, walnut oil and soy. In the USA, women are advised to limit their seafood intake during pregnancy to 340 g per week. According to a recent study published in an esteemed journal, maternal seafood consumption should be more than 340 g per week. A lower seafood intake during pregnancy was in the study associated with an increased risk of suboptimum developmental outcome.[41] Further, the findings suggest a protective effect of fish intake during pregnancy against the risk of atopy and asthma.[42] Consumption of apples during pregnancy may also have a protective effect against the development of childhood asthma and allergic diseases.[43]

Healthy and varied diet during pregnancy is required for normal fetal growth and development. Most pregnant women need 2,200–2,900 kcal a day.[44] If appropriate nutritional elements are not present in a pregnant woman's diet, a number of maternal deficiencies can occur, especially in calcium, phosphates, iron and vitamins.[19]

Fetal Cardiovascular System

The cardiovascular system is the first embryonic system to start functioning. The need for substrates which facilitate fast growth and development of the embryo requires an early development of the mechanism that supplies the cells with nutrients and removes the metabolic products from them. Cardiovascular development begins when the process of diffusion becomes inadequate to supply the fetus with nutrients and oxygen. Blood circulation can be observed in the "body" of the embryo as early as at the end of the third week of the intrauterine life.[45]

Between the 27–35th day of intrauterine life, during which the embryo grows from 5 mm in length to about 16–17 mm, cardiac septum and endocardial cushions begin to form. The endocardial cushions will give rise to mitral and tricuspid valves. By the end of 7th week, they are short and thick, but over the next few weeks they are becoming longer and thinner, and achieve their final shape. Impairments in cardiac septum development lead to the existence of pathological communication between the heart chambers **(Fig. 11)**, which can be more or less life-threatening condition for newborn child. Some of these anomalies, such as ventricular septal defect, are among common congenital anomalies and can occur independently or as a part of different syndromes.[46,47] Fetal echocardiography is a powerful tool and many cardiac malformations can be successfully diagnosed before birth.

The human heart starts beating between the 21–23rd day after fertilization, at a heart rate of 65 beats/min.[48] In that period, the heart is a tube-like structure with a single lumen. Between the 5–9th week of gestation the heart rate accelerates from 80 beats/min to 165 beats/min.[49,50] It has been shown that a continuous decrease in the heart rate during this period is associated with miscarriages occurring in the first trimester.[50] By the 10th week after fertilization, the heart rate has reached its highest value (approximately 170/min), it starts decreasing **(Fig. 12)**. Before birth, the human heart contracts at a rate of about 140 beats/min.

The fetal circulatory system operates much differently than the circulatory system of the newborn baby, which is not surprising considering the specific features of fetal environment. After the birth, the individual components of the circulatory system are in serial connection. However, the fetal circulatory system is organized in parallel circle.[51] Further, fetal values of cardiac output and blood pressure are significantly different from values in adults.

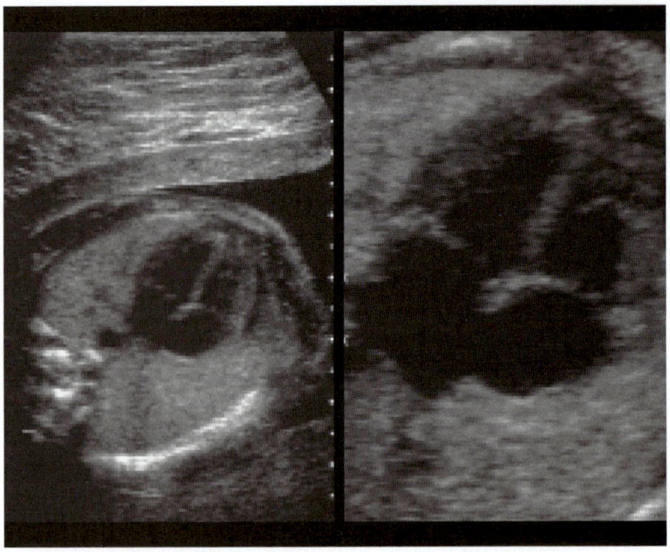

Fig. 11: Four chamber view of the fetal heart.

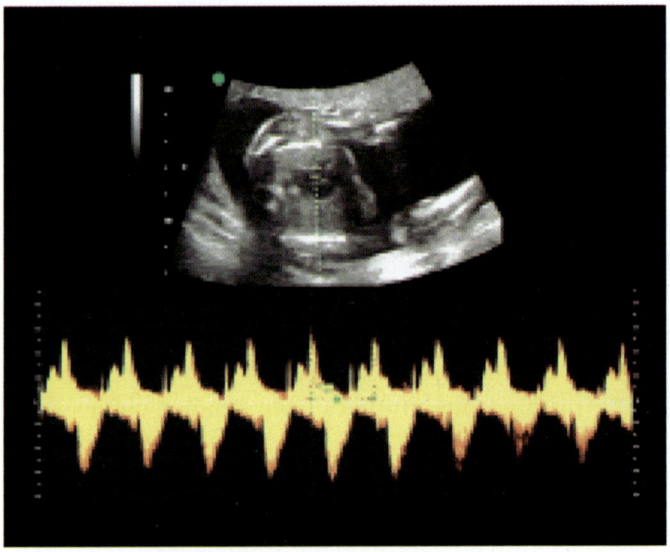

Fig. 12: Fetal cardiac activity with a heart rate of 150 bpm.

During intrauterine life, blood returning from the placenta through the umbilical vein passes through the ductus venosus, mainly bypassing the liver. Then most of the blood entering the right atrium from the inferior vena cava is directed in a straight pathway across the posterior aspect of the right atrium and through the foramen ovale directly into the left atrium. Thus, the well-oxygenated blood from the placenta enters mainly the left side of the heart, rather than the right side and is pumped by the left ventricle mainly into the arteries of the head and forelimbs. The blood entering the right atrium from the superior vena cava is directed downward through the tricuspid valve into the right ventricle. This blood is mainly deoxygenated blood from the head region of the fetus and it is pumped by the right ventricle into the pulmonary artery. Since, the pressure in the pulmonary artery is about 0.7 kPa higher than the pressure in the aorta, almost all the blood from the pulmonary artery goes through the arterial duct (ductus Botallijev) into the descending aorta, then through the two umbilical arteries into the placenta, where the deoxygenated blood becomes oxygenated. Only a small portion of blood from the descending aorta portion goes to the visceral organs and lower extremities.[19]

Blood carrying the highest oxygen saturation goes to the fetal heart, the brain, the upper extremities while the other parts of fetal body receive blood with lower oxygen saturation. Also, fetal blood pO_2 is much lower than maternal blood pO_2. At term pO_2 of fetal blood after the oxygenation in the placenta amounts 30 mm Hg.[2] Such low pO_2 levels can be observed in adults at altitudes between 6000–8000 meters, at which human life is barely possible. Therefore, fetal environment has long been considered "the Mount Everest in utero".[52] Despite the low pO_2 in the fetal blood, the fetus does not live in hypoxic environment. Due to adaptive mechanisms, the amount of oxygen delivered to the fetal tissue is similar to the amount of oxygen delivered to maternal tissue by maternal blood.[19] In addition, the hemoglobin concentration of fetal blood is about 50% greater than that of the mother. Furthermore, fetal hemoglobin can carry more oxygen at a low than it can at a high PCO_2. The fetal blood entering the placenta carries large amounts of carbon dioxide, but much of this carbon dioxide diffuses from the fetal blood into the maternal blood. Loss of the carbon dioxide makes the fetal blood more alkaline, whereas the increased carbon dioxide in the maternal blood makes it more acidic. These changes cause the capacity of fetal blood to combine with oxygen to increase and that of maternal blood to decrease. This forces more oxygen from the maternal blood, while enhancing oxygen uptake by the fetal blood. Thus, the Bohr shift operates in one direction in the maternal blood and in the other direction in the fetal blood. These two effects make the Bohr shift twice as important here as it is for oxygen exchange in the lungs; therefore, it is called the double Bohr effect. These mechanisms, as well as a large cardiac output, ensure adequate supply of oxygen of fetal tissues, despite its low partial pressure.[19]

Maintenance of normal cardiovascular function, blood pressure, heart rate and the flow distribution through the placenta and fetal tissue are influenced by the local vascular and reflex mechanisms. Further, the autonomic nervous system and hormones also have an effect on the fetal heart and circulation. The potential regulators can be identified by measuring their concentration and dynamics of secretion in states in which a redistribution of the blood flow occurs, such as fetal hypoxia. The first line of supervision over the circulation of the fetus are the carotid chemoreceptors, but not the aortic chemoreceptors. They mediate the fetal cardiovascular response (redistribution of circulation in favor of vital organs like the heart, brain and adrenal glands to acute hypoxemia).[53] Slower regulators, the second line of control, are hormones antidiuretic hormone (ADH), angiotensin II, catecholamines and cortisol.[54-56] ADH and angiotensin II are released independently of the carotid chemoreceptors, whereas the secretion of cortisol and catecholamines is partially under the control of these neural mechanisms. After carotid sinus denervation or splanchnic blockade, rapid secretion of cortisol in response to hypoxia or a sudden drop in blood pressure, is decreased. While the secretion of ACTH does not change and occurs about 15 minutes after stimulation.[57,58] Thus, the rapid rise in cortisol secretion is the result of neural mechanisms and not as a result of ACTH stimulation. However, the role and purpose of such regulation is unclear. Medullary, hypothalamic and cerebral cortical activity also affect fetal cardiovascular function.[59] Furthermore, in control of fetal circulation autocrine and paracrine mechanisms play important role. Some of the possible regulators of the peripheral resistance, at least in the sheep fetuses, are endothelin-1 and nitrogen-(II)-oxide (NO).[60,61] They allow an increase of cerebral flow in fetal hypoxia. Several other factors such as sleeping of the fetus or uterine contractions, can also have a temporary influence on the cardiovascular system.[62]

One of the most important events after the delivery is the adjustment of the circulation of new conditions. The transitional period of circulation, which lasts 4–12 hours after birth, is characterized by a large increase of the blood flow through the lungs and by the establishment of the pulmonary circulation. The primary change in the circulation at birth is loss of the tremendous blood flow through the placenta, which approximately doubles the systemic vascular resistance at birth. This increases the aortic pressure as well as the pressures in the left ventricle and left atrium. Furthermore, in the unexpanded fetal lungs, the blood vessels are compressed because of the small volume of the lungs. After birth, the pulmonary vascular resistance greatly decreases as a result of expansion of the lungs. Also, in fetal life, the hypoxia of the lungs causes considerable tonic vasoconstriction of the lung blood vessels but when aeration of the lungs eliminates the hypoxia, the capillary endothelial cells produce vasoactive substances such as NO and prostaglandin I2, which have a strong vasodilatory effect and vasodilation takes place.[19] All these changes together reduce the resistance to blood flow through the lungs as much as fivefold, which reduces the pulmonary arterial pressure, right ventricular pressure and right atrial pressure. Changes in pulmonary and systemic resistances at birth cause blood now to attempt to flow from the left atrium into the right atrium, through the foramen ovale. Consequently, the small valve that lies over the foramen ovale on the left side of the atrial septum closes over this opening, thereby preventing further flow through the foramen ovale. Arterial ductus begins to close around four hours after birth and is usually completely closed after 24 hours. Its closing marks the end of the transitional period of the newborn circulation. After birth, blood begins to flow backward from the aorta into the pulmonary artery through the ductus arteriosus, rather than in the other direction as in fetal life. However, after only a few hours, the muscle wall of the ductus arteriosus constricts markedly. This is called functional closure of the ductus arteriosus. Then, during the next 1–4 months, the ductus arteriosus ordinarily becomes anatomically occluded by growth of fibrous tissue into its lumen. The cause of ductus arteriosus closure relates to the increased oxygenation of the blood flowing through the ductus. In fetal life, the PO_2 of the ductus blood is only 15–20 mm Hg, but it increases to about 100 mm Hg within a few hours after birth. Furthermore, many experiments have shown that the degree of contraction of the smooth muscle in the ductus wall is highly related to this availability of oxygen.[19] The reason for the closure of the venous duct is still unknown. Immediately after birth, blood flow through the umbilical vein ceases, but most of the portal blood still flows through the ductus venosus, with only a small amount passing through the channels of the liver. However, within 1–3 hours the muscle wall of the ductus venosus contracts strongly and closes this avenue of flow. As a consequence, the portal venous pressure rises from near 0 to 6 to 10 mm Hg, which is enough to force portal venous blood flow through the liver sinuses. Although, the ductus venosus rarely fails to close, we know almost nothing about what causes the closure. Knowing the characteristics of this transitional phase of circulation is very important because the postnatal increase of the resistance in the pulmonary capillaries, for example caused by hypoxia or respiratory distress syndrome, if exceeds the value of systemic resistance, can restore conditions as they existed in the fetal life, greater resistance in the pulmonary circulation than in systemic and pulmonary-aortic or right-left flow of blood through the arterial duct.[19]

Fetal Gastrointestinal System, Development of Appetite and Satiety Mechanisms

The primitive gut forms during the fourth week of the embryonic development. The primitive gut is divided into three parts: the foregut, midgut and hindgut. The derivatives of the foregut are the pharynx and its derivatives, the lower respiratory tract, the esophagus, the stomach, the duodenum, proximal to the common bile duct, and the liver, biliary tract, gallbladder, and pancreas. The derivatives of the midgut are the small intestines [except for the duodenum from the stomach **(Fig. 13)** to the entry of the common bile duct], cecum and appendix, ascending colon, and proximal one-half to two-thirds of the transverse colon. The derivatives of the hindgut are the distal one-third to one-half of the transverse colon, descending colon, sigmoid colon, rectum and upper portion of the anal canal, and part of the urogenital system.[63] Activity of the gastrointestinal system begins during an early stage of pregnancy. By 10 weeks, peristalsis begins in the large intestine[64] and by 11 weeks in the small intestine.[65] Also, fetal swallowing activity was observed from the 11th week of gestation.[66]

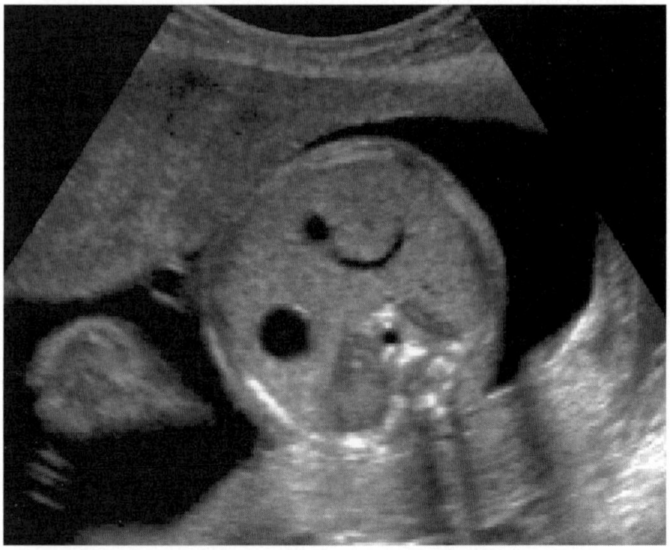

Fig. 13: Transverse scan of the fetal abdomen showing the stomach, liver, and intrahepatic part of the umbilical vein.

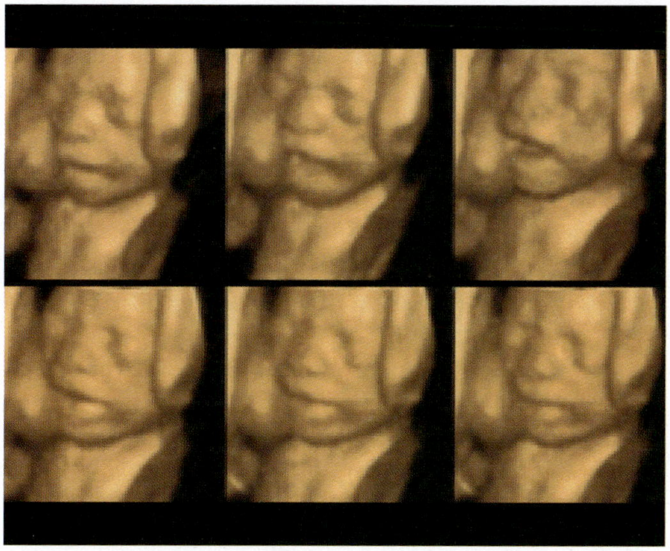

Fig. 14: A sequence of images of the fetus recorded by 4D sonography showing swallowing movements.

Swallowing amniotic fluid reflects fetal CNS maturation and has numerous, although not entirely understood roles **(Fig. 14)**. Fetal swallowing activity contributes to somatic growth, development and maturation of the fetal gastrointestinal tract. It has been estimated that swallowing of amniotic fluid proteins provides 10–15% of nitrogen requirements in the normal fetus. Upper gastrointestinal tract obstructions in human fetuses are associated with significantly greater occurrence of fetal growth restriction as compared with lower gastrointestinal obstructions. Studies have demonstrated that impairment of fetal swallowing in rabbits near term induces weight decrease. Esophageal ligation of ovine fetuses during midgestation induces a 30% decrease of small intestine villus height and a reduction in the liver, pancreas and intestinal weight.[67] Fetal swallowing is an important, yet not the only mechanism of amniotic fluid volume regulation. Altered fetal swallowing has been associated with both a decrease and an increase in the amniotic fluid volume.[68] These conditions are associated with a higher risk of perinatal morbidity and mortality. Furthermore, in some fetuses with esophageal atresia, the volume of amniotic fluid is increased. It is important to note that this is the case in some, but not all fetuses with esophageal atresia. Namely, this anomaly is often accompanied by tracheoesophageal fistula, a shortcut to the gastrointestinal tract. Therefore, intake of liquid during the respiratory movements might explain the nonappearance of polyhydramnios in some of these cases.[67] Polyhydramnios sometimes, although not always, develops in anencephalic fetuses. Some of these fetuses have an intact swallowing reflex. Cases of a normal amniotic fluid volume and reduced fetal swallowing have also been described. Assessment of fetal swallowing using gray-scale and color Doppler sonography has demonstrated that there is a fetal trend towards the development of more coordinated swallow-related movements and more functional nose-mouth flow with the advancement of gestational age. These investigators have postulated that knowledge of the physiologic mechanism involving swallowing development could contribute to identification of altered swallow-related movements in fetuses with malformations of the gastrointestinal tract or with neurological disorders.[69] Our investigation, performed by 4D ultrasound, has shown that swallowing pattern displays a peak frequency at the end of the second trimester. At the beginning of the third trimester, a decreasing incidence of this pattern was recorded.[70] Some studies have shown that fetal swallowing activity may be modulated in accordance with neurobehavioral state alterations (stimulation of swallowing with shifts from quiet to active sleep). Furthermore, fetal swallowing is influenced by the volume of amniotic fluid, hypoxia, hypotension and plasma osmolality changes.[67] Experiments in fetal lambs have indicated that dipsogenic mechanisms begin to regulate swallowing during intrauterine life. Swallowing and arginine-vasopressin (AVP) secretion increase, following the central administration of hypertonic saline solution and angiotensin II.[71,72] However, the fetus seems to have an extensively reduced sensitivity to osmotic stimuli when compared to the adult,[73-75] despite the intact dipsogenic nuclei. The fetus swallows about six times more liquid in comparison to the adult. Mechanisms underlying the high rate of human fetal swallowing are regulated, in part, by tonic activity of central angiotensin II, glutamate N-methyl-D-aspartate (NMDA) receptors and neuronal production of the nitric oxide.[68] A reduced NMDA receptor expression within the forebrain dipsogenic neurons contributes to observed differences in drinking activities between the fetus/neonate and the adult.[76] Reduced swallowing activity during the systemic hypotension, despite elevated renin levels in plasma, provides further evidence that the fetal dipsogenic response is markedly different from that of the adult.[77] It is possible that dipsogenic responses develop *in utero* in the human fetus to provide thirst stimulation for appropriate water intake during the immediate neonatal period.[67]

According to some studies, altered intrauterine osmotic environment may modulate not only fetal swallowing activity, but also the development of adult sensitivities for thirst, AVP secretion and AVP responsiveness.[67,68,78] An animal study demonstrated that extracellular dehydration during pregnancy (commonly observed during pregnancy after vomiting or diarrhea) can enhance the natriophilic propensity in offspring and suggested that vomiting during pregnancy may contribute to the epidemiological factors of hypertension.[78] Furthermore, mothers consuming excessive amounts of salt and water during pregnancy increase salt preference in adult offspring.[79] Similar to dipsogenic mechanisms, peripheral and central fetal orexic mechanism also develop during intrauterine life. Prenatal ingestive behavior is manifested as swallowing and intake of amniotic fluid. By swallowing amniotic fluid, the fetus explores a wide variety of tastes even before birth. By the 7th week of gestation, taste buds develop in human embryos.[80] Fetal taste bud cells are spread over a wider surface than in the neonate or the adult.[81] It has been shown that sweet taste, such as that of a low-concentration sucrose solution, stimulates swallowing in the human fetus, whereas the incidence of swallowing movements decreases following the injection of Lipiodol—a bitter extract of poppy seeds used as a contrast—into the amniotic fluid.[81] Sweet taste is already *in utero* the favorite taste. It has been found that although oral sucrose significantly stimulates near term ovine fetal ingestive behavior, sweet taste adaptation or habituation does not occur, in contrast to that observed in adult animals and humans. Absence of taste adaptation in the fetus/newborn may facilitate increased neonatal food intake and accelerated growth.[82] Increased or decreased glucose level in the serum does not affect the swallowing activity.[81] The main feeding regulatory factors, neuropeptide Y (NPY) and leptin, are secreted in the human fetuses as early as at 16–18 weeks, respectively.[83-85] NPY is the most potent known inducer of food intake and leptin is a satiety factor. In some animal experiments, increased fetal swallowing has been demonstrated upon central NPY administration.[86] The role of leptin in regulating ingestive behavior is interesting because, as opposed to its function in adults, leptin does not suppress fetal ingestive behavior.[68] Fetal swallowing was significantly increased following the injection of leptin.[87] Therefore, some investigators have postulated that the absence of leptin-inhibitory response potentiates feeding and facilitates weight gain in newborns, despite high body fat levels.[88] Some findings suggest a possible role of leptin in the development of the fetal gastrointestinal tract.[89] Apart from determined high leptin concentration in amniotic fluid and in the gastrointestinal mucosa at the time when the fetus starts swallowing an early presence of Ob-Rb (functional receptor of leptin) has been found in mucosa. This suggests a possible role for leptin, exerted endoluminally and in a paracrine pathway, in the developmental process (growth and/or maturation) of the human digestive tract.[89] According to some other studies, the potential *in utero* imprinting of appetite and satiety mechanisms may affect infant, childhood and ultimately adult appetite "set-points". An adverse intrauterine environment, with altered fetal orexic factors, could change the normal set-points of appetitive behavior and potentially lead to programming of adulthood hyperphagia and obesity.[68,88] In a paper, prenatal exposure to over or undernutrition, rapid growth in early infancy, an early adiposity rebound in childhood and early pubertal development have all been implicated in the development of obesity.[90] Further investigations are needed to delineate precisely the relationship between the intrauterine environment and the development of the set-points of adult appetite and thirst.

It is important to note that the function of the fetal digestive system also begins at an early stage of pregnancy. Water, electrolytes and other small molecules, such as glucose are absorbed through the small bowel.[21] By 13 weeks, the intestine starts to absorb glucose and water swallowed by the fetus.[65] Salivary amylase activity was found in the amniotic fluid in the late first trimester pregnancies. Enzyme activity breaking down peptone is present in the small intestine of 7–10 week old fetuses and rises slightly after the 14th week of gestation. Lipase was found in the stomachs of fetuses in the 4th month of gestation, its activity increased with subsequent development. In addition, the pH of the gastric fluid in newborns is usually neutral or slightly acidic and the acidity increases shortly after birth, within several hours. The first traces of gastric acidity appear in four month old fetuses.[91] Generally, during the last 2–3 months, fetal gastrointestinal function approaches that of the normal neonate. However, if the infant is more than two months premature, the digestive and absorptive systems are almost always inadequate. The absorption of fat is so poor that the premature infant must have low-fat diet.[19] Insufficient fat absorption can cause problem to newborns that were fed milk that contains more fat than breast milk, such as undiluted cow milk.[81]

Fetal Respiratory System

Fetal lungs begin to develop in the 4th week after fertilization. At this time, the respiratory diverticulum (lung bud) appears ventrally to the caudal portion of the foregut. Angiogenesis in the lungs begins at the 5th week after fertilization. From the 16–26th week of pregnancy, formation of early respiratory units occurs and pneumocytes types II appear. From 26th week until birth, thinning of the respiratory membrane takes place, primitive alveoli dilate and establish close relationship with the capillaries. From 36th week onwards, secondary alveolar septa, with rich capillary network, develop. Hence, respiratory surface enlarges. Further thinning of the respiratory membrane happens.[46] Mature neonate has 50% lower number of alveoli than an adult. Final number of alveoli is reached at 2nd year of postnatal life.[92] Normal fetal lung development requires the presence of lung liquid as well as fetal movements, like breathing. In the regulation of the lung liquid volume fetal breathing-like movements have a very important role. Other functions of breathing-like movements **(Fig. 15)** during intrauterine life are the development of respiratory muscles, widening of the alveolar spaces, maintenance of the lung liquid volume and lung organogenesis.[93-95] Animal investigation has shown that absence of respiratory movements (due to destruction of the brainstem nuclei above the phrenic nucleus) leads to hypoplasia of the lungs.[96] Breathing-like movements appear at the 10th week.[97] Early in gestation, fetal breathing activity is variable and isolated event but the frequency and complexity of the breathing patterns change over the following weeks and months. Changes in breathing-like patterns are consequences of the maturation of the fetal lungs as well as the respiratory and sleep centers in the CNS. During the 38–39th week of gestation, the frequency of movements decrease to 41 respirations per minute and the movements become as regular as in the postnatal period.[98] A number of internal and external factors can influence fetal breathing-like movements during the second half of pregnancy. At 24–28 weeks, the fetal respiratory rate can rise as high as 44 inhale/exhale cycles per minute.[99] This rate changes according to maternal carbon dioxide (CO_2) levels, strongly suggesting that respiratory center in the brainstem of the fetus already detects and responds to changes in CO_2 levels in the blood. This respiratory response to CO_2 is similar to that seen in newborns and adults.[100] Furthermore, an increased number of fetal respiratory movements following the elevation of the glucose concentration in the maternal blood have been observed at the 34th week of gestation.[101,102] Recent investigation has shown that intermittent maternal fasting is connected with a considerable alteration in the frequency and pattern of fetal breathing-like movements from the 30th week of gestation onwards.[103] Following premature rupture of membranes,[104,105] during the three days prior to the initiation of labor, a decrease in fetal breathing-like has been recorded.[106,107] However, similar maturation patterns in breathing and spontaneous fetal body movements were demonstrated among low-and high-risk fetuses threatening to deliver prematurely, which suggests normal functional development in the high-risk fetal group.[108] Some studies have shown that maternal consumption of alcohol, methadone, as well as cigarette smoking decrease the incidence of breathing-like movements.[109-111] On the contrary, aminophylline, conjugated estrogens and betamethasone are responsible for an increase in its frequency.[112,113]

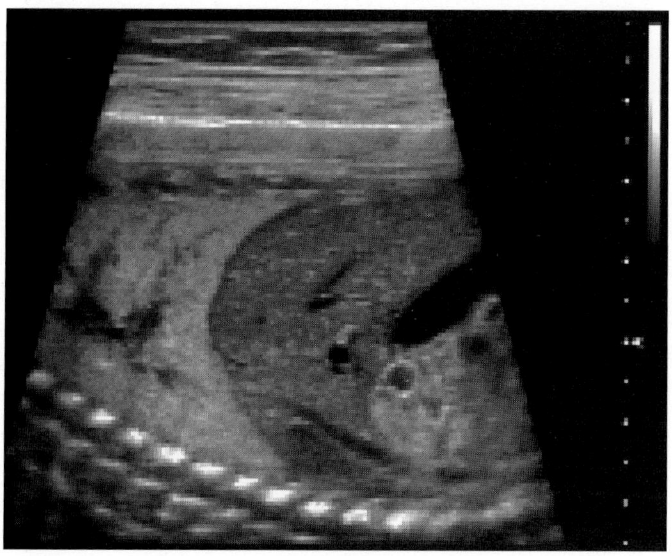

Fig. 15: Image of the fetus recorded by 2D sonography showing fetal lung and liver.

One of the most important events in the lung development is production and secretion of surfactant. At the end of 6th month, alveolar cells pneumocytes type II appear and begin to secrete surfactant. These cells differ from pneumocytes type I by the presence of numerous surfactant containing granules, lamellar bodies. By adsorbing to the air-water interface of alveoli during the first breath, with the hydrophilic head-groups in the water and the hydrophobic tails facing towards the air, the main lipid component of surfactant, dipalmitoyl-phosphatidyl-choline, reduces surface tension. In this way, surfactant prevents the closure of the alveoli, with each expiration.[46] The composition of surfactant changes during fetal life. Mature surfactant, rich with dipalmitoylphosphatidylcholine, is detectable after 35 weeks of gestation and indicates the functional maturity of fetal lungs. It is important to emphasize that the secretion of pulmonary surfactant in the lung liquid occurs only in the last weeks of fetal life.[114] Besides phospholipids, surfactant contains proteins. Four types of surfactant-associated proteins have been described, SP-A, SP-B, SP-C and SP-D. They differ in structure, as well as in the function. SP-A and SP-D are hydrophilic molecules, they stimulate the secretion and removal of phospholipids and participate in maintaining of the homeostasis of surfactant. SP-B and SP-C are hydrophobic molecules as they enable the spreading of the phospholipid bilayer along the alveoli and improve the stability of surfactant. However, most important role of all proteins is the defense as they are participating in innate immune defense of the lung. In addition, they bind and react with many micro-organisms, allergens and mitogens, and their receptors have been detected in alveolar macrophages.[115] Various hormones and inflammatory mediators affect the synthesis and secretion of surfactant. There are convincing data to support the use of antenatal corticosteroids in improving the respiratory outcome of newborn infants, especially those at greatest risk of developing respiratory failure. The current data suggest that this improvement may be due to enhanced expression of proteins and phospholipids of the surfactant system and enzymes of the antioxidant systems. Nevertheless, caution is needed, as the scanty data that are available in animal models suggest that lung growth, especially the development of capillary network and secondary alveolar septa, as well as somatic growth may be adversely affected.[116] The existence of receptors for triiodothyronine, thyroid hormone in the fetal lung, as well as certain studies conducted in animal models, suggest that this hormone also participates in the development of the fetal lung. Data have shown that thyroid hormones promote morphogenesis of lung histotypic structures but have a negative effect on surfactant synthesis.[117,118] However, it seems that the role of prolactin, which increases in the serum of fetuses just before birth, is important for lung maturation.[119] It is known that children of mothers who are heroin abusers have lower incidence of neonatal respiratory distress syndrome and heroin stimulates prolactin secretion.[120] Studies conducted on experimental animals have shown that estrogen also stimulates the synthesis of surfactant in the fetal lungs too.[121,122] Insulin and androgens play a role in inhibition of surfactant secretion. Higher incidence of neonatal respiratory distress in children of diabetic mother and in normal male neonates has been confirmed. Insulin and androgens inhibit synthesis of the surfactant. Chronic hyperglycemia with hyperinsulinemia have been connected with the delayed appearance of surfactant in the fetal lung tissue.[123] The hypothesis that insulin achieves its inhibitory effect primarily by disruption of protein synthesis of surfactant was confirmed by studies on cell cultures of human pneumocytes type II.[124] However, it is interesting, that insulin, administered together with cortisol stimulates the synthesis of surfactant more than cortisol alone.[124] Respiratory distress syndrome of new-born is more common in male than in female children, possibly due to later start of surfactant production in male fetuses. This difference could be influenced by androgen effects, but definitely genetic factors have a certain role in it.[125,126] Further, powerful modulators of lung maturation are inflammatory mediators, particularly interleukin 1, tumor necrosis factor-á and bacterial endotoxin. Maternal chorioamnionitis, in which the fetus is exposed to inflammatory agents, is a common cause of premature birth. However, these children, rarely suffer from respiratory distress syndrome. Still, although these cytokines enhance the maturation of the lungs and allow the survival of the child, their long-term effect is negative because they affect lung growth and development, especially vascularization.[127] Therefore, in these children the respiratory surface is decreased. In addition, due to insufficient vascularization, vascular resistance in the lungs remains high after birth. This prevents the increase in flow through the lungs and leads to pulmonary arterial hypertension.[128]

Although, the fetal lungs are functionally inactive during the entire period of intrauterine life, respiratory function becomes essential for survival of the infant immediately after birth. Breathing is initiated by sudden exposure to the exterior world and it is a consequence of slightly asphyxiated state due to the birth process and sensory impulses that originate from the suddenly cooled skin. If an infant doesn't begin to breathe immediately, progressive hypoxia and hypercapnia develop, and additionally stimulate the respiratory center. At birth, the walls of alveoli are collapsed due to the viscid fluid that fills them. More than 25 mm Hg of negative inspiratory pressure is required to oppose the effect of surface tension.

First inspirations of the neonate are extremely powerful and capable of creating as much as 60 mm Hg negative pressure in the intrapleural space. During first inspiration, about 40 milliliters of air enters the lungs. To deflate the lungs, considerable positive pressure is required because of viscous resistance offered by the fluid in the bronchioles. Expansion of the alveoli and increased concentration of oxygen in them stimulates the release of vasodilator substances from the endothelium of capillaries. This, together with the mechanical stretching of the alveoli, leads to the dilatation of the lung capillaries and the resistance to blood flow in the pulmonary circulation decreases several fold. Development of a nearly normal compliance curve and normal postnatal breathing establishes within 40 minutes after birth.[19]

In addition to allowing gas exchange, increased blood flows through the lungs probably accelerate reabsorption of the lung liquid. Although, the existence of lung liquid is necessary for the development of the lung, it must be quickly removed during delivery to allow normal breathing of the newborn. Most of the lung liquid reabsorbs in the pulmonary circulation and only a small part of it removes through the upper airway during passage through the birth canal. Infusions of norepinephrine in concentrations, similar to those present at the delivery, prevent the lung liquid secretion. Hormones and factors that facilitate the removal of liquid from the lungs are arginine–vasopressin, catecholamine, prostaglandin-E_2, prolactin, surfactant, some growth factors and increase of the concentration of oxygen in the lungs, originating from the first breath.[19]

Fetal Urinary System

At the beginning of the 4th week, the intermediate mesoderm forms the nephrogenic cords. From the nephrogenic cords, three successive sets of excretory organs develop: the pronephros, the mesonephros and the metanephros. The first two, i.e., the pronephros and mesonephros, persist over a period of time and then regress, while the third, the metanephros, forms the definitive kidney. The permanent adult kidney, the metanephros, begins to develop early in the fifth week and is functional 2–3 weeks later. The ureteric bud develops as an outgrowth from the mesonephric duct. The ureteric bud forms the ureter, renal pelvis, calyces and collecting tubules. The nephrons are derived from the metanephric blastema.[63] First nephrons appear in the kidney medulla, around 20–22 weeks of gestation, later they can be found in the periphery of the kidney. Formation of nephrons ends around the 35th week of gestation and further development occurs due to the growth of existing nephrons.[129] At birth, the nephrons, approximately one million in each kidney, are formed but are still short. No new nephrons are formed after birth. During infancy, the nephrons complete their differentiation and increase in size until adulthood.[63] Enlargement of the glomeruli, enlargement and elongation of the tubules, as well as enlargement of the vascular and connective tissue contribute to the growth of kidneys.[130] Failure in the maturation of the primitive kidneys can lead to the abnormal development of the genital system, adrenal glands and lungs.[129] Various anomalies of the urinary tract can be caused by developmental disorders of pronephros and mesonephros. Developmental anomalies of the urinary tract account for about 40% of all anomalies. Frequent occurrence of the urinary tract anomalies is due to complicated ontogenesis of this system.[130] Recently, attention has been given to less noticeable but potentially very harmful consequences of impaired kidney development, such as a congenital nephron deficit. Since, the lack of nephrons after birth is unrecoverable, numerous studies have been conducted to detect factors that in some way may impair the process of nephrogenesis.[131] Studies conducted on the cell cultures of the fetal kidney showed that retinoids, metabolites of vitamin A, have a significant impact on the number of nephrons and that this effect is dose-dependent. Vitamin A deficiency in pregnant women is rare in developed countries but is more frequently observed in underdeveloped countries as a result of insufficient food intake. Even in a healthy population, concentrations of vitamin A and retinoids in the plasma considerably vary. Habits that are most commonly associated with its low plasma values are cigarette smoking, alcoholism and unbalanced diets.[131] Unfortunately, lack of vitamin A is not the only factor that can lead to a nephron deficit. Experiments on animals have proved that fetal growth restriction,[132] maternal hyperglycemia[133] and some medications, such as gentamicin,[134] cause a reduced number of nephrons, which cannot be fully compensated for after birth. If we remember that nephrogenesis in the humans ends before birth, we can assume that the harmful effects of these factors on the human fetus may be even more dangerous. Even a slight deficit of nephrons, often unrecognized after the birth, could be associated with diseases that occur later in the life, such as renal failure or hypertension. Therefore, more and more scientists believe that congenital nephron deficit could be a "missing link" in understanding of the etiology of essential hypertension.[131]

For many years, data on fetal renal function have been insufficient and indirect. Investigations were carried out mainly in experimental animals and aborted fetuses. The insertion of a catheter into the fetal blood vessels and bladder allowed the testing under physiological conditions, and brought new insights about the function of the fetal kidneys, and the application of ultrasonic methods, enabled the noninvasive and easy way to study the physiology and pathophysiology of fetal urinary tract. Glomerular filtration rate in term-fetuses, measured by ultrasound and biochemical measurements, is 0.73–5.25 mL/min, which amounts to 1/29–1/4 values in adults. After birth, during the first four days of life, glomerular filtration rate rapidly increases.[135] It was found that the time of umbilical cord ligation influences on the value of glomerular filtration rate. In the newborns in which umbilical cord ligation was performed relatively late after the birth, a circulating blood volume and glomerular filtration was 40–50% greater than in the newborns in which the umbilical cord ligation was done immediately after birth.[129] Further, values of tubular reabsorption in fetal kidneys at term range between 55–97% of the adult values.[135,136] Although histologically, kidney tubules seem well developed, at the time of delivery, the surface of transporting cells and the number of transporters is small. Reabsorption and excretory function are not completely developed. Immature cells tubules have low concentration of Na^+/K^+ ATPase, an enzyme that provides energy for active transport of sodium.[137,138] Therefore, capacity of renal tubular cells for sodium transport is limited. Consequently, reabsorption of bicarbonates, glucose and phosphates is also limited.[139-141] Due to low glucose threshold, tendency of excretion of glucose and consequently of the water and sodium is increased. Because of that in neonate, dehydration can develop more rapidly than in an adult. Further, it was found that term-fetus is not capable to respond on dehydration or hypertonic solution by creating concentrated urine, like adult. Sodium overload of the mature newborn and increase of plasmatic concentration of sodium can cause increase of the body mass due to generalized edema. If the newborn gets a cow's milk, which contains four times more sodium, protein and phosphate than mother's breast milk, signs of salt and fluid retention may occur.[129] The fetus usually produces hypotonic urine and in case of dehydration, ability to concentrate urine does not exceed the limit of 600–700 mOsm/L. Antidiuretic hormone (ADH), whose role is to preserve water in the body by concentrating the urine, the fetus begins to produce in the 11th week of pregnancy and its concentration in fetal blood is almost equal to the concentration in adults. Infusion of hypertonic NaCl solution, hypoxia or hypovolemia can increase concentration of ADH in fetal plasma.[142,143] Therefore, we cannot talk about lack of ADH, as a cause of low osmolarity of fetal urine. However, it is possible to assume that the kidney is insensitive to ADH. The fetus cannot concentrate urine before appearing of specific water channels called aquaporin. They occur in human fetuses in the 12–15th week of pregnancy but their expression in the fetus and newborn is much lower than in adults.[142] Insensitivity of the fetal kidney to ADH could be explained by the slow emergence of these water channels.[81] Further, hydrogen ion secretion in the fetus and newborn is sufficient to allow bicarbonate reabsorption and excretion of metabolic acids. Filtered phosphate and synthesized ammonia are in quantities sufficient for buffering excessive hydrogen ions.[81] However, it is important to note that the fetal kidneys do not play a major role in the regulation of acid-base balance. Even in fetuses with renal agenesis, acid-base balance may be normal.[129] In fetus, the acid-base balance is regulated by maternal lungs and kidneys. CO_2 is quickly removed through the placenta into the mother's bloodstream and then mother exhaled it.[144] Large amounts of CO_2 can be effectively removed if the mother's respiration, the uteroplacental flow and the umbilical flow are normal. Somewhat, more slowly, metabolic acids are transferred through the placental barrier and they are excreted through the mother's kidneys.[145] Thus, regulation of fetal acid-base balance depends on many interrelated factors, which include state of the mother, placenta and the fetus.

Fetal kidneys **(Fig. 16)** excrete urine from the 3rd month of pregnancy. This can be confirmed by the existence of urine in the bladder of the fetus **(Fig. 17)**.[146,147] Urine extracted from the fetal kidney is hypotonic and that is not surprising because the main excretion function is performed by the placenta. Due to this fact, electrolyte composition of fetal urine is poor.[146-148] The pH of fetal urine is about 6.[149] By the midgestation, fetal urine becomes the main source of amniotic fluid and swallowing the main way of its removal. These two processes are essential elements in the production and regulation of amniotic fluid in the middle trimester. The term-fetus excretes in the amniotic fluid about 400–1,200 mL of urine daily. The fact that fetal urine is the main component of the amniotic fluid

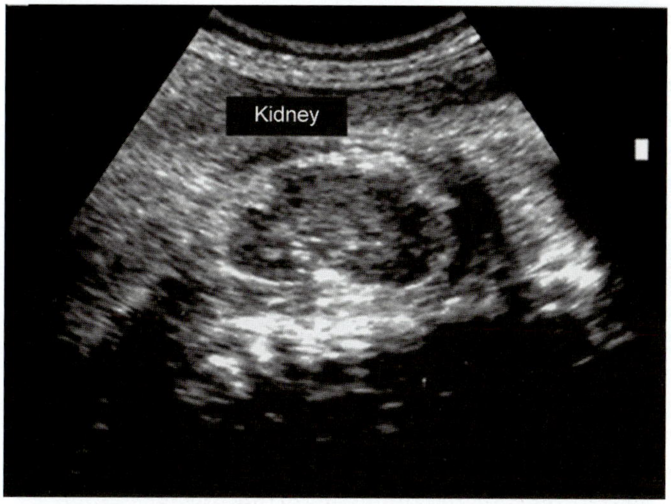

Fig. 16: 2D ultrasound image showing fetal kidney.

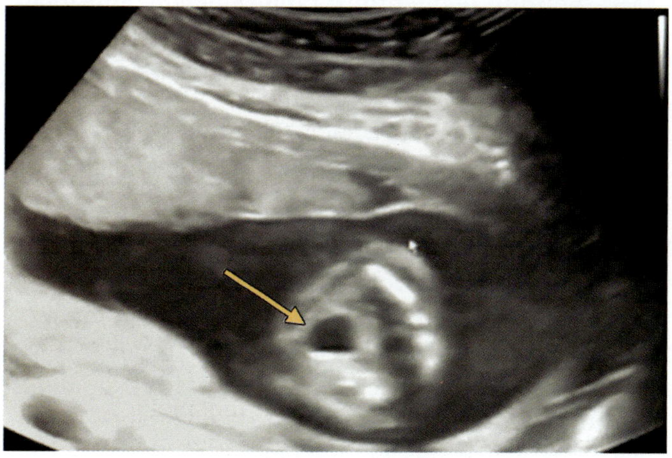

Fig. 17: 2D ultrasound image showing fetal bladder.

in the second half of pregnancy, allows us to determine the concentrations of electrolytes, creatinine, protein or glucose. Further, recording of their changes enables us to study the functional development and maturation of the fetal kidney during this period.[81] After birth, the kidneys are still immature, more accurately, their functional capacity is limited. Due to this, disorders in the maintenance of homeostasis can easily develop. Exchange of fluid in the newborn is very large and the intensity of metabolism and acid production are higher than in the adult. Taking into account immaturity of the kidney, we can easily understand that in this period acidosis, dehydration and sometimes excessive hydration frequently develop. The disruption in the maintenance of homeostasis is more often if the child is born before term, in hypoxia or infection. Fetal kidneys and kidneys of newborn do not perform their functions poorly, indeed, they work impressively, but they need time to achieve the perfect harmony of their functions.

Fetal Central Nervous System

Development of the human CNS begins in the early embryonic period and proceeds through a sequence of very complicated processes long after delivery. CNS develops from the embryonic ectoderm. Cells that will become neurons and glial cells originate from the neural plate, which is located within the ectoderm and contains about 125,000 cells. The neural plate is formed in the early third week of pregnancy. Its lateral edges are gradually rising and approaching one another, forming first a concave area known as the neural groove and then the neural tube. Cranial and caudal opening of the neural tube are closing between the 25–27th day of pregnancy.[150] Failure of these openings to close contributes a major class of neural abnormalities. Further development is characterized by changes in size, shape and internal structure of the neural tube wall, which reflect the complex histogenetic processes. Since some parts of the neural tube grow and develop at different speeds and intensities, it bends and changes its shape, forming the major subdivisions of the CNS. There are three subdivisions of the cranial part of the neural tube: prosencephalon, the mesencephalon, and the rhombencephalon. They will each eventually develop into distinct regions of the central nervous system: the forebrain (the cerebral cortex and basal ganglia), midbrain and posterior brain (the cerebellum, pons and medulla oblongata). From the caudal part of the neural tube develops the spinal cord.[46]

Early embryonic development is characterized by its immobilization. Prerequisite for fetal movements is the existence of interneuronal and neuromuscular connections. The earliest interneuronal connections—the synapses, can be detected in the spinal cord shortly before the onset of embryonic motility, at 6–7 weeks of gestation.[151] Therefore, the neural activity leading to the first detectable movements is considered to originate from the spinal motoneurons.[152] Another important prerequisite for the motility is the development and innervation of muscular fibers. It is well-known that primitive muscle fibers (myotubes) are able to contract as soon as they are innervated by motor neurons.[153] Between 6–8 weeks of gestation, muscle fibers have formed by fusion of myoblasts, efferent and afferent neuromuscular connections have developed, and spontaneous neural activity causing motility can begin. The first spontaneous embryonic movements are gross body movements and they can be observed at the 7–7.5th weeks of gestation. They consist of slow flexion and extension of the fetal trunk, accompanied by the passive displacement of arms and legs.[154] These, so called, "vermicular" movements appear in irregular sequences.[155] Simultaneously, with the onset of spontaneous movements, at the 7.5th week of gestation, the earliest motor reflex activity can be observed, indicating the existence of the first afferent-efferent circuits in the spinal cord.[156] The first reflex movements are massive and indicate a limited number of synapses in a reflex pathway. General movements are the first complex, well-organized movement pattern, which involve head, trunk and limb movements. This pattern has been interpreted as the first sign of a supraspinal control on motor activity[157,158] and can be recognized from 8–9 weeks of gestation onwards **(Fig. 18)**.[158,159]

The brainstem is fashioned around the 7th week of gestation[157] and basic structures of the diencephalon and cerebral hemispheres are formed by the end of the 8th gestational week.[159] The remarkable expansion of the cerebral hemispheres follows during the remainder of gestation. The development of synapses in the human cerebral cortex begins after the formation of the cortical plate, at the end of the 10th week of gestation.[160,161] The brainstem consists of the medulla oblongata, pons and midbrain. It forms and matures in a caudal to rostral direction. That means that the fillogenetically older structures, such as the medulla oblongata, will form and mature earlier in the gestation. In addition to its many subnuclei, the medulla gives rise to a variety of descending spinal motor tracts which reflexively trigger limb and body movements. It also hosts the five cranial nerves (VIII–XII), which exert tremendous influences on gross body movements, heart rate, respiration and the head turning. As the medulla matures in advance of more rostral structures of the brainstem, reflexive movements of the head, body, extremities, as well as breathing movements and alterations in heart rate, appear in advance of other functions.

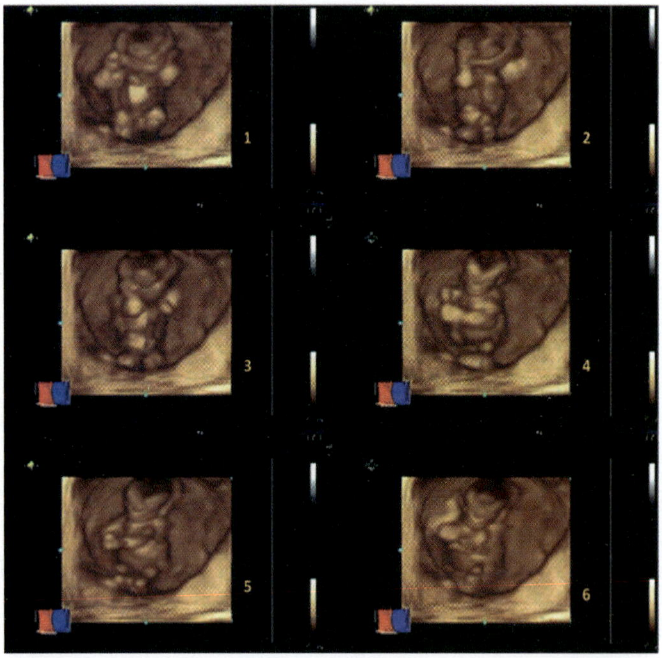

Fig. 18: A sequence of images of the fetus at 9 weeks of gestation recorded by 4D sonography, showing general movements.

The formation of pons begins almost simultaneously, but its maturation is more prolonged. The structures of the pons include the V-VIII cranial nerves (vestibular nuclei of the nerve VIII) and the medial longitudinal fasciculus (MLF), pontine tegmentum, raphe nucleus and locus coeruleus, which exert widespread influences on arousal, including the sleep-wake cycles. Facial movements, which are also controlled by V and VII cranial nerve, appear around 10–11 weeks.[157] The brain stem gradually begins to take the control over fetal movements and behavioral patterns during the first trimester and continues its maturation in the second trimester, resulting in expansion and complexity of the behavioral repertoires.[157]

From 10 weeks onwards, the number and frequency of fetal movements increase and the repertoire of movements begins to expand. Qualitative changes in general movements can be also observed. These movements, which are slow and limited amplitude during 8–9 weeks, become more forceful at 10–12 weeks. After the 12th week, they become more variable in speed and amplitude.[162] Using four dimensional (4D) sonography, Kurjak and collaborators have found that from 13 gestational weeks onwards, a "goal orientation" of hand movements appears and a target point can be recognized for each hand movement.[163] According to the spatial orientation, they classified the hand movements into several subtypes: hand to head, hand to mouth **(Fig. 19)**, hand near mouth, hand to face, hand near face, hand to eye and hand to ear. Our longitudinal study, performed by 4D ultrasound in 100 fetuses from all trimesters of normal pregnancies, has shown increasing frequency of various movement patterns, such as general movements, isolated arm and leg movements, stretching, as well as head movements, during the first trimester.[164] Using 4D sonography, general movements were found to be the most frequent movement pattern between 9–14 weeks of

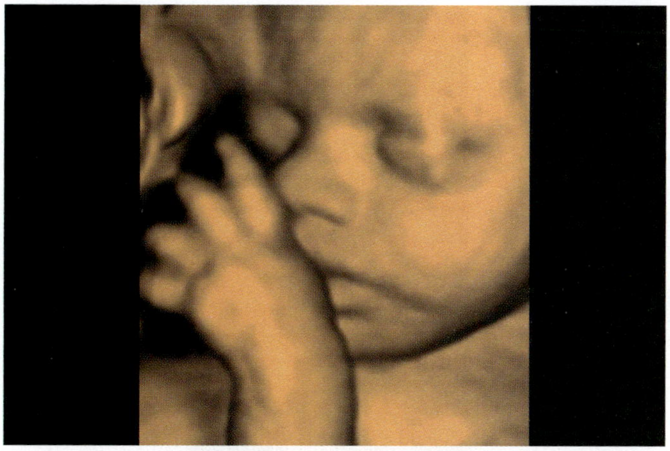

Fig. 19: Image of the fetus recorded by 3D/4D sonography, showing hand-to-mouth movement.

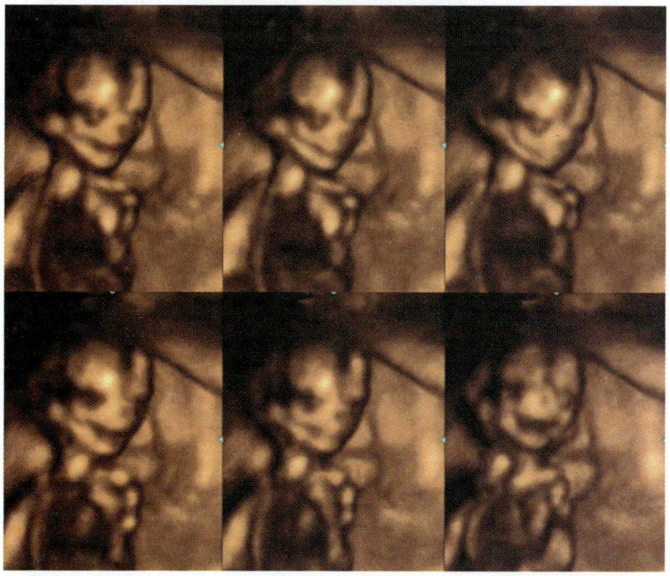

Fig. 20: A sequence of images recorded by 4D sonography showing fetal mouth opening movements at 16 weeks of gestation.

gestation.[165] From 14–19 weeks of gestation, fetuses are highly active and the longest period between movements last only 5–6 minutes. In the 15th week, 16 different types of movements can be observed. Besides the general body movements and isolated limb movements, retroflection, anteflextion and rotation of the head can be easily seen. Moreover, facial movements such as mouthing **(Fig. 20)**, yawning, hiccups, suckling and swallowing, can be added to the wide repertoire of fetal motor activity in this period.[158] The earliest eye movements appear as sporadic movements with a limited frequency, at 16–18th weeks of gestation.[166,167] The delayed onset of eye movements can be explained with later onset of midbrain maturation.

Although, the midbrain begins to form at almost the same time as the pons, its maturation does not even begin until the second trimester. It consists of the dopamine producing substantia nigra, the inferior-auditory and superior-visual colliculus, and cranial nerves III–IV, which, together with MLF and cranial nerve VI, control eye movements.[166,167]

Fetal human brain has a number of transitory structures, which cannot be observed in the adult human brain. One of the very important zone in the developing cortex is the subplate zone, that is a site for transient synapses and neuronal interactions. The development of subplate zone, between the 15–17th weeks of gestation, is accompanied with an increase in the number of cortical synapses, which probably form the substrate for the earliest cortical electric activity at 19 weeks of gestation.[168] Subplate zone can play a major role in the developmental plasticity following perinatal brain damage.[169]

The second half of pregnancy is characterized by organization of fetal movement patterns and increase in complexity of movements. The periods of fetal quiescence begin to increase and the rest-activity cycles become recognizable. Hardly any new movement pattern emerges in this period. The number of general body movements, which tends to increase from the 9th week onwards, gradually declines during the last 10 weeks of the pregnancy.[170-172] Although this decrease was first explained as a consequence of the decrease in amniotic fluid volume, it is now considered to be a result of cerebral maturation processes. As the medulla oblongata matures, myelinates and stabilizes, these spontaneous movements are less easily triggered, and begin to be controlled by more stable intrinsic activities generated within the brainstem.[157] It is very important to point out that general movements are characterized by large variation and complexity in the third trimester.[173] Revolutionary improvement in the study of fetal facial movements came with the development of 3D and 4D sonography. Our results confirmed the potential of 3D/4D sonography for the investigation of structural and functional development of the fetal face.[174] The application of 4D sonography in the examination of fetal facial movements has revealed the existence of a full range of facial expressions, including smiling, crying and eyelid movements,[164,175] similar to emotional expressions in adults, in the 2nd and 3rd trimesters. Other facial movements, such as yawning, suckling, swallowing and jaw opening can also be observed in this period by 4D ultrasound. Recent study demonstrated that

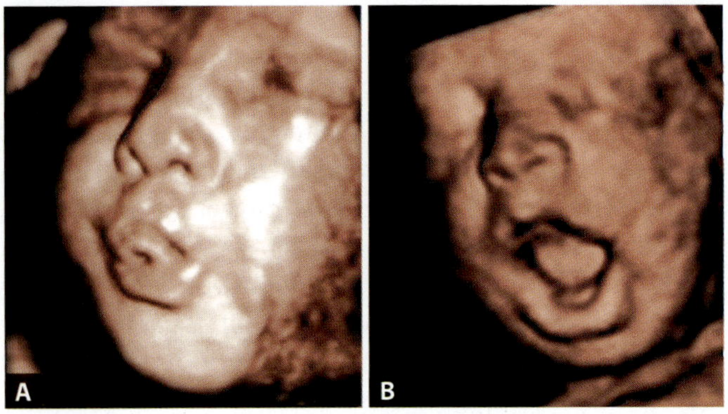

Figs. 21A and B: Images of the fetus in the 3rd trimester recorded by 3D/4D sonography, exhibiting mouthing movements.

the most frequent facial movement patterns in the 2nd trimester were isolated eye blinking, grimacing, suckling and swallowing, whereas mouthing, yawning, tongue expulsion and smiling could be seen less frequently. Mouthing was the most frequent facial movement during early third trimester[176] **(Figs. 21A and B)**. Our longitudinal analysis of the frequencies of different facial movements in the 2nd and 3rd trimester revealed some interesting results. Contrary to the declining trend of head movement and hand movement patterns from the beginning of the second trimester to the end of the third trimester, a constant increase in the frequencies of almost all facial movement patterns was observed during the 2nd trimester. Various types of facial expression patterns displayed a peak frequency at the end of 2nd trimester, except eye blinking pattern **(Fig. 22)**, which displayed a peak frequency at 28 weeks of gestation. During the remainder of pregnancy, decreasing or stagnant incidence of facial expression patterns was noted.[164] Obviously, this developmental trend provides yet another example of the maturation of the medulla oblongata, pons and midbrain, or perhaps even the establishment of control of more cranial structures. The facts that even in the embryonic period same inductive forces that cause the growth and reshaping of the neural tube influence the development of facial structures and that many genetic disorders affecting the CNS are also characterized by dysmorphology and dysfunction of facial structures, emphasize the importance of structural and functional evaluation of the fetal face.[159,177] Our study has demonstrated that there were no movements observed in fetal life that were not present in neonatal life. Furthermore, prenatal—neonatal continuity exists even in subtle, fine movements such as facial mimics.[178]

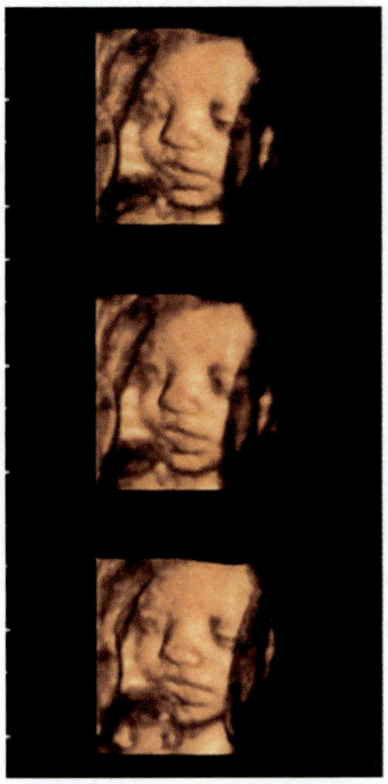

Fig. 22: A sequence of images of the fetus in the 3rd trimester recorded by 4D sonography, showing eye blinking.

In addition to morphological studies of the development of the central nervous system and studies about fetal behavior that provide insight into the functional development of central nervous system of fetuses, attention of researchers attracts the development of the fetal senses. For a long time, experts from different fields of science debate about whether the fetus feels pain. In humans, it is possible to distinguish several different reactions to pain. The simplest is reflex motor reaction, removal of stimulated body parts from painful stimuli. Next unconscious reaction involves the secretion of the so-called stress hormones—cortisol and catecholamines. The most complex reaction is conscious perception of pain and emotional reaction to it. We can claim with certainty that the first two are already present in the fetal period. The earliest reactions to painful stimuli are motor reflexes, resembling withdrawal reflexes. They appear early in gestation. Reflex threshold is remarkably low and various kinds of stimuli may induce very holistic and unspecific reactions. It is important to emphasize that these reactions are completely reflexive, directed by the spinal cord, and higher perception or processing of painful sensation does not exist at this stage.[179] Further, as early as 16–18 weeks of gestation, fetal cerebral blood flow increases during invasive procedures.[180,181] This increase of blood flow towards the brain may be mediated by the sympathetic system or by other undetermined mechanisms.[181] With regard to the autonomic and endocrine responses to pain, an elevation of noradrenaline, cortisol and beta-endorphin plasma levels, in response to needle pricking of the innervated hepatic vein for intrauterine transfusion, was registered in a 23-week-old fetus. Pricking of the noninnervated placental cord insertion for the same purpose had no effect.[182,183] Obviously, painful stimuli trigger a wide spectrum of reactions, such as activation of the hypothalamo-hypophyseal axis or autonomic nervous system, without reaching the cortex. It has been suggested that neither motor reflexes nor hormonal stress responses to invasive procedures prove the existence of fetal pain.[184] It is unknown whether and when the fetus begins consciously to feel pain. Functional thalamocortical connections are required for fetal awareness of noxious stimuli. Thalamocortical path is formed between 22–26 weeks and after this period, the fetus is probably capable of consciously perceiving painful stimuli. Evidence for conscious pain perception during intrauterine life is indirect, but evidence for the subconscious incorporation of fetal pain into neurological development and plasticity is incontrovertible.[185] Despite the great interest in conscious experience and memory of pain, unconscious reactions like the secretion of stress hormones and their far-reaching detrimental effect, are probably more dangerous for the development of fetus than terrifying memories.

Reflex arcs involving the brainstem, such as vestibular, auditory and olfactory, mature early in fetal life. Vestibular nerve cells mature earlier than neurons of the lateral and inferior vestibular nuclei, which begin to function during the 9th week of pregnancy. It is believed that vestibular stimulation has a role in the emerging fetal movements. Nearly weightless state of the fetus in the uterus provides a particularly convenient medium for the vestibular reflexes. According to electrophysiological examinations of evoked potentials in prematurely delivered healthy infants, cochlear function develops between 22–25 weeks of gestation and its maturation continues during the first six months after delivery.[186-188] However, fluid in the fetal ear as well as the immaturity of the cochlea, complicate the sound transmission, so that only strong acoustic stimuli can be registered by the fetus.[157] Due to this reason and because of the immaturity of the cochlea, a very strong stimuli is needed for fetus to notice it. Maternal heartbeats and motility of gastrointestinal tract during digestion appear to generate 60–90 decibels of sound in utero, which is comparable to noise of the busiest street.[189] During the last weeks of pregnancy, from the 36th gestational week onwards, the fetus reacts to extremely loud sounds and even the mother's voice with reflex movements of the body, by turning his head, and increased heart rate. More fascinating is the notion that a fetus at this age not only hears sounds but also can discriminate between different sounds. This finding is explained by the tonotopic organization of the cochlear nuclei and by the maturation of the brainstem during the last weeks of pregnancy. It was noted that the development of the auditory system can be disrupted by the influence of adverse factors (cigarette consumption) and also in some pathological conditions (intrauterine growth restriction, maternal hypertension).[190-192] It is important to mention also that development of the auditory system affects the subsequent learning of speech and language acquisition.

Animal experiments have indicated that the intrauterine environment is not completely deprived of light. Although, the developing fetus cannot distinguish objects clearly, the intensity of light is equal to the splendor that occurs through the cheek when mouth is highlighted by the powerful batteries. Furthermore, according to some experimental results, the development of visual and auditory organs could not be possible without any light or auditory stimulation.[193,194] The structural development of sensory pathways is a prerequisite for functional development, but the final organization of the brain circuitries depends mainly on guidance from external inputs.[169] A histological study of the human visual pathway has shown that thalamic projections reach the visual cortex between 23–27 weeks of gestation.[195] The primary visual cortex can be clearly delineated in the occipital lobe by immunohistochemical staining even before the 25th week. In this cortical area, synaptogenesis persists between 24 weeks of gestation and 8 months after delivery,[193] while myelination of the optical tract begins at 32 weeks of gestation.[194] Cortical visual evoked potentials indicate the development and maturation of the primary visual cortex. Maturation of the visual cortex is characterized by the appearance of surface-positive evoked potentials, which occurs between the 36–40th weeks.[169] New data have shown that the amplitude of visual evoked responses can be used in the assessment of fetal and neonatal habituation to light stimuli.[196] Flash stimuli over the maternal abdomen can cause the visual evoked brain activity in the human fetus, recorded by magnetoencephalography. The latency of the fetal response falls with increasing gestational age and begins to approach the adult latency near term.[197] Experimental findings have demonstrated the importance of fetal eye motility in retinal (neuronal) cell differentiation, as well as eye functional maturation.[198]

Fetal life in utero is organized in cyclical patterns. From the midgestation onwards, periods of activity begin to alternate with the periods of rest. Between 30–38 weeks of pregnancy the difference between quiet and paradoxical, "active" sleep can be seen. In advanced pregnancy, the fetus usually sleeps at the same time as the mother. In fetal animals, simultaneous measurements of fetal electrocortical activity, eye and body movements have shown that deep sleep, characterized by high-voltage waves and decreased fetal activity, occurred during 54% of a day. The total length of the rapid eye movement (REM) sleep period, characterized by low-voltage waves and REMs, lasted 40% of a day. The wakeful state (6% of a day) is characterized by low-voltage waves.[199] In human premature newborns, born four weeks prior to term, 60–65% of the total sleeping period is REM sleeping, whereas in term-newborns, the REM sleeping period includes 50% of the total 16 hours of sleep.[200] During delivery, fetal EEG shows waves characteristic for quiet sleep, active sleep and wakefulness of the newborn.[201] It is thought that REM sleep plays a role in the development of the nervous system, similar as physical activity helps to develop muscles. REM sleep is probably caused by intense activity of neural circuits and thus participates in the development of the central nervous system.[202]

The human brain is intricately designed to execute cognitive functions, such as perception, attention, memory and learning. Psychobiologic investigations inspired the hypothesis that the acoustically rich environment in the uterus contributes to fetal learning.[203] The intrauterine origin of learning and memory processes has been investigated extensively employing habituation methods, classical conditioning or exposure learning to assess fetal learning.

It was also found that the fetus has the ability to remember tastes to which it was exposed during the intrauterine period. Flavors from the mother's diet during pregnancy are transmitted to amniotic fluid and are swallowed by the fetus. Consequently, the type of food eaten by the mother during pregnancy is experienced by the infants before their first exposure to solid food. For instance, garlic ingestion by pregnant women significantly alters the odor of their amniotic fluid, barely 45 minutes after ingestion.[204] Prenatal experience of taste greatly affects the newborn child. It prepares it for the taste of the mother's milk, whose taste also depends on the mother's diet. Prenatal and early postnatal exposure to a flavor enhances the infant's enjoyment of that flavor in solid foods during weaning.[205] A study has shown that the infants who have been exposed to the flavor of carrots in either amniotic fluid or breast milk behaved differently in response to that flavor in food than did the nonexposed control infants. Specifically, previously exposed infants exhibited fewer negative facial expressions while being fed the carrot-flavored cereal compared to the plain cereal, whereas control infants whose mothers drank water during pregnancy and lactation exhibited no such difference.[205] According to data, the neonate strongly reacts to fragrant signals of mother's breasts.[206,207] In the close proximity of mother's breasts, in the first minutes after birth, the newborn spontaneously turns towards the breast and starts making the movement of sucking even before coming in the direct contact with the breast.[208] In the first days of life, it demonstrates a similar reaction to its own amniotic fluid.[209] To some extent, the chemical profile of breast secretions overlaps with that of amniotic fluid. Therefore, early postnatal attraction to odors associated with the nipple/areola may reflect prenatal exposure and familiarization.[210]

The development of human brain is not completed at the time of delivery. Only subcortical formations and primary cortical areas are well-developed in a newborn. Associative cortex, barely visible in a newborn, is scantily developed in a 6 months old infant. Postnatal formation of synapses in associative cortical areas, which intensifies between the 8th month and the 2nd year of life, precedes the onset of first cognitive functions, such as speech. Following the 2nd year of life, many redundant synapses are eliminated. Elimination of synapses begins very rapidly and continues slowly until puberty, when the same number of synapses as seen in adults is reached.[211]

Fetal Stress

A large number of environmental factors can trigger the fetal stress response. For instance, maternal under-nutrition or placental insufficiency can alter the intra-uterine environment, causing fetal stress.[212] Painful stimuli also lead to the fetal stress response.[213] Even severe maternal emotional stress or stressful life events, according to some investigations, may influence the fetal environment.[214-216] The primary role of stress is the protection of organism but fetal exposure to stress may affect neurodevelopment, as well as the development of many other organ systems and have lifelong consequences. Many adaptive changes induced by fetal stress increase the chance of fetal survival by creating a short-term protection. However, these changes can leave profound alterations in the structure and functions of the organism.[212] It is a known fact that fetal cardiovascular adaptation to hypoxia is manifested by the redistribution of blood flow primarily towards the fetal brain. However, our latest investigations have shown that severe brain damage can develop despite the fetal blood flow redistribution and increased brain perfusion, even earlier than it was previously thought.[217] The neuroendocrine stress axis includes the production of the corticotropin releasing hormone (CRH), adrenocorticotropic hormone (ACTH) and cortisol. Fetal CRH has been shown to influence the timing of birth. These findings have pointed to an active role of the fetus in the initiation of parturition.[81] Furthermore, ACTH impairs motor coordination and muscle tonicity, reduces attention span and increases irritability.[212] Recently, epidemiological and experimental investigations have shown that chronic exposure to high levels of cortisol during intrauterine life, occurring either as a result of its exogenous application or the fetal stress, has a very adverse effect in the long run. Unfortunately, it has been established that cortisol, which accelerates lung and brain maturation and enables survival of premature infants, may have an adverse effect on growth of the lungs, development of the secondary alveolar septa and even on the growth of the whole organism.[218] Accelerated maturation of the brain is also associated with the structural as well as behavioral changes. Stress induces structural changes of the hippocampus[219-222] that are associated with memory impairment and learning disabilities. Behavioral changes associated with accelerated maturation of the brain include hyperalertness and impaired fetal responsiveness to novel stimuli.[223] Retrospective studies on children whose mothers experienced severe psychological stress or adverse life events during their pregnancy have suggested long-term neurodevelopment effects on the infant.[224-227] Such children exhibited symptoms of attention deficit hyperactivity disorder, sleep disorders, unsociable and inconsiderate behavior, as well as psychiatric disorders, including schizophrenic episodes, depressive and neurotic symptoms, drug abuse and anxiety.[228] Increased maternal stress during pregnancy seems to influence infant temperament and cognitive functions.[229,230] Moreover, stressful maternal life events measured during the first part of pregnancy negatively affected the child's attention/concentration index measured at the age of six.[231] The adverse health effects of stress may also include an increased risk of certain birth defects (cleft palate, cleft lip with or without cleft palate, d-transposition of the great arteries and tetralogy of Fallot).[214] Chronic high glucocorticoid exposure in utero is associated with adult hypertension and according to some data with coronary disease. Impaired glucose tolerance has also been noticed.[232-234] We can conclude that some of the most common diseases of the modern society may have their origins in prenatal life.

CONCLUSION

Fetal developmental potential is determined at the moment of conception by genetic inheritance. However, this development is modulated by environmental factors. Basic and clinical researches into fetal life present us with ever deeper understandings of important role that the environment plays in prenatal and postnatal life. It is important to recognize that both, the mother and the fetus, actively participate in the maintenance of the physiological intrauterine environment. Unfortunately, the fetus is not entirely protected from harmful influences of the external factors. By altering the intrauterine environment, these factors can have a long-term effect on fetal health. Finally, physiological fetal growth and development is the precondition for optimal child development.

REFERENCES

1. Stables D. Physiology in childbearing with anatomy and related biosciences. Edinburgh: Bailliere Tindall; 1999. pp. 73-148.
2. Wong KHH, Adashi EY. Early conceptus growth and immunobiologic adaptations of pregnancy. In: Reece EA, Hobbins JC, Gant NF (Eds). Clinical obstetrics: the fetus and mother. Oxford: Blackwell Publishing Ltd; 2007. pp. 3-19.
3. Huppertz B, Kingdom JCP. The placenta and fetal membranes. In: Edmonds KD (Ed). Dewhurst's Textbook of Obstetrics and Gynaecology. Oxford: Blackwell Publishing Ltd; 2007. pp. 19-28.
4. http://www.centrus.com.br/DiplomaFMF/SeriesFMF/doppler/capitulos-html/chapter_03.htm
5. Kahn BF, Hobbins JC, Galan HL. Intrauterine growth restriction. In: Gibbs RS, Karlan BY, Haney AF, Nygaard (Eds). Danforth's Obstetrics and Gynecology. Philadelphia: Lippincott Williams and Wilkins; 2008. pp. 198-220.
6. Baschat AA. Fetal growth restriction—from observation to intervention. J Perinat Med. 2010;38(3):239-46.
7. Harrington K, Goldfrad C, Carpenter RG, et al. Transvaginal uterine and umbilical artery Doppler examination of 12-16 weeks and the subsequent development of pre-eclampsia

and intrauterine growth retardation. Ultrasound Obstet Gynecol. 1997;9(2):94-100.
8. Rizzo G, Arduini D, Romanini C. Umbilical vein pulsations: a physiologic finding in early gestation. Am J Obstet Gynecol. 1992;167(3):675-7.
9. Giles WB, Trudinger BJ, Baird PJ. Fetal umbilical artery flow velocity waveforms and placental resistance: pathological correlation. Br J Obstet Gynaecol. 1985;92(1):31-8.
10. Karsdorp VH, Dirks BK, van der Linden JC, et al. Placenta morphology and absent or reversed end diastolic flow velocities in the umbilical artery: a clinical and morphometrical study. Placenta. 1996;17(7):393-9.
11. Baschat AA. Fetal responses to placental insufficiency: an update. BJOG. 2004;111(10):1031-41.
12. Arbeille P, Maulik D, Fignon A, et al. Assessment of the fetal PO_2 changes by cerebral and umbilical Doppler on lamb fetuses during acute hypoxia. Ultrasound Med Biol. 1995;21(7):861-70.
13. Arbeille P, Roncin A, Berson M, et al. Exploration of the fetal cerebral blood flow by duplex Doppler linear array system in normal and pathological pregnancies. Ultrasound Med Biol. 1987;13(6):329-37.
14. Gramellini D, Folli MC, Raboni S, et al. Cerebral-umbilical Doppler ratio as predictor of adverse perinatal outcome. Obstet Gynecol. 1992;79:416-20.
15. Arbeille P, Maulik D, Salihagic' A, et al. Effect of long-term cocaine administration to pregnant ewes on fetal hemodynamics, oxygenation, and growth. Obstet Gynecol. 1997;90(5):795-802.
16. Fignon A, Salihagic A, Akoka S, et al. Twenty-day cerebral and umbilical Doppler monitoring on a growth retarded and hypoxic fetus. Eur J Obstet Gynecol Reprod Biol. 1996;66(1):83-6.
17. Laurini RN, Arbeille B, Gemberg C, et al. Brain damage and hypoxia in an ovine fetal chronic cocaine model. Eur J Obstet Gynecol Reprod Biol. 1999;86(1):15-22.
18. Salihagic A, Georgescus M, Perrotin F, et al. Daily Doppler assessment of the fetal hemodynamic response to chronic hypoxia: a five case report. Prenat Neonat Med. 2000;5:35-41.
19. Guyton i Hall. Medicinska fiziologija. 11. Izdanje. Zagreb: Medicinska naklada; 2006. pp. 1042-52, 1027-41, 918-30.
20. Marieb EN. Human Anatomy and Physiology. 5th edn. San Francisco: Benjamin Cummings; 2000. pp. 1118-48.
21. Johnson MH, Everitt BI. Essential Reproduction. 5th edn. Oxford: Blackwell Science; 2000. pp. 203-22.
22. Ross MG, Ervin MG, Novak D. Fetal Physiology. In: Gabbe SG, Niebyl JR, Simpson JL (Eds). Obstetrics Normal and Problem Pregnancies. Philadelphia: Churchill Livingston Elsevier; 2007. pp. 26-54.
23. Handwerger S, Freemark M. The role of placental growth hormone and placental lactogen in the regulation of human fetal growth and development. J Pediatric Endocrinol Metabol. 2000;13(4):343-56.
24. Lovinger RD, Kaplan SL, Grumbach MMJ. Congenital hypopituitarism associated with neonatal hypoglycemia and microphallus: four cases secondary to hypothalamic hormone deficiencies. Pediatr. 1975;87(6 Pt 2):1171-81.
25. Goodman HG, Grumbach MM, Kapaln SL. Growth and growth hormone. II. A comparison of isolated growth hormone deficiency and multiple pituitary hormone deficiencies in 35 patients with idiopathic hypopituitary dwarfism. N Eng J Med. 1968;278(2):57-68.
26. Lemons JA, Ridenour R, Orsini EN. Congenital absence of the pancreas and intrauterine growth retardation. Pediatr. 1979;64(2):255-7.
27. Lassare C, Hardouin S, Daffos F, et al. Serum insulin-like growth factors and insulin-like growth factors binding protein in the human fetus. Relationships with growth in normal subjects and in subjects with intrauterine growth retardation. Pediatr Res. 1991;29(3):219-25.
28. Ashton IK, Zapf J, Einschenk I, et al. Insulin-like growth factors IGF 1 and 2 in human fetal plasma and relationship to gestational age and fetal size during mid pregnancy. Acta Endocrinol. 1985;110:558-63.
29. Basset NS, et al. The effect of maternal starvation on plasma insulin-like growth factor I concentration in the late gestation ovine fetus. Pediatr Res. 1990;27:401-4.
30. Oliver MH, et al. Glucose but not a mixed amino acid infusion regulates insulin like growth factor-I concentration in fetal sheep. Pediatr Res. 1993;34:62-5.
31. Prada JA, Tsang RC. Biological mechanisms of environmentally induced causes of IUGR. Eur J Clin Nutr. 1998;52 (Suppl 1):S21-7;discussion S27-8.
32. Mirlesse V, et al. Placental growth hormone levels in normal pregnancy and in pregnancies with intrauterine growth retardation. Pediatr Res. 1993;34:439-42.
33. Gluckman PD, Grumbach MM, Kaplan SL. The human fetal hypothalamus and pituitary gland. In: Tulchinsky D, Ryan KJ (Eds). Maternal-fetal endocrinology. Philadelphia: WB Saunders Company 1980; str 196.
34. Czeizel AE. Folic acid in the prevention of neural tube defects. J Pediatr Gastroenterol Nutr. 1995;20(1):4-16.
35. Canfield MA, Collins JS, Botto LD, et al. Changes in the birth prevalence of selected birth defects after grain fortification with folic acid in the United States: findings from a multi-state population-based study. Birth Defects Res A Clin Mol Teratol. 2005;73(10):679-89.
36. Bower C, Miller M, Payne J, Serna P. Folate intake and the primary prevention of non-neural birth defects. Aust N Z J Public Health. 2006;30(3):258-61.
37. Czeizel AE, Puhó E. Maternal use of nutritional supplements during the first month of pregnancy and decreased risk of Down's syndrome: case-control study. Nutrition. 2005;21(6):698-704.
38. Judge MP, Harel O, Lammi-Keefe CJ. A docosahexaenoic acid-functional food during pregnancy benefits infant visual acuity at four but not six months of age. Lipids. 2007;42(2):117-22.

39. Judge MP, Harel O, Lammi-Keefe CJ. Maternal consumption of a docosahexaenoic acid-containing functional food during pregnancy: benefit for infant performance on problem-solving but not on recognition memory tasks at age 9 mo. Am J Clin Nutr. 2007;85(6):1572-7.
40. Helland IB, Smith L, Saarem K, et al. Maternal supplementation with very-long-chain n-3 fatty acids during pregnancy and lactation augments children's IQ at 4 years of age. Pediatrics. 2003;111(1):e39-44.
41. Hibbeln JR, Davis JM, Steer C, et al. Maternal seafood consumption in pregnancy and neurodevelopmental outcomes in childhood (ALSPAC study): an observational cohort study. Lancet. 2007;369(9561):578-85.
42. Romieu I, Torrent M, Garcia-Esteban R, et al. Maternal fish intake during pregnancy and atopy and asthma in infancy. Clin Exp Allergy. 2007;37(4):518-25.
43. Willers SM, Devereux G, Craig LC, et al. Maternal food consumption during pregnancy and asthma, respiratory and atopic symptoms in 5-year-old children. Thorax. 2007;62(9):773-9.
44. Kaiser L, Allen LH. Position of the American Dietetic Association: nutrition and lifestyle for a healthy pregnancy outcome. J Am Diet Assoc. 2008;102(10):553-61.
45. Tucker Blackburn S, Lee Loper D. Maternal, fetal and neonatal physiology. A clinical perspective. Philadelphia-London-Toronto-Montreal-Sydney-Tokyo: WB Saunders Company; 1992. pp. 228-47.
46. Sadler TW. Langmanova Medicinska embriologija. Zagreb: Školska knjiga; 1996. pp. 183-231, 232-41,272-311,374-415.
47. Azhar M, Wave SM. Genetic and developmental basis of cardiovascular malformations. Clin Perinatol. 2016;43(1): 39-53.
48. Sutton MJ, Gill T, Plappert P. Functional anatomic development in the fetal heart. In: Polin RA, Fox WW (Eds). Fetal and neonatal physiology. Philadelphia-London-Toronto-Montreal-Sydney-Tokyo: WB Saunders Company; 1992. pp. 598-607.
49. Schats R, Jansen CAM, Wladimiroff JW. Embryonic heart activity: appearance and development in early human pregnancy. Br J Obstet Gynecol. 1990,97(11):989-94.
50. Merchiers EH, Dhont M, De Sutter PA, et al. Predictive value of early embryonic cardiac activity for pregnancy outcome. Am J Obstet Gynecol. 1991;165(1):11-4.
51. Berne RM, Levy MN. Fiziologija. 3. izd. Zagreb: Medicinska naklada; 1996. pp. 489-91,831-63,879-907,908-48.
52. Bancroft J. Researches in prenatal life. Oxford: Blackwell; 1946.
53. Bartelds B, van Bel F, Teitel DF, et al. Carotid, not aortic, chemoreceptors mediate the fetal cardiovascular response to acute hypoxemia in lambs. Pediatr Res. 1993;34(1):51-5.
54. Jones CT, Robinson RO. Plasma catecholamines in fetal and adult sheep. J Physiol. 1975;248:15-33.
55. Guissani DA, McGrrigle HHG, Spencer JA, et al. Effect of carotid denervation on plasma vasopressin level during acute hypoxia in late gestation sheep fetus. J Physiol. 1994;477(1):81-7.
56. Green LR, McGarrigle HHG, Bennet L, et al. The effect of acute hypoxaemia on plasma angiotensin II in intact and carotid sinus-denervated fetal sheep. J Physiol. 1994;470(P):81P.
57. Richardson B, Korkola S, Assano H, et al. Regional blood flow and the endocrine response to sustained hypoxaemia in the preterm ovine fetus. Ped Res. 1996;40(2):337-43.
58. Myers DA, Robertshow D, Nathanielsz PW. Effect of bilateral splanchnic nerve section on adrenal function in the ovine fetus. Endocrinology. 1990;127:2328-35.
59. Tucker Blackburn S, Lee Loper D. Maternal, fetal and neonatal physiology. A clinical perspective. Philadelphia-London-Toronto-Montreal-Sydney-Tokyo: WB Saunders Company; 1992. pp. 228-47.
60. Green LR, McGrrigle HHG, Bennet L, et al. Effect of carotid sinus denervation on plasma endothelin-1 during acute isocapnic hypoxaemia im the late gestation ovine fetus (sažetak). J Soc Gynaecol Inv. 1995;2(2):159.
61. Green LR, Bennet L, Hanson MA. The role of nitric oxide synthesis in cardiovascular response to acute hypoxia in the late gestation sheep fetus. J Physiol. 1996;497(Pt 1):271-7.
62. Heymann MA. Fetal cerebrovascular physiology. In: Creasy RK, Resnik R. Maternal-fetal medicine: principles and practice. 2 izd. Philadelphia-London-Toronto-Montreal-Sydney-Tokyo: WB Saunders Company; 1989. pp. 288-300.
63. Trivedi VN, Hay P, Hay JC. Normal embryonic and fetal development. In: Reece EA, Hobbins JC, Gant NF (Eds). Clinical obstetrics: the fetus and mother. Oxford: Blackwell Publishing Ltd; 2007. pp. 19-35.
64. Grand RJ, Watkins JB, Torti FM. Development of the human gastrointestinal tract: a review. Gastroenterology. 1976;70(5 PT. 1):790-810.
65. Cunningham FG, MacDonald PC, Gant NF, et al. Williams Obstetrics, 20th edition. Stamford: Appleton and Lange; 1997.
66. Diamant NE. Development of esophageal function. Am Rev Respir Dis. 1985;131:S29-32.
67. Ross MG, Nijland JM. Development of ingestive behavior. Am J Physiol. 1998;274:R879-93.
68. El-Haddad MA, Desai M, Gayle D, et al. In utero development of fetal thirst and appetite: potential for programming. J Soc Gynecol Investig. 2004;11(3):123-30.
69. Grassi R, Farina R, Floriani I, et al. Assessment of fetal swallowing with gray-scale and color Doppler sonography. AJR Am J Roentgenol. 2005;185(5):1322-7.
70. Kurjak A, Andonotopo W, Hafner T, et al. Normal standards for fetal neurobehavioral developments—longitudinal quantification by four-dimensional sonography. J Perinat Med. 2006;34(1):56-65.
71. Ross MG, Kullama LK, Ogundipe OA, et al. Ovine fetal swallowing response to intracerebroventricular hypertonic saline. J Appl Physiol. 1995;78(6):2267-71.

72. Ross MG, Kullama LK, Ogundipe OA, et al. Central angiotensin II stimulation of ovine fetal swallowing. J Appl Physiol. 1994;76(3):1340-5.
73. Davison JM, Gilmore EA, Dürr J. Altered osmotic thresholds for vasopressin secretion and thirst in human pregnancy. Am J Physiol. 1984;246:105-9.
74. Ross MG, Sherman DJ, Schreyer P, et al. Fetal rehydration via amniotic fluid: contribution of fetal swallowing. Pediat Res. 1991;29(2):214-7.
75. Nijland MJ, Kullama LK, Ross MG. Maternal plasma hypo-osmolality: effects on spontaneous and stimulated ovine fetal swallowing. J Mater-Fetal Med. 1998;7(4):165-71.
76. El-Haddad MA, Chao CR, Ross MG. N-methyl-D-aspartate glutamate receptor mediates spontaneous and angiotensin II-stimulated ovine fetal swallowing. J Soc Gynecol Investig. 2005;12(7):504-9.
77. Ross MG, Sherman DJ, Ervin MG, et al. Fetal swallowing: response to systemic hypotension. Am J Physiol. 1990;257:R130-4.
78. Nicolaidis S, Galaverna O, Meltzer CH. Extracellular dehydration during pregnancy increases salt appetite of offspring. Am J Physiol. 1990;258(1 Pt 2):R281-3.
79. Vijande M, Brime JI, López-Sela P, et al. Increased salt preference in adult offspring raised by mother rats consuming excessive amounts of salt and water. Regul Pept. 1996;66(1-2):105-8.
80. Bradley RM, Mistretta CM. The developing sense of taste. In: Olfaction and Taste VDA, Denton and JP Coghlan (Eds). New York: Academic; 1975. pp. 91-8.
81. Salihagic' A, Kurjak A, Medic' M. Novije spoznaje o fiziologiji fetusa. In: Kurjak A, Đelemiš J (Eds). Ginekologija i perinatologija II. Varaždin:Tonomir; 2003. pp. 112-52.
82. El-Haddad MA, Jia Y, Ross MG. Persistent sucrose stimulation of ovine fetal ingestion: lack of adaptation responses. J Matern Fetal Neonatal Med. 2005;18(2):123-7.
83. Kawamura K, Takebayashi S. The development of noradrenaline-, acetylcholinesterase-, neuropeptide Y- and vasoactive intestinal polypeptide-containing nerves in human cerebral arteries. Neurosci Lett. 1994;175(1-2):1-4.
84. Cetin I, Morpurgo PS, Radaelli T, et al. Fetal plasma leptin concentrations: relationship with different intrauterine growth patterns from 19 weeks to term. Pediatr Res. 2000;48(5):646-51.
85. Jaquet D, Leger J, Levy-Marchal C, et al. Ontogeny of leptin in human fetuses and newborns: effect of intrauterine growth retardation on serum leptin concentrations. J Clin Endocrinol Metab. 1998;83(4):1243-6.
86. Roberts TJ, Caston-Balderrama A, Nijland MJ, et al. Central neuropeptide Y stimulates ingestive behavior and increases urine output in the ovine fetus. Am J Physiol Endocrinol Metab. 2000;279:E494-500.
87. Roberts TJ, Nijland MJ, Caston-Balderrama A, et al. Central leptin stimulates ingestive behavior and urine flow in the near term ovine fetus. Horm Metab Res. 2001;33(3):144-50.
88. Ross MG, El-Haddad M, Desai M, et al. Unopposed orexic pathways in the developing fetus. Physiol Behav. 2003;79(1):79-88.
89. Aparicio T, Kermorgant S, Darmoul D, et al. Leptin and Ob-Rb receptor isoform in the human digestive tract during fetal development. J Clin Endocrinol Metab. 2005;90(11): 6177-84.
90. Adair LS. Child and adolescent obesity: epidemiology and developmental perspectives. Physiol Behav. 2008;94(1):8-16.
91. Cunningham FG, Gant NF, Leveno KJ, et al. Williams Obstetrics. 21st edn. New York: McGraw-Hill; 2001.
92. Kotecha S. Lung growth: implications for the newborn infant. Arch Dis Child Neonatal Ed. 2000;82(1):F69-74.
93. Dawes GS. Breathing before birth in animals and man. An essay in developmental medicine. N Engl J Med. 1974;290(10):557-9.
94. Olver RE, Strang LB. Ion fluxes across the pulmonary epithelium and the secretion of lung liquid in the fetal lamb. J Physiol. 1974;241(2):327-57.
95. Jain L. Alveolar fluid clearance in developing lungs and its role in neonatal transition. Clin Perinatol. 1999;26(3):585-99.
96. Wigglesworth JS, Desai R. Effects on lung growth of cervical cord section in the rabbit fetus. Early Hum Dev. 1979;3(1):51-65.
97. de Vries JI, Visser GH, Prechtl HF. The emergence of fetal behavior. In: Qualitative aspects. Early Human Dev. 1982;7(4):301-22.
98. Patrick J, Campbell K, Carmichael L, et al. A definition of human fetal apnea and the distribution of fetal apneic intervals during the last 10 weeks of pregnancy. Am J Obstet Gynecol. 1978;136(4):471-7.
99. Natale R, Nasello-Paterson C, Connors G. Patterns of fetal breathing activity in the human fetus at 24 to 28 weeks of gestation. Am J Obstet Gynecol. 1988;158(2):317-21.
100. Connors G, Hunse C, Carmichael L, et al. Control of fetal breathing in the human fetus between 24 and 34 weeks gestation. Am J Obstet Gynecol. 1989;160(4):932-8.
101. Natale R, Patrick J, Richardson B. Effects of maternal venous plasma glucose concentrations on fetal breathing movements. Am J Obstet Gynecol. 1978;132(1):36-41.
102. Patrick J, Natale R, Richardson B. Patterns of human fetal breathing activity at 34 to 35 weeks gestational age. Am J Obstet Gynecol. 1978;132(5):507-13.
103. Mirghani HM, Weerasinghe SD, Smith JR, et al. The effect of intermittent maternal fasting on human fetal breathing movements. Obstet Gynaecol. 2004;24(6):635-7.
104. Roberts AB, Goldstein I, Romero R, et al. Fetal breathing movements after preterm premature rupture of membranes. Am J Obstet Gynecol. 1991;164(3):821-5.
105. Kivikoski A, Amon E, Vaalamo PO, et al. Effect of third-trimester premature rupture of membranes on fetal breathing movements: a prospective case-control study. Am J Obstet Gynecol. 1988;159(6):1474-7.

106. Richardson B, Natale R, Patrick J. Human fetal breathing activity during induced labor at term. Am J Obstet Gynecol. 1979;133(3):247-55.
107. Besinger RE, Compton AA, Hayashi RH. The presence or absence of fetal breathing movements as a predictor of outcome in preterm labor. Am J Obstet Gynecol. 1987;157(3):753-7.
108. Kisilevsky BS, Hains SMJ, Low JA. Maturation of body and breathing movements in 24-33 week-old fetuses threatening to deliver prematurely. Early Hum Dev. 1999;55(1):25-38.
109. Fox HE, Steinbrecher M, Pessel D, et al. Maternal ethanol ingestion and occurrence of human breathing movements. Am J Obstet Gynecol. 1978;132(4):354-61.
110. Richardson B, O'Grady JP, Olsen GD. Fetal breathing movements in response to carbon dioxide in patients on methadone maintenance. Am J Obstet Gynecol. 1984;150(4):400-4.
111. Manning FA, Wym Pugh E, Boddy K. Effect of cigarette smoking on fetal breathing movements in normal pregnancy. Br Med J. 1975;1(5957):552-8.
112. Ishigava M, Yoneyama Y, Power GG, et al. Maternal teophylline administration and breathing movements in late gestation human fetus. Obstet Gynecol. 1996;88(6):973-8.
113. Cosmi EV, Cosmi E, La Torre R. The effect of fetal breathing movements on the utero-placental circulation. Early Pregnancy. 2001;5(1):51-2.
114. Jobe A. Development of the fetal lung. U: Creasy RK, Resnik R. Maternal- fetal medicine: principles and practice. 2 izd. Philadelphia-London-Toronto-Montreal-Sydney-Tokyo: WB Saunders Company; 1989. pp. 288-300.
115. Haagsman HP, Demiel RV. Surfactant associated proteins: functions and structural variations. Comp Biochem A Mol Integr Physiol. 2001;129(1):91-108.
116. Vyas JR, Kotecha S. The effect of antenatal and postnatal corticosteroids on the preterm lung. Arch Dis Child Fetal Neonatal Ed. 1997;77:F147-50.
117. Hundertmark S, Ragosch V, Zimmermann B, et al. Effect of dexametasone, triiodothyronine and dimetyl-isopropyl-thyronine on the maturation of the fetal lung. J Perinat Med. 1999;27(4):309-15.
118. Chan L, Miller TF, Yuxin J, et al. Antenatal triiodothyronine improves neonatal pulmonary function in preterm lambs. J Soc Gynecol Investig. 1998;5(3):122-6.
119. Debieve F, Beerlandt S, Hubinot C, et al. Gonadotropines, prolactin, inhibin A, inhibin B, and activin A in human fetal serum from midpregnancy and term pregnancy. J Clin Endocrin Metab. 1997;85(1):270-4.
120. Glass L, Rajegowda BK, Evans HE. Absence of respiratory distress syndrome in premature infants of heroin-addicted mothers. Lancet. 1971;2(7726):685-6.
121. Thuresson-Klein A, Moawad AH, Hedqvust P. Estrogen stimulates formation of lamellar bodies in the rat fetal lung. Am J Obstet Gynecol. 1985;151(4):506-14.
122. Adamson IY, Bakowska J, Mc Millan E, et al. Accelerated fetal lung maturation by estrogen is associated with an epithelial-fibroblast interaction. In Vitro Cell Dev Biol. 1990;26 (8):784-90.
123. Warburton D. Chronic hyperglycemia reduces surface active maternal flux in tracheal fluid of fetal lambs. J Clin Invest. 1983;71(3):550-5.
124. Dekowski SA, Snyder JM. The combined effect of insulin and cortisol on surfactant protein mRNA levels. Pediatr Res. 1995;38(4):513-21.
125. Klein JM, Nielsen HC. Androgen regulation of epidermal growth factor receptor binding activity during rabbit fetal development. J Clin Invest. 1993;91(2):425-31.
126. Hallman M, Glumoff V, Ramet M. Surfactant in respiratory distress syndrome and lung injury. Comp Biochem Physiol A Mol Integr Physiol. 2001;1:287-94.
127. Jobe AH, Ikegami M. Antenatal infection/inflammation and postnatal lung maturation and injury. Resp Res. 2001;2(1):27-32.
128. Mardešic' D i sur. Pedijatrija. 6. izd. Zagreb: Školska knjiga; 2000. pp. 303-94.
129. Kleinmann LI. The kidney. In: Stave U (Ed). Perinatal physiology. New York-London: Plenum Medical Book Company; 1978. pp. 589-616.
130. Çvoric' A. Razvoj bubrega i bubrežnih funkcija. In: Koraè D. Pedijatrija. Beograd. Zagreb: Medicinska knjiga; 1983. pp. 441-3.
131. Gilbert T, Merlet-Bénichou C. Retinoids and nephron mass control. Pediatr Nephrol. 2000; 14(12):1137-44.
132. Merlet-Benichou C, Gilbert M, Muffet-Joly M, et al. Intrauterine growth development leads to a permanent nephron deficit in the rat. Pediatr Nephrol. 1994;8(2):175-80.
133. Amri K, Freund N, Vilar J, et al. Adverse effects of hyperglycemia on kidney development in rats: in vivo and in vitro studies. Diabetes. 1999;48(11):2240-5.
134. Gilbert T, Gaonach S, Moreau E, et al. Defect of nephrogenesis induced by gentamicin in rat metanephric organ culture. Lab Invest. 1994;70(5):656-66.
135. Kurjak A, Kirkinen P, Latin V, et al. Ultrasonic assessment of fetal kidney function in normal and complicated pregnancies. Am J Obstet Gynecol. 1981;141(3):266-70.
136. Wladimiroff JW. Effect of furosemide on fetal urine production. Br J Obstet Gynaecol. 1975;82(3):221-4.
137. Aperia A, Larsson L, Zetterström R. Hormonal induction of Na^{+}/K^{+} ATPase in developing proximal tubular cells. Am J Physiol. 1981;241(4):F356-60.
138. Schmidt U, Horster M. Na^{+} -K^{+} - activated ATPase: Activity maturation in rabbit nephron segments dissected in vitro. Am J Physiol. 1977;233:F55-61.
139. Arant BS Jr. Developmental patterns of renal function maturation compared in the human neonate. J Pediatr. 1978;92(5):705-12.
140. Karlen J, Paeria A, Zetterström R. Renal excretion of calcium and phosphate in preterm and fullterm infants. J Pediatr. 1985;106:814-9.

141. Schwartz GJ, Evan AP. Development of solute transport in rabbit proximal tubule. In: HCO_3^- and glucose absorption. Am J Physol. 1983;245:F382-6.
142. Battaglia FC, Meschia IG. An introduction to fetal physiology. Orlando: Academic Press; 1986. pp. 154-67, 184-5.
143. Devuyst O, Burrow CR, Smith BL, et al. Expression of aquaporins -1 and -2 during nephrogenesis and in autosomal dominant polycystic kidney disease. Am J Physiol. 1996;271(1 Pt 2):F169-83.
144. Boylan PC, Parisi VM. Fetal acido-base balance. In: Creasy RK, Resnik R (Eds). Maternal-fetal medicine: principles and practice. Philadelphia-London-Toronto-Montreal-Sydeny-Tokyo: WB Saunders Company; 1989. pp. 362-73.
145. Winkler CA, Kittelberger AM, Watkins RH. Maturation of carbonic anchidrase IV expression in rabbit kidney. Am J Physiol Renal Physiol. 2001;280(5):F895-903.
146. McCance RA, Widdowson EM. Renal function before birth. In: Widdowson EM (Ed). Studies in perinatal physiology. 1. izd. Bath: Pitman press; 1980. pp. 94-103.
147. McGroy WW. Development of renal function in utero. Cambridge:Harvard University Press; 1972. pp. 51-78.
148. McCance RA, Young WF. The secretion of urine by newborn infants. In: Widdowson EM (Ed). Studies in perinatal physiology. 1. izd. Bath: Pitman press; 1980. pp. 45-50.
149. McCance RA, Von Fimck MA. The titratable acidity, pH, ammonia and phosphates in the urine of very young infants. In: Widdowson EM (Ed). Studies in perinatal physiology. 1. izd. Bath: Pitman press; 1980. pp. 81-8.
150. Judaš M, Kostovic' I. Temelji neuroznanosti. 1. izd. MD Zagreb;1997. pp. 24-31,622-42,353-60.
151. Okado N, Kakimi S, Kojima T. Synaptogenesis in the cervical cord of the human embryo: sequence of synapse formation in a spinal reflex pathway. J Comp Neurol. 1979;184(3):491-518.
152. Okado N, Kojima T. Ontogeny of the central nervous system: neurogenesis, fibre connection, synaptogenesis and myelination in the spinal cord. In: Prechtl HFR (Ed). Continuity of neural function from prenatal to postnatal life. Oxford: Blackwell Science; 1984. pp. 31-5.
153. Landmesser LT, Morris DG. The development of functional innervation in the hind limb of the chick embryo. J Physiol. 1975;249(2):301-26.
154. Prechtl HFR. Ultrasound studies of human fetal behaviour. Early Hum Dev. 1985;12(2):91-8.
155. Ianniruberto A, Tajani E. Ultrasonographic study of fetal movements. Semin Perinatol. 1981;4:175-81.
156. Okado N. Onset of synapse formation in the human spinal cord. J Comp Neurol. 1981;201(2):211-9.
157. Joseph R. Fetal brain and cognitive development. Dev Rev. 1999;20:81-98.
158. de Vries JIP, Visser GHA, Prechtl HFR. The emergence of fetal behavior. I. Qualitative aspects. Early Human Dev. 1982;7(4):301-22.
159. Pomeroy SL, Volpe JJ. Development of the nervous system. In: Polin RA, Fox, WW (Eds): fetal and neonatal physiology. Philadelphia: London-Toronto-Montreal-Sydney-Tokyo: WB Saunders Company; 1992. pp. 1491-509.
160. Kostovic' I, Judas M. Transient patterns of cortical lamination during prenatal life: do they have implications for treatment? Neurosci Biobehav Rev. 2007;31(8): 1157-68.
161. Molliver ME, Kostovic I, Van der Loos H. The development of synapses in cerebral cortex of the human fetus. Brain Res. 1973;50(2):403-7.
162. Lüchinger AB, Hadders-Algra M, van Kan CM, et al. Fetal onset of general movements. Pediatr Res. 2008;63(2):191-5.
163. Kurjak A, Azumendi G, Vecek N, et al. Fetal hand movements and facial expression in normal pregnancy studied by four-dimensional sonography. J Perinat Med. 2003;31(6):496-508.
164. Kurjak A, Andonotopo W, Hafner T, et al. Normal standards for fetal neurobehavioral developments—longitudinal quantification by four-dimensional sonography. J Perinat Med. 2006;34(1):56-65.
165. Andonotopo W, Medic M, Salihagic-Kadic A, et al. The assessment of fetal behavior in early pregnancy: comparison between 2D and 4D sonographic scanning. J Perinat Med. 2005;33(5):406-14.
166. Awoust J, Levi S. Neurological maturation of the human fetus. Ultrasound Med Biol. 1983; Suppl 2:583-7.
167. Inoue M, Koyanagi T, Nakahara H. Functional development of human eye-movement in utero assessed quantitatively with real-time ultrasound. Am J Obstet Gynecol. 1986;155(1): 170-4.
168. Kostovic' I, Rakic P. Developmental history of the transient subplate zone in the visual and somatosensory cortex of the macaque monkey and human brain. J Comp Neurol. 1990;274(3):441-70.
169. Kostovic' I, Judas M, Petanjek Z, et al. Ontogenesis of goal-directed behavior: anatomo-functional considerations. Int J Psychophysiol. 1995;19(2):85-102.
170. D'Elia A, Pighetti M, Moccia G, et al. Spontaneous motor activity in normal fetus. Early Human Dev. 2001;65(2):139-44.
171. Natale R, Nasello-Paterson C, Turlink R. Longitudinal measurements of fetal breathing, body movements, and heart rate accelerations, and decelerations at 24 and 32 weeks of gestation. Am J Obstet Gynecol. 1985;151(2):256-63.
172. Eller DP, Stramm SL, Newman RB. The effect of maternal intravenous glucose administration on fetal activity. Am J Obstet Gynecol. 1992;167(4 Pt 1):1071-4.
173. Haddres-Algra M. Putative neural substrate of normal and abnormal general movements. Neurosci Biobehav Rev. 2007;31(8):1181-90.
174. Kurjak A, Azumendi G, Andonotopo W, et al. Three- and four-dimensional ultrasonography for the structural and

functional evaluation of the fetal face. Am J Obstet Gynecol. 2007;196(1):16-28.
175. Kozuma S, Baba K, Okai T, et al. Dynamic observation of the fetal face by three-dimensional ultrasound. Ultrasound Obstet Gynecol. 1999;13(4):283-4.
176. Yan F, Dai SY, Akther N, et al. Four-dimensional sonographic assessment of fetal facial expression early in the third trimester. Int J Gynaecol Obstet. 2006;94(2):108-13.
177. Merz E, C Weller. 2D and 3D Ultrasound in the evaluation of normal and abnormal fetal anatomy in the second and third trimesters in a level III center. Ultraschall Med. 2005;26(1): 9-16.
178. Kurjak A, Stanojevic M, Andonotopo W, et al. Behavioral pattern continuity from prenatal to postnatal life: a study by four-dimensional (4D) ultrasonography. J Perinat Med. 2004;32(4):346-53.
179. Vanhatalo S, van Nieuvenhuizen O. Fetal pain? Brain Dev. 2000;22(3):145-50.
180. Teixeira JM, Glover V, Fisk NM. Acute cerebral redistribution in response to invasive procedures in the human fetus. Am J Obstet Gynecol. 1999;181(4):1018-25.
181. Smith RP, Gitau R, Glover V, et al. Pain and stress in the human fetus. Eur J Obstet Gynecol Reprod Biol. 2000;92(1):161-5.
182. Giannakoulopoulos X, Sepulveda W, Kourtis P, et al. Fetal plasma cortisol and beta endorphin response to intrauterine needling. Lancet. 1994;344(8915):77-81.
183. Giannakoulopolous X, Teixeira J, Fisk N, et al. Human fetal and maternal noradernaline responses to invasive procedures. Pediatr Res. 1999;45(4 Pt 1):494-9.
184. Lee SJ, Ralston HJ, Drey EA, et al. Fetal pain: a systematic multidisciplinary review of the evidence. JAMA. 2005; 294(8):947-54.
185. Lowery CL, Hardman MP, Manning N, et al. Neurodevelopmental changes of fetal pain. Semin Perinatol. 2007;31(5):275-82.
186. Morlet T, Collet L, Salle B, et al. Functional maturation of cochlear active mechanisms and of the medial olivocochlear system in humans. Acta Otolaryngol. 1993;113(3):271-7.
187. Morlet T, Collet L, Duclaux R, et al. Spontaneous and evoked otoacustical emissions in preterm and full term neonates, Is there a clinical application? Int J Ped OtoRhinoLaryngol. 1995;33(3):207-11.
188. Leader LR, Baille P, Martin B, et al. The assessment and significance of habituation to a repeated stimulus by the human fetus. Early Human Dev. 1982;7(3):211-9.
189. Liley AW. Fetus as a person. Speech held at the 8th meeting of the psychiatric societies of Australia and New Zealand. Fetal therapy. 1986;1:8-17.
190. Sun W, Hansen A, Zhang L, et al. Neonatal nicotine exposure impairs development of auditory temporal processing. Hear Res. 2008;245(1-2):58-64.
191. Kiefer I, Siegel E, Preissl H, et al. Delayed maturation of auditory-evoked responses in growth-restricted fetuses revealed by magnetoencephalographic recordings. Am J Obstet Gynecol. 2008;199(5):503.e1-7.
192. Lee CT, Brown CA, Hains SM, et al. Fetal development: voice processing in normotensive and hypertensive pregnancies. Biol Res Nurs. 2007;8(4):272-82.
193. Huttenlocher PR, de Courten CH. The development of synapses in striate cortex of man. Human Neurobiol. 1987;6(1):1-9.
194. Magoon EH, Robb RM. Development of myelin in human optic nerve tract. A light and electron microscopic study. Arch Ophtalmol. 1981;99(4):655-9.
195. Kostovic I, Rakic P. Development of prestriate visual projections in the monkey and human fetal cerebrum revealed by transient cholinesterase staining. J Neurosci. 1984;4(1):25-42.
196. Sheridan CJ, Preissl H, Siegel ER, et al. Neonatal and fetal response decrement of evoked responses: A MEG study. Clin Neurophysiol. 2008;119(4):796-804.
197. Eswaran H, Wilson J, Preissl H, et al. Magnetoencephalographic recordings of visual evoked brain activity in the human fetus. Lancet. 2002;360(9335):779-80.
198. Kablar B. Determination of retinal cell fates is affected in the absence of extraocular striated muscles. Dev Dyn. 2000;226(3):478-90.
199. Ruckenbush Y, Gaujoux M, Eghbali B. Sleep cycles and kinesis in the fetal lamb. Electroenceph Clin Neurophysiol. 1977;42(2):226-37.
200. Kelly DD. Sleep and dreaming. In: Kandell ER, Schwartz JH (Eds). Principles of neural science. 2nd edn. New York-Amsterdam-Oxford: Elsevier Science Publishing; 1985. p. 651.
201. Rosen MG, Scibetta JJ, Chik L, et al. An approach to the study of brain damage: the principles of fetal FEEG. Am J Obstet Gynecol. 1973;115:37-47.
202. Roffag HP, Muzio JN, Dement WC. Ontogenetic development of the human sleep-dream cycle. Science. 1966;152(3722):604-19.
203. Abrams RM, Gerhardt KJ. The acoustic environment and physiological responses of the fetus. J Perinatol. 2000;20(8 Pt 2):S31-6.
204. Mennella JA, Johnson A, Beauchamp GK. Garlic ingestion by pregnant women alters the odor of amniotic fluid. Chem Senses. 1995;20(2):207-9.
205. Mennella JA, Jagnow CP, Beauchamp GK. Prenatal and postnatal flavor learning by human infants. Pediatrics. 2001;107(6):E88.
206. Varendi H, Porter RH, Winberg J. Does the newborn baby find the nipple by smell? Lancet. 1994;334(8928):989-90.
207. Varendi H, Porter RH, Winberg J. Natural odour preference of newborn change over time. Acta Pediatrica. 1997;86:985-90.
208. Widstrom AM, Ransjö-Arvidson AB, Christensson K, et al. Gastric suction in healthy newborn infant. Effects on

circulation and developing feeding behavior. Acta Paediatr Scand. 1987;76(4):556-72.
209. Varendi H, Porter RH, Winberg J. Attractiveness of amniotic fluid odor: evidence of prenatal olfactory learning? Acta Paediatr. 1996;85(10):1223-7.
210. Porter RH, Winberg J. Unique salience of maternal breast odors for newborn infants. Neurosci Biobehav Rev. 1999;23(3):439-49.
211. Kostovic I. Prenatal development of nucleus basalis complex and related fiber system in man: a histochemical study. Neuroscience. 1986;17(4):1047-77.
212. Salihagic Kadic A, Medic M, Kurjak A. Recent advances in neurophysiology. In: Kurjak A, Azumendi G (Eds). The fetus in three dimensions. London: Informa Healtcare; 2007. pp. 411-33.
213. Anand KJ. Clinical importance of pain and stress in preterm neonates. Biol Neonate. 1998;73(1):1-9.
214. Carmichael SL, Shaw GM, Yang W, et al. Maternal stressful life events and risks of birth defects. Epidemiology. 2007;18(3):356-61.
215. Monk C, Fifer WP, Myers MM, et al. Maternal stress responses and anxiety during pregnancy: effects on fetal heart rate. Dev Psychobiol. 2000;36(1):67-77.
216. DiPietro JA, Hilton SC, Hawkins M, et al. Maternal stress and affect influence fetal neurobehavioral development. Dev Psychol. 2002;38(5):659-68.
217. Jugovic' D, Tumbri J, Medic' M, et al. New Doppler index for prediction of perinatal brain damage in growth-restricted and hypoxic fetuses. Ultrasound Obstet Gynecol. 2007;30(3):303-11.
218. Hundertmark S, Ragosch V, Zimmermann B, et al. Effect of dexamethasone, triiodothyronine and dimethyl-isopropyl-thyronine on lung maturation of the fetal rat lung. J Perinat Med. 1999;27(4):309-15.
219. Uno H, Lohmiller L, Thieme C, et al. Brain damage induced by prenatal exposure to dexamethasone in fetal rhesus macaques. I. Hippocampus. Brain Res Dev Brain Res. 1990;53(2):157-67.
220. Barbazanges A, Piazza PV, Le Moal M, et al. Maternal glucocorticoid secretion mediates long-term effects of prenatal stress. J Neurosci. 1996;16(12):3943-9.
221. Hayashi A, Nagaoka M, Yamada K, et al. Maternal stress induces synaptic loss and developmental disabilities of offspring. Int J Dev Neurosci. 1998;16(3-4):209-16.
222. Rees S, Harding R. Brain development during fetal life: influences of the intra-uterine environment. Neurosci Lett. 2004;361(1-3):111-4.
223. Sandman CA, Wadhwa PD, Chicz-Demet A, et al. Maternal corticortropin-releasing hormone and habituation in human fetus. Dev Psychobiol. 1999;34(3):163-73.
224. Glover V. Maternal stress or anxiety in pregnancy and emotional development of the child. Br J Psychiatry. 1997;171:105-6.
225. Graham YP, Heim C, Goodman SH, et al. The effects of neonatal stress on brain development: implications for psychopathology. Dev Psychopathol. 1999;11(3):545-65.
226. Weinstock M. Does prenatal stress impair coping and regulation of hypothalamic-pituitary-adrenal axis. Neurosci Biobehav Rev. 1997;21(1):1-10.
227. Weinstock M. Alterations induced by gestational stress in brain morphology and behavior of the off-spring. Prog Neurobiol. 2001;65(5):427-51.
228. Amiel-Tison C, Cabrol D, Denver R, et al. Fetal adaptation to stress: Part II. Evolutionary aspects; stress induced hippocampal damage; long-term effects on behavior; consequences on adult health. Early Human Dev. 2004;78(2):81-94.
229. Buitelaar JK, Huizink AC, Mulder EJ, et al. Prenatal stress and cognitive development and temperament in infants. Neurobiol Aging. 2003;24 (Suppl 1):S53-60; discussion S67-8.
230. Davis EP, Glynn LM, Schetter CD, et al. Prenatal exposure to maternal depression and cortisol influences infant temperament. J Am Acad Child Adolesc Psychiatry. 2007;46(6):737-46.
231. Gutteling BM, de Weerth C, Zandbelt N, et al. Does maternal prenatal stress adversely affect the child's learning and memory at age six? J Abnorm Child Psychol. 2006;34(6):789-98.
232. Benediktsson R, Lindsay RS, Noble J, et al. Glucocorticoid exposure in utero: a new model of adult hypertension. Lancet. 1993;341(8841):339-41.
233. Edward CR, Benediktsson R, Lindsay RS, et al. Dysfunction of placental glucocorticoid barrier: link between fetal environment and adult hypertension? Lancet. 1993;341(8841):355-7.
234. Hales CN, Barker DJ, Clark PM, et al. Fetal and infant growth and impaired glucose tolerance at age 64. BMJ. 1991;303(6809):1019-22.

CHAPTER 7

HDlive Silhouette and HDlive Flow: New Application of 3D Ultrasound in Prenatal Diagnosis

Ritsuko K Pooh

INTRODUCTION

Owing to prenatal ultrasound technology, there has been an immense acceleration in understanding of early human development. The anatomy and physiology of embryonic development is a field where medicine exerts greatest impact on early pregnancy at present, and it opens fascinating aspects of embryonic differentiation. Advances of fetal ultrasound technology have established a field of sonoembryology[1,2] which is still evolving. Recent development of three-dimensional(3D)/four-dimensional (4D) sonography has revealed structural and functional early human development in utero.[3-6] 3D/4D sonography moved prenatal diagnosis of fetal anomalies from the second to the first trimester of pregnancy.[7] The 3D transducers take several hundreds or thousands of two-dimensional (2D) ultrasound images over a short (30–40 degree) arc. These images are then transferred to a computer that integrates them into a single image. The first generation of 3D ultrasound lacked the capability to reconstruct images rapidly and with high resolution. These limitations could explain why the method was not very popular initially.[8] With current clinically available equipment, 3D sonographic reconstruction is fast, with high resolution, giving ultrasound the ability to image in real time. Also, 3D ultrasound allows volume data to be stored and manipulated long after the patient has left the examination room. Storage of a single volume of data is easy and quick, yet the stored volume permits interpretation of the scanned region in multiple planes.[8] 3D/4D ultrasound has improved its functions with high definition live (HDlive) technology and furthermore, great advances of ultrasound technology have produced new applications of HDlive silhouette and HDlive flow.

This chapter demonstrates detailed and comprehensive fetal structural images and angiogram of normal and abnormal fetuses from the first trimester depicted by 3D HDlive silhouette and flows, which closely resemble those from anatomy atlases or scientific documentaries, and describes clinical significance and pitfalls of those novel applications.

HDLIVE (HIGH DEFINITION LIVE) TECHNIQUE

Both 3D and 4D ultrasound have improved our knowledge regarding the development of the embryo and fetus and of a great number of fetal anomalies.[8] The great achievement in the field of 3D/4D ultrasound is HDlive technology. This technology is a novel ultrasound technique that improves the 3D/4D images. HDlive ultrasound has resulted in remarkable progress in visualization of early embryos and fetuses and in the development of sonoembryology.[9] With HDlive ultrasound, both structural and functional developments can be assessed from early pregnancy more objectively and reliably and indeed, those new technologies have moved embryology from postmortem studies to the in vivo environment.[8]

HDlive uses an adjustable light source and software that calculates the propagation of light through surface structures in relation to the light direction.[10] The virtual light source produces selective illumination, and the respective shadows are created by the structures where the light is reflected. This combination of light and shadows increases depth perception and produces remarkable images that are more natural than those obtained with classic 3D ultrasound. The virtual light can be placed in the front, back, or lateral sides, where viewing is desired until the best image is achieved. A great advantage is that the soft can be applied to all images stored in the machine's memory.[9] As shown in **Figure 1**, HDlive image of the fetus in **Figure 1B** is more clearly demonstrating the fetus as well as intrauterine structure surrounding the fetus by shadowing with virtual light than classic 3D image

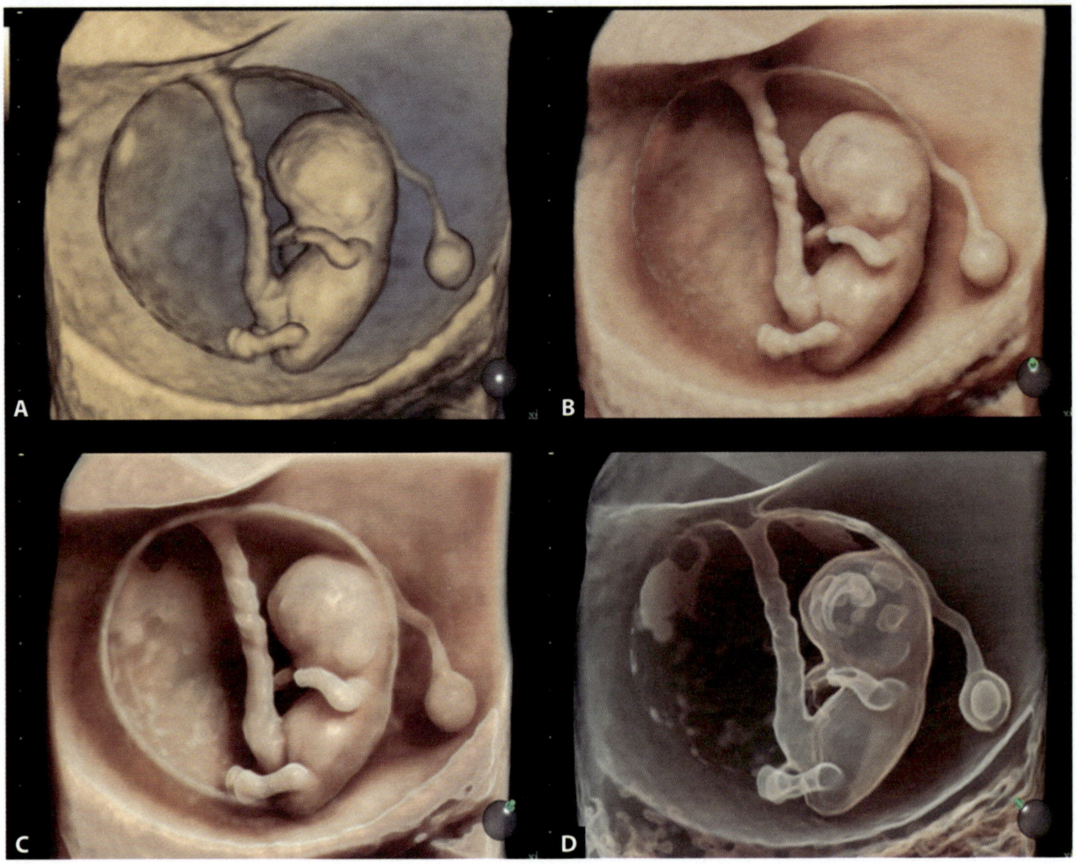

Figs. 1A to D: Different image demonstration with using the same 3D volume dataset of 9-week-fetus; (A) Classic 3D imaging of 9-week-fetus; (B) Conventional HDlive imaging; (C) HDlive silhouette image with surface smoothing; (D) HDlive silhouette image with demonstration of both inner and outer structure.

in **Figure1A**. **Figure 2A and B** are the dichorionic twinning images rendered with HDlive. The render direction (position of the "virtual light") in the image **(Fig. 2A)** is in the front and the image **(Fig. 2B)** is processed with the light position in the back.

Practically in obstetrical ultrasound, HDlive could be used during all three trimesters of pregnancy. There have been several reports on HDlive demonstration of fetal surface.[9,11-13] Three-dimensional HDlive further "humanizes" the fetus, enables detailed observation of the fetal face in the first trimester, and reveals that a small fetus is not more a fetus but a "person" from the first trimester.[13] Detailed structural abnormalities of face, fingers, toes and even amniotic membranes in the first trimester could be well-demonstrated by HDlive technique.[13,14]

HDlive Silhouette Imaging Technology

New applications of HDlive silhouette and HDlive flow were released at the end of 2014. The algorithm of HDlive silhouette creates a gradient at organ boundaries, fluid filled cavity and vessels walls, where an abrupt change of the acoustic impedance exists within tissues.[15,16] By HDlive silhouette mode, an inner cystic structure with fluid collection can be depicted through the outer surface structure of the body and it can be appropriately named as 'see-through fashion'.[15] The examiner can adjust HDlive silhouette percentage with controlling threshold and gain simultaneously for visualizing target organs of interest.

HDlive silhouette emphasizes the borderlines between organs with different echogenicity, therefore, both the target of interest floating within fluid correction and cystic area in echogenic organs are simultaneously demonstrated. By HDlive silhouette mode, an inner cystic structure with fluid collection can be depicted through the outer surface structure of the body and it can be appropriately named as *'see-through fashion.'*[15, 17,18]

The placental surface is demonstrated through the amniotic fluid and report on HDlive silhouette imaging of circumvallate placenta was recently published.[19]

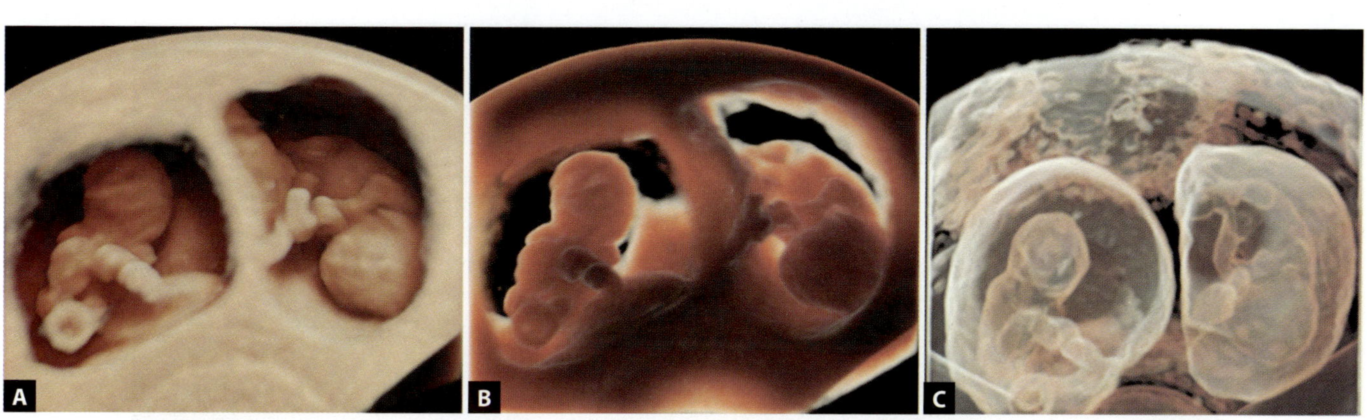

Figs. 2A to C: Different HDlive imaging of 8-week dichorionic twin; (A) and (B) HDlive images with different light sources; (C) HDlive silhouette image of the same volume dataset.

HDlive Silhouette Imaging of Hypoechoic Structures

Figure 1C is rendered with slight degree of silhouette ultrasound for surface smoothing and image (D) is high-degree silhouette ultrasound for demonstrating brain vesicles within outer surface of the fetus. **Figure 2C** shows the twin gestational sacs with fetuses inside the sacs.

Thus, any cystic area or hypoechoic part can be target of interest by HDlive silhouette imaging.

During the early embryonic period, the central nervous system anatomy rapidly changes in appearance. 3D sonography using transvaginal sonography with high-resolution probes allows imaging of early structures in the embryonic brain. **Figure 3** is the schematic picture of the embryonal brain which contains three parts: (1) Forebrain (prosencephalon), (2) midbrain (mesencephalon), and (3) hindbrain (rhombencephalon). The forebrain (prosencephalon) includes the telencephalon containing cerebral hemispheres and diencephalon containing thalamus, hypothalamus, epithalamus, and subthalamus. The midbrain (mesencephalon) is the most rostral part of the brainstem, and locates above the pons, and adjoins rostrally to the thalamus. The hindbrain (rhombencephalon) is the posterior part of the three primary divisions, which includes metencephalon containing pons and cerebellum and myelencephalon containing medulla oblongata. In 1998, Blaas et al.[20] sensationally demonstrated early human brain vesicles in different colors and measured their volumes by 3D scanning embryos ranged between 9.3 and 39 mm, and performed post-processing procedure. Thereafter, embryonic brain structure was demonstrated by advancing 3D technology of inversion-rendering mode[21,22] and sonoembryology has become more sophisticated and objective. Advancing imaging techniques allow the definition of in-vivo anatomy including visualization of the embryonic features that could not be characterized in fixed specimens.[23] 3D images of embryos were generated using the high-frequency transvaginal transducer (Voluson® E10 with 6 to 12 MHz/256 element 3D/4D transvaginal transducer, GE Healthcare, Milwaukee, USA). Transvaginal

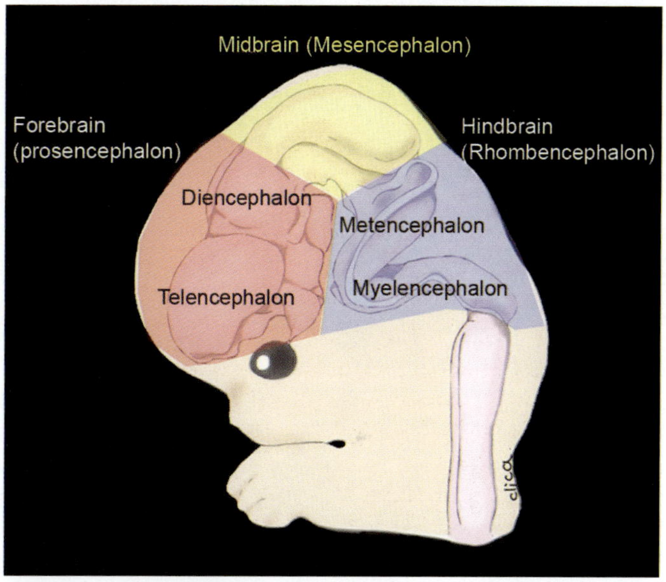

Fig. 3: Schematic picture of embryonal brain. (Drawn by Clica@ CRIFM). The forebrain (prosencephalon) includes the telencephalon containing cerebral hemispheres and diencephalon containing thalamus, hypothalamus, epithalamus and subthalamus. The midbrain (mesencephalon) is the most rostral part of the brainstem and located above the pons, and adjoined rostrally to the thalamus. The hindbrain (rhombencephalon) is the posterior part of the three primary divisions, which includes metencephalon containing pons and cerebellum and myelencephalon containing medulla oblongata.

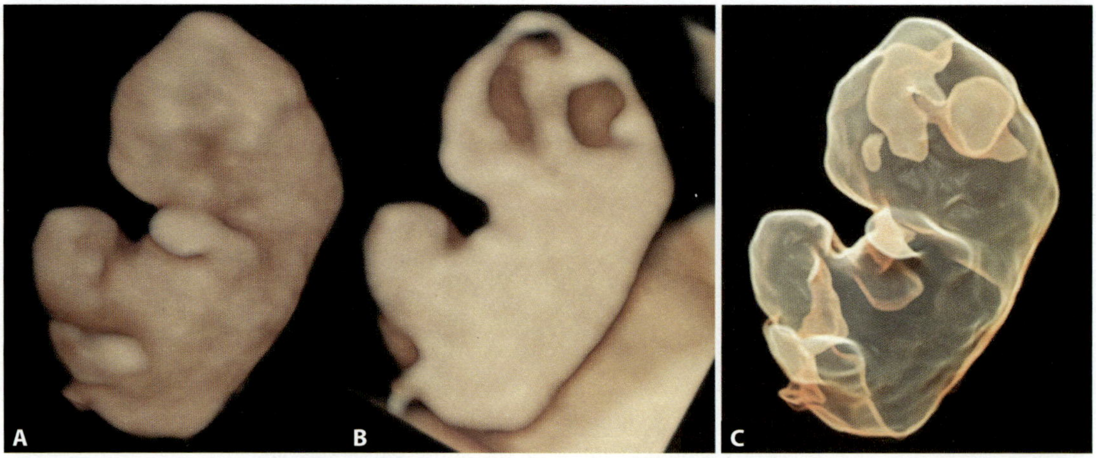

Figs. 4A to C: 3D images of CRL 19.3 mm normal embryo; (A) Surface image of embryo with HDlive; (B) Median cutting image of the same embryo; (C) HDlive silhouette image of the same embryo. The premature brain vesicles are well-demonstrated.

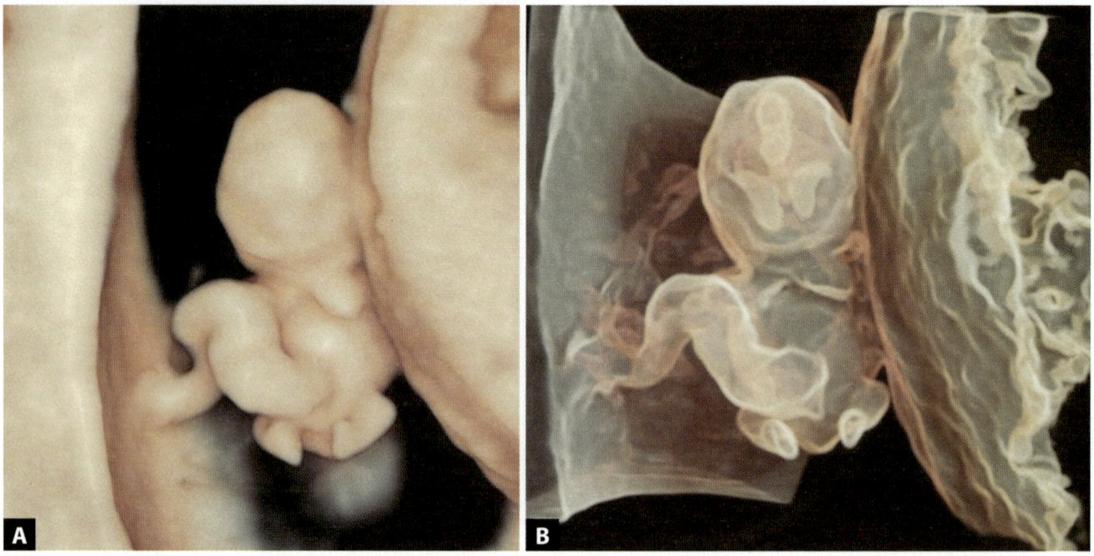

Figs. 5A and B: 8-week-embryo with HDlive silhouette; (A) Conventional HDlive image. Surface rendering with shadow demonstrates the outer surface of the embryo and umbilical cord; (B) Same image with HDlive silhouette. Premature brain cavity is well-demonstrated within outer surface of embryo.

approach combined with high frequency of 12 MHz with a harmonic phase inversion method can provide us images with high quality and high resolution demonstrating detailed embryonal structures, especially brain vesicles. As shown in **Figs. 4 and 5**, inside structure of the brain vesicles of normal embryos is well-demonstrated by HDlive silhouette mode. **Figs. 6 and 7** show rapid change of the developing brain vesicles by HDlive silhouette mode in different stages. Abnormal brain structure at 10 weeks is comprehensively detected by HDlive silhouette mode in **Fig. 8**. Not only brain cavity in early pregnancy but megacystis **(Fig. 9)** huge bladder in a case of prune belly syndrome **(Fig. 10)**, pleural effusion **(Fig. 11)**, the fused ventricle and the single ventricle in semilobar/alobar holoprosencephaly **(Fig. 12)** are well-visualized. **Figure 13** demonstrates enlarged bilateral ventricles and third and forth ventricles in a single volume dataset in a case of Dandy Walker malformation. Eyeball with outer surface of fetal face in a case with exophthalmos is depicted in **Figure 14**. Thus, any cystic area or hypoechoic part can be target of interest by HDlive silhouette imaging.

The eyeball including lens and the vitreous body is bilaterally created in early embryological stage **(Fig. 15)**. The eyeball is visualized by silhouette ultrasound as shown

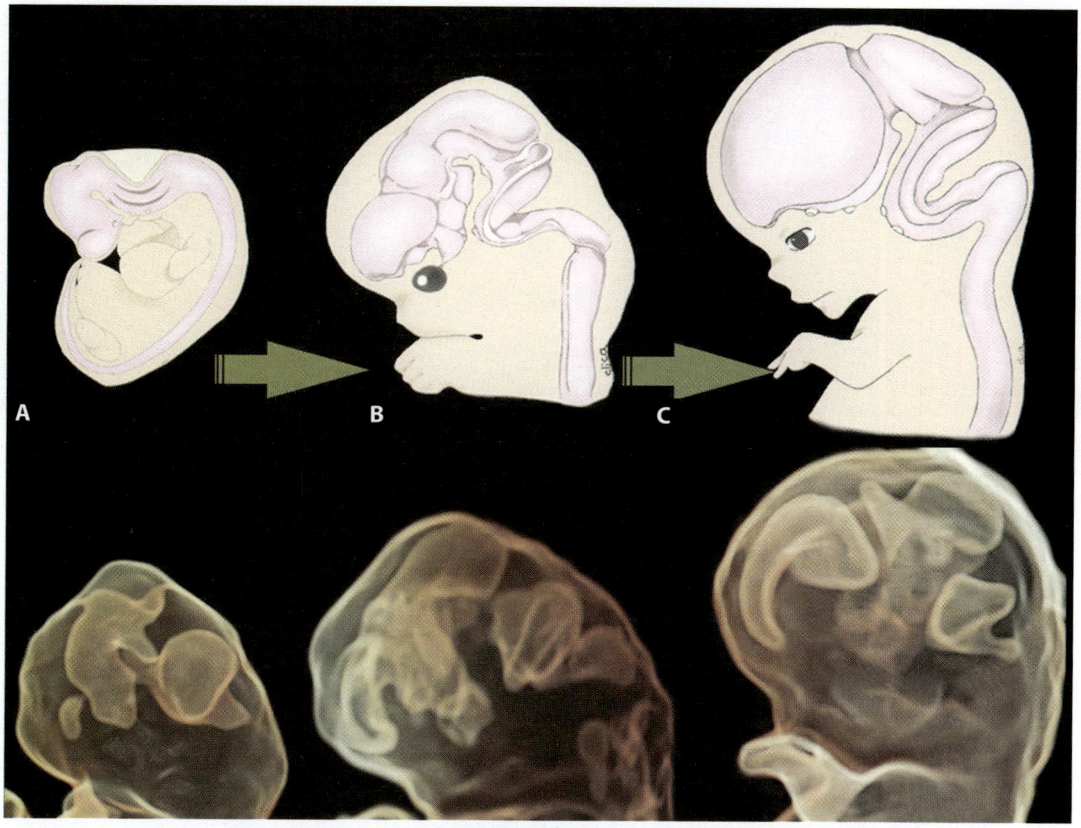

Figs. 6A to C: Lateral view of early brain development by HDlive silhouette mode; (A) Embryo with CRL 19.3 mm; (B) Embryo with CRL 22.3 mm; (C) Fetus with CRL 23.9 mm upper; schematic illustration showing early brain development. (Drawn by Clica@CRIFM). The development of three primary brain divisions of forebrain, midbrain and hindbrain is well-demonstrated.

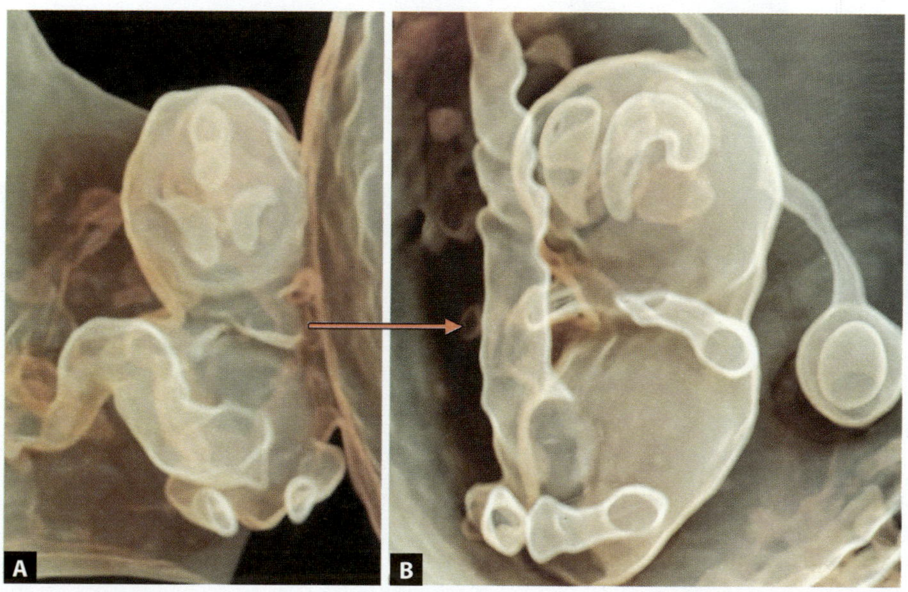

Figs. 7A and B: Frontal view of brain development by HDlive silhouette mode; (A) Fetus with CRL 22.3 mm. Bilateral telencephalon (forebrain) and midbrain are well-demonstrated; (B) Frontal-oblique view of fetus with CRL 23.9 mm. Rapid development of early brain is comprehensively depicted.

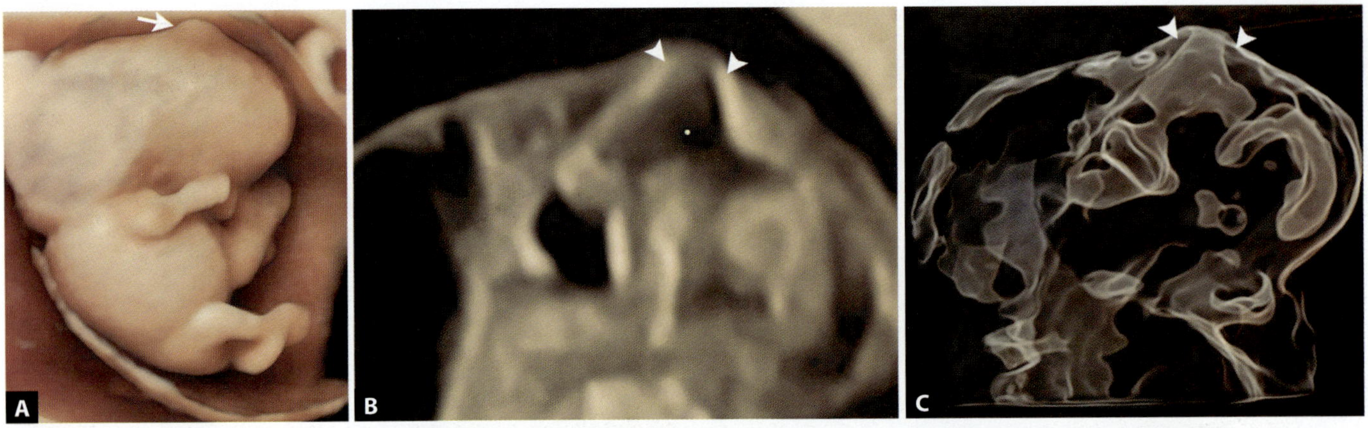

Figs. 8A to C: Abnormal midbrain cavity at 10 weeks of gestation; (A) 3D HDlive image of the fetus. Note the prominent top of the fetal head (arrow) due to abnormal midbrain; (B) Midsagittal cutting section of the brain. Abnormal appearance of midbrain (arrowheads) is visible; (C) HDlive silhouette image of the fetal head. Abnormal prominent midbrain (arrowheads) is depicted between forebrain and hindbrain.

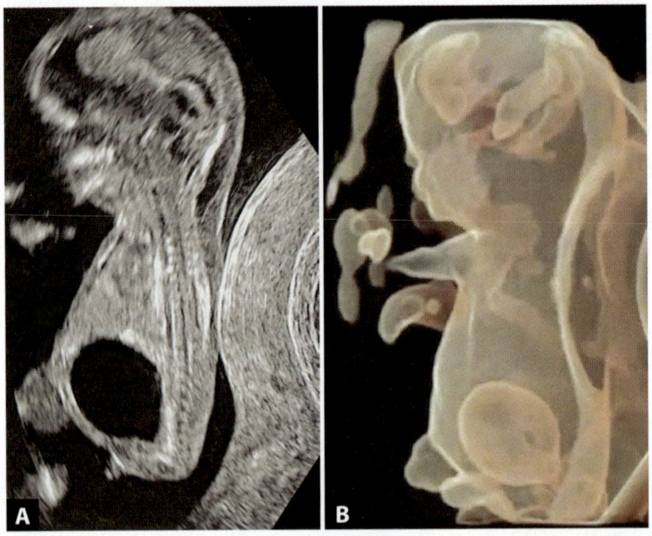

Figs. 9A and B: Megacystis at 13 weeks of gestation in a case of trisomy 18; (A) 2D sagittal cutting section. Enlarged bladder is demonstrated; (B) HDlive silhouette image. Enlarged bladder is depicted simultaneously with fetal surface.

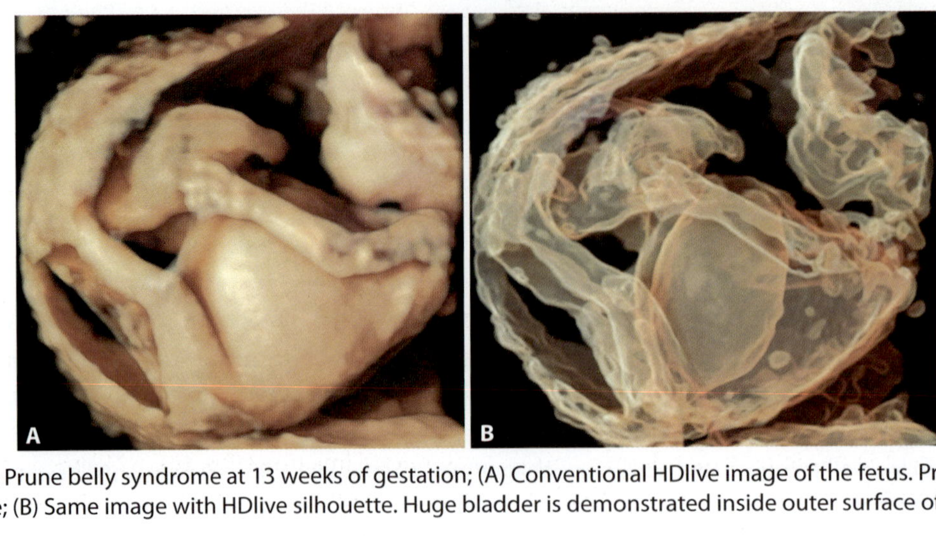

Figs. 10A and B: Prune belly syndrome at 13 weeks of gestation; (A) Conventional HDlive image of the fetus. Prominent abdomen is visible; (B) Same image with HDlive silhouette. Huge bladder is demonstrated inside outer surface of the fetus.

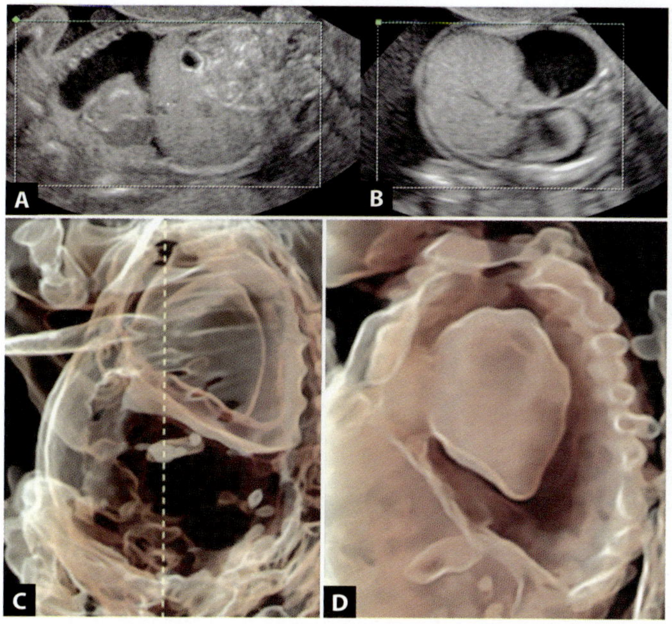

Figs. 11A to D: Fetal hydrothorax at 17 weeks of gestation; (A and B) 2D coronal and axial images of fetal thorax. Pleural effusion is more prominent in the left side; (C) HDlive silhouette image. Pleural effusion and lung floating in the fluid correction are well-demonstrated; (D) Same image with different HDlive silhouette degree and gain. Lung is more emphasized than image C.

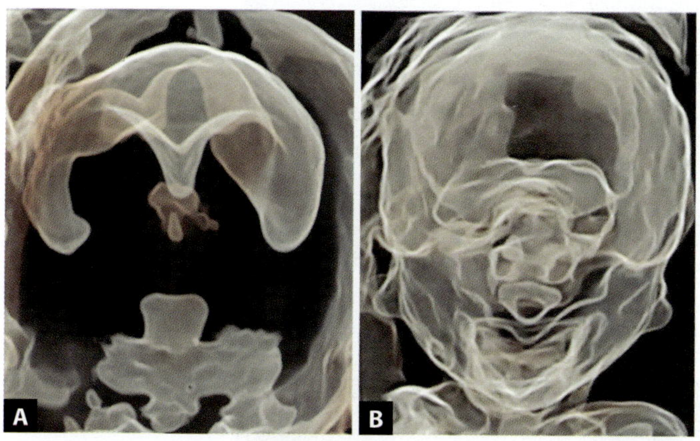

Figs. 12A and B: Brain ventricular shape of semilobar and alobar holoprosencephaly by HDlive silhouette imaging at 14 weeks of gestation; (A) Fused ventricle of semilobar holoprosencephaly demonstrated with HDlive silhouette; (B) Single ventricle of alobar holoprosencephaly demonstrated with HDlive silhouette.

in **Figure 16**, demonstrating the visualization of eyeball development between 12 an 13 weeks. At the beginning of 12 weeks, a small cystic part appears and at the middle of 12 weeks, the eyeball is depicted much larger and at 13 weeks, the lens and vitreous body in the eyeball can

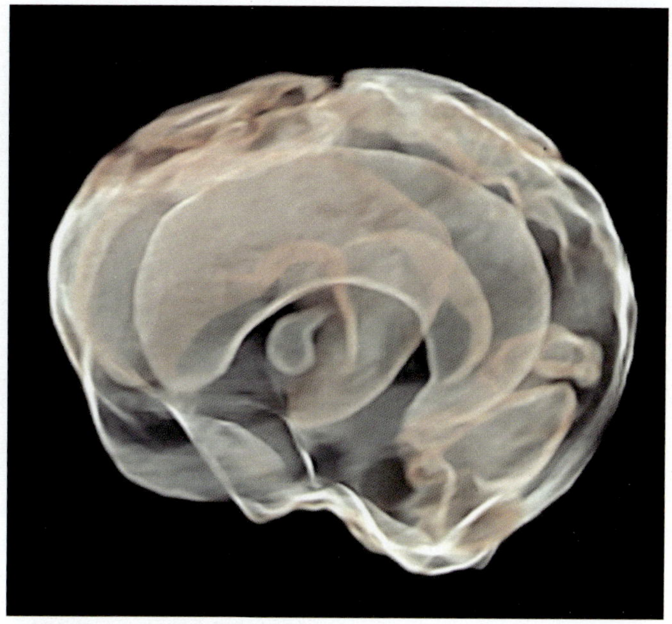

Fig. 13: Ventriculomegaly associated with Dandy Walker syndrome by HDlive silhouette imaging at 16 weeks of gestation. Enlargement of bilateral lateral ventricles, third ventricle and forth ventricle is well-demonstrated inside the brain.

be identified and thereafter the lens and vitreous body are continuously demonstrated by silhouette ultrasound. The author demonstrated fetal eye and ocular vascularity three-dimensionally in the second trimester.[17] This new technology has a great potential to open a new field of 'fetal 3D sono-ophthalmology', which has been never invented by conventional ultrasound technology.[17]

Thus, silhouette ultrasound shows comprehensive structure demonstrating inner and outer morphology simultaneously. However, it occasionally appears to demonstrate too many inner structures overlapping one another to understand their relations. The author has cut the volume dataset with a rectangle cube and rendered the cut slice with silhouette ultrasound. The author calls this silhouette ultrasound demonstration of thick slice of 3D volume dataset as 'thick-slice silhouette'.[24] Normal brain image in the coronal cutting section by tomographic ultrasound imaging and the thick-slice silhouette image from the same 3D volume dataset are shown in **Figure 17**. In **Figure 18A**, although it is difficult to grasp the abnormal structure by silhouette ultrasound image **(Fig. 18B)**, it is easy to understand by demonstrating the dorsal sac associated with holoprosencephaly by thick-slice silhouette imaging **(Fig. 18C)**. **Figure 19** shows thick-slice images of hydrocephalus at 19 weeks of gestation.

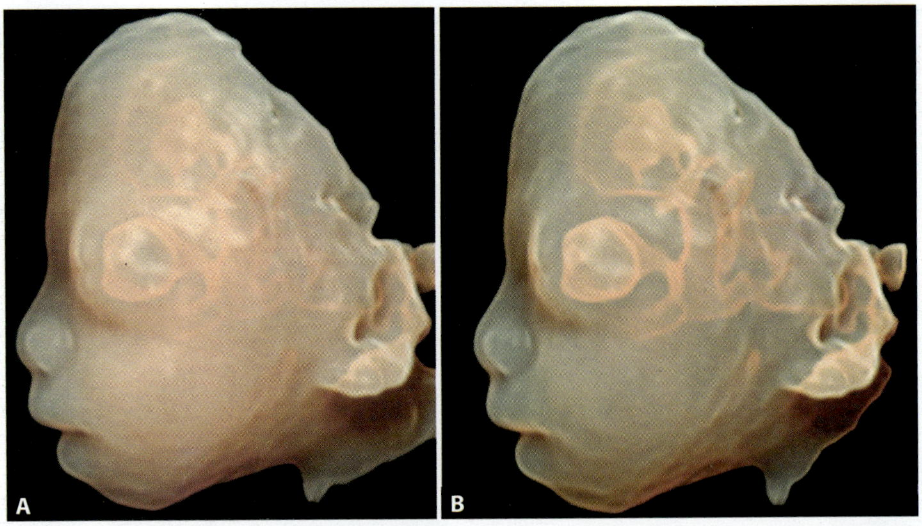

Figs. 14A and B: Exophthalmos by HDlive silhouette imaging at 20 weeks of gestation; (A) Profile image with HDlive silhouette. Exophthalmos is demonstrated; (B) Same image with different HDlive silhouette degree. Inner eyeball is well-depicted.

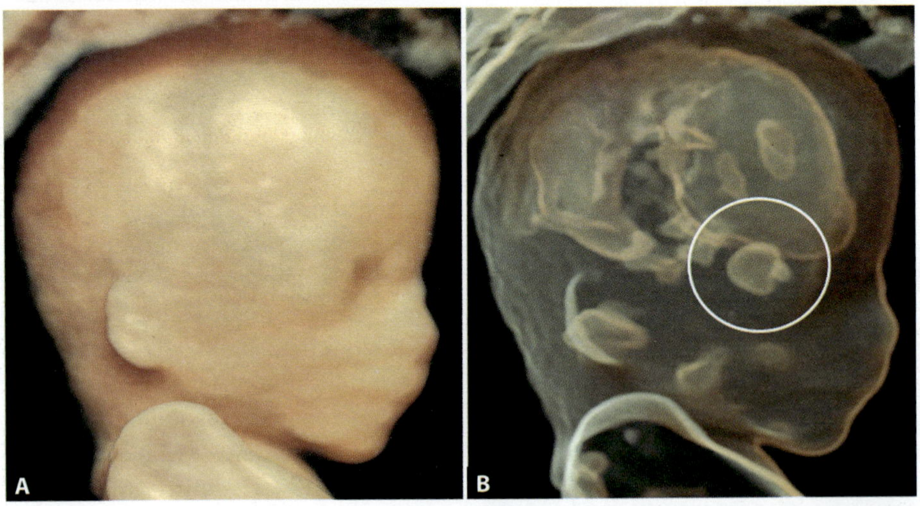

Figs. 15A and B: Eye lens and vitreous body at 13 weeks of gestation. Both images are the same volume dataset. Left image is HDlive image and right image is HDlive silhouette image. Silhouette ultrasound demonstrates eye lens and vitreous body (in circle).

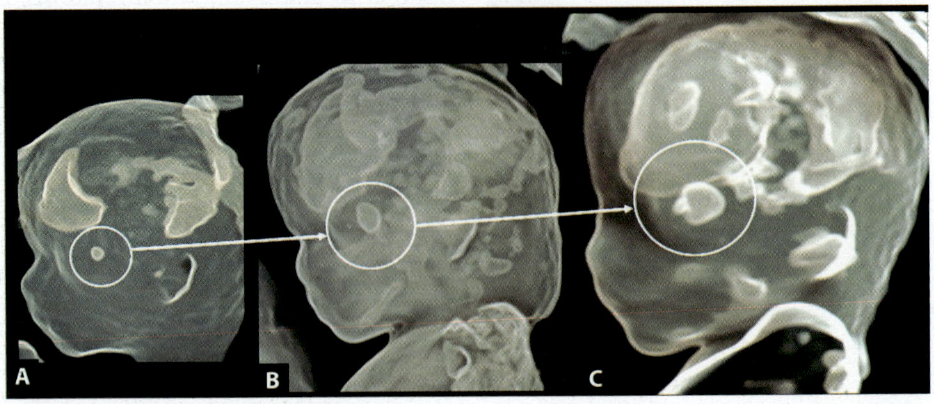

Figs. 16A to C: Silhouette visualization of eyeball development between 12 and 13 weeks; (A) At the beginning of 12 weeks, a small cystic part appears (white circle); (B) At the middle of 12 weeks, the eyeball is depicted much larger than the figure (A); (C) At 13 weeks, the lens and vitreous body in the eyeball can be identified in most normal cases.

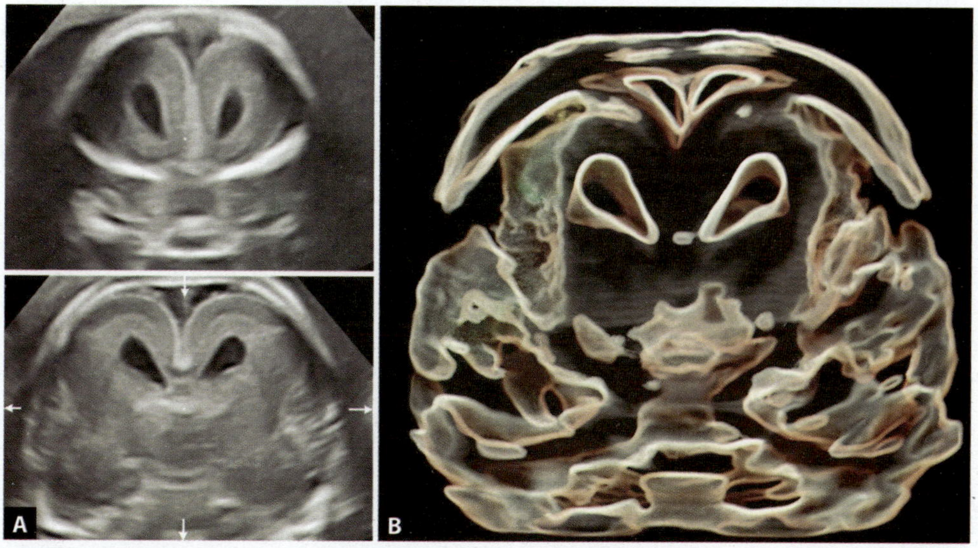

Figs. 17A and B: Thick-slice silhouette of normal brain at 18 weeks of gestation; (A) 2 images are from 3D coronal tomographic images; (B) Thick-slice image from the same 3D volume dataset as the left image.

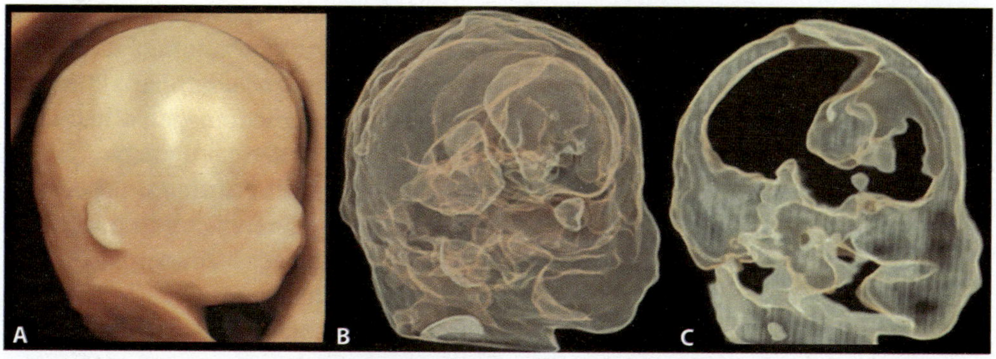

Figs. 18A to C: Different demonstration with HDlive silhouette of holoprosencephaly at 13 weeks of gestation; (A) Surface image of fetal head and face; (B) See-through image of fetal head and intracerebral structure. Abnormally enlarged ventricle with abnormal cystic structure is visible; (C) Thick-slice silhouette demonstration of sagittal sectioned brain. The huge cystic area continued to ventricle was confirmed as the dorsal sac associated with holoprosencephaly.

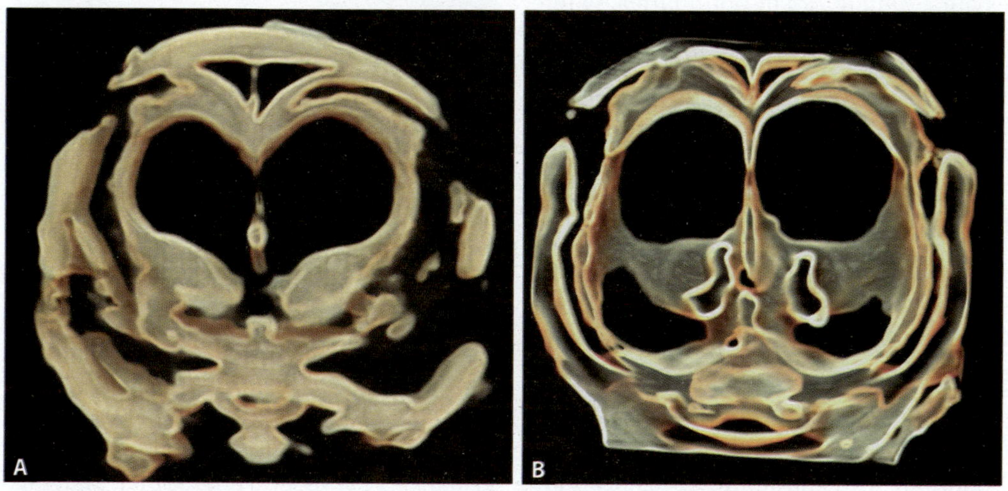

Figs. 19A and B: Hydrocephalus at 19 weeks of gestation by thick-slice imaging; (A) anterior cutting section of coronal section; (B) Posterior cutting section of coronal section.

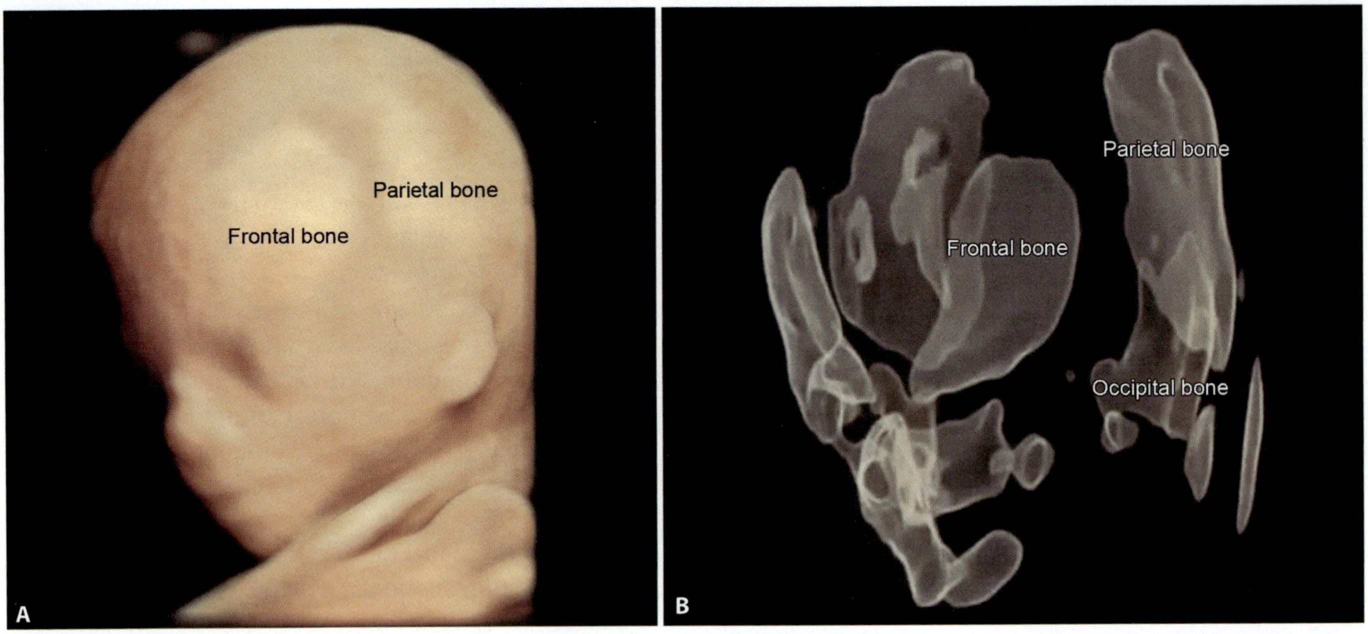

Figs. 20A and B: Cranial bones of 13-week fetus with HDlive silhouette mode; (A) HDlive image of fetal head. Frontal bone and parietal bone are demonstrated through thin skin; (B) Same image with HDlive silhouette mode as the left. Cranial bones (frontal bone, parietal bone, and occipital bone) and facial bones are extracted.

HDlive Silhouette Imaging of Hyperechoic Structures

The utilization of post-processing algorithms such as maximum mode can be used to demonstrate the fetal skeleton. Chaoui et al.[25] reported clear 3D images for the identification of an abnormally wide metopic suture in the second trimester of pregnancy. However, rapid ossification of the craniofacial bones occurs during the first trimester of pregnancy. As described above, HDlive silhouette algorithm creates a gradient at organ boundaries, where an abrupt change of the acoustic impedance exists within tissues. Therefore, silhouette mode can depict not only hypoechoic structure but also hyperechoic structure such as bones.[16] **Figure 20** shows HDlive silhouette image extracting frontal, parietal and occipital bones and **Figure 21** shows the anterior fontanelle at 16 weeks. The vertebrae and ribs can be visualized from small fetus **Figure 22** and interestingly extracted skeletal system is demonstrated in the early second trimester as shown in **Figure 23**. The image showing extracted bony structure is comprehensive as 3D-CT or X-ray. **Figure 24** shows lumber spina bifida by silhouette ultrasound. Limb abnormalities such as polydactyly and clubfoot with silhouette ultrasound are demonstrated in **Figures 25 and 26**.

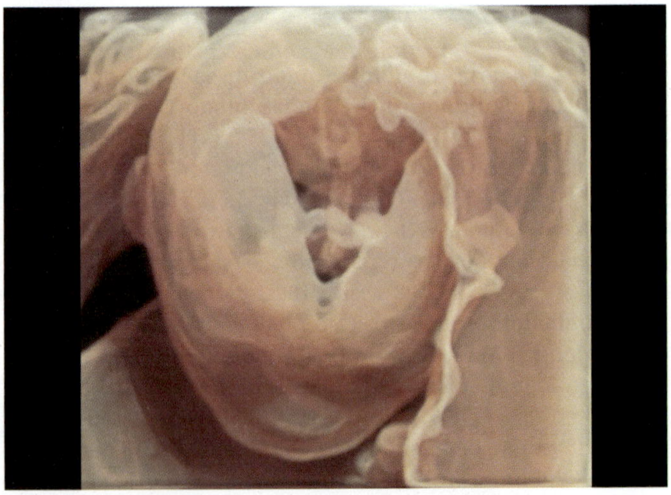

Fig. 21: Anterior fontanelle at 16 weeks by HDlive silhouette imaging.

Thus, silhouette ultrasound can demonstrate the bony structure and may possess a great potential of investigating skeletal dysplasia from early pregnancy.

HDLIVE FLOW IMAGING TECHNOLOGY

The development of the embryonic circulation became visualized by 3D power Doppler imaging technology.[3] In 1993 and 1994, color Doppler detection and assessment

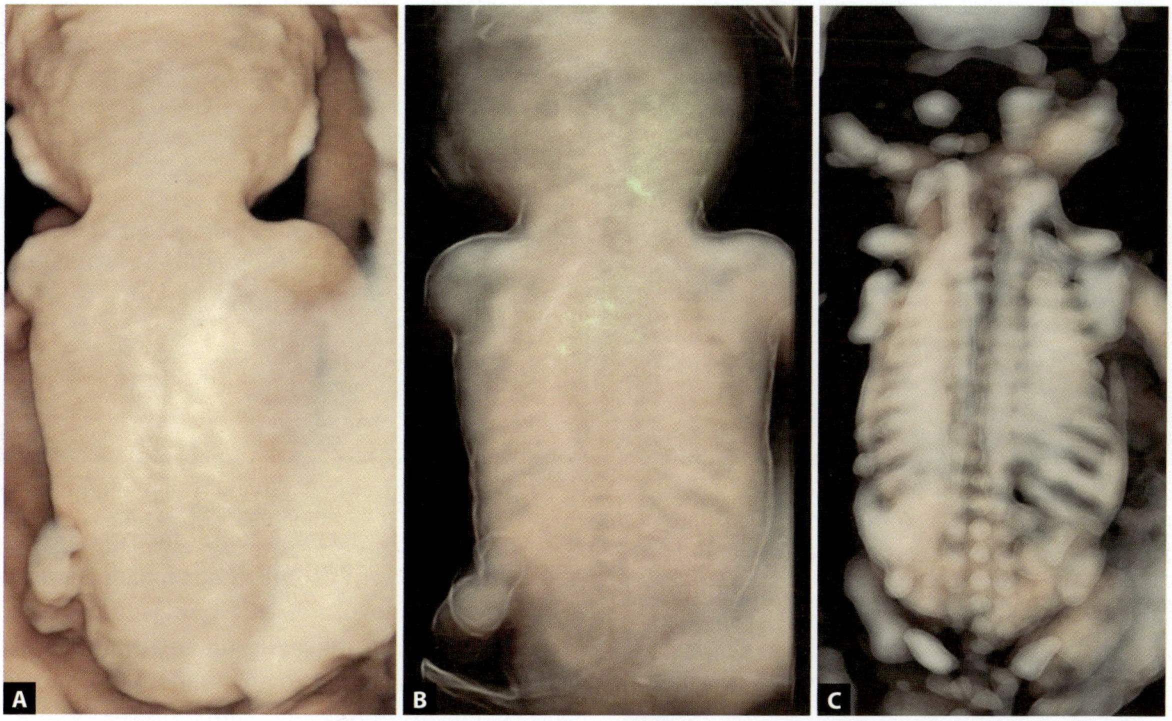

Figs. 22A to C: Vertebrae and ribs of 12-week-fetus with HDlive silhouette; (A) HDlive image of fetal back; (B and C) Same volume dataset with HDlive silhouette. Skeletal structure is emphasized by silhouette mode.

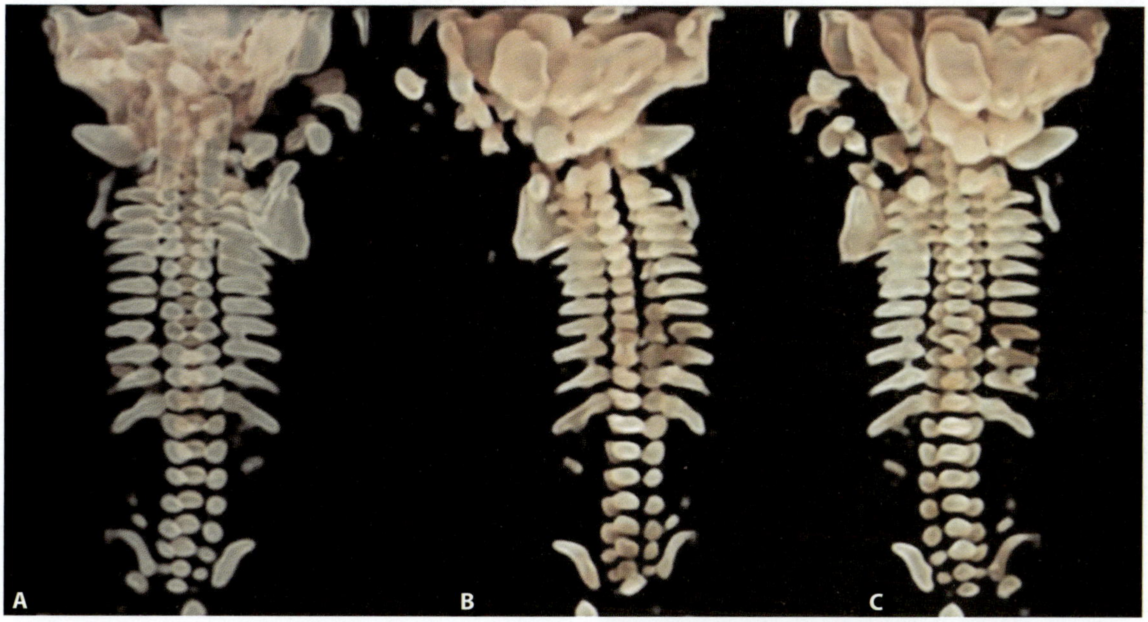

Figs. 23A to C: Vertebrae, ribs and illia by HDlive silhouette imaging at 18 weeks of gestation; (A) Posterior-anterior view; (B) Oblique-anterior view; (C) Anterior-posterior view.

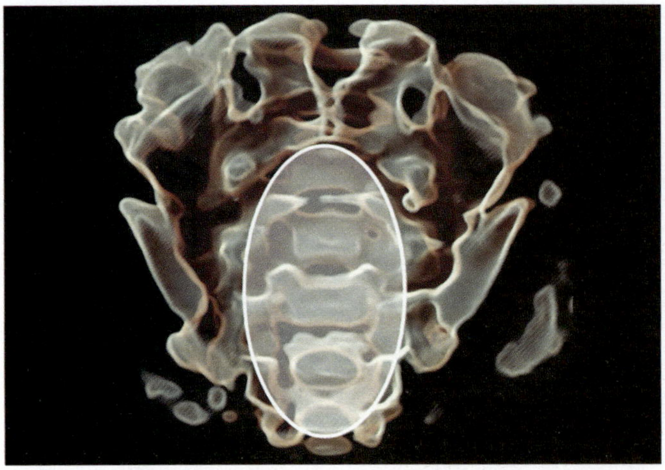

Fig. 24: Spina bifida at 31 weeks of gestation by HDlive silhouette. Vertebral structure is well-demonstrated by HDlive silhouette imaging. The lamina opening (white circle) indicates spina bifida.

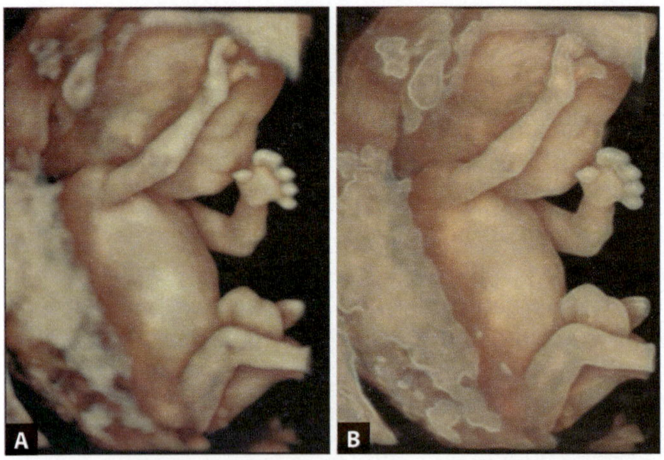

Figs. 25A and B: Polydactyly of the fetus with trisomy 13 by HDlive silhouette at 13 weeks of gestation; (A) Conventional HDlive image. 6 fingers are well-demonstrated; (B) Same image with HDlive silhouette image. Finger bones are demonstrated.

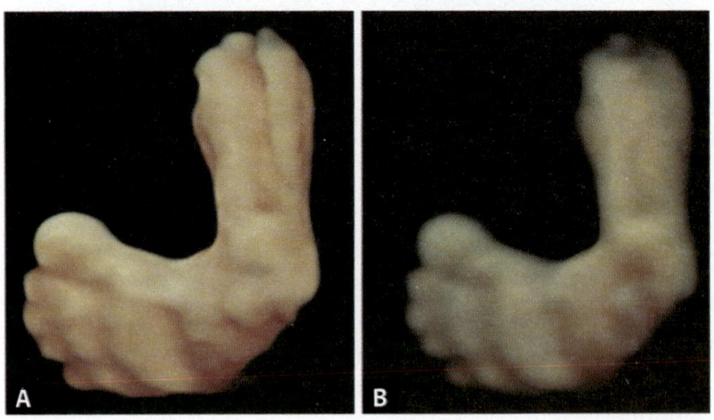

Figs. 26A and B: Clubfoot by HDlive silhouette imaging at 18 weeks of gestation; (A) Conventional HDlive image; (B) Same image with HDlive silhouette showing bony structure of the toe.

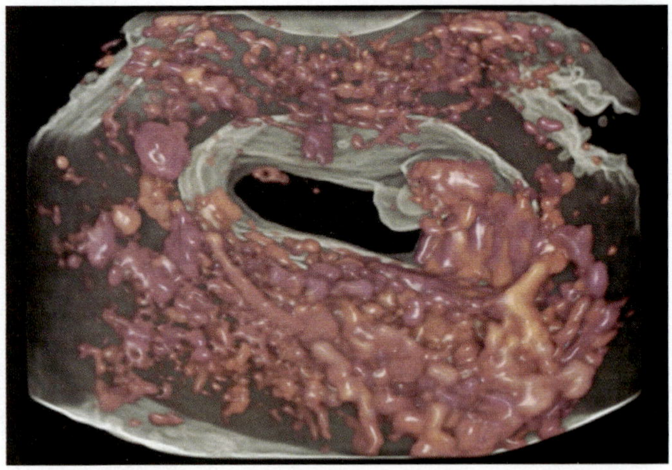

Fig. 27: Intrauterine vascularity by HDlive silhouette and flow imaging at 6 weeks of gestation. Inside of gestational sac, embryonal vascularity and rich vascularity area on the sac wall are well-demonstrated. This rich vascularized area will become the placenta.

of brain vessels in the early fetus using a transvaginal approach was reported.[26,27] In 1996, the author reported clear visualization by transvaginal power Doppler of the common carotid arteries, internal/external carotid arteries and middle cerebral arteries at 12 weeks of gestation.[28]

HDlive flow[14-18] is a recent application of three-dimensional (3D) ultrasound technology generating a 3D-view of the blood flow and providing a realistic rendering of fine vascular structure. Combination of HDlive silhouette and HDlive flow can be described as a 'see-through fashion,'[14] because of its comprehensive orientation and persuasive localization of inner structure as well as of fetal angiostructure inside the morphological structure.

By using advanced technology of HDlive flow combined with HDlive silhouette, intrauterine vascularity imaging at 6 weeks of gestation is clearly demonstrated **(Fig. 27)**. Fetal intracorporeal hemodynamic structure can be demonstrated from early embryo **(Fig. 28)**, showing premature vessels toward the midbrain at 8 weeks of gestation. **Figures 29 and 30** demonstrate normal intracorporeal angiostructure by 3D HDlive silhouette/flow imaging with bidirectional power Doppler at 13 and 20 weeks of gestation respectively. The umbilical arteries, umbilical vein, ductus venosus, inferior vena cava, descending aorta as well as rich pulmonary vascularity are clearly demonstrated in a single 3D reconstructed image. Those images indicate existence of rich pulmonary vascularity from even before lung maturation from the first trimester.[18] Cord insertion and coiling of the cord and

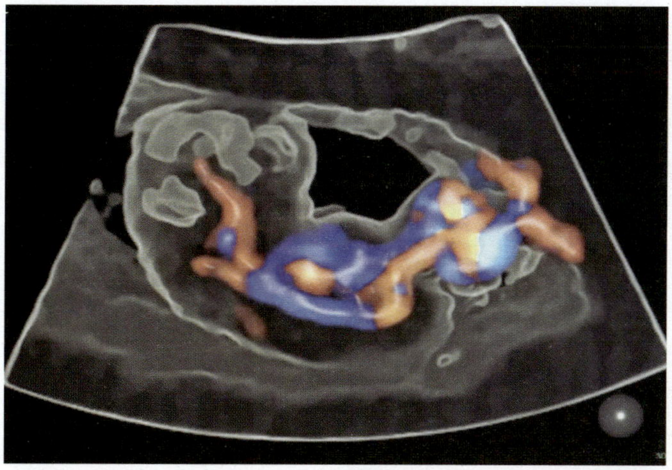

Fig. 28: Intracorporeal hemodynamic structure by HDlive silhouette and flow imaging at 8 weeks of gestation. Vascular structure is demonstrated with fetal body surface by silhouette mode. Premature brain cavities of forebrain, midbrain and hindbrain as well as fetal whole vascular structure are simultaneously demonstrated in the fetal body. Note the premature blood vessel of the central nervous system towards the brain cavity.

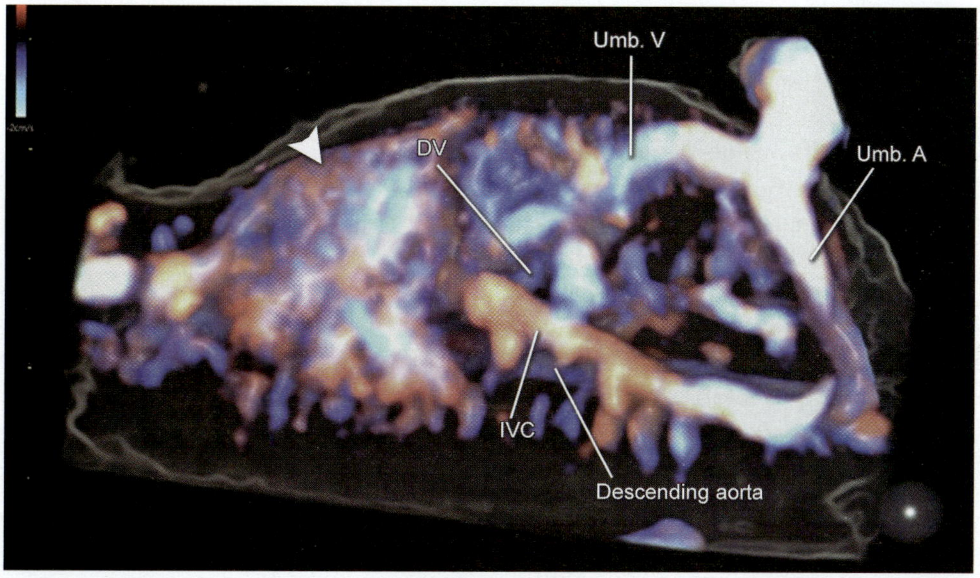

Fig. 29: 13-week-fetal thoracoabdominal vascular structure demonstrated by HDlive flow imaging. Pulmonary arteries and veins (arrowhead) are well-demonstrated. Recent advanced imaging technology of HDlive flow showing pulmonary vasculature from the first trimester may have a great potential to investigate fetal lung development and maturity from early gestation. (DV: ductus venosus; IVC: inferior vena cava; Umb. V: umbilical vein; Umb. A: umbilical artery)

cord abnormality can be easily demonstrated as shown in **Figures 31 and 32**. Intracardiac vascular structure at 12 weeks of gestation is also well demonstrated in **Figure 33**, showing dynamic flows in each right and left heart and crossing of the great arteries. **Figure 34** demonstrates intracardiac HDlive flow image in a case of tetralogy of Fallot at 15 weeks of gestation. Brain vascularity network is created rapidly and precisely. **Figure 35** shows comprehensive cervicocranial vascular hemodynamic structure with internal carotid artery, anterior and middle cerebral arteries at 13 weeks of gestation. By 20 weeks of gestation, brain develops remarkably according to vascular networking **(Figs. 36 and 37)**. Medullary veins are well-demonstrated between pia matter and subependymal zone at 29 weeks of gestation **(Fig. 38)**. As mentioned above, silhouette ultrasound will contribute to a new field

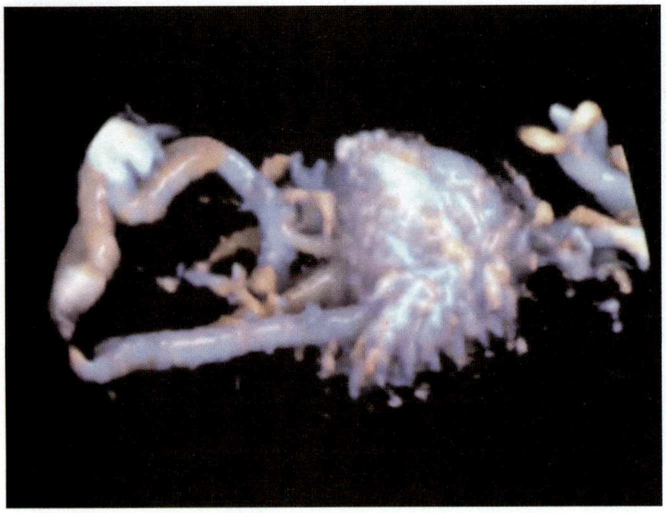

Fig. 30: Thoracoabdominal vascular structure by HDlive flow at 20 weeks of gestation. Pulmonary vascular structure, descending aorta, umbilical artery, umbilical vein, ductus venosus and inferior vena cava are well-demonstrated. Note rich vascularity of the lung.

of "sono-ophthalmology". HDlive flow furthermore adds the vascular information such as the hyaloid artery inside eyeball **(Fig. 39)**. The hyaloid artery is retrogressing during pregnancy and no remnant hyaloid artery is visible in most of mature neonates. Therefore, hyaloid artery can be observed in only young fetuses and immature neonates.

Thus, HDlive flow imaging provides us much more detailed clinical information on the fetal vascularity and hemodynamics than conventional sonoangiogram.

Clinical Significance and Pitfalls of HDlive Silhouette and Flow Imaging

By using HDlive silhouette imaging, inner structure can be demonstrated with outer surface without cutting the image. Furthermore non-cystic structure as well as cystic structure can be demonstrated, such as bony structure. Skeletal image by HDlive silhouette may be similar to 3D-CT therefore investigation of skeletal system

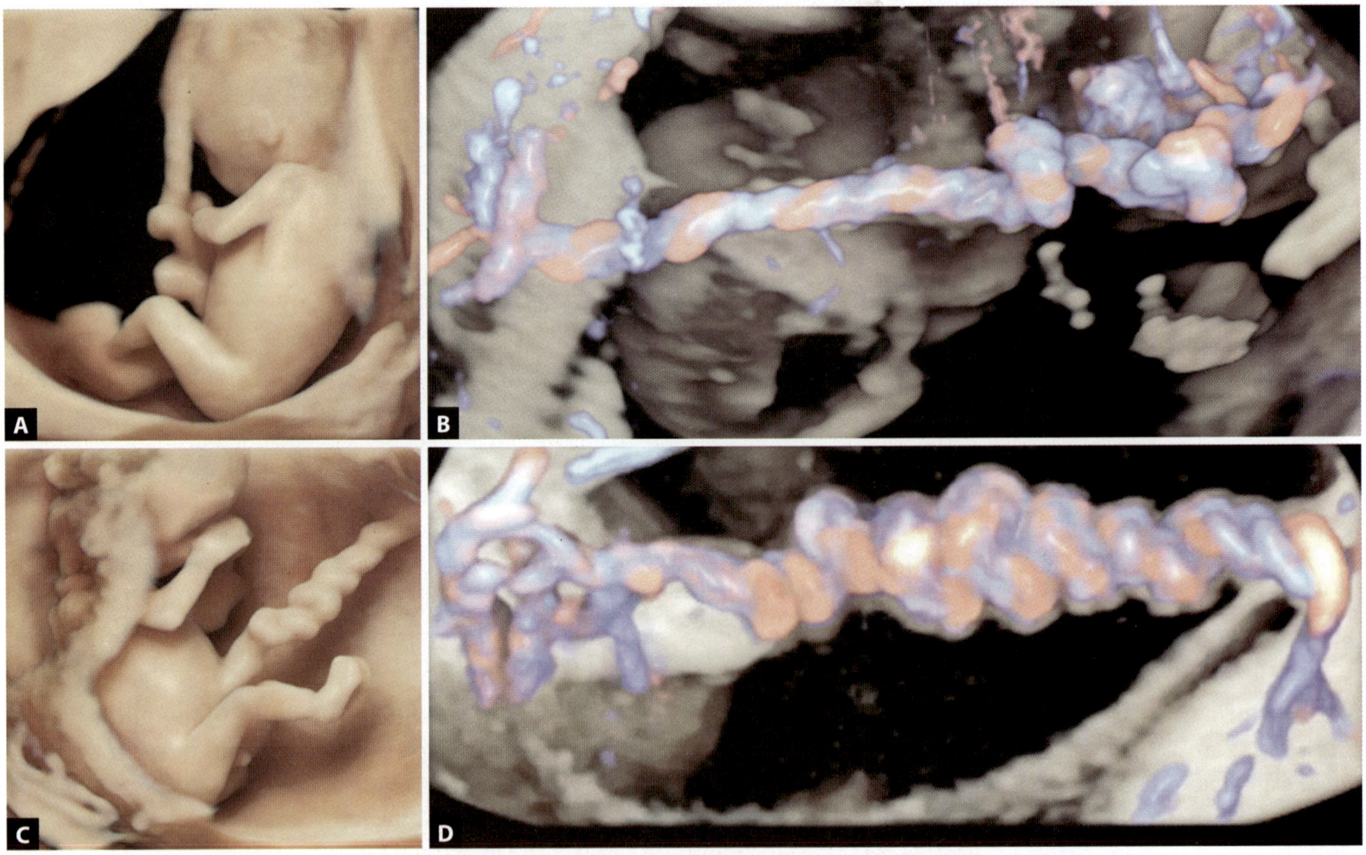

Figs. 31A to D: Normal umbilical cord and excessive coiling cord by HDlive silhouette and flow imaging at 12 weeks of gestation; (A) HDlive fetal and umbilical cord image; (B) HDlive silhouette and flow image of the cord of fetus A; (C) HDlive fetal and excessive coiling cord image; (D) HDlive silhouette and flow image of the cord of fetus C. Note the high-pitch of coils seen in image D compared to image B.

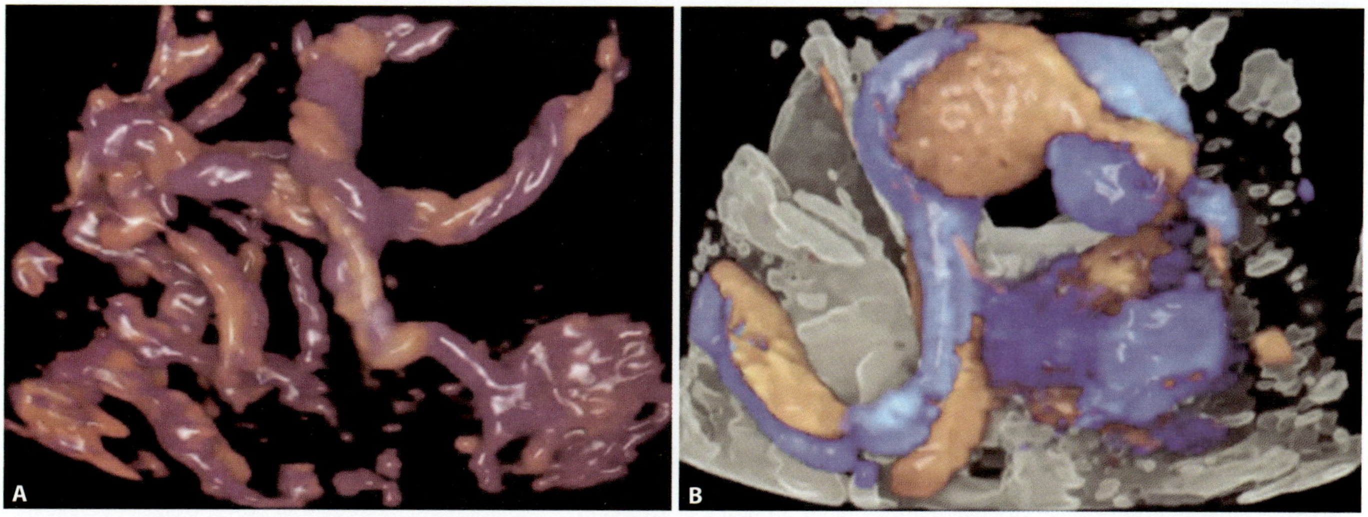

Figs. 32A and B: Normal floating cord and umbilical arterial aneurysm by HDlive silhouette and flow imaging at 19–20 weeks of gestation; (A) Normal floating cord at 19 weeks; (B) Umbilical arterial aneurysm at 20 weeks. Note the dilated umbilical artery with straight cord.

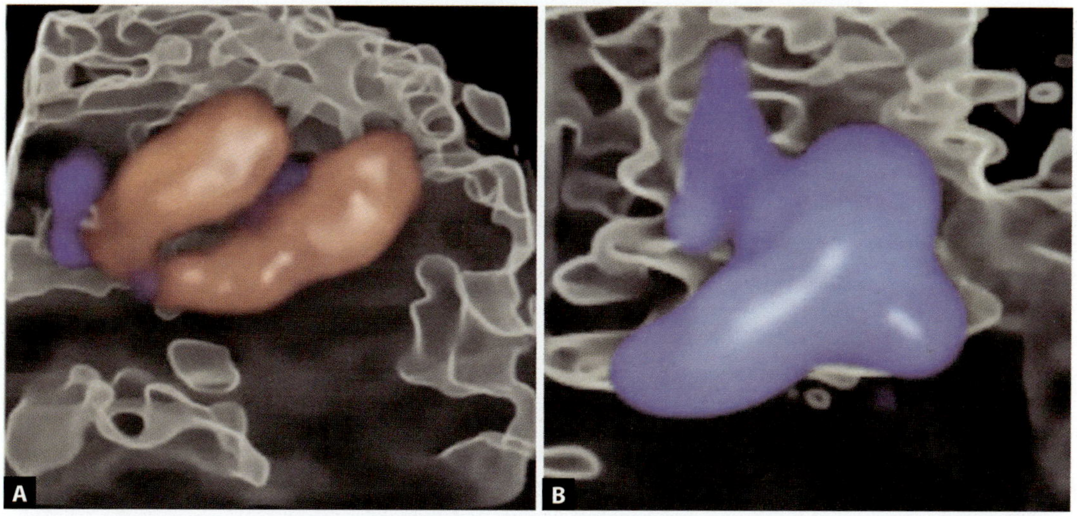

Figs. 33A and B: Normal cardiac hemodynamic imaging by HDlive silhouette and flow at 12 weeks of gestation; (A) Intracardiac angiostructure. Flows of right and left heart are visible; (B) Crossing of great arteries are well-demonstrated.

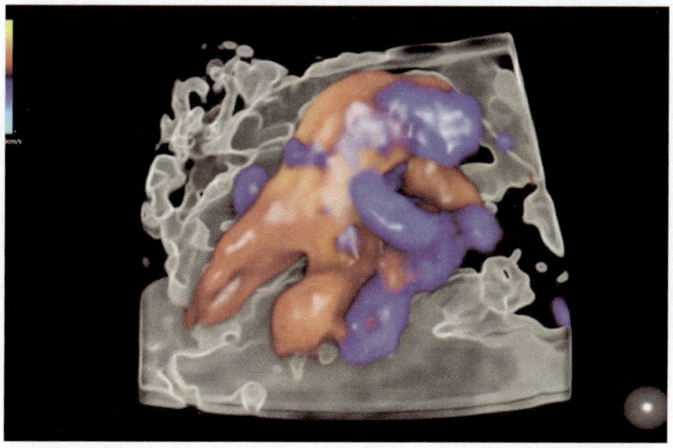

Fig. 34: Tetralogy of Fallot by HDlive silhouette and flow imaging at 15 weeks of gestation: Note the overriding aortic flow from both right and left ventricles.

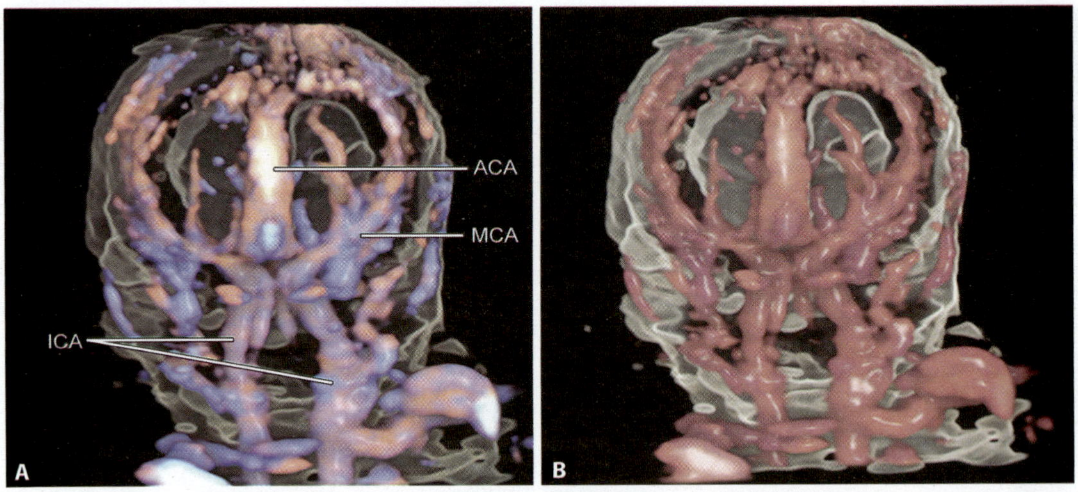

Figs. 35A and B: Cervicocranial vascular hemodynamic structure at 13 weeks of gestation; (A) Bidirectional power Doppler HDlive flow image of brain vasculature of 12-week-fetus; (B) The same ultrasound angiogram dataset with unicolor demonstration. (ACA: anterior cerebral artery; MCA: middle cerebral artery; ICA: internal carotid artery)

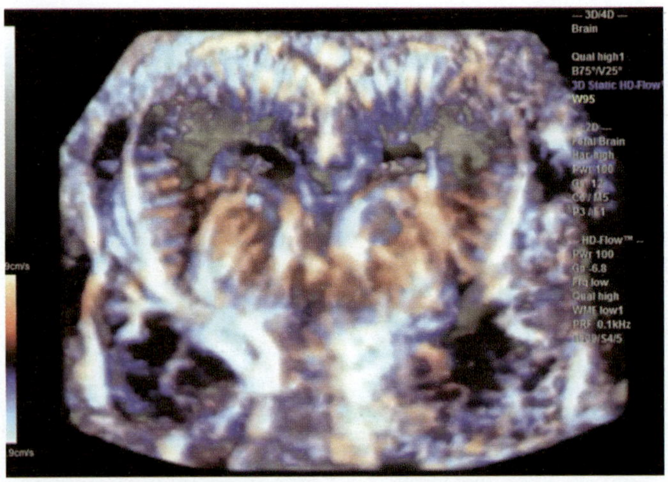

Fig. 36: Normal intracranial sonoangiogram at 19 weeks by HDlive flow imaging: Brain vascular networking is well-created as early as 19 weeks.

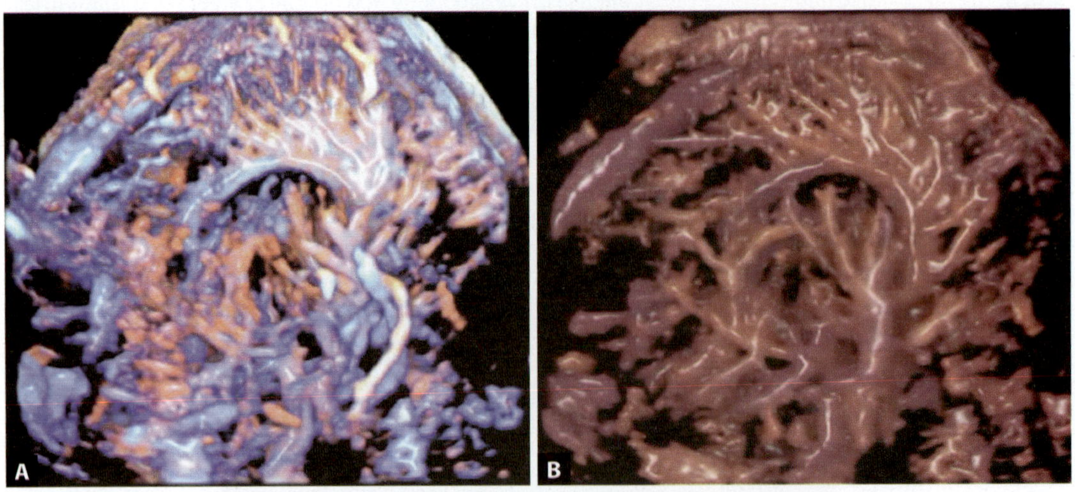

Figs. 37A and B: Normal brain vascular structure by HDlive flow imaging at 20 weeks of gestation; (A) Bidirectional power Doppler 3D HDlive flow image of fetal vascular structure; (B) Monocolor HDlive flow image.

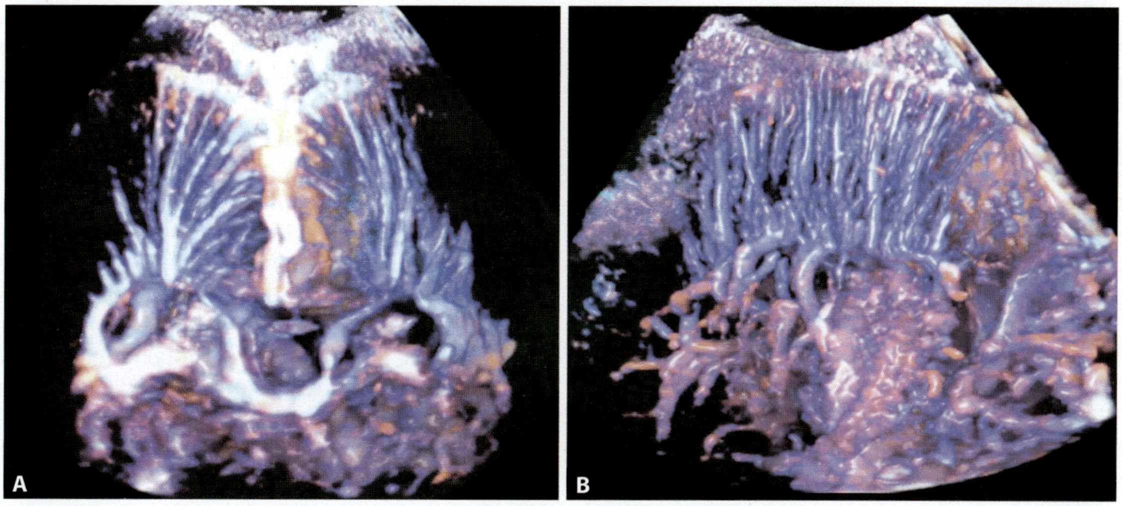

Figs. 38A and B: Normal cerebral medullary veins by HDlive flow imaging at 29 weeks of gestation; (A) Coronal image; (B) Sagittal image. Numerous fine medullary veins between cerebral surface and subependymal zone are well-demonstrated.

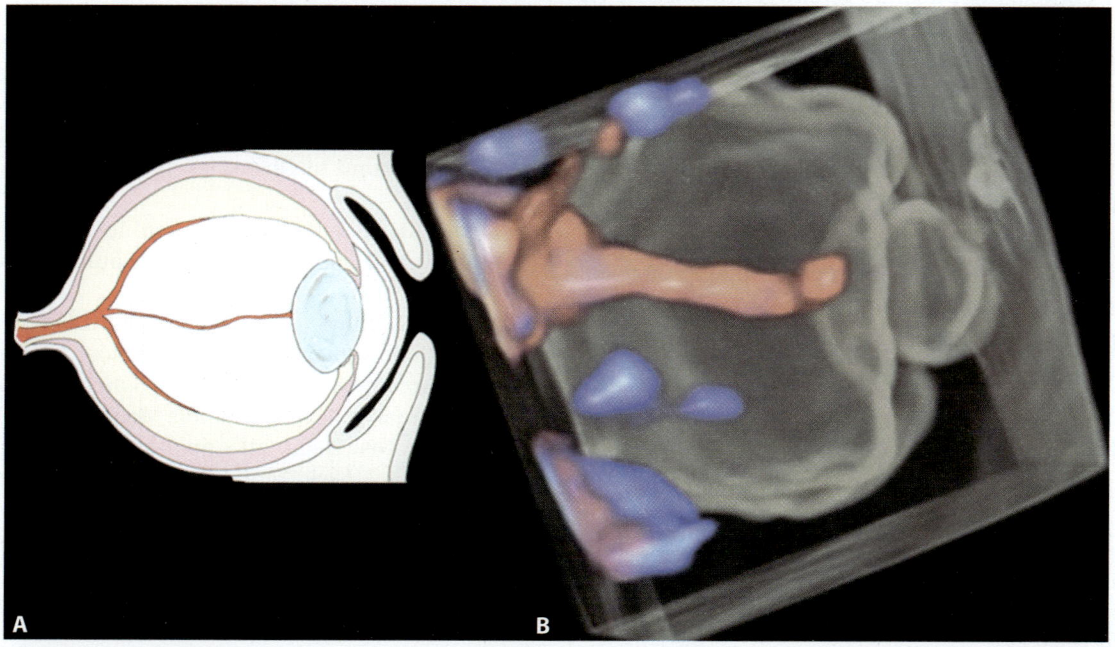

Figs. 39A and B: Vitreous humor, lens and hyaloid artery by HDlive silhouette and flow imaging at 19 weeks of gestation; (A) Schematic picture of the fetal eyeball. Hyaloid artery runs to the lens along with central canal inside vitreous humor; (B) HDlive silhouette and flow imaging of the eye at 19 weeks. Vitreous humor, lens and hyaloid artery are well-demonstrated.

diseases by HDlive silhouette imaging with noninvasive technology will be one of our challenges in prenatal imaging diagnosis. HDlive flow imaging demonstrated fine peripheral blood vessels such as vascularity of the lung, brain and eyeballs. Moreover, HDlive flow combined with silhouette mode demonstrates the precise location of vascularity inside fetal organs and may add further clinical information of vascularization. However, examiners should consider pitfalls of HDlive silhouette imaging. The degree of gain, threshold, and silhouette or combination of those, it is possible to create completely different images with different clinical information from a single volume dataset.[14] This fact expands flexibility of imaging and demonstration, however, can create virtual reality. For obtaining accurate clinical information, examiners should consider that they might create false images and incorrect clinical information.

CONCLUSION

As described in this article, 'see-through fashion' imaging technology provides us comprehensive orientation and persuasive localization of inner morphological structure as well as of angiostructure inside the fetal organs. Conventional technology has detected morphological structure and angiostructure independently, however simultaneous demonstration of both morphology and circulation can potentially provide more accurate clinical information for prenatal diagnoses and proper perinatal management.[12]

Prenatal ultrasound has established sonoembryology and neurosonology. HDlive silhouette and flow imaging add further clinical significance to conventional 3D/4D imaging in those fields and may open up a new field of *sono-ophthalmology*.[17,24]

HDlive silhouette and flow technologies allow extending the detection of congenital anomalies to an earlier gestational age, and it is beyond description that non-invasive direct viewing of the embryo/fetus by all-inclusive ultrasound technology is definitely the first modality in a field of prenatal diagnosis and help our goal of proper perinatal care and management, even in the era of molecular genetics and advanced sequencing of fetal DNA in the maternal blood.[24]

REFERENCES

1. Timor-Tritsch IE, Peisner DB, Raju S. Sonoembryology: an organ-oriented approach using a high-frequency vaginal probe. J Clin Ultrasound. 1990;18(4):286-98.
2. Benoit B, Hafner T, Kurjak A, Kupesic S, Bekavac I, Bozek T. Three-dimensional sonoembryology. J Perinat Med. 2002;30(1):63-73.
3. Kurjak A, Pooh RK, Merce LT, Carrera JM, Salihagic-Kadic A, Andonotopo W. Structural and functional early human development assessed by three-dimensional (3D) and four-dimensional (4D) sonography. Fertil Steril. 2005;84(5):1285-99.
4. Pooh RK, Shiota K, Kurjak A. Imaging of the human embryo with magnetic resonance imaging microscopy and high-resolution transvaginal 3-dimensional sonography: human embryology in the 21st century. Am J Obstet Gynecol. 2011;204(1):77.e1-16.
5. Pooh RK. 3D Sonoembryology. DSJUOG. 2011;5(1):7-15.
6. Pooh RK. Early detection of fetal abnormality. DSJUOG. 2013;7(1):46-50.
7. Pooh RK, Kurjak A. Editorial. 3D/4D sonography moved prenatal diagnosis of fetal anomalies from the second to the first trimester of pregnancy. The Journal of Maternal-Fetal and Neonatal Medicine. 2012;25(5):433-55.
8. Grigore M, Cojocaru C, Lazar T. The role of HD Live Technology in Obstetrics and Gynecology, Present and Future. DSJUOG. 2014;8(3):234-8.
9. Bonilla-Musoles F, Raga F, Castillo JC, Bonilla F Jr, Climent MT, Caballero O. High definition Real-Time Ultrasound (HDlive) of embryonic and fetal malformations before week 16. DSJUOG. 2013;7(1):1-8.
10. Nebeker J, Nelson R. Imaging of sound speed reflection ultrasound tomography. JUM. 2012;31(9):1389-404.
11. Kagan KO, Pintoffl K, Hoopmann M. First-trimester ultrasound images using HDlive. Ultrasound Obstet Gynecol. 2011;38(5):607.
12. Hata T, Hanaoka U, Tenkumo C, Sato M, Tanaka H, Ishimura M. Three- and four-dimensional HDlive rendering images of normal and abnormal fetuses: pictorial essay. Arch Gynecol Obstet. 2012;286(6):1431-5.
13. Pooh RK, Kurjak A. Novel application of three-dimensional HDlive imaging in prenatal diagnosis from the first trimester. Journal of Perinatal Medicine. 2015;43(2):147-58.
14. Pooh RK. First Trimester Scan by 3D, 3D HDlive and HDlive Silhouette/Flow Ultrasound Imaging. Donald School Journal of Ultrasound in Obstetrics and Gynecology. 2015;9(4):361-71.
15. Pooh RK. 'See-through Fashion' in Prenatal Diagnostic Imaging. Donald School J Ultrasound Obstet Gynecol. 2015;9(2):111.
16. Pooh RK. Brand new technology of HDlive silhouette and HDlive flow images. In Donald School Atlas of Advanced Ultrasound in Obstetrics and Gynecology by Pooh RK and Kurjak A. Jaypee Brothers Medical Publishers Private Limited, New Delhi, 2015. pp. 1-39.
17. Pooh RK. A New Field of 'Fetal Sono-ophthalmology by 3D HDlive Silhouette and Flow. Donald School Journal of Ultrasound in Obstetrics and Gynecology. July-September 2015;9(3):221-2.
18. Pooh RK. 13-week Pulmonary Sonoangiogram by 3D HDlive Flow. Donald School Journal of Ultrasound in Obstetrics and Gynecology, October-December 2015;9(4):355-6.
19. AboEllail MAM, Kanenishi K, Mori N, Kurobe A, Hata T. HDlive imaging of circumvallate placenta. Ultrasound Obstet Gynecol. 2015;46:513-4.
20. Blaas HG, Eik-Nes SH, Berg S, Torp H. In-vivo three-dimensional ultrasound reconstructions of embryos and early fetuses. Lancet. 1998;352(9135):1182-86.
21. Kim MS, Jeanty P, Turner C, Benoit B. Three-dimensional sonographic evaluations of embryonic brain development. J Ultrasound Med. 2008;27(1):119-24.
22. Hata T, Dai SY, Kanenishi K, Tanaka H. Three-dimensional volume-rendered imaging of embryonic brain vesicles using inversion mode. J Obstet Gynaecol Res. 2009;35(2):258-61.

23. Pooh RK. Neurosonoembryology by three-dimensional ultrasound. Semin Fetal Neonatal Med 2012;17(5):261-8.
24. Pooh RK. Sonoembryology by 3D HDlive silhouette ultrasound. What is added by the 'see-through fashion'? J Perinat Med in press, 2016.
25. Chaoui R, Levaillant JM, Benoit B, Faro C, Wegrzyn P, Nicolaides KH. Three-dimensional sonographic description of abnormal metopic suture in second- and third-trimester fetuses. Ultrasound Obstet Gynecol. 2005;26(7): 761-4.
26. Kurjak A, Zudenigo D, Predanic M, Kupesic S. Recent advances in the Doppler study of early fetomaternal circulation. J Perinat Med. 1993;21(6):419-39.
27. Kurjak A, Schulman H, Predanic A, Predanic M, Kupesic S, Zalud I. Fetal choroid plexus vascularization assessed by color flow ultrasonography. J Ultrasound Med. 1994; 13(11):841-4.
28. Pooh RK, Aono T. Transvaginal power Doppler angiography of the fetal brain. Ultrasound Obstet Gynecol 1996;8(6):417-21.

8

CHAPTER

Normal and Abnormal Early Pregnancy

Tamara Illescas, Waldo Sepulveda

INTRODUCTION

Ultrasound (US) is nowadays an integral part of antenatal care and, due to the wide availability of transvaginal (TV) probes and dramatic improvement in image resolution, its use during the first trimester of pregnancy is the standard of care worldwide.

Early pregnancy is a period of uncertainty, especially during the first three postconceptional weeks, since the size of the structures will not be within the range for US evaluation. Vaginal bleeding is the main physical sign associated to pathology in early pregnancy; in this scenario, a TV US scan is mandatory to ascertain the location and viability of the pregnancy and to rule out conditions such as miscarriage, ectopic pregnancy, or trophoblastic disease.

The first-trimester US examination must be performed by adequately trained and accredited professionals. A deep knowledge of embryology and pregnancy development features is needed to identify and distinguish normal from abnormal findings. Determination of maternal serum β-hCG levels is an important complementary diagnostic tool for the evaluation of early pregnancy and the detection of pathological conditions.

It is important to keep in mind that no therapeutic decisions must be taken until the clinician is certain of the location and viability of the pregnancy, as long as the mother remains clinically stable. This means that sometimes the only option to reach a definitive diagnosis is watchful waiting and follow-up scans.

The aim of this chapter is to review the main features leading to a safe interpretation of US findings in early pregnancy in order to distinguish the different clinical conditions including definite normal findings, definite abnormal findings, and uncertain findings that will require further evaluation.

Before starting the US scan, we should obtain some information from the patient's background, such as age, parity, mode of conception, previous gynecological diseases, and other medical conditions. The last menstrual period (LMP) is an especially important piece of information, which should be correlated to the sonographically estimated date of delivery [by measuring the crown-rump length (CRL) if the embryo is visible]. In countries where it is available, pregnant women should be routinely offered a first-trimester US scan between 11 weeks and 13 weeks and 6 days to accurately estimate the gestational age and screen for chromosomal and anatomical fetal abnormalities.[1,2]

In early first trimester, the use of TV US probes is of paramount importance, since the structures to be studied are tiny and may be beyond the resolution limits of transabdominal (TA) probes. Nevertheless, the combined use of both probes can be helpful to first achieve a good survey of the pelvic anatomy and then to proceed into the detailed study of smaller structures with TV US.[3]

- *TA:* Curvilinear transducer (4–7 MHz probe) to obtain a global view of the pelvis and exclude any pelvic pathology (fibroids, ovarian cysts, suspicion of ectopic pregnancy):
  - Look for any obvious myometrial or cervical pathology.
  - Describe any uterine malformation.
  - Scan both adnexa entirely, searching for any obvious ovarian pathology or adnexal masses.
  - Document any amount of free abdominal fluid.
- *TV:* Curvilinear high-frequency transducer (9–12 MHz probe). Closer proximity of the transducer to the structures results in a better display of the pelvic anatomy.

INTRAUTERINE PREGNANCY OF UNKNOWN VIABILITY

During the earliest stages of pregnancy, there are some definitive findings that easily lead to the confirmatory diagnoses of viable intrauterine pregnancy (IUP), ectopic pregnancy, or pregnancy failure. However, other findings are uncertain and would lead to two possibilities, both of which must be handled conservatively until the diagnosis is certain.[4]

Pregnancy of Unknown Location (PUL)

This is the term given to a transient state of early pregnancy during which no definite image of an IUP can be identified by TV US and the adnexa look normal, overall conforming a normal pelvic US scan. In this situation, the three main diagnostic possibilities include:

1. Intrauterine pregnancy.
2. Occult ectopic pregnancy.
3. Pregnancy failure.

Unfortunately, a single determination of β-hCG maternal serum level does not allow reliable differentiation among the three possibilities, thus close surveillance with follow-up US scans and repeated determination of β-hCG maternal serum levels is indicated.

Intrauterine Pregnancy of Unknown Viability

This term can apply to normal situations before development of an embryo with detectable cardiac activity, including:[4]

- An empty intrauterine gestational sac **(Fig. 1)**.
- A gestational sac with a yolk sac but no embryo.
- A gestational sac with a yolk sac and an embryo with a CRL <7 mm but not yet displaying cardiac activity **(Fig. 2)**.

At any of these stages, we can look for signs of poor prognosis on the US scan (see below). Although these signs are suspicious for adverse outcomes, they are not definite and no therapeutic decisions should be taken on its basis.

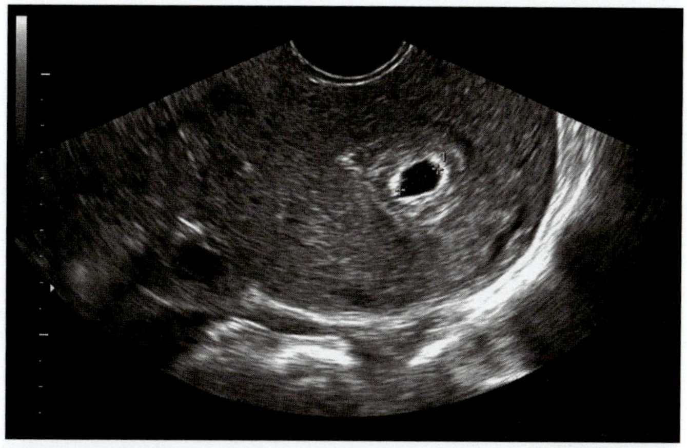

Fig. 1: 'Double-ring' image: The trophoblast appears as an echogenic rim surrounding the gestational sac. The inner ring corresponds to the decidua capsularis, the chorionic villi and the chorion itself; the outer ring is the decidua parietalis. Outside the uterus we can see the corpus luteum.
Source: Delta Ultrasound Diagnostic Center in Obstetrics and Gynecology, Madrid, Spain.

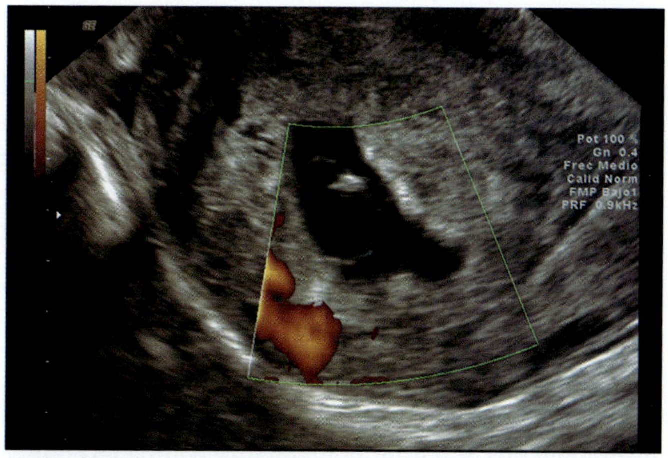

Fig. 2: Intrauterine pregnancy of unknown viability: There is a gestational sac with a yolk sac and an embryo with a CRL of 3 mm, not displaying cardiac activity. There are certain signs indicating a poor prognosis: the CRL is smaller than expected for the LMP and the gestational sac shape is irregular.
Source: Delta Ultrasound Diagnostic Center in Obstetrics and Gynecology, Madrid, Spain.

NORMAL EARLY PREGNANCY

Events Following Implantation

Decidual Reaction

At 31 postmenstrual days the gestational sac is not yet visible. The main intrauterine finding is the identification of a thickened endometrium of 14–16 mm that is hyperechogenic and homogeneous in texture, corresponding to the decidual reaction. It presents sonographically with posterior acoustic enhancement, the middle line between the two endometrial layers is hardly visible, and the limit with the adjacent myometrium is blurry. The decidual reaction is the result of increased hormonal serum levels that, at this early stage of development are independent of pregnancy location.

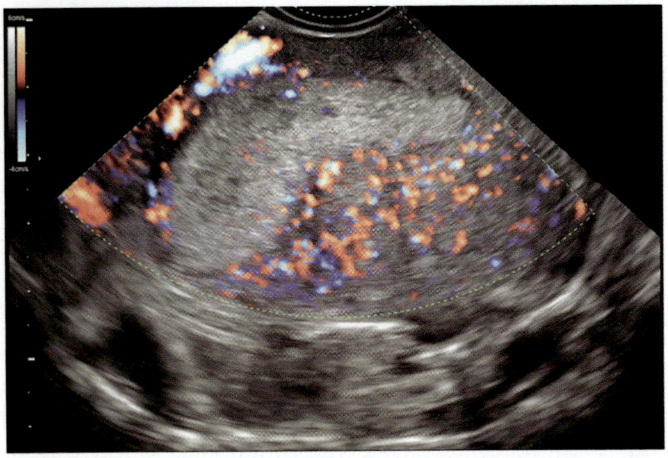

Fig. 3: Pregnancy of unknown location: The gestational sac is not visible yet. There is a thickened hyperechogenic endometrium, corresponding to the decidual reaction. The decidual reaction will manifest, under the hormonal influence, regardless the location of the gestational sac thus the first days after a positive pregnancy test are uncertain and sonographically correspond to a PUL.
Source: Delta Ultrasound Diagnostic Center in Obstetrics and Gynecology, Madrid, Spain.

Forty-eight hours later, direct visualization of a gestational sac (mean diameter of 2.5 mm), eccentrically placed in one of the endometrial leafs, allows the confirmation of an IUP. The decidual reaction can be present regardless the location of the gestational sac; that's why the first days after a positive pregnancy test are uncertain and, sonographically, this finding is classified as a PUL **(Fig. 3)**.[5]

Doppler Changes

The uterine artery resistance index gradually decreases during the first trimester of pregnancy, with a leveling of the protodiastolic notch and an increase of the diastolic flow velocities. These changes are the result of the conversion of spiral arteries into non-muscular dilated tortuous channels with the subsequent decrease in total peripheral resistance to flow (first wave of trophoblast invasion).[6]

The dilated spiral arteries are easily detected with color or power Doppler close to the chorion. They are characterized by relatively lower resistance and higher peak velocities followed by turbulent flow (comet sign) and this finding may be helpful to confirm the placental implantation site. However, the spread use of spectral Doppler is not recommended in the early first trimester, if there is a possibility of a normal viable IUP.[4,6]

Gestational Sac

The gestational sac is expected to be visualized by TV US at 4.5–5 weeks of gestation (β-hCG serum levels >1500 mUI/mL). It is an anechoic image of 1–2 mm surrounded by an echogenic rim, the trophoblast. It is embedded in one of the layers of the decidua, usually in the upper half of the uterine cavity.

In the first weeks of pregnancy, the gestational sac is expected to be round-shaped thus its diameter accurately corresponds to the gestational age: 12, 18, 25, and 35 mm corresponding to 5, 6, 7, and 8 gestational weeks, respectively. After this time, the sac will adapt to the cavity, taking a more irregular shape; the CRL will be the most accurate measurement to establish the probable date of delivery from now on until the end of the first trimester.[5]

Trophoblast Reaction

The trophoblast appears as an echogenic rim, 1–1.5 mm wide, surrounding the gestational sac. From 25 to 28 postconceptional days a 'double-ring' image can be identified: the inner ring corresponds to the decidua capsularis, the chorionic villi, and the chorion itself; the outer ring corresponds to the decidua parietalis **(*see* Fig. 1)**. There is a narrow anechoic band between the two rings, corresponding to the uterine cavity which is not yet obliterated.[7]

The double ring is interrupted in the zone where the chorionic villi join the decidua basalis to form the chorion frondosum, just by the yolk sac. On the opposite side, in the area of the decidua capsularis, the chorionic villi will transform into an avascular shell (chorion laeve) **(Fig. 4)**.[6]

At 8.4 postmenstrual weeks the uterine cavity will be completely obliterated and the double-ring image would transform into a single echogenic and homogeneous ring, 8-mm thick. At 10 weeks of gestation the thickness will vary from 5 mm at the chorion laeve to 20 mm at the chorion frondosum.

In a normal placentation process, the spiral arteries' changes progressively go deep into the inner third of the myometrium, until at the end of the first half of pregnancy all the spiral arteries are transformed into wide blood channels (second wave of trophoblast invasion) **(Fig. 5)**.[6]

Yolk Sac

This is the first structure to be identified within the gestational sac. When the gestational sac is first identified with US, this corresponds almost entirely to the yolk sac

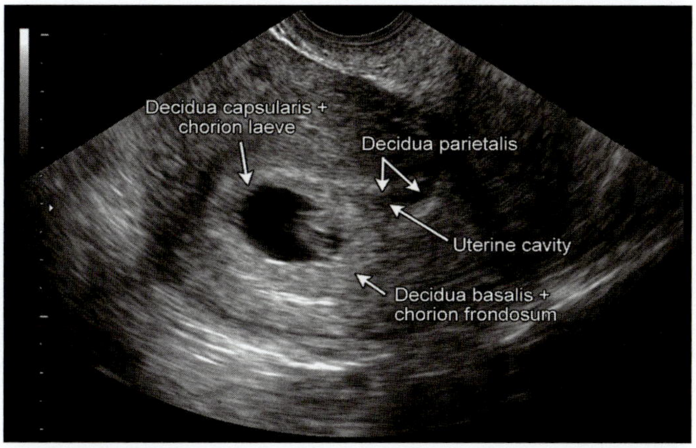

Fig. 4: 7-week pregnancy to illustrate the different decidual and chorionic layers: The characteristic double ring is interrupted in the zone where the chorionic villi join the decidua basalis to form the chorion frondosum near the yolk sac. On the opposite side, in the area of the decidua capsularis, the chorionic villi will transform into an avascular shell (chorion laeve). There is a triangular anechoic area corresponding to the uterine cavity which is not yet obliterated. The patient had a former C-section and the uterine scar on the anterior wall of the uterus casts some acoustic shadowing.
Source: Hospital Universitari Vall d'Hebron, Barcelona, Spain.

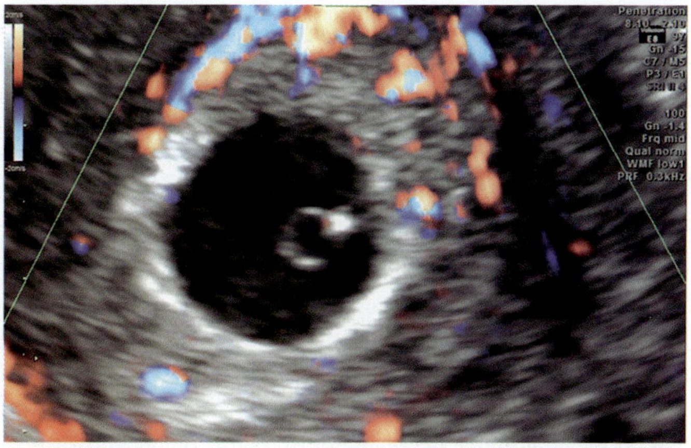

Fig. 5: Early pregnancy: Gestational sac with a yolk sac inside and an embryo smaller than 1 mm. The amnion is hardly discernible and the cardiac activity is not clearly visible yet. The dilated spiral arteries are easily detected with color Doppler close to the chorion frondosum.
Source: Delta Ultrasound Diagnostic Center in Obstetrics and Gynecology, Madrid, Spain.

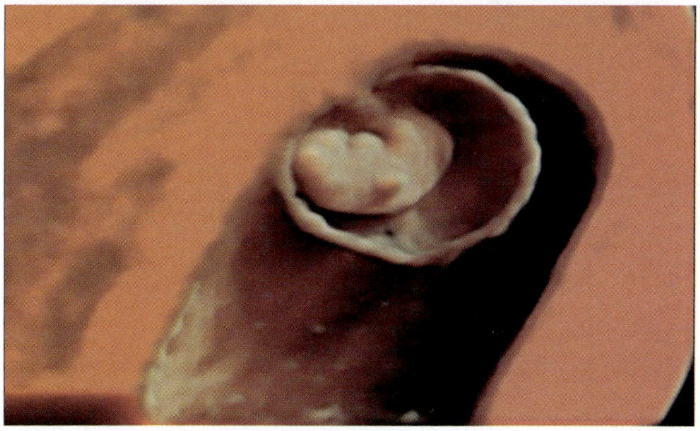

Fig. 6: HD live 3D US: Amnion encircling an embryo; the extraembryonic coelom is still large.
Source: Delta Ultrasound Diagnostic Center in Obstetrics and Gynecology, Madrid, Spain.

surrounded by a thin band of extraembryonic coelom. The yolk sac is the source of pluripotential stem cells, which migrate to the embryo through the vitelline duct, a tubular structure that connects the yolk sac and the embryonic midgut.[6]

The visualization of the yolk sac confirms an IUP and rules out the possibility of an ectopic pregnancy pseudosac. It is visible from the 5th postmenstrual week, with a diameter of 1.5–2 mm, as a round structure of hyperechoic rim and sonoluscent content. It clearly separates from the embryo during the 6th week and is located outside the amniotic cavity, floating in the extraembryonic coelom. Its mean diameter is 5 mm and usually disappears between the 10th and 12th weeks **(Fig. 5)**.[5]

Amnion

At 6–8 weeks of gestation the amnion is visualized as a thin rounded structure encircling the embryo **(Fig. 6)**. Mean amniotic sac diameter is approximately equal to the CRL in normal very early pregnancies[6] so, at these stages, it is not unusual that the embryo is identified before the amnion can be visualized **(Fig. 7)**.

The amniotic cavity size increases with gestation and the distance between the amnion and the chorion is progressively reduced until they are fused in a process that finishes from 10 to 14 weeks of gestation.

Embryo

The Carnegie development stages describe the correlation between gestational age, size, and morphologic characteristics of the embryo. The 8 embryonic weeks (56 days) are divided into 23 stages. According to this classification, it would be possible to know the gestational age by examining the features and matching them with the corresponding Carnegie stages. Theoretically, this might be even more accurate than the CRL, especially during the

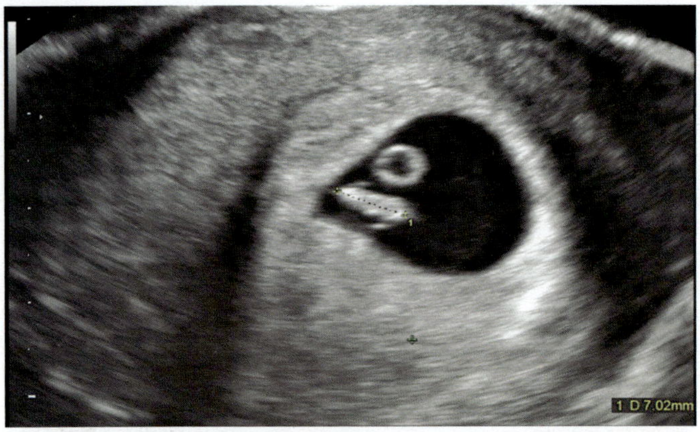

Fig. 7: Mean amniotic sac diameter is approximately equal to the CRL in normal very early pregnancies: The CRL is 7 mm, projecting to a gestational age of 6 weeks 4 days. The yolk sac is patent, while the amnion is hardly visible.
Source: Delta Ultrasound Diagnostic Center in Obstetrics and Gynecology, Madrid, Spain.

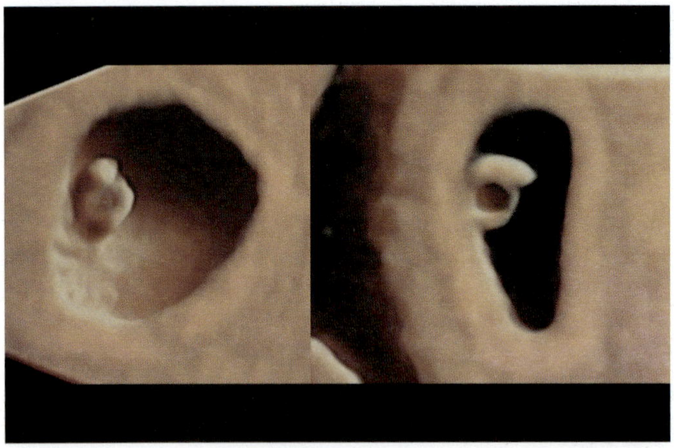

Fig. 8: HDlive 3D US (representation of 2 orthogonal planes): The CRL is 2 mm (consistent with 5 weeks of gestation) and the embryo can be first seen as a thickening on the yolk sac wall (the 'engagement ring' sign), near the trophoblast (12th Carnegie stage). The amnion is not yet discernible.
Source: Delta Ultrasound Diagnostic Center in Obstetrics and Gynecology, Madrid, Spain.

embryonic period. The comparative sonographic study of the embryonic anatomy (sonoembryology) is feasible from the 15th Carnegie stage.[7,8]

When the gestational sac is first identified at 4.5–5 weeks, the embryo measures 0.2 mm and it is beyond reach of the current US resolution so it is sonographically undetectable. At 5.5 weeks (12th Carnegie stage) the embryo's size is 2 mm and we can first see it as a thickening on the yolk sac wall, near the trophoblast (the 'engagement ring' sign, **Fig. 8**).

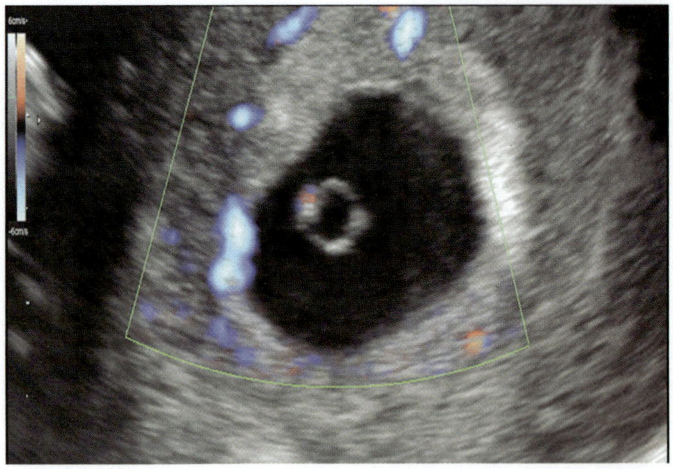

Fig. 9: Embryonic heart activity can be demonstrated from the 3rd post-ovulation week, when the cardiac primordium appears. In a significant proportion of the cases the heart activity cannot be ascertained before the CRL is 3–4 mm; however in this case the cardiac activity can be demonstrated with the use of color Doppler.
Source: Delta Ultrasound Diagnostic Center in Obstetrics and Gynecology, Madrid, Spain.

Embryonic heart activity can be demonstrated from the 3rd post-ovulation week, when the cardiac primordium appears, but in a significant proportion of cases the heart activity cannot be ascertained before the embryo's size gets 3–4 mm at least **(Fig. 9)**.

A summary of the main features to be identified in the main Carnegie stages is described below:

- **15th Carnegie stage** (*7th postmenstrual week, CRL of 7–9 mm*): the embryo is in strong ventral flexion; the cephalic pole and the neural groove are discernible; the four limb buds are visible **(Fig. 10)**.
- **17th and 18th Carnegie stages** (*8–8.4th postmenstrual week, CRL of 13–17 mm*): The body is quite cuboidal and progressively straightens out; the head is relatively large **(Fig. 11)**. Nasofrontal groove and auricular hillocks are distinct **(Fig. 12)**. The digital plate of hand is patent; finger and toe rays appear. Chondrification begins in humerus, radius, and some vertebral centers. The umbilical cord insertion is now discernible. The rhombencephalon is visible as an anechoic vesicle at the top of the head **(Fig. 13)**.
- **20th and 21st Carnegie stages** (*9.3–9.5th postmenstrual week, CRL of 21–24 mm*): The cervical angle widens. The limb segments are distinct and the elbow is flexed. The hands have short and thick fingers and they barely reach one another in front of the trunk, although they approach the thorax and

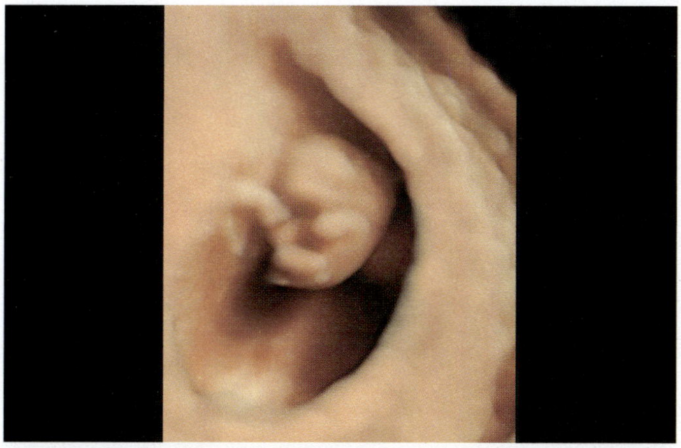

Fig. 10: HDlive 3D US: 15th Carnegie stage (7th postmenstrual week, CRL of 7–9 mm). The embryo is in strong ventral flexion; the cephalic pole and the four limb buds are visible.
Source: Delta Ultrasound Diagnostic Center in Obstetrics and Gynecology, Madrid, Spain.

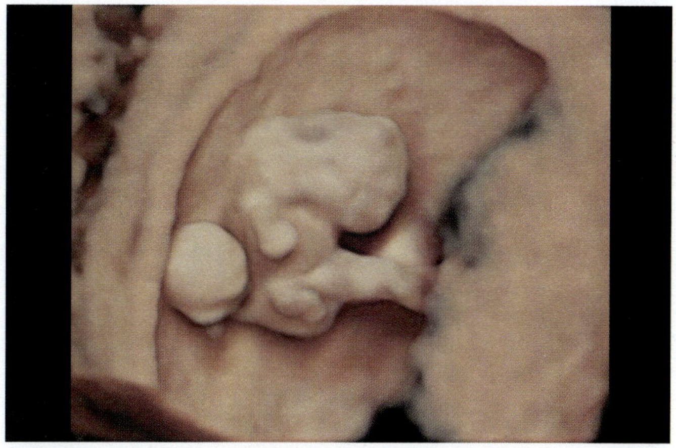

Fig. 11: HDlive 3D US; 8th postmenstrual weeks, CRL of 15 mm: The body is quite cuboidal and the head is relatively large. The umbilical cord insertion is discernible.
Source: Delta Ultrasound Diagnostic Center in Obstetrics and Gynecology, Madrid, Spain.

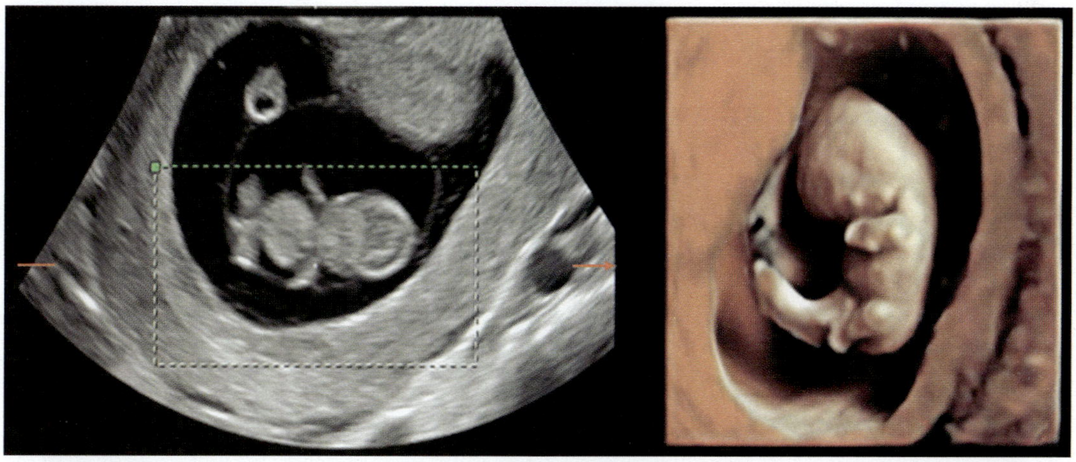

Fig. 12: HDlive 3D US; 8 weeks and 3 days, CRL of 19 mm: The nasofrontal groove and the auricular hillocks are distinct. The digital plate of hand is patent; finger and toe rays begin to appear. The umbilical cord insertion is discernible. The yolk sac is visible out of the amnion, floating in the extraembryonic coelom.
Source: Delta Ultrasound Diagnostic Center in Obstetrics and Gynecology, Madrid, Spain.

the nose. Fingers are long and remain extended; feet approach with toes eventually touching each other. Toe rays are prominent, but interdigital notches have not yet appeared. The physiological midgut herniation is now discernible by TV US, although it is present from the 17th stage on (the liver and the mesenterium grow faster than the abdomen, making the bowel migrate to the cord abdominal insertion). The developing spine is visible as two echogenic parallel lines on the back of the embryo. The lateral ventricles of the brain can be seen at this stage **(Figs. 14 to 16)**.

- **22nd Carnegie stage** (*10th postmenstrual week, CRL of 24–28 mm*): Toes are longer, the embryo can separate its hand from the trunk and the fingers of one hand can overlap the other hand's fingers.
- **23rd Carnegie stage** (*10.4th postmenstrual week, CRL of 28-31 mm*): The head is rounder. The limbs are longer and better developed. The physiological midgut herniation measures 6 mm. The forearm can reach or even surpass the level of the shoulder. The fingers are usually aligned although the embryo sometimes closes them and makes a fist. The gender cannot yet

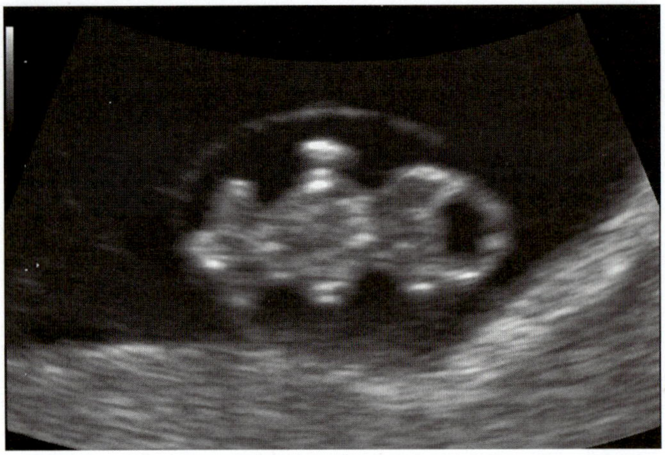

Fig. 13: 7 weeks and 6 days, CRL of 15 mm: The rhombencephalon if visible as an anechoic vesicle at the top of the head.
Source: Delta Ultrasound Diagnostic Center in Obstetrics and Gynecology, Madrid, Spain.

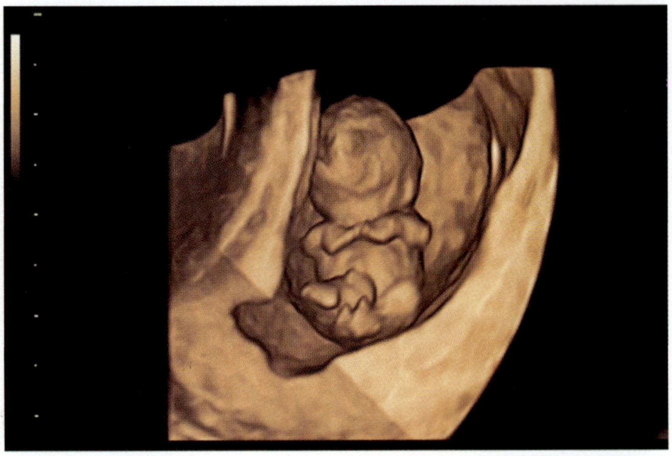

Fig. 14: 20th and 21st Carnegie stages; the CRL is 22.6 mm, consistent with a gestational age of 9 weeks 1 day. 3D US: The cervical angle widens. The hands have short and thick fingers and barely reach one another in front of the trunk, while they approach the thorax and the nose. Fingers remain extended; feet approach with toes eventually touching each other. Toe rays are prominent, but interdigital notches have not yet appeared. The physiological midgut herniation is discernible.
Source: Delta Ultrasound Diagnostic Center in Obstetrics and Gynecology, Madrid, Spain.

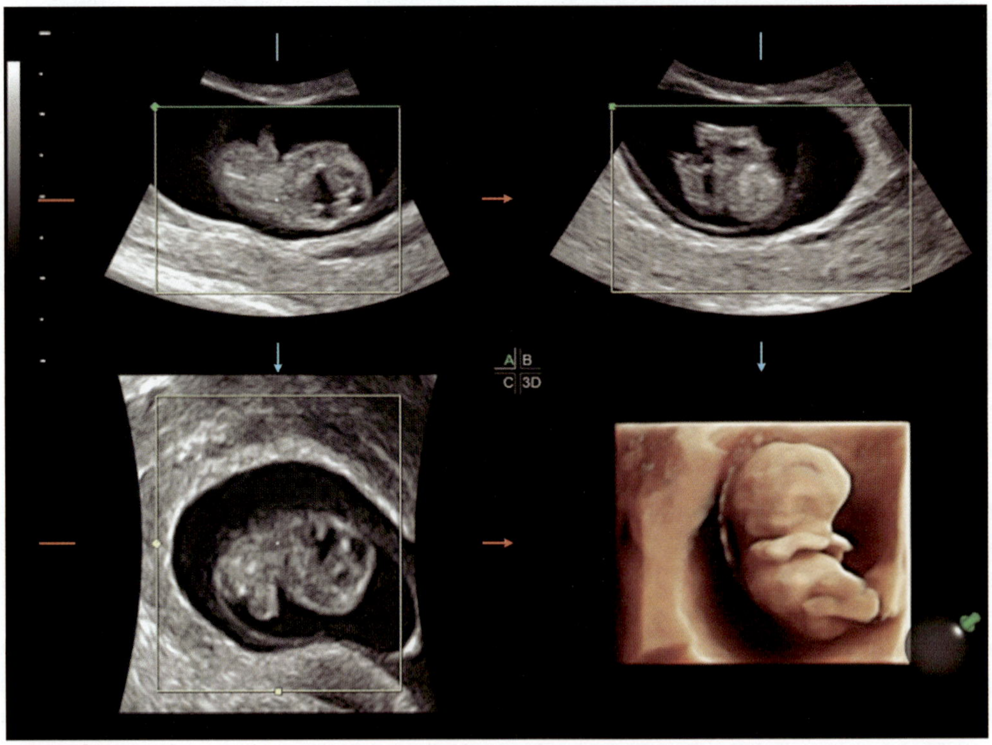

Fig. 15: 20th and 21st Carnegie stages; the CRL is 22.6 mm, consistent with a gestational age of 9 weeks 1 day. HDlive 3D US: The elbow is flexed. The hands barely reach one another in front of the trunk. The physiological midgut herniation and the cerebral ventricles are now discernible by transvaginal US.
Source: Delta Ultrasound Diagnostic Center in Obstetrics and Gynecology, Madrid, Spain.

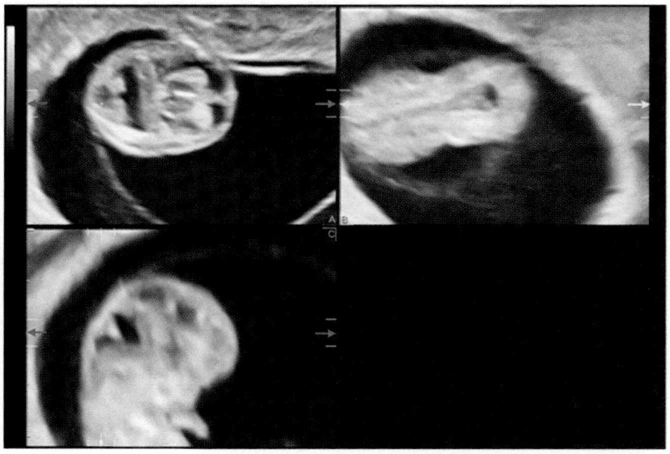

Fig. 16: 20th and 21st Carnegie stages; the CRL is 22.6 mm, consistent with a gestational age of 9 weeks 1 day. Multiplanar 3D image shows the cerebral ventricles and the developing spine (two echogenic parallel lines on the back of the embryo).
Source: Delta Ultrasound Diagnostic Center in Obstetrics and Gynecology, Madrid, Spain.

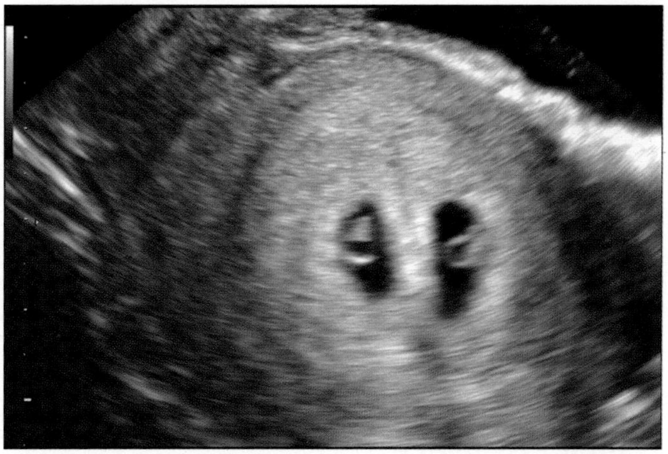

Fig. 17: Lambda sign in early twin pregnancy (6 weeks 4 days): Two embryos with its correspondent yolk sac can be ascertained. Their separating wall is thick, indicating that there are both amnion and chorion between the two twins. This stands for a dichorionic diamniotic twin pregnancy.
Source: Delta Ultrasound Diagnostic Center in Obstetrics and Gynecology, Madrid, Spain.

be ascertained by US. This is the end of the embryonic period (10–10.4 weeks).

- **Fetal period**:
  - *Week 11*: The limbs, their segments and joints are entirely developed. The thumb opposition to the rest of the fingers starts. The umbilical cord is 4 cm long and 0.5 cm wide and the vessels and the blood flow are identifiable. The physiological midgut herniation progressively regresses and this is considered by some authors as the sonographic milestone indicating the end of the embryonic period.[9]
  - *Week 12*: Fetal gender can be determined with 80-90% accuracy by studying the position of the genital tubercle.[10] The relative proportions and length of the limbs are not yet definitive, the lower limbs still being a bit shorter.

The 11–13 weeks of gestation period is the optimal one for the early evaluation of fetal anatomy and assessment of risk for aneuploidies:[2]

- US evaluation of risk for aneuploidies is based on the nuchal translucency measurement and other complementary markers, such as the presence/absence of the nasal bone, blood flow through the ductus venosus and presence/absence of tricuspid regurgitation.[11]
- The anatomical study can be ensured by routine assessment of certain fetal planes during the first trimester of pregnancy, briefly:[2,3,12]
  - Mid-sagittal view of the fetus.
  - *Sagittal view of the fetal head:* Evaluation of the nuchal translucency, nasal bone, and certain structures of the mid-brain.[13]
  - *Axial plane of the fetal head:* 'Butterfly sign' for the evaluation of the developing brain.[14]
  - Coronal view of the fetal face to evaluate the primary palate, nasal bones, and mandibular bones.[15-17]
  - *Thorax:* 4-chamber view of the fetal heart displaying heart activity.
  - *Abdomen:* Visualization of the stomach in the left upper quadrant and the bladder in the pelvis.
  - Abdominal wall and insertion of the umbilical cord.
  - Upper and lower limbs.

Multiple pregnancy

The number of fetuses must be ascertained as soon as possible, especially in those pregnancies achieved by assisted reproductive techniques. Early scanning will easily confirm fetal number and the position of each fetus in the case of a multiple pregnancy **(Fig. 17)**. The number and position of placentas should be determined, in particular by examining the placental-membrane junction for the presence or absence of the *lambda sign* (chorionicity). In monochorionic twins, the amniotic membranes should be further assessed to determine if the fetuses are in separate amniotic sacs (amnionicity). The first trimester is the optimal gestation to investigate all these aspects.[2,3]

ABNORMAL EARLY PREGNANCY

Location and viability are the two main issues when assessing an US scan in early pregnancy.

Before 11 weeks of gestation, there is no justification for routine scanning if the patient remains asymptomatic: the likelihood for the diagnosis of a PUL would be higher the earlier the pregnancy thus increasing the anxiety of the patient, the risk for iatrogenic interventions, and the cost of repeated investigations. However, in cases of vaginal bleeding or abdominal pain, an US scan must be done to rule out miscarriage, ectopic pregnancy, or trophoblastic disease.[1]

Ectopic Pregnancy

In cases when the decidual reaction is present but no gestational sac is visualized inside the uterine cavity by TV US, an ectopic pregnancy must be suspected, especially when the maternal serum β-hCG levels are >1500 mUI/mL and the patient presents with vaginal bleeding and/or abdominal pain.[4]

Sometimes an indeterminate intrauterine fluid collection can be visualized. The image of a pseudosac may be difficult to distinguish from a true gestational sac, although the gestational sac is rounder, eccentric with respect to the uterine cavity midline, and shows the trophoblastic echogenic enhancement ('double-ring' sign). The pseudosac usually consists of a small amount of blood trapped between the two layers of a thickened endometrium, therefore it usually takes the shape of a spindle. Color Doppler US will show either absent or very low velocity blood flow with moderate resistance index (whereas an IUP shows high velocity and low resistance flow around the gestational sac).[6]

The adnexa must be carefully scanned in search for any suspicious signs of an ectopic pregnancy. If no diagnostic image can be ascertained in the US scan, then monitoring with serial determinations of maternal serum β-hCG levels and US examinations may be of help for the confirmation.

In recent years, the treatment options for ectopic pregnancy have evolved from surgery to medical treatment with methotrexate in selected cases. However, it is of paramount importance to remember that, as long as there is any possibility of an IUP, methotrexate must be never administered to the patient.

Trophoblastic Disease or Molar Pregnancy

In the first weeks of pregnancy, the implantation of the embryo will determine the site of the uterus where the placenta will be located. Usually the placental echostructure is homogeneous and hypoechoic. In the first trimester of pregnancy, it is possible to notice anechoic cystic areas within the placenta, which would raise the suspicion for a partial or total molar pregnancy.

In molar pregnancy, the uterus is enlarged and the maternal serum β-hCG levels are very increased and not correlating with gestational age. The classic US features of a complete molar pregnancy are the display of vesicles ('snowstorm' or 'honey-comb' pattern) and the presence of theca-lutein ovarian cysts.[18]

Early Pregnancy Failure—Miscarriage

Miscarriage, also called spontaneous abortion, is an event that results in the loss of the products of conception during early pregnancy, usually in the first half of gestation, with a fetal weight <500 g. This is a frequent event in human pregnancies, especially if we consider the first weeks of gestation. The rate of miscarriage can be up to 30–40% if only very early pregnancies are taking into account, i.e. the ones confirmed biochemically but not yet visible by US (preclinical o biochemical miscarriage). Once the pregnancy can be ascertained by US the rate of miscarriage decreases to 10–15%. After confirming the presence of a live embryo, the possibility of a miscarriage is only 3-4%.[5]

The main causes for first-trimester miscarriage, accounting for at least 80-90% of the cases, are:

- Aneuploidies, trisomy 16 and triploidy being the most common ones.
- Structural anomalies.

After the 10 weeks of gestation, the predominant factors are maternal or environmental. In fact, miscarriage is considered as a natural selection process that would spontaneously clear 95% of morphological and genetic errors.

The following represents a classification of the different types of miscarriage:

Threatened Miscarriage

It presents with abnormal vaginal bleeding in up to 25% of pregnancies, which can be associated to mild hypogastric pain. Some of these episodes would actually correspond to implantation hemorrhage, but these cases are not definitely discernible from actual threatened miscarriage episodes.

Most of these pregnancies will go on if US can be ascertained the embryonic/fetal cardiac activity with US.

The uterine cervix does not appear dilated on physical examination.

Incomplete Miscarriage

Part of the products of conception, but not all, have been expelled from the body thus the cervix is dilated. Sonographic confirmation is sometimes difficult: the decidual thickness is usually more than 15 mm and the uterine content often looks heterogeneous.

Complete Miscarriage

All the products of conception are expelled from the body thus the cervix is not dilated anymore. The pain and the bleeding subside. By US, the decidual thickness is less than 15 mm.

Missed Abortion

The pregnancy is no longer developing but there are not yet any clinical manifestations. US is necessary for the diagnosis demonstrating an embryo or a fetus without cardiac activity. Clinical examination shows that the cervix is closed.

Blighted Ovum (Anembryonic Pregnancy)

There is a gestational sac of ≥25 mm diameter, with no embryo inside. Sometimes a missed abortion is misdiagnosed as a blighted ovum since there are pregnancies interrupted very early in which the embryo was very small and may not be identifiable by US anymore. If we see the amnion or the yolk sac inside the gestational sac, we should rule out the possibility of a blighted ovum because these structures need the presence of an embryo to develop.

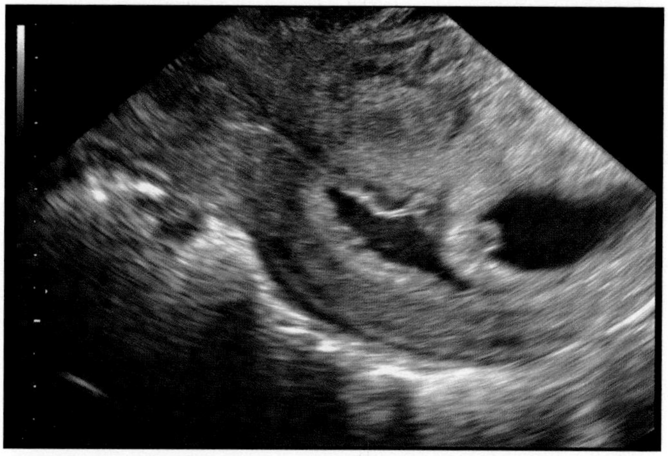

Fig. 18: Supracervical hematoma in early pregnancy.
Source: Delta Ultrasound Diagnostic Center in Obstetrics and Gynecology, Madrid, Spain.

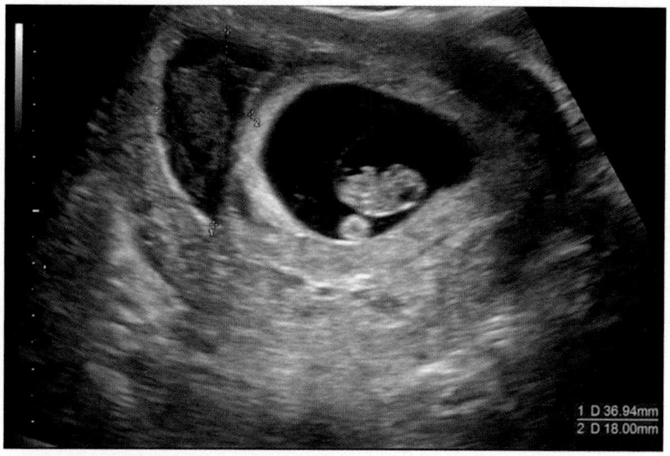

Fig. 19: Retrochorionic hematoma in an 8-week pregnancy.
Source: Delta Ultrasound Diagnostic Center in Obstetrics and Gynecology, Madrid, Spain.

Intrauterine Hematomas

Intrauterine hematomas are a quite common finding during the first-trimester scan. They consist of a collection of blood between the uterine wall and the gestational sac. They can be asymptomatic or associated to vaginal bleeding and it usually increases the risk of miscarriage.

The main prognostic factor is location (rather than the volume of the hematoma). The supracervical hematomas **(Fig. 18)** are the milder ones since they are easily drained through the vagina whereas the retroplacental collections are the worst due to the risk of placental detachment.[6,19] The prognosis worsens if the hematoma appears early in pregnancy (before 8 weeks) **(Fig. 19)**.

In the presence of hematomas, there will be an increase in the spiral arteries impedance along with a decrease in the flow velocity, both due to mechanical compression. With the progression of pregnancy and growth of the trophoblastic tissue, most of the hematomas will gradually disappear and blood circulation will normalize.[20]

A close follow-up is needed, not only by US but also checking the clinical symptoms (amount of vaginal bleeding). Intrauterine hematomas must be differentiated from a nonevolving second gestational sac (blighted twin): the hematomas are usually crescent-shaped whereas a gestational sac tends to be round and appears as an echogenic trophoblast ring **(Fig. 20)**.

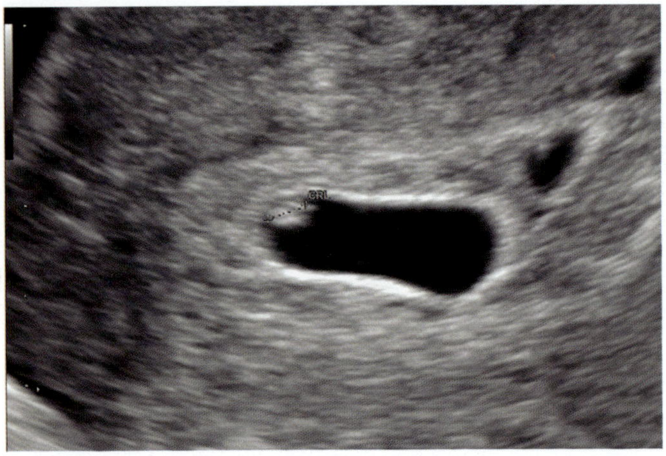

Fig. 20: Early pregnancy with poor prognostic signs. The CRL is smaller than expected and the gestational sac is slightly irregular. To the right of the picture there is a smaller sac image, probably corresponding to a blighted twin.
Source: Delta Ultrasound Diagnostic Center in Obstetrics and Gynecology, Madrid, Spain.

TABLE 1: Diagnostic ultrasound criteria for early pregnancy loss

- Absent embryonic cardiac activity when the CRL is ≥7 mm
- Absent embryonic cardiac activity on two US scans, 7 days apart
- Absence of an embryo with heart activity 10 days after the initial scan showed a gestational sac ≥12 mm or a gestational sac with a yolk sac inside
- Absence of an embryo with heart activity and no significant growth of the gestational sac 14 days after the initial scan showed a gestational sac <12 mm or a gestational sac without a yolk sac inside

Blighted ovum: Gestational sac ≥25 mm with no evidence of an embryo

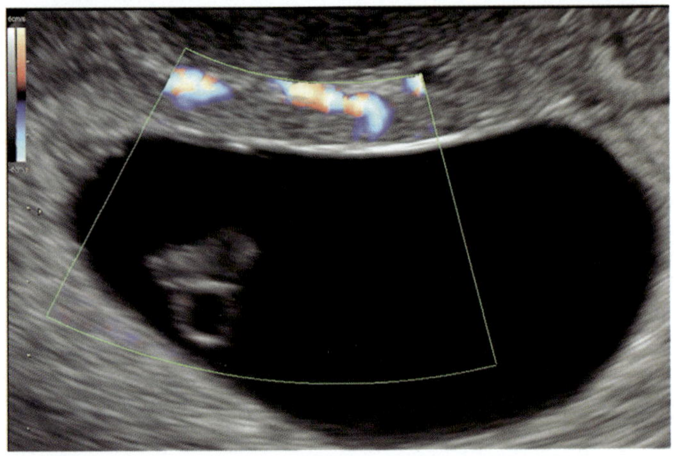

Fig. 21: Missed abortion: The CRL is 8 mm, consistent with a gestational age of 6 weeks 5 days; no cardiac activity can be demonstrated with color Doppler.
Source: Delta Ultrasound Diagnostic Center in Obstetrics and Gynecology, Madrid, Spain.

Prediction and Diagnosis of Miscarriage

The anamnesis and the physical examination are mandatory to get to the diagnosis of a miscarriage. Sometimes the findings would be evident enough to ascertain the diagnosis (significant vaginal bleeding, dilated cervix, products of conception expelled through the vagina). Most of the times, though, an US examination is needed for confirmation; furthermore, repeat US examination is often required, especially in very early pregnancies. To avoid misinterpretation of the physical examination and the US scan, we need certain information for the right estimation of the gestational age:[5]

- Last menstrual period.
- Duration and regularity of the menstrual periods.
- Use and type of contraception.
- Date of the first positive pregnancy test.

In cases where the US findings are not definitive and the gestational age cannot be confidently ascertained, it is always preferable to rescan the patient one week later to confirm the diagnosis of a miscarriage.

DIAGNOSTIC ULTRASOUND CRITERIA FOR EARLY PREGNANCY LOSS

The US findings that allow diagnostic confirmation of a pregnancy loss are described below **(Table 1)**:[5,21]

- **Absent cardiac activity in an embryo with a CRL ≥7 mm:** The embryonic cardiac activity is present several days before it can actually be ascertained by US. The previous reported cutoff of ≥5 mm has been proven unsafe thus more recent publications[4,21] recommend to reschedule the patient for a new scan 7 days later in cases with a CRL <7 mm and no evidence of cardiac activity, as long as the clinical conditions are stable **(Fig. 21)**.
- **Subsequent US scans with no significant changes in the sac's size or embryonic development:**[4,21]
  - Absent embryonic cardiac activity on two US scans, 7 days apart.
  - Absence of an embryo with heart activity 10 days after the initial scan showed a gestational sac ≥12 mm or a gestational sac with a yolk sac inside.
  - Absence of an embryo with heart activity and no significant growth of the gestational sac 14 days after

the initial scan showed a gestational sac <12 mm or a gestational sac without a yolk sac inside.

- **Anembryonic pregnancy (blighted ovum):** There is a gestational sac of ≥25 mm with no evidence of an embryo.

We emphasize that these are general recommendations so in case the operator's expertise, equipment resolution, and conditions for the scan are suboptimal, the patient should be rescheduled for a follow-up scan some days later in order to confirm or rule out the diagnosis.

Monitoring the maternal serum β-hCG levels can be useful as a complement for diagnosis and follow-up, especially at the stage of PUL. Once the pregnancy has been located by US, subsequent determination of maternal serum β-hCG levels is no longer necessary. With serum β-hCG levels below 1000 mUI/mL, the pregnancy is not supposedly amenable to US visualization; when the levels are over 1,500 mUI/mL, intrauterine pregnancies can be ascertained by transvaginal US in >90% of cases. The yolk sac should be observed inside the gestational sac with levels of 7,000–10,000 mUI/mL. An embryo with positive heart activity should be seen when the levels are over 10,800 mUI/mL.[5] These levels must not be considered absolutely discriminatory, thus no definite diagnosis must be made on its basis: even though the likelihood of an ectopic pregnancy is very high if an empty uterus is found in association with maternal serum β-hCG levels are higher than 3,000 mUI/mL, there is still a 0.5% likelihood of a viable IUP in this case.[4]

TABLE 2: Risk US indicators for early pregnancy loss. These findings work as markers for a high risk of miscarriage, but they are not the cause of it. They usually appear some days before the pregnancy stops evolving, but the definitive confirmation of a missed abortion requires any of the diagnostic criteria mentioned in Table 1. The best predictive features are indicated in bold.

Trophoblast	*Thickness:* Discrepancies >3 mm Abnormal US appearance, with multiple small vesicles Poor trophoblastic vascularization (scarce signal with color Doppler US)
Gestational sac	*Abnormal size:* Less than expected for gestational age *Early oligohydramnios:* Difference between the CRL and the mean sac diameter <5 mm **Sac not growing in subsequent scans** **'Two-bubble' sign or 'empty amnion'** Irregular shape Low-set gestational sac Absent double-ring sign Too thin decidual reaction
Yolk sac	Nonvisible yolk sac Too large or too small yolk sac Irregular shape Calcification of the yolk sac Double yolk sac in a singleton pregnancy
Embryo	**CRL smaller than expected for gestational age** (especially if >1 week) Slow or absent embryonic movements **Bradycardia** (<80–90 bpm below the 7th week and <100 bpm beyond the 7th week) **or arrhythmia**

ULTRASOUND HIGH-RISK INDICATORS FOR EARLY PREGNANCY LOSS

There are some findings in the first trimester that, although not diagnostic, are strongly predictive of poor pregnancy outcomes. These findings work as markers for a high risk of miscarriage, but they are not the cause of it **(Table 2)**. They usually appear some days before the pregnancy stops evolving, but the definitive confirmation of a missed abortion requires any of the aforementioned diagnostic criteria. Among these signs, the best predictors for a miscarriage are embryonic bradycardia and the discrepancies in size (gestational sac to CRL) and gestation (US vs LMP).

Trophoblast

- **Thickness:** The trophoblast thickness in millimeters should be equal to the number of weeks of gestation. Discrepancies larger than 3 mm imply a bad prognosis. If the trophoblast is too thick or edematous it is an ominous sign since it can correspond to a molar pregnancy.
- **Abnormal US appearance,** with multiple small vesicles. This is highly suspicious of a molar pregnancy.
- **Poor trophoblastic vascularization** (scarce blood flow signal with color Doppler US). This is sometimes conditioned by the so-called phenomenon of 'inverse placentation': if the chorion frondosum does not develop on the decidua basalis, but on the decidua capsularis instead, the blood flow is poorer and the risk of a miscarriage increases.

Gestational Sac

- **Abnormal size:** Less than expected for gestational age.
- **Early oligohydramnios**: From 6 to 10 weeks, if the difference between the CRL and the mean diameter of

the gestational sac is less than 5 mm (this difference is usually above 15–20 mm), the risk for miscarriage is >80%.[22]

- **Sac not growing in subsequent scans:** The gestational sac should normally grow 1–2 mm in size per day.[6]
- **Empty amnion:** In normal pregnancies, it is not unusual that the embryo is identified before the amnion can be visualized. The opposite situation, though, is abnormal. The combination of the amnion with the yolk sac, identified as two round adjacent structures, with no image corresponding to the embryo, is abnormal. It has been described as the 'two-bubble' sign or 'empty amnion' and the suspicion of a missed abortion must be raised, especially when the gestational sac diameter is >16 mm **(Fig. 22).**[23,24]
- **Irregular shape (Figs. 2 and 22).**
- **Low-set gestational sac.**
- **Absent double ring sign.**
- **Too thin decidual reaction:** <2 mm.

Yolk Sac

The yolk sac is the first visible structure inside the gestational sac. A certain predictive value for adverse outcomes in early pregnancy has been attributed to the following features:[6,25]

- Nonvisible yolk sac.
- Too large or too small yolk sac (the normal range being 3–7 mm) **(Fig. 23)**.
- Irregular shape.
- Calcification of the yolk sac.
- Double yolk sac in a singleton pregnancy.

However, the relevance of these changes is not definitely established. Differences in size and shape are less relevant if we can ascertain the embryo heart activity.[5]

Embryo

- **CRL smaller than expected for gestational age:** The CRL is measured in a midsagittal section from the top of the head (crown) to the end of the rump of the embryo by TV US;[3] the evaluation of the CRL is more reliable when the longest diameter of the embryo reaches 18–22 mm.[6] Especially in women with regular menstrual periods, when the difference between the observed and the expected CRL is >1 week, there is a 3-fold increase in the risk for miscarriage **(see Fig. 2).**[26]
- **Slow or absent embryonic movements,** especially after the 8th week.
- **Low embryonic heart rate:** The embryonic heart rate progressively increases from the 6th to the 9th post-menstrual weeks, from 100 to 170 bpm. It stabilizes at the 11th week and then it starts decreasing to get to 145–150 bpm around the 20th week. Low heart rates (<80–90 bpm below the 7th week and <100 bpm from the 7th week on) or arrhythmia are usually ominous signs with a high risk of miscarriage, but only the

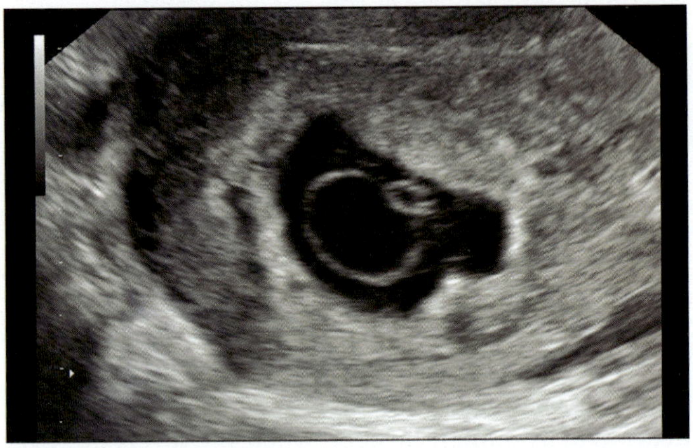

Fig. 22: 'Two-bubble' sign or 'empty amnion': The combination of the amnion with the yolk sac, identified as two round adjacent structures, with no image corresponding to the embryo, is abnormal. The suspicion of a missed abortion must be raised especially when the gestational sac diameter is >16 mm. In this case, the sac has also an irregular shape.
Source: Delta Ultrasound Diagnostic Center in Obstetrics and Gynecology, Madrid, Spain.

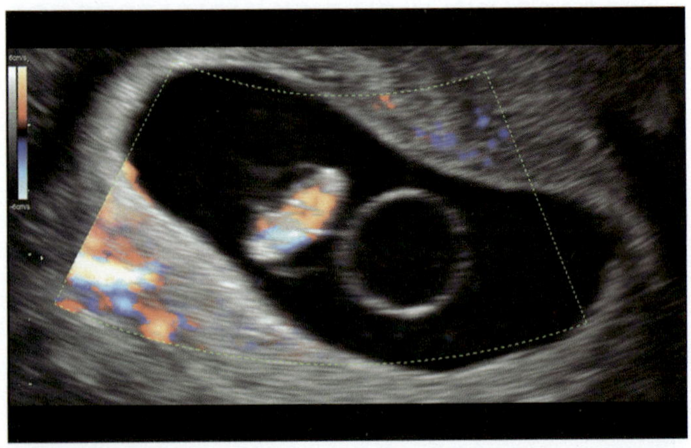

Fig. 23: The CRL is 7 mm and the yolk sac is almost 9 mm. Although a large yolk sac is a sign for poor prognosis, this is not a definitive diagnostic sign. In fact, heart activity is patent with color Doppler thus the embryo is alive.
Source: Delta Ultrasound Diagnostic Center in Obstetrics and Gynecology, Madrid, Spain.

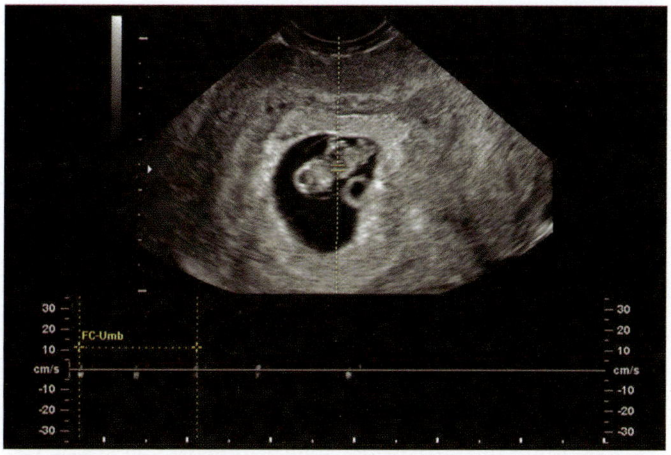

Fig. 24: Bradycardia (85 bpm) in a clearly dsymorphic embryo. The CRL is 16 mm, consistent with a gestational age of 8 weeks. Low heart rates (<80-90 bpm below the 7th week and <100 bpm from the 7th week on) or arrhythmia are ominous signs with a high risk of miscarriage, but only the absence of the heart rate permits to ascertain the diagnosis of a dead embryo.
Source: Delta Ultrasound Diagnostic Center in Obstetrics and Gynecology, Madrid, Spain.

absence of the heart rate permits to ascertain the diagnosis of a dead embryo **(Fig. 24)**.[27]

Clinical Factors

These are some clinical factors associated to a poor prognosis for the pregnancy:[5]

- Maternal age >35 years.
- (Early) vaginal bleeding.
- Maternal serum β-hCG levels not properly increasing.
- History of recurrent miscarriage.
- Other associated maternal conditions:
  - Uterine fibroids, especially if multiple or submucous.
  - Uterine malformations.

CONCLUSION: PRACTICAL CONSIDERATIONS

TV US and determination of maternal serum β-hCG levels are the two main tools for evaluation of early pregnancy.[4] The diagnosis of early pregnancy loss must be based only on diagnostic features to 100% ascertain the confirmation since, after this point, irreversible therapeutic decisions are to be made. If the findings are not definitive the patient must be reevaluated, as long as she is clinically stable, until a definitive diagnosis is reached.

The recommendations to be followed after an early-pregnancy US scan are summarized below:[4,5,21]

1. *The gestational sac cannot be ascertained yet (PUL):* The actual gestation may be less than the weeks calculated from the LMP. If there are no clinical signs and no US suspicion of an ectopic pregnancy, another US scan should be scheduled in 1–2 weeks. Sometimes serial determination of maternal serum β-hCG levels can provide additional useful information.
2. *An intrauterine gestational sac is visible, but neither an embryo nor the yolk sac can be ascertained (IUP of unknown viability):* The diagnosis of a blighted ovum can only be confirmed with a single US scan if the average gestational sac diameter is ≥25 mm. Otherwise, a follow-up US scan should be scheduled in 14 days. If the mean sac diameter is ≥12 mm or a yolk sac is visible, then the second scan may be in 7–10 days instead.[4,21]
3. *The gestational sac and the yolk sac are visible, and there is an embryo without evidence of cardiac activity (IUP of unknown viability):* Unless the CRL is ≥7 mm, a follow-up US scan should be scheduled in 7 days for confirmation of viability.[4,21]
4. *The gestational sac and the yolk sac are visible, and there is an embryo with cardiac activity present:* The pregnancy is ongoing. We can check for prognostic signs and schedule the next scan according to the background, US and clinical findings, and local protocols.

REFERENCES

1. Salomon LJ, Alfirevic Z, Bilardo CM, Chalouhi GE, Ghi T, Kagan KO, et al. ISUOG Practice Guidelines: performance of first-trimester fetal ultrasound scan. Ultrasound Obstet Gynecol. 2013;41(1):102-13.
2. Illescas T. Rational use of ultrasound in normal and abnormal early pregnancy. DSJUOG. 2015;9(2):205-10.
3. Illescas T. 11 to 14 Weeks' Scan. In: Donald School Textbook of Power Point Presentations on Advanced Ultrasound in Obstetrics and Gynecology. 1st edn. 2015. Jaypee Brothers Medical Publishers. ISBN 978-93-515-2920-0.
4. Rodgers SK, Chang C, DeBardeleben JT, Horrow MM. Normal and Abnormal US Findings in Early First-Trimester Pregnancy: Review of the Society of Radiologists in Ultrasound 2012 Consensus Panel Recommendations. Radiographics. 2015;35(7):2135-48.
5. Illescas Molina T, Martínez Ten P, Bajo Arenas JM. Miscarriage and threatened miscarriage. In: Ecografía Obstétrica. SEGO. Madrid; 2011.

6. Honemeyer H, Kurjak A, Monni G. Normal and Abnormal Early Pregnancy. In: Donald School Textbook of Ultrasound in Obstetrics and Gynecology. 3rd edn. Jaypee Brothers Medical Publishers; 2011.
7. Sadler TW. Langman's medical embryology. 12th edn. Lippincott Williams and Wilkins. Wolters Kluwer Health; 2012.
8. Persaud M. Clinical embryology. 6th edn. McGraw-Hill Interamericana; 1999.
9. Blaas HG. The examination of the embryo and early fetus: how and by whom? Ultrasound Obstet Gynecol. 1999; 14(3):153-8.
10. Begoña Adiego B, Pilar Martínez T, Javier Pérez P, Alicia Crespo R, Belén Santacruz M, Tamara Illescas M, et al. Determination of fetal gender in the first trimester of pregnancy: prospective study. Rev Chil Obstet Ginecol. 2010;0(2):117-23.
11. Molina TI, Martín BS. Other markers in the first trimester and its clinical significance. In: Ecografía en el primer trimestre de la gestación. Curso teórico-práctico de ecografía y Doppler SESEGO. SESEGO. Madrid; 2012.
12. Sepulveda W, Illescas T, Adiego B, Martinez-Ten P. Prenatal Detection of Fetal Anomalies at the 11- to 13-Week Scan – Part I: Brain, Face and Neck. Donald School J Ultrasound Obstet Gynecol. 2013;7(4):359-68.
13. Burgos BA, Ten PM, Molina. Embryology of the fetal brain: sonographic assessment. In: Neurosonografía fetal normal. Editorial Glosa. Barcelona; 2012.
14. Sepulveda W, Dezerega V, Be C. First-trimester sonographic diagnosis of holoprosencephaly: value of the 'butterfly sign'. J Ultrasound Med. 204;23(6):761-5.
15. Sepulveda W, Wong AE, Martinez-Ten P, Perez-Pedregosa J. Retronasal triangle: a sonographic landmark for the screening of cleft palate in the first trimester. Ultrasound Obstet Gynecol. 2010;35(1):7-13.
16. Adiego B, Martinez-Ten P, Illescas T, Bermejo C, Sepulveda W. First-trimester assessment of the nasal bone using the retronasal triangle view. A prospective study. Ultrasound Obstet Gynecol. 2014;43:272-6.
17. Sepulveda W, Wong AE, Viñals F, Andreeva E, Adzehova N, Martinez-Ten P. Absent mandibular gap in the retronasal triangle view: a clue to the diagnosis of micrognathia in the first trimester. Ultrasound Obstet Gynecol. 2012;39(2):152-6.
18. Stevens FT, Katzorke N, Tempfer C, Kreimer U, Bizjak GI, Fleisch MC, et al. Gestational Trophoblastic Disorders: An Update in 2015. Geburtshilfe Frauenheilkd. 2015;75(10): 1043-50.
19. Kurjak A, Schulman H, Zudenigo D, Kupesic S, Kos M, Goldenberg M. Subchorionic hematomas in early pregnancy: clinical outcome and blood flow patterns. J Matern Fetal Med. 1996;5:41-4.
20. Kurjak A, Zudenigo D, Predanic M, Kupesic S, Funduk B. Assessment of the fetomaternal circulation in threatened abortion by transvaginal color Doppler. Fetal Diagn Ther. 1994;9:341-7.
21. Preisler J, Kopeika J, Ismail L, Vathanan V, Farren J, Abdallah Y, et al. Defining safe criteria to diagnose miscarriage: prospective observational multicentre study. BMJ. 2015;351:h4579.
22. Dickey RP, Olar TT, Taylor SN, Curole DN, Matulich EM. Relationship of small gestational sac-crown-rump length differences to abortion and abortus karyotypes. Obstet Gynecol. 1992;79:554-7.
23. McKenna KM, Feldstein VA, Goldstein RB, Filly RA. The empty amnion: a sign of early pregnancy failure. J Ultrasound Med. 1995;14:117-21.
24. Yegul NT, Filly RA. Further observations on the empty "amnion sign". J Cllin Ultrasound. 2010;38:113-7.
25. Varelas, FK, Prapas, NM, Liang RI, Prapas IM, Makedos GA. Yolk sac size and embryonic heart rate as prognostic factors of first trimester pregnancy outcome. Eur J Obstet Gynecol Reprod Biol. 2008;138:10-3.
26. Koornstra G, Exalto N. Echography in the first pregnancy trimester has prognostic value. Ned Tijdschr Geneeskd 1991;135:2231-5.
27. Doubilet PM, Benson CB, Chow JS. Long-term prognosis of pregnancies complicated by slow embryonic heart rates in the early first trimester. J Ultrasound Med. 1999;18:537-41.

9

CHAPTER

Ectopic Pregnancy: Diagnosing and Treating the Challenge*

Sanja Kupesic Plavsic, Sonal Panchal, Ulrich Honemeyer

INTRODUCTION

Ectopic pregnancy represents implantation of the fertilized ovum outside the uterine cavity. In 95% of the cases, it is localized in the Fallopian tube (95%). Other sites such as the abdominal cavity, ovary, intraligamentous location, cornual, intramural or cervical sites are not unusual.[1-4] The exact cause of blastocyst implantation and development outside the endometrial cavity is not fully understood. The increased incidence of ectopic pregnancy found during the last decades,[5,6] are mainly attributed to the greater degree of socially acceptable sexual behavior, which has led to an increased incidence of pelvic inflammatory disease (PID). Fortunately, fatal outcomes have been reduced by up to 75% due to early diagnosis and less invasive treatment techniques. The mechanical factors predisposing towards pathomorphological site of implantation include: low-grade pelvic infection (the main cause for the faulty implantation), peritubal adhesions (resulting from a previous history of PID), and salpingitis with the partial or total destruction of the tubal mucosa. It has been reported that ectopic pregnancies do occur in totally normal tubes, suggesting that abnormalities of the conceptus or maternal hormonal changes may act as etiological factors.[7,8]

Risk factors for ectopic pregnancy are STD-PID (sexually transmitted diseases-pelvic inflammatory disease),[9,10] assisted reproductive techniques, abnormalities of the conceptus, maternal hormonal changes, surgical procedures in pelvis,[11] IUD (intrauterine device),[12,13] previous ectopic pregnancy, fibroids, uterine malformations, cigarette smoking, etc. It is essential to identify risk factors so we can provide patients with adequate information to diagnose and treat an ectopic pregnancy early and in addition possibly to develop preventive strategies.[14-16] The main challenge of an ectopic pregnancy is the clinical presentation.[17] Symptoms can vary from vaginal spotting to vasomotor shock with hemoperitoneum.[18,19] The classic triad of delayed menses, irregular vaginal bleeding and abdominal pain is not commonly encountered and the exact frequency of these clinical symptoms and signs is hard to assess.[1] Both the typical and atypical clinical presentations can mimic various diseases. These dieseases may have no connection with pathology of reproductive system examples of such are appendicitis, diverticulitis, nonspecific mesenterial lymphadenitis, or diseases of the urinary system. Most commonly an ectopic pregnancy is confused with an early spontaneous abortion because of the similar symptoms in both processes (delayed menses, enlarged and softened uterus and bleeding). Other conditions that should be considered in the differential diagnosis of an ectopic pregnancy are: normal intrauterine pregnancy, salpingitis, torsion or rupture of the ovarian cyst, adnexal torsion, bleeding corpus luteum, endometriosis, appendicitis, gastroenteritis, diverticulitis, conditions affecting urinary tract, etc. Therefore, early and reliable diagnosis of an ectopic pregnancy is a major challenge for every clinician. Significance of the early diagnosis renders the possibility of conservative methods of treatment. This is crucial for preserving further reproductive capability and in severe cases life itself.[20] Diagnostic procedures are divided into two groups:

Noninvasive: History, general clinical and gynecological examination, hormonal and other laboratory markers and ultrasound diagnostics.

Invasive: Culdocentesis,[21] curettage[22] and laparoscopy.

*"*Ectopic Pregnancy:* Diagnosing and Treating the Challenge". It includes updated bibliography, and additional high resolution ultrasound images. After reading this chapter, the interested reader should be able to gain an objective point of view on the role of transabdominal, transvaginal, color Doppler and three-dimensional ultrasound in the assessment of ectopic pregnancy.

THE ROLE OF BIOCHEMICAL MARKERS IN ECTOPIC PREGNANCY

Beta hCG (human chorionic gonadotropin) is the glycoprotein hormone released into circulation as soon as implantation occurs. Beta hCG is produced by the human placental trophoblastic cells from the 8th day post conception. Its blood concentration rises 1.7 times every 24 hours.[23] The commonly used urine beta hCG tests react at concentrations equal to or higher than 1000 IU/L of urine, which means that they become positive 10–14 days after conception.[1] False positive results are mainly obtained in the case of proteinuria, erythrocyturia, gynecological tumors, tuboovarian abscess,[24] or some drug intake (e.g. tranquilizers). In cases of an ectopic pregnancy, the embryo usually disappears by getting resorbed. In such cases, the ultrasound visualizes an empty gestational sac which produces smaller amounts of beta hCG. Normal levels of beta hCG can only be found in cases of a live embryo. This occurs in 5–8% of ectopic pregnancies.[23] Because of the low concentrations of human chorionic gonadotropin, only 40–60% of ectopic pregnancies have a positive urine test. Therefore, the more sensitive blood test should be performed, which becomes positive 10 days after conception.[23] In an ectopic pregnancy, the absolute values of beta hCG levels in circulation are much lower than in normal intrauterine pregnancies of the same gestational age.[25,26] The dynamics of the titer show a slower increase of circulating concentrations and a prolonged time for the doubling values. The most important use of the quantitative beta hCG determination is in conjunction with ultrasonography in order to understand the value of "the discriminatory zone" of beta hCG. The discriminatory zone represents that level of beta hCG above which all normal intrauterine chorionic sacs will be detected by ultrasound. There is now almost a consensus in considering the discriminatory zone to be about 1000 mIU/mL with the use of transvaginal probe of at least 5 MHz.[27-30]

THE ROLE OF ULTRASOUND IN THE DIAGNOSIS OF AN ECTOPIC PREGNANCY

With recent technological development, ultrasonography (but more precisely, transvaginal sonography) has become the "gold standard" diagnostic modality for the effective and fast detection of an ectopic pregnancy. An important advantage of most currently used transvaginal transducers is the ability to perform simultaneous B-mode and spectral Doppler studies, allowing easy identification of the ectopic peritrophoblastic flow. In comparison to transvaginal sonography, transabdominal ultrasound, as a method for detecting ectopic gestation is restricted for a very small number of oddly located ectopic pregnancies, mainly high up in the pelvis—outside the effective reach of 5 MHz vaginal probe.[31]

Transabdominal Ultrasound

The absence of a gestational sac inside the intrauterine cavity at 6 weeks of gestation raises the suspicion of an ectopic pregnancy. Transabdominal ultrasonography cannot reliably diagnose ectopic pregnancy, except when a live fetus is demonstrated in the abdominal cavity. In only 3–5% of the cases, an ectopic gestational sac with embryonic echoes and clear heart activity can be demonstrated.[32] A probe with frequency of 3.5 MHz and large contact area is used for transabdominal ultrasonographic imaging. A full bladder plays the role of an acoustic window. Resolution of this probe is somewhat lower, but the penetration is much deeper than one of the transvaginal probe.

The best results in confirming the intrauterine pregnancy are achieved using following criteria:

- Normal size, shape and location of the gestational sac in the uterine cavity.
- Double ring surrounding the gestational sac.
- Embryonic parts with an eventual heart action.
- Heart action.

Signs of an ectopic pregnancy can be divided into uterine and extrauterine, some of which are just suggestive or diagnostic.

Diagnostic signs include—absence of the intrauterine gestational sac surrounded by a double ring, absence of the yolk sac and/or fetal structures inside the gestational sac and presence of extraovarian adnexal structure.

Suggestive signs include—uterine enlargement with a thickened endometrium and blood or coagulum in the retrouterine space.[32]

Low sensitivity, specificity, positive and negative predictive values for detection of an ectopic pregnancy are shortcomings of transabdominal ultrasound.[33,34] This modality still has some value in successful detection of a small proportion of ectopic pregnancies with bizarre location, such as the high pelvis.

Transvaginal Ultrasound

In comparison with the transabdominal approach, the transvaginal ultrasound enables a much better image of the morphological features in pelvis, thanks to the higher frequencies and probe location in the immediate vicinity of the examined area. The sensitivity of transvaginal sonography was found to be 96%, the specificity reached 88%, the positive predictive value 89% and the negative predictive value is 95%.[35] An intrauterine gestational sac surrounded by a double ring with clear embryonic echo is considered to be strong evidence against an ectopic pregnancy because a heterotopic pregnancy (intrauterine and ectopic), coincide rarely. This must be taken into consideration, especially in the patients undergoing some of the methods of assisted reproduction.[36]

Intrauterine sonographic findings in women with ectopic pregnancy are variable **(Fig. 1A)**. These include:

- Empty uterus, with or without increased endometrial thickness.
- Central hypoechoic area or a sac-like structure inside the cavity—the so called pseudogestational sac.
- Concurrent intrauterine pregnancy.

Early intrauterine pregnancy and recent spontaneous abortion may present themselves on transvaginal sonography with an empty uterus and an endometrial layer of variable thickness.[3] Therefore, they are considered to be suggestive signs. A pseudogestational sac can be demonstrated in 10–20% of patients with an ectopic pregnancy[3] as a mixed echo pattern of endometrium that results from a decidual reaction, fluid or both. Careful examination of the uterine cavity usually allows a reliable distinction to be made between the pseudogestational sac and a normal gestational sac. The pseudogestational sac is detected in the middle of the uterine cavity, with a changing shape, due to myometrial contractions. In differentiating a real gestational sac from a pseudogestational one, transvaginal color and pulsed Doppler ultrasound proved to be very useful.

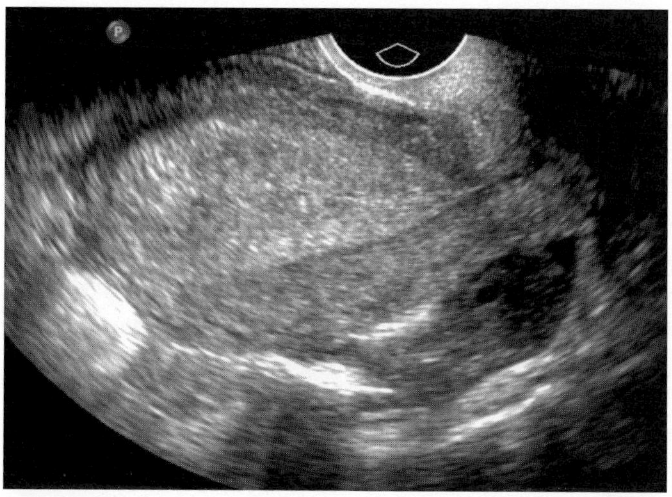

Fig. 1A: Key to the diagnosis of ectopic pregnancy is determination of the presence or absence of an intrauterine gestational sac correlated with quantitative serum beta-subunit hCG (β-hCG) levels. An ectopic pregnancy should be suspected if transvaginal ultrasonography does not show an intrauterine gestational sac when the beta hCG level is higher than 1,500 mIU/mL. Here is an example of a thickened endometrium and empty uterus in a patient with ectopic pregnancy.

Adnexal sonographic findings in women with ectopic pregnancy are variable. A gestational sac located inside adnexa with a clear embryonic echo and heart activity directly proves an ectopic pregnancy. This is seen only in 15–28% of the cases. Less rare is visualization of an adnexal gestational sac with or without embryonic echo (without heart activity) **(Figs. 1B and C)**.[37] Such a finding is detected in 46–71% of reported cases if tube is unruptured.[38] The most common finding is an unspecific adnexal tumor. Free fluid in the retrouterine space is seen in 40–83% of cases.

Accurate ultrasound diagnosis of ectopic pregnancy depends strongly on the examiner's experience. Adnexal abnormalities may be difficult to identify because of confusion with loops of bowel or other pelvic structures.[39]

There are four adnexal structures that may resemble an ectopic pregnancy and should be correctly identified.[40] One is the corpus luteum, which is eccentrically located within the ovary, surrounded by ovarian tissue and possibly creating the impression of a sac-like structure. About 85% of ectopic pregnancies are formed on the same side as the corpus luteum.[41] This is important to bear in mind while trying to distinguish a tubal pregnancy from the ipsilateral corpus luteum. When the corpus luteum is found in

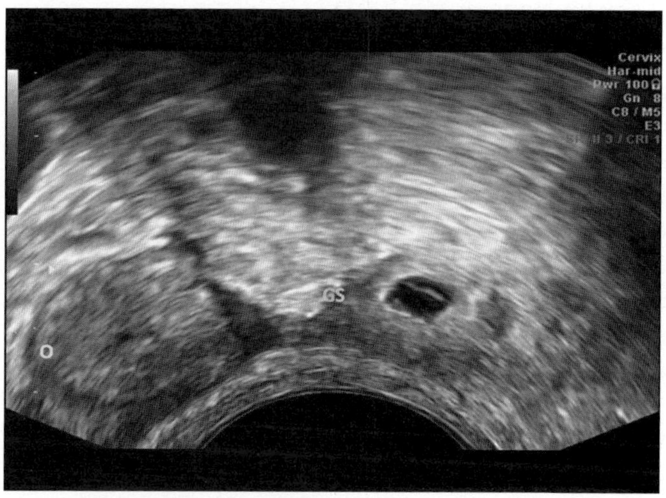

Fig. 1B: Transvaginal ultrasound of ectopic pregnancy. Gestational sac (GS) is visualized adjacent to the ovary (O).

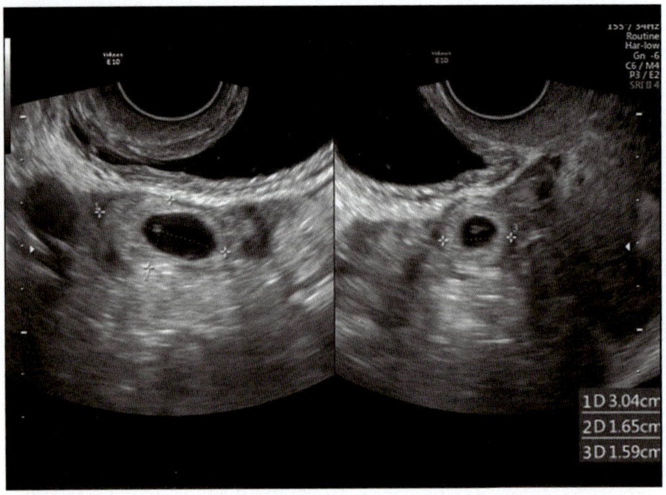

Fig. 1C: B mode ultrasound image of the right adnexa showing a gestational sac (central anechoic area with thick hyperechoic rim and the anechoic area showing yolk sac and a tiny fetal pole), between the uterus and the ovary. Sonographic findings indicate right tubal ectopic pregnancy.

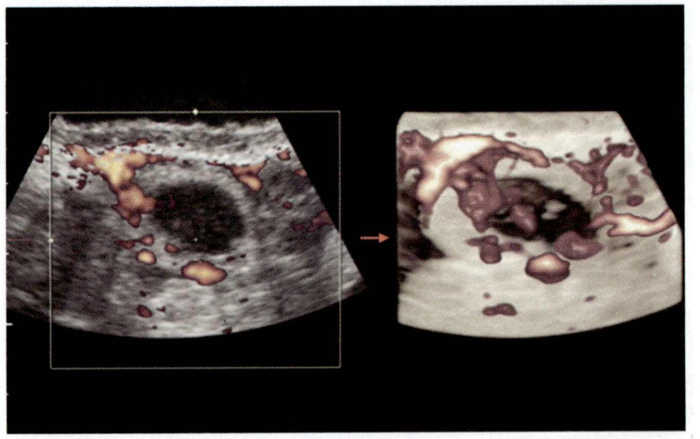

Fig. 1D: The same case as in the previous figure. 3D power Doppler image demonstrates vascularization surrounding the gestational sac. Power Doppler signals are also visualized in the tiny embryonic pole.

the ovary, its echogenicity is slightly (or at times even substantially) lower than that of trophoblastic tissue of the tubal ring. Furthermore, the hemorrhagic corpus luteum usually shows a hypoechoic rather than a cystic central region.[42] Three other conditions that need to be correctly differentiated from an ectopic gestation are a thick-walled ovarian follicle, the small intestine, and pathological tubal conditions, such as hydrosalpinx containing fluid.

Using the protocol of a combination of clinical examination, serum beta hCG assay and transvaginal ultrasound examination, it is possible to diagnose ectopic pregnancy with a sensitivity of 100% and specificity of 99%.[43]

Another problem in the detection of an ectopic pregnancy in the adnexal region arises in patients undergoing assisted reproductive procedures or simple hormonal superovulation. Besides the increased risk for ectopic pregnancy in these patients, a large number of artificial corpora lutea will be seen that resemble the tubal ring of an ectopic pregnancy. Sometimes cystic adnexal masses (ovarian cystadenoma, cystadenofibroma, endometrioma, teratoma and pedunculated fibroids) may also raise differential diagnostic problems.

Although free intraperitoneal fluid is seen in 40–83% of women with an ectopic pregnancy, it can also be seen in up to 20% of normal intrauterine pregnancies.[38] In a case of tubal abortion, echogenic echoes suggesting the presence of blood clots are demonstrated, while tubal rupture is associated with a homogeneous, hypoechoic retrouterine echo that represents blood collection. The possibility of an ectopic pregnancy increases if the amount of fluid is moderate-to-large, but the absence of blood does not exclude its diagnosis.

A serial serum beta hCG assay may raise the suspicion of an ectopic pregnancy at a very early gestational age, when the transvaginal ultrasound scan may not be able to demonstrate the site of the pregnancy. Under these circumstances, sometimes it is necessary to perform a laparoscopic examination to exclude the possibility of an ectopic pregnancy. However, even laparoscopic examination may not be able to achieve a precise diagnosis, especially when the ectopic pregnancy is very small or when there are coexisting pathologies such as hydrosalpinges, adhesions or fibroids. Some reports demonstrated that a laparoscopic ultrasound can facilitate the diagnosis of the site of an ectopic pregnancy intraoperatively, even if it is as small as 3.9 mm.[44] The number of negative laparoscopies can be decreased and a repeat laparoscopy avoided. Therefore, laparoscopic ultrasound should be used when the site of the ectopic pregnancy cannot be determined or is obscured by other pathologies during the laparoscopic examination.

Color Doppler Ultrasound

The ultrasound machine with color Doppler facility is an excellent guide to search for blood flow signals within the entire pelvis. The color flow pattern associated with an ectopic pregnancy is variable **(Figs. 1D and E)**. It usually

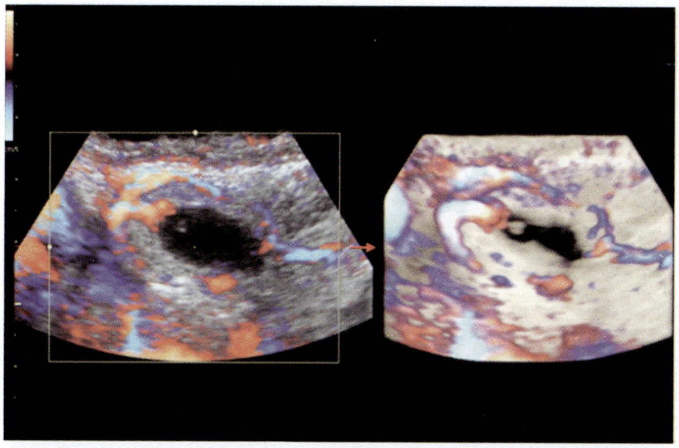

Fig. 1E: The same case assessed by high definition flow. Prominent vascularization is noticed surrounding the gestational sac. Doppler findings indicate trophoblast vitality.

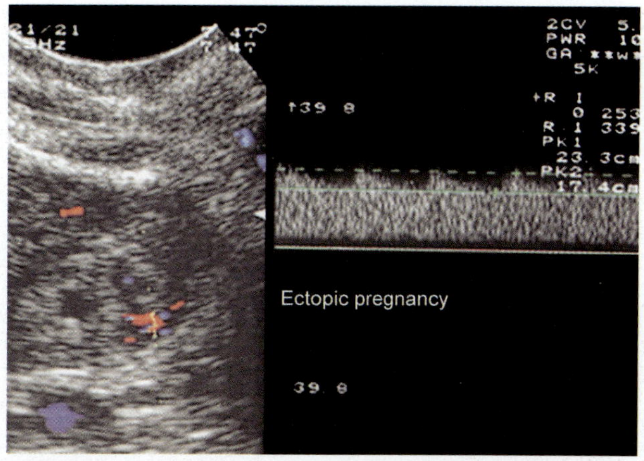

Fig. 2B: The same patient as in previous figure. Blood flow velocity waveforms depicted from the area of peritrophoblastic flow show high velocity (23.3 cm/s) and low vascular resistance (RI = 0.25).

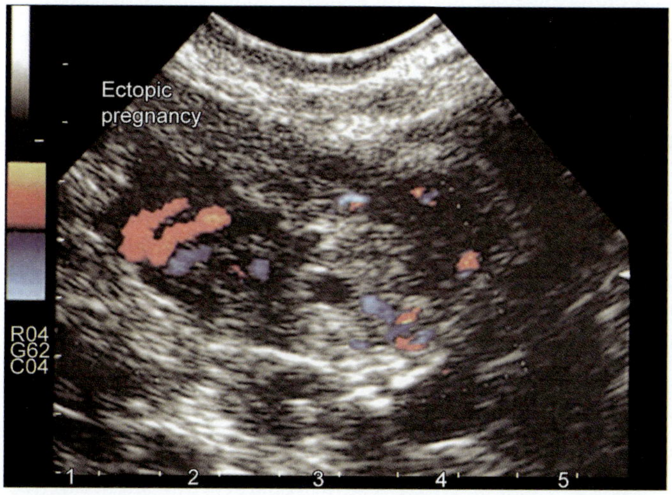

Fig. 2A: Transvaginal color Doppler scan of a small gestational sac in the adnexal region measuring 8–10 mm. Note the dilated tubal vessels, indicating the pathophysiological site of the pregnancy (within the tube).

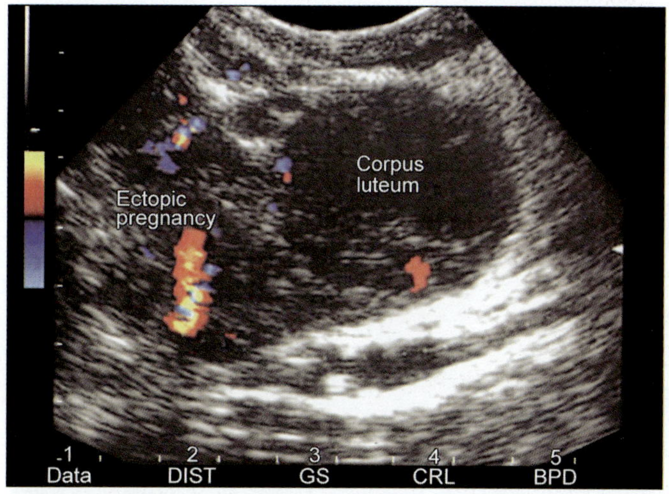

Fig. 2C: The same patient as in **Figures 2A and B**. An ipsilateral corpus luteum is demonstrated laterally to the ectopic gestational sac.

presents as randomly dispersed multiple small vessels within the adnexa **(Fig. 2A)**, showing high velocity and low impedance signals (RI = 0.36–0.45) which are clearly separated from the ovarian tissue and corpus luteum **(Fig. 2B)**. The sensitivity of the transvaginal color and pulsed Doppler in the diagnosis of an ectopic pregnancy has been reported by several studies and ranges from 73–96%, and the specificity ranges from 87–100%.[3,4,38,45]

Visualization of the ipsilateral corpus luteum blood flow may aid in the diagnosis of an ectopic pregnancy **(Fig. 2C)**. The RI of luteal flow in cases of ectopic pregnancy has been reported to be 0.48 ± 0.07, which is between the values of a non-pregnant women (0.42 ± 0.12) and those with normal early intrauterine pregnancy (0.53 ± 0.09).[46] In majority of patients with a proven ectopic pregnancy, luteal flow is detected on the same side as the ectopic pregnancy. This observation could be used as a guide when searching for an ectopic pregnancy **(Fig. 2D)**.

The between-side difference in the tubal artery blood flow was also documented. There was a significant increase in the tubal artery blood flow on the side of the tubal gestation. The mean reduction of the RI on the side with the ectopic pregnancy compared to the opposite side was 15.5%.[4] These changes appear to be due to trophoblastic invasion and showed no dependence on the gestational age. A bright color when visualized on the

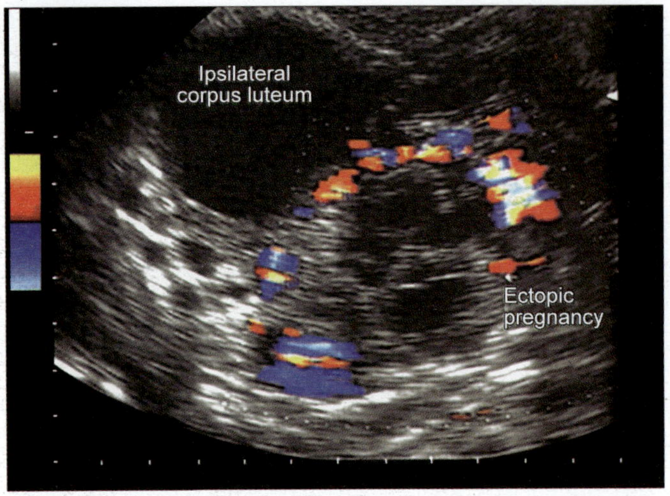

Fig. 2D: Color Doppler facilitates visualization of randomly dispersed tubal arteries indicating prominent trophoblastic vitality and invasiveness. Note the ipsilateral corpus luteum.

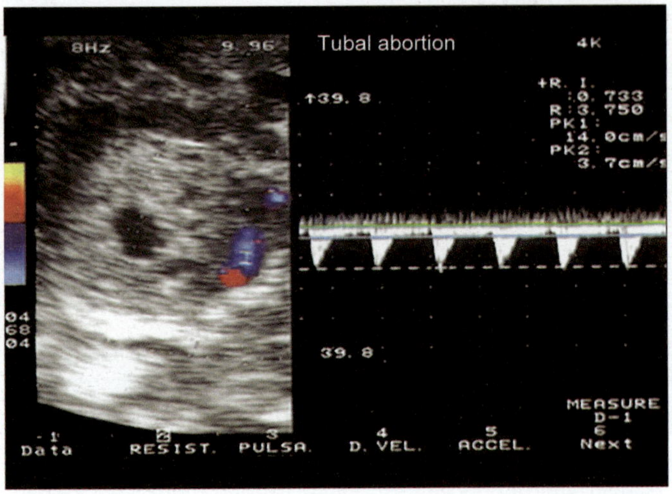

Fig. 4: Gestational sac measuring 12 mm in the left adnexal region. Color Doppler depicts a small area of angiogenesis characterized by a high resistance index (RI = 0.73). This finding is indicative of tubal abortion.

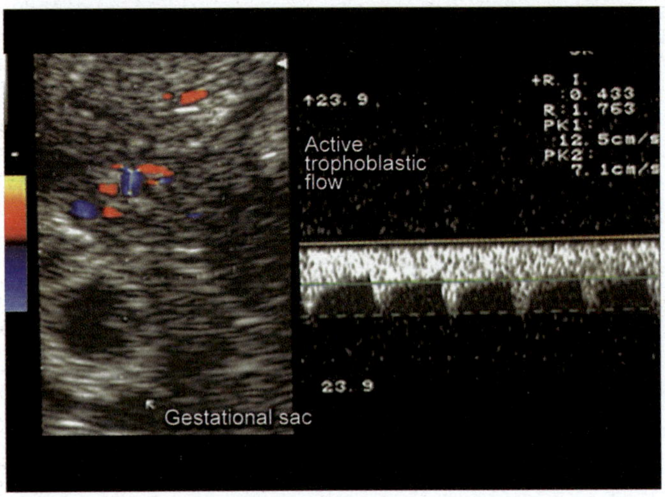

Fig. 3: Transvaginal color Doppler imaging of a left-sided ectopic pregnancy. Note the color signals indicative of invasive trophoblast (left). Pulsed Doppler waveform analysis (right) demonstrates low resistance index (RI = 0.43).

screen while using the pulsed Doppler facility is due to the very high speed of the peritrophoblastic blood flow and low impedance **(Fig. 3)**. It should be stressed that patients with tubal abortion demonstrate significantly higher vascular impedance of peritrophoblastic flow (RI >0.60), and less prominent color signals **(Fig. 4)**.

The main diagnostic importance of transvaginal color and pulsed Doppler is in differentiating the nature of a nonspecific adnexal mass. Doppler blood flow indices in the uterine, spiral arteries and corpus luteum arteries in ectopic and intrauterine pregnancies showed that the mean uterine and spiral artery RI decreased with an increased gestational age of the intrauterine pregnancies, but remained constantly high in ectopic pregnancies.[47] The peak systolic blood flow velocity in the uterine artery increased with an increasing gestational age in intrauterine pregnancies and the values were significantly higher than in ectopic pregnancies.[48] The difference in peak systolic velocity reflects a decreased blood supply to the ectopic pregnancy. An intrauterine gestational sac shows prominent peritrophoblastic vascular signals (RI = 0.44–0.45), while pseudogestational sacs do not demonstrate increased blood flow (RI >0.55). It has been suggested that velocities below 21 cm/s are diagnostic for pseudogestational sac and can successfully rule out trophoblastic flow of a normal intrauterine pregnancy.[49]

The intravascular ultrasound contrast agent has a recognizable effect on Doppler ultrasonographic examination of the adnexal circulation. It appears to be helpful when the finding in the color flow imaging is ambiguous. The use of the contrast agent may also facilitate localization of trophoblastic tissue in hemorrhagic adnexal lesions.[50]

As with other diagnostic methods, transvaginal color and pulsed Doppler studies include both, false-positive and false-negative findings. A false-positive diagnosis arises predominantly from the corpus luteum, but in exceptional cases some adnexal lesions may mimic an ectopic pregnancy. A false-negative result may arise

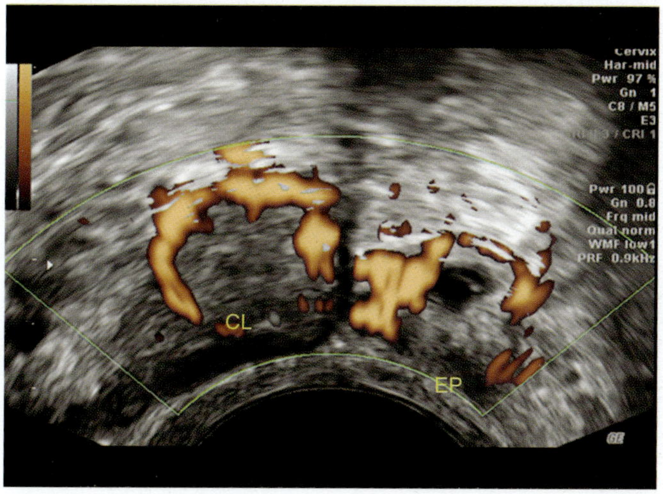

Fig. 5A: Transvaginal power Doppler of tubal ectopic pregnancy (EP) and ipsilateral corpus luteum (CL).

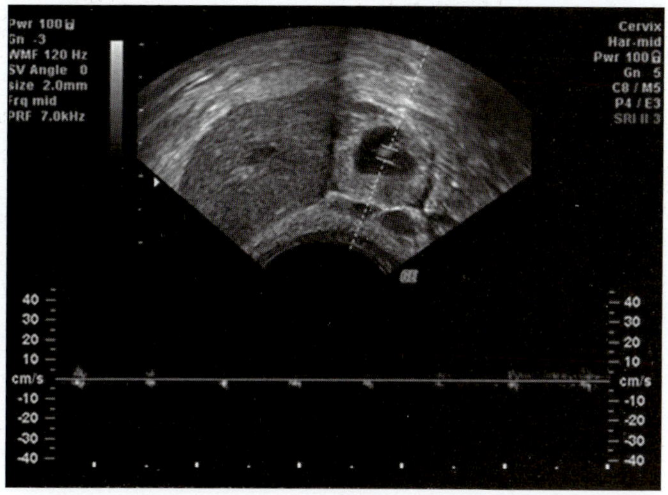

Fig. 5B: The same patient as in **Figure 5A**. Irregular heart activity is obtained from the ectopic gestational sac.

from technical inadequacy, lack of experience or the patients' noncompliance. The other possibility of a faulty diagnosis is a nonvascularized ectopic gestation, as these are associated with low beta hCG values.

Some authors compared technical errors with improper setting of color flow parameters.[51] The color velocity scale, color priority, color gain, color sensitivity and color wall filter should be adjusted to optimize color flow information. Technical errors may result in the false diagnosis of an ovarian torsion, malignancy and an ectopic pregnancy.

The diagnosis of ectopic pregnancy still remains a challenge to the clinician despite advances in ultrasound and biochemical technology. Frequently, the diagnosis remains uncertain until a laparoscopy or D&C are performed. With the increasing tendency towards conservative therapy, the distinction between ectopic pregnancies that will resolve spontaneously and those that will rupture is essential.[52] Usually patients without any acute symptoms and with declining beta hCG values are treated conservatively.[53] However, secondary ruptures have been reported in patients with low initial beta hCG concentrations.[54] The differentiation between viable ectopic pregnancies with trophoblastic activity and dissolving tubal abortions could facilitate the decision to proceed with conservative or operative treatment.

After implantation in the mucosa of endosalpinx, the lamina propria and then the muscularis of the oviduct, the blastocyst grows mainly between the lumen of the tube and its peritoneal covering.[55] Growth occurs both parallel to the long axis of the tube and circumferentially around it. As the trophoblast invades surrounding vessels, intensive blood flow and/or intraperitoneal bleeding occurs **(Figs. 5 and 6).** The intensive ring of vascular signals could be a criterion for viability of an ectopic pregnancy that can be determined rapidly and easily and seems to be independent of beta hCG values.[56] In patients with a viable ectopic pregnancy, especially in those cases where beta hCG levels slowly normalize who demand a conservative treatment, this method could provide an aid in addition to beta hCG values for supervising the efficiency of treatment. This way duration of the hospitalization

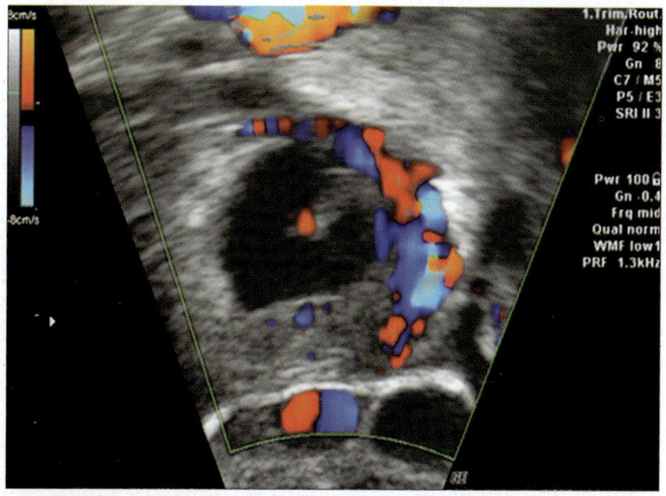

Fig. 6A: Prominent blood flow signals indicate vital trophoblast. In addition to peritrophoblastic flow, color Doppler can depict embryonic cardiac activity.

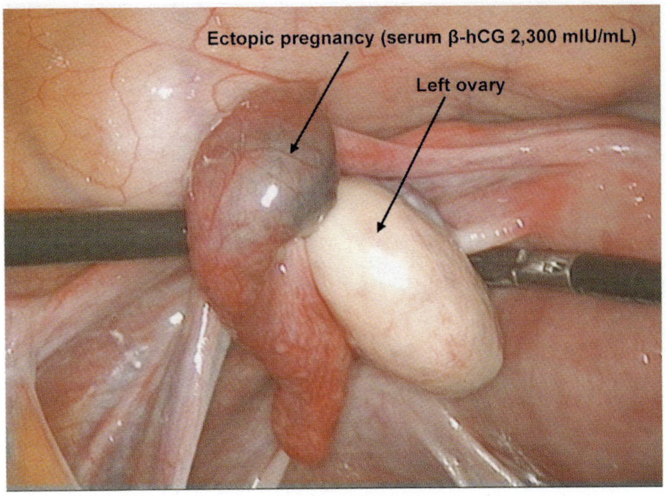

Fig. 6B: Laparoscopic image of ectopic pregnancy. Note ipsilateral corpus luteum.

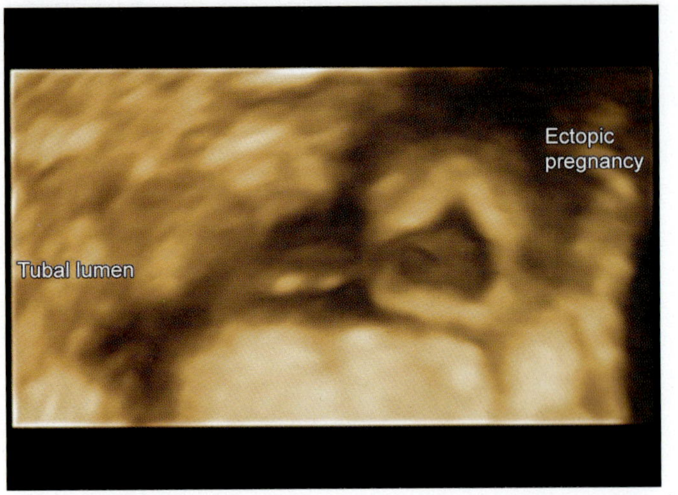

Fig. 7A: 3D ultrasound acquired volume rendered in surface mode of the dilated tube, seen as a hypoechoic area. The lumen shows ballooning laterally—probably in the fimbrial end of the tube. This ballooned up end shows gestational sac with yolk sac and decidual reaction. Tubal ectopic, still retained in the fimbrial end of the tube.

could be shortened, the patients uncertainty diminished and the cost of the treatment reduced. In cases of persistent high beta hCG levels after operative removal of the ectopic pregnancy, color Doppler sonography can provide evidence for the presence of viable trophoblast remnants. On the contrary, in asymptomatic patients with hypoperfused and/or avascular ectopic gestational sac and decreased values of beta hCG, expectant treatment can be established.

3D Ultrasound in the Assessment of Tubal Ectopic Pregnancy

Three-dimensional (3D) ultrasound technology offers some advantages over conventional two-dimensional (2D) sonographic imaging.[57, 58] Modern systems are capable of generating surface and transparent views depicting the sculpture-like reconstruction of surfaces or the transparent images structure's content **(Figs. 7A to D)**.

Planar mode tomograms are helpful in distinguishing the early intraendometrial gestational sac from a collection of the fluid between the endometrial leaves (pseudogestational sac).

A prospective follow-up study was conducted in order to evaluate the potential utility of 3D ultrasound to differentiate the intrauterine from ectopic gestations.[59] Fifty-four pregnancies with a gestational age <10 weeks and with an intrauterine gestational sac <5 mm in diameter formed the study group. The configuration of the endometrium in the frontal plane of the uterus was correlated with pregnancy outcome. After exclusion of three patients with a poor 3D image quality, the

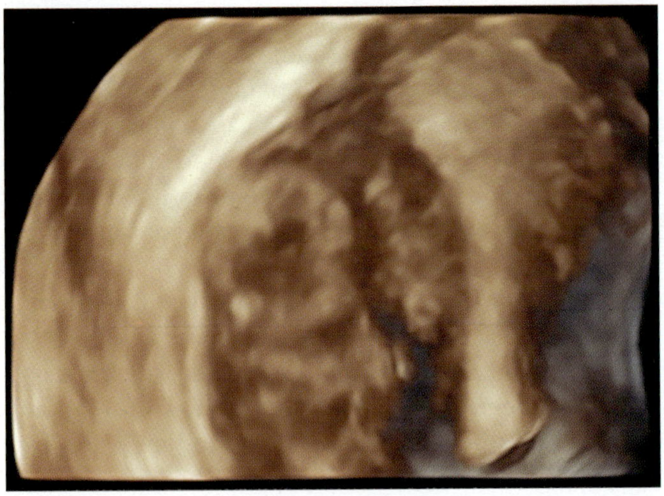

Fig. 7B: 3D ultrasound, surface rendered image showing coronal view of the endometrium—empty endometrial cavity. Two anechoic areas, both surrounded with hyperechoic thick rim. 3D ultrasound indicates twin ectopic pregnancy.

endometrial shape was found to be asymmetrical with regard to the median longitudinal axis of the uterus in 84% of intrauterine pregnancies, whereas endometrium showed symmetry in the frontal plane in 90% of ectopic pregnancies. Intrauterine fluid accumulation may distort the uterine cavity, thus being responsible for false-positive, as well as false-negative results. The evaluation of the endometrial shape in the frontal plane appeared to

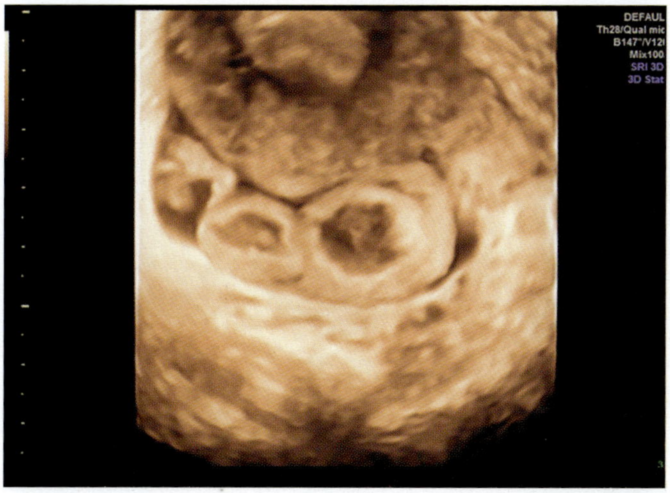

Fig. 7C: 3D ultrasound image of the uterus in transverse plane. Posterior to the uterus are two gestational sacs. Minimal fluid is seen around these gestational sacs in which a floating fimbrial end of the tube is seen (to the left). Surface rendering indicates twin tubal pregnancy.

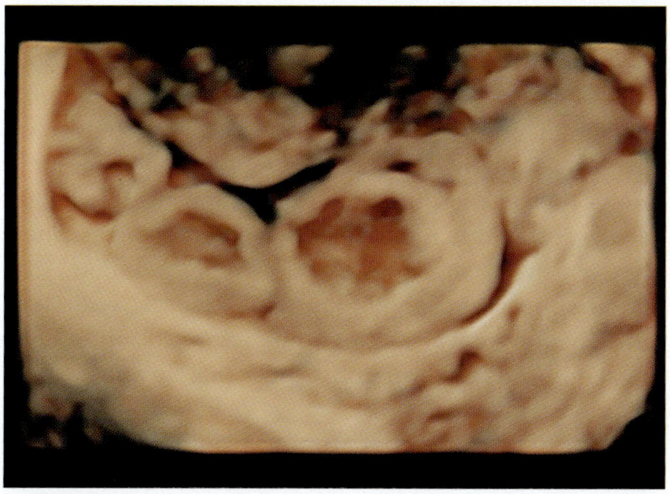

Fig. 7D: The same patient assessed by HDlive mode. Two ectopic gestational sacs and fimbrial end of the tube are visualized posterior to the uterus.

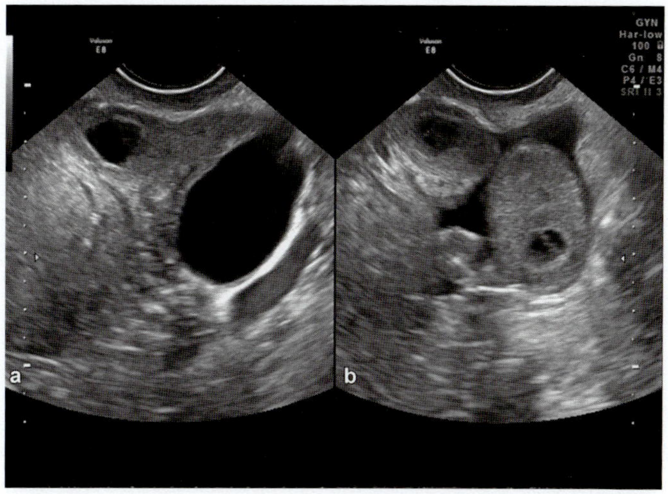

Fig. 8A: B mode ultrasound image of the adnexa shows two anechoic lesions with thick walls. The lesion which is farther to the probe shows thick hyperechoic rim, which is typical for a gestational sac, with free fluid around. The anechoic lesion which is closer to the probe has thick walls, but does not show typical hyperechoic rim of decidual reaction on the right side of image a. On image b the lesion appears intraovarian. Laparoscopy confirmed right ectopic pregnancy. Cystic lesion medially from ectopic pregnancy was proven to be corpus luteum.

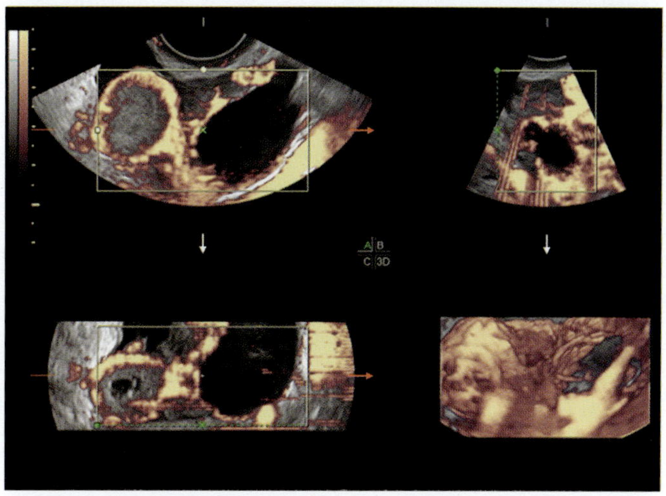

Fig. 8B: 3D power Doppler image of the same patient. Rim of vascularity around the ectopic pregnancy, as well as around the corpus luteum of the ipsilateral ovary is demonstrated both in multiplanar images and on the rendered image (right lower image).

be a useful additional means of distinguishing intrauterine from ectopic pregnancies, especially when a gestational sac was not clearly demonstrated with the conventional ultrasound. Similarly, preliminary data of other authors suggested that 3D sonography is an effective procedure for early diagnosis of ectopic pregnancy in asymptomatic patients before 6 weeks of amenorrhea.[60]

The possible use of 3D power Doppler is the monitoring of the vascularity of an ectopic pregnancy **(Figs. 8A and B)**. In case of hyperperfusion, the patients should be subjected to laparoscopy or medical treatment immediately. The hypoperfusion, quantified by indices of vascularity (VI) and flow (FI) could indicate that the ectopic pregnancy is spontaneously being resolved, and that laparoscopy should be postponed. This way, the

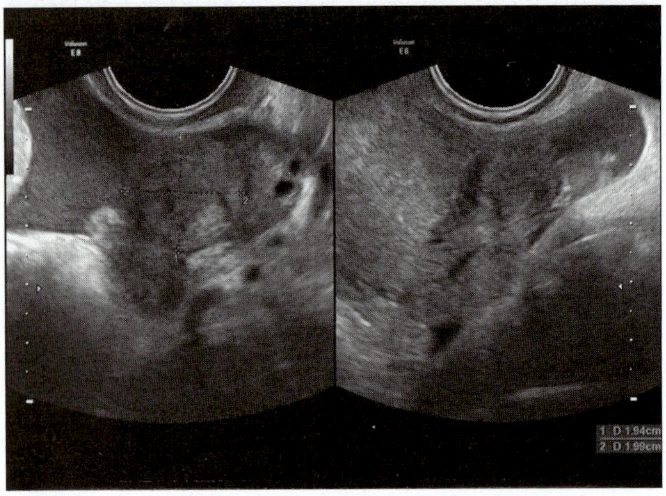

Fig. 9A: B mode ultrasound image of the pelvis showing a round isoechoic, extraovarian mass. Fluid with low level echogenicities is seen around the mass and the ovary. The image on the right side shows soft tissue echogenicity with irregular margin—fimbrial end of the tube. Findings are suggestive of ectopic pregnancy.

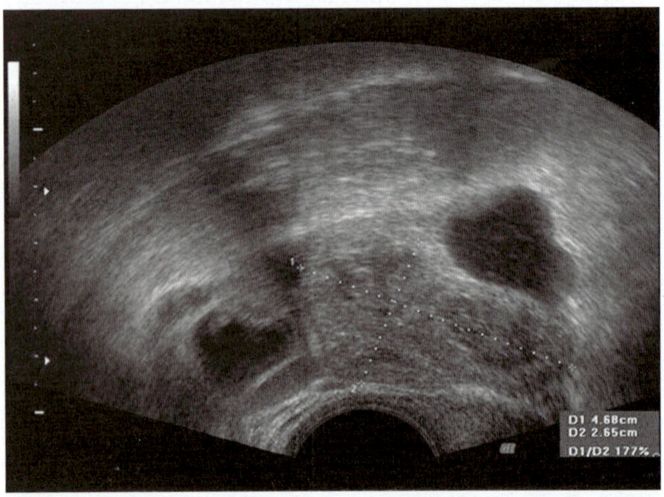

Fig. 9B: Transvaginal ultrasound of a complex adnexal mass in a patient with positive pregnancy test. Note tubular structure with solid part measuring 4.6 x 2.7 cm.

conservative approach to an ectopic pregnancy would rely on more precise and easily obtainable data. **Figures 9A to C** illustrate two cases of chronic ectopic pregnancy, both manifested as complex adnexal mass. Because of its echogenicity and varying sonographic appearances the mass may be confused for pelvic inflammatory disease and complex cystic lesions such as endometrioma or hemorrhagic cyst.

Shih and colleagues[61] described the use of 3D color/power angiography in two cases in which an

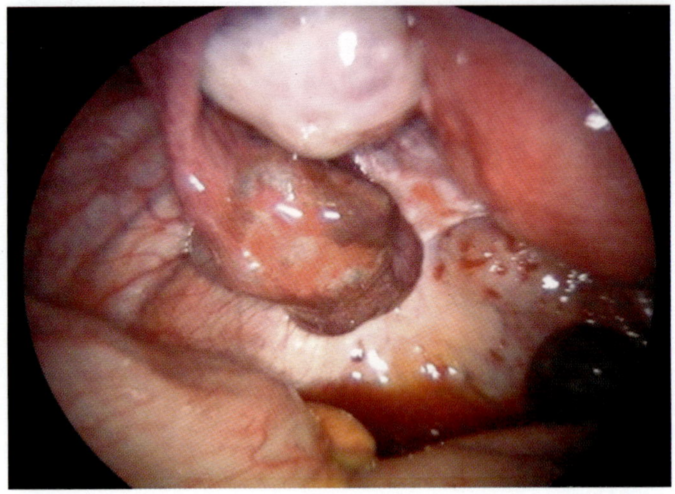

Fig. 9C: Laparoscopy revealed chronic tubal pregnancy and free fluid in the cul-de-sac.

arteriovenous malformation of the mesosalpinx was diagnosed following involution of an anembryonic ectopic gestation. The diagnosis of arteriovenous malformations has traditionally been made by arteriography. Recently, it has also been diagnosed by noninvasive methods such as contrast enhanced CT, MRI and color Doppler ultrasound. The advantage of 3D reconstruction of color/power angiography images is a better spatial and anatomic orientation and a quick demonstration of the vessels, usually within one minute, especially in the areas where complex structures are present. Therefore, unlike MRI, digital subtraction angiography or contrast enhanced CT, 3D color/power angiography allows the physician to examine vascular anatomy immediately and without radiation exposure.

Most tubal gestations are not ongoing viable gestations. They are usually in the involutional phase of abortion within a confined area which results in the extrusion of products of conception through a ruptured site or fimbriae. In the two reported cases, the serum assays of beta hCG in both patients increased to significant levels which precluded intrauterine missed abortion.[61] Besides, there were neither retained products of conception in utero nor heavy vaginal bleeding (indicating process of abortion in progress) prior to the diagnosis of arteriovenous malformation. Therefore, the authors speculated that there might be an ectopic gestation occurring somewhere, although they could only find a pelvic arteriovenous malformation rather than an adnexal gestational sac.

The major difference between uterine implantation and tubal gestation is that endosalpingeal stroma usually fails to undergo decidualization. The chorionic villi of the tubal implantation may then invade into the tubal wall and mesentery (mesosalpinx) more directly and rapidly. The vascularization within the ectopic pregnancy is an analog of placenta increta.[55] In such situations, cytotrophoblast may invade the contiguous artery and vein of the mesosalpinx with destruction of these vessels' walls, and thus, may induce an arteriovenous malformation in situ or nearby. Possibly, the secretion of angiogenic factors (by trophoblast) and the increasing afterload of an arterioventricular shunt existing in the tubal gestation can induce the rapid growth of a small pre-existing congenital arteriovenous malformation. However, two unusual cases of adnexal arteriovenous malformations associated with "vanishing" ectopic gestation where congenital etiology seemed unlikely have also been reported.[61] B-mode ultrasound and color Doppler provided information on the hemodynamics of the vascular tumor and led to the diagnosis of the arteriovenous malformation. Three-dimensional color/power angiography further improved the understanding of the complex vascular anatomy and refined the diagnosis.

Even though the exact role of 3D ultrasound in the pathology of early pregnancy is yet to be established, promising results in already published papers are encouraging. Unlimited numbers of sections are easily obtained without the need for excessive manipulation of the probe. Additional progress has been made, owing to the permanent possibility or repeated analysis of previous stored 3D volumes and Cartesian elimination of surrounding structures and artifacts. A three-dimensional reconstruction of stored images without any degradation is the most impressive benefit of 3D scanning.

OTHER SITES OF IMPLANTATION

About 5% of ectopic pregnancies implant in sites other than the tubes.[1] These are at times more difficult to detect and some, owing to their specific sites of implantation, may cause rupture, significant bleeding and higher morbidity and mortality than the tubal gestations.

Angular Pregnancy

Angular pregnancy is defined as a pregnancy implanted in one of the lateral angles of the uterine cavity **(Figs. 10A and B)**. It is associated with increased risk of miscarriage, preterm labor, massive hemorrhage, placenta accreta and post-partum placental retention.[62]

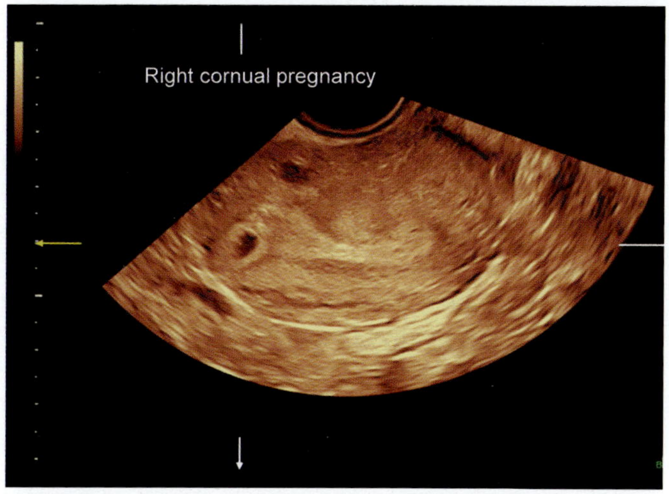

Fig. 10A: B-mode ultrasound image of the uterus in transverse section, showing an anechoic roundish area with hyperechoic rim (early gestation sac) at the right end of the endometrial cavity. The gestational sac is covered by endometrium medially but laterally it shows only a myometrial cover suggesting an angular pregnancy.

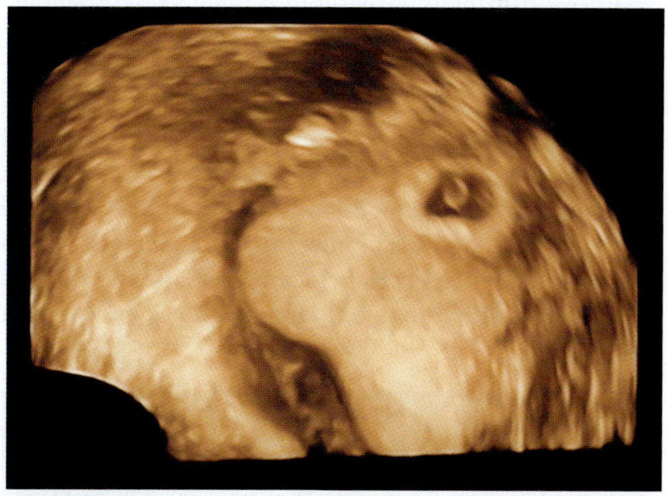

Fig. 10B: 3D ultrasound acquired volume of the uterus. The gestational sac with yolk sac and fetal pole is seen lateral to the endometrial cavity, with myometrial mantle laterally. 3D sonographic findings are suggestive of angular pregnancy.

Interstitial (Cornual) Pregnancy

Interstitial pregnancy occurs in 1.1–6.3% of all ectopic pregnancies.[1,63] This location of the ectopic pregnancy usually occurs following in vitro fertilization (IVF) and previous salpingectomy,[63] but in most cases there are no apparent risk factors. Interstitial pregnancy clinically presents with abdominal pain and a tender asymmetrically enlarged uterus. The major problem of this location lies in late diagnosis, because it is commonly diagnosed after the rupture of the cornu has occurred and this may result in massive hemorrhage. Previously, interstitial pregnancies were diagnosed only at laparotomy following the rupture. For the reason of major hemorrhage, hysterectomy rate was as high as 40%.[60] In recent years, the routine use of ultrasound for the assessment of women with early pregnancy complications has enabled a noninvasive diagnosis of interstitial pregnancy to be made. Earlier diagnosis made before serious complications, allows the use of more conservative management, such as medical treatment or laparoscopic surgery.

A viable interstitial pregnancy may occasionally be misinterpreted as a normal intrauterine pregnancy. Therefore, it is important that strict diagnostic criteria are used in every case:[64]

- Empty uterine cavity.
- Chorionic sac that is seen separately and more than 1 cm from the most lateral edge of the uterine cavity and surrounded by a thin myometrial layer **(Fig. 11A)**.

It is worth to mention that approximately 15% of patients with interstitial pregnancy have heterotopic pregnancy.[64] In these cases, intrauterine findings may be misleading and should be interpreted with caution, rather than being used as primary diagnostic criterion. Visualization of the interstitial part of the tube in close proximity of the endometrium and depiction of the trophoblastic tissue improves the diagnosis of interstitial pregnancy.[65] It also confirms that pregnancy is located outside the uterine cavity, facilitating the differential diagnosis between an interstitial pregnancy and unusual forms of intrauterine pregnancy such as angular pregnancy or pregnancy in the cornu of an anomalous uterus. This sign is particularly helpful in women with small intramural fibroids located in vicinity of the interstitial part of the tube, which may be misinterpreted as a solid interstitial pregnancy.[66] In women with fibroids, the intramural part of the tube is displaced and can be visualized bypassing the mass, thus preventing the false-positive diagnosis of the interstitial pregnancy. Color Doppler facilitates the diagnosis of a cornual pregnancy by exposing low resistance peritrophoblastic flow **(Fig. 11B)**.

Three-dimensional ultrasound has the advantage of providing views of the uterus, which can rarely be obtained by conventional 2D ultrasound scan.[67] In the coronal section, the position of the interstitial pregnancy in relation to the uterine cavity can be studied in detail **(Fig. 11C)**. Visualization of the proximal section of the interstitial tube is also facilitated, which increases the diagnostic confidence.[67] It is believed that 3D ultrasound is a helpful diagnostic tool in women with suspected interstitial pregnancy and should be considered in the cases where the diagnosis is not certain on conventional 2D transvaginal ultrasound scan [65,68] **(Figs. 11D and E)**. It has been demonstrated that 3D color and/or power Doppler may aid in early diagnosis of cornual/interstitial pregnancy **(Fig. 11F)**.

Most cornual/interstitial ectopic pregnancies are treated by laparoscopy and laparotomy using various

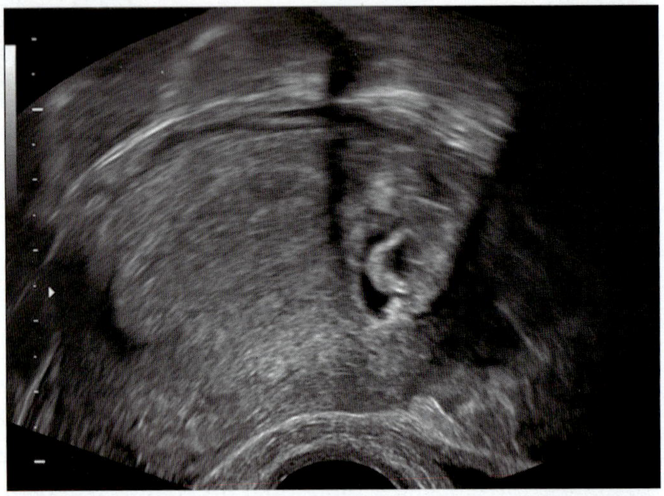

Fig. 11A: Transvaginal ultrasound demonstrates empty uterine cavity and a chorionic sac seen separately and more than 1 cm from the most lateral edge of the uterine cavity and surrounded by a thin myometrial layer.

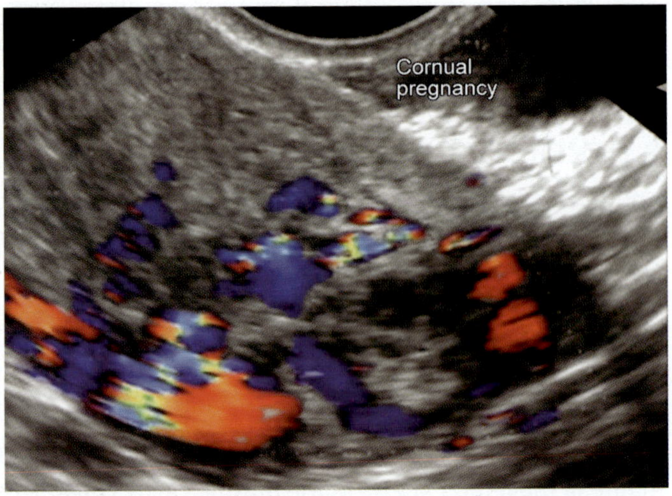

Fig. 11B: Transvaginal color Doppler scan of interstitial pregnancy. Color signals facilitate early diagnosis of this ectopic pregnancy location by exposing prominent peritrophoblastic flow.

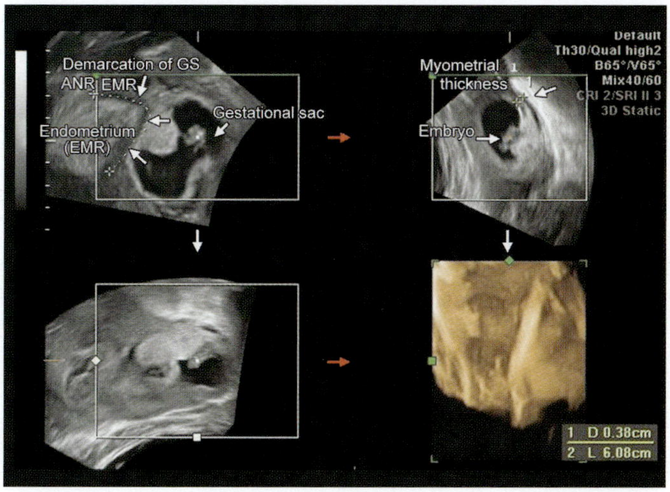

Fig. 11C: Three-dimensional ultrasound provides views of the uterus, which cannot be obtained by conventional 2D ultrasound scan. Coronal section (upper left image), and surface rendering (lower right image) enable visualization of the cornual ectopic pregnancy.

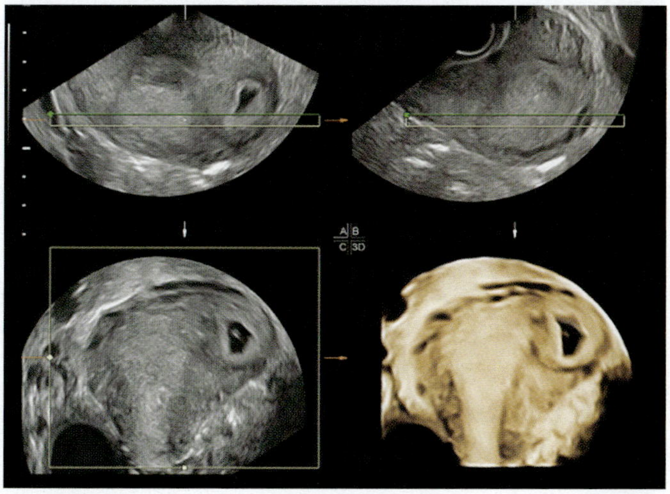

Fig. 11D: 3D ultrasound acquired volume of the uterus, showing the gestational sac in the acquisition planes and the coronal plane. The gestational sac does not show any continuity with the endometrial cavity. Gestational sac is not seen in the B plane because the reference dot is not on the gestational sac. The rendered image (right lower image) shows empty endometrial cavity and the gestational sac laterally from the endometrial cavity, with myometrial mantle between the endometrial cavity and the gestational sac. 3D sonographic findings are typical for cornual or interstial pregnancy.

surgical procedures (excision, suturing, etc.) **(Figs. 12A to E)**. Lately, transvaginal sonographic puncture and local injection of methotrexate, has been used to treat both viable and non-viable interstitial pregnancies.[64] There have

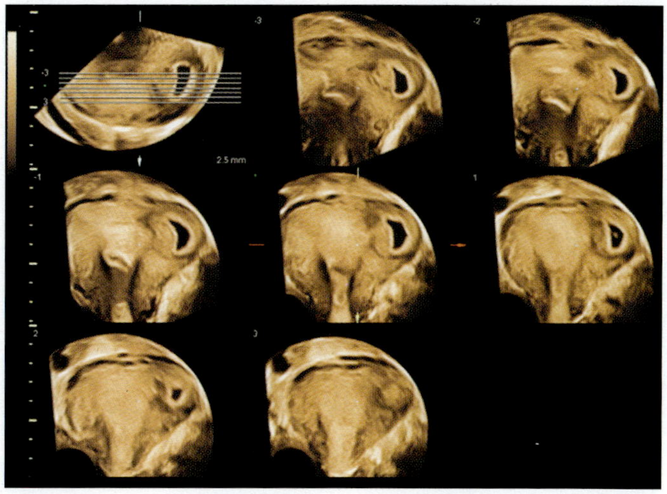

Fig. 11E: Tomographic ultrasound image of the same patient as in the previous figure, confirms the findings of cornual ectopic pregnancy.

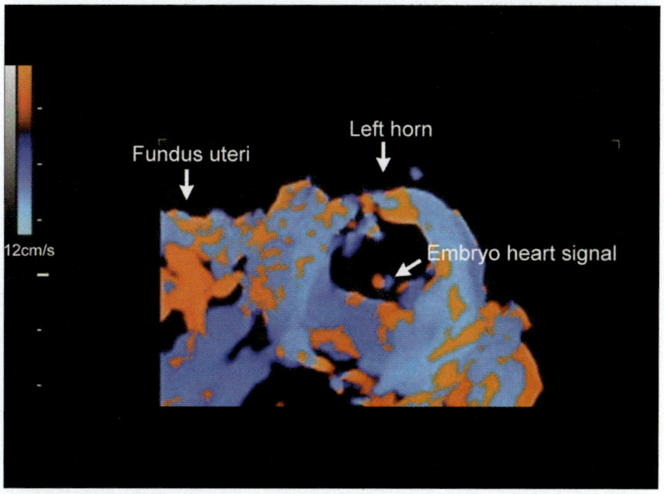

Fig. 11F: Three-dimensional color Doppler ultrasound of cornual pregnancy. Prominent peritrophoblastic flow indicates vital trophoblast.

been very few reported side-effects after treatment with low dose local injection of methotrexate.[69] Data reported in the literature suggest the superiority of local therapy, with regard to both the safety aspect and the success rates. In general, a likely explanation for the increased effectiveness of local injection is a higher concentration of therapeutic agent achieved at the target tissue. Although absorption of methotrexate into the circulation occurs after both local and systemic administration, a lower dose of methotrexate is used locally, leading to lower

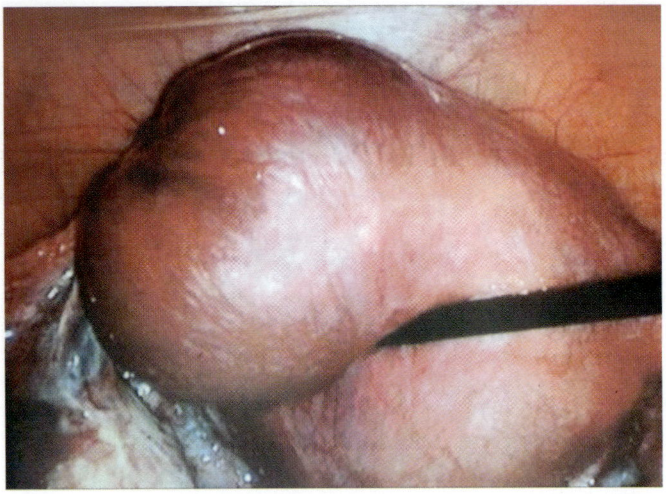

Fig. 12A: Laparaoscopic view of cornual pregnancy. Note swelling and hypervascularity of the cornual area.

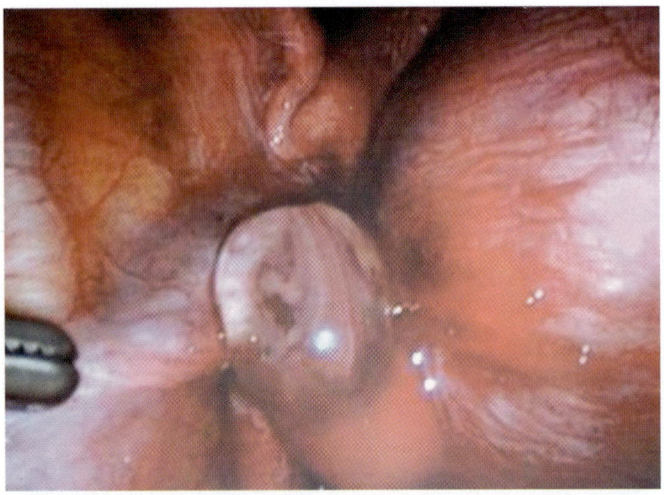

Fig. 12B: Laparoscopic image demonstrates the gestational sac with an embryo at the site of cornual pregnancy rupture.

systemic levels, and therefore, fewer side-effects.[70] Color Doppler plays an extremely important role providing an aid in approaching the cornual pregnancy from the medial aspect and traversing the thicker myometrial layer so rupture or bleeding are less likely to occur.[71] In these cases, color Doppler guidance during the instillation of methotrexate enables better visualization of blood vessels and avoidance of intraprocedural complications.

Viable heterotopic/interstitial pregnancies are often treated by local injection of potassium chloride, as this is not teratogenic. All six reported cases of heterotopic pregnancies in the literature were successfully treated in this way, with three (50%) intrauterine pregnancies progressing normally to full term.[4]

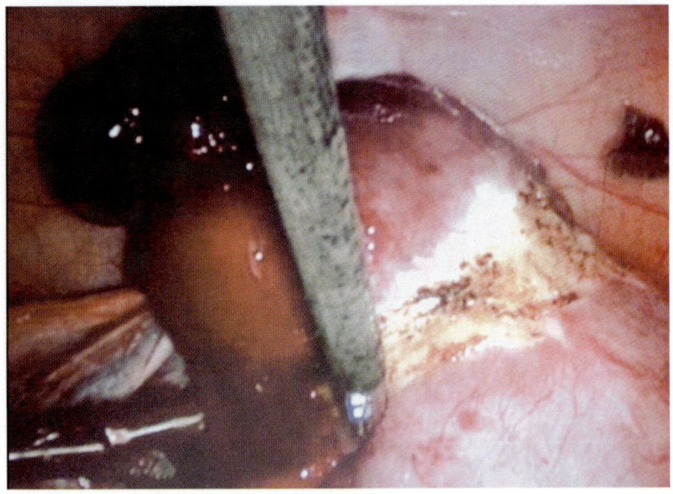

Fig. 12C: Resection of the cornual pregnancy after infiltration with vasopressin.

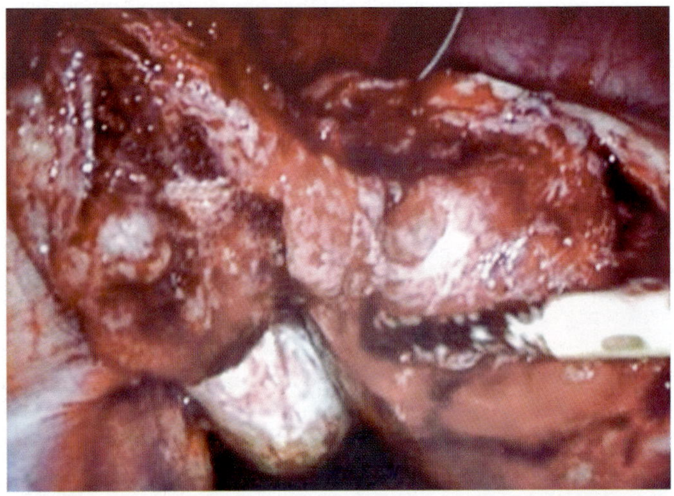

Fig. 12D: Cornual pregnancy at the time of excision.

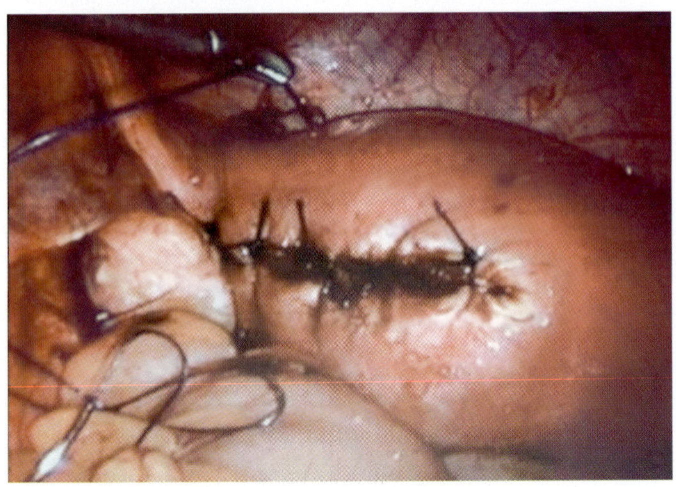

Fig. 12E: Closure of the cornual region with sutures.

Expectant management of the interstitial pregnancy has also been reported.[64,66] All three nonviable interstitial pregnancies managed in this way were resolved spontaneously without any need for intervention. Expectant management can, therefore, be useful option in selected cases.

Cervical Pregnancy

Cervical pregnancy is defined as the implantation of the conceptus below the level of the internal os. It is the rare condition that occurs in one in 50,000.[4] Intrauterine adhesions, uterine anomalies, previous cesarean sections, fibroids, previous therapeutic abortions and IVF treatment have all been associated with cervical implantation. Traditionally, the diagnosis of cervical pregnancy was based solely on clinical findings and history reports after hysterectomy. Therefore, it is likely that only the most severe cases were diagnosed, and a number of cervical pregnancies went undiagnosed or were treated as incomplete miscarriages. In the past two decades, ultrasound has become the method of choice for diagnosis of early pregnancy disorders and certainly contributed to the recent increase in number of reported cervical pregnancies.

The diagnosis of cervical pregnancy can be made using the following criteria:

- No evidence on intrauterine pregnancy.
- An hour glass uterine shape with ballooned cervical canal.
- Presence of a gestational sac or placental tissue within the cervical canal, and a closed internal os **(Fig. 13A)**.

Early diagnosis may also explain the milder clinical symptoms and better prognosis of cervical pregnancy today as compared to preultrasound era.

Transvaginal ultrasound approach has become the accepted standard for the examination of patients with suspected early pregnancy abnormalities. Apart from providing superior images of pelvic anatomy, the addition of color Doppler enables simultaneous visualization of the pelvic blood vessels and embryonic heart action **(Figs. 13B and C)**. The level of the insertion of the uterine arteries should be used to identify the internal os, and thus, facilitate the diagnosis of a cervical pregnancy.[71] The extensive vascular blood supply to the trophoblastic tissue originating from the adjacent maternal arteries at the implantation site (within the cervix) is easily visualized by transvaginal color Doppler. The products of conception in transit through the cervix after the failure of a normally implanted pregnancy are detached from their implantation site and maternal vascular supply. It is, therefore, impossible to detect any peritrophoblastic blood flow in these cases.[72] Conversely, even a small amount of placental tissue in a true cervical pregnancy remains highly vascularized on color Doppler examination.[73] This facilitates the differential diagnosis between the cervical pregnancy and incomplete miscarriage. Color Doppler analysis may also improve selection of the patients for primary surgical removal of cervical pregnancy and assist in planning D&C following medical treatment. It is necessary to stress the potential of 3D sonography in diagnosis of cervical gestation and include the better anatomic orientation and multiplanar sections of the investigated area.

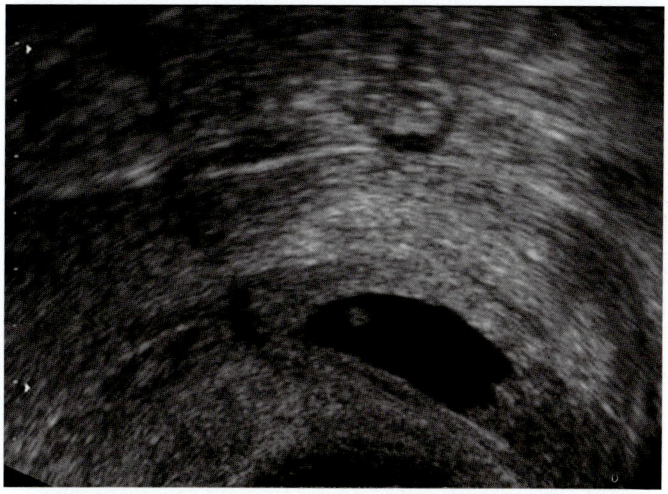

Fig. 13A: Transvaginal ultrasound demonstrates a cervical pregnancy. Both internal and external cervical os are closed.

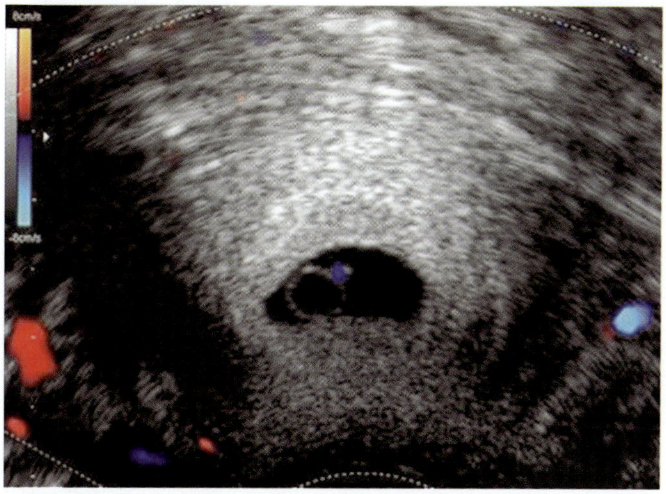

Fig. 13B: Transvaginal color Doppler scan of a cervical pregnancy. Note yolk sac and embryonic heart activity.

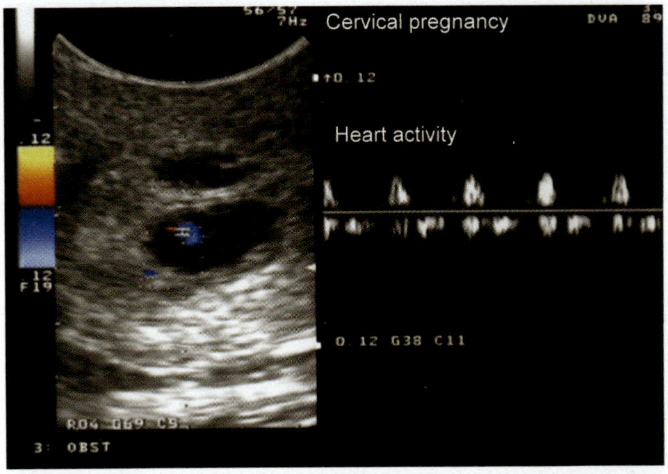

Fig. 13C: Transvaginal color Doppler scan of a cervical pregnancy. Blood flow signals are derived from the fetal heart and demonstrate regular heart action.

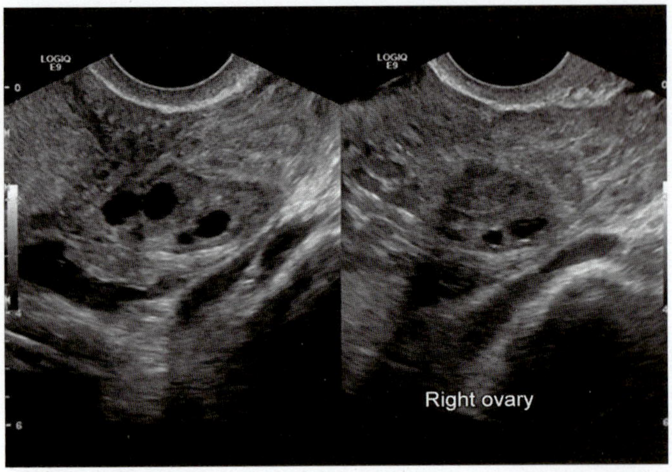

Fig. 14A: Transvaginal ultrasound scan of a complex ovarian mass in a patient with positive pregnancy test and no evidence of intrauterine pregnancy.

Local injection of methotrexate or potassium chloride appears to be the most effective way of treating an early viable cervical pregnancy regardless of the gestational age. There are no data on the use of local injection in nonviable pregnancies and it is uncertain whether the treatment would be as effective as in viable pregnancies. Systemic use of methotrexate in non-viable pregnancies is simple and highly effective.

The regiments and dosages of methotrexate used for systemic therapy have varied considerably. There is no clear correlation between the dose and therapeutic success and it is, therefore, logical to use as little methotrexate as possible to minimize side-effects. The usual regiment should be two intramuscular injections of 1 mg/kg methotrexate followed by folic acid. For local injection, 25 mg methotrexate into gestation sac appears to be sufficient. Potassium chloride 3–5 mEq is equally successful and less likely to cause side-effects.[4]

The place of surgery should be limited to those cases where medical treatment has failed. Dilatation and curettage in combination with cervical cerclage or the insertion of a Foley catheter is probably the best choice for a general gynecologist and is as effective as more complicated and expensive methods for the prevention of uncontrollable hemorrhage.[71]

The sonographic diagnosis of an **ovarian pregnancy** is extremely difficult to establish. It has been calculated that ovarian pregnancy accounts for less than 3% of ectopic pregnancies.[1,2] The sonographic diagnosis is made upon the finding of a hyperechoic trophoblastic ring detected

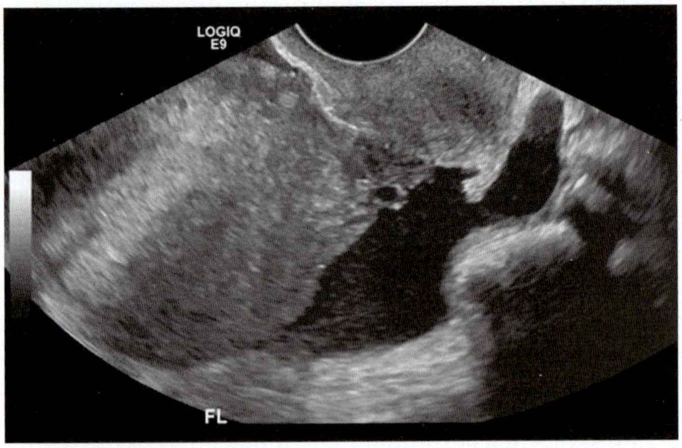

Fig. 14B: The same patient as in **Figure14A**. Free fluid is visualized in the cul-de-sac.

within the ovarian tissue **(Figs. 14A to C)**, and the fact that it is impossible to separate the ectopic gestational sac from the ovary by transabdominal pressure from either examiner's hand or transvaginal ultrasound probe.[2] Color Doppler facilitates detection of the peritrophoblastic flow, which can speed up the entire diagnostic procedure.

Intra-abdominal Pregnancy

It is a rare condition, constituting only 1% of all ectopic gestations.[74] Its complications, however, can be devastating. These include massive hemorrhage due to disseminated intravascular coagulation (DIC) and placental separation complicating fetal demise, or infection with abscess formation. The outlook for the fetus is even worse, and perinatal mortality may reach 75%, with up to 90% of

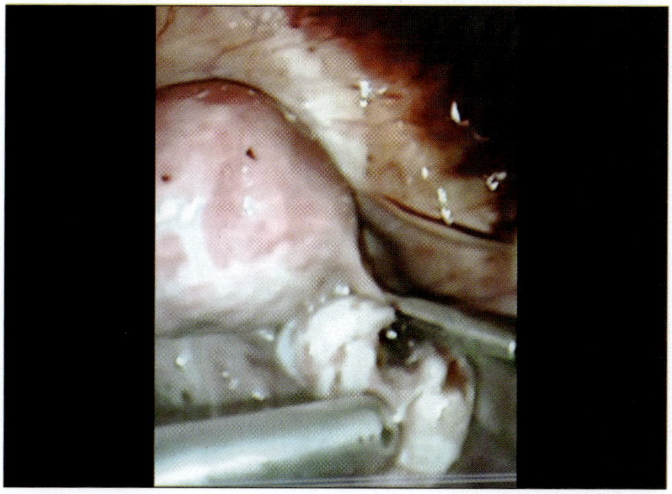

Fig. 14C: The same patient as in **Figures 14A and B**. Laparoscopy confirmed the diagnosis of ovarian pregnancy.

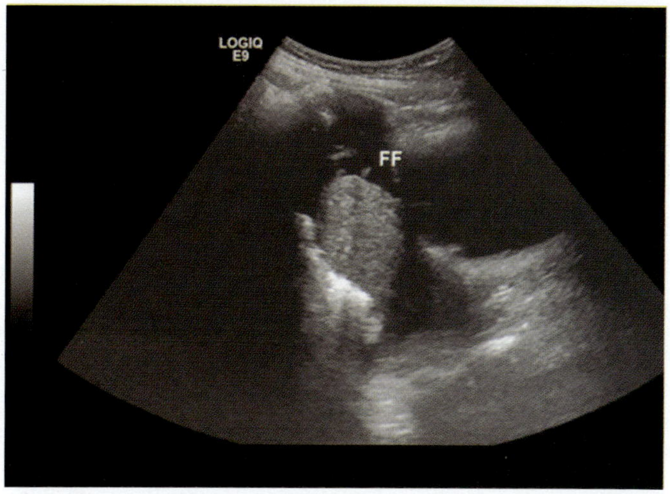

Fig. 15A: Transabdominal ultrasound shows empty uterus and free fluid in the pelvis. Patient presented with abnormal genital tract bleeding and abdominal/pelvic pain at 15 weeks gestation.

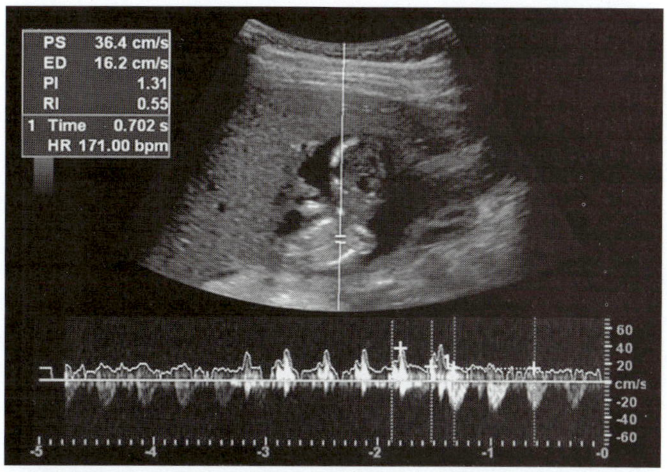

Fig. 15B: Transabdominal pulsed Doppler ultrasound demonstrates regular heart activity with frequency of 171 beats per minute.

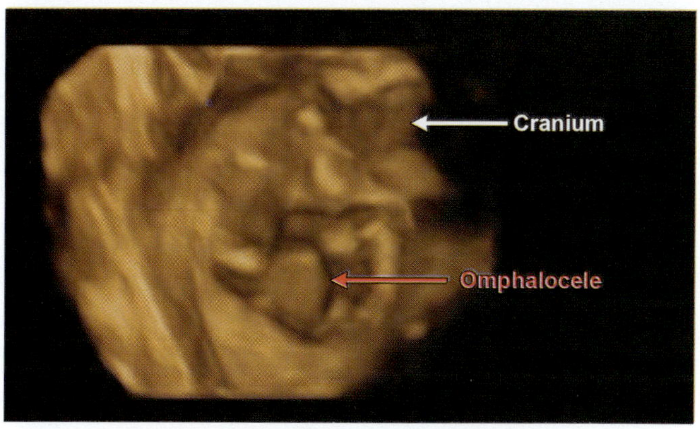

Fig. 15C: Three-dimensional ultrasound of the same fetus demonstrates an omphalocele.

the surviving infants having serious malformations.[75] The diagnosis of the abdominal pregnancy is not easy, especially in the early stages. Characteristically, patients present with abdominal pain, vaginal bleeding and gastrointestinal complaints. Ultrasonography combined with beta hCG estimations have made early diagnosis easier. The problem still exists, because as a patient subgroup, an ambiguous clinical presentation still remains.[76]

Ultrasound seems to be the most valuable diagnostic tool to localize this rare type of ectopic pregnancy.[2] Primary abdominal pregnancy is condition where fertilized egg implants itself directly into the peritoneal surface of abdominal cavity. If, however, an early tubal pregnancy dislodges and aborts into the pelvis, adhering to peritoneal surface, it is termed as a secondary abdominal pregnancy through the secondary nidation. The sonographic presentation of abdominal pregnancy is no different from any other ectopic pregnancy, i.e. showing no evidence of intrauterine pregnancy **(Fig. 15A)**, presence of a hyperechoic ectopic gestational sac containing embryonic/fetal structures and extraembryonic structures with or without active heart beats **(Figs.15B and C)**. Oligohydramnion is the rule and there is no uterine mantle around the fetus.

Surgery is a time-honored treatment for abdominal pregnancy following its diagnosis, with placenta left in situ **(Figs. 15D and E)**. This is mainly because, in many instances, the placenta is attached to vital organs or vascular sites, which could be seriously damaged during placental separation. No serious complications occur when it is left in situ.[77] An additional important factor is that

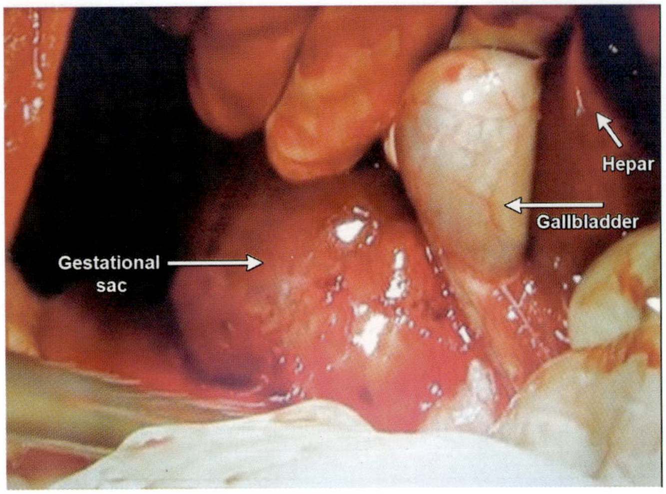

Fig. 15D: Laparoscopy revealed abdominal pregnancy. Gestational sac was implanted below the liver and gallbladder.

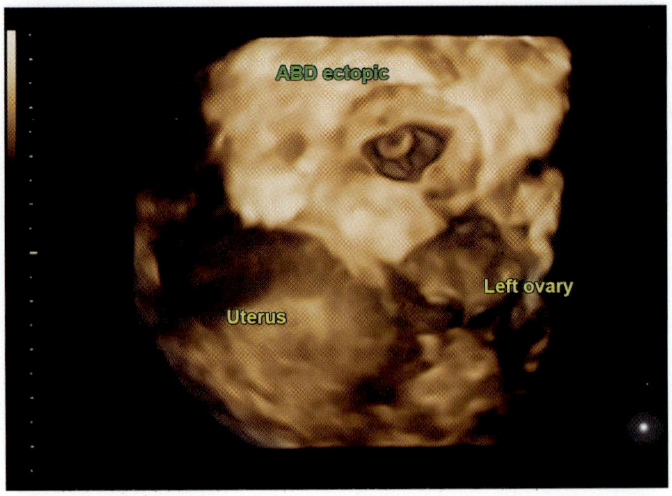

Fig. 15F: 3D ultrasound image showing surface rendered volume of the uterus and left ovary. A hypoechoic tubular structure is seen between the uterus and the ovary. A gestational sac with yolk sac and the fetal pole is seen away from these pelvic organs. 3D imaging is suggestive of abdominal pregnancy, which was confirmed by laparoscopy.

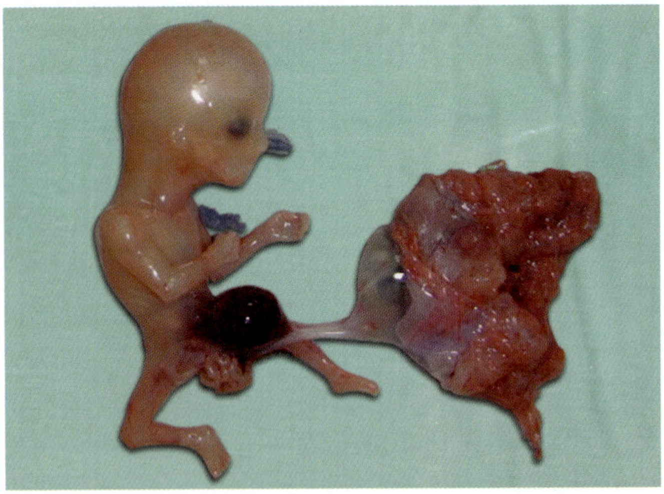

Fig. 15E: Gross anatomy of the fetus with evidence of an omphalocele. Compare the image with **Figure 14C**.

most abdominal pregnancies are diagnosed relatively late in pregnancy, when the placenta and its area of attachment are larger. Recently, abdominal pregnancies have been diagnosed earlier and in one case the diagnosis was made at 6 weeks of amenorrhea.[74] This made it possible for these pregnancies to be removed laparoscopically. The possible advantages of such therapeutic approach include lower morbidity and mortality, as well as better fertility outcome. However, only a limited number of cases of abdominal pregnancy have been reported early in pregnancy and the safety of operative laparoscopy can be guaranteed only in appropriately selected cases.[74] Similar cases demonstrate the further importance of first-trimester ultrasound examination in diagnosing early pregnancy complications. The importance of sonographic imaging in cases of acute abdomen in pregnancy cannot be over-stressed.[78]

Although there are no available data on the use of color Doppler and 3D ultrasound in this field, we believe that these modalities may add additional information on the implantation site and attachment of the placenta to the surrounding structures **(Fig. 15F)**.

Cesarean Section Scar

Ectopic pregnancy represents a rare, though growing subset of potentially life-threatening conditions **(Figs. 16A to D)**. Transvaginal ultrasound has a reported sensitivity of 85% for detection of CS scar ectopic pregnancy **(Fig. 17A)**.[79,80] An accurate and prompt diagnosis is crucial to avoid catastrophic complications such as uterine rupture, placenta accreta and massive bleeding, which might lead to hysterectomy.[81] Color Doppler, 3D and 3D power Doppler ultrasound may aid in early diagnosis of this condition **(Figs. 17B and C)**. Various therapeutic approaches have been reported for this rare type of ectopic pregnancy such as systemic use of methotrexate, hysteroscopic treatment, uterine arterial embolization, uterine curettage, transabdominal uterine scar incision or laparoscopic hysterotomy.[82]

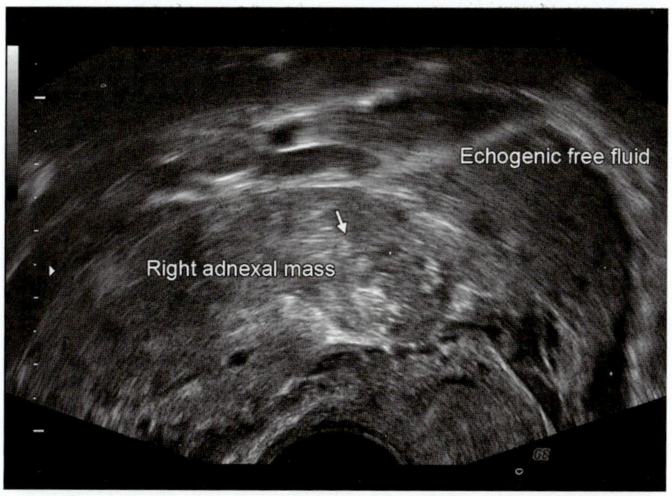

Fig. 16A: Transvaginal ultrasound scan demonstrates a complex adnexal mass in a patient presenting with amenorrhea, pelvic pain and positive pregnancy test.

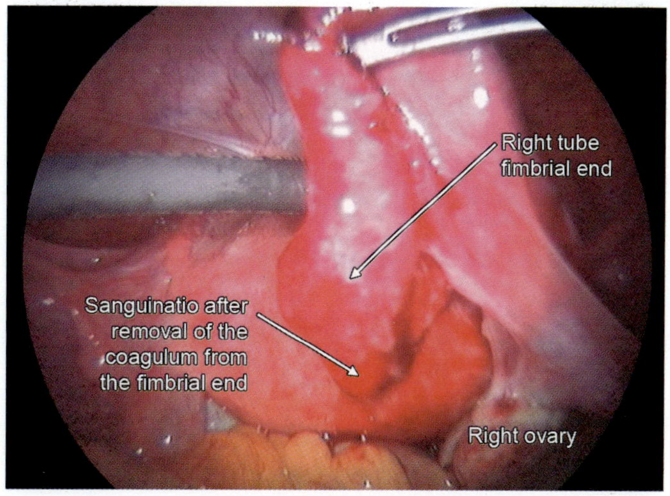

Fig. 16C: Laparoscopy revealed ectopic pregnancy in the ampular part of the tube, hematosalpynx and bleeding from the fimbrial end.

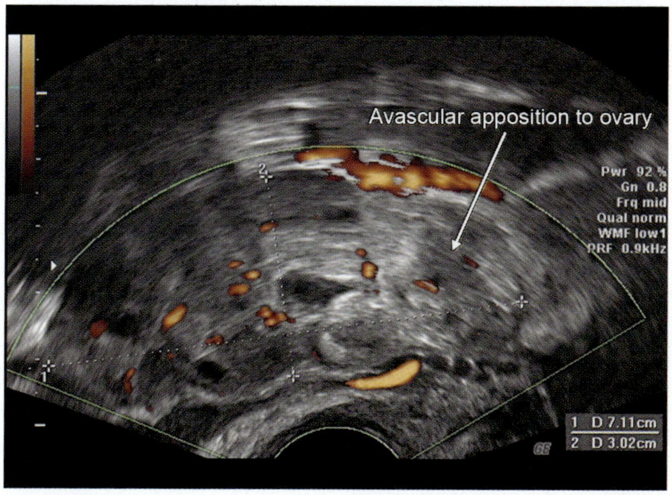

Fig. 16B: Color Doppler ultrasound demonstrates increased vascularity suggestive of ectopic pregnancy with vital trophoblast.

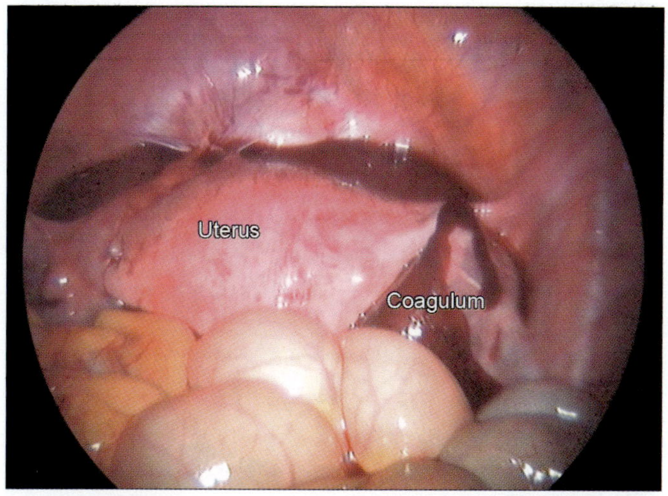

Fig. 16D: Free fluid and coagulum in the cul-de-sac.

THERAPY

Throughout the years, the treatment of ectopic pregnancy has been emergency laparotomy, including salpingectomy. In order to preserve fertility, alternatives to laparotomy and salpingectomy include observation, laparoscopic removal of ectopic pregnancy and systemic or local use of methotrexate or other feticidal agents. As medical therapy for ectopic pregnancy becomes a common practice, familiarity with its side effects may lead to greater success rates. The decision to abandon medical treatment and proceed with surgery should be based on defined guidelines, such as development of peritoneal signs, decreasing hemoglobin levels, or hemodynamic instability.[83]

Methotrexate may be administered systemically, locally or in combination.[84-86] Local application is performed either laparoscopically or transvaginally under ultrasound needle puncture.[40] In the latter approach, methotrexate is injected directly into the gestational sac. The success rate of systemic, single dose methotrexate (83–96%) is similar to that of local administration under laparoscopic guidance (89–100%), but the success rate of methotrexate under ultrasound guidance seems to be lower (70–83%).[87] Local injection of methotrexate under control of color

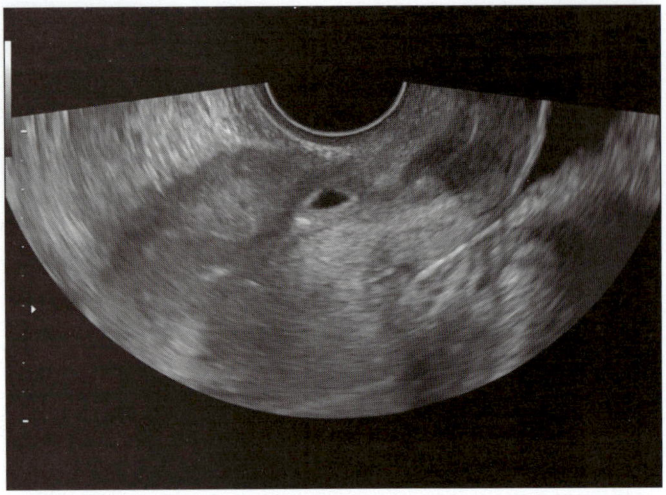

Fig. 17A: B-mode ultrasound image of the uterus in longitudinal, sagittal section. Endometrium appears thin and ill-defined. Patient had a history of previous cesarean section. An anechoic oval structure with hyperechoic rim is seen anterior to the endometrium, with only myometrium between the sac and the serosa. Sonographic findings are suggestive of post C-section scar pregnancy.

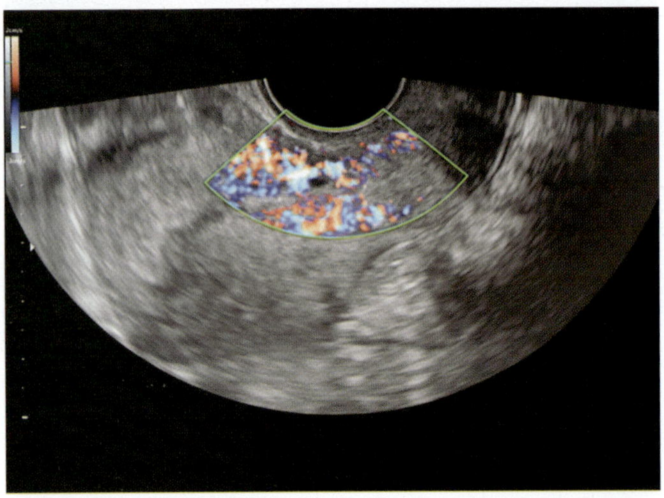

Fig. 17B: The same patient as in the previous image assessed by high definition Doppler. Note a rim of vascularity around the gestational sac, indicating vital trophoblast.

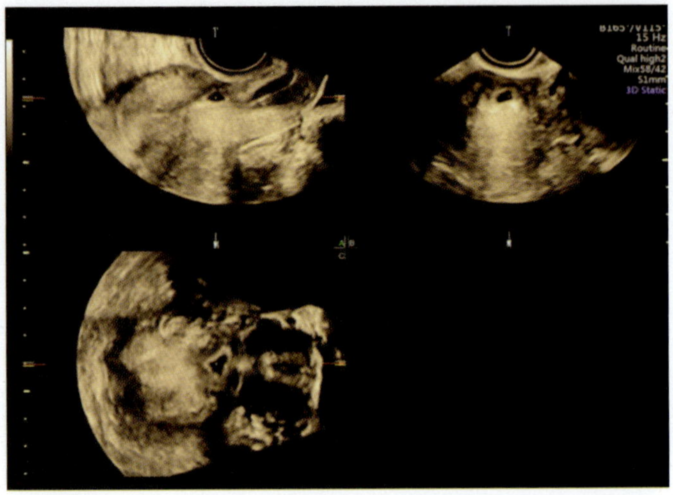

Fig. 17C: 3D ultrasound acquisition revealed the final diagnosis of the post C-section scar pregnancy in all three (sagittal, coronal and axial) planes.

Doppler imaging may increase the success rate.[4] The use of color and pulsed Doppler enables visualization of the trophoblastic adnexal flow with high velocity and low impedance pulsed Doppler (RI < 0.40). The needle can be inserted into the area of maximum color signal, which marks trophoblastic invasiveness and vitality.

Pharmacological management of an unruptured, size-appropriate ectopic pregnancy is now an established standard of care. The present protocol recommends systemic use of methotrexate in a single-dose.[88] This form of methotrexate has proven to be successful and cost-effective alternative to traditional surgical management of ectopic pregnancy.[89] In view of the risk of standard therapy and the patients' desire for fertility, methotrexate treatment may be a therapeutic alternative in cervical pregnancy as well. Recent reports have affirmed that ectopic pregnancy has become, a medical rather than a surgical disease.[2,4,69,72,79,87,88,90]

Puncture injections are valid and reasonable alternative to a traditional surgical approach, especially in patients with an interstitial, cervical or heterotopic pregnancy. In these particular cases, puncture procedures guided by transvaginal ultrasound can efficiently replace surgical treatment and save the patient from unnecessary hysterectomy.

Early diagnosis is the key to effective nonsurgical treatment. Diagnostic algorithms using serial beta hCG measurements and transvaginal ultrasound examinations make definitive diagnosis possible without laparoscopy **(Fig. 16A)**. As stated before, with help of color Doppler it is possible to identify the activity, invasiveness and vitality of trophoblasts. **(Fig. 16B)** These represent the most important characteristics for making the decision for more selective management of an ectopic pregnancy. Three-dimensional ultrasound seems to be an even more effective procedure for early diagnosis of ectopic pregnancy in asymptomatic patients, even before 6 weeks of amenorrhea.[59]

Laparoscopic salpingostomy, the surgical gold standard, is an effective therapy in patients who are hemodynamically stable and wish to preserve their fertility **(Figs. 16C and D)**. The reproductive performance after salpingostomy appears to be equal to, or better than salpingectomy, but the recurrent ectopic pregnancy rate is slightly higher.[3] A variable systemic dose of methotrexate produces outcomes close to those of laparoscopic salpingostomy in similar patients.[91] Methotrexate treatment is recommended in the asymptomatic patient with serum beta hCG levels of less than 2,000 IU/mL, a tubal diameter of <2 cm and absence of fetal heart activity. The patient's understanding of her condition and compliance are mandatory. However, in many cases, the ectopic pregnancy does not meet suitable medical criteria and still requires surgery. In cases suspicious of tubal abortion with a high impedance signal (RI >0.55) and beta hCG below 1,000 IU/mL, local administration of methotrexate is not advised. A recent paper assessed the protocol of a single dose methotrexate for the treatment of ectopic pregnancy and confirmed that 15% decrease in serum hCG between day 4 and 7 is a very good predictor of the likely success of medical treatment.[92] A recent meta-analysis including data from 26 trials demonstrated the success with the single-dose regimen to be 88.1%, while the success with the multiple dose regimen was 92.7%.[93] A small randomized clinical trial also demonstrated the single-dose regimen to have a slightly higher failure rate.[94] Barnhart et al. more recently reported that the minimum rise in beta hCG for a potentially viable pregnancy in women who present with vaginal bleeding or pain is 53% per 2 days (up to 5,000 IU/L).[95] A hybrid protocol, involving 2 equal doses of methotrexate (50 mg/m^2) given on days 1 and 4 without the use of leucovorin has been shown to be an effective and convenient alternative to the existing regimens.[96]

CONCLUSION

With the use of beta hCG testing and transvaginal ultrasound our approach to the patient with a suspected ectopic pregnancy has been vastly improved. An important advantage of the most currently used transvaginal transducers is the ability to perform simultaneous color and spectral Doppler studies, allowing easy identification of the ectopic peritrophoblastic flow. Therefore, color should be applied whenever a finding is suggestive of ectopic pregnancy.

Further progresses in diagnostic procedures were made when 3D ultrasound was introduced. Transvaginal 3D ultrasound enables the clinician to perceive the true spatial relations, and thus, easily distinguish the origin of an ectopic pregnancy, while 3D power Doppler allows detailed analysis of the vascularization.

Transvaginal color and pulsed Doppler imaging may be potentially used for detection of the patients with less prominent tubal perfusion, suitable for the expectant management of an ectopic pregnancy. It is expected that the increased sensitivity of the serum beta hCG immunoassay and the quality of transvaginal B-mode, color Doppler ultrasound and more recently 3D with color and power Doppler facilities will allow even earlier detection and conservative management of ectopic pregnancies. Furthermore, it seems that the fertility outcomes and the number of women attempting to conceive after an ectopic pregnancy will increase even more.

REFERENCES

1. Ectopic pregnancy. In: Speroff L, Glass R H, Kase NG (Eds). Clinical Gynecologic Endocrinology and Infertility. London: Williams and Wilkins; 1999.pp.1149-67.
2. Timor-Tristch IE, Monteagudo A. Ectopic pregnancy. In: Kupesic S, de Ziegler D (Eds). Ultrasound and infertility. UK: Partenon Publishing Group, 2000.pp.215-39.
3. Kurjak A, Kupesic S. Ectopic pregnancy. In: Kurjak A (Ed). Ultrasound in Obstetrics and Gynecology. Boston: CRC Press; 1990.pp.225-35.
4. Kupesic S, Kurjak A. Color Doppler assessment of ectopic pregnancy. In: Kurjak A, Kupesic S (Eds). An Atlas of Transvaginal Color Doppler. London: Parthenon Publishing; 2000.pp.137-47.
5. Boufous S, Quartararo M, Mohsin M, Parker J. Trends in the incidence of ectopic pregnancy in New South Wales between 1990-1998. Aust N Z J Obstet Gynaecol. 2001;41:436-8.
6. Rajkhowa M, Glass MR, Rutherford AJ, Balen AH, Sharma V, Cuckle HS. Trends in the incidence of ectopic pregnancy in England and Wales from 1966 to 1996. BJOG. 2000;107: 369-74.
7. Nederlof KP, Lawson HW, Saftlas AF, Atrash HK, Finch EL. Ectopic pregnancy surveillance. Morbid Mortal Weekly Rep 1990;39:9.
8. Strandell A, Thorburn J, Hamberger L. Risk factors for ectopic pregnancy in assisted reproduction. Fertil Steril. 1999;2:282-6.
9. Kamwendo F, Forslin L, Bodin L, Danielsson D. Epidemiology of ectopic pregnancy during a 28 year period and the role of pelvic inflammatory disease. Sex Transm Infect. 2000;76: 28-32.

10. Barlow RE, Cooke ID, Odukoya O, Heatley MK, Jenkins J, Narayansingh G, et al. The prevalence of *Chlamydia trachomatis* in fresh tissue specimens from patients with ectopic pregnancy or tubal factor infertility as determined by PCR and in-situ hybridisation. J Med Microbiol. 2001;50: 902-8.
11. Brown WD, Burrows L, Todd CS. Ectopic pregnancy after cesarean hysterectomy. Obstet Gynecol. 2002;99:933-4.
12. Bouyer J, Rachou E, Germain E, Fernandez H, Coste J, Pouly JL, et al. Risk factors for extrauterine pregnancy in women using an intrauterine device. Fertil Steril. 2000;74:899-908.
13. Bouyer J, Coste J, Fernandez H, Pouly JL, Job-Spira N. Sites of ectopic pregnancy: a 10 year population-based study of 1800 cases. Hum Reprod. 2002;17:3224-30.
14. Mol BW, van der Veen F, Bossuyt PM. Symptom-free women at increased risk of ectopic pregnancy: should we screen? Acta Obstet Gynecol Scand. 2002;81:661-72.
15. Kalinski MA, Guss DA. Hemorrhagic shock from a ruptured ectopic pregnancy in a patient with a negative urine pregnancy test result. Ann Emerg Med. 2002;40:102-5.
16. Mertz HL, Yalcinkaya TM. Early diagnosis of ectopic pregnancy. Does use of a strict algorithm decrease the incidence of tubal rupture? Reprod Med. 2001;46:29-33.
17. Sagaster P, Zojer N, Dekan G, Ludwig HA. Paraneoplastic syndrome mimicking extrauterine pregnancy. Ann Oncol. 2002;13:170-2.
18. Hick JL, Rodgerson JD, Heegaard WG, Sterner S. Vital signs fail to correlate with hemoperitoneum from ruptured ectopic pregnancy. Am J Emerg Med. 2001;19:488-91.
19. Birkhahn RH, Gaeta TJ, Bei R, Bove JJ. Shock index in the first trimester of pregnancy and its relationship to ruptured ectopic pregnancy. Acad Emerg Med. 2002;9:115-9.
20. Wong E, Suat SO. Ectopic pregnancy-a diagnostic challenge in the emergency department. Eur J Emerg Med. 2000;7: 189-94
21. Dart R, McLean SA, Dart L. Isolated fluid in the cul-de-sac: how well does it predict ectopic pregnancy? Am J Emerg Med. 2002;20:1-4.
22. Barnhart KT, Katz I, Hummel A, Gracia CR. Presumed diagnosis of ectopic pregnancy. Obstet Gynecol. 2002; 100:505-10.
23. Sheppard RW, Patton PE, Novy MJ. Serial beta hCG measurements in the early detection of ectopic pregnancy. Obstet. Gynecol. 1990;7:417-20.
24. Levsky ME, Handler JA, Suarez RD, Esrig ET. False-positive urine beta-HCG in a woman with a tubo-ovarian abscess. J Emerg Med. 2001;21:407-9.
25. Dumps P, Meisser A, Pons D, Morales MA, Anguenot JL, Campana A, et al. Accuracy of single measurements of pregnancy-associated plasma protein-A, human chorionic gonadotropin and progesterone in the diagnosis of early pregnancy failure. Eur J Obstet Gynecol Reprod Biol. 2002;100:174-80.
26. Poppe WA, Vandenbussche N. Eur Postoperative day 3 serum human chorionic gonadotropin decline as a predictor of persistent ectopic pregnancy after linear salpingotomy. J Obstet Gynecol Reprod Biol. 2001;99:249-52.
27. Timor-Tristch IE, Rottem S, Thale I. Review of transvaginal ultrasonography: description with clinical application. Ultrasound. Q 1988;6:1-32.
28. Peisner DB, Timor-Tritsch IE. The discriminatory zone of beta hCG for vaginal probes. J Clin Ultrasound. 1990;18:280-5.
29. Fossum GT, Dvajan V, Kletzky DA. Early detection of pregnancy with transvaginal ultrasound. Fertil Steril. 1988;49:788-91.
30. Bernascheck G, Euaelstorfer R, Csaicsich P. Vaginal sonography versus serum human chorionic gonadotropin in early detection of pregnancy. Am J Obstet. 1988;158: 608-12.
31. Albayram F, Hamper UM. First-trimester obstetric emergencies: spectrum of sonographic findings. J Clin Ultrasound. 2002;30:161-77.
32. Kurjak A, Zalud I, Volpe G. Conventional B-mode and transvaginal color Doppler on ultrasound assessment of ectopic pregnancy. Acta Med. 1990;44:91-103.
33. Rubin GL, Petersin HB, Dorfman SF. Ectopic pregnancy in the United States 1970-1978. J Am Med Assoc. 1983;249:1725-9.
34. Bolton G, Cohen F. Detecting and treating ectopic pregnancy. Contemp Obstet Gynecol. 1981;18:101-4.
35. Hopp H, Schaar P, Entezami M. Diagnostic reliability of vaginal ultrasound in ectopic pregnancy. Geburtshilfe Frauen. 1995;55:666-70.
36. Hertzberg BS, Kliewer MA. Ectopic pregnancy: ultrasound diagnosis and interpretive pitfalls. South Med J. 1995;88: 1191-8.
37. Thoma ME. Early detection of ectopic pregnancy visualizing the presence of a tubal ring with ultrasonography performed by emergency physicians. Am J Emerg Med. 2000;18:444-8.
38. Nyberg D. Ectopic pregnancy. In: Nyberg DA, Hill LM, Bohm-Velez M, (Eds). Transvaginal Sonography. St. Luis: Mosby Year Book; 1992.pp.105-35.
39. Wojak JC, Clayton MJ, Nolan TE. Outcomes of ultrasound diagnosis of ectopic pregnancy. Dependence on observer experience. Invest Radiol. 1995;30:115-7.
40. Timor-Tritsch IE, Yeh MN, Peisner DB, Lesser KB, Slavik TA. The use of transvaginal ultrasonography in the diagnosis of ectopic pregnancy. Am J Obstet Gynecol. 1989;161:167-70.
41. Pellerito JS, Taylor KJW, Quedens-Case C. Ectopic pregnancy: evaluation with endovaginal color flow imaging. Radiology. 1992;183:831-3.
42. Fleischer AC, Pennell RG, McKee MS. Ectopic pregnancy: features at transvaginal sonography. Radiology. 1990;174:375-8.
43. Bernhart K, Mennuti MT, Benjamin D, Jacobson S, Goodman D, Contifaris C. Prompt diagnosis of ectopic

pregnancy in an emergency department setting. Obstet Gynecol. 1994;84:1010-5.
44. Leung TY, Ng PS, Fung TY. Ectopic pregnancy diagnosed by laparoscopic ultrasound scan. Ultrasound Obstet Gynecol. 1999;13:281-6.
45. Kurjak A, Zalud I, Shulman H. Ectopic pregnancy: transvaginal color Doppler of trophoblastic flow in questionable adnexa. J Ultrasound Med. 1991;10:685-9.
46. Zalud I, Kurjak A. The assessment of luteal blood flow in pregnant and non-pregnant women by transvaginal color Doppler. J Perinat Med. 1990;18:215-21.
47. Jurkovic D, Bourne TH, Jauniaux E, Campbell S, Collins WP. Transvaginal color Doppler study of blood flow in ectopic pregnancies. Fertil Steril. 1992;57:68-73.
48. Wherry KL, Dubinsky TJ, Waitches GM, Richardson ML, Reed S. Low-resistance endometrial arterial flow in the exclusion of ectopic pregnancy revisited. J Ultrasound Med. 2001;20:335-42.
49. Dillon EH, Feyock AL, Taylor KJW. Pseudogestational sacs: Doppler US differentiation from normal or abnormal intrauterine pregnancies. Radiology. 1990;176:359-64.
50. Orden MR, Gudmundsson S, Helin HL, Kirkinen P. Intravascular contrast agent in the ultrasonography of ectopic pregnancy. Ultrasound Obstet Gynecol. 1999;14:348-52.
51. Pellerito JS, Troiano RN, Quedens-Case C, Taylor KJW. Common pitfalls of endovaginal color Doppler flow imaging. Radiographics. 1995;15:37-47.
52. Lurie S, Katz Z. Where a pendulum of expectant management of ectopic pregnancy should rest? Gynecol Obstet Invest. 1996;45:145.
53. Stovall TG, Link WF. Expectant management of ectopic pregnancy. Obstet Gynecol Clin North Am. 1991;18:135-44.
54. Laurie S, Insler V. Can the serum beta hCG level reliably predict likelihood of a ruptured tubal pregnancy? Isr J Obstet Gynecol. 1992;3:152-544.
55. Budowich M, Johnson TRB, Genadry R. The histopathology of developing tubal ectopic pregnancy. Fertil Steril. 1980;34: 169-73.
56. Kemp B, Funk A, Hauptmann S, Rath W. Doppler sonographic criteria for viability in symptomless ectopic pregnancies. Lancet. 1997;349:1220-1.
57. Baba K, Stach K, Sakamoto S, Okai T, Shiego I. Development of an ultrasonic system for three dimensional reconstruction of the fetus. J Perinat Med. 1989;17:19-24.
58. Fredfelt KE, Holm HH, Pedersen JF. Three dimensional ultrasonic scanning. Acta Radiol Diagn. 1995;25:237-40.
59. Rempen A. The shape of the endometrium evaluated with three-dimensional ultrasound: an additional predictor of extrauterine pregnancy. Hum Reprod. 1998;13:450-4.
60. Harika G, Gabriel R, Carre-Pigeon F, Alemany L, Quereux C, Wahl P. Primary application of three-dimensional ultrasonography to early diagnosis of ectopic pregnancy. Eur J Obstet Gynecol Reprod Biol. 1995;60:117-20.
61. Shih JC, Shyu MK, Cheng WF, Lee CN, Jou HJ, Wang RM, et al. Arteriovenous malformation of mesosalpinx associated with a vanishing ectopic pregnancy: diagnosis with three-dimensional color power angiography. Ultrasound Obstet Gynecol. 1999;13:63-6.
62. Mancino D, Carbone L, Ragucci V, et al. Angular pregnancy at 6th week of pregnancy treated with minimally invasive surgery preceded by systemic and local medical therapy with methotrexate. Case report. Giorn It Ostet Gin. 2013; 35(3):462-65.
63. Agarwal SK, Wisot AL, Garzo G, Meldrum DR. Cornual pregnancies in patients with prior salpingectomy undergoing in vitro fertilization and embryo transfer. Fertil Steril. 1996;65:659-60.
64. Timor-Tritsch IE, Monteagudo A, Matera C, Veit C. Sonographic evaluation of cornual pregnancies treated without surgery. Obstet Gynecol. 1992;79:1044-9.
65. Honemeyer U, Kupesic Plavsic S, Kurjak A. Interstitial ectopic pregnancy: the essential role of ultrasound diagnosis. Donald School Journal of Ultrasound in Obstetrics and Gynecology, 2010;4(3):321-25.
66. Hafner T, Aslam N, Ros JA, Zosmer N, Jurkovic D. The effectiveness of non-surgical management of early interstitial pregnancy: a report of ten cases and review of the literature. Ultrasound Obstet Gynecol. 1999;13:131-6.
67. Jurkovic D, Geipel A, Gruboeck K, Jauniaux E, Natucci M, Campbell S. Three-dimensional ultrasound for the assessment of uterine anatomy and detection of congenital uterine anomalies. A comparison with hysterosalpingography and two dimensional sonography. Ultrasound Obstet Gynecol. 1995;5:233-7.
68. Lawrence A, Jurkovic D. Three-dimensional ultrasound diagnosis of interstitial pregnancy. Ultrasound Obstet Gynecol. 1999;14:292-3.
69. Ben-Sholmo I, Eliyahu S, Yanai N, Shalev E. Methotrexate as a possible cause of ovarian cyst formation: experience with women treated for ectopic pregnancies. Fertil Steril. 1997;67:786-8.
70. Schiff E, Tsabari A, Shalev E, Maschiach S, Bustan M, Weiner E. Pharmacokinetics of methotrexate after local tubal injection for conservative treatment of ectopic pregnancy. Fertil Steril. 1992;57:688-90.
71. Timor-Tritsch IE, Monteagudo A, Mandeville EO, Peisner DB, Parra-Anaya G, Pirrone EC. Successful management of viable cervical pregnancy by local injection of methotrexate guided by transvaginal ultrasonography. Am J Obstet Gynecol. 1994;170:737-9.
72. Jurkovic D, Hacket E, Campbell S. Diagnosis and treatment of early cervical pregnancy: a review and a report of two cases treated conservatively. Ultrasound Obstet Gynecol. 1996;8:373-80.
73. Jauniaux E, Taidi J, Jurkovic D, Campbell S, Hustin J. Comparison of color Doppler features and pathological findings in complicated early pregnancy. Hum Reprod. 1994;9:2432-7.

74. Morita Y, Tsutsumi O, Kurmochi K, Momoeda M, Yoshikawa H, Taketeani Y. Successful laparoscopic management of primary abdominal pregnancy. Hum Reprod. 1996;11:2546-7.
75. Ahmed B, Fawzi HW, Abushama M. Advanced abdominal pregnancy in the developing countries. J Obstet Gynecol. 1996;16:400-5.
76. Angtuaco TL, Shah HR, Meal MR, Quirk JG. Ultrasound evaluation of abdominal pregnancy. Crit Rev Diagn Imaging. 1994;35:1-59.
77. Bajo JM, Garcia FA, Huertas MA. Sonographic follow-up of a placenta left in situ after delivery of the fetus in abdominal pregnancy. Ultrasound Obstet Gynecol. 1996;7:285-8.
78. Zaki ZMS. An unusual presentation of ectopic pregnancy. Ultrasound Obstet Gynecol. 1998;11:456-8.
79. Rheinbolt M, Osborn D, Delprosto Z. Cesarean section scar ectopic pregnancy: a clinical case series. J Ultrasound. 2015; 21:18(2):191-95.
80. Riaz RM, Williams TR, Craig BM, Myers DT. Cesarean section ectopic pregnancy: imaging features, current treatment options and clinical outcomes. Abdom Imaging. 2015;40(7):2589-99.
81. Qian ZD, Guo QY, Huang LL. Identifying risk factors for recurrent cesarean scar pregnancy: a case control study. Fertil Steril. 2014;102(1):129-34.
82. Wang Z, Le A, Shan L, et al. Assessment of transvaginal hysterotomy combined with medication for Cesarean Scar ectopic pregnancy. J Minim Invasive Gynecol. 2012: 19(5):639-42.
83. Thoen LD, Crenin MD. Medical treatment of ectopic pregnancy with methotrexate. Fertil Steril. 1997;68:727-30.
84. Lipscomb GH, Meyer NL, Flynn DE, Peterson M, Ling FW. Oral methotrexate for treatment of ectopic pregnancy. Am J Obstet Gynecol. 2002;186:1192-5.
85. Haimov-Kochman R, Sciaky-Tamir Y, Yanai N, Yagel S. Conservative management of two ectopic pregnancies implanted in previous uterine scars. Ultrasound Obstet Gynecol. 2002;19:616-9.
86. El-Lamie IK, Shehata NA, Kamel HA. Intramuscular methotrexate for tubal pregnancy. J Reprod Med. 2002;47:144-50.
87. Yao M, Tulandi T. Current status of surgical and non-surgical management of ectopic pregnancy. Fertil Steril. 1997;67: 421-33.
88. Powell MP, Spellman JR. Medical management of the patient with an ectopic pregnancy. J Perinat Neonat Nurs. 1997;9:31-43.
89. Luciano AA, Roy G, Solima E, Ann NY. Ectopic pregnancy from surgical emergency to medical management. Acad Sci. 2001;943:235-54.
90. Morlock RJ, Lafata JE, Eisenstein D. Cost-effectiveness of single-dose methotrexate compared with laparoscopic treatment of ectopic pregnancy. Obstet Gynecol. 2000;95:407-12.
91. Tulandi T, Sammour A. Evidence-based management of ectopic pregnancy. Curr Opin Obstet Gynecol. 2000; 12:289-92.
92. Stovall TG, Ling FW, Carson SA, Buster JE. Serum progesterone and uterine curettage in differential diagnosis of ectopic pregnancy. Fertil Steril. 1992; 57(2):456-7.
93. Kirk E, Condous G, van Calster B, Haider Z, van Huffel S, Timmerman D, et al. A validation of the most commonly used protocol to predict the success of single dose metotrexate in the treatment of ectopic pregnancy. Hum Reprod. 2004;19:1900-10.
94. Van Den Eeden SK, Shan J, Bruce C, Glasser M. Ectopic pregnancy rate and treatment utilization in a large managed care organization. Obstet Gynecol. 2005;105:1052-7.
95. Barnhart KT, Sammel MD, Hummel A, Jain J, Chakhtoura N, Strauss J. A novel "two dose" regimen of methotrexate to treat ectopic pregnancy. Fertil Steril. 2005;84(Suppl):S130.
96. Alleyassin A, Khademi A, Aghahosseini M, Safdarian L, Badenoosh B, Hamed EA. Comparison of success rates in the medical management of ectopic pregnancy with single-dose and multiple-dose administration of methotrexate: a prospective, randomized clinical trial. Fertil Steril. 2006;85(6):1661-6.

10

CHAPTER

Sonographic Determination of Gestational Age

Robin B Kalish, Frank A Chervenak

INTRODUCTION

Importance of Accurate Gestational Age Assessment

Accurate assessment of gestational age is fundamental in managing both low- and high-risk pregnancies. In particular, uncertain gestational age has been associated with adverse pregnancy outcomes including low birth weight, spontaneous preterm delivery and perinatal mortality, independent of maternal characteristics.[1] Making appropriate management decisions and delivering optimal obstetric care necessitates accurate appraisal of gestational age. For example, proper diagnosis and management of preterm labor and post-term pregnancy requires an accurate estimation of fetal age. Many pregnancies considered to be preterm or post-term are wrongly classified. Unnecessary testing, such as fetal monitoring and unwarranted interventions, including induction for supposed post-term pregnancies may lead to an increased risk of maternal and neonatal morbidity. In addition, pregnancies erroneously thought to be preterm may be subject to avoidable and expensive hospitalization stays as well as excessive and potentially dangerous medication use including tocolytic therapy. In one study by Kramer et al. that assessed over 11,000 pregnant women who underwent early ultrasound, one-fourth of all infants who would be classified as premature and one-eighth of all infants who would be classified as post-term by menstrual history alone would be misdiagnosed.[2] Accurate pregnancy dating may also assist obstetricians in appropriately counseling women who are at imminent risk of a preterm delivery about likely neonatal outcomes.

Precise knowledge of gestational age is also essential in the evaluation of fetal growth and the detection of intrauterine growth restriction. During the third trimester, fundal height assessment may be helpful in determining appropriate fetal growth by comparing the measurement to a known gestational age. In addition, dating a pregnancy is imperative for scheduling invasive diagnostic tests, such as chorionic villus sampling (CVS) or amniocentesis, as appropriate timing can influence the safety of the procedure. Certainty of gestational age is also important in the interpretation of biochemical serum screening test results and may help avoid undue parental anxiety from miscalculations and superfluous invasive procedures, which may increase the risk of pregnancy loss. Assessment of gestational age is also crucial for counseling patients regarding the option of pregnancy termination.

ASSESSMENT OF GESTATIONAL AGE BY LAST MENSTRUAL PERIOD

Traditionally, the first day of the last menstrual period (LMP) has been used as a reference point, with a predicted delivery date 280 days later. The estimated date of confinement (EDC) can also be calculated by Nägele's rule by subtracting three months and adding seven days to the first day of the last normal menstrual period. However, there are inherent problems in assessing gestational age using the menstrual cycle. One obstacle in using the LMP is the varying length of the follicular phase and the fact that many women do not have regular menstrual cycles. Walker et al. evaluated 75 ovulatory cycles using luteinizing hormone levels as a biochemical marker and found that ovulation occurred within a wide range of 8–31 days after the LMP.[3] Similarly, Chiazze et al. collected over 30,000 recorded menstrual cycles from 2,316 women and found that only 77% of women have average cycle lengths between 25 and 31 days.[4] Another barrier in using a menstrual history is that many women do not routinely document or remember their LMP. Campbell et al. demonstrated that of more than 4,000 pregnant women, 45% were not certain about their LMP as a result of poor recall, irregular cycles, bleeding in early pregnancy or oral contraceptive use within two months of conception.[5]

Clinical Methods for Determining Gestational Age

Other methods used to assess gestational age have included uterine size assessment, time at quickening and fundal height measurements. However, these clinical methods are often suboptimal. Robinson noted that uterine size determination by bimanual examination produced incorrect assessments by more than 2 weeks in over 30% of patients.[6] Similarly, fundal height estimation does not provide a reliable guide to predicting gestational age. Beazly et al. found up to eight weeks variation in gestational age for any particular fundal height measurement during the second and third trimesters.[7] In addition, quickening or initial perception of fetal movement can vary greatly among women. While these modalities may be useful adjuncts, they are unreliable as the sole tool for the precise dating of a pregnancy.

Ultrasound Assessment of Gestational Age

In recent years, ultrasound assessment of gestational age has become an integral part of obstetric practice.[8] Correspondingly, prediction of gestational age is a central element of obstetric ultrasonography. Fetal biometry has been used to predict gestational age since the time of A-mode ultrasound.[9] Currently, the sonographic estimation is derived from calculations based on fetal measurements and serves as an indirect indicator of gestational age. Over the past three decades, numerous equations regarding the relationship between fetal biometric parameters and gestational age have been described and have proven early antenatal ultrasound to be an objective and accurate means of establishing gestational age.[10-15]

First Trimester Ultrasound

Ultrasound assessment of gestational age is most accurate in the first trimester of pregnancy.[16] During this time, biological variation in fetal size is minimal. The gestational sac is the earliest unequivocal sonographic sign of pregnancy.[17-20] Historically, gestational sac size and volume had been used as a means to estimate gestational age.[21,22] This structure sonographically resembles a fluid filled sac surrounded by a bright echogenic ring, the developing chorionic villi, within the endometrial cavity **(Fig. 1)**. This sac can be visualized as early as five menstrual

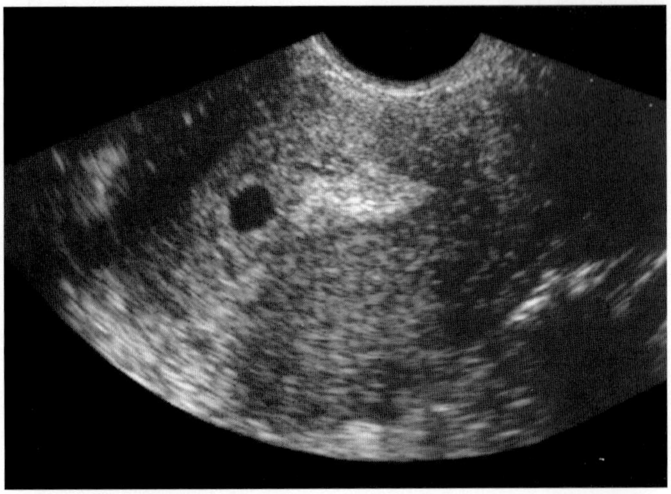

Fig. 1: Transvaginal ultrasound image demonstrating an early gestational sac prior to the visualization of a fetal pole.

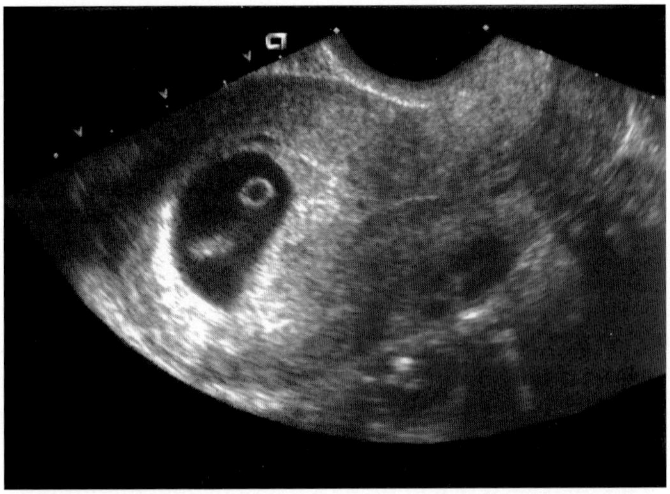

Fig. 2: Transvaginal ultrasound image demonstrating an early embryo with a visible yolk sac at approximately 7 weeks gestation.

weeks using transvaginal sonography.[23-25] More recently, studies have shown that fetal age assessment by gestation sac measurement is not reliable, with a prediction error up to 2 weeks.[6,26] Another imprecise yet often used modality is the sonographic visualization of distinct developing structures.[27] During the fifth menstrual week, the yolk sac—the earliest embryonic structure detectable by sonography, can be visualized prior to the appearance of the fetal pole. And, by the end of the 6th menstrual week, a fetal pole with cardiac activity should be present **(Fig. 2)**. Subsequently, the presence of limb buds and midgut herniation can be seen at approximately 8 weeks of gestation. However, these developmental landmarks can only provide rough estimates to the actual fetal age.

In 1973, Robinson reported using the CRL for determining gestational age.[28] Since that time, ultrasound equipment, techniques and prediction formulas have substantially improved and allow for more rapid and precise measurement of the CRL and determination of gestational age.[29,30] For the best results, the fetus should be imaged in a longitudinal plane. The greatest embryonic length should be measured by placing the calipers at the head and rump of the fetus **(Fig. 3)**. Three adequate CRL measurements should be taken and the average used for gestational age determination.[31] The accuracy of the CRL measurement has been well documented in the medical literature. Specifically, gestational age can be estimated safely with a maximal error of 3–5 days in the first trimester.[6,16,32,33]

In summary, first trimester ultrasound is a useful and reliable tool in the assessment of gestational age. In particular, sonographic measurement of the CRL during the first trimester is the best parameter for estimating gestational age and is accurate within five days of the actual conception date.[16,32]

Second Trimester Ultrasound

Although routine ultrasonography at 18–20 weeks gestation historically has been controversial,[34] it is currently practiced by most obstetricians in the United States.[35] In addition to screening for fetal anomalies, sonographic gestational age assessment may be of clinical value in that it has been shown to decrease the incidence of post-term as well as preterm diagnoses and thus the administration of tocolytic agents.[36,37] In addition, uncertain gestational age has been associated with higher perinatal mortality rates and an increase of low birth weight and spontaneous preterm delivery.[1]

Ultrasound parameters: When choosing the optimal parameter for estimating gestational age, it is essential that the structure has little biologic variation, is growing at a rapid pace and can be measured with a high degree of reproducibility.[38] In the past, the biparietal diameter (BPD) had been described as a reliable method of determining gestational age.[9,12] While the BPD was the first fetal parameter to be clinically utilized in the determination of fetal age in the second trimester, more recent studies have evaluated the use of several other biometric parameters including head circumference (HC),[39] abdominal circumference (AC),[40] femur length (FL),[41] foot length,[42] ear size,[43] orbital diameters,[44,45] cerebellum diameter[46,47] and others. In a large study by Chervenak et al. that evaluated pregnancies conceived by IVF and thus had known conception dates, HC was found to be the best predictor of gestational age compared with other commonly used parameters **(Table 1)**.[48] This finding is in agreement with that of Hadlock,[10] Ott[11] and Benson[49] who compared the performance of HC, BPD, FL and AC in different populations.

The HC should be measured in a plane that is perpendicular to the parietal bones and traverses the third ventricle and thalami **(Fig. 4)**.[31] The image should

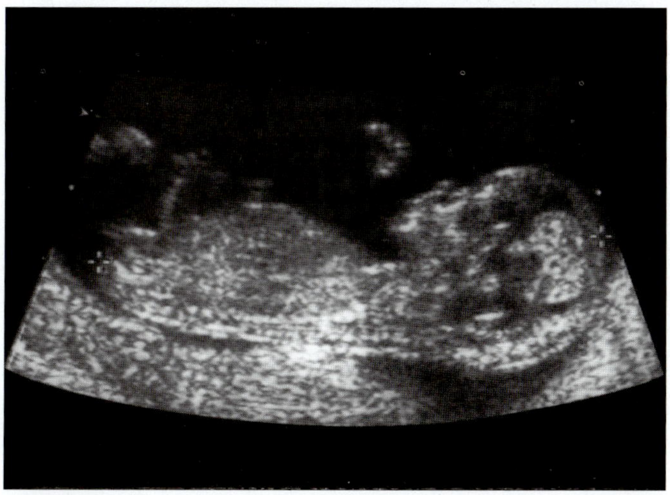

Fig. 3: Ultrasound image demonstrating the fetal crown-rump length measurement in the first trimester.

TABLE 1: Comparison of stepwise multiple linear regression in estimation of fetal age for singletons using different second trimester biometric parameters by Chervenak et al.[47]

Biometric parameters	*Random error (days)*
HC	3.77
AC	3.96
BPD	4.26
FL	4.35
HC+AC	3.44
HC+FL	3.55
HC+AC+FL	3.35

[*Adapted from:* Chervenak FA, Skupski DW, Romero R, et al. How accurate is fetal biometry in the assessment of fetal age? Am J Obstet Gynecol. 1998;178(4):678-87.]

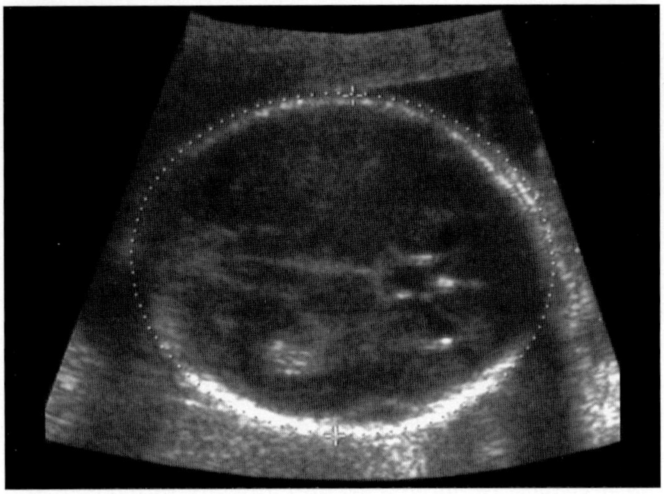

Fig. 4: Ultrasound image demonstrating the head circumference measurement in a second trimester fetus.

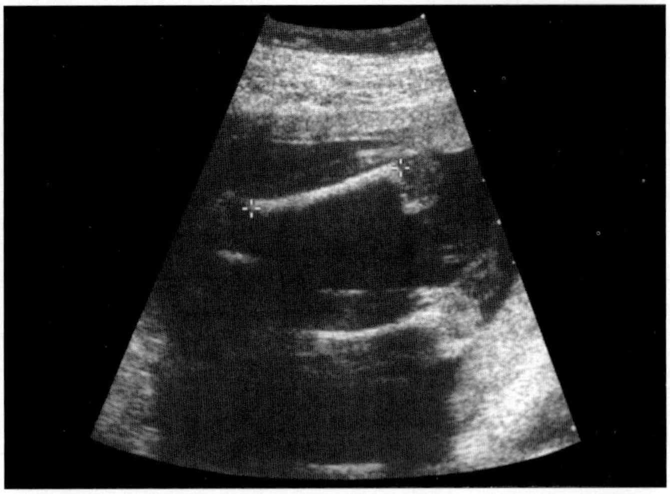

Fig. 5: Ultrasound image demonstrating the femur length measurement in a second trimester fetus.

also demonstrate smooth, symmetrical calvaria and the presence of a cavum septum pellucidum. The calipers should be placed on the outer edges of the calvaria and a computer-generated ellipse should be adjusted to fit around the fetal head without including the scalp. The BPD can be taken in the same plane by placing the calipers on the outer edge of the proximal calvarium wall and on the inner edge of the distal calvarium wall.[50] The BPD, while highly correlated with HC, is less accurate as a predictor of gestational age as a result of variation in head shape.[48]

Multiple parameters have been shown to improve the accuracy of gestational age assessment.[48] Along with HC, the addition of one parameter (AC or FL) or two parameters (AC and FL) is slightly superior to HC alone in the prediction of fetal age. **Table 1** demonstrates the relative error associated with the use of different biometric parameters. The use of multiple parameters also reduces the effect of outliers caused by biologic phenomena (i.e., congenital anomalies or growth variation) or technical error in measurement of a single structure. Still, with multiple parameters, it is important to take the images in the proper plane and place the calipers appropriately. For example, when assessing FL, the long axis of the femur should be aligned with the transducer measuring only the osseous portions of the diaphysis and metaphysis of the proximal femur. While not included in the FL measurement, the proximal epiphyseal cartilage (future greater trochanter) and the distal femoral epiphyseal cartilage (future distal femoral condyle) should be visualized to assure that the entire osseous femur can be measured without foreshortening or elongation **(Fig. 5)**.[31,51] Similarly, the AC must be measured appropriately in order to obtain an accurate estimate. The image should be taken in a plane slightly superior to the umbilicus at the greatest transverse abdominal diameter, with the liver, stomach, spleen and junction of the right and left portal veins visualized **(Fig. 6)**.[31]

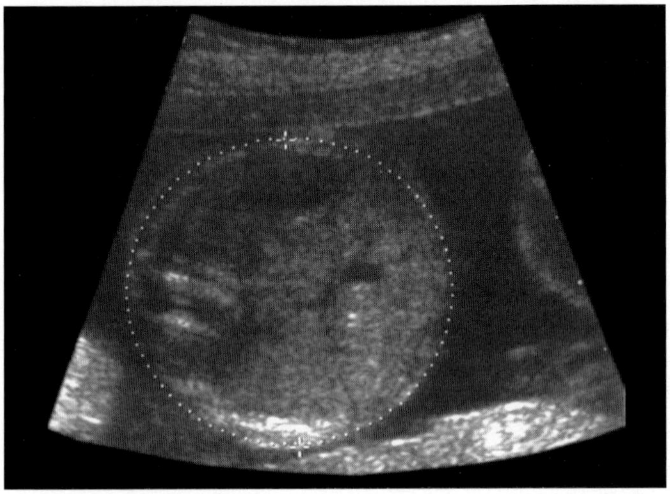

Fig. 6: Ultrasound image demonstrating the abdominal circumference measurement in a second trimester fetus.

Most modern ultrasound machines are equipped with computer software that will automatically calculate the estimated gestational age based on the entered measurements. Using a large singleton IVF population from 14–22 weeks, Chervenak et al. derived an optimal gestational age prediction formula using stepwise linear regression with a standard deviation (SD) of 3.5 days between the predicted and true gestational age.[48]

This formula was compared to 38 previously published equations. Nearly all equations produced a prediction within 1 week demonstrating that fetal biometry in the midtrimester for assessment of gestational age is applicable and accurate across populations and institutions. Clinically, when a discrepancy greater than 7 days (2SD) exists between the menstrual and ultrasound dating in the second trimester, the biometric prediction should be given preference.

Recently, we published a study evaluating and comparing the accuracy of first- and second-trimester ultrasound assessment of gestational age using pregnancies conceived with IVF.[16] Our data showed that first- and second-trimester estimates of gestational age had small differences in the systematic and random error components for an estimated gestational age that was based on fetal CRL or biometry. On the basis of this data derived from pregnancies with known conception dates, ultrasound scanning can determine fetal age to within less than 5 days in the first trimester and less than 7 days in the second trimester in more than 95% of cases. This data further confirms the findings of Wisser et al.[32] and Chervenak et al.[48] regarding the precision of ultrasound scans to assess gestational age in the first and second trimester, respectively.

Third Trimester Ultrasound

While ultrasound has proven to be useful in the assessment of gestational age in the first and second trimesters, accuracy in the third trimester is not as reliable. Biologic variation can be a major factor that affects accuracy in gestational age prediction, and this variability greatly increases with advancing pregnancy. Doubilet and Benson evaluated late third-trimester ultrasound examinations of women who had also received a first-trimester examination and found the disparity in gestational age assessments to be 3 weeks or greater.[52] Thus, third-trimester sonographic estimates of gestational age should be used with caution, if at all.

MULTIFETAL PREGNANCIES

Dating equations generated for singletons can be applied to twins and triplets in order to accurately predict fetal age. Chervenak et al. used multiple linear regression to determine an optimal dating formula for multiple gestations.[48] In twin pregnancies, a single averaged prediction of the gestational age of each fetus is appropriate and was found to yield the most accurate results. This approach of averaging the two fetal age estimates is reasonable as the combined biologic and measurement variability among twins is larger than the decrease in average size of twins relative to singletons. In contrast, using the maximum or minimum estimate in a twin set yielded a slightly larger systematic error than an averaged prediction **(Table 2)**. In the case of triplets, one day can be added to the average of the largest and shortest gestational age prediction among these fetuses for the most accurate gestational age assessment.

TABLE 2: Application of a singleton multiple linear regression formula for estimation of fetal age to multiple gestations by Chervenak et al.

Pregnancy type	*Prediction type*	*Mean error (days)*
Twins	GA of larger twin GA of smaller twin Mean GA of both fetuses GA of larger twin GA of smaller twin	0.8 –1.3 –0.3 2.2
Triplets	GA of largest triplet GA of smallest triplet Mean GA of all fetuses GA of largest triplet GA of smallest triplet	0.8 –3.4 –1.3 4.2

(GA: gestational age)

[*Adapted from:* Chervenak FA, Skupski DW, Romero R, et al. How accurate is fetal biometry in the assessment of fetal age? Am J Obstet Gynecol. 1998;178(4):678-87.]

Slightly larger deviations in the predictions are not unexpected for individual twins or triplets as the formulae have been derived from a singleton population. However, this imprecision is partially compensated for by the fact that multiple pregnancy predictions are based on more information, namely two or three times as many measurements as for singletons. As singleton and multiple gestations grow at similar rates during the second trimester, the difference in the uncertainty of the prediction for gestational age is small using a singleton gestation formula. Indeed, using IVF pregnancies with known conception dates, we have published data confirming that gestational age predictions for twin and triplet gestations have similar accuracy as singleton gestations **(Table 3)**.[16]

CHOOSING A DUE DATE

When the date of conception is unequivocal, as in cases of IVF, the estimated date of confinement should not

TABLE 3: Discrepancies between ultrasound estimates and true gestational age for the first and second trimester in singleton, twin, and triplet pregnancies.

	Systematic error[a]		Random error[b]		Absolute error[a]		
	First trimester	Second trimester	First trimester	Second trimester	First trimester	Second trimester	Second|– |first|[c]
Singleton	+1.3 ± 0.2 days	–0.1 ± 0.4 days	2.4 days	3.5 days	2.3 ± 0.1 days	2.8 ± 0.2 days	0.5 ± 0.3 days
Twin	+1.4 ± 0.2 days	–0.6 ± 0.3 days	1.7 days	2.7 days	1.8 ± 0.1 days	2.1 ± 0.2 days	0.3 ± 0.3 days
Triplet	+0.8 ± 0.4 days	–0.6 ± 0.5 days	2.1 days	2.8 days	1.7 ± 0.2 days	2.2 ± 0.3 days	0.5 ± 0.3 days

Systematic error, average difference between estimated and true gestational age; Random error, residual standard deviation between estimated and true gestational age; Absolute error, average absolute value of the discrepancy between estimated and true gestational age.

[a]Mean ± standard error of the mean

[b]Standard deviation

[c]For gestations with both assessments

[*Adapted from:* Kalish RB, Thaler HT, Chasen ST, Gupta M, et al. First- and second-trimester ultrasound assessment of gestational age. Am J Obstet Gynecol. 2004;191(3):975-8.]

Flowchart 1: Gestational age assessment using first trimester ultrasound.

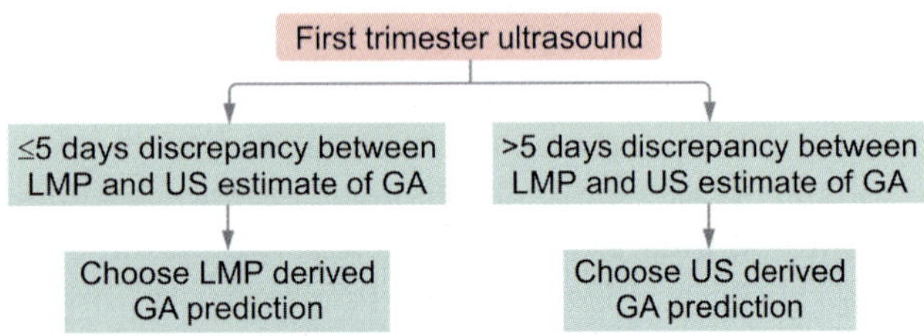

(LMP: last menstrual period; US: ultrasound; GA: gestational age)

Flowchart 2: Gestational age assessment using second trimester ultrasound.

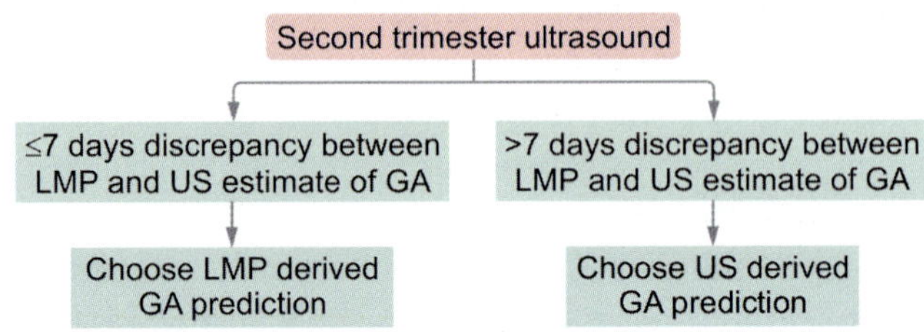

(LMP: last menstrual period; US: ultrasound; GA: gestational age)

be changed based on ultrasound. However, more often than not, this is not the case. In the first trimester, an estimated date of confinement (EDC) based on the LMP that is greater than 5 days different from the CRL measurement should be changed to the sonographically derived EDC **(Flowchart 1)**.[28,32,33] In the second trimester, a combination of biometric parameters that includes the HC should be used to predict the EDC. In the face of a discrepancy of more than seven days in the second trimester, the sonographic biometric prediction should be given preference, provided there is no anomaly or severe growth delay **(Flowchart 2)**.[48] In fact, some authors argue that biometric prediction in the first and second trimesters should be given preference in every case.[53-55]

One of the most common and serious mistakes made when determining gestational age is changing the due date based on a second or subsequent ultrasound examination. The inaccuracy of ultrasound dating increases with gestational age. If the LMP and clinical findings suggest a gestational age within 5 days of a first trimester scan or within 7 days of a second trimester scan, no further investigation is necessary. If the initial first or second trimester sonographically determined gestational age is outside these ranges, the due date should be changed. However, as the pregnancy progresses, revision of a due date that was based on a previous ultrasound is never warranted. If there is a discrepancy between the gestational age assessments of two ultrasound examinations, considering explanations such as intrauterine growth restriction (IUGR), macrosomia or other pathological conditions may be appropriate.

ULTRASOUND PITFALLS

Recent advances in ultrasound image quality and the wide availability of accurate biometric formulas have greatly improved physicians' ability to calculate gestational age. However, properly dating a pregnancy sonographically still depends on adherence to good ultrasound technique. Obtaining a clear and precise image of each biometric indicator is essential. Errors in estimation may arise from technical difficulties including obtaining the proper axis for measurement, movement of the mother or fetus, machine sensitivity settings or caliper placement. If a certain biometric indicator is not well visualized or is difficult to measure, it is better to use an alternative indicator rather than include a suboptimal measurement. In addition, it is helpful to obtain several measurements of each indicator and use an average to ensure a more precise calculation of fetal age.

CONCLUSION

Knowledge of gestational age is of great importance in obstetric practice. Optimal assessment requires good judgment by the obstetrician caring for the patient. Since clinical data such as the menstrual cycle or uterine size are often not reliable, the most precise parameter for pregnancy dating should be determined by the obstetrician early in the pregnancy. Ultrasound is an accurate and useful modality for the assessment of gestational age in the first and second trimester of pregnancy and, as a routine part of prenatal care, can greatly impact obstetric management and improve antepartum care.

REFERENCES

1. Hall MH, Carr-Hill RA. The significance of uncertain gestation for obstetric outcome. Br J Obstet Gynaecol. 1985;92(5):452-60.
2. Kramer MS, McLean FH, Boyd ME, et al. The validity of gestational age estimation by menstrual dating in term, preterm and post-term pregnancies. JAMA. 1988;260(22): 3306-8.
3. Walker EM, Lewis M, Cooper W, et al. Occult biochemical pregnancy: fact or fiction? Br J Obstet Gynaecol. 1988;95(7):659-63.
4. Chiazze L Jr, Brayer FT, Macisco JJ Jr, et al. The length and variability of the human menstrual cycle. JAMA. 1968; 203(6):377-80.
5. Campbell S, Warsof SL, Little D, et al. Routine ultrasound screening for the prediction of gestational age. Obstet Gynecol. 1985;65(5):613-20.
6. Robinson HP. Gestational age determination: first trimester. In: Chervenak FA, Isaacson GC, Campbell S (Eds). Ultrasound in Obstetrics and Gynecology. Boston: Little, Brown and Company; 1993. pp. 295-304.
7. Beazley JM, Underhill RA. Fallacy of the fundal height. Br Med J. 1970;4(5732):404-6.
8. Kalish RB, Chervenak FA. Ultrasound assessment of gestational age. Optimal Obstetrics. 2002;1:1-6.
9. Campbell S. The prediction of fetal maturity by ultrasonic measurement of the biparietal diameter. J Obstet Gynaecol Br Commonw. 1969;76(7):603-6.
10. Hadlock FP, Deter RL, Harrist RB, et al. Estimating fetal age: computer assisted analysis of multiple fetal growth parameters. Radiology. 1984;152(2):497-501.
11. Ott WJ. Accurate gestational dating revisited. Am J Perinatol. 1994;11(6):404-8.
12. Kurtz AB, Wapner RJ, Kurtz RJ, et al. Analysis of biparietal diameter as an accurate indicator of gestational age. J Clin Ultrasound. 1980;8(4):319-26.
13. Mul T, Mongelli M, Gardosi J. A comparative analysis of second-trimester ultrasound dating formulas in pregnancies conceived with artificial reproductive techniques. Ultrasound Obstet Gynecol. 1996;8(6):397-402.
14. Campbell S, Newman GB. Growth of the fetal biparietal diameter during normal pregnancy. J Obstet Gynaecol Br Commonw. 1971;78(6):513-9.
15. Persson PH, Weldner BM. Reliability of ultrasound fetometry in estimating gestational age in the second trimester. Acta Obstet Gynecol Scand. 1986;65(5):481-3.
16. Kalish RB, Thaler HT, Chasen ST, et al. First- and second-trimester ultrasound assessment of gestational age. Am J Obstet Gynecol. 2004;191(3):975-8.
17. Goldstein I, Zimmer EA, Tamir A, et al. Evaluation of normal gestational sac growth: appearance of embryonic heartbeat and embryo body movements using the transvaginal technique. Obstet Gynecol. 1991;77(6):885-8.
18. Yeh HC, Rabinowitz JG. Amniotic sac development: ultrasound features of early pregnancy—the double bleb sign. Radiology. 1988;166:97-103.
19. Selbing A. Gestational age and ultrasonic measurement of gestational sac, crown-rump length and biparietal diameter during the first 15 weeks of pregnancy. Acta Obstet Gynecol Scand. 1982;61(3):233-5.
20. Bernaschek G, Rudelstorfer R, Csaicsich P. Vaginal sonography versus human chorionic gonadotropin in early detection of pregnancy. Am J Obstet Gynecol. 1988;158 (3 Pt. 1):608-12.
21. Kohorn EI, Kaufman M. Sonar in the first trimester of pregnancy. Obstet Gynecol. 1974;44(4):473-83.
22. Donald I, Abdulla U. Ultrasonics in obstetrics and gynaecology. Br J Rad. 1967;40:604-11.
23. Hellman LM, Kobayashi M, Fillitri L, et al. Growth and development of the human fetus prior to the twentieth week of gestation. Am J Obstet Gynecol. 1969;103(6):789-800.
24. Nyberg DA, Filly RA, Mahony BS, et al. Early gestation: correlation of HCG levels and sonographic identification. AJR. 1985;144(5):951-4.
25. De Crispigny LC, Cooper D, McKenna M. Early detection of intrauterine pregnancy with ultrasound. J Ultrasound Med. 1988;7(3):7-10.
26. Warren WB, Timor-Tritsch I, Peisner DB, et al. Dating the early pregnancy by sequential appearance of embryonic structures. Am J Obstet Gynecol. 1989;161(3):747-53.
27. Steinkampf MP, Guzick DS, Hammond KR, et al. Identification of early pregnancy landmarks by transvaginal sonography: analysis by logistic regression. Fertility and Sterility. 1997;68(1):168-70.

28. Robinson HP, Fleming JE. A critical evaluation of sonar "crown-rump length" measurements. Br J Obstet Gynaecol. 1975;82(9):702-10.
29. Daya S. Accuracy of gestational age estimation by means of fetal crown-rump length measurement. Am J Obstet Gynecol. 1993;168(3 Pt. 1):903-8.
30. MacGregor SN, Tamura RK, Sabbagha RE, et al. Underestimation of gestational age by conventional crown-rump length curves. Obstet Gynecol. 1987;70(3 Pt. 1):344-8.
31. Filly RA, Hadlock FP. Sonographic determination of menstrual age. In: Callen PW (Ed). Ultrasonography in Obstetrics and Gynecology. Philadelphia: WB Saunders; 2000. pp. 146-70.
32. Wisser J, Dirschedl P, Krone S. Estimation of gestational age by transvaginal sonographic measurement of greatest embryonic length in dated human embryos. Ultrasound in Obstetrics and Gynecology. 1994;4(6):457-62.
33. Drumm JE, Clinch J, MacKenzie G. The ultrasonic measurement of fetal crown-rump length as a method of assessing gestational age. Br J Obstet Gynaecol. 1976;83(6):417-21.
34. Ewigman BG, Crane JP, Frigoletto FD, et al. Effect of prenatal ultrasound screening on perinatal outcome. N Engl J Med. 1993;329(12):821-7.
35. Chervenak FA, McCullough LB. Should all pregnant women have an ultrasound examination? Ultrasound Obstet Gynecol. 1994;4(3):177-9.
36. Whitworth M, Brisker L, Neilson JP, et al. Ultrasound for fetal assessment in early pregnancy. Cochrane Database Syst Rev. 2010;(4):CD007058. (PMID 20393955).
37. Taipale P, Hiilesmaa V. Predicting delivery date by ultrasound and last menstrual period in early gestation. Obstet Gynecol. 2001;97(2):189-94.
38. Campbell S. Gestational age determination: second trimester. In: Chervenak FA, Isaacson GC, Campbell S (Eds). Ultrasound in Obstetrics and Gynecology. Boston: Little, Brown and Company; 1993. pp. 305-10.
39. Hadlock FP, Deter RL, Harrist RB, et al. Fetal head circumference: relation to menstrual age. Am J Radiol. 1982;138(4): 649-53.
40. Hadlock FP, Deter RL, Harrist RB, et al. Fetal abdominal circumference as a predictor of menstrual age. Am J Radiol. 1982;139(2):367-70.
41. O'Brien G, Queenan JT, Campbell S. Assessment of gestational age in the second trimester by real-time ultrasound measurement of the femur length. Am J Obstet Gynecol. 1981;139(5):540-5.
42. Mercer BM, Sklar S, Shariatmadar A, et al. Fetal foot length as a predictor of gestational age. Am J Obstet Gynecol. 1987;156(2):350-5.
43. Chitkara U, Lee L, El-Sayed YY, et al. Ultrasonographic ear length measurement in normal second- and third-trimester fetuses. Am J Obstet Gynecol. 2000;183(1):230-4.
44. Mayden KL, Tortora M, Berkowitz RL, et al. Orbital diameters: a new parameter for prenatal diagnosis and dating. Am J Obstet Gynecol. 1982;144(3):289-97.
45. Goldstein I, Tamir A, Zimmer EZ, et al. Growth of the fetal orbit and lens in normal pregnancies. Ultrasound Obstet Gynecol. 1998;12(3):175-9.
46. Davies MW, Swaminathan M, Betheras FR. Measurement of the transverse cerebellar diameter in preterm neonates and its use in assessment of gestational age. Australasian Radiology. 2001;45(3):309-12.
47. Smith PA, Johansson D, Tzannatos C, et al. Prenatal measurement of the fetal cerebellum and cisterna cerebellomedullaris by ultrasound. Prenat Diagn. 1986;6(2):133-41.
48. Chervenak FA, Skupski DW, Romero R, et al. How accurate is fetal biometry in the assessment of fetal age? Am J Obstet Gynecol. 1998;178(4):678-87.
49. Benson CB, Doubilet PM. Sonographic prediction of gestational age: accuracy of second- and third-trimester fetal measurements. AJR. 1991;157(6):1275-7.
50. Manning FA. General principles and applications of ultrasonography. In: Creasy RK, Resnik R (Eds). Maternal-Fetal Medicine. Philadelphia: WB Saunders Company; 1999. pp. 169-206.
51. Goldstein RB, Filly RA, Simpson G. Pitfalls in femur length measurements. J Ultrasound Med. 1987;6(4):203-7.
52. Doubilet PM, Benson CB. Improved prediction of gestational age in the late third trimester. J Ultrasound Med. 1993;12(11):647-53.
53. Geirsson RT. Ultrasound: the rational way to determine gestational age. Fetal and Maternal Medicine. 1997;9(3):133-46.
54. Geirsson RT, Have G. Comparison of actual and ultrasound estimated second trimester gestational length in in-vitro fertilized pregnancies. Acta Obstet Gynecol Scand. 1993;72(5):344-6.
55. Geirsson RT. Ultrasound instead of last menstrual period as the basis of gestational age assignment. Ultrasound Obstet Gynecol. 1991;1(3):212-9.

11

CHAPTER

Trophoblastic Diseases

Kazuo Maeda, Asim Kurjak

INTRODUCTION

Although trophoblastic diseases were frequent in East Asia in the past, choriocarcinoma is rare at present after the introduction of effective chemotherapy and postmolar management in Japan. Molar pregnancy is also decreased, possibly due to ultrasound diagnosis and termination in early pregnancy. Outcome of disease has greatly improved by ultrasound diagnosis including real-time B-mode, color/power Doppler flow images and pulsed Doppler tumor blood flow studies.

TABLE 1: Pathological classification of trophoblastic diseases.[1]

- Gestational trophoblastic disease
- Hydatidiform mole
- Complete hydatidiform mole
- Partial hydatidiform mole
- Invasive hydatidiform mole
- Choriocarcinoma
- Placental site trophoblastic tumor (PSTT)
- Persistent trophoblastic disease (PTD)
- Nongestational choriocarcinoma

CLASSIFICATION, DEVELOPMENT AND PATHOLOGY

Trophoblastic diseases are grossly classified into gestational trophoblastic disease and nongestational choriocarcinoma. Gestational diseases are pathologically classified[1] into hydatidiform mole, choriocarcinoma and placental site trophoblastic tumor (PSTT) and epithelioid trophoblastic tumor (ETT). There is also persistent trophoblastic disease that is a particular clinical entity. Hydatidiform mole is subdivided into complete mole, partial mole and invasive mole. There is definite outcome difference between choriocarcinoma and invasive mole which are classified by pathological changes in spite of their symptomatic resemblance. There are also clinical National Cancer Institute (NCL)/National Institute of Health (NIH) classification and Federation Internatiole de Gynecologie et d' Obstetrique (FIGO) staging **(Table 1)**.

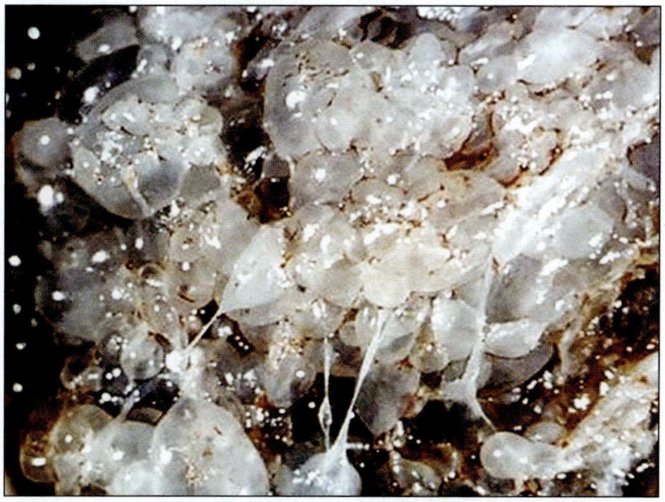

Fig. 1: Molar vesicles in a complete hydatidiform mole in situ in the uterus.

COMPLETE HYDATIDIFORM MOLE

Complete (total) hydatidiform mole is an abnormal pregnancy, where placental villi change into molar vesicles, there is neither embryo or fetus, nor umbilical cord **(Fig. 1)**. Amnion is, however, found in some cases.[2] No capillary vessel is found in molar vesicles covered by proliferated trophoblasts. With an intravascular mole the vesicles spread into blood vessels. The metastasis rarely appears in distant organs.

The chromosome is usually diploid 46,XX, where the XX are both of male origin (androgenesis) and the mechanism is two X sperms fertilized in a vacant ovum without a nucleus[3] or single X is fertilized and divided into two after the fertilization. The chromosome is rarely

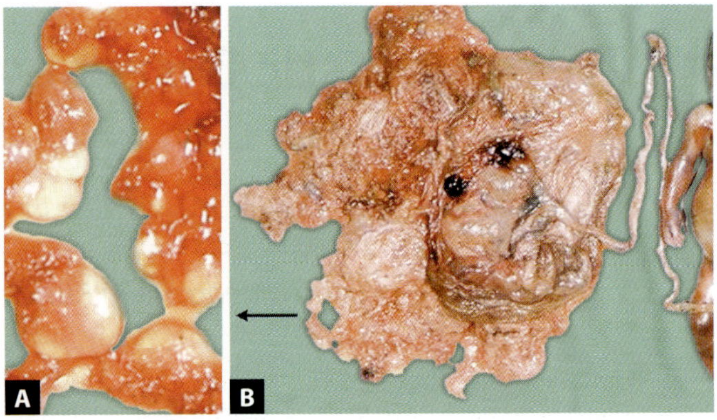

Figs. 2A and B: Partial hydatidiform mole in the placenta with an anomalous fetus in 6 months of pregnancy. Left enclosed figure is of enlarged molar vesicles.

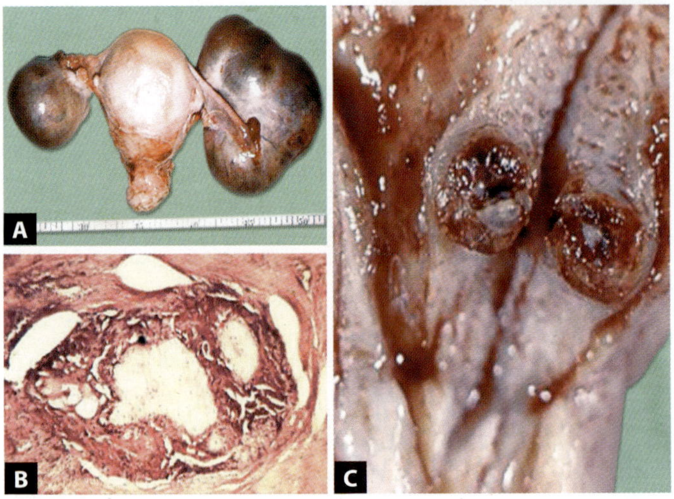

Figs. 3A to C: (A) A case 01 invasive mole in removed uterus and theca lutein cysts before 1960; (B) Invaded molar vesicle was found in the myometrium and (C) Histology was invasive—mole surrounded by proliferated trophoblasts.

46,XY, where X and Y are of male origin.[4] Complete mole can also develop in one of the twins or triplets. The risk of repeated mole is less than 1%, while it is not indicated for chemotherapy.[5] Telomerase activity in complete mole may progress to an invasive mole or choriocarcinoma.[6]

Ovarian theca lutein cysts are frequent in developed complete mole and invasive moles **(Figs. 3A to C)**, while its incidence is low in the first trimester.[7] Since the lutein cyst is not a trophoblastic disease and disappears after remission, surgical removal is not appropriate.

PARTIAL HYDATIDIFORM MOLE

A partial hydatidiform mole is partial change of placental villi into molar vesicles, associated with embryo, fetus or fetal parts **(Figs. 2A and B)**. Fetal anomalies are common. Chromosomes are usually triploids, 69,XXX, 69,XXY or 69,XYY.[8] DNA analysis confirmed the androgenic mechanism.[9] Capillary vessels are found in the interstitium of molar vesicles.

INVASIVE HYDATIDIFORM MOLE

Invasive hydatidiform mole is the invasion of molar vesicles into the myometrium with destruction and hemorrhage. The lesion is found either in total or partial moles, usually after molar evacuation. The change is visually noted in a surgical specimen and microscopically confirmed, where the trophoblasts proliferate, hemorrhage and necrosis occur in the myometrium **(Figs. 3A to C)**. An invasive mole rarely metastasized and has low malignancy, e.g., pulmonary focus spontaneously disappeared after hysterectomy in an invasive mole case. The outcome is more favorable than choriocarcinoma.

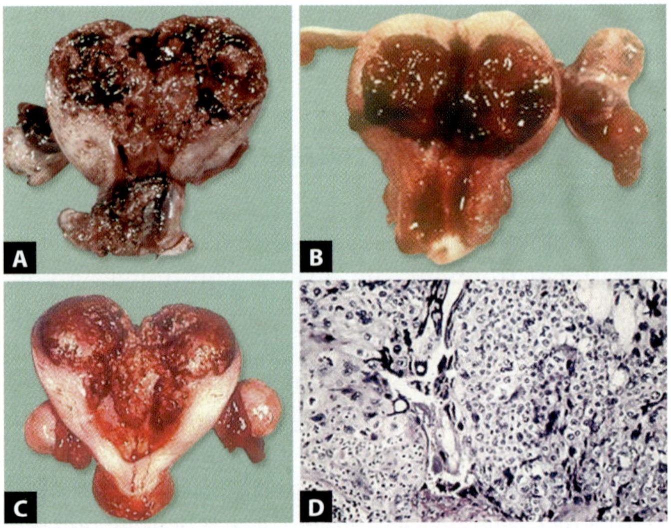

Figs. 4A to D: (A to C) Three cases of choriocarcinoma surgically removed around at 1960 before the introduction of effective chemotherapy. The color of intrauterine tumor was dark red characteristic in the choriocarcinoma; (D) Histology of choriocarcinoma where syncytio and cytotrophoblasts actively proliferated but no villus pattern was detected.

CHORIOCARCINOMA

Choriocarcinoma is solid trophoblastic tumor developed primarily in the myometrium **(Figs. 4A to D)** or in distant organs and tissues,[10-15] usually after the removal of a complete or partial hydatidiform mole and also infrequently after abortion or normal delivery. They are defined as gestational choriocarcinoma or trophoblastic disease (GTD).

Nongestational choriocarcinoma develops from germ cells in the ovary[10] or testis, or from other cancer cells. Primary choriocarcinomas are also reported in reproductive as well as in nonreproductive organs, e.g., vulva,[11] uterine cervix,[12] lung, stomach, pancreas,[13,14] gallbladder[15] and urinary bladder.[16] Uterine cervical choriocarcinoma was also experienced.[17] Choriocarcinoma is constructed of syncytia and cytotrophoblasts and shows no villus pattern at all (**Figs. 4A to D**). Since, the villus pattern is a characteristic sign of an invasive mole (**Figs. 3A to C**) and its outcome is less ominous than choriocarcinoma, microscopic studies should be detailed on the whole specimen if the uterus is removed.

Widespread distant metastases of choriocarcinoma was common before the introduction of effective chemotherapy. The interval of diagnosis and metastasis was about half to 1 year. Early metastases were dark red tumors on the external genitalia and vaginal wall. Subsequent frequent spread was the lung, where typical radiographic foci showed round shapes of various sizes (**Figs. 5A to G**), while a diffuse pulmonary shadow is found in multiple trophoblast emboli in pulmonary arterioles. Organs or tissues were affected after pulmonary metastasis, e.g., skin,[18] subcutaneous tissue, intestine, liver, spleen, kidney, heart,[19,20] spinal cord, coronary artery[21] and finally in brain (**Figs. 5A to G**). Every organ is damaged by the trophoblasts and hemorrhage. Patients died from brain and multiple metastases due to damage and dysfunction occurring before effective chemotherapy.

Choriocarcinomas are divided into three subtypes:

1. Gestational choriocarcinoma is related to pregnancy and three categories are further classified:
   a. Uterine choriocarcinoma is the most common, which develops in the uterus after a hydatidiform mole and rarely after abortion or normal delivery. Choriocarcinoma with an intact pregnancy has been reported.[22]
   b. Extrauterine choriocarcinoma develops primarily at the place of ectopic pregnancy; there is no tumor in the uterus.
   c. Intraplacental choriocarcinoma is found in the placenta mainly after delivery. These cases were reported to be associated with viable pregnancy.[23]

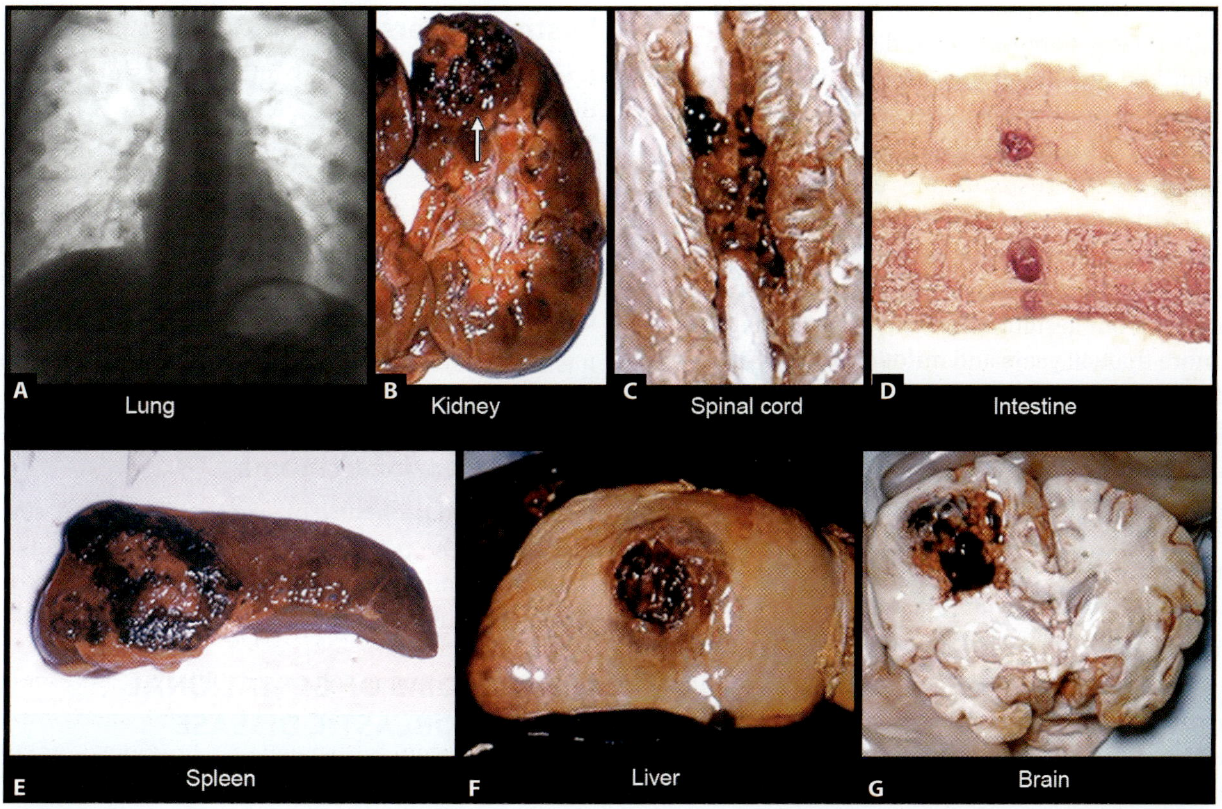

Figs. 5A to G: Radiogram shows typically round foci of choriocarcinoma metastases. Dark red choriocarcinoma metastases in the lung, kidney, spinal cord, intestine, spleen, liver and brain (photographed after autopsies).

2. Nongestational choriocarcinoma is divided into two categories:
   a. Choriocarcinoma of germ cell origin is a subtype of the germ cell tumor which develops in the ovary of the woman before marriage or the testis of an adult male. This tumor is more resistant to chemotherapy than a gestational tumor.
   b. Choriocarcinoma derived from other carcinomas involves choriocarcinomatous change of other cancers that may excrete human chorionic gonadotropin (hCG).
3. Unclassified choriocarcinoma is unclassified into gestational or nongestational.

PLACENTAL SITE TROPHOBLASTIC TUMOR

The placental site trophoblastic tumor (PSTT) is a rare uterine tumor of proliferated intermediate trophoblasts.[24] The tumor is preceded by a hydatidiform mole, abortion or delivery. The levels of hCG are low and the human placental lactogen (HPL) is higher than β-hCG.[25] Final diagnosis is made by histological study. Metastasis and recurrence are commonplace.[24-28] A case of PSTT was reported in both mother and child.[29] PSTT produces less β-hCG and is less sensitive to chemotherapy. More than half of patients present with disease confined in the uterus and the remainder present with disease extension beyond the uterus. Simple hysterectomy is the mainstay of treatment. The outcome of patients with disease confined in the uterus is usually excellent, while most patients with the extension beyond the uterus experience progression of disease and die despite surgery and intense chemotherapy. Other adverse prognostic factors are, interval from gestational events is more than 2 years, age is more than 40 years and mitotic count is higher than 5 mf/10 HPF. The EP/EMA regimen seems to be the most effective chemotherapy.[30] In another report[31] of 55 PSTT cases, statistically significant adverse survival factors were over 35 years of age, interval since the last pregnancy over 2 years, deep myometrial invasion, stage III or IV, maximum hCG level more than 1,000 mIU/mL, extensive coagulative necrosis, high mitotic rate and the presence of cells with clear cytoplasm.

EPITHELIOID TROPHOBLASTIC TUMOR

The epithelioid trophoblastic tumor (ETT) is rare trophoblastic disease which represented vaginal bleeding, associated with a gestational event. Serum hCG was elevated. Two out of fourteen presented extrauterine lesions. In the uterus, ETT was presented as a discrete, hemorrhagic solid and cystic lesion. Microscopically, it was composed of intermediate trophoblastic cells forming nests and solid masses; typically islands of trophoblastic cells were surrounded by necrotic masses; mean mitosis was 2/10 HPF; it was immunohistochemically positive for inhibin-alpha, cytokeratin, hPL, placental alkaline phosphatase and Mel-CAM(CD-148),[32] its monomorphic growth pattern was more close to PSTT than choriocarcinoma. ETT grows in a nodular fashion compared to the infiltrative pattern of PSTT; it appears to be less aggressive than choriocarcinoma, more closely resembling to the behavior of PSTT, where histological and immunohistochemical features were characteristic of EPTT,[33] although a report[34] included ETT in the category of PSTT.

PERSISTENT TROPHOBLASTIC DISEASE

The persistent trophoblastic disease (PTD) is a postmolar metastatic mole, disseminated trophoblasts in tissues, invasive mole or choriocarcinoma; no specimen has been obtained and a pathological finding is unknown.

Postmolar Persistent hCG

It shows abnormal type II hCG regression pattern after the hydatidiform mole, i.e., urinary hCG greater than 100 mIU/mL after 5 weeks, serum hCG greater than 100 mIU/mL after 8 weeks, or serum hCG greater than β 1.0 mIU/mL (hCG β CTP 0.5 mIU/mL) after 20 weeks, where the focus is unknown.

Clinical Invasive Mole or Metastatic Mole

It is estimated by the modified Ishizuka[1] scoring system or by the suspected focus.

Clinical Choriocarcinoma

It is estimated from the Ishizuka scoring system, suspected focus or by the postmolar state where hCG levels elevate again after complete remission; this is confirmed by lower than cut-off hCG level, except for new pregnancies.

SYMPTOMS OF GESTATIONAL TROPHOBLASTIC DISEASE

Complete Hydatidiform Mole

Typical symptoms of well-developed complete hydatidiform moles are hyperemesis, hypertension, no fetal movement, no fetal heart beat with Doppler detector, larger uterus than in normal pregnancy, abdominal pain, hemorrhage after amenorrhea, expelled molar vesicles and urinary hCG levels usually higher than 100,000 mIU/mL. Typical symptoms are infrequently detected by ultrasonic screening in the first trimester of pregnancy; with transvaginal scan, an early stage hydatidiform mole can be detected and evacuated before its development. Ovarian theca lutein cysts are also detected by ultrasound.

Partial Hydatidiform Mole

Symptoms of the mole associated with living fetus are similar to common pregnancy except for hyperemesis, enlarged uterus and high titer hCG. Ultrasonic screening of pregnancy detects partial molar changes of the placenta with the embryo, fetus or fetal particles being present. Twenty percent of complete moles are followed by sequelae and choriocarcinoma develops in 2% of cases with a complete mole, whereas partial moles show sequelae in 5% of cases and rarely progress to choriocarcinoma.[25]

Invasive Hydatidiform Mole

An invasive mole is found after a mole and presents with vaginal bleeding, enlarged uterus, bilaterally enlarged ovaries and high urinary or serum hCG levels. The symptoms resemble those of choriocarcinoma and differential diagnosis is needed. The interval from antecedent molar pregnancy is usually within half a year and it is shorter than choriocarcinoma. Urinary hCG is continuously elevated after molar curettage, but the titer is lower than choriocarcinoma. Ultrasonic study discloses the presence of molar vesicles in the myometrial mass.

Choriocarcinoma

Gestational choriocarcinoma is usually preceded by a molar pregnancy and rarely by abortion or term delivery. The interval from antecedent pregnancy can be longer than 1 year and longer than with an invasive mole. There may be a period of partial remission and it can exist for more than 10 years as an extrauterine choriocarcinoma. The symptoms are vaginal bleeding, enlarged uterus, high hCG titer, ovarian masses and irregular basal body temperature (BBT). Choriocarcinoma is often diagnosed by the presence of metastasis. Multiple pulmonary foci show the progress of malignancy. The hCG titer should be checked even in nongynecological cases when pulmonary round foci are found in the female patient. The symptoms resulting from distant metastases suggest choriocarcinoma, e.g., abdominal pain and hemorrhage in hepatic lesion, or persistent headache and vomiting followed by unconciousness and apnea in the brain metastasis.

Placental Site Trophoblastic Tumor

It can be preceded by any gestational process. Enlarged uterus and vaginal bleeding are the clinical symptoms. Metastasis is frequent. The disease often recurs after treatment. PSTT is malignant and can be fatal.[25]

Persistent Trophoblastic Disease

It includes postmolar hCG persistence, clinically invasive or metastatic moles choriocarcinoma. Although the focus is unknown, all three show persistence of abnormally high hCG titers.

DIAGNOSIS OF GESTATIONAL TROPHOBLASTIC DISEASE

Complete Hydatidiform Mole

Complete hydatidiform mole is diagnosed by symptoms, such as high urinary and serum hCG titers, and particularly by ultrasonic B-mode, color Doppler and Doppler flowmetry. Transvaginal scan is useful in the first trimester. Ultrasonic B-mode detects molar vesicles in the uterine cavity without detecting a fetus or embryo or its particles **(Figs. 6A and B)**. Amniotic membrane and fluid are, however, occasionally detected by the B-mode. A characteristic molar pattern is composed of multiple small cysts, but not a snowstorm pattern **(Fig. 7)** with a modern real-time B-mode device.

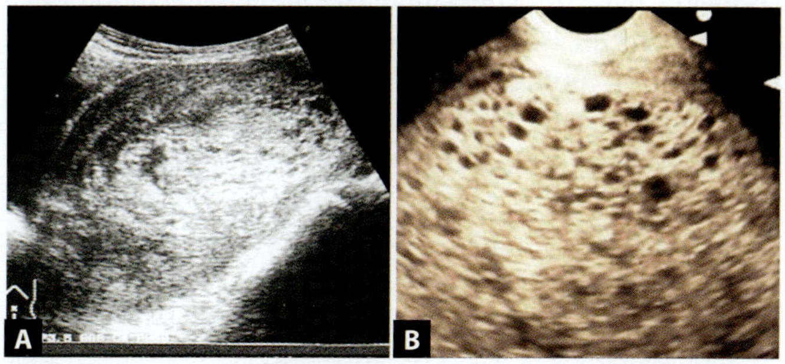

Figs. 6A and B: Typical vesicular images in grown-up complete moles imaged by real-time B-mode.
Courtesy: (A) M Utsu Seirei Mikatahara Hospital, Japan (11 weeks of pregnancy); (B) S Kupesic, University of Zagreb, Croatia

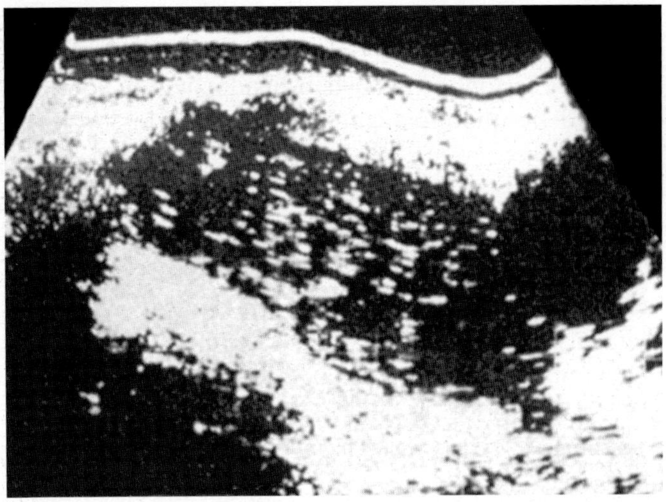

Fig. 7: Erroneous artifact of complete hydatidiform mole imaged by contact-compound scan B-mode in old time. It was called "snow-storm pattern" which was thought typical image of complete mole in old time but a heavy artifact caused by bad resolution of old transducer of single unit without suitable focusing. Modern real-time scanner does not produce snow-storm pattern but round vesicular images in the mole.

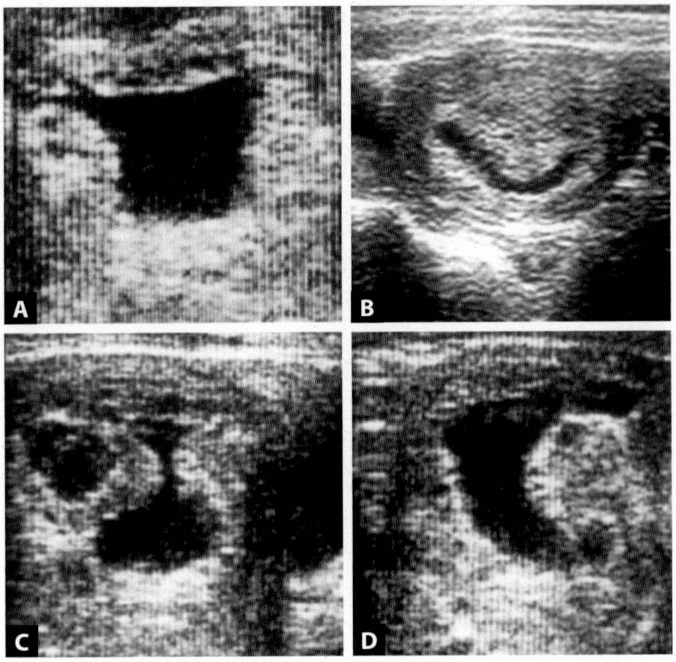

Figs. 8A to D: (A and B) Complete molar images detected by real-time B-mode in early first trimester resembled a blighted ovum. Empty but thick gestational sac without embryo nor yolk sac was characteristic; (C and D) The chorion became thick and irregular, then produced molar vesicles in the irregular mass 2–3 weeks later.

Characteristic changes are found in complete hydatidiform moles by various ultrasonic imaging techniques.

Real-Time B-Mode

A complete hydatidiform mole is detected in its early stages by screening during the first trimester. An empty gestational sac, where the wall showed small cystic changes without an embryo was ultrasonically detected before typical growth of the complete hydatidiform mole **(Figs. 8A to D)**. An early complete mole resembles a blighted ovum, whereas vomiting and high urinary hCG titer of molar case are contradictory to the presence of a blighted ovum. The chorionic plate thickness increases and typical molar cysts develop within 1–2 weeks in early pregnancy. Complete hydatidiform mole develops in one of the twins or triplets. It is diagnosed by the septum that has originated from the fetus **(Figs. 9 and 10)**. A partial mole in a singleton pregnancy is differentiated from the complete mole of a multiple pregnancy by the partial molar change of the placental villi without separating the septum, or by the presence of triploid chromosome.

The specimen of atypical blighted ovum should be carefully examined by histology after curettages and suspicious cases should be monitored by urinary hCG and transvaginal scan 8-mode.

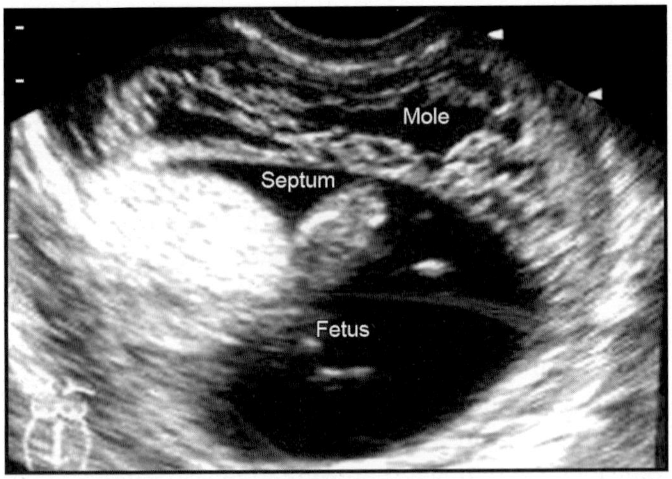

Fig. 9: Complete mole of a twin is differentiated from partial mole by the clear formation of the septum between the fetus and molar vesicles in the B-mode examination of twin pregnancy.
Courtesy: M Utsu, Japan

Color and Power Doppler Flow Mapping

The diagnosis of molar pregnancy is difficult with simple B-mode when the uterine cavity is filled with homogeneous image without typical vesicular changes.

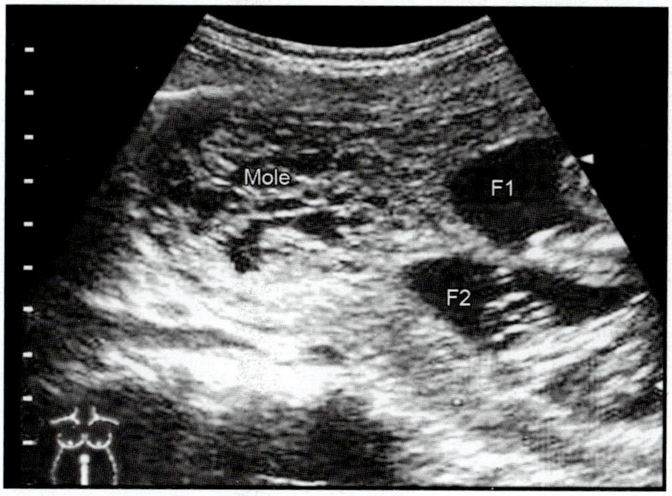

Fig. 10: The complete mole in a triplet pregnancy was also determined by the clear septum between the mole and other fetuses.
Courtesy: M Utsu, Japan

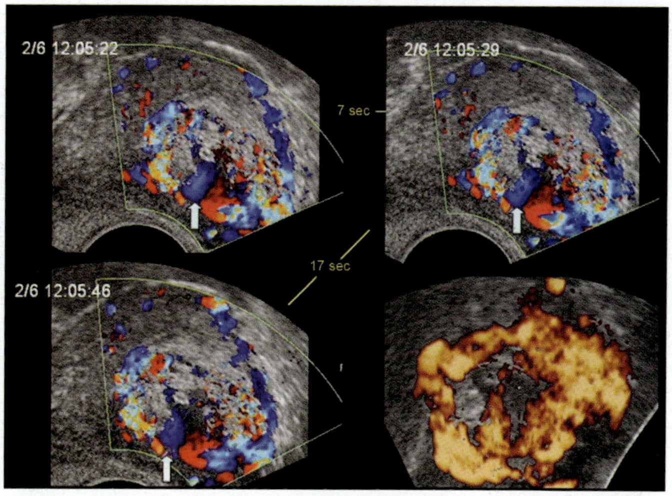

Fig. 11: Three static color Doppler and power Doppler images were recorded in a complete hydatidiform mole. Color Doppler images were almost identical in spite of time differences, i.e., particular blood flow existed in the uterus. Red and blue color images suggested blood streams taking opposite directions, i.e., arterial jet stream into intervesicular spaces and venous drainage. Multiple small round images in the images can be molar vesicles. Power Doppler also showed rich intrauterine blood flow. The blue color flow (arrows) beated about 80 times per minute in the real-time color images. These findings are new diagnostic marker of complete hydatidiform mole.
Courtesy: G Varga

The difficulty may be caused by identical ultrasonic density of molar vesicles to that of intervesicular blood. The two materials, molar vesicles and the blood are unable to be differentiated in the case. The detection of blood flow in the uterine cavity in complete molar pregnancy is the answer to the difficult diagnosis with real-time B-mode. A complete hydatidiform mole was studied by 2D color Doppler, power Doppler, pulsed Doppler flow wave with flow impedance and by 3D power Doppler flow mapping.

The static color Doppler flow mapping visualized rich color flow pattern of various direction in the uterine cavity without detecting fetal or placental blood flow. The color pattern was almost stable in the repeated color Doppler images of which interval was 7 and 17 seconds, when ultrasound probe was held at fixed position. The fixed blood flow was confirmed in the uterus by the color images which probably show jet streams of spiral arteries located at the uterine wall and the draining of the blood into the vein located at the other part **(Fig. 11)**. Round low-intensity images found among the blood flow images indicated the presence of molar vesicles floated among maternal intrauterine blood flow. The real-time color Doppler flow mapping visualized a jet blood flow streaming into the uterine cavity of which pulse rate was about 80 beats/min. It was confirmed by pulsed Doppler arterial flow velocity wave, of which pulse rate was 83 beats/min **(Fig. 12)**.

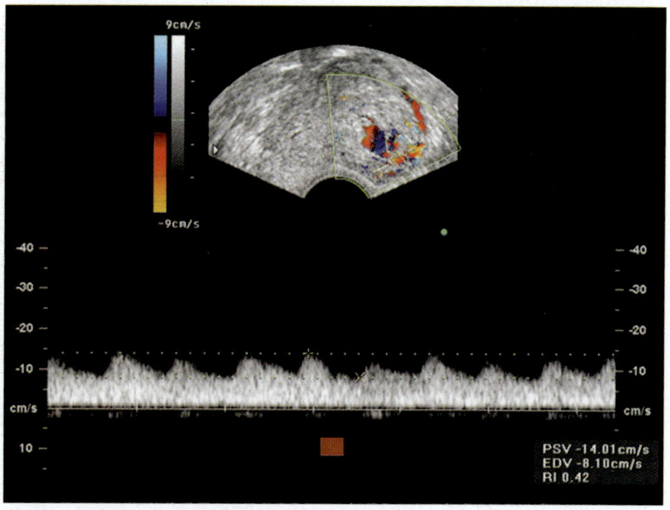

Fig. 12: Pulsed Doppler flow velocity wave in the complete mole showed 83 beats/min flow which coincided with the real-time color Doppler observation. RI was as low as 0.42 and systolic flow velocity was as slow as 14 cm/sec.
Courtesy: G Varga

Power Doppler now mapping detected molar vesicles more clearly and furthermore, 3D power Doppler image revealed rich intrauterine blood now **(Fig. 13)**. From these results, it was confirmed that 2D color and power Doppler flow image and 3D power Doppler image

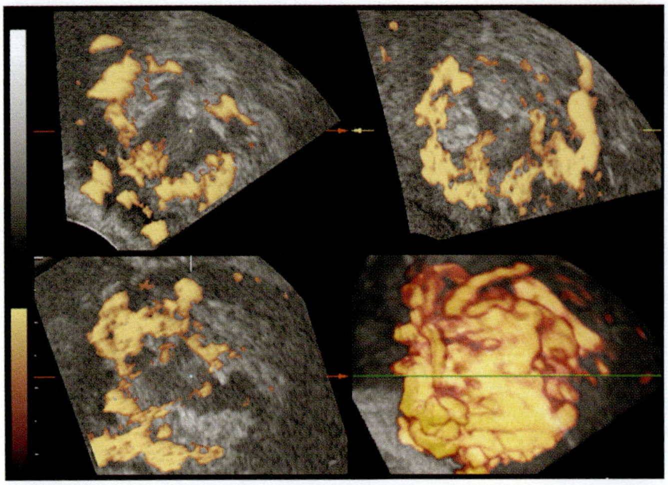

Fig. 13: Orthogonal three planes of 2D power Doppler showed clear molar vesicles and the 3D power Doppler showed rich intreuterine blood flow of various directions. There was no image of the fetus or fetal blood flow or any fetal particle through all images of these Doppler studies.
Courtesy: G Varga

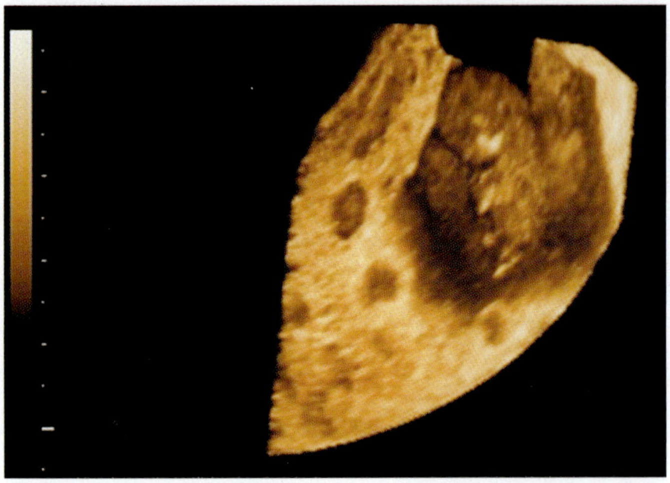

Fig. 14: A partial hydatidiform mole was diagnosed by placental molar vesicles and a fetus by the 3D ultrasound.
Courtesy: JR Benitez, Clinics Gutenberg, Spain

are new diagnostic technique of complete hydatidiform mole. Further, progress is expected in the flow characters of a hydatidiform mole by 4D ultrasound images.

Pulsed Doppler Flow Wave and Flow Impedance

Diastolic flow is larger and the resistance index (RI) was lower in uterine, arcuate, radial and spiral arteries in the mole than in normal pregnancy.[35] Also, RI was low in the molar flow.[36] In the present study, in the intervesicular space of the complete mole, peak systolic velocity of maternal arterial blood is as slow as 14 cm/sec and the RI is as low as 0.42 **(Fig. 12)**. Theoretically, fetal blood flow is not recorded, because there is no fetal capillary in the complete mole vesicle.

hCG and Other Diagnostic Methods

Complete hydatidiform mole is estimated when urinary or serum hCG levels are higher than 10,000 mIU/mL, which is within the higher normal range of early pregnancy. A complete mole can, however, be present with lower hCG levels. The postmolar state is monitored every 1–2 weeks by hCG levels, ultrasound and local conditions after the mole removal by repeated curettages, until the hCG reaches a low cut-off level. Abnormal regression of hCG or persistent trophoblastic disease is treated with chemotherapy for the prophylaxis of choriocarcinoma.[37] Chromosomal diploidy and DNA analysis reports androgenic origin.

Partial Hydatidiform Mole

Partial hydatidiform mole is diagnosed by symptoms, such as high urinary hCG and presence of fetus, or the partial image of the fetus and partial changes of the placenta into molar vesicles. 3D ultrasound shows the diagnosis of a particle mole in early pregnancy **(Fig. 14)**. Anomalies are frequent in the fetus. Chromosomal examination shows triploidy. Postmolar changes of urinary and serum hCG are the same as with a complete hydatidiform mole. Chemotherapy in the case of abnormal regression and persistent trophoblastic disease is also the same as for a complete hydatidiform mole.

Microscopically Diagnosed Hydatidiform Mole

The cases of blighted ovum or common pregnancy microscopically diagnosed as hydatidiform mole after the termination should receive postmolar monitoring as detailed as the mole diagnosed by the other diagnostic methods.

Invasive Hydatidiform Mole

Invasive hydatidiform moles are mainly found within half a year after the termination of a complete or partial molar pregnancy, although the molar tissue can invade the myometrium during pregnancy. Myometrial invasion may be detected by detailed and hard study with B-mode and color or power Doppler flow mapping of the uterine wall before the termination.

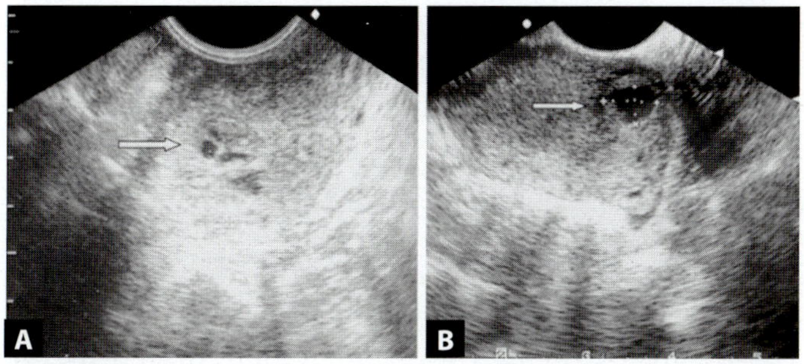

Figs. 15A and B: Invasive mole was confirmed by the detection of cystic villus pattern—arrows imaged by real-time B-mode ultrasound. Focus size was 1.23 × 0.88 cm in the right sonogram.
Courtesy: S Yoshida, Tottori University Hospital, Japan

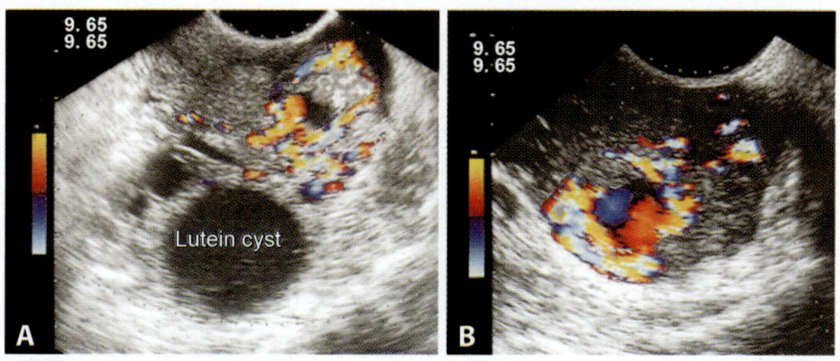

Figs. 16A and B: Rich blood flow was detected by color Doppler flow mapping around the villus patterns of invasive mole. A theca lutein cyst was confirmed to be avascular in **Figure16A**.
Courtesy: S Yoshida

The symptoms of invasive mole are similar to those of choriocarcinoma, i.e., postmolar development, vaginal bleeding, enlarged uterus and possible metastasis. Urinary or serum hCG is positive, but the levels are lower than with choriocarcinoma. Ultrasound B-mode shows a uterine mass. An invasive mole is usually diagnosed if molar cysts are imaged in the tumor **(Figs. 15A and B)**. Rich blood flow is found by color flow mapping **(Figs. 16A and B)** and power Doppler imaging. Flow impedance is low with an invasive mole. In contrast, flow impedance is high in the wall artery of a theca lutein cyst.

Gestational Choriocarcinoma

Gestational choriocarcinoma develops after a hydatidiform mole, abortion or normal delivery. Clinical symptoms are vaginal bleeding, enlarged uterus, ovarian masses, high hCG titer and is similar to an early stage invasive mole before metastasis. The interval of its development is usually more than half a year after the mole, and longer than that of an invasive mole which is mainly within half a year. Metastases are found in external genitalia and the vaginal wall in its early stage, and then in the lung. An invasive mole rarely develops the metastasis.

TABLE 2: Clinical differentiation of choriocarcinoma and invasive mole.

	Choriocarcinoma	*Invasive mole*
Antecedent pregnancy	Mole, abortion, term delivery	Mole
Vaginal bleeding	Yes	Yes
Enlarged uterus	Yes	Yes
High hCG titer	Yes	Yes
Postmolar period	> 6 months, years, >10 years	Usually <6 months
Metastasis	Frequent and wide, until brain	Rare
Uterine B-mode image	Solid mass	Villus pattern
Pelvic angiography	Pooling focus	Villus pattern
Distribution	Whole body, systemic disease	Local in the uterus
Outcome	Fatal without chemotherapy	Less malignant

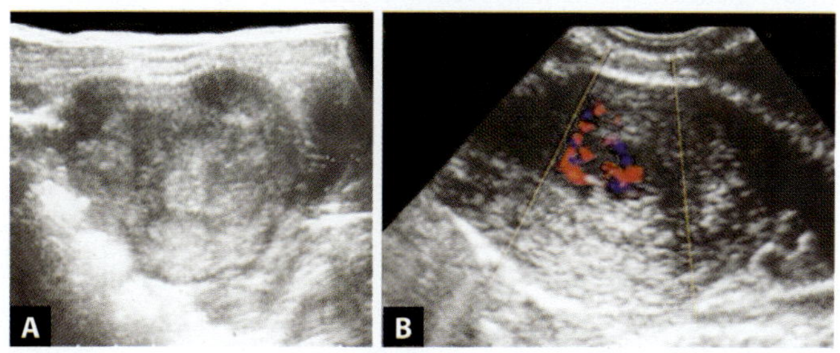

Figs. 17A and B: There is no villus pattern in ultrasound images of choriocarcinoma.
Courtesy: (A) B-mode—M Terahara, Imakyurei Hospital, Japan; (B) Color Doppler—S Kondo, Saitama University Hospital, Japan

Differential diagnosis of choriocarcinoma from an invasive mole is important, because the outcome is ominous in the former and less risky in the latter, in spite of the similarity of clinical symptoms **(Table 2)**. Ultrasonic detection of a cystic pattern in the focus **(Figs. 15 and 16)** is decisive evidence for an invasive mole, while a cystic villus pattern is not detected by various ultrasound imaging techniques in a choriocarcinoma, while color Doppler flow mapping shows a rich blood flow **(Figs. 17A and B)**. Flow impedance is usually low in both diseases, but it is lower in choriocarcinoma than in an invasive mole.[38] The RI of uterine artery is significantly lower in a choriocarcinoma than in a hydatidiform mole.[38] A differential gene expression pattern is reported between normal trophoblast and choriocarcinoma cells.[39] Although, the risk was clinically suspected by FIGO staging, NIC/NIH classification, Ishizuka's and WHO's scoring tables, it is important to examine the trophoblastic disease with objective imaging techniques, particularly with various ultrasound methods. Pelvic angiography has been used in the past, but ultrasound is an alternative to the angiography at present.

Nongestational Choriocarcinoma

Nongestational choriocarcinoma of germ cell origin develops in the ovary or testis without precedence of gestation. Urinary and serum hCG levels are positive and palpation and ultrasound imaging reveal the tumor. DNA polymorphism analysis is reported in pure non-gestational choriocarcinoma.[40] Metamorphosed cancer to choriocarcinoma is diagnosed by its own symptoms and findings associated with hCG excretion.

Persistent Trophoblastic Disease

Since, the persistent trophoblastic disease patients receive chemotherapy that may lead to complete remission without surgical removal of the foci, no histological diagnosis is made and the clinical diagnosis is final in the case of complete remission.

Placental Site Trophoblastic Tumor

The long interval after antecedent gestation and symptoms including vaginal bleeding and enlarged uterus and the lack of high hCG titer, suggest the presence of the disease. Differential diagnosis from other malignant trophoblastic disease is required. Also, due to its rarity, the diagnosis tends to be incorrect. Final diagnosis is made by histology of the removed specimen. Other than common examination and B-mode, color Doppler documents indicated uterine vascularity that is characterized by low resistance flow, its persistence after the chemotherapy and negative plasma β-hCG. Serial transvaginal color Doppler is useful for monitoring chemotherapy and residual tumor.[41] Savelli, et al. (2009)[42] reported a PSTT case who was 34-year-old woman who complained persistent vaginal bleeding and raised β-hCG (308–546 mIU/mL) 6 months after the 2nd cesarean section showed enlarged uterus, presence of inhomogeneous lesion with 3 cm diameter and ill-defined outer borders by transvaginal ultrasound (TVS) and several blood vessels within the mass by power Doppler imaging. The MRI revealed similar intramyometrial mass. Histological diagnosis of violet colored tissue obtained by an operative hysteroscopy was PSTT. The patient underwent total laparoscopic hysterectomy and peritoneal washing which revealed no malignancy. The final diagnosis was PSTT confined within the uterus (FIGO stage I). No adjuvant chemotherapy was performed. The diagnosis on TVS was largely determined by the inhomogeneous mass with undefined borders. Power Doppler imaging strengthened the diagnosis by showing irregularly dispersed blood vessels within the mass.

Our case reported by U Honemeyer, a 32-year-old woman who received C-section for the 1st pregnancy in March 2009, complained intermittent vaginal bleeding in February and 5 months amenorrhea since March, 2010. She was suspected to be suffering from choriocarcinoma but β-hCG was low at 64 mIU/mL. Her uterus had enlarged to the size of 12 weeks pregnancy, and normal cervix and adnexal region. Transvaginal ultrasound (TVS) disclosed 6.09 × 6.68 cm tumor with multiple lacunae and undistinct margin within the uterus **(Figs. 18 and 19)**. Color flow was remarkable surrounding the tumor and in the lacunae by color Doppler flow mapping and the flow signal was surrounding the surface of the tumor **(Figs. 20 to 25)**. Tumor malignancy was supposed due to the very low resistance index of pulsed Doppler flow velocity wave **(Fig. 23)**, but the tumor seemed not to invade the myometrium and surrounding tissues. No distant metastasis was found

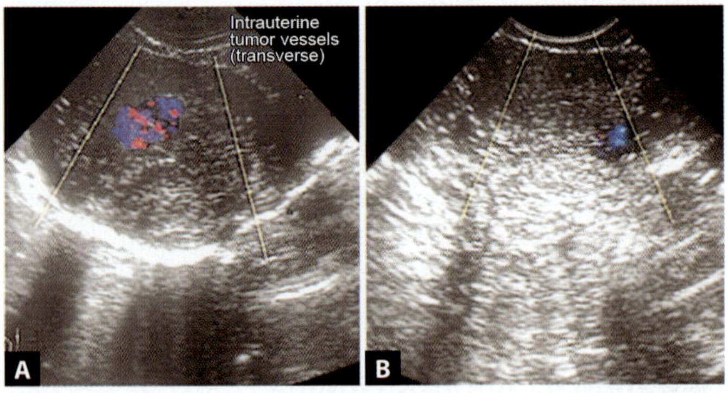

Figs. 18A and B: Chemotherapy of choriocarcinoma with MTX. (A) Adriamycin and cyclophosphamide was monitored by hCG, B-mode ultrasound, color Doppler and pulsed Doppler flow indices; (B) Tumor flow RI and PI sharply increased in the first course of chemotherapy. Color Doppler image and hCG decreased after two chemotherapeutic courses and complete remission was achieved. The flow indices can be useful for early estimation of choriocarcinoma sensitivity to chemotherapy.
Courtesy: S Kondo[21]

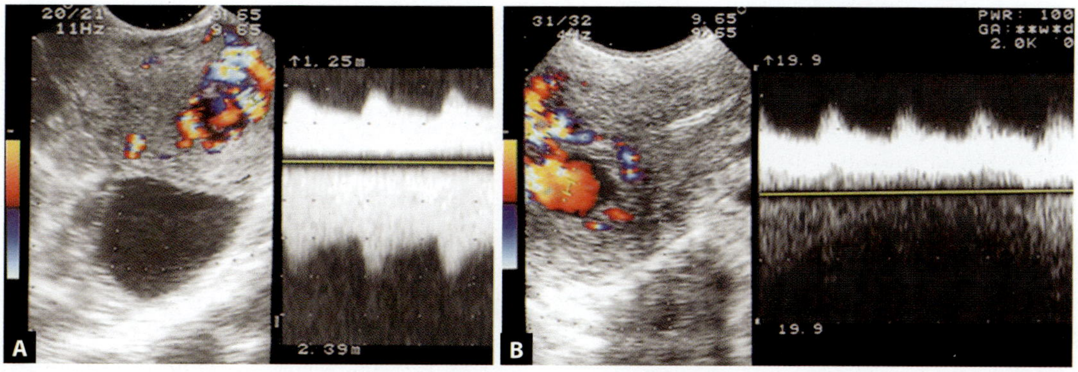

Figs. 19A and B: Pulsed Doppler RI and color Doppler did not significantly change in an invasive mole refractory to chemotherapy. (A) Tumor flow RI was 0.23 before MTX chemotherapy; (B) 0.36 after two MTX courses.
Courtesy: S Yoshida

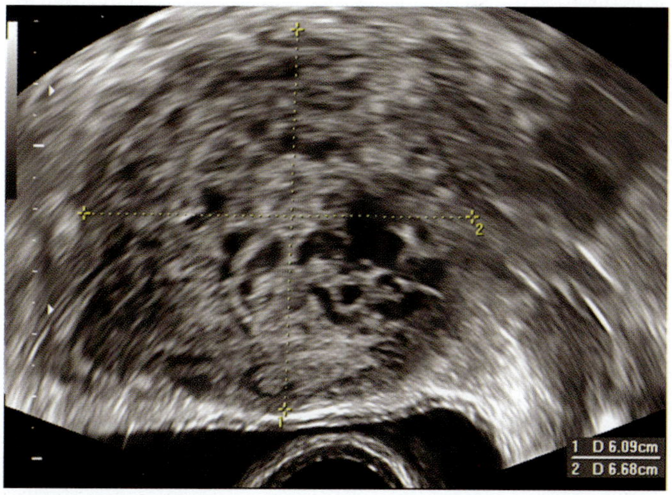

Fig. 20: 2D B-mode of Honemeyer's case shows intrauterine tumor with multiple lacunae and indistinct border of the tumor.
Courtesy: U Honemeyer

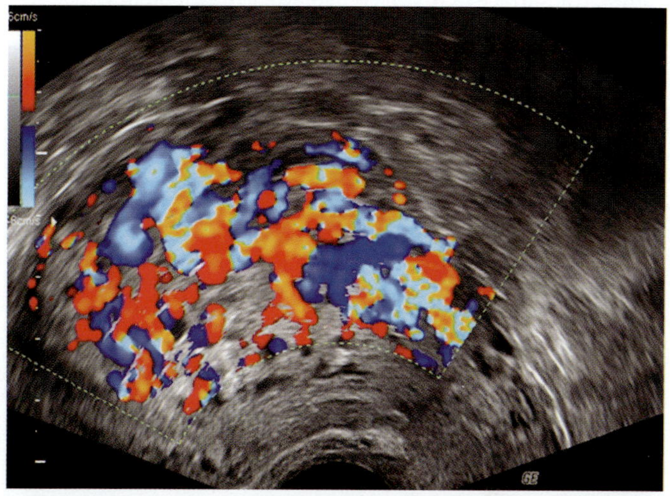

Fig. 21: 3D multiple section image of **Figure 20** tumor. Many lacunae and moderately distinct border of the tumor are revealed.
Courtesy: U Honemeyer

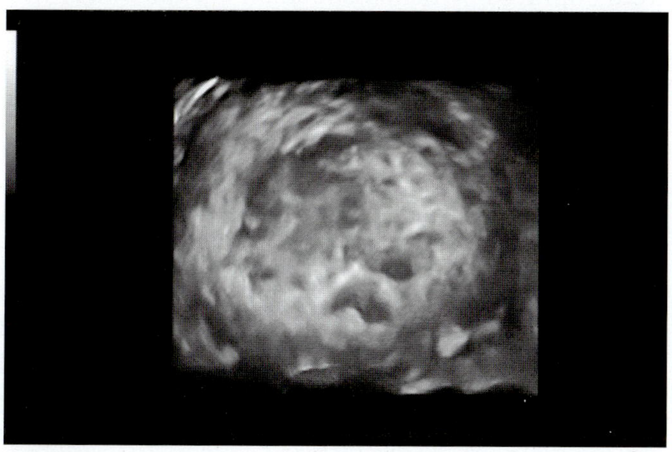

Fig. 22: 2D color Doppler flow mapping of the tumor shown in **Figure 20**. Rich blood flow is recognized in the tumor and its lacunae.
Courtesy: U Honemeyer

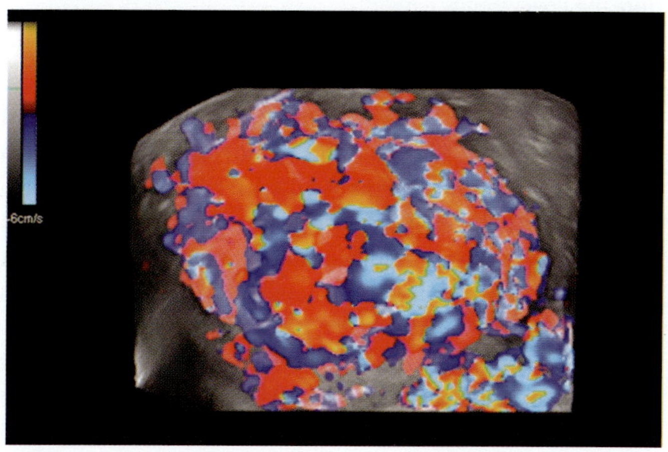

Fig. 23: 3D color Doppler flow mapping of **Figure 20** tumor which shows rich blood flow covering the surface of tumor.
Courtesy: U Honemeyer

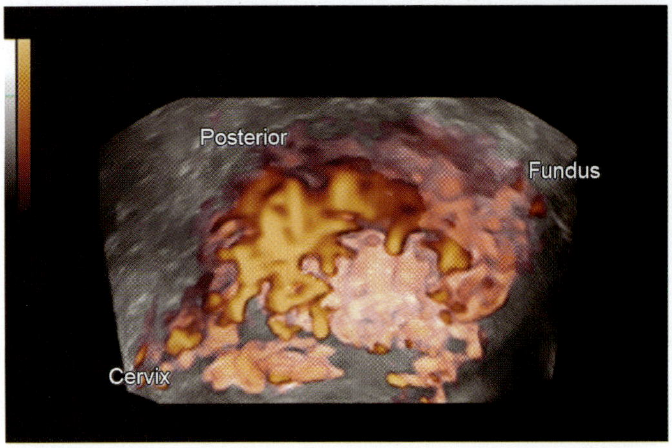

Fig. 24: 3D power Doppler flow mapping of the **Figures 20** and 21 tumor. The surface of tumor is covered by the blood flow.
Courtesy: U Honemeyer

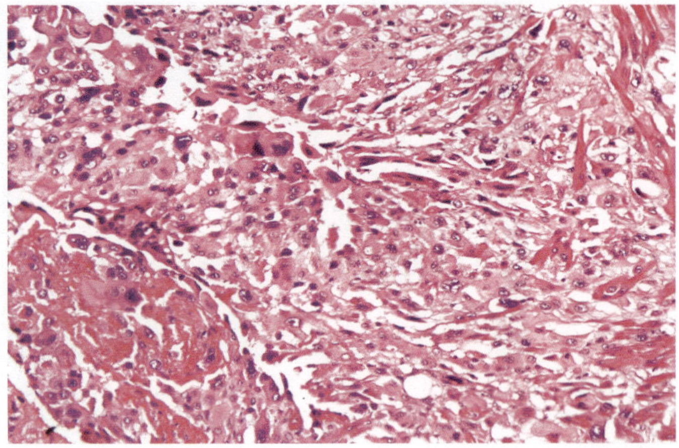

Fig. 26: The H-E stain histology of excised uterine tumor of which pathological diagnosis was "Feature are of placental site trophoblastic tumor".

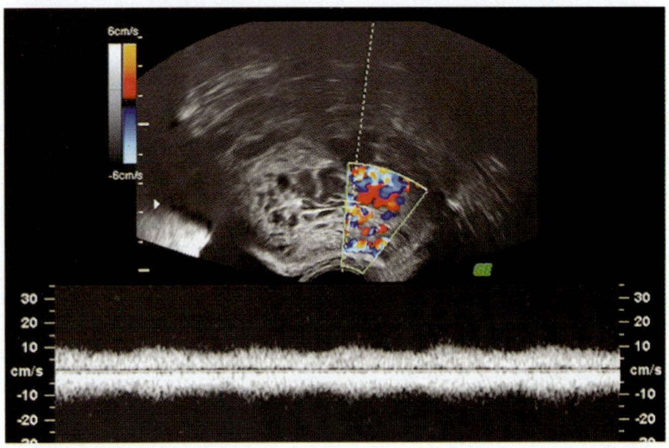

Fig. 25: The pulsed Doppler blood flow velocity wave of **Figure 20** tumor. The resistance index is very small because of rich blood flow in the diastolic phase. Malignant feature of tumor was supposed from the flow velocity curve.
Courtesy: U Honemeyer

outside the uterus. She was sent to the other hospital and received surgery to excise the tumor of about 4 × 4 cm from the posterior uterine wall which was supposed to be a PSTT. The uterine and abdominal walls were closed in layers. The uterus and vagina was packed with ribbon gauges. No active bleeding was seen. The patient was treated in ICU after the surgery. β-hCG level was 54, and the patient received 50 mg methotrexate injection. The tumor micro-scopically examined by a pathologist showed in two sections myometrial smooth muscle bundles infiltrated by tumor cells (morphologically intermediate cells) which had pleomorphic and hyperchromatic nucleus with multiple prominent nucleoli, cytoplasm was eosinophilic, tumor giant cells were invading blood vessels also seen on areas of necrosis and hemorrhage. The impression was "Features are of placental site trophoblastic tumor **(Fig. 26)**". Advised immunohistochemistry was hPL and hCG. The serum β-hCG level was dropping and about 20 mIU/mL 2 months after the surgery when color Doppler still revealed intrauterine tumor.

Epithelioid Trophoblastic Tumor

An epithelioid trophoblastic tumor (ETT) case was reported by Okumura et al.[43] with its transvaginal sonogram and color flow mapping, where rich color flow revealed surrounding intrauterine tumor with multiple lacunae.

Vaginal bleeding, uterine tumor and serum β-hCG were improved by the combination chemotherapy with MTX, actinomycin D, etoposide and cysplatin, and later the patient received hysterectomy. Its histology was intermediate trophoblasts with epithelioid appearance and nuclear pleomorphism.

THERAPY OF TROPHOBLASTIC DISEASES

Complete Hydatidiform Mole

Complete hydatidiform mole is treated primarily by curettage, where the well-developed massive mole should be carefully treated, i.e., the cervix is slowly dilated and uterine contraction is induced by prostaglandin before expulsion and curettage to prevent excessive hemorrhage and uterine damage. Ultrasonically diagnosed early stage evacuation is easier than treating the developed mole in later stages. Curettage is repeated for complete evacuation.

Ultrasound monitoring of intrauterine maneuver is useful for successful curettage and the prevention of uterine damage.

Partial Hydatidiform Mole

In the treatment of a partial hydatidiform mole, labor is induced by prostaglandin, followed by curettage for expulsion of the fetus and removal of the mole.

Postmolar Monitoring

Postmolar monitoring is indispensable for the detection of any sequelae and prevention of malignant trophoblastic disease. After ultrasonically confirmed complete evacuation of the uterus, ultrasonic transvaginal scan and urinary or serum hCG are studied every 1–2 weeks until hCG decreases to normal cut-off levels, then every 1–2 months for a year.[25] An X-ray image is studied when there is any suspicion of pulmonary change. Clinical care, however, lasts for 3 years, because 85% of choriocarcinomas develop at 3 years after the mole.

It is type I when the postmolar hCG regression pattern is normal and when urinary hCG is decreased to 1,000 mIU/mL or less after 5 weeks, serum hCG is 100 mIU/mL or less after 8 weeks and serum hCG is 1 mIU/mL or less with an hCG β-CTP system 0.5 mIU/mL which is the cut-off level after 20 weeks. Type II is abnormal regression, where the hCG level is higher than type I regression. Type II or hCG re-relevation after transient remission should be treated by prophylactic chemotherapy[44] for prevention of the development of choriocarcinoma, where the use of methotrexate (MTX) is common. Prophylactic chemotherapy was tried in our controlled study,[37] where significantly less choriocarcinoma (actually zero) developed in the study group than in the control group.

Choriocarcinoma

Choriocarcinoma is treated by primary chemotherapy, which means the first choice of treatment for choriocarcinoma is chemotherapy, because choriocarcinoma is not a local tumor but systemic disease and the tumor is sensitive to chemotherapy. Hysterectomy was common in the old ages, but was frequently followed by metastases. Radiation was also a local therapy. MTX was the first primary chemotherapy in 1960s. It was systemic chemotherapy because choriocarcinoma was recognized as a systemic disease, the effect is further improved by combined chemotherapy, which is EMA (Etoposide, MTX, Actinomycin-D),[45] or further combination of CO (cyclophosphamide and vincristine), forming the EMA/CO regimen.[46,47] The most intensive therapy may be salvage chemotherapy including etoposide or cisplatine.[48] Chemotherapy-resistant metastasis or recurrence is associated with surgery, e.g., pulmonary lobectomy or craniotomy,[49] and when severe vaginal bleeding accompanies uterine removal. Active combination of hysterectomy[50] or endoscopic surgery[51] and chemotherapy resulted in favorable remission.

Serum hCG level should be lower than the cut-off level for complete remission, i.e., disappearance of primary and metastatic foci and lower hCG levels than the cut-off level. Since, there is cross-sensitivity of hCG antibody to pituitary luteinizing hormone (LH), hCG β or hCG β-CTP antibody that is more specific for hCG is in common use in trophoblastic disease, particularly low-level hCG. However, recent studies reported the presence of false positive tests in some hCG antibodies including hCG β and hCG β-CTP.[52,53] The reports suggested repeated tests, urine test instead of serum, serial dilution test or removal of interfering substances if there is any discrepancy among clinical condition and the test results.

The systemic side effects of intensive chemotherapy are stomatitis, skin eruption, hair-fall, fever, reduced granulocytes, bone marrow damage, hepatic lesion, gastrointestinal tract damage, etc. Heavily life-threatening is bone marrow damage and its expression is leukopenia in peripheral blood. Mild leukopenia is cured by steroids, while severe damage is treated by bone marrow transplantation and stem cell support.[50]

Intra-arterial infusion chemotherapy was used in the treatment of liver metastases, which decreased by using this treatment.[54] We[17] tried internal iliac arterial infusion in the chemotherapy of uterine cervical choriocarcinoma, followed by tumor regression and necrotic change. Pregnancy outcome after complete remission obtained by intensive chemotherapy was favorable and the treatment showed minimal impact.[55] As for further long-term influence of chemotherapy treatment, menopause was 3 years earlier than in control women.[56]

The Role of Ultrasound in the Chemotherapy of Choriocarcinoma

Tumor size and blood flow are effectively monitored in chemotherapy by various ultrasound techniques. Primary or metastatic tumor reduces the size of the ultrasound image and the tumoral blood flow reduces by color or power flow imaging when chemotherapy is effective **(Figs. 18 and 19)**. Early estimation of the tumor sensitivity to systemic chemotherapy is requested in actual chemotherapy.

Pulsed Doppler for the Early Detection of Sensitivity to Chemotherapy

Impedance to flow in the tumor, e.g., RI and PI, clearly elevated immediately after initiation of chemotherapy in the first course, when the choriocarcinoma was sensitive to chemotherapy,[21] before later reduction of hCG and color Doppler flow image and tumor reduction. The changes of flow indices may be caused by tumor shrinkage by the effective chemotherapy. In contrast, a chemotherapy-resistant invasive mole showed no change of RI and PI in tumor flow.[21] Another chemotherapy resistant invasive mole also showed only mild increase of RI at the end of systemic chemotherapy. Therefore, tumor blood flow impedance can be the indicator of tumor sensitivity in the early period of chemotherapy. This method can also be tried in other malignancy chemotherapy treatments.

Germ cell origin choriocarcinoma is treated by its original therapy, usually resection followed by adjuvant chemotherapy. Metastasis surgically removed and followed by chemotherapy. Resistive cases receive multiple adjuvant therapy, usually EMA/CO therapy. Cancer which has metamorphosed to choriocarcinoma may receive its own therapy and chemotherapy.

Persistent Trophoblastic Disease

Postmolar hCG persistence receives prophylactic chemotherapy for the choriocarcinoma, usually single MTX. The courses are repeated until hCG reaches normal levels. Clinical choriocarcinoma receives common chemotherapy treatment as described previously. Clinically, invasive mole also receive chemotherapy treatment, but hysterectomy when it is refractory.

Invasive Mole

Invasive moles are treated by systemic chemotherapy, although they tend to be refractory. An invasive mole is a molar vesicle which is more differentiated than choriocarcinoma. A higher local dose of agents may be needed for invasive moles than choriocarcinomas. Local therapy before hysterectomy in the future may be tumor resection or laser evaporation in the open uterus, or possibly less invasive focused ultrasound hyperthermia.

Placental Site Trophoblastic Tumor

The PSTT was treated by hysterectomy when it was limited in the uterus, while chemotherapy was used when it was spread further than the uterus, although clinical outcome was poor when the precedent pregnancy was more than 2 years before the PSTT.[57] Janni et al.[58] recommended a cytostatic-surgical approach for metastatic PSTT. Furthermore, Tsuji et al.[59] reported that resection of tumor and EMA/CO chemotherapy could achieve long-term remission and save the fertility of young patients. Other reports[60-63] also obtained favorable results mainly by EMA/CO chemotherapy and further use of the etoposide-cisplatin cycle.[63] The outcome of patients with FIGO stage I-II disease were excellent after hysterectomy, but for III-IV stage patients the survival rate was only for 30%.[62] In these reports, PSTT responds to chemotherapy, and complete remission can be expected.

Other Reported Treatment

Wantanebe et al.[64] reported choriocarcinoma in the pulmonary artery which needed treatment with emergency pulmonary embolectomy under cardiopulmonary bypass. Kohyama et al.[65] reported the stereotactic radiation therapy of the choriocarcinoma in the cranium followed by conventional craniospinal irradiation. Bohlmann et al.[19] reported intracardiac resection of a metastatic choriocarcinoma. Brain metastasis is usually treated in intensive chemotherapy.[66] We also experienced massive MTX treatment in a case of brain metastasis; the patient was successfully treated and has survived for more than 20 years.

CONCLUSION

Classification, clinical course, pathological change, diagnosis and chemotherapy of trophoblastic disease were studied, particularly ultrasound diagnosis with real-time B-mode, 3D image, color/power Doppler flow mapping and 3D power Doppler was analyzed. Complete hydatidiform mole in the first trimester and in multiple pregnancy were diagnosed by real-time B-mode. It was new discovery that 2D and 3D color/power Doppler detected a characteristic blood flow pattern in the complete hydatidiform mole. 3D ultrasound was used in the diagnosis of partial mole. Ultrasound imaging was important in the postmolar monitoring. Invasive mole and choriocarcinoma were differentiated by real-time B-mode and color Doppler images. Effective primary chemotherapy and preventive chemotherapy for choriocarcinoma were proposed. The sensitivity of choriocarcinoma to chemotherapy was proved by elevated RI and PI in pulsed Doppler flowmetry. Ultrasound was useful in the diagnosis of trophoblastic disease and also for the monitoring of its treatments.

REFERENCES

1. Japan Society of Obstetrics and Gynecology and Japanese Pathological Society. The general rules for clinical and pathological management of trophoblastic diseases. 2nd edition. Tokyo: Kanehara Shuppan,1995.
2. Weaver DT, Fisher RA, Newlands ES, et al. Amniotic tissue in complete hydatidiform moles can be androgenetic. J Pathol. 2000;191:67-70.
3. Kajii T, Ohama K. Androgenetic origin of hydatidiform mole. Nature. 1977;268(5621):633-4.
4. Ohama K, Kajii T, Okamoto E, et al. Dispermic origin of XY hydatidiform mole. Nature. 1981;292(5823):551-2.
5. Lorigan PC, Sharma S, Bright N, et al. Characteristics of women with recurrent molar pregnancies. Gynecol Oncol. 2000;78(3 pt. 1):288-92.
6. Bae SN, Kim SJ. Telomerase activity in complete hydatidiform mole. Am J Obstet Gynecol. 1999;180(2 Pt. 1):328-33.
7. Lazarus E, Hulka C, Siewert B, et al. Sonographic appearance of early complete molar pregnancy. J Ultrasound Med. 1999;18:589-94.
8. Szulman AE. Philippe E, Boue JG, et al. Human triploidy association with partial hydatidiform moles and nonmolar conceptuses. Hum Pathol. 1981;12(11):1016-21.
9. Hirose M, Kimura T, Mitsuno N, et al. DNA flow cytometric quantification and DNA polymorphism analysis in the case of, a complete mole with a coexisting fetus. J Ass Reprod Genet. 1999;16(5):263-7.
10. Suita S, Sono K, Tajiri T, et al. Malignant germ cell tumors: clinical characteristics, treatment and outcome. A report from the study group for pediatric solid malignant Tumors in the Kyushu area, Japa J Pediatr Surg. 2002;37:1703-6.
11. Weiss S, Amit A, Schwarz MR, et al. Primary choriocarcinoma of the vulva. Int J Gynecol Cancer. 2001;11(3):251-4.
12. Yahata T, Kodama S, Kase H, et al. Primary choriocarcinoma of the uterine cervix: clinical, MRI, and color Doppler ultrasonographic study. Gynecol Oncol. 1997; 64(2):274-8.
13. Coskun M, Agildere AM, Boyvart F, et al. Primary choriocarcinoma of the stomach and pancreas: CT findings. Eur Radiol. 1988;8(8):1425-8.
14. Liu Z, Mira JL, Cruz-Caudilo JC. Primary gastric choriocarcinoma:a case report and review of the literature. Arch Pathol Lab Med. 2001;125(12):1601-4.
15. Wang JC, Angeles S, Chak P, et al. Choriocarcinoma of the gallbladder: treated with cisplatine-based chemotherapy. Med Oncol. 2001;18:165-9.
16. Sievert K, Weber EA, Herwig R, et al. Pure primary choriocarcinoma of the urinary bladder with long-term survival. Urology. 2000;56(5):856.
17. Koga K, Izuchi S, Maed K, et al. Treatment of chorionepithelioma of uterine cervix with hypogastric arterial infusion of amethopterin. J Jpn Obstet Gynecol Soc. 1966;13:245-9.
18. Chama CM, Nggada HA, Nuhu A. Cutaneous metastasis of gestational choriocarcinoma. Int J Gynecol Obstet. 2002;77(3):249-50.
19. Bohlmann MK, Eckstein FS, Allemann Y, et al. Intracardiac, resection of a metastatic choriocarcinoma. Gynecol Oncol. 2002;84:157-80.
20. Gersak B, Lakic N, Gorjup V, et al. Right ventricular metastatic, choriocarcinoma obstructing inflow and outflow tract. Ann Thorac Surg. 2002;73(5):1631-3.
21. Kondo S. Personal communication. In: Maeda K (Ed). Gestational trophoblastic disease, Lecture in the Ian Donald Inter-University School of Medical Ultrasound, Dubrovnik; 1995.
22. Steigrad SM, Cheung AP, Oshborn RA. Choriocarcinoma coexistent with and intact, pregnancy: case report and review of the literature. J Obstet Gynecol Res. 1999;25:197-203.
23. Jacque SM, Quershi F, Doss BJ, et al. Intraplacental choriocarcinoma associated with viable pregnancy: pathologic features and implications for the mother and infant. Pediatr Dev Pathol. 1998;1(5):380-7.
24. Feltmate CM, Genset DR, Goldstein DP, et al. Advances in the understanding of placental site trophoblastic tumor. J Reprod Med. 2002;47:337-41.
25. Santoso JT, Coleman RI (Eds). Handbook of Gyn Oncology. New York: McGraw Hill; 2001.
26. Mangili G, Garavaglia E, De Marzi P, et al. Metastatic placental site trophoblastic tumor. Report of a case with complete response to chemotherapy. J Reprod Med. 2001;46(3):259-62.
27. Remadi S, Lifschita-Mercer B, Ben-Hur H, et al. Metastasizing placental site trophoblastic tumor: immunohistochemical and DNA analysis. 2 case reports and a review of the literature. Arch Gynecol Obstet. 1997;259(2):97-103.
28. Feltmate CM, Genest DR, Wise L, et al. Placental site trophoblastic tumor: a 17-year experience at the New England Trophoblastic Disease Center. Gynecol Oncol. 2001;82(3):415-9.
29. Monclair T, Abeler VM, Kren J, et al. Placental site trophoblastic tumor (PSTT) in mother and child: first report of PSTT in infancy. Med Pediatr Oncol. 2002;38(3):187-91.
30. Piura B. Placental site trophoblastic tumor: a challenging rare entity. Eur J Gynaecol Oncol. 2006;27(6):545-51.
31. Baergen RN, Rutgers JL, Young RH, et al. Placental site trophoblastic tumor: a study of 55 cases and review of the literature emphasizing factors of prognostic significance. Gynecol Oncol. 2006;100(3):511-20. Epub 2005 Oct 21.

32. Allison KH, Love JE, Garcia RL. Epithelioid trophoblastic tumor: review of a rare neoplasm of the chorionic-type intermediate trophoblast. Arch Pathol Lab Med. 2006;130(12):1875-7.
33. Shih IM, Kurman RJ. Epithelioid trophoblastic tumor: a neoplasm distinct from choriocarcinoma and placental site trophoblastic tumor simulating carcinoma. Am J Surg Pathol. 1998;22(11):1393-403.
34. Sebire NJ, Lindsay I. Current issues in the histopathology of gestational trophoblastic tumors. Fetal Pediatr Pathol. 2010;29(1):30-44.
35. Kurjak A, Zalud I, Predanic M, et al. Transvaginal color and pulsed Doppler study of uterine blood flow in the first and early second trimesters of pregnancy: normal versus abnormal. J Ultrasound Med. 1994;13(1):43-7.
36. Kurjak A, Zalud L, Salihagic A, et al. Transvaginal color Doppler in the assessment of abnormal early pregnancy. J Perinat Med. 1991;19(3):155-65.
37. Koga K, Maeda K. Prophylactic chemotherapy with amethopterin for the prevention if choriocarcinoma following removal of hydatidiform mole. Am J Obstet Gyncol. 1968;100:270-5.
38. Gungor T, Ekin M, Dumanli H, et al. Color Doppler ultrasonography in the earlier differentiation of benign molehydatidiform from malignant gestational trophoblastic disease. Acta Obstet Gynecol Scand. 1998;77(8):860-2.
39. Vegh GL, Fulop V, Liu Y, et al. Differential gene expression pattern between normal human trophoblast and choriocarcinoma cell lines: downregulation of heat shock protein-27 in choriocarcinoma in vitro and in vivo. Gynecol Oncol. 1999;75(3):391-6.
40. Shigematsu T, Kamura T, Wake N, et al. DNA polymorphism analysis of a pure polymorphism non-gestational choriocarcinoma of the ovary: case report. Eur J Gynecol Oncol. 2000;21:153-4.
41. Bettencourt E, Pinto E, Abreul E, et al. Placental site trophoblastic tumor: the value of transvaginal colour and pulsed Doppler sonography (TV-CGS) in its diagnosis: case report. Eur J Gynecol Oncol. 1997;18:461-4.
42. Savelli L, Pollastri P, Mabrouk M, et al. Placental site trophoblastic tumor diagnosed on transvaginal sonography. Ultrasound Obstet Gynecol. 2009;34(2):235-6.
43. Okumura M, Fushida K, Rezende WW, et al. Sonographic appearance of gestational trophoblastic disease evolving into epithelioid trophoblastic tumor. Ultrasound Obstet Gynecol. 2010;36(2):249-51.
44. PMK TK, Kim SN, Lee SK. Analysis of risk factors for postmolar trophoblastic disease: categorization of risk factors and effect of prophylactic chemotherapy. Yonsei Med J. 1996;37:412-9.
45. Soto-Wright V, Goldstein DP, Bernstein MR, et al. The management of gestational trophoblastic tumors with etoposide, methotrexate, and actinomycin D. Gynecol Oncol. 1997;64(1):156-9.
46. Newlands ES, Oaradubas FJ, Fisher RA. Recent, advances in gestational trophoblast disease. Hematol Oncol Clin. North Am. 1999;13(1):225-44.
47. Nozue A, Ichikawa Y, Minami R, et al. Postpartum choriocarcinoma complicated by brain and lung metastases treated successfully with EMA/CO regimen. BJOG. 2000;107(9):1171-2.
48. Okamoto T, Goto S. Resistance to multiple agent chemotherapy including cisplatin after chronic low-dosage oral etoposide. Administration in gestational choriocarcinoma. Gynecol Obstet Invest. 2001;52(2):139-41.
49. Kang SB, Lee CM, Kim JW, et al. Chemoresistant choriocarcinoma cured by pulmonary lobectomy and craniotomy. Int J Gynecol Cancer. 2000;10(2):165-9.
50. Knox S, Brooke SE, Wog-You cheong J, et al. Choriocarcinoma and epithelial trophoblastic tumor: successful treatment of relapse with hysterectomy and high dose chemotherapy with peripheral stem cell support: a case report. Gynecol Oncol. 2002;85(1):204-8.
51. Chou HH, Lai CH, Wang PN, et al. Combination of high-dose chemotherapy, autologous bone marrow/peripheral blood stem cell transplantation, and thoracoscopic surgery in refractory nongestational choriocarcinoma of a 45XO/46XY female: a case report. Gynecol Oncol. 1997;64(3):521-5.
52. Cole LA, Butler S. Detection of hCG in trophoblastic disease. The USA hCG reference service experience. J Reprod Med. 2002;47(6):433-44.
53. ACOG Committee opinion. Avoiding inappropriate clinical decisions based on false-positive human chorionic gonadotropin test results. Obstet Gyecol. 2002;100(5 Pt 1): 1057-9.
54. Tanase K, Tawada M, Moriyama N, et al. Intra-arterial infusion chemotherapy for liver metastases of testicular tumors: report of two cases. Hinyokika Kiyo. 2000;46(11): 823-7.
55. Woolas RP, Bower M, Newlands ES, et al. Influence of chemotherapy for gestational trophoblastic disease on subsequent pregnancy outcome. Br J Obstet Gynaecol. 1998;105(9):1032-5.
56. Bower M, Rustin GJ, Newlands ES, et al. Chemotherapy for gestational trophoblastic tumours hastens menopause by 3 years. Eur J Cancer. 1998;34(8):1204-7.
57. Newlands ES, Bower M, Fisher RA, et al. Management of placental site trophoblastic tumors. J Reprod Med. 1995;43(1):53-9.
58. Janni W, Hantschmann P, Rehbock J, et al. Successful treatment of malignant placental site trophoblastic tumor with combined cytostatic-surgical approach: case report and review of literature. Gynecol Oncol. 1999;75(1):164-9.
59. Tsuji Y, Tsubamoto H, Hori M, et al. Case of PSTT treated with chemotherapy followed by open uterine tumor resection to preserve fertility. Gynecol Oncol. 2002;87(3): 303-7.

60. Twigs LB, Hartenbach E, Saltzman AK, et al. Metastatic placental site trophoblastic tumor. Int J Gynecol Obst. 1998;60(Suppl. l):S51-5.
61. Swisher E, Drescher CW. Metastatic placental site trophoblastic tumor: long-term remission in a patient treated with EMA/CO chemotherapy. Gynecol Oncol. 1998;68(1):62-5.
62. Chang YL, Chang TC, Hsuen KG, et al. Prognostic factors and treatment for placental site trophoblastic tumor report of 3 cases and analysis of 88 cases. Gynecol Oncol. 1999;73(2):216-22.
63. Randall TC, Coukos G, Wheeler JE, et al. Prolonged remission of recurrent, metastatic placental site trophoblastic tumor after chemotherapy. Gynecol Oncol. 2000;76(1):115-7.
64. Watanbe S, Shimokawa K, Sakasegawa K, et al. Choriocarcinoma in the pulmonary artery treated with emergency pulmonary embolectomy. Chest. 2002;121(2):654-6.
65. Kohyama S, Uematsu M, Ishihara S, et al. An experience of stereotactic radiation therapy for primary intracranial choriocarcinoma. Tumori. 2001;87(3):162-5.
66. Landanio G, Sartore-Bianchi A, Giannetta L, et al. Controversies in the management of brain metastases: the role of chemotherapy. Forum (Genova). 2001;11(1):59-74.

12

CHAPTER

First-trimester Ultrasound Screening for Fetal Anomalies and Adverse Pregnancy Outcomes

Jon Hyett, Jiri Sonek

INTRODUCTION

The utility of the first-trimester ultrasound examination of the gravid uterus and its contents continues to expand. Improvements in the resolution of ultrasound equipment and better understanding of normal and abnormal fetal development now enable us to perform a highly reliable fetal anatomic evaluation even at a relatively early gestational age (11–13^{+6} weeks). Furthermore, first-trimester evaluation of the fetus, maternal pelvic vasculature, and maternal serum in conjunction with maternal history and physical examination may be used to establish the risk of fetal aneuploidy and certain pregnancy complications that do not become clinically evident until later in gestation. In this chapter, we will discuss current information regarding the benefits and limitations of this approach.

Gray-scale examination of the fetal head and neck yields a great amount of information regarding the risk of trisomy 21 and other aneuploidies. Many of the ultrasound markers that are used in the first trimester to establish the risk of trisomy 21 have their equivalents in the postnatal phenotype. In 1866, Langdon Down[1] described individuals with a syndrome that later came to bear his name as "having skin that appears to be too large for their bodies" [recognized as increased nuchal translucency (NT) thickness],[2] having a "small nose" [recognized as an absent or hypoplastic nasal bone (NB)],[3] and having a "flat face" [recognized as a shallow frontomaxillary facial (FMF) angle].[4]

Gray-scale and color Doppler examination of the fetal heart in the first trimester may yield evidence of a cardiac defect, which is the most common structural anomaly seen in individuals with trisomy 21.[5] However, even in the absence of an overt structural defect, cardiac function may be altered. There is ample evidence that the microscopic and ultrastructural anatomy of the myocardium and valve leaflets is abnormal in trisomy 21.[6-8] These findings were exploited to develop a second type of ultrasound marker through Doppler evaluation of the cardiovascular system. Cardiac function can be assessed through evaluation of blood flow across the tricuspid valve (TCV)[9-11] or through the ductus venosus (DV).[12-19] Additionally, a measure of fetal heart rate (FHR) may also be helpful. Whilst this marker is of marginal benefit in screening for trisomy 21, it has significant value when screening for other types of aneuploidy.[2,20]

Pregnancy and the development of the placenta are associated with the appearance of novel proteins in maternal blood, and alteration in the levels of already extant proteins. Through empirical observation followed by prospective studies, it has been noted that the concentration of some proteins differs between aneuploid and chromosomally normal pregnancies. At 12 weeks of gestation, two proteins have significant discriminative power between populations of trisomic and chromosomally normal fetuses: Free beta-human chorionic gonadotropin (free β-hCG) and pregnancy-associated plasma protein-A (PAPP-A).[21] It should be stressed that it is the free β-hCG rather than other forms of hCG that has been tested most rigorously and performs best.

First-trimester screening has been shown to be useful not only for trisomy 21 but for other types of aneuploidy (trisomies 18 and 13, monosomy X, other aneuploidies involving the sex chromosomes and triploidy).[2,3,22-24] Some of these conditions are associated with median nuchal translucencies that are even thicker than that seen with trisomy 21 and are also more likely to have other major or minor structural defects. As a result, in some cases, detection rates are even higher than for trisomy 21.[2,22]

Other first-trimester markers have been described that facilitate earlier detection of structural anomalies. Changes to the brainstem and intercranial translucency can be visualized in the same midsagittal plane as is used for assessment of NT and enable detection of the majority of cases of spina bifida.[25] Similarly, the midsagittal plane can be used to identify cleft palate, often exceedingly difficult at later gestations.[26]

First-trimester Doppler evaluation of the maternal uterine arteries coupled with measurement of maternal serum biomarkers and maternal blood pressure measurement has been shown to be useful in estimating the risk of preterm preeclampsia.[27-29] Up to 90% of cases of early, severe preeclampsia can be identified, which are frequently associated with growth restriction. Identification of a high-risk cohort allows effective prophylactic intervention through prescription of aspirin, with a 62% reduction in prevalence of preeclampsia leading to preterm delivery (<37 weeks).[30]

The Fetal Medicine Foundation played an active role in the development and implementation of these first-trimester markers. They are included in the current Fetal Medicine Foundation's algorithm for first-trimester pregnancy evaluation.

AN ARGUMENT FOR SCREENING IN THE FIRST TRIMESTER

Evaluating pregnancies formally in the first trimester has a number of potential benefits. The combination of ultrasound (NT) and maternal serum markers (PAPP-A and free β-hCG) provides the best method of screening for fetal aneuploidy with a high (approximately 90%) detection rate and positive predictive value.[31] Ultrasound measurements are helpful in establishing the risk of a number of fetal disorders in addition to aneuploidy.[32-78] Fetal anatomy can be systematically examined even at this early gestation, and the majority of major structural anomalies can be detected at this stage.[79-90]

The majority of women have a normal pregnancy and can be appropriately reassured, relieving the anxiety that many feel about the risk of fetal abnormality. In the minority of cases where a problem is detected, first-trimester diagnosis preserves maximum privacy and autonomy as well as safety with regards to reproductive choices. An added advantage of first-trimester ultrasound evaluation lies in accurate pregnancy dating through measurement of the crown–rump length (CRL).[91] Accurate gestational age is one of the most important pieces of information in the management of both high-risk and normal pregnancies.

First-trimester ultrasound is particularly valuable in multiple gestations as chorionicity can be determined most accurately at an early stage.[92-94] A distinct thickening of the dividing membrane ("lambda" or "twin peak" sign) as it approaches the placental surface indicates that the pregnancy is dichorionic (DC), whereas a thin, "T-shaped" insertion of the membrane into the placental surface is indicative of monochorionic placentation. The accurate determination of chorionicity is fundamental for successful management of twin pregnancies: Monochorionicity is associated with a risk of adverse perinatal outcome that is higher than in DC pregnancies.[95] Therefore, monochorionic pregnancies merit a significantly increased level of antenatal surveillance.

Algorithms used to calculate risks for aneuploidy vary in monochorionic and DC pregnancies. This is to account for the fact that the monochorionic twins are monozygous as well as the fact that biochemical parameters vary according to the type of placentation.[96-98] Unlike maternal serum biochemistries, the use of ultrasound markers in multiple gestations allows risk to be assigned to each individual fetus, rather than establishing a risk for the pregnancy overall. Maternal serum markers in higher order multiple gestations (triplets and greater) are unreliable and first-trimester ultrasound screening is the best option.

In monochorionic/diamniotic gestations, the risk of developing twin-to-twin transfusion syndrome (TTTS) later in pregnancy may be estimated by measuring the NT's (the likelihood of TTTS increases with increasing difference in the NT measurements between the two fetuses),[99] and by evaluating the DV with Doppler (presence of reversed a-wave increases the risk of TTTS).[100]

An Argument for Confining the First-trimester Ultrasound Examination to 11–13^{+6} Weeks of Gestation

The benefits of a first-trimester ultrasound examination are best realized between 11 and 13^{+6} weeks of gestation. Visualization of normal anatomical structures is easier after the process of embryonic development is more complete,[101] allowing the identification of anomalies that are not necessarily visible at an earlier stage. For example, physiologic extra-abdominal herniation of the bowel continues to 11 weeks of gestation making the diagnosis of an omphalocele difficult prior to this time.[102,103] The cranial vault is not ossified prior to 11 weeks of gestation, which reduces the accuracy of first-trimester diagnosis of exencephaly/anencephaly sequence.[104] Finally, aside from NT measurement, the effectiveness of first-trimester markers prior to 11 weeks of gestation is likely reduced. For example, the NB is not normally ossified prior to 11 weeks of gestation[105] and almost 50% of normal fetuses have an incompetent TCV at 10 weeks of gestation.[106]

The effectiveness of NT measurement as a marker of aneuploidy diminishes beyond 13^{+6} weeks—a gestation where image acquisition also becomes more difficult due to fetal lie.[107-109] Estimation of gestational age by measurement of CRL becomes inaccurate beyond this gestational age, and the potential benefits of early diagnosis with regard to complications of interrupting the pregnancy are reduced.

ELEMENTS OF FIRST-TRIMESTER FETAL SCREENING

General Principles of Screening

The development of a credible screening protocol has a number of essential components. Firstly, markers (ultrasound or maternal serum) need to be identified. A marker for aneuploidy is defined as an observation that has a different prevalence in euploid and aneuploid populations. Each marker can be ascribed a specific mathematical value, known as a likelihood ratio, which is based on the ratio of prevalence of the observation in the two populations. For any individual, the absolute risk of having aneuploidy is then calculated by multiplying the background risk of the disease by this likelihood ratio.

Likelihood ratios can be calculated to reflect the presence or absence of the observation—positive and negative likelihood ratios, respectively. Both are important as the negative likelihood ratio also impacts the overall risk for aneuploidy, improving test specificity. The strength of a marker depends on the degree of difference in the prevalence of the observation in normal and aneuploid fetuses. Some markers are affected by other maternal and fetal factors (e.g., the effect of maternal weight, smoking, and ethnicity on maternal serum biochemistry).[2] These effects need to be accounted for mathematically when generating likelihood ratios. Similarly, if more than one marker is used it needs to be established whether or not they are interdependent. A weak association between markers usually may be compensated for mathematically. If the association is strong, it may be best not to use them together. The manner in which the marker is examined must be standardized, so that it is reproducible and may be implemented in more than one center.

The implementation of a credible screening protocol also has a number of essential components. Above all, only those operators that have the appropriate background and training should be involved in the performance of screening. It is equally important to establish a quality assurance system that reviews the performance of the screening on an ongoing basis.

General Principles of the Use of Ultrasound and Biochemical Markers

Two techniques are used to generate likelihood ratios for the markers used in first-trimester screening: By the use of continuous variables and categorical variables.

Nuchal translucency thickness, maternal serum free β-hCG and PAPP-A, the FMF angle, and FHR are all continuous variables. Generally, normal ranges of continuous variables change with gestational age in both euploid and aneuploid populations. The likelihood ratio is based on the measurement itself while considering any changes associated with gestational age. Small variations in measurement lead to small changes in the likelihood ratio and in the calculated risk for aneuploidy. This contrasts with markers like the absent NB, tricuspid regurgitation, an abnormal DV a-wave and other structural anomalies that are categorical: They are either present or not—and the likelihood ratio is either positive or negative. The result of the assessment (positive or negative) is generally associated with a large change in risk.

The final risk for Down syndrome is calculated by multiplying an "a priori risk" by these likelihood ratios. The "a priori" risk is based on maternal age but must also take into account gestational age and any history of a previous affected pregnancy.[110,111] Of note is that while the history of a previous affected pregnancy is a categorical variable, the "a priori" risk based on maternal and gestational age is a continuous variable. Therefore, the addition of either categorical or continuous type of markers results in a continuous spectrum of risks across the screened population.

The final risk can be viewed in two ways: From an individual's perspective and from the public health perspective. From the individual perspective, the value of risk assessment is to help the patient with the decision whether or not to proceed with diagnostic testing. However, the decision to proceed with diagnostic testing depends on a number of other factors including the individual's attitude toward having an affected child, the stress that a miscarriage would create, and whether or not termination of pregnancy is an acceptable option. Even though, the patient is provided with numerical risks of aneuploidy based on the individual risk assessment and procedure-related loss rate, the significance that she attaches to these adverse events varies from individual to individual. Nondirective counseling and honoring patient autonomy are paramount.

From a public health perspective, it is the detection and false-positive (FP) rates that are important. To that end, it is necessary to define a "risk cut-off," which divides the population into "high-risk" and "low-risk" group, i.e., those that are screen positive and those that are screen negative. Generally, it is only those women that fall into the "high-risk" category that are offered an invasive diagnostic test. However, in accordance with the dictum of patient autonomy, even patients who are in the low-risk category and who understand the risks of an invasive procedure may choose to have an invasive procedure done. The cut-off is somewhat arbitrary, but over the past 30 years, it has been set so the false-positive rate is 5%. Recently, due to the effectiveness of combined first-trimester screening, some programs have adjusted this cut-off to reduce the false-positive rate while maintaining the high levels of detection.[112] Reduction in the false-positive rate results in a reduction of invasive procedures. This in turn decreases the overall cost and the number of normal fetuses lost as a result of invasive procedures.

In order to appropriately compare screening algorithms and programs, it is critical to evaluate them while holding either the false-positive rate or the detection rate constant (e.g., holding the false-positive rate at 5% and looking at the detection rates that two or more separate screening approaches produce or holding the detection rate at 90% and looking at the various false-positive rates).

Crown–rump Length

The background prevalence of Down syndrome, normal ranges of continuously variable markers (NT and FMF angle measurements, serum free β-hCG, and PAPP-A), and prevalence of categorical markers (NB absence, tricuspid regurgitation, and abnormal DV a-wave) are all dependent on gestational age. Consequently, it is critical to establish the gestational age as accurately as possible in order for the correct "a priori" risk and likelihood ratios to be used.[91] Measurement of fetal CRL appears to be the most reliable method for determining gestational age.[113] To measure the CRL, a midline longitudinal view of the fetus is obtained and the image is magnified so that the fetus fills the screen. The fetus is measured from the top of the head to the rump. The measurement should be done with the fetus in a neutral position, i.e., not hyperflexed or extended. Salomon et al. developed a model, which simulates the effect of inaccurate CRL measurements on Down syndrome risks based on the combination of first-trimester NT and second-trimester biochemical markers.[114] They showed that even small (5 mm) changes in CRL led to significant changes in risk and concluded that quality assurance of CRL measurements may be as important as methods currently used to standardize measurements of NT. At the present time, development of a CRL measurement quality assurance program is hampered by the fact that there is no gold standard that can be used for comparison of acquired datasets.

Nuchal Translucency

Nuchal translucency describes a sonographically echolucent space beneath the skin at the nape of the neck.[111] This sonolucent area can be seen in all fetuses between 11 and 13^{+6} weeks of gestation. As NT thickness increases, there is an increasing chance of the fetus being affected by a chromosomal or structural abnormality, a genetic syndrome, or intrauterine death.[53] Despite this, a proportion of fetuses with increased NT will be normal, underscoring the fact that this finding is not diagnostic and serves merely as a marker for a potential fetal anomaly.[115]

Possible Mechanisms for Increased Nuchal Translucency

A number of mechanisms for increased NT have been proposed: Structural cardiovascular abnormalities and/or abnormalities of myocardial performance,[6,116-119] abnormalities of connective tissue composition,[7,8,120-122] abnormalities or delay in lymphatic system formation,[65,66,123,124] increase in intrathoracic pressure,[47,54-60] decrease in fetal movement,[50,69-71] fetal hypoproteinemia,[68,125] fetal anemia,[72-75] and fetal infection.[76-78,126] It is likely that under different clinical circumstances, different mechanisms are in effect. It is also likely that in many cases, especially in fetuses with chromosomal defects, the thickened NT is caused by more than one mechanism. The latter is exemplified by trisomy 21 where abnormalities of the connective tissue and lymphatic system along with cardiovascular defects are commonly seen in the same fetus.

Nuchal Translucency Measurement

A standardized method for measurement of NT thickness has been described by the Fetal Medicine Foundation

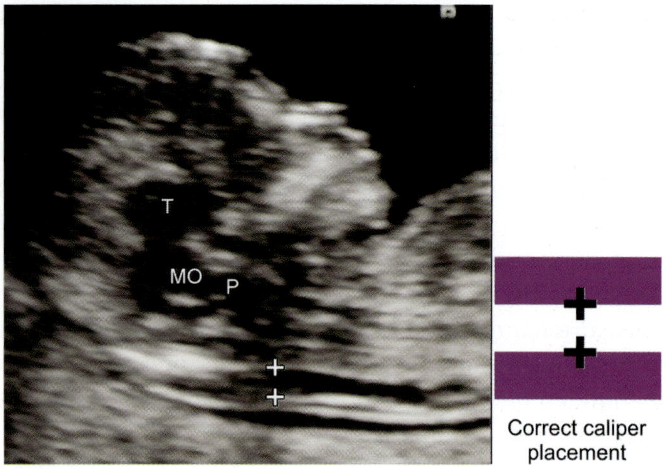

Fig. 1: Nuchal translucency measurement that meets Fetal Medicine Foundation criteria. The correct caliper placement is "on-to-on". (MO: medulla oblongata; P: pons; T: thalamus)

BOX 1: The Fetal Medicine Foundation criteria for the measurement of NT.

- *CRL:* 45–84 mm (11^{+0}–13^{+6} weeks of gestation)
- Midsagittal view (fetus may either be facing toward or away from the transducer)
- Landmarks of the profile—skin over the nasal bridge and the nasal tip
- *Intracranial structures:* Thalamus, pons, and medulla oblongata
- Image size—head and upper thorax occupies most of the screen (measurement degree of precision—1 mm)
- Neutral fetal position (avoid neck extension or flexion)
- Skin line needs to be seen separately from the amnion
- Nuchal cord (5% of the cases measure NT above and below the nuchal cord and average the measurements)
- "On-to-on" caliper placement
- Motivated sonographer

(CRL: crown–rump length; NT: nuchal translucency)

(Fig. 1 and Box 1). The software that has been developed by the foundation to generate likelihood ratios and to provide individual risk assessment is based on this method of assessment.[127] Nuchal measurements are made at 11–13^{+6} weeks of gestation, corresponding to a CRL measurement of 45–84 mm. The fetus is assessed in a midsagittal section with the head and neck in a neutral position. There are a number of anatomic landmarks that help to establish that the ultrasound plane is in the midline: Delineation of the fetal profile with echogenic lines representing the skin over the nasal bridge and nasal tip being visible in the same view (only if the fetus is facing the transducer) and the intracranial hypoechoic regions of the thalamus, the pons, and the medulla oblongata (if the fetus is either facing toward or away from the transducer). Extension of the neck artificially increases the NT measurement and hyperflexion decreases it.[128] The image should be magnified such that the fetal head and the upper thorax occupy the majority of the image, so that caliper measurements are accurate to an interval of 0.1 mm. Square calipers should be used to measure the NT at its widest point, placing the calipers so that the inner aspect of the caliper cross hatch is flush with the inner aspect of the echodense lines bracketing the nuchal fluid. The ultrasound settings should be adjusted so that these lines are as thin and sharply delineated as possible. This view is optimized by keeping the face of the transducer parallel to the longitudinal axis of the fetus, i.e., insonating the nuchal skin at 90°. The NT must be clearly differentiated from the amniotic membrane, which has a similar ultrasound appearance to the skin line. The measurement should be repeated on at least three separate images and the largest measurement that meets the criteria should be used for risk assessment.

In approximately 5% of cases, a nuchal cord is identified.[129] The initial suspicion of a nuchal cord being present is often raised when a segment of NT cannot be clearly visualized or an indentation in the NT is noted. Commonly, faint echodense lines are seen in this region, which represent walls of the tortuous umbilical vessels in cross section. The presence of a nuchal cord is best confirmed with color Doppler. In this circumstance, the NT should be measured both above and below the nuchal cord and risk assessment is based on the average of these two measurements.

Risk assessment is based on NT thickness alone, not the subjective appearance of this region. On close inspection, septations may be seen in all thickened nuchal translucencies; attempting to differentiate between simple NT and a "cystic hygroma" is not useful.[130] Assigning different risks based on the appearance of NT was proposed as a part of the FASTER study.[131] The statistical analysis used in this article was questioned by some.[132] Additionally, subsequent analysis of the same data by the FASTER group did suggest that NT size rather than appearance is the most important.[133]

Nuchal Translucency and Fetal Aneuploidy

The prevalence of chromosomal defects increases with increasing NT thickness.[134,135] The relation between fetal NT and chromosomal defects was initially derived from a multicenter screening study involving[95,125] singleton pregnancies.[134] The distribution of NT measurements has changed since that time due to minor adjustments in measurement technique and improvements in ultrasound equipment. The distribution of normal measurements that is currently used for risk estimation is based on 37,078 fetuses examined in a standardized fashion at the Fetal Medicine Centre in London between 1999 and 2005.[107]

The mathematical descriptions of the NT measurement distribution and the manner in which the likelihood ratios are generated have evolved over the past 15 years. Recently, a mixture model of the NT measurement distributions has been introduced.[107] This model is based on the observation that the NT measurement distributions in both euploid and aneuploid fetuses follow two distinct patterns. In a certain population of fetuses, NT measurement ranges increase between 11 and 13^{+6} weeks of gestation, whereas in a second population, NT measurements are independent of gestational age and remain constant over this time period. The percentage of fetuses that fit into these two categories varies according to the chromosomal complement. Recent changes to the statistical methodology used for risk assessment have improved both the sensitivity and specificity of screening for chromosomal abnormality—particularly for trisomies 13 and 18.

When measured correctly, NT is arguably the most robust single marker for chromosomal abnormality.[31] The NT measurement is therefore the "foundation stone" of any screening protocol that includes first-trimester ultrasound examination. Using just the combination of maternal age and NT measurement, the detection rates for a 5% false-positive rate are about 75% for trisomies 21, 18, and 13, and are 90% and 60% for monosomy X and triploidy, respectively.[134,136,137]

The maternal serum analytes that have been shown to be most effective in first-trimester screening for aneuploidy are free β-hCG and PAPP-A. As NT measurements and the serum analytes are independent of one another, they can all be used to adjust the "a priori" maternal age-related risk (combined first-trimester screen) without the need for additional mathematical manipulation.[21,138-142] Combined screening improves the detection rate for trisomies 21, 18, and 13, monosomy X and triploidy to 90% or more for a 5% false-positive rate.[2,143,144]

Nasal Bone

The logic behind using the prenatal NB evaluation in screening for trisomy 21 is based on the characteristic facial features found in individuals with Down syndrome and on anthropometric, radiological, and histological studies.[145-149] All of these studies demonstrate a significant difference in either the size of the NB or in the degree of ossification between euploid individuals and those with trisomy 21.[150]

This phenomenon is also apparent on prenatal ultrasound,[151] and a number of studies have been published indicating that absence of the NB is highly associated with trisomy 21 in both the first and the second trimesters.

Mechanism for the Nasal Bone Absence in Trisomy 21

The exact mechanism leading to the NB abnormalities seen in trisomy 21 is unknown. However, it is likely that the changes in connective tissue known to exist in trisomy 21 are at least in part responsible.[120-122,148,149]

Ultrasound Evaluation of the Fetal Nasal Bone

In the first trimester, the nasal bridge is evaluated only for the presence or absence of the NB.[150,152-157] Measuring the NB does not appear to improve screening performance at this gestational age.[150,158]

The protocol for ultrasound evaluation of the NB is shown in **Figures 2A and B and Box 2**. A midline section of the fetal profile is obtained by visualizing the following fetal structures: The hypoechoic region of the thalamus, pons, and medulla oblongata, the echogenic line over the nasal bridge representing the skin, and an echogenic line that is located anteriorly and slightly superiorly to the nasal bridge represent the skin over the nasal tip. If the NB is present, an echogenic line is also seen within the substance of the nasal bridge. This line is approximately parallel to the line representing the nasal bridge skin. These two lines form a so-called "equal sign". The echogenicity of the NB needs to be greater than that of the skin in order for the NB to be identified as present. The reason for this requirement is that even if the NB is not ossified (i.e., sonographically absent), a very faint echodense line may be seen within the nasal bridge.

In order to visualize these anatomic landmarks and identify the NB as a separate structure from the nasal skin, the image needs to be magnified so that the fetal head and upper thorax occupy the majority of the screen. The angle of insonation is extremely important in evaluation of the NB. The face of the transducer should be parallel to the longitudinal axis of the nasal bridge and the NB

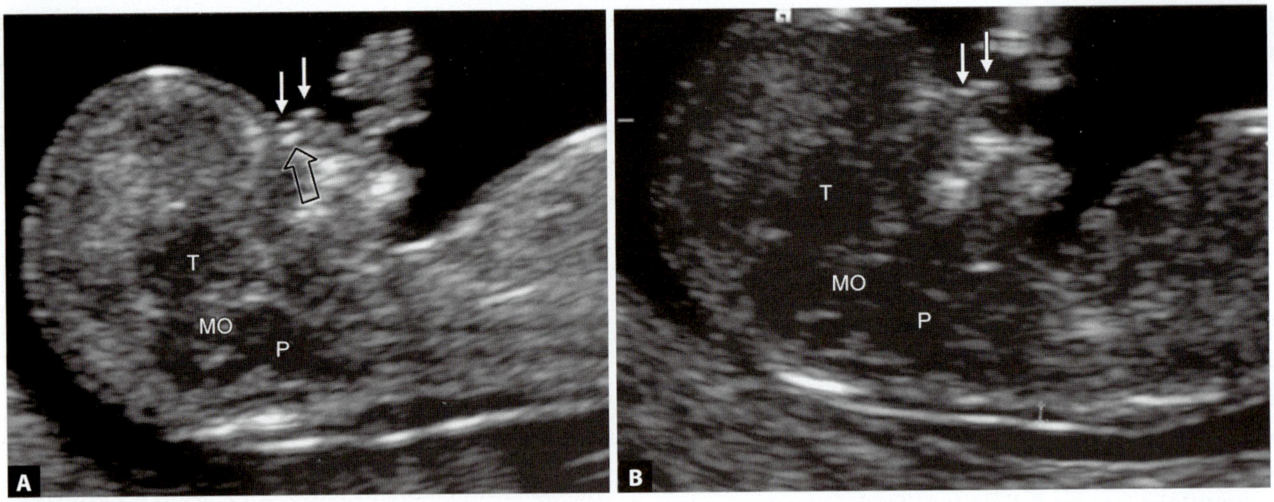

Figs. 2A and B: Nasal bone evaluation that meets Fetal Medicine Foundation criteria (solid arrows = skin over the nasal bridge and the tip of the nose, open arrow = nasal bone). (A) The nasal bone is present (note the "equal sign" formed by the echogenic lines of the skin of the nasal bridge and the nasal bone); (B) The nasal bone is absent (note the absence of the "equal sign"). (MO: medulla oblongata; P: pons; T: thalamus)

BOX 2: The Fetal Medicine Foundation criteria for evaluation of the nasal bone.

- *CRL:* 45–84 mm (11^{+0}–13^{+6} weeks of gestation)
- Midsagittal view (fetus must be facing toward the transducer)
- Image size—head and upper thorax occupies most of the screen
- The face of the transducer is parallel to the long axis of the nasal bone and the skin over the nasal bridge
- Fetal profile must include an echogenic line representing the skin over nasal bridge and an echogenic line in front of it representing the skin over the nasal tip
- Intracranial structures—hypoechoic areas representing the region of the thalamus, pons, and the medulla oblongata
- If the nasal bone is present, a line that is more echogenic than the skin is seen within the nasal bridge. This line is approximately parallel to the skin over the nasal bridge; the two lines form the so called "equal sign"

(CRL: crown–rump length)

(90° angle of insonation). The NB may become sonographically invisible if there is a significant deviation from this angle. This is due to the fact that the NB is an extremely thin structure and the lateral resolution of ultrasound equipment is insufficient to visualize the NB if it is viewed "end-on" (close to 0° angle of insonation). NB evaluation may be done only if the fetus is facing the transducer.

Three-dimensional (3D) ultrasound does not appear to significantly improve the success of examination of the NB.[159] However, one advantage that it holds over the two-dimensional (2D) examination is that it can reliably identify unilateral absence of the NB.[159] The exact likelihood ratio associated with this finding has not been established. However, since it has been seen in association with trisomy 21, unilateral absence of the NB has been assigned the same significance as the bilateral finding.

Nasal Bone and Fetal Aneuploidy

A review of several major studies including approximately 50,000 fetuses found that the NB was absent in 2% of euploid and 65% of trisomy 21 fetuses.[150] The prevalence of an absent NB is also increased in trisomy 18 (55%), trisomy 13 (34%), monosomy X (11%) but not in triploidy.[160] The presence or absence of the NB is independent of the maternal serum free β-hCG and PAPP-A levels.[3,152,161,162] However, likelihood ratios do need to be adjusted for gestational age, ethnicity, and NT thickness.[161] A higher proportion of euploid fetuses have an absent NB at early (11 weeks) gestation and the prevalence of this marker is higher in Africans than Asians and Caucasians with resultant changes in the likelihood ratios. The relationship between an absent NB and NT measurement is not significant until the NT measurement exceeds the 99th percentile (equating to approximately 3.5 mm at any point between 11 and 13^{+6} weeks of gestation).[160] The consequence of this is that in most circumstances, the likelihood ratio for an absent NB does not have to be adjusted for the NT measurement.

A study of 19,614 fetuses demonstrated that the addition of NB evaluation to traditional combined first-trimester screening led to a decrease in the false-positive

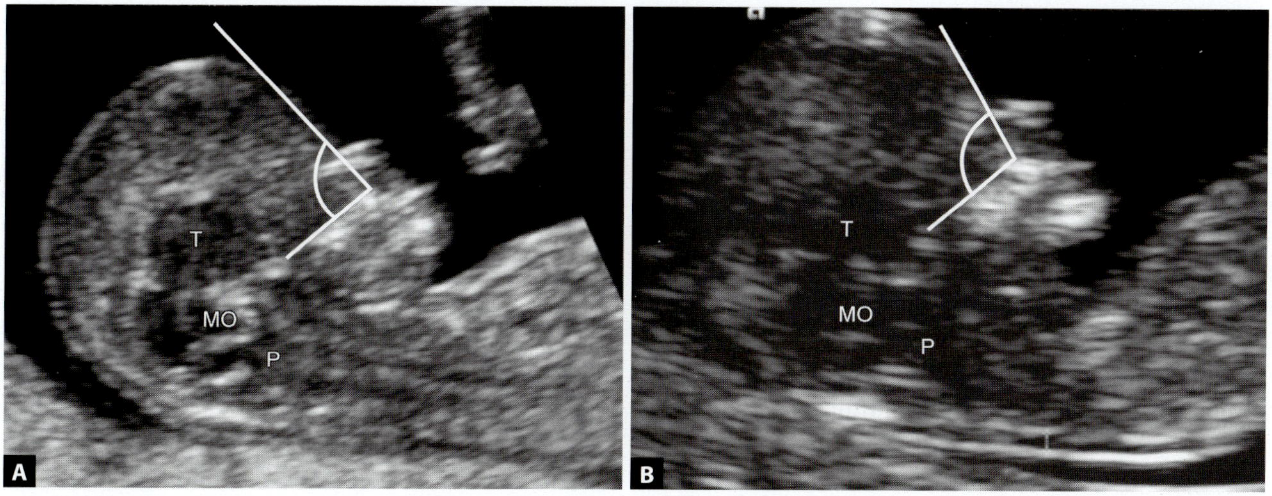

Figs. 3A and B: Frontomaxillary angle measurement that meets Fetal Medicine Foundation criteria. Note the absence of the frontal process of the maxilla between the hard palate and the nasal bone, which helps to assure that plane of insonation is precisely in the midline. (A) The frontomaxillary angle is acute and within normal limits; (B) The frontomaxillary angle is obtuse and is above the normal range. (MO: medulla oblongata; P: pons; T: thalamus)

rate (to 3%) and increase in the detection rate (92%) of trisomy 21. In this series, inclusion of the NB in the screening algorithm gave a 100% detection rate for trisomies 18, 13, and for monosomy X.[3] Inclusion of the NB is the screening algorithm which may be of particular value in an environment where biochemistry is not readily available or is expensive as this will improve sensitivity and specificity of the first-trimester ultrasound assessment. Alternatively, in an environment where biochemistry is readily available, the addition of the NB as an ultrasound marker for trisomy 21 predominantly allows improved specificity at a high level of sensitivity.

Frontomaxillary Facial Angle

A flat face is recognized as a common dysmorphic feature in individuals with Down syndrome. This may be subjectively assessed even on prenatal ultrasound by examining the fetal profile. However, in order for this facial feature to be exploited for screening purposes, a method had to be developed to evaluate it using a standardized measurement. The FMF angle measurement is an objective way to estimate mid-face hypoplasia; the deeper the location of the front edge of the maxilla is with respect to the forehead, the shallower the FMF angle.[163] The reason for mid-face hypoplasia in trisomy 21 also appears to be the presence of abnormal connective tissue. Theoretically, abnormal bone modeling due to hypotonia of the tongue may also be a contributing factor.

BOX 3: Fetal Medicine Foundation criteria for measurement of the frontomaxillary angle.

- *CRL:* 45–84 mm (11^{+0}–13^{+6} weeks of gestation)
- Midsagittal view (fetus must be facing toward the transducer)
- Image size—head and upper thorax occupies most of the screen
- Face of the transducer is approximately parallel to the long axis of the nasal bone
- Fetal profile must include an echogenic line representing the skin over nasal bridge and an echogenic line in front of it representing the skin over the nasal tip
- Intracranial structures—hypoechoic areas representing the region of the thalamus, pons, and the medulla oblongata
- Space between the upper palate and the nose should be devoid of echogenic structures (frontal process of the maxilla)
- FMF angle—first ray is drawn along the upper edge of the hard palate, apex of the angle is at the anterior edge of the maxilla, second ray from the apex upward resting on the echogenic line beneath the skin (the noncalcified metopic suture)

(CRL: crown–rump length; FMF: frontomaxillary facial)

Frontomaxillary Facial Angle Measurement

The image requirements for FMF angle measurement **(Figs. 3A and B and Box 3)** are very similar to those for NB evaluation. The head and the upper thorax should fill the majority of the image and the fetus needs to be facing the transducer. The greatest of care must be taken to obtain a precise midline section, as the smallest deviation has a significant effect on measurement.[164] The landmarks used to determine this are the same as those used for NB evaluation: Echogenic skin over the nasal bridge and nasal tip seen in the same view on the surface of the profile and the intracranial hypoechoic regions of the thalamus, pons, and the medulla oblongata.[164] Additionally, in the precise midline view, the area between the upper edge of the hard palate and the NB is relatively echo free. As the plane of insonation deviates slightly from the midline, an echogenic structure comes into view. This represents the frontal process of the maxilla, a finding that should be absent in the correct view. The use of 3D ultrasound may be helpful in establishing the precise midline section.[164]

The angle of insonation is also similar to the one required for NB evaluation: The face of the transducer should be roughly parallel to the long axis of the NB and the skin over the nasal bridge. The hard palate, which is composed of the maxilla and the vomer bones, is seen as a roughly trapezoid echogenic structure with the posterior portion being slightly thicker than the anterior one.

In order to measure the frontomaxillary angle, the following lines are generated: The first one runs along the upper edge of the hard palate. The vertex of the angle is at the anterior-most portion of the maxilla. The second line of the angle runs upward from the vertex toward the forehead. It is positioned so its inner edge rests upon the metopic suture, which lies a short distance beneath the skin. In the first trimester, the metopic suture is not yet ossified. Therefore, it is seen as a line of similar echogenicity as the skin.

The deep position of the front edge of the maxilla in fetuses with trisomy 21 may be due to maxillary hypoplasia, dorsal displacement of the maxilla, or a combination of the two. **Figures 3A and B** illustrate the difference between FMF measurements in a fetus with trisomy 21 and in a euploid fetus.

In the first trimester, the division between the vomer bones and the maxilla is usually difficult to see. However, toward the end of the first trimester, this division may become evident as an oblique hypoechoic line running from the upper edge of the hard palate anteriorly to the lower edge of the hard palate posteriorly.[165] This line should not be used to form the lower boundary of the FMF angle.

Frontomaxillary Angle and Fetal Aneuploidy

The normal range of frontomaxillary angle measurements decreases with advancing gestational age.[166] They are independent of NT measurements, presence or absence of the NB, and maternal serum biochemistries.[4,163]

Shallow FMF angles are seen not only in trisomy 21 but also in trisomies 18 and 13. Fetuses with trisomies 21, 18, and 13 have FMF angle measurements that are above the 95th percentile in 45%, 58%, and 48% cases, respectively.[4,167,168] In a study, which included 782 euploid fetuses and 108 fetuses with trisomy 21, a 92% detection rate for a 3% false-positive rate was achieved by adding FMF angle measurement to the combined screen.[4] This marker has not been widely adopted in combined first-trimester screening programs.

Doppler Evaluations of Fetal Blood Flow as Markers for Aneuploidy

The fetal cardiovascular system has a number of structural and functional features that differentiate it from the cardiovascular system ex utero. The arrangement of the myocytes within the fetal heart is less well organized and there are fewer sarcomeres per unit mass.[6] The fetal myocardium has lower compliance resulting in a higher intraventricular pressure at any cardiac volume. Early in pregnancy, placental vascular resistance is relatively high, placing additional strain on the heart. As a consequence, the fetal heart functions at the upper limits of the Frank–Starling curve. In the first trimester, abnormalities of cardiac structure and/or performance may lead to detectable changes in blood flow through certain structures. The two structures that have been investigated the most and hold promise in screening for aneuploidy are the TCV[169] and the DV.[170]

The DV is strictly a fetal structure that carries 50% of the oxygenated blood from the umbilical vein (UV) and empties into the inferior vena cava at a point that is very close to the right atrium. Its proximity to the right side of the heart makes it susceptible to changes in cardiac function.[171-182] TCV flow is considered abnormal in the presence of regurgitation and DV flow is considered abnormal if the a-wave is reversed (see below). The temporal relationship between Doppler flow patterns (normal and abnormal) across the TCV and DV is demonstrated in **Figure 4**.

These hemodynamic markers are very useful as a component of combined first-trimester screening as they improve screening efficacy but also highlight cardiovascular changes that may be associated with other forms of structural heart disease that are not associated with aneuploidy.

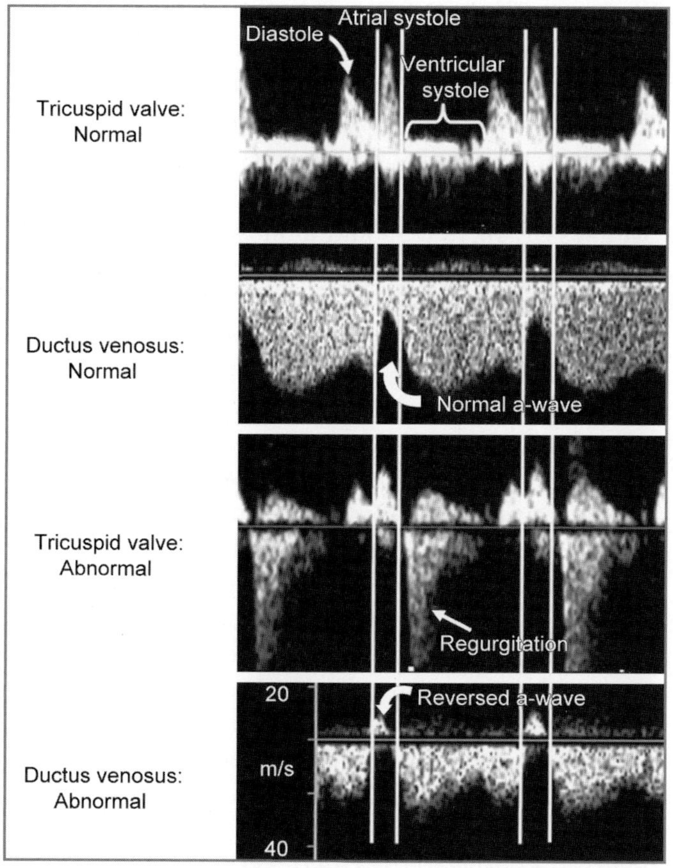

Fig. 4: Tricuspid valve and ductus venosus Doppler waveforms demonstrating temporal relationship between normal and abnormal findings during the cardiac cycle.[126]

Tricuspid Valve Regurgitation

The exact reason for the increased prevalence of TCV regurgitation in fetuses with trisomy 21 is not completely clear. However, it is likely that it is related to the structural and ultrastructural changes in the heart that are known to be associated with trisomy 21: Decreased number of myocytes, abnormal orientation of myocytes and myofibrils, and abnormal connective tissue.[6,8,120-122] It may be that these changes result in a relative dilatation of the right ventricle. It is also recognized that dilatation of the right ventricle may lead to tricuspid regurgitation by dilating the TCV annulus. Finally, the connective tissue abnormalities that affect the myocardium are also present in the valve itself.[8] It may be that both of these mechanisms are involved in causing TCV incompetence and regurgitation.

Pulsed Doppler Evaluation of Blood Flow Across the Tricuspid Valve

The protocol for TCV evaluation using pulsed Doppler is shown in **Figures 5A and B and Box 4**. A magnified transverse section of the fetal thorax containing a four-chamber view is obtained. The angle of insonation is important. The heart view should be apical so that the angle of insonation with respect to the ventricular septum is less than 30°. The Doppler gate is placed across the TCV. The gate should be relatively large (2–3 mm) to make certain that it covers both sides of the valve. It should be kept in

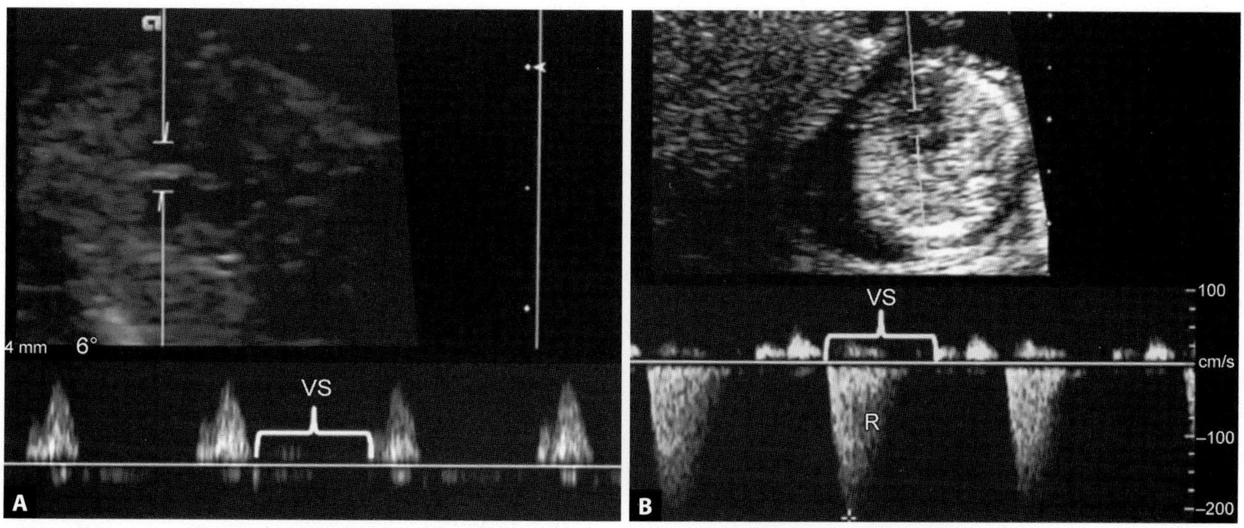

Figs. 5A and B: Evaluation of the flow across the tricuspid valve (TCV) using Doppler: (A) Normal flow pattern across the TCV with no regurgitant flow during ventricular systole (VS); (B) Abnormal flow pattern across the TCV with regurgitant flow (R) present during VS.

BOX 4: The Fetal Medicine Foundation criteria for the evaluation of flow across the tricuspid valve using Doppler.

- *CRL:* 45–84 mm (11^{+0} –13^{+6} weeks of gestation)
- Apical four-chamber heart view (fetus may be facing toward or away from the transducer)
- Image size—thorax occupies most of the screen
- Pulsed-wave Doppler—the sample gate should be large (2–3 mm in width) and is positioned across the tricuspid valve, the angle formed by the ventricular septum and Doppler beam must be <30°
- True tricuspid regurgitation (R)—(1) velocity >60 cm/sec (in order to differentiate from a great vessel waveform where the velocity is generally 50 cm/sec); (2) duration >30% of the ventricular systole (VS)
- At least three sample volumes need to be obtained as the insufficiency may not be present in all three cusps

(CRL: crown–rump length)

mind that not all of the leaflets of the TCV are necessarily incompetent. Therefore, at least three Doppler evaluations should be obtained. It is also helpful to interrogate the TCV flow in real-time sweeping through the valve to make sure that it is interrogated in its entirety. If tricuspid regurgitation is present, color Doppler may occasionally demonstrate a small discrete jet within the right atrium.

The normal TCV waveform demonstrates a biphasic pattern of blood flow into the right ventricle. The first peak represents filling during ventricular diastole and the second peak represents filling in atrial systole **(Figs. 4 and 5)**. If the TCV is competent, there should be no flow during ventricular systole. Since the size of the first-trimester heart is quite small and a relatively large Doppler gate is used, the waveform may be contaminated by flow through the left ventricular outflow tract. The direction of blood flow through the aortic root is the same as that of the regurgitant jet and they are seen at the same point in the cardiac cycle; therefore, it is imperative to be able to differentiate between the two. There are two consistent differences in their flow pattern. Firstly, the velocity in the great vessel is typically <40 cm/sec, whereas the velocity of the regurgitant jet is always >60 cm/sec. Therefore, in order to diagnose TCV regurgitation, the blood flow velocity has to be in excess of 60 cm/sec. Secondly, unlike flow through the left ventricular outflow tract, the regurgitant jet has a distinctive high-pitched hissing sound on Doppler. Indeed, it is often this sound that first alerts the sonographer to the presence of TCV regurgitation. Since a signal from a closing TCV and trivial tricuspid regurgitation are fairly common findings and are of no clinical significance; regurgitation must last at least 30% of the ventricular systole to be defined as an abnormal finding.

Tricuspid Valve Doppler and Fetal Aneuploidy

Tricuspid regurgitation is more prevalent in aneuploid than euploid fetuses. The prevalence in fetuses with trisomies 21, 18, and 13 and monosomy X is 56%, 33%, 30%, and 38%, respectively. The prevalence of tricuspid regurgitation in euploid fetuses is 1%.[11] In a study of 19,614 fetuses where TCV evaluation was added to combined first-trimester screening, a 96% detection rate for trisomy 21 was achieved while maintaining a 3% false-positive rate. The detection rates for trisomies 18 and 13 and monosomy X were 92%, 100% and 100%, respectively.[11]

The prevalence of tricuspid regurgitation decreases with advancing gestational age and increases with NT thickness.[11] These associations are factored into the risk algorithm developed by the Fetal Medicine Foundation. It should be noted that tricuspid regurgitation is also associated with an increased risk of congenital heart defects (CHDs).[10] A careful examination of the fetal heart should be performed at the time when TCV regurgitation is noted and repeated in the mid-second trimester.

Reversed A-wave in the Ductus Venosus

The exact reason for a reversal of the a-wave in the DV in association with trisomy 21 is also not clear. However, it is likely that this abnormality is not a result of a change in the DV itself but rather due to a change in the fetal heart performance. Therefore, the ultrastructural changes in the cardiac anatomy described earlier in the "TCV regurgitation" section may also be responsible for this phenomenon.[6,8,120-122] However, the a-wave abnormality is likely to be the result of decreased compliance of the ventricular walls rather than ventricular dilatation. The mechanical explanation for a-wave reversal may be that the atrial wall is contracting against a relatively stiffer wall and has to generate more pressure to push the blood across the TCV. The increased back pressure, which would be inevitably generated in this situation, may be sufficient to either stop or reverse the blood flow during atrial systole (absent or reversed a-wave).

Pulsed Doppler Evaluation of Blood Flow through the Ductus Venosus

The fetus is examined in right parasagittal section **(Figs. 6A and B and Box 5)**. The DV is seen as a short continuation

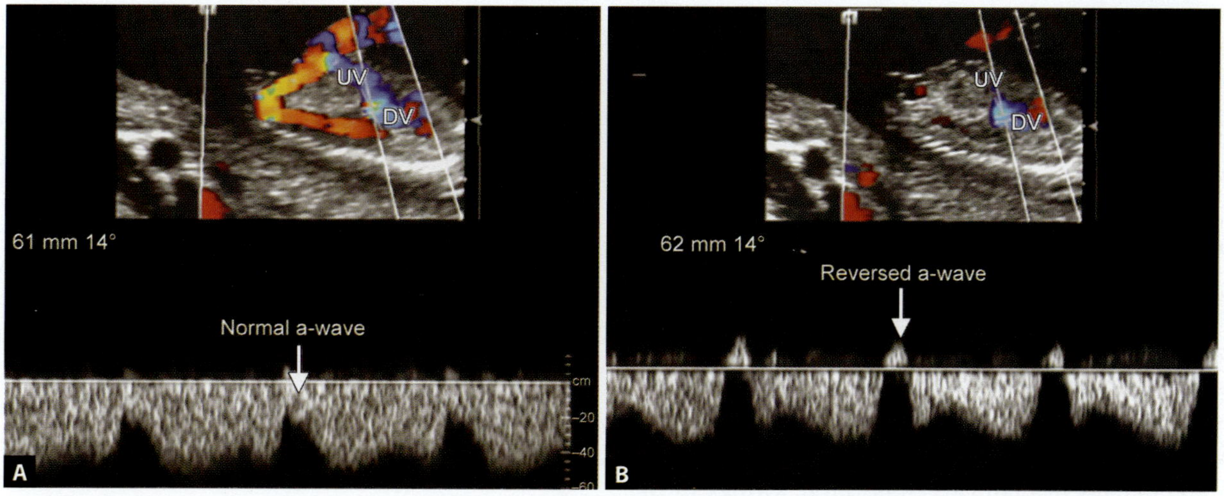

Figs. 6A and B: Evaluation of the ductus venosus flow using Doppler. (A) Normal DV flow pattern with antegrade flow during the entire cardiac cycle, including during the atrial contraction (a-wave); (B) Abnormal DV flow pattern with reversed flow during the atrial contraction (a-wave). (DV: ductus venosus; UV: umbilical vein)

BOX 5: The Fetal Medicine Foundation criteria for the evaluation of DV flow using Doppler.

- *CRL:* 45–84 mm (11^{+0}–13^{+6} weeks of gestation)
- Right ventral midsagittal view
- Image size—thorax and abdomen occupy most of the screen
- Color flow Doppler is used to identify the hepatic portion of the umbilical vein and the DV, which appears as a continuation of the umbilical vein. Since the flow velocity in the DV is significantly higher than in the rest of the venous system, aliasing will be seen on color Doppler
- Pulsed-wave Doppler—angle of insonation with respect to the longitudinal axis of the DV must be <30° and the sample gate must be small (0.5–1 mm)
- The filter should be set at a low frequency (50–70 Hz), so the a-wave is not obscured
- The sweep speed should be high (2–3 cm/sec); the spreading of the waveforms allows better assessment of the a-wave

(CRL: crown–rump length; DV: ductus venosus)

of the hepatic portion of the UV and is best identified using color Doppler. The DV is distinguishable from the UV as it has a distinctly higher velocity and aliasing of flow can be seen. The pulsed Doppler gate is placed within the lumen of the DV. The gate needs to be small (0.5–1 mm) to minimize contamination of the signal by venous structures such as the hepatic veins and the inferior vena cava, which are in close proximity. The magnification should be such that the fetal abdomen and thorax fill the majority of the image. The angle of insonation of the Doppler beam should be <30° with respect to the longitudinal axis of the DV.

On pulsed Doppler, a normal DV waveform demonstrates forward blood flow throughout the cardiac cycle. There are two adjoining peaks of increased flow representing ventricular systole and the diastole. Normally, blood flow is diminished during atrial systole but forward flow is maintained **(Figs. 4 and 6)**.

Ductus Venosus Doppler Flow and Fetal Aneuploidy

A reversed A-wave is seen not only in fetuses affected by trisomy 21 but also in those with trisomies 18 and 13 and monosomy X. The prevalence of reversed flow in the A-wave of the DV in fetuses with trisomies 21, 18, and 13 and monosomy X is 66%, 58%, 55%, and 75%, respectively. The prevalence of a reversed A-wave in euploid fetuses is 3%.[17] In a study of 19,614 fetuses where evaluation of the DV was added to combined first-trimester screening, 96% of fetuses affected by trisomy 21 were detected while maintaining a 3% false-positive rate. The detection rates for trisomies 18 and 13 and monosomy X were 92%, 100% and 100%, respectively.[17]

The prevalence of A-wave reversal decreases with advancing gestational age and increases with NT thickness. These associations are mathematically accounted for in the FMF risk algorithm.[17] A-wave abnormalities are also associated with an increased risk of cardiac anomalies.[18,19,180] A careful examination of the fetal heart should be performed at the time when the reversed A-wave is noted and be repeated in the mid-second trimester.

Fetal Heart Rate in Screening for Aneuploidy

It has been noted that aneuploid fetuses tend to have different heart rates from euploid fetuses at the time of first-trimester screening.[2,20] The largest difference is seen in trisomy 13 and monosomy X where the heart rate is >95th percentile in 69% and 53% of cases, respectively. The heart rate also tends to be increased in trisomy 21 but much less so (14% are >95th percentile). Both trisomy 18 and triploid fetuses tend to be bradycardic (19% and 36% <5th percentile, respectively). If FHR is included in first-trimester screening, it needs to be adjusted for gestational age as the normal ranges decrease between 11 and 13^{+6} weeks of gestation.[2,20]

Small changes in FHR can cause large swings in the risks calculated for aneuploidy. If the heart rate is identified as being outside of the normal range, it is best to repeat the assessment later in the ultrasound examination to ensure the accuracy of this finding.

QUALITY ASSURANCE IN FIRST-TRIMESTER ULTRASOUND

All the ultrasound markers for aneuploidy listed above can be used to generate likelihood ratios in risk assessment for trisomy 21 and other chromosomal abnormalities. The likelihood ratios are based on the described prevalence of these anomalies in normal and aneuploid populations. It is, therefore, extremely important to standardize techniques for measurement to ensure that accurate risks are produced. Sonographers must have adequate opportunity for training and to develop experience in first-trimester ultrasound before they begin to employ any of the ultrasound markers for risk assessment. It is equally important to have a method of audit in place that provides operators with feedback about their performance. The Fetal Medicine Foundation provides sonographers with an opportunity to complete an annual audit cycle to review their performance. This involves comparison of an individual's NT measurement data with the internationally established normal ranges. Undermeasurement of NT has the potential to decrease both the false-positive rate and the detection rate of screening while overmeasurement will lead to an increase in both of these parameters.[179]

For example, review of the audit process in Australia, using the methods described by the FMF, has shown that while the national range of NT measurements is almost identical to that described in a UK population, there is a significant minority of operators who either under- or overmeasure NT.[180] This process of review of the audit system has allowed the NT accreditation program to identify operators that have widely differing NT distributions and provide them with additional education and assist them with development of practical skills in first-trimester ultrasound.

Studies examining the introduction of additional markers, such as examination of the NB and of the DV, have shown that a sonographer needs to perform approximately 60–80 ultrasound examinations in order to be able to evaluate each of the first-trimester markers correctly on a consistent basis.[181-183] These markers are categorical, i.e., they are either present or absent, and their prevalence is high in the aneuploid population and low in the euploid population. Consequently, the likelihood ratios (positive and negative) are large and have a significant effect on risk evaluation. This underscores the fact that adequate training and experience before employing these markers is critical. Methods for auditing categorical markers on an ongoing basis are less well developed. One approach currently available is to monitor the overall screen positive rate as this is a reflection of the false-positive rate. If the false-positive rate deviates significantly from that reported in the reference population, one of the explanations may be inappropriate examination of the additional ultrasound markers. This is especially true if the sonographer's distribution of NT measurements is adequate. Evaluating first-trimester ultrasound markers in a manner that is not in accordance with the standard method not only affects the performance of the screening program overall but also provides individual patients with inaccurate risk assessments.

First-trimester Screening for Aneuploidy Using Multiple Ultrasound Markers

Assessment of these additional ultrasound markers is best performed within the context of an overall risk algorithm rather than independently as the latter approach risks increasing the false-positive rate. The ultrasound and maternal serum biochemical markers described above are sufficiently independent of each other to be used in combination. This can be either done by evaluating and using all markers in the calculation of risks for every fetus or on a contingent basis. The latter approach includes the use of three categories: High, intermediate, and low risk. It begins by calculation of the risk for aneuploidy from a more limited combination of markers. Evaluation of additional markers is done only in fetuses that fall into the intermediate risk group, i.e., it is contingent on the initial findings. The contingent approach allows the extra markers to be used selectively but still increases the detection rate whilst maintaining a low false-positive rate. Furthermore, mathematical modeling predicts that the detection and false-positive rates are identical whether the contingent approach is used or if all markers are examined in every fetus.

An algorithm using ultrasound markers for aneuploidy on a contingent basis in the first trimester was developed by the Fetal Medicine Foundation.[141] The first step taken in using this approach is to perform the combined screen (maternal age, NT measurement, free β-hCG level, and PAPP-A level) in every patient. Based on the results of the combined screen, the patients are divided into the three categories described above: High-risk (trisomy 21 risk of >1:50), intermediate-risk (trisomy 21 risk of 1:51 to 1:1,000), and low-risk category (trisomy 21 risk <1:1,000). The patients that fall into the high-risk category are offered an invasive diagnostic procedure without any additional screening. This category constitutes only 1.3% of the total screened population but contains 82% of the fetuses with trisomy 21. The low-risk group constitutes the majority of the screened population (86.7%) but contains only 4% of fetuses with trisomy 21. These patients are reassured and invasive diagnostic testing is limited to women requesting it, despite the screening result. The intermediate risk category constitutes 12% of the screened population and includes 14% of trisomy 21 fetuses. Women in this group undergo additional screening by evaluating the additional ultrasound markers (NB, FMF angle, TCV, and DV). If the resultant risk of trisomy 21 exceeds 1:100, an invasive diagnostic test is offered. If it is less than that, they are treated in the same way as the low-risk group. A careful mid-second trimester ultrasound examination is indicated for patients who reach that point in all three categories. For a 2% false-positive rate, the detection rate for trisomy 21 using one, two, three or four additional marker are 90%, 94%, 95% and 96%, respectively. These detection rates are the same whether the contingent approach is used or if all additional markers are used in every patient.[3,4,11,17,140]

Structural Abnormalities as Markers of Aneuploidy

Some structural anomalies, seen on first-trimester ultrasound, also increase the risk of aneuploidy. As such they play a dual role: They serve as markers and they are of clinical significance even in the absence of aneuploidy. Structural abnormalities that have well-defined fixed risks associated with them include holoprosencephaly (risk of 1 in 2 for trisomy 13), diaphragmatic hernia (risk of 1 in 4 for trisomy 18), atrioventricular septal defect (risk of 1 in 2 for trisomy 21), omphalocele (risk of 1 in 4 for trisomy 18 and risk of 1 in 10 for trisomy 13), megacystis defined as bladder length of >7 mm (risk of 1 in 10 for either trisomy 18 or 13).[184-186] The fixed risks associated with these anomalies are included in the FMF risk algorithm.

"Soft" Ultrasound Markers for Aneuploidy

Some ultrasound markers that have been shown to increase the risk of fetal aneuploidy in the second trimester appear to do so in the first trimester as well. "Soft" or "pure" ultrasound markers are defined as those findings that, in the absence of aneuploidy, have no clinical significance. These include choroid plexus cysts (>1.5 mm), echogenic intracardiac foci, hyperechogenic bowel, and hydronephrosis (anteroposterior diameter of the renal pelvis >1.5 mm).[187] These markers are also included in the FMF algorithm in screening for trisomy 21. The presence of these markers should be interpreted in the context of the presence/absence of other markers or anomalies: An isolated minor marker probably does not increase the risk of aneuploidy as the absence of other markers acts as a counterbalance and decreases the risk sufficiently to negate the effect of the presence of a single marker.[187]

Incorporating Noninvasive Prenatal Testing in a Screening Program for Common Chromosomal Abnormalities

Noninvasive prenatal testing (NIPT) analyses fragments of chromosomes in cell-free DNA. There are a variety of technologies that are commercially available for clinical use and the screening efficacy of this test is very high, with high detection rates for trisomies 21, 18, 13, low screen positive rates, and the potential to expand to other chromosomal abnormalities.[188] There is one "head to head" study comparing combined first-trimester screening to NIPT, which shows significantly higher screening efficacy for cell-free DNA analysis—although, importantly, these data were assessed after exclusion of 3% of the population who had an unreportable NIPT test—including three pregnancies where the fetus was affected by Down syndrome.[189] There are few jurisdictions that currently offer NIPT as a population screening tool that is free to women at the point of care. The cost has a significant cost which raises issues of enfranchisement at a population screening level. One method of combining both tools is to offer NIPT contingent to the combined first-trimester screening test result.[190] If NIPT replaces first-trimester ultrasound assessment then a number of additional benefits of a first-trimester scan (identifying multiples, pregnancy viability and dating, structural anomalies, and screening for preeclampsia) will be lost. From the perspective of identifying pregnancies affected by aneuploidy, there is good evidence to show that a portion of fetuses that have an atypical chromosomal abnormality are currently detected on the basis of polarized NT or biochemical measurements, and these are not typically identified by NIPT.[191]

SCREENING MULTIPLE PREGNANCIES FOR DOWN SYNDROME

The calculation of the risk of aneuploidy in a twin pregnancy is complicated by a number of factors. Ultrasound is very effective at determining chorionicity. Monochorionic twins can be defined as being monozygotic, which almost universally have the same karyotype. DC twins, on the other hand, may be either dizygotic (majority) or monozygotic (minority). In dizygotic twins, development of abnormalities in one or the other fetus is an essentially independent event. The result is that if an abnormality is present, it generally affects only one fetus. Both fetuses may also be affected, though the statistical chance of this happening is invariably very small. In the small proportion of DC twins that are monozygotic, if aneuploidy is present, generally both the fetuses are affected.

Placentation also affects the performance of biochemical markers, as the presence of a "normal" twin placenta partially masks any changes in serum markers seen in the placenta of the affected cotwin. The situation becomes more complex in higher order multiples, and currently there is no data to support the use of serum screening in these groups. Due to these difficulties, it is tempting to rely on markers for aneuploidy that are expressed by the fetus, namely those that can be assessed with ultrasound: NT thickness, the NB, FMF angle, and the hemodynamic markers.

In singleton pregnancies, the calculation of risks generated by combined first-trimester screening first involves defining a background risk based on maternal age, gestational age, and taking account of a previous history of a pregnancy affected by aneuploidy. Maternal age-related risks for twins have been calculated and published and suggest that the presence of two fetuses compounds the risk for the mother.[192,193] The first consequence of this is that a 32-year-old woman carrying twins effectively has the same background risk as a 35-year-old woman pregnancy. Therefore, maternal age potentially has a greater impact on the final risk generated through screening in twins and may lead to an increase in the false-positive rate for any age group compared to singleton pregnancies. There is a little prospective data to support this proposed increase in risk and some concern over the methodology by which these risks were calculated and it has been suggested that the overall level of risk in a dizygotic twin pregnancy is in fact similar to that seen in a singleton pregnancy.[194]

Gestational age, which also affects the background level of risk, may be harder to calculate in a twin pregnancy. Since it is rare to find both twins that have the same CRL measurement, a decision must be made as to which CRL should be used for gestational age assessment. It is likely that if a pathologic process affects fetal growth in the first trimester, it will do so by restricting it. Therefore, it appears to be sensible to use the larger CRL measurement for dating purposes. It should be remembered that likelihood ratios for all ultrasound and biochemical findings are generated on the basis of CRL and relatively small changes in CRL can affect risks significantly.[114] Similarly, large CRL discrepancies are associated with poor pregnancy outcome[195,196] and include pathologies, which may also impact the markers being assessed for aneuploidy.

There is some evidence that points to an association between the NT measurements in twin pairs. Interestingly, this appears to be present in both monochorionic and DC twin pregnancies. Therefore, it has been suggested that likelihood ratio generated in one twin should be based not only on its own NT measurement but be also adjusted by a correction factor based on the cotwin's NT measurement.[197,198]

Most importantly, there is a good evidence to suggest that NT measurements in monochorionic twins may be affected by an early form of TTTS.[99,199] It is thought that the inequity in the circulating blood volumes of the twins results in nuchal thickening in the recipient. Since this condition affects up to 15% of monochorionic twins, a significant discordance in fetal NT's is more likely an early sign of TTTS than of aneuploidy.[99] Vandencrus et al. examined a number of options for the incorporation of NT in risk assessment in monochorionic twins.[200] The method that appears to produce the best result is to calculate risks based on CRL and NT for each individual fetus and assign the overall risk for the whole pregnancy by averaging the two. This is, however, likely associated with an increase in the screen positive rate of screening.

There are a few studies that have examined the incorporation of additional ultrasound markers in a screening strategy for twins. Matias et al. have shown that the hemodynamic marker of an absent or reversed a-wave in the DV is strongly associated with TTTS.[182] To date, there is no data on the performance of TCV regurgitation in this cohort of pregnancies. The NB is an attractive and potentially powerful marker in twins—as pathologies related to fetal growth and/or TTTS are unlikely to affect the presence of the NB. Sepulveda et al. have demonstrated that the technical difficulties the sonographer faces in assessing twins can be overcome and that the NB can be assessed effectively in 95% of cases.[201] Early data examining the effectiveness of a variety of screening combinations suggests that using NT and NB may be more effective than using NT and biochemistry.[202] Effective screening of twins appears to be possible. However, limitations inherent to the calculation of risk under these circumstances and the potential influence by pathologies other than aneuploidy need to be recognized.

FIRST-TRIMESTER SCREENING FOR FETAL ANOMALIES OTHER THAN CHROMOSOMAL DEFECTS

Nuchal Translucency Measurement as a Marker for Fetal Abnormalities in Chromosomally Normal Fetuses

Nuchal translucency thickening is associated with an increase in poor pregnancy outcome even if the fetus is chromosomally normal.[203-212] This increase does not become statistically significant until the NT measurement exceeds the 99th percentile. Conveniently, the 99th percentile cutoff remains constant at 3.5 mm across the 11–13^{+6} weeks of gestational period.[208]

A number of different fetal conditions may result in NT thickening making this measurement a useful test across a broad range of fetal anomalies.

Nuchal Translucency Thickening and Fetal Structural Defects

The prevalence of major fetal abnormalities increases exponentially as the NT measurement increases beyond the 99th percentile (>3.5 mm). The prevalence is approximately 2.5% for an NT of 3.5 mm and reaches 45% for an NT of 6.5 mm or more.[50,205]

One of the most important areas where NT screening appears to offer an advantage is the prenatal diagnosis of cardiac defects. Cardiac defects are some of the most common congenital structural anomalies, but their prenatal diagnosis is in many cases challenging. However, if an accurate prenatal diagnosis of CHD is made, the overall outcome is improved by allowing for the fetus to be delivered in a setting where appropriate neonatal treatment is available. Combined data from a number of screening studies demonstrates that the prevalence of major cardiac defects is 1–2% in fetuses with a <3.5 mm NT measurement. A significant increase in the prevalence of CHD is noted with NT measurements ≥3.5 mm: 3% (3.5–4.5 mm), 7% (4.5–5.4 mm), 20% (5.4–6.4 mm), and 30% (≥6.5 mm).[36,39,41-43,203]

A meta-analysis of screening studies showed a detection rate of 31% for CHD using an NT measurement of 3.5 mm as the cutoff. It is estimated that fetal echocardiography in all chromosomally normal fetuses with NT above the 99th percentile would identify one major cardiac defect in every 16 patients' examined.[46] Furthermore, this analysis showed that increased NT measurements increase the risk of a variety of heart defects. Results of another study arrived at the same conclusion.[213] In this multicenter study, nuchal thickening was found to be present in all types of heart defects: Left as well as right heart lesions, septal defects, outflow tract disorders, laterality disorders, and complex heart lesions.

With improvements in the resolution of ultrasound equipment, a detailed fetal cardiac evaluation may be performed even in the first trimester of pregnancy. Many of the major cardiac defects may now be diagnosed at the time of the 11–13^{+6} week scan.[37,51,88,214,215] Even if a specific diagnosis cannot be made, the cardiac examination often indicates whether or not a cardiac structural defect is present.

There are a number of other types of fetal defects that are seen more commonly in fetuses with NT measurements of >3.5 mm than in fetuses with normal NT measurements.[51-53,198] These include diaphragmatic hernia,[48] omphalocele,[47] body stalk anomaly,[49] skeletal defects,[54-64] and certain genetic syndromes such as congenital adrenal hyperplasia,[67] fetal akinesia deformation sequence,[69] Noonan syndrome,[65] Smith-Lemli-Opitz syndrome,[216] and spinal muscular atrophy.[70,71]

There are many additional disorders that have been reported in association with a thickened NT that are quite rare. Because of their rarity, a definite association with a thickened NT is difficult to prove in many of these.[52]

Finally, the prevalence of fetal demise is increased in chromosomally normal fetuses in which the NT measurement ≥3.5 mm even if a specific fetal defect cannot be diagnosed. An analysis of 4,540 fetuses categorized based on the NT measurement showed an increase in intrauterine loss from 1.3% in the 95th–99th percentile group to 20% in those that had NT measurements ≥6.5 mm.[51,205] The majority of fetal losses occur by 20 weeks of gestation. In fetuses that survive to the midsecond trimester and in which a targeted ultrasound fails to reveal any anomalies or increased nuchal fold thickness, the risk for perinatal or long-term morbidity and mortality does not appear to be increased.[208,209,217,218]

Sequential and systematic review of fetal anatomy at the time of the 11–13^{+6} week scan will detect up to 50% of major structural anomalies.[219,220] Structural anomalies often have a different appearance in early pregnancy compared to the midtrimester. Screening for spina bifida, for example, relies on a different set of markers when screening at 12 rather than 18–22 weeks.

Screening for Open Neural Tube Defects

One of the major failings of the first-trimester fetal ultrasound examination had been the inability to consistently diagnose open neural tube defects (ONTD) other than the exencephaly/anencephaly sequence. However, a recently described intracranial marker [intracerebral translucency (IT)] may overcome this deficiency.[25] The fetal image required to evaluate the IT is identical to those needed for the NT, NB, and FMF angle evaluation. A magnified midline view of the fetal head and upper thorax is obtained and the following intracranial structures need to be visualized: Hypoechoic regions of the thalamus, the pons (brainstem), and the medulla oblongata **(Fig. 7 and Box 6)**. Intracranial translucency represents the fluid-filled fourth ventricle, which is located posterior to the pons. The combination of the posterior border of the pons and the floor of the fourth ventricle is seen as a single, thin echogenic line, which forms the anterior border of the IT. The posterior border of the IT is the roof of the fourth ventricle. This is also seen as a relatively thin echogenic line accentuated by the choroid plexus of the fourth ventricle.

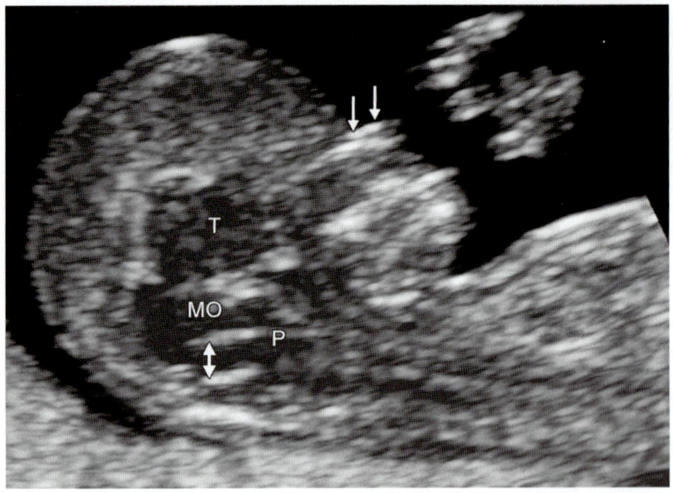

Fig. 7: Evaluation of the intracranial translucency (double arrow) that meets Fetal Medicine Foundation criteria. (MO: medulla oblongata; P: pons; T: thalamus; solid arrows: skin of the nasal bridge and the tip of the nose)

BOX 6: The Fetal Medicine Foundation criteria for evaluation of the IT.

- *CRL:* 45–84 mm (11^{+0}–13^{+6} weeks of gestation)
- Midsagittal view (fetus may either be facing toward or away from the transducer, but the IT is more difficult to see with the fetus facing away from the transducer due to shadowing from the occipital bone)
- Intracranial structures—thalamus, pons, and medulla oblongata
- Image size—head and upper thorax occupies most of the screen
- The IT represents fluid within the developing fourth ventricle. The anterior echogenic line is formed by the combination of the posterior border of the pons and the floor of the fourth ventricle. The posterior echogenic line is the roof of the fourth ventricle accentuated by the presence of the choroid plexus

(CRL: crown–rump length; IT: intracranial translucency)

The IT was consistently visualized and was found to be normal at the 11–13^{+6} week scan in the 200 consecutive fetuses that were subsequently shown not to have an ONTD.[25] In the same study, each of the four fetuses that were diagnosed with an ONTD in the second trimester had an absent first trimester IT (i.e., the fourth ventricle was obliterated).[25] The proposed mechanism for this finding is similar to that of the Chiari type II malformation ("banana sign") seen in second trimester fetuses with spina bifida aperta: Decreased pressure in the subarachnoid spaces leading to the caudal displacement of the brain. In the initial study dealing with IT, it appeared that measuring the IT does not provide additional information. However, this needs to be evaluated in prospective studies.

Another recent publication looked at the difference in FMF angle measurements in 20 fetuses with ONTD and 100 fetuses with a normal spine at 11 and 13 weeks of gestation. 90% of the fetuses with ONTD had a FMF angle measurement below the 5th percentile. The FMF angle measurements in the fetuses with ONTD were on average 10° smaller than in fetuses with normal spine.

It would be premature to state that obliteration of IT and/or an unusually small FMF angle measurement have the same predictive value as the Chiari type II malformation or the bifrontal scalloping in the second trimester. However, detection of either one of these findings at the time of the first-trimester ultrasound should lead to an extremely careful ultrasound evaluation of the spine. If the appearance of the spine is normal on the initial scan, the fetus should be reexamined at approximately 16 weeks. A 20-week scan should also be performed if the 16-week scan is normal.

First-trimester Screening for Preeclampsia

Preeclampsia is associated with vascular problems within the placental bed often described as placental insufficiency. Even though the diagnosis of preeclampsia is not made until the second-half of the pregnancy, maldevelopment of the placental bed vessels occurs well before that time.[221] Vascular resistance to the placenta and placental bed normally decreases as the pregnancy progresses. This process is inhibited in many of those patients who are destined to develop preeclampsia. Different degrees of severity of placental insufficiency appear to be associated with various pregnancy-associated hypertensive disorders, including early-onset preeclampsia [<34 weeks of gestation, very often associated with intrauterine growth restriction (IUGR)], late-onset preeclampsia (≥34 weeks of gestation), and gestational hypertension.[29]

Pulsed Doppler Evaluation of Blood Flow through the Uterine Arteries

The impedance of the maternal blood supply to the placental bed may be estimated by measuring the pulsatility index (PI) of the uterine arteries using Doppler ultrasound. It has been shown that the risk of developing preeclampsia increases with uterine artery PI.[27-29]

First-trimester Doppler examination of the uterine artery involves obtaining a sagittal view of the cervix and the lower uterine segment where the cervical canal and the endocervix are identified. The transducer is then tilted from side-to-side to locate the uterine arteries at the level of the endocervix with the aid of color Doppler **(Fig. 8 and Box 7)**. The PI is measured using pulsed Doppler with the sample gate set at 2 mm. The angle of insonation with respect to the longitudinal axis of the uterine artery should be <30°. Magnification needs to be such that the uterine artery can be identified with confidence and the Doppler may be placed accurately within the lumen. In addition to identifying the artery in its proper location, there are two main ways to confirm that the vessel being interrogated with Doppler is the uterine artery. Firstly, the direction of the blood flow should be toward the transducer (i.e., toward the uterine fundus) when the transabdominal approach is used; this assures that the cervical branches are not being insonated. Secondly, the peak velocity of the insonated vessel should be >60 cm/sec. This assures that the main uterine artery is being insonated rather one of its branches. At least three waveforms similar in shape should be obtained and the PI should be measured in both uterine arteries. The lowest PI is used for risk assessment.

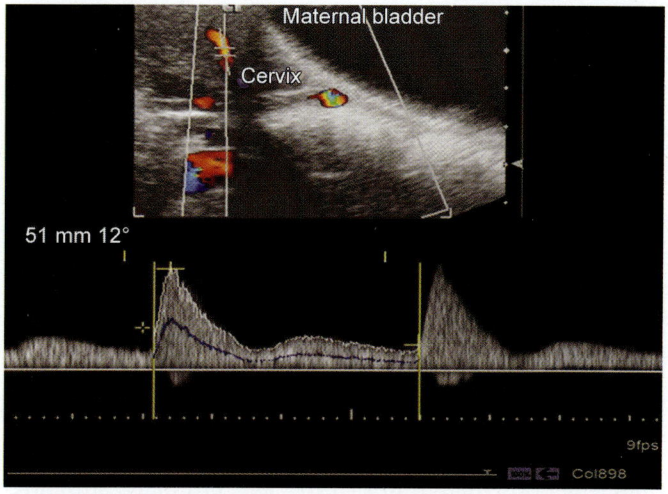

Fig. 8: Evaluation of the uterine artery blood flow using Doppler.

BOX 7: The Fetal Medicine Foundation criteria for the evaluation of uterine artery blood flow using Doppler.

- Location of the uterine artery—just lateral to the cervix at the level of the endocervix
- Doppler gate—2 mm
- Angle of insonation—<30°
- *Direction of flow:* Toward the uterine fundus
- Peak systolic velocity—>60 cm/sec
- The lowest PI is used for risk assessment

(PI: pulsatility index)

Uterine Artery Doppler and Preeclampsia

The initial publication reporting a multivariate screening algorithm included 7,797 patients. The risk parameters were maternal history, uterine artery PI (increased PI increases the risk of preeclampsia), mean arterial pressure (MAP) (increased MAP increases the risk of preeclampsia), PAPP-A (decreased PAPP-A increases the risk of preeclampsia), and placental growth factor (PlGF) (decreased PlGF increases the risk of preeclampsia).[27] The risk algorithm has been refined to use a Bayesian statistical approach.[28] Features of maternal history that appear to make a significant independent contribution to preeclampsia risk assessment include maternal body mass index (BMI), age, ethnicity, smoking, and parity. Combining all these risk factors was shown to predict 90% of early preeclampsia, 70% of preterm preeclampsia, and 40% of late preeclampsia for a 10% false-positive rate.[27] This compares favorably with screening based on maternal history alone where only 30% of early and 20% of late preeclampsia are predicted for a 5% false-positive rate.

Women deemed high risk through first-trimester screening for preterm preeclampsia should be offered aspirin, which has been shown to reduce the prevalence of preterm disease by 62%.[30] The original randomized controlled trial is supported by the findings of a number of other groups who have demonstrated that both the screening algorithm and the intervention are effective.[222] This intervention is very cost-effective, primarily due to a significant reduction in the length of neonatal stay.[223]

Risk algorithms are being developed for other adverse pregnancy outcomes, such as fetal growth restriction, spontaneous preterm delivery, preterm prelabor rupture of membranes, and gestational diabetes.[224-227] These require further enhancement to improve screening efficacy and validate use in different populations. These screening tools will then need to be assessed in combination with treatments designed to mitigate risk.

CONCLUSION

Over the past 40 years, ultrasound has become established as an invaluable tool in obstetric management. There has been a steady increase in our understanding of normal and abnormal fetal physiology along with an improvement in the quality of ultrasound equipment. This has not only led to our ability to diagnose an ever-increasing number of fetal conditions but has also moved the point of diagnosis to an earlier gestation. This benefits the patient in a number of ways not the least of which is maintaining the maximum level of privacy and preservation of reproductive choices.

Advances in the screening capabilities of the first-trimester scan have led to an improved detection of fetal abnormalities, especially aneuploidy and resulted in a decreased false-positive rate. The latter has two very important benefits: Fewer women have to go through the stress of being told that they fall into the "increased risk" category and fewer women undergo invasive diagnostic procedures. The decrease in the number of invasive diagnostic procedures being performed in turn leads to a decrease in both miscarriage and cost related to invasive procedures.

As our understanding of risk assessment improves, we are able to screen pregnancies for complications other than those caused by the genetic makeup of the fetus. This includes the use of ultrasound assessment of maternal uterine artery flow which can be combined with other clinical and biochemical parameters to accurately estimate the risk of developing preeclampsia and fetal growth restriction later in pregnancy. By improving the selection of high-risk patients, we may be able to manipulate placental development therapeutically and reduce the prevalence of this disease in the future.

As the utility of ultrasound expands and this tool is used in predictive models, our responsibility to perform a quality assured examination increases. This can be achieved only with proper training followed by an ongoing and rigorous quality assurance program. A factor that is difficult to quantify but is nonetheless crucial in performing a high-quality ultrasound examination is the level of commitment on the part of each individual sonographer.

REFERENCES

1. Down LJ. Observations on an ethnic classification of idiots. Clin Lectures and Reports. London Hospital. 1866;3:259-62.
2. Kagan KO, Wright D, Valencia C, et al. Screening for trisomies 21, 18 and 13 by maternal age, fetal nuchal translucency, fetal heart rate free beta-hCG and pregnancy-associated plasma protein-A. Human Reprod. 2008;23:1968-75.
3. Kagan KO, Cicero S, Staboulidou I, et al. Fetal nasal bone in screening for trisomy 21, 18, 13 and Turner syndrome at 11-13 weeks of gestation. Ultrasound in Obstet Gynecol. 2009;33:259-64.
4. Borenstein M, Persico N, Kagan KO, et al. Frontomaxillary facial angle in screening for trisomy 21 at 11+0 to 13+6 weeks. Ultrasound Obstet Gynecol. 2008;32(1):5-11.

5. Vis JC, Duffels MGJ, Winter MM, et al. Down syndrome: a cardiovascular perspective. J Intellect Disabil Res. 2009;53(5):419-25.
6. Recalde AL, Landing BH, Lipsey AI. Increased cardiac muscle size and reduced cell number in Down syndrome: heart muscle cell number in Down syndrome. Pediatric Pathol. 1986;6(1):47-53.
7. Gittenberger-De Groot AC, Bartram U, Oosthoek PW, et al. Collagen type VI expression during cardiac development and in human fetuses with trisomy 21. Anat Rec A Discov Mol Cell Evol Bio. 2003;275(2):1109-16.
8. Carvalhaes LS, Gervásio OL, Guatimosim C, et al. Collagen XVIII/endostatin is associated with the epithelial-mesenchymal transformation in the atrioventricular valves during cardiac development. Dev Dynamics. 2006;235(1):132-42.
9. Huggon IC, DeFigueiredo DB, Allan LD. Tricuspid regurgitation in the diagnosis of chromosomal anomalies in the fetus at 11–14 weeks of gestation. Heart. 2003;89(9):1071-3.
10. Faiola S, Tsoi E, Huggon IC, et al. Likelihood ratio for trisomy 21 in fetuses with tricuspid regurgitation at the 11 to 13+6 week scan. Ultrasound Obstet Gynecol. 2005;26(1):22-7.
11. Kagan KO, Valencia C, Livanos P, et al. Tricuspid regurgitation in screening for trisomies 21, 18 and 13 and Turner syndrome at 11+0 to 13+6 weeks of gestation. Ultrasound Obstet Gynecol. 2009;33(1):18-22.
12. Maiz N, Valencia C, Emmanuel EE, et al. Screening for adverse pregnancy outcome by ductus venosus Doppler at 11-13+6 weeks of gestation. Obstet Gynecol. 2008;112(3):598-605.
13. Mavrides E, Sairam S, Hollis B, et al. Screening for aneuploidy in the first trimester by assessment of blood flow in the ductus venosus. BJOG. 2002;109(9):1015-9.
14. Murta CG, Moron AF, Avila MA, et al. Application of ductus venosus Doppler elocimetry for the detection of fetal aneuploidy in the first trimester of pregnancy. Fetal Diagn Ther. 2002;17(5):308-14.
15. Zoppi MA, Putzolu M, Ibba RM, et al. First-trimester ductus venosus velocimetry in relation to nuchal translucency thickness and fetal karyotype. Fetal Diagn Ther. 2002;17(1):52-7.
16. Borrell A, Martinez JM, Seres A, et al. Ductus venosus assessment at the time of nuchal translucency measurement in the detection of fetal aneuploidy. Prenat Diagn. 2003;23(11):921-6.
17. Maiz N, Valencia C, Kagan KO, et al. Ductus venosus Doppler in screening for trisomies 21, 18, and 13 and Turner syndrome at 11–13 weeks of gestation. Ultrasound Obstet Gynecol. 2009;33(5):512-7.
18. Bilardo CM, Müller MA, Zikulnig L, et al. Ductus venosus studies in fetuses at high risk for chromosomal or heart abnormalities: relationship with nuchal translucency measurement and fetal outcome. Ultrasound Obstet Gynecol. 2001;17(4):288-94.
19. Maiz N, Plasencia W, Daklis T, et al. Ductus venosus Doppler in fetuses with cardiac defects and increased nuchal translucency thickness. Ultrasound Obstet Gynecol. 2008;31(3):256-60.
20. Liao AW, Snijders R, Geerts L, et al. Fetal heart rate in chromosomally abnormal fetuses. Ultrasound Obstet Gynecol. 2000;16(7):610-3.
21. Spencer K, Souter V, Tul N, et al. A screening program for trisomy 21 at 10–14 weeks using fetal nuchal translucency, maternal serum free beta-human chorionic gonadotropin and pregnancy-associated plasma protein-A. Ultrasound Obstet Gynecol. 1999;13(4):231-7.
22. Wagner P, Sonek J, Hoopmann M, et al. First-trimester screening for trisomies 18 and 13, triploidy and Turner syndrome by detailed early anomaly scan. Ultrasound Obstet Gynecol. 2016;48:446-51.
23. Syngelaki A, Pergament E, Homfray T, et al. Replacing the combined test by cell-free DNA testing in screening for trisomies 21, 18 and 13: impact on the diagnosis of other chromosomal abnormalities. Fetal Diagn Ther. 2014;35:174-84.
24. Vogel I, Tabor A, Ekelund C, et al.; The Danish Fetal Medicine Study Group, and the Danish Cytogenetic Study Group. Population-Based Screening for Trisomies and Atypical Chromosomal Abnormalities: Improving Efficacy using the Combined First Trimester Screening Algorithm as well as Individual Risk Parameters. Fetal Diagn Ther. 2019;45:424-9.
25. Chen FC, Gerhardt J, Entezami M, et al. Detection of Spina Bifida by First Trimester Screening - Results of the Prospective Multicenter Berlin IT-Study. Ultraschall Med. 2017;38(2):151-7.
26. Chaoui R, Orosz G, Heling KS, et al. Maxillary gap at 11-13 weeks' gestation: marker of cleft lip and palate. Ultrasound Obstet Gynecol. 2015;46(6):665-9.
27. Poon LC, Kametas NA, Maiz N, et al. First-trimester prediction of hypertensive disorders in pregnancy. Hypertension. 2009;53(5):812-8.
28. Wright D, Tan MY, O'Gorman N, et al. Predictive performance of the competing risk model in screening for preeclampsia. Am J Obstet Gynecol. 2019;220(2):199.e1-199.e13.
29. Poon LC, Shennan A, Hyett JA, et al. The International Federation of Gynecology and Obstetrics (FIGO) initiative on pre-eclampsia: A pragmatic guide for first-trimester screening and prevention. Int J Gynaecol Obstet. 2019;145 Suppl 1(Suppl 1):1-33.
30. Rolnik DL, Wright D, Poon LC, et al. Aspirin versus Placebo in Pregnancies at High Risk for Preterm Preeclampsia. N Engl J Med. 2017;377(7):613-22.
31. Cuckle H, Benn P, Wright D. Down syndrome screening in the first and/or second trimester: model predicted

performance using meta-analysis parameters. Semin Perinatol. 2005;29(4):252-7.
32. Hyett J, Moscoso G, Papapanagiotou G, et al. Abnormalities of the heart and great arteries in chromosomally normal fetuses with increased nuchal translucency thickness at 11–13 weeks of gestation. Ultrasound Obstet Gynecol. 1996;7(4):245-50.
33. Schwarzler P, Carvalho JS, Senat MV, et al. Screening for fetal aneuploidies and fetal cardiac abnormalities by nuchal translucency thickness measurement at 10–14 weeks of gestation as part of routine antenatal care in an unselected population. Br J Obstet Gynaecol. 1999;106(10):1029-34.
34. Bahado-Singh RO, Wapner R, Thom E, et al. Elevated first-trimester nuchal translucency increases the risk of congenital heart defects. Am J Obstet Gynecol. 2005;192(5):1357-61.
35. Moselhi M, Thilaganathan B. Nuchal translucency: a marker for the antenatal diagnosis of aortic coarctation. Br J Obstet Gynaecol. 1996;103(10):1044-5.
36. Hyett JA, Perdu M, Sharland GK, et al. Increased nuchal translucency at 10–14 weeks of gestation as a marker for major cardiac defects. Ultrasound Obstet Gynecol. 1997;10(4):242-6.
37. Zosmer N, Souter VL, Chan CSY, et al. Early diagnosis of major cardiac defects in chromosomally normal fetuses with increased nuchal translucency. Br J Obstet Gynaecol. 1999;106(8):829-33.
38. Ghi T, Huggon IC, Zosmer N, et al. Incidence of major structural cardiac defects associated with increased nuchal translucency but normal karyotype. Ultrasound Obstet Gynecol. 2001;18(6):610-4.
39. Lopes LM, Brizot ML, Lopes MA, et al. Structural and functional cardiac abnormalities identified prior to 16 weeks of gestation in fetuses with increased nuchal translucency. Ultrasound Obstet Gynecol. 2003;22(5):470-8.
40. Galindo A, Comas C, Martinez JM, et al. Cardiac defects in chromosomally normal fetuses with increased nuchal translucency at 10-14 weeks of gestation. J Matern Fetal Neonatal Med. 2003;13(3):163-70.
41. McAuliffe F, Winsor S, Hornberger LK, et al. Fetal cardiac defects and increased nuchal translucency thickness. Am J Obstet Gynecol. 2003;189, Abstract 571.
42. Hyett J, Perdu M, Sharland G, et al. Using fetal nuchal translucency to screen for major congenital cardiac defects at 10–14 weeks of gestation: population-based cohort study. BMJ. 1999;318(7176):81-5.
43. Mavrides E, Cobian-Sanchez F, Tekay A, et al. Limitations of using first trimester nuchal translucency measurement in routine screening for major congenital heart defects. Ultrasound Obstet Gynecol. 2001;17(2):106-10.
44. Orvos H, Wayda K, Kozinszky Z, et al. Increased nuchal translucency and congenital heart defects in euploid fetuses. The Szeged experience. Eur J Obstet Gynecol Reprod Biol. 2002;101(2):124-8.
45. Hafner E, Schuller T, Metzenbauer M, et al. Increased nuchal translucency and congenital heart defects in a low-risk population. Prenat Diagn. 2003;23(12):985-9.
46. Makrydimas G, Sotiriadis A, Ioannidis JP. Screening performance of first-trimester nuchal translucency for major cardiac defects: a meta-analysis. Am J Obstet Gynecol. 2003;189(5):1330-5.
47. Schemm S, Gembruch U, Germer U, et al. Omphalocele-exstrophy-imperforate anus-spinal defects (OEIS) complex associated with increased nuchal translucency. Ultrasound Obstet Gynecol. 2003;22(1):95-7.
48. Sebire NJ, Snijders RJM, Davenport M, et al. Fetal nuchal translucency thickness at 10–14 weeks of gestation and congenital diaphragmatic hernia. Obstet Gynecol. 1997;90(6):943-6.
49. Smrcek JM, Germer U, Krokowski M, et al. Prenatal ultrasound diagnosis and management of body stalk anomaly: analysis of nine singleton and two multiple pregnancies. Ultrasound Obstet Gynecol. 2003;21(4):322-8.
50. Monteagudo A, Mayberry P, Rebarber A, et al. Sirenomelia sequence: first-trimester diagnosis with both two- and three-dimensional sonography. J Ultrasound Med. 2002; 21(8):915-20.
51. Souka AP, Snidjers RJM, Novakov A, et al. Defects and syndromes in chromosomally normal fetuses with increased nuchal translucency at 10–14 weeks of gestation. Ultrasound Obstet Gynecol. 1998;11(6):391-400.
52. Souka A, Heath V. Increased nuchal translucency with normal karyotype. In: Sebire NJ, Snijders RJM, Nicolaides KH (Eds). The 11–14 week scan: diagnosis of fetal abnormalities. Carnforth, UK: Parthenon Publishing; 1999. pp. 67-88.
53. Souka AP, Von Kaisenberg CS, Hyett JA, et al. Increased nuchal translucency with normal karyotype. Am J Obstet Gynecol. 2005;192(4):1005-21.
54. Ben Ami M, Perlitz Y, Haddad S, et al. Increased nuchal translucency is associated with asphyxiating thoracic dysplasia. Ultrasound Obstet Gynecol. 1997;10(4):297-8.
55. Soothill PW, Vuthiwong C, Rees H. Achondrogenesis type 2 diagnosed by transvaginal ultrasound at 12 weeks of gestation. Prenat Diagn. 1993;13(6):523-8.
56. Makrydimas G, Souka A, Skentou H, et al. Osteogenesis imperfecta and other skeletal dysplasias presenting with increased nuchal translucency in the first trimester. Am J Med Genet. 2001;98(2):117-20.
57. Meizner I, Barnhard Y. Achondrogenesis type I diagnosed by transvaginal ultrasonography at 13 weeks of gestation. Am J Obstet Gynecol. 1995;173(5):1620-2.
58. den Hollander NS, van der Harten HJ, Vermeij-Keers C, et al. First trimester diagnosis of Blomstrand lethal osteochondrodysplasia. Am J Med Genet. 1997;73(3):345-50.
59. Souka AP, Raymond FL, Mornet E, et al. Hypophosphatasia associated with increased nuchal translucency: a report of

three consecutive pregnancies. Ultrasound Obstet Gynecol. 2002;20:294-5.
60. Eliyahu S, Weiner E, Lahav D, et al. Early sonographic diagnosis of Jarcho-Levin syndrome: a prospective screening program in one family. Ultrasound Obstet Gynecol. 1997;9(5):314-8.
61. Souter V, Nyberg D, Siebert JR, et al. Upper limb phocomelia associated with increased nuchal translucency in a monochorionic twin pregnancy. J Ultrasound Med. 2002;21(3):355-60.
62. Petrikovsky BM, Gross B, Bialer M, et al. Prenatal diagnosis of pseudothalidomide syndrome in consecutive pregnancies of a consanguineous couple. Ultrasound Obstet Gynecol. 1997;10(6):425-8.
63. Percin EF, Guvenal T, Cetin A, et al. First-trimester diagnosis of Robinow syndrome. Fetal Diagn Ther. 2001;16(5):308-11.
64. Hill LM, Leary J. Transvaginal sonographic diagnosis of short-rib polydactyly dysplasia at 13 weeks of gestation. Prenat Diagn. 1998;18(11):1198-201.
65. Achiron R, Heggesh J, Grisaru D, et al. Noonan syndrome: a cryptic condition in early gestation. Am J Med Genet. 2000;92(3):159-65.
66. Souka AP, Krampl E, Geerts L, et al. Congenital lymphedema presenting with increased nuchal translucency at 13 weeks of gestation. Prenat Diagn. 2002;22(2):91-2.
67. Fincham J, Pandya PP, Yuksel B, et al. Increased first-trimester nuchal translucency as a prenatal manifestation of salt-wasting congenital adrenal hyperplasia. Ultrasound Obstet Gynecol. 2002;20(4):392-4.
68. Souka AP, Skentou H, Geerts L, et al. Congenital nephrotic syndrome presenting with increased nuchal translucency in the first trimester. Prenat Diagn. 2002;22(2):93-5.
69. Hyett J, Noble P, Sebire NJ, et al. Lethal congenital arthrogryposis presents with increased nuchal translucency at 10–14 weeks of gestation. Ultrasound Obstet Gynecol. 1997;9(5):310-3.
70. Rijhsinghani A, Yankowitz J, Howser D, et al. Sonographic and maternal serum screening abnormalities in fetuses affected by spinal muscular atrophy. Prenat Diagn. 1997;17(2):166-9.
71. de Jong-Pleij EA, Stoutenbecek P, van der Mark-Batseva NN, et al. The association of spinal muscular atrophy type II and increased nuchal translucency. Ultrasound Obstet Gynecol. 2002;19(3):312-3.
72. Lam YH, Tang MH, Lee CP, et al. Nuchal translucency in fetuses affected by homozygous a-thalassemia-1 at 12–13 weeks of gestation. Ultrasound Obstet Gynecol. 1999;13(4):238-40.
73. Souka AP, Bower S, Geerts L, et al. Blackfan-Diamond anemia and dyserythropoietic anemia presenting with increased nuchal translucency at 12 weeks of gestation. Ultrasound Obstet Gynecol. 2002;20(2):197-9.
74. Pannier E, Viot G, Aubry MC, et al. Congenital erythropoietic porphyria (Gunther's disease): two cases with very early prenatal manifestation and cystic hydroma. Prenat Diagn. 2003;23(1):25-30.
75. Tercanli S, Miny P, Siebert MS, et al. Fanconi anemia associated with increased nuchal translucency detected by first-trimester ultrasound. Ultrasound Obstet Gynecol. 2001;17(2):160-2.
76. Petrikovsky BM, Baker D, Schneider E. Fetal hydrops secondary to human parvovirus infection in early pregnancy. Prenat Diagn. 1996;16(4):342-4.
77. Markenson G, Correia LA, Cohn G, et al. Parvoviral infection associated with increased nuchal translucency: a case report. J Perinatol. 2000;20(2):129-31.
78. Smulian JC, Egan JF, Rodis JF. Fetal hydrops in the first trimester associated with maternal parvovirus infection. J Clin Ultrasound. 1998;26(6):314-6.
79. Becker R, Wegner RD. Detailed screening for fetal anomalies and cardiac defects at the 11–13 week scan. Ultrasound Obstet Gynecol. 2006;27(6):613-8.
80. Green JJ, Hobbins JC. Abdominal ultrasound examination of the first trimester fetus. Am J Obstet Gynecol. 1988;159(1):165-75.
81. Rottem S, Bronshtein M, Thaler I, et al. First trimester transvaginal sonographic diagnosis of fetal anomalies. Lancet. 1989;1(8635):444-5.
82. Johnson P, Sharland G, Maxwell D, et al. The role of transvaginal sonography in the early detection of congenital heart disease. Ultrasound Obstet Gynecol. 1992;2(4):248-51.
83. Braithwaite JM, Armstrong MA, Economides DL. Assessment of fetal anatomy at 12 to 13 weeks of gestation by transabdominal and transvaginal sonography. Br J Obstet Gynaecol. 1996;103(1):82-5.
84. Hernadi L, Torocsik M. Screening for fetal anomalies in the 12th week of pregnancy by transvaginal sonography in an unselected population. Prenat Diagn. 1997;17(8):753-9.
85. Economides DL, Braithwaite JM. First trimester ultrasonographic diagnosis of fetal structural abnormalities in a low risk population. Br J Obstet Gynaecol. 1998; 105(1):53-7.
86. Carvalho MH, Brizot ML, Lopes LM, et al. Detection of fetal structural abnormalities at the 11–14 week ultrasound scan. Prenat Diagn. 2002;22(1):1-4.
87. Souka AP, Pilalis A, Kavalakis I, et al. Screening for major structural abnormalities at the 11- to 14-week ultrasound scan. Am J Obstet Gynecol. 2006;194(2):393-6.
88. Gembruch U, Knöpfle G, Bald R, et al. Early diagnosis of fetal congenital heart disease by transvaginal echocardiography. Ultrasound Obstet Gynecol. 1993;3(5):310-7.
89. Achiron R, Rotstein Z, Lipitz S, et al. First-trimester diagnosis of fetal congenital heart disease by transvaginal ultrasonography. Obstet Gynecol. 1994;84(1):69-72.
90. Smrcek JM, Gembruch U, Krokowski M, et al. The evaluation of cardiac biometry in major cardiac defects detected in early pregnancy. Arch Gynecol Obstet. 2003;268(2):94-101.

91. Wisser J, Dirschedl P, Krone S. Estimation of gestational age by transvaginal sonographic measurements of greatest embryonic length in dated human embryos. Ultrasound Obstet Gynecol. 1994;4(6):457-62.
92. Monteagudo A, Timor-Tritsch I, Sharma S. Early and simple determination of chorionic and amniotic type in multifetal gestations in the first 14 weeks by high frequency transvaginal ultrasound. Am J Obstet Gynecol. 1994;170(3):824-9.
93. Sepulveda W, Sebire NJ, Hughes K, et al. The lambda sign at 10–14 weeks of gestation as a predictor of chorionicity in twin pregnancies. Ultrasound Obstet Gynecol. 1996; 7(6):421-3.
94. Selpuveda W, Sebire NJ, Hughes K, et al. Evolution of the lambda or twin/chorionic peak sign in dichorionic twin pregnancies. Obstet Gynecol. 1997;89(3):439-41.
95. Sebire NJ, Snijders RJ, Hughes K, et al. The hidden mortality of monochorinic twin pregnancies. Br J Obstet Gynaecol. 1997;104(10):1203-7.
96. Noble PL, Snijders RJ, Abraha HD, et al. Maternal serum free beta-hCG at 10 to 14 weeks in trisomic twin pregnancies. Br J Obstet Gynaecol. 1997;104(6):741-3.
97. Spencer K. Screening for trisomy 21 in twin pregnancies in the first trimester using free beta-hCG and PAPP-A, combined with fetal nuchal translucency thickness. Prenat Diagn. 2000;20(2):91-5.
98. Spencer K, Nicolaides KH. Screening for trisomy 21 in twins using first trimester ultrasound and maternal serum biochemistry in a one-stop clinic: a review of three years experience. BJOG. 2003;110(3):276-80.
99. Kagan KO, Gassoni A, Selpuveda-Gonzalez G, et al. Discordance in nuchal translucency thickness in the prediction of severe twin-to-twin transfusion syndrome. Ultrasound Obstet Gynecol. 2007;29(5):527-32.
100. Maiz N, Staboulidou I, Leal AM, et al. Ductus venosus Doppler at 11 to 13 weeks of gestation in the prediction of outcome in twin pregnancies. Obstet Gynecol. 2009;113(4):860-5.
101. Souka AP, Pilalis A, Kavalakis Y, et al. Assessment of fetal anatomy at the 11–14 week ultrasound examination. 2004;24(7):730-4.
102. van Zalen-Sprock RM, van Vugt JMG, van Geijn HP. First-trimester sonography of physiological midgut herniation and early diagnosis of omphalocele. Prenat Diagn. 1997;17(6):511-8.
103. Snijders RJ, Sebire NJ, Souka A, et al. Fetal exomphalos and chromosomal defects: relationship to maternal age and gestation. Ultrasound Obstet Gynecol. 1995;6(4):250-5.
104. Johnson SP, Sebire NJ, Snijders RJ, et al. Ultrasound screening for anecephaly at 10–14 weeks of gestation. Ultrasound Obstet Gynecol. 1997;9(1):14-16.
105. Sandikcioglu M, Molsted K, Kjaer I. The prenatal development of the human nasal and vomeral bones. J Craniofac Genet Dev Biol. 1994;14(2):124-34.
106. Makikallio K, Jouppila P, Rasanen J. Human fetal cardiac function during the first trimester of pregnancy. Heart. 2005;91(3):334-8.
107. Wright D, Kagan KO, Molina FS, et al. A mixture model of nuchal translucency thickness in screening for chromosomal defects. Ultrasound Obstet Gynecol. 2008;31(4):376-83.
108. Whitlow BJ, Economides DL. The optimal gestational age to examine fetal anatomy and measure nuchal translucency in the first trimester. Ultrasound Obstet Gynecol. 1998;11(4):258-61.
109. Mulvey S, Baker L, Edwards A, et al. Optimizing the timing for nuchal translucency measurement. Prenat Diagn. 2002;22(9):775-7.
110. Nicolaides KH, Brizot ML, Snijders RJ. Fetal nuchal translucency: ultrasound screening for fetal trisomy in the first trimester. Br J Obstet Gynaecol. 1994;101(9):782-6.
111. Uehara S, Yaegashi N, Maeda T, et al. Risk of recurrence of fetal chromosomal aberration: analysis of trisomy 21, trisomy 18, trisomy 13, and 45 X, in 1,076 Japanese mothers. J Obstet Gynaecol Res. 1999;25(6):373-9.
112. UK National Screening Committee Policy. Down's Syndrome Screening. Compiled by the National Screening Committee, 2006. Available from: http://www.library.nhs.uk/screening. [Last accessed February, 2011].
113. Chalouhi GE, Bernard JP, Ville Y, et al. A comparison of first trimester measurements for prediction of delivery date. J Matern Fetal Neonatal Med. 2011;24(1):51-7.
114. Salomon LJ, Bernard M, Amarsy R, et al. The impact of crown-rump length measurement error on combined Down syndrome screening: a simulation study. Ultrasound Obstet Gynecol. 2009;33(5):506-11.
115. Nicolaides KH, Azar G, Byrne D, et al. Fetal nuchal translucency: ultrasound screening for chromosomal defects in first trimester of pregnancy. BMJ. 1992;304 (6831):867-9.
116. Simpson JM, Sharland GK. Nuchal translucency and congenital heart defects: heart failure or not? Ultrasound Obstet Gynecol. 2000;16(1):30-6.
117. Rizzo G, Muscatello A, Angelini E, et al. Abnormal cardiac function in fetuses with increased nuchal translucency. Ultrasound Obstet Gynecol. 2003;21(6):539-42.
118. Hyett JA, Brizot ML, von Kaisenberg CS, et al. Cardiac gene expression of atrial natriuretic peptide and brain natriuretic peptide in trisomic fetuses. Obstet Gynecol. 1996;87(4):506-10.
119. Tsuchimochi H, Kurimoto F, Leki K, et al. Atrial natriuretic peptide distribution in fetal and failed adult human hearts. Circulation. 1988;78(4):920-7.
120. von Kaisenberg CS, Krenn V, Ludwig M, et al. Morphological classification of nuchal skin in fetuses with trisomy 21, 18 and 13 at 12–18 weeks and in a trisomy 16 mouse. Anat Embryol (Berl). 1998;197(2):105-24.

121. von Kaisenberg CS, Brand-Saberi B, Christ B, et al. Collagen type VI gene expression in the skin of trisomy 21 fetuses. Obstet Gynecol. 1998;91(3):319-23.
122. Böhlandt S, von Kaisenberg CS, Wewetzer K, et al. Hyaluronan in the nuchal skin of chromosomally abnormal fetuses. Hum Reprod. 2000;15(5):1155-8.
123. Chitayat D, Kalousek DK, Bamforth JS. Lymphatic abnormalities in fetuses with posterior cervical cystic hygroma. Am J Med Genet. 1989;33(3):352-6.
124. von Kaisenberg CS, Nicolaides KH, Brand-Siberi B. Lymphatic vessel hypoplasia in fetuses with Turner syndrome. Hum Reprod. 1999;14(3):823-6.
125. Nicolaides KH, Rodeck CH, Lange I, et al. Fetoscopy in the assessment of unexplained fetal hydrops. Br J Obstet Gynaecol. 1985;92(7):671-9.
126. Sohan K, Carroll S, Byrne D, et al. Parvovirus as a differential diagnosis of hydrops fetalis in the first trimester. Fetal Diagn Ther. 2000;15(4):234-6.
127. Pandya PP, Snijders RJ, Johnson SP, et al. Screening for fetal trisomies by maternal age and fetal nuchal translucency thickness at 10 to 14 weeks of gestation. Br J Obstet Gynaecol. 1995;102(12):957-62.
128. Whitlow BJ, Chatzipapas IK, Economides DL. The effect of fetal neck position on nuchal translucency measurement at 10–14 weeks. Br J Obstet Gynaecol. 1998;105:872-6.
129. Shaefer M, Laurichesse-Delmas H, Ville Y. The effect of nuchal cord on nuchal translucency measurement at 10–14 weeks. Ultrasound Obstet Gynecol. 1998;11(4):271-3.
130. Molina F, Avgidou K, Kagan K, et al. Cystic hygromas, nuchal edema, and nuchal translucency at 11–14 weeks of gestation. Obstet Gynecol. 2006;107(3):678-83.
131. Malone FD, Ball RH, Nyberg DA, et al. First-trimester septated cystic hygroma: prevalence, natural history, and pediatric outcome. Obstet Gynecol. 2005;106(2):288-94.
132. Sonek J, Croom C, McKenna D, et al. Letter to the Editor. Obstet Gynecol. 2006;107:424.
133. Comstock CH, Malone FD, Ball RH, et al. Is there a nuchal translucency millimeter measurement above which there is no added benefit from first trimester serum screening? Am J Obstet Gynecol. 2006;195:843-7.
134. Snijders RJ, Noble P, Sebire N, et al. UK multicentre project on assessment of risk of trisomy 21 by maternal age and fetal nuchal translucency thickness at 10–14 weeks of gestation. Lancet. 1998;352(9125):343-6.
135. Hewitt BG, de Crespigny L, Sampson AJ, et al. Correlation between nuchal thickness and abnormal karyotype in first trimester fetuses. Med J Aust. 1996;165(7):365-8.
136. Snijders RJ, Johnson S, Sebire NJ, et al. First-trimester ultrasound screening for chromosomal defects. Ultrasound Obstet Gynecol. 1996;7:216-26.
137. Pajkrt E, van Lith JM, Mol BW, et al. Screening for Down's syndrome by fetal nuchal translucency measurement in a general obstetric population. Ultrasound Obstet Gynecol. 1998;12:163-9.
138. Spencer K, Spencer DE, Power M, et al. Screening for chromosomal abnormalities in the first trimester using ultrasound and maternal serum biochemistry and in a one-stop clinic: a review of three years prospective experience. Br J Obstet Gynaecol. 2003;110(3):281-6.
139. Kagan KO, Wright D, Baker A, et al. Screening for trisomy 21 by maternal age, fetal nuchal translucency thickness, free beta human chorionic gonadotropin and pregnancy-associated plasma protein-A. Ultrasound Obstet Gynecol. 2008;31(6):618-24.
140. Kagan KO, Etchegaray A, Zhou Y, et al. Prospective validation of first-trimester combined screening for trisomy 21. Ultrasound Obstet Gynecol. 2009;34(1):14-8.
141. Nicolaides KH, Spencer K, Avgidou K, et al. Multicenter study of first-trimester screening for trisomy 21 in 75,821 pregnancies: results and estimation of the potential impact of individual risk-orientated two-stage first-trimester screening. Ultrasound Obstet Gynecol. 2005;25(3):221-6.
142. Avgidou K, Papageorghiou A, Bindra R, et al. Prospective first-trimester screening for trisomy 21 in 30,564 pregnancies. Am J Obstet Gynecol. 2005;192(6):1761-7.
143. Kagan KO, Anderson JM, Anwandter G, et al. Screening for triploidy by the risk algorithms for trisomies 21, 18 and 13 at 11–13 weeks and 6 days of gestation. Prenat Diagn. 2008;28(13):1209-13.
144. Kagan KO, Wright D, Maiz N, et al. Screening for trisomy 18 by maternal age, fetal nuchal translucency, free beta-human chorionic gonadotropin and pregnancy-associated plasma protein-A. Ultrasound Obstet Gynecol. 2008;32(4):488-92.
145. Farkas LG, Katic MJ, Forrest CR, et al. Surface anatomy of the face in Down's syndrome: linear and angular measurements in the craniofacial regions. J Craniofac Surg. 2001;12(4):373-9.
146. Keeling JW, Hansen BF, Kjaer I. Pattern of malformation in the axial skeleton in human trisomy 21 fetuses. Am J Med Genet. 1997;68(4):466-71.
147. Stempfle N, Huten Y, Fredouille C, et al. Skeletal abnormalities in fetuses with Down's syndrome: A radiologic postmortem study. Pediatr Radiol. 1999;29:682-8.
148. Tuxen A, Keeling JW, Reintoft I, et al. A histological and radiological investigation of the nasal bone in fetuses with Down syndrome. Ultrasound Obstet Gynecol. 2003;22(1):22-6.
149. Minderer S, Gloning KP, Henrich W, et al. The nasal bone in fetuses with trisomy 21: sonographic versus pathomorphological findings. Ultrasound Obstet Gynecol. 2003;22(1):16-21.
150. Sonek J, Cicero S, Neiger R, et al. Nasal bone assessment in prenatal screening for trisomy 21. Am J Obstet Gynecol. 2006;195:1219-30.
151. Sonek J, Nicolaides K. Prenatal ultrasonographic diagnosis of nasal bone abnormalities in three fetuses with Down syndrome. Am J Obstet Gynecol. 2002;186(1):139-41.

152. Cicero S, Curcio P, Papageorghiou A, et al. Absence of nasal bone in fetuses with Trisomy 21 at 11–14 weeks of gestation: an observational study. Lancet. 2001;358(9294):1665-7.
153. Otano L, Aiello H, Igarzabal L, et al. Association between first trimester absence of fetal nasal bone on ultrasound and Down's syndrome. Prenat Diagn. 2002;22(10):930-2.
154. Zoppi MA, Ibba RM, Axinan C, et al. Absence of fetal nasal bone and aneuploidies at first-trimester nuchal translucency screening in unselected pregnancies. Prenat Diagn. 2003;23(6):496-500.
155. Viora E, Masturzo B, Errante G, et al. Ultrasound evaluation of fetal nasal bone at 11 to 14 weeks in a consecutive series of 1906 fetuses. Prenat Diagn. 2003;23(10):784-7.
156. Wong SF, Choi H, Ho LC. Nasal bone hypoplasia: is it a common finding amongst chromosomally normal fetuses of southern Chinese women? Gynecol Obstet Invest. 2003;56(2):99-101.
157. Cicero S, Longo D, Rembouskos G, et al. Absent nasal bone at 11–14 weeks of gestation and chromosomal defects. Ultrasound Obstet Gynecol. 2003;22(1):31-5.
158. Cicero S, Bindra R, Rembouskos G, et al. Fetal nasal bone length in chromosomally normal and abnormal fetuses at 11–14 weeks of gestation. J Matern Fetal Neonatal Med. 2002;11(6):400-2.
159. Rembouskos G, Cicero S, Longo D, et al. Assessment of the fetal nasal bone at 11–14 weeks of gestation by three-dimensional ultrasound. Ultrasound Obstet Gynecol. 2004;23(3):232-6.
160. Cicero S, Rembouskos G, Vandecruys H, et al. Likelihood ratio for trisomy 21 in fetuses with absent nasal bone at the 11–14 weeks scan. Ultrasound Obstet Gynecol. 2004;23(3):218-23.
161. Cicero S, Bindra R, Rembouskos G, et al. Integrated ultrasound and biochemical screening for trisomy 21 using nuchal translucency, absent fetal nasal bone, free beta-hCG, and PAPP-A at 11 to 14 weeks of gestation. Prenat Diagn. 2003;23(4):306-10.
162. Cicero S, Avgidu K, Rembouskos G, et al. Nasal bone assessment in prenatal screening for trisomy 21. Am J Obstet Gynecol. 2006;195(1):109-14.
163. Sonek J, Borenstein M, Dagklis T, et al. Frontomaxillary facial angle in fetuses with trisomy 21 at 11-13 (+6) Weeks'. Am J Obstet Gynecol. 2007;196(3):271.e1-4.
164. Plasencia W, Dagklis T, Pachoumi C, et al. Frontomaxillary facial angle at 11+0 to 13+6 weeks: effect of plane of acquisition. Ultrasound Obstet Gynecol. 2007;29(6):660-5.
165. Sonek J, Borenstein M, Downing C, et al. Frontomaxillary facial angles in screening for trisomy 21 at 14-23 weeks of gestation. Am J Obstet Gynecol. 2007;197(2):160.e1-5.
166. Borenstein M, Persico N, Kaihura C, et al. Frontomaxillary facial angle in chromosomally normal fetuses at 11+0 to 13+6 weeks. Ultrasound Obstet Gynecol. 2007;30(7):737-41.
167. Borenstein M, Persico N, Dagklis T, et al. Frontomaxillary facial angle in fetuses with trisomy 13 at 11+0 to 13+6 weeks. Ultrasound Obstet Gynecol. 2007;30(6):819-23.
168. Borenstein M, Persico N, Strobl I, et al. Frontomaxillary and mandibulomaxillary facial angles at 11+0 to 13+6 weeks in fetuses with trisomy 18. Ultrasound Obstet Gynecol. 2007;30(7):928-33.
169. Falcon O, Auer M, Gerovassili A, et al. Screening for trisomy 21 by tricuspid regurgitation, nuchal translucency and maternal serum free β-hCG and PAPP-A at 11+0 to 13+6 weeks. Ultrasound Obstet Gynecol. 2006;27(2):151-5.
170. Antolin E, Comas C, Torrents M, et al. The role of ductus venosus blood flow assessment in screening for chromosomal abnormalities at 10–16 weeks of gestation. Ultrasound Obstet Gynecol. 2001;17(4):295-300.
171. Huisman TW, Bilardo CM. Transient increase in nuchal translucency thickness and reversed end-diastolic ductus venosus flow in a fetus with trisomy 18. Ultrasound Obstet Gynecol. 1997;10(6):397-9.
172. Montenegro N, Matias A, Areias JC, et al. Ductus venosus revisited: a Doppler blood flow evaluation in the first trimester of pregnancy. Ultrasound in Med and Biol. 1997;23:171-6.
173. Borrell A, Antolin E, Costa D, et al. Abnormal ductus venosus blood flow in trisomy 21 fetuses during early pregnancy. Am J Obstet Gynecol. 1998;179(6 Pt 1):1612-7.
174. Matias A, Gomes C, Flack N, et al. Screening for chromosomal abnormalities at 10–14 weeks: the role of ductus venosus blood flow. Ultrasound Obstet Gynecol. 1998;12(6):380-4.
175. Matias A, Montenegro N, Areias JC, et al. Anomalous fetal venous return associated with major chormosomopathies in the late first trimester of pregnancy. Ultrasound Obstet Gynecol. 1998;11(3):209-13.
176. Matias A, Huggon I, Areias JC, et al. Cardiac defects in chromosomally normal fetuses with abnormal ductus venosus blood flow at 10–14 weeks. Ultrasound Obstet Gynecol. 1999;14(5):307-10.
177. Matias A, Montenegro N, Areias JC, et al. Haemodynamic evaluation of the first trimester fetus with special emphasis on venous return. Hum Reprod Update. 2000;6(2):177-89.
178. Matias A, Ramalho C, Montenegro N. Search for hemodynamic compromise at 11–14 weeks in monochorionic twin pregnancy: Is abnormal flow in the ductus venosus predictive of twin-twin transfusion syndrome? J Matern Fetal Neonatal Med. 2005;18(2):79-86.
179. Kagan KO, Wright D, Etchegaray A, et al. Effect of deviation of nuchal translucency measurements on the performance of screening for trisomy 21. Ultrasound Obstet Gynecol. 2009;33(6):657-64.
180. Nisbet DL, Robertson AC, Schluter PJ, et al. Auditing ultrasound assessment of fetal nuchal translucency thickness: a review of Australian National Data 2002-2008. Aust N Z J Obstet Gynaecol. 2010;50(5):450-5.

181. Braithwaite JM, Kadir RA, Pepera TA, et al. Nuchal translucency measurement: training of potential examiners. Ultrasound Obstet Gynecol. 1996;8(3):192-5.
182. Cicero S, Dezerega V, Andrade E, et al. Learning curve for sonographic examination of the fetal nasal bone at 11–14 weeks. Ultrasound Obstet Gynecol. 2003;22(2):135-7.
183. Maiz N, Kagan KO, Milovanovic A, et al. Learning curve for Doppler assessment of ductus venosus flow at 11-13+6 weeks of gestation. Ultrasound Obstet Gynecol. 2008;31:503-6.
184. Nicolaides KH, Snijders RJ, Gosden CM, et al. Ultrasonographically detectable markers of fetal chromosomal abnormalities. Lancet. 1992;340(8821):704-7.
185. Liao A, Sebire N, Geerts L, et al. Megacystis at 10–14 weeks of gestation: chromosomal defects and outcome according to bladder length. Ultrasound Obstet Gynecol. 2003;21(4):338-41.
186. Sebire NJ, Von Kaisenberg C, Rubio C, et al. Fetal megacystis at 10–14 weeks of gestation. Ultrasound Obstet Gynecol. 1996;8(6):387-90.
187. Dagklis T, Plasencia W, Maiz N, et al. Choroid plexus cyst, intracranial echogenic focus, hyperechoic bowel and hydronephrosis in screening for trisomy 21 at 11+0 to 13+6 weeks. Ultrasound Obstet Gynecol. 2008;31:132-5.
188. Gil MM, Accurti V, Santacruz B, et al. Analysis of cell-free DNA in maternal blood in screening for aneuploidies: updated meta-analysis. Ultrasound Obstet Gynecol. 2017;50:302-14.
189. Norton ME, Jacobsson B, Swamy GK, et al. Cell-free DNA analysis for noninvasive examination of trisomy. N Engl J Med. 2015;372:1589-97.
190. Gil MM, Revello R, Poon LC, et al. Clinical implementation of routine screening for fetal trisomies in the UK NHS: cell-free DNA test contingent on results from first-trimester combined test. Ultrasound Obstet Gynecol. 2016;47:45-52.
191. Petersen OB, Vogel I, Ekelund C, et al.; Danish Fetal Medicine Study Group; Danish Clinical Genetics Study Group. Potential diagnostic consequences of applying non-invasive prenatal testing: population-based study from a country with existing first-trimester screening. Ultrasound Obstet Gynecol. 2014;43:265-71.
192. Rodis JF, Egan JF, Craffey A, et al. Calculated risk of chromosomal abnormalities in twin gestations. Obstet Gynecol. 1990;76(6):1037-41.
193. Odibo AO, Elkousy MH, Ural SH, et al. Screening for aneuploidy in twin pregnancies: maternal age- and race-specific risk assessment between 9–14 weeks. Twin Res. 2003;6(4):251-6.
194. Cuckle H. Down's syndrome screening in twins. J Med Screen. 1998;5(1):3-4.
195. Bartha JL, Ling Y, Kyle P, et al. Clinical consequences of first- trimester growth discordance in twins. Eur J Obstet Gynecol Reprod Biol. 2005;119(1):56-9.
196. Kalish RB, Gupta M, Perni SC, et al. Clinical significance of first-trimester crown rump length disparity in dichorionic twin gestations. Am J Obstet Gynecol. 2004;191(4):1437-40.
197. Wøjdemann KR, Larsen SO, Shalmi AC, et al. Nuchal translucency measurements are highly correlated in both mono- and dichorionic twin pairs. Prenat Diagn. 2006;26(3):218-20.
198. Cuckle H, Maymon R. Down syndrome risk calculation for a twin fetus taking account of the nuchal translucency in the co-twin. Prenat Diagn. 2010;30(9):827-33.
199. Sebire NJ, D'Ercole C, Hughes K, et al. Increased nuchal translucency thickness at 10–14 weeks of gestation as a predictor of severe twin-to-twin transfusion syndrome. Ultrasound Obstet Gynecol. 1997;10(2):86-9.
200. Vandecruys H, Faiola S, Auer M, et al. Screening for trisomy 21 in monochorionic twins by measurement of fetal nuchal translucency thickness. Ultrasound Obstet Gynecol. 2005;25(6):551-3.
201. Sepulveda W, Wong AE, Casasbuenas A. Nuchal translucency and nasal bone in first-trimester ultrasound screening for aneuploidy in multiple pregnancies. Ultrasound Obstet Gynecol. 2009;33(2):152-6.
202. Cleary-Goldman J, Rebarber A, Krantz D, et al. First-trimester screening with nasal bone in twins. Am J Obstet Gynecol. 2008;199(3):283.e1-3.
203. Ville Y, Lalondrelle C, Doumerc S, et al. First-trimester diagnosis of nuchal anomalies: significance and fetal outcome. Ultrasound Obstet Gynecol. 1992;2(5):314-6.
204. Brady AF, Pandya PP, Yuksel B, et al. Outcome of chromosomally normal livebirths with increased fetal nuchal translucency at 10–14 weeks of gestation. J Med Genet. 1998;35(3):222-4.
205. Souka AP, Krampl E, Bakalis S, et al. Outcome of pregnancy in chromosomally normal fetuses with increased nuchal translucency in the first trimester. Ultrasound Obstet Gynecol. 2001;18(1):9-17.
206. Mangione R, Guyon F, Taine L, et al. Pregnancy outcome and prognosis in fetuses with increased first-trimester nuchal translucency. Fetal Diagn Ther. 2001;16(6):360-3.
207. Bilardo CM, Pajkrt E, de Graaf I, et al. Outcome of fetuses with enlarged nuchal translucency and normal karyotype. Ultrasound Obstet Gynecol. 1998;11(6):401-6.
208. Michailidis GD, Economides DL. Nuchal translucency measurement and pregnancy outcome in karyotypically normal fetuses. Ultrasound Obstet Gynecol. 2001;17(2):102-5.
209. Shulman LP, Emerson DS, Grevengood C, et al. Clinical course and outcome of fetuses with isolated cystic nuchal lesions and normal karyotypes detected in the first trimester. Am J Obstet Gynecol. 1994;171(5):1278-81.
210. Cheng C, Bahado-Singh RO, Chen S, et al. Pregnancy outcomes with increased nuchal translucency after routine Down syndrome screening. Int J Gynaecol Obstet. 2004;84(1):5-9.

211. Senat MV, De Keersmaecker B, Audibert F, et al. Pregnancy outcome in fetuses with increased nuchal translucency and normal karyotype. Prenat Diagn. 2002;22(5):345-9.
212. Cha'Ban FK, van Splunder P, Los FJ, et al. Fetal outcome in nuchal translucency with emphasis on normal fetal karyotype. Prenat Diagn. 1996;16(6):537-41.
213. Makrymidas G, Sotiradis A, Huggon IC, et al. Nuchal translucency and fetal cardiac defects: a pooled analysis of major fetal echocardiography centers. Am J Obstet Gynecol. 2005;192(1):89-5.
214. Carvalho JS, Moscoso G, Ville Y. First trimester transabdominal fetal echocardiography. Lancet. 1998;351(9108):1023-7.
215. Simpson JM, Jones A, Callaghan N, et al. Accuracy and limitations of transabdominal fetal echocardiography at 12–15 weeks of gestation in a population at high risk for congenital heart disease. Br J Obstet Gynaecol. 2000;16:30-6.
216. Hyett JA, Clayton PT, Moscoso G, et al. Increased first trimester nuchal translucency as a prenatal manifestation of Smith-Lemli-Opitz syndrome. Am J Med Genet. 1995;58(4):374-6.
217. Maymon R, Jauniaux E, Cohen O, et al. Pregnancy outcome and infant follow-up of fetuses with abnormally increased first trimester nuchal translucency. Hum Reprod. 2000;15(9):2023-7.
218. Hiippala A, Eronen M, Taipale P, et al. Fetal nuchal translucency and normal chromosomes: a long-term follow-up study. Ultrasound Obstet Gynecol. 2001;18(1):18-22.
219. Khong TY, De Wolf F, Robertson F, et al. Inadequate maternal vascular response to placentation in pregnancies complicated by preeclampsia and by small-for-gestational age infants. Brit J Obstet Gynaecol. 1986;93:1049-59.
220. Salomon LJ, Alfirevic Z, Bilardo CM, et al. ISUOG practice guidelines: performance of first-trimester fetal ultrasound scan. Ultrasound Obstet Gynecol. 2013;41:102-13.
221. Syngelaki A, Hammami A, Bower S, et al. Diagnosis of fetal non-chromosomal abnormalities on routine ultrasound examination at 11-13 weeks' gestation. Ultrasound Obstet Gynecol. 2019;54:468-76.
222. Foster AB, Park F, Hyett J. Do first-trimester screening algorithms for preeclampsia aligned to use of preventative therapies reduce the prevalence of pre-term preeclampsia: A systematic review and meta-analysis. Prenat Diagn. 2023;43(7):950-8.
223. Wright D, Rolnik DL, Syngelaki A, et al. Aspirin for Evidence-Based Preeclampsia Prevention trial: effect of aspirin on length of stay in the neonatal intensive care unit. Am J Obstet Gynecol. 2018;218(6):612.e1-612.e6.
224. Crovetto F, Crispi F, Scazzocchio E, et al. First-trimester screening for early and late small-for-gestational-age neonates using maternal serum biochemistry, blood pressure and uterine artery Doppler. Ultrasound Obstet Gynecol. 2014;43(1):34-40.
225. Sweeting AN, Wong J, Appelblom H, et al. A Novel Early Pregnancy Risk Prediction Model for Gestational Diabetes Mellitus. Fetal Diagn Ther. 2019;45(2):76-84.
226. El-Achi V, de Vries B, O'Brien C, et al. First-Trimester Prediction of Preterm Prelabour Rupture of Membranes. Fetal Diagn Ther. 2020;47(8):624-9.
227. Greco E, Gupta R, Syngelaki A, et al. First-trimester screening for spontaneous preterm delivery with maternal characteristics and cervical length. Fetal Diagn Ther. 2012;31(3):154-61.

13

CHAPTER

Fetal Biometry

Frederico Rocha, Ivica Zalud

INTRODUCTION

It is important to understand some definitions applied to fetal biometry. Conceptional age is the age of the fetus from the day of fertilization. In obstetrics, we conventionally use the term gestational age as the fetal age. However, gestational age is the conceptional age plus 14 days, and it is also called menstrual age. For clinical and ultrasound purposes, we use the term gestational age when referring to the measurements of the embryo or fetus.

Ultrasound permits an accurate determination of gestational age and is also an important tool for the assessment of fetal growth and diagnosis of fetal growth disorders. When the gestational age is established, the pregnancy should not be redated.[1]

Accurate dating is essential for the proper timing of chorionic villi sampling and nuchal translucency (NT) assessment in the first trimester, amniocentesis in the second trimester as well as relating the various maternal blood serum levels to risk factors and timing for elective cesarean section.[1]

The focus of this chapter is to review the methods of biometric measurements and estimation of gestational age and fetal growth.

FIRST-TRIMESTER MEASUREMENTS

Gestational Sac

The first definitive sonographic sign to suggest early pregnancy is visualization of the gestational sac **(Fig. 1)**. Gestational sac size measurement should be determined by calculating the mean sac diameter (MSD). This value is obtained by adding the three orthogonal sac diameter dimensions of the chorionic cavity and dividing by three. To correctly measure sac diameter, the cursors should be placed on the sac itself and should not include the echogenic region surrounding the gestational sac.[2] Gestational sac grows 1–2 mm in early pregnancy, but it is less accurate when the embryonic or fetal pole is identified.[2] Gestational sac measurements have only moderate accuracy in establishing gestational age. Intraobserver variability is significant and alternative measurements (e.g., CRL) are more superior. We use gestational sac measurements only in the case when the embryo is not visualized, and the last menstrual period is unknown.

Crown–Rump Length

The crown–rump length (CRL) is considered the standard biometric measurement of the embryo in the first trimester.[3] By definition, the crown-rump length is the longest straight-line measurement of the embryo measured from the outer margin of the cephalic pole to the rump **(Fig. 2)**. Tables have been formulated to estimate gestational age for each numeric measurement of CRL up to 120 mm.[3-5] In general, when the CRL is under 25 mm, the GA (in days) is CRL+42.[4]

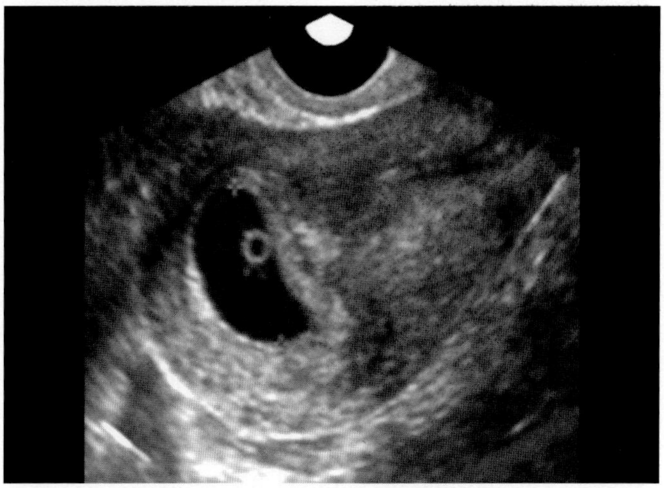

Fig. 1: Gestational sac measurements. Yolk sac is also visible.

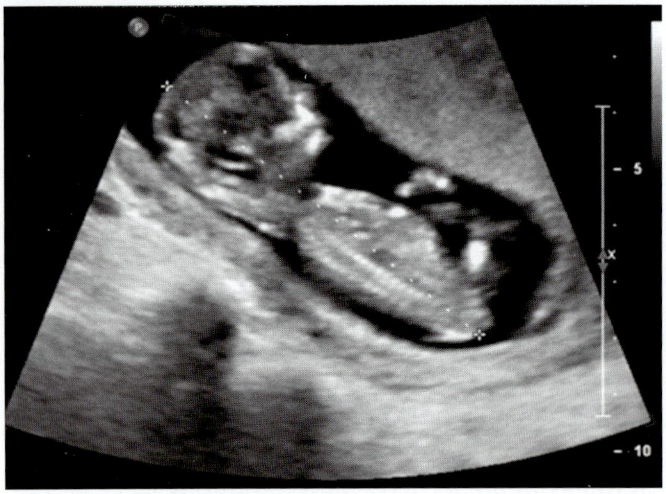

Fig. 2: Crown–rump length measurement in a 13 weeks 1 day fetus.

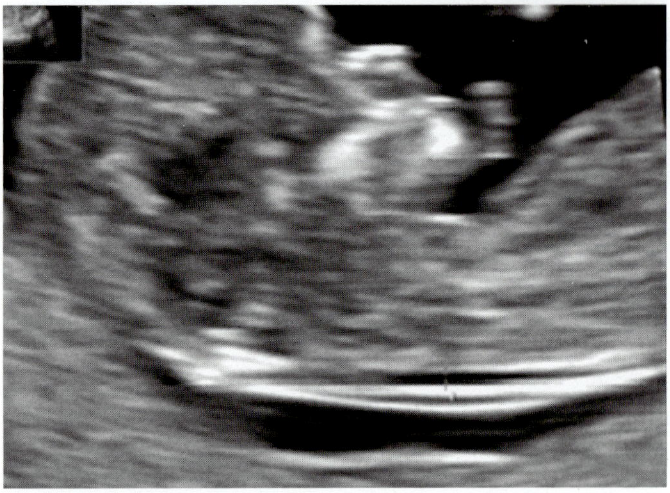

Fig. 3: Nuchal translucency measurement.

Standard practice for determining gestational age is to take the mean of three CRL measurements.[6] When CRL is measured between 7 and 10 weeks, this method is accurate within 3 days.[3,6] However, accuracy wanes as the gestation progresses. Estimation of gestational age by CRL between 10 and 14 weeks is accurate within ±5 days.[7,8] The CRL remains the standard biometric measurement for first-trimester estimation of gestational age up to 14 weeks. In our practice, if CRL is more than 5 mm, embryonic cardiac activity has to be documented; otherwise, the diagnosis of missed abortion is made.

Nuchal Translucency

Nuchal translucency is the subcutaneous collection of fluid behind the fetal back and neck. This hypoechoic space is presumed to represent mesenchymal edema and is often associated with distended jugular lymphatic.[9] An NT >95th percentile is strongly associated with fetal chromosomal abnormalities, isolated heart defects, intrauterine fetal demise, structural malformations and rare genetic syndromes.[10] The optimal gestational age for measurement of fetal NT is 11 weeks to 13 weeks and 6 days. The minimum fetal crown-rump length should be 45 mm and the maximum 84 mm.[11,12] This gestational time frame might vary between different clinical practices and genetic laboratories. In our practice, we use NT measurement as a part of the sequential screen in the risk assessment for aneuploidy. Genetic counseling is integrated in evaluation process. The optimal time for NT assessment is between 10 weeks 3 days and 13 weeks and 6 days of gestation or CRL 39–84 mm. The use of NT measurements in assessment of aneuploidy has been studied excessively. In order to perform NT measurements, individuals need to possess ultrasound proficiency certified by appropriate authority or society with constant quality assurance and improvement processes in place. The NT measurements in combination with serum analytes is excellent screening test for aneuploidy.

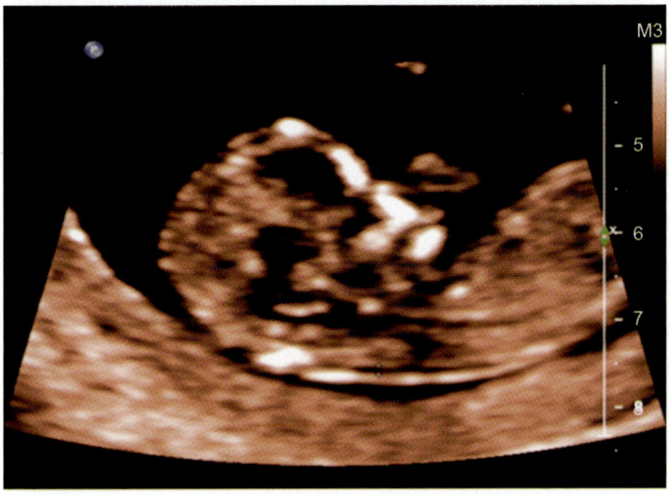

Fig. 4: Another normal nuchal translucency measurement.

Only the fetal head and upper thorax should be included in the image for the measurement of NT **(Figs. 3 and 4)**. A sagittal section of the fetus, as for measurement of fetal crown-rump length, should be obtained and the NT should be measured with the fetus in the neutral position. The maximum thickness of the subcutaneous

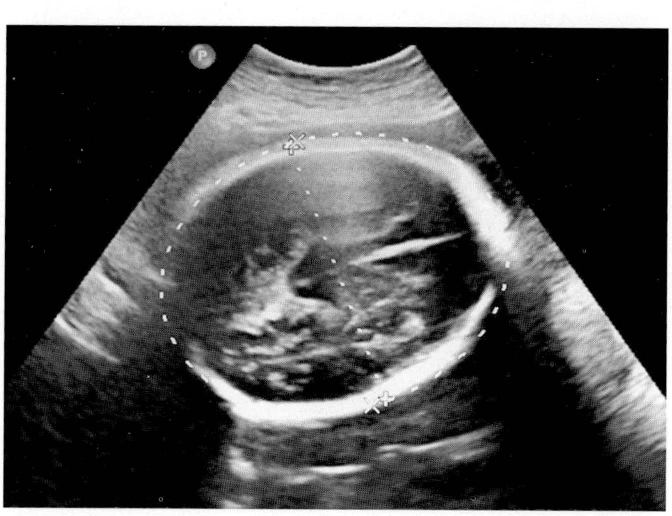

Fig. 5: Head circumference and biparietal diameter measurement.

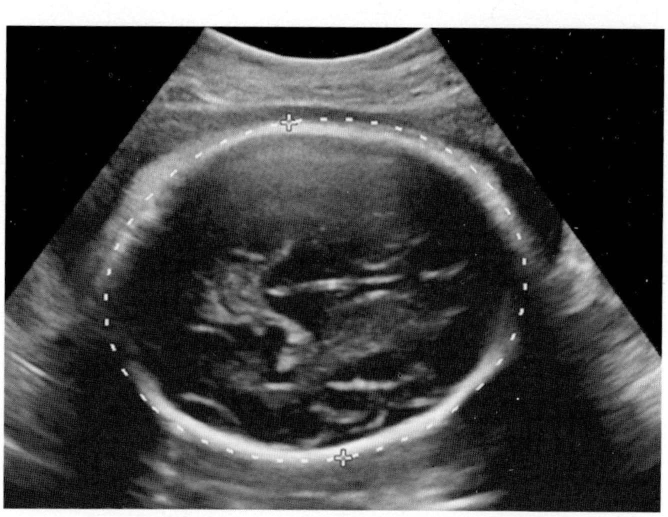

Fig. 6: Head circumference measurement.

translucency between the skin and the soft tissue overlying the cervical spine should be measured. The calipers should be placed on the lines that define the NT thickness from its inner-to-inner borders. Care must be taken to distinguish between fetal skin and amnion because, at this gestation, both structures appear as thin membranes.[11,12]

SECOND-TRIMESTER MEASUREMENTS

The four standard biometric parameters commonly used to estimate gestational age and/or fetal weight in the second and third trimesters are biparietal diameter (BPD), head circumference (HC), abdominal circumference (AC) and femur length (FL).

Biparietal Diameter

Biparietal diameter is measured at the level of the thalami and cavum septum pellucidum (CSP) **(Fig. 5)**. The cerebellar hemispheres should not be visible in this scanning plane. The measurement is taken from the outer edge of the proximal skull to the inner edge of the distal skull.[11] It is the best studied biometric parameter because it is highly reproducible and can predict gestational age within ±7 days when measured between 14 and 20 weeks of gestation.[13-15] By the mid to late third trimester, the margin of error is 3–4 weeks. This significant variation is likely due to a large normal biological variation in fetal shape and size near term.[13-15]

In late pregnancy, it can be difficult to obtain the ideal imaging plane due to the head lying low in the pelvis. A change in head shape due to molding can cause dolichocephaly (flattened and elongated) or brachycephaly which can affect the BPD measurement.[16,17] When this occurs the cephalic index (CI) should be measured. Cephalic index refers to the ratio of the BPD and the occipitofrontal diameter (OFD) multiplied by 100 [CI = (BPD/OFD) × 100%].[16-18]

The standard CI range for normal shaped craniums approximates one standard deviation from the mean (>74 or <83). Therefore, if the CI measurement approaches the outer limits of the normal range, the use of the BPD for estimation of gestational age is not accurate.[16-18]

Head Circumference

Head circumference is measured at the same level as the biparietal diameter, around the outer perimeter of the calvarium **(Figs. 5 and 6)**. This measurement is not affected by shape of the head. It is important to avoid measuring the outer margin of the skin overlying the scalp, since doing so will falsely increase the HC.[11]

Femur Length

Femoral diaphysis length can be reliably used after 14 weeks' gestational age **(Fig. 7)**. The long axis of the femoral shaft is most accurately measured with the beam of insonation being perpendicular to the shaft, excluding the distal femoral epiphysis.[11]

Abdominal Circumference

Abdominal circumference or average abdominal diameter should be determined at the skin line on a true transverse

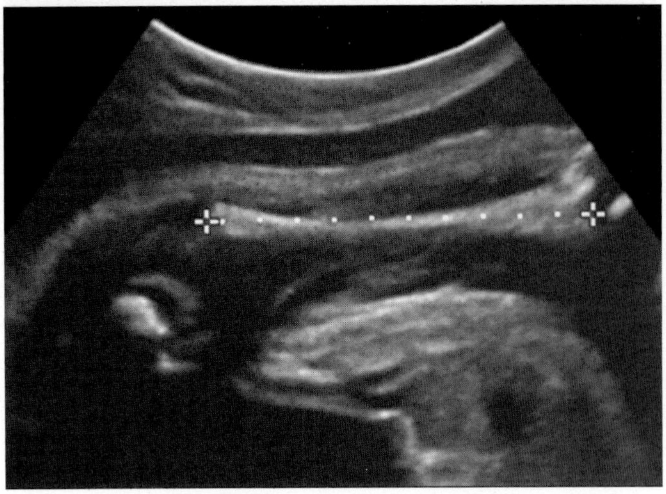

Fig. 7: Femur length measurement.

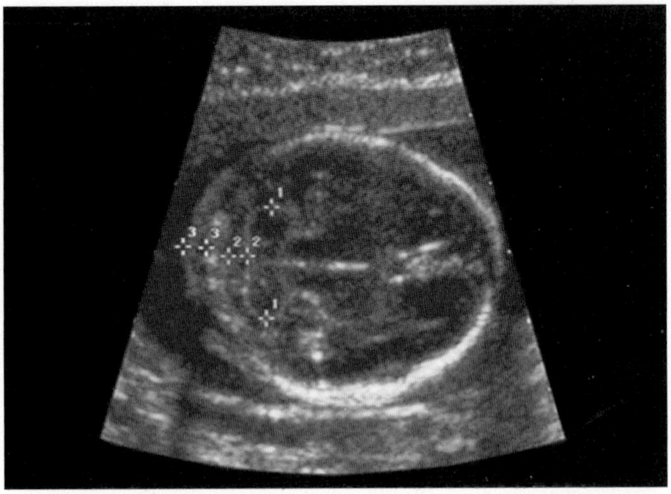

Fig. 9: Measurement of the cerebellum, posterior fossa and nuchal fold.

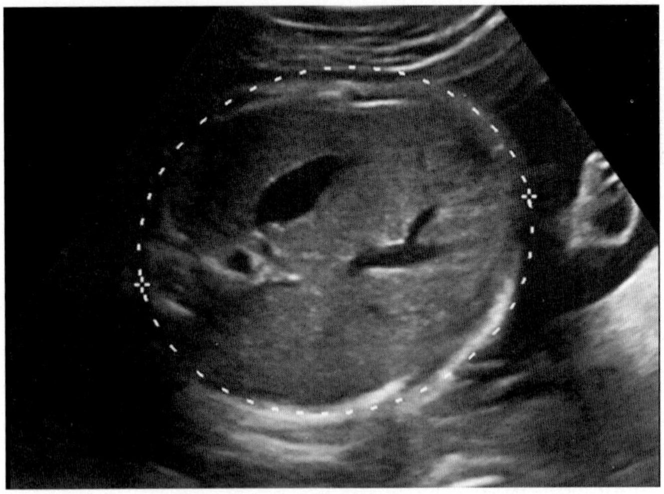

Fig. 8: Abdominal circumference.

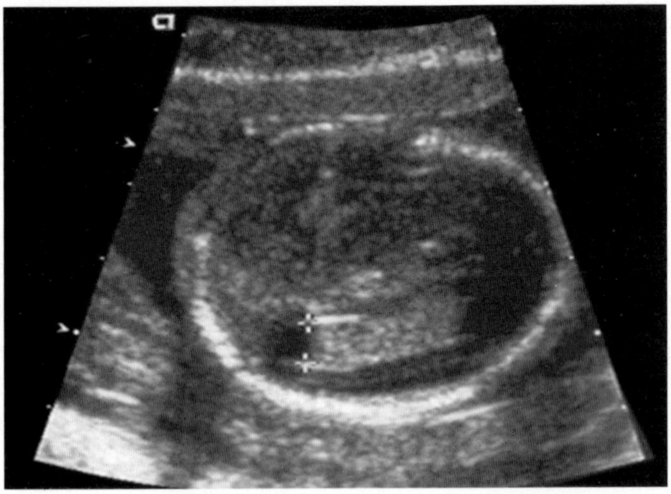

Fig. 10: Posterior horn of the lateral ventricles.

view at the level of the junction of the umbilical vein, portal sinus and fetal stomach when visible **(Fig. 8)**.[11] Several studies have stated that this imaging plane is the most difficult to obtain, especially in late pregnancy and yet is one of the most essential for inclusion in a fetal weight formula.[11]

Other Measurements

Ultrasound evaluation and measurements of cerebellum, posterior fossa, nuchal fold, posterior horn of the lateral ventricle and renal pelvis are part of detailed anatomical survey **(Figs. 9 to 11)**. Those measurements have role in anatomical integrity and aneuploidy assessment and are not routinely used for gestational age or fetal growth evaluation. For more details, please see other chapters in the book.

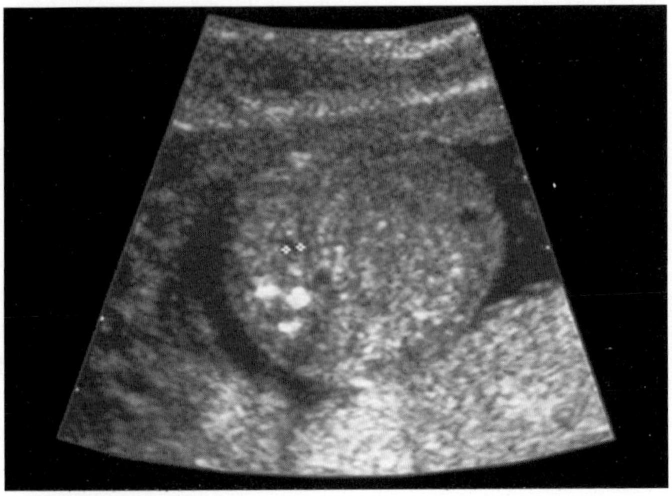

Fig. 11: Anterior-posterior diameter of the renal pelvis.

Estimating Fetal Age Using Multiple Markers

A number of combinations of fetal parameters, including the combination of head circumference and femur length, provided age estimates that were significantly better than those using any single parameter alone.[19,20] Hadlock and colleagues showed that in 177 normal pregnancies, there was significant improvement in the ultrasound estimation of estimated date of delivery when two or more parameters were used to make that estimate, rather than just BPD alone.[19] Before 36 weeks' gestation, the optimal combination of parameters included the BPD, AC and FL. However, after 36 weeks, the HC, AC and FL gave the best estimate with significant reduction in the mean errors, standard deviation, and size of maximum error.

Chervenak et al. published a large study of patients conceived by IVF, to assess the accuracy of fetal biometry in the second trimester of pregnancy for assignment of fetal age. Results showed that head circumference was the best individual predictor of fetal age. The addition of abdominal circumference and femur length to head circumference improved the overall accuracy of dating compared with any individual measurement. The study concluded that the use of fetal biometry in the second trimester is also an accurate means of establishing gestational age within 7 days.[21]

Third-trimester sonographic estimation of gestational age has been proven to be an inaccurate method with median error of plus or minus three weeks after 30 weeks gestation.[21,22] The imprecision of the measurements occur primarily because of the normal variability among fetuses. The accuracy of third-trimester biometric measurements is also impaired by fetal crowding, shadowing from other fetal bony parts, diminished amniotic fluid volumes and descent of the presenting part into the pelvis.[23]

Other non-traditional methods of biometry have been attempted as an alternative to aid in the determination of the gestational age in late gestation. Those include transverse cerebellar diameter, fetal foot length epiphyseal ossification centers.[24] Among those the transverse cerebellar diameter in millimeters correlates well with the gestational age up to 22–24 weeks.[24-26]

Ultrasound fetal biometry requires training and it can be time consuming. A new concept that could improve efficiency and limit the measurement errors by inexperienced sonographers is the automatic fetal measurements by the pattern recognition **(Fig. 12)**. This approach could reduce keystrokes and therefore reduce repetitive stress injuries. It could also improve everyday work-flow to increase patient productivity.[22]

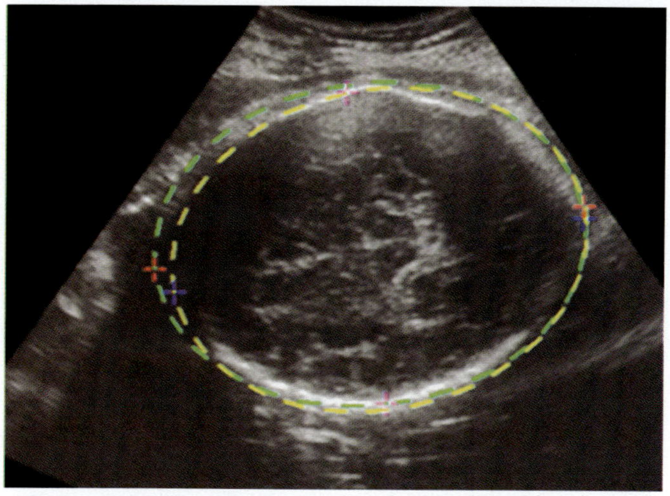

Fig. 12: Automatic measurements of the head circumference generated by pattern recognition software.

Estimating Fetal Weight

A variety of formulas are used for prediction of fetal weight. Not all authorities agree on any formula derived from fetal parts measurements.[27] Fetuses from different populations may show different growth patterns. Race and parity are important parameters to consider when applying general population growth curves.[28-31] Birth weight standards vary from one population to another, depending upon ethnicity and environmental and socioeconomic circumstances.[28,30] Fetal growth formulas provide weight estimates with errors of up to 20% when compared with actual birth weights.[11,13-15] A study reported a general tendency to underestimate the weight in fetuses with high birth weight (>4,000 g).[32-34]

Three-dimensional Biometry

The introduction of three-dimensional (3D) ultrasound imaging has allowed the accurate and reliable calculation of fetal organ volumes. Some authors have demonstrated that the prediction of birth weight using fetal limb volumetry is more precise than that obtained using conventional 2D ultrasound parameters.[29] Different organ volumes have been used, including kidneys, adrenal gland, brain, cerebellum and fetal thigh. The 3D ultrasound techniques require technically advanced and expensive equipment, special operator training and skills, and are time consuming.[35] At present, it does not seem reasonable to abandon the 2D ultrasound methods in favor of 3D ultrasound imaging for fetal weight estimation.[35]

CONCLUSION

The application of fetal biometric measurements in routine obstetrical care has definitely become part of the standard of care. Ultrasound evaluation is essential to confirm or establish gestational age. In the first trimester, its use has optimized the establishment of an accurate pregnancy dating and also as an important tool in the screening for chromosomal anomalies. Later in gestation, the biometric measurements of a fetus help estimate fetal weight and follow the growth. The use of customized growth curves appropriate for local population may help improve the accuracy of the biometric estimates for the fetus.

REFERENCES

1. ACOG Practice Bulletin No. 101: Ultrasonography in pregnancy. Obstet Gynecol. 2009;113(2 Pt 1):451-61.
2. Laing FC, Frates MC. Ultrasound evaluation during the first trimester of pregnancy. In: Callen PW (Ed): Ultrasonography in Obstetrics and Gynecology. 4th edn. Philadelphia: WB Saunders; 2000.
3. Robinson HP, Fleming JE. A critical evaluation of sonar "crown-rump length" measurements. Br J Obstet Gynaecol. 1975;82(9):702-10.
4. Goldstein SR, Wolfson R. Endovaginal ultrasonographic measurement of early embryonic size as a means of assessing gestational age. J Ultrasound Med. 1994;13(1):27-31.
5. Daya S. Accuracy of gestational age estimation by means of fetal crown-rump length measurement. Am J Obstet Gynecol. 1993;168(3):903-8.
6. Kalish RB. Sonographic determination of the gestational age. In: Asim Kurjak (Ed): Donald School Textbook of Ultrasound in Obstetrics and Gynecology, 2nd edn. New Delhi: Jaypee Brothers Medical Publishers; 2008.
7. Hadlock FP, Shah YP, Kanon DJ, et al. Fetal crown-rump length: reevaluation of relation to menstrual age (5-18 weeks) with high-resolution real-time US. Radiology. 1992;182(2):501-5.
8. MacGregor SN, Tamura RK, Sabbagha RE, et al. Underestimation of gestational age by conventional crown-rump length dating curves. Obstet Gynecol. 1987;70(3 Pt 1):344-8.
9. Bekker MN, Haak MC, Rekoert-Hollander M, et al. Increased nuchal translucency and distended jugular lymphatic sacs on first-trimester ultrasound. Ultrasound Obstet Gynecol. 2005;25(3):239-45.
10. Haak MC, van Vugt JM. Pathophysiology of increased nuchal translucency: a review of the literature. Human Reproduction Update. 2003;9(2):175-84.
11. AIUM Practice Guideline for the Performance of Obstetric Ultrasound Examinations. AIUM 2007 http://www.aium.org/publications/guidelines/obstetric.pdf (Accessed October 31, 2010).
12. Sebire NJ, Snijders RJM, Hughes K, et al. Screening for trisomy 21 in twin pregnancies by maternal age and fetal nuchal translucency thickness at 10-14 weeks of gestation. BJOG. 1996;103(10):999-1003.
13. Hadlock FP, Harrist RB, Martinez-Poyer J. How accurate is second trimester fetal dating? J Ultrasound Med. 1991;10(10):557-61.
14. Rossavik IK, Fishburne JI. Conceptional age, menstrual age, and ultrasound age: a second-trimester comparison of pregnancies of known conception date with pregnancies dated from the last menstrual period. Obstet Gynecol. 1989;73(2):243-9.
15. Hadlock FP, Deter RL, Harrist RB, et al. Fetal biparietal diameter: rational choice of plane of section for sonographic measurement. AJR A J Roentgenol. 1982;138(5):871-4.
16. O'Keeffe DF, Garite TJ, Elliott JP, et al. The accuracy of estimated gestational age based on ultrasound measurement of biparietal diameter in preterm premature rupture of the membranes. Am J Obstet Gynecol. 1985;151(3): 309-12.
17. Hadlock FP, Deter RL, Carpenter RJ, et al. Estimating fetal age: effect of head shape on BPD. AJR Am J Roentgenol. 1981;137(1):83-5.
18. Gray DL, Songster GS, Parvin CA, et al. Cephalic index: a gestational age-dependent biometric parameter. Obstet Gynecol. 1989;74(4):600-3.
19. Hadlock FP, Deter RL, Harrist RB, et al. Estimating fetal age: computer assisted analysis of multiple fetal growth parameters. Radiology. 1984;152(2):497-501.
20. Hadlock FP, Harrist RB, Shah YP, et al. Estimating fetal age using multiple parameters: a prospective evaluation in a racially mixed population. Am J Obstet Gynecol. 1987;156(4):955-7.
21. Chervenak FA, Skupski DW, Romero R, et al. How accurate is fetal biometry in the assessment of fetal age? Am J Obstet Gynecol. 1998;178(4):678-87.
22. Zalud I, Good S, Carneiro G, et al. Fetal biometry: a comparison between experienced sonographers and automated measurements. J Matern Fetal Neonat Med. 2009;22(1):43-50.
23. Platz E, Newman R. Diagnosis of IUGR: traditional biometry. Semin Perinatol. 2008;32(3):140-7.
24. Gottlieb AG, Galan HL. Nontraditional sonographic pearls in estimating gestational age. Semin Perinatol. 2008;32(3):154-60.
25. Doubilet PM, Benson CB. Improved prediction of gestational age in the late third trimester. J Ultrasound Med. 1993;12(11):647-53.
26. Goldstein I, Reece EA, Pilu G, et al. Cerebellar measurements with ultrasonography in the evaluation of fetal growth and development. Am J Obstet Gynecol. 1987;156(5):1065-9.

27. Degani S. Fetal biometry: clinical, pathological, and technical considerations. Obstet Gynecol Surv. 2001;56(3):159-67.
28. Brenner WE, Edelman DA, Hendricks CH. A standard of fetal growth for the United States of America. Am J Obstet Gynecol. 1976;126(5):555-64.
29. Raju TNK, Winegar A, Seifert L, et al. Birth weight and gestational age standards based on regional perinatal network data: an analysis of risk factors. Am J Perinatol. 1987;4(3):253-8.
30. Mongelli M, Gardosi J. Reduction of false-positive diagnosis of fetal growth restriction by application of customized fetal growth standards. Obstet Gynecol. 1996;88(5):844-8.
31. Zhang J, Bowes WA. Birth-weight-for-gestational-age patterns by race, sex, and parity in the United States population. Obstet Gynecol. 1995;86(2):200-8.
32. Miller JM Jr, Korndorf FA 3rd, Gabert HA. Fetal weight estimates in late pregnancy with emphasis on macrosomia. J Clin Ultrasound. 1986;14(6):437-42.
33. Bennini JR, et al. Birth-weight prediction by two- and three-dimensional ultrasound imaging. Ultrasound Obstet Gynecol. 2010;35(4):426-33.
34. Dudley NJ. A systematic review of the ultrasound estimation of fetal weight. Ultrasound Obstet Gynecol. 2005;25(1): 80-9.
35. Lindell G, Marsál K. Sonographic fetal weight estimation in prolonged pregnancy: comparative study of two- and three-dimensional methods. Ultrasound Obstet Gynecol. 2009;33(3):295-300.

14

CHAPTER

Doppler Ultrasound: State of the Art

William Goh, Ivica Zalud

INTRODUCTION

Christian Doppler first reported on the Doppler effect in 1842 describing the changes in the frequency of a light or sound wave produced by a changing relationship between two objects.[1] The traditional example given to describe the Doppler principle is the sound level when a train approaches and then departs from a station. The frequency of the sound is higher in pitch when the train approaches the station and lower when it departs. The change in sound pitch is also termed a frequency shift and is proportional to the speed of movement of the sound (or light) emitting source.[2] Clinically, the combination of real-time ultrasound with pulse wave Doppler allows the identification of a specific area or blood vessel for sampling. When an ultrasound beam with a certain frequency is used to insonate a blood vessel, the reflected frequency shift is proportional to blood flow velocity within that blood vessel. The frequency shift is highest in systole when blood flow is the fastest and lowest in diastole when flow is slowest. The frequency shift is also angle dependent and velocity is measured accurately when the angle of incidence (cosine Θ) is as small as possible. When a sound beam is perpendicular to the direction of flow, the measured velocity is zero since the cosine of 90° is zero. Using ratios of frequency shifts of flows in systole and diastole, Doppler indices can be made independent of the effects of the angle of the ultrasound beam. The indices used in Doppler ultrasound reflect vascular resistance and include the systolic/diastolic (S/D ratio), the resistance index (RI = systolic velocity-diastolic velocity/systolic velocity) and the pulsatility index (PI = systolic velocity-diastolic velocity/mean velocity).[3] The S/D ratios are used frequently in the United States to assess arterial waveforms though some experts feel that the PI is a more reproducible index.

PULSED DOPPLER ULTRASOUND IN MATERNAL FETAL MEDICINE

Umbilical Artery Doppler

Umbilical artery Doppler is easy to obtain **(Figs. 1 and 2)**. Using a combination of pulsed echo and continuous wave Doppler ultrasound, Stuart et al. first characterized umbilical artery (UA) velocity waveforms in normal pregnancies from 16 to 20 weeks of gestation and showed that umbilical artery angle independent indices decreased with advancing gestation.[4] Trudinger et al. then showed that ratios of peak systolic to least diastolic flow velocities in umbilical arteries became abnormal in pathologic conditions, such as intrauterine growth restriction (IUGR).[5] A meta-analysis of UA Doppler in the management of high-risk pregnancies for preeclampsia and IUGR has been shown to reduce antenatal admissions by 44%, labor induction by 29%, cesarean section for non-reassuring fetal heart tracings by 52% and more importantly perinatal mortality by 38%.[6] Absent or reverse

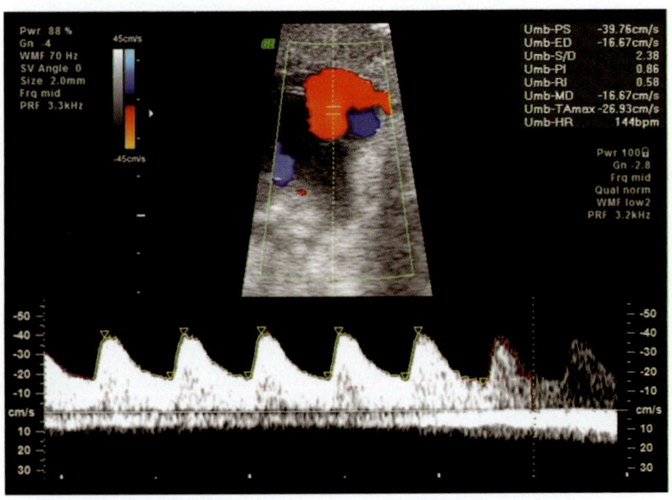

Fig. 1: Umbilical artery Doppler: Normal blood flow.

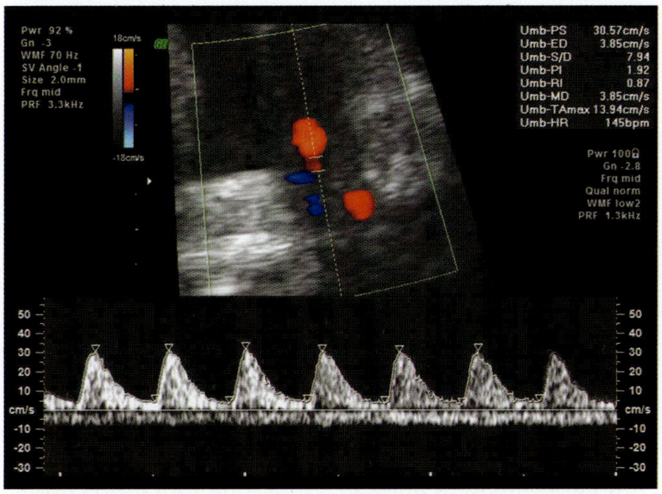

Fig. 2: Umbilical artery Doppler: Abnormal blood flow with increased resistance.

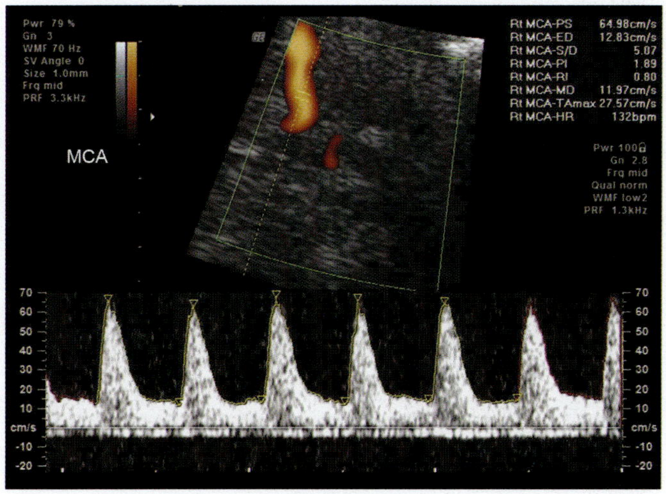

Fig. 3: Abnormal MCA Doppler with high peak velocity blood flow.

end-diastolic flow in the UA is now clearly shown to be associated with advanced fetal compromise and associated with increased perinatal morbidity and mortality and is an indication for delivery. The measurement of Doppler flow in the UA is also an excellent tool to aid in prognosis in pregnancies complicated by twin-twin transfusion syndrome (TTTS). Absent end-diastolic flow in the donor twin is associated with a higher risk of intrauterine fetal demise of the donor when patients are undergoing either amnioreduction or laser therapy for TTTS. Kontopoulos et al. have recommended assessment of AEDV in the preoperative evaluation of TTTS patients.[7]

Middle Cerebral Artery Doppler

The middle cerebral artery (MCA) is the most studied cerebral artery because it is the most accessible cerebral vessel and it carries 80% of the cerebral blood flow. It can be sampled at an angle of 0° between the ultrasound beam and the direction of blood flow and the real velocity of blood flow is actually measured in the form of a peak systolic velocity (PSV). One of the most important applications of Doppler technology in obstetrics has been the detection of fetal anemia in pregnancies complicated by red cell isoimmunization or other causes **(Fig. 3)**. There appears to be excellent reproducibility when the proximal vessel is sampled after its origin from the internal carotid artery. A PSV above 1.5 MoM for the fetus' gestational age has been shown to have a 100% sensitivity for detecting fetal anemia.[8] The MCA PSV is actually more reliable than the delta OD450 in the diagnosis of fetal anemia leading ACOG to issue a statement that Doppler ultrasound evaluation in the management of alloimmunization allows for a more thorough and less invasive workup with fewer risks to mother and fetus.[9] Besides diagnosis and management of fetal anemia, MCA PSV may also be helpful in the management of monochorionic diamniotic pregnancies complicated by twin anemia polycythemia sequence (TAPS). Five percent of monochorionic diamniotic pregnancies are complicated by large intertwin hemoglobin differences in the absence of amniotic fluid discordances. Slaghekke et al. have shown that the recipient twin in these pregnancies have MCA PSV's <0.8 MoM.[10] In addition to donor anemia, the diagnosis of TAPS is important because the recipient twin is at risk for thrombocytopenia and polycythemia-hyperviscosity syndrome. The MCA PSV is also a new parameter in the assessment of IUGR. Mari et al. showed that MCA waveforms change in growth restricted fetuses and is a more significantly related to fetal hypoxemia and hypercapnia.[11] These changes are suggestive of fetal brain autoregulation.

Uterine Artery Doppler

The uterine artery can be assessed as it crosses over the external iliac artery **(Fig. 4)**. Inter- and intraobserver variability has been reported to be about 10%.[12] Significant decrease in the S/D ratio of the uterine artery (UtA) occurs with advancing gestation until 26 weeks as diastolic velocities increase.[3] This is a result of normal trophoblastic invasion leading to spiral artery remodeling

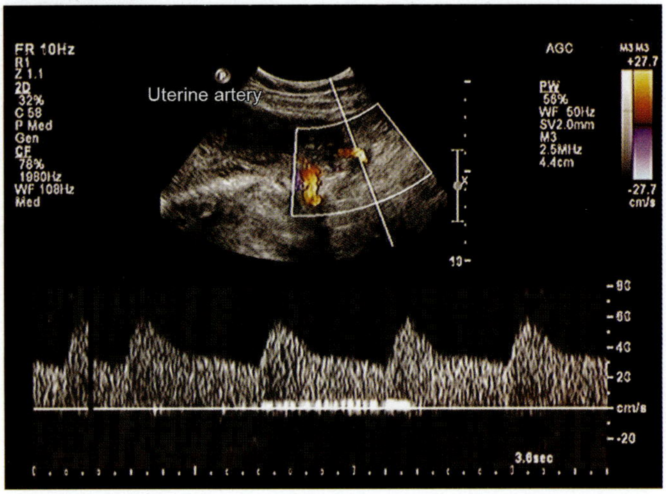

Fig. 4: Uterine artery Doppler in normal pregnancy.

resulting in a low-resistance system that allows for the normal maternal-fetal exchange of nutrients, waste and metabolites. Phupong and Dejthevaporn showed that a disruption of this transition from high to low impedance was associated with an increased risk of preeclampsia and small for gestational age infants in previously healthy nulliparous women.[13] Onwudiwe et al. also showed that UtA Doppler screening played a significant role in the prediction of a small for gestational age (SGA) neonate, preeclampsia and also gestational hypertension.[14] In the presence of obstetric complications, such as fetal growth restriction, UtA Doppler identifies the fetus at higher risk for preterm delivery and lower birth weight. Li et al. showed that bilateral UtA notching was a more significant predictor of adverse pregnancy outcome when compared to umbilical artery Doppler.[15] Ferrazzi et al. showed that abnormal UtA Doppler in pregnancies complicated by IUGR was an important indicator of hypoxic or ischemic placental lesions.[16] Abnormal UtA Dopplers in fetus with growth restriction also identify mothers with an increased risk of the development of preeclampsia later in pregnancy.[17] In addition, abnormal UtA Doppler in high-risk pregnancies appears to be a significant predicator of the need for cesarean section, SGA neonate and prematurity that was independent and superior to that of umbilical artery Doppler.[18] UtA Doppler studies are considered investigational in the USA.

Umbilical Cord Compression

Abnormalities of the umbilical cord (e.g., velamentous insertions, true knots and strictures) are usually only noted postpartum. Abuhamad et al. first showed the umbilical artery Doppler waveforms can be abnormal in monoamniotic twin pregnancies complicated by cord entanglement.[19] In a prospective trial, Abuhamad et al. showed that UA waveform notching appears to be a strong predictor of cord entanglement, true knots, cord stricture, velamentous insertion, tight nuchal cords and abnormal cord coiling.[20]

Venous Doppler

Doppler applications in obstetrics have largely focused on arterial flow profiles which give information on downstream impedance and upstream pressure. Venous Doppler evaluation allows estimation of forward cardiac function and venous distribution.[21] With the exception of the umbilical vein, all veins have a 4-phase flow pattern. Forward velocity are highest during ventricular systole (S) and early diastole (D). Velocity are lower during the ascent of the atrioventricular ring (v) and especially during atrial systole (A).

Ductus Venosus

The fetal circulation consists of two parallel blood streams that are uniquely partitioned. The single umbilical vein carries oxygenated blood from the placenta to the fetus reaching the fetal liver as the first major organ. A 55% of the blood flow is diverted to the left lobe, 20% to the right lobe and 25% to the ductus venosus (DV) towards the heart. The DV acts as the first partition determining the proportion of umbilical venous blood diverted to the heart and it carries the most rapidly moving blood in the venous system and is thus easily identifiable on Doppler ultrasound **(Fig. 5)**. Rizzo et al. studied Doppler indices from both the inferior vena cava (IVC) and DV and compared these values to cordocentesis derived blood sampling in IUGR fetuses and showed that abnormal DV S/A ratios could predict hypoxemia in this subgroup.[22] Several authors have reported on the use of DV studies in the prediction of fetal compromise in IUGR and other vascular abnormalities allowing for delivery prior to changes in biophysical profile scores. Baschat et al. showed that DV Doppler parameters combined with IVC and UV Doppler measurements correctly predicted acid-base status in a significant proportion of IUGR neonates.[23] Similarly, Schwarze et al. showed that abnormal DV waveforms in preterm IUGR fetuses along with ARED was strongly associated with adverse fetal and perinatal

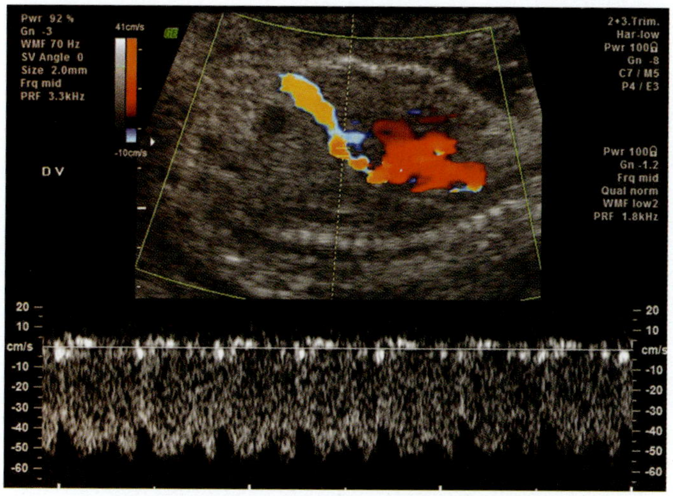

Fig. 5: Normal ductus venosus blood flow.

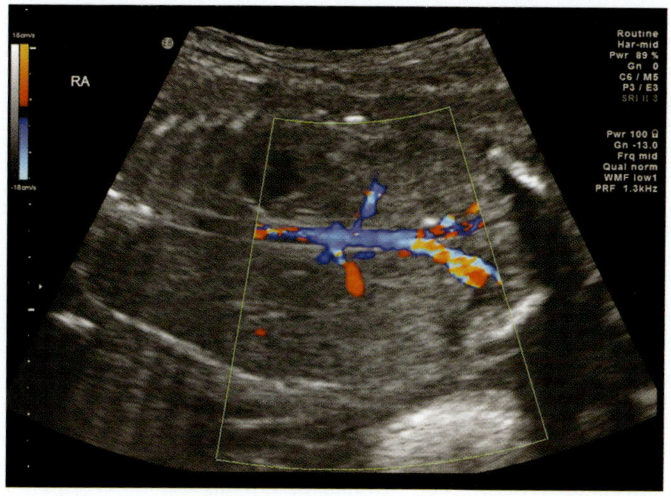

Fig. 6: Renal artery color Doppler.

outcome less than 32 weeks allowing for better timing of delivery.[24] Mari et al. caution that DV waveforms alone cannot be used as the sole indicator for delivery, especially in the IUGR fetus less than 30 weeks.[25] They recommend using MCA PSV along with DV reversed flow as indicators for delivery, given the high perinatal mortality rates when IUGR fetuses are delivered less than 29 weeks of gestation.

Umbilical Vein

Umbilical vein Doppler provide information on fetal forward cardiac flow. Until 15 weeks, the umbilical vein has pulsations which are related to IVC patterns.[26] After this gestational age, pulsations may be associated with fetal heart accelerations, breathing and cord constriction. Pulsations may also be seen in the presence of severe IUGR and fetal hydrops.[27] Hofstaetter et al. showed umbilical vein pulsations were a more sensitive indicator of heart failure in fetal hydrops compared to heart size, cardiac function, arterial Doppler and DV measurements.[28]

Other Veins

The hepatic veins and IVC share characteristics with the DV but is not easily interpreted. The portal veins have no pulsations, and respond to fetal hypoxemia.[29] The ease of measuring the DV however makes it the vessel of choice in venous Doppler measurements currently.

COLOR AND POWER DOPPLER IMAGING

Doppler imaging has provided velocity information when their beams are directed at blood vessels, and this technology has been available for many years. However, real-time Doppler imaging only became available with fast signal processing which produces several images per second of the scanned region.[30] Fast signal processing allows for the production of color Doppler velocity images and Power Doppler image. Color Doppler shows the direction of flow information extracted by the electronics from the sequence of returning echoes (red denoting flow toward the transducer and blue away). Power Doppler images are generated when the power level at each image pixel is presented as a level of brightness. Image brightness is uniform except at vessel walls or in turbulent areas making power Doppler a sensitive technique for depicting flow in small vessels.

Color and power Doppler ultrasound has been used to image the vasculature of the fetal lung, kidney and brain **(Fig. 6)**.[31] Since Power Doppler has the advantage of displaying intensity of a returning Doppler signal, it is less dependent on the orientation of the blood vessel and is a useful technology to use in obstetrical imaging. Guerriero et al. used transvaginal color Doppler imaging to diagnose prenatal intracranial hemorrhage in the second trimester[32] and Pilu et al. have used this technology to correctly identify discrepant intracranial vasculature allowing for prenatal microcephaly diagnosis.[33] Fetal sacrococcygeal teratomas have been diagnosed prenatally using amplitude-based color Doppler sonography.[34] Other applications of color Doppler imaging in pregnancy include fetal echocardiography[35] and the identification of renal arteries in pregnancies complicated by oligohydramnios.[36]

A major application of color Doppler in obstetrics is the evaluation of the placenta and is useful for the antenatal diagnosis of placenta previa, placenta accreta and vasa previa.[37,38] The accuracy of in vivo detection of arterioarterial anastomoses in monochorionic twins and its protection against the development of twin-to-twin transfusion syndrome was found to be highly specific with the use of power Doppler ultrasound technology and has been advocated as having a role in the stratification of antenatal assessment of monochorionic twins.[39]

DOPPLER ULTRASOUND IN THREE-DIMENSIONS

Three-dimension (3D) ultrasound is a natural development in the evolution of ultrasound technology. The acquisition of data points throughout an entire volume of interest is required to produce a 3D ultrasound picture.[31] Slow acquisition speeds yield more scanned slices and volume data points and is used to image static organs whereas fast speeds are used for imaging moving structures, such as fetuses. Ultra fast acquisition allow for four-dimensional (4D) real-time imaging. 3D imaging reconstruction is voxel-based with the voxel being the smallest 3D picture unit. This allows for each pixel (smallest 2D picture unit) to be placed in the correct position in 3D volume reconstruction.

3D Power Doppler

This technology allows for the three-dimensional reconstruction of vessels after their visualization using power Doppler ultrasound **(Fig. 7)**. Instead of frequency shifts, 3D power Doppler analyzes amplitude signals and has been shown to be three to five times more sensitive than conventional color Doppler in visualizing small vessels and slower flows.[39] Additionally, vessel visualization is not affected by angle of insonation and is not susceptible to aliasing. Three-dimensional quantification of blood flow from color Doppler is not possible. A new method for blood flow and vascularization has been developed to better depict overall blood flow in 3D power Doppler studies.[40] The vascularization index (VI) = color voxels/(total voxels - background voxels) and measures flow in a region of interest. Flow index (FI) = weighted color voxels/(color voxels - border voxels) and measures the intensity of color flow in a region of interest and is not an indicator of perfusion. The vascularization flow Index (VFI) = weighted color voxels/(total voxels - background voxels) and combines the percent of color voxels and intensity in a region of interest and therefore represents both blood flow and vascularization.

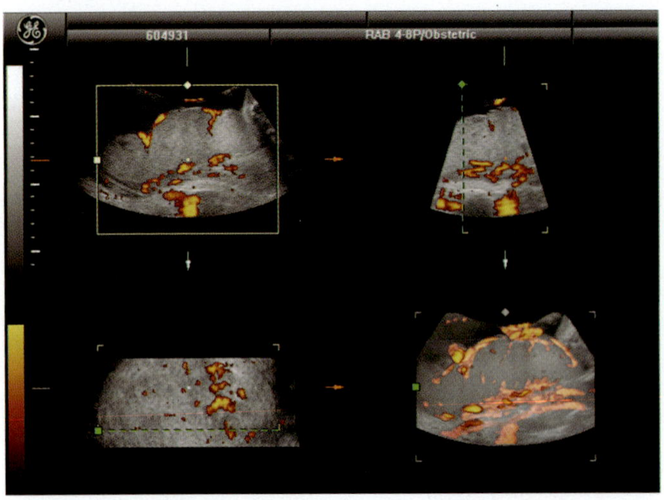

Fig. 7: 3D Doppler of normal placenta.

3D Doppler ultrasound is advantageous for the study of normal uterine, placental and fetal cardiovascular development. The 3D Doppler reconstruction of ultrasound images has become an available option on ultrasound equipments. Several clinical applications are feasible in all parenchymatous organs (mainly the liver and kidneys), peripheral vessels (supra-aortic trunks and limb vessels) and central (the aorta and iliac arteries) or cerebral vessels. Moreover, tumoral vessels in parenchymatous organs can be reconstructed, and the fetal blood flow can be seen with excellent detailing. The introduction of 3D has permitted to study normal and abnormal peripheral, central and parenchymatous vessels, with similar patterns to those obtained with digital angiography. The spatial relationships between the vascular structures of the placenta were studied with 3D ultrasound angiograms. The applications of this new technique include the analysis of vascular anatomy and the potential assessment of organ perfusion in the future.

Doppler ultrasound waveform analysis of the maternal-fetal circulation has emerged to add useful information in the determination of fetal wellbeing. One of potential application of 3D Doppler could be in the study of vascular changes in patients with IUGR and preeclampsia. It is a known fact that IUGR and preeclampsia is commonly associated with deficient trophoblastic invasion of the maternal spiral arteries during the first and second trimester. This problem can produce abnormally increased resistance to flow through the uterine circulation, and the resulting placental insufficiency can significantly reduce the delivery of oxygen to the fetus. Abnormal placental development is associated with fetal and neonatal morbidity, growth impairment, incidence of major congenital anomalies, increased incidence of preterm birth, fetal non-reassuring status in labor, neonatal intensive care admissions, and overall mortality. If proven clinically useful in large scale prospective studies, 3D Doppler evaluation of placenta could establish a foundation for earlier in vivo recognition of homodynamic changes in preeclampsia and possibly in IUGR. Three-dimensional power Doppler sonography has the potential to study the process of placentation and evaluate the development of the embryonic and fetal cardiovascular system.[41,42]

Matijevic and Kurjak compared the performance of 2D and 3D power Doppler ultrasound in the visualization of the placental vascular network during ongoing pregnancy.[43] There was no difference in the visualization of primary placental stem vessels by 2D and 3D power Doppler. However, 3D power Doppler performed better distally, with statistically significant differences at the level of secondary stem, and even more prominent differences at the level of tertiary stem vessels. There was no difference in the visualization rate of radial and spiral arteries. The authors concluded that 3D Doppler was superior to 2D Doppler in the determination of the distal vascular branches of the fetal placental blood vessels.

The relationship of large and vascularized chorioangiomas and adverse pregnancy outcome is well recognized. Shih et al. studied a patient with a large placental tumor and signs of impending fetal cardiac failure.[44] The angioarchitecture of the tumor depicted by three-dimensional (3D) power Doppler ultrasound enabled them to accurately diagnose a placental chorioangioma. During the follow-up period, quantitative flow data obtained using 3D power Doppler indicated altered hemodynamics in the tumor and concomitant improvement in the condition of the fetus, enabling them to manage the mother conservatively. Spontaneous delivery occurred at 38 weeks without any complications. This report demonstrates the potential value of 3D power Doppler in prenatal diagnosis and monitoring of pregnancies complicated by large, vascularized chorioangioma.

3D Doppler ultrasound is a new method which allows the spatial presentation of fetal vessels in utero. Hartung et al. have examined the feasibility of this technique in prenatal diagnosis.[45] The aim of their study with normal human fetuses was to determine the adjustment of the system presets, the optimal insonation planes and the regions of interest. Seven regions of interest were examined in three different planes. Best examinations were achieved in the vessels of the umbilical cord (successful rate 100%), followed by the placental and abdominal (84% each), cerebral (80%), pulmonary (64%), and renal vessels (51%). The most difficult conditions for examination and the most unreliable results were found for the fetal heart with a success rate of only 31% of the cases. Similar to the experience in 2D power Doppler, a plane with blood flow towards the transducer was the best insonation plane. In this study the authors were able to show that 3D Doppler of fetal vessels is possible. The feasibility is limited by fetal movements and unfavorable fetal positioning. The possible benefit of the method is to diagnose complex fetal vascular malformations in the future.

Ritchie et al. have developed a system for producing 3D angiograms from a series of two-dimensional power-mode Doppler ultrasound.[46] Two-dimensional Doppler scans were acquired using a commercial scanner and image-registration hardware. Two-dimensional images were then digitized, and specially designed software reconstructed 3D volumes and displayed volume-rendered images. Scanning a flow phantom constructed from tubing assessed the geometric accuracy of their system. The system was tested on patients by scanning native and transplanted kidneys, and placentas. Three-dimensional images of the phantoms depicted the spatial relationships between blood flows within the tubing segments and contained less than 1 mm of geometric distortion. Three-dimensional images of the kidney and placenta demonstrated that spatial relationships between vasculature structures could be visualized with 3D Doppler ultrasound. Applications of this new technique include analysis of vascular anatomy and the potential assessment of organ perfusion.

Chaoui et al. wanted to assess the fetal cardiovascular system using 3D power Doppler in normal and abnormal conditions during the second half of pregnancy. The following regions of interest were assessed: placental, umbilical, abdominal, renal, pulmonary and intracranial vessels together with the heart and great arteries. Satisfactory visualization of the fetal vascular system using 3D Doppler could be achieved in normal pregnancies. The main difficulty during the learning curve was the optimization of the power Doppler image prior to 3D data acquisition. Despite good visualization conditions, the reconstruction of satisfactory images was only possible in 56 out of the 87 (64%) pregnancies with abnormal vascular anatomy. These were abnormalities of placenta and umbilical vessels, intra-abdominal and intrathoracic anomalies, renal malformations, central nervous system and cardiac defects. The main reasons for the lack of information were fetal position and movements, overlapping with signals from neighboring vessels as well as technical limitations of the online system.

Zalud and Shaha have evaluated uteroplacental circulation using 3D power Doppler and established norms for placental and spiral artery blood flow in normal pregnancies between 14 and 25 weeks of gestation.[47] They showed that VI, FI and VFI all increased slowly in placental and spiral arteries with advancing gestation though these indices were all elevated with increasing parity.[48] Merce et al. note that the use of 3D power Doppler is akin to a "vascular biopsy" and is an appropriate tool for the routine evaluation of the placenta vascular tree during gestation and that these indices are significantly related to fetal biometry and umbilical artery Doppler velocimetry.[49] Bartha et al. used 3D power Doppler to evaluate fetal cerebral circulation in both normal and IUGR fetuses and showed that on average, VI, FI and VFI were all increased in fetuses with growth restriction suggesting hemodynamic redistribution that was higher than expected by conventional Doppler flow studies.[50] Even the fetal hepatic and portal system can be evaluated by 3D power Doppler. Kalache et al. identified absent ductus venosus, direct connection of the umbilical vein to the right atrium and umbilical vein to the inferior vena cava using 3D power Doppler.[51]

Placenta accreta has become the leading cause of emergency peripartum hysterectomy and the rates have increased markedly in the last few decades.[52] The resulting blood loss and surgery results in significant maternal and neonatal morbidity and occasionally mortality and is becoming a significant problem in obstetrics today. The antepartum diagnosis of accreta is essential and has been shown to result less blood transfusions, intensive care unit (ICU) admissions, genitourinary tract injuries and a decrease in neonatal intensive care unit (NICU) length of stay, respiratory distress syndrome (RDS) and surfactant use.[53] The addition of 3D power Doppler imaging of the placenta, especially in the basal view may be a useful complementary technique for the antenatal diagnosis or exclusion of placenta accreta **(Fig. 8)**.[54]

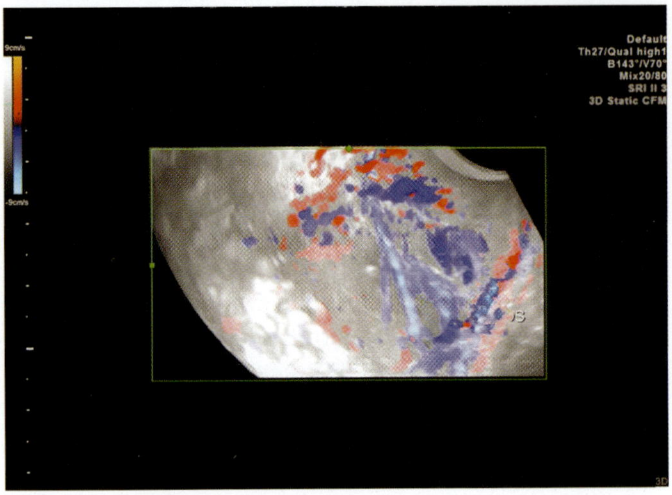

Fig. 8: 3D Doppler of placenta accreta.

CONCLUSION

Doppler ultrasound of the umbilical artery plays an important role in the management of IUGR and preeclampsia and aids in prognostication in twin-to-twin transfusion syndrome while notching in the waveform is a predictor of umbilical cord abnormalities. Middle cerebral artery Doppler reliably detects fetal anemia and may be useful in the assessment of IUGR as well. Abnormal uterine artery Doppler may play a role in predicting growth restriction, hypertensive disorders of pregnancy and preterm delivery. Abnormal ductus venosus waveforms can also be used to predict adverse fetal outcome and may allow for better timing of delivery while umbilical venous pulsations may be a sensitive marker for fetal heart failure in hydropic pregnancies. 3D power Doppler allows better small vessel visualization that is not affected by angle of insonation and has been used to diagnose placental and cord abnormalities. As clinical experience with these new technologies increase and as the technology improves further, it is reasonable to expect that 3D Doppler and 4D ultrasound will be complementary addition to well established 2D Doppler ultrasound imaging.

REFERENCES

1. Doppler C. Uber das farbige. Licht der Dopplersterne und einigr anderer Gestirne des Himmels. (On the coloured light of double stars and certain other stars of the heavens). Royal Bohemian Society. 1842;2:465.
2. Callen P. Ultrasonography in Obstetrics and Gynecology. 5th edition. Saunders Elsevier; 2008.

3. Hoffman S, Galan H. Assessing the 'at-risk' fetus: Doppler ultrasound. Curr Opin Obstet Gynecol. 2009;21:161-6.
4. Stuart B, Drumm J, Fitzgerald D, Duignan N. Fetal blood velocity waveforms in normal pregnancy. Br J Obstet Gynaecol. 1980;87(9):780-5.
5. Trudinger B, Giles W, Cook C, et al. Fetal umbilical artery flow velocity waveforms and placental resistance: clinical significance. Br J Obstet Gynaecol. 1985;92(1):23-30.
6. Alfirevic Z, Neilson J. Doppler ultrasonography in high-risk pregnancies: systematic review with meta-analysis. Am J Obstet Gynecol. 1995;172(5):1379-87.
7. Kontopoulous E, Quintero R, Chmait R, Bornick P, Russell Z, Allen M. Percent absent end-diastolic velocity in the umbilical artery waveform as a predictor of intrauterine fetal demise of the donor twin after selective laser photocoagulation of communicating vessels in twin-twin transfusions syndrome. Ultrasound Obstet Gynecol. 2007;30(1):35-9.
8. Mari G, Adrignolo A, Abuhamad Z, Pirhonen J, Jones D, Ludomirsky A, et al. Diagnosis of fetal anemia with Doppler ultrasound in the pregnancy complicated by maternal blood group isoimmunization. Ultrasound Obstet Gynecol. 1995;5(6):400-5.
9. ACOG Practice Bulletin No. 75: management of alloimmunization. Obstet Gynecol. 2006;108(2):457-64.
10. Slaghekke F, Kist W, Oepkes D, Pasman S, Middeldorp J, Klumper F, et al. Twin Anemia-Polycythemia Sequence: Diagnostic criteria, classification, perinatal management and outcome. Fetal Diagn Ther. 2010.
11. Mari G, Hanif F, Kruger M, Cosmi E, Santolaya-Forgas J, Treadwell M. Middle cerebral artery peak systolic velocity: a new Doppler parameter in the assessment of growth-restricted fetuses. Ultrasound Obstet Gynecol. 2007;29(3):310-6.
12. Ghidini A, Locatelli A. Monitoring of Fetal well-being: Role of uterine artery Doppler. Semin Perinatol. 2008;32:258-62.
13. Phupong V, Dejthevaporn T. Predicting risks of preeclampsia and small for gestational age infant by uterine artery Doppler. Hypertens Pregnancy. 2008;27:387-95.
14. Onwudiwe N, Yu C, Poon L, et al. Prediction of preeclampsia by a combination of maternal history, uterine artery Doppler and mean arterial pressure. Ultrasound Obstet Gynecol. 2008;32(7):877-83.
15. Li H, Gudnason H, Olofsson P, et al. Increased uterine artery vascular impedance is related to adverse outcome of pregnancy but is present in only one-third of late third-trimester pre-eclamptic women. Ultrasound Obstet Gynecol. 2005;25(5):459-63.
16. Ferrazzi E, Bulfamante G, Mezzopane R, Barbera A, Ghidini A, Pardi G. Uterine Doppler velocimetry and placental hypoxic-ischemic lesion in pregnancies with fetal intrauterine growth restriction. Placenta. 1999;20(5-6):389-94.
17. McCowan L, North R, Harding J. Abnormal uterine artery Doppler in small-for-gestational-age pregnancies is associated with later hypertension. Aust NZJ Obstet Gynaecol. 2001;41(1):56-60.
18. Gudmundsson S, Korszun P, Olofsson P, Dubiel M. New score indicating placental vascular resistance. Acta Obstet Gynecol Scand. 2003;82(9):807-12.
19. Abuhamad A, Mari G, Copel J, et al. Umbilical artery flow velocity waveforms in monoamniotic twins with cord entanglement. Obstet Gyencol. 1995;86(4 Pt 2):674-7.
20. Abuhamad A, Sclater A, Carlson E, Moriarity R, Aguiar M. Umbilical artery Doppler waveform notching: is it a marker for cord and placental abnormalities? J Ultrasound Med. 2002;21(8):857-60.
21. Baschat A, Harman C. Venous Doppler in the assessment of fetal cardiovascular status. Curr Opin Obstet Gynecol. 2006;18:156-63.
22. Rizzo G, Capponi A, Talone P, et al. Doppler indices from inferior vena cava and ductus venosus in predicting pH and oxygen tension in umbilical blood at cordocentesis in growth retarded fetuses. Ultrasound Obstet Gynecol. 1996;7(6):401-10.
23. Baschat A, Guclu S, Kush M, Gembruch U, Weiner C, Harman C. Venous Doppler in the prediction of acid-base status of growth-restriction fetuses with elevated placental blood flow resistance. Am J Obstet Gynecol. 2004;191(1):277-84.
24. Schawarze A, Gembruch U, Krapp M, Katalinic A, Germer U, Axt-Fliedner R. Qualitative venous Doppler flow waveform analysis in preterm intrauterine growth-restricted fetuses with ARED flow in the umbilical artery—correlation with short term outcome. Ultrasound Obstet Gynecol. 2005;25(6):573-9.
25. Mari G, Hanif F, Treadwell M, Kruger M. Gestational age at delivery and Doppler waveforms in very preterm intrauterine growth-restricted fetuses as predicators of perinatal mortality. J Ultrasound Med. 2007;26(5):555-9.
26. Rizzo G, Arduini D, Romanini C. Umbilical vein pulsations: a physiologic finding in early gestation. Am J Obstet Gynecol. 1992;167(3):675-7.
27. Mari G, Hanif F. Fetal Doppler: Umbilical artery, middle cerebral artery and venous system. Semin Perinatol. 2008;32(4):253-7.
28. Hofstaetter C, Hansmann M, Eik-Nes S, et al. A cardiovascular profile score in the surveillance of fetal hydrops. J Matern Fetal Neonatal Med. 2006;19(7):407-1330.
29. Bellotti M, Pennati G, De Gasperi C, Bozzo M, Battaglia F, Ferrazzi E. Simultaneous measurements of umbilical venous, fetal hepatic and ductus venosus blood flow in growth-restricted human fetuses. Am J Obstet Gynecol. 2004;190(5):1347-58.
30. McDicken W, Anderson T. The difference between colour Doppler velocity imaging and power Doppler imaging. Eur J Echocardiography. 2002;3:240-4.

31. Fortunato S. The use of power Doppler and color power angiography in fetal imaging. Am J Obstet Gynecol. 1996;174:1828-33.
32. Guerriero S, Ajossa S, Mais V, Risalvato A, Angiolucci M, Labate F, et al. Color Doppler energy imaging in the diagnosis of fetal intracranial hemorrhage in the second trimester. Ultrasound Obstet Gynecol. 1997;10(3):205-8.
33. Pilu G, Falco P, Milani V, Perolo A, Bovicelli L. Prenatal diagnosis of micrcophaly assisted by vaginal sonography and power Doppler. Ultrasound Obstet Gynecol. 1998;11(5):357-60.
34. Fox D, Bruner J, Fleischer A. Amplitude-based color Doppler sonography of fetus with sacrococcygeal teratoma. J Ultrasound Med. 1996;15:785-7.
35. Chua L, Twining P. A comparison of power colour flow with frequency based color flow Doppler fetal echocardiography. Clin Radiol. 1997;52(9):712-4.
36. DeVore G. The value of color Doppler sonography in the diagnosis of renal agenesis. J Ultrasound Med. 1995;14(6):443-9.
37. Chou M, Ho E, Lee Y. Prenatal diagnosis of placenta previa accreta by transabdominal color Doppler ultrasound. Ultrasound Obstet Gynecol. 2000;15(1):28-35.
38. Devesa R, Munoz A, Torrents M, et al. Prenatal diagnosis of vasa previa with transvaginal color Doppler ultrasound. Ultrasound Obstet Gynecol. 1996;8(2):139-41.
39. Chaoui R, Kalache K, Hartung J. Application of three-dimensional power Doppler ultrasound in prenatal diagnosis. Ultrasound Obstet Gynecol. 2001;17:22-9.
40. Pairleitner H, Steiner H, Hasenoehrl G, Staudach A. Three-dimensional power Doppler sonography: imaging and quantifying blood flow and vascularization. Ultrasound Obstet Gynecol. 1999;14:139-43.
41. Pretorius DH, Nelson TR, Baergen RN, et al. Imaging of placental vasculature using three-dimensional ultrasound and color power Doppler: a preliminary study. J Perinat Med. 2002;30:48-56.
42. Chaoui R, Hoffmann J, Heling KS. Three-dimensional (3D) and 4D color Doppler fetal echocardiography using spatio-temporal image correlation (STIC). Ultrasound Obstet Gynecol. 2004;23:535-45.
43. Matijevic R, Kurjak A. The assessment of placental blood vessels by three-dimensional power Doppler ultrasound. J Perinat Med. 2002;30:26-32.
44. Shih JC, Ko TL, Lin MC, et al. Quantitative three-dimensional power Doppler ultrasound predicts the outcome of placental chorioangioma. Ultrasound Obstet Gynecol. 2004;24:202-6.
45. Hartung J, Kalache KD, Chaoui R. Three-dimensional power Doppler ultrasonography (3D-PDU) in fetal diagnosis. Ultraschall Med. 2004;25:200-5.
46. Ritchie CJ, Edwards WS, Mack LA, et al. Three-dimensional ultrasonic angiography using power-mode Doppler. Ultrasound Med Biol. 1996;22:277-86.
47. Zalud I, Shaha S. Evaluation of the uteroplacental circulation by three-dimensional Doppler ultrasound in the second trimester of normal pregnancy. J Matern Fetal Neonatal Med. 2007;20(4):299-305.
48. Zalud I, Shaha S. Three-dimensional sonography of the placenta and uterine spiral vasculature: influence of maternal age and parity. J Clin Ultrasound. 2008;36(7):391-6.
49. Merce L, Barco M, Bau S, Kupesic S, Kurjak A. Assessment of placental vascularization by three-dimensional power Doppler "Vascular Biospy" in normal pregnancies. Croat Med J. 2005;465):765-71.
50. Bartha J, Moya E, Hervias-Vivancos B. Three-dimensional power Doppler analysis of cerebral circulation in normal and growth restricted fetuses. J Cereb Blood Flow Metab. 2009;29(9):1609-18.
51. Kalache K, Romero R, Goncalves L, Chaiworapongsa T, Espinoza J, Schoen M, et al. Three-dimensional color power imaging of the fetal hepatic circulation. Am J Obstet Gynecol. 2003;189(3):1401-6.
52. Miller D, Chollet J, Goodwin T. Clinical risk factors for placenta previa-placenta accreta. Am J Obstet Gynecol. 1997;177:210-4.
53. Warhak C, Ramos G, Eskander R, Benirschke K, Saenz C, Kelly T, et al. Effect of predelivery diagnosis in 99 consecutive cases of placenta accreta. Obstet Gynecol. 2010;115(1):65-9.
54. Shih J, Jaraquemada P, Su Y, Shyu M, Lin C, Lin S, et al. Role of three-dimensional power Doppler in the antenatal diagnosis of placenta accreta: comparison with gray-scale and color Doppler techniques. Ultrasound Obstet Gynecol. 2009;33:193-203.

15

CHAPTER

Guidelines for the Doppler Assessment of the Umbilical and Middle Cerebral Arteries in Obstetrics

Autumn Broady, Ivica Zalud

INTRODUCTION

The use of Doppler ultrasound is an important tool in the obstetrical assessment of an at-risk fetus. Principles of the Doppler effect can be used to monitor placental and fetal blood flow in pregnancies complicated by fetal growth restriction or in the surveillance for fetal anemia from maternal alloimmunization. Indications and techniques for umbilical artery and middle cerebral artery Doppler assessment are reviewed.

UMBILICAL ARTERY

Blood flow in the umbilical cord is usually high-flow and low-resistance with increasing end-diastolic flow as gestation advances.[1] This low-impedance system can be seen as early as 14 weeks gestation.[2] The umbilical arteries carry deoxygenated blood from the fetus to the placenta, and changes in their blood flow are indicative of placental compromise. Doppler evaluation of the umbilical artery is to be performed in the presence of fetal growth restriction (IUGR), as it has not been shown to be a reliable screening tool in the prediction of development of IUGR.[3]

A biphasic waveform corresponding to systole and diastole is produced when the umbilical artery is evaluated by pulsed Doppler.[4] Forward flow of blood should occur during both phases of the cardiac cycle. Qualitative assessment of the direction of end-diastolic flow in the umbilical artery is a reproducible method to evaluate the presence of placental compromise, particularly in the setting of IUGR and placental insufficiency. Reduction followed by reversal of end-diastolic blood flow in the umbilical artery has been shown to correlate with the degree of placental dysfunction, particularly the obliteration of small arteries in the tertiary stem villi. Reversed flow represents more advanced dysfunction, with more than 70% of placental arteries compromised.[2,5]

The most commonly used quantitative assessments of the umbilical artery using Doppler are the pulsatility index and S/D ratio.[3] These ratios are independent of the alterations of measured blood flow due to changes in the angle on insonation of the ultrasound beam.[4] The pulsatility index should be used in cases of absent end-diastolic flow as the S/D will be immeasurable.

Standard technique should be employed in obtaining the umbilical artery waveform to ensure reproducibility and accuracy of measurements **(Table 1 and Fig. 1)**. Doppler measurements should be taken from a free-floating loop of umbilical cord near the abdominal insertion site. Care should be taken to ensure the loop of cord is not compressed between the uterine wall or the fetus, as this can alter cord resistance and blood flow. Measurements taken near the placental insertion have a lower resistance than sites close to the abdominal insertion.[6] Measurements should be taken in the absence of fetal breathing and while the waveform is uniform. The umbilical artery is identified on color Doppler using the number of vessels identified, pulsatile color flow pattern, caliber and blood flow direction.[7] The pulsed Doppler gate should be placed over the targeted area of

TABLE 1: Methodological guidelines for Doppler assessment of the umbilical artery blood flow.

- Locate a free loop of uncompressed cord
- Identify umbilical artery, using color Doppler as necessary
- Magnify until the loop of cord fills the majority of the image
- Pulsed Doppler gate 1–2 mm
- Adjust caliper gate over single umbilical artery
- Adjust power Doppler scale to fit velocity
- Obtain at least 5 uniform waveforms for measurement of indices
- Ensure absence of fetal breathing and movement during measurement
- Observe the As Low as Reasonably Achievable (ALARA) Principle during evaluation

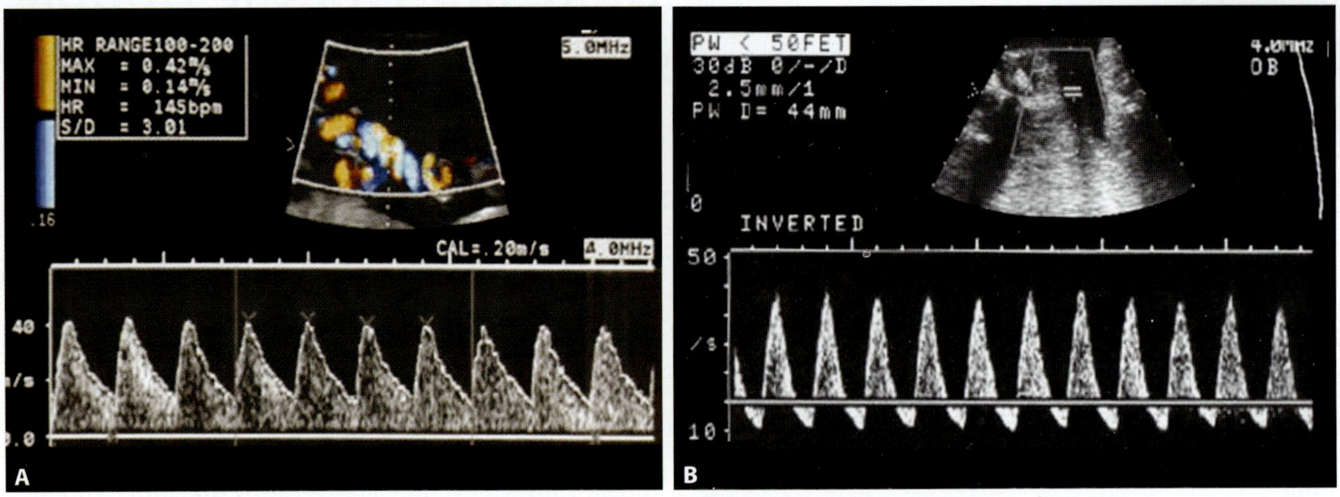

Figs.1A and B: Doppler waveform of the umbilical artery: (A) Normal umbilical artery waveform; (B) Abnormal (reversed) end diastolic waveform.

the umbilical artery and the gate should be sized to ensure that only the artery is sampled. Adjustments in the gain and pulsed Doppler scale should be made to ensure the flow velocity is within the measured scale. The angle of insonation should be kept as low as possible to maximize systolic and diastolic flow.[7]

Middle Cerebral Artery

In contrast to the umbilical artery, fetal cerebral circulation is a high-impedance system. The middle cerebral artery (MCA) is the most accessible cerebral vessel to visualize via ultrasound and carries the majority of cerebral fetal blood flow.[8] The MCA is a terminal branch of the carotid artery and arises from the circle of Willis within the fetal brain.

A biphasic waveform corresponding to systole and diastole is produced when the MCA is evaluated by pulsed Doppler.[4] Forward flow of blood should occur during both phases of the cardiac cycle. Commonly used quantitative measurements of blood flow in the MCA include the peak systolic velocity (PSV) and resistance index. Currently, assessment of and screening for fetal anemia in pregnancies complicated by maternal alloimmunization or congenital infections (e.g. parvo virus) is the accepted use of MCA Doppler evaluation. Normally, PSV increases with advancing gestation, necessitating the conversion of values of multiples of the median (MoM) to evaluate for pathological increases. PSV increases in the presence of fetal anemia due to increased cardiac output and lower blood viscosity.[4]

Measurement of cerebral blood flow has also been investigated in fetal growth restriction, based on the physiologic redistribution of blood flow that occurs in the presence of fetal hypoxemia. Hypoxemia results in fetal adaptations in blood flow, with the preservation of flow to the brain, heart, and adrenal glands, producing the so-called "Brain-sparing" effect.[9,10] The cerebroplacental ratio (CPR) is calculated by dividing Doppler indices of the MCA by the indices of the umbilical artery. The pulsatility index is the most commonly used index in calculating the CPR, although other indices have been studied. This ratio accounts for the interaction of blood flow changes in the fetal brain as a result of increased placental resistance.[11] Abnormal CPR values <1 are typically defined as abnormal, although conversion of values to multiples of the median has also been reported. Recently, abnormal CPR values have been associated with increased risk of adverse perinatal outcomes including stillbirth, perinatal mortality, fetal distress, neonatal intensive care admission, and poor neonatal neurologic outcomes.[11-14] Further investigation is needed before MCA assessment is incorporated into standard clinical practice in the setting of fetal growth restriction.

Precise methodology is paramount in measurement of MCA indices. The Society for Maternal-Fetal Medicine recently published step-by-step guidelines for the proper technique of measurement of the MCA PSV, which are reviewed in detail in **Table 2** and **Figure 2**. The measurements should be performed when the fetus is at rest and MCA measurements should be repeated at

TABLE 2: Methodological guidelines for Doppler assessment of the middle cerebral artery blood flow.

- Obtain a transverse view of the fetal head at the level of the sphenoid bones. Brain landmarks include visualization of the thalami and cavum septum pellucidum
- Visualize the circle of Willis using color Doppler
- Visualize the middle cerebral artery originating off the circle of Willis. The entire length of the MCA should be seen
- Select MCA closest to the transducer if feasible
- Magnify the image such that the MCA occupies >50% of the image
- Pulsed Doppler gate 1–2 mm
- Adjust caliper gate over MCA. The PSV should be sampled close to its origin from the internal carotid artery
- Adjust pulse wave Doppler scale to fit velocity
- The angle between the ultrasound beam and the direction of blood flow should be as close to 0 degrees as possible, ideally <10 degrees, and parallel to the entire vessel length. If this is not possible, the angle of insonation should be <30 degrees
- Obtain at least 5 uniform waveforms for measurement of PSV. The highest waveform should be used to measure the PSV
- Ensure absence of fetal breathing and movement during measurement
- Repeat sequence at least 3 times. The highest PSV value should be used for clinical care
- Observe the As Low as Reasonably Achievable (ALARA) Principle during evaluation

Adapted from: SMFM; 2015.

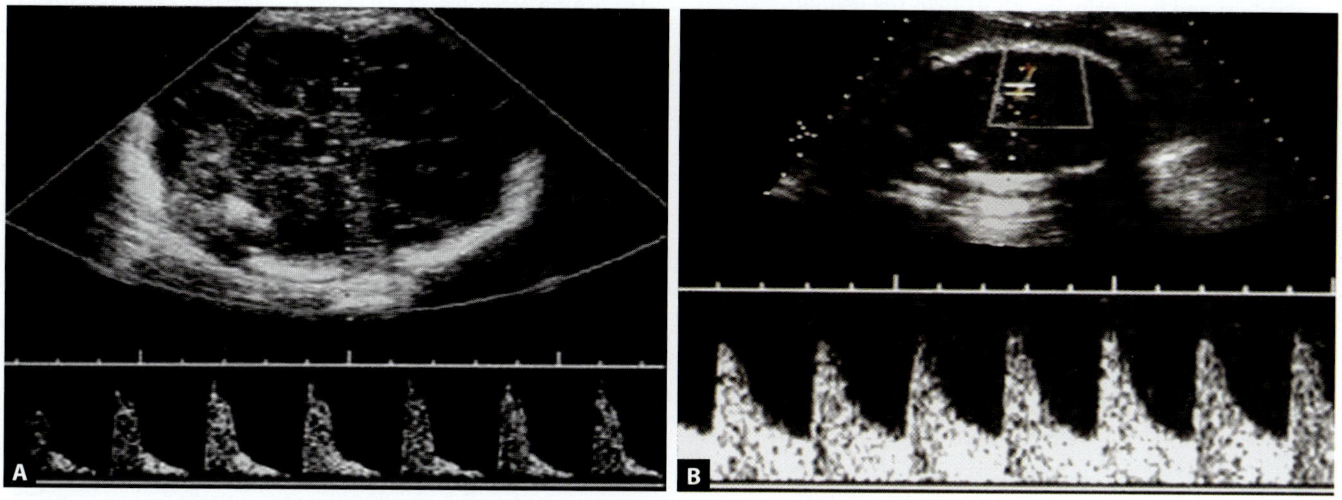

Figs.2A and B: Doppler waveform of the middle cerebral artery (MCA): (A) Normal MCA Doppler waveform; (B) Abnormal MCA Doppler waveform.

least three times to minimize effects of fetal heart rate change on MCA indices.[15] Care should also be taken not to put excessive pressure on the fetal head during the measurement as this may falsely reduce end-diastolic flow.[7] Measurements should be taken from the proximal portion of the MCA, near its origin at the circle of Willis, as PSV decreases with increasing distance from the origin.[7] The angle of insonation should be as close to 0 degrees as possible for most accurate estimations of blood flow velocity, although angle correction is possible and accurate if fetal positioning does not allow for this angle.[16] The highest point of the pulsed Doppler waveform is then measured to obtain the PSV and other indices.

REFERENCES

1. Fleischer A, Schulman H, Farmakides G, Bracero L, Blattner P, Randolph G. Umbilical artery waveforms and intrauterine growth retardation. AJOG. 1985;151:502-5.
2. Trudinger BJ, Stevens D, Connelly A, Hales JR, Alexander G, Bradley L, Fawcett A, Thrompson RS. The effect of embolizations of the umbilical circulation. AJOG. 1987;157:1443-8.
3. Society for Maternal-Fetal Medicine Publications Committee, Berkley E, Chauhan SP, Abuhamad A. Doppler assessment of the fetus with intrauterine growth restriction. AJOG. 2012;206:300-8.
4. Callen PW. Ultrasonography in Obstetrics and Gynecology. Philadelphia, PA: Elsevier; 2008.

5. Thompson RS, Trudinger BJ. Doppler waveform pulsatility index and resistance, pressure and flow in the umbilical placental circulation: an investigation using a mathematical model. Ultrasound in Med Biol. 1990;16:449-58.
6. Trudinger BJ. Doppler ultrasonography and fetal well being. In: Reece EA, Hobbins JC, Mahoney M, Petrie RH (Eds). Medicine of the fetus and mother. Philadelphia, PA: JB Lipincott Co; 1992.
7. Creasy RK, Resnik R, Iams JD, Lockwood CJ, Moore TR, Greene MF. Maternal-Fetal Medicine Principles and Practice. Philadelphia, PA: Elsevier; 2014.
8. Veille JC, Hanson R, Tatum K. Longitudinal quantitation of middle cerebral artery blood flow in normal human fetuses. AJOG. 1993;169:1393-8.
9. Mari G, Deter RL. Middle cerebral artery flow velocity waveforms in normal and small-for-gestational age fetuses. AJOG. 1992;166:1262-70.
10. Behrman RE, Lees MH, Peterson EN, De Lan- noy CW, Seeds AE. Distribution of the circulation in the normal and asphyxiated fetal primate. AJOG.1970;108:956-69.
11. DeVore GR. The importance of the cerebroplacental ratio in the evaluation of fetal well-being in SGA and AGA fetuses. AJOG. 2015;213:5-15.
12. Kahlil AA, Morales-Rosello J, Elsaddig M, Khan N, Papageorghiou A, Bhide A, et al. The association between fetal Doppler and admission to the neonatal unit at term. AJOG. 2015; 213: 57.e1-7. doi: 10.1016/j.ajog.2014.10.013. Epub 2014 Oct 15.
13. Kahlil A, Morales-Rosello J, Townsend R, Morlando M, Papageorghiou A, Bhide A, et al. Are fetal cerebroplacental ratio and impaired placental perfusion recorded in the third trimester predictors of stillbirth and perinatal loss? Ultrasound Obstet Gynecol. 2015; doi: 10.1002/uog.15729.
14. Jugović D, Tumbri J, Medić M, Jukić MK, Kurjak A, Arbeille P, et al. New Doppler index for prediction of perinatal brain damage in growth-restricted and hypoxic fetuses. Ultrasound Obstet Gynecol. 2007;30:303-11.
15. Society for Maternal-Fetal Medicine, Mari G, Norton ME, Stone J, Berghella V, Sciscione AC, Tate D, et al. SMFM Clinical Guideline #8: the fetus at risk for anemia—diagnosis and management. AJOG. 2015;212:697-710. doi: 10.1016/j. ajog.2015.01.059. Epub 2015 Mar 27.
16. Ruma MS, Swartz AE, Kim E, Herring AH, Menard MK, Moise KJ Jr. Angle correction can be used to measure peak systolic velocity in the fetal middle cerebral artery. AJOG. 2009;200:397.e1-3.

16

CHAPTER

Ultrasound and Doppler Management of Intrauterine Growth Restriction

José M Carrera, Francesc Figueras, Eva Meler Barrabés

INTRODUCTION

Intrauterine growth restriction (IUGR) undoubtedly is one of the most challenging areas of research for obstetricians today. It is considered as a major contributor to perinatal morbidity and mortality, and has been described as etiologically responsible of about a 50% of perinatal deaths occurring preterm and 20% at term.[1] In addition, growth restriction is associated with intrapartum distress and metabolic acidosis, which are in turn contributors to hypoxic encephalopathy and cerebral palsy.[2] Furthermore, there is increasing evidence of the association between fetal growth restriction and infant death[3] and metabolic syndrome in adulthood.[4] Despite marked progress made over the past two decades in both diagnostic procedures and management strategies, the question of what causes growth restriction still remains unanswered in 30–40% of all cases of IUGR.

DEFINITIONS

It is necessary to make a difference between three different concepts: growth, development and maturity. "Growth" is usually defined as the process whereby the body mass of a living being increases in size as a result of the increase in number and/or size of its cells. "Development" should be understood as the process by which the organs acquire their particular anatomy and their specific functions in living beings, and consequently the progressive anatomical and functional "Maturity" of all of them, as well as its physiological regulations. Thanks to these three processes, which are going on in a parallel way, the fetus reach at the gestation terminus maturity enough to face the extrauterine life.

Regarding the fetal weight anomalies, a clear distinction should be made between the meanings of three different terms: Low-birth-weight (LBW), small-for-gestational age (SGA), and intrauterine growth restriction (IUGR). The LBW refers only to newborn infants weighing less than 2,500 grams independently of gestational age. Some of these newborns will be premature and others will be newborns with a growth restriction. The SGA is a term based on a statistical definition, which includes all newborn infants found below the lower range limit of normal weight by gestational age. Hence, is a term that comprises a heterogeneous group of fetuses and newborns with several etiologic conditions. The IUGR theoretically refers to any process that is capable of limiting intrinsic fetal growth potential in utero, but is mainly used to define those cases in which a placental insufficiency is responsible for the growth deficit.

Unfortunately, in literature, the terms IUGR and SGA are frequently considered as synonymous. This confusion was increased even more when the National Institute of Child Health and Human Development in the USA stated that for "both medical and research purposes, IUGR should be defined as a situation which results in a newborn weight that is lower than 10th percentile for its gestational age".

CLASSIFICATION

Most Fetal Medicine Units classify SGA in three main categories according to what Soothill published in a breaking editorial.[5] Firstly, the "IUGR", that is limited to those fetuses in which a reduction in their growth potential is believed to be due to placental insufficiency. Secondly, the "Normal-SGA", which includes those SGA fetuses, which are believed to be constitutionally small. And, finally, the "Abnormal-SGA", which comprises other pathological causes of SGA as infections, congenital malformations, chromosomopathies, etc. Despite that in the past, SGA fetuses and neonates were classified according to the relationship between abdominal and cephalic biometries as symmetrical or asymmetrical, this classification has demonstrated to be poorly correlated with the underlying etiological condition,[6] with the gasometric status of the fetus at cordocentesis[7] or with any of the perinatal events that define an adverse perinatal outcome,[8-9] and, therefore, is no longer recommended as a primary tool in managing SGA fetuses.

INCIDENCE

While the incidence of SGA depends upon the used threshold for normality (10th, 5th or 2.5th centile) resulting in a 10%, 5% or 2.5%, respectively, the incidence of IUGR varies greatly in the literature, with reports of figures ranging from 1–12%. The reason for this may be found in different factors, including the social and economic status of the population studied; different criteria used for discrimination (10th percentile, 5th percentile, etc.), different ways in which standard curves are drawn, data obtained from transverse or longitudinal studies, etc.[10] Approximately, only a 20–30% of all SGA fetuses are true growth-restricted fetuses,[11] whereas only a 10–20% are patho logical-SGA.[12] Hence, most of the cases of SGA are constitutionally small, i.e. normal-SGA.

SCREENING

"Traditional" maternal serum screening have proved disappointing for IUGR: elevated levels of alphafeto protein and human chorionic gonadotrophin are associated with IUGR but are very poor screening tests (sensitivity about 5%).[13] For the time being, the bio chemi cal markers that are more promising candidates for antenatal screening are FMSlike tyrosine kinase 1 and placental growth factor. Despite that, there exists evidence of the association between the plasmatic maternal levels of these markers and the occurrence of preeclampsia and growth-restriction,[14] new clinical studies are required before its clinical application.

Since IUGR is caused by uteroplacental insufficiency and it shares some common physiopathological paths with preeclampsia leading to a poor trophoblast invasion, IUGR has been associated with an increased resistance in the uterine arteries. Doppler evaluation of this vessel constitutes the main screening method for IUGR. Evaluation of this tool has been hampered by different criteria for growth-restriction and for abnormal Doppler waveform, by discrepancies in the targeted population and by differences in instrumentation (use of color Doppler, transvaginal versus transabdominal approach) among the studies. Nevertheless, a multicentric and massive-population based study[15] aimed to evaluate the role of transvaginal uterine artery at 23 weeks, has demonstrated an overall sensitivity for growth-restriction of 16%. Nevertheless, when the event of interest is the occurrence of disease requiring delivery before 32 weeks (which represents the subgroup with significant perinatal morbidity and mortality), the sensitivity for preeclampsia-associated and no-preeclampsia-associated growth restriction is 93% and 56%, respectively, with specificities of 95%. It would be appealing to move the screening into early pregnancy, but despite the fact that it seems a promising strategy for preeclampsia, the sensitivity of uterine artery Doppler evaluation in early second trimester for growth restriction requiring delivery before 32 is only of 28% (12% for growth restriction without preeclampsia).[16] Hence, it seems that uterine artery evaluation identifies a subgroup with an increased risk for developing severe growth-restriction.

Screening strategies which combine epidemiological, biochemical and Doppler parameters are being tested to enhance the low sensitivity of each individual parameter.

DIAGNOSIS

The antenatal detection of IUGR is of utmost importance and constitutes a major challenge for modern obstetrics. SGA neonates not antenatally detected had a 4-fold risk of adverse outcome.[17] Furthermore, it has been reported that a suboptimal antenatal management is the most common finding in cases of unexplained stillborns.[18]

Anamnesis

Antenatal risk factors include a previous history of SGA or stillbirth, toxic substances such as tobacco, alcohol and other drugs, fetal infections (CMV and Rubeola are the most associated ones) and maternal diseases (mainly renal and vascular). Other risk factors are preeclampsia related such as thrombophilic conditions, obesity and chronic hypertension. Although, these risk factors are multiple and not always well-defined, a correct anamnesis remains a key step to select a population of high-risk on which a close follow-up may be warranted. Nevertheless, only 10% of this high-risk group will develop IUGR.

Fundal Height Measurement

Both the fundal height measurement and the abdominal palpation have sensitivities of about 30% to detect SGA[19] and therefore, could not be recommended. Nevertheless, it has been reported that customized standards for fundal height, which adjust for parity, maternal height and weight, ethnicity and fetal gender, and a longitudinal evaluation allow sensitivities of about 50%,[20] comparable to the detection rate of routine third trimester fetal biometry in low-risk pregnancies. In settings where a policy of third-trimester ultrasound is not in place, fundal height measurements remain common practice.

Ultrasound Diagnosis

An accurate antenatal detection of SGA fetuses remains the key process to subsequently detect and manage IUGR. This ultrasound assessment require three consecutive steps:

1. Pregnancy Dating
2. Biometric evaluation
3. Assessing growth as normal or abnormal.

Pregnancy Dating

Pregnancy dating based upon the last menstrual period provides inaccurate estimates of the gestational age, since up to a 20% of women with regular cycles ovulate later than expected.[21] Hence, in clinical settings where a policy of first or early second trimester scan is in place, it seems to be more appropriate to systematically use the fetal biometries to date the pregnancy and ensure a reliable fetal age assessment for most purposes, for example, Down's syndrome screening. There are several formulae to date the pregnancy from early biometries, with low systematic and random errors. Crown-rump length (CRL) is a biometric parameter that can be measured in the early stages of gestation. Technically, the main limitation is the progressive bending of the embryo, which makes measurements less reliable beyond 12–13 weeks of gestation (or 60–70 mm). Normal reference ranges to date the pregnancy are published elsewhere.[22] If possible, below the 14 weeks, all obstetric ultrasound units are currently recommended to adopt this method of assessing gestational age from crownrump length. From then on, it seems conceptually more appropriate to use cephalic (head circumference) and/or femur (femur length) biometries. Series in which different formulas have been tested in pregnancies conceived with artificial reproductive techniques provide comprehensive recommendations on this matter.[23] Once the pregnancy has been dated by an early scan, further adjustments must not be performed.

Biometric Evaluation

Initially and still in many places, the biparietal diameter (BPD) was the only measurement that was routinely taken for the assessment of fetal growth. When pregnancy is normal, this parameter falls within the normal range and can be considered as a representative indicator of the growth of other fetal organs and tissues, but when pregnancy is abnormal it may still fall within the normal range (head size is rarely affected in many cases of IUGR) although in this case, it is not representative indicator of the growth of other fetal structures. On the other hand, misdiagnoses have been on many occasions in fetuses with marked brachycephalism or dolichocephalism in association with normal develop ment of the rest of the body. In addition, measurement of the BPD does not permit determination of fetal weight with acceptable reliability. The substitution of BPD by head circumference or cephalic area does not substantially improve the sensitivity of the method. With the purpose of improving the screening method, measurement of the length of the femur was introduced. It has the advantage that it measures a component of fetal longitudinal growth and does not suffer the sudden flattening out characteristic of cephalic parameters at term, although it has the disadvantage of not being a useful parameter for establishing the diagnosis of IUGR early stages. Abdominal circumference (AC) is the most accurate single biometry to predict SGA at birth.[24] In high-risk women, AC at less than the tenth centile has sensitivities of 72.9–94.5% and specificities of 50.6–83.8% in the prediction of fetuses with birthweight at less than the tenth centile. The use of cross-sectional reference charts for each biometry with the closest distribution to that of the screened population remains the gold standard and some studies alert to the impact of choice of reference charts in the assessment of fetal biometry. In that sense they recommend to use Z-scores in order to choose the most appropriate chart.[25] Moreover, many charts require the average of at least three repeated measurements in order to control random error. By increasing the number of measurements to four, the 95% error span is reduced to half.

Fetal biometries could be used to estimate the fetal weight. The estimated fetal weight (EFW) predicts the occurrence of SGA at birth with sensitivities of 33.3–89.2% and specificities of 53.7–90.9%.[24] A prospective study[26] comparing several formulas concluded that Shepard formula[27] have the best interclass correlation coefficient, with smallest mean difference from actual birthweight.

Nevertheless, for fetuses weighting less than 2,000 gm, this formula has not been validated. The Hadlock formula[28] may be more appropriate when the fetus is expected to be very small.[29]

Controversy exists regarding using AC or EFW for the antenatal assessment of fetal growth. Whereas AC, the simplest method, has in high-pregnancies higher sensitivities, EFW has a stronger association with birthweight below the 10th centile.[24] We prefer using EFW since it is more consistent with the neonatal assessment, which is mainly performed by weight. In addition, the accuracy of the individual fetal parameters cannot be checked as there is no gold standard. On the contrary, estimated fetal weight could be assessed against birthweight and has a random error of about 8%.[28]

Since, growth is a dynamic process, it seems logical that its quantification requires the evaluation of serial measurements. In fact, serial measurements of AC and EFW are superior to single estimates in the prediction of neonatal growth restriction defined by ponderal index or skin-fold thickness[30] and in the prediction of adverse outcome.[31] Nevertheless, from our point of view, there are major concerns regarding the use of serial measurements. Firstly, there is a scarcity of published normal ranges for growth velocity and is common practice to use normal ranges derived from transversal series to evaluate serial measurements, and use of standards across population may be misleading. Secondly, there is no agreement regarding the optimal methodology. Theoretically, conditional centiles, whereby the EFW or AC of each individual fetus at a first ultrasound examination is extrapolated to give a range of normal ranges (expressed as centiles) at a later scan, appears to be the most appropriate method for longitudinal growth assessment.[33] Compared to the ranges for the entire population, the conditional ranges for small fetus would be narrower and skewed in the direction of the initial measurement.[33] However, this approach has not demonstrated to be superior to other methodologically more straightforward alternatives, such as z-velocity.[34] In addition, the interval between scan is of paramount importance since two-week intervals are associated with false-positive rates for growth restriction in excess of 10%, increasing to much higher rates late in the third trimester.[35] A four-week interval, which is a too long interval for clinical purposes in high-risk pregnancies, has been reported to optimize the prediction.[36]

Individualized growth standards could be inferred in a forward direction on the basis of ultrasound biometry in early pregnancy. The Rossavik model[37] calculates an expected growth curve from two scans at about 18 and 24–26 weeks. In addition to have failed to demonstrate an improvement in the prediction of fetal weight,[38] there are several concerns regarding its conceptual framework. First, ultrasound error at each of the sequential scans can lead to substantial variation when forward projecting the growth curve that has been calculated from these measurements. Second, the fetus could already be affected by early-onset growth restriction, especially at the latter of the two scans, which would result in depressed values being projected as a "norm".

Assessing Growth

The normal ranges used when evaluating fetal growth is a question of utmost importance. When evaluating single measurements, such as AC, it is recommended to use local standards since differences between populations could be a source of unaccuracy. Nevertheless, strict methodological requirements are needed for normal ranges: a transversal design (each fetus is measured only once), reliable dating, enough sample size at the extremes of the gestational age and correct exclusion criteria. With regard to the question of selection criteria for the development of fetal size, only conditions for which information is available at the time of scanning for fetal growth should be excluded, such as fetal malformations and maternal diseases frequently associated with IUGR.[39] A comprehensive review of several reference ranges is provided elsewhere.[40]

For AC, a systematic review[24] found that a threshold of the tenth centile had better sensitivities and specificities than other commonly used centiles.

Regarding normal ranges for fetal weight, neonatal weight is frequently used as a proxy for fetal weight. Nevertheless, due to the fact that an epidemiological association exists between IUGR and preterm delivery, the birthweight distribution in preterm gestations is negatively skewed, while the distribution of fetal weight at the same gestation is close to normal.[41] As a consequence, population-based standards fail to identify a significant proportion of cases of preterm intrauterine SGA.[42]

For EFW, a systematic review[24] found that a threshold of the tenth centile had better sensitivities and specificities than other commonly used centiles.

Due to the fact that several maternal (height, weight, race, age, parity) and fetal (number, gender) variables play a significant role in fetal growth both in low- and high-risk pregnancies, population-based birth weight standards result in misclassification of a large proportion of cases.[43] Individually adjusted or customized growth charts aim to optimize the assessment of fetal growth by taking individual variation into account and by projecting an optimal curve which delineates the potential weight gain in each pregnancy. The use of customized birthweight standards, which take these factors into account, has demonstrated to improve the definition of SGA and the prediction of abnormal five-minute Apgar score, hospital stay length, admission to the intensive care unit, hypoglycemia, need for neonatal resuscitation and perinatal death, both in high-risk[44] and low-risk[45-48] populations. On the other hand, those neonates with a normal customized birthweight have been found to have a perinatal outcome comparable to the general population, regardless of being SGA according population-based centiles.[44-47] The inference of these findings are that SGA according to customized standards and growth restriction are equivalent, and it has been claimed that customized SGA could be used as reliable proxy of growth restriction.[43]

Regarding the customized fetal weight assessment, it has been found that a threshold of the tenth centile had better sensitivities and specificities than other used centiles for the prediction of adverse outcome.[44]

Three-dimensional Fetal Growth Assessment

The advent of three-dimensional sonography has allowed a new insight into fetal growth. The upper arm[49] or thigh[50] volumes are parameters for detecting IUGR,[49] but need further validation. Calculation of organ volumes could also be made reliably and in a noninvasive way using this new technology. Interestingly, the fetal brain/liver volume ratio has been described[51] as a predictor of fetal outcome in the growth-restricted fetus. An inverse relationship exists in small-for-gestational age fetuses between brain/liver volume ratio and fetal weight-related umbilical venous blood flow. The benefit of prospectively assessing organ values also requires further studies and could not be recommended.

DIAGNOSIS OF THE TYPE OF SGA

Following the diagnosis of a SGA fetus, further evaluation is warranted to determine the type of SGA.

Abnormal SGA

- *Anatomical ultrasound:* An anatomical study is mandatory to rule out the presence of malformations (up to 25% of malformed fetuses are SGA) or the presence of signs of fetal infection (ventriculomegaly, microcephalia, brain or intra-abdominal calcifications, placentomegaly, hydramnios). Most cases of congenital cytomegalovirus infection have oligo hydramnios and therefore should be considered in the differential diagnosis.
- *Karyotyping:* Up to 15% of the abnormal SGA fetuses have some associated syndrome,[47] being either aneuploidy and nonaneuploidy syndromes. Some of them are recognized to be related to imprinting/methylation defects, e.g. the Silver Rusell, a clinically heterogeneous syndrome characterized by intrauterine and postnatal growth retardation with spared cranial growth, dysmorphic features and frequent body asymmetry. The risk of association is greater when there are associated structural abnormalities, a normal liquor volume or a normal uterine or umbilical artery Doppler. Therefore, it may also be appropriate to offer some genetic studies in selected cases.
- *Infectious study:* Although less than 5% of the cases are associated with infection, a TORCH serology seems reasonable to rule out this etiology. In most of the developed countries, the most prevalent infectious etiology of SGA is the cytomegalovirus. In cases, where an early infection is suspected, an amniotic fluid PCR determination for cytomegalo virus may be useful even in the presence of a negative maternal IgM.

IUGR versus Normal SGA

The differentiation between growth-restricted and constitutionally small fetuses is essential for clinical practice: whereas the former are those who have failed to reach its genetically endowed growth potential, the latter are considered to represent one end of the normal size spectrum. The benchmark for this differentiation is the Doppler evaluation.

Umbilical Artery Doppler

Vasoconstriction phenomena of the tertiary stem villi[52] are considered responsible for the up river modifications in the normal wave flow velocity of the umbilical artery with a decrease in the diastolic velocities and an increase in the resistance and impedance indices. From the pioneering research in Doppler, it has been clearly demonstrated that abnormal umbilical Doppler correlates with histological evidence of placental vascular pathology. As a result, Doppler umbilical artery indices correlate with fetal levels of glucose, amino acids and blood gases[53,54] and therefore, it could be considered as a surrogate measurement of the placental functionality. Moreover, a decreased flow in the umbilical vein has also been demonstrated in an asymptomatic stage of the disease related to a decrease of the placental volume. SGA with abnormal umbilical artery Doppler are smaller.[55-57] There is an extensive body of evidence that those SGA fetuses with abnormal umbilical artery flow are at higher risk of adverse perinatal outcome than those with normal flow.[31,45,55-60] Even when controlling for gestational age at delivery some series have reported a significant association between the abnormal umbilical artery flow and the perinatal results.[31,55,60] In addition, the occurrence of perinatal death in the presence of a normal umbilical flow is very uncommon.[55,57,61] Thus, Doppler of the umbilical artery flow could be considered as a risk discriminator tool in the management of SGA fetuses. Evidence supports those SGA fetuses with normal Doppler benefit from a nonintensive follow-up.[62] As a consequence of this evidence, SGA fetuses with normal Doppler have been claimed normal SGA fetuses, representing the lowest spectrum of healthy fetuses and to manage them accordingly.[6,63] Some recent studies would suggest that even those normal-SGA would have a suboptimal perinatal and neurodevelopmental outcome,[64-66] suggesting that a proportion of these SGA fetuses are, in reality, late-onset mild IUGR cases.

Cerebroumbilical Ratio

It has been claimed that the relationship between the umbilical and cerebral flow provides a more sensitive tool to discriminate between constitutional SGA and IUGR as it may be decreased even when UA and MCA are very close to normal. In fact, animal models have demonstrated that this ratio is better correlated with hypoxia than its individual components.[64] Furthermore, it has also been extensively reported that the prediction of adverse outcome is improved using umbilical and cerebral parameters in a combined ratio,[66-73] with sensitivities of about 70%.[68,74] This initial redistribution would also be reflected in an impaired flow in the fetal aorta.

Uterine Artery

A defective trophoblast invasion is a common pattern in early and severe cases of growth restriction,[75] and this phenomenon is responsible for the presence of abnormal flow patterns in the uterine artery.

It has been suggested that uterine artery Doppler provide additional value to the umbilical and cerebral arteries to predict the occurrence of adverse outcome media,[76,77] and some management protocols consider this parameter as a criteria for IUGR independently to the fetal Doppler parameters. Nevertheless, a systematic review with metaanalysis[78] found that uterine artery Doppler had limited accuracy in predicting IUGR and perinatal death, and, therefore, its use needs to be evaluated further in studies.

STUDY OF FETAL DETERIORATION

Assessment of fetal well-being and delivery when the risks of leaving the fetus in an intrauterine hostile environment are considered to be greater than the risks of prematurity, remains the main management strategy for IUGR fetuses. Fetal well-being tests could be classified as chronic or acute. Whilst the former become progressively abnormal due to increasing hypoxemia and/or hypoxia, the latter correlate with acute changes occurring in advanced stages of fetal compromise, characterized by severe hypoxia and metabolic acidosis, and usually precede fetal death in few days. Since, there does not exist a fixed sequence of fetal deterioration, integration of several well-being tests into comprehen sive management protocols seems to be warranted.

Chronic Tests

Umbilical Artery

Vasoconstriction changes of the tertiary stem villi[52] are considered responsible for the upriver modifications in the wave flow velocity of the umbilical artery with a decrease in the diastolic velocities and an increase in the resistance and impedance indices. In advanced stages of placental histological and functional damage, diastolic velocities will become absent or even reversed. It has not been demonstrated qualitative differences in placental histological changes between the cases of IUGR with abnormal but positive diastolic flow and cases with reversed end-diastolic flow,[52] and therefore, the latter is considered the end of the spectrum of placental damage and is associated with an increased risk of perinatal death. As suggested by animal[79] and mathematical[80] experimental models of chronic placental embolization, it is required the obliteration of more than a 50% of the placental vessels before absent or reversed end-diastolic velocities appear.

Studies where IUGR fetuses were followed longitudinally[81] have reported that up to 80% of the fetuses have abnormal umbilical artery indices two weeks before the fetal acute deterioration, and, therefore, this parameter could be considered a chronic marker. End-diastolic velocities have been reported to be present on an average one week before the acute deterioration.[81] Up to 40% of fetuses with acidosis show this umbilical flow pattern.[81] Despite the fact that an association exists between the presence of reversed enddiastolic flow in the umbilical artery and adverse perinatal outcome (with a sensitivity and specificity of about 60%), it is not clear whether this association is due to the confounding effect of prematurity and abnormal precordial venous flows.[82] Recent series[83,84] of severely compromised IUGR suggest an independent value of this pattern to predict perinatal morbidity and mortality, with a relative risk of 4.0 and 10.6 for those fetuses with absent or reversed enddiastolic flow, respectively. In addition to increased fetal and neonatal mortality, this finding is also associated with increased risk of long-term abnormal neurodevelopment.

However, a multicenter randomized trial,[85] the Growth Restriction Intervention Trial (GRIT), found that early delivery prompted by umbilical artery reversed enddiastolic flow does not improve the mortality rate or the neurological outcome in preterm IUGR fetuses, supporting the concept that a safe interval of 24–48 hours exists to allow for corticoid administration for lung maturation.

Middle Cerebral Artery

The reduction in the number of functional arterioles in the tertiary villi leads to a decrease in the PO_2 in the fetal blood. This event sets into motion a phenomena of circulatory redistribution principally characterized by the redistribution and centralization of blood flow. The better oxygenated blood goes towards the most vital organs (brain, heart, adrenals), whilst vasoconstriction limits the blood supply at the organs considered less indispensable (digestive system, lungs, skin, skeleton, etc.). As a consequence, a vasodilatation in the cerebral arteries occurs, known as a "brain-sparing" effect. This vasodilatation leads to an increase in the diastolic velocities and a decrease in the resistance and impe dance indices in these vessels. The middle cerebral artery has become the standard for the clinical evaluation of the centralization of flow in IUGR fetuses. MCA pulsatility index steadily decrease through gestational age in preterm IUGR fetuses, suggesting a progressive redistribution.[86]

Moreover, longitudinal studies on deteriorating IUGR fetuses have reported that the pulsatility index in the MCA progressively becomes abnormal.[86] Up to a 80% of fetuses have vasodilatation 2 weeks before the acute deterioration,[81] although other series have found this figure to be less than 50%.[83] Preliminary findings of an acute loss of the MCA vasodilatation in advanced stages of fetal compromise have not been confirmed in more recent series,[81,83,86,87] and therefore, this sign does not seem to be clinically relevant for management purposes.

The value of cerebral Doppler to predict adverse outcome in the overall population of SGA fetuses is limited, with low sensitivities.[68,74] It has been suggested[88,89] that in near term SGA fetuses, the MCA could be useful to predict adverse outcome, independently of the umbilical artery Doppler. In addition, controversy exists whether cerebral vasodilatation is a merely protective mechanism or on the contrary is associated with suboptimal neurological development.70 In a longitudinal cohort of infants born preterm (26–33 weeks), accelerated visual maturation was found using visual evoked cortical potentials at 3 years. At 5 years, these series demonstrated that both the changes in cerebral Doppler and the acceleration of visual maturation were associated with a deficit in cognitive scores. Recently, studies in the same cohort confirmed that brain sparing was associated with impaired visual function and visual motor capabilities at 11 years of age.[70,71] In consequence, further evidence is required before recommending its use as an isolated surveillance tool.

Amniotic Fluid

The pathways leading to oligohydramnios in fetuses with IUGR is not well-understood. A renal hypo perfusion caused by redistribution phenomena and resulting in a decrease in the urinary production explains only partially this finding. A meta-analysis[90] of 18 randomized studies demonstrated that an amniotic fluid index less than 5 is associated with abnormal 5-minute Apgar score, but failed to demonstrate an association with acidosis. Longitudinal studies IUGR fetuses have shown that the amniotic fluid index progressively decrease.[83,84,86] Nowadays, amniotic fluid volume in believed to be a chronic parameter. In fact, among the components of biophysical profile, it is the only one that is not consi dered acute. One week before the acute deterioration, a 20–30% of cases have oligohydramnios.[84,87]

Acute Markers

Precordial Veins (Ductus Venosus, Inferior Vena Cava and Umbilical Vein)

There is a growing evidence that the fetal heart contributes to the hemodynamic redistribution by shifting the main cardiac output to the left ventricle, maximizing the oxygen supply to the brain. Animal studies have confirmed this adaptative mechanism.[91] Nevertheless, with increasingly adverse condition, these cardiac adaptive mechanisms have been suggested to become overburdened and a progressive impairment of cardiac function has been reported in longitudinal studies.[91] Secondary to severe tissue hypoxia, anerobic metabolism is required for energy production. Chronically, this anerobic metabolism leads to metabolic acidemia and acidosis. The fetal myocardium responds to this acidosis with myocardial cell necrosis phenomena, with replacement by fibroid tissue, which affects the myocardial compliance and therefore increase teledia stolic pressure at both ventricles. The increased concentrations of troponin-T in neonates with pulsatile umbilical vein[92] suggests that myocardial cell destruction is the underlying cause of precordial veins flow abnormalities, with a decrease in velocities during atrial contraction and a consequent increase in pulsatility indices.

The association between abnormal precordial veins flows and adverse perinatal outcome has been extensively reported and has been demonstrated to be independent of the gestational age at delivery.[82] It has also been shown a correlation with acidosis by cordocentesis.[93]

The ductus venosus would allow the diversion of highly oxygenated blood from the umbilical vein into the right atria. This preferential blood flow crosses the foramen ovale to the left cavities and hence to irrigate the fetal brain. There are two possible mechanisms for abnormal venous blood flow waveforms in severe hypoxemia. Firstly, the flow redistribution in the umbilical venous blood towards the DV at the expense of hepatic blood flow, and secondly, there may be a myocardial failure. Whereas ductus venous pulsatility index above the 95th centile is an earlier sign, reversed velocities during atrial contraction represents the end of the spectrum of abnormal flow. It has been reported[94] that in these preterm fetuses, a 3SD cut-off optimize the combination of sensitivity and specificity. Moreover, a recent multicentric prospective study demonstrated that ductus venosus Doppler parameters emerge as the primary cardiovascular factor in predicting neonatal outcome in those preterm early-onset IUGR fetuses below 28 weeks. The perinatal mortality when there an absent or reversed flow in the a-wave was present ranged from 60–100%.[94] However, its sensitivity for perinatal death is still 40–70%.

Although each precordial vein correctly predicts acidbase status in a significant proportion of IUGR neonates, combination, rather than single vessel assessment provides the best predictive accuracy. Doppler abnormality in either vessel identified about a 90% of newborns with acidosis.[95,96]

Longitudinal studies have demonstrated that precordial vein flow waveforms become abnormal in advanced stages of fetal compromise.[81,83,86,87] The temporal relation with other acute markers are variable: whereas in about a 50% of cases, abnormal ductus venosus precedes the loss of short-term variability in the fetal heart rate, this later sign is the first to become abnormal in the other cases.[86] In about a 90% of cases, the ductus venosus become abnormal only 48–72 hours before the biophysical profile shows changes.[87] Debate exists regarding the advantages of DV Doppler investigation over the biophysical profile. However, observational studies suggest that to integrate both DV Doppler investigation and biophysical profile in the management of preterm IUGR seems to more effectively stratify IUGR fetuses into risk categories. Further research is warranted to investigate how they are best combined.

Other Cardiac Doppler Parameters

The aortic isthmus is a link between the right and left ventricles which perfuse the lower body and placental circulation, and upper body, respectively. Consequently, its blood flow pattern reflects the balance between both ventricular outputs and the existence of differences in the vascular impedance in either vascular system. The clinical use of aortic isthmus waveforms for monitoring fetal deterioration in IUGR has been limited, but preliminary work suggests that abnormal AoI impedance indices are an intermediate step between placental insufficiency hypoxemia and cardiac decompensation.[96,97] A prospective study in severe early-onset IUGR demonstrated that a retrograde flow in the AoI in growth-restricted fetuses correlated strongly with adverse perinatal outcome.[98]

Hypoxemia and acidosis may also impair cardiac contractility directly. The myocardial performance index (MPI) is a novel method in fetal medicine that assesses both systolic and diastolic functions by including the measurement of isovolumetric and ejection times and would be useful in assessing the progressive hemodynamic deterioration. It has been recently reported to be independently associated with perinatal mortality, mainly in very preterm IUGR fetuses,[99] although its role as a surveillance tool needs to be further elucidated.

Fetal Heart Rate

Due to severe hypoxemia, signal from peripheral chemoreceptors and baroreceptors triggers a para sympathetic response that results in fetal heart decelerations. In advanced stages of fetal compromise, the direct effect of acidosis on the nervous system and on the myocardium results in a loss of the fetal heart rate variability as well as deceleration.

Early studies on high-risk demonstrated that though highly sensitive, a 50% rate of false positive hampers its clinical usefulness. In addition, a meta-analysis[100] on highrisk pregnancies failed to demonstrate any beneficial effect in reducing perinatal mortality. Hence, there is no evidence to support the use of traditional fetal heart rate in IUGR fetuses.

Computerized fetal heart rate analyses has provided new insight into the pathophysiology of IUGR. It has been demonstrated by cordocentesis that the short-term variability closely correlates with acidosis and severe hypoxia. Despite the fact that Bracero et al.[101] demons trated non-significant perinatal outcome differences between visual and computerized FHR, more recent longitudinal series pointed out a potential role as acute marker.[86] Short-term variability becomes abnormal coinciding with the ductus venosus: whereas in about a 50% of cases abnormal ductus venosus precedes the loss of short-term variability in the fetal heart rate, this later sign is the first to become abnormal in the other cases.[86] Both parameters are considered acute responses to fetal acidosis.

Biophysical Profile

Among the components of the Manning[102] biophysical profile, amniotic fluid volume is the more chronic parameter. With increasing fetal compromise, the amniotic fluid volume progressively decreases.[83,86] In advanced stages of hypoxia, a decrease in the breathing movements is observed and finally, mainly acidosis accounts for the loss of fetal tone and gross body movements.

Observational studies demonstrated an association between abnormal biophysical profile and perinatal mortality and cerebral palsy.[103] Studies in which a cordocentesis was performed demonstrated a good correlation with acidosis,[104] being the fetal tone and gross motor movements the best correlated components. However, similarly to the fetal heart rate, although highly sensitive, a 50% rate of false positive limits the clinical usefulness of the biophysical profile.[105] A meta-analysis[106] showed no significant benefit of biophysical profile in highrisk pregnancies, but more recent series[107] on IUGR have suggested that both Doppler and BPS effectively stratify IUGR fetuses into risk categories. Since, fetal deterioration appears to be independently reflected by both tests, further studies are warranted to prove the usefulness of combined both testing modalities. The above mentioned study uses a cut-off of 4 (or 6 if oligohydramnios exists), for the time being these are the more comprehensive criteria for decision-making.

Longitudinal series[87] have demonstrated that except for the amniotic fluid volume and the fetal heart rate, the other components of the biophysical profile become abnormal in advanced stages of fetal compromise. In about 90% of cases, the ductus venosus become abnormal only 48–72 hours before the biophysical profile.[87]

OBSTETRIC MANAGEMENT

Despite clear guidelines supported by strong evidence cannot be provided, protocols for management of SGA fetus may be developed according to current knowledge. It is evident that an integrated approach seems most appropriate when using any Doppler algorithm in management. Our protocol is as follows:

- Normal-SGA (estimated fetal weight below the 10th centile with normal cerebroplacental ratio and normal uterine artery Doppler flow): Excluding infectious and genetic causes, the perinatal results are good. Fortnightly Doppler and biophysical profile are performed. Delivery should only be indicated for obstetrics or maternal factors. A vaginal delivery with continuous fetal monitoring is recommended. Delivery should not be postponed more than 40 weeks of gestation.
- The IUGR with normal fetal well-being tests (estimated fetal weight below the 10th centile with abnormal cerebroplacental ratio but no presence of vasodilation or uterine artery Doppler flow): Weekly Doppler and biophysical profiles are performed. Delivery beyond 37 weeks or when pulmonary maturity is proven, could be considered. A vaginal delivery with continuous fetal monitoring is recommended.

- The IUGR (estimated fetal weight below the 10th centile with abnormal cerebroplacental ratio or uterine artery Doppler flow) with significant placental insufficiency (absent end-diastolic flow in the umbilical artery) or centralization (persistent vasodilatation of middle cerebral artery):
  a. Beyond 34 weeks: A vaginal delivery is accepted. A cesarean section would be required in absent enddiastolic umbilical flow.
  b. Between 32 and 34 weeks:
     i. Reversed end-diastolic flow: Steroids and delivery in 24-48 hours by cesarean section
     ii. Absent end-diastolic flow: Steroids, daily Doppler and biophysical profile until 34 weeks.
  c. Below 32 weeks: Steroids, daily Doppler and biophysical profile until 34 weeks.
- The IUGR (estimated fetal weight below the 10th centile with abnormal cerebroplacental ratio or uterine artery Doppler flow) with suspected fetal compromise (persistent increased ductus venosus waveforms pulsatility, low short-term variability, abnormal biophysical profile):
  a. Beyond 32 weeks: Delivery by cesarean section
  b. Below 32 weeks: Hospital admission, steroids, daily Doppler and biophysical profile/12 hours until 32 weeks.
- The IUGR (estimated fetal weight below the 10th centile with abnormal cerebroplacental ratio or uterine artery Doppler flow) with fetal decompensation (persistent absent or reversed a-wave in the ductus venosus or persistent pulsatile umbilical vein or persistent abnormal biophysical profile or decelerative cardiotocography): delivery by cesarean section at a tertiary care center. In the subgroup under 28 weeks, each case should be evaluated by a multidisciplinary committee composed by an obstetrician and a neonatologist with experience in those case, and taking into account the opinion of the parents: expectant management could be an option in these extremely preterm and compromised fetuses.

REFERENCES

1. Kady S, Gardosi J. Perinatal mortality and fetal growth restriction. Best Pract Res Clin Obstet Gynaecol. 2004;18(3):397-410.
2. Jarvis S, Glinianaia SV, Torrioli MG, et al. Cerebral palsy and intrauterine growth in single births: European collaborative study. Lancet. 2003;362(9390):1106-11.
3. Smith GC, Wood AM, Pell JP, et al. Sudden infant death syndrome and complications in other pregnancies. Lancet. 2005;366(9503):2107-11.
4. Godfrey KM, Barker DJ. Fetal nutrition and adult disease. Am J Clin Nutr. 2000;71(5 Suppl):1344S-52S.
5. Todros T, Plazzotta C, Pastorin L. Body proportionality of the small-for-date fetus: is it related to aetiological factors? Early Hum Dev. 1996;45(1-2):1-9.
6. Soothill PW, Bobrow CS, Holmes R. Small for gestational age is not a diagnosis. Ultrasound Obstet Gynecol. 1999; 13(4):225-8.
7. Blackwell SC, Moldenhauer J, Redman M, et al. Relationship between the sonographic pattern of intrauterine growth restriction and acid-base status at the time of cordocentensis. Arch Gynecol Obstet. 2001;264(4):191-3.
8. Lin CC, Su SJ, River LP. Comparison of associated highrisk factors and perinatal outcome between symmetric and asymmetric fetal intrauterine growth retardation. Am J Obstet Gynecol. 1991;164(6 Pt 1):1535-41; discussion 1541-2.
9. Kramer MS, Olivier M, McLean FH, et al. Impact of intrauterine growth retardation and body proportionality on fetal and neonatal outcome. Pediatrics. 1990;86(5):707-13.
10. Carrera J. Definitions, etiology and clinical implications. Ultrasound and Fetal Growth. London: The Parthenon Publish; 1999. pp. 17-34.
11. Wilcox AJ. Intrauterine growth retardation: beyond birthweight criteria. Early Hum Dev. 1983;8(3-4):189-93.
12. Snijders RJ, Sherrod C, Gosden CM, et al. Fetal growth retardation: associated malformations and chromosomal abnormalities. Am J Obstet Gynecol. 1993;168(2):547-55.
13. Yaron Y, Ochshorn Y, Heifetz S, et al. First trimester maternal serum free human chorionic gonadotropin as a predictor of adverse pregnancy outcome. Fetal Diagn Ther. 2002;17(6):352-6.
14. Levine RJ, Lam C, Qian C, et al. Soluble endoglin and other circulating antiangiogenic factors in preeclampsia. N Engl J Med. 2006;355(10):992-1005.
15. Papageorghiou AT, Yu CK, Bindra R, et al. Multicenter screening for pre-eclampsia and fetal growth restriction by transvaginal uterine artery Doppler at 23 weeks of gestation. Ultrasound Obstet Gynecol. 2001;18(5):441-9.
16. Martin AM, Bindra R, Curcio P, et al. Screening for preeclampsia and fetal growth restriction by uterine artery Doppler at 11-14 weeks of gestation. Ultrasound Obstet Gynecol. 2001;18(6):583-6.
17. Lindqvist PG, Molin J. Does antenatal identification of small-for-gestational age fetuses significantly improve their outcome? Ultrasound Obstet Gynecol. 2005;25(3):258-64.
18. European comparison of perinatal care—the Euronatal Study. Maternal and Child Health Consortium. CESDI 8th Annual Report: Confidential Inquiry of Sitllbirth and Deaths in Infancy. 2001.

19. British College of Obstetricians and Gynaecologist. The Investigation and Management of The Small-for-Gesta tional Age Fetus. Geen-Top Guidelines 2002 (Guideline No.31).
20. Gardosi J, Francis A. Controlled trial of fundal height measurement plotted on customised antenatal growth charts. Br J Obstet Gynaecol. 1999;106(4):309-17.
21. Mongelli M, Wilcox M, Gardosi J. Estimating the date of confinement: ultrasonographic biometry versus certain menstrual dates. Am J Obstet Gynecol. 1996;174(1 Pt 1): 278-81.
22. Robinson HP, Fleming JE. A critical evaluation of sonar "crown-rump length" measurements. Br J Obstet Gynaecol. 1975;82(9):702-10.
23. Mul T, Mongelli M, Gardosi J. A comparative analysis of second-trimester ultrasound dating formulae in pregnan cies conceived with artificial reproductive techniques. Ultrasound Obstet Gynecol. 1996;8(6):397-402.
24. Chang TC, Robson SC, Boys RJ, et al. Prediction of the small for gestational age infant: which ultrasonic measurement is best? Obstet Gynecol. 1992;80(6):1030-8.
25. Chien PF, Owen P, Khan KS. Validity of ultrasound estima tion of fetal weight. Obstet Gynecol. 2000;95(6 Pt 1):856-60.
26. Salomon LJ, Bernard JP, Duyme M, et al. The impact of choice of reference charts and equations on the assessment of fetal biometry. Ultrasound Obstet Gynecol. 2005;25(6): 559-65.
27. Shepard MJ, Richards VA, Berkowitz RL, et al. An evaluation of two equations for predicting fetal weight by ultrasound. Am J Obstet Gynecol. 1982;142(1):47-54.
28. Hadlock FP, Harrist RB, Sharman RS, et al. Estimation of fetal weight with the use of head, body, and femur measurements—a prospective study. Am J Obstet Gynecol. 1985;151(3):333-7.
29. Kaaij MW, Struijk PC, Lotgering FK. Accuracy of sonographic estimates of fetal weight in very small infants. Ultrasound Obstet Gynecol. 1999;13(2):99-102.
30. Chang TC, Robson SC, Spencer JA, et al. Identification of fetal growth retardation: comparison of Doppler waveform indices and serial ultrasound measurements of abdominal circumference and fetal weight. Obstet Gynecol. 1993;82(2):230-6.
31. Chang TC, Robson SC, Spencer JA, et al. Prediction of perinatal morbidity at term in small fetuses: comparison of fetal growth and Doppler ultrasound. Br J Obstet Gynaecol. 1994;101(5):422-7.
32. Royston P, Altman DG. Design and analysis of longitudinal studies of fetal size. Ultrasound Obstet Gynecol. 1995;6(5):307-12.
33. Kiserud T, Lian S. Biometric assessment. Best practice and Research Clinical Obstetrics and gynecology. 2009;23: 819-31.
34. Owen P, Donnet ML, Ogston SA, et al. Standards for ultrasound fetal growth velocity. Br J Obstet Gynaecol. 1996;103(1):60-9.
35. Mongelli M, Ek S, Tambyrajia R. Screening for fetal growth restriction: a mathematical model of the effect of time interval and ultrasound error. Obstet Gynecol. 1998;92(6): 908-12.
36. Mondry A, Pengbo L, Loh M, Mongelli M. Z-velocity in screening for intrauterine growth restriction. Ultrasound Obstet Gynecol. 2005;26(6):634-8.
37. Deter RL, Rossavik IK, Harrist RB, et al. Mathematic modeling of fetal growth: development of individual growth curve standards. Obstet Gynecol. 1986;68(2):156-61.
38. Shields LE, Huff RW, Jackson GM, et al. Fetal growth: a comparison of growth curves with mathematical modeling. J Ultrasound Med. 1993;12(5):271-4.
39. Altman DG, Chitty LS. Charts of fetal size: 1. Methodology. Br J Obstet Gynaecol. 1994;101(1):29-34.
40. Figueras F, Torrents M, Munoz A, et al. References intervals for fetal biometrical parameters. Eur J Obstet Gynecol Reprod Biol. 2002;105(1):25-30.
41. Wilcox M, Gardosi J, Mongelli M, et al. Birth weight from pregnancies dated by ultrasonography in a multicultural British population. BMJ. 1993;307(6904):588-91.
42. Gardosi JO. Prematurity and fetal growth restriction. Early Hum Dev. 2005;81(1):43-9.
43. Gardosi J. Customized fetal growth standards: rationale and clinical application. Semin Perinatol. 2004;28(1):33-40.
44. De Jong CL, Francis A, Van Geijn HP, et al. Customized fetal weight limits for antenatal detection of fetal growth restriction. Ultrasound Obstet Gynecol. 2000;15(1):36-40.
45. McCowan LM, Harding JE, Stewart AW. Customized birthweight centiles predict SGA pregnancies with perinatal morbidity. BJOG. 2005;112(8):1026-33.
46. Clausson B, Gardosi J, Francis A, et al. Perinatal outcome in SGA births defined by customised versus population-based birthweight standards. BJOG. 2001;108(8):830-4.
47. Ego A, Subtil D, Grange G, et al. Customized versus population-based birth weight standards for identifying growth restricted infants: a French multicenter study. Am J Obstet Gynecol. 2006;194(4):1042-9.
48. Sciscione AC, Gorman R, Callan NA. Adjustment of birth weight standards for maternal and infant characteristics improves the prediction of outcome in the small-forgestational- age infant. Am J Obstet Gynecol. 1996;175(3 Pt 1):544-7.
49. Chang CH, Yu CH, Ko HC, et al. Fetal upper arm volume in predicting intrauterine growth restriction: a three-dimensional ultrasound study. Ultrasound Med Biol. 2005;31(11):1435-9.
50. Chang CH, Yu CH, Ko HC, et al. The efficacy assessment of thigh volume in predicting intrauterine fetal growth restriction by three-dimensional ultrasound. Ultrasound Med Biol. 2005;31(7):883-7.
51. Chang CH, Yu CH, Chang FM, et al. The assessment of normal fetal liver volume by three-dimensional ultrasound. Ultrasound Med Biol. 2003;29(8):1123-9.

52. Sebire NJ. Umbilical artery Doppler revisited: patho physiology of changes in intrauterine growth restriction revealed. Ultrasound Obstet Gynecol. 2003;21(5):419-22.
53. Nicolaides KH, Bilardo CM, Soothill PW, et al. Absence of end diastolic frequencies in umbilical artery: a sign of fetal hypoxia and acidosis. BMJ. 1988;297(6655):1026-7.
54. Karsdorp VH, van Vugt JM, Jakobs C, et al. Amino acids, glucose and lactate concentrations in umbilical cord blood in relation to umbilical artery flow patterns. Eur J Obstet Gynecol Reprod Biol. 1994;57(2):117-22.
55. Trudinger BJ, Cook CM, Giles WB, et al. Fetal umbilical artery velocity waveforms and subsequent neonatal outcome. Br J Obstet Gynaecol. 1991;98(4):378-84.
56. James DK, Parker MJ, Smoleniec JS. Comprehensive fetal assessment with three ultrasonographic characteristics. Am J Obstet Gynecol. 1992;166(5):1486-95.
57. Burke G, Stuart B, Crowley P, et al. Is intrauterine growth retardation with normal umbilical artery blood flow a benign condition? BMJ. 1990;300(6731):1044-5.
58. Gaziano EP, Knox H, Ferrera B, et al. Is it time to reassess the risk for the growth-retarded fetus with normal Doppler velocimetry of the umbilical artery? Am J Obstet Gynecol. 1994;170(6):1734-41; discussion 1741-3.
59. Reuwer PJ, Sijmons EA, Rietman GW, et al. Intrauterine growth retardation: prediction of perinatal distress by Doppler ultrasound. Lancet. 1987;2(8556):415-8.
60. Yoon BH, Lee CM, Kim SW. An abnormal umbilical artery waveform: a strong and independent predictor of adverse perinatal outcome in patients with preeclampsia. Am J Obstet Gynecol. 1994;171(3):713-21.
61. McCowan LM, Harding JE, Stewart AW. Umbilical artery Doppler studies in small for gestational age babies reflect disease severity. BJOG. 2000;107(7):916-25.
62. McCowan LM, Harding JE, Roberts AB, et al. A pilot randomized controlled trial of two regimens of fetal surveillance for small-for-gestational-age fetuses with normal results of umbilical artery doppler velocimetry. Am J Obstet Gynecol. 2000;182(1 Pt 1):81-6.
63. Bobrow CS, Soothill PW. Fetal growth velocity: a cautionary tale. Lancet. 1999;353(9163):1460.
64. Arbeille P, Maulik D, Fignon A, et al. Assessment of the fetal PO2 changes by cerebral and umbilical Doppler on lamb fetuses during acute hypoxia. Ultrasound Med Biol. 1995;21(7):861-70.
65. Figueras F, Eixarch E, Meler E, et al. Small-for-gestationalage fetuses with normal umbilical artery Doppler have suboptimal perinatal and neurodevelopmental outcome. Eur J Obstet Gynecol Reprod Biol. 2008;136(1):34-8.
66. Leitner Y, Fattal-Valevski A, Geva R, et al. Neurodevelopmental outcome of children with intrauterine growth retardation: a longitudinal, 10-year prospective study. J Child Neurol. 2007;22(5);580-7.
67. Arias F. Accuracy of the middle-cerebral-to-umbilical-artery resistance index ratio in the prediction of neonatal outcome in patients at high risk for fetal and neonatal complications. Am J Obstet Gynecol. 1994;171(6):1541-5.
68. Bahado-Singh RO, Kovanci E, Jeffres A, et al. The Doppler cerebroplacental ratio and perinatal outcome in intrauterine growth restriction. Am J Obstet Gynecol. 1999;180(3 Pt 1):750-6.
69. Gramellini D, Folli MC, Raboni S, et al. Cerebral-umbilical Doppler ratio as a predictor of adverse perinatal outcome. Obstet Gynecol. 1992;79(3):416-20.
70. Scherjon S, Briet J, Oosting H, et al. The discrepancy between maturation of visual-evoked potentials and cognitive outcome at five years in very preterm infants with and without hemodynamic signs of fetal brain-sparing. Pediatrics. 2000;105(2):385-91.
71. Kok JH, Prick L, Merckel E, et al. Visual function at 11 years of age in preterm-born children with and without fetal brain sparing. Pediatrics. 2007;119(6):e1342-50.
72. Devine PA, Bracero LA, Lysikiewicz A, et al. Middle cerebral to umbilical artery Doppler ratio in post-date pregnancies. Obstet Gynecol. 1994;84(5):856-60.
73. Makhseed M, Jirous J, Ahmed MA, et al. Middle cerebral artery to umbilical artery resistance index ratio in the prediction of neonatal outcome. Int J Gynaecol Obstet. 2000;71(2):119-25.
74. Odibo AO, Riddick C, Pare E, et al. Cerebroplacental Doppler ratio and adverse perinatal outcomes in intrauterine growth restriction: evaluating the impact of using gestational agespecific reference values. J Ultrasound Med. 2005;24(9):1223- 8.
75. Madazli R, Somunkiran A, Calay Z, et al. Histomorphology of the placenta and the placental bed of growth restricted foetuses and correlation with the Doppler velocimetries of the uterine and umbilical arteries. Placenta. 2003;24(5):510-6.
76. Severi FM, Bocchi C, Visentin A, et al. Uterine and fetal cerebral Doppler predict the outcome of third-trimester small-for-gestational age fetuses with normal umbilical artery Doppler. Ultrasound Obstet Gynecol. 2002;19(3):225-8.
77. Vergani P, Roncaglia N, Andreotti C, et al. Prognostic value of uterine artery Doppler velocimetry in growth-restricted fetuses delivered near term. Am J Obstet Gynecol. 2002;187(4):932- 6.
78. Chien PF, Arnott N, Gordon A, et al. How useful is uterine artery Doppler flow velocimetry in the prediction of preeclampsia, intrauterine growth retardation and perinatal death? An overview. BJOG. 2000;107(2):196-208.
79. Morrow RJ, Adamson SL, Bull SB, et al. Effect of placental embolization on the umbilical arterial velocity waveform in fetal sheep. Am J Obstet Gynecol. 1989;161(4):1055-60.
80. Thompson RS, Trudinger BJ. Doppler waveform pulsatility index and resistance, pressure and flow in the umbilical placental circulation: an investigation using a mathematical model. Ultrasound Med Biol. 1990;16(5):449-58.

81. Ferrazzi E, Bozzo M, Rigano S, et al. Temporal sequence of abnormal Doppler changes in the peripheral and central circulatory systems of the severely growth-restricted fetus. Ultrasound Obstet Gynecol. 2002;19(2):140-6.
82. Schwarze A, Gembruch U, Krapp M, et al. Qualitative venous Doppler flow waveform analysis in preterm intrauterine growth-restricted fetuses with ARED flow in the umbilical artery—correlation with short-term outcome. Ultrasound Obstet Gynecol. 2005;25(6):573-9.
83. Cosmi E, Ambrosini G, D'Antona D, et al. Doppler, cardiotocography, and biophysical profile changes in growthrestricted fetuses. Obstet Gynecol. 2005;106(6): 1240-5.
84. Valcamonico A, Danti L, Frusca T, et al. Absent end-diastolic velocity in umbilical artery: risk of neonatal morbidity and brain damage. Am J Obstet Gynecol. 1994;170(3):796-801.
85. Thornton JG, Hornbuckle J, Vail A, et al. Infant wellbeing at 2 years of age in the Growth Restriction Intervention Trial (GRIT): multicentred randomised controlled trial. Lancet. 2004;364(9433):513-20.
86. Hecher K, Bilardo CM, Stigter RH, et al. Monitoring of fetuses with intrauterine growth restriction: a longitudinal study. Ultrasound Obstet Gynecol. 2001;18(6):564-70.
87. Baschat AA, Gembruch U, Harman CR. The sequence of changes in Doppler and biophysical parameters as severe fetal growth restriction worsens. Ultrasound Obstet Gynecol. 2001;18(6):571-7.
88. Hershkovitz R, Kingdom JC, Geary M, et al. Fetal cerebral blood flow redistribution in late gestation: identification of compromise in small fetuses with normal umbilical artery Doppler. Ultrasound Obstet Gynecol. 2000;15(3):209-12.
89. To WW, Chan AM, Mok KM. Use of umbilical-cerebral Doppler ratios in predicting fetal growth restriction in near-term fetuses. Aust N Z J Obstet Gynaecol. 2005;45(2):130-6.
90. Chauhan SP, Sanderson M, Hendrix NW, et al. Perinatal outcome and amniotic fluid index in the antepartum and intrapartum periods: a meta-analysis. Am J Obstet Gynecol. 1999;181(6):1473-8.
91. Gilbert RD. Fetal myocardial responses to long-term hypoxemia. Comp Biochem Physiol A Mol Integr Physiol. 1998;119(3):669-74.
92. Makikallio K, Vuolteenaho O, Jouppila P, et al. Association of severe placental insufficiency and systemic venous pressure rise in the fetus with increased neonatal cardiac troponin T levels. Am J Obstet Gynecol. 2000;183(3):726-31.
93. Hecher K, Snijders R, Campbell S, et al. Fetal venous, intracardiac, and arterial blood flow measurements in intrauterine growth retardation: relationship with fetal blood gases. Am J Obstet Gynecol. 1995;173(1):10-5.
94. Bilardo CM, Wolf H, Stigter RH, et al. Relationship between monitoring parameters and perinatal outcome in severe, early intrauterine growth restriction. Ultrasound Obstet Gynecol. 2004;23(2):119-25.
95. Bashat AA, Cosmi E, Bilardo C, et al. Predictors of neonatal outcome in early-onset placental dysfunction. Obstet Gynecol. 2007;109(2 Pt 1):253-61.
96. Baschat AA, Guclu S, Kush ML, Gembruch U, Weiner CP, Harman CR. Venous Doppler in the prediction of acid-base status of growth-restricted fetuses with elevated placental blood flow resistance. Am J Obstet Gynecol. 2004;191(1):277-84.
97. Kennelly MM, Farah N, Turner MJ, et al. Aortic isthmus Doppler velocimetry: role in assessment of preterm fetal growth restriction. Prenat Diagn. 2010;30(5):395-401.
98. Del Río M, Martínez JM, Figueras F, et al. Doppler assessment of the aortic isthmus and perinatal outcome in preterm fetuses with severe intrauterine growth restriction. Ultrasound Obstet Gynecol. 2008;31(1):41-7.
99. Hernandez-Andrade E, Crispi F, Benavides-Serralde A, et al. Contribution of the modified myocardial performance index and aortic isthmus blood flow index to refine predic tion of mortality in preterm intrauterine growth restricted fetuses. Ultrasound Obstet Gynecol. 2009;34(4):430-6.
100. Pattison N, McCowan L. Cardiotocography for antepartum fetal assessment. Cochrane Database Syst Rev. 2000(2): CD001068.
101. Bracero LA, Morgan S, Byrne DW. Comparison of visual and computerized interpretation of nonstress test results in a randomized controlled trial. Am J Obstet Gynecol. 1999;181(5 Pt 1):1254-8.
102. Manning FA, Platt LD, Sipos L. Antepartum fetal evaluation: development of a fetal biophysical profile. Am J Obstet Gynecol. 1980;136(6):787-95.
103. Manning FA, Bondaji N, Harman CR, et al. Fetal assessment based on fetal biophysical profile scoring. VIII. The incidence of cerebral palsy in tested and untested perinates. Am J Obstet Gynecol. 1998;178(4):696-706.
104. Manning FA, Snijders R, Harman CR, et al. Fetal biophysical profile score. VI. Correlation with antepartum umbilical venous fetal pH. Am J Obstet Gynecol. 1993;169(4): 755-63.
105. Miller DA, Rabello YA, Paul RH. The modified biophysical profile: antepartum testing in the 1990s. Am J Obstet Gynecol. 1996;174(3):812-7.
106. Alfirevic Z, Neilson JP. Biophysical profile for fetal assessment in high risk pregnancies. Cochrane Database Syst Rev. 2000(2):CD000038.
107. Baschat AA, Galan HL, Bhide A, et al. Doppler and biophysical assessment in growth restricted fetuses: distribution of test results. Ultrasound Obstet Gynecol. 2006; 27(1):41-7.

CHAPTER 17

Fetal Central Nervous System

Ritsuko K Pooh

INTRODUCTION

The brain is three-dimensional structure and should be assessed in basic three planes of sagittal, coronal, and axial sections. Transvaginal observation of the fetal brain offers sagittal and coronal views of the brain from fetal parietal direction through the fontanelles and/or the sagittal suture as ultrasound windows. This method has contributed to the prenatal assessment of congenital CNS anomalies and acquired brain damage in utero.

Three-dimensional (3D) ultrasound is one of the most attractive modalities in the field of fetal ultrasound imaging. By recent advances of 3D HDlive, HDlive silhouette and flow, the brain morphology and vascular structure can be demonstrated more objectively and accurately.

The combination of transvaginal approach and 3D ultrasound technologies provides us more and more information of fetal brain development, congenital anomalies as well as intrauterine acquired injuries.

TRANSVAGINAL NEUROSONOGRAPHY

Imaging technologies have been remarkably improved and contributed to prenatal evaluation of fetal central nervous system (CNS) development and assessment of CNS abnormalities in utero.

Conventional transabdominal ultrasonography, by which it is possible to observe fetuses through maternal abdominal wall, uterine wall and sometimes placenta, has been most widely utilized for antenatal imaging diagnosis. By transabdominal approach, the whole central nervous system of fetuses can be well demonstrated, for instance, the brain in the axial section and the spine in the sagittal section. However, transabdominal approach to the fetal central nervous system has several obstacles such as maternal abdominal wall, placenta and fetal cranial bones and it is difficult to obtain clear and detailed images of fetal CNS structure.

Introduction of high-frequency transvaginal transducer has contributed to establishing "sonoembryology"[1] and recent general use of transvaginal sonography in early pregnancy enabled early diagnoses of major fetal anomalies.[2] In the middle and late pregnancy, fetal CNS is generally evaluated through maternal abdominal wall. The brain, however, is three-dimensional structure, and should be assessed in basic three planes of sagittal, coronal, and axial sections. Sonographic assessment of the fetal brain in the sagittal and coronal section requires an approach from fetal parietal direction. Transvaginal sonography of the fetal brain opened a new field in medicine, "neurosonography".[3] Transvaginal approach to the normal fetal brain during the second and third trimester was introduced in the beginning of 1990s. It was the first practical application of three-dimensional central nervous system assessment by two-dimensional (2D) ultrasound.[4] Transvaginal observation of the fetal brain offers sagittal and coronal views of the brain from fetal parietal direction[5-8] through the fontanelles and/or the sagittal suture as ultrasound windows. Serial oblique sections[3] via the same ultrasound window reveal the intracranial morphology in detail. This method has contributed to the prenatal assessment of congenital CNS anomalies and acquired brain damage in utero.

BASIC ANATOMICAL KNOWLEDGE OF THE BRAIN

As described above, the brain should be understood as a three-dimensional structure. It is generally believed that the brain anatomy is complicated and there must be lots of terms to remember. However, in order to demonstrate the brain structure and evaluate fetal CNS disorders, it is not necessary to remember all of detailed structure. Here, essential anatomical structures are selected for neuroimaging and comprehension of fetal CNS diseases.

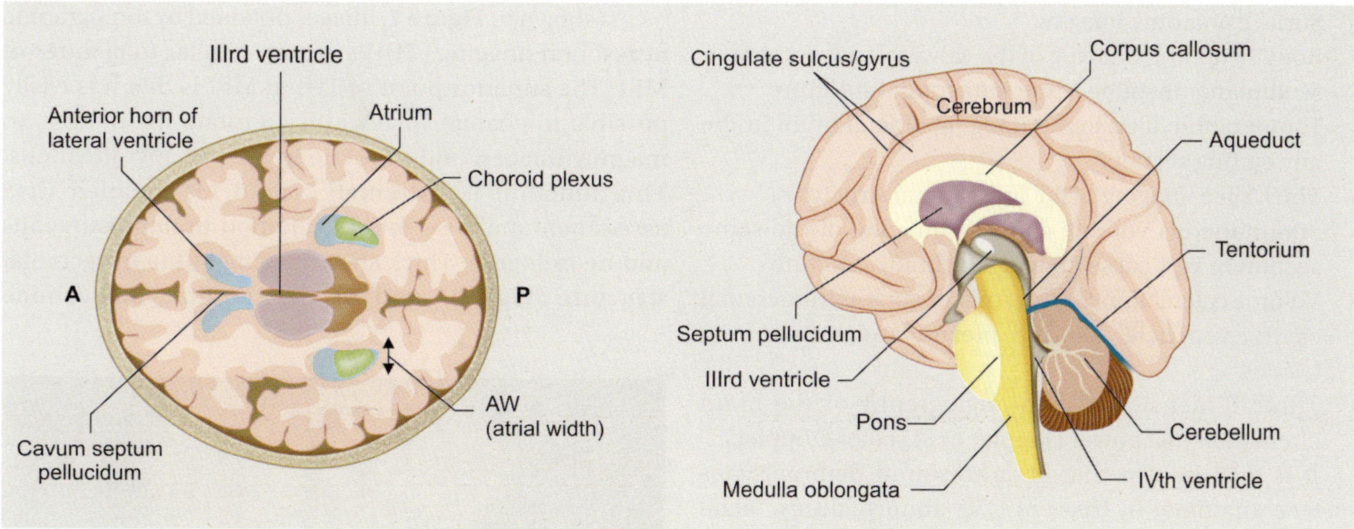

Fig. 1: Basic anatomy of the fetal brain (Axial and sagittal sections).

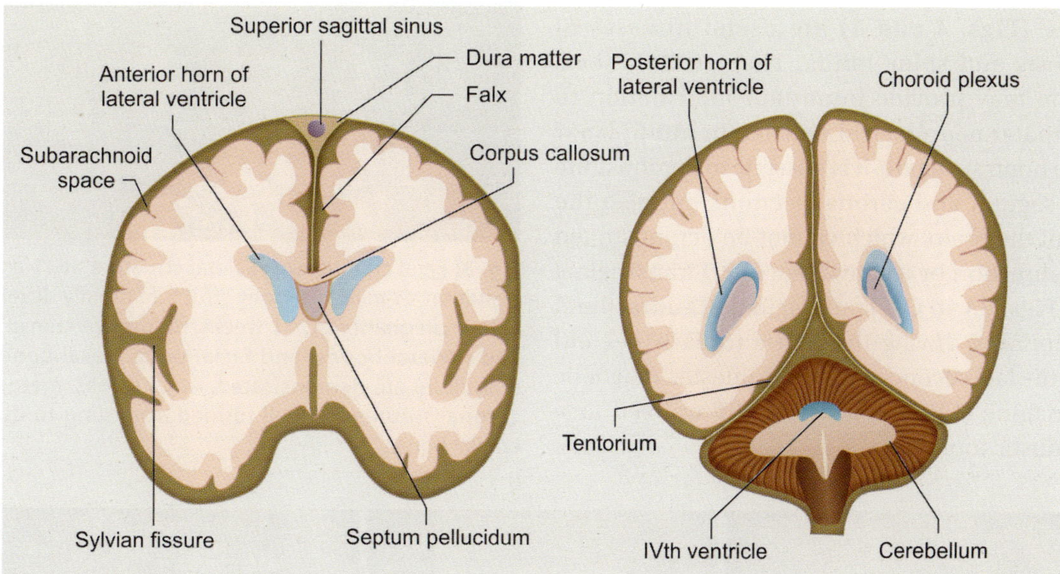

Fig. 2: Basic anatomy of the fetal brain (Coronal section).

Figure 1 shows the basic brain anatomy in the axial and sagittal sections and **Figure 2** shows the anterior coronal and posterior coronal sections.

TRANSVAGINAL 3D SONOGRAPHIC ASSESSMENT OF FETAL CNS

Three-dimensional (3D) ultrasound is one of the most attractive modalities in the field of fetal ultrasound imaging. There are two scanning methods of free-hand scan and automatic scan. Automatic scan by dedicated 3D transducer produces motor driven automatic sweeping and is called as a fan scan. With this method, a shift and/or angle-change of the transducer is not required during scanning and scan duration needs only several seconds. After acquisition of the target organ, multiplanar imaging analysis, and tomographic imaging analysis are possible. The combination of both transvaginal sonography and 3D ultrasound[9-12] may be a great diagnostic tool for evaluation of three-dimensional structure of fetal CNS. Recent advanced 3D ultrasound equipment have several useful functions as below:

- Surface anatomy imaging
- Bony structural imaging of the calvaria and vertebrae
- Multiplanar imaging of the intracranial structure
- Tomographic ultrasound imaging of fetal brain in the any cutting section
- Thick slice imaging of the intracranial structure
- Simultaneous volume contrast imaging of the same section or vertical section of fetal brain structure
- Volume calculation of target organs such as intracranial cavity, ventricle, choroid plexus, and intracranial lesions
- Three-dimensional sono-angiography of the brain circulation (3D power Doppler or 3D color Doppler).

It is well known that 3D ultrasound demonstrates surface anatomy. In cases of CNS abnormalities, facial abnormalities and extremities anomalies are often complicated. Therefore, surface reconstructed images are helpful. Bony structural imaging of the calvaria **(Fig. 3)** and vertebrae **(Figs. 4 and 5)** are useful in cases of craniosynostosis and spina bifida. The vertebral level of spina bifida may provide important information to prospect postnatal neurological deficits. In multiplanar imaging of the brain structure, it is possible to demonstrate not only the sagittal and coronal sections but also the axial section of the brain, which cannot be demonstrated from parietal direction by a conventional 2D transvaginal sonography **(Figs. 6A to C)**. Transvaginal 3D ultrasound is the first modality during the first and early second trimesters. In the late second and third trimester, magnetic resonance imaging (MRI) is occasionally utilized as a prenatal diagnostic tool.[13]

As shown in **Figure 7**, images obtained by tomographic ultrasound imaging (TUI) are quite similar to pictures of MRI. The superior point of TUI to MRI is that it is easily possible to change slice width, to rotate the images, to magnify images, and to rotate images to any directions. This function is extremely useful for detailed CNS assessment and also for consultation to neurosurgeons and neurologists. Thick slice imaging of the intracranial structure **(Figs. 8A and B)** and simultaneous volume

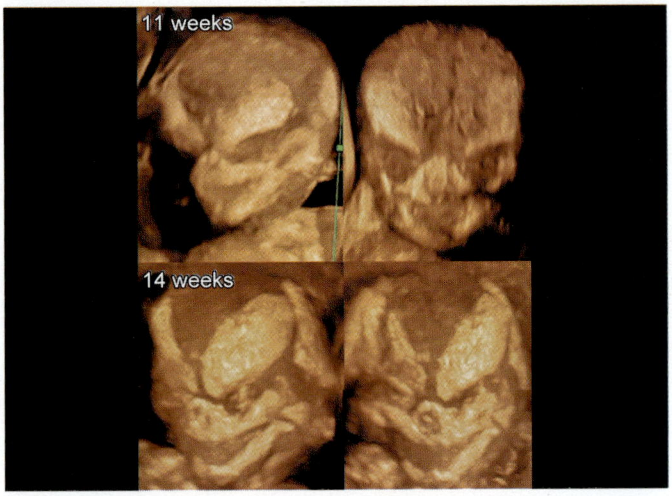

Fig. 3: Fetal craniofacial skeletal structure at 11 and 14 weeks of gestation. Craniofacial bony structure rapidly develops in the first half of pregnancy. At 11 weeks, premature cranial bones (frontal and parietal bones) and facial bone (nasal bone, maxilla, and mandible) are demonstrated. At 14 weeks, metopic suture and coronal sutures are well formed according to development of cranial bones.

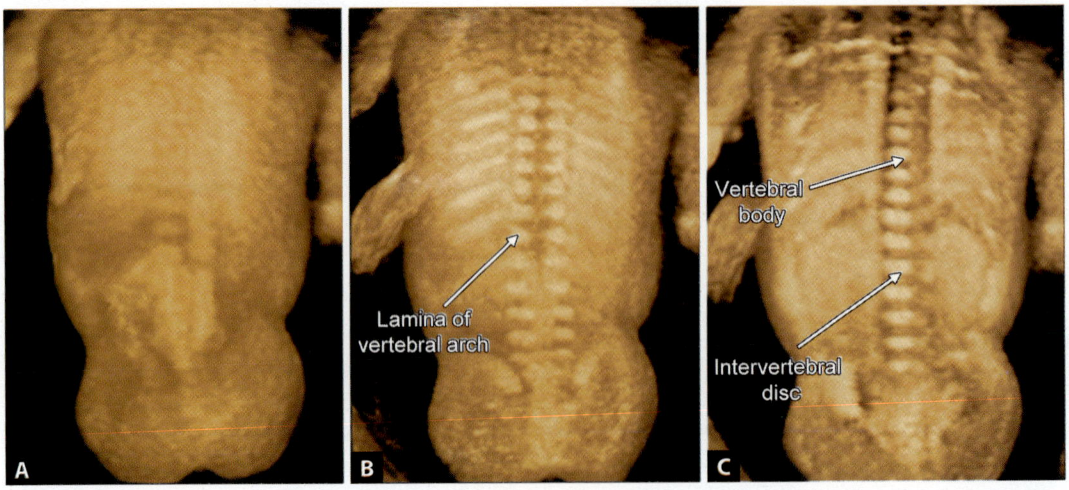

Figs. 4A to C: 3D image of normal vertebral structure at 16 weeks of gestation. 3D reconstructed image of the surface level (A), vertebral arch level (B) and vertebral body level (C). Intervertebral disc spaces are well demonstrated.

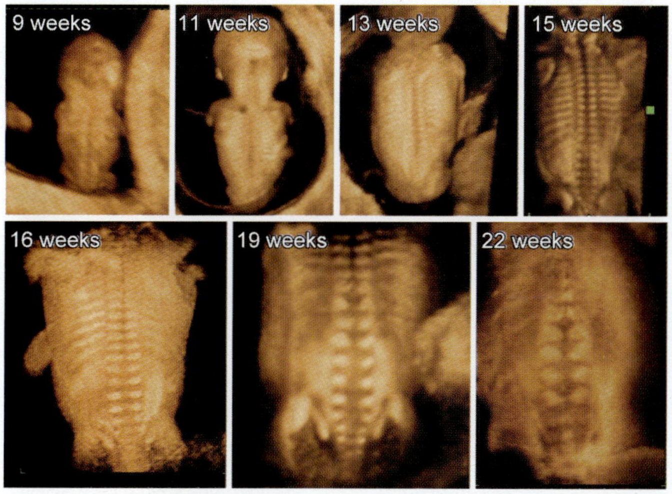

Fig. 5: Fetal vertebral development by 3D-US from 9 to 22 weeks of gestation. Approaching stage of bilateral vertebral lamina according to neural tube closure is visible with advanced gestational weeks.

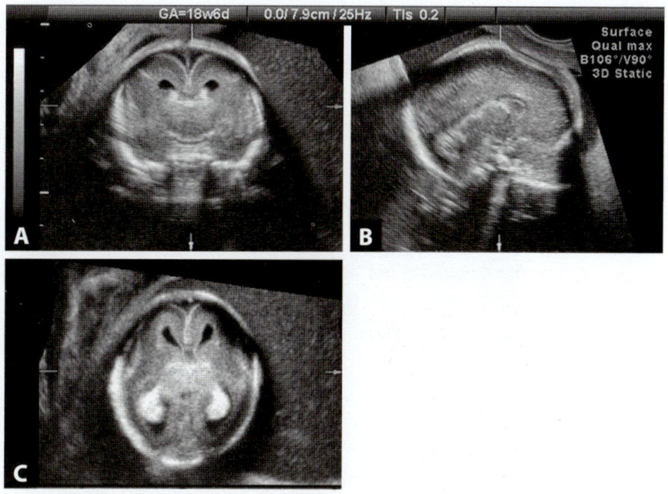

Figs. 6A to C: 3D orthogonal view of normal brain at 18 weeks of gestation. Three-orthogonal view is useful to obtain orientation of the brain structure. Coronal (A), sagittal (B), and axial (C) images can be visualized on a single screen. Any rotation of the brain image around any (x, y, z) axis is possible.

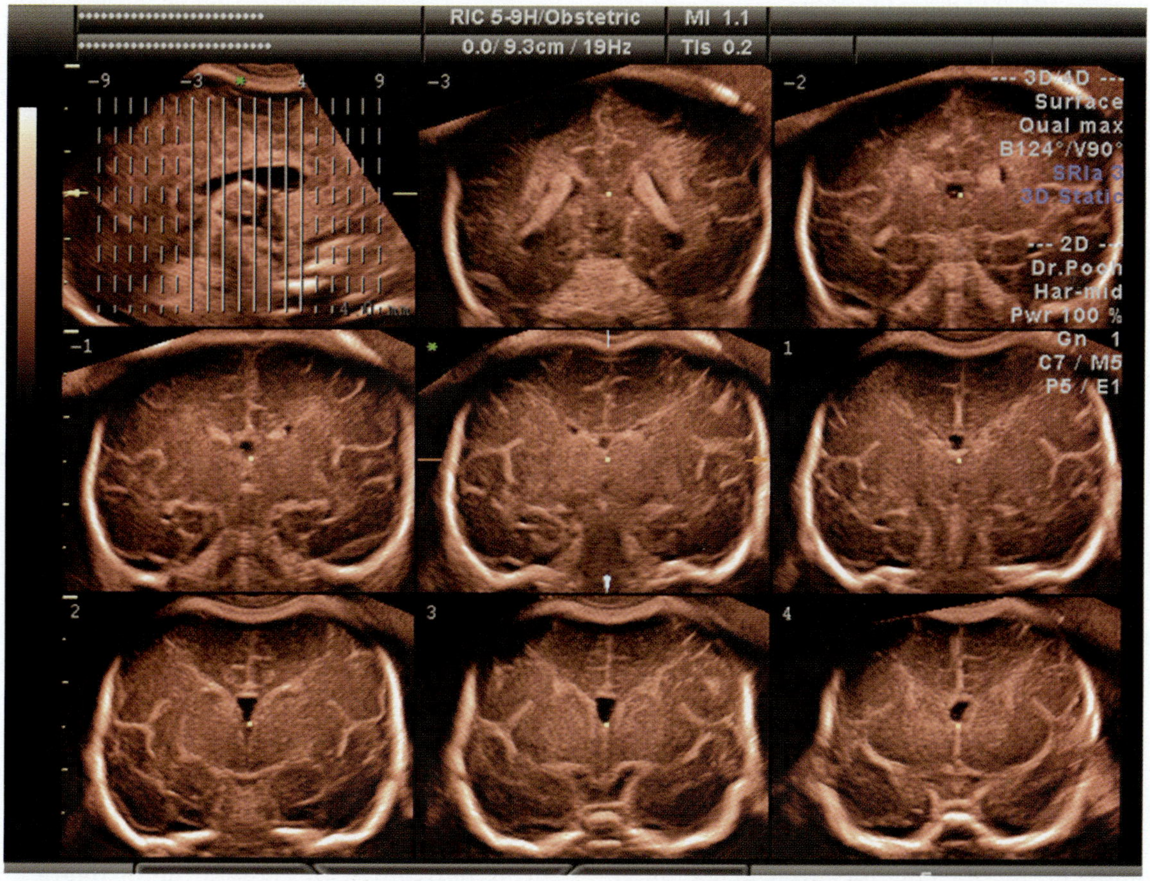

Fig. 7: Tomographic ultrasound imaging (TUI) of the fetal brain. Normal brain in the coronal cutting section at 31 weeks of gestation. Intracranial structure including gyral formation is clearly demonstrated.

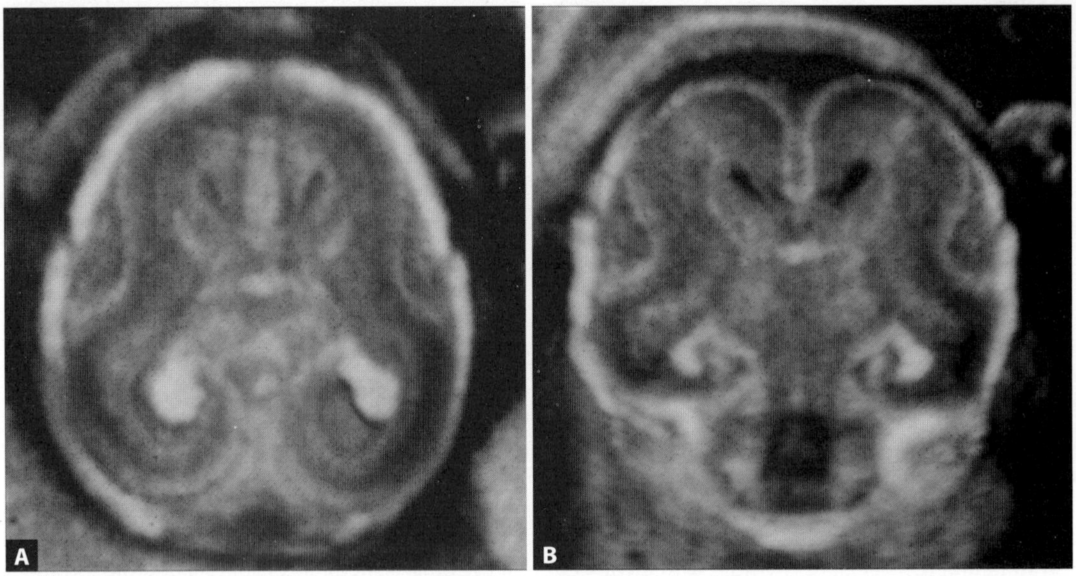

Figs. 8A and B: 3D thick slices of the brain (20 weeks of gestation). Axial thick slice (A) and coronal thick slice (B) of the premature brain. Observation by those 3D thick slices, anatomy of cortical structure and inside of ventricles become comprehensive.

contrast imaging (VCI) of the same plane or vertical plane of conventional 2D image are often convenient to observe the gyral formation and inside lateral ventricles.[14] The premature brain image obtained by use of VCI clearly demonstrates anatomical CNS structure.

Volume extracted image and volume calculation of the fetal brain in early pregnancy was reported in 1990s.[15,16] In our institute, VOLUSON 730 Expert (GE Medical Systems, Milwaukee, USA) with transvaginal 3D transducer and 3D View or 4D View software (Kretztechnik AG, Zipf, Austria) has been used for volume extraction and volume estimation of the brain structure.[17-19] On three orthogonal images, the target organ can be traced automatically or manually with rotation of volume imaging data. After tracing, volume extracted image is demonstrated and volume calculation data is shown **(Figs. 9A and B)**. 3D fetal brain volume measurements have a good intraobserver and interobserver reliability[20,21] and could be used to determine estimated gestational age.[20] Volume analysis by 3D ultrasound provides exceedingly informative imaging data. Volume analysis of the structure of interest provides an intelligible evaluation of the brain structure in total, and longitudinal and objective assessment of enlarged ventricles and intracranial occupying lesions **(Fig. 10)**. Any intracranial organ can be chosen as a target for volumetry no matter how distorted its shape and appearance may be. In new method of inversion mode, the cystic portions within the volume are displayed in their entirety as an echogenic area, while the gray-scale portions of the image are rendered as transparent[22] and recently it has been applied in fetal diagnosis.[23,24] **Figure 11** shows inversion-mode images of enlarged ventricles seen at 19 weeks of gestation.

The brain circulation demonstrated by transvaginal 2D power Doppler was first reported in 1996.[25] Thereafter, transvaginal 3D power Doppler assessment of fetal brain vascularity was successful.[18,26] Recently, by advanced technology of directional power Doppler, 3D angiostructural image has become furthermore sophisticated **(Figs. 12A to C)**. Recent high-frequent transvaginal neuroscan has been able to demonstrate the medullary veins from the cortex towards subependymal area **(Figs. 13A to C)**.

The three primary brain vesicles of forebrain (prosencephalon), midbrain (mesencephalon) and hindbrain (rhombencephalon) are formed in early embryonal period. At 7 and 8 weeks of gestation, those three primary brain vesicles are demonstrated on the mid-sagittal plane. The forebrain partly divides into two secondary brain vesicles of the telencephalon and diencephalons, and the hindbrain partly divides into the metencephalon and myelencephalon. The five secondary brain vesicles are consequently formed. The telencephalon forms derivatives of cerebral hemisphere and lateral ventricles.[27] At 9 weeks of gestation, those secondary vesicles are detected by sonography. Thereafter, the

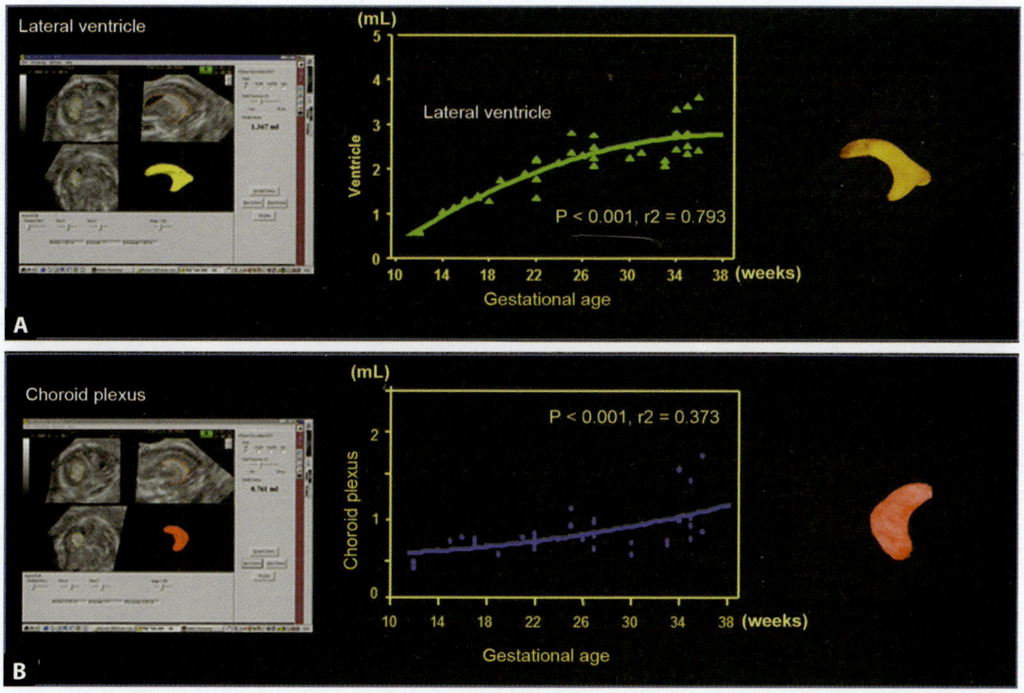

Figs. 9A and B: 3D volume extraction and volumetric analysis of lateral ventricle and choroid plexus. On three orthogonal sections, the target organ can be traced automatically or manually with rotation of volume imaging data. After tracing, volume extracted image (right) is demonstrated and volume calculation data is shown. Middle graphs show normograms of ventricular size (A) and choroid plexus size (B) during pregnancy.

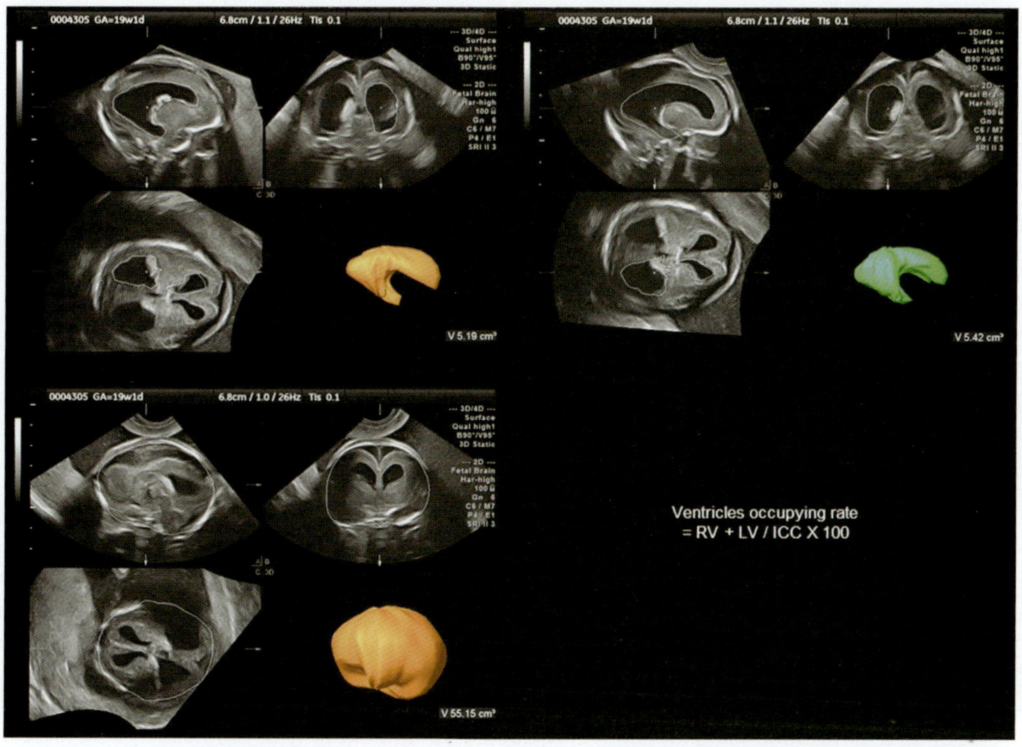

Fig. 10: 3D volume extraction and volumetric analysis of lateral ventricle and intracranial cavity. Each volume of right ventricle (RV) and left ventricle (LV) and intracranial cavity volume can be calculated by 3D volumetry. Total ventricular volume/intracranial cavity (ICC) volume shows ventricles occupying rate and it is useful for longitudinal assessment of ventriculomegaly cases.

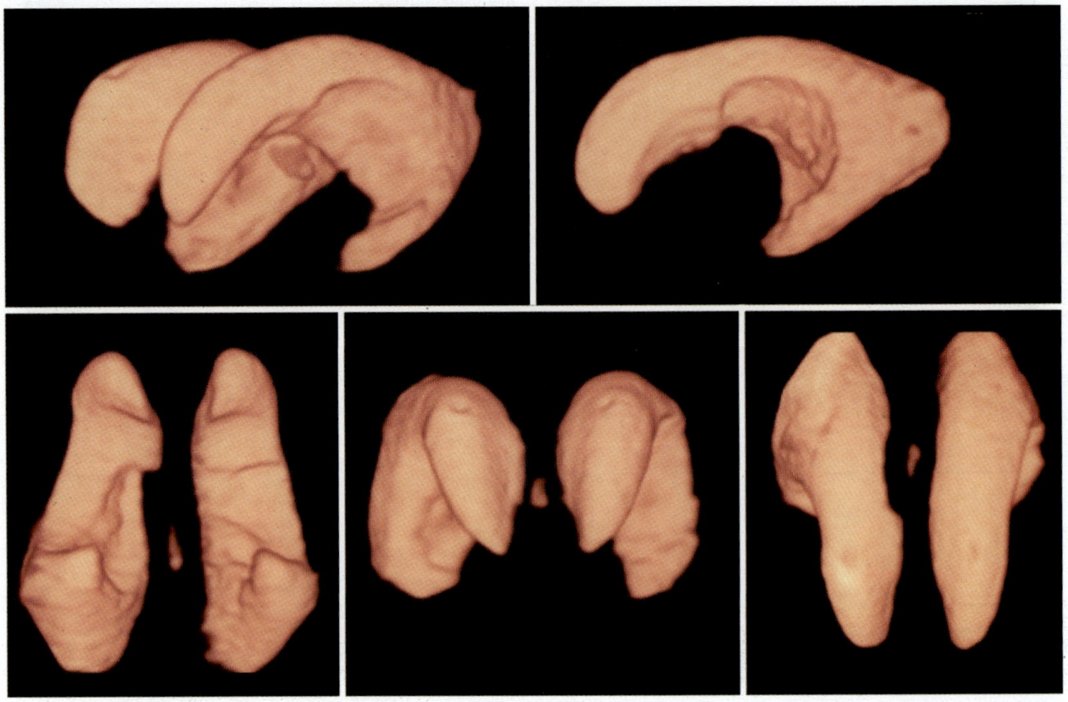

Fig. 11: 3D extraction volume imaging of bilateral ventricles by inversion mode. Ventricle appearance is objectively demonstratable by inversion mode. Those images were from ventriculomegaly case at 19 weeks of gestation.

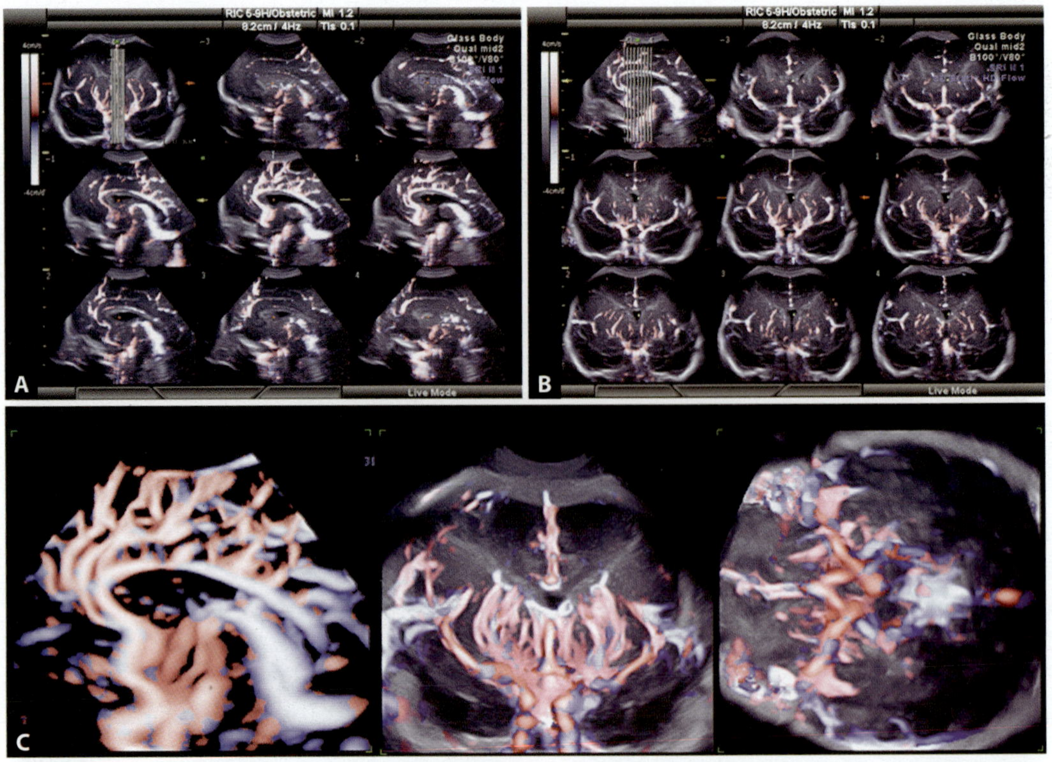

Figs. 12A to C: Tomographic ultrasound imaging and reconstructed 3D angiography of normal cerebral circulation at 31 weeks. Tomographic directional power Doppler imaging of sagittal (A), coronal (B) sections. Anterior cerebral arteries and their branches are seen on the sagittal plane, middle cerebral arteries, and their branches on the coronal plane; (C) 3D sonoangiogram of sagittal, coronal, and axial sections from left.

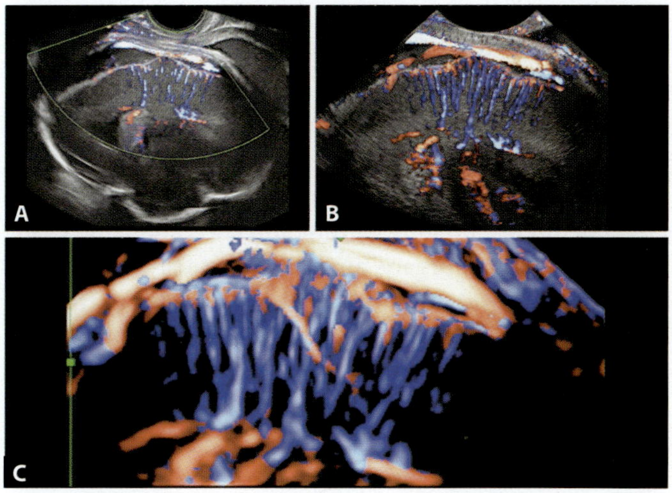

Figs. 13A to C: Normal medullary veins at 28 weeks. (A) Intracerebral peripheral vessels by 2D directional power Doppler; (B) Parasagittal plane from 3D orthogonal view. The upper large vessel is the superior sagittal sinus. Cerebral superficial vessels are on the surface of cerebrum. Numerous linear vessels run down from the cortex towards subependymal region are medurally veins; (C) 3D reconstructed image.

premature brain vesicles rapidly develop during the first half of pregnancy. The choroid plexuses develop in the roof of the third ventricle, in the medial walls of the lateral ventricles and in the roof of the fourth ventricle.[27] The choroid plexuses secrete ventricular fluid, which becomes cerebrospinal fluid (CSF). The choroid plexuses are high echogenic structure, detectable from ninth gestational week and conspicuous during the first trimester. From the beginning of the second trimester, the choroid plexuses of lateral ventricle gradually change its location backward. As the cerebral cortex develops, the commissures connect corresponding areas of the cerebral hemispheres with one another. The largest cerebral commissure is the corpus callosum, connecting neocortical areas. The corpus callosum initially lies in the lamina terminalis, but fibers are added to it as the cortex enlarges; as a result, it gradually extends beyond the lamina terminalis. The rest of the lamina terminalis lies between the corpus callosum and the fornix. It becomes stretched to form the thin septum pellucidum, a thin plate of brain tissue. The corpus callosum extends over the roof of the diencephalon.[27] The corpus callosum is detectable by ultrasound from around 16 weeks of gestation in some cases and at 18 weeks in most cases. **Figures 14A to C** show normal 17-week-brain. Neuroimaging in the third trimester, gyral formation is a main change of brain development **(Fig. 7)**.

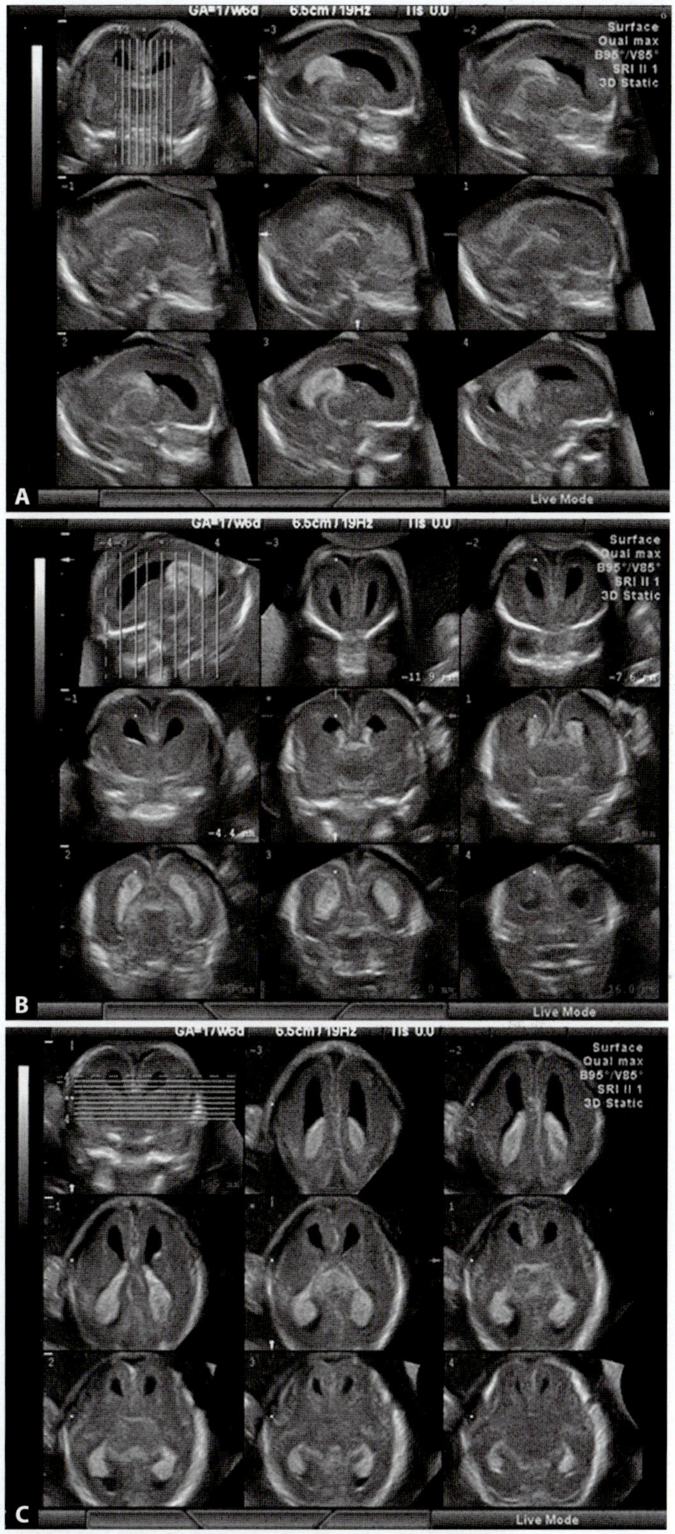

Figs. 14A to C: Normal brain at 17 weeks. Tomographic ultrasound imaging of sagittal (A); coronal (B); and axial (C) sections. Choroid plexus (echogenic part) shifts its position to posterior half of the lateral ventricles.

Initially the surface of the hemispheres is smooth, however, as growth proceeds, sulci (grooves or furrows) and gyri (convolutions or elevations) develop. The sulci and gyri permit a considerable increase in the surface area of the cerebral cortex without requiring an extensive increase in cranial size. As each cerebral hemisphere grows, the cortex covering the external surface of the corpus striatum grows relatively slowly and is soon overgrown. This buried cortex, hidden from view in the depths of the lateral sulcus (fissure) of the cerebral hemisphere, is the insula.[27]

NEW APPLICATION OF HDLIVE SILHOUETTE AND FLOW IN FETAL NEUROLOGY

The great achievement in the field of 3D/4D ultrasound is HDlive technology.[28] This technology is a novel ultrasound technique that improves the 3D/4D images. HDlive uses an adjustable light source and software that calculates the propagation of light through surface structures in relation to the light direction.[29] The virtual light source produces selective illumination, and the respective shadows are created by the structures where the light is reflected. There have been several reports on HDlive demonstration of fetal surface.[30-32]

Moreover, new applications of HDlive silhouette and HDlive flow[33] were released at the end of 2014. The algorithm of HDlive silhouette creates a gradient at organ boundaries, fluid-filled cavity and vessels walls, where an abrupt change of the acoustic impedance exists within tissues.[33-35] The examiner can adjust HDlive silhouette percentage with controlling threshold and gain simultaneously for visualizing target organs of interest. HDlive silhouette emphasizes the borderlines between organs with different echogenicity, therefore, both the target of interest floating within fluid correction and cystic area in echogenic organs are simultaneously demonstrated. By HDlive silhouette mode, an inner cystic structure with fluid collection can be depicted through the outer surface structure of the body and it can be appropriately named as *'see-through fashion.'*[33,35-37] The placental surface is demonstrated through the amniotic fluid and report on HDlive silhouette imaging of circumvallate placenta was recently published.[38] Silhouette ultrasound shows comprehensive structure demonstrating inner and outer morphology simultaneously. However, it occasionally appears to demonstrate too many inner structures overlapping one another to understand their relations. The author has cut the volume dataset with a rectangle cube and rendered the cut slice with silhouette ultrasound. The author calls this silhouette ultrasound demonstration of thick slice of 3D volume dataset as 'thick-slice silhouette.'[39] Normal brain image in the coronal cutting section by tomographic ultrasound imaging and the thick-slice silhouette image from the same 3D volume dataset are shown in **Figures 15A to C**. Silhouette mode can depict not only hypoechoic structure but also hyperechoic structure

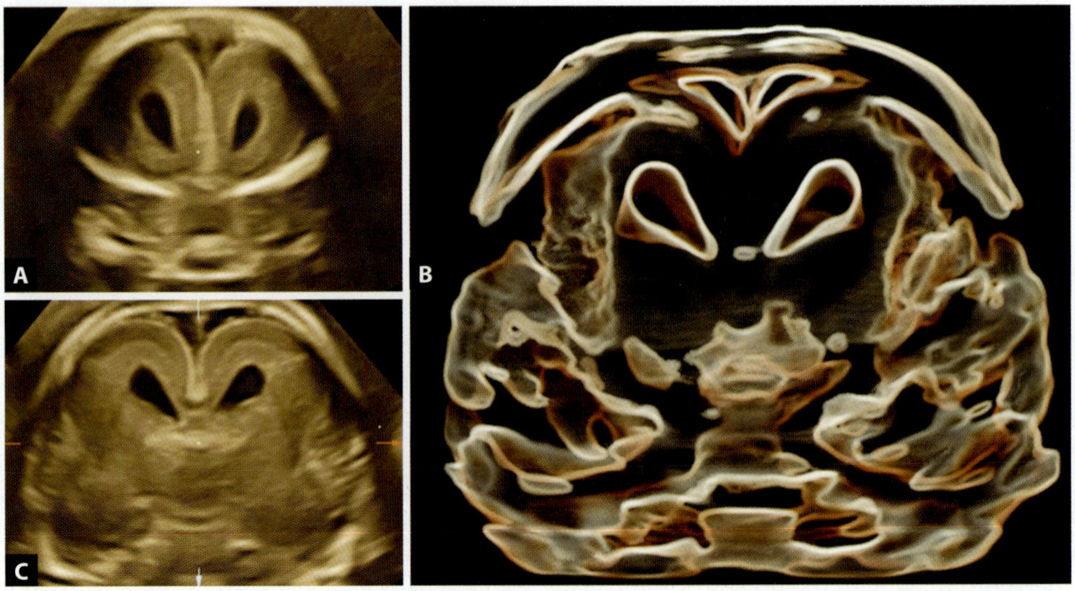

Figs. 15A to C: Thick-slice silhouette of normal brain at 18 weeks of gestation. (A and B) Images are from 3D coronal tomographic images; (C) Thick-slice image from the same 3D volume dataset as A and B.

such as bones.[35,38,41] **Figure 16** shows the anterior fontanelle at 16 weeks. The vertebrae and ribs can be visualized from a small fetus and interestingly extracted skeletal system is demonstrated in the early second trimester as shown in **Figures 17A to C**. The image showing extracted bony structure is comprehensive as 3D-CT or X-ray.

HDlive flow.[33-38,41] is a recent application of three-dimensional (3D) ultrasound technology generating a 3D-view of the blood flow and providing a realistic rendering of fine vascular structure. Combination of HDlive silhouette and HDlive flow can be described as a 'see-through fashion,'[33] because of its comprehensive orientation and persuasive localization of inner structure as well as of fetal angiostructure inside the morphological structure. **Figures 18A and B** demonstrate the normal intracorporeal angiostructure by 3D HDlive silhouette/flow imaging with bidirectional power Doppler at 20 weeks of gestation respectively. Medullary veins are well demonstrated between pia matter and subependymal zone **(Figs. 19A and B)**.

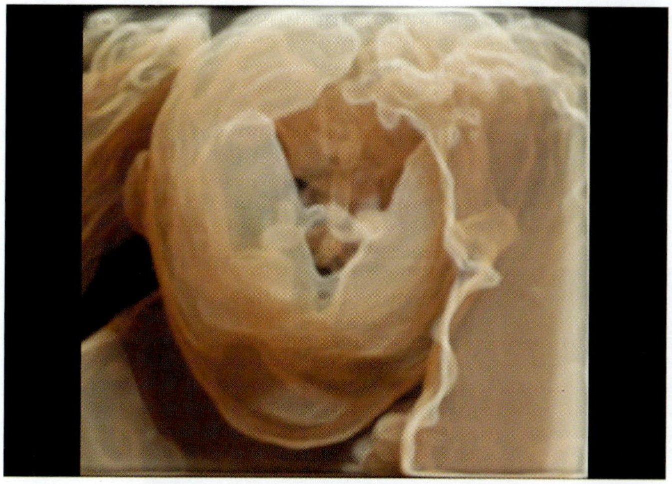

Fig. 16: Anterior fontanelle at 16 weeks by HDlive silhouette imaging.

3D/4D SONOGRAPHY AND MRI: ALTERNATIVES OR COMPLEMENTARIES

In multiplanar imaging of the brain structure, it is possible to demonstrate not only the sagittal and coronal sections but also the axial section of the brain, which cannot be demonstrated from parietal direction by a conventional 2D transvaginal sonography. Parallel slicing provides a tomographic visualization of internal morphology similar to MR imaging. Parallel slices used to be obtained on translating the cutting plane, however, recent advanced technology can produce tomographic ultrasound images and demonstrate a series of parallel cutting slices on a single screen as well as MRI does.[14] As described above, images obtained by tomographic ultrasound imaging (TUI) are quite similar to pictures of MRI. The superior point of TUI to MRI is easy off-line analysis, with changing

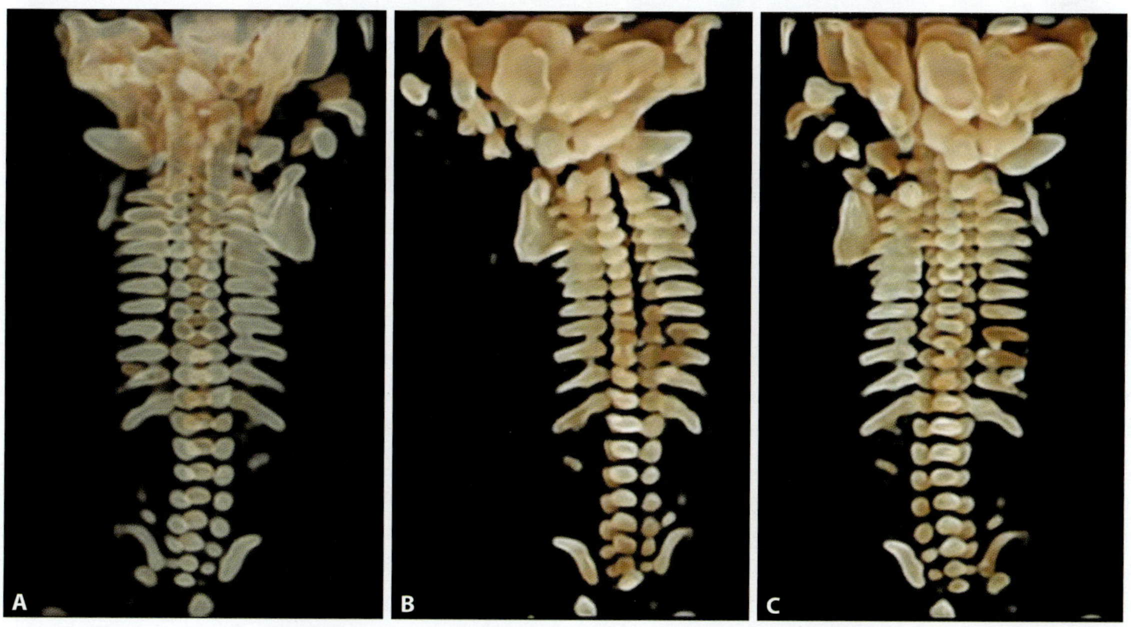

Figs. 17A to C: Vertebrae, ribs, and iliac by HDlive silhouette imaging at 18 weeks of gestation: (A) Posterior-anterior view; (B) Oblique-anterior view; (C) Anterior-posterior view.

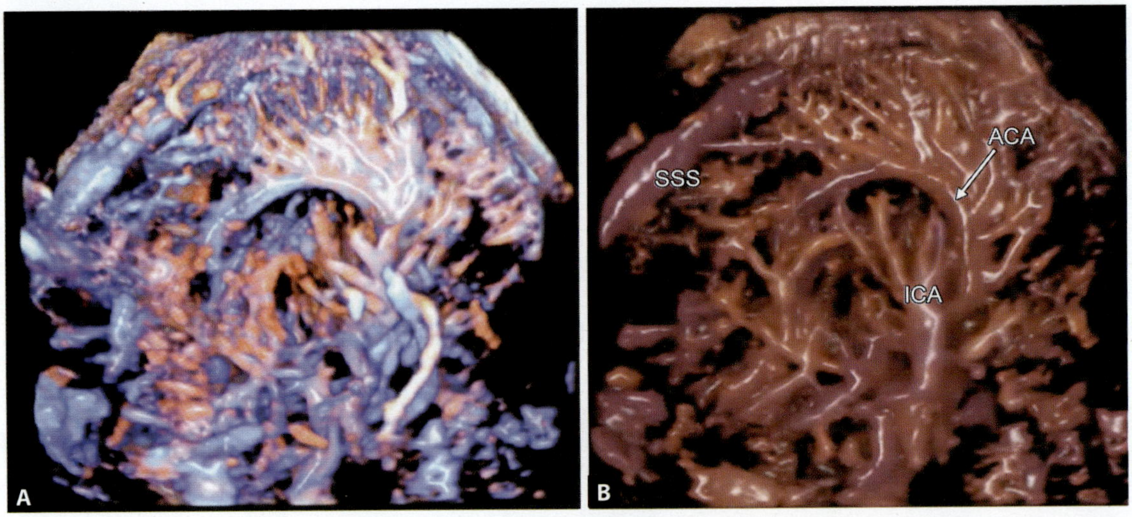

Figs. 18A and B: Normal brain vascular structure by HDlive flow imaging at 20 weeks of gestation. (A) Bidirectional power Doppler 3D HDlive flow image of fetal vascular structure; (B) Mono-color HDlive flow image. (ACA: anterior cerebral artery; ICA: internal carotid artery; SSS: superior sagittal sinus)

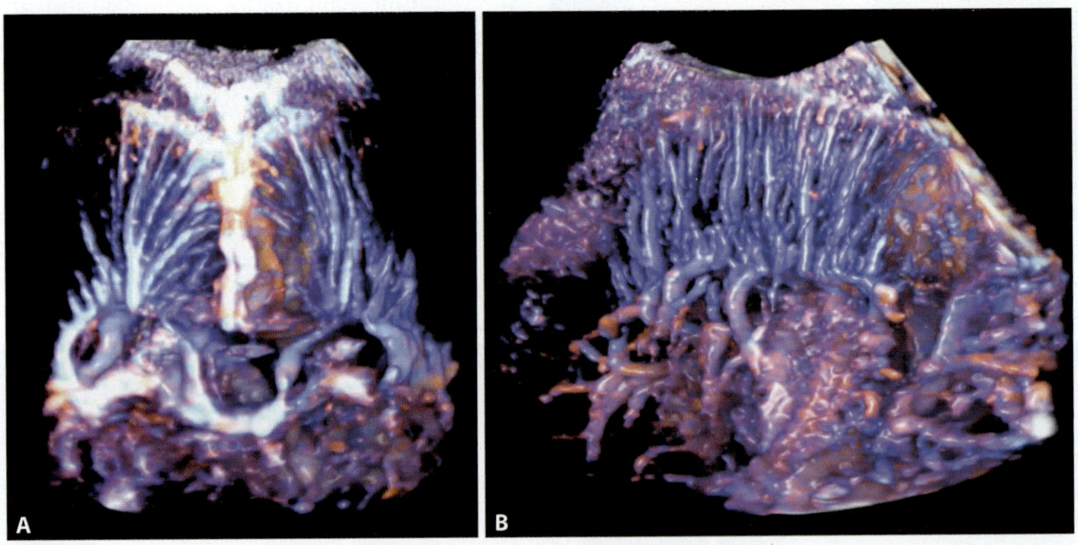

Figs. 19A and B: Normal cerebral medullary veins by HDlive flow imaging at 29 weeks of gestation. (A) Coronal image; (B) Sagittal image. Numerous fine medullary veins between cerebral surface and subependymal zone are well demonstrated.

slice width, magnifying images, and rotating images to any directions. This function is extremely useful for detailed CNS assessment and also for consultation to neurosurgeons and neurologists. As shown in **Figures 20A and B** (hydrocephalus at 21 weeks of gestation, ultrasound, and MRI) and **Figures 21A and B** (hydrocephalus ex vacuo, ultrasound and MRI), the transvaginal 3D tomographic ultrasound imaging demonstrates the detailed intracranial structures and seems not to require the further imaging modality.

Fetal neuroimaging with advanced 3D ultrasound technology is an easy, noninvasive, and reproducible methods. It produces not only comprehensible images but also objective imaging data. Easy storage/extraction of raw volume data set enables easy off-line analysis and consultation to neurologists and neurosurgeons. 3D technology also provides us a longitudinal study of maldevelopment of CNS diseases by a serial neuroscan through a whole gestational period. Dedicated transvaginal 3D ultrasound is no doubt the first modality suitable for

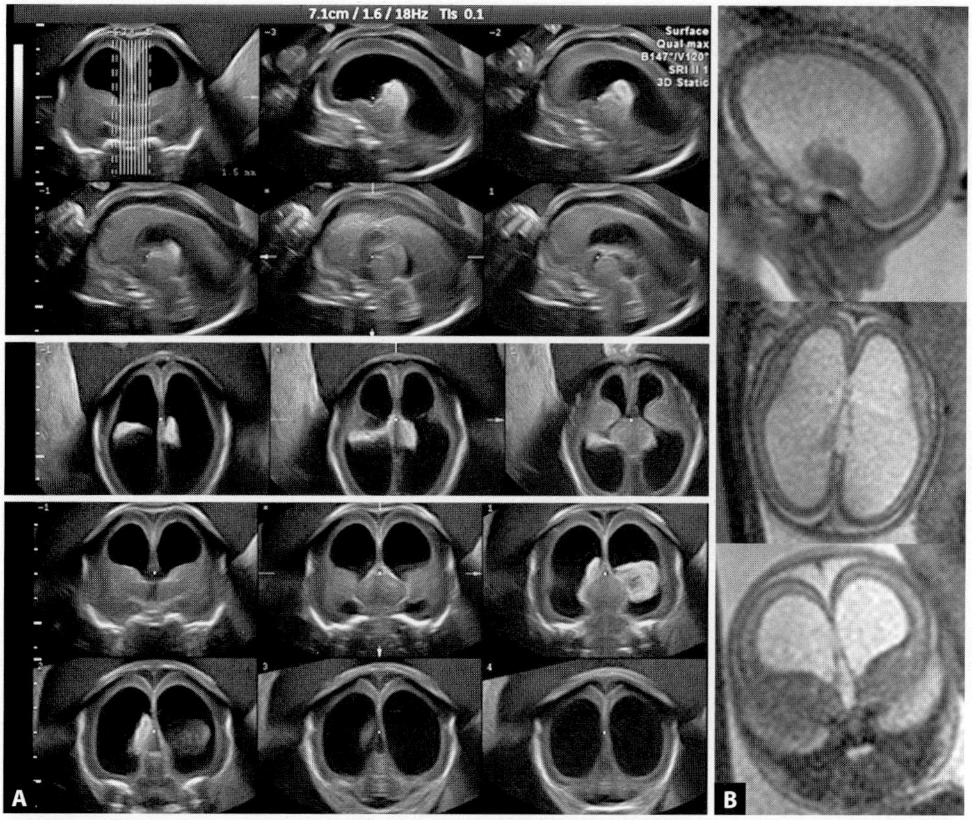

Figs. 20A and B: Tomographic ultrasound imaging (TUI) and MR imaging of hydrocephalus at 21 weeks of gestation. (A) Sagittal, axial, and coronal parallel cutting sections by sonography well demonstrated ventriculomegaly. Partial agenesis of the corpus callosum is detected in the mid-sagittal section; (B) MRI images of the same case. No significant difference between sonography and MRI.

visualization and assessment of fetal CNS. Although the first introduction of transvaginal fetal neurosonography, which has revolutionized the visualization of the fetal brain, was almost 20 years ago, this approach has still not gained popularity in the world. Malinger et al.[42] described that this fact may be due to the relatively complex brain anatomy and pathology that is usually not familiar enough to most obstetricians and to reluctance to use transvaginal sonography in many countries.

Recent advances in fast MRI technology have remarkably improved the T2-weighted image resolution despite a short acquisition time, and minimized artifacts due to fetal movement and/or maternal respiratory motion. MR imaging is not influenced by physical factors such as fetal location, fetal head position and ossification of fetal cranial bones, which sometimes obstruct transvaginal ultrasound approach. Magnetic resonance imaging is playing an increasingly prominent role in depicting brain maturation, especially cortical formation that follows a temporospatial pattern, and in detecting developmental abnormalities of the cortex and other brain sectors.[43] MR imaging of fetal CNS possesses less abilities in detecting bony structure and angioarchitectonics and in volumetric assessment, compared with transvaginal 3D ultrasound imaging. However, in multiplanar imaging, MRI has much superiority in the assessment of a whole intracranial structure including the brainstem **(Figs. 22 and 23)**, posterior fossa and gyral formation **(Figs. 24A to C)** with better contrast between different tissue. In cases of microcephaly, with difficulty of obtaining ultrasound windows of fontanelles and sutures, intracranial observation by MRI is much more helpful than transfontanelle ultrasound neuroscan.

It has been controversial whether ultrasound or MRI is more practical and effective in prenatal assessment of fetal CNS abnormalities. Several previous studies[44-47] on MRI in diagnosis of fetal brain anomalies have reported that MRI added more valuable information than ultrasound. Kubik-Huch et al.[48] published the statistical analysis study with the result finding no statistically significant

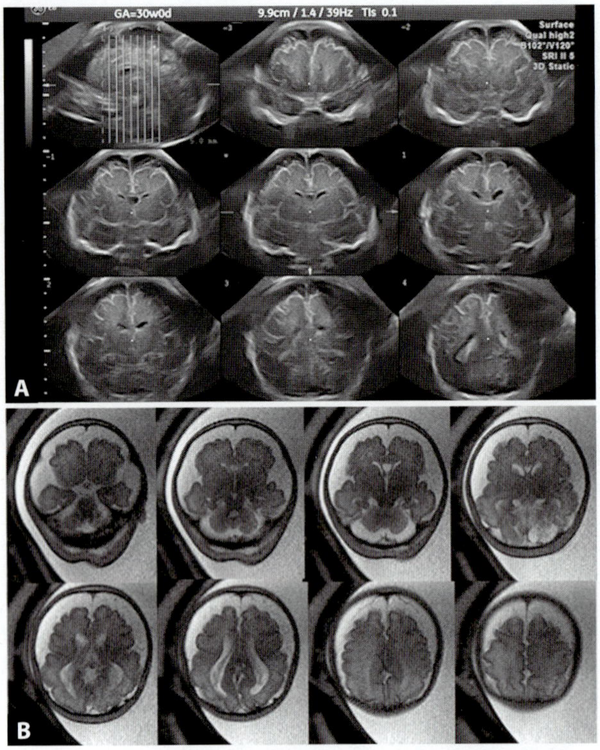

Figs. 21A and B: Tomographic ultrasound imaging (TUI) and MR imaging of hydrocephalus ex vacuo at 30 weeks of gestation. (A) TUI coronal image of the brain. Note the conspicuous external subarachnoid/subdural space around hemispheres; (B) MR images of the same case. The cause of this phenomenon was unknown, and this space spontaneously disappeared three weeks later. Array CGH of amnio cells was normal but postnatal neurological prognosis has been progressively deteriorated.

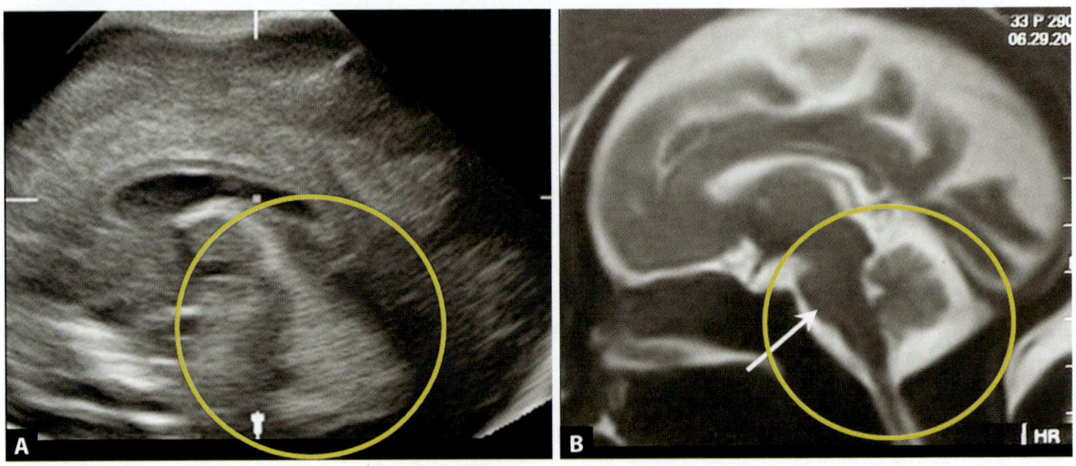

Figs. 22A and B: Comparison of transvaginal 3D US and MRI in demonstrating the brainstem and posterior fossa. Median cutting section images of normal fetal brain by transvaginal sonography (A) and MRI (B) at 30 weeks of gestation. Inside circles, the brainstem and posterior fossa are demonstrated. Although ultrasound image shows the cerebellum and fourth ventricle, MR image reveals much clearer appearance of brainstem (arrow) and detailed cerebellar structure than sonogram, because of MR feature of higher contrast between different tissues.

difference between sonography and MR imaging for the detection of abnormality in any organ system. Malinger et al.[42] criticized that the past reports describing superiority of MRI over ultrasound may have been biased because a comparison had been done with routine transabdominal ultrasound examinations, without insistence on an additional confirmatory tertiary level ultrasound examination, especially by transvaginal sonography. Their opinion seems to be right to the point. In their other article, they described that dedicated neurosonography by transvaginal sonography is equal to MRI in the diagnosis of fetal brain anomalies, in most cases MRI confirmed the

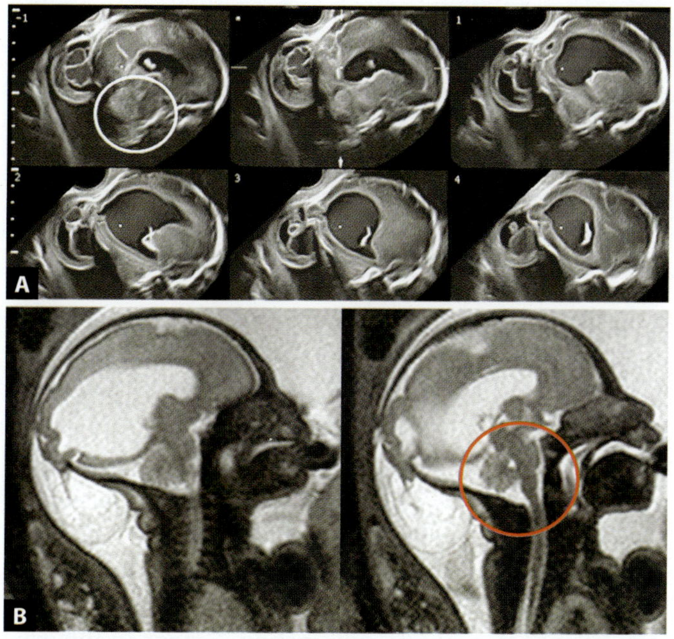

Figs. 23A and B: Tomographic ultrasound imaging (TUI) and MR imaging of the brain in a case of encephalomeningocele at 28 weeks of gestation. Prolapsed cerebral tissue with meninges are well demonstrated by both TUI (A) and MRI (B), but MRI indicates that the amount of cerebral tissue inside encephalomeningocele is quite little. Furthermore, in cases with encephalocele, it is important the existence of Chiari malformation, and the brainstem and posterior fossa is more clearly depicted by MRI (red circle) than sonography (white circle). This case had no Chiari malformation.

ultrasonographic diagnosis and in a minority of cases each modality provided additional/different information.[49] They also concluded that the major role of MRI was in reassurance of the parents regarding the presence or absence of brain anomalies. This is an easily acceptable observation for sonographers with expertise.

In fact, as shown in **Figures 20 and 21**, no significant difference between dedicated neurosonography and MRI in detection of intracranial structure. In late pregnancy with developed calvarium and vertebrae, MRI is superior in detection of the spinal cord inside the spinal canal and cerebellar herniation with Chiari malformation **(Figs. 25C and D)**, however, detection of the accurate vertebral level of spina bifida and associated lower limb abnormality can be easily assessed by 3D ultrasound **(Figs. 25A and B)**. In cases with CMV infection, intracranial calcification can be detected only by dedicated neurosonography **(Figs. 26A and B)**, not visualized by MR imaging. The vascular anomaly such as Galen's aneurismal malformation or intratumoral vascularity **(Figs. 27A to F)** is much more

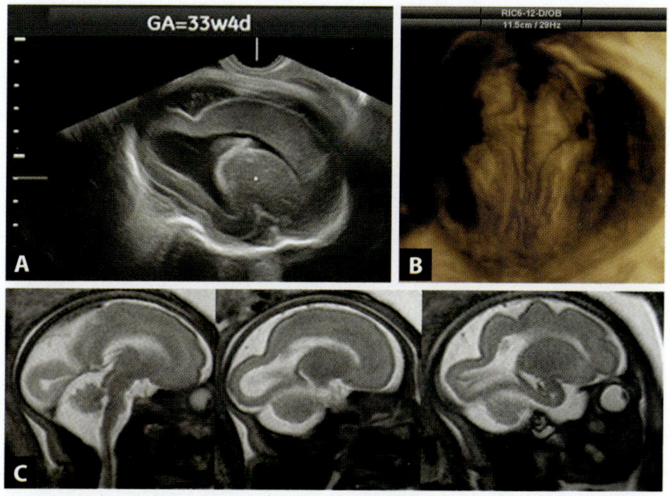

Figs. 24A to C: Cortical development by sonography and MRI in a case of pachygyria at 33 weeks of gestation. Cortical development with gyral/sulcal formation should be remarkably demonstrated after 29 weeks by parasagittal plane. In this case, sonography shows less gyri/sulci on the parasagittal sonographic image (A) and 3D sonographic surface anatomical view (B). (C) MRI images of midsagittal and parasagittal sections. In late pregnancy, transfontanelle/trans-sutural sonography is getting more difficult because of cranial ossification. MRI greatly helps in demonstration of cortical development after 30 weeks of gestation.

clearly detectable by using 3D power Doppler or 3D B flow images. An additional advantage of 3D sonography is demonstration of extra CNS anomalies strongly associated with CNS abnormalities, such as fetal face and extremities **(Figs. 28A to E)**. The advantages of both MRI and dedicated sonography are summarized in **Table 1**.

Regarding objectives of accurate prenatal diagnosis for proper management, any less-invasive modalities can be used. For CNS anomaly screening scan, ultrasound is no doubt the first modality, and once CNS abnormality is suspicious, after considering each advantage and disadvantage of transvaginal 3D ultrasound and MR imaging, it is suggested to use those different technologies according to what to be detected and evaluated in each abnormal CNS case. Of course, those two technologies should be utilized as alternatives and complementaries as well.[50]

VENTRICULOMEGALY AND HYDROCEPHALUS

"Hydrocephalus" and "ventriculomegaly" are both the terms used to describe dilatation of the lateral ventricles. However, those two should be distinguished from each

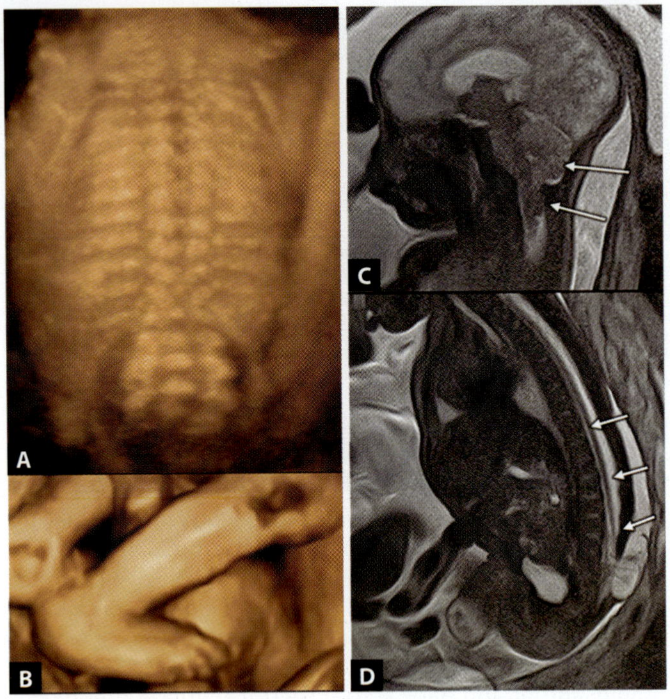

Figs. 25A to D: Features of 3D sonography and MRI in cases of myelomeningocele. In cases of myelomeningocele, 3D ultrasound can demonstrate the accurate vertebral level of spina bifida (A) and affected foot joint appearance (B). MRI can demonstrate the condition of Chiari type II malformation (C, arrows) and spinal cord inside the spinal canal (D, arrows) in detail. In late pregnancy, cerebrospinal region and intravertebral structure cannot be depicted by sonography because of cranial/vertebral ossification, therefore, MR imaging is more reliable in demonstrating those structures.

other. Hydrocephalus signifies dilated lateral ventricles resulted from increased amount of CSF inside the ventricles and increased intracranial pressure, while ventriculomegaly is a dilatation of lateral ventricles without increased intracranial pressure, due to cerebral hypoplasia or CNS anomaly such as agenesis of the corpus callosum.[8,51] Of course, ventriculomegaly can sometimes change into hydrocephalic state. In sonographic imaging, those two intracranial conditions can be differentiated by visualization of subarachnoid space and appearance of choroid plexus. In normal conditions, subarachnoid space, visualized around the both cerebral hemispheres is well preserved during pregnancy **(Figs. 29A and B)**. Choroid plexus is a soft tissue and easily affected by external pressure. Obliterated subarachnoid space and dangling choroid plexus are observed in the case of hydrocephalus. In contrast, the subarachnoid space and choroid plexus are well preserved in cases of ventriculomegaly **(Fig. 30)**. It is difficult to evaluate subarachnoid space in the axial plane because the subarachnoid space is observed in the parietal side of the hemispheres. Therefore, transabdominal approach may not differentiate accurately hydrocephalus with increased intracranial pressure from ventriculomegaly without pressure. It is suggested that the evaluation of enlarged ventricles should be done in the parasagittal and coronal views by transvaginal approach to the fetal brain or 3D multidimensional analysis. As a screening examination, the measurement of AW **(Fig. 31)** is useful with a cut-off value of 10 mm[52,53] although isolated

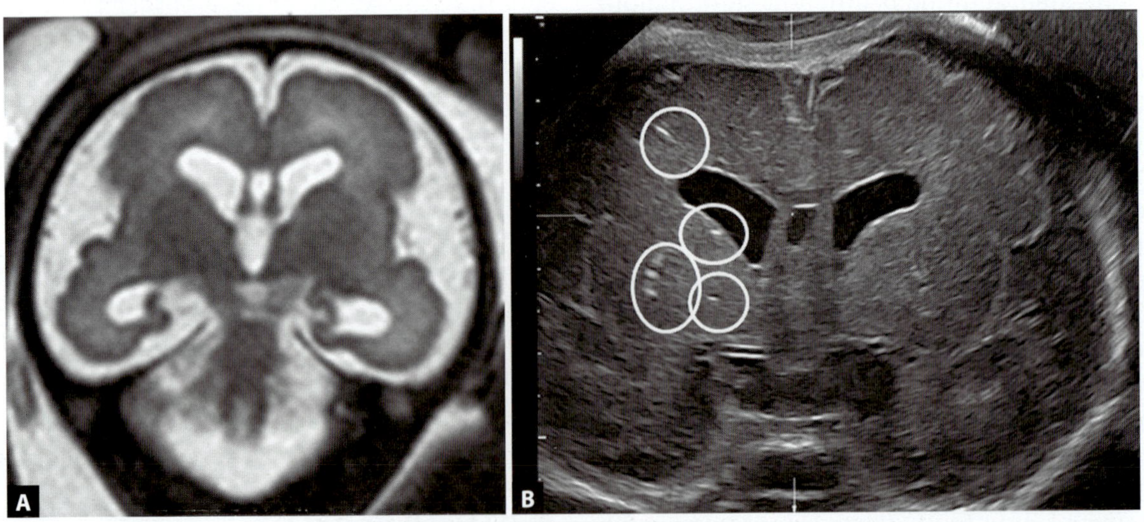

Figs. 26A and B: Comparison of MR and sonographic images in a case of cytomegaloviral infection. Cytomegaloviral infection often affects the brain development and representative features of the affected brain are ventriculomegaly, cortical maldevelopment and intracranial calcification. MR image at 34 weeks (A) well shows ventriculomegaly and cortical maldevelopment. Sonographic image at the same gestation (B) add the information of multiple intracranial calcification (inside circles), which is never demonstratable by MRI.

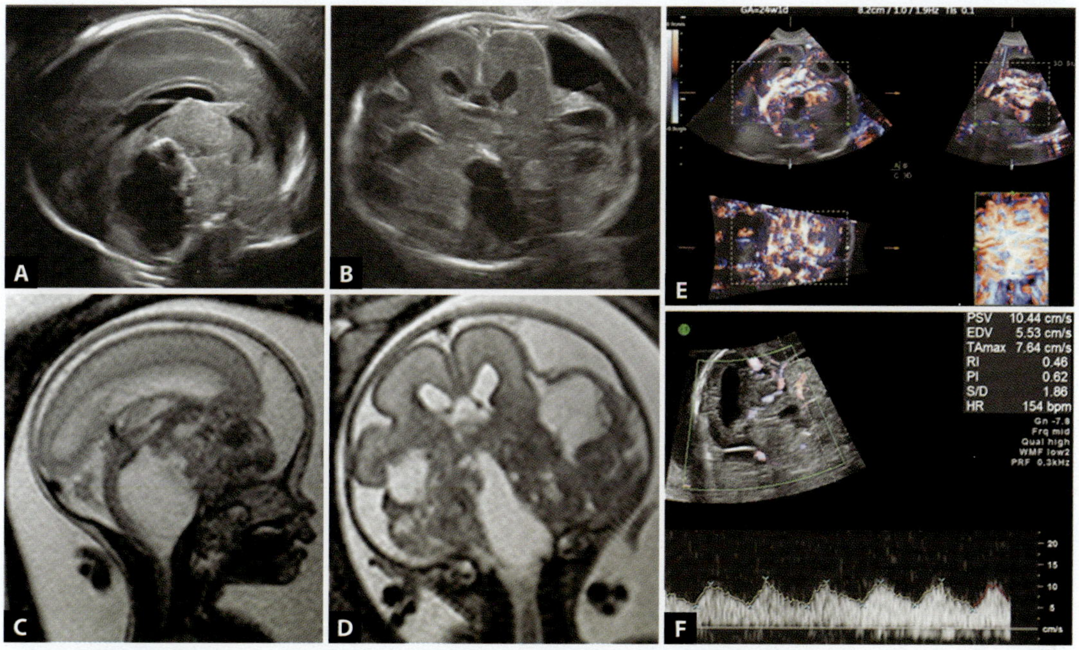

Figs. 27A to F: Comparison of MR and sonographic images in a case of brain tumor at 26 weeks of gestation. (A and B) Sonographic median and anterior-coronal images; (C and D) MR median and anterior-coronal images. Note the huge tumor below the oppressed bilateral hemispheres and oppressed brainstem; (E) Three-orthogonal view and reconstructed image by 3D bidirectional power Doppler; (F) Intratumoral blood flow with low resistance is demonstrated. Intracranial morphology is more comprehensive by MRI than sonography due to MR feature of more contrast between different tissues, however, sonography is much more helpful in assessment of intratumoral vasculature and blood flow analysis.

mild ventriculomegaly with AW of 10–12 mm may be normal variant.[54] In normal fetuses, blood flow waveforms of dural sinuses, such as the superior sagittal sinus, vein of Galen and straight sinus have pulsatile pattern.[55] However, in cases with progressive hydrocephalus, normal pulsation disappears and blood flow waveforms become flat pattern.[55] Intracranial venous blood flow may be related to increased intracranial pressure.

Variety of Mild Ventriculomegaly with AW 10–15 mm

Mild ventriculomegaly is defined as the width of the atrium of the lateral cerebral ventricles of 10–15 mm. It has been reported that mild ventriculomegaly with atrial width 10–15 mm resolves in 29%, remains stable in 57%, progresses in 14% of the cases during pregnancy.[56] **Figures 32 to 35** show the prenatal diagnostic imaging of the cases with mild ventriculomegaly and associated abnormalities such as craniosynostosis, micrognathia, vein of Galen aneurysmal malformation and multiple intracerebral bleeding. These cases were referred due to ventriculomegaly and atrial width was 10–13 mm at referral. Various outcomes and prognosis followed according to complicated abnormalities.

Table 2 summarizes 23 cases of ventriculomegaly with atrial width 10–15 mm; 13 cases with additional anomaly and 10 cases without other abnormality. More than 30% of cases with other abnormalities had chromosomal aberration or genetic disorder. However, among the cases with other complications, 30% of them have had no neurological deficit in short-term. It is difficult to estimate postnatal prognosis simply by intrauterine progression or resolution of ventricular enlargement during pregnancy. Normalization of ventricular enlargement during fetal period was seen in 70% of cases with no other complications. In our series, all cases with both no complications and spontaneous resolution of enlargement have had favorable prognosis in short-term.

Generally, in cases of mild fetal ventriculomegaly with a normal karyotype and an absence of malformations, the outcome appears to be favorable.[57] Pilu, et al.[58] reviewed 234 cases of borderline ventriculomegaly including an abnormal outcome in 22.8% and concluded that borderline ventriculomegaly carries an increased risk of cerebral maldevelopment, delayed neurological development

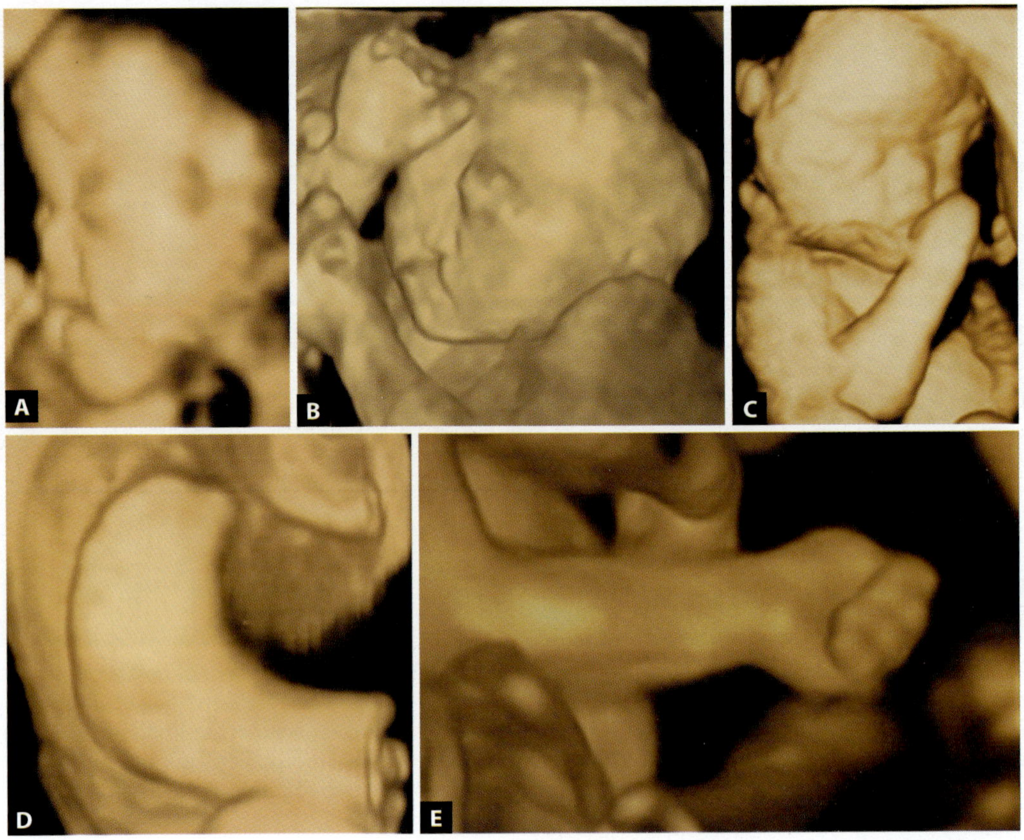

Figs. 28A to E: 3D sonographic feature of extra CNS abnormality assessment. 3D sonographic surface anatomy can demonstrate extra CNS abnormalities which are strongly associated or affected with brain anomalies, such as facial abnormalities and limb abnormalities. (A) Facial anomaly with exophthalmos and prominent forehead in a case of Apert syndrome; (B) Exophthalmos, nasal aplasia, and cleft lip in a case of holoprosencephaly; (C and D) Syndactyly in a case of Apert syndrome; (E) Adducted thumb in a case of X-linked hydrocephalus.

TABLE 1: Advantages of magnetic resonance imaging (MRI) and dedicated 3D transvaginal sonography in CNS assessment.

MRI	*3D-TVS*
• Whole brain assessment • Brainstem development • Posterior fossa assessment • Cortical development	• Intracranial calcification • Vascular anomaly • Intratumoral vascularity • Bony structure assessment • Extra CNS abnormality detection

and, possibly, chromosomal aberrations. Isolated mild ventriculomegaly with atrial width of 10–12 mm may be normal variation. Signorelli, et al.[54] described that their data of normal neurodevelopment between 18 months and 10 years after birth in cases of isolated mild ventriculomegaly (atrial width of 10-12 mm), should provide a basis for reassuring counseling. Ouahba et al.[59] recently reported the outcome of 167 cases of isolated mild ventriculomegaly and concluded that in addition to associated anomalies, three criteria are often associated with an unfavorable outcome: atrial width greater than 12 mm, progression of the enlargement, and asymmetrical and bilateral ventriculomegaly.

Moderate-to-severe Ventriculomegaly with AW >15 mm

The term *'Hydrocephalus'* does not identify a specified disease but is a generic term which means a serial pathologic condition because of abnormal circulation of CSF. Treatment method of hydrocephalus should be selected according to age of onset and symptoms. Congenital hydrocephalus is classified into three categories by causes which disturb CSF circulation pathway; simple hydrocehalus, dysgenetic hydrocephalus, and secondary hydrocephalus.[51]

a. *Simple hydrocephalus:* Simple hydrocephalus caused by developmental abnormality which is

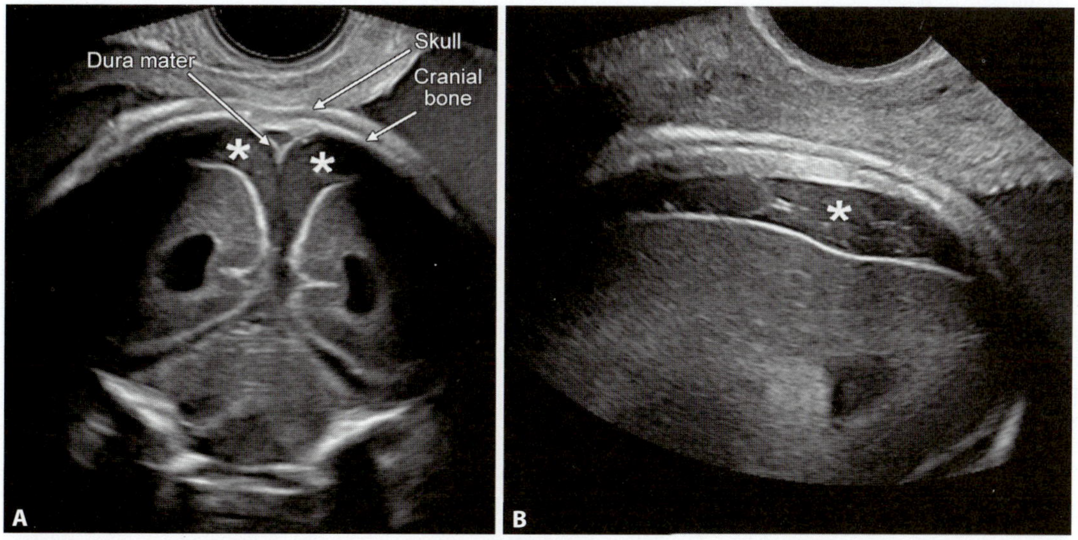

Figs. 29A and B: Subarachnoid space in normal 25-week-brain. (A) Posterior coronal image. Asterisks indicate subarachnoid space; (B) Parasagittal image.

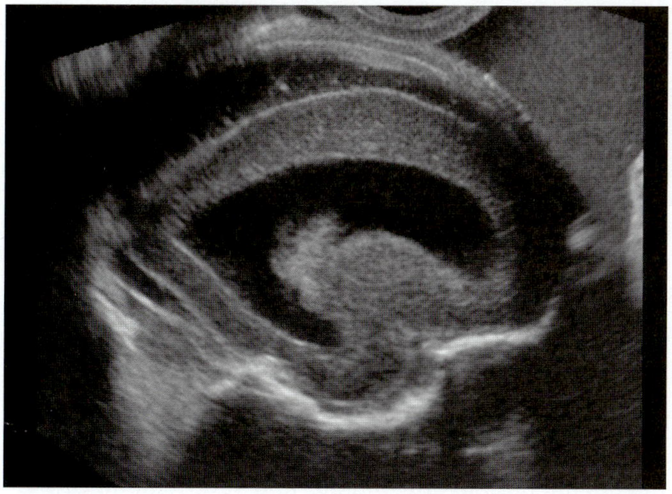

Fig. 30: Ventriculomegaly due to cerebral hypoplasia at 29 weeks of gestation. Enlarged ventricle exists but subarachnoid space is well preserved, and no dangling choroid plexus is seen. From those findings, non-increased intercranial pressure (ICP) is estimated. This condition should be differentiated from hydrocephalus with increased ICP.

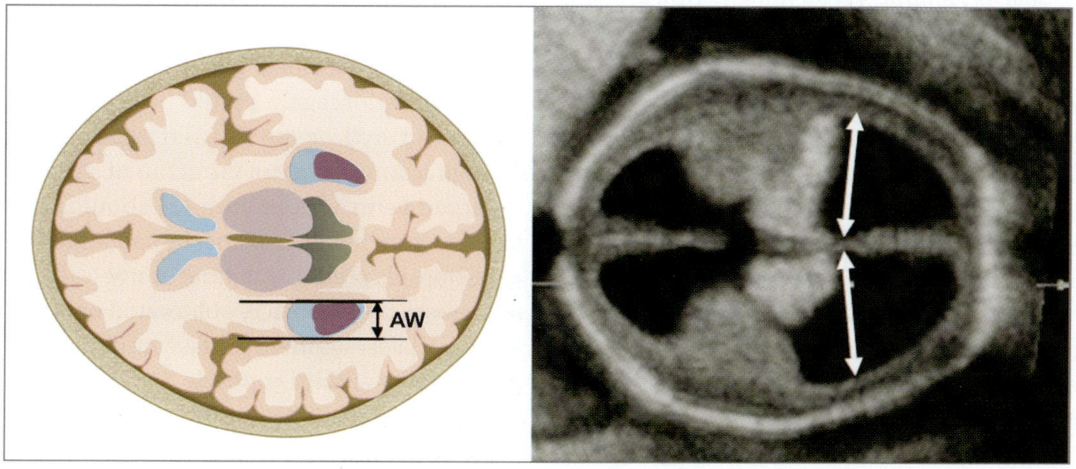

Fig. 31: Atrial width (AW) measurement.

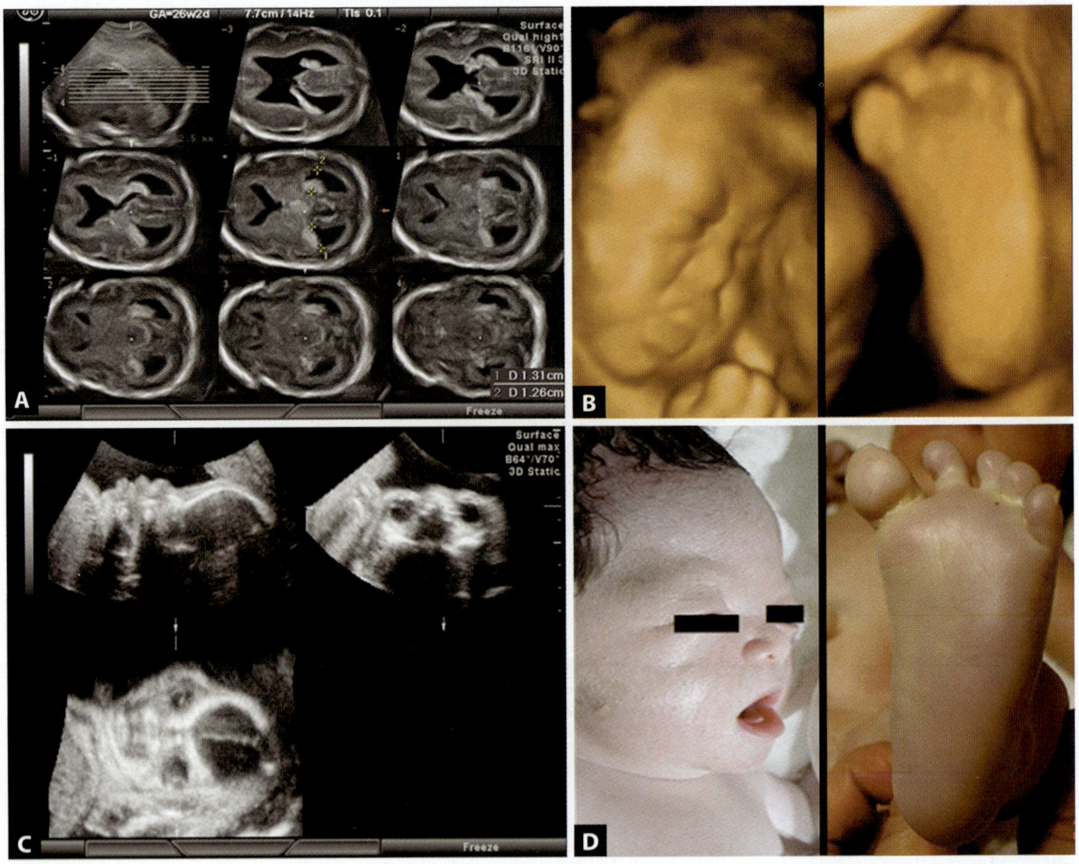

Figs. 32A to D: Mild ventriculomegaly due to craniosynostosis (Pfeiffer syndrome). (A) Tomographic ultrasound imaging of the brain at 26 weeks. Fused ventricle with mild enlargement is demonstrated. Atrial width measurement shows 12–13 mm; (B) 3D surface images of fetal face and foot. Exophthalmos with flat face and large thumb are seen; (C) Three orthogonal view of fetal face; (D) Abnormal facial expression and foot appearance after birth.

localized within CSF circulation pathway, includes aqueductal stenosis, atresia of foramen Monro, and maldevelopment of arachnoid granulation.

b. *Dysgenetic hydrocephalus:* Dysgenetic hydrocephalus indicates hydrocephalus as a result of cerebral developmental disorder in early developmental stage and includes hydranencephaly, holoprosencephaly, porencephaly, schizencephaly, Dandy-Walker malformation, dysraphism, and Chiari malformation.
c. *Secondary hydrocephalus:* Secondary hydrocephalus is a generic term indicating hydrocephalus caused by intracranial pathologic condition, such as brain tumor, intracranial infection and intracranial hemorrhage.

In cases with progressive hydrocephalus, there may be seven stages of progression: (1) Increased fluid collection of lateral ventricles; (2) Increased intracranial pressure; (3) Dangling choroids plexus; (4) Disappearance of subarachnoid space; (5) Excessive extension of the dura and superior sagittal sinus; (6) Disappearance of venous pulsation, and finally; (7) Enlarged skull.[51] In general, both hydrocephalus and ventriculomegaly are still evaluated by the measurement of biparietal diameter (BPD) and atrial width (AW) in transabdominal axial section. As described above, however, hydrocephalus and ventriculomegaly should be differentiated from each other and hydrocephalic state should be assessed by changing appearance of intracranial structure. To evaluate enlarged ventricles, examiners should carefully observe the structure below and specify causes of hydrocephalus:

- Choroids plexus, dangling or not
- Subarachnoid space, obliterated or not
- Ventricles, symmetry, or asymmetry
- Visibility of third ventricle
- Pulsation of dural sinuses
- Ventricular size (3D volume calculation if possible)
- Other abnormalities.

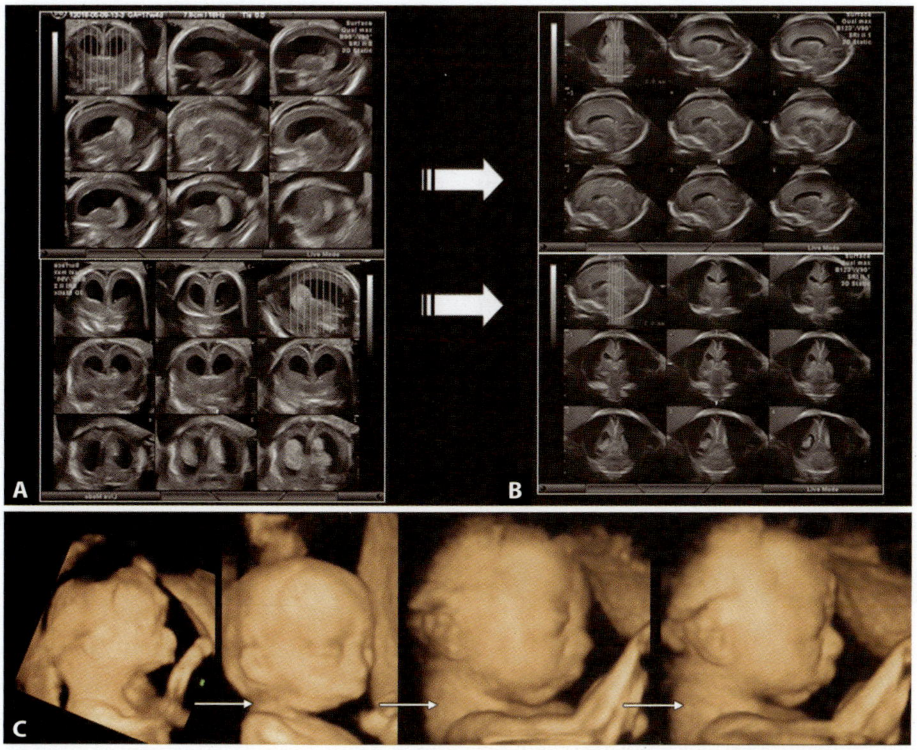

Figs. 33A to C: Mild ventriculomegaly and micrognathia with spontaneous resolution (Pierre-Robin syndrome). (A) Tomographic ultrasound imaging of the brain at 17 weeks. Atrial width measurement shows 10–11 mm; (B) Tomographic brain imaging at 25 weeks. Spontaneous resolution of ventriculomegaly is seen; (C) Slow mandiblar development between 17 and 28 weeks of gestation was demonstrated by 3D reconstructed images.

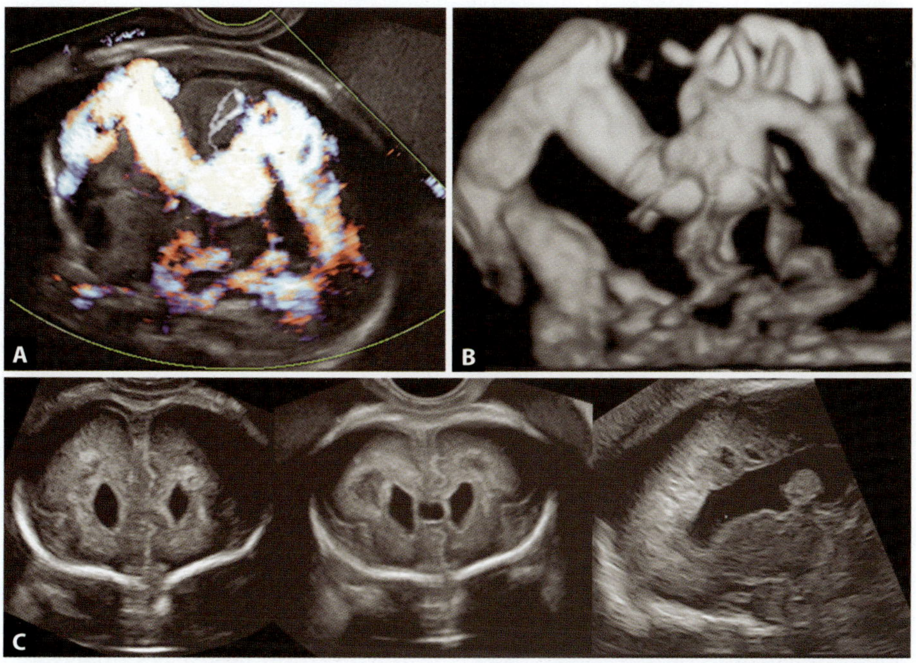

Figs. 34A to C: Mild ventriculomegaly and brain damage due to vein of Galen aneurysmal malformation (28 weeks). (A) Bidirectional power Doppler image of sagittal section. Enlarged sinus is seen; (B) 3D B-flow image of vascular structure. Many arteries run directly toward aneurysmal sac; (C) Anterior coronal slices and parasagittal sections of the brain. Note multiple brain damage with low and high echogenicity around mildly enlarged ventricles. Atrial width measurement was just 10 mm at this stage.

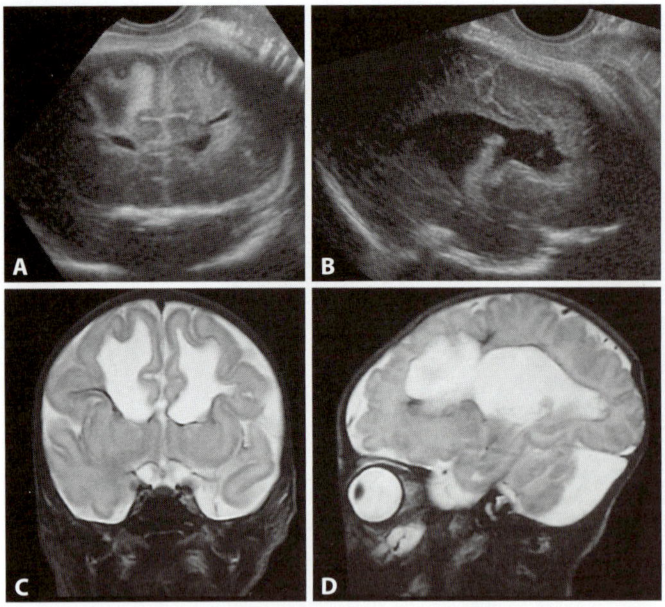

Figs. 35A to D: Mild ventriculomegaly to postnatal porencephaly due to multiple cerebral hemorrhage. (A) Anterior coronal section at 36 weeks. Note the low echogenic parts inside high echogenicity, which indicate brain hemorrhage; (B) Parasagittal section. Note the irregular ventricular wall indicating the beginning of porencephaly. At this stage, atrial width measurement was 10–12 mm; (C) MR coronal image at 17 postnatal day. Conspicuous bilateral porencephalic parts fused with lateral ventricles are seen; (D) Parasagittal section of MRI. Porencephalic cyst was clearly formed for 4 weeks.

TABLE 2: Twenty-three cases of ventriculomegaly with atrial width of 10–15 mm.

With additional abnormality	***13/23 cases (56.5%)***
• Chromosomal/genetic abnormality	31%
• Other brain abnormality	69%
• Extra CNS abnormality	31%
• MR, CP, neurological deficits	40%
• No neurological deficit (<2 years)	30%
• IUFD, TOP	30%
• *Ventriculomegaly during pregnancy:*	
– Resolved	31%
– Remain stable	31%
– Progressive	23%
– Uncertain	15%
No other abnormality	***10/23 cases (43.5%)***
• Cerebral palsy	10%
• Epilepsy	10%
• No neurological deficit (<2 years)	80%
• *Ventriculomegaly during pregnancy:*	
– Resolved	70%
– Remain stable	20%
– Progressive	10%

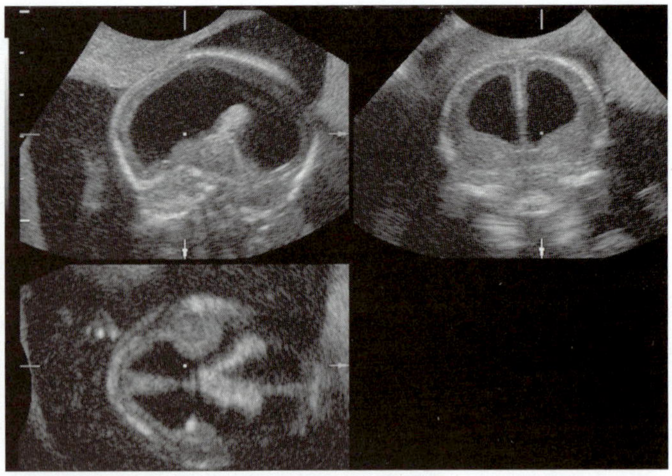

Fig. 36: Hydrocephalus due to myelomeningocele and Chiari type II malformation at 17 weeks. Severe hydrocephalus with dangling choroid plexus and disappearing subarachnoid space.

Figures 36 to 39 show the prenatal sonographic imaging of fetal ventriculomegaly with atrial width of over 15 mm. Although all cases have similar ventricular appearance, the causes of ventriculomegaly vary, such as Chiari type II malformation **(Fig. 36)**, aquedactal obstruction **(Figs. 37A to G)**, aquedactal stenosis and cerebral hypoplasia **(Figs. 38A to D)**, and amniotic band syndrome (ABS)**(Figs. 39A to C)**. In the case of ABS, amniotic band attached to the scalp resulted in partial cranial bone defect and a small cephalocele, which may have caused Monro obstruction and enlarged ventricles.

Table 3 shows the summary of 23 ventriculomegaly cases with atrial width >15 mm.

Nine cases (39.1%) had no other CNS abnormality but two out of those 9 were complicated with chromosomal aberration. Among the rest of 14 cases, holoprosencephaly was detected in 5 cases and myelomeningocele in 5 cases. Four cases out of 7 without any complication had favorable postnatal prognosis after ventricular-peritoneal shunting procedure.

CONGENITAL CNS ANOMALIES

During fetal period, the embryonal premature CNS structure rapidly develops into the mature structure with gyral formation. Within this rapid change of development, various developmental disorders and/or insults result in various phenotypes of fetal CNS abnormalities. For understanding fetal CNS diseases, basic knowledge of the development of the nervous system is essential. The developmental stages and their major disorders are described as **Table 4**.

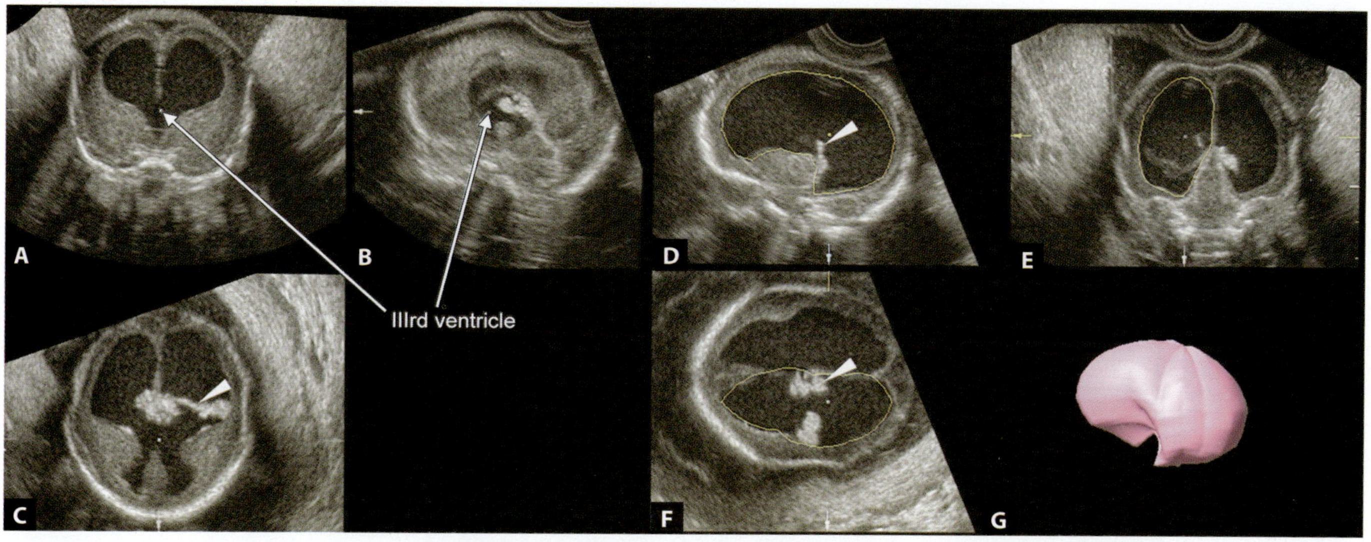

Figs. 37A to G: Hydrocephalus due to aqueductal obstruction at 19 weeks of gestation. (A to C) Three-orghogonal views with anterior coronal (A) and median sagittal (B) and axial (C) slices. Bilateral ventriculomegaly and third ventriculomegaly (IIIrd ventricle) are seen. No enlargement of the fourth ventricle indicates obstruction of the aqueduct; (D to G) Three orthogonal views with parasagittal (D) and posterior coronal (E) and axial (F) slices. Subarachnoid space is already obliterated and dangling choroid plexus (arrowheads) is seen; (G) Shows extracted 3D ventricular image by VOCAL mode. The ventricle in this case was 10-fold size of normal 19-week-ventricle.

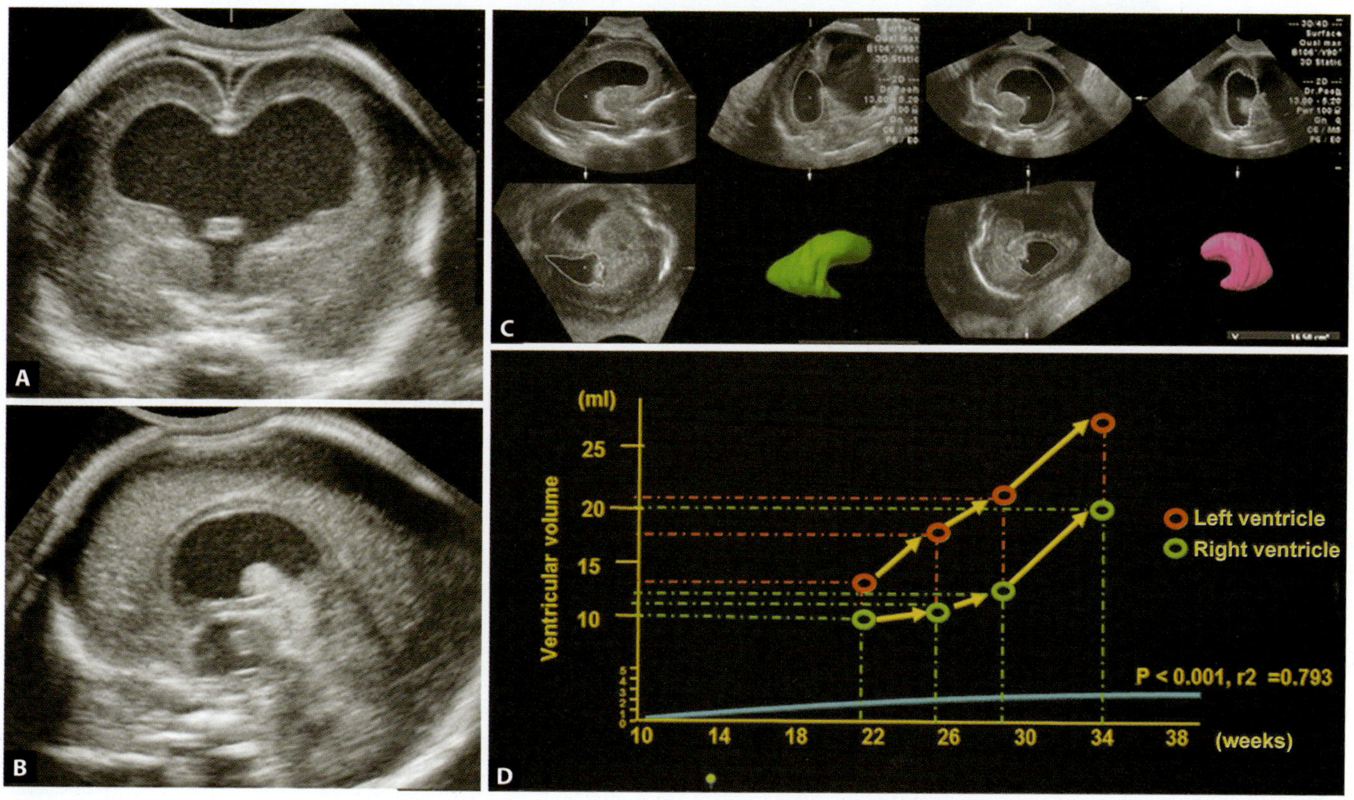

Figs. 38A to D: Moderate ventriculomegaly (21 weeks). (A and B) Ultrasound images in the coronal and sagittal sections. Fused ventriculomegaly, enlarged foramen of Monro, mild IIIrd ventriculomegaly are demonstrated in the coronal section, and no enlargement of IVth ventricle was seen in the sagittal section. Therefore, aqueductal stenosis and cerebral hypoplasia were suspected; (C) 3D images with volume calculation of bilateral ventricles; (D) Longitudinal study of ventricular size was on the graph. This case shows moderate increase of ventricular size during pregnancy.

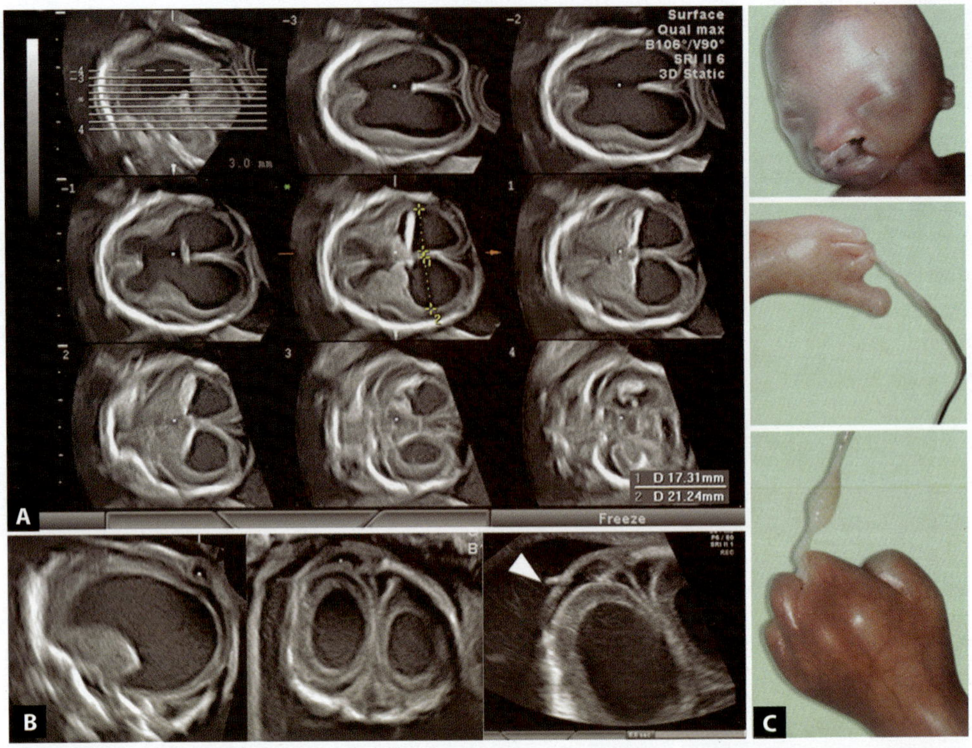

Figs. 39A to C: Hydrocephalus due to amniotic band syndrome (20 weeks). (A) Tomographic ultrasound imaging in the axial section of fetal brain at referral. Bilateral atrial width was 17 and 21 mm respectively. From the observation of enlarged ventricles, simple hydrocephalus due to Monro obstruction was suspected. However, the fetus was complicated with cleft lip, amputation of fingers and amniotic band was detected by extra CNS scan; (B) Small cephalocele (arrows) were seen with remnant of the amniotic band (arrowhead). (C) Macroscopic view of the face and extremities after termination of pregnancy.

TABLE 3: Twenty-three cases of ventriculomegaly of atrial width more than 15 mm.

• *Isolated ventriculomegaly:*	9
– Normal karyotypes	7
– Abnormal	2
• Holoprosencephaly	5
• Myelomeningocele	5
• Dandy–Walker syndrome	1
• Agenesis of CC	1
• ACC + IHC	1
• Multiple porencephaly	1
• Total	23

Cranium Bifidum

Prevalence: Anencephaly; 0.29/1,000 births,[60] overall neural tube defect (NTD); 0.58–1.17/1,000 births.[47-49] Many reported remarkable reduction of prevalence of NTDs after using folic acid supplementation and fortification,[60-63] although some reported no decline of anencephaly rate.[64]

Definition: As in spina bifida, cranium bifidum is classified into four types of encephaloschisis (including anencephaly and exencephaly), meningocele, encephalomeningocele, encephalocystocele, and cranium bifidum occultum. Encephalocele occurs in the occipital region in 70–80%. Acrania, exencephaly and anencephaly are not independent anomalies. It is considered that dysraphia (absent cranial vault, acrania) occurs in very early stage and disintegration of the exposed brain (exencephaly) during the fetal period results in anencephaly.[65]

Etiology: Multifactorial inheritance, single mutant genes, specific teratogens (valproic acid), maternal diabetes, environmental factors, predominant in females.

Pathogenesis: Failure of anterior neural tube closure or a restricted disorder of neurulation.

Associated anomalies: Open spina bifida (iniencephaly), Chiari type III malformation, bilateral renal cystic dysplasia, and postaxial polydactyly with occipital cephalocele (Meckel-Gruber syndrome), hydrocephalus, polyhydramnios.

Prenatal diagnosis: Acrania in **Figures 40A to C**, anencephaly in **Figures 41A to D**, encephalocele in

TABLE 4: Developmental stages and major disorders.

Developmental stage	*Disorders*
Primary neurulation (3–4 weeks of gestation)	• Spina bifida aperta • Cranium bifidum
Caudal neural tube formation (secondary neurulation, from 4 weeks of gestation)	Occult dysraphic states
Procencephalic development (2–3 months of gestation)	Holoprosencephaly Agenesis of the corpus callosum, agenesis of the septum pellucidum, septo-optic dysplasia
Neuronal proliferation (3–4 months of gestation)	Micrencephaly, macrencephaly
Neuronal migration (3–5 months of gestation)	• Schizencephaly • Lissencephaly, pachygyria • Polymicrogyria
Organization (5 months of gestation—years postnatal)	Idiopathic mental retardation
Myelination (Birth—years postnatal)	Cerebral white matter hypoplasia

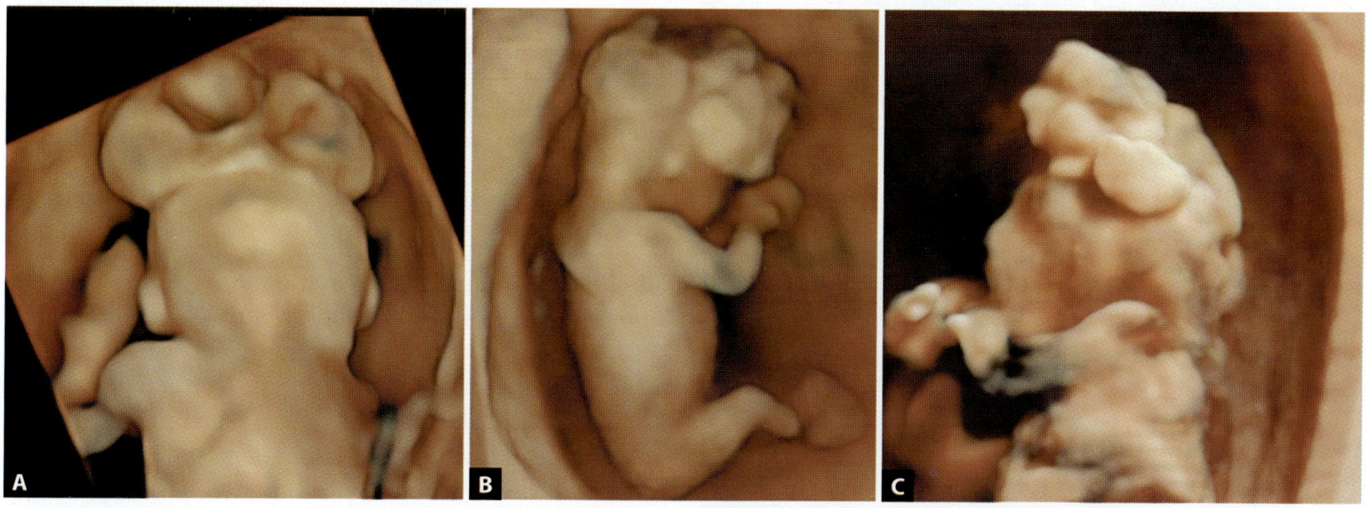

Figs. 40A to C: Acrania at 12 weeks of gestation. HDlive images show various patterns of acrania in the first trimester.

Figures 42A to D, and early detection of iniencephaly in **Figures 43A to C**.

Differential diagnosis: Amniotic band syndrome (ABS). In cases of ABS, cranial destruction occurs secondarily to an amniotic band, similar appearance is observed. However, ABS has completely different pathogenesis from acrania/excencephaly.

Prognosis: Anencephaly is a uniformly lethal anomaly. Other types of cranium bifidum, various neurological deficits may occur, depending on types and degrees.

Recurrence risk: Used to be high recurrence risk of 5–13%, however, recently declined by use of folic acid supplementation and fortification.

Obstetrical management: Termination of pregnancy can be offered in cases with anencephaly.

Neurosurgical management: For other cranium bifidum, surgical operation aims at transposition of cerebral tissue into the intracranial cavity. Ventriculoperitoneal shunt for hydrocephalus.

Spina Bifida

Prevalence: 0.22/1000 births,[60] overall neural tube defect (NTD); 0.58–1.17/1000 births.[47-49] Many reported remarkable reduction of prevalence of NTDs after using folic acid supplementation and fortification.[60-63]

Definition: Spina bifida aperta, manifest form of spina bifida is classified into four types: meningocele,

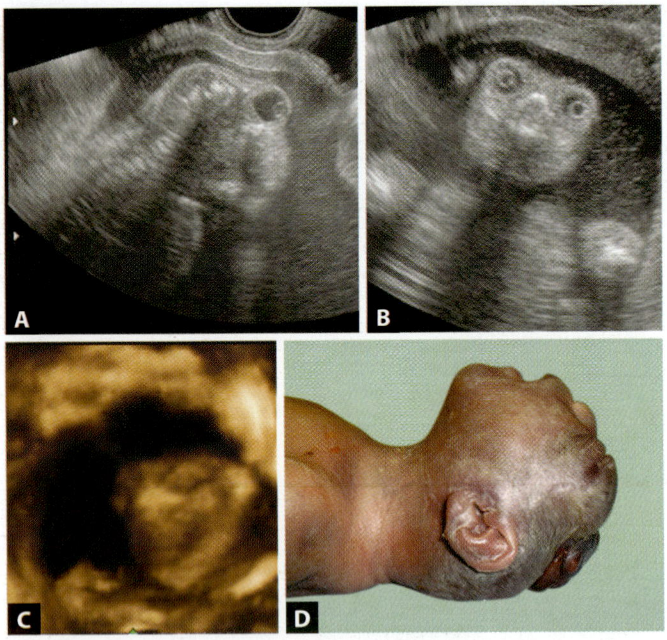

Figs. 41A to D: Anencephaly in middle gestation (same case as **Figure 25**). (A) US sagittal image at 23 weeks of gestation; (B) US coronal image; (C) 3D US image; (D) External appearances of stillborn fetus at 25 weeks of gestation. It is clear that excencephalic brain tissue which had existed for 10 weeks scattered in the amniotic space.

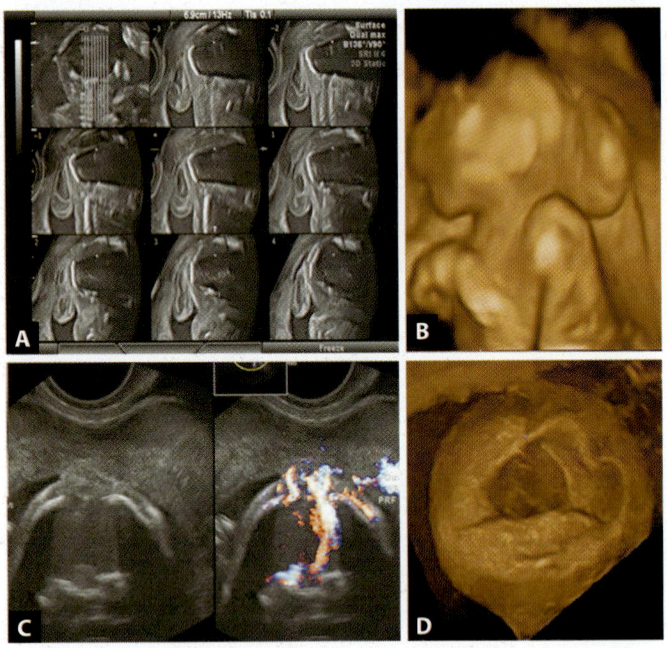

Figs. 42A to D: Encephalocele at 18 weeks of gestation. (A) Tomographic sagittal imaging of encephalocele; (B) 3D reconstructed image. Microcephaly and occipital encephalocele are demonstrated; (C) Gray scale mode and bidirectional power Doppler image of connection between intracranial brain and extracranial brain. Cerebral vessels between them are clearly visualized. (D) 3D maximum mode of the occipital bone defect.

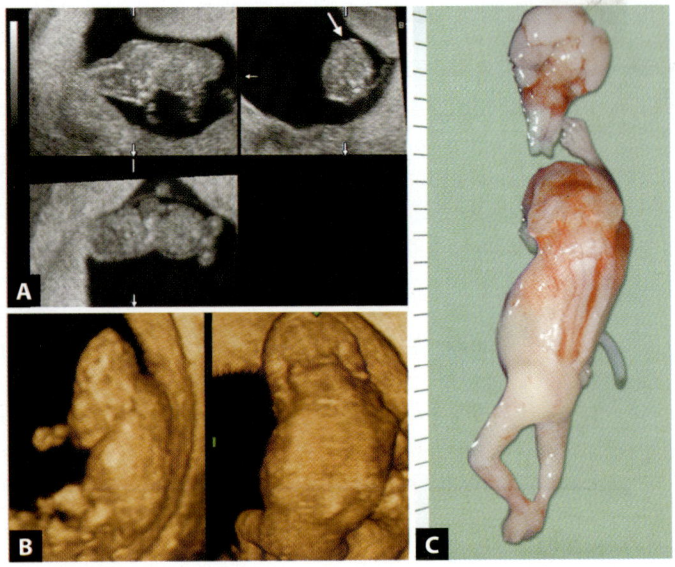

Figs. 43A to C: 3D detection of a fetus with iniencephaly and acrania at 10 weeks of gestation. (A) Three orthogonal views of the fetus. Spina bifida (arrow) was demonstrated in the coronal section; (B) 3D images show the fetal lateral and dorsal views; (C) External appearance of aborted fetus at the end of 11 weeks of gestation. The brain and a part of spinal cord was detached at delivery.

myelomeningocele, myelocystocele, myeloschisis. *Spina bifida occuluta* is a generic term of spinal diseases covered with normal skin tissue and does not indicate spinal diseases which cannot be diagnosed by external appearance, cutaneous abnormalities near the spinal lesion are found; skin bulge (subcutaneous lipoma), dimple, hair tuft, pigmentation, skin appendage and hemangioma. In case with thickened film terminale, dermal sinus, or diastematomyelia (split cord malformation), abnormal tethering and fixation of the spinal cord occur.

Etiology: Multifactorial inheritance, single mutant genes, autosomal recessive, chromosomal abnormalities (trisomy 18, 13), specific teratogens (valproic acid), maternal diabetes, environmental factors, predominant in females.

Pathogenesis:

- *Spina bifida aperta:* An impairment of neural tube closure
- *Spina bifida occuluta:* Caudal neural tube malformation by the processes of canalization and retrogressive differentiation.

Associated anomalies: Chiari type II malformation, hydrocephalus, scoliosis (above L2), kyphosis, polyhydramnios, additional non-CNS anomalies.

Prenatal diagnosis: **Figures 44 to 47**.

Differential diagnosis: Sacrococcygeal teratoma.

Prognosis: Disturbance of motor, sensory, and sphincter function. Depends on lesion levels. Below S1; enable to walk unaided, above L2; wheelchair dependent, variable at intermediate level.

Recurrence risk: Decreased, almost no recurrence rate[66] by use of folic acid supplementation and fortification.

Obstetrical management: In case with spina bifida aperta, especially with defect of skin, cesarean section is preferable to protect the spinal cord and nerves and prevent infection.

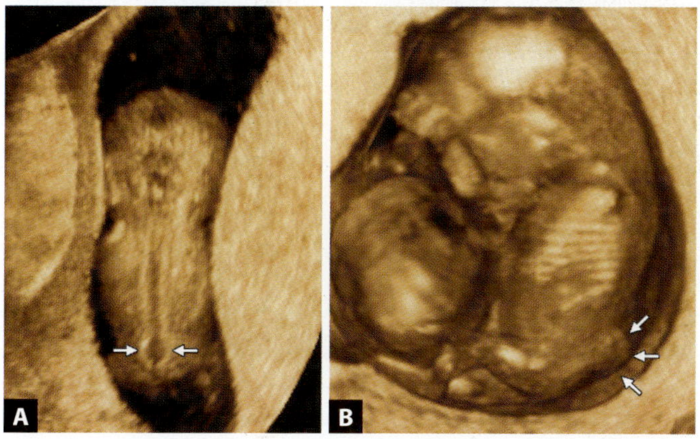

Figs. 44A and B: Myelomeningocele in the first trimester. Three-dimensional dorsal view at 9 weeks (A) clearly demonstrates a neural tube defect at the lower lumbar and sacral level (arrows); (B) Shows the same fetus at 12 weeks of gestation. Arrows indicate the lumbosacral myelomeningocele.

Neurosurgical management:

- *Spina bifida aperta:* In cases with defects of normal skin tissue, immediate closure of spina bifida after birth reduces spinal infection. Spinal cord reconstruction is the most important role of operation. Miniature Ommaya reservoir placement and subsequent ventriculoperitoneal shunt are required for hydrocephalus. For symptomatic Chiari malformation, posterior fossa decompressive craniectomy and/or tonsillectomy is performed.
- *Spina bifida occuluta:* The aim of surgical treatment for is decompression of the spinal cord and cutting off tethering to the spinal cord.

Chiari Malformation

Prevalence: Depends on prevalence of spina bifida (Chiari type II malformation). According to the recent remarkable reduction of prevalence of NTDs after using folic acid supplementation and fortification, prevalence has declined. Other types are rare.

Definition: Chiari classified anomalies with cerebellar herniation in the spinal canal into three types by contents of herniated tissue; contents of type I is a lip of cerebellum, type II part of cerebellum, fourth ventricle and medulla oblongata, pons, and type III large herniation of the posterior fossa. Thereafter, type IV with just cerebellar hypogenesis was added. However, this classification occasionally leads to confusion in neuroimaging diagnosis.

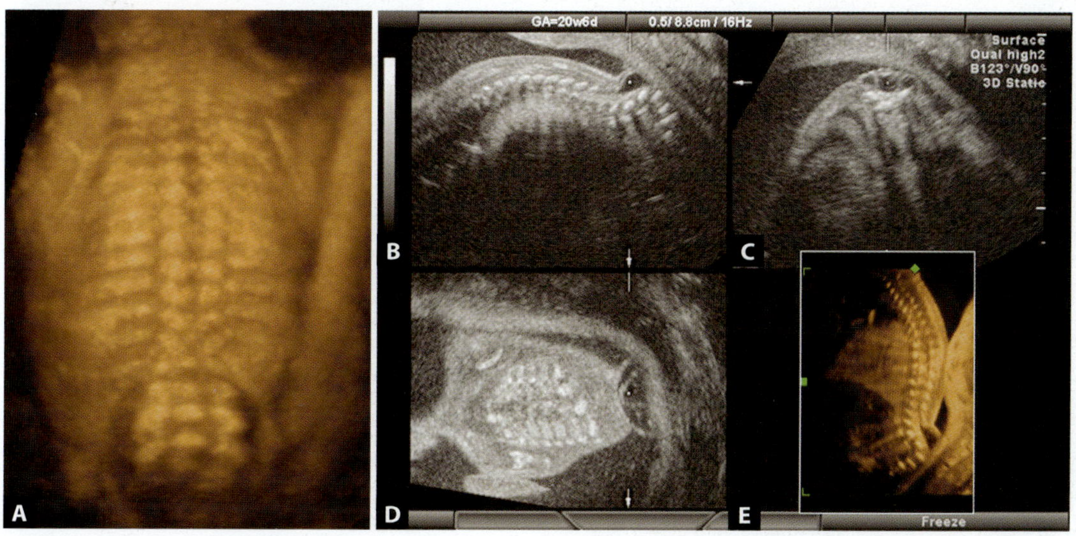

Figs. 45A to E: Myelomeningocele with severe kphosis at 20 weeks of gestation. (A) 3D surface reconstruction image shows the large myelomeningocele from T12. Black-white pictures (B to D) show three orthogonal views of vertebral structure and myelomeningocele with severe kyphosis; (E) Image demonstrates the 3D thick slice of vertebral structure.

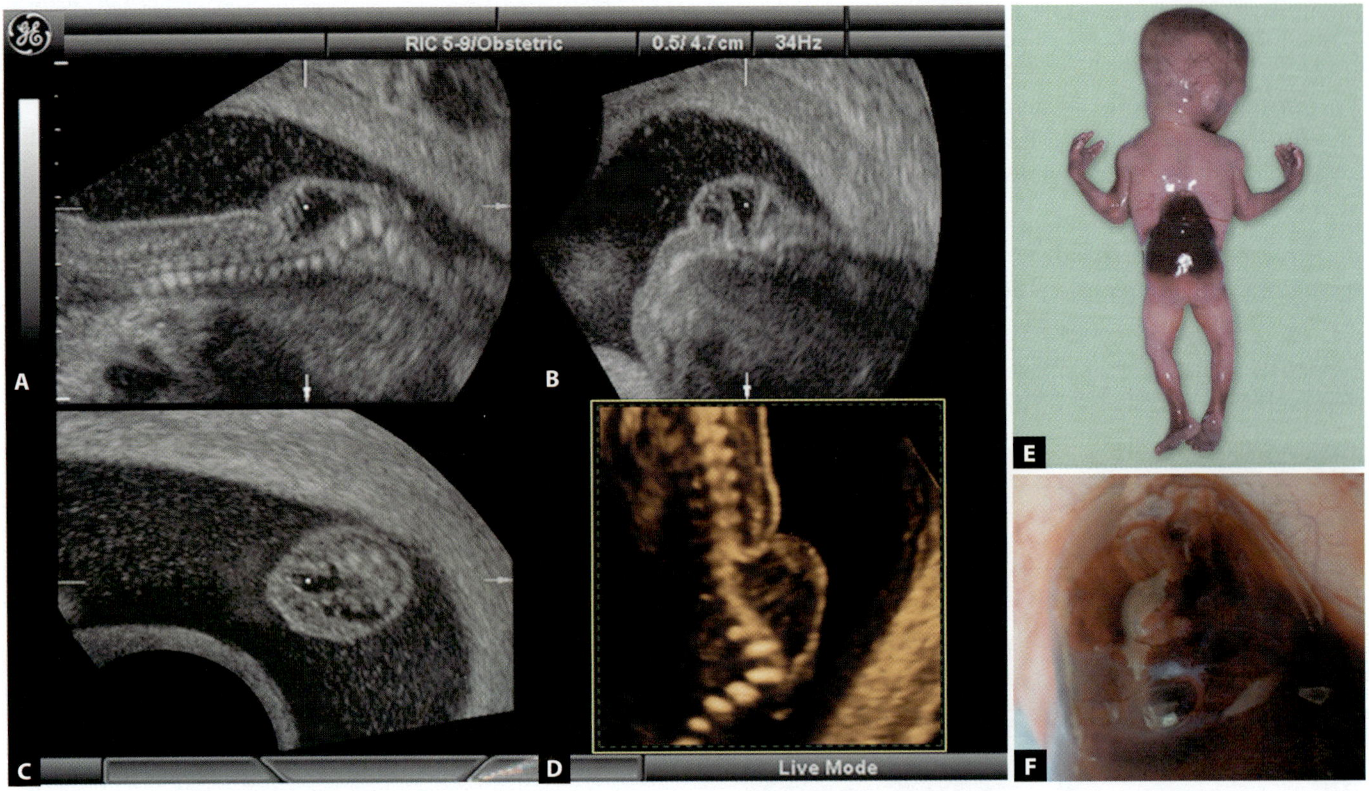

Figs. 46A to F: 3D US image of myelomeningocele with kyphosis at 16 weeks of gestation. Three orthogonal views and surface reconstruction image. (A) Sagittal US image. Spinal cord completely protrude into the sac surface from spinal canal and severe kyphosis are seen; (B) Axial US view; (C) Coronal US view of myelomeningocele; (D) Figure demonstrates the sagittal vertebral bony structure by 3D thick slice; (E) Image shows aborted fetus at 17 weeks; (F) Image shows tortuous structure of spinal cord.

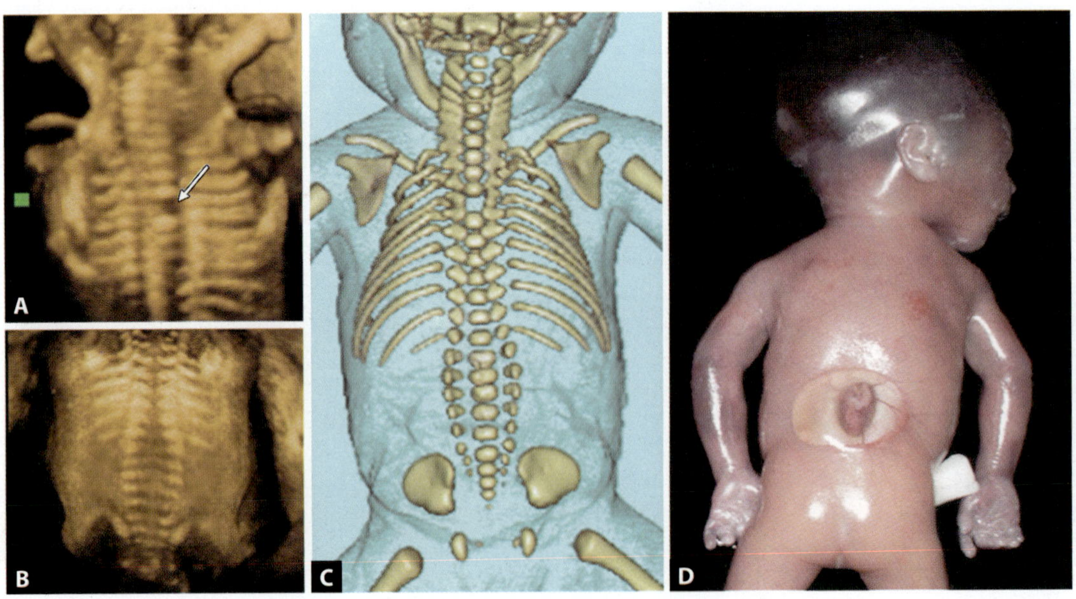

Figs. 47A to D: Myelomeningocele with vertebral body defect at 17 weeks. (A) Image demonstrates vertebral body defect of T4 and T5 (arrow); (B) Image demonstrates spina bifida from T11 level; (C) 3D-CT image of aborted fetus at 20 weeks of gestation. L4 and L5 vertebral body defect and spina bifida are well demonstrated; (D) Shows the myelomeningocele of aborted fetus.

Therefore, at present, the classification as below is advocated.

- *Type I:* Herniation of only cerebellar tonsil, not associated by myelomeningocele
- *Type II (**Figs. 48A and B**):* Herniation of cerebellar tonsil and brainstem. Medullary kink, tentorial dysplasia, associated with myelomeningocele
- *Type III:* Associated with cephalocele or craniocervical meningocele, in which cerebellum and brainstem herniated.

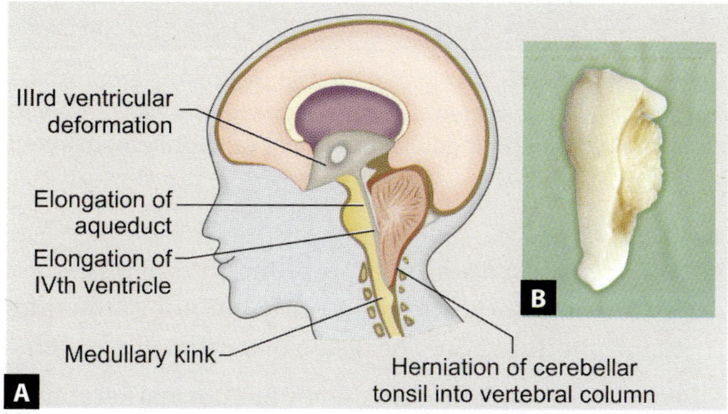

Figs. 48A and B: (A) Schema and macroscopic finding of Chiari type II malformation. Chiari type II malformation is characterized by inferior displacement of the lower cerebellum through the foramen magnum with obliteration of the cisterna magna, inferior displacement of the medulla into the spinal canal, and elongation of the fourth ventricle and aqueduct; (B) Shows the macroscopic view of the elongated aqueduct, IVth ventricle and cerebellum from the specimen of an aborted fetus at 21 weeks of gestation.

- *Type IV:* Associated with marked cerebellar hypogenesis and posterior fossa shrinking.

Synonyms: Arnold-Chiari malformation

Etiology: Depends on the types.

Pathogenesis: Chiari malformation occurs according to: (1) Inferior displacement of the medulla and the fourth ventricle into the upper cervical canal; (2) Elongation and thinning of the upper medulla and lower pons and persistence of the embryonic flexure of these structures; (3) Inferior displacement of the lower cerebellum through the foramen magnum into the upper cervical region; and (4) A variety of bony defects of the foramen magnum, occiput, and upper cervical vertebrae.[67]

Associated anomalies: Hydrocephalus caused by obstruction of fourth ventricular outflow or associated aqueductal stenosis. Myelomeningocele or myeloschisis (type II), cephalocele or craniocervical meningocele (type III), cerebellar hypogenesis (type IV), and syringomyelia (type I).

Prenatal diagnosis: Prenatal US diagnosis by features; lemon sign which indicates deformity of the frontal bone, banana sign which indicates abnormal shape of cerebellum without cisterna magna space **(Figs. 49A to C)**, medullary kink, small clivus-supraocciput angle.[68] Lemon and banana signs are circumstantial evidences of Chiari malformation. Sonographic detection of Chiari malformation itself is occasionally possible **(Figs. 50A and B)**.

Differential diagnosis: Craniosynostosis.

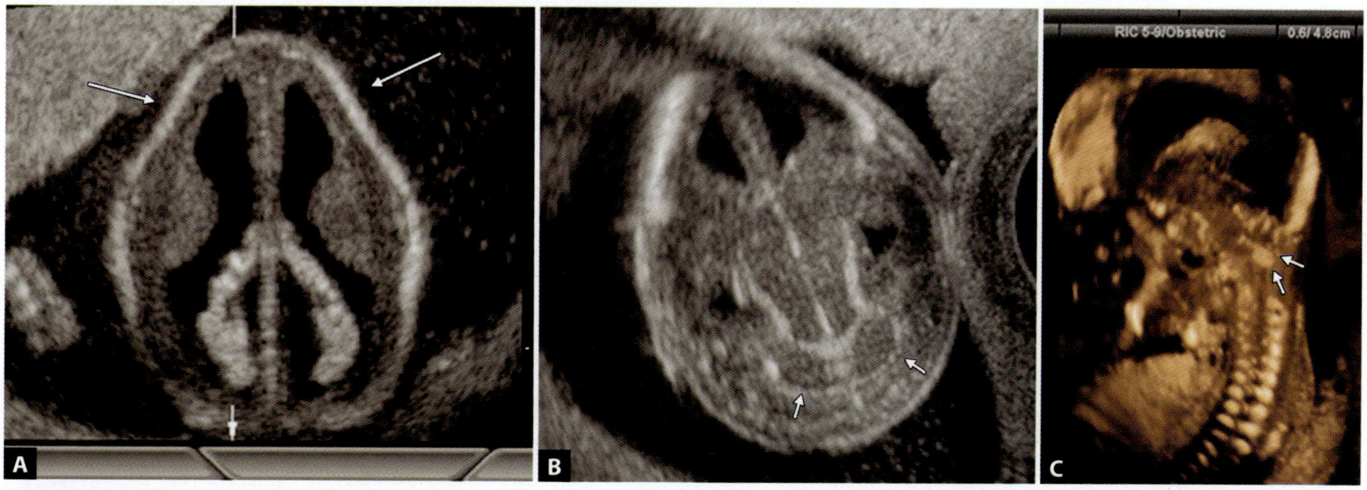

Figs. 49A to C: Chiari type II malformation at 16 weeks of gestation. Chiari type II malformation is observed in most cases with myelomeningocele and myeloschisis. (A) Typical lemon sign (arrows); (B) Typical banana sign (arrows); (C) 3D reconstruction internal image of Chiari type II malformation (arrows).

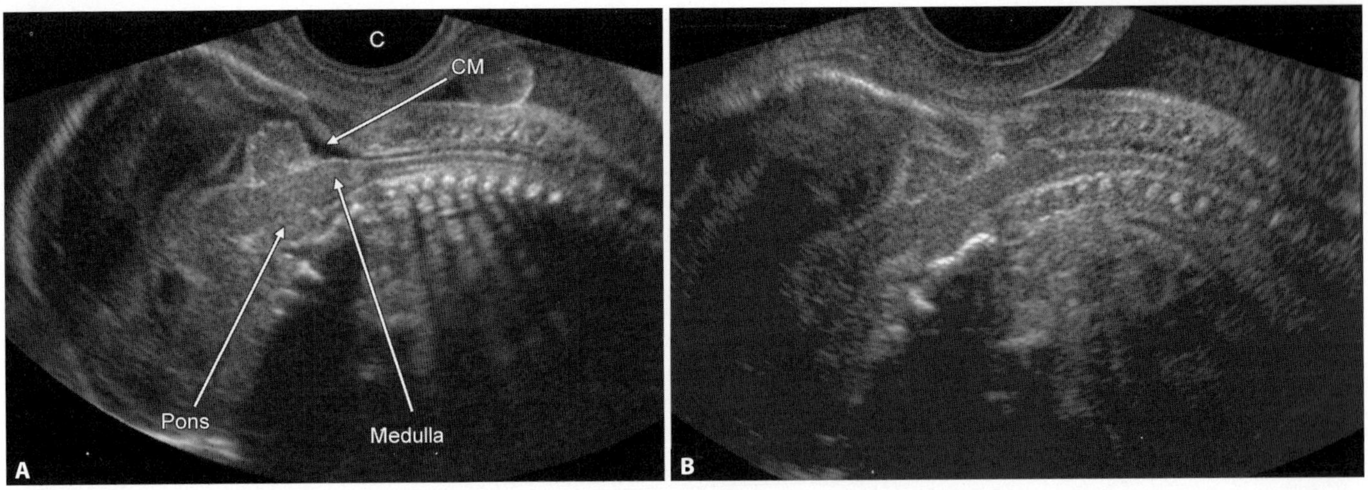

Figs. 50A and B: Ultrasound imaging of Chiari II malformation at 20 weeks of gestation. (A) Normal sagittal section of cerebrospinal region at 20 weeks. The brainstem (pons and medulla) and cerebellum (C) are well demonstrated. Cisterna magna (CM) is well preserved. (B) The same cutting section of Chiari II malformation. Herniation of the cerebellum and medulla into spinal canal is demonstrated. Posterior fossa including cisterna magna is compressed.

Prognosis: Nearly every case of myelomeningocele is accompanied morphological Chiari II malformation. Many cases with Chiari II are asymptomatic. However, clinical features due to Chiari malformation, such as feeding disturbances, laryngeal stridor, or apneic episode, are found in approximately 9–30% of cases. In cases with these clinical features, vital prognosis is often poor.

Recurrence risk: Depends on types of Chiari malformation. Decreased according to decline of NTD recurrence rate by use of folic acid supplementation and fortification.

Neurosurgical management: Neurosurgical decompression of foramen magnum (FMD) for any types of Chiari malformation. Syringo-subarachnoid shunt for Chiari type I.

Holoprosencephaly

Incidence: 1 in 15,000–20,000 live births, however, initial incidence may be more than sixty-fold greater in aborted human embryos.[69,70]

Classification: Holoprosencephalies are classified into three varieties:

1. *Alobar type:* A single-sphered cerebral structure with a single common ventricle, posterior large cyst of third ventricle (dorsal sac), absence of olfactory bulbs and tracts and a single optic nerve.
2. *Semilobar type:* With formation of a posterior portion of the interhemispheric fissure.
3. *Lobar type:* With formation of the interhemispheric fissure anteriorly and posteriorly but not in the mid-hemispheric region. The fusion of the fornices is seen.[71]

Etiology: 75% of holoprosencephaly has normal karyotype, but chromosomes 2, 3, 7, 13, 18 and 21 have been implicated in holoprosencephaly.[61] Particularly, trisomy 13 has most commonly been observed. Autosomal dominant transmission is rare.

Pathogenesis: Failure of cleavage of the prosencephalon and diencephalon during early first trimester (5–6 weeks) results in holoprosencephaly.

Associated anomalies: Facial abnormalities such as cyclopia, ethmocephaly, cebocephaly, flat nose, cleft lip, and palate are invariably associated with holoprosencephaly. Extracerebral abnormalities are also invariably associated, such as renal cysts/dysplasia, omphalocele, cardiac disease and or myelomeningocele.

Prenatal diagnosis: Alobar type in the first trimester and at 15 weeks of gestation are shown in **Figures 51 and 52**, and semilobar type in late pregnancy in **Figures 53 and 54** show facial appearance in cases of holoprosencephaly.

Differential diagnosis: Hydrocephalus, hydranencephaly.

Prognosis: Extremely poor in alobar holoprosencephaly. Uncertain in lobar type. Various but poor in semilobar type.

Recurrence risk: 6%,[72] but much lower in sporadic or trisomy cases, much higher in genetic cases.

Management: Chromosomal evaluation is offered.

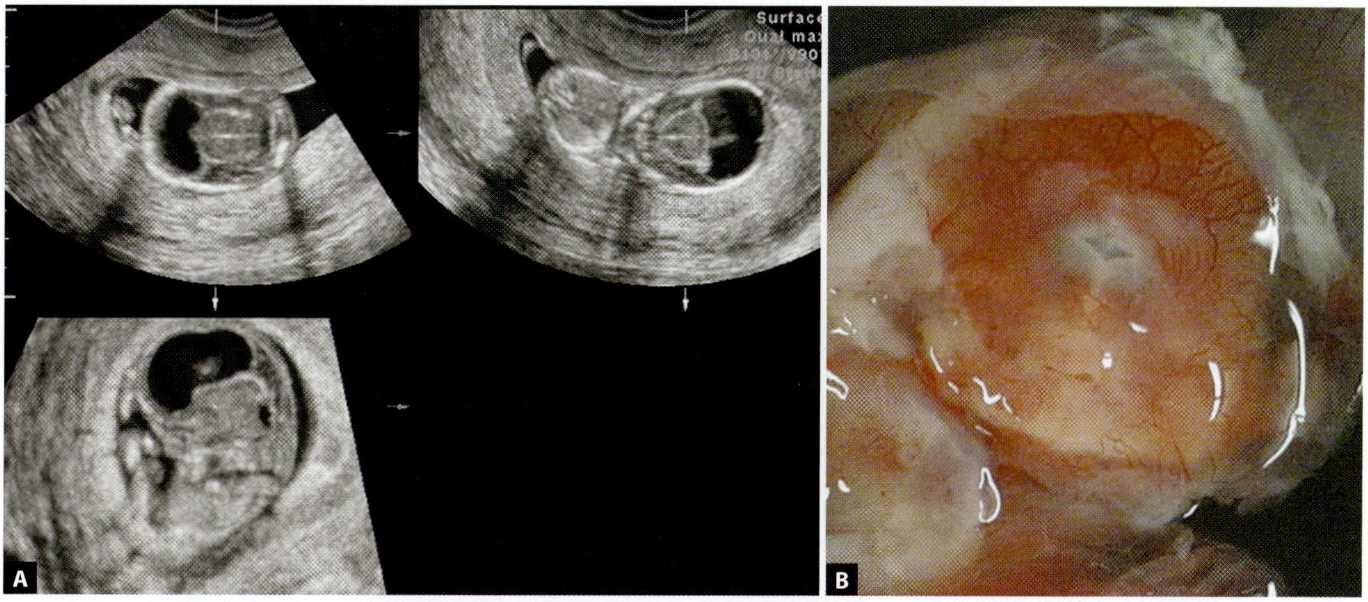

Figs. 51A and B: Alobar holoprocencephaly in the first trimester. (A) Three orthogonal views demonstrate holoprocencephaly at 13 weeks. CRL was compatible to 10 weeks of gestation; (B) Shows the face of aborted fetus with cyclopia, arhinia, and small mouth.

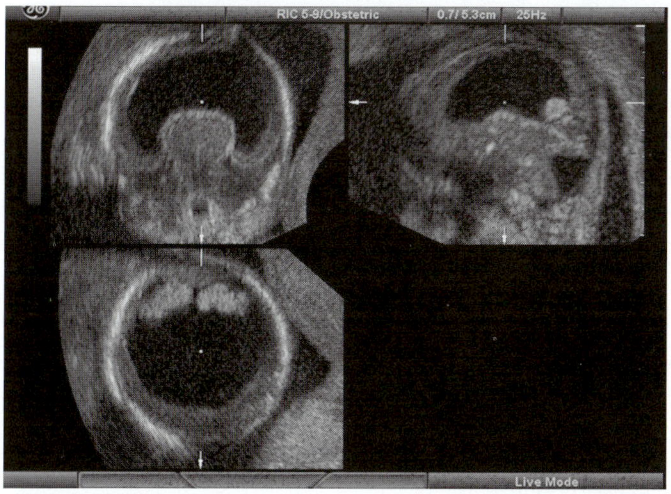

Fig. 52: Alobar holoprosencephaly at 15 weeks of gestation. Three orthogonal images of intracranial structure show a complete single ventricle within a single-sphered cerebral structure.

Agenesis of the Corpus Callosum

Prevalence: Uncertain, but 3–7:1,000 in the general population is estimated.

Definition: Absence of the corpus callosum, which may be divided into (complete) agenesis, partial agenesis or hypogenesis of the corpus callosum.

- *Complete agenesis:* Complete absence of the corpus callosum
- *Partial agenesis (hypogenesis)*: Absence of splenium or posterior portion in various degrees.

Etiology: Chromosomal aberration in 20% of affected cases, such as trisomy 18, 8 and 13. Autosomal dominant, autosomal recessive, X-linked recessive, part of mendelian syndromes such as Walker-Warburg syndrome, and X-linked dominant such as Aicardi syndrome.

Pathogenesis: Uncertain, but callosal formation may be associated with migration disorder.

Associated anomalies: Colpocephaly (ventriculomegaly with disproportionate enlargement of trigones, occipital horns and temporal horns, not hydrocephaly), superior elongation of the third ventricle, interhemispheric cyst, lipoma of the corpus callosum.

Prenatal diagnosis: Prenatal features of agenesis of the corpus callosum are shown in **Figure 55** and sonographic and MRI images are shown in **Figures 56A to H**. Abnormal brain vessels in a case of agenesis of the corpus callosum is demonstrated in **Figures 57A to D**.

Diagnosis: As the corpus callosum is depicted after 17 or 18 weeks of gestation by ultrasound, it is impossible to diagnose agenesis of the corpus callosum prior to this age.[73]

Prognosis: Various. Depends on associated anomalies. Most cases with isolated agenesis of the corpus callosum without other abnormalities are asymptomatic and prognosis is good. Complete agenesis has a worse prognosis than partial agenesis.[74] Epilepsy, intellectual impairment or psychiatric disorder[75] may occur later on.

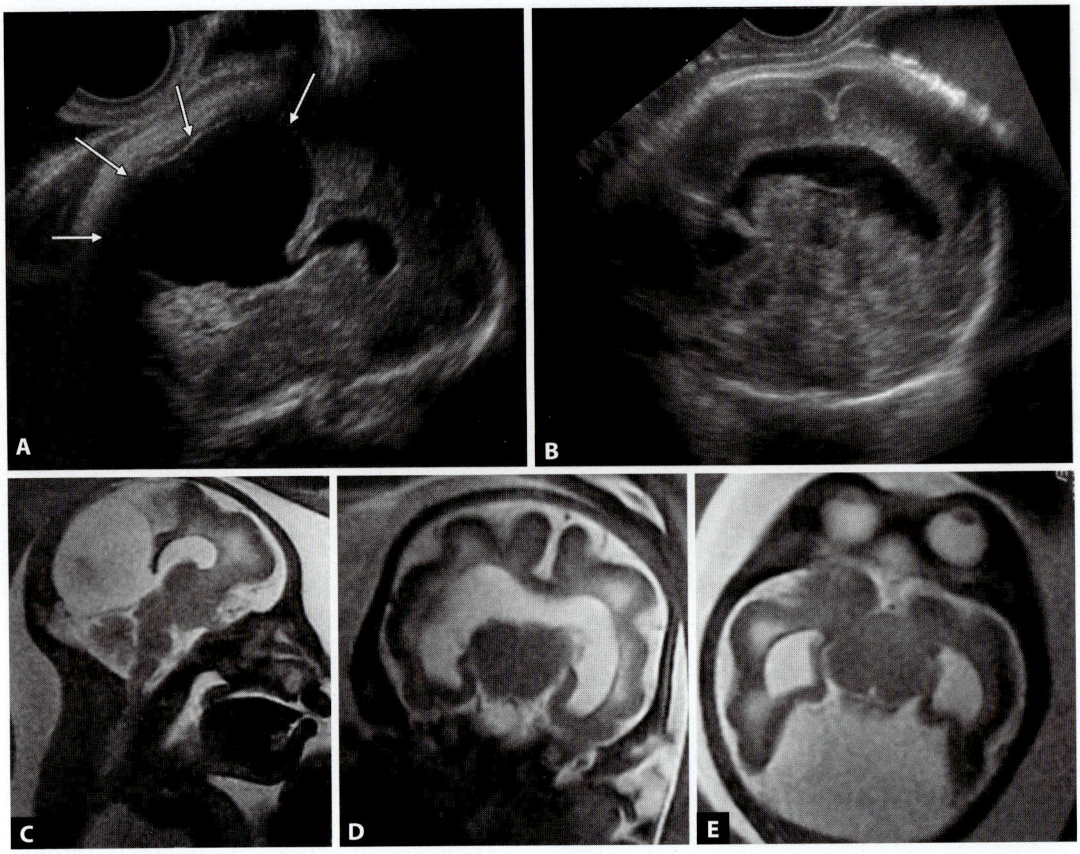

Figs. 53A to E: Semilobar holoprosencephaly at 33 weeks of gestation. (A) Shows dorsal sac (arrows) in the median section; (B)Demonstrates the fused ventricle; (C to E) Fetal MR images. Sagittal (C); coronal (D); and axial (E) sections. A blind end of nasal cavity and hypotelorism are seen in the sagittal and axial MR images, respectively.

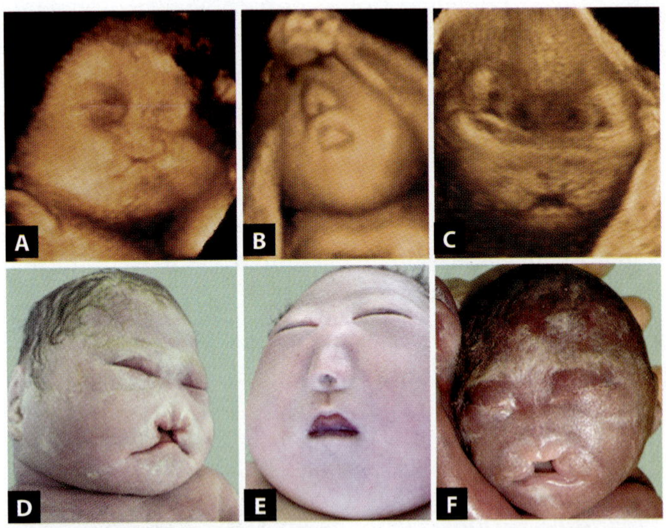

Figs. 54A to F: Facial abnormality in cases of holoprosencephaly. (A to C) Prenatal 3D facial images and (D to F) show postpartum face appearance of each baby. (A) Alobar holoprosencephaly at 20 weeks; (B and C) Semilobar type in late pregnancy. Hypotelorism, and exophthalmos are common; (D and E) Cases had cleft lip and palate and obstruction of the nasal cavity; (F) Case had a single and obstructed nasal cavity.

Recurrence risk: Depends on etiology. Chromosomal; 1%, autosomal recessive; 25%, X-linked recessive male; 50%.

Management: Standard obstetrical care. Chromosomal evaluation is offered. In cases with interhemispheric cysts, postnatal fenestration or shunt procedure may be performed.

Absent Septum Pellucidum and Septo-optic Dysplasia

Incidence: Unknown, rare.

Definition:

- *Absent septum pellucidum:* Absence of the septum pellucidum with or without associated anomalies. The septum pellucidum can be destroyed by concomitant hydrocephalus or by contiguous ischemic lesions such as porencephaly. An isolated absent septum pellucidum[76] exists but rare.
- *Septo-optic dysplasia:* Absence of the septum pellucidum and unilateral or bilateral hypoplasia of the optic nerve.

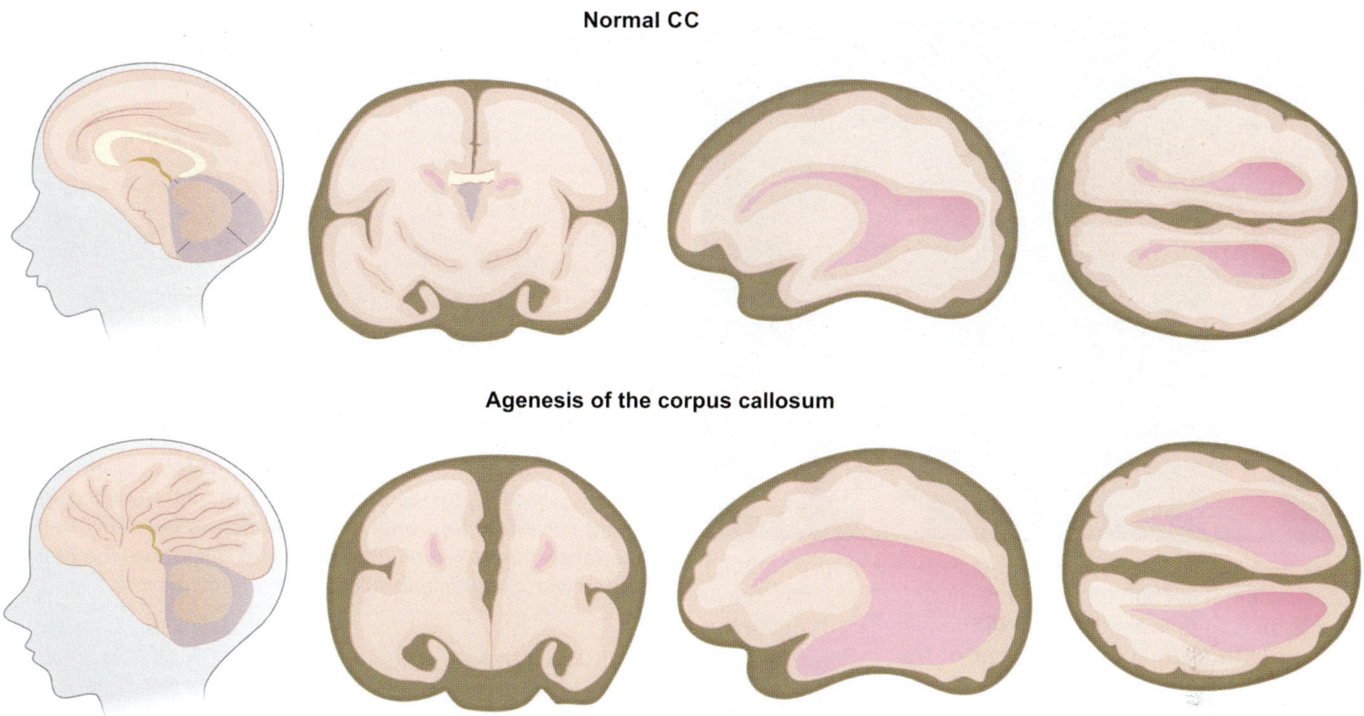

Fig. 55: Schematic diagrams showing four major features of agenesis of the corpus callosum (AOCC). Midsagittal, anterior coronal, parasagittal and axial views from the left. Upper pictures are normal structure for comparison.

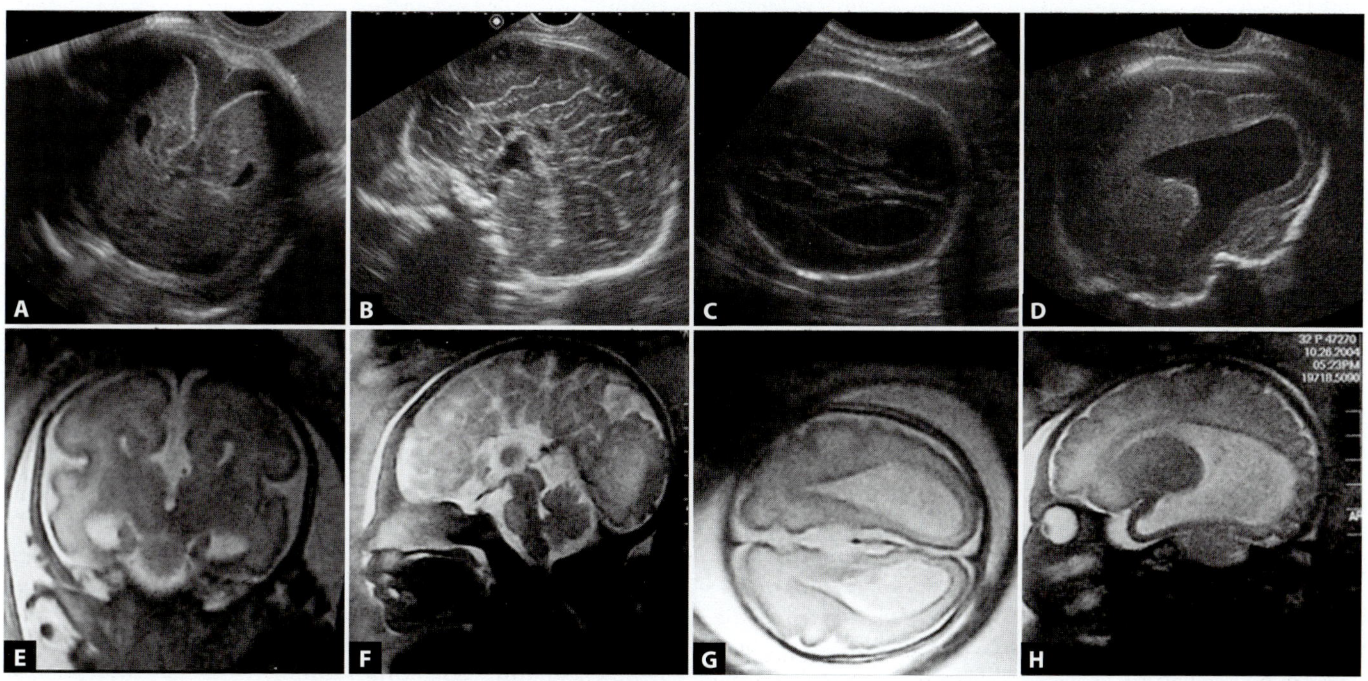

Figs. 56A to H: Fetal US and MR images of complete agenesis of the corpus callosum. Sonographic images (A to D) and MR images (E to H). Anterior coronal, midsagittal, axial, and parasagittal sections from the left. No communicated bridge is between bilateral hemispheres. Note the bull's horn-like appearance of the anterior horns of lateral ventricle in the coronal image. Typical ventricular shape of colpocephaly is demonstrated on the axial and parasagittal sections.

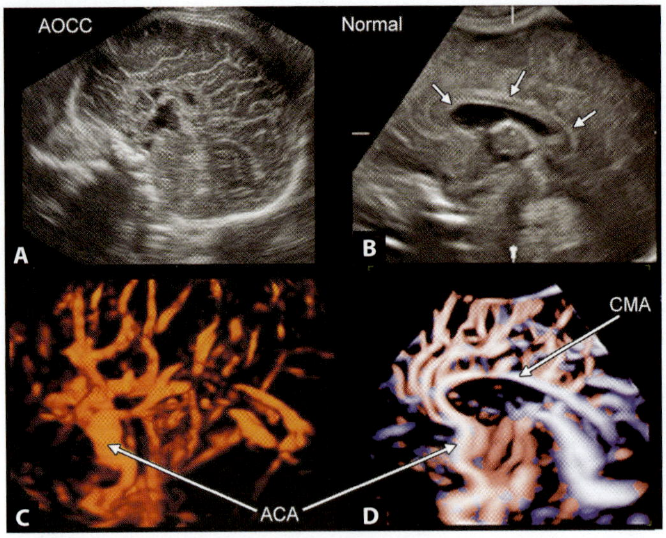

Figs. 57A to D: Agenesis of the corpus callosum (AOCC). (A) Midsagittal section in a case of AOCC. Typical radial sulcus formation is seen instead of normal cingulate sulcus and gyrus formed with normal development of the corpus callosum (B, arrows) seen; (C) Angiostructure by 3D power Doppler. Normal callosomarginal artery (CMA, D) does not exist and radial formation of the branches of anterior cerebral arteries (ACA) is seen.

Synonyms: de Morsier syndrome (septo-optic dysplasia).

Etiology: Maternal drug (multidrug, valproic acid,[77] cocaine),[78] autosomal recessive, *HESX1* homeodomain gene mutation.[79]

Pathogenesis: May occur as a vascular disruption sequence, with other prosencephalic or neuronal migration disorders.

Associated anomalies: Schizencephaly, gyral abnormalities, heterotopias, hypotelorism, ventriculomegaly, communicating lateral ventricles, bilateral cleft lip and palate, hypopituitarism.

Differential diagnosis: Dysgenesis of the corpus callosum, lobar holoprosencephaly.

Prognosis: Depends on associated anomalies. Variable degree of mental deficit, multiple endocrine dysfunction. In cases with isolated absence of septum pellucidum, prognosis may be good.

Recurrence risk: Unknown.

Management: Confirmation of diagnosis after birth is important for genetic counseling. Endocrine dysfunction should be searched and corrected. Shunt procedure in cases with progressive ventriculomegaly.

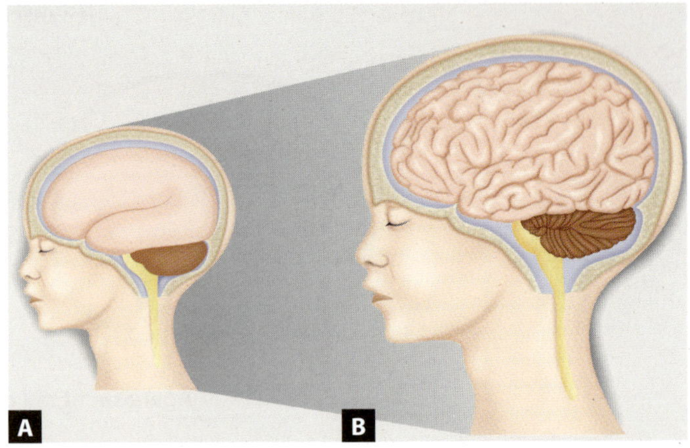

Figs. 58A and B: Changing appearance of fetal brain during pregnancy. In the early second trimester (A), smooth brain surface without sulcation. Neuronal migration occurs between 3 and 5 gestational months. As a consequence of migration, the brain is matured with gyration and sulcation (B) after 8 months.

Migration Disorder

Incidence: Rare

Definition: Arise specifically from defective formation of the central nervous system.

Etiology: Thought to be genetic in cause.

Pathogenesis: The abnormal migration of neurons in the developing brain and nervous system. In the developing brain, neurons must migrate from the areas where they are born to the areas where they will settle into their proper neural circuits. Neuronal migration, which occurs as early as the third month of gestation, is controlled by a complex assortment of chemical guides and signals. As a consequence of migration, the brain is matured with gyration and sulcation after eight months **(Figs. 58A and B)**. When these signals are absent or incorrect, neurons do not end up where they belong. This can result in structurally abnormal or missing areas of the brain in the cerebral hemispheres, cerebellum, brainstem, or hippocampus, including schizencephaly, porencephaly, lissencephaly, agyria, macrogyria, pachygyria, microgyria, micropolygyria, neuronal heterotopias (including band heterotopia), agenesis of the corpus callosum, and agenesis of the cranial nerves.

Differential diagnosis: Brain tumor.

Prenatal diagnosis: Phenotype due to migration disorder on the surface of cerebral hemispheres appears in the late pregnancy, therefore, it seems to be not possible to detect migration disorder before gyration. Toi, et al.[80] reported normal sulcation pattern during pregnancy depicted by transabdominal ultrasound imaging. During pregnancy, the first evidence indicating the consequence of migration is the Sylvian fissure[81-83] and the most comprehensive cutting section, in which bilateral Sylvian fissures are well demonstrated, as shown in **Figure 59**. This cutting section is taken by sonogram via anterior fontanelle as an ultrasound window. During the latter half of the second trimester, the cortical structure macroscopically develops, and the most distinct morphological difference appears to be the different structure of Sylvian fissure. Thus, the Sylvian fissure is one of the landmarks indicating cortical development by normal migration. **Figures 60A and B** demonstrated migration disorder at 24 weeks and 5 days of gestation in a case of microdeletion/microduplication chromosomal disorder, showing abnormal development of Sylvian fissures. Occasionally migration disorder occurs unilaterally. **Figures 61 and 62** show unilateral migration disorder detected by ultrasonography and MRI at 18 and 29 weeks of gestation respectively. **Figures 63A to F** are pachygyria at 33 weeks detected by ultrasounography and MRI.

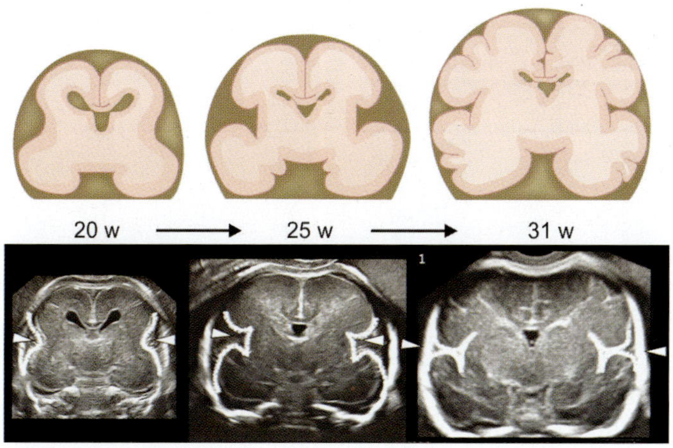

Fig. 59: Changing appearance of Sylvian fissure in the anterior coronal section by transvaginal sonography. At 20 weeks of gestation, bilateral Sylvian fissures (arrowheads) appear to be indentations (left). With cortical development, Sylvian fissures are formed with sharp edges during the latter half of second trimester (middle) and become as lateral sulci in late pregnancy. Sylvian fissure appearance is one of the most reliable ultrasound markers for the assessment of cortical development.

Prognosis: Symptoms vary according to the specific disorder and the degree of brain abnormality and subsequent neurological losses, but often feature poor muscle tone and motor function, seizures, developmental delays, mental retardation, failure to grow and thrive, difficulties with feeding, swelling in the extremities, and a smaller than normal head. Most infants with a neuronal migration disorder appear normal, but some disorders have characteristic facial or skull features.

Recurrence risk: Unknown

Treatment: Treatment is symptomatic and may include antiseizure medication and special or supplemental education consisting of physical, occupational, and speech therapies.

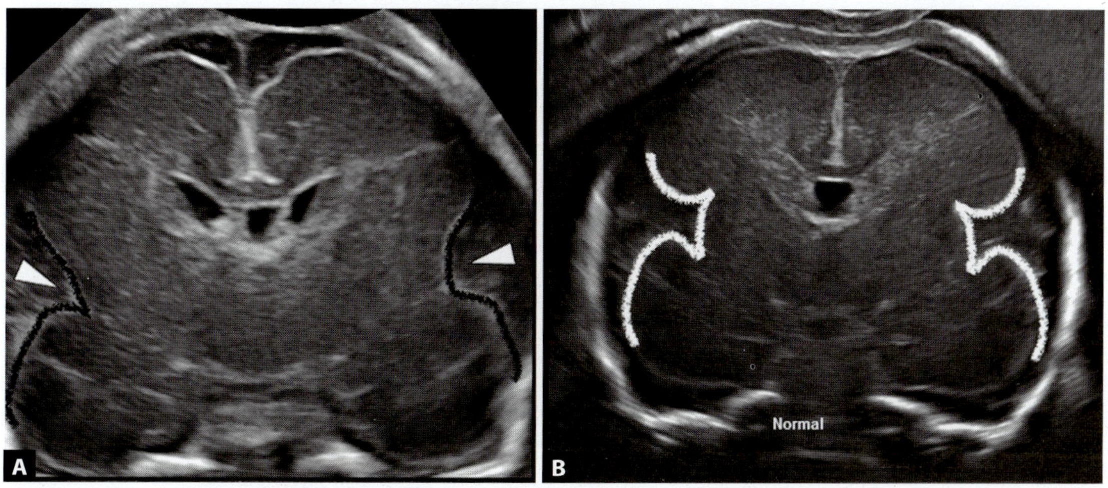

Figs. 60A and B: A case of migration disorder at 25 weeks of gestation. (A) Ultrasound image of anterior coronal section. Abnormal Sylvian fissures (arrowheads) are demonstrated; (B) The normal Sylvian fissures at the same gestational age.

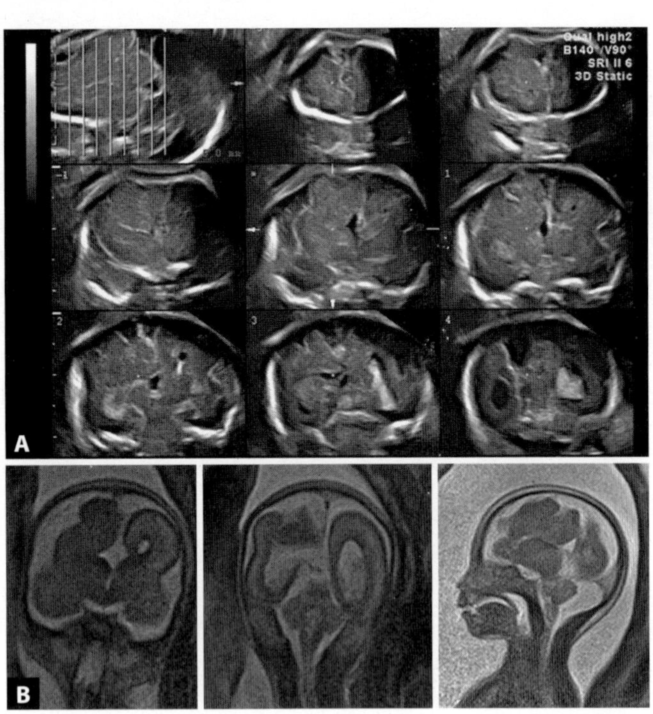

Figs. 61A and B: Migration disorder at 18 weeks of gestation. (A) Tomographic coronal image of the brain. Note the different development between bilateral hemispheres; (B) MR images. Anterior-coronal, posterior-coronal, and sagittal sections from the left. Unilateral abnormal brain development was caused according to migration disorder.

Lissencephaly

Incidence: Unknown, rare

Definition: Characterized by a lack of gyral development and conventionally divided into two types:

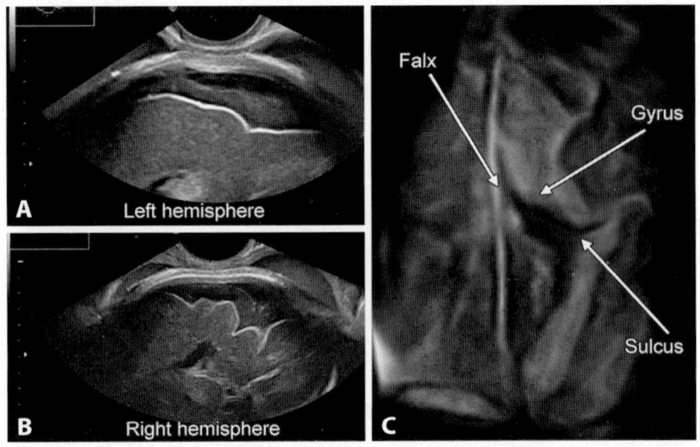

Figs. 62A to C: Ultrasound images of abnormal cortical formation at 29 weeks of gestation. Parasagittal image of the surface of left hemisphere (A) and right hemisphere (B). Note the marked difference of cortical formation between hemispheres; (C) 3D ultrasound image demonstrating the surface anatomy of hemispheres in parietal view. The different formation of gyri and sulci between hemispheres is clearly depicted.

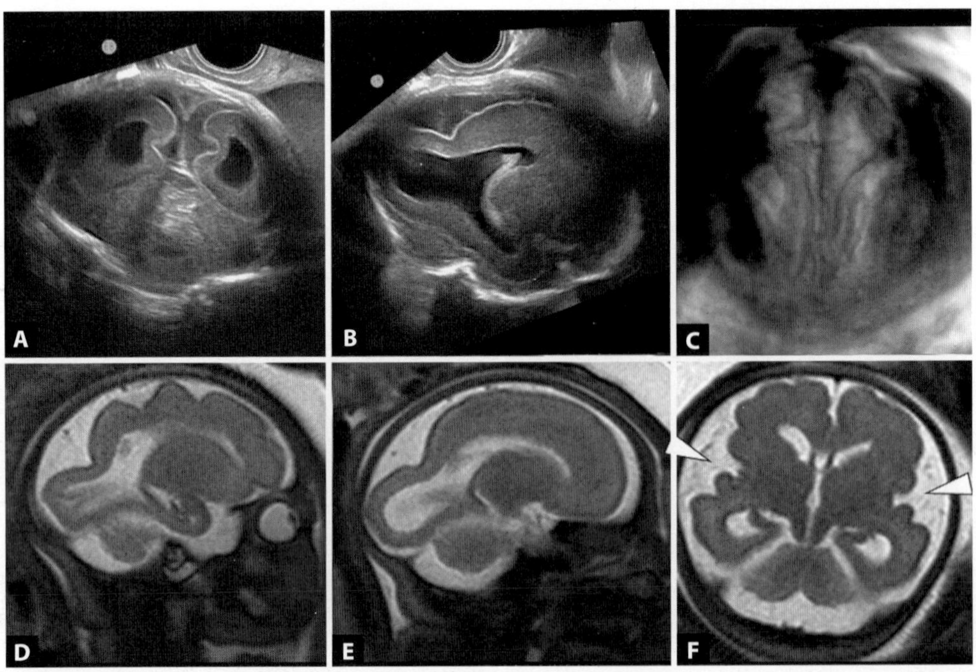

Figs. 63A to F: Pachygyria at 33 weeks of gestation. Ultrasound images (A to C) and MR images (D to F). (A to C) Transvaginal ultrasound images. Posterior coronal (A) and parasagittal (B) sections show the smooth surface of the cerebral hemispheres; (C) Surface anatomy by 3D ultrasound of the cerebral superficial structure in parietal view; (D to F) MR images at the same gestation. Parasagittal sections (D and E) show pachygyria. Anterior coronal section (F) shows bilateral premature and shallow Sylvian fissures (arrowheads) are demonstrated.

1. *Lissencephaly type I:* A smooth surface of the brain. Cerebral wall is similar to that of an approximately 12-week-old fetus.[84]
2. *Lissencephaly type II:* Cobblestone appearance.
   - *Walker-Warburg syndrome* with macrocephaly, congenital muscular dystrophy, cerebellar malformation, retinal malformation. *Fukuyama congenital muscular dystrophy* with microcephaly and congenital muscular dystrophy.

Recently, many of responsible genes were clarified and classification has been changed by etiology **(Table 5)**.

Synonyms: Agyria, pachygyria, Walker-Warburg syndrome was known as HARD±E syndrome (hydrocephalus, agyria, retinal dysplasia, with or without encephalocele).

Etiology: Isolated lissencephaly is linked to chromosome 17p13.3 and chromosome Xq24-q24. Miller-Dieker syndrome is also linked to chromosome 17p13.3. Walker-Warburg syndrome is autosomal recessive inheritance. Fukuyama congenital muscular dystrophy is link to chromosome 9q31, fukutin.[85]

Pathogenesis: Defective neuronal migration with four, rather than six, layers in the cortex.

Associated anomalies: Polyhydramnios, less fetal movement, colpocephaly, agenesis of the corpus callosum, Dandy-Walker malformation, in Miller-Dieker syndrome, micrognathia, flat nose, high forehead, low-set ears, cardiac anomalies, genital anomalies in male are often observed.

TABLE 5: Classification of lissencephaly

Category	***Types***
Classic (or Type 1) lissencephaly	• *LIS1 (17p13.3):* Lissencephaly due to *PAFAH1B1* gene mutation, which subdivides into: – Type 1 isolated lissencephaly – Miller-Dieker syndrome • *LISX1:* Lissencephaly due to doublecortin *(DCX)* gene (Xq23) mutation • lissencephaly, type 1, isolated, without other known genetic defects
Cobblestone (or Type 2) lissencephaly	• Walker-Warburg syndrome, also called HARD (E) syndrome • Fukuyama syndrome • Muscle-eye-brain (MEB) disease
X-linked lissencephaly	*ARX* gene (Xq22.13) mutation
Lissencephaly with cerebellar hypoplasia	Norman-Roberts syndrome (reelin gene (7q22.1) mutation)
Microlissencephaly	Lissencephaly + Microcephaly

Prenatal diagnosis: A few reports of prenatal diagnosis of lissencephaly have been published.[86-88] Without previous history of an affected child probably it is difficult to make diagnosis of lissencephaly until 26–28 weeks of gestation.

Prognosis:

- *Classical type I:* Hypotonia, paucity of movements, feeding disturbance, seizures. The prognosis is poor, and death occurs.
- *Classical type II:* Severe seizures, mental disorders, severe muscle disease with hypotonia. Death in the first year is common.

Recurrence risk: Depends on etiology.

Management: Karyotyping is recommended to detect the chromosomal defects.

Schizencephaly

Incidence: Rare

Definition: A disorder characterized by congenital clefts in the cerebral mantle, lined by pia-ependyma, with communication between the subarachnoid space laterally and the ventricular system medially **(Fig. 64)**. 63% is unilateral and 37% bilateral. Frontal region in 44% and frontoparietal 30%.[84]

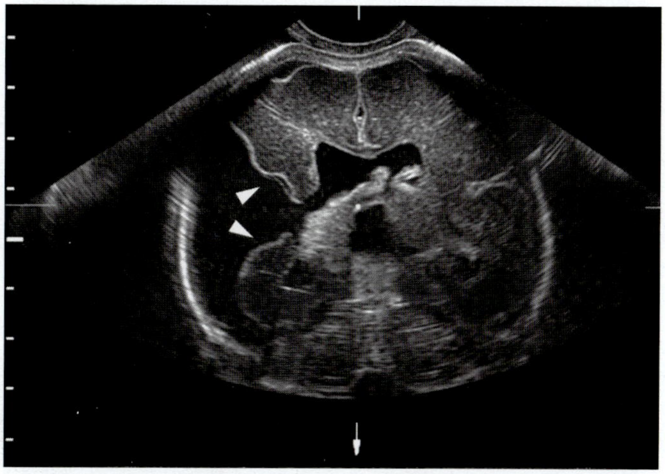

Fig. 64: Schizencephaly at 27 weeks of gestation. Coronal section of the fetal brain. Arrowheads indicate congenital lined by pia-ependyma, with communication between the subarachnoid space laterally and the lateral ventricle.

Etiology: Uncertain. In certain familial case, a point mutation in the homeobox gene, EMX2 was found.[89,90] Cytomegalovirus infection was also related in some cases.[91]

Pathogenesis: Neuronal migration disorder.

Associated anomalies: Ventriculomegaly, microcephaly, polymicrogyria, gray matter heterotopias, dysgenesis of the corpus callosum, absence of the septum pellucidum, and optic nerve hypoplasia.

Differential diagnosis: Porencephaly, arachnoid cyst or other intracranial cystic masses. MR imaging is useful in diagnosis of schizencephaly.[92]

Prognosis: Variable. Generally suffer from mental retardation, seizures, developmental delay and motor disturbances.

Recurrence risk: Unknown.

Management: Ventriculoperitoneal shunt for progressive hydrocephalus.

Dandy-Walker Malformation, Dandy-Walker Variant and Megacisterna Magna

Incidence: Dandy-Walker malformation has an estimated prevalence of about 1:30,000 births, and is found in 4–12% of all cases of infantile hydrocephalus.[93] Incidence of Dandy-Walker variant and megacisterna magna is unknown.

Definition: At present, the term Dandy-Walker complex[94] is used to indicate a spectrum of anomalies of the posterior fossa that are classified by axial CT scans as it follows. Dandy-Walker malformation, hypoplastic vermis, and megacisterna magna seem to represent a continuum of developmental anomalies of the posterior fossa.[76] **Figure 65** shows the differential diagnosis of hypoechoic lesion of the posterior fossa.

- *Dandy-Walker malformation (classic):* Cystic dilatation of fourth ventricle, enlarged posterior fossa, elevated tentorium and complete or partial agenesis of the cerebellar vermis.
- *Hypoplastic vermis:* Variable hypoplasia of the cerebellar vermis with or without enlargement of the posterior fossa.
- *Megacisterna magna:* Enlarged cisterna magna with integrity of both cerebellar vermis and fourth ventricle.

Etiology: Mendelian disorders such as Warburg, chromosomal aberration such as 45,X, partial monosomy/trisomy, viral infections and diabetes.

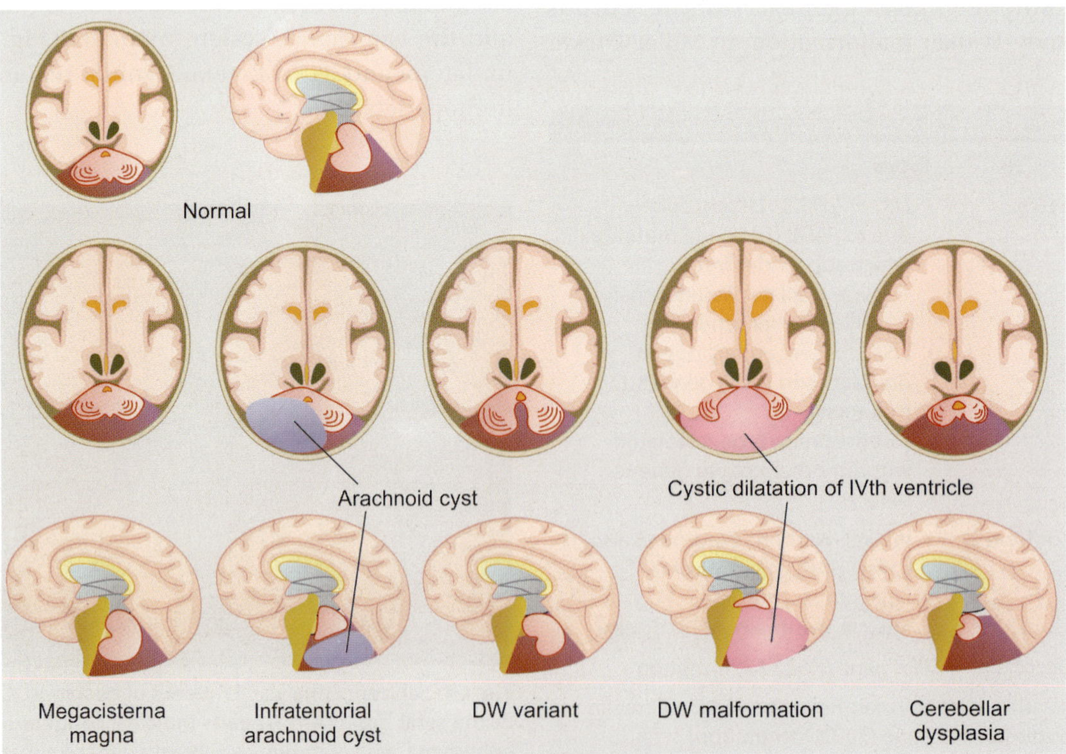

Fig. 65: Differential diagnosis of "hypoechoic lesion" of the posterior fossa.

Pathogenesis: During development of the fourth ventricular roof, a delay or total failure of the foramen of Magendie to open occurs, allowing a buildup of CSF and development of the cystic dilation of the fourth ventricle. Despite the subsequent opening of the foramina of Luschka (usually patent in Dandy-Walker malformation), cystic dilatation of the fourth ventricle persists, and CSF flow is impaired.

Associated anomalies of Dandy-Walker malformation: Hydrocephalus. Other midline anomalies, such as agenesis of the corpus callosum, holoprosencephaly and occipital encephalocele. Extracranial abnormalities such as congenital heart diseases, neural tube defects, and cleft lip/palate. The frequency of additional anomalies ranges between 50 and 70%.

Prenatal diagnosis: Dandy-Walker malformation is shown in **Figures 66 and 67**, and hypoplastic vermis is shown in **Figures 68 and 69**. To observe the agenesis of the cerebellar vermis, axial cutting section is preferable. To observe the elevated tentorium, sagittal section is preferable.

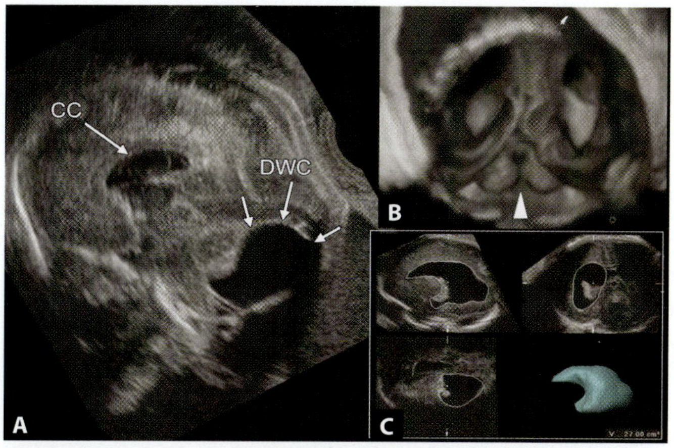

Figs. 66A to C: Dandy-Walker malformation at 28 weeks of gestation. (A) Shows the median section of the brain. Corpus callosum (CC) is normally demonstrated and Dandy-Walker cyst (DWC, arrows) is seen in the posterior fossa; (B) 3D view in the posterior coronal section. Hypoplastic vermis of the cerebellum (arrowhead) is seen; (C) Three orthogonal views and an extracted ventricular appearance demonstrate moderate ventriculomegaly in this case.

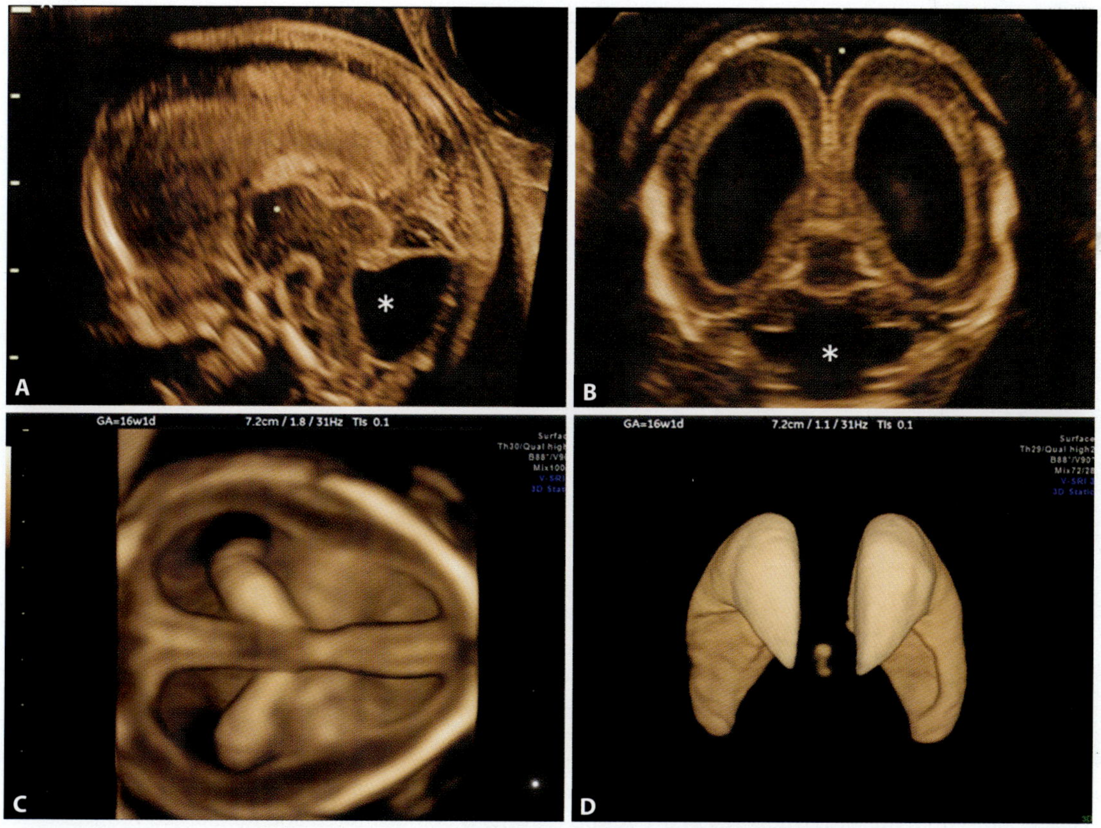

Figs. 67A to D: Dandy-Walker malformation at 16 weeks of gestation. (A) Midsagittal section of the brain. Asterisk indicates cystic dilatation of fourth ventricle; (B) Posterior coronal section of the brain; (C) Axial section of 3D volume dataset, showing ventriculomegaly with dangling choroid plexus; (D) Extracted ventricules by 3D inversion mode.

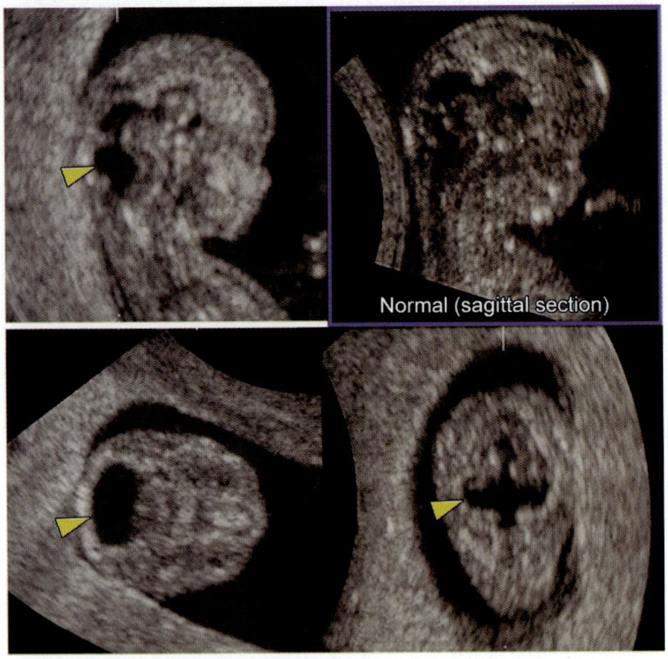

Fig. 68: Early stage of Dandy-Walker malformation or variant at 11 weeks of gestation. Abnormal dilatation of the posterior fossa (arrowheads). Upper right Figure is a sagittal image at the same gestational age in a normal case. Amniocentesis revealed trisomy 9 mosaicism and the fetus died in utero at 19 weeks.

Differential diagnosis: Infratentorial arachnoid cyst, other intracranial cystic tumor, hydrocephalus, cerebellar dysplasia.

Prognosis: Progressive hydrocephalus, not observed in neonates but often progressive during the first one month. Cases diagnosed in utero or neonatal period; outcome is generally unfavorable. Nearly 40% die, and 75% of survivors exhibit cognitive deficits. The prognosis of Dandy-Walker variant is good. The clinical significance of megacisterna magna is uncertain.

Recurrence risk: Depends on etiology. Generally, 1–5% (Dandy-Walker malformation).

Management: Cyst-peritoneal shunt, cyst-ventriculoperitoneal shunt.

Arachnoid Cyst and Interhemispheric Cyst

Prevalence: 1% of intracranial masses in newborns.

Definition: Congenital or acquired cyst, lined by arachnoid membranes, and filled with fluid collection which is the same character as the cerebrospinal fluid. The number of cysts is mostly single, but two or more cysts can be occasionally observed. Location of

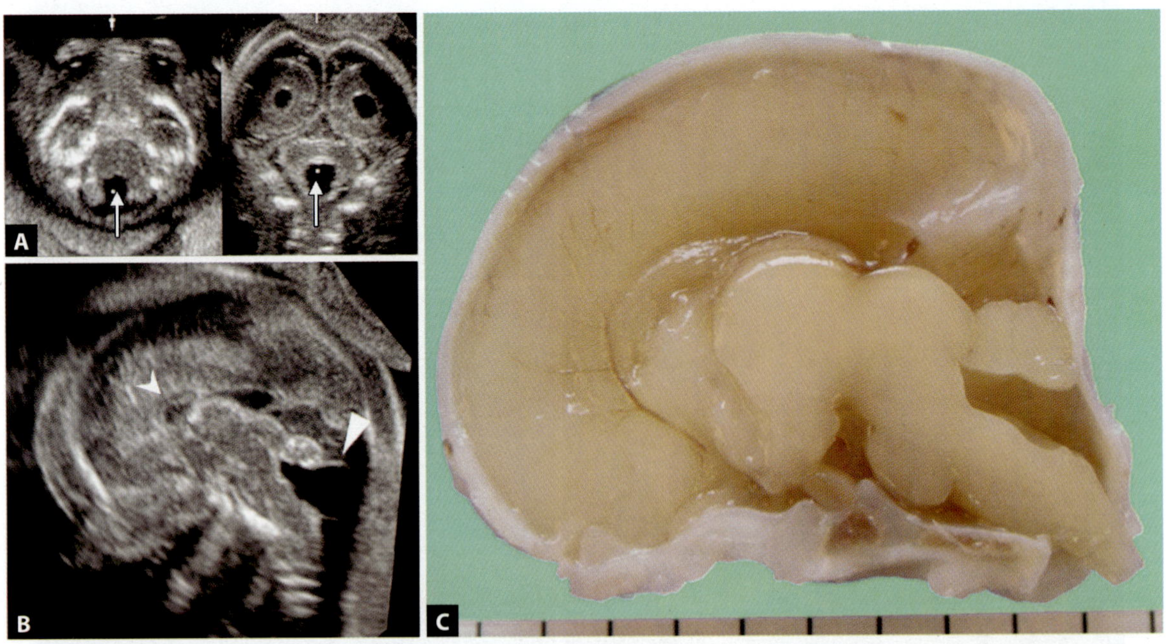

Figs. 69A to C: Dandy-Walker variant at 20 weeks of gestation. (A) Shows the 2D axial, 2D posterior coronal, 3D thick slices of oblique coronal and axial sections from the left. Hypoplasia of the vermis (arrows) is demonstrated and no marked ventriculomegaly was seen; (B) Shows the median section. Partial agenesis of the corpus callosum (arrowhead), floated cerebellum and cystic formation of the posterior fossa (triangle arrowhead) are seen; (C) Shows the median cutting section of the specimen of an aborted fetus at 21 weeks of gestation. This case had other complicated anomalies and the karyotype was partial trisomy of chromosome 10.

arachnoid cyst is various; approximately 50% of cysts occur from the Sylvian fissure (middle fossa), 20% from the posterior fossa, and 10–20% each from the convexity, suprasellar, interhemisphere, and quadrigeminal cistern. Interhemisperic cysts are often associated with agenesis or hypogenesis of the corpus callosum.

Etiology: Unknown

Pathogenesis: Congenital arachnoid cyst is formed by maldevelopment of the arachnoid membrane. CSF accumulation in the subarachnoid space or intra-arachnoid layers from a choroid plexus-like tissue within the cyst wall, leads to a progressive distension of the lesion.

Associated anomalies: Unilateral or bilateral hydrocephalus, macrocrania.

Prenatal diagnosis: Interhemispheric cyst is shown in **Figures 70A to D**, suprasellar arachnoid cyst is shown in **Figures 71A to F**. Intrauterine spontaneous resolution or changing cyst size are often detected. Detection in the first trimester was reported.[95]

Differential diagnosis: Porencephaly, schizencephaly, third ventriculomegaly, intracranial cystic type tumor, vein of Galen aneurysm, Dandy-Walker malformation, large cisterna magna, external hydrocephalus.

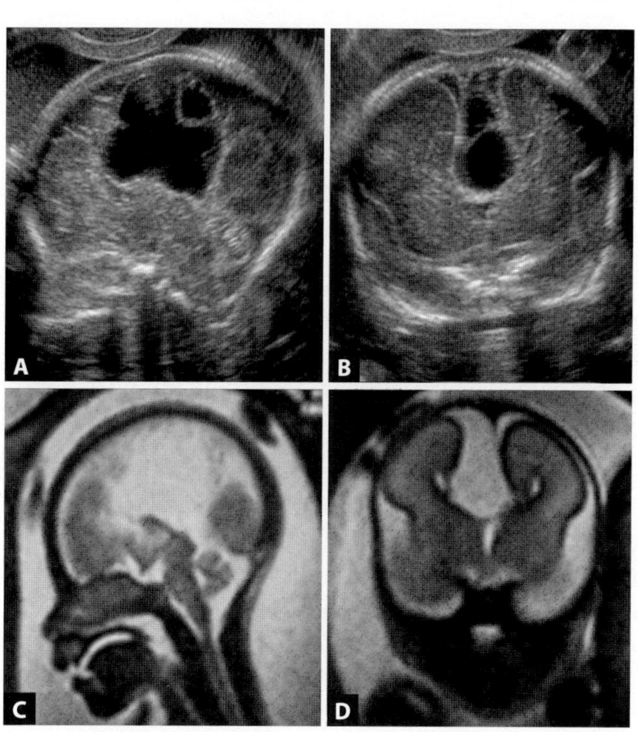

Figs. 70A to D: US and MR images of interhemispheric cyst at 24 weeks of gestation. (A) US median section; (B) US anterior coronal section; (C) MR median section; (D) MR anterior coronal section. Cystic lesion exists between hemispheres. Intracystic cysts are visible on US images.

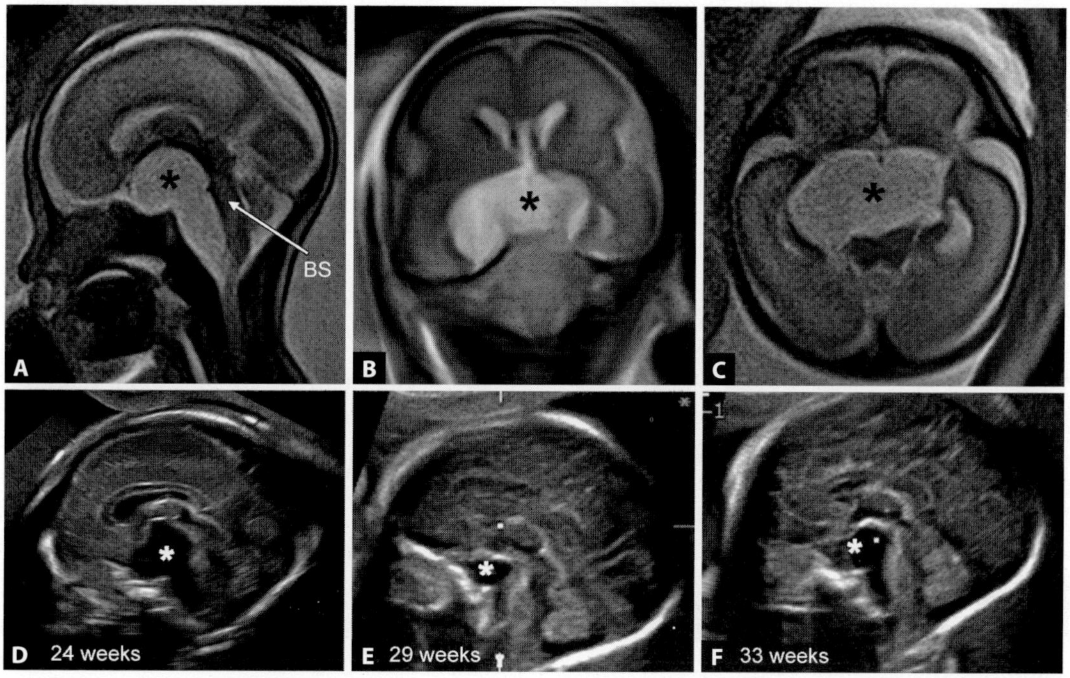

Figs. 71A to F: MR images and serial US scan images of suprasellar arachnoid cyst. (A to C) MRI at 24 weeks of gestation. Sagittal, coronal, and axial planes from the left. Suprasellar arachnoid cyst oppressing the brainstem (BS) and bilateral hemispheres; (D to F) Serial scan images of the midsagittal section. Spontaneous size decrease from 24 to 29 weeks and increase from 29 to 33 weeks are well demonstrated. Asterisks indicate the arachnoid cyst.

Prognosis: Generally good. Postnatally, many are asymptomatic and remain quiescent for years, although others expand and cause neurological symptoms by compressing adjacent brain, ventriculomegaly, and/or expanding the overlying skull.

Recurrence risk: Unknown

Obstetrical management: Arachnoid cysts may increase or decrease its size. Therefore, expectant management of antenatally diagnosed cases is suggested.[96] In cases with accompanied hydrocephalus, mode and timing of delivery may be modified.

Postnatal management: In cases with those symptoms or with prospects of neurological symptoms, treatment should be considered. Operation methods includes:

- Cyst fenestration by craniotomy
- Cyst fenestration by neuroendoscopy
- Cyst-peritoneal shunt.

Craniotomy, shunting or neuroendoscopic method has been still controversial.[97,98]

Craniosynostosis

Incidence: Unknown

Definition: Premature closure of cranial suture, which may affect one or more cranial sutures. Simple sagittal synostosis is most common. Various cranial shapes depend on affected suture(s) **(Table 6)**.

Etiology: Crouzon (AD, variable), Apert (AD, usually new mutation), Pfeiffer (AD), Antley-Bixler (AR). In five autosomal dominant craniosynostosis syndromes (Apert, Crouzon, Pfeiffer, Jackson-Weiss and Crouzon syndrome with acanthosis nigricans) result from mutations in *FGFR* genes.[99]

Pathogenesis:[100] (1) Cranial vault bones with decreased growth potential; (2) Asymmetrical bone deposition at perimeter sutures; (3) Sutures adjacent to the prematurely fused suture compensate in growth more than those sutures not contiguous with the closed suture; (4) Enhanced symmetrical bone deposition occurs along both sides of a non-perimeter suture continuing prematurely closed suture.

Associated anomalies: Hypertelorism, syndactyly, polydactyly, exophthalmos.

Prenatal diagnosis: Facial abnormality and intracranial structure with abnormal shape of ventricles in a case of Pfeiffer syndrome are demonstrated in **Figure 22**.

TABLE 6: Affected sutures, cranial shape, and craniosynostosis syndromes.

Sagittal suture	Scaphocephaly or dolichocephaly
Bilateral coronal suture	Brachycephaly
Unilateral coronal suture	Anterior plagiocephaly
Metopic suture	Trigonocephaly
Lambdoid suture	Acrocephaly
Unilateral lambdoid suture	Posterior plagiocephaly
Coronal/lambdoid/ metopic or squamous/ sagittal suture	Cloverleaf skull
Total cranial sutures	Oxycephaly
Syndromes:	
Crouzon syndrome	• Acrocephaly, synostosis of coronal, sagittal, and lambdoid sutures • With ocular proptosis, maxillary hypoplasia
Apert syndrome	• Brachycephaly, irregular synostosis, especially coronal suture • With midfacial hypoplasia, syndactyly, broad distal phalanx of thumb and big toe
Pfeiffer syndrome	• Brachycephaly, synostosis of coronal and/or sagittal sutures • With hypertelorism, broad thumbs and toes, partial syndactyly
Antley-Bixler syndrome	• Brachycephaly, multiple synostosis, especially of coronal suture • With maxillary hypoplasia, radiohumeral synostosis, choanal atresia, arthrogryposis

Abnormal craniofacial appearance can be detected by 2D/3D ultrasound.[101,102]

Prognosis: Various. In some of trigonocephaly and syndromic types, prognosis is poor.

Recurrence risk: Depends on etiology.

Management: Operative aim of cranioplasty is improvement of intracranial pressure and cosmetic change.

Vein of Galen Aneurysm

Incidence: Rare.

Definition: Direct arteriovenous fistulas between choroidal and/or quadrigeminal arteries and an overlying single median venous sac.

Synonyms: Vein of Galen malformation

Etiology: Unknown.

Pathogenesis: Venous sac most probably represents persistence of the embryonic median prosencephalic vein of Markowski, not the vein of Galen, per se.[103]

Associated anomalies: Cardiomegaly, high cardiac output, secondary hydrocephalus, macrocrania, cerebral ischemia (intracranial steal phenomenon), subarachnoid/cerebral/intraventricular hemorrhages.

Prenatal diagnosis: 2D and 3D color/power Doppler and 3D B-flow detection of VGAM and brain damage caused by cerebral ischemia or hemorrhage with mild ventriculomegaly are shown in **Figure 24**.

Differential diagnosis: Arachnoid cyst, porencephalic cyst, intracranial teratoma. Color/power Doppler is helpful for differential diagnosis.

Prognosis: According to earlier review, outcome did not differ between treated and nontreated group and over 80% of cases died.[104] However, recent advances in treatment have improved outcome, such that 60–100% survive and over 60% have a good neurological outcome.[105,106]

Recurrence risk: Unknown

Management: Evaluation of the fetal high-output cardiac state for the proper obstetrical management. Percutaneous embolization by microcoils is a recent main postnatal treatment and remarkably improved outcome.

Choroid Plexus Cysts

Incidence: 0.61–2.89% of all fetuses scanned.[107-113]

Definition: Cysts with fluid collection within the choroids plexus, which may exist unilaterally or bilaterally. They are depicted in the second trimester and usually resolve by the 24th week.

Etiology: Normal variant.

Pathogenesis: Choroid plexus is located within the ventricular system and produces cerebrospinal fluid. Within the choroidal villi, choroid plexus cysts exist, surrounded by the loose stroma of the choroid plexus.[110] Choroid plexus cysts probably result from entrapment of cerebrospinal fluid within tangled villi of the fetal ventricular system.[114]

Associated anomalies: In cases of trisomy 18, associated anomalies include growth retardation, congenital heart diseases such as ventricular septum defect and double outlet right ventricle, overlapping finger, facial anomaly, cerebellar dysplasia and others.

Prenatal diagnosis: It is impossible to distinguish normal from abnormal karyotypes only by location and appearance of choroid plexus cyst. Detection of additional anomalies is important for differential diagnosis.

Differential diagnosis: Intraventricular hemorrhage

Prognosis: Choroid plexus cysts, per se, are usually asymptomatic and benign, but rarely, symptomatic and disturbs CSF flow.[115,116] Isolated choroids plexus cysts may be normal variation.

Recurrence risk: Unknown

Management: An isolated choroid plexus cyst is an indication to perform a detailed and accurate examination of other markers of aneuploid. If the choroid plexus cyst is an isolated finding, there is no reason to perform amniocentesis.[111]

ACQUIRED BRAIN ABNORMALITIES IN UTERO

In terms of encephalopathy or cerebral palsy, *'timing of brain insult, antepartum, intrapartum or postpartum?'* is one of the serious controversial issues including medico-socio-legal-ethical problems.[51] Although brain insults may relate to antepartum events in a substantial number of term infants with hypoxic-ischemic encephalopathy, the timing of insult cannot always be clarified. It is a hard task to give antepartum evidences of brain injury predictive of cerebral palsy. Fetal heart rate monitoring cannot reveal the presence of encephalopathy, and neuroimaging by ultrasound and MR imaging is the most reliable modality for disclosure of silent encephalopathy. In many cases with cerebral palsy with acquired brain insults, especially, term-delivered infants with reactive fetal heart rate tracing and good Apgar score at delivery, are not suspected having encephalopathy and often overlooked for months or years. Recent imaging technology has revealed brain insult in utero.

Brain Tumors

Incidence: Extremely rare.

Definition: Tumors located in the intracranial cavity.

Histological types: Brain tumors are divided into teratoma, most commonly reported and nonteratomatous tumor. Nonteratomatous tumors includes neuroepithelial tumor, such as medulloblastoma, astrocytoma, choroids plexus papilloma, choroids plexus carcinoma, ependymoma, ependymoblastoma, and mesenchymal tumor such as craniopharyngioma, sarcoma, fibroma, hemangioblastoma, hemangioma and meningioma, and others of lipoma of the corpus callosum, subependymal giant-cell astrocytoma associated with tuberous sclerosis (often accompanied by cardiac rhabdomyoma).[117,118]

Location of tumor: Supratentorial predominance in neonatal tumor. Infratentorial predominance in medulloblastoma. Choroid plexus papilloma is located within the lateral ventricles.

Associated abnormalities: Macrocrania or local skull swelling, epignathus, secondary hydrocephalus, intracranial hemorrhage, intraventricular hemorrhage, polyhydramnios, heart failure by high-cardiac output[119] and/or hydrops.

Diagnosis: Intracranial masses with solid, cystic or mixture pattern with or without visualization of hypervascularity by ultrasound and fetal MRI. Brain tumors should be considered in cases with unexplained intracranial hemorrhage.

Prenatal diagnosis: Prenatal diagnosis of intracranial tumor and its vascularization by 3D power Doppler is shown in **Figures 72A to E**, glioma at 18 weeks in **Figures 73A to D**.

Differential diagnosis: Arachnoid cyst, vein of Galen aneurysm, porencephaly, schizencephaly, periventricular leukomalacia, subdural hemorrhage.

Prognosis: Fetal demise, stillborn may occur. Prognosis in neonates is generally poor but depends on timing of diagnosis and the histological type of tumor. Choroid plexus papilloma has a minimal mortality rate and high likelihood of neonatal outcome. The mortality rate of teratomas is over 90%, medulloblastoma over 80%. Other tumors have various prognosis.

Recurrence risk: Unknown

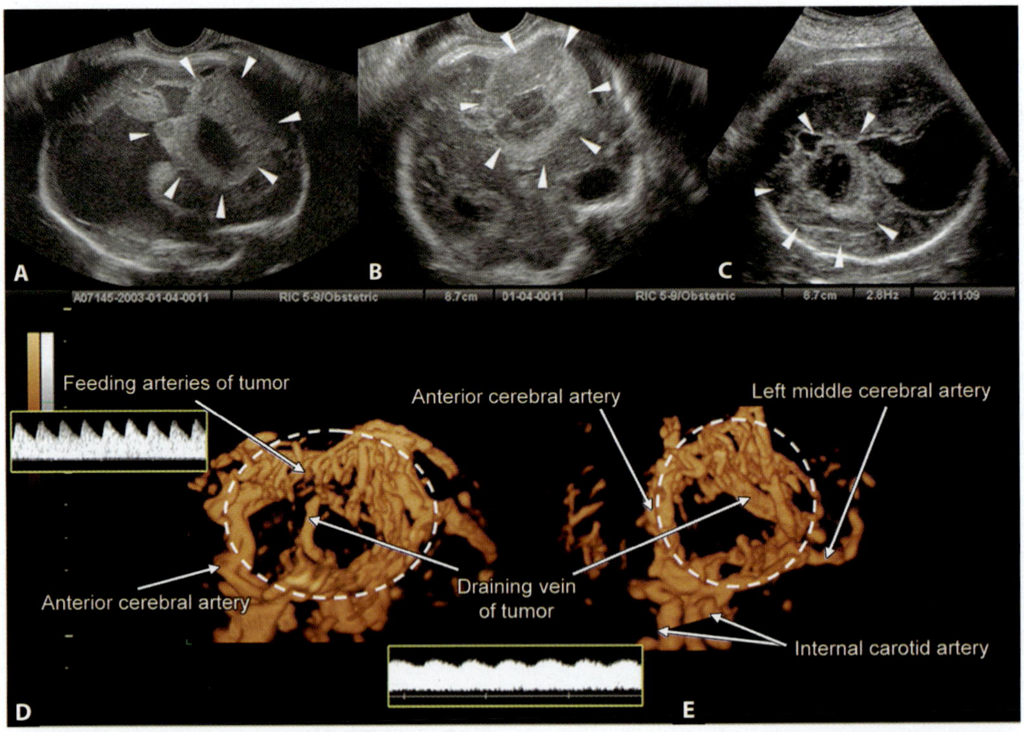

Figs. 72A to E: Ultrasound images and tumoral vascular visualization by 3D power Doppler in a fetus of intracranial tumor with interventricular hemorrhage (35 weeks and 5 days of gestation). (A to C) Sagittal, coronal, and axial US images. Huge tumor (arrowheads) with hemorrhage within the tumor in the frontoparietal lobe complicated with unilateral hydrocephalus with intraventricular hemorrhage (arrow); (D) Oblique sagittal view from fetal left side; (E) Oblique coronal view from fetal frontal side. Tumor is fed by numerous feeding arteries from anterior cerebral artery. Feeder arteries have low resistant flow waveform. One large vein which drains blood from tumor is visible. The draining vein has pulsatile flow.

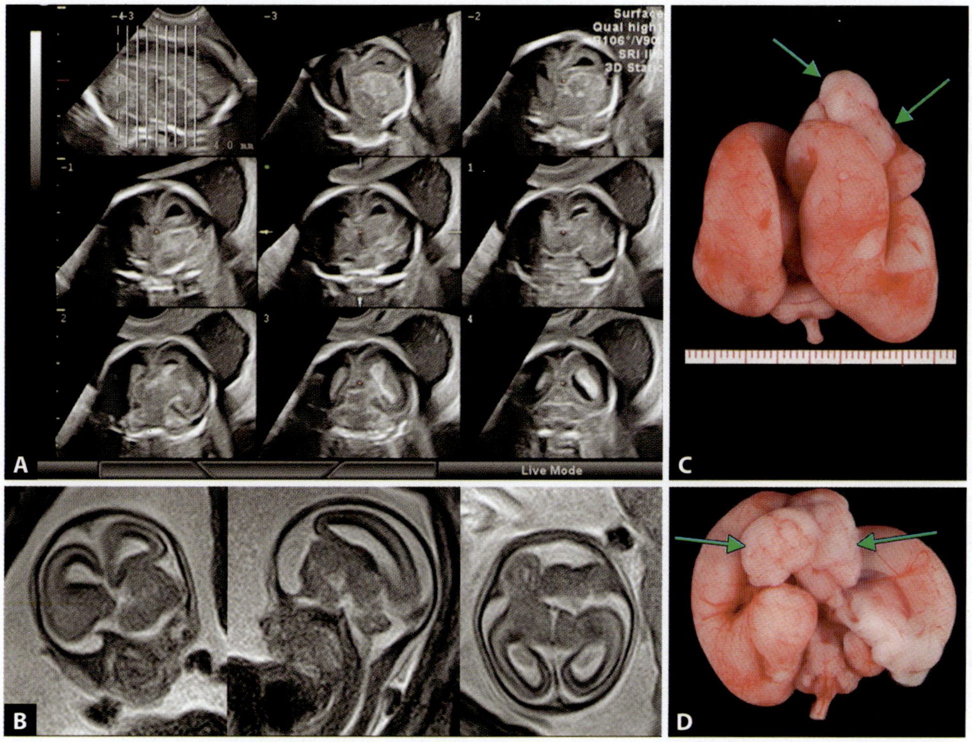

Figs. 73A to D: Brain tumor at 18 weeks of gestation. (A) Tomographic coronal image of the brain. Unilateral hemisphere is oppressed by echogenic mass; (B) MR images. Coronal, sagittal, and axial planes from the left; (C) Brain specimen from the parietal direction. The tumor is indicated by green arrows; (D) View from the bottom. The tumor was easily detachable from the brain.

Management: Cesarean section may be considered. Neurosurgical tumor resection including subtotal hemispherectomy by craniotomy and chemotherapy are possible treatments for neonatal tumors. Radiation therapy is usually not indicated in neonates.

Subependymal Pseudocysts

Prevalence: 2.6–5% of all neonates, 1% of premature newborns, unknown in fetuses.

Definition: Cystic formation, which is located in the caudothalamic groove or in the caudate nucleus, lateral to the wall of the anterior horns of lateral ventricles.

Synonyms: Periventricular pseudocysts.[120,121]

Etiology: Infection (cytomegalovirus, rubella), subependymal hemorrhage, metabolic diseases, chromosomal deletions (del q6, del p4) cocaine exposure and others.

Pathogenesis: Cystic cavity is lined by a pseudocapsule, consisting of aggregates of germinal cells and glial tissue, but no epithelium can be found. Origin of pseudocysts is uncertain. May be cystic matrix regression or germinolysis.

Associated anomalies: Congenital infection such as cytomegalovirus, congenital heart diseases, associated CNS abnormalities.

Prenatal diagnosis: Often detectable by transvaginal sonography in the sagittal and anterior-coronal sections.

Differential diagnosis: Periventricular leukomalacia.

Prognosis: Good in cases with isolated subependymal pseudocysts. In cases with accompanied abnormalities, such as cardiac disease, cytomegalovirus infection, other intracranial abnormalities, or cases with atypical pseudocysts, prognosis may be poor.[120-122]

Recurrence risk: Unknown.

Management: In many cases, cysts regress in several months after birth. Normal obstetrical/neonatal care.

Porencephaly

Incidence: Unknown.

Definition: Fluid-filled spaces replacing normal brain parenchyma and may or may not communicate with the lateral ventricles or subarachnoid space.

Synonyms: Porencephalic cyst.

Etiology: Ischemic episode, trauma[123] demise of one twin, intercerebral hemorrhage, infection.

Pathogenesis:[124] Easy to occur when immature cerebrum has some factors with propensity of dissolution and cavitation (high content of water, myelinated fiber bundles, deficient astroglial response). The timing of ischemic injury (may be as early as second trimester) is strongly related to porencephaly, hydranencephaly.

Associated anomalies: Intercerebral hemorrhage, interventricular hemorrhage, hydrocephalus.

Prenatal diagnosis: **Figures 74A to F** show porencephaly after intracerebral hemorrhage at 25 weeks. Some cases in utero have been reported.[125,126]

Differential diagnosis: Schizencephaly, arachnoid cyst, intracranial cystic tumor, other cysts. Porencephalic cyst never causes a mass effect, which is observed in cases with arachnoid cyst or other cystic mass lesions. This condition is acquired brain insult and differentiated from schizencephaly of migration disorder.

Prognosis: Various, depends on timing and size of lesion. Seizures, neurological deficits, cerebral palsy often occur.[127]

Recurrence risk: Unknown.

Management: Ventriculoperitoneal shunt if hydrocephalus progresses.

Hydranencephaly

Incidence: 1–2.5:10,000 births.

Definition: Absence of the cerebral hemispheres and a sac-like structure containing cerebral spinal fluid surrounding the brainstem and basal ganglia.

Etiology: Ischemic episode, trauma, demise of one twin, intercerebral hemorrhage, infection. There are several theories but bilateral occlusion of the supraclinoid segment of the internal carotid arteries[128] or of the middle cerebral arteries is one of the cause of subtotal defects of cerebral hemisphere.

Pathogenesis: Easy to occur when immature cerebrum has some factors with propensity of dissolution and cavitation (high content of water, myelinated fiber bundles, deficient astroglial response). The timing of ischemic injury (may be as early as second trimester) is strongly related to porencephaly and hydranencephaly.

Prenatal diagnosis: Recently hydranencephaly from 11 weeks of gestation has been reported.[129]

Differential diagnosis: Massive hydrocephalus, alobar holoprosencephaly, porencephaly.

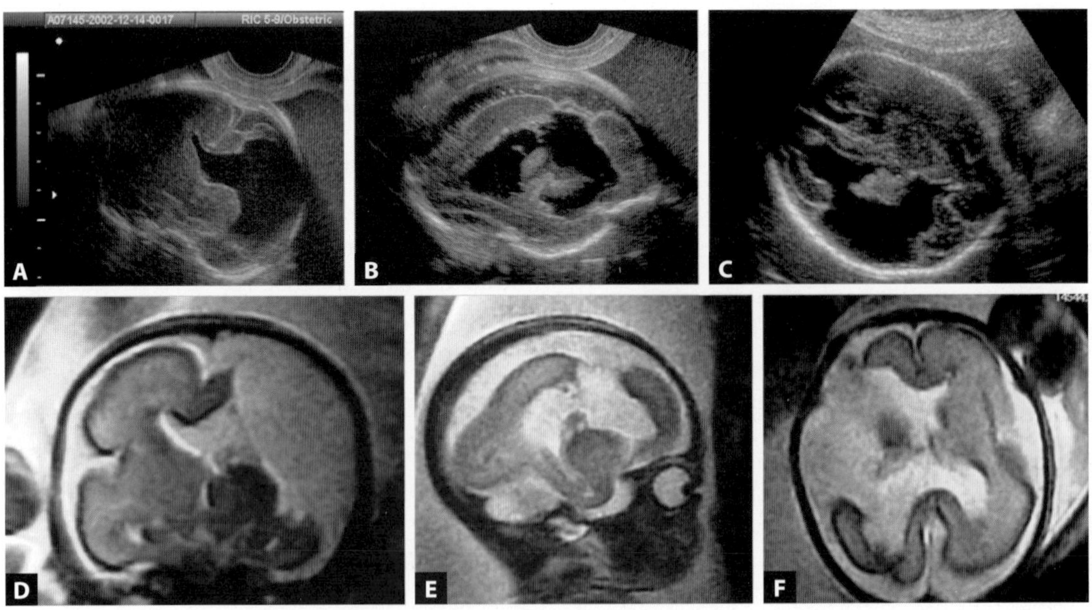

Figs. 74A to F: Fetal US and MR images of porencephaly at 25 weeks of gestation. (A) Transvaginal US coronal image. Defect of parietolateral part of the unilateral cerebrum. This case has also absent septum pellucidum; (B) Parasagittal US image. Porencephalic part is fused with the unilateral ventricle. Echogenicity of inside ventricular wall indicates intraventricular hemorrhage; (C) Transabdominal US axial image; (D to F) Fetal MR images at the same day. Coronal, parasagittal, and axial sections from the left side.

Prognosis: Extremely poor

Recurrence risk: Unknown

Management: No active treatment. Shunt procedure for progressive increase of infant's head.

Intracranial Hemorrhage

Incidence: Unknown, rare in utero.

Definition: Hemorrhage, bleeding inside of the cranium. Intracranial hemorrhage includes subdural hemorrhage, primary subarachnoid hemorrhage, intracerebellar hemorrhage, intraventricular hemorrhage and intraparenchymal hemorrhage other than cerebellar hemorrhage.[130]

Etiology: Trauma, alloimmune and idiopathic thrombocytopenia, von Willebrand's disease, specific medications (warfarin) or illicit drug (cocaine) abuse, seizure, fetal conditions including congenital factor-X and factor-V deficiencies, intracranial tumor, twin-twin transfusion, demise of a co-twin, vascular diseases, or fetomaternal hemorrhage, extracorporeal membrane oxygenation (ECMO).[131] Recent reports have described intracranial hemorrhage associated with *COL4A1* gene mutation.[132-136]

Associated anomalies: Hydrocephalus, hydranencephaly, porencephaly, or microcephaly.

Prenatal diagnosis: **Figures 75A to D** show multiple intracerebral hemorrhage at 35 weeks.

Differential diagnosis: Intracranial tumor.

Prognosis: Poor in premature infants. Apnea, seizures, and other neurological symptoms.

Recurrence risk: Depends on etiology.

Management: Ventriculoperitoneal shunt if hydrocephalus progresses.

Fetal Periventricular Leukomalacia

Incidence: 25–75% of premature infants at autopsy are complicated with periventricular white matter injury. However, clinically, incidence may be much lower. 5 to 10% of infants less than 1500 g birth weight. In at term infants, periventricular leukomalacia (PVL) is very rare.

Definition: Multifocal areas of necrosis found deep in the cortical white matter, which are often symmetrical and occur adjacent to the lateral ventricles. Periventricular leukomalacia represents a major precursor for neurological and intellectual impairment, and cerebral palsy in later life.

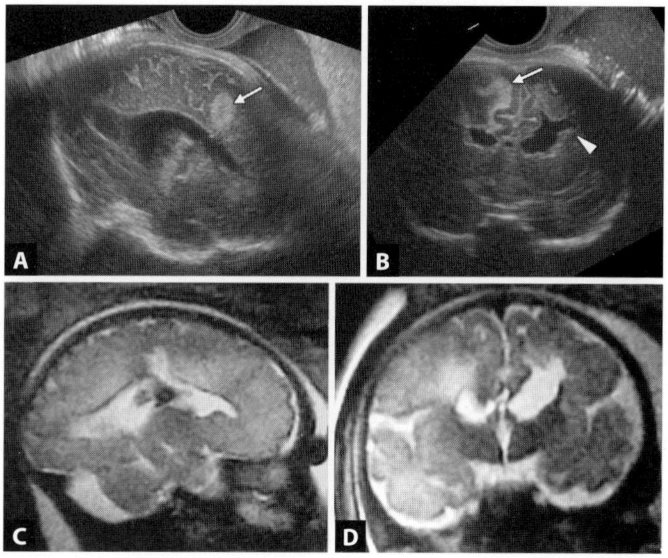

Figs. 75A to D: US and MR images in a fetus with cerebral hemorrhage and mild ventriculomegaly at 35 weeks of gestation. Ultrasound parasagittal (A) and anterior coronal (B) images of the brain. Arrows indicate intracerebral hemorrhage. Arrowhead shows a porencephalic part fused with the lateral ventricle; (C and D) MR images showing the same cutting sections as upper US images.

Etiology: Birth trauma, asphyxia and respiratory failure, cardiopulmonary defects, premature birth/low birth weight, associated immature cerebrovascular development and lack of appropriate autoregulation of cerebral blood flow in response to hypoxic-ischemic insults.[137]

Pathogenesis: Distinctive and consist primarily of both focal periventricular necrosis and more diffuse cerebral white matter injury. The two most common sites are at the level of the cerebral white matter near the trigone of the lateral ventricles and around the foramen of Monro. Volpe[124] describes three factors, such as: (1) periventricular vascular anatomical and physiological factors, (2) cerebral ischemia, (3) intrinsic vulnerability of cerebral white matter of premature newborn, are strongly related to PVL.

Differential diagnosis: Subarachnoid (periventricular) pseudocysts, porencephaly, other intracranial cystic formation.

Prognosis: Neurological features of PVL in neonatal period is probable lower limb weakness and as features of long-term sequelae, spastic diplegia, Intellectual deficits and visual deficits are observed.[124]

Recurrence risk: Unknown.

Management: Early rehabilitation.

Microcephaly

Incidence: Unknown

Definition: A head circumference that is more than two standard deviations below the normal mean for age, sex, race, and gestation (Some authorities define microcephaly as more than three standard deviations below the mean).

Etiology: Infections such as rubella, cytomegalovirus (CMV), varicella (chickenpox) virus and toxoplasmosis, radiation, medications, chromosomal abnormalities, and genetic diseases. It is part of many chromosomal abnormalities and other syndromes including:

- Chromosomal abnormalities—trisomy 18 (Edwards syndome), trisomy 13 (Patau syndrome), the Wolf-Hirschhorn syndrome, the cat cry syndrome, and partial deletion of long arm of chromosome 13.
- Contiguous gene syndromes—Miller-Dieker syndrome, Langer-Giedion syndrome, Prader-Willi syndrome, and the aniridia—Wilms, tumor syndrome.
- Genetic disorders—Johanson-Blizzard syndrome, Seckel syndrome, and the Smith-Lemli-Opitz syndrome.
- Environmental insults—maternal PKU (mothers who have poorly controlled PKU during pregnancy) and the fetal alcohol syndrome.

Pathogenesis: May be caused by a disturbance in the proliferation of nerve cells. Abnormalities of neurocranial architecture occur in approximately two-thirds of cases.[138]

Differential diagnosis: Craniosynostosis.

Prenatal diagnosis: Ultrasonograms and MR images of typical microcephaly are shown in **Figures 76A to F**. Occasionally, microcephaly occur with late onset during pregnancy.[139]

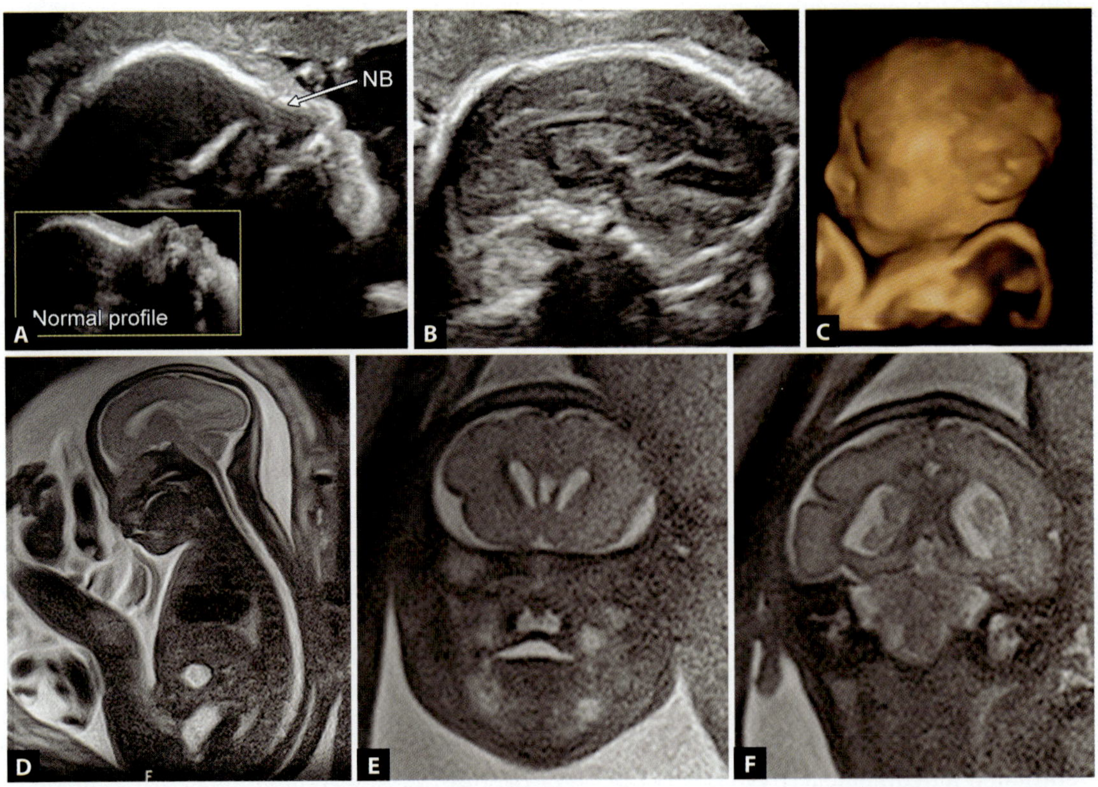

Figs. 76A to F: Microcephaly at 28 weeks of gestation. (A) Fetal face in the sagittal section. Note the flat face with the frontal bone and nasal bone (NB) on a single line, comparing to the normal face in the yellow box; (B) Sagittal section of the brain. Microcephaly and micro-brain are detectable; (C) 3D reconstruction image of fetal craniofacial expression; (D to F) MR image in the sagittal, anteror-coronal, and posterocoronal sections from the left.

Prognosis: Development of motor functions and speech may be delayed. Hyperactivity and mental retardation are common occurrences, although the degree of each varies. Convulsions may also occur. Motor ability varies, ranging from clumsiness in some to spastic quadriplegia in others.

Recurrence risk: Unknown.

Treatment: No specific treatment for microcephaly. Treatment is symptomatic and supportive.

FUTURE ASPECTS

Prenatal ultrasound has established neuro-sonoembryology and neurosonology. By using 3D/4D ultrasound, HDlive and HDlive silhouette imaging, more and more information in fetal neurology can be obtained from mysterious intrauterine world.

Those up-to-date 3D technologies allow extending the detection of congenital anomalies to an earlier gestational age, and it is beyond description that non-invasive direct viewing of the embryo/fetus by all-inclusive ultrasound technology is definitely the first modality in a field of prenatal diagnosis and help our goal of proper perinatal care and management, even in the era of molecular genetics and advanced sequencing of fetal DNA in the maternal blood.[38,41]

REFERENCES

1. Timor-Tritsch IE, Peisner, DB, Raju S. Sonoembryology: an organ-oriented approach using a high-frequency vaginal probe. J Clin Ultrasound. 1990;18:286-98.
2. Pooh RK. B-mode and Doppler studies of the abnormal fetus in the first trimester. In: Chervenak FA, Kurjak A (Eds). Fetal Medicine. Parthenon Publishing, Carnforth; 1999. pp.46-51.
3. Timor-Tritsch IE, Monteagudo A. Transvaginal fetal neurosonography: standardization of the planes and sections by anatomic landmarks. Ultrasound Obstet Gynecol. 1996;8:42-7.
4. Monteagudo A, Reuss ML, Timor-Tritsch IE. Imaging the fetal brain in the second and third trimesters using transvaginal sonography. Obstet Gynecol. 1991;77:27-32.
5. Monteagudo A, Timor-Tritsch IE, Moomjy M. In utero detection of ventriculomegaly during the second and third trimesters by transvaginal sonography. Ultrasound Obstet Gynecol. 1994;4:193-8.
6. Monteagudo A, Timor-Tritsch IE. Development of fetal gyri, sulci and fissures: a transvaginal sonographic study. Ultrasound Obstet Gynecol. 1997;9:222-8.
7. Pooh RK, Nakagawa Y, Nagamachi N, Pooh KH, Nakagawa Y, Maeda K, et al. Transvaginal sonography of the fetal brain: detection of abnormal morphology and circulation. Croat Med J. 1998;39:147-57.
8. Pooh RK, Maeda K, Pooh KH, Kurjak A. Sonographic assessment of the fetal brain morphology. Prenat Neonat Med. 1999;4:18-38.
9. Pooh RK. Three-dimensional ultrasound of the fetal brain. In: Kurjak A (Ed). Clinical application of 3D ultrasonography. Parthenon Publishing, Carnforth; 2000. pp.176-80.
10. Pooh RK, Pooh KH, Nakagawa Y, Nishida S, Ohno Y. Clinical application of Three-dimensional ultrasound in fetal brain assessment. Croat Med J. 2000;41:245-51.
11. Timor-Tritsch IE, Monteagudo A, Mayberry P. Three-dimensional ultrasound evaluation of the fetal brain: the three horn view. Ultrasound Obstet Gynecol. 2000;16:302-6.
12. Monteagudo A, Timor-Tritsch IE, Mayberry P. Three-dimensional transvaginal neurosonography of the fetal brain: 'navigating' in the volume scan. Ultrasound Obstet Gynecol. 2000;16:307-13.
13. Pooh RK, Nagao Y, Pooh KH. Fetal neuroimaging by transvaginal 3D ultrasound and MRI. Ultrasound Rev Obstet Gynecol. 2006;6:123-34.
14. Pooh RK, Pooh KH. Fetal neuroimaging with new technology. Ultrasound Review Obstet Gynecol. 2002; 2:178-81.
15. Blaas HG, Eik-Nes SH, Kiserud T, Berg S, Angelsen B, Olstad B. Three-dimensional imaging of the brain cavities in human embryos. Ultrasound Obstet Gynecol. 1995;5:228-32.
16. Blaas HG, Eik-Nes SH, Berg S, Torp H. In-vivo three-dimensional ultrasound reconstructions of embryos and early fetuses. Lancet. 1998;352:1182-6.
17. Pooh RK. Fetal brain assessment by three-dimensional ultrasound. In: Kurjak A, Kupesic S (Eds). Clinical Application of 3D Sonography. Carnforth, UK: Parthenon Publishing; 2000. pp.171-9.
18. Pooh RK, Pooh KH. Transvaginal 3D and Doppler ultrasonography of the fetal brain. Semin Perinatol. 2001;25:38-43.
19. Pooh RK, Pooh KH. The assessment of fetal brain morphology and circulation by transvaginal 3D sonography and power Doppler. J Perinat Med. 2002;30:48-56.
20. Endres LK, Cohen L. Reliability and validity of three-dimensional fetal brain volumes. J Ultrasound Med. 2001;20:1265-9.
21. Roelfsema NM, Hop WC, Boito SM, Wladimiroff JW. Three-dimensional sonographic measurement of normal fetal brain volume during the second half of pregnancy. Am J Obstet Gynecol. 2004;190(1):275-80.
22. Benacerraf BR. Inversion mode display of 3D sonography: applications in obstetric and gynecologic imaging. Am J Roentgenol. 2006;187(4):965-71.
23. Kusanovic JP, Nien JK, Gonçalves LF, Espinoza J, Lee W, Balasubramaniam M, et al. The use of inversion mode and 3D manual segmentation in volume measurement of fetal fluid-filled structures: comparison with virtual organ

computer-aided anaLysis (VOCAL). Ultrasound Obstet Gynecol. 2008;31(2):177-86.
24. Hata T, Dai SY, Kanenishi K, Tanaka H. Three-dimensional volume-rendered imaging of embryonic brain vesicles using inversion mode. J Obstet Gynaecol Res. 2009;35(2):258-61.
25. Pooh RK, Aono T. Transvaginal power Doppler angiography of the fetal brain. Ultrasound Obstet Gynecol. 1996;8:417-21.
26. Pooh RK. Two-dimensional and three-dimensional Doppler angiography in fetal brain circulation. In: Kurjak A (Ed). 3D Power Doppler in Obstetrics and Gynecology. Parthenon Publishing, Carnforth; 1999. pp.105-111.
27. Moore KL, Persaud TVN. The developing human: clinically-oriented embryology, 7th edition. Saunders, Pensylvania; 2003.
28. Pooh RK, Kurjak A. Novel application of three-dimensional HD-live imaging in prenatal diagnosis from the first trimester. Journal of Perinatal Medicine. 2015:43(2);147-58.
29. Nebeker J, Nelson R. Imaging of sound speed reflection ultrasound tomography. JUM. 2012;31(9):1389-404.
30. Bonilla-Musoles F, Raga F, Castillo JC, Bonilla F Jr, Climent MT, Caballero O. High definition real-time ultrasound (HDlive) of embryonic and fetal malformations before week 16. DSJUOG. 2013;7(1):1-8.
31. Kagan KO, Pintoffl K, Hoopmann M. First-trimester ultrasound images using HDlive. Ultrasound Obstet Gynecol. 2011;38(5):607.
32. Hata T, Hanaoka U, Tenkumo C, Sato M, Tanaka H, Ishimura M. Three- and four-dimensional HDlive rendering images of normal and abnormal fetuses: pictorial essay. Arch Gynecol Obstet. 2012;286(6):1431-5.
33. Pooh RK. First Trimester Scan by 3D, 3D HDlive and HDlive Silhouette/Flow Ultrasound Imaging. Donald School Journal of Ultrasound in Obstetrics and Gynecology. October-December 2015;9(4):361-71.
34. Pooh RK. 'See-through Fashion' in Prenatal Diagnostic Imaging. Donald School J Ultrasound Obstet Gynecol. 2015;9(2):111.
35. Pooh RK. Brand new technology of HDlive silhouette and HDlive flow images. In: Pooh RK and Kurjak A (Eds). Donald School Atlas of Advanced Ultrasound in Obstetrics and Gynecology. New Delhi Jaypee Brothers Medical Publishers (P) Ltd, New Delhi. 2015. p. 1-39.
36. Pooh RK. A New Field of 'Fetal Sono-ophthalmology by 3D HDlive Silhouette and Flow. Donald School Journal of Ultrasound in Obstetrics and Gynecology. July-September 2015;9(3):221-2.
37. Pooh RK. 13-week Pulmonary Sonoangiogram by 3D HDlive Flow. Donald School Journal of Ultrasound in Obstetrics and Gynecology. 2015;9(4):355-6.
38. Pooh RK. Sonoembryology by 3D HDlive silhouette ultrasound. What is added by the 'see-through fashion'? J Perinat Med, in press; 2016.
39. AboEllail MAM, Kanenishi K, Mori N, Kurobe A, Hata T. HDlive imaging of circumvallate placenta. Ultrasound Obstet Gynecol. 2015;46:513-4.
40. Pooh RK. Three-dimensional HDlive Thick-Slice Silhouette of Fetal Brain. Donald School Journal of Ultrasound in Obstetrics and Gynecology. January-March. 2016.
41. Pooh RK. Recent advances of 3D ultrasound, silhouette ultrasound and sonoangiogram in fetal neurology. Donald School Journal of Ultrasound in Obstetrics and Gynecology. 2016.
42. Malinger G, Lev D, Lerman-Sagie T. Is fetal magnetic resonance imaging superior to neurosonography for detection of brain anomalies? Ultrasound Obstet Gynecol. 2002; 20:317-21.
43. Girard N, Chaumoitre K, Confort-Gouny S, Viola A, Levrier O. Magnetic resonance imaging and the detection of fetal brain anomalies, injury, and physiologic adaptations. Curr Opin Obstet Gynecol. 2006;18:164-76.
44. Levine D, Barnes PD, Madsen JR, Abbott J, Metha T, Edelman RR. Central nervous system abnormalities assessed with prenatal magnetic resonance imaging. Obstet Gynecol. 1999;94:1011-9.
45. Simon EM, Goldstein RB, Coakley FV, Filly RA, Broderick KC, Musci TJ, et al. Fast MR imaging of fetal CNS anomalies in utero. Am J Neuroradiol. 2000;21:1688-98.
46. Sonigo PC, Rypens FF, Carteret M, Delezoide AL, Brunelle FO. MR imaging of fetal cerebral anomalies. Pediatr Radiol. 1998;28:212-22.
47. Wagenvoort AM, Bekker MN, Go ATJI, Vandenbussche FPHA, Van Buchem MA, Valk J, et al. Ultrafast scan magnetic resonance in prenatal diagnosis. Fetal Diagn Ther. 2000;15:364-72.
48. Kubik-Huch RA, Huisman TAGM, Wisser J, Gottstein-Aalame N, Debatin JF, Seifert B, et al. Ultrafast MR imaging of the fetus. AJR. 2000;174:1599-606.
49. Malinger G, Ben-Sira L, Lev D, Ben-Aroya Z, Kidron D, Lerman-Sagie T. Fetal brain imaging: a comparison between magnetic resonance imaging and dedicated neurosonography. Ultrasound Obstet Gynecol. 2004;23:333-40.
50. Pooh RK, Kurjak A. 3D and 4D sonography and magnetic resonance in the assessment of normal and abnormal CNS development: alternative or complementary. J Perinat Med. 2010 Oct 27. [Epub ahead of print]
51. Pooh RK, Maeda K, Pooh KH. An atlas of fetal central nervous system disease: diagnosis and management. Parthenon CRC Press, London, New York; 2003.
52. Alagappan R, Browning PD, Laorr A, McGahan JP. Distal lateral ventricular atrium: reevaluation of normal range. Radiology. 1994;193:405-8.
53. Almog B, Gamzu R, Achiron R, et al. Fetal lateral ventricular width: what should be its upper limit? A prospective cohort study and reanalysis of the current and previous data. J Ultrasound Med. 2003;22:39-43.
54. Signorelli M, Tiberti A, Valseriati D, Molin E, Cerri V, Groli C, et al. Width of the fetal lateral ventricular atrium between 10 and 12 mm: a simple variation of the norm? Ultrasound Obstet Gynecol. 2004;23:14-8.

55. Pooh RK, Pooh KH, Nakagawa Y, Maeda K, Fukui R, Aono T. Transvaginal Doppler assessment of fetal intracranial venous flow. Obstet Gynecol. 1999;93:697-701.
56. Kelly EN, Allen VM, Seaward G, Windrim R, Ryan G. Mild ventriculomegaly in the fetus, natural history, associated findings and outcome of isolated mild ventriculomegaly: a literature review. Prenat Diagn. 2001;21:697-700.
57. Goldstein I, Copel JA, Makhoul IR. Mild cerebral ventriculomegaly in fetuses: characteristics and outcome. Fetal Diagn Ther. 2005;20:281-4.
58. Pilu G, Falco P, Gabrielli S, Perolo A, Sandri F, Bovicelli L. The clinical significance of fetal isolated cerebral borderline ventriculomegaly: report of 31 cases and review of the literature. Ultrasound Obstet Gynecol. 1999;14:320-6.
59. Ouahba J, Luton D, Vuillard E, Garel C, Gressens P, Blanc N, et al. Prenatal isolated mild ventriculomegaly: outcome in 167 cases. BJOG. 2006;113:1072-9.
60. Martinez de Villarreal L, Perez JZ, Vazquez PA, Herrera RH, Campos Mdel R, Lopez RA, et al. Decline of neural tube defects cases after a folic acid campaign in Nuevo Leon, Mexico. Teratology. 2002;66:249-56.
61. Ray JG, Meier C, Vermeulen MJ, Boss S, Wyatt PR, Cole DE. Association of neural tube defects and folic acid food fortification in Canada. Lancet. 2002;360:2047-8.
62. Persad VL, Van den Hof MC, Dube JM, Zimmer P. Incidence of open neural tube defects in Nova Scotia after folic acid fortification. CMAJ. 2002;167:241-5.
63. Mathews TJ, Honein MA, Erickson JD. Spina bifida and anencephaly prevalence—United States, 1991-2001. MMWR Recomm Rep. 2002;51:9-11.
64. Green NS. Folic acid supplementation and prevention of birth defects. J Nutr. 2002;132:2356S-60S.
65. Monteagudo A, Timor-Tritsch IE. Fetal neurosonography of congenital brain anomalies. In: Timor-Tritsch IE, Monteagudo A, Cohen HL (Eds). Ultrasonography of the prenatal and neonatal brain. 2nd edition. McGraw-Hill, New York; 2001. pp.151-258.
66. Stevenson RE, Allen WP, Pai GS, Best R, Seaver LH, Dean J, Thompson S. Decline in prevalence of neural tube defects in a high-risk region of the United States. Pediatrics. 2000;106:677-83.
67. Volpe JJ. Neural tube formation and prosencephalic development. Neurology of the Newborn, 4th edition, Philadelphia; WB Saunders; 2001. pp.3-44.
68. D'Addario V, Pinto V, Del Bianco A, Di Naro E, Tartagni M, Miniello G, et al. The clivus-supraocciput angle: a useful measurement to evaluate the shape and size of the fetal posterior fossa and to diagnose Chiari II malformation. Ultrasound Obstet Gynecol. 2001;18:146-9.
69. Matsunaga E, Shiota K. Holoprosencephaly in hyman embryos: epidemiologic studies of 150 cases. Teratology. 1977;16:261-72.
70. Cohen MM Jr. Perspectives on holoprosencephaly-I. Epidemiology, genetics and syndromology. Teratology. 1989;40:211-35.
71. Pilu G, Ambrosetto P, Sandri F, et al. Intraventricular fused fornices: a specific sign of fetal lobar holoprosencephaly. Ultrasound Obstet Gynecol. 1994;34:259-62.
72. Cohen MM. An update on the holoprosencephalic disorders. J Pediatr. 1982;101:865-9.
73. Pilu G, Porelo A, Falco P, Visentin A. Median anomalies of the brain. In: Timor-Tritsch IE, Monteagudo A, Cohen HL (Eds). Ultrasonography of the prenatal and neonatal brain. 2nd edition. McGraw-Hill, New York; 2001. pp.259-76.
74. Goodyear PW, Bannister CM, Russell S, Rimmer S. Outcome in prenatally diagnosed fetal agenesis of the corpus callosum. Fetal Diagn Ther. 2001;16:139-45.
75. Taylor M, David AS. Agenesis of the corpus callosum: a United Kingdom series of 56 cases. J Neurol Neurosurg Psychiatry. 1998;64:131-4.
76. Schmidt-Riese U, Zieger M. Ultrasound diagnosis of isolated aplasia of the septum pellucidum. Ultraschall Med. 1994;15:286-92.
77. McMahon CL, Braddock SR. Septo-optic dysplasia as a manifestation of valproic acid embryopathy. Teratology. 2001;64:83-6.
78. Dominguez R, Aguirre Vila-Coro A, Slopis JM, Bohan TP. Brain and ocular abnormalities in infants with in utero exposure to cocaine and other street drugs. Am J Dis Child. 1991;145:688-95.
79. Dattani MT, Martinez-Barbera JP, Thomas PQ, Brickman JM, Gupta R, Martensson IL, et al. Mutations in the homeobox gene *HESX1/Hesx1* associated with septo-optic dysplasia in human and mouse. Nat Genet. 1998;19:125-33.
80. Toi AL, Lister WS, Fong KW. How early are fetal cerebral sulci visible at prenatal ultrasound and what is the normal pattern of early fetal sulcal development? Ultrasound Obstet Gynecol. 2004;24(7):706-15.
81. Pooh RK. Fetal Neuroimaging of Neural Migration Disorder. In: Lazebnik N, Lazebnik RS (Eds). Ultrasound Clinics, Elsevier. 2008;3(4):541-52.
82. Lerman-Sagie T, Malinger G. Focus on the fetal Sylvian fissure. Ultrasound Obstet Gynecol. 2008;32(1):3-4.
83. Guibaud L, Selleret L, Larroche JC, Buenerd A, Alias F, Gaucherand P, et al. Abnormal Sylvian fissure on prenatal cerebral imaging: significance and correlation with neuropathological and postnatal data. Ultrasound Obstet Gynecol. 2008;32(1):50-60.
84. Volpe JJ. Neuronal proliferation, migration, organization and myelination. Neurology of the newborn. 4th edition. WB Saunders, USA; 2001. pp.45-99.
85. Kobayashi K, Nakahori Y, Miyake M, Matsumura K, Kondo-Iida E, Nomura Y, et al. An ancient retrotransposal insertion causes Fukuyama-type congenital muscular dystrophy. Nature. 1998;394(6691):388-92.
86. McGahan JP, Grix A, Gerscovich EO. Prenatal diagnosis of lissencephaly: Miller-Dieker syndrome. J Clin Ultrasound. 1994;22:560-3.

87. Greco P, Resta M, Vimercati A, Dicuonzo F, Loverro G, Vicino M, et al. Antenatal diagnosis of isolated lissencephaly by ultrasound and magnetic resonance imaging. Ultrasound Obstet Gynecol. 1998;12:276-9.
88. Kojima K, Suzuki Y, Seki K, Yamamoto T, Sato T, Tanaka T, Suzumori K. Prenatal diagnosis of lissencephaly (type II) by ultrasound and fast magnetic resonance imaging. Fetal Diagn Ther. 2002;17:34-6.
89. Granata T, Farina L, Faiella A, Cardini R, D'Incerti L, Boncinelli E, et al. Familial schizencephaly associated with EMX2 mutation. Neurology. 1997;48:1403-6.
90. Brunelli S, Faiella A, Capra V, Nigro V, Simeone A, Cama A, et al. Germline mutations in the homeobox gene EMX2 in patients with severe schizencephaly. Nat Genet. 1996;12: 94-6.
91. Iannetti P, Nigro G, Spalice A, Faiella A, Boncinelli E. Cytomegalovirus infection and schizencephaly: case reports. Ann Neurol. 1998;43:123-7.
92. Denis D, Maugey-Laulom B, Carles D, Pedespan JM, Brun M, Chateil JF. Prenatal diagnosis of schizencephaly by fetal magnetic resonance imaging. Fetal Diagn Ther. 2001;16: 354-9.
93. Osenbach RK, Menezes AH. Diagnosis and management of the Dandy-Walker malformation: 30 years of experience. Pediatr Neurosurg. 1991;18:179-85.
94. Barkovich AJ, Kjos BO, Normal D, et al. Revised classification of the posterior fossa cysts and cyst-like malformations based on the results of multiplanar MR imaging. AJNR. 1989;10:977-88.
95. Bretelle F, Senat MV, Bernard JP, Hillion Y, Ville Y. First-trimester diagnosis of fetal arachnoid cyst: prenatal implication. Ultrasound Obstet Gynecol. 2002;20:400-2.
96. Elbers SE, Furness ME. Resolution of presumed arachnoid cyst in utero. Ultrasound Obstet Gynecol. 1999;14:353-5
97. Ciricillo SF, Cogen PH, Harsh GR, et al. Intracranial arachnoid cysts in children: a comparison of the effects of fenestration and shunting. J Neurosurg. 1991;74:230-5.
98. Nakamura Y, Mizukawa K, Yamamoto K, Nagashima T. Endoscopic treatment for a huge neonatal prepontine-suprasellar arachnoid cyst: a case report. Pediatr Neurosurg. 2001;35:220-4.
99. Hollway GE, Suthers GK, Haan EA, Thompson E, David DJ, Gecz J, et al. Mutation detection in FGFR2 craniosynostosis syndromes. Hum Genet. 1997;99:251-5.
100. Delashaw JB, Persing JA, Broaddus WC, Jane JA. Cranial vault growth in craniosynostosis. J Neurosurg. 1989;70:159-65.
101. Benacerraf BR, Spiro R, Mitchell AG. Using three-dimensional ultrasound to detect craniosynostosis in a fetus with Pfeiffer syndrome. Ultrasound Obstet Gynecol. 2000;16:391-4.
102. Pooh RK, Nakagawa Y, Pooh KH, Nakagawa Y, Nagamachi N. Fetal craniofacial structure and intracranial morphology in a case of Apert syndrome. Ultrasound Obstet Gynecol. 1999;13:274-80.
103. Raybaud CA, Strother CM, Hald JK. Aneurysms of the vein of Galen: embryonic considerations and anatomical features relating to the pathogenesis of the malformation. Neuroradiology. 1989;31:109-28.
104. Hoffman HJ, Chuang S, Hendrick EB, Humphreys RP. Aneurysms of the vein of Galen. Experience at The Hospital for Sick Children, Toronto. J Neurosurg. 1982;57(3):316-22.
105. Campi A, Rodesch G, Scotti G, Lasjaunias P. Aneurysmal malformation of the vein of Galen in three patients: clinical and radiological follow-up. Neuroradiology. 1998;40(12):816-21.
106. Friedman DM, Verma R, Madrid M, Wisoff JH, Berenstein A. Recent improvement in outcome using transcatheter embolization techniques for neonatal aneurysmal malformations of the vein of Galen. Pediatrics. 1993;91(3): 583-6.
107. Kupferminc MJ, Tamura RK, Sabbagha RE, Parilla BV, Cohen LS, Pergament E. Isolated choroid plexus cyst(s): an indication for amniocentesis. Am J Obstet Gynecol. 1994;171:1068-71.
108. Reinsch R. Choroid plexus cysts—association with trisomy: prospective review of 16,059 patients. Am J Obstet Gynecol. 1997;176:1381-3.
109. Snijders RJ, Shawa L, Nicolaides KH. Fetal choroid plexus cysts and trisomy 18: assessment of risk based on ultrasound findings and maternal age. Prenat Diagn. 1994;14:1119-27.
110. Nadel AS, Bromley BS, Frigoletto FD Jr, Estroff JA, Benacerraf BR. Isolated choroid plexus cysts in the second-trimester fetus: is amniocentesis really indicated? Radiology. 1992;185:545-8.
111. Coco C, Jeanty P. Karyotyping of fetuses with isolated choroid plexus cysts is not justified in an unselected Population. J Ultrasound Med. 2004;23:899-906.
112. Morcos CL, Platt LD, Carlson DE, Gregory KD, Greene NH, Korst LM. The isolated choroid plexus cyst. Obstet Gynecol. 1998;92:232-6.
113. Geary M, Patel S, Lamont R. Isolated choroid plexus cysts and association with fetal aneuploidy in an unselected population. Ultrasound Obstet Gynecol. 1997;10:171-3.
114. Kennedy KA, Carey JC. Choroid plexus cysts: significance and current management practices. Semin Ultrasound CT MR. 1993;14:23-30.
115. Lam AH, Villanueva AC. Symptomatic third ventricular choroid plexus cysts. Pediatr Radiol. 1992;22:413-6.
116. Parizek J, Jakubec J, Hobza V, Nemeckova J, Cernoch Z, Sercl M, et al. Choroid plexus cyst of the left lateral ventricle with intermittent blockage of the foramen of Monro, and initial invagination into the III ventricle in a child. Childs Nerv Syst. 1998;14:700-8.
117. Wakai S, Arai T, Nagai M. Congenital brain tumors. Surg Neurol. 1984;21:597-609.
118. Volpe JJ. Brain tumors and vein of Galen malformation. Neurology of the Newborn, 4th edition, Philadelphia; WB Saunders; 2001. pp.841-56.

119. Sherer DM, Abramowicz JS, Eggers PC, Metlay LA, Sinkin RA, Woods JR Jr. Prenatal ultrasonographic diagnosis of intracranial teratoma and massive craniomegaly with associated high-output cardiac failure. Am J Obstet Gynecol. 1993;168:97-9.
120. Lu JH, Emons D, Kowalewski S. Connatal periventricular pseudocysts in the neonate. Pediatr Radiol. 1992;22(1):55-8.
121. Malinger G, Lev D, Ben Sira L, Kidron D, Tamarkin M, Lerman-Sagie T. Congenital periventricular pseudocysts: prenatal sonographic appearance and clinical implications. Ultrasound Obstet Gynecol. 2002;20(5):447-51.
122. Bats AS, Molho M, Senat MV, Paupe A, Bernard JP, Ville Y. Subependymal pseudocysts in the fetal brain: prenatal diagnosis of two cases and review of the literature. Ultrasound Obstet Gynecol. 2002;20(5):502-5.
123. Eller KM, Kuller JA. Porencephaly secondary to fetal trauma during amniocentesis. Obstet Gynecol. 1995;85:865-7.
124. Volpe JJ. Hypoxic-Ischemic Encephalopathy: Neuropathology and pathogenesis. Neurology of the Neuborn, 4th edition, Philadelphia; WB Saunders; 2001. pp.296-330.
125. Meizner I, Elchalal U. Prenatal sonographic diagnosis of anterior fossa porencephaly. J Clin Ultrasound. 1996;24:96-9.
126. de Laveaucoupet J, Audibert F, Guis F, Rambaud C, Suarez B, Boithias-Guerot C, et al. Fetal magnetic resonance imaging (MRI) of ischemic brain injury. Prenat Diagn. 2001;21:729-36.
127. Scher MS, Belfar H, Martin J, Painter MJ. Destructive brain lesions of presumed fetal onset: antepartum causes of cerebral palsy. Pediatrics. 1991;88:898-906.
128. Stevenson DA, Hart BL, Clericuzio CL. Hydranencephaly in an infant with vascular malformations. Am J Med Genet. 2001;104:295-8.
129. Lam YH, Tang MH. Serial sonographic features of a fetus with hydranencephaly from 11 weeks to term. Ultrasound Obstet Gynecol. 2000;16:77-9.
130. Sherer DM, Anyaegbunam A, Onyeije C. Antepartum fetal intracranial hemorrhage, predisposing factors and prenatal sonography: a review. Am J Perinatol. 1998; 15:431-41.
131. Hardart GE, Fackler JC. Predictors of intracranial hemorrhage during neonatal extracorporeal membrane oxygenation. J Pediatr. 1999;134:156-9.
132. Gould DB, Phalan FC, Breedveld GJ, van Mil SE, Smith RS, Schimenti JC, et al. Mutations in COL4A1 cause perinatal cerebral hemorrhage and porencephaly. Science. 2005;308:1167-71.
133. de Vries LS, Koopman C, Groenendaal F, Van Schooneveld M, Verheijen FW, Verbeek E, et al. COL4A1 mutation in two preterm siblings with antenatal onset of parenchymal hemorrhage. Ann Neurol. 2009;65:12-8.
134. Meuwissen ME, de Vries LS, Verbeek HA, Lequin MH, Govaert PP, Schot R, et al. Sporadic COL4A1 mutations with extensive prenatal porencephaly resembling hydranencephaly. Neurology. 2011;76:844-6.
135. Vermeulen RJ, Peeters-Scholte C, Van Vught JJ, Barkhof F, Rizzu P, van der Schoor SR, et al. Fetal origin of brain damage in 2 infants with a COL4A1 mutation: fetal and neonatal MRI. Neuropediatrics. 2011;42:1-3.
136. Lichtenbelt KD, Pistorius LR, De Tollenaer SM, Mancini GM, De Vries LS. Prenatal genetic confirmation of a COL4A1 mutation presenting with sonographic fetal intracranial hemorrhage. Ultrasound Obstet Gynecol. 2012;39(6):726-7.
137. Rezaie P, Dean A. Periventricular leukomalacia, inflammation and white matter lesions within the developing nervous system. Neuropathology. 2002;22:106-32.
138. Persutte WH. Microcephaly—no small deal. Ultrasound Obstet Gynecol. 1998;11(5):317-8.
139. Schwarzler P, Homfray T, Bernard JP, Bland JM, Ville Y. Late onset microcephaly: failure of prenatal diagnosis. Ultrasound Obstet Gynecol. 2003;22(6):640-2.

18

CHAPTER

Corpus Callosum and Three-dimensional Ultrasound

Sonila Pashaj, Eberhard Merz

INTRODUCTION

The brain's complexity arises from its connectivity.[1] The corpus callosum (CC), named due to its anatomical compactness, is the major telencephalic commissure.[2] It is made of over 190 million nerve fibers that connect the left and right hemispheres of the brain[3] and is responsible for the transfer of motor, sensorial and cognitive information between the two brain hemispheres.[4] Each hemisphere of the brain is specialized in controlling movement and feeling in the opposite half of the body, as well as in processing certain types of information (such as language or spatial patterns). Thus, to coordinate movement or to process complex information, the hemispheres must communicate with each other.

In a human fetus, rudimentary corpus callosum fibers cross the midline by 12 embryonic weeks.[5,6] Development of its anatomical structure is considered to be complete at a crown-rump length of 150–200 mm.[7, 8] The adult form of the corpus callosum is achieved by 18 weeks of gestation and its height will increase with myelination. During the 3rd month after birth, the size decreases as a large proportion of the huge population of the callosal axons (over 109 billion) is eliminated. This weeding out confines contacts between the hemispheres to certain cortical zones.[9]

While the entire structure develops prior to birth, the axons of the corpus callosum continue to become more and more effective and efficient on into adolescence. The anterior and posterior corpus callosum sectors are among the most rapidly developing white matter structures in humans.[10] By the time, a child is approximately 12 years of age, the corpus callosum functions essentially as it will do in adulthood, allowing rapid interaction between the two sides of the brain. Parents report that children with absent corpus callosum (ACC) and intact early motor development (i.e. sitting and walking within the normal age range) are significantly likely to display clinically relevant behavior problems as far as they reach the 6- to 11-year-old age range. They may exhibit somatic complaints, attention problems, aggressive behavior, social problems and thought problems.[10]

The answer to the question frequently asked by parents as to whether the corpus callosum represents the only path between the hemispheres of the brain is as follows: although it does not represent the only path, it is by far the most important one. A number of much smaller connections are usually present in corpus callosum pathologies with the anterior commissure being the largest and most useful of these pathways. However, the anterior commissure is comprised of only about 50,000 axons that connect the temporal lobes, which is significantly less than the over 190 million axons contained in the corpus callosum.[11]

THREE-DIMENSIONAL OVER TWO-DIMENSIONAL SONOGRAPHY IN THE DEMONSTRATION OF THE CORPUS CALLOSUM

Fetal neurosonography with imaging of the corpus callosum can be performed using two- and three-dimensional ultrasound.[12,13] The corpus callosum is considered to be fully developed in ultrasound, when it overlies the quadrigeminal plate of the mesencephalon in the median view of the fetal brain.[14,15] Corpus callosum is displaced as an anechogenic band, demarcated superiorly and inferiorly by two echogenic lines. The presence of hyperechogenicity signifies possible pathology, chiefly callosal lipoma.[16, 17]

Clear sonographic visualization of the corpus callosum requires scanning planes that are difficult to obtain in utero with 2D ultrasound. Due to its arch-shape, the structure cannot be demonstrated using standard axial

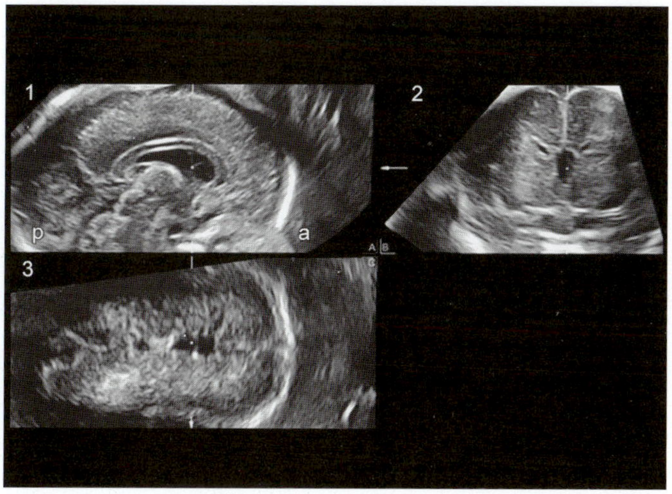

Fig. 1: Multiplanar 3D view of the normal fetal brain acquired transvaginally through the anterior fontanel at 27 weeks of gestation, showing the three orthogonal planes. Plane A (1) represents the median plane, Plane B (2) the coronal plane and Plane C (3) the axial plane of the fetal brain.

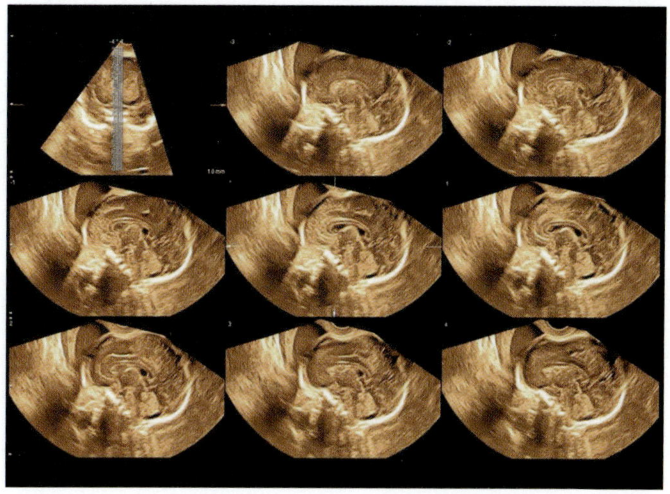

Fig. 2: The tomographic display is useful because it allows the visualization of multiple parallel slices at different spacing through a volume at the same time on the screen. The planes are similar to those seen by CT or MRI.

planes, while coronal planes enable the visualization on screen of only a small portion at a time.[16]

The cephalic presentation enables the use of endovaginal probes to study the fetal brain, but even with this technique the examination can be difficult in cases of asynclitism of the fetal head. Furthermore, this approach has a limited range in terms of lateral movement of the intravaginal probe.[12] In the presence of breech presentation the corpus callosum can be demonstrated only with an abdominal scan.[18]

Due to the limitations of 2D ultrasound,[9,16,19] new techniques for evaluation of the fetal median plane have been developed using the different display modes available with 3D ultrasonography.

In contrast to 2D sonography 3D ultrasound provides many advantages in imaging of the fetal brain anatomy, because the different cerebral planes can be shown using various display modes. Different display modes, including the 3D orthogonal-plane mode **(Fig. 1)**, parallel-plane mode **(Fig. 2)** and surface mode **(Fig. 3)**[20] makes possible to obtain not only a detailed view of the fetal face,[21] but also, to enable a rapid and easy evaluation of intracranial structures anatomy such as the corpus callosum.[22,23]

There are also differences between the planes obtained by 2D or 3D transabdominal or transvaginal ultrasound examination. Using a 2D ultrasound probe, all sections arise from a single point usually at the anterior fontanel and fan-out in a radial fashion, the planes are oblique to each other **(Figs. 4A and B)**. However, using 3D sonography enables the sections derived from the volume to be reconstructed so that they are parallel to each other similar to those obtained by computer tomography or magnetic resonance imaging.[13]

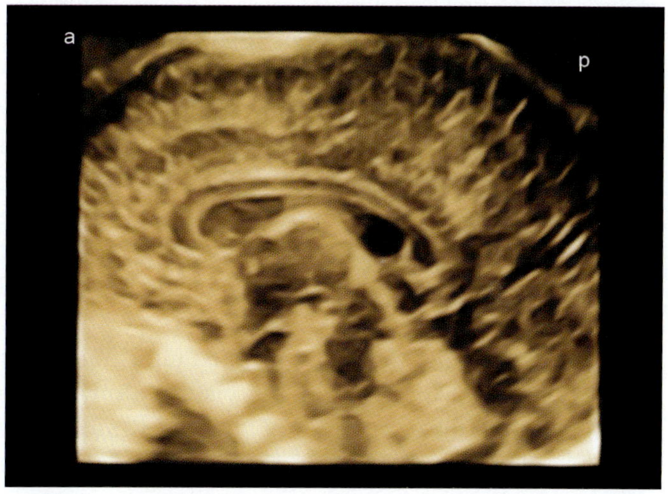

Fig. 3: Surface demonstration of the hypoechogenic corpus callosum in a thick slice's technique. (a, anterior; p, posterior)

The images of the sections that are below the fontanel and or the sutures have higher resolution than those located more lateral or distal from the acquisition plane.[13] When acquisition of the volume is performed by aligning the 3D probe at the anterior fontanel or the sagittal

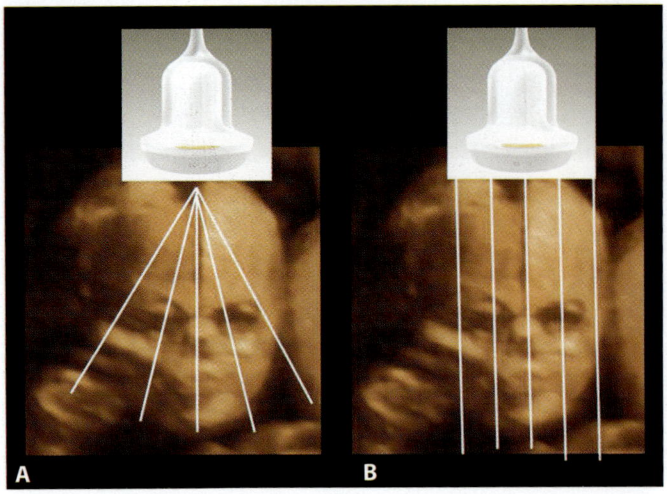

Figs. 4A and B: (A) Two-dimensional ultrasound planes arise from a single point usually through the anterior fontanel and radiate in angled planes. (B) The planes reconstructed by three-dimensional ultrasounds are parallel to each other in the tomographic mode.

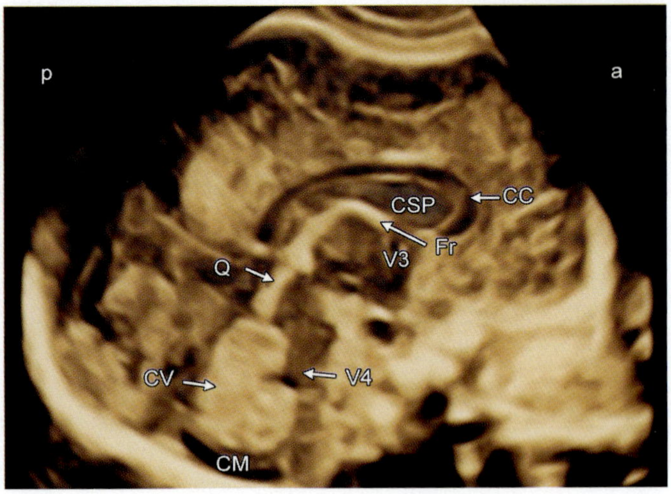

Fig. 5: Surface-rendered 3D image of the median plane, with visualization of cavum septi pellucidi (CSP), quadrigeminal plate (Q), cisterna magna (CM), cerebellar vermix (CV), fornix (Fr) and third (V3) and fourth (V4) ventricles. (a: anterior; p: posterior)

sutures, the frontal and parietal areas of the brain are well visualized including the superior subarachnoid cisterns, the convexity of the brain, the corpus callosum and the lateral ventricles, but the fossa posterior is suboptimally visualized **(Fig. 5)**. In contrast, the volume taken from the small posterior fontanel allowed a good demonstration of the posterior fossa, but not the other structures of the midbrain. This is due to the shadow caused by the ossified parts of the fetal head, observed especially in the third trimester of pregnancy.

The advantage of three-dimensional ultrasound over two-dimensional imaging for the visualization of the corpus callosum is significant. Three-dimensional ultrasound does not only reduce the time of the examination but also enhances the quality of the image.[15]

As an alternative method for the study of the midline structures, some authors have proposed using 3D multiplanar display mode or volume contrast imaging to reconstruct the median plane from the axial plane of the fetal brain.[23-28] However, these techniques have two important limitations for clinical use: first, the corpus callosum is demonstrated incorrectly as a hyperechoic structure,[26] making the differential diagnosis of corpus callosal lipoma difficult; second, the corpus callosum cannot be differentiated clearly from the cavum septi pellucidi, which leads to difficulties in the diagnoses of septo-optic dysplasia or syndromes related to an absent cavum septi pellucidi (e.g., Apert syndrome, De Grouchy syndrome).

The most appropriate method for clinical decision is the acquisition of such a volume from the median plane, the parasagittal planes or the oblique planes. By rotating the volume into a standard orientation, it is possible to achieve a symmetric demonstration of the fetal brain in the axial and coronal view. The simultaneous demonstration of the three orthogonal planes is used to visualize the brain in all three planes, while the user can scroll to navigate through the volume in a continuous fashion.[29] This enables all three scanning planes to be simultaneously displayed on the screen which allows the demonstration of the entire corpus callosum structure in the median plane and shortens the process of obtaining the correct sagittal and coronal section.[15,30,31] According to our experience, the 3D demonstration of the corpus callosum is possible even in difficult cases. Under such conditions the sonographer can exert manual control by using the free hand to manipulate the fetal head from outside the abdomen to permit visualization of the corpus callosum.[15]

Use of 3D technique enables even the less experienced sonographer to visualize the corpus callosum. The sonographic information can be stored as a volume data set, enabling not only the offline analysis with the potential to revise and obtain additional images in the different display modes, but also the consultation with an expert. This will facilitate the introduction of corpus callosum demonstration in every guideline.

Indications for Displaying the Corpus Callosum

Since the central nervous system malformations are one of the most common of all congenital anomalies, detailed evaluation of the fetal brain helps diagnose these malformations. The demonstration of corpus callosum anatomy, as an important landmark for brain development is performed just in cases of fetal, maternal indication or suspected familial disorder.[32]

a. Fetal indications
   1. Dilatation of the lateral ventricles,
   2. Absence of the cavum septi pellucidi and widely separated parallel frontal horns,
   3. Abnormal head circumference,
   4. Fetal brain or spinal masses,
   5. Twin pregnancy,
   6. Fetuses presenting with extracerebral multiple malformations that can be associated with brain lesions, e.g., thoracic lymphangioma and megalencephaly, cardiac malformation and leukomalacia.

b. Maternal
   1. Infections,
   2. Coagulation disorders,
   3. Metabolic disorders.

c. Suspected familial disorder
   1. X-linked hydrocephalus,
   2. Tuberous sclerosis,
   3. Neurofibromatosis type 1.

The indirect signs of corpus callosum pathologies are not always present at the time of the anatomic survey and may be apparent only in the mid and third trimester. 3D neurosonography transabdominally or transvaginally facilitates the demonstration of the corpus callosum allowing introducing it as an integral part of routine anatomic examination as some guidelines recommend.[33]

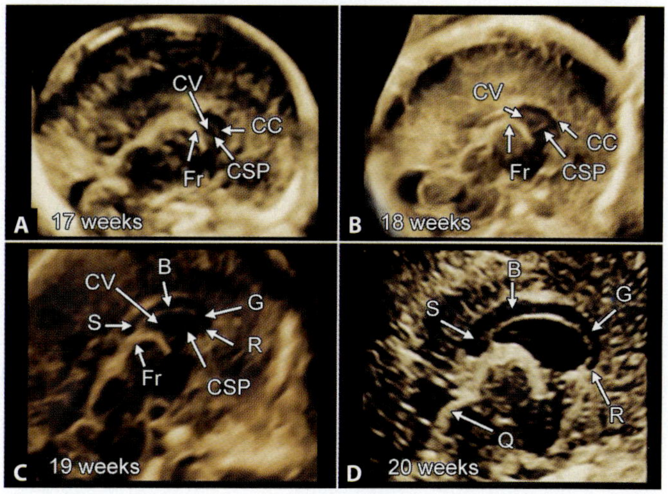

Figs. 6A to D: (A) 3D surface rendering of the corpus callosum (CC) at 17 weeks of gestation (median plane of the fetal head). In this plane the corpus callosum is seen as an anechoic structure. The rostrum is oriented vertically. There is no clear differentiation between the four anatomical parts of the corpus callosum nor is a clear structure of CSP and CV to be seen. Note that the corpus callosum is overlying the fornix (Fr); (B) The corpus callosum at 18 weeks of gestation. Although the length of the corpus callosum is markedly increased, it is still a very thin structure. No clear structure of CSP and CV is seen. The corpus callosum overlies the fornix (Fr); (C) The corpus callosum at 19 weeks of gestation. The structure has markedly increased in length and the four anatomical parts are recognizable: the rostum (R), the genu (G), the body (B), and the splenium (S). The rostrum remains to be vertically oriented and all the structure begins to assume a curved shape. At this gestational week, the anechoic structure below the corpus callosum (= CSP and CV) can be identified in the form of one cavity; (D) The corpus callosum at 20 weeks of gestation demonstrating the beaked segment of the rostrum (R) and the genu (G) below the callosal sulcus. The body (B) and the splenium (S) are elongated. There is no isthmus between the body and the splenium. At this time the corpus callosum is fully developed (Q, quadrigeminal plate).

DEMONSTRATION OF THE NORMAL DEVELOPMENT OF THE CORPUS CALLOSUM USING 3D ULTRASONOGRAPHY

Using 3D ultrasound, we were able to demonstrate the corpus callosum as a small anechoic structure starting from 17 weeks of gestation[15] **(Figs. 6A to D)**. However, at this time point, the corpus callosum is too small to enable a precise differentiation among the four anatomical parts and is overlying the fornix (Fr). At this gestational week the anechoic structure below the corpus callosum known as cavum septi pellucidi (CSP) and cavum vergae (CV) can be identified in the form of one cavity. After 20 weeks of gestation, the corpus callosum should be routinely visualizable in its regular structure on sonography. The corpus callosum development involves horizontal and vertical changes. The horizontal changes show a nonlinear growth of the corpus callosum length which is more rapid in the second trimester, followed by a slower growth in the third trimester. Vertical changes comprise the orientation of the rostrum and the flexion of the genu. At 19 gestational weeks the rostrum shows a more semivertical orientation, followed by a more semihorizontal orientation starting from 23 weeks of

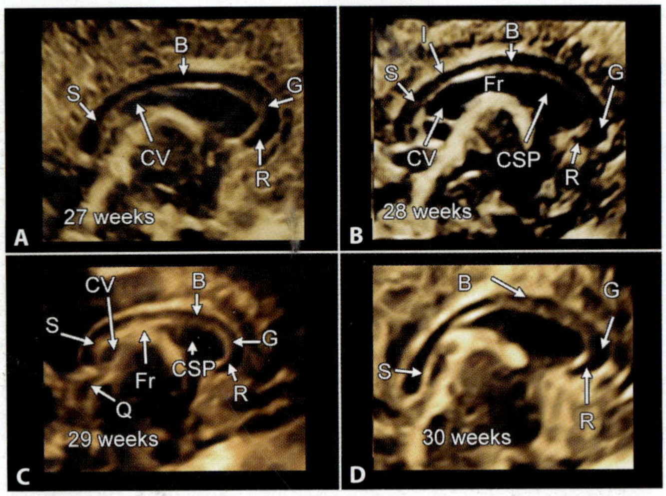

Figs. 7A to D: (A) The corpus callosum at 27 weeks of gestation revealing the four anatomical parts of the corpus callosum. The cavum vergae (CV) is relatively closed. The structure of corpus callosum is thicker at this time. R, rostrum; G, genu; B, body; S, splenium; (B) The corpus callosum at 28 weeks of gestation. Here the isthmus (I) can be identified. There is a marked separation between the cavum vergae (CV) and the cavum septi pellucidi (CSP). Fr, fornix; R, rostrum; G, genu; B, body; S, splenium; (C) The corpus callosum at 29 weeks of gestation. Note the horizontal orientation of the rostrum (R). Moreover, the anterior part of the corpus callosum progresses in its flexion. The splenium (S) reaches the quadrigeminal plate (Q) and the fornix (Fr) has contact to the inferior margin of the corpus callosum, isolating the cavum vergae (CV) from cavum septi pellucidi (CSP); (D) The corpus callosum at 30 weeks of gestation. The flexion of the genu (G) of the corpus callosum increases, being more prominent than the posterior part. The length of the corpus callosum continues to increase and the cavum vergae is completely closed. (R: rostrum; B: body; S: splenium)

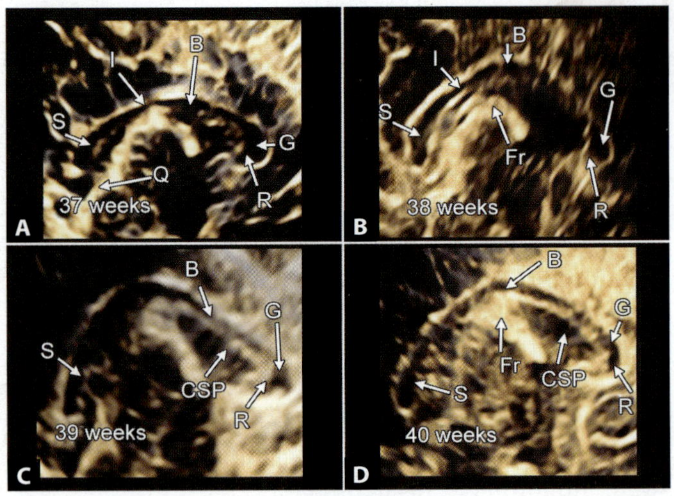

Figs. 8A to D: (A) The corpus callosum at 37 weeks of gestation. There is a marked slowing down of the length growth. Moreover, the height (= thickness) of the body (B) of the corpus callosum regresses. The anterior part is thicker and curved, while the posterior part elongates until the quadrigeminal plate (Q). The isthmus (I) appears as an anatomical region between splenium (S) and body (B). R, rostrum; (B) The corpus callosum at 38 weeks of gestation. The body (B) is becoming thinner, while the splenium (S) is increasing in its height (= thickness). The isthmus (I) is a consistent finding. The posterior part of the corpus callosum has a clearly defined relationship with the fornix (Fr). G, genu; R, rostrum; (C) The corpus callosum at 39 weeks of gestation. The rostrum (R) is horizontally oriented. The genu (G) has reached its full flexion. The body (B) is thinner, while the splenium (S) continues to elongate posteriorly. The cavum septi pellucidi (CSP) is viewed as a small anechoic structure below the anterior part of the corpus callosum; (D) The corpus callosum at 40 weeks of gestation, revealing a thinner structure, which has reached its comma shape adult form. The cavum septi pellucidi (CSP) is presented as a hypoechoic structure below the anterior part of the corpus callosum. The body (B) takes contact with the fornix (Fr). (G: genu; R: rostrum; S: splenium)

gestation. The flexion of the genu can already be visualized at 19 weeks of gestation and increases continuously from 23 weeks until term. At 23 weeks of gestations, there is a more pronounced demarcation between the two cavities below the corpus callosum, namely CSP and CV. During the period from 26 to 28 gestational weeks the corpus callosum shows an increase in height (= thickness) and a progressive flexion of the genu as well as a semihorizontally oriented rostrum, while the splenium overlies nearly the quadrigeminal plate, in order to achieve the comma-shape adult form **(Figs. 7A to D)**. The length of the corpus callosum is marked by a gradual increase during this period. The anechoic cavity below the corpus callosum is divided into two cavities: The cavum vergae and the cavum septi pellucidi, which can be partially or well differentiated from each other.

The corpus callosum at 29 weeks of gestation has a horizontal orientation of the rostrum (R) and the anterior part of it progresses in its flexion. The splenium (S) reaches the quadrigeminal plate (Q) and the fornix (Fr) has contact to the inferior margin of the corpus callosum, isolating the cavum vergae (CV) from the cavum septi pellucidi (CSP). After 32 weeks of gestations a closed cavum vergae is a persistent finding **(Figs. 8A to D)**.

Regarding the echogenicity of the corpus callosum, we found a hypoechoic structure of the corpus callosum with a clear demarcation from the cavum septi pellucidi throughout the entire observation time **(Figs. 6 to 8)**.

Magnetic Resonance Imaging (MRI) or 3D Neurosonography

It is widely accepted that MRI can supply higher diagnostic accuracy in the fetus compared with ultrasound. MRI is not influenced by physical factors, such as fetal presentation, fetal head position and ossification of fetal cranial bones, which may sometimes obstruct the view to the fetal brain using transvaginal ultrasound. MRI plays an important role in the demonstration of brain maturation, especially in normal and abnormal cortical development.[32] Fetal magnetic resonance imaging is particularly useful for certain fetal brain disorders[32,34] demonstrating possible additional cerebral anomalies, such as late sulcation, migration anomalies and heterotopias. Moreover, MRI has a better contrast between different tissues[32] while the diffusion-weighted magnetic resonance imaging (dMRI)[35] allows the clarification of callosal microstructure and connectivity.[3]

There is no clear evidence that MRI is superior to ultrasound in the diagnoses of most common brain anomalies. MRI is gaining popularity because of a lack of expertise in most ultrasound units in visualizing all parts of the brain and to pass the responsibility over to radiologists and their high-tech equipment.[36]

In contrast to 3D ultrasound, MRI is an expensive procedure, requires special radiological knowledge as well as a separate appointment in order to be performed and is time consuming. In addition, MRI is less sensitive in detecting bony structure and angioarchitectonics as well as in volumetric assessment, compared with 3D ultrasound imaging. MRI gives additional information in rare cases with migration disorder. As a result, we can say that MRI is a complementary examination in complicated cases or when the high 3D ultrasonographic technology is not available.

BIOMETRY OF THE FETAL CORPUS CALLOSUM BY THREE-DIMENSIONAL ULTRASOUND

The visualization and biometry of the corpus callosum has been of considerable interest to many researchers using magnetic resonance imaging (MRI) and 2D as well as 3D ultrasound.[6,9,12,13,19,22,23,25-28,37-40]

In a recent published article with data from three- dimensional fetal head volumes of 466 normal pregnancies, between 17+0 and 41+6 weeks of gestation, a nonlinear growth of corpus callosum was reported.[15]

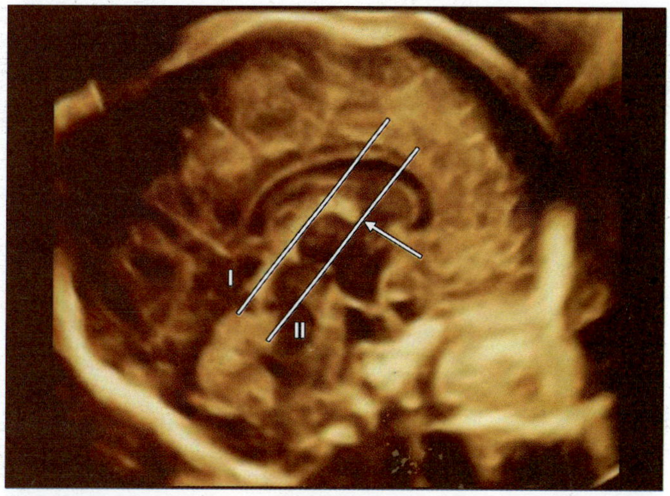

Fig. 9: Normal corpus callosal development with flexion of the genu. The flexion of the genu can be evaluated by drawing a reference line (line I) between the fornix and the quadrigeminal plate. On shifting this line parallel to the most anterior part of the fornix (arrow, line II), the genu is in front of this line and the body behind this line.

Each three- dimensional volume of the fetal head acquired from sagittal planes was assessed for clear representation of the entire hypoechoic corpus callosum, including rostrum, genu, body and splenium. The rostrum is the bill-shaped segment at the front part of the corpus callosum oriented posteriorly or posteroinferiorly. The genu is the curved anterior portion of the corpus callosum, projecting anteriorly to a line drawn parallel to the posterior part of the fornix and the quadrigeminal plate and starting at the most anterior part of the fornix **(Fig. 9)**. The body is the slightly curved horizontal structure, while the splenium is the portion oriented posteriorly and located at the rear of the corpus callosum.[15]

In this article corpus callosal measurements included three different lengths of this structure **(Fig. 10A)** and the height (thickness) of the rostrum, genu, body and splenium **(Fig. 10B)**. All measurements were made in the median plane. The first of the three corpus callosal length measurements, the 'curved corpus callosal length' (CCL-C), was performed using a trace length; the second, the 'inner-inner corpus callosal length' (CCL-II), was made from the innermost part of the rostrum to the innermost part of the splenium; the final one, the 'outer–outer corpus callosal length' (CCL-OO), was performed from the most anterior part of the genu to the most posterior part of the splenium, tracing a straight rostrocaudal line. All measurements

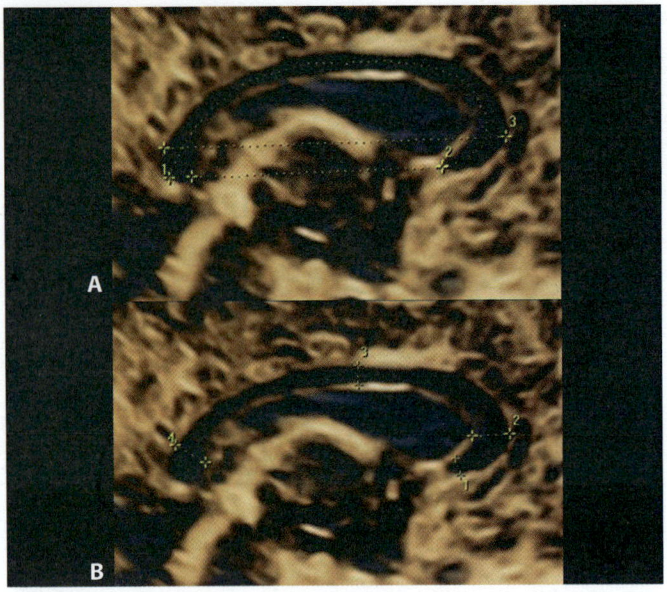

Figs. 10A and B: Three-dimensional surface-rendered median views of the fetal corpus callosum at 27 gestational weeks. (A) Corpus callosal length measurements: curved corpus callosal length (CCL-C; calipers 1), inner–inner corpus callosal length (CCL-II; calipers 2) and outer–outer corpus callosal length (CCL-OO; calipers 3); (B) Height measurements of the four different parts of the corpus callosum: rostrum (calipers 1), genu (calipers 2), body (calipers 3) and splenium (calipers 4).

of the corpus callosum related to the length and height of the hypoechoic area, excluding the hyperechoic sulcus of the corpus callosum and the cingulate gyrus superiorly, as well as the cavum septi pellucidi and cavum vergae inferiorly. A cross-shaped caliper with 0.1 mm resolution was used for these measurements.[15]

During gestation an approximately fourfold increase in the different corpus callosum lengths can be observed, a threefold increase in the rostrum height (= thickness), a fourfold increase in the genu height, a twofold increase in the body height and a threefold increase in the splenium height. The growth pattern of the rostrum and the body height seems to be similar and is characterized by a rapid development up to 24 and 22 gestational weeks, respectively, before entering into a period of stagnation. The growth pattern of the genu and the splenium height were also noted to be similar.[15]

In cases of abnormally thin or thick corpus callosum, the availability of reference ranges for corpus callosal length and the height of the four different parts of the structure is very helpful, as illustrated by the pathological cases reported in the literature.[15,41]

DETECTION OF FETAL CORPUS CALLOSUM ABNORMALITIES BY MEANS OF 3D ULTRASOUND

Abnormalities of the corpus callosum include agenesis, partial agenesis, hypoplasia, hyperplasia and lipoma with enhanced echogenicity.[41]

Complete agenesis of the corpus callosum (ACC) is the nondevelopment of the corpus callosum from as early as 12 weeks of gestation.[42] Hypogenesis of the corpus callosum, also known as partial agenesis, is characterized by congenital partial absence of the corpus callosum.[11] Corpus callosum thickness reflects the volume of the hemispheres and responds to changes through direct effects or Wallerian degeneration.[43] Hypoplasia or thinning of the corpus callosum is a condition characterized by a fully formed corpus callosum but thin for expected age and sex of individuals.[11] Hyperplasia (= abnormal thickening) of the corpus callosum might be part of a primary disorder in which the corpus callosum finding is essential to diagnosis: abnormal thickening can also be secondary to inflammation, infection and trauma.[43] Corpus callosum hypertrophy has been first described in adults with schizophrenia.[44] A thick corpus callosum may also be seen in patients with neurofibromatosis,[45] in patients with the macrocephaly-capillary malformation syndrome[46] and in Cohen syndrome.[47]

Agenesis of the corpus callosum was the first pathology of the corpus callosum to be reported prenatally.[17,48]

In a study of 31 cases of corpus callosum pathologies such as agenesis, partial agenesis, hypoplasia and hyperplasia or mixed form of hypo- and hyperplasia and lipoma with enhanced echogenicity[41] additional information was provided for use in prenatal parental counseling, as well as to demonstrate the clinical relevance of the new reference ranges published recently,[15] which allow the accurate diagnosis of corpus callosum pathologies. According to this article, the corpus callosum pathologies were defined as follows:[41]

1. Agenesis of the corpus callosum was determined following identification of the direct signs and comprised the demonstration of the absence of the corpus callosum in the median plane, as well as in the axial and coronal views.
2. Partial agenesis of the corpus callosum was diagnosed when at least one of the anatomical segments was missing, while the height of the remaining parts was within the normal range and all three lengths of the

corpus callosum were less than the 5th percentiles according to growth charts.

3. Hypoplasia was diagnosed when all anatomical segments were present and the height of at least one corpus callosum segment was less than the 5th percentile according to growth charts, while all 3 lengths were normal or reduced.
4. Hyperplasia was defined when all anatomical segments were present and the height of at least one corpus callosum segment was found above the 95th percentile according to our growth charts, while all 3 lengths were normal or out of the normal range.
5. A combination of hypo- and hyperplasia (= mixed abnormal thickening) was diagnosed when all anatomical segments were present and the height of at least one segment was found above the 95th percentile and another segment below the 5th percentile, independent of the length range.

Corpus callosum malformations are diagnosed in a large number of conditions that interfere with early cerebral development, including chromosomal and metabolic disorders, as well as intrauterine exposure to teratogen substances and infections.[11]

In prenatal diagnosis 3D ultrasound offers a number of advantages over conventional 2D ultrasound in the assessment of fetal neuroanatomy.[20,49]

Complete agenesis represents a complex condition which can result from a disruption in any one of the multiple steps of callosal development, such as cellular proliferation and migration, axon growth, or glial patterning at the midline.[11]

Prenatal diagnosis of complete agenesis is feasible by expert sonography from 18 to 20 weeks of gestation onwards and relies on the recognition of direct and/or indirect signs.[17,50-52] Although the prenatal diagnosis of complete agenesis was first described by Comstock et al. in 1985,[48] until today it continues to be regarded as a malformation of uncertain prevalence and clinical significance. Direct signs consist of the demonstration of the absence of the corpus callosum in the median and coronal views of the fetal brain. Furthermore, the median plane shows an atypical radiating appearance of the median sulci, which converge toward the third ventricle. In the majority of cases the cingulated gyrus is absent or may be incomplete.[50]

Indirect signs include the so-called tear-drop-shaped ventricles[53] as well as colpocephaly,[54] which is characterized by dilatation of the atria and occipital horns of the lateral ventricles. All of these signs were consistently observed in our series of fetuses with corpus callosum agenesis. Additional sonographic findings are diagnosed due to the presence of underlying chromosomal anomalies or genetic syndromes.[55,56] In our series over 75% of the cases had additional sonographic findings and showed a poor prognosis.[41]

In isolated agenesis of the corpus callosum a wide variety of outcomes has been reported, ranging from completely normal[50-52,57-58] to severely impaired neurodevelopment,[59] to epilepsy or behavioral disorders.[60] Termination of pregnancies is often demanded by the parents, as reported by a recent article.[41] From three fetuses with isolated corpus callosum agenesis in two of these cases a termination of pregnancy was required by the parents and in the remaining case the meanwhile 5-years-old child shows a normal development.

Partial agenesis of the corpus callosum results from growth arrest which occurs between 12 and 18 weeks of gestation and usually involves the dorsal part of the splenium, with the more anterior part being preserved.[14]

It remains uncertain whether partial agenesis of the corpus callosum represents a true malformation or is the consequence of a disruptive event. In prenatal ultrasound the measurements of all three corpus callosum lengths must be below the 5th percentile **(Figs. 11A to C)**.

The precise visualization of the median plane of the fetal brain and the known reference ranges of the corpus callosum segments enable a more accurate diagnosis of corpus callosum underdevelopment and is therefore most relevant for prenatal management and counseling.

As reported in the literature the most frequently affected parts in partial agenesis of the corpus callosum were the body and the splenium.[41] Splenial structure have a correlation with language skills.[11] In developmentally impaired populations both over- and underdevelopment of the splenium result in the impairment of visuospatial skills, attention, and motor coordination. Furthermore, individuals with reduced posterior callosal connections were found to also have impairments in excitatory interhemispheric transfer, diminished processing speed during complex tasks, and social skill impairments. A general observation is that the callosal area is positively correlated with attention, regardless of how other comorbid conditions may impact callosal structure.[11]

Hypoplasia of the corpus callosum is related to a decrease in thickness or to a decrease in both thickness and length. Hypoplasia occurs as a result of the late destruction

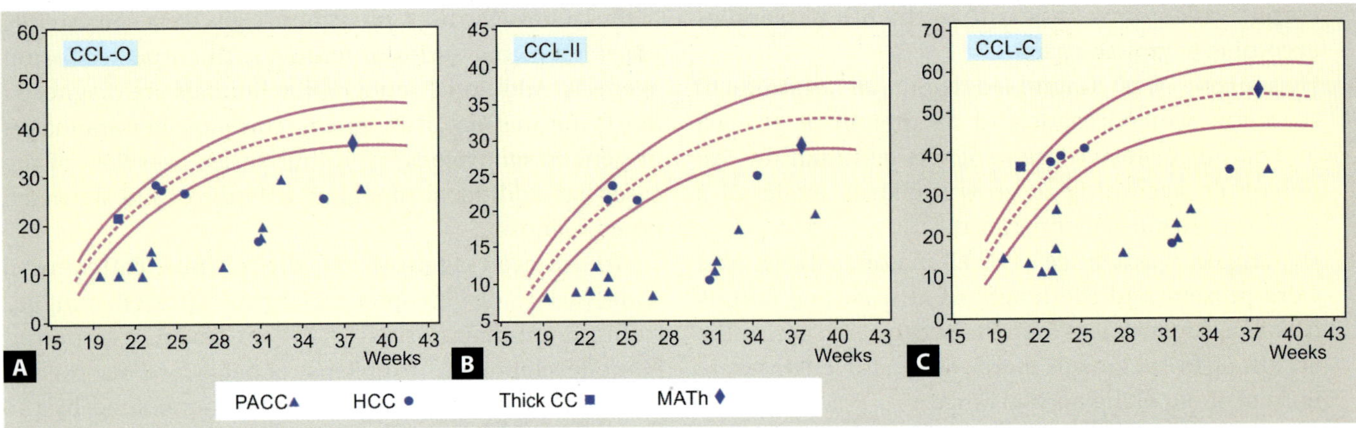

Figs. 11A to C: The graphs shows the 90% reference band for the three corpus callosum length measurements in relation to the gestational age from 18 to 41 gestational weeks. The lines represent the 5th, 50th and 95th percentiles. (A) Outer corpus callosum length (CCL-O); (B) Inner corpus callosum length (CCL-II); (C) Curved corpus callosum length (CCL-C). Furthermore, demonstration of 18 cases of corpus callosum pathologies: partial corpus callosum agenesis (PACC) (n = 11), corpus callosum hypoplasia (HCC) (n = 5), thick corpus callosum (ThickCC) (n = 1) and mixed abnormal thickness (MATh) (n = 1). All CCL-O, CCL-II, CCL-C measurements for partial corpus callosum agenesis are found below the 5th percentile of the growth charts.

(Adapted after Pashaj and Merz).[41]

of the corpus callosum owing to a metabolic, infectious or ischemic origin.[42] In contrast to a primary malformation, callosal hypoplasia is more likely to depend upon an external factor affecting the number and size of callosal axons.[42] Recent reports of corpus callosum hypoplasia were found to have additional sonographic findings, due to the underlying genetic or chromosomal syndromes.[41] Prenatal diagnosis is still challenging and relies on a clear demonstration of the corpus callosum structure in the median plane, as well as on a precise measurement that can be compared with normal values observed at the corresponding gestational age.

In cases of hyperplasia of corpus callosum, the knowledge of growth charts of corpus callosum length and height of the four different segments of the corpus callosum is of great importance **(Figs. 12A to D)**. Hyperplasia and a combined form of hypo- and hyperplasia of corpus callosum were found in association with fetal syndromes.[41]

In the presence of a prenatally detected corpus callosum anomaly, counseling of the parents remains the major problem. Although we are able to demonstrate structural abnormalities of the corpus callosum accurately with 3D ultrasound and the new reference ranges for the seven different corpus callosum measurements, the precise prognosis in the different corpus callosum anomalies continues to be challenging.

DISCUSSION

Research on corpus callosum will be of major importance for a variety of scientific disciplines in the future. In the field of embryology conflicting data have been reported in regard to corpus callosum development. In 1968, Rakic and Yakovlev[5] published an article on the development of the cerebral commissures and the septum pellucidum. According to this report, the corpus callosum grows from front to rear with the genu developing more prenatally and the splenium more postnatally. Furthermore, the rostrum is known to be the last part to be formed in utero.[5] Whereas clinical observation appears to indicate that the rostrum represents the last portion to develop, recent studies based on diffusion tensor magnetic resonance imaging were able to demonstrate that callosal connections begin more centrally in the hippocampal primordium and the subsequent growth progresses bidirectionally both anterior and posterior, with more prominent anterior growth.[6,35] The rostrum together with the genu and the anterior part of the body were found to be present as early as around 15 gestational weeks, while the caudal portion of the corpus callosum, known as the splenium, does not become prominent until 18-19 gestational weeks.[6,61]

Among the pathological findings in the literature there were two cases of partial corpus callosum agenesis that support the reported bidirectional development of the

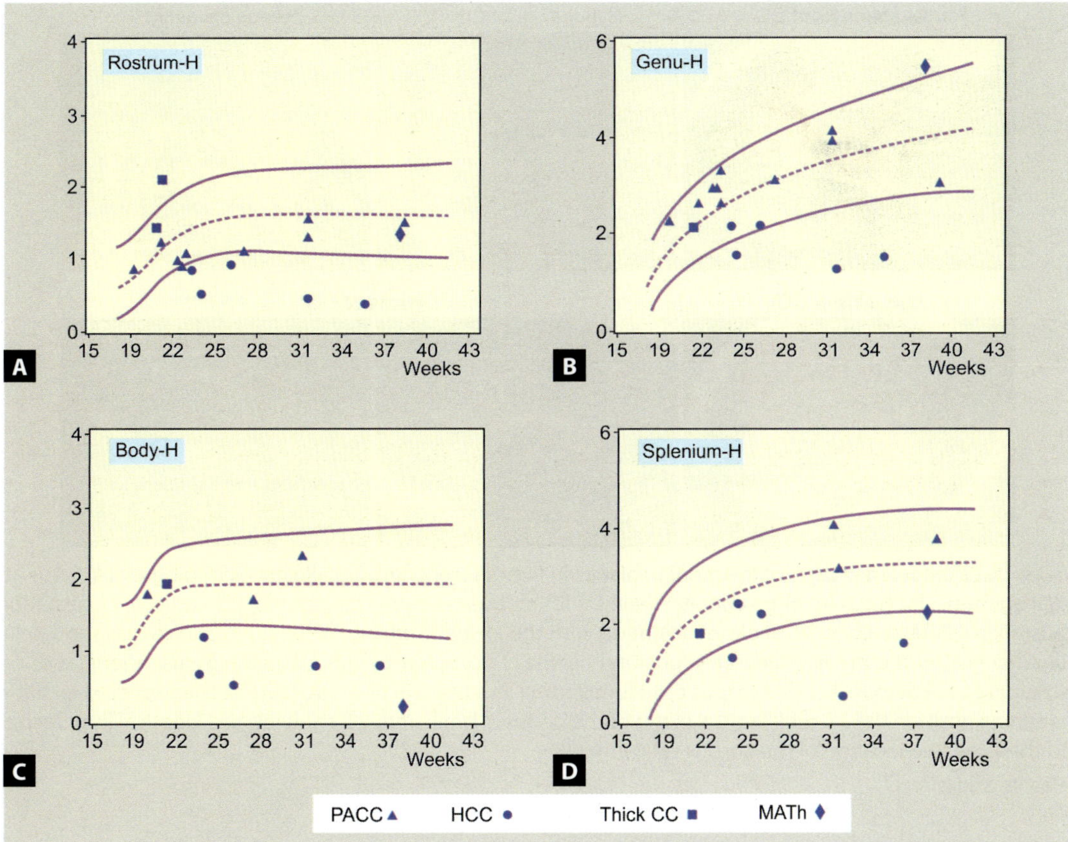

Figs. 12A to D: The graphs show the 90% reference band for the rostrum, genu, body and splenium height in relation to the gestational age from 18 to 41 gestational weeks. The lines represent the 5th, 50th and 95th percentiles; (A) Rostrum height (Rostrum-H): Demonstration of 16 cases diagnosed with corpus callosum pathologies: partial corpus callosum agenesis (PACC) (n = 9), corpus callosum hypoplasia (HCC) (n = 5), thick corpus callosum (Thick CC) (n = 1) and mixed abnormal thickness (MATh) (n = 1). In nine cases of partial corpus callosum agenesis, the measurements of the rostrum heights were found to be within the normal range, whereas the rostrum was absent in the other two cases; (B) Genu height (Genu-H): Demonstration of 17 cases with corpus callosum pathologies: partial corpus callosum agenesis (n = 10), corpus callosum hypoplasia (n = 5), thick corpus callosum (n = 1) and mixed abnormal thickness (MATh) (n = 1); (C) Body height (Body-H): Demonstration of the 10 cases with corpus callosum pathologies: partial corpus callosum agenesis (n = 3), corpus callosum hypoplasia (n = 5), thick corpus callosum (n = 1) and mixed abnormal thickness (MATh) (n = 1); (D) Splenium height (Splenium-H): Demonstration of 10 cases of corpus callosum pathologies: partial corpus callosum agenesis (n = 3), corpus callosum hypoplasia (n = 5), thick corpus callosum (n = 1) and mixed abnormal thickness (MATh) (n = 1).

(Adapted after Pashaj and Merz).[41]

corpus callosum.[15,41] In these cases, we were able to demonstrate the anterior and posterior part of the corpus callosum with the absence of the central part of the body. These pathological cases can be explained by a fusion failure of the anterior and posterior part of the corpus callosum, resulting in an absent body.

3D ultrasound is not able to distinguish the callosal microstructure during the embryological development of corpus callosum. In contrast to 3D ultrasound, diffusion-weighted magnetic resonance imaging (d-MRI) can provide information on the topographic organization of the corpus callosum, thus gaining further insights into the embryology of the corpus callosum.[35]

A vast amount of work is required in the field of genetics with regard to the mode of inheritance. More recently reported data suggest a sporadic to polygenic inheritance.[11] The biological basis of disorders of corpus callosum is complex. Understanding the biological basis of many other pathologies associated with corpus callosum disorders, such as schizophrenia and autismus, requires not only the identification of genes that regulate each process but also the knowledge of how they work together, to produce the

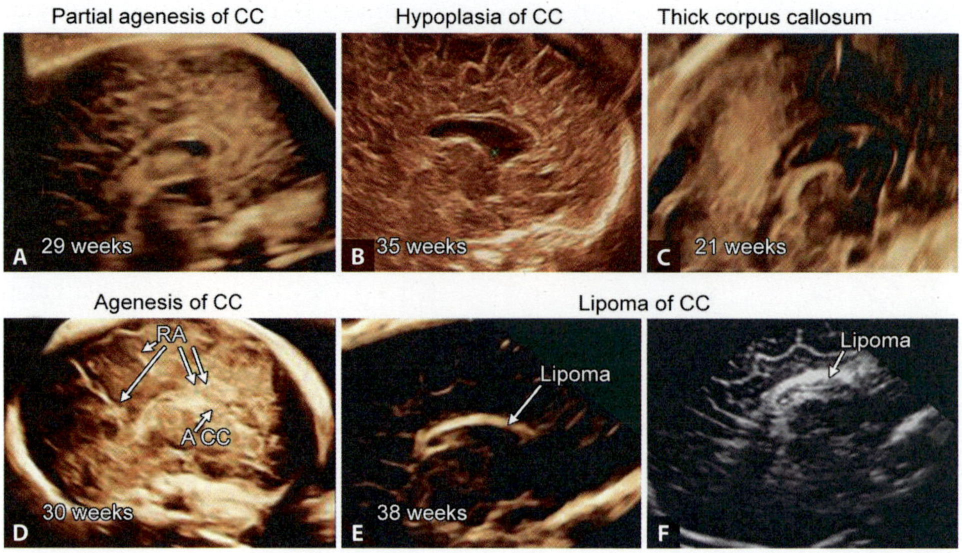

Figs. 13A to F: 3D surface rendered images of the median planes in five different corpus callosum pathologies: (A) Fetus at 29 gestational weeks with partial agenesis; (B) Fetus at 35 gestational weeks with corpus callosum hypoplasia; (C) Fetus at 21 gestational weeks with thick corpus callosum; (D) Fetal brain at 30 weeks of gestation with the absence of corpus callosum and cavum septi pellucidi. This view shows the radial array (RA) of the medial gyri in the position normally occupied by the cingulate gyrus. Agenesis of corpus callosum (ACC); (E) The remaining case demonstrates a corpus callosum lipoma as a hyperechoic structure at the expected location of the corpus callosum; (F) The same lipoma in the 2D mid-sagittal plane of the neonate brain at day 3 showing the identical hyperechoic sonographic structure around the expected location of the corpus callosum.
(Adapted after Pashaj and Merz).[41]

corpus callosum. These complex biological basis is reflected by the large numbers of human congenital syndromes associated with pathological corpus callosum.[62-64] In some patients the agenesis of corpus callosum may be entirely asymptomatic, without apparent associated clinical deficits and with only mild intellectual difficulties, such as problems in visual processing and higher order language functions, with social deficits becoming clearly apparent only on psychomotor testing.[11,65,66] Many individuals with callosal agenesis also carry a diagnosis of attention deficit or autistic spectrum disorders.[67,68] For this reason infants with ACC need to see a variety of different specialists. Some of the physicians and other professionals who may have to be consulted include: neurologists, endocrinologists, geneticists, ophthalmologists, speech-language therapists, occupational therapists, physical therapists, early intervention specialists, and social workers.

In the field of prenatal diagnosis there is an underestimation of corpus calllosum pathologies. While ACC is well-demonstrated in the literature, reports on the diagnosis of partial agenesis, hypoplasia and hypertrophia of corpus callosum are scarce **(Figs. 13A to F)**. Different guidelines for routine fetal brain examinations recommend the transabdominal approach using axial brain planes to visualize the falx, thalami, cavum septi pellucidi, lateral ventricles with the choroid plexus, cerebellum and cistern magna. The use of these axial planes is, however, not sufficient to display the corpus callosum. Currently the evaluation of the corpus callosum is not officially recommended as an integral part of the basic ultrasound routine examination. Therefore, corpus callosum pathologies are only suspected in the presence of indirect signs. Agenesis of corpus callosum can be well diagnosed with 2D and 3D ultrasound according to the known indirect sonographic signs, such as abnormal ventricular configuration, upward displacement of the 3rd ventricle, absence of cavum septi pellucidi, radial array of medial sulci and bullhorn shape of the lateral ventricles.[17] In addition, indirect signs are not always present at the time of anatomic survey and may appear only later in the mid and late third trimester. Moreover, these indirect signs are not always detectable in some of the corpus callosum pathologies.

Thus, the accurate diagnoses of partial agenesis, hypoplasia, hyperplasia or mixed abnormal thickening of corpus callosum not only require a precise demonstration of the corpus callosum in the median plane of the fetal head, but also an exact knowledge of the normal reference ranges of the corpus callosum (length and height).

CONCLUSION

In summary, 3D ultrasound enables a precise demonstration of the normal and abnormal corpus callosum in the median plane. Due to the complex anatomy of the fetal brain, it is helpful to have reference views, tables and charts of the dimensions of the corpus callosum for the accurate diagnosis of abnormalities of the corpus callosum. When an unusual image is encountered, the question should then be 'What is the specific anomaly?' instead of just: 'Is this abnormal anatomy?' The knowledge gained from this chapter allows detection of abnormal size of the fetal corpus callosum, and can provide additional information for the counseling of parents confronted with corpus callosum pathology in their unborn baby. As in pediatric central nervous system disease, it is not only important to evaluate the presence or absence of the corpus callosum for congenital anomalies but also to evaluate the thickness of the different segments. By correlating the prenatal corpus callosum abnormalities with the known functions of the different corpus callosum segments, we can attempt to gain insight into the impact not only on prenatal neurological development, but also on postnatal neurological outcome. This presents a challenging area for future research studies.

REFERENCES

1. Schoenemann PT, Sheehan M J, Glotzer LD. Prefrontal white matter volume is disproportionately larger in humans than in other primates. Nature Neurosci. 2005:8;242-52.
2. Raybaud C. The corpus callosum, the other great forebrain commissures and the septum pellucidum: anatomy, development and malformation. Neuroradiology. 2010; 52:447-77.
3. Tomasch J. Size, distribution, and number of fibres in the human corpus callosum. The Anat. Rec. 1954:119,119-35.
4. Mangione R, Fries N, Godard P, et al. Neurodevelopment outcome following prenatal diagnoses of an isolated anomaly of the corpus callosum. Ultrasound Obstet Gynecol. 2011;37:290-5.
5. Rakic P, Yakovlev PI. Development of the corpus callosum and cavum septi in man. J Comp Neurol. 1968;132:45-72.
6. Kier L, Truwit CL. The normal and abnormal genu of the corpus callosum: an evolutionary, embryologic, anatomic and MR analysis. Am J Neuroradiol. 1996;17:1631-41.
7. Streeter G. Development of the central nervous system. Ch. II. In. Keibel and Mall's Manual of Human Embryology. JB Lippincott & Co; 1912.
8. Hamilton WJ, Boyd JD and Mossman HW. Human Embryology. Cambridge: W Heffer and Sons; 1952.
9. Achiron R, Achiron A. Development of the human fetal corpus callosum: a high-resolution, cross-sectional sonographic study. Ultrasound Obstet Gynecol. 2001; 18:343-7.
10. Paul LK. Developmental malformation of the corpus callosum: a review of typical callosal development and examples of developmental disorders with callosal involvement. J Neurodev Disord. 2011;3:3-37.
11. Paul LK, Brown WS, Adolphs R, Tiszka JM, Richards LJ, Mukherjee P, et al. Agenesis of the corpus callosum: genetic, developmental and functional aspects of connectivity. Nat Rev Neurosci. 2007;8:287-99.
12. Monteagudo A, Reuss M L, Timor-Tritsch IE. Imaging the fetal brain in the second and third trimester using transvaginal sonography. Obstet Gynecol. 1991;77:27-32.
13. Monteagudo A, Timor-Tritsch IE. Normal sonographic development of the central nervous system from the second trimester onwards using 2-D, 3-D and transvaginal sonography. Prenat Diag. 2009;29:326-39.
14. Ghi T, Carletti E, Cera E, Falco P, Tagliavini G, Michelacci L, et al. Prenatal diagnosis and outcome of partial agenesis and hypoplasia of the corpus callosum. Ultrasound Obstet Gynecol. 2010;35,35-41.
15. Pashaj S, Merz E, Wellek S. Biometric measurements of the fetal corpus callosum by three-dimensional ultrasound. Ultrasound Obstet Gynecol. 2013;42:691-8.
16. Malinger G, Lerman-Sagie T, Viñals F. Three-dimensional sagittal reconstruction of the corpus callosum: fact or artifact? Ultrasound Obstet Gynecol. 2006;28:742-3.
17. Pilu G, Sandri F, Perolo A, Pittalis G, Grisolia G, Cocchi G, et al. Sonography of fetal agenesis of the corpus callosum: a survey of 35 cases. Ultrasound Obstet Gynecol. 1993;3:318-29.
18. Pilu G, De Palma L, Romero R, et al. The fetal subarachnoid cisterns. An ultrasound study with report of a case of congenital communicating hydrocephalus. J Ultrasound Med. 1986;5:365-72.
19. Malinger G, Zakut H. The corpus callosum: Normal Fetal development as shown by transvaginal sonography. Am J Roentgenol. 1993;161;1041-3.
20. Merz E, Abramowicz JS. 3D/4D ultrasound in prenatal diagnosis: is it time for routine use? Clin Obstet Gynecol. 2012;55:336-51.
21. Merz E, Abramovicz J, Baba K, Blass HG, Deng J, Gindes L, et al. 3D imaging of the fetal face – recommendations from the International 3D Focus Group. Ultraschall Med. 2012;33:175-82.
22. Merz E. Targeted depiction of the fetal corpus callosum with 3D ultrasound. Ultraschall Med. 2010;31:441.

23. Bornstein E, Monteagudo A, Santos R, et al. IE. A systematic technique using 3-dimensional ultrasound provides a simple and reproducible mode to evaluate the corpus callosum. Am J Obstet Gynecol. 2010;202(2):201.e1-5.
24. Viñals F, Munoz M, Naveas R, Schalper J, Giuliano S. The fetal cerebellar vermis: anatomy and biometry assessment using 4D volume contrast imaging in the C-plane (VCI-C). Ultrasound Obstet Gynecol. 2005;26:622-7.
25. Correa FF, Lara C, Bellver J, Remohi J, Pellicer A, Serra V. Examination of the fetal brain by transabdominal threedimensional ultrasound: potential for routine neurosonographic studies. Ultrasound Obstet Gynecol. 2006;27:503-8.
26. Pilu G, Segata M, Ghi T, Carletti A, Perolo A, Santini D, et al. Diagnosis of midline anomalies of the fetal brain with the three-dimensional median view. Ultrasound Obstet Gynecol. 2006.27:522-9.
27. Miguelote FR, Vides B, Santos FR, Palha AJ, Matias A, Sousa N. The role of tridimensional imaging reconstruction to measure the corpus callosum: comparison with direct mid-sagittal views. Prenat Diagn. 2011:DOI:10.1002/pd.2794.
28. Rizzo G, Pietrolucci ME, Capponi A, et al. Assessment of corpus callosum Biometric measurement at 18 to 32 weeks´gestation by 3-dimensional sonography. J Ultrasound Med. 2011;30:47-53.
29. Merz E, Benoit B, Blass GH, Baba K, Kratochwil A, Nelson T, et al. Standardization of three-dimensional images in obstetrics and gynecology: consensus statement. Ultrasound Obstet Gynecol. 2007;29:697-703.
30. Monteagudo A, Timor-Tritsch IE, Mayberry P. Three-dimensional transvaginal neurosonography of the fetal brain: "navigating" in the volume scan. Ultrasound Obstet Gynecol. 2000;16:307-313.
31. Timor-Tritsch IE, Monteagudo A, Mayberry P. Three-dimensional ultrasound evaluation of the fetal brain: the three horn view. Ultrasound Obstet Gynecol 2000a;16:302-6.
32. Girard N, Chaumoitre K, Confort-Gouny S, et al. Magnetic resonance imaging and the detection of the fetal brain anomalies, injury and physiologic adaptations. Curr Opin Obstet Gynecol. 2006;18:164-76.
33. Sonographic examination of the fetal brain central nervous system: guidelines for performing basic examination and the fetal neurosonogram. Ultrasound Obstetric Gynecol 2007:29:109-16.
34. Girard NJ, Raybaud CA. Ventriculomegaly and pericerebral collection in the fetus: early stage of benign external hydrocephalus? Childs Nerv Syst. 2001;17:239-45.
35. Huang H, Xue R, Zhang J, Ren T, Richards LJ, Yarowsky P, et al. Anatomical characterization of human fetal brain development with diffusion tensor magnetic resonance imaging. J Neurosci. 2009;29:4263-73.
36. Malinger G, Lev D, Lerman-Sagie T. Is fetal magnetic resonance imaging superior to neurosonography for detection of brain anomalies? Ultrasound Obstet Gynecol. 2002; 20:317-321
37. Chasen S, Birnholz J, Gurewitsch E, et al. Antenatal growth of the corpus callosum. Am J Obstet Gynecol. 1997;176:S66.
38. Aboitiz F, Scheibel AB, Fisher RS, Zaidel E. Fiber composition of the corpus callosum. Brain Res. 1992;598:143-53.
39. Harreld JH, Bhore R, Chason DP, et al. Corpus callosum length by gestational age as evaluated by fetal MR imaging. Am J Neuroradiol. 2011;32:490-94.
40. Araujo Júnior E, Visentainer M, Simioni C, Ruano R, Nardozza LM, Moron AF. Reference values for the length and area of the fetal corpus callosum on 3-dimensional sonography using the transfrontal view. J Ultrasound Med. 2012;31:205-12.
41. Pashaj S, Merz E. Detection of fetal corpus callosum abnormalities by means of 3D ultrasound. Ultraschall in Med. 2016;37:185-94.
42. Paupe A, Bidat L, Sonigo P, Lenclen R, Molho M, Ville Y. Prenatal diagnosis of hypoplasia of the corpus callosum in association with non-ketotic hyperglycinemia. Ultrasound Obstet Gynecol. 2002;20:616-9.
43. Andronikou S, Pillay T, Gabuza L, Mahomed N, Naidoo J, Hlabangana LT, et al. Corpus callosum thickness in children: an MRI pattern-recognition approach on the midsagittal image. Pediatr Radiol. 2015;45:258-72. doi: 10. 1007 s00247-014-2998-9. Epub 2014.
44. Nasrallah NA, Andreasen NC, Coffman JA, Olson SC, Dunn VD, Ehrhardt JC, et al. Controlled magnetic resonance imaging study of corpus callosum thickness in schizophrenia. Biol Psychiatry. 1986;21:274-82.
45. Margariti PN, Blekas K, Katzioti FG, Zikou AK, Tzoufi M, Argyropoulou MI. Magnetization transfer ratio and volumetric analysis of the brain in macrocephalic patients with neurofibromatosis type 1. Eur Radiol. 2007;17:433-8.
46. Conway RL, Pressman BD, Dobyns WB, Danielpour M, Lee J, Sanchez-Lara PA, et al. Neuroimaging findings in macrocephaly-capillary malformation: a longitudinal study of 17 patients. Am J Med Genet A. 2007;143A: 2981-3008.
47. Kivitie-Kallio S, Norio R. Cohen syndrome: essential features, natural history, and heterogeneity. Am J Med Genet. 2001;102:125-35.
48. Comstock CH, Culp D, Gonzalez J, Boal DB. Agenesis of the corpus callosum in the fetus: its evolution and significance. J Ultrasound Med. 1985;4:613-6.
49. Merz E, Pashaj S. Current role of 3-D/4D sonography in obstetrics and gynecology. Donald School. J Ultrasound Obstetrics Gynecology 2013;7:400-8.
50. Pisani F, Bianchi ME, Piantelli G, et al. Prenatal diagnosis of agenesis of corpus callosum: what is the neuro-developmental outcome? Pediatr Int 2006;48:298-304.
51. Moutard ML, Kieffer V, Feingold J, et al. Isolated corpus callosm agenesis: a ten-year follow-up after prenatal diagnosis [how are the children without corpus callosum at 10 years of age?]. Prenat Diagn. 2012;32:277-83.

52. Moutard ML, Kieffer V, Feingold J, et al. Agenesis of corpus callosum: prenatal diagnosis and prognosis. Childs Nerv Syst. 2003;19:471-6.
53. D'Addario V, Pinto V, Di Cagno L, et al. The midsagittal view of the fetal brain: a useful landmark in recognizing the cause of fetal cerebral ventriculomegaly. J Perinat Med. 2005;33:423-7.
54. Volpe P, Paladini D, Resta M, et al. Characteristics, associations and outcome of partial agenesis of the corpus callosum in the fetus. Ultrasound Obstet Gynecol. 2006;27:509-16.
55. Volpe P, Campobasso G, De Robertis V, Rembouskos G. Disorders of the prosencephalic development. Prenat Diagn. 2009;29:340-54.
56. Bedeschi MF, Bonaglia MC, Grasso R, et al. Agenesis of the corpus callosum: clinical and genetic study in 63 young patients. Pediatr Neurol. 2006;34:186-93.
57. Sotiriadis A, Makrydimas G. Neurodevelopment after prenatal diagnosis of isolated agenesis of the corpus callosum: an integrative review. Am J Obstet Gynecol. 2012;206: 337.e1-5.
58. Moutard ML, Lewin F, Adamsbaum C, Gelot A, Rodriguez D, Ponsot G. Role of neuropediatrics in prenatal diagnosis. Arch Pediatr. 2011; 8 [Suppl 2]: 442-444s.
59. Fratelli N, Papageorghiou AT, Prefumo F, Bakalis S, Homfray T, Thilaganathan B. Outcome of prenatally diagnosed agenesis of the corpus callosum. Prenat Diagn. 2007;27: 512-7.
60. Moes P, Schilmoeller K, Schillmoer G. Physical, motor, sensory and developmental features associated with agenesis of the corpus callosum. Child Care Health Dev. 2009;5:656-72.
61. Ren T, Anderson A, Shen WB, Huang H, Plachez C, Zhang J, et al. Imaging, anatomical and molecular analysis of the callosal formation in the developing human fetal brain. Anat Rec A Discov Mol Cell Evol Biol. 2006:288:191-204.
62. Barkovich AJ. Pediatric Neuroimaging. Congenital Malformations of the Brain and Skull. 4th ed. Lippincott Philadelphia: Williams & Wilkins. 2005:296-304.
63. Barkovich AJ, Norman D. Anomalies of the corpus callosum: correlation with further anomalies of the brain. Am J Roentgenol. 1988;151:171-9.
64. Hetts SW, Sherr EH, Chao S, et al. Anomalies of the corpus callosum: an MR analysis of the phenotypic spectrum of associated malformations. Am J Roentgenol. 2006;187:1343-8.
65. Bayard S, Gosselin N, Robert M, et al. Inter- and intra-hemispheric processing of visual event-related potentials in the absence of the corpus callosum. J Cogn Neurosci. 2004;16:401-14.
66. Huber-Okrainec J, Blaser SE, Dennis M. Idiom comprehension deficits in relation to corpus callosum agenesis and hypoplasia in children with spina bifida meningomyelocele. Brain Lang. 2005;93:349-68.
67. Badaruddin DH, Andrews GL, Bolte S, Schilmoeller KJ, Schilmoeller G, Paul LK, et al. Social and Behavioral Problems of Children with Agenesis of the Corpus Callosum. Child Psychiatry Hum Dev. 2007.
68. Doherty D, Tu S, Schilmoeller K, et al. Health-related issues in individuals with agenesis of the corpus callosum. Child Care Health Dev. 2006;32:333-42.

19

CHAPTER

Detection of Limb Malformations: Role of 3D/4D Ultrasound

Eberhard Merz

INTRODUCTION

The 3D/4D ultrasound has evolved into a powerful and effective adjunct to conventional 2D ultrasound and has become a part of daily clinical routine in prenatal diagnosis. Once a suspicious finding has been detected in a 2D examination of the fetus, 3D/4D ultrasound is applied as a helpful adjunct in establishing the final diagnosis. Particularly in the diagnosis of fetal limb/skeletal anomalies, which increasingly involves the detection of different surface and bone abnormalities, the various display options offered by 3D ultrasound provide an excellent means of detecting these defects. The 4D ultrasound additionally provides a real-time three-dimensional display of normal and abnormal fetal movements of the extremities. The sequentially stored volumes allow a detailed examination from the memory, similar to a 2D cine loop. The operator can thus rapidly locate the volume which gives the best 3D view of a particular movement phase or anatomical area.

In cases with a high recurrence risk of a particular malformation, 3D/4D rendered images of the normal anatomy give worried parents a greater degree of reassurance than 2D images can provide.

INCIDENCE OF LIMB ANOMALIES

Anomalies of the limbs occur in approximately 2.2% of all newborns.[1]

ETIOLOGY

Limb abnormalities are characterized by a heterogeneous etiology. Possible defects include genetic defects, defects due to exposure to exogenous agents or an amniotic band syndrome or defects due to a severe reduction in amniotic fluid (oligohydramnios). A number of the abnormalities are associated with specific genetic syndromes or chromosomal aberrations.

Different Types of Limb Malformations

Fetal limb malformations can generally be divided into the three following groups:

1. Abnormalities representing a generalized disorder of bone and cartilage growth (osteochondrodysplasias).
2. Abnormalities confined to individual bones or limb segments (e.g., peromelia).
3. Limb malformations impairing fetal mobility (e.g., arthrogryposis multiplex congenita).

3D ULTRASOUND APPEARANCE OF THE LIMBS/FETAL SKELETON

In contrast to 2D ultrasound, which permits images to be displayed in one plane only, 3D ultrasound offers various display options.

Multiplanar View

This view demonstrates the three orthogonal planes at the same time on the monitor **(Figs. 1A to C)**.[2] All planes can be translated or rotated, allowing the operator to conduct a detailed survey of the stored volume. Any arbitrary 2D plane can be reconstructed from a stored volume and displayed.

Tomographic View

This view demonstrates a certain volume in parallel planes as in CT or MRI **(Fig. 2)**.[3,4] The distance between the parallel slices as well as the direction of the slices can be chosen by the operator.

Surface View

Surface imaging is used to demonstrate fetal body surfaces **(Figs. 3A and B)**.[2]

In conventional 3D surface reconstruction, the fetal skin surface is illuminated by a fixed virtual light source

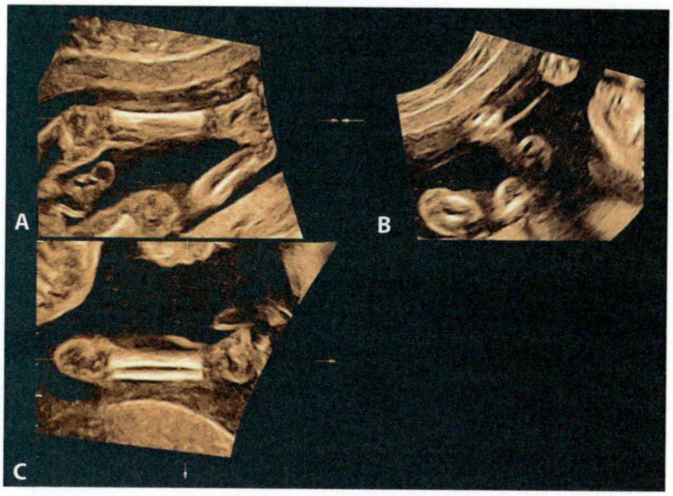

Figs 1A to C: Multiplanar (= triplanar) display of the right lower limb (20 weeks of gestation). (A) Sagittal scan plane, showing tibia; (B) Transverse scan plane, showing tibia and fibula; (C) Coronal scan plane, demonstrating tibia and fibula.

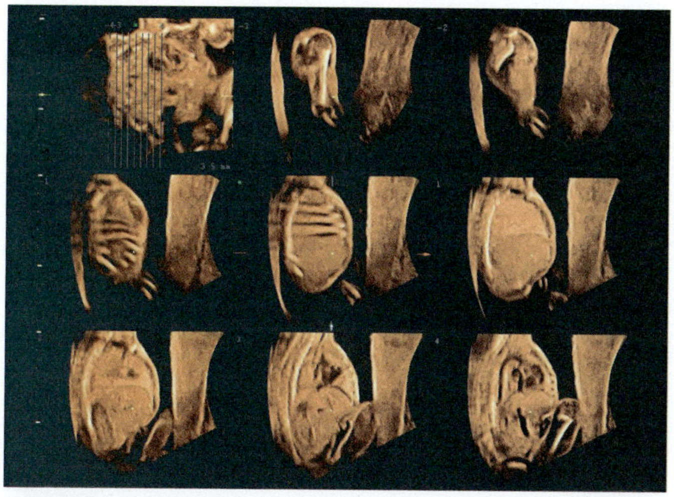

Fig. 2: Tomographic views of the right arm and the right half of the thorax (sagittal planes with a distance of 3.5 mm) (20 weeks).

and the fetus is typically visualized in a shade of yellow **(Figs. 3A and B)**. The brightness of the surface details of the fetal structures is derived directly from the grayscale values of the echoes from the acquired volume. The latest technology "HDlive" uses a movable virtual light source that can illuminate the examination object from all sides **(Figs. 4A to C)**.[5] The brightness and shadow of the fetal surface are calculated from the reflection and scattering behavior of the structures in relation to the light direction, i.e. the original ultrasound grayscale values no longer apply. The human skin-based color spectrum and the movable virtual light source allow almost photographic imaging of fetuses. In the case of optimal positioning of the virtual light source, this technique can be used to detect normal anatomical structures as well as pathological changes, particularly surface defects, with greater detail and clarity than possible with the previous 3D surface technique. This technique provides such extraordinarily realistic imaging of

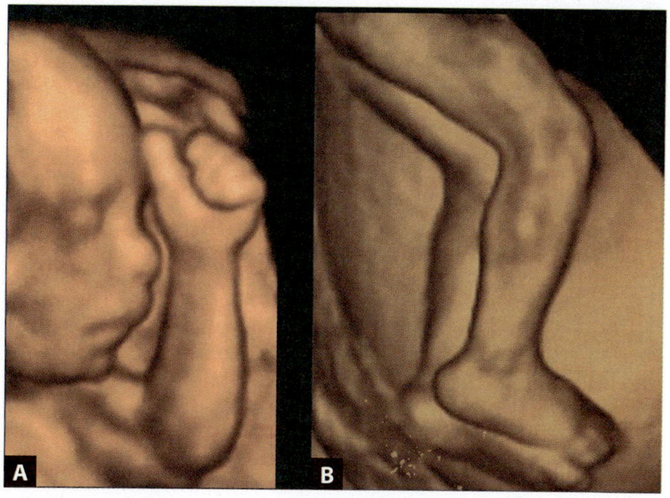

Figs. 3A and B: Surface-rendered views. (A) Lateral view of a fetal face and left forearm (20 weeks); (B) Lateral view of fetal legs (21 weeks).

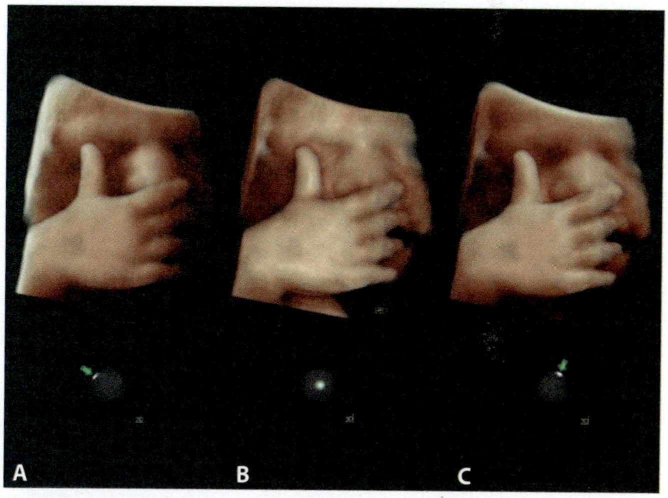

Figs. 4A to C: Surface reconstruction of a fetus (27+2 weeks) using HDlive technology with a movable virtual light source. In Figure 4A the light source illuminates the fetal face and hand from the upper right side of the fetus, in Figure 4B from a front view and in Figure 4C from the upper left side of the fetus. Depending on the position of the virtual light source, the particular anatomical structures (face, hand with fingers) are visualized in a more accentuated manner. The different light and shadow effects also enhances the three-dimensionality of the object to be visualized.

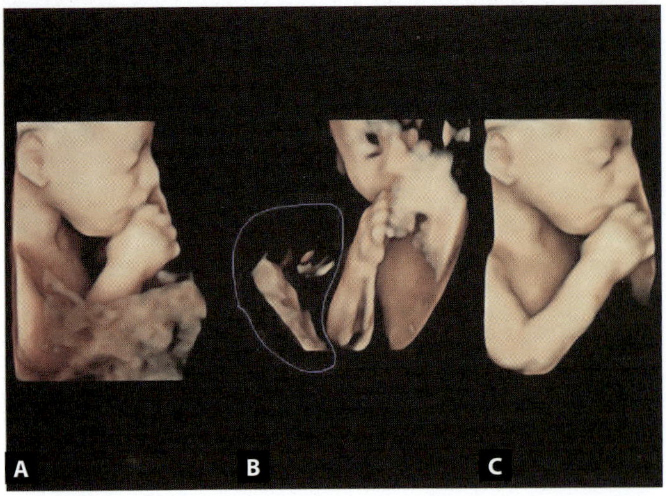

Figs. 5A to C: Use of the electronic scalpel. (A) Image after volume acquisition with overlying structures; (B) Rotating of the volume and removing the overlaying structures by use of the "inside contour mode" (blue line); (C) Final result after re-rotating the volume in the starting position. HDlive (27 weeks).

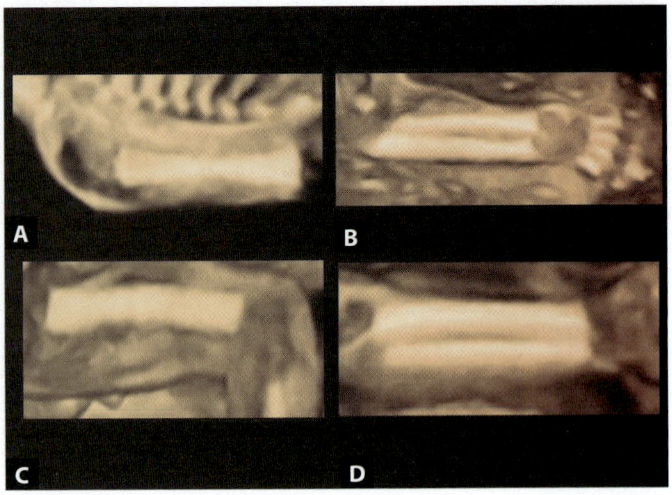

Figs. 6A to D: Rendered views of cut surfaces revealing the normal long bones at 20 weeks of gestation. (A) Humerus; (B) Radius and ulna; (C) Femur; (D) Tibia and fibula.

fetuses that it is almost impossible to differentiate between actual photographs and ultrasound scans.[5]

A basic requirement of all 3D surface rendering is the presence of an adequate fluid pocket in front of the region of interest (ROI) and the absence of overlying or abutting structures. All structures obscuring the ROI have to be removed electronically using an "electronic scalpel" **(Figs. 5A to C)**.[6]

Transparent View

The maximum mode preferentially displays hyperechoic structures like bones, while markedly attenuating less echogenic structures, such as the soft tissue **(Figs. 6 and 7)**.[2] The transparent view is capable of displaying all ossified regions of the fetal skeleton.

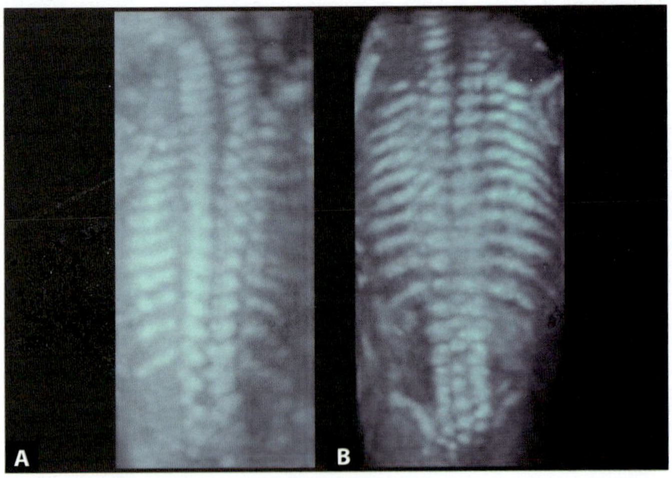

Figs. 7A and B: Transparent (maximum mode) view of normal fetal skeletons. (A) 16 weeks; (B) 20 weeks.

Animated Rotating Display

Entire series of images can be reconstructed within a few seconds with both the surface and the transparent mode. This enables viewing the object of interest from multiple angles in the form of an animated, rotating display[2] **(Figs. 8A to E)**.

4D ULTRASOUND APPEARANCE OF THE LIMBS/FETAL SKELETON

In contrast to 3D ultrasound, which can acquire only static pictures, 4D ultrasound can depict fetal movements in real time **(Figs. 9A to D)**.[7,8] This provides an excellent opportunity to observe limb movements in the surface and the transparent mode.

TRANSVAGINAL/TRANSABDOMINAL ULTRASOUND EXAMINATION OF THE LIMBS/FETAL SKELETON

All phases of embryologic limb development during the first trimester can be depicted with transvaginal 3D/4D ultrasound.[9,10] A targeted search for severe limb anomalies can already be conducted at this stage. However, most of

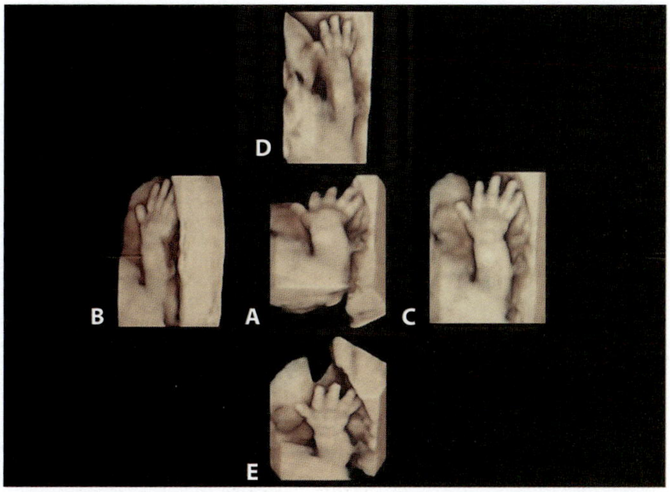

Figs. 8A to E: Cine mode with demonstration of the region of interest from different angles by rotating the volume around the Y-axis (A to B and C) or X-axis (A to D and E). (A) Starting position, (B) rotating 50° to the left, (C) rotating 50° to the right, (D) rotating up 50°, (E) rotating down 50°. HDlive (26+5 weeks).

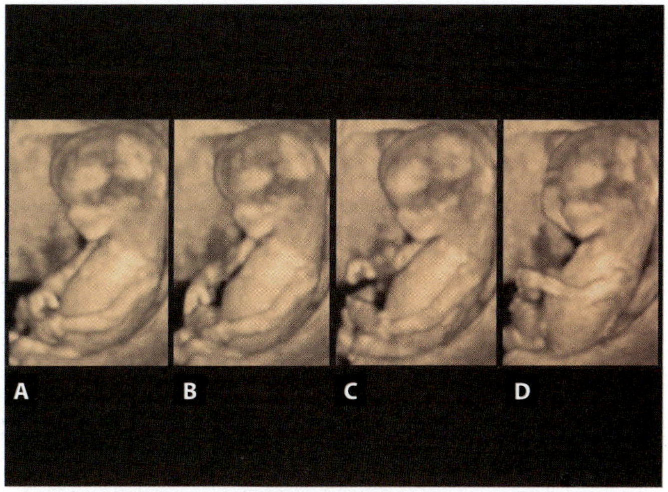

Figs. 9A to D: 4D rendering: Surface demonstration of limb movements (12 weeks).

the antenatal diagnoses will be done using transabdominal 3D/4D ultrasound starting at approximately 13 weeks of gestation.

GENERAL ASPECTS OF THE SONOGRAPHIC DETECTION OF LIMB MALFORMATIONS

During the second trimester, a large number of fetal malformations are detectable by conventional two-dimensional ultrasound.[11,12] This technology can, however, provide only two-dimensional sectional views of the fetus, while individual sectional planes of the region of interest cannot be achieved in the presence of an unfavorable position of the fetus. Furthermore, complex anomalies require an evaluation not only in one, but in multiple planes.[2]

The 3D/4D ultrasound technology with its different display modes facilitates the demonstration of skeletal/limb malformations.[13-27] In particular surface anomalies can be communicated to the parents or the pediatric surgeon. Conversely, in cases where fetal surface defects have been excluded, a key advantage of 3D ultrasound may be seen in its ability to give the worried parents a greater degree of reassurance than 2D images can provide.[28]

In a study comparing 2D and 3D ultrasound for the diagnosis of limb malformations, Merz et al. reported an advantage of 3D over 2D ultrasound in 90.3% of cases.[20]

The fact that the majority of skeletal anomalies occur in a low risk population makes a thorough prenatal

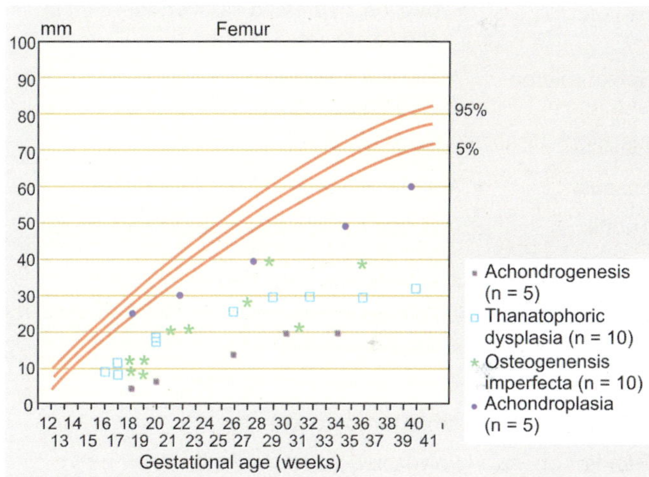

Fig. 10: Femur length in various osteochondrodysplasias. The degree of bone shortening is highest in achondrogenesis and smallest in achondroplasia
(Adapted from Merz E.[12])

ultrasound examination a precondition for the detection of limb malformations. A definitive diagnosis of a limb malformation requires not only the measurement of the fetal head, abdomen and femur but of all long bones. All data should be plotted on nomograms to obtain a precise profile of the fetal growth and to determine the severity of bone shortening **(Fig. 10 and Table 1)**.

In cases where fetal bone length cannot be accurately interpreted due to uncertain data, it can be helpful to compare the length of the femur and the foot. At least during the second trimester, the femur and the foot have

TABLE 1: Bone parameters for the differential diagnosis of limb anomalies.
Bone length
Pattern of bone shortening (rhizomelia, mesomelia, micromelia)
Absence or hypoplasia of a bone (e.g., radial or fibular aplasia)
Abnormal bone structure (diaphysis, metaphysis)
Degree of bowing
Detection of bone fractures

(Adapted from Merz E.[12])

TABLE 2: Parameters for the differentiation of skeletal anomalies.	
Head	• Head size (macrocephaly) • Abnormal head shape (cloverleaf) • Ossification of calvaria • Deformable calvaria • Hypertelorism • Abnormal facial profile (flat profile, frontal bossing, depressed nasal bridge, cleft lip and palate, retrognathia)
Spinal column	Abnormal curvature Hypomineralization
Clavicle	Aplasia, hypoplasia
Scapula	Aplasia, hypoplasia
Thorax	• Thoracic shape (champagne-cork thorax, bell-shaped) • Hypoplasia of the bony thorax • Pulmonary hypoplasia • Cardiac anomaly
Pelvic bones	Absent or delayed ossification
Gender	Ambiguous gender
Hands	Polydactyly
Feet	Foot length, pes equinovarus, polydactyly
Movement pattern	Decreased motor activity

(Adapted from Merz E.[12])

similar lengths. A femur which is measured considerably shorter than the foot is always suspicious for skeletal dysplasia.[12]

In all cases of suspected bone dysplasia additional anatomic details have to be checked to enable a differential diagnosis **(Table 2)**.

Osteochondrodysplasias

The incidence of skeletal dysplasias is approximately 1:4,100 newborns, including stillbirths.[29] The incidence of lethal osteochondrodysplasias is approximately 1:19,000 live births.[30]

TABLE 3: Patterns of limb shortening.	
Rhizomelia	Shortening of the proximal long bones (femur, humerus)
Mesomelia	Shortening of the distal long bones (tibia, fibula, radius, ulna)
Acromelia	Shortening of the distal segments (hands, feet)
Micromelia	Shortening of the proximal and distal long bones

(Adapted from Merz E.[12])

TABLE 19.4: Fatal osteochondrodysplasias with narrow thorax.
Achondrogenesis **(Figs. 10, 11 and 14)**
Hypochondrogenesis
Thanatophoric dysplasia **(Figs. 10, 12 and 14)**
Osteogenesis imperfecta II **(Figs. 10, 13 and 15)**
Camptomelic dysplasia **(Fig. 16)**
Homozygous achondroplasia
Short rib polydactyly syndrome I–VII **(Fig. 17)**

The most common skeletal dysplasias are:

- Thanatophoric dysplasia
- Achondroplasia
- Achondrogenesis
- Osteogenesis imperfecta.

All of these dysplasias are characterized by severe limb shortening. The degree and type of shortening as well as the demonstration of fractures or bowing of the long bones are used to differentiate between the different osteochondrodysplasias **(Fig. 10 and Table 3)**.

The lethal group of skeletal dysplasias is characterized by short limb bones, a narrow thorax and hypoplastic lungs **(Table 4)**.[12,31]

The photorealistic view of the fetus in the surface display provides valuable opportunities for the detection of disproportional growth of short limbs **(Fig. 11)**, frontal bossing **(Fig. 12)**, narrow thorax **(Fig. 12)**, or axis deviation of the limbs **(Fig. 13)**. The transparent display facilitates the detection of ossification defects involving the long limb bones, the skull, the bony thorax and the spine, scapula and pelvis. Not only shortening but also bowing or the presence of fractures can be observed in the long bones **(Figs 14 to 16)**.

The interactive shift from one display mode to the other is particularly useful for the detection or exclusion of specific abnormalities, making it possible to identify

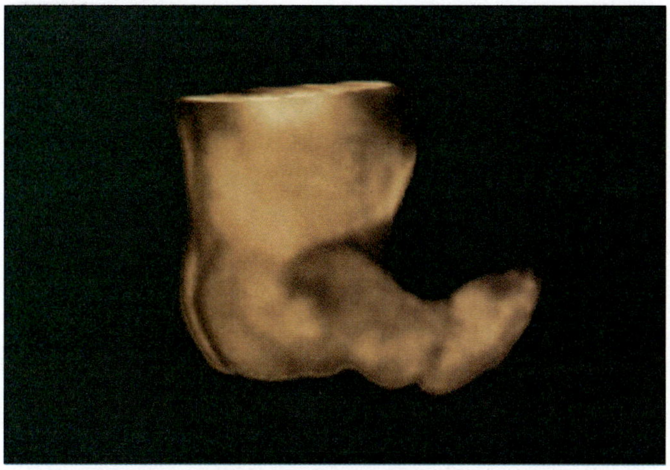

Fig. 11: Surface-rendered view of a fetus with achondrogenesis (22 weeks).

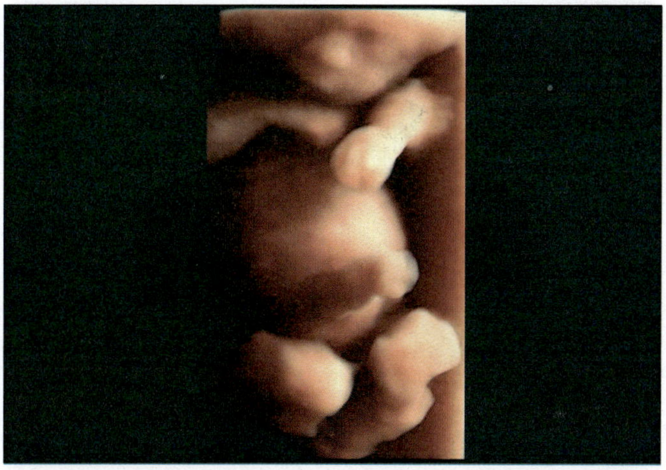

Fig. 13: Surface-rendered view of a fetus with osteogenesis imperfecta II. Severe bowing of the limbs due to several fractures of the long bones (20 weeks).

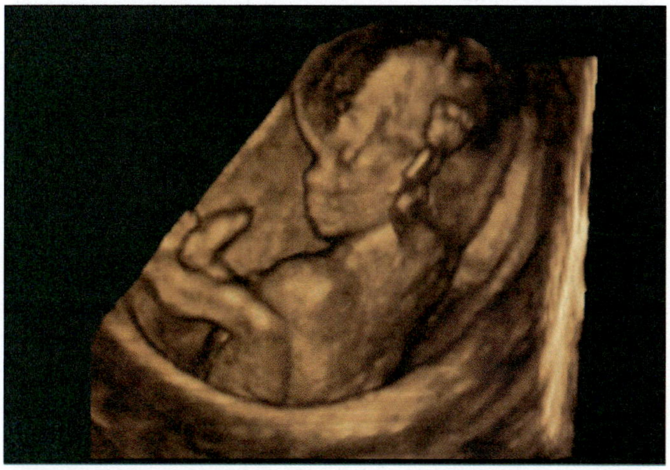

Fig. 12: Surface-rendered view of thanatophoric dysplasia with short limbs, frontal bossing and narrow thorax (16+2 weeks).

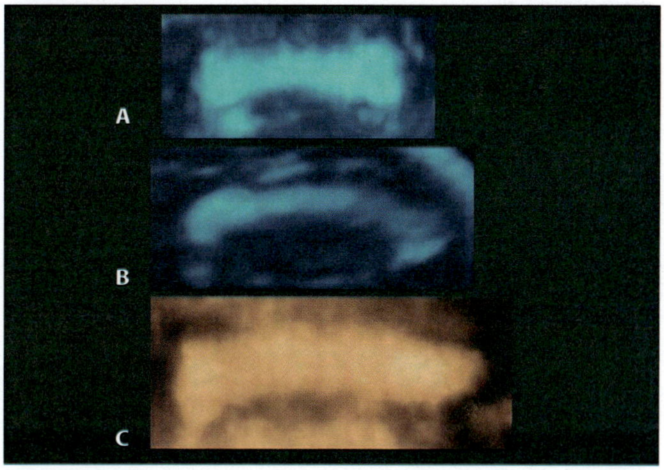

Figs. 14A to C: Transparent views of different femurs; (A) Very short femur in a fetus with achondrogenesis; (B) Short and bowed femur in a fetus with thanatophoric dysplasia; (C) Slightly shortened femur in a fetus with achondroplasia.

even subtle fetal abnormalities and to define the extent of a defect in all dimensions.

An essential aim of prenatal diagnosis is the early detection or exclusion of lethal forms of skeletal dysplasia. However, it has to be taken into account that some osteochondrodysplasias, in particular nonlethal dysplasias such as heterozygous achondroplasia **(Fig. 14C)**, are not detectable before 20 weeks of gestation.

Limb Anomalies Involving Specific Segments Only

Isolated limb defects can be detected only by critical comparison of the right and left limb.

Surface rendering has created new capabilities in the diagnosis of limb anomalies which involve specific segments only **(Table 5)**.[32] Since the examination is not performed on a live, moving fetus but on a digitally stored limb that can be rotated freely in space, isolated limb defects, such as amelia **(Figs. 18A and B)** or peromelia **(Fig. 19)** can readily be detected. Nevertheless, the examiner needs to be very careful in establishing the diagnosis. If the arm or the leg is not completely within the volume box, the distal part of the limb will be electronically cut by the volume box and may thus falsely be interpreted as a malformation, e.g., peromelia **(Figs. 20A and B)**. In all cases of uncertainty the

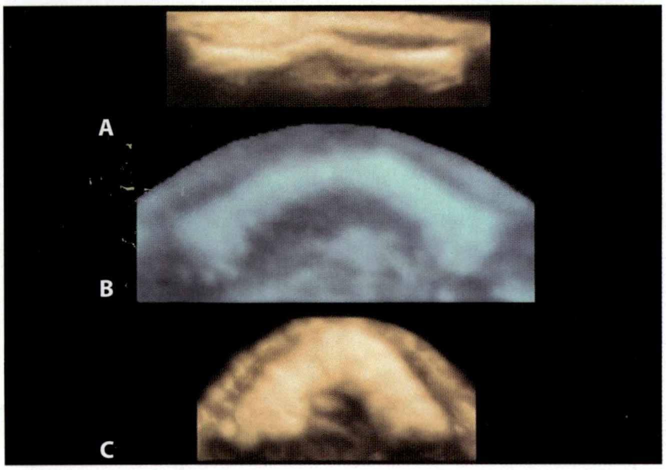

Figs. 15A to C: Transparent views of different femurs with deviation of the bone axis due to fractures (osteogenesis imperfecta II); (A) Angulation; (B) Moderate bowing; (C) Severe bowing.

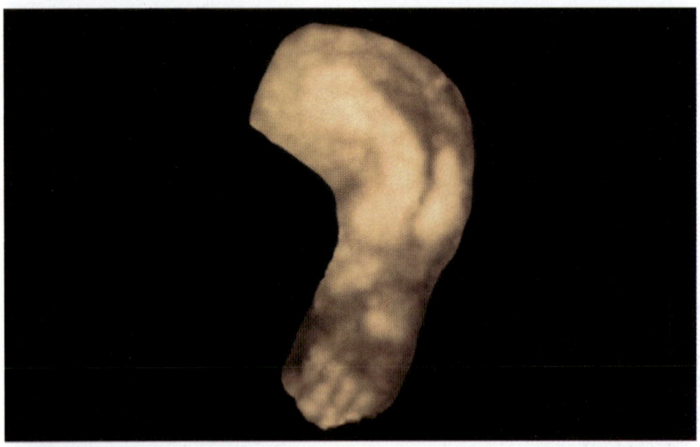

Fig. 16: Severe bowing of the lower limb bones in camptomelic dysplasia (20 weeks).

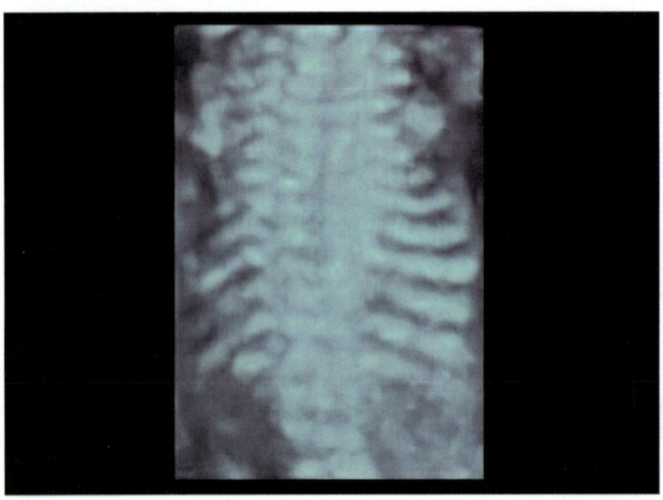

Fig. 17: Short rib polydactyly syndrome. The maximum mode reveals the poorly ossified short ribs (22 weeks).

TABLE 5: Nomenclature for limb abnormalities

Term	Definition
Amelia	Absence of one or more limbs
Peromelia	Absence or deformity of the terminal part of a limb or limbs
Hemimelia	Absence of the distal portion of one limb (form of peromelia)
Meromelia	Partial absence of a limb
Acheira	Absence of one or both hands
Apodia	Absence of one or both feet
Acheiropodia	Absence of hands and feet
Adactyly	Absence of fingers or toes
Phocomelia	A malformation in which the proximal portions of the extremities are poorly developed or absent. Hands and feet are directly attached to the trunk
Ectromelia	Hypoplasia of the long bones of the limbs
Oligodactylia	Subnormal number of fingers or toes
Polydactyly • preaxial • postaxial	Condition of having supernumerary fingers or toes • Extradigit on radial or tibial side • Extradigit on ulnar or fibular side
Brachydactylia	Abnormal shortness of the fingers or toes
Ectrodactylism	Absence of all or part of a digit (split hand, lobster claw)
Sirenomelia	Anomaly in which the lower extremities are fused
Syndactylism	A fusion of two or more fingers or toes
Clinodactyly	Permanent medial or lateral deflection of one or more fingers
Camptodactylia	Permanent flexion of fingers or toes
Talipes • valgus • varus	Clubfoot • Heel and foot are turned outward • Heel and foot are turned inward

false-positive defect can be excluded in an animated rotating image display.

Axis deviations of the limbs **(Figs. 21A and B)** are always suspicious of fractures in the long bones or aplasia of one bone (e.g., radius aplasia). The absence of radius and angular deviation of the hand serve as an indication of a Holt–Oram syndrome **(Figs. 21A and B).** Surface demonstration of the fetal hand further permits the detection of ectrodactylism **(Fig. 22)**, oligodactylia, brachydactylia or syndactylism **(Fig. 23)**. Moreover, the 3D surface analysis of the stored hand can conclusively demonstrate the presence of polydactylia, such as pre- or postaxial hexadactyly

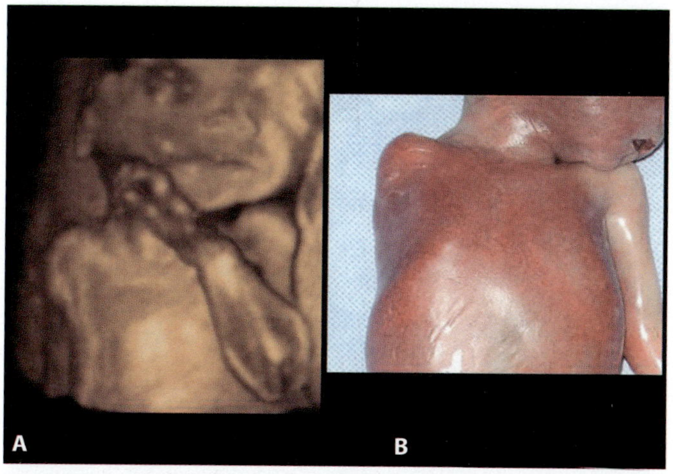

Figs. 18A and B: (A) Surface-rendered view of amelia on the right side (22 weeks); (B) Specimen after abortion.

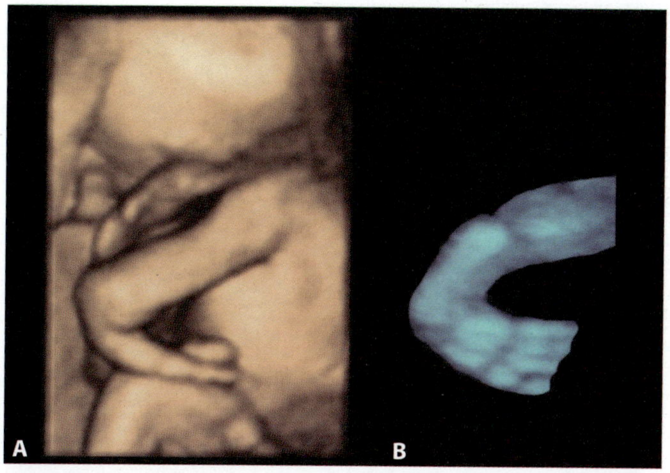

Figs. 21A and B: Fetus with Holt–Oram syndrome (19 weeks). (A) Surface-rendered view of the left arm with severe deviation of the forearm; (B) Transparent view of the same arm showing radial aplasia and severe angulation of the hand with only 4 fingers.

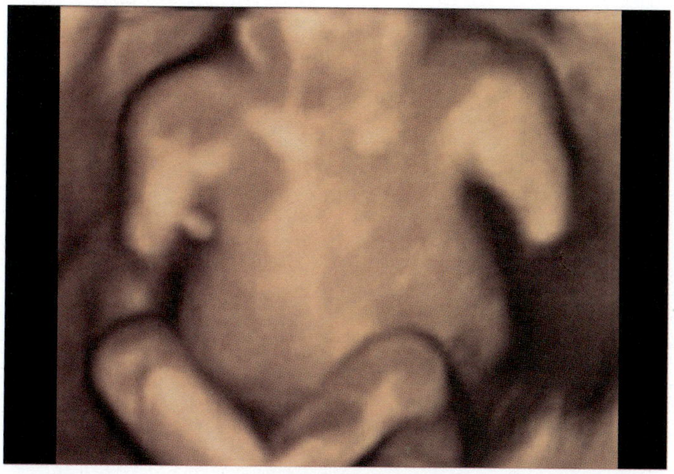

Fig. 19: Surface-rendered view of bilateral peromelia (17+1 weeks).

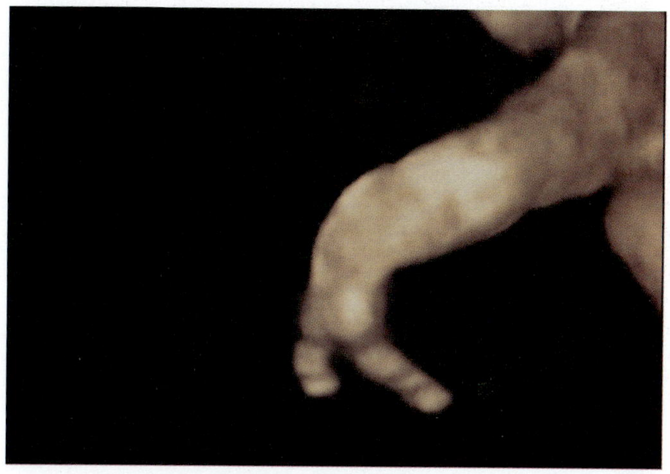

Fig. 22: Surface-rendered view of a fetus with ectrodactylism (22 weeks).

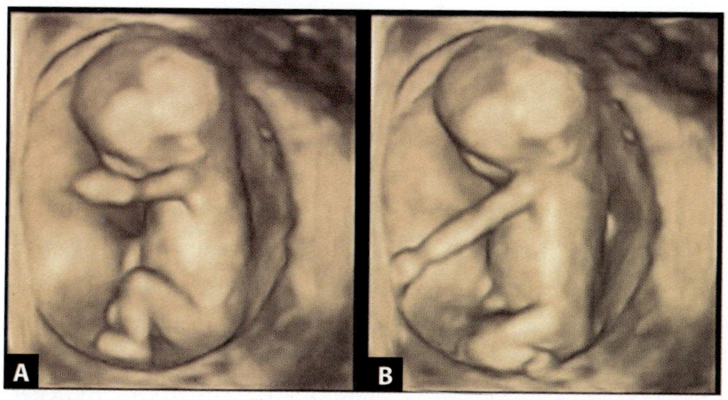

Fig. 20A and B: (A) Surface-rendered view mimicking a peromelia, due to placement of the distal forearm outside the volume box; (B) Same fetus with demonstration of the entire arm inside the volume box (17+4 weeks).

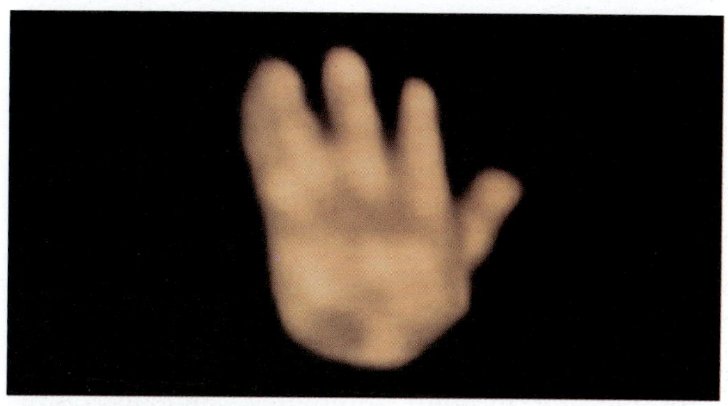

Fig. 23: Surface-rendered view of syndactylism between finger 4 and 5 (21+6 weeks).

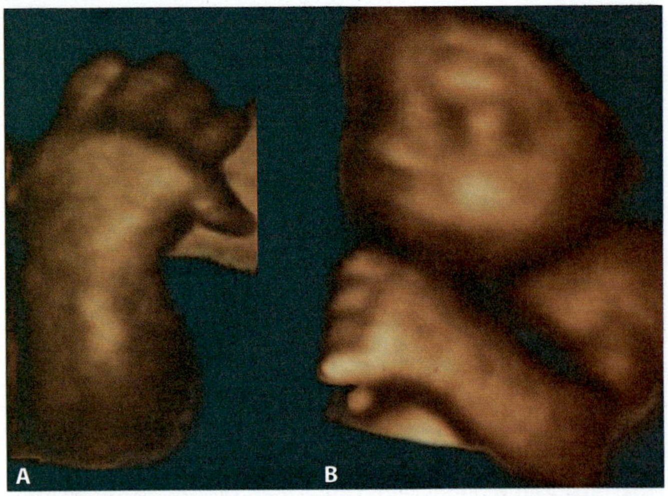

Figs. 24A and B: Surface-rendered views of hexadactyly. (A) Postaxial hexadactyly right (31 weeks); (B) Postaxial hexadactyly left (31 weeks).

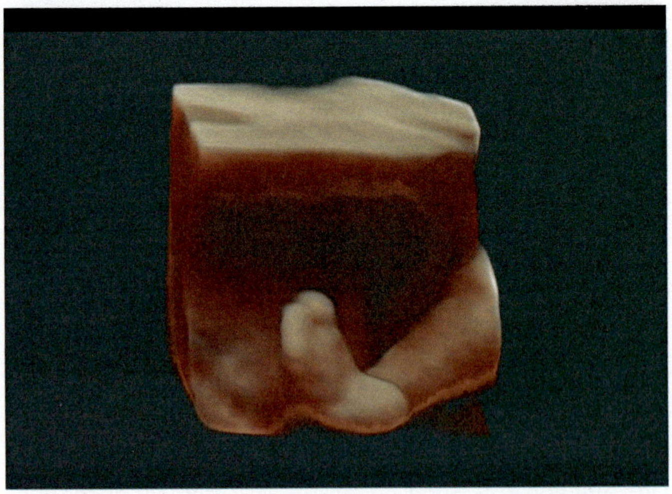

Fig. 26: Surface-rendered view of a club foot (31+6 weeks).

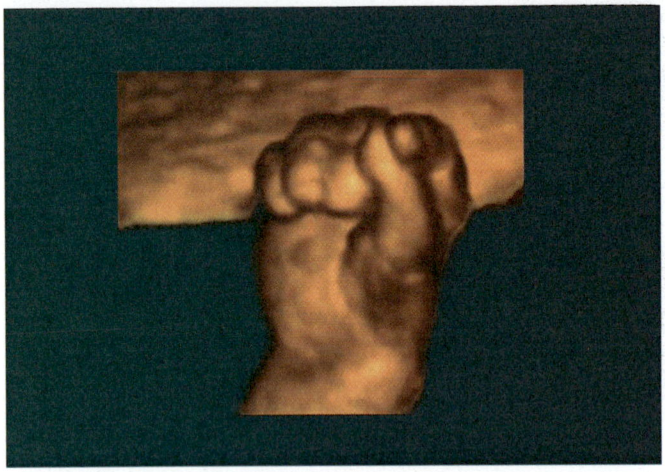

Fig. 25: Overlapping fingers, indicating the presence of a chromosomal defect (here trisomy 18) (29 weeks).

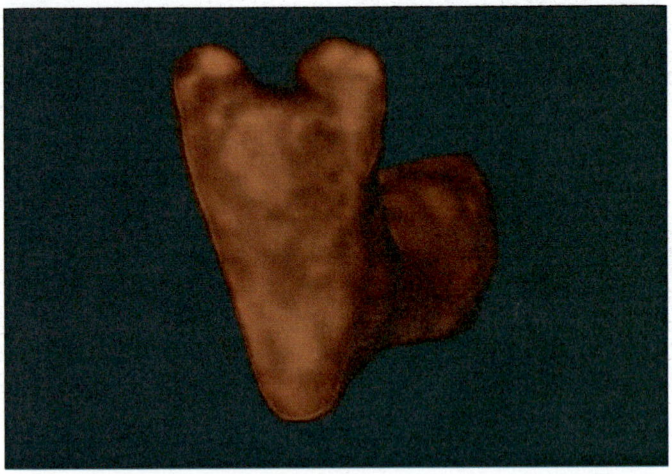

Fig. 27: Surface-rendered view of a split foot with only two toes (21+2 weeks).

(Figs. 24A and B). Clinodactyly, camptodactylia or overlapping fingers **(Fig. 25)** are also easily detectable.

This also applies to a detailed examination of the foot. Angular deformities, such as club foot **(Fig. 26)** or oligodactylia of the foot **(Fig. 27)** can be readily demonstrated.[15,17]

In all limb anomalies involving only specific segments of the foot, the use of the transparent mode is mandatory to display the bone defects **(Fig. 21B)**.

A number of limb anomalies, such as radius aplasia or overlapping fingers **(Fig. 25)**, are indicators of chromosomal aberrations and should serve as an indication for karyotyping.

Limb Malformations which Impair Fetal Mobility

4D ultrasound with its acquisition rate of up to 35 volumes/s provides an excellent means of detecting abnormal fetal movement patterns.[28] All grades of intrauterine flexion or extension contractures affecting a variable number of joints can occur in arthrogryposis multiplex congenita (AMC) **(Fig. 28)**. Polyhydramnios combined with the absence of fetal movement and clubfeet invariably gives rise to the suspicion of AMC with CNS involvement.[12] The combination of AMC with pulmonary hypoplasia serves as an indication of a Pena-Shokeir syndrome[12] with a grave prognosis.

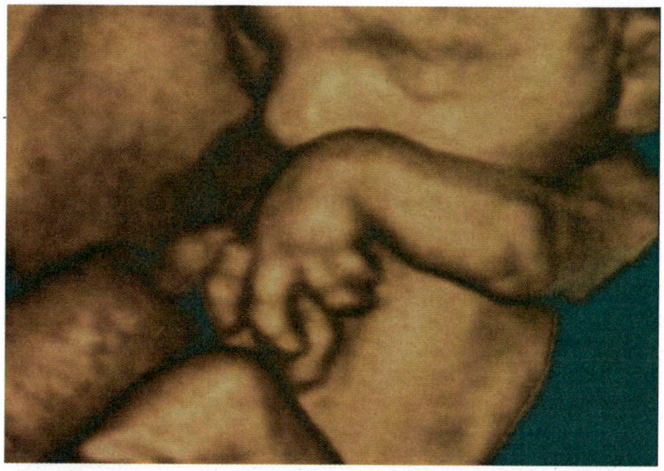

Fig. 28: Surface-rendered view of a fetus with arthrogryposis multipex congenita (21+6 weeks). Despite the acute polyhydramnios the fetus shows no arm movement due to contractures of the wrist and fingers.

A neural tube defect has to be excluded in all cases of abnormal movement patterns of the fetal limbs.

REFERENCES

1. Schaller A. Geburtsmedizinische Teratologie: Extremitätenfehlbildungen. Urban & Schwarzenberg, München; 1975. p. 138.
2. Merz E. 3D Ultrasound in prenatal diagnosis. In. Merz E (ed): Ultrasound in Obstetrics. Thieme, Stuttgart - New York; 2005. pp. 516-8.
3. Kalache KD, Bamberg C, Proquitte H, Sarioglu N, Lebek H, Esser T. Three-dimensional multi-slice view: new prospects for evaluation of congenital anomalies in the fetus. J Ultrasound Med. 2006;25(8):1041-9.
4. Merz E. Tomographic ultrasound imaging. Ultraschall in Med. 2006;27(4):307-8.
5. Merz E. Surface reconstruction of a fetus (28+2 GW) using HDlive technology. Ultraschall in Med. 2012;33(3):211-2.
6. Merz E, Miric-Tesanic D, Welter C. Value of the electronic scalpel (cut mode) in the evaluation of the fetal face. Ultrasound Obstet Gynecol. 2000;16(6):564-8.
7. Kurjak A, Carrera J, Medic M, Azumendi G, Andonotopo W, Stanojevic M. The antenatal development of fetal behavioral patterns assessed by four-dimensional sonography. J Matern Fetal Neonatal Med. 2005;17(6):401-16.
8. Hata T, Kanenishi K, Tanaka H, Marumo G, Sasaki M. Four-dimensional ultrasound evaluation of fetal neurobehavioral development. Donald School Journal of Ultrasound in Obstetrics and Gynecology. 2010;4:233-48.
9. Benoit B. The value of three-dimensional ultrasonography in the screening of the fetal skeleton. Childs Nerv Syst. 2003;19(7-8):403-9.
10. Benoit B, Hafner T, Kurjak A, Kupesic S, Bekavac I, Bozek T. Three-dimensional sonoembryology. J Perinat Med. 2002;30(1):63-73.
11. Goncalves L, Jeanty P. Fetal biometry of skeletal dysplasias: a multicentric study. J. Ultrasound Med. 1994;13(12):977-85.
12. Merz E. Anomalies of the extremities. In: Merz E (Ed.). Ultrasound in Obstetrics. Thieme, Stuttgart - New York: 2005. pp. 336-58.
13. Steiner H, Spitzer D, Weiss-Wichert PH, Graf AH, Staudach A. Three-dimensional ultrasound in prenatal diagnosis of skeletal dysplasia. Prenat Diagn. 1995;15(4):373-7.
14. Lee A, Kratochwil A, Deutinger J, Bernaschek G. Three dimensional ultrasound in diagnosing phocomelia. Ultrasound Obstet Gynecol. 1995;5(4):238-40.
15. Merz E, Bahlmann F, Weber G. Volume (3D)-scanning in the evaluation of fetal malformations: a new dimension in prenatal diagnosis. Ultrasound Obstet Gynecol. 1995;5(4):222-7.
16. Dyson RL, Pretorius DH, Dudorick NE, Jophnson DD, Sklansky MS, Cantrell CJ, et al. Three-dimensional ultrasound in the evaluation of fetal anomalies. Ultrasound Obstet Gynecol. 2000;16(4):321-8.
17. Kos M, Hafner T, Funduk-Kurjak B, Bozek T, Kurjak A. Limb deformities and three-dimensional ultrasound. J Perinat Med. 2002;30(1):40-7.
18. Krakow D, Williams J 3rd, Poehl M, Rimoin DL, Platt LD. Use of three-dimensional ultrasound imaging in the diagnosis of prenatal-onset skeletal dysplasias. Ultrasound Obstet Gynecol. 2003;21(5):467-72.
19. Ruano R, Molho M, Roume J, Ville Y. Prenatal diagnosis of fetal skeletal dysplasias by combining two-dimensional and three-dimensional ultrasound and intrauterine three-dimensional helical computer tomography. Ultrasound Obstet Gynecol. 2004;24(2):134-40.
20. Merz E, Welter C. 2D and 3D ultrasound in the evaluation of normal and abnormal fetal anatomy in the second and third trimesters in a level III center. Ultraschall in Med. 2005;26(1):9-16.
21. Chen CP, Chang TY, Su YN, Hsu CY, Wang W. Prenatal two- and three-dimensional ultrasound diagnosis of limb reduction defects associated with homozygous alpha-thalassemia. Fetal Diagn Ther. 2006;21(4):374-9.
22. David AL, Turnbull C, Scott R, Freeman J, Bilardo CM, van Maarle M, Chitty LS. Diagnosis of Apert syndrome in the second-trimester using 2D and 3D ultrasound. Prenat Diagn. 2007;27(7):629-32.
23. Kennelly MM, Moran P. A clinical algorithm of prenatal diagnosis of radial ray defects with two and three dimensional ultrasound. Prenat Diagn. 2007;27(8):730-7.
24. Lin IW, Chueh, HY, Chang SD, Cheng PJ. The application of three-dimensional ultrasonography in the prenatal diagnosis of arthrogryposis. Taiwan J Obstet Gynecol. 2008;47(1):75-8.

25. Kang A, Visca E, Bruder E, Holzgreve W, Struben H, Tercanli S. Prenatal diagnosis of a case of ectrodactyly in 2D and 3D ultrasound. Ultraschall Med. 2009;30(2):121-3.
26. Tsai PY, Chang CH, Yu CH, Cheng YC, Chang FM. Thanatophoric dysplasia: role of 3D imensional sonography. J Clin Ultrasound. 2009;37(1):31-4.
27. Bashiri A, Sheizaf B, Burstein E, Landau D, Hershkovitz R, Mazor M. Three dimensional ultrasound diagnosis of caudal regression syndrome at 14 gestational weeks. Arch Gynecol Obstet. 2009;280(3):505-7.
28. Merz E. 3D and 4D ultrasonography. In: Twining P, McHugo JM, Pilling DW (Eds): Textbook of fetal abnormalities. Churchill Livingstone: Elsevier; 2007. pp. 483-93.
29. Camera G, Mastroiacovo P. Birth prevalence of skeletal dysplasias in the Italian multicentric monitoring system for birth defects. In: Papadatos CJ, Bartsocas CS (Eds): Skeletal Dysplasias. New York: Alan R. Liss; 1982; pp. 441-9.
30. Curran JP, Sigman BA, Opitz, JM. Lethal forms of chondrodysplastic dwarfism. Pediatrics. 1974;53(1):76-85.
31. Merz E, Miric-Tesanic D, Bahlmann F, Weber G, Hallermann C. Prenatal sonographic chest and lung measurements for predicting severe pulmonary hypoplasia. Prenat Diagn. 1999;19(7):614-9.
32. Merz E, Oberstein A, Welter C. 3D/4D ultrasound - diagnostic value in the assessment of anomalies affecting specific limb segments or bones. Ultrasound Obstet Gynecol. 2009;34 (Suppl. 1)178.

20

CHAPTER

The Fetal Thorax

Aleksandar Ljubic, Tatjana Bozanovic

INTRODUCTION

Although relatively uncommon, congenital abnormalities in the thorax are important because of the potential effect on lung growth as well as the effect of the intrinsic abnormality.

DEVELOPMENTAL ANATOMY AND ULTRASONOGRAPHIC CORRELATIONS

The ossification of the thoracic cage/ribs begins at the end of the first trimester.[1] The lower aperture of the thorax with the lower ribs is one of the landmarks for measurement of the abdomen. The thoracic transverse diameter, the mean abdominal diameter and the abdominal circumference are measurements taken at virtually the same level of the fetal body. Measurement of the thoracic length in a long axis of the midline section is done from the superior end of the sternum to the level of the diaphragm.

The rib length is measured by tracing the lateral edge of a rib at the level of the four-chamber view. Its size correlates well with fetal age, thus this parameter can be useful in management of a pregnancy with fetal skeletal dysplasia.[2]

The sternum shows extremely individual variation in its development: the number of sonographically visible ossification centers varies (up to six), and the first 2 to 3 ossification centers appear at the 19 weeks of gestation, a fourth center during weeks 22 to 23, and five ossification centers are usually visible from 29 weeks onwards.[1]

The main structures in the fetal thorax that are subject to examination are the heart, the lungs and eventually the esophagus. The anatomy of the heart is of interest because it can be influenced by extracardiac anomalies within thorax, e.g., unilateral pulmonal hypoplasia or cystic adenomatoid lung malformation. While the heart occupies approximately half of the size of the thorax, during the embryonic period it occupies one-third of the thoracic area positioned in the middle of the thorax with the apex pointing towards the left during the second and the third trimester.[2] The lungs are homogeneously echogenic and largely isoechoic comparing to other mediastinal structures. The left lung is limited in its extent by the heart. Because of its complex anatomy and importance, the detailed anatomy and anomalies of the heart are discussed in a different chapter.

Diaphragm

The borderline between the thorax (lungs, heart) and the abdominal content is the diaphragm. Sonographically, the diaphragm appears as a thin, dark, arched line; it usually shows a dome on each side, where the right side seems higher than the left side. However, a recent anatomical studies[3] did not find any difference between the height of the left and the right diaphragmatic dome. The costodiaphragmatic recess is most commonly located at the level of the 9th rib.[3] The *function of the diaphragm*, namely breathing, has been the subject of extensive ultrasound research. As early as the 1970s, ultrasound studies of fetal breathing movements (FBM) in human fetuses showed that their presence was indicative of well-being, while the absence of FBM, though less reliably, was a sign of pregnancy disorder. Movements of the diaphragm start as early as 9 to 10 weeks.[4] Hiccups can be registered first, followed by breathing movements during week 10.

At 8 weeks of gestation, clear identification of the difference between thoracic and abdominal content is already possible, especially in those cases with a mild fluid accumulation in the thorax or pericardiac cavity, however, at that stage the pleuroperitoneal canals are still open. The diaphragm, or rather the dividing line between the thoracic and abdominal content, becomes detectable at approximately 10 to11 weeks.

Lungs

The development of the vertebrate lung has been subdivided into five distinct periods based on the anatomical changes that occur in lung architecture: embryonic (3–7 weeks), pseudoglandular (7–17 weeks), canalicular (17–29 weeks), saccular (24–36 weeks), and alveolar (36 weeks to maturity). Initially, the tracheobronchial tubules are formed from the pulmonary diverticulum that forms at the medial tracheolaryngeal sulcus in the ventral wall of the foregut. Branching of the trachea produces two lobar bronchi on the left and three on the right side, defining the lobar anatomy of the human lung. The esophagus and trachea separate, bronchial tubules subdivide to form the bronchial pulmonary segments, and the splanchnic mesenchyme undergoes differentiation and organization to form blood vessels, lymphatics, and other supporting structures. In the pseudoglandular period (7–17 weeks) there is rapid expansion of the conducting airways and peripheral lung tubules, which continue to branch and bud to form acinar tubules. The expansion of these small tubules in the periphery of the lung produces a glandular appearance. The peripheral lung mesenchyme thins and becomes increasingly vascularized. Neuroendocrine bodies, nerves and organized smooth muscle are observed in the developing areas. Cartilage rings form around the segmental bronchi. The pleura and peritoneal cavity closes, the diaphragm thickens and becomes increasingly muscularized.[5]

The *echogenicity of the lungs* usually appears somewhat brighter than the echogenicity of the liver; this becomes clearer by applying harmonic imaging **(Figs. 1A and B)**.[6] Tekesin and co-workers tried to quantify this subjective assessment of the tissue appearance by quantitative ultrasonic tissue characterization.[6] They concluded that the echogenicity of the fetal lung showed a particular changing pattern during pregnancy. The mean gray value of the lungs was almost the same as that of the liver at 22 to 23 weeks gestation, decreased between 23 and 31 weeks, and increased again later in pregnancy. They thought that these changes of echogenicity coincided with the saccular and alveolar phases of fetal lung development. Normal data for the *pulmonal size* are important to assess lung development in a fetus at risk for pulmonary hypoplasia such as congenital diaphragmatic hernia, cystic adenomatoid lung malformation or pleural effusions.

During the recent 10 years, 2D ultrasound[7,8] and 3D ultrasound assessment[6,9,10] of normal and abnormal lungs has been studied *in extenso*. The significance of *3D ultrasound volumetry versus 2D measurements* in the prenatal assessment of lung hypoplasia still remains to be evaluated in studies on a larger scale. For example, in diaphragmatic hernia the identification of the lung contours is very difficult, especially on the side of the diaphragmatic defect. The potential of lung volumetry in the prenatal assessment of fetal lung anomalies has already been indicated.[10,11]

Esophagus

The examination of the fetal *esophagus* has received little attention in the medical literature. The esophagus is a tube permitting the passage of fluid to the stomach during the process of swallowing. The esophagus is usually empty except in pathological conditions such as duodenal obstruction, when an increased fluid volume dilates the duodenum, the stomach, and in several cases the

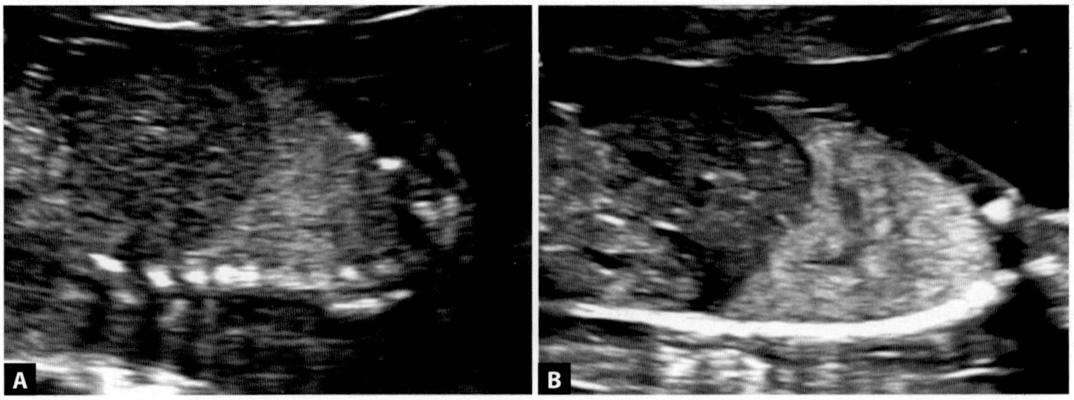

Figs. 1A and B: Sagittal section through right lung, diaphragm, liver and bowel at 18 weeks; (A) standard gray scale; (B) by using harmonic imaging a better distinction between liver and lungs is achieved.

esophagus as well. The esophagus has a tubular echogenic appearance consisting of four parallel echogenic lines, and can be seen in the thorax in close contact with the posterior aspect of the heart.[2] These lines represent the outer and luminal borders of the esophageal wall. In early pregnancy, these echogenic lines melt together on the ultrasound screen into two or one echogenic line.

Malinger et al.,[12] examined 60 fetuses of between 19 and 25 weeks to demonstrate luminal patency and peristaltic waves of the esophagus. They obtained complete anatomical visualization of the entire esophagus throughout its course in 87% of the cases, and at least partial visualization was possible in 97%. Passage of fluid through the esophageal lumen was recorded during 5 minutes of examination in 90% of the fetuses. Thus, it is possible to evaluate the esophagus in fetuses with suspected obstruction.[13]

Thymus

The 3-vessel view is a parallel plan to the 4-chamber view, but a little bit more cranial which is a plan also for evaluation of thymus. The thymus is just in front of the great arteries at the 3-vessel plan. It is easier to recognize from the late 2nd trimester onwards, when it starts to undergo significant hypertrophy. It appears as a well-defined roundish solid structure interposed between the great vessels, just behind the sternum and weakly hypoechoic in which this different echogenicity is not easy to pick up, especially if not high-frequency (>5 MHz) transducer is used. The thymus is located on top of the heart and unlike the lungs, shows movements synchronous with the cardiac cycle.

SCANNING TECHNIQUES

The fetus is usually scanned with a 3.5 to 5.0 MHz probe. The thorax is scanned in a transaxial plane, supplemented by sagittal and coronal planes as needed. The four chamber heart scan is useful to assess chest size and lung status. Color flow Doppler is a valuable adjunct to assess vascular structures and their connections.

Before doing the detailed examination of the thoracic contents, an overall view of the whole trunk should be obtained to make sure that the relative proportions are correct.

At the transverse section of the thoracic circumference at the level of the heart should be roughly similar to the abdominal circumference at the level of umbilical vein.

The ribs should enclose about two-thirds of the thorax which should be almost circular in transverse section.

The major thoracic contents are the heart and great vessels and the lungs. The heart occupys about one-third of the chest and is situated with the apex towards the left side, the left ventricle lying posterolaterally and the right anteromedially.

The left lung lies behind the heart and is smaller than the right. The continuity of the diaphragm should be checked in sagittal and coronal views, thus confirming that liver and bowels are separated from heart and lungs.

The echogenicity of the lungs is usually brighter than the liver which becomes more distinctive by harmonic imaging. The echogenicity of the fetal lung showed a particular characteristic pattern during the course of pregnancy. It is almost the same as that of the liver at 22–23 weeks gestation, but later on decreased between 23 and 31 weeks and increased again later in pregnancy. Lungs volume estimation is important to assess lung development in a fetus at risk for pulmonary hypoplasia such as congenital diaphragmatic hernia, cystic adenomatoid lung malformation or hydrothorax.

Lung echogenicity does not correlate with lung maturity. Although well-studied, lung lengths are not easily reproducible. Thoracic perimeter measurements are made at the level of the four-chamber view and do not include the soft tissue areas beyond the ribs. The thoracic circumference/abdominal circumference ratio is constant through the late second trimester and in the third trimester: >0.80. 3D reconstruction techniques are reliable and reproducible for fetal lung volumes. During recent years, two-(2D) and three-dimensional (3D) ultrasound assessment of normal and abnormal structure of lungs has been studied extensively. The significance of 3D ultrasound volumetry in the antenatal assessment of lung hypoplasia still remains on discussion.

PATHOLOGY

Diaphragmatic Hernia

The diaphragm is a borderline between the thorax and the abdominal cavity. Sonographically, the diaphragm appears as a thin, dark, hypoechoic, arched line **(Fig. 2)**. Continuity of this thin and dark line is actually a kind of demarcation between abdominal and thoracic contents. If this line is interrupted or cannot be seen clearly, then diaphragmatic hernia should be questioned. The costo-diaphragmatic recess is most commonly located at the level of the ninth rib. The function of the diaphragm has been studied extensively by ultrasound. Movements of the diaphragm start as early as 9–10 weeks. Hiccups can be seen first, followed by breathing movements at 10th week of gestation.

Diaphragmatic hernia represents herniation of the abdominal contents into the chest, through a defect in the diaphragm. The defect in diaphragm exists from the tenth week of gestation, but the herniation of the gut into the chest in about 50% of the cases may not occur before the 24th week and this is probably the cause of the relatively low detection rate at the 18–20 weeks scan, though the evidence suggests that the marker for those cases where the prognosis is likely to be poor is increased nuchal translucency at the 11–14 weeks scan.[14]

The incidence of diaphragmatic hernia on birth is 1/2500–4000. There are three types of hernias **(Fig. 3)**:

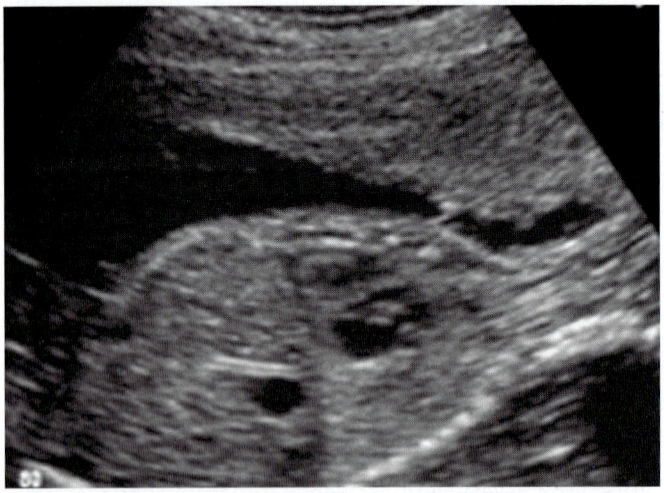

Fig. 2: Normal appearance of heart and lungs. There is clear demarcation zone—diaphragm as a vertical anechoic line between the abdomen, on the left side of the picture, and thorax, on the right side.

1. Posterolateral defect, or Bochdalek's hernia, which accounts for about 90% of cases found in the neonatal period. It occurs on the left side in 80% of cases, on the right in 15% and may be bilateral in approximately 5%. The commonest contents of a left-sided hernia are stomach, bowel and spleen **(Fig. 4)**. If the defect is right-sided the usual intrathoracic organs are liver and gallbladder.
2. Parasternal defect, or Morgagni's hernia—it accounts for 1-2% of cases and is more often right-sided or bilateral. It usually contains liver.
3. Eventration of the diaphragm occurs in 5% of cases and it is more commonly reported on the right.

Prenatal diagnosis by ultrasound is based on:

- Demonstration of abdominal organs within the thoracic cavity. On longitudinal scanning, a defect in the posterior aspect of the diaphragm may be seen, at least for the most common Bochdalek type of hernia. For left side congenital diaphragmatic hernia (CDH), mediastinal shift and rightwards displacement of the heart can be seen, and in most cases, a fluid-filled stomach or bowels are later on present within the thoracic cavity **(Figs 5 to 7)**. An important feature to look for is presence of (a portion of) the liver in the thorax. Doppler interrogation of the umbilical vein and hepatic vessels may be helpful in this respect. With right side CDH, the right lobe of the liver usually herniates into the chest, combined with mediastinal shift to the left
- Shift in the position of the heart or cardiac compression
- Polyhydramnion is a common associated finding. It is rarely observed before 24 weeks of gestation and is thought to be due to either esophageal compression or reduced absorption of fluid by the hypoplastic lungs.

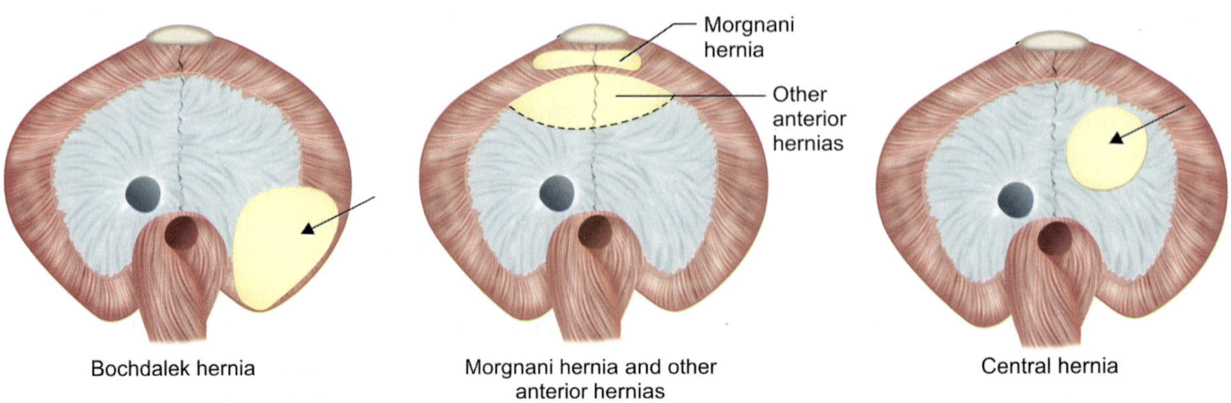

Fig. 3: Anatomic descriptions of diaphragmatic defects.

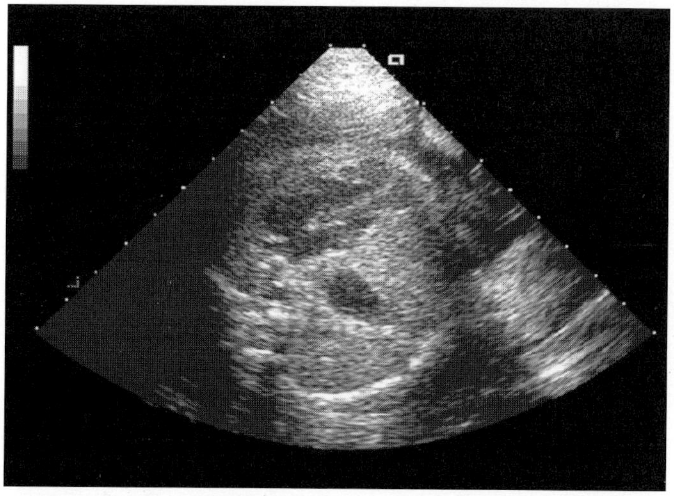

Fig. 4: Left-sided diaphragmatic hernia. The displacement of the heart to the right.

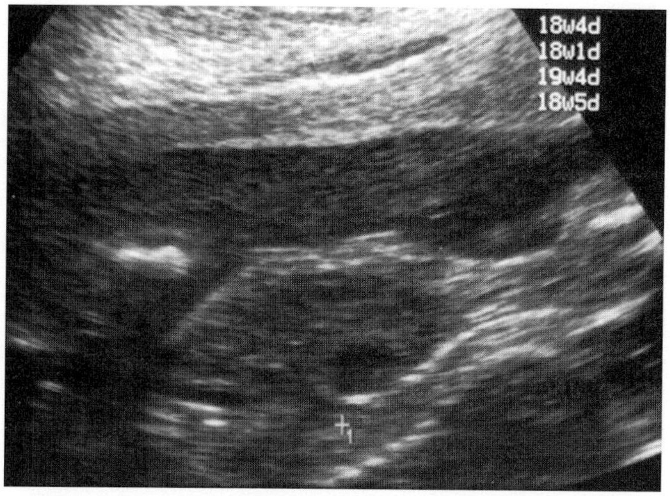

Fig. 6: Left-sided diaphragmatic hernia. Oblique sagittal view with the absence of diaphragm.

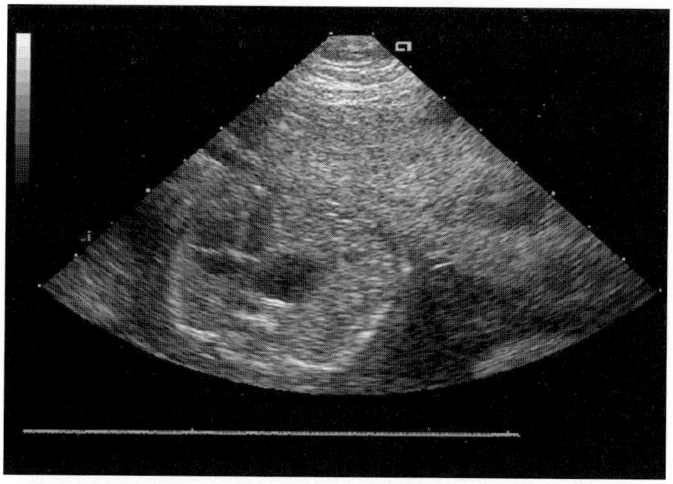

Fig. 5: Left-sided diaphragmatic hernia. Diaphragmatic hernia with the gaster in the thoracic cavity.

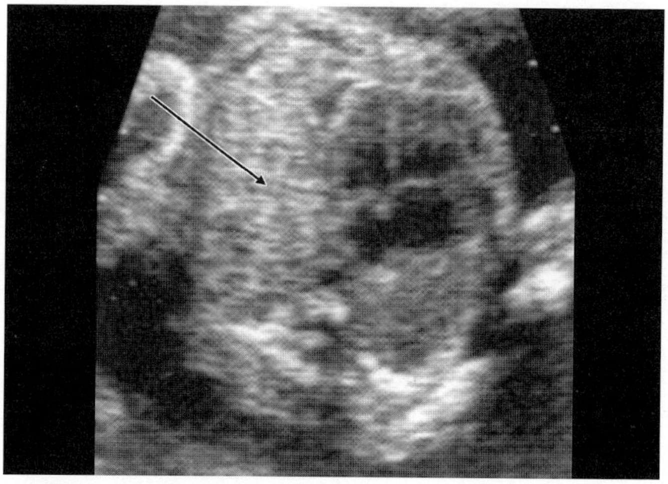

Fig. 7: Left-sided diaphragmatic hernia. Diaphragmatic hernia with the intestines in the thoracic cavity.

A right-sided hernia may be harder to diagnose because of the similar echogenicity of the lung and liver tissue, but the condition should be suspected by the presence of mediastinal shift or hydrothorax.

Differential Diagnosis

The differential diagnosis includes other cystic chest lesions such as cystic adenomatoid malformation, bronchogenic cysts or tumors of the chest.

Associated Anomalies

In prenatal series, about 50% of fetuses have an isolated diaphragmatic defect and in the rest a chromosomal abnormality may be found, usually trisomy 18, as well as a major defect including congenital heart disease, exomphalos, renal anomalies, brain anomalies and spinal abnormalities.

The incidence of aneuploidy was reported that is overall 14% of pregnancies, particularly trisomy's 13 and 18. Comprehensive anatomy scanning including fetal echocardiography is essential to detect other structural anomalies because at least 33% of cases will have other anomalies including cardiac defects.

Syndromes Associated with Diaphragmatic Hernia

- *Pallister-Killian syndrome* (Tetrasomy 12p): Polyhydramnios, rhizomelic limb shortening, abnormal facial profile with prominent philtrum, fetal somatic overgrowth in addition to diaphragmatic hernia. These are variable and even absent. Pallister-Killian syndrome is a mosaicism for an isochromosome of 12p, which is an extra two short arms of chromosome-12. Therefore, the fetus has four copies of 12p in some cell lines. In a case of a highly suspicion of Pallister-Killian Syndrome, the amniocentesis should be done for correct diagnosis because the cytogenetic abnormality may not be detected in either chorionic villi or fetal blood.

- *Fryns syndrome* is a rare autosomal recessive disorder of multiple congenital abnormalities, but can be found in about 4% of fetuses in CDH cases with normal chromosomes. Main criteria for diagnosis include CDH, hypoplasia of distal limb and nail, and abnormal facies. Cataracts may be detected later in gestation. IUGR, an increased nuchal fold together with CDH are the cases to be suspected for Fryns syndrome. Prognosis is very poor and 86% with an early lethal outcome. This is a difficult diagnosis in a fetus in the absence history for a previously affected child or parental consanguinity, therefore it is important to have genetic consultation when a diaphragmatic hernia is found together with other anomalies and normal karyotype.
- *Simpson-Golabi-Behmel syndrome:* It is an X-linked recessive disorder due to mutations in glypican 3 (Xq26). There is overlap with the features of Pallister-Killian syndrome and Beckwith Wideman syndrome (BWS) with overgrowth of somatic organs antenatally and postnatally. The birth weight and birth head circumference of affected males are usually both >97th centile. Cardiac defects and gastrointestinal malformations and polydactyly can be found with elevated maternal AFP. Unless there are life threatening malformations, this is not a lethal condition with most male fetuses with learning difficulties and overgrowth later in life. As in the case of BWS, males require screening for Wilms tumor. There may be a family history of X-linked development problems and carrier mothers may have distinctive facial features which a genetic consultation can be useful for definitive diagnosis antenatally.
- *Cornelia de Lange syndrome* is a rare sporadic syndrome with a birth incidence of about 1 in 50,000 and caused by new mutations in NIPBL. The fetus has IUGR (usually apparent in the third trimester), with upper limb anomalies such as short forearms with small hands and tapering fingers to oligodactily, severe limb reduction defects. The features are distinctive with brachycephaly, depressed nasal bridge, long philtrum and micrognathia can be seen by antenatal ultrasound and clearly seen at birth. Maternal serum pregnancy associated plasma protein-A is significantly reduced in Cornelia de Lange syndrome.
- *Wilms tumor (WT1) related conditions* [Wilms associated genital anomalies retardation (WAGR), del 11p13 Wilms tumor, Aniridia, Frasier syndrome, Meacham syndrome, Denys-Drash syndrome]: Predisposition to Wilms tumor and male pseudohermaphroditism together with other external and internal genital anomalies are clinical features. A 46, XY karyotype in a phenotypic female with a diaphragmatic hernia would suggest one of these conditions. Denys-Drash, Frasier and Meacham syndromes are all caused by mutations in WT1, but WAGR is a microdeletion syndrome requiring specific FISH analysis.
- *Donnai-Barrow syndrome* is caused by mutations in the gene LRP2 and a rare condition with corpus callosum agenesis, sensorineural deafness and developmental delay, dysmorphic facies with hypertelorism, CDH.

About 50% of fetuses have an isolated diaphragmatic defect and in the rest associated anomalies such as chromosomal abnormality usually trisomy 18, as well as a major defect, including congenital heart disease, exomphalos, renal anomalies, brain anomalies and spinal abnormalities, Fryns, Goldenhar, Beckwith-Wiedemann, Cornelia de Lange, Aperts and lethal pterygium.

Management of Pregnancy

When diaphragmatic hernia is diagnosed antenatally fetal karyotyping and detailed ultrasound examination of the fetus (in particular the heart) should be undertaken. Fetal echocardiography should be arranged as well as consultation with pediatric surgeon.

Prediction of Outcome

In neonates with isolated diaphragmatic hernia the primary determinant of survival is the presence of pulmonary hypoplasia and hypertension. The mortality has remained high despite optimal postnatal management and the introduction of extracorporal membrane oxygenation.

Antenatal prediction of pulmonary hypoplasia is difficult and it is the most important part in counseling parents and selecting those cases that may benefit from prenatal surgery. In isolated cases of CDH, prognosis is poor when the liver is intrathoracic[15] and the lung-to-head ratio (LHR) is less than 1.[16]

When making a measurement of the LHR, a transverse section of the chest is taken at the level of the 4-chamber view. The contralateral lung is measured—the longest axis is measured and multiplied by the longest measurement perpendicular to it. This is placed over the head circumference, which is measured at the standard biparietal view, typically showing 2 equal hemispheres, the septum cavum pellucidum, one-third of the way from the front to the back, and the posterior horns of the lateral ventricles.[17]

Recent research show that in isolated congenital diaphragmatic hernia, fetal lung volume measurement by three-dimensional ultrasound may be a potential predictor for pulmonary hypoplasia and postnatal outcome.[11,18]

Fetal surgery can be a reasonable approach in the treatment of CDH. The aim of surgery is to prevent lung hypoplasia. Although fetal surgery initially involved reduction of the hernia by open repair in utero, current practice involves ballooning of the trachea. Tracheal occlusion results in increased lung volume and accelerated lung maturity.

The initial fetal surgery was a patch closure of the diaphragmatic defect with abdominal silo with an open fetal surgery. Also fetuses with herniation of the left lobe of the liver could not be solved by this way because of that reduction of the herniated liver led to kinking of the umbilical vein which compromise the blood flow.

More recently, fetal tracheal occlusion (TO) has been used as a treatment modality for CDH. It has been shown that the dynamics of fetal lung fluid affect lung growth. Although tracheal occlusion might offer a relatively simple approach to accelerate lung growth in human fetuses with CDH, on the other hand further experimental studies in the sheep model also demonstrated that tracheal occlusion had a detrimental effect on lung maturation because of disappearance of type II pneumocytes, but other studies demonstrated that released tracheal occlusion at an interval prior to delivery could induce type II pneumocytes and significant lung growth, although there was evidence that lung function was not restored to normal because abnormally thick wall causing in a limited gas exchange.

A minimally invasive approach to tracheal occlusion in the sheep model utilizing a deployable balloon technology placed via a single small trocar has been proposed. Overall outcomes in 210 FETO interventions increased survival from 24% to 49% in severe cases with left-sided CDH and from 0% to 35% in right CDH when compared to expectantly managed cases.

The risk of prematurity and preterm premature rupture of membranes was high, despite the use of small-diameter fetoscopes with a high incidence of prematurity (50.0%), extreme prematurity (15.0%) and preterm premature rupture of the membranes (35.0%). Infant survival to 6 months was 10% in FETO group and 4.8% in controls, and severe pulmonary arterial hypertension is 50% in FETO group and 85.7% in controls.

CYSTIC ADENOMATOID MALFORMATION

Cystic adenomatoid malformation (CAM) of the lung is a developmental abnormality of the lung characterized by a cystic mass of disordered pulmonary parenchyma with proliferation of terminal respiratory bronchioles and a lack of normal alveoli.[19] CCAMs occur as a result of failure of induction of mesenchyme by bronchiolar epithelium. The lesion is characterized by focal abnormal proliferation of bronchiolar like air spaces and absence of alveoli. CAM usually arise from a single pulmonary lobe and multilobar or bilateral lung involvement is rare. The prenatal natural history of CAM is quite variable, forming a spectrum in severity extending from cases that present in utero as a rapidly growing intrathoracic mass resulting in non-immune hydrops and in utero demise to lesions which, despite achieving a significant size, spontaneously regress and disappear during the third trimester.[20] As many as 40% of CAMs will progress to hydrops and without fetal surgery, this is almost uniformly fatal, while as many as 15% of CAMs will regress and may disappear completely.[20] Unfortunately, no predictor has been available to determine into which category a particular fetus will fall. Studies of large CAMs that were resected in utero because they resulted in non immune hydrops have shown a higher rate of cellular proliferation and lower rate of apoptosis than normal fetal lung of equivalent gestational age.[21] The rapid growth of some CAMs during the late second and early third trimesters may be caused by disregulation of mesenchymal platelet-derived growth factor gene expression driving cellular proliferation.[19]

The diagnosis of CAM relies on the demonstration of a solid or cystic, nonpulsatile intrathoracic tumor.

Stocker et al. proposed a classification of CAM into three subtypes according to the size of the cysts—type I has large cysts, type II has multiple small cysts of less than 1.2 cm in diameter, and type III consists of a noncystic lesion producing mediastinal shift.[22] The worst prognosis

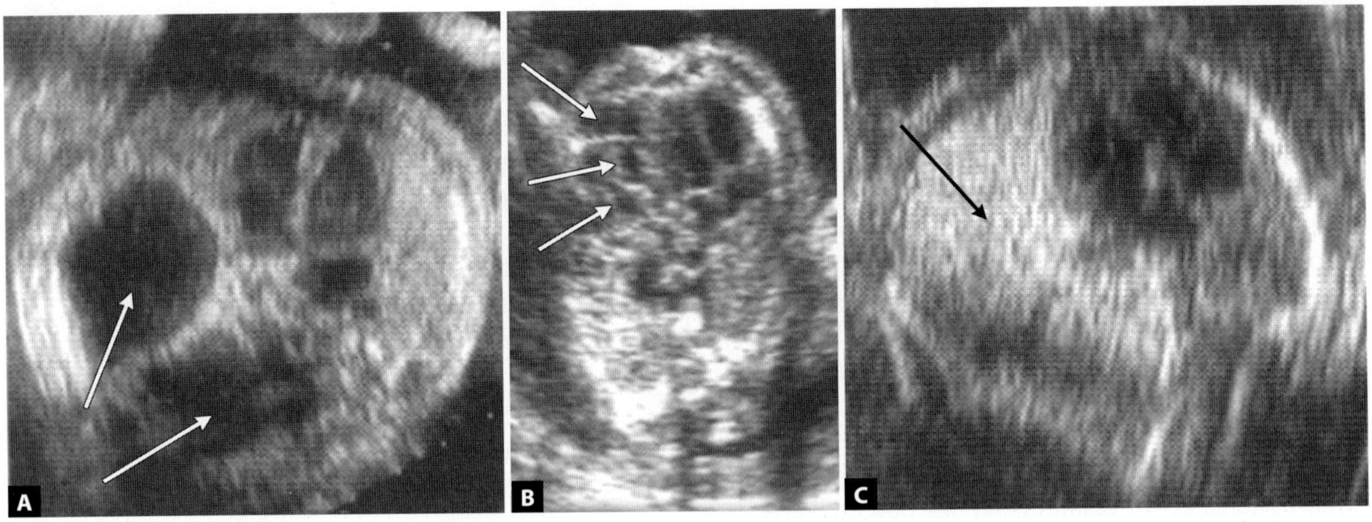

Figs. 8A to C: Three different subtypes of CAM according to the size of the cysts (A) CAM I; (B) CAM II and (C) CAM III.

is seen in type III lesions. Associated anomalies are frequently present in type II. Prenatally, the more useful characterization is to identify CAM as either cystic or solid as these provide more useful categories for determining options and prognosis **(Figs. 8A to C)**.[23]

Unilateral lesions are often associated with deviation of the mediastinum in the contralateral side. In bilateral disease, the heart may be severely compressed, and this is usually associated with ascites from venocaval obstruction or cardiac compression.

In about 85% of cases, CAM is unilateral and approximately half are microcystic and the other half macrocystic. During the third trimester polyhydramnios may develop, which is likely to be due to decreased fetal swallowing, the consequence of esophageal compression by the mass or there may be increased fetal lung fluid production by the abnormal tissue.

Associated Anomalies

The condition is usually isolated but in about 10% of cases there are additional malformations, usually renal, abdominal wall or central nervous system. There is no significant association with chromosomal defects.

Prognosis

Bilateral CAM is a lethal condition while unilateral CAM is associated with a good prognosis:

- In about 40% of cases, there is apparent spontaneous antenatal resolution of the lesion
- In 50% it remains the same
- In 10% it enlarges.

In majority of cases, it either remains the same in size or there is an apparent spontaneous antenatal resolution, and in a minority of cases, it enlarges. Good prognosis has been shown in recent studies, with about half of cases in pregnancies that were allowed to continue resulting in spontaneous regression.[24,25]

In the majority of cases with antenatal resolution, postnatal investigation with chest X-ray, computed tomography and magnetic resonance imaging will demonstrate residual lung disease.

Serial ultrasonographic evaluation is important to follow fetal lung lesions for its gowing pattern and the early occurrence of fetal hydrops. For the prediction of fetal hydrops, a prognostic tool using sonographic measurement of the CCAM volume was developed. The CCAM volume ratio (CVR) is calculated by dividing the CCAM volume (length × width × height × 0.52) by head circumference. A greater ratio more than 1.6 is predictive of increased (75%) risk of the development of fetal hydrops.

Unilateral lesions are usually associated with the shift of the mediastinum into the contralateral side. In bilateral disease, the heart can be severely compressed and is usually associated with ascites due to venocaval obstruction or cardiac compression. In about 85% of cases, CCAM is unilateral. During the third trimester, polyhydramnios may develop, which is likely to be due to decreased fetal swallowing, the consequence of esophageal compression by the mass.

The majority of fetuses with CCAM have a decreased size in the third trimester and undergo normal vaginal delivery with postnatal resection at 5–8 weeks of life (no respiratory symptoms at birth; resection of lesion due to risks of infections, pneumothorax, and malignant degeneration), but some fetuses require more extensive evaluation and treatment in utero.

Open fetal surgical resection was originally suggested in case of poor prognosis for hydropic fetuses with large cystic lung lesions. Subsequently, it has become clear that these fetuses can be successfully treated with the minimal invasive approach of thoracoamniotic shunting. Insertion of such a catheter in a large cyst of a CCAM has been successful. Thereafter, several case reports and small series describe the results of this technique in hydraulic and nonhydropic fetuses with CCAM or BPS.

Controversy about the role of thoracoamniotic shunting in nonhydropic fetuses remains for several reasons. It may be difficult to predict the evolution of a macrocystic lung lesion and timing of development of hydrops. Also, there are no randomized studies comparing treatment vs. non-treatment in non-hydropic fetuses. The shunting procedure is preferable before going to hydrops in appropriate case such as mediastinal or cardiac shift with a large cystic CCAM.

In microcystic lesions (CCAM type-2 or CCAM type-3), cysts are too small for drainage. When a systemic feeding vessel is found which is very easy after technological advancement, percutaneous laser coagulation or injection of a sclerosing agent can be successful. Percutaneous ablation of a microcystic CCAM in a hydropic case using laser have been described **(Figs. 9A to C)**.

Resolution of a large CCAM after steroid therapy given for lung maturation was described. In the mean time, current evidence suggests that in large CCAMs with hydrops, steroids therapy appears to be a reasonably first line therapy, also because of the virtual absence of maternal side-effects. Whether steroids should also be used in CCAMs without hydrops is more questionable, as the prognosis without intervention is generally good and spontaneous regression can often occur.

FETAL HYDROTHORAX

Antenatal diagnosis can be made by an anechoic space surrounding the lungs and majority bilateral. Pleural effusions sonographically appear as anechogenic fluid in the thorax. When unilateral and large, the hydrothorax can demonstrate considerable mass effect on the diaphragm, inverting the diaphragm and displacing the heart and mediastinal structures into contralateral hemithorax. If it is bilateral, it shows an ultrasound appearence with two moon-shaped anechoic areas surrounding the mediastinum.

FETAL PLEURAL EFFUSIONS

Fetal pleural effusions can be primary or secondary, with an estimated incidence of 1:10,000–15,000 pregnancies. Primary pleural effusions, correctly termed 'hydrothorax' antenatally are due to lymphatic leakage and can be unilateral or bilateral. Secondary pleural effusions are usually part of a generalized picture of fluid retention in nonimmune hydrops and their prognosis is mainly dependent on the underlying pathology. Secondary hydrothorax is more symmetric in size with little mediastinal shift. If there is septation or solid component within fluid it should be taken into account with other differential diagnoses. Pleural effusions were first reported antenatally in 1977.[26]

Their optimal antenatal management is controversial because some fetuses are not significantly compromised, whereas others either die in utero from secondary hydrops or at birth from pulmonary hypoplasia.

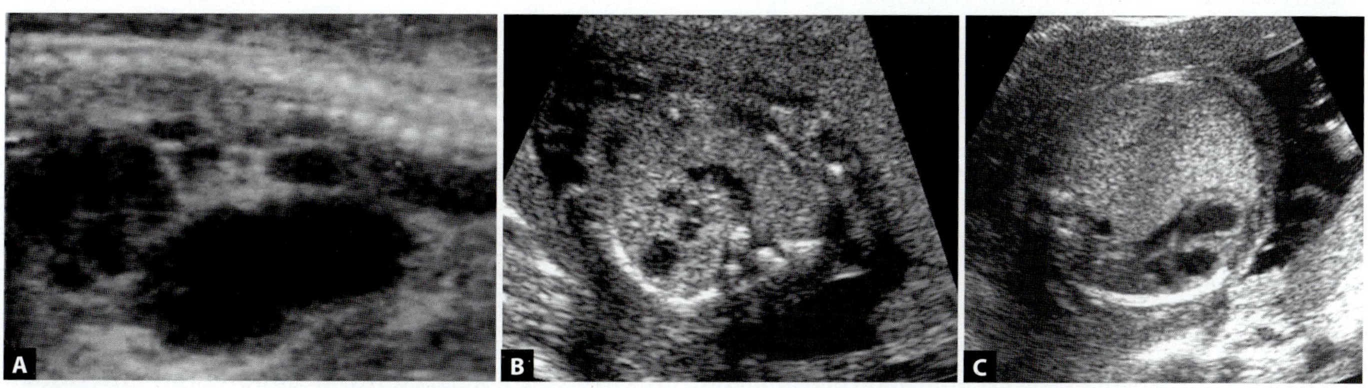

Figs. 9A to C: (A) Microcystic (cysts <5 mm in diameter); (B) Mixed and (C) Macrocystic (cysts >5 mm in diameter) form of CAM.

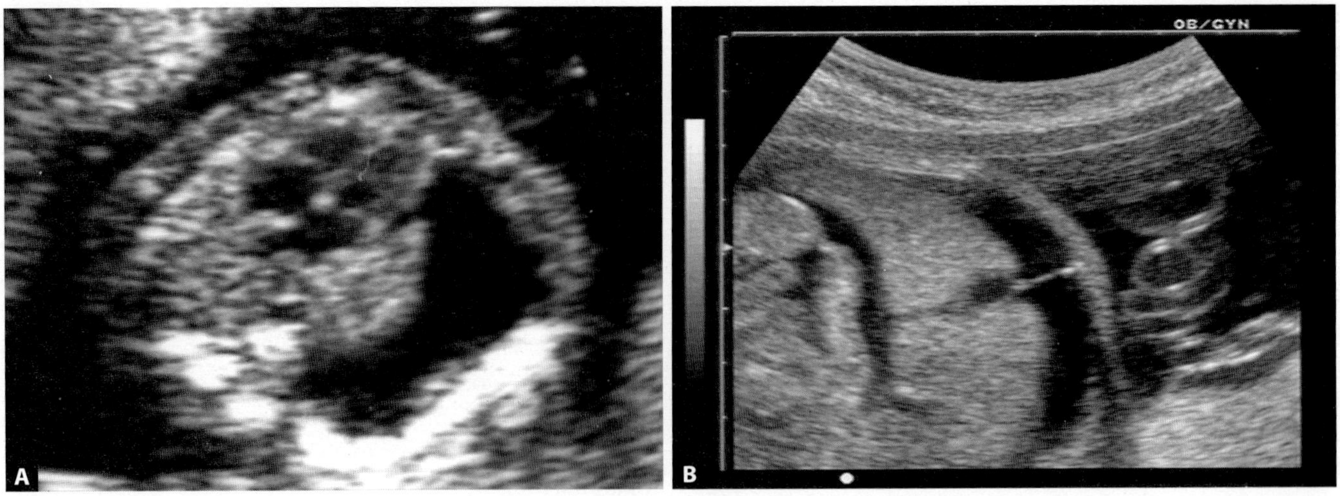

Figs. 10A and B: Ultrasound appearances of pleural effusion.

The first step on detecting a fetal pleural effusion should be to determine whether it is primary or secondary. Primary fetal hydrothorax is a diagnosis of exclusion and the workup is similar to that for hydrops: maternal serology to exclude congenital infections (toxoplasmosis, rubella, cytomegalovirus, syphilis, herpes and parvovirus B195); blood type and antibody screen to rule-out immune hydrops; Kleihauer–Betke test to exclude fetomaternal hemorrhage and Doppler evaluation of the peak systolic velocity (PSV) in the middle cerebral artery (MCA) to exclude fetal anemia. Fetal anemia will always present with ascites before a pleural effusion appears. Fetal karyotype is recommended because aneuploidy (predominantly trisomy 21 and 45,X) has been reported in 6–17% of fetuses with hydrothorax, the vast majority of which are hydropic.[27]

The fact that pleural effusions are associated with structural fetal malformations in 25% of cases highlights the importance of meticulous ultrasound and echocardiographic evaluations. Pulmonary causes of secondary hydrothorax, such as congenital cystic adenomatoid malformation (CCAM), bronchopulmonary sequestration (BPS) or congenital diaphragmatic hernia (CDH), should be excluded **(Figs. 10 and 11)**.[28]

Unlike a small amount of pericardial fluid which may be physiological, a fetal pleural fluid collection is always abnormal. Primary hydrothorax may be idiopathic or consequent to thoracic duct malformations. Primary pleural effusions are generally chylous in origin, which occurs as a consequence of an accumulation of lymphatic fluid due to atresia, agenesis or fistulas of the lymphatic duct. In the feeding infant or adult, aspirated fluid of a chylous effusion is characteristically milky because of the presence of chylomicrons in the lymph fluid. But aspirates of fetal chylothorax is clear and yellowish colored because of that the lymph fluid does not contain chylomicrons as a consequence of the fasting state of the fetus. Analysis of chylous effusion in the fetus typically shows a large number of lymphocytes, and >80% lymphocytes in the fluid is pathognomonic for a chylous effusion. Congenital pulmonary lymphangiectasia is another rare cause of isolated fetal hydrothorax. This is a congenital pulmonary disease,characterized by a subpleural, interlobar, perivascular or peribronchial lymphatic dilatation.

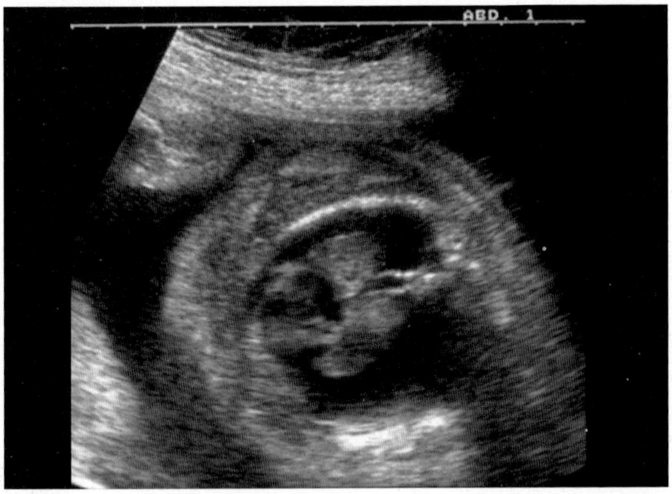

Fig. 11: Thoracic shunting of pleural effusion. Shunt can be seen at the posterior paraspinal site.

On the other hand, fetal hydrthorax is thought to be one of the earliest signs of hydrops fetalis. The causes of fetal hydrothorax with hydrops include cardiac and vascular diseases (50%), chromosomal abnormality (more frequently trisomy 21 and Turner syndrome with the rate of 7 to 10%), anemia and hematological diseases, pulmonary abnormalities, skeletal dysplasia, hepatic or metabolic diseases and infections including TORCH, parvovirus B19. Other major congenital abnormalities such as congenital diaphragmatic hernia, extralobar sequestration, Congenital cystic adenomatoid malformation, thyroid teratoma or fetal goiter are found in 25–40% of fetuses with nonimmune hydrops fetalis. Perinatal mortality is about >90% in hydropic fetuses with hydrothorax if another structural abnormality is identified. Therefore, it is important to make a complete anatomic survey in any hydropic fetus with hydrothorax.

Prognosis

Irrespective of the underlying cause, infants affected by pleural effusions usually present in the neonatal period with severe, and often fatal, respiratory insufficiency. This is either a direct result of pulmonary compression caused by the effusions, or due to pulmonary hypoplasia secondary to chronic intrathoracic compression. The overall mortality of neonates with pleural effusions increases from low in infants with isolated pleural effusions to very high in those with gross hydrops.[26] Chromosomal abnormalities, mainly trisomy 21, are found in about 5% of fetuses with apparently isolated pleural effusions.

In the human, isolated fetal pleural effusions may resolve spontaneously antenatally, or they may persist. In some cases, postnatal thoracocentesis may be sufficient, but in others the chronic compression of the fetal lungs can result in pulmonary hypoplasia and neonatal death. Additionally, mediastinal compression may lead to the development of fetal hydrops and polyhydramnios which are associated with a high risk of premature delivery and subsequent perinatal death.[26]

Unilateral fetal hydrothorax can occur more sporadically and is caused by a congenital malformation of the thoracic duct or the pulmonary lymphatic system. It is usually diagnosed in the second or early third trimester. The prognosis of fetal hydrothorax is difficult to predict with expected perinatal mortality rates between 22 and 53%. Therefore, counseling on perinatal outcome is very hard for the selection of cases for fetal intervention or early delivery.

Irrespective of the underlying cause, fetal hydrothorax is potentially responsible for fetal and neonatal death due to pulmonary hypoplasia caused by chronic intrathoracic compression and due to hydrops caused by mediastinal shift, cardiac compression and vena caval obstruction with low cardiac output and also due to the prematurity as a consequence of polyhydramnios caused by esophagus compression (mediasitnal shift) and/or low amnitoic fluid uptake of the lungs. Infants affected by fetal hydrothorax present usually severe respiratory problem and insufficiency. Sometimes, it can be seen as an associated maternal morbidity, as in the mirror syndrome characterized by a generalized edema, due to the hydropic placenta that produces vasoactive substances.

Parameters associated with a better prognostic include later gestational age at diagnosis, spontaneous resolution of the effusion prior to delivery, lack of hydrops, isolated effusion and unilateral effusion.

For prognostic features, several investigators reported outcomes of fetuses with antenatally diagnosed hydrothorax. Adverse prognostic indicators included bilaterality, presence of hydrops, absence of spontaneous resolution and premature delivery. Polyhydramnios has also prognostic significance, with the uterine overdistention, predisposing to preterm labor and delivery. Even without hydrops, large pleural effusions can cause pulmonary hypoplasia due to compression. The time of onset, size and duration of the pleural effusion influence the development of pulmonary hypoplasia. The most common cause of neonatal mortality with fetal hydrothorax is respiratory insufficiency due to pulmonary hypoplasia.

Therapy

There are several options in the management of fetuses with isolated hydrothorax for which the options depend on gestational age, severity of effusion, evidence of progression, hydrops, polyhydramnios or mediastinal shift. The outcome of fetal hydrothorax is significantly worsened by prematurity (less than 32 weeks of gestation), the presence of hydrops and lack of fetal therapy. When the hydrothorax is small, isolated and well-tolerated, expectant management with frequent follow-up may be most benefical because of the possibility of spontaneous resolution. If the fetal pleural effusion is very large or increases by gestational age, then a fetal intervention is needed. Fetal intervention for pleural effusion can include a single and serial thoracocentesis (less effective)

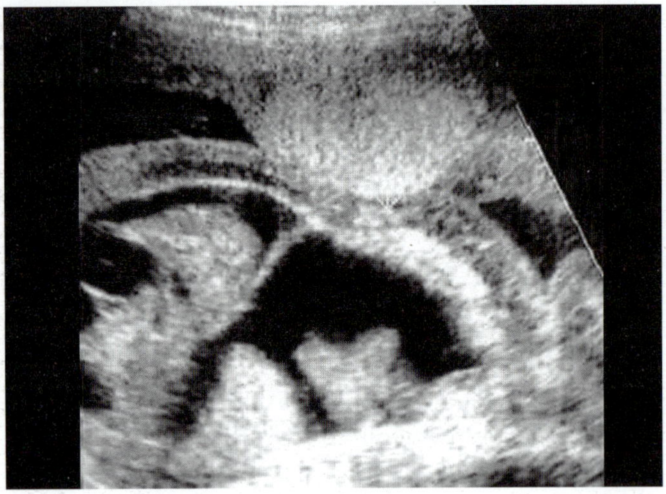

Fig. 12: Sagittal scan of the fetal thorax demonstrating bilateral hydrothorax and the sequestered lung. Note also the evidence of ascites and subcutaneous edema.

or thoracoamniotic shunting to allow the drainage of fetal fluid into the amniotic fluid **(Fig. 12)**.

Thoracocentesis is a diagnostic procedure to obtain pleural fluid for cell count, culture and to establish whether the effusion is chylous. Additionally and importantly, ultrasound evaluation should be done again after decompression because undiagnosed cardiac abnormality or other intrathoracic lesion may become apparent which cannot be seen easily due to compressed organs and anatomy.

When hydrothorax reaccumulates after the initial thoracocentesis and with the development of mediastinal shift or fetal hydrops, a thoracoamniotic shunt should be done.

LUNG SEQUESTRATION/PULMONARY SEQUESTRATION

Pulmonary sequestration (PS) is a rare developmental abnormality in which a segment of lung parenchyma is isolated from the normal lung tissue. It receives its blood supply from the systemic circulation, rather than the pulmonary artery. Also known as accessory lung, the sequestration is a congenital malformation consisting of lung parenchyma which is separated from normal lung and does not communicate with the normal tracheobronchial tree.

If it happens prior to closure of the pleura they have no separate pleural and are called intralobar sequestrations and after closure of the pleura, they are called extralobar sequestrations and have its own pleura. The sequestered lung tissue may either be adjacent to the normal lung and covered by the same pleura (intralobar sequestration) or it may have its own pleura (extralobar sequestration). Intralobar sequestration typically affects the lower lobes.[29] In extralobar sequestration, the lung is most commonly located between the lower lobe and diaphragm but it can also be found below the diaphragm in the abdomen.

Ultrasonically, the abnormal lung appears as an echogenic intrathoracic or intraabdominal mass. Typical sonographic pictures include a lobar or triangular echogenic lesion in the lung base, usually left side. Color Doppler shows that an atypical arterial blood supply from the descending aorta and occasionally from the intercostal, celiac or splenic arteries. Extralobar sequestrations may be thoracic or extrathoracic **(Figs 13A to D)**.

Pulmonary sequestration seems to be roughly triangular in shape, with the apex pointing towards the mediastinum. Intralobar sequestrations drain into pulmonary veins and extralobar sequestrations usually into a systemic vein, occasionally the azygos, hemiazygos or inferior vena cava. As with CCAM, pulmonary sequestration is virtually always unilateral usually on the left side. Unilateral, and involves the left lower lobe in 90% of cases. Pulmonary sequestration seems to be roughly triangular in shape, with the apex pointing towards the mediastinum. In about 50% of cases there is an associated pleural effusion. Polyhydramnios is a frequent complication. There is a variable mediastinal shift and hydrops. Several sequestrations regress spontaneously. No specific features indicate which sequestrations are likely to resolve. Persistent sequestrations may stabilize or may need surgical resection (postnatal).

Associated Anomalies

Extrapulmonary anomalies are found in about 60% of cases with extralobar sequestration and 10% of those with intralobar sequestration. Pulmonary sequestrations are occasionally associated with other thoracic and foregut anomalies such a CDH, CCAMs, bronchogenic cysts, neurenteric cysts and also including congenital heart disease, renal anomalies and hydrocephalus. They can show ipsilateral hydrothorax.

Prognosis

The condition carries a very poor prognosis, due to pulmonary hypoplasia or the associated malformations.

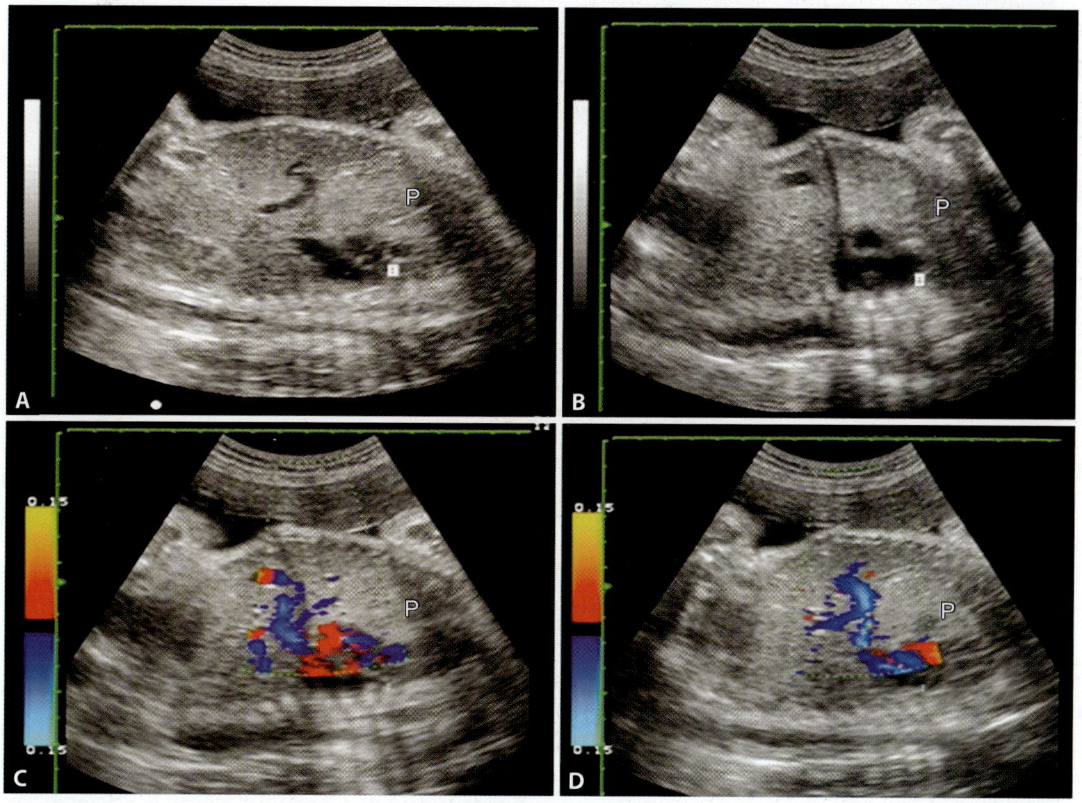

Figs. 13A to D: Pulmonary sequestration: (A) The echogenic intrathoracic mass; (B) Intralobar sequestration affects the lower lobes. Triangular echogenic lesion in the lung base; (C) Color Doppler shows that an atypical arterial blood supply from the descending aorta; (D) Vascularization can also be found below the diaphragm in the abdomen.

Some cases may not become apparent until later in life, the individual complaining of repeated chest infections or hemorrhage.[29]

Therapy

In some cases, pulmonary sequestration is associated with hydrops. In these cases, a single tap or the placement of a thoracoamniotic shunt may resolve the hydrops due to venous compression. Minimally invasive ultrasound-guided interventions for pulmonary sequestration include thoracoamniotic shunting with associated hydrothorax as well as occlusion of the vascular supply to the lung mass, either by vascular injection of a sclerosing agent, laser ablation, radiofrequency ablation. Still the optimal fetal therapeutic strategy remains controversial.

Interruption of blood flow in the feeding vessel of BPS has been described using pure alcohol in one case, polidocanol in three cases and N-butyl-2-cyanoacrylate in one case. The sclerosing agent was injected directly into the feeding vessel of BPS in all cases. Hydrops resolved in all cases after treatment modalities. But one child, treated with polidocanol sclerotherapy, died in the neonatal period from operative complications after resection of the remaining lesion.

Interruption of blood flow in the feeding vessel of a BPS by intrafetal laser has been described as a treatment modality in hydropic fetuses with BPS. Successful ultrasound guided laser coagulation of the feeding vessel of BPS using laser through a 18G-needle was described.[35] In two cases, hydrops have been dissolved after laser surgery and the fetuses survived uneventfully.

Preliminary results on ultrasound-guided intrafetal laser ablation of the abnormal systemic blood supply of BPS have been reported.[34,35] This technique might be more effective than drainage of pleural effusion as it targets the tumor rather than its symptoms. Laser therapy can also reduce the need for postnatal surgery; in cases treated only with drainage of the fetal hydrothorax, postnatal surgery was necessary to resect the tumor in five out of six liveborn cases, whereas, in cases treated with antenatal occlusion of the feeding vessel, postnatal surgery was necessary in only one out of five cases.

Syndromic Associations with Congenital Anomalies of the Fetal Thorax

Conditions to Consider in the Presence of a Congenital Diaphragmatic Hernia (CDH)

Pallister-Killian syndrome (Tetrasomy 12p): In addition to diaphragmatic hernia, polyhydramnios, rhizomelic limb shortening and an abnormal facial profile with prominent philtrum are found in association with fetal somatic overgrowth. These features are variable and may even be absent. Pallister-Killian syndrome is a chromosomal abnormality with mosaicism for an isochromosome of 12p, which is an extrachromosome comprising the two short arms of 12. Thus, the fetus has four copies of 12p in some cell lines. In the neonate, this chromosome abnormality is usually present in skin fibroblasts but not usually in blood. For this reason, the cytogenetic abnormality may not be detected in either chorionic villi or fetal blood, the latter being the least indicated method because of the low frequency of the iso-chromosome in lymphocytes. In cases thought to have a normal karyotype following CVS, amniocentesis should be considered if this diagnosis is suspected, as this is most likely to reveal the mosaicism, particularly if fluorescent in situ hybridisation (FISH) and especially interphase FISH on noncultured cells is performed.[29]

Fryns syndrome: Fryns syndrome is a rare autosomal recessive disorder of multiple congenital abnormalities, but can occur in around 4% of fetuses with CDH and multiple anomalies with normal chromosomes. Major diagnostic criteria include CDH, distal limb and nail hypoplasia and abnormal facies.[30]

Prenatally, suspicion of this condition is raised in fetuses with a CDH, IUGR and an increased nuchal fold. Cataracts may be detected later in gestation .

Simpson-Golabi-Behmel syndrome: This X-linked recessive disorder is due to mutations in *glypican 3* (Xq26). There is overlap with the features of Pallister-Killian syndrome and BWS, with overgrowth of prenatal onset that continues postnatally. The birth weight and birth occipital-frontal circumference (OFC) of affected males are usually both >97th centile. They may have cardiac and gastrointestinal malformations and polydactyly.

Maternal AFP is elevated. Unless there are life-threatening malformations, this is not a lethal condition with most boys presenting at later age with other manifestations of the syndrome, such as learning difficulties and overgrowth.[31]

Cornelia de Lange syndrome: Cornelia de Lange (de Lange) syndrome is a rare sporadic syndrome with a birth incidence of about 1 in 50,000 and is caused by new mutations in *NIPBL*.[31] The fetus has IUGR (often developing in the third trimester), with upper limb anomalies ranging from short forearms with small hands and tapering fingers to oligodactyly and severe limb reduction defects. Diaphragmatic hernia is a recognized but relatively rare feature, although may be more frequently represented in cases presenting prenatally.

There are distinctive craniofacial features (micro-brachycephaly, depressed nasal bridge with anteverted nares, long smooth overhanging philtrum and micrognathia) which may be recognized with prenatal ultrasound and are clearly seen at birth.[32] Maternal serum pregnancy-associated plasma protein-A is reported to be significantly reduced in de Lange syndrome.

CONGENITAL CYSTIC LUNG LESIONS

If a cystic lung lesion is isolated and unilateral karyotyping is not obsolutely indicated. 'Bilateral' lesions may represent laryngeal/tracheal atresia, thus consideration should be given to the autosomal recessive Fraser-cryptophthalmos syndrome where the likely mechanism for pulmonary hyperplasia is retention of fetal lung fluid by laryngeal or tracheal obstruction.

Fraser (Cryptophthalmos) Syndrome

Fraser syndrome is inherited in an autosomal recessive fashion and can be caused by mutation in the *FRAS1* gene or in the *FREM2* gene and there may be yet further unidentified gene(s). The classic features are a combination of cryptophthalmos, laryngeal stenosis, syndactyly, renal agenesis and genital abnormalities (fused labia and enlarged clitoris).[32] It is now recognized that not all infants with Fraser syndrome have cryptophalmos. Some authors observed pulmonary hyperplasia and laryngeal stenosis in two siblings with Fraser syndrome. Markedly enlarged echogenic lungs may be demonstrable on ultrasound in this condition.

Esophageal/Tracheoesophageal Atresia

Tracheoesophageal atresia (TOF) results from incomplete separation of the foregut into the trachea and esophagus, and 85% of TOF is associated with esophageal atresia.

Laryngeal/tracheal atresia are rare congenital anomalies which are associated with demise soon after birth, unless treated antenatally. These arise consequent to either subglottic laryngeal atresia, tracheal stenosis or atresia, or, tracheal webs or cysts and are also known as congenital high airways obstruction (CHAOS). Pathologically, failure of efflux of fluid from the fetal lung results in exaggerated lung development. Ultrasound features include symmetric enlargement of both lungs with squeezed and anterior displacement of the heart and reduced cardiac angle (sometimes to zero) by high intrathoracic pressure. The lungs are homogeneously echogenic, often similar to autosomal recessive infantile polycystic kidneys, since the underlying lesion consists of numerous fluid-filled spaces. The diaphragm is flat or inverted and cutaneous edema is common as is hydrops. Polyhydramnios is seen consequent to esophageal compression. The distal trachea and bronchii may be identified as tubular bulging fluid-filled structures in the mediastinum.

The risk of chromosomal abnormality is extremely low, but extremely high risk for Fraser syndrome with extremely unfavorable outcome (laryngeal atresia, cleft lip/palate, congenital heart disease, microphthalmia, syndactyly, external ear anomalies, and bilateral renal agenesis, genital abnormalities with fused labia and enlarged clitoris). Fraser syndrome shows autosomal recessive inheritance caused by mutation in the FRAS1 gene or in the FREM2 gene. Postnatal therapy is the only available option to manage the fetus with laryngeal atresia in the EXIT procedure (ex utero intrapartum treatment).

About half the number of infants with a TOF will have other malformations, in particular anomalies of the heart, limbs and vertebrae. Chromosomal anomalies, including trisomy 21, trisomy 18 and deletion of 22q11, developmental and genetic syndromes are relatively frequent and need to be carefully considered and investigated.[33] If the pregnancy is terminated, a detailed postmortem examination should be performed to establish if the malformation is isolated or part of a syndrome or association. This should include cytogenetic testing and consent for tissue/DNA storage.

We can conclude that in the majority of pregnancies where the fetus is diagnosed with an isolated lung lesion, the parents can be reassured that the outcome is likely favorable. In the absence of hydrops, even large lesions can be treated expectantly with weekly or bi-weekly monitoring. Also, selection of an appropriate site for delivery is another important point which is crucial for better outcome. If there is a growing pattern of the pathology by gestational age, especially with a mediastinal shift and displacement of the heart, there is indication for fetal surgery. In microcystic-CCAMs with hydrops, a course of steroids may be beneficial less than 32 weeks of gestational age. Although promising, more evidence is needed to establish its role.[34,35] Minimally invasive fetal interventions such as thoracoamniotic shunting of fetal hydorthorax and large cysts, or occlusion of the feeding artery of microcystic-CCAM or pulmonary sequestrations should be taken into account in appropriate cases. Therefore, those cases should be taken care of in a fetal or perinatal center where this surgery is performed because it is not so easy and possible sometimes to predict the prognosis for expectant or interventional management.

REFERENCES

1. Zalel Y, Lipitz S, Soriano D. The development of the fetal sternum: a cross-sectional sonography. Ultrasound Obstet Gynecol. 1999;13:187-90.
2. Blaas HGK, Eik-Nes SH. Sonographic development of the normal foetal thorax and abdomen across gestation. Prenat Diagn. 2008;28:568-80.
3. Malas MA, Evcil EH, Desdicioglu K. Size and location of the fetal diaphragm during the fetal period in human fetuses. Surg Radiol Anat. 2007;29:155-64.
4. de Vries JIP, Fong BF. Normal fetal motility: an overview. Ultrasound Obstet Gynecol. 2006;27:701-11.
5. Whitsett JA, Wert SE, Trapnell BC. Genetic disorders influencing lung formation and function at birth. Human Mol Genet. 2004;13:207-15.
6. Kalache KD, Espinoza J, Chgaiworapongsa T. Three-dimensional ultrasound fetal lung volumen measurment: a systematic study comparing the multiplanar method with the rotational technique. Ultrasound Obstet Gynecol. 2003;21:111-8.
7. Peralta CFA, Cavoretto P, Csapo B, et al. Assessment of lung area in normal fetuses at 12-32 weeks. Ultrasound Obstet Gynecol. 2005;26:718-24.
8. Jani J, Peralta CFA, Benachi A, et al. Assessment of lung area in fetuses with congenital diaphragmatic hernia. Ultrasound Obstet. 2007;30:72-6.
9. Chang CH, Yu CH, Chang FM, et al. Volumetric assessment of normal fetal lungs using three-dimensional ultrasound. Ultrasound Med Bio. 2003;29:935-42.
10. Peralta CFA, Cavoretto P, Csapo B, et al. Lung and heart volumes by three-dimensional ultrasound in normal fetuses at 12-32 weeks' gestation. Ultrasound Obstet Gynecol. 2006; 27:128-33.
11. Osada H, Iitsuka Y, Masuda K, et al. Application of lung volume measurement by three-dimensional ultrasonography for clinical assessment of fetal lung development. J Ultrasound Med. 2002;21:841-47.

12. Malinger G, Levine A, Rotmensch S. The fetal esophagus: anatomical and physiological ultrasonographic characterization using a high-resolution linear transducer. Ultrasound Obstet Gynecol. 2004;24:500-5.
13. Brantberg A, Blaas HGK, Haugen SE, et al. Esophageal obstruction—prenatal detection rate and outcome. Ultrasound Obstet Gynecol. 2007;30:180-7.
14. Variet F, Bousquet F, Clemenson A, Chauleur C, Kopp Dutour N, Tronchet M, et al. Congenital diaphragmatic hernia. Two cases with early prenatal diagnosis and increased nuchal translucency. Fetal Diagn Ther. 2003;18(1):33-5.
15. Kitano Y, Nakagawa S, Kuroda T, Honna T, Itoh Y, Nakamura T, et al. Liver position in fetal congenital diaphragmatic hernia retains a prognostic value in the era of lung-protective strategy. J Pediatr Surg. 2005;40(12):1827-32.
16. Jani J, Benachi A, Favre R, et al. Lung-to-head ratio and liver position to predict outcome in early diagnosed isolated left-sided diaphragmatic hernia fetuses: a multicenter study. Am J Obstet Gynecol. 2004;191:176-82.
17. Deprest J, Jani J, Van Schoubroeck D, Cannie M, Gallot D, Dymarkowski S, et al. Current consequences of prenatal diagnosis of congenital diaphragmatic hernia. Journal of Pediatric Surgery. 2006;41(2):423-30.
18. Ruano R, Benachi A, Joubin L, Aubry MC, Thalabard JC, Dumez Y, et al. Three-dimensional ultrasonographic assessment of fetal lung volume as prognostic factor in isolated congenital diaphragmatic hernia. BJOG. 2004;111(5):423-29.
19. Crombleholme T, Coleman B, Hedrick H, Liechty K, Howell L, et al. Cystic adenomatoid malformation volume ratio predicts outcome in prenatally diagnosed cystic adenomatoid malformation of the Lung. J Pediatric Surg. 2002;37(3):331-8.
20. Winters WD, Effmann EL, Nghiam HV, et al. Disappearing fetal lung masses: Importance of postnatal imaging studies. Pediatr Radiol. 1997;27:535-9.
21. Cass DL, Quinn TM, Yang EY, et al. Increased cell proliferation and decreased apoptosis characterizes congenital cystic adenomatoid malformation of the lung. J Pediatr Surg. 1998;33:1043-7.
22. Stocker JT, Madewell JE, Drake RM. Congenital cystic adenomatoid malformation of the lung. Classification and morphologic spectrum. Hum Pathol. 1977;8:155-71.
23. Gilbert-Barness E, Debich-Spicer D. Respiratory system. In: Gilbert-Barness E, Debich-Spicer D, (Eds). Embryo and fetal pathology. Cambridge, UK: Cambridge University Press. 2004;470-89.
24. Duncombe G, Dickinson J, Kikiros C. Prenatal diagnosis and management of congenital cystic adenomatoid malformation of the lung. Am J Obstet Gynecol. 2002; 187:950-4.
25. Laberge JM, Flageole H, Pugash D, Khalife S, Blair G, Filiatrault D, et al. Congenital cystic adenomatoid malformation of the lung: prognosis when diagnosed in utero. Saudi Med J. 2004;24(5 Suppl):S33.
26. Yinon Y, Kelly E, Rzan G. Fetal pleural effusions. Best Practice & Research Clin Obstet and Gynaecol. 2008;22(1): 77-96.
27. Waller K, Chaithongwongwatthana S, Yamasmit W, et al. Chromosomal abnormalities among 246 fetuses with pleural effusions detected on prenatal ultrasound examination: factors associated with an increased risk of aneuploidy. Genet Med. 2005;7(6):417-21.
28. Frazier AA, Dosado DE, Cristenson ML, et al. Intralobar seqestration: radiologic-pathologic correlation. Radiographics 1997;17:725-45.
29. Doray B, Girard-Lemaire F, Gasser B, et al. Pallister-Killian syndrome: difficulties of prenatal diagnosis. Prenat Diagn 2002;22(6):470-7.
30. Slavotinek A. Fryns syndrome: a review of the phenotype and diagnostic guidelines. Am J Med Genet 2004;124:427-33.
31. Slavotinek AM. 2007. Single gene disorders associated with congenital diaphragmatic hernia. Am J Med Genet C Semin Med Genet. 2007;145:172-83.
32. Hurst J, Firth H, Chitty L. Syndromic associations with congenital anomalies of the fetal thorax and abdomen Prenat Diagn. 2008;28:676-84.
33. Shaw-Smith C. 2006. Esophageal atresia, tracheo-esophageal fistula, and the VACTERL association: review of genetics and epidemiology. J Med Genet. 2006;43:545-54
34. Ruano R, da Silva MM, Salustiano EM, Kilby MD, Tannuri U, Zugaib M. Percutaneous laser ablation under ultrasound guidance for fetal hyperechogenic microcystic lung lesions with hydrops: A single center cohort and a literature review. Prenat Diagn. 2012;32:1127-32.
35. Mallmann MR, Geipel A, Bludau M, Matil K, Gottschalk I, Hoopmann M, et al. Bronchopulmonary sequestration with massive pleural effusion: pleuroamniotic shunting vs. intrafetal vascular laser ablation. Ultrasound Obstet Gynecol. 2014;44:441-6.

21

CHAPTER

Three-dimensional and Four-dimensional Evaluation of the Fetal Heart

Carmen Comas Gabriel

INTRODUCTION

During the past 25 years, two-dimensional (2D) imaging of the fetal heart has evolved into a sophisticated and widely practiced clinical tool, but most heart diseases still go prenatally undetected despite routine fetal ultrasound evaluations. Over the next few years, tremendous advances in fetal cardiac imaging, including three-dimensional (3D) imaging, promise to revolutionize both the prenatal detection and diagnosis of congenital heart diseases. Image resolution continues to improve year after year, allowing earlier and better visualization of cardiac structures. This chapter reviews the possibilities of the 3D and four-dimensional (4D) fetal echocardiography. Three-dimensional imaging of the fetal heart may improve the detection of outflow tract abnormalities and facilitate comprehension of complex forms of congenital heart diseases (CHDs). This review highlights the potential of acquiring a digital volume data set of a heart cycle for later offline examination, either for an offline diagnosis, a second opinion (e.g. via Internet link) or for teaching fetal echocardiography to trainees and sonographers. On the other hand, other imaging modalities, such as Doppler tissue imaging and magnetic resonance imaging, continue to evolve and to complement two- and three-dimensional sonographic imaging of the fetal heart. As a result of these ongoing advances in prenatal detection and assessment of CHD, this is an exciting and promising time for the field of fetal cardiac imaging.[1]

IMPACT OF CONGENITAL HEART DISEASES: EPIDEMIOLOGY AND POPULATION AT RISK

Prenatal detection of fetal congenital heart defects remains the most problematic issue of prenatal diagnosis.[2] Major CHDs are the most common severe congenital malformations, with an incidence of about five in a thousand live births, whenever complete ascertainment is done and minor lesions are excluded.[2,3] Congenital heart anomalies have a significant effect on affected children's life with up to 25–35% mortality rate during pregnancy and the postnatal period and it is during the first year of life when 60% of this mortality occurs. Moreover, major CHDs are responsible for nearly 50% of all neonatal and infant deaths due to congenital anomalies and it is likely to be significantly higher if spontaneous abortions are considered. Although CHDs used to appear isolated, they are frequently associated with other defects, such as chromosomal anomalies and genetic syndromes. Their incidence is six times greater than chromosomal abnormalities and four times greater than neural tube defects.[2-4] Nonetheless, structural cardiac defects are among the most frequently missed abnormalities by prenatal ultrasound.[5] Although, the at-risk population-based approach has been crucial in decreasing disease, prenatal diagnosis of CHD remains largely a scenario of too much effort for too few diagnoses. Clinicians need to re-examine the reasons for this shortfall and redefine new strategies to improve the efficacy of our effort.

It must be remembered that 90% of congenital heart defects occur in low-risk mothers. The way forward to increase detection of CHD is to improve the effectiveness of screening programs so that a higher number of cases from low-risk populations are referred for a specialized scan. The positive aspect of screening for cardiac defects compared with other anomalies (e.g., Down syndrome, neural tube defects) is that it does not automatically result in the termination of pregnancy in most cases. It is one of the anomalies where optimizing management of the neonate in the perinatal period could improve outcome. Improved morbidity/mortality has been clearly shown as a result of prenatal diagnosis in the outcome of all forms of CHD, which are dependent on the patency of the arterial duct in the immediate postnatal period, being the transposition of the great arteries, the single most important lesion to diagnose prenatally.[6]

All these reasons emphasize the role of sonography in prenatal diagnosis of congenital heart abnormalities.

PRENATAL DIAGNOSIS OF CONGENITAL HEART DISEASES: CURRENT SITUATION

Screening Techniques

Most major CHDs can be prenatally diagnosed by detailed transabdominal second-trimester echocardiography at 20–22 weeks' gestation.[2,4,7-9] The identification of pregnancies at high risk for CHD needing referral to specialist centers is of paramount importance in order to reduce the rate of overlooked defects.[9,10] However, the main problem in prenatal diagnosis of CHD is that the majority of cases take place in pregnancies with no identifiable risk factors. Therefore, there is wide agreement that cardiac ultrasound screening should be introduced as an integral part of the routine scan at 20–22 week. In the 1990s, the American Institute of Ultrasound in Medicine and the American College of Radiology incorporated the four-chamber view into their formal guidelines for the screening fetal ultrasound.[11,12] Although early investigators found the four-chamber view to have a high sensitivity for the prenatal detection of CHD, subsequent studies have found this view to be far less sensitive. Even in the best hands, this plane may fail to detect significant percentage of major frequently ductal-dependent CHD. Many investigators have demonstrated an incremental value of adding outflow tracts to the routine screening fetal ultrasound.[13,14] When applied to low-risk population, scrutiny of the four-chamber view allows only the detection of 40% of the anomalies, while additional visualization of the outflow tracts and the great arteries increase the rate up to 60–70%.[4,7,8] The systematic incorporation of the four-chamber view and outflow tracts into the routine screening, fetal ultrasound represents an important advance in fetal cardiac image.

The Standard Fetal Cardiac Examination Protocol

The basic fetal cardiac screening examination entails an analysis of the four-chamber view, obtained from an axial plane across the fetal thorax. If technically feasible, optional views of the outflow tracts can be obtained as a part of an extended cardiac screening examination. The systematic incorporation of the four-chamber view and outflow tracts into the routine screening fetal ultrasound represents an important advance in fetal cardiac image. Summarizing the data from screening studies, a detection rate of less than 10% can be expected if the heart is not explicitly examined, a rate of 10–40% detection if the four-chamber view is visualized and a rate of 40–80% if the visualization of the great vessels is added.[4,7,8]

In a high-risk pregnancy, in addition to the information provided by the basic screening exam, a detailed analysis of cardiac structure and function may further characterize visceroatrial situs, systemic and pulmonary venous connections, foramen ovale mechanism, atrioventricular connections, ventriculoarterial connections, great vessels relationship and sagittal views of the aortic and ductal arches. Additional sonographic techniques can be used for this purpose, as Doppler ultrasonography or M-mode modality.

Color Doppler is an essential tool for the fetal cardiologist, but is not considered standard of care for a routine obstetric scan. Color Doppler findings can substantially increase the likelihood of prenatal diagnosis and decrease the incidence of false-positive diagnosis. Spectral power Doppler can also add important information to normal and abnormal color flow patterns.

Recently, a sequential segmental approach for the complete evaluation of fetal heart disease as a screening technique has been described using five or six short-axis views from the fetal upper abdomen to the mediastinum.[15,16] The transverse view of the fetal upper abdomen is obtained to determine the arrangement of the abdominal organs, which, in most cases, provides the important clues to the determination of the atrial arrangement. The four-chamber view is obtained to evaluate the atrioventricular junctions. The views of the left and right ventricular outflow tracts are obtained to evaluate the ventriculoarterial junctions. The three-vessel view and the aortic arch view are obtained for the evaluation of the arrangement and size of the great arteries, which provides the additional clues to the diagnosis of the abnormalities involving the ventriculo-arterial junctions and the great arteries.

Suggestions to Improve Detection Rate of Congenital Heart Defects

Inadequate examination is likely to be the most common cause of heart defects being overlooked in the four-chamber view. Chaoui have suggested some hints to improve visualization of the heart.[17] Examination of the fetal heart should be carried out at every second-trimester screening examination. This should ideally be performed at 20–22 weeks' gestation, using a 5-MHz transducer. Optimal analysis of the heart may be achieved by magnification of the image, using the zoom function, so that the heart fills a third to half of the screen and by the use of the cine-loop to assess the different phases of the cardiac cycle. Established ultrasound screening programs also increase detection rates.[5] They have to focus on equivocal prenatal signs of the heart abnormality, so called borderline findings, which should raise suspicion for referral to a specialist, as echogenic foci, small pericardial effusions, mild discrepancy in ventricular size, tricuspid regurgitation or deviation of the cardiac axis. Since heart anomalies developing *in utero* can be missed at second-trimester scan, fetal heart should be examined if third-trimester scanning is performed. The use of color Doppler during cardiac scanning will also improve detection rates, increasing the speed and the accuracy of the fetal cardiac scan, although it is controversial to use this modality for screening purposes.

Finally, introduction of 3D technology in the field of the prenatal diagnosis has allowed a better evaluation of the static anatomical structures. Nevertheless, its application in the study of the fetal heart has not involved a significant advance up to now, since the fetal heart being a structure in rapid movement, the conventional 3D image appeared distorted without providing significant diagnostic information.

HISTORY OF FETAL ECHOCARDIOGRAPHY

The birth of fetal echocardiography occurred in the late 1970s, when fetal heart movements were first visualized by primitive A-scan ultrasound or by M-mode techniques. Since then, different technologies and modalities have been incorporated in order to improve the diagnostic accuracy and possibilities in this field. We review the diagnostic tools that are available and the potential roles of fetal echocardiography in the field of fetal medicine.[18]

Real-time ultrasound is still the gold standard for the structural evaluation of the fetal heart. In the most sophisticated ultrasound machines, there is an ideal setting for fetal heart evaluation which is based on a high image resolution, a high frame rate and good penetration. Two main features have facilitated the prenatal assessment of the fetal heart: the use of transducers with a high frequency (5–7 MHz transducers) and the incorporation of the cine-loop and the zoom functions. Tissue harmonic imaging (THI) has recently been introduced to enhance diagnostic performance in individuals with limited acoustic window mainly due to obesity or abdominal scarring.[19] Their different behavior from the fundamental frequency ultrasound, the energy of which decreases linearly with depth, is the reason why the use of THI has been shown to improve image quality in some circumstances, particularly in obese individuals.

Time motion (M-mode) was a revolutionary tool in fetal cardiology when simultaneous real-time visualization became available. First used for cardiac biometry, it was soon relegated to a second line since such measurements became easier using the cine-loop techniques to selectively image diastole and systole. Two main fields of interest are still in the domain of M-mode: the assessment and classification of fetal arrhythmias (where this mode can document the atrioventricular conduction by putting the cursor simultaneously in an atrial and ventricular structure) and to assess myocardial contractility (calculating indices such as shortening fraction, ejection fraction, etc.).

The acquisition of flow velocity waveforms from different fetal cardiac structures and vessels by using *pulsed or continuous wave Doppler* ultrasound enables a noninvasive quantification of perfusion: Evaluation of peak velocities in different sites of the circulatory system, measurement of contractility indices, stroke volume and the recent incorporation of the assessment of coronary and venous system are some examples. The pathological conditions investigated are no longer confined to fetal heart defects but have expanded to include other fetal conditions involving the cardiovascular system. Investigation of intracardiac flow in severe intrauterine growth restriction, diabetes or fetal anemia represents some examples of the big potential of this technical modality.

In addition to grayscale examination of the fetal heart, *color Doppler* is now considered to be a second-line investigation for cardiac evaluation. This method allows rapid orientation within the fetal heart and completes the evaluation supplied by grayscale information. Once abnormal flow is suspected, quantification by Doppler flow velocities waveforms becomes mandatory.

Color Doppler is an essential tool for the fetal cardiologist, but is not considered standard of care for a routine obstetric scan.

Power Doppler ultrasound is a technique introduced in the early 1990s using the information from the amplitude of the Doppler signal rather than the frequency shift and direction, opening the possibility of displaying flow independently of its velocity and direction. Since this technique is significantly more sensitive than conventional color Doppler, it has been applied in regions with low flow and small vessels. This technique can be used in fetal cardiology, facilitating the detection of some CHD (such as small ventricular septal defects) and enabling spatial orientation of the great vessels. On the other hand, we cannot be informed about the blood direction or turbulences. However, these characteristics make it suitable for the 3D power Doppler evaluation of the cardiovascular system.

In *tissue Doppler echocardiography (TDE)*, color-coding is used to visualize wall movements rather than blood flow. Tissue Doppler echocardiography has only recently been applied to the fetus, with promising preliminary results.[20,21] Color and power Doppler mapping could be applied on a regular high-resolution ultrasound machine by sampling the relatively high reflected acoustic energy from cardiac walls. Fetal TDE is a new technique that can provide additional insights into fetal cardiac function that are not available with the conventional approach.

Although *fetal 3D* imaging currently faces important image resolution concerns, the technique has the potential to improve markedly both the prenatal detection and diagnosis of CHD. Already demonstrated to improve the diagnosis of CHD in infants, children and adults, 3D imaging of the fetal heart offers important potential advantages over conventional 2D imaging. By acquiring volumetric data within a few seconds from a single window, 3D imaging may reduce scanning time and operator dependence. For screening the low-risk pregnancy, 3D imaging may facilitate visualization of the four-chamber view and outflow tracts, particularly when 2D imaging fails because of time constraint, limited window or sonographer inexperience. Volume data sets could be transmitted electronically to experts for further evaluation. For teaching purposes, the volumetric data sets could be sent to a remote virtual scanning station. Finally, quantitative measurements using 3D imaging promise to be more accurate and reproducible than those derived from 2D imaging. Sophisticated volume processing algorithms that allow quantitative measurements of volume and function may offer additional insights into cardiac function and development. Recently, *spatiotemporal image correlation (STIC)* has been introduced as a new 3D technique allowing the automatic acquisition of a volume of data from the fetal heart, being displayed as a cineloop of a single cardiac cycle. This technique allows dynamic multiplanar slicing and surface rendering of heart anatomy. Spatiotemporal imaging correlation, in combination with color or power Doppler ultrasound, is a promising new tool for multiplanar and 3D/4D rendering of the fetal heart, making possible the assessment of hemodynamics changes throughout the cardiac cycle. Since its commercial introduction in 2002, some foreign authors have published their experience in the management and application of this new technology. In the following section, we deeply review this topic and present the first study on a nationwide scale with the introduction of the new technology in our environment.

Telemedicine represents an emerging but potentially critical advance in prenatal screening for CHD.[22,23] Telemedicine, like 3D ultrasound, may enable fetuses to be scanned in remote sites, with their respective studies reviewed instantaneously or within minutes at more centrally located, highly specialized centers, avoiding the need to transport the pregnant patient.

NEW PERSPECTIVES IN THREE- AND FOUR-DIMENSIONAL FETAL ECHOCARDIOGRAPHY

Rapid advances in graphics computing and micro-engineering have offered new techniques for prenatal cardiac imaging. Some of them can be noninvasively applied to both clinical and laboratory settings, including dynamic 3D echocardiography, myocardial Doppler imaging, harmonic ultrasound imaging and B-flow sonography. Appropriate use of these new tools will not only provide unique information for better clinical assessment of fetal cardiac disease but also offer new ways to improved understanding of cardiovascular development and pathogenesis.[24] This improvement in imaging technology combined with new sophisticated computer processing systems promise to revolutionize both prenatal detection and diagnosis of CHD.[25] Even 2D imaging still remains the principal diagnostic modality to confirm normal cardiac development and in cases of congenital heart abnormalities, new techniques (dynamic 3D color Doppler ultrasound, Doppler-gated 3D fetal echocardiography and 3D multiplanar time-motion ultrasound) are now technically feasible for a wide range of lesions and may provide additional information of clinical value in some selected cases. In this sense, new terms have been recently incorporated in our practice, for describing various multidimensional imaging features, including "three-dimensional", "four-dimensional", "real-time", "cardiac gating", "online" or "offline".[26] This chapter reviews the possibilities of 3D and 4D fetal echocardiography, where a volume data set can be acquired as a static volume, as a real-time 3D volume or as an offline 4D volume cine using STIC software.[27] Spatial-temporal image correlation is explained and the potentials of this modality are particularly emphasized in the next section.

Fetal Cardiac Screening

As current methods to screen the fetus for cardiac abnormalities continue to miss most CHD, a more effective approach to screening the low-risk population for fetal heart disease would represent an important clinical advance. In this sense, preliminary results suggest that 3D and 4D technologies applied to prenatal diagnosis have the potential to function as a screening tool for fetal heart diseases. Investigators are trying to demonstrate the feasibility and applications of different modalities, such as real-time,[28] gated reconstructive 3D imaging[29] or fetal real-time 3D echocardiography (RT3DE).[30]

Feasibility to Obtain Greater Number of Cardiac Views

Three-dimensional ultrasonography permits a greater number of cardiac planes to be extracted from volume data than does 2D standard ultrasonography. Bega's study compares the percentage of cardiac planes obtained by conventional 2D or 3D ultrasonography, demonstrating higher successful view by the latter technique for the left and right outflow tracts and ductal and aortic arches.[31]

Improvement of Basic Cardiac Views in Unfavorable Fetal Positions

Among the basic cardiac views in fetuses in anterior spine positions, 3D ultrasound improves the visualization of pulmonary outflow tracts and provides reliable alternate technique for clinical use.[32]

Evaluation of Fetal Cardiac Function

Three-dimensional echocardiography can provide estimates of ventricular volume and function.[33] Particularly, 3D imaging can provide estimates of ventricular volume changes in fetal hearts with abnormal ventricular morphology that cannot be easily performed by 2D echocardiography.[34] This technique is a promising tool for the evaluation of fetuses with CHD and cardiac dysfunction, and it may provide insight into evolving CHDs.

Dynamic Three-dimensional Color Doppler Ultrasound

By using simultaneously two ultrasound machines, one grayscale and color Doppler echocardiography and another one for spectral Doppler ultrasound, a novel technique has made possible the prenatal visualization of the spatial distribution and the true direction of intracardiac flow of blood in 4D in the absence of motion artifacts. This technique suggests that diagnosis of cardiac malformations can be made on the basis of morphological and hemodynamics changes throughout the entire cardiac cycle, offering significant information complementary to conventional techniques.[35]

Doppler-gated Three-dimensional Fetal Echocardiography

Even 2D imaging remains the principal diagnostic modality to confirm normal or abnormal cardiac development, Doppler-gated 3D fetal echocardiography is technically feasible for a wide range of lesions and may provide additional information of clinical value in some selected cases.[36] Gated 3D fetal echocardiography provides significantly better visualization and comprehension of cardiac anatomy than nongated 3D fetal echocardiography. The superiority of gated over nongated 3D fetal echocardiography appears to come from both improved image quality and the anatomic clues that derive from the ability to view cardiac motion.[29]

Real-time Three-dimensional Echocardiography

Conventional prenatal screening for CHD involves a time-consuming and highly operator-dependent acquisition of the four-chamber view and outflow tracts. In response, many investigators have demonstrated the potential for gated, reconstructive 3D echocardiography to evaluate the fetal heart. Reconstructive 3D echocardiography has been shown to simplify and shorten the acquisition component of fetal cardiac imaging. However, reconstructive 3D fetal cardiac imaging reconstructs a volume of data following the sequential acquisition of a series of planes. As a result, reconstructive approaches suffer from artifacts related to cardiac gating and random fetal and maternal motion. In contrast, RT3DE acquires a volume of data virtually instantaneously, without the need for cardiac gating and with less potential for artifacts. By acquiring the entire fetal heart instantaneously as a single volume, RT3DE may facilitate fetal cardiac screening. In this sense, preliminary studies suggest a high sensitivity for detecting CHD (93%), although specificity is low (45%), with a high rate of "cannot determine" responses and false-positive artifacts.[30] These preliminary results suggest that RT3DE has the potential to function as a screening tool for fetal heart disease. However, artifacts must be recognized and minimized, resolution must improve and substantial training will be necessary prior to widespread clinical use.

Three-dimensional Power Doppler Ultrasound

In the recent years few reports and studies demonstrated that the 3D power Doppler ultrasound (3D-PDU) helps in the reconstruction of the vessels of interest, and thus, improves the understanding of the spatial appearance of the vascular tree.[37]

Three-dimensional Multiplanar Time-motion Ultrasound

This new technique enables the easy acquisition of optimal M-mode traces from different heart structures. Because offline plane positioning is possible on 3D multiplanar reconstruction, M-mode traces can be obtained from different stored cardiac structures independently of the fetal position.[38]

Spatiotemporal Image Correlation

Spatiotemporal image correlation is a new approach for clinical assessment of the fetal heart. This feature offers an easy-to-use technique to acquire data from the fetal heart and its visualization in a 4D sequence. The acquisition is performed in two steps. First, data is acquired by a single, automatic volume sweep. In the second step, the system analyzes the data according to their spatial and temporal domain and processes a 4D sequence. This sequence presents the heart beating in real-time in a multiplanar display. The examiner can navigate within the heart, re-slice and produce all the standard planes necessary for comprehensive diagnosis.

The acquisition of the 3D volume information is based on initial application of 2D imaging techniques including grayscale, Doppler, power Doppler and B-flow modalities. Once the cardiac volume is obtained, a combination of postprocessing tools such as surface mode, minimal mode, transverse rendering, inversion and glass body modes allow preferential display of various features of the fetal heart. Motion display modes including cineloop and STIC in combination with automated and semi-automated display of examination planes opens a whole new array of diagnostic possibilities in clinical practice.[39]

New Reconstructive Approaches

Real-time 3D echocardiography with instantaneous volume-rendered displays of the fetal heart represents a new approach to fetal cardiac imaging with tremendous clinical potential.[28] New plans and views, not visualized in conventional fetal 2D echocardiography, can be generated with minimal processing of rendered image displays.

Virtual Echocardiography by Internet Link

A complete virtual cardiological examination can be achieved in stored 3D volumes of the fetal heart and transmitted to a tertiary fetal cardiology center via the Internet. Previous experiences have demonstrated that 3D virtual cardiac examination is possible.[40,41] The use of the internet link has major implications, particularly for situations in which the scanning center is geographically remote from the tertiary center, or facilitating a second opinion diagnosis.

CLINICAL APPLICATION OF 3D OR 4D IN FETAL CARDIOVASCULAR SYSTEM

The clinical application of 3D or 4D in prenatal visualization of the fetal cardiovascular system is closely related to the regions of interest known from the application of color and power Doppler ultrasound: vessels of the placenta, umbilical cord, abdomen, kidneys, lung, brain and fetal tumors as well as the heart and great vessels.[37]

Peripheral Vascular System in 3D

Umbilical Cord and Placenta

From Chaoui experience, it seems to be the structure most easily accessible to 3D throughout pregnancy. Intraplacental vessel network architecture can be visualized with this method. Abnormalities such as placenta previa, vasa previa or velamentous insertion can be demonstrated as well as single umbilical artery or less important conditions as the connecting vessels in twin pregnancies, nuchal cord or true or false knot.[37,42]

Intra-abdominal Vessels

The vessels of interest are the umbilical vein, the ductus venosus, the portal vein, the hepatic veins, splenic vessels, inferior vena cava and abdominal aorta. Since the application of color Doppler and the recent intensive study of the ductus venosus, abnormalities of intrahepatic venous system were detected to be more common as expected. Conditions to study by 3D power Doppler could involve the abnormal cord insertion on the abdomen (omphalocele, gastroschisis), abnormal umbilical vein size (varix or ectasia) and absence of the ductus venosus or abnormal course of vessels in isomerism conditions.

Renal Vessels

The visualization of renal vessels is known to increase the accuracy of the diagnosis of kidney malformations in the fetus. The renal vascular tree is well visualized in a coronal plane with the descending aorta showing a horizontal course. Conditions with possible benefit of 3D-PDU application are agenesis of one or both kidneys, arteries in duplex kidney, horseshoe or pelvic kidney.

Intracerebral Vessels

A transversal insonation easily allows the reconstruction of the circulus of Willis, whereas a more sagittal approach enables the visualization of the pericallosal artery with its ramifications. Choosing a lower velocity scale flow, the cerebral veins and sagittal sinus can be imaged as well. Main fields of interest are the abnormal anterior cerebral artery in agenesis of corpus callosum, the aneurysm of the vein of Galen and disturbed vascular anatomy in cerebral malformations.

Lung Vessels

Fields of interest are the analysis of the 3D vessel architecture in cystic lung malformation, congenital diaphragmatic hernia and bronchopulmonary sequestration. The role of color or power Doppler in predicting pulmonary hypoplasia failed and it is not expected that the 3D demonstration of the vessels could be in this field of great interest in the near future.[37]

Fetal Tumors or Aberrant Vessels

Aberrant vessels can be visualized in the presence of several malformations like lung sequestration, chorioangioma, lymphangioma or in sacrococcygeal teratoma, acardiac twin, etc. In this sense, fetal tumors can be of interest to be visualized not only for their risk of cardiac failure due to the presence of arteriovenous fistulae, but also to assess compression of shifting of neighboring organs.

The Fetal Heart in 3D and 4D

In the last decade, 3D and 4D fetal echocardiography was investigated intensively in laboratories using external work stations, static volume sweep, matrix transducers and recently a new ultrasound equipment with integrated software (STIC™) was introduced allowing a reliable 3D and 4D fetal echocardiography.[39]

SPATIOTEMPORAL IMAGING CORRELATION: A NEW APPROACH TO THREE- AND FOUR-DIMENSIONAL EVALUATION OF THE FETAL HEART

In 2002, Voluson Expert 730 (GE Medical Systems, Kretz Ultrasound, Zipf, Austria) introduced a new technological concept called Spatiotemporal Image Correlation (STIC). This technology enables to review, handle and store digitally volume data of the fetal heart in a looped cine sequence. The aim for the development of the STIC technique was to create a useful screening tool that is easy to use and facilitates the detection of the fetal heart anomalies during the routine obstetrical scan. In several studies, 4D fetal echocardiography proves to offer a more comprehensive assessment of the fetal heart morphology and relationship of the great vessels,[29,36,43] even if the fetus is in an unfavorable scanning position.[32]

Spatiotemporal image correlation basically displays three different imaging modalities, in a grayscale, in color Doppler and in power Doppler **(Figs. 1A to C)**. Each of them can display two possible formats, multiplanar (showing perpendicular planes to each other) or rendered (reconstruction of the plane A) **(Figs. 2A to D)**. The rendered format can be displayed in different algorithms (gray, color and glass body) **(Figs. 3A to D)**. The multiplanar format is the first system that allows a simultaneous and dynamic multiplanar evaluation of several 2D planes. The volumetric format is a technique process in which the 3D structures of the scanned volume are transferred to a 2D image.

TECHNICAL BASES

The main aspects that have to be considered when evaluating a 3D imaging system are the volume data acquisition and the image rendering display. The acquisition can be achieved either in 3D static mode (a volume consisting of series of still images) or in 4D mode (which reflects the beating character of the heart).

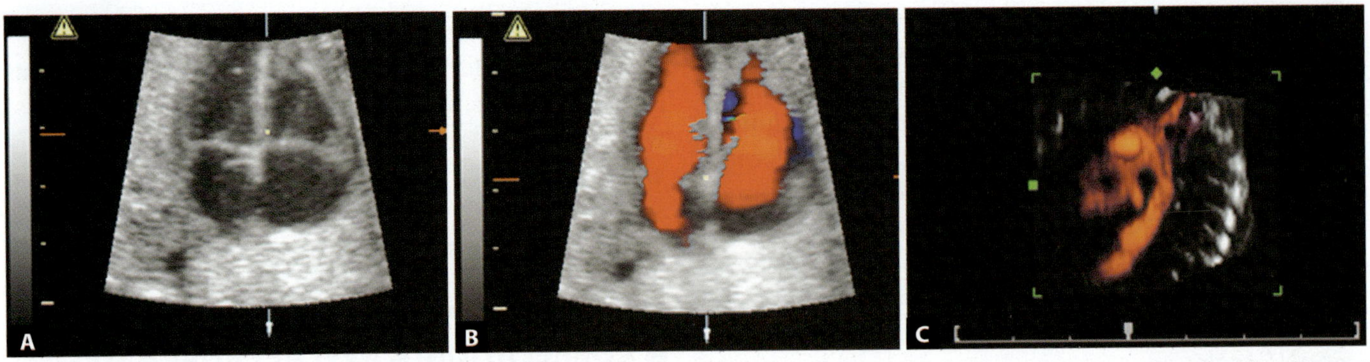

Figs. 1A to C: Spatiotemporal image correlation technique offers different display formats, in grayscale or combined with color and power Doppler. (A) Display format in grayscale; (B) Display format in grayscale combined with color Doppler; (C) Display format in grayscale combined with power Doppler.

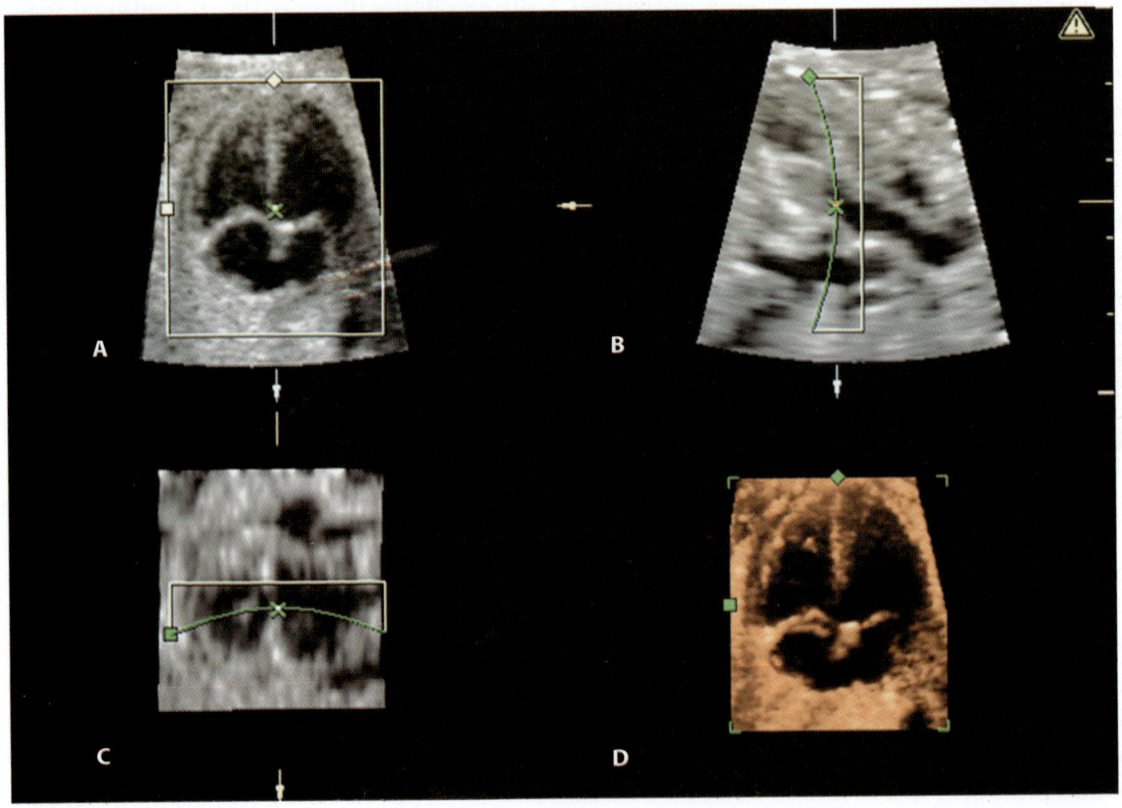

Figs. 2A to D: (A) Plane A demonstrates the acquired image obtained during the STIC sweep; (B) Plane B is the orthogonal plane vertical to the plane A (sagittal plane); (C) Plane C is the orthogonal plane horizontal to the plane A (coronal plane); (D) Volume rendering image.

The latter can be acquired either in live real-time 3D or as offline 4D, which is possible by the recent advent of the new software of STIC. In these acquisitions heart and vessels can be visualized either in grayscale mode or in combination with color Doppler,[44] power Doppler or B-flow.[37] Image rendering is the process of creating a 3D visual representation of the parameters of interest.

The STIC technology enables the automatic and sequential acquisition of 2D images in a volume digitally stored, performing a single sweep in slow motion over a limited area of interest, which provides a high-resolution image (150 frames/second). It is possible to optimize the image changing the acquisition time (between 7, 5 and 15 seconds, with intervals of 2, 5 seconds) and the sweep

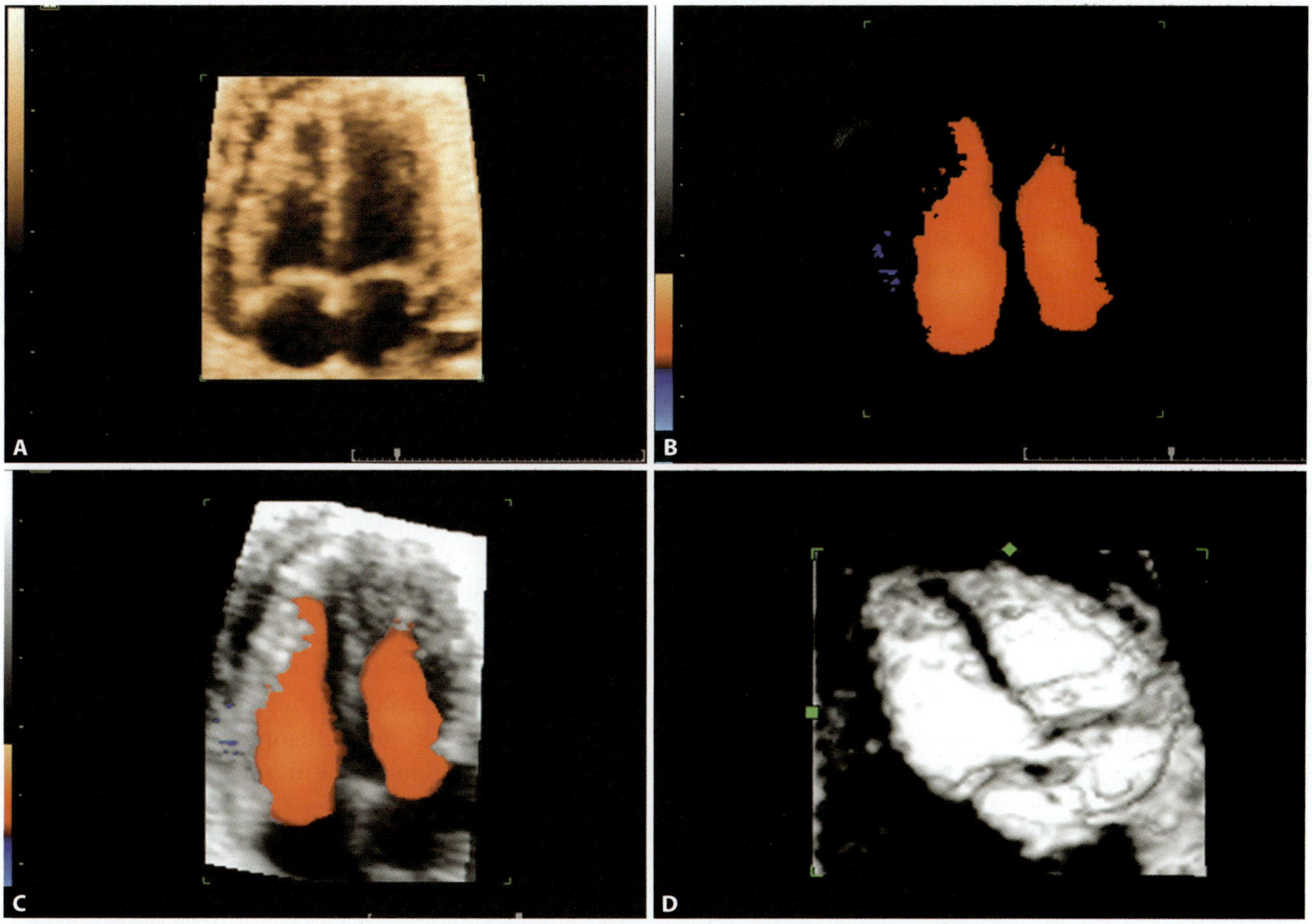

Figs. 3A to D: The heart volume dataset can be displayed as a single image of a 3D/4D surface or a transparent volume, in which grayscale or color Doppler information or both can be demonstrated (so called "glass body" mode). Inversed mode has been recently described as a new rendering algorithm that transforms echolucent structures into echogenic voxels. (A) Gray rendering volume; (B) Color rendering volume; (C) Glass body rendering volume; (D) Inversed mode rendering volume.

angle (from 15 to 40°, with intervals of 5°). The steps are defined as follows:

Acquisition

Automatic volume acquisition: It means the array inside the transducer housing performs an automatic slow single sweep, recording one single 3D data set. This volume consists of a high number of 2D frames, one behind the other. Due to the small region of interest, the B-mode frame rate during the volume scan is very high, in the range of approximately 150 frames per second, which means that 2D images are stored in high resolution.

Post Processing

After the volume scan is acquired, the system runs a spatial and temporal correlation of the recorded data. This technology identifies the rhythmical movements and depending on their periodicity, the fetal heart rate can be calculated. Based on the exact timing of the systolic peak and the time fraction between one systole and the next, the system rearranges the 2D images, obtaining consecutive volumes presenting a complete and "synchronized" cardiac cycle (it correlates the images of different cardiac cycles obtained in the slow sweep rearranging the events according to their spatial and temporal domain).

Visualization

These volumes are displayed in an endless cine sequence (showing the heart cycle in real-time in cine-loop), which can be played in different possibilities [slow motion, frame-by-frame, stopped at any stage during the cycle, rotation in the three planes of the space (x, y and z planes), multiplanar view, single plane, volumetric reconstruction, etc.]. Similarly, it is possible to perform postprocessing adjustments, such as the gamma curve correction to optimize the contrast resolution, the modification of color threshold (balance to control and modify the color intensity over the grayscale) or grayscale threshold, etc.

Summarizing, thanks to this algorithm, following a dynamic acquisition of a volume dataset including the fetal heart, a single cardiac cycle is virtually reconstructed according to heart rate with fundamental section planes being displayed in multiplanar fashion or integrated into a moving volume (4D echocardiography). In this sense, STIC can be defined as an "online" system with an "indirect volume scan" and "post-3D/4D-acquisition correlation".[44] Thanks to this technique, a more comprehensive investigation of fetal heart is feasible since all structures are amenable to exploration along any view angle, irrespective of fetal position.

ADVANTAGES

Improved Temporal Resolution

Due to the increased number of frames acquired for a specific anatomical region using STIC technique, this method results in improved temporal resolution of the online dynamic 3D image sequence that is displayed in the multiplanar or the rendered display.[45] As a result, the difficult or nonidentifiable cardiac images in the conventional 2D mode can improve with this new approach.

Dynamic Evaluation of the Four-chamber View

It enables a dynamic evaluation of the four-chamber view. It does not examine a single static four-chamber plane at a time but it allows a dynamic study of this view in the three planes, in anteroposterior sense as well as laterolateral and superoinferior, letting in this way the planes rotate around a 360° axis.

Evaluation of the Outflow Tracts

The 2D evaluation of the outflow tracts may be difficult due to an inadequate fetal orientation or the own fetal movement. The STIC technology facilitates the assessment of the outflow tracts since it enables the rotation of the data volume around a single reference point.[32,44]

Multiplanar Dynamic Display and Navigation

The volume acquired by 3D ultrasonography can be displayed on a monitor in three orthogonal planes, representing the transverse, sagittal and coronal planes of a representative 2D plane within the volume. Such a display of three orthogonal planes from the 3D volume acquisition is termed "multiplanar display". Spatiotemporal imaging correlation is the first system with a simultaneous dynamic multiplanar view in the three planes.[45,46] Using multiplanar slicing, examiners can dynamically visualize the heart in three orthogonal planes at the same time. The reference dot can be employed to "navigate" the volume in any direction, placing the reference dot at any location in planes a, b or c and observing the corresponding plane changes in their respective images **(Figs. 4 to 6)**.

Reconstruction of a Three-dimensional Rendered Image

It enables the reconstruction of a 3D rendered image that contains depth and volume which may provide additional information that is not available from the multiplanar image slices.[44,46] Thanks to multiplanar volume rendering of the cardiac structures, some CHDs, traditionally proven inaccurate in prenatal diagnosis, can be accurately documented, such as small ventricular defects[47] or abnormal venous connections.[48]

Online Acquisition (Patient in the Room)

It reduces the online exploration time. Moreover, acquisition is less operator-dependent compared to 2D conventional sonography.

Offline Analysis

This technique allows recreating again the examination of the heart. Through the 2D mode, the static images or videotapes can only be reviewed in a retrospective way. Undoubtedly, this is one of the most promising applications of this technique, opening up new opportunities for consultation, clinical diagnoses or new screening strategies.[45,49]

Timing

It can be theoretically applied at any time during the gestation. However, some limitations may be found later in gestation in fetuses with large hearts and early in gestation as a result of low discrimination of signals.[44]

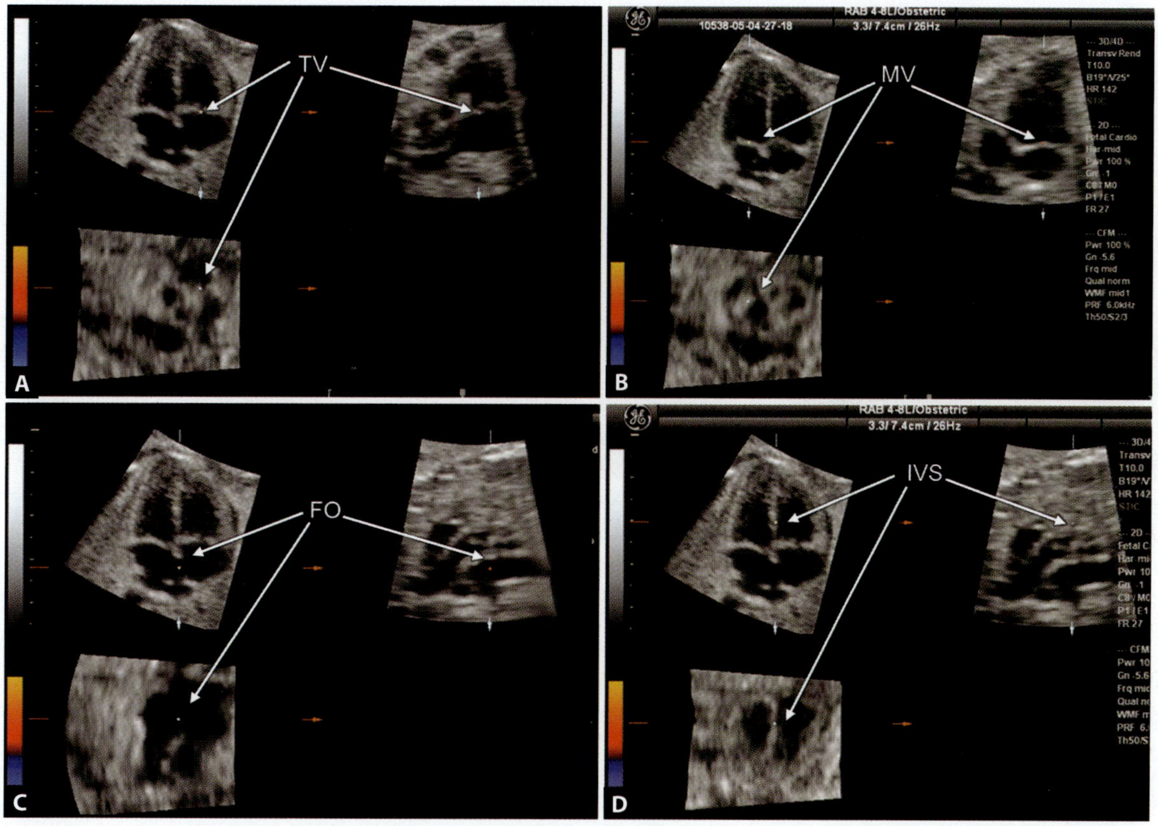

Figs. 4A to D: Three-dimensional multiplanar slicing of the four-chamber view. The examiner can place the reference dot at any location in planes A, B or C and observe the corresponding plane change their respective images. By using the cineloop the examiner can choose within the volume the heart cycle phase of interest. (A) The reference dot is positioned at the level of the tricuspid valve during systole. The valves can be visualized simultaneously in the three orthogonal planes: transverse (left upper panel), sagittal (right upper panel) and coronal (left lower panel); (B) The reference dot is positioned at the level of the mitral valve, during systole. The valves can be visualized simultaneously in the three orthogonal planes: transverse (left upper panel), sagittal (right upper panel) and coronal (left lower panel); (C) The reference dot is positioned at the level of the foramen ovale. Both atria can be visualized in the coronal plane (left lower panel) and a sagittal view of the foramen ovale is provided on the right upper panel; (D) The reference dot is positioned at the level of the interventricular septum. A sagittal view of the interventricular septum can be visualized simultaneously in the right upper panel. (FO: foramen ovale; IVS: interventricular septum; MV: mitral valve; TV: tricuspid valve)

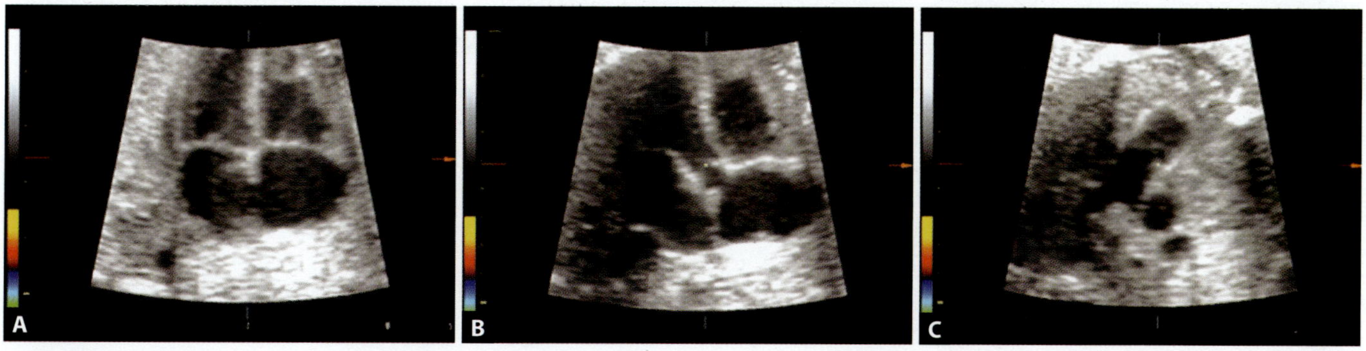

Figs. 5A to C: The examiner can magnify and visualize the plane A in a single format. By scrolling through the volume we can visualize any plane. In this case, the most important planes are presented: (A) the four-chamber view; (B) the five-chamber view; (C) The three vessels and trachea view. By using the cineloop, the examiner can choose within the volume the heart cycle phase of interest.

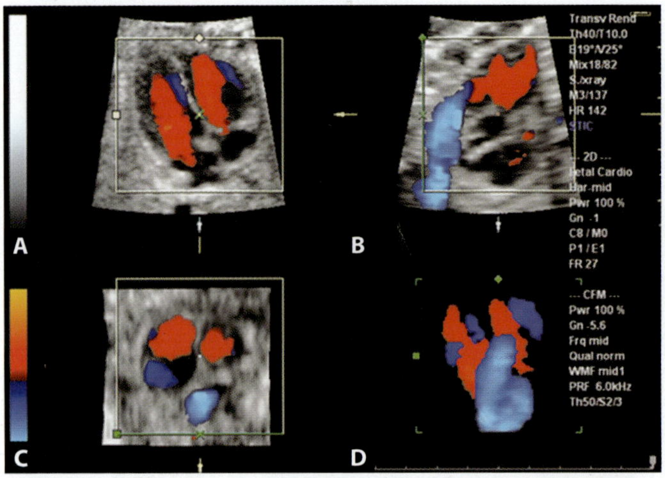

Figs. 6A to D: Color Doppler spatiotemporal image correlation (STIC) volume of a 27-week fetus displayed in multiplanar (A to C) and render mode (D). By scrolling through the cineloop the different phases of the cardiac cycle can be visualized as the diastolic filling of the ventricles, the beginning of the systole with blood flow streaming in the outflow tracts and late systole with blood still recognizable in both great vessels. In this view the criss-crossing of the great vessels can be appreciated in a way not seen before in prenatal diagnosis. Due to the presetting of color persistence the volume in D plane shows simultaneously late diastole and early systole. Additionally, in C plane we can appreciate a new anatomical view, the en-face view of the AV valves, with both mitral and tricuspid valve demonstrated during diastolic flow (red).

New Anatomical Planes

It presents new anatomical planes, which can be difficult or impossible to obtain through the conventional 2D mode. Such views could focus on demonstrating the AV-valves, the so called "en-face view" of the atrioventricular valves",[44] or the interventricular or atrial septum. The future will show which views are appropriate for clinical application.

New Promising Technology

New promising technology can be introduced, in combination with STIC technique, such as Speckle Reduction System or Tomographic Ultrasound Imaging. Speckle Reduction System allows us to improve image resolution, particularly in difficult scan conditions **(Fig. 7)**. Tomographic Ultrasound Imaging (TUI) allows the diagnosis in one unique screen of multiples images **(Fig. 8)**.

High Intra- and Interobserver Repeatability

Cardiac examination from 4D-STIC volumes has showed a high repeatability between and within observers in each trimester of pregnancy.[50]

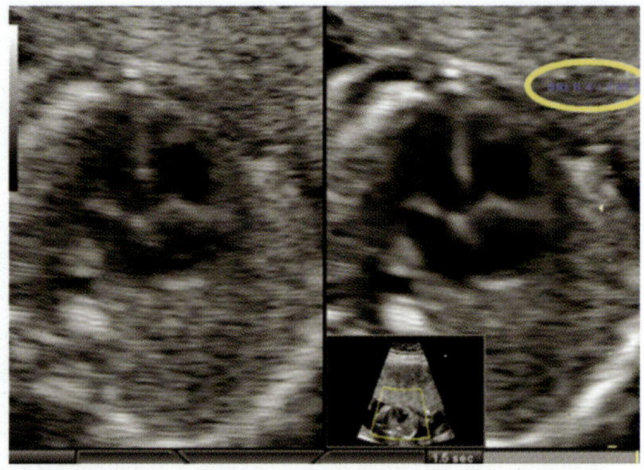

Fig. 7: The speckle reduction system (SRI II) may reduce the artifacts, improving the image resolution, particularly in difficult quality image cases.

Volume Measurements

Four-dimensional ultrasonography with STIC is a feasible and accurate method for calculating volumes of 0.30 mL upwards. In an in vitro model, the 3D slice method proved accurate, was the least time consuming, had the best reliability and had the smallest LOA. This method may prove useful when applied to *in vivo* investigations.[51]

Telestic

It lends itself to storage and review of volume data by the examiner or by experts at remote sites. Volume datasets can be transmitted to remote sites via Internet in order to facilitate the access to the reference experts located in difficult geographical areas with the possibility of seeking advice from them. TELESTIC facilitates asking them for a second diagnostic opinion. Moreover, TELESTIC can be used as a filter in order to relieve the workload in these reference centers. Likewise, this modality offers a wide range of possibilities and new applications in the teaching field.[40,41,52]

LIMITATIONS

There are potential limitations to this technique. Some factors are inherent to conventional ultrasonography, some others are specifically dependent on 3D technology, some of them are inherent to Color Doppler technology and a few ones are related to STIC method.

Specific Limitations of Two-dimensional Technology

- Resolution limitations typical of 2D image
- Low resolution of the reconstructed planes (planes B and C)

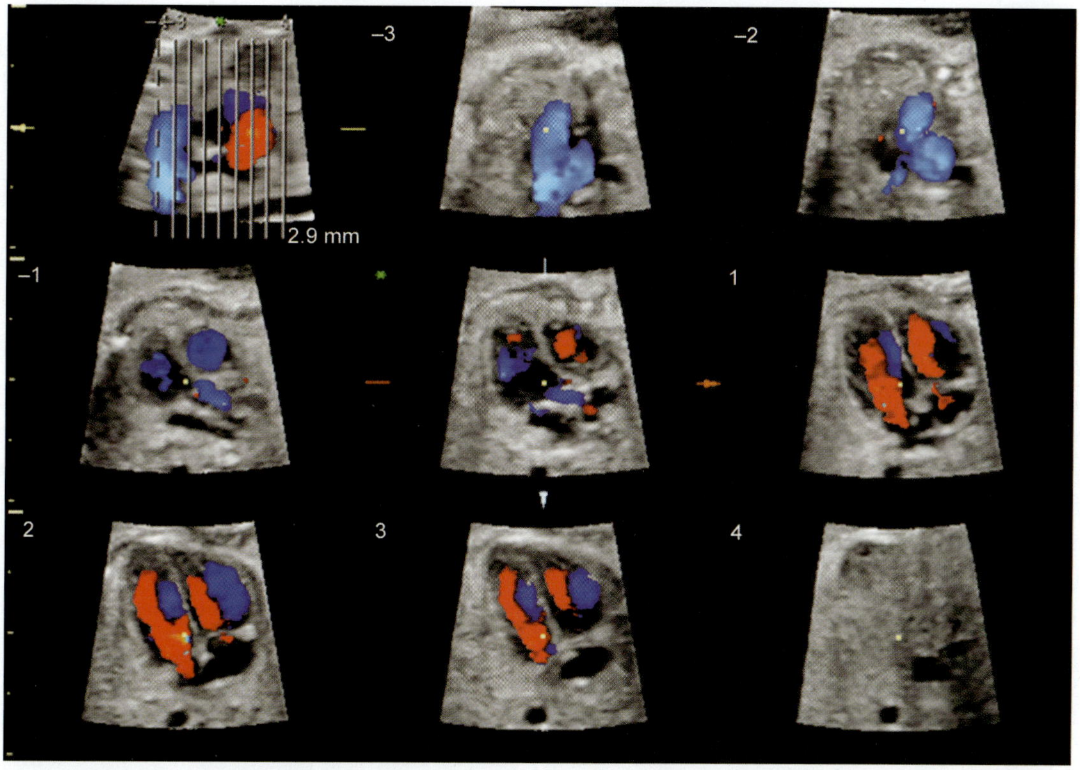

Fig. 8: Tomographic ultrasound imaging (TUI) in a normal fetal heart at 20 weeks of gestation. TUI allows the diagnosis in one unique screen of multiples images.

- Low resolution of the image, especially at early gestational ages.

Specific Limitations of Three-dimensional Technology

During the volume acquisition time, the maternal and fetal movements produce artifacts, especially in B and C planes. Whenever possible, acquisition must be performed in the absence of maternal and fetal movements.

Specific Limitations of Color Doppler Technology

- Lack of color signal when the region of interest is perpendicular to the ultrasounds (in these cases it is advisable to modify the angle of insonation)
- Adding the color, as it happens in conventional 2D modality, the resolution is reduced, in comparison with the image on a grayscale.

Specific Limitations of STIC Technology

- The fetal arrhythmias are the main limitation of this technology, since a synchronization of the cardiac cycle is not permitted in these cases. When important changes are detected in the fetal heart rate during the volume acquisition, the calculation of such rate may not be accurate or valuable enough with the appearance of artifacts caused by the difficulty in synchronizing the 2D images at the right time within the cycle
- Learning curve required managing this technology as well as the extra-time involving the image post-processing
- Economical expenses and current commercial monopoly of this technology. It is expected that in the near future other companies will provide new software with new possibilities of 3D/4D acquisition and rendering.

CURRENT APPLICATIONS AND NEW PERSPECTIVES

Nowadays, different work groups have published their initial experience with this new technology. The current lines of research are focused in the following points:

- *Clinical application in unselected population and also in population at-risk*: Preliminary studies suggest that real-time 3D echocardiography has the potential to function as a screening tool for fetal heart disease, by introducing new screening strategies and new concepts, such as "offline echocardiography" or "screening echocardiography" or "tele-echocardiography".[30,49] Some studies of 4D echocardiography using STIC have focused on the acquisition of volume data sets by operators with limited experience in echocardiography and subsequent analysis by an expert.[49]

- *Systematization of the multiplanar technique*: Some studies of 4D echocardiography using STIC have focused on the development of a multiplanar technique to systematically examine the four-chamber view and the outflow tracts.
    - In this sense, Gonçalves has recently described a four-step technique to simultaneously display the right and left ventricular outflow tracts.[46] By the use of the four-chamber view as the starting point, the heart is rotated approximately 45° around the z-axis and the reference dot placed at the center of the interventricular septum. Next, the volume is rotated clockwise around the y-axis until the left ventricular outflow tract is visualized. The reference dot is repositioned at the center of the outflow tract, above the aortic valve. A short-axis view of the right ventricular outflow tract is displayed simultaneously in the right upper panel **(Figs. 9A to D)**
    - With the same purpose, DeVore describes a new technique using 3D multiplanar imaging that allows the examiner to identify the outflow tracts within a few minutes of acquiring the 3D volume dataset by rotating the volume dataset around the x- and y- axes.[53] It is called "the spin technique". The full length of the main pulmonary artery,

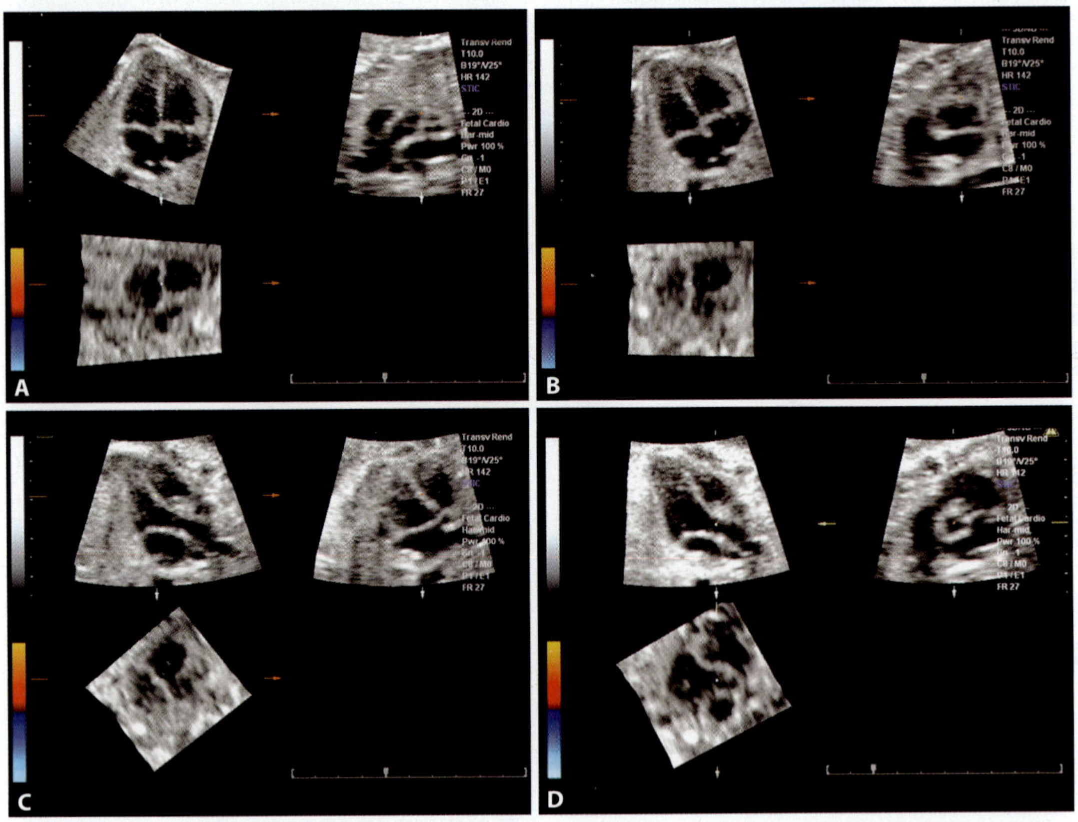

Figs. 9A to D: Systematization of the multiplanar technique: Four-step technique. Some studies of four-dimensional echocardiography using STIC have focused on the development of a multiplanar technique to systematically examine the four-chamber view and the outflow tracts. Gonçalves has recently described a four-step technique to simultaneously display the right and left ventricular outflow tracts.[46] (A) By the use of the four-chamber view as the starting point; (B) The heart is rotated approximately 45° around the z-axis and the reference dot placed at the center of the interventricular septum; (C) Next, the volume is rotated clockwise around the y-axis until the left ventricular outflow tract is visualized. The reference dot is repositioned at the center of the outflow tract, above the aortic valve; (D) A short-axis view of the right ventricular outflow tract is displayed simultaneously in the right upper panel.

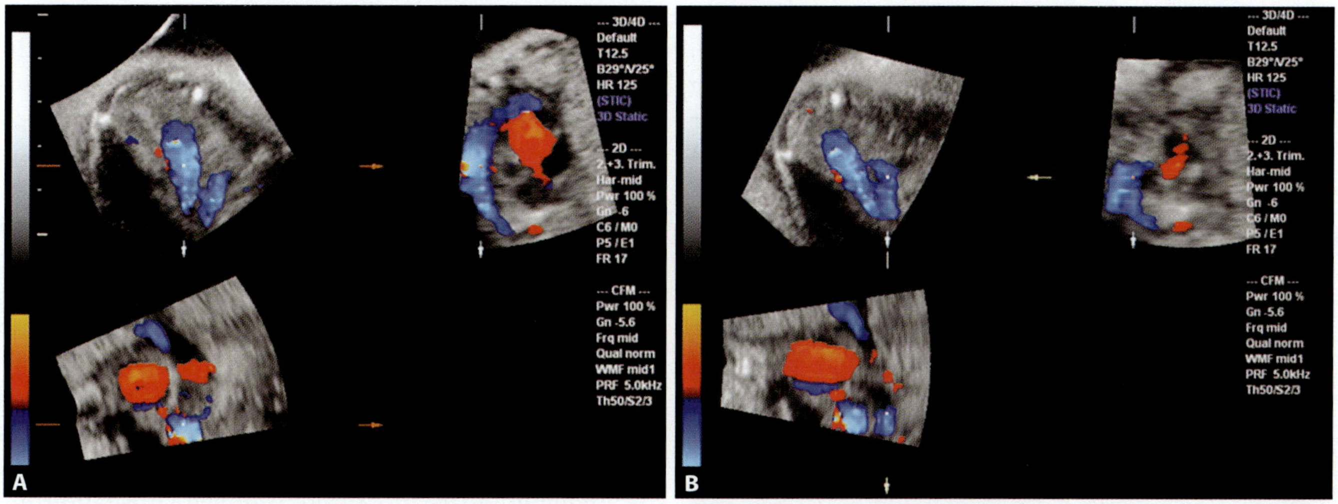

Figs. 10A and B: Systematization of the multiplanar technique: The spin technique. Some studies of four-dimensional echocardiography using spatiotemporal image correlation have focused on the development of a multiplanar technique to systematically examine the four-chamber view and the outflow tracts. DeVore described a new technique using 3D multiplanar imaging that allows the examiner to identify the outflow tracts within a few minutes of acquiring the three-dimensional volume dataset by rotating the volume dataset around the x- and y-axes.[53] It is called "the spin technique". (A) The full length of the main pulmonary artery and ductus arteriosus, and (B) Aortic arch can be easily identified in the normal fetus by rotating the volume dataset along the x- and y-axes.

ductus arteriosus, aortic arch and superior vena cava can be easily identified in the normal fetus by rotating the volume dataset along the x- and y-axes. Three-dimensional multiplanar evaluation of the fetal heart allows the examiner to identify the outflow tracts using a simple and reproducible technique that requires only rotation around x- and y- axes from reference images obtained in a transverse sweep through the fetal chest **(Figs. 10A and B)**.

- *Reproducibility study*: In this sense, recent studies suggest the reproducibility of this technique, in the terms of intraobserver and interobserver variability, although these studies are still referred to as small series[50]. Gonçalves, including a series of 20 volume datasets acquired from fetuses with normal cardiac anatomy, concludes that STIC can be reproducibly used to evaluate fetal cardiac outflow tracts by independent examiners.[54]
- *Assessment of the diagnosis ability referred to as heart diseases*: Thanks to multiplanar volume rendering of the cardiac structures, some congenital heart diseases, traditionally proven inaccurate in prenatal diagnosis, can be accurately documented, such as small ventricular defects,[47] abnormal venous connections[48] or right aortic arch. Additionally, Color Doppler STIC has the potential to simplify visualization of the outflow tracts and may improve the diagnosis of some congenital heart abnormalities[43,44] **(Figs. 11 to 14)**.

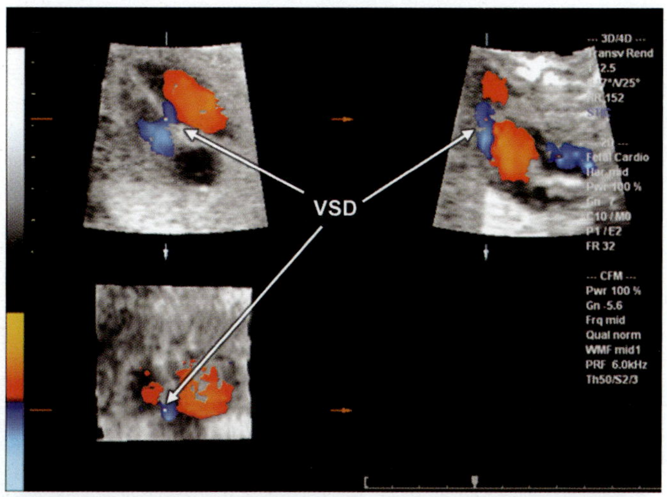

Fig. 11: One application of the multiplanar mode is demonstrated in this fetus of 22 weeks of gestation with a ventricular septal defect (VSD) showing shunting from the left to the right ventricle (blue color crossing the septum). The arrows point to the dot present in all three planes, which shows the intersection point of these planes. The examiner can place the dot in the region of interest (here in the plane A) and see its position in both the other planes.

- *Specific applications in the prenatal diagnosis of congenital heart diseases*: Four-dimensional grayscale and power Doppler STIC can be used to systematically visualize the abnormal relationship of the outflow tracts in fetuses with transposition of the great arteries (TGA)[44,55] **(Figs. 13A and B)**. The detection rate of TGA by standard obstetrical scan evaluation is low and this disappointing performance has been attributed to issues related to technical difficulties in consistently imaging the outflow tracts. In this sense, 4D ultrasonography may overcome technical limitations related to the skills required to obtain appropriate planes of section. Recently, a new sign seems to help to identify additional cases of TGA. The en-face view of both AV valves and great vessels in fetuses with TGA displayed the main pulmonary artery situated side-by-side with the aorta ("big-eyed frog" sign). In contrast, fetuses with normal hearts did not have this characteristic sonographic sign. This novel sonographic sign may prove helpful in the prenatal diagnosis of TGA.[56] Finally, the "starfish" sign has been described as a novel sonographic finding with B-flow imaging and spatiotemporal image correlation in a fetus with total anomalous pulmonary venous return.[57]

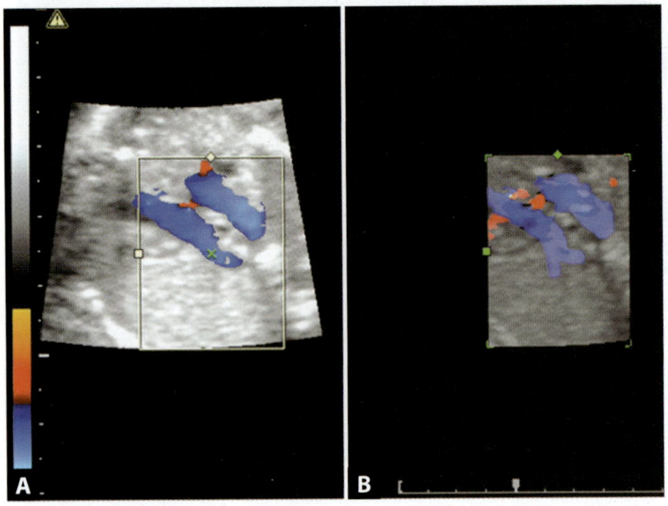

Figs. 12A and B: A 22 weeks of gestation fetus with a right aortic arch. Two simultaneous image displays. (A) The axial plane, the plane of the acquired image obtained during the spatiotemporal image correlation sweep, corresponding to an axial plane at the level of upper mediastinum; (B) Glass-body rendered image corresponding to the acquisition plane. In both images, we can appreciate the anechoic area representing the trachea surrounded by the ductal arch (on the left side of the trachea) and the aortic arch (on the right side of the trachea).

- *Estimation of volumes and masses in animal experimental models*: Estimation of ventricular volume and mass is important for baseline and serial evaluation of fetuses with normal and abnormal hearts. Direct measurement of chamber wall volumes and mass can be made without geometric assumptions by 3D fetal echocardiography. Recent studies have established the feasibility of fetal ventricular mass measurements with 3D ultrasound technology and have developed normal values from 15 weeks' gestation to term.[51,58] Non-gated fast 3D fetal echocardiography is an acceptable modality for determination of cardiac chamber wall volume and mass with good accuracy and acceptable

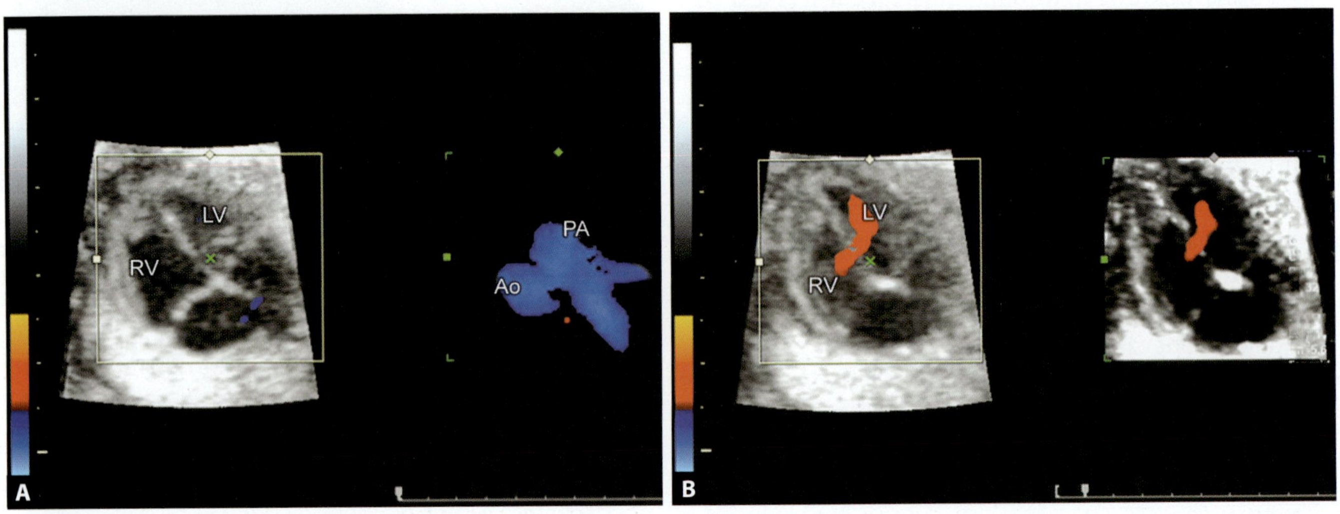

Figs. 13A and B: A fetus with transposition of the great arteries and interventricular septum defect at 22 weeks of gestation. (A) Note the parallel course of both ventricles. The three-dimensional color rendering demonstrates the bifurcation of the pulmonary artery connecting to the left ventricle; (B) Note the additional ventricular septal defect (red color crossing the septum), in both two-dimensional four-chamber view and glass body rendered image. (Ao: aorta; LV: left ventricle; PA: pulmonary artery; RV: right ventricle)

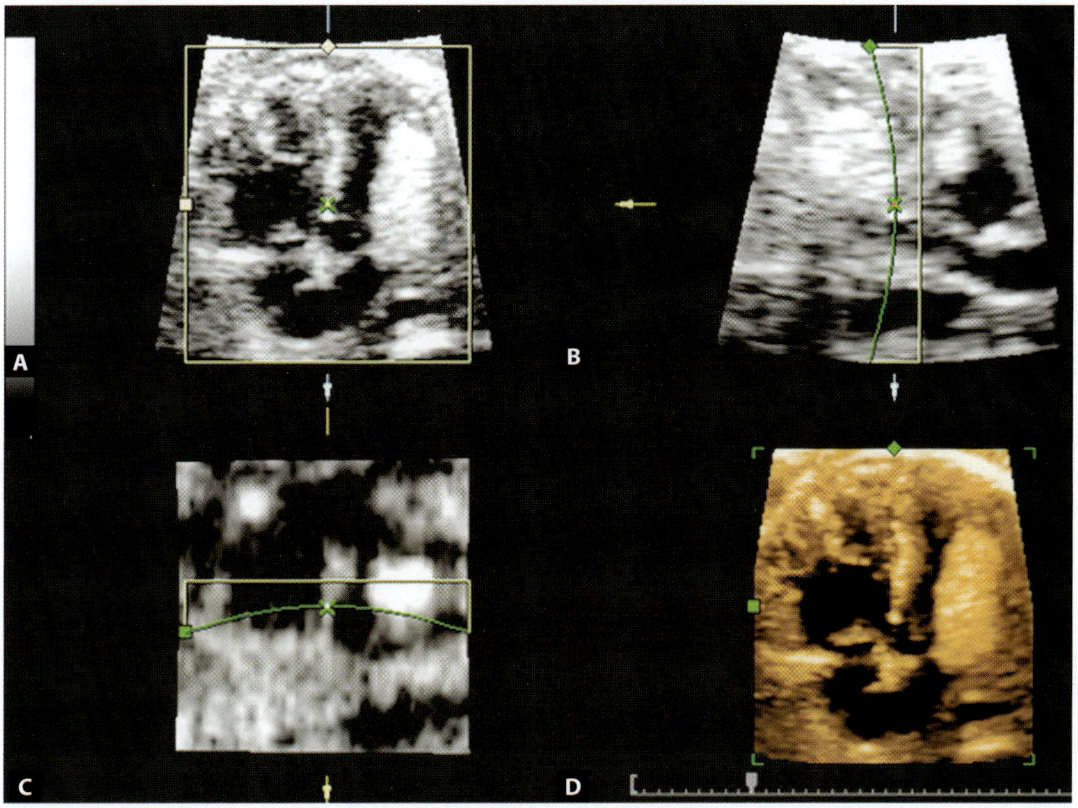

Figs. 14A to D: A fetus with multiple solid cardiac tumors at 29 weeks of gestation, postnatally diagnosed as sclerosis tuberosa. Four simultaneous image displays. (A) The axial plane, the plane of the acquired image obtained during the spatiotemporal image correlation sweep; (B) The orthogonal plane vertical to the plane A (the sagittal plane); (C) The orthogonal plane horizontal to the plane a (coronal plane); (D) Gray rendered image.

interobserver variability. This method should be especially valuable as an objective serial measurement in clinical fetal studies with structurally or functionally abnormal hearts **(Figs. 14A to D)**.

- *Algorithms for the automated obtaining of the standard anatomical slices from the stored volume*: It is anticipated that algorithms developed to image specific cardiac structures with 3D or 4D volume datasets may eventually become automated by computer software.[59-61] Despite the recent advances in ultrasonographic imaging, the acquisition, display and manipulation of 3D volumes is a technique that requires a substantial learning curve. It is theoretically possible to obtain a volume of a specific organ, such as the fetal heart and to allow an automatic program to display out of this volume all the 2D planes that are required for a complete anatomic evaluation of this organ. Abuhamad termed this new concept as automatic multiplanar imaging (AMI). Once a 3D volume of the fetal heart is obtained from the level of a standardized plane, such as the four-chamber view, for instance, AMI will automatically generate all other standardized planes from the acquired volume in an operator-independent method, improving the reproducibility of AMI-generated ultrasonographic images. Automatic multiplanar imaging allows for a complete evaluation of anatomically complex organs with a standardized and operator-independent approach. A software with this purpose, called Sonography-based Volume Computer Aided Diagnosis (Sono VCAD) has been recently commercialized. By standardizing the approach to image acquisition and display and by substantially reducing the possibility of human error and reducing scan time, SonoVCAD will improve the diagnostic acumen of ultrasound imaging, and thus, prove advantageous to clinical practice.
- *Application of this technology in the telemedicine field (TELESTIC)*: Preliminary studies suggest that a telemedicine link via Internet combined with STIC technology (TELESTIC) is technically feasible.[40,41,52,62]

TELESTIC permits a second diagnostic opinion and also generates a link between different centers resultant in a new virtual tool for teaching and training in fetal heart.

- *Application in early fetal echocardiography*: Offline evaluation of 4D-STIC acquired volumes of the fetal heart in the first and early second trimester of pregnancy is reliable not only for early reassurance of normal cardiac anatomy but also to diagnose most major structural heart defects.[50,62,63]
- *New diagnostic algorithms* (Minimum Projection Mode, Inversed mode, B-flow).
  - The Minimum Projection Mode (MPM) is a rendering algorithm available in some 3D and 4D ultrasonography systems that, in one image, allows the visualization of vessels and cystic anatomic structures located in different scanning planes. This algorithm is an alternative rendering modality that facilitates visualization of normal and abnormal vascular connections to the fetal heart particularly at the level of the three-vessel view.[64] This technique may be useful in prenatal diagnosis of conotruncal abnormalities and in the assessment of the spatial relationships of abnormal vascular connections in the upper mediastinum.
  - The "inversion mode" algorithm has been recently introduced in fetal imaging as a new tool for 3D rendering of fluid-filled structures.[47,65,66] This novel 3D post-processing algorithm enables any fetal structure with an anechoic content to be converted into an echogenic volume. Numerous fetal disorders have been accurately described using inversion mode 3D ultrasound, such as urinary tract anomalies, gastrointestinal obstructions, hydrocephalus, cysts, and more recently, the inversion mode has been employed to display the fetal heart. Using this approach the beating heart is dynamically transformed into a hyperechogenic 3D structure due to signal conversion of the blood flowing within the cardiac structures. Since this technique does not use color or power Doppler sonography as a "digital contrast" to highlight the blood vessels, it does not have the inherent limitations to image reconstruction related to the angle of insonation, temporal resolution or intensity of the Doppler signal. This new rendering modality allows a better documentation of some cardiac defects, traditionally proven inaccurate in prenatal diagnosis, such as small ventricular defects,[47] or abnormal systemic venous connections,[48] as well as prenatal evaluation of complex disorders requiring precise definition of visceral situs, such as heterotaxy syndromes.[65]
  - Recently, B-flow imaging and STIC have been demonstrated to improve the visualization of small vessels with low-flow velocity. In fact, when applied to 3D fetal echocardiography, the B-flow modality is a direct volume non-gated scanning method that is able to show blood flow in the heart and in the vessels in real-time, without color Doppler flow. When compared with color and power Doppler sonography, B-flow sonography has a higher frame rate and better spatial resolution. It allows angle-independent detection of weak blood reflectors from vessels. Consequently, this approach theoretically has the potential to facilitate the prenatal diagnosis of TAPVC, and might be especially important in identifying and tracking the route of thin vessels with low blood flow velocity.[57,67,68]

FIRST SPANISH STUDY IN SPATIOTEMPORAL IMAGE CORRELATION TECHNOLOGY

Introduction

Since the origin of the fetal echocardiography at the end of 1970, new techniques and applications have been appearing forming a field whose present situation and future perspectives are widely different from the original ones. The recent introduction of the 3D and 4D ultrasonography opens a promising perspective in prenatal diagnosis, especially in certain types of surface pathologies. Nevertheless, the application of this technology is complex in echocardiography considering the movement and the dynamics itself in the cardio-vascular system, being this the main limitation in the 3D and 4D reconstruction. Nowadays, this limitation has been overcome with the incorporation of a new technological appliance called STIC.

Objective

To assess the use and performance of the STIC technique in order to perform a "basic and extended cardiac fetal evaluation", with an online acquisition of the cardiac volume during the morphological scan by a general sonographer and offline analysis by an expert in fetal cardiology.

Methods and Material

A number of 58 volumes are prospectively obtained during the routine morphological scan, by a general sonographer, in 28 patients randomly selected among the ones attending our unit. Afterwards, an experimented examiner in fetal echocardiography proceeds to their offline analysis. The acquisition is made from a four-chamber view on a gray scale in an automated single sweep in a slow motion, by standardizing the acquisition time in 10 seconds (7'5–12'5) and the sweep angle in 25° (20–30), depending on the gestational age. The criteria defining a basic cardiac fetal study are the evaluation of the inflow tracts (four-chamber view) and the evaluation of the outflow tracts (five-chamber view, three-vessel view or three-vessel view and traquea). The criteria defining an extended cardiac fetal study are the evaluation of the inflow tracts, the evaluation of the outflow tracts and the situs visceral. The successful rate of volume acquisition and analysis is evaluated, as well as the percentage of cases in which it is possible a basic or extended cardiac evaluation, through the single sweep and multiplanar navigation. Cases with normal morphological scan at 20–22 weeks' gestation are included, excluding those cases with chromosomal anomalies or extracardiac malformations.

Results

Cases with gestational ages ranging between 17 and 35 weeks are included. A basic cardiac examination according to set criteria was achieved in 100% of cases, while an extended cardiac examination was achieved in 86% of them. Multiplanar study improved the visualization of those structures not identifiable through the initial acquisition single plane in all cases.

CONCLUSION

We present the first study on a nationwide scale about the introduction and applications of the STIC technology. The introduction of this new technique, surpassing the limitation of the cardiac movement in the volumetric reconstruction, enables a fast and easy online acquisition of a cardiac volume, during the routine morphological scan, suggesting the possibility of carrying out a more complete offline analysis of the cardiovascular structures. Spatiotemporal image correlation volumes can be obtained by operators inexperienced in fetal echocardiography and their offline analysis enables recognition of most of the structures and views necessary to assess fetal cardiac anatomy. It is emphasized that the high rate of success in the volume acquisition and offline analysis, allowing the possibility of an extended cardiac evaluation, in what we would call, "Screening Offline Extended Cardiac Examination" or "Basic Offline Echocardiography".

Methodology

Cardiac volumes were prospectively stored according to the STIC technology[52] during the screening morphological ultrasound examination, by a general sonographer, in an aleatory selection of obstetric patients attending our unit in the period between December 2004 and February 2005 (Gutenberg Centre, Malaga, Spain). A number of 28 fetal explorations were included, all of them randomly distributed in our program, depending on the pressure attendance and the availability of ultrasound machine equipped with the STIC technology. Only fetal explorations considered as normal were included, excluding those cases with cardiac, extracardiac or chromosomal anomalies. A number between 1 and 4 volumes were acquired per patient on a grayscale (online acquisition). Afterwards, a second examiner expert in fetal echocardiography assessed the collected volumes in order to make a cardiac "basic" evaluation and an "extended" evaluation, in a limited time of 15 minutes per patient (offline analysis).

Firstly, only the initial acquisition single plane is examined, followed by a multiplanar study in order to improve the visualization of those structures not identifiable through the initial acquisition plane. The offline analysis includes the assessment of the situs visceral, the cardiac size, the cardiac axis, the myocardial contractility, the symmetry of cavities, the cardiac crux, the insertion of the atrioventricular (AV) valves and the opening of these ones, the moderator band, the foramen ovale, the crossing of great arteries, the outflow tracts of both ventricles and the pulmonary and aortic valves. These structures are assessed in the four-chamber view (4C view), five-chamber view (5C view), three-vessel view (3VV) and the three-vessel view including trachea (3VVT). The criteria defining the assessment of the situs visceral are the abdominal identification of the position and location of the stomach, abdominal aorta and inferior vena cava and the identification of the thoracic aorta and the cardiac atrial cavities. The criteria defining

TABLE 1: Methodological data from our study. The characteristics of the patients and volumes in our study are reported in this table.

Period of study	December 2004 to February 2005
Number of patients (n)	28
Number of analyzed volumes	58
GA (average and range)	23 weeks (17–35)
Acquisition conditions: • Time (average and range) • Angle (average and range)	 10 seconds (7.5–12.5) 25° (20–30)
Acquisition plane: • apical 4C • lateral 4C • basal 4C	 68% 14% 18%
Offline analysis (average time)	15 minutes/ patient

(4C: four-chamber view); GA: gestational age in completed weeks; n: number of cases in the serial;)

TABLE 2: Visualization rate of the cardiac structures (STIC). Success rate of visualizing different cardiac structures and plans using spatiotemporal image correlation (STIC).

Cardiac structures checklist	***Visualization rate %***
Situs visceral	86
Cardiac size	100
Cardiac axis	100
Myocardiac contractility	100
Cavities symmetry	100
Cardiac crux	96
AV valves insertion	93
AV valves opening	100
Moderator band	100
Foramen ovale	100
Crossing of great arteries	100
Outflow tract LV	100
Outflow tract RV	100
Pulmonary valve	100
Aortic valve	100
4C **5C** **3VV** **3VVT**	100 100 100 64
Extended cardiac study*	86

(AV: Atrioventricular; LV: left ventricle; RV: right ventricle; 4C: four-chamber view; 5C: five-chamber view; 3VV: three-vessel view; 3VVT: three-vessel and trachea view)

*The extended cardiac study includes the evaluation of the inflow tracts, the outflow tracts and the situs visceral.

a basic fetal cardiac study are both the evaluation of the inflow tracts view (4C view) and the evaluation of the outflow tracts view (5C view and 3VV or 3VVT) **(Figs. 5A to C)**. The criteria defining an extended cardiac fetal study are the following: the evaluation of the inflow tracts (4C view), the evaluation of the outflow tracts (5C view and 3VV or 3VVT) and the situs visceral evaluation.

In our study we standardized the volume acquisition in a time of 10 seconds, with a sweep angle of 25°, modifying these variables according to the cardiac size and the conditions in the exploration (fetal movements). The acquisition was achieved from the 4C view, apical (preferable), basal or lateral depending on the fetal position, in a sweep covering the initial slice, going under and over it (including superior abdomen and thorax). Offline analysis was performed by a single investigator using the 4D View Software Version 2.1 (GE Medical Systems, Kretz Ultrasound, Zipf, Austria).

Results

A total amount of 58 explorations of fetal cardiac volumes in 28 patients have been included, with gestational ages ranging between 17 and 35 weeks. The characteristics of the patients and volumes are reported in **Table 1**. The mean visualization scores for the different structures and views are shown in **Tables 2 and 3**. We evaluate the successful rate in visualizing the fetal cardiac structures through the single sweep and the multiplanar format view.

TABLE 3: Contribution of the multiplanar study. Contribution of the multiplanar study in visualizing different cardiac structures and plans using spatiotemporal image correlation (STIC).

Multiplanar contribution	***%***
4-step technique GA	71
IVC-RA	93
SVC-RA	79
Ao arch (sagittal)	54
Ductal arch (sagittal)	71
Additional contribution*	100

4-step technique: A four step technique to evaluate the outflow tracts from the four-chamber view

(Ao arch: aortic arch; GA: great arteries; IVC-RA: inferior vena cava to right atrium; SVC-RA: superior vena cava to right atrium)

*Percentage of cases in which the multiplanar examination has contributed to get some additional information.

COMMENT

The detection of CHD is still considered as one of the most problematic areas in the prenatal diagnosis field. Inspite of being the most frequent and severe congenital malformation in neonates, nowadays it is still one of the least diagnosed pathologies during fetal life. Besides, it is well known that the prognosis of most of them, particularly the ductus-dependent anomalies, is meaningfully better in terms of morbidity and mortality when the anomaly is prenatally detected. Their prevalence and impact are the essential factors motivating the interest to improve the prenatal detection strategies.

In this sense, the incorporation of the 4C view during the morphological scan at 20 weeks of gestation, in the so called basic cardiac scan, has improved the prenatal detection of CHD.[11,12] Recently, the inclusion of the outflow tracts evaluation in the so-called extended cardiac scan has been highly recommended in order to improve the detection of conotruncal abnormalities.[13,14] Nevertheless, conventional prenatal screening for congenital heart disease still involves a time-consuming and highly operator-dependent acquisition of the four-chamber view and outflow tracts. As routine prenatal screening in the general obstetric setting is unsatisfactory, the main objective of this technique is to propose a method that is able to identify or exclude major CHD in a screening policy. It has been recently demonstrated that STIC acquisition of the fetal heart is feasible with high success rates in visualizing the heart structures. According to our experience and a few published studies,[46,49,52] the anatomy of the fetal heart can be confidentially demonstrated by the means of STIC acquisition carried out by an operator unskilled in fetal cardiology. We point out the high success rate for visualizing the structures and views included in our checklist, suggesting that most of the relevant ultrasonographic data of the fetal heart can be obtained in one STIC volume. By acquiring the entire fetal heart instantaneously as a single volume, STIC technology may facilitate fetal cardiac screening. The STIC data volume acquired by a non-expert sonographer or general obstetrician can be subsequently be used by a fetal echocardiologist for prenatal confirmation of a normal heart anatomy or exclusion of major cardiac defects.[49] That could be particularly true if the dataset volume for analysis is automatically acquired, thus reducing the need for technical skills and expertise from the sonographers. In this sense, artifacts must also be recognized and minimized, resolution must improve, and substantial training will be necessary prior to widespread clinical use. Real-time 3D examination of the fetal heart with the use of matrix phased-array probes may help to overcome such difficulties in the future.

In summary, the introduction of the STIC technology, surpassing the limitation of the cardiac movement in the volumetric reconstruction, provides a fast and easy online acquisition of the cardiac volume in the context of a routine ultrasound examination with the possibility of carrying out a more complete offline analysis of the cardiovascular structures. Potential advantages include the possibility of offline analysis in the patient's absence, remote diagnosis, novel scanning planes and new approaches for medical education. It has emphasized on the high rate of success in the volume acquisition and offline analysis, allowing the possibility of an extended cardiac evaluation, in what we would call "*Screening offline extended cardiac scan*" or "*Basic offline echocardiography*". This concept can be introduced as a new promising strategy that can be implemented in the general population in order to improve the prenatal detection rate of congenital heart abnormalities.

REFERENCES

1. Sklansky M. Advances in fetal cardiac imaging. Pediatr Cardiol. 2004;25(3):307-21.
2. Allan L, Benacerraf B, Copel JA, et al. Isolated major congenital heart disease. Ultrasound Obstet Gynecol. 2001;17(5):370-9.
3. Mitchell SC, Korones SB, Berendes HW. Congenital heart disease in 56,109 births. Incidence and natural history. Circulation. 1971;43(3):323-32.
4. Allan L, Sharland G, Milburn A, et al. Prospective diagnosis of 1,006 consecutive cases of congenital heart disease in the fetus. J Am Coll Cardiol. 1994;23(6):1452-8.
5. Garne E, Stoll C, Clementi M; Euroscan Group. Evaluation of prenatal diagnosis of congenital heart diseases by ultrasound: experience from 20 European registries. Ultrasound Obstet Gynecol. 2001;17(5):386-91.
6. Bonnet D, Coltri A, Butera G, et al. Detection of transposition of the great arteries in fetuses reduces neonatal morbidity and mortality. Circulation. 1999;99(7):916-8.
7. Allan LD. Fetal cardiology. Curr Opin Obstet Gynecol. 1996;8(2):142-7.
8. Gembruch U. Prenatal diagnosis of congenital heart disease. Prenat Diagn. 1997;17(13):1283-98.
9. Todros T. Prenatal diagnosis and management of fetal cardiovascular malformations. Curr Opin Obstet Gynecol. 2000;12(2):105-9.
10. Levi S, Schaaps JP, De Havay P, Coulon R, Defoort P. End result of routine ultrasound screening for congenital anomalies. The Belgian Multicentric study 1984-92. Ultrasound Obstet Gynecol. 1995;5(6):366-71.

11. Lee W. Performance of the basic fetal cardiac ultrasound examination. J Ultrasound Med. 1998;17(9):601-7.
12. Royal College of Obstetricians and Gynaecologists. Ultrasound Screening. Royal College of Obstetricians and Gynaecologists 2000. [online] Available from: http://www.rcog.org.uk/mainpages.asp?PageID=439#20week. [Accessed in February, 2011]
13. Carvalho JS, Mavrides E, Shinebourne EA, et al. Improving the effectiveness of routine prenatal screening for major congenital heart defects. Heart. 2002;88(4):387-91.
14. Kirk JS, Riggs TW, Comstock CH, et al. Prenatal screening for cardiac anomalies: the value of routine addition of the aortic root to the four-chamber view. Obstet Gynecol. 1994;84(3):427-31.
15. Yagel S, Cohen SM, Achiron R. Examination of the fetal heart by five short-axis views: a proposed screening method for comprehensive cardiac evaluation. Ultrasound Obstet Gynecol. 2001;17(5):367-9.
16. Yoo SJ, Lee YH, Cho KS, et al. Sequential segmental approach to fetal congenital heart disease. Cardiol Young. 1999;9(4):430-44.
17. Chaoui R. The four-chamber view: four reasons why it seems to fail in screening for cardiac abnormalities and suggestions to improve detection rate. Ultrasound Obstet Gynecol. 2003;22(1):3-10.
18. Chaoui R. Fetal echocardiography: state of art. Ultrasound Obstet Gynecol. 2001;17(4):277-84.
19. Paladini D, Vasallo M, Tartaglione A, et al. The role of tissue harmonic imaging in fetal echocardiography. Ultrasound Obstet Gynecol. 2004;23(2):159-64.
20. Tutschek B, Zimmermann T, Buck T, et al. Fetal tissue Doppler echocardiography: detection rates of cardiac structures and quantitative assessment of the fetal heart. Ultrasound Obstet Gynecol. 2003;21(1):26-32.
21. Paladini D, Lamberti A, Teodoro A, et al. Tissue Doppler imaging of the fetal heart. Ultrasound Obstet Gynecol. 2000;16(6):530-5.
22. Sharma S, Parness IA, Kamenir SA, et al. Screening fetal echocardiography by telemedicine: efficacy and clinical acceptance. J Am Soc Echocardiogr. 2003;16(3):202-8.
23. Nelson TR, Pretorius DH, Lev-Toaff A, et al. Feasibility of performing a virtual patient examination using three-dimensional ultrasonographic data acquired at remote locations. J Ultrasound Med. 2001;20(9):941-52.
24. Deng J, Rodeck CH. New fetal cardiac imaging techniques. Prenat Diagn. 2004;24(13):1092-103.
25. Sklansky M. New dimensions and directions in fetal cardiology. Curr Opin Pediatr. 2003;15(5):463-71.
26. Deng J. Terminology of three-dimensional and four-dimensional ultrasound imaging of the fetal heart and other moving body parts. Ultrasound Obstet Gynecol. 2003;22(4):336-44.
27. Chaoui R, Heling KS. New developments in fetal heart scanning: three- and four-dimensional fetal echocardiography. Semin Fetal Neonat Med. 2005;10(6):567-77.
28. Sklansky MS, DeVore GR, Wong PC. Real-time 3-dimensional fetal echocardiography with and instantaneous volume-rendered display: early description and pictorial essay. J Ultrasound Med. 2004;23(2):283-9.
29. Sklansky MS, Nelson TR, Pretorius DH. Three-dimensional fetal echocardiography: gated versus nongated techniques. J Ultrasound Med. 1998;17(7):451-7.
30. Sklansky M, Miller D, DeVore G, et al. Prenatal screening for congenital heart disease using real-time three-dimensional echocardiography and a novel 'sweep volume' acquisition technique. Ultrasound Obstet Gynecol. 2005;25(5):435-43.
31. Bega G, Kuhlman K, Lev-Toaff A, et al. Application of three-dimensional ultrasonography in the evaluation of the fetal heart. J Ultrasound Med. 2001;20(4):307-13.
32. Wang PH, Chen GD, Lin LY. Imaging comparison of basic cardiac views between two- and three-dimensional ultrasound in normal fetuses in anterior spine positions. Int J Cardiovasc Imaging. 2002;18(1):17-23.
33. Esh-Broder E, Ushakov FB, Imbar T, et al. Application of free-hand three-dimensional echocardiography in the evaluation of fetal cardiac ejection fraction: a preliminary study. Ultrasound Obstet Gynecol. 2004;23(6):546-51.
34. Meyer-Wittkopf M, Cole A, Cooper SG, et al. Three-dimensional quantitative echocardiographic assessment of ventricular volume in healthy human fetuses and in fetuses with congenital heart disease. J Ultrasound Med. 2001;20(4):317-27.
35. Deng J, Yates R, Sullivan ID, et al. Dynamic three-dimensional color Doppler ultrasound of human fetal intracardiac flow. Ultrasound Obstet Gynecol. 2002;20(2):131-6.
36. Meyer-Wittkopf M, Cooper S, Vaughan J, et al. Three-dimensional (3D) echocardiographic analysis of congenital heart disease in the fetus: comparison with cross-sectional (2D) fetal echocardiography. Ultrasound Obstet Gynecol. 2001;17(6):485-92.
37. Chaoui R. Three-dimensional ultrasound of the blood flow in the fetal cardiovascular system. In: Kurjak A (Ed). Textbook of Perinatal Medicine. New Delhi, India: Jaypee Brothers Medical Publishers; 2005. pp. 644-53.
38. Jürgens J, Chaoui R. Three-dimensional multiplanar time-motion ultrasound or anatomical M-mode of the fetal heart: a new technique in fetal echocardiography. Ultrasound Obstet Gynecol. 2003;21(2):119-23.
39. Turan S, Turan O, Baschat AA. Three- and four-dimensional fetal echocardiography. Fetal Diagn Ther. 2009;25(4):361-72.
40. Michailidis GD, Simpson JM, Karidas C, et al. Detailed three-dimensional fetal echocardiography facilitated by an Internet link. Ultrasound Obstet Gynecol. 2001;18(4):325-8.
41. Viñals F, Mandujano L, Vargas G, et al. Prenatal diagnosis of congenital heart disease using four-dimensional spatio-temporal image correlation (STIC) telemedicine via an Internet link: a pilot study. Ultrasound Obstet Gynecol. 2005;25(1):25-31.
42. Lee W, Kirk JS, Comstock CH, et al. Vasa previa: prenatal detection by three-dimensional ultrasonography. Ultrasound Obstet Gynecol. 2000;16(4):384-7.

43. Gonçalves LF, Romero R, Espinoza J, et al. Four-dimensional ultrasonography of the fetal heart using color Doppler spatiotemporal image correlation. J Ultrasound Med. 2004;23(4):473-81.
44. Chaoui R, Hoffmann J, Heling KS. Three-dimensional (3D) and 4D color Doppler fetal echocardiography using spatio-temporal image correlation (STIC). Ultrasound Obstet Gynecol. 2004;23(6):535-45.
45. DeVore GR, Falkensammer P, Sklansky MS, et al. Spatio-temporal image correlation (STIC): new technology for evaluation of the fetal heart. Ultrasound Obstet Gynecol. 2003;22(4):380-7.
46. Gonçalves LF, Lee W, Chaiworapongsa T, et al. Four-dimensional ultrasonography of the fetal heart with spatiotemporal image correlation. Am J Obstet Gynecol. 2003;189(6):1792-802.
47. Ghi T, Cera E, Segata M, et al. Inversion mode spatio-temporal image correlation (STIC) echocardiography in three-dimensional rendering of fetal ventricular septal defects. Ultrasound Obstet Gynecol. 2005;26(6):679-80.
48. Espinoza J, Gonçalves LF, Lee W, et al. A novel method to improve prenatal diagnosis of abnormal systemic venous connections using three- and four-dimensional ultrasonography and 'inversion mode'. Ultrasound Obstet Gynecol. 2005;25(5):428-34.
49. Viñals F, Poblete P, Giuliano A. Spatiotemporal image correlation (STIC): a new tool for the prenatal screening of congenital heart defects. Ultrasound Obstet Gynecol. 2003;22(4):388-94.
50. Bennasar M, Martínez JM, Olivella A, et al. Feasibility and accuracy of fetal echocardiography using four-dimensional spatiotemporal image correlation technology before 16 weeks' gestation. Ultrasound Obstet Gynecol. 2009;33(6): 645-51.
51. Uittenbogaard LB, Haak MC, Peters RJ, et al. Validation of volume measurements for fetal echocardiography using four-dimensional ultrasound imaging and spatiotemporal image correlation. Ultrasound Obstet Gynecol. 2010; 35(3):324-31.
52. Viñals F, Mandujano L, Vargas G, et al. Prenatal diagnosis of congenital heart disease using four-dimensional spatio-temporal image correlation (STIC) telemedicine via an Internet link: a pilot study. Ultrasound Obstet Gynecol. 2005;25(1):25-31.
53. DeVore GR, Polanco B, Sklansky MS, et al. The 'spin' technique: a new method for examination of the fetal outflow tracts using three-dimensional ultrasound. Ultrasound Obstet Gynecol. 2004;24(1):72-82.
54. Gonçalves LF, Espinoza J, Romero R, et al. Four-dimensional fetal echocardiography with spatiotemporal image correlation (STIC): a systematic study of standard cardiac views assessed by different observers. J Matern Fetal Neonatal Med. 2005;17(5):323-31.
55. Gonçalves LF, Espinoza J, Romero R, et al. A systematic approach to prenatal diagnosis of transposition of the great arteries using 4-dimensional ultrasonography with spatiotemporal image correlation. J Ultrasound Med. 2004;23(9):1225-31.
56. Shih JC, Shyu MK, Su YN, et al. 'Big-eyed frog' sign on spatiotemporal image correlation (STIC) in the antenatal diagnosis of transposition of the great arteries. Ultrasound Obstet Gynecol. 2008;32(6):762-8.
57. Lee W, Espinoza J, Cutler N, et al. The 'starfish' sign: a novel sonographic finding with B-flow imaging and spatiotemporal image correlation in a fetus with total anomalous pulmonary venous return. Ultrasound Obstet Gynecol. 2010;35(1):124-5.
58. Bhat AH, Corbett V, Carpenter N, et al. Fetal ventricular mass determination on three-dimensional echocardiography: studies in normal fetuses and validation experiments. Circulation. 2004;110(9):1054-60.
59. Abuhamad A. Automated Multiplanar Imaging. A novel approach to Ultrasonography. J Ultrasound Med. 2004;23(5):573-6.
60. Abuhamad A, Falkensammer P, Reichartseder F, et al. Automated retrieval of standard diagnostic fetal cardiac ultrasound planes in the second trimester of pregnancy: a prospective evaluation of software. Ultrasound Obstet Gynecol. 2008;31(1):30-6.
61. Tutschek B, Sahn DJ. Semi-automatic segmentation of fetal cardiac cavities: progress towards an automatic fetal echocardiogram. Ultrasound Obstet Gynecol. 2008;32(2): 176-80.
62. Viñals F, Ascenzo R, Naveas R, et al. Fetal echocardiography at 11 + 0 to 13 + 6 weeks using four-dimensional spatiotemporal image correlation telemedicine via an Internet link: a pilot study. Ultrasound Obstet Gynecol. 2008;31(6):633-8.
63. Turan S, Turan OM, Ty-Torredes K, et al. Standardization of the first-trimester fetal cardiac examination using spatiotemporal image correlation with tomographic ultrasound and color Doppler imaging. Ultrasound Obstet Gynecol. 2009;33(6):652-6.
64. Espinoza J, Gonçalves LF, Lee W, et al. The use of the minimum projection mode in 4-dimensional examination of the fetal heart with spatiotemporal image correlation. J Ultrasound Med. 2004;23(10):1337-48.
65. Gonçalves LF, Espinoza J, Lee W, et al. Three- and four-dimensional reconstruction of the aortic and ductal arches using inversion mode: a new rendering algorithm for visualization of fluid-filled anatomical structures. Ultrasound Obstet Gynecol. 2004;24(6):696-8.
66. Lee W, Gonçalves LF, Espinoza J, et al. Inversion mode: a new volume analysis tool for 3-dimensional ultrasonography. J Ultrasound Med. 2005;24(2):201-7.
67. Zhang M, Pu DR, Zhou QC, et al. Four-dimensional echocardiography with B-flow imaging and spatiotemporal image correlation in the assessment of congenital heart defects. Prenat Diagn. 2010;30(5):443-8.
68. Volpe P, Campobasso G, De Robertis V, et al. Two- and four-dimensional echocardiography with B-flow imaging and spatiotemporal image correlation in prenatal diagnosis of isolated total anomalous pulmonary venous connection. Ultrasound Obstet Gynecol. 2007;30(6):830-7.

CHAPTER 22

Spatial and Temporal Image Correlation and Other Volume Ultrasound Techniques in the Fetal Heart Evaluation After 10 Years of Practice

Marcin Wiechec, Agnieszka Nocun

INTRODUCTION

It has been over 10 years since the first attempts of using three-dimensional (3D) ultrasound in fetal echocardiography were made.[1-5] At first, there were hopes that with the use of this method, we would be able to obtain more accurate images and would have access to cardiac views impossible to visualize with the use of two-dimensional (2D) ultrasound.[2] From the very beginning of applying 3D methods, new teleconsulting opportunities have been created in this field.[6,7] In the recent years, there was a progress in shortening of the acquisition time of 3D volume data with the use of matrix transducers.[8,9] From the time perspective, the authors of this chapter, being modern imaging techniques practitioners, reached the conclusion that the greatest achievement of utilizing those methods is the possibility of understanding of complex anatomy of a normal fetal heart and a heart with congenital defects by a noncardiologist. Because of this fact, fetal heart examination is easier to systematize and standardize. Taking the above into consideration, 3D techniques are of a priceless didactic value. Owing to them, it is possible to simulate the evaluation of congenital heart disease and compare this situation with the 3D datasets during the training sessions and workshops. On the basis of 3D fetal echocardiography, three-dimensional printouts used for learning to diagnose fetal heart diseases have been worked out.[10] However, a wider application of these methods in screening is more difficult because of obvious limitations of volume ultrasound like motion artifacts, shadowing behind fetal skeletal structures and changing scanning conditions even in the same patient.[11,12] All these elements, which are essential factors of ultrasound examination, limit reproducibility of volume ultrasound in fetal heart evaluation. A number of methods based on automated mapping of fetal heart views from 3D volume datasets have been developed.[13-15] Nevertheless, all these methods are based on the analysis of normal heart geometry and their diagnostic application, according to the authors, is very limited. In terms of scan duration these techniques are most of the time inferior to simple 2D sweeps in grey scale and color mapping. However, the producers of ultrasound equipment are still developing automated methods and taking into account the progress in the aspect of shortening the acquisition duration, under the condition of considering differences among geometric hearts with congenital diseases, those methods may bring the expected diagnostic results in the future.

TECHNICAL ASPECTS

At this point in time, among 3D techniques used for assessment of fetal heart, it is possible to distinguish the following acquisition techniques:

- Static 3D
- Spatial and temporal image correlation (STIC)
- 4D real time/3D live in multiplanar view and biplanar view.

Static 3D

Due to the dynamic character of examined organ, which contracts with a great frequency, 3D static acquisition is done in exceptional cases. It is usually used for acquisition of the whole fetal trunk in order to obtain information about the visceral situs and both thoracic and abdominal organs considering their structure **(Figs. 1 and 2)**.

With this method, it is possible to detect situs abnormalities and severe abnormalities in the cardiac structure.

The main cause of its limited use is the fact that static examination does not include the functional aspect. Therefore, the most often-used volume technique to examine a fetal heart is STIC because of fast fetal heart rate, which is about 150 BPM.

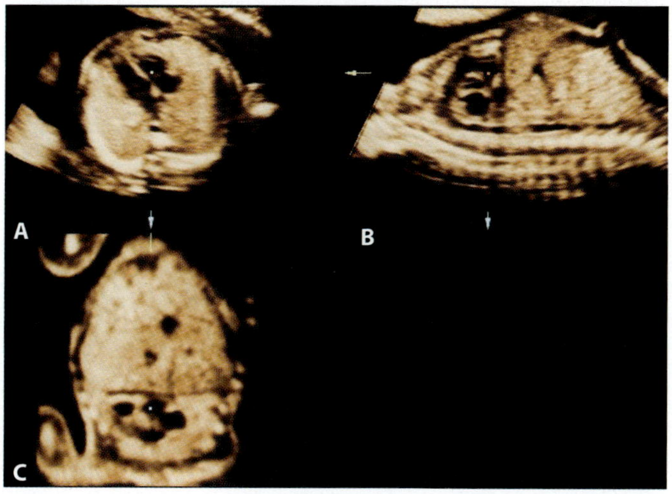

Fig. 1: A 3D static dataset presenting the multiplanar view of the fetal heart with the correct arrangement of viscera (situs solitus). This is a properly oriented volume dataset. In the A plane (upper left image) the axis of the heart is directed to the left. In the B plane the section is through the ductal arch (the heart seen on the left). In the C plane the coronal section through the fetal chest in shown.

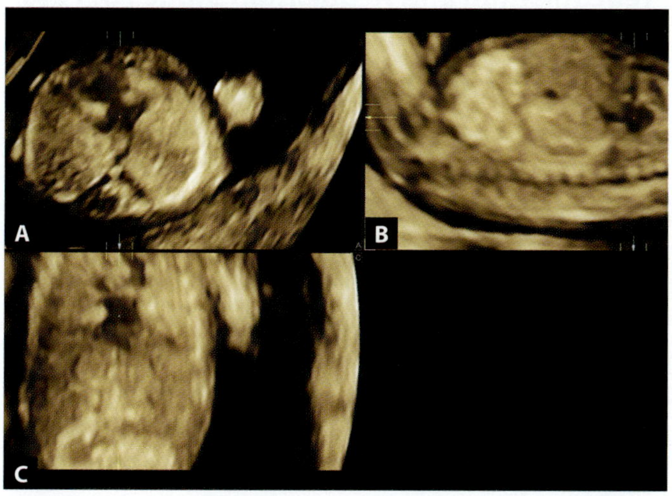

Fig. 2: A 3D static dataset presenting the multiplanar view of the fetal heart with the abnormal arrangement of viscera (situs inversus). This is a properly oriented volume dataset. In the A plane (upper left image) the axis of the heart is directed to the left. In the B plane the heart is seen on the right. In the C plane the coronal section through the fetal chest in shown.

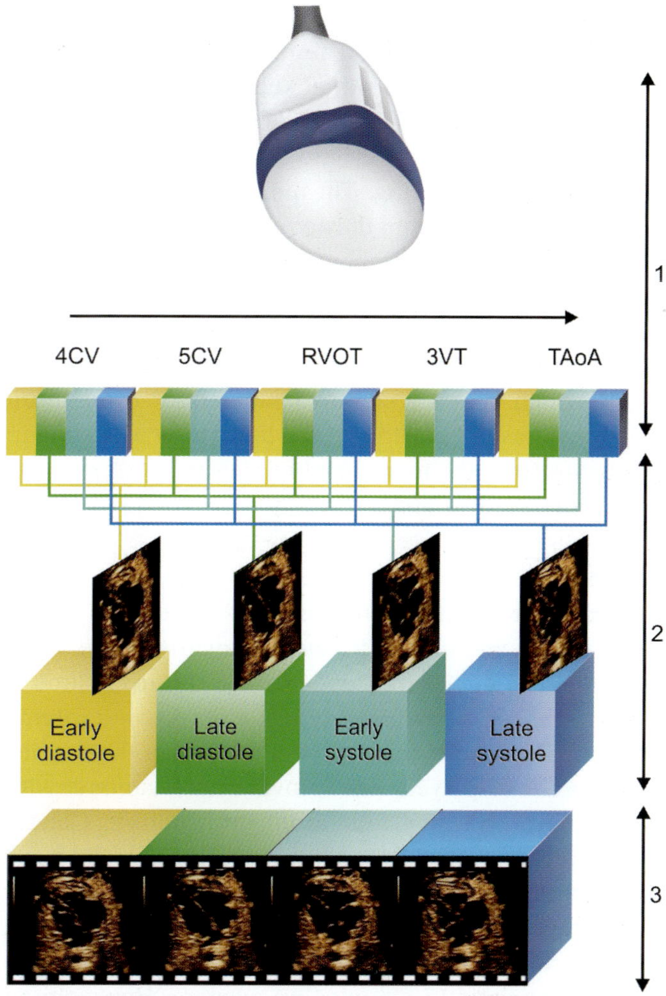

Fig. 3: STIC acquisition and processing is presented: One slow 3D sweep. The machine detects the location and timing of each systolic beat and calculates the heart rate. Then the system determines the time frame between each beat which allows for rearranging of the B-mode frames into a new order depending on their temporal event within the heart cycle. Since, the machine knows the length of the sweep and the heart rate it can calculate the location of each peak systolic frame and other points in the cardiac cycle and combine the information in it with all the other frames of the corresponding times. Because many frames at the exact time reference are averaged together the temporal resolution compares to a high frame rate B-mode image. The rearranging results in a final product of one heart cycle replayed in a continuous cine loop.

Spatial and Temporal Image Correlation

The concept of spatial and temporal image correlation (STIC) consists of a slower static 3D acquisition of the fetal heart, encompassing approximately 25 cycles. During the process of acquisition, the beam is swept through the heart capturing diastole and systole in tiny subphases (**Fig. 3**).[2,16] For example, as the beam sweeps into the four chamber view it is recorded in the phase of early then mid and late diastole, then early mid and late systole. As the sweep continues into the five chamber view it is also captured in the phase of early mid and late diastole, then early mid and late systole, and so on, until the sweep reaches the most superior part of the heart, the transverse section of the aortic arch. The result is one large static volume block. Each individual subphase of the cardiac cycle is then rearranged temporally and grouped into new separate volume blocks. Eventually, approximately 20 to 40 blocks come into being.[2] The quality of the final product depends on the speed of the acquisition sweep. A slower sweep allows for more subphases of the cardiac cycle to be obtained, grouped together and rearranged, which adds spatial information to the final product. The final product is presented in the form of an orderly dynamic sequence, a clip, which is arranged into 1 full cardiac cycle, from the early phase of diastole to the late phase of systole in all planes, from the four-chamber view to the transverse section of the aortic arch.

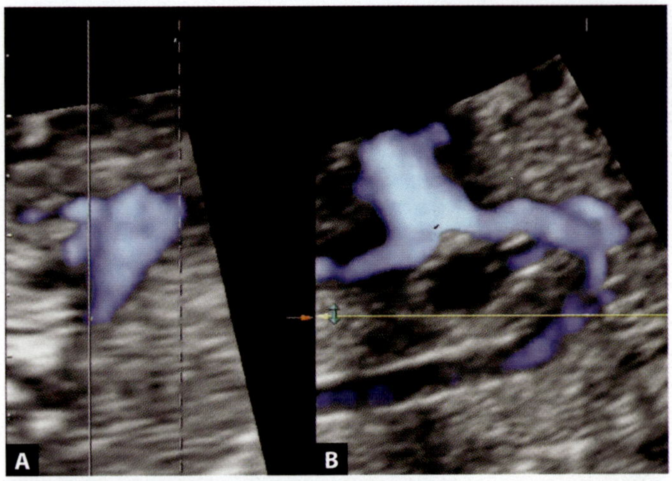

Figs. 4A and B: Biplanar view. (A) Three-vessel and trachea view presenting a tiny aortic arch; (B) Sagittal view of the hypoplastic aortic arch.

4D Real Time

Despite technological progress, 4D technique is still of worse quality than the STIC and even with the use of the most modern matrix transducers the STIC acquisition is preferred because of higher frequency of recorded volume datasets. Because of that more subphases of the cardiac cycle can be displayed, what provides the examiner with more comprehensive functional information. Classic hybrid volume transducers allow capturing the fetal heart in 4D mode on the level of a few volumes per second on average, which is not to be accepted in fetal heart examination. Matrix transducers allow recording with the frequency of 15 volumes on average. However, an average of STIC acquisition in B-mode has better results with the frequency of approximately 40 volumes per second. However, if the examiner considers an analysis of a particular part of the heart, like, e.g., the aortic arch or systemic veins, 4D offers a unique method of biplanar view in real time.[9] With the use of this technique, the examiner is able to follow aortic arch in axial and sagittal views at the same time. Such imaging may be of a great importance in the assessment of aortic coarctation, aortic arch hypoplasia, or aortic arch interruption **(Figs. 4A and B)**.

Because of above-mentioned facts, the authors will focus on STIC mode in the further part of the chapter.

THE PROCESS OF STIC ACQUISITION

It is to be divided into two fundamental stages:

1. The first one is connected to the preparation to the acquisition and the acquisition itself
2. The second one consists of the verification of conducted acquisition, saving volume dataset in the scanner memory and volume dataset review by the use of wide spectrum of visualization modes.

Preacquisition and Acquisition Stages of Fetal Heart Assessment in STIC Mode

Before Acquisition

Every volume dataset irrespective of applied method should be preceded by a series of preparatory proceedings. The first and the most important is the choice of acoustic window, which is the shortest way to the examined organ, which reduces the number of artifacts.

There are two most often used techniques of acquisition: axial and sagittal one. This is the reason why the preparatory proceedings should be explained for each of these techniques separately.

Axial Acquisition

At this stage, the examiner is forced to find the most optimal place to apply the transducer, which allows for the sweep of cardiac views presenting lack or minimal shadowing resulting from fetal skeletal structures. “Escaping” from acoustic shadows is of utmost importance and every sonologist and sonographer must assure that shadows are not encountered in any section of the heart. So before the STIC acquisition is initiated, it is prudent to make a 2D sweep through the heart imitating the STIC acquisition. If on some sections shadows are visible, one should seek a better acoustic window. It must be remembered that shadows from 2D images will always be rewritten on the three-dimensional dataset.

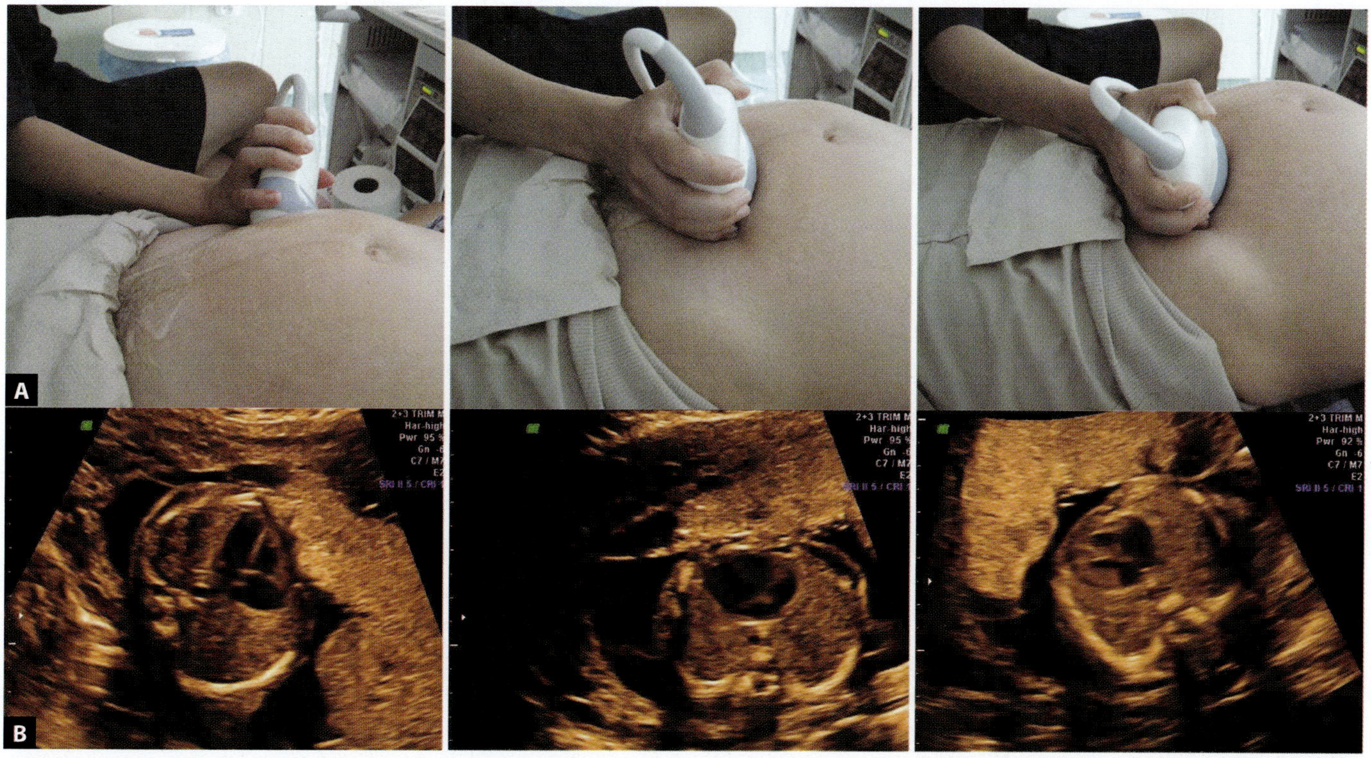

Figs. 5A and B: Translation technique is shown, which is actually nothing more than changing the application point of the transducer. At the time of translation the same section through the fetal chest is displayed on the monitor, but the relationship between the transducer and the target changes. Translation is used for identifying the most suitable insonation angle. (A) Movements with the probe on the patient's abdomen; (B) Effect of translation on the image.

On account of that, on the basis of the authors' experience, the preferred insonation angle to interventricular septum (IVS) should reach about 45 degrees. Apical view with the apex at the 12 o'clock position is better to be avoided due to the suboptimal insonation to the IVS. The same situation concerns basal view, which is always connected with moderate shadowing from fetal ribs. The correction of the insonation angle may be conducted with the use of the transducer—by translation maneuver **(Figs. 5A and B)**.

It should be also emphasized, especially for beginners, that the examiner should avoid oblique views during the acquisition. The acquisition should be conducted in possibly most accurate axial views. To maintain "clear" axial view it is helpful to make fetal ribs, which are a perfect landmark of symmetric cross-section through the fetal thorax. If on the screen there are a few ribs visible on one side, it means that the view should be corrected before the acquisition. Watch carefully for the ribs in the fetal chest to appear similar on both the right and left sides, and that the fetal abdomen and chest are round and not elongated. Keep your image angle wide enough to view the entire width of the fetus so you can easily identify structures that will help you recognize that you are in a true transverse section of the fetus.

Sagittal Acquisition

It is best if acoustic window allows clear visualization of sagittal views, without shadowing. Perpendicular insonation to the anterior thoracic wall is preferable, what minimizes shadowing artifacts.

B-mode Settings, Zooming and Framing

The next stage in the preparation for acquisition is a correct setting of the scanner, which equals to applying the highest transducer frequency, which does not enhance shadowing artifacts. Furthermore, in order to prepare for the STIC acquisition, the authors successfully apply presets based on the combination of harmonic imaging, compounding and speckle reduction. In addition, it reduces artifacts resulting from excessive ultrasound dispersion in fetal tissues. Together with the presented basic rules of setting

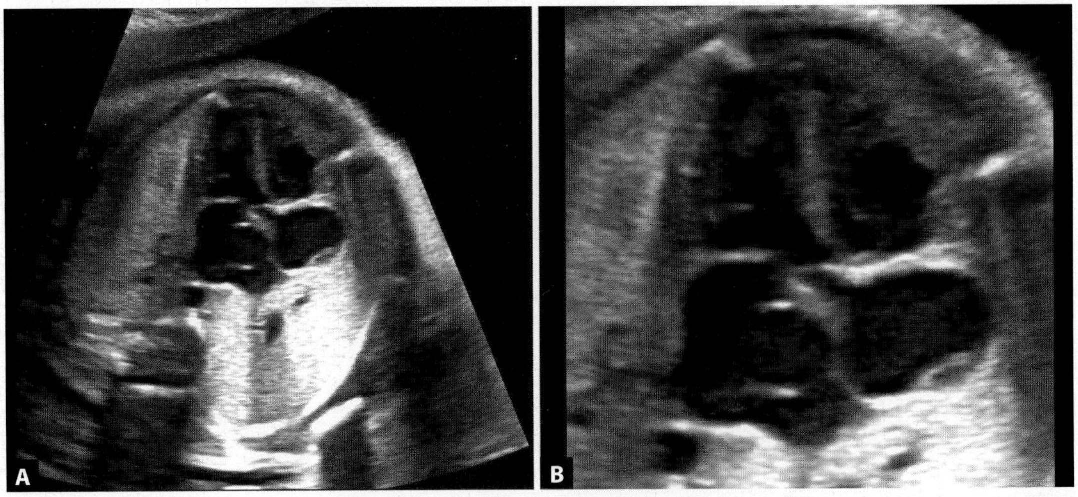

Figs. 6A and B: 2D image preparation for STIC acquisition—framing and zooming. (A) A frame covers the whole chest with small magnification; (B) A frame covers only the heart and includes the descending aorta, high magnification.

the scanner in B-mode, paying special attention to saving volume datasets of fetal heart, HD zooming and framing is of a great importance. At the beginning, it is advised to set zooming and framing which cover the whole fetal chest. After going through basic learning process, which includes about 200 acquisitions, when the examiner is able to maintain the symmetry of axial and sagittal sections correctly, it is possible to apply HD zooming and set framing in such a way to show only the heart and descending aorta **(Figs. 6A and B)**.

Such a manipulation increases the frame rate in 2D-mode, which in turn, leads to higher frequency of captured volumes in STIC mode. As a result, it gives a greater number of saved subphases of the heart cycle in the analyzed sequence of volumes. At this point, it should be emphasized that it is very useful in acquisition including information with color Doppler mapping, Power Doppler and bidirectional power Doppler. The minimum frame rate before volume acquisition in 2D when vascular mapping is on is 20 Hz. If it is lower, then the acquired color information is strongly disturbed.

Acquisition Settings

Now after a proper acoustic window has been selected it is time to make decisions regarding 2 important STIC parameters, the STIC volume angle and the STIC acquisition time.

The STIC volume angle refers to the length of the sweep. One should determine how large of an area that you want to acquire information within. The decision to set the volume angle is dependent on the size of the heart. The greater the size of the heart (gestational age of the fetus) the greater volume angle you will need. A rule of thumb for setting the degree of the angle coincidently coincides with the gestational age in weeks of the fetus.

When acquiring your volume from a transverse plane pick a volume angle that is bigger of 5 to 10 degrees than the gestational age in weeks. Example: an angle of 25 degrees is a good choice for a 20 week fetus. Use a 35 to 40 degree angle for a 30 weeks fetus.

When acquiring your volume from a sagittal plane pick a volume angle that is the same as the gestational age in weeks plus 10 degrees. Example: an angle of 30 degrees is a good choice for a 20 weeks fetus. Use a 40 degree angle for a 30 weeks fetus.

Of course these numbers need to be adjusted larger in cases of cardiomegaly. A minimum angle size, which is acceptable for STIC use is 15 degrees.

The STIC acquisition time determines the length of the duration of the acquisition. Your choice in setting the acquisition time should depend on how active the fetus is at the time that you are trying to do your STIC acquisition. A longer time will create a sweep, which has more time to obtain information thus adding to the quality of the volume dataset. However, with a longer time also comes more opportunity for the fetus to move creating motion artifacts. You of course will have the opportunity to delete the volume and try again if the fetus moves during the acquisition. A minimum time for a STIC acquisition is 2 seconds and a maximum time is 15 seconds depending on the applied probe.

STIC Acquisition

After setting the equipment, the examiner should possibly quickly find the starting view (SV), which refers to the center point of the volume of information, which you are trying to create. It is the midpoint of the volume angle. The SV is the place on the image that you locate from which the sweep will back up ½ the distance of the angle that you have decided on and begin the sweep. The sweep will begin, come to the midpoint (the SV) and continue past the SV for another ½ of the sweep angle. This is the same way in which classic three-dimensional volume acquisition is performed. See the diagram below **(Fig. 7)**.

The recommended SV for acquisitions done in the axial view is five-chamber view and in the sagittal plane is the ventricular short axis view just below the level of the atrio-ventricular valves **(Figs. 8 and 9)**.

In case of acquisition conducted with the use of matrix transducers, the acquisition preview shown on the screen is unimportant because of its short duration of about 2–4 seconds.

However, in case of classic volume transducers during about 10-second acquisition, the acquisition you can watch as the sweep moves through the different levels of the heart. The acquisition is conveniently played at a slow speed so you can watch to make sure the sweep encompassed the stomach on one end and the transverse section of the aortic arch on the other end. You can also watch to see that the fetus did not move and that the proper positioning was maintained to visualize the common views. The experienced eye can detect even the smallest movements of the fetus such as hiccups or respiratory movements, which can cause artifacts **(Figs. 10 and 11)**.

Postacquisition Stages of Fetal Heart Assessment in STIC Mode

Verifying the Machines Calculation of the Heart Rate

The machine detects the location and timing of each systolic beat and calculates the heart rate. After the

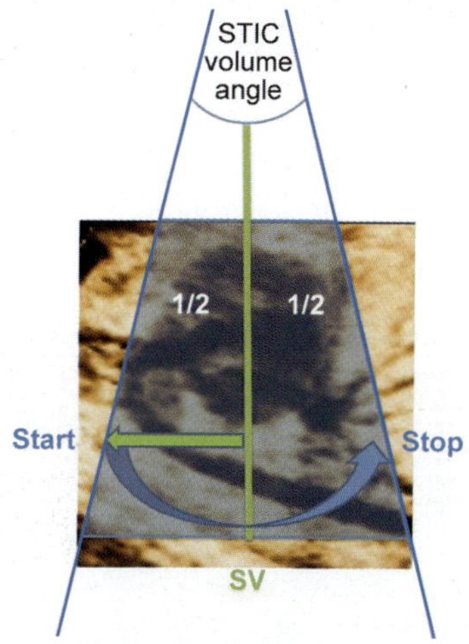

Fig. 7: Volume acquisition. The starting view (SV) is the mid point of the selected volume angle and thus the central section of the volume dataset. The SV is chosen and the transducer automatically sweeps 50% of the chosen volume angle away from the SV. The sweep then begins acquiring information towards the OPA, the sweep continues past the OPA and ends at the equidistance away from the SV at which it began.

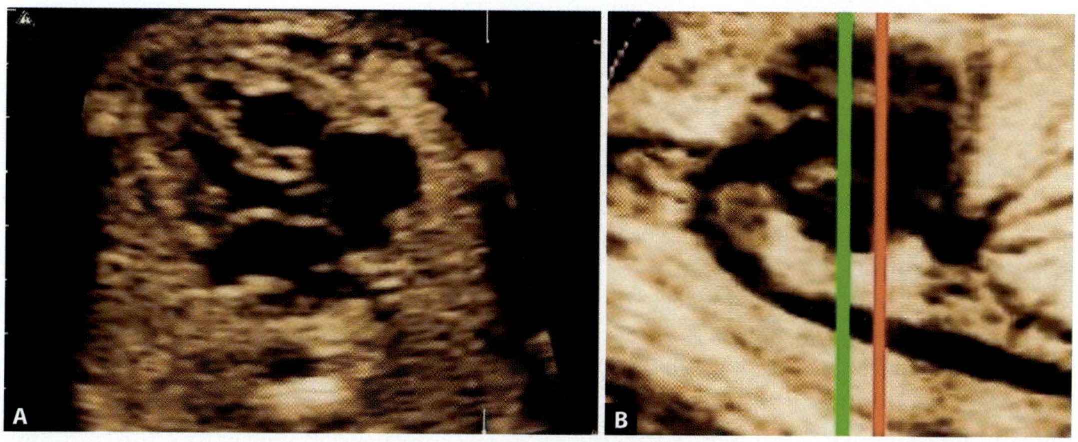

Figs. 8A and B: The starting view (SV) in transverse STIC technique; (A) The five chamber view; (B) A reconstructed image of the heart in the sagittal plane. The green line demonstrates the level of the SV for the transverse STIC acquisition, which is the level of the five chamber view. The red line demonstrates the level of the 4-chamber view. As you can see, the green line (the 5-chamber view) depicts the midpoint of the information which we would like to include in the sweep. The red line (the 4-chamber view) is located too inferior.

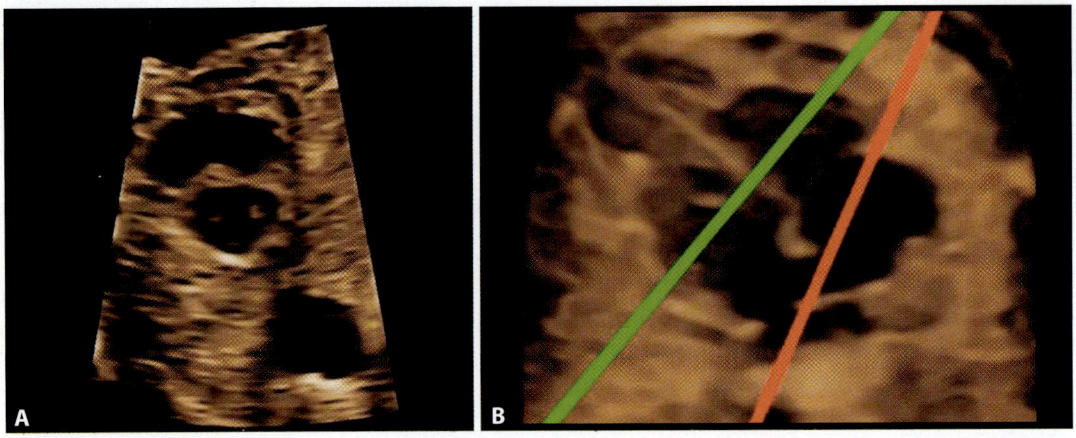

Figs. 9A and B: The starting view (SV) in sagittal STIC technique: (A) Ventricular short axis view just below the atrioventricular valves; (B) A reconstructed image of the heart in the transverse plane. The green line demonstrates the level of the SV for the sagittal STIC acquisition, which is at the level of the ventricular short axis view. The red line demonstrates the level of the aortic arch which would be too far to the right for an optimal STIC acquisition.

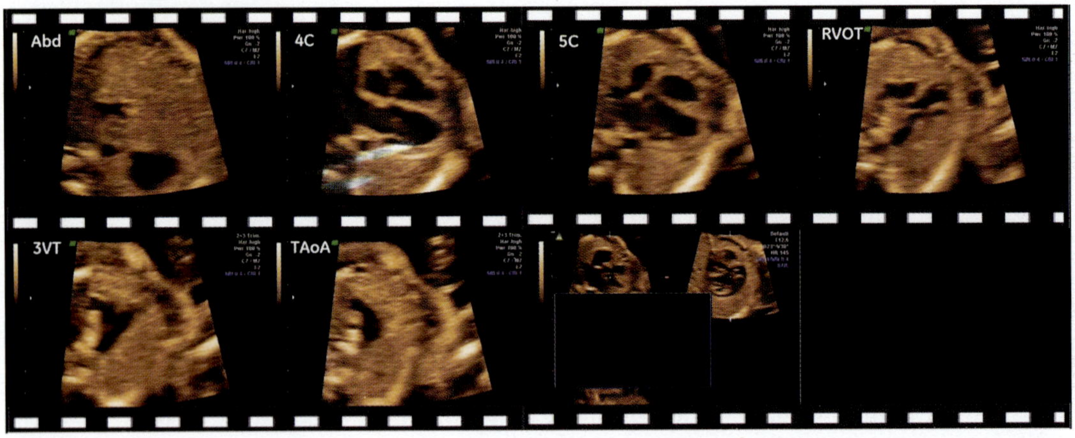

Fig. 10: The static illustration of the preview in progress of the transverse, transabdominal STIC acquisition. The viewing permits the examiner to watch each transverse section of the fetal heart during the acquisition and to check whether or not artifacts occurred. (Abd: upper abdominal view; 4C: four-chamber view; 5C: five-chamber view; RVOT: right outflow tract; 3VT: three vessels and trachea view; TAoA: the transverse section through the aortic arch)

acquisition of the volume, a box will appear telling you the machines calculation of the estimated fetal heart rate. If the machines estimated heart rate is not consistent with what you observed while imaging the heart you must cancel the acquisition and try again.

Initial Review of the Volume Dataset

A following element of the estimation of the quality of a newly acquired volume sequence of datasets is the quick review. You will be looking for any reason to reject this particular dataset sequence or to decide whether or not you will save it to the machine hard drive for later review and manipulation. The most obvious reasons for rejection of the STIC dataset are motion and/or shadowing artifacts. Using the multiplanar imaging option easily does this quick review. Here you will want to activate the reference image B and look for breaks in the reconstruction, which signify motion by the fetus during the acquisition **(Fig. 12)**.

Then, within the same reference image B, which is the sagittal plane, one can move the pivot point horizontally, to the right and left, while watching the A plane. Each of the recommended views from the transverse aortic arch view to the level of the stomach in the abdomen will come into view and can be evaluated for motion or shadowing artifacts, or any other undesirable quality.

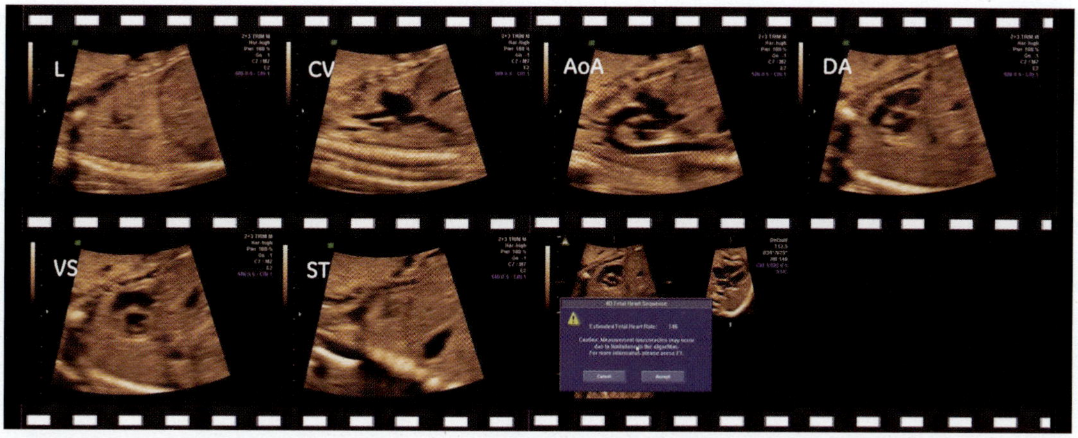

Fig. 11: The static illustration of the preview in progress of the sagittal, transabdominal STIC acquisition. The viewing permits the examiner to watch each sagittal section of the fetal heart during the acquisition and to check whether or not artifacts occurred. (L: section through right lung; CV: long axis caval view; AoA: aortic arch; DA: ductal arch; VS: ventricular short axis view; ST: sagittal section through the fetal trunk at the level of the stomach)

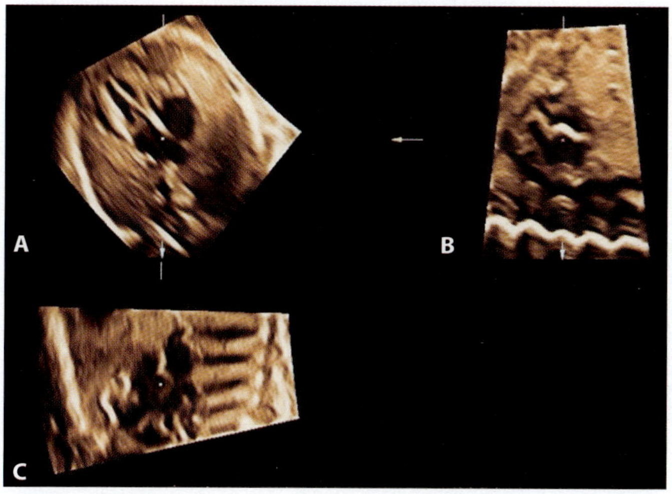

Fig. 12: Quality rating of a new STIC dataset-motion artifacts. The multiplanar view of the fetal heart. Reference images B and C demonstrate numerous breaks in the reconstruction signifying motion of the fetus during the progress of acquisition.

If after previewing the quality of the volume dataset and verifying that the fetal heart rate is correct then the STIC volume dataset should be stored to the hard drive of the ultrasound machine. If you forget to store the volume this information will be unavailable later for review and manipulation.

STIC Dataset Anatomic Orientation

Similarly as in 2D, 3D fetal echocardiography is based on standardized cardiac sections.[17-20] An innovation and advantage in STIC is the ability to always review the STIC images in the identical orientation from one exam to the next, one institution to the next, and even one country to the next. This is possible due to the ability to manipulate the images by means of rotational knobs, which are standardized among equipment manufactures. This takes away the variability of fetal lie and promotes a continuity and unification of the prenatal diagnoses of congenital heart disease by the use of STIC.

The orientation of STIC volumes is a completely new sonographic skill.[21] It exists in the consistent anatomical arrangement of every heart, stored in STIC mode, according to the same repeatable rules, so as to prepare the volume block for review in a well-organized and reproducible manner.

Foundations of the three-dimensional orientation of the fetal heart were laid in 2001 by Bega and co-authors on static 3D volumes.[17] In the following years it was refined by other authors.[18,20,22,23]

For correct orientation of STIC volumes, knobs are available which rotate images on the x, y and z axis. Coupled with the parallel shift control knob virtually any acquired position of the fetal heart can be manipulated into standard orientations. The image below represents a correctly oriented volume data block of the heart, ready for review and interpretation.

Above is a multiplanar view of a STIC volume dataset. The examiner has arranged the anatomy in the standard viewing planes first described by Bega and coworkers which is, in the A plane, with the apex of the heart to the left of the screen.[17] If the heart is normal the B plane will show the aortic or ductal arch to the left of the image also. Some others have proposed orientating STIC images with

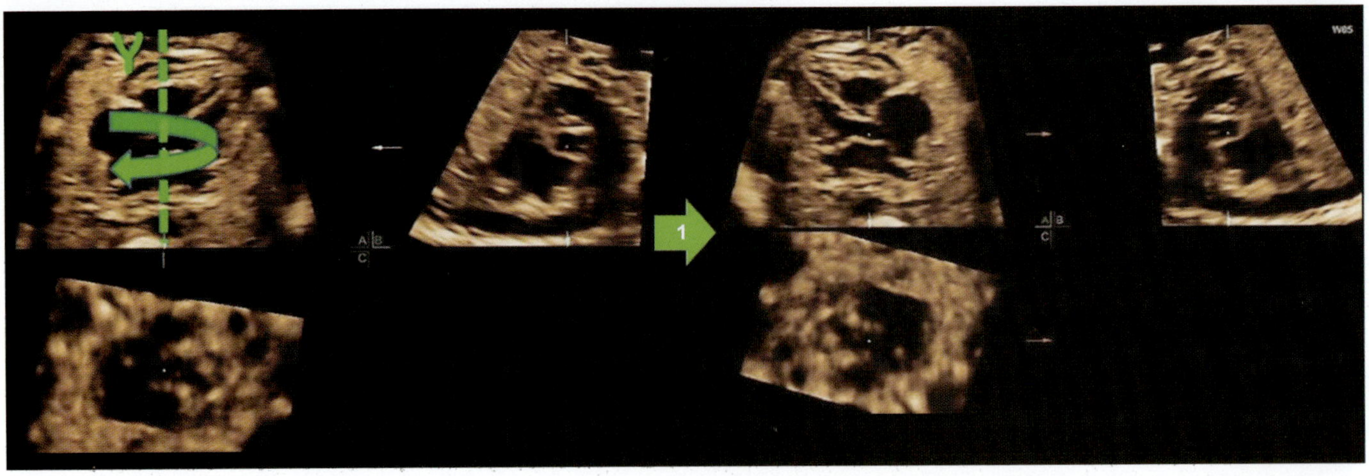

Fig. 13: The dataset in the top picture was acquired with the apex of the heart to the right of the image. Since we always want to view our volumes with the apex to the left one must turn the image of 4CV in the reference plane A by 180 degrees using the Y-axis rotation knob. The result is the bottom picture.

the apex of the heart to the right rather than the left. We believe that orientation with the apex to the left of the image is a good standard and will use this orientation throughout the remainder of this chapter.

Orientating a STIC volume is the process of image orientation in which the operator utilizes the x, y and z knobs and the parallel shift knob on the machine to twist, rotate or flip the images until they end up in a standardized viewing layout whereas the A plane is a transverse 4-chamber image of the heart with the apex to the left of the image. The B plane is a reconstructed sagittal image showing superior to the left and inferior to the right, and the C place is a reconstructed coronal image. This will place the images in planes, which will make review and manipulation easy and predictable.

There are several ways to arrive at this standard orientation of the apex to the left in the A plane. These methods all are based on the utilization of linear structures, situated in the anatomical neighborhood of the heart. These structures include: the spine, the descending aorta, the interventricular septum and the ductal arch. The orientation should be always performed in the multiplanar view. In multiplanar mode each image has a small dot, which is called the pivot point. By utilizing the x, y and z knobs the image will rotate on this pivot point allowing you to align structures within the image to a standardized orientation.

In **Figures 13 to 17** manipulation of the images into a standard viewing orientation is shown.

Any of the above methods will work to manipulate the volume into the standard viewing orientation in which the apex of the heart is on the left in the A plane.

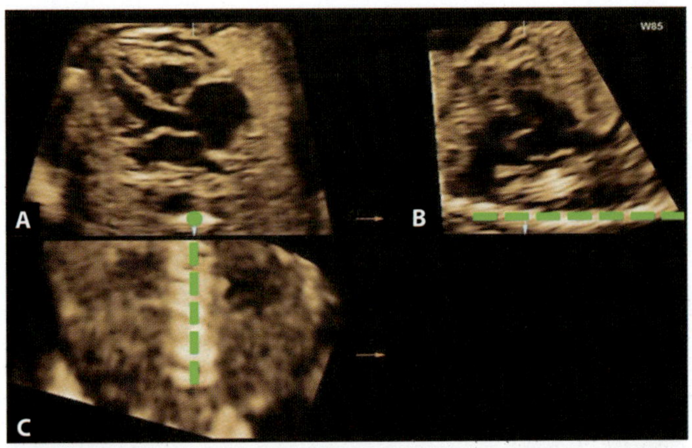

Fig. 14: The pivot point in the A plane on the spine. The spine was used in the B and C planes to line up the images horizontally in B, and vertically in C. This resulted in an optimal orientation of the volume which can now be reviewed.

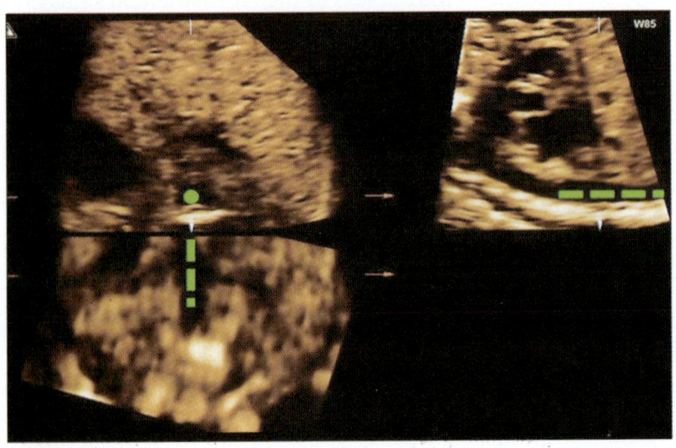

Fig. 15: In this picture the descending aorta was used in like manner as the spine.

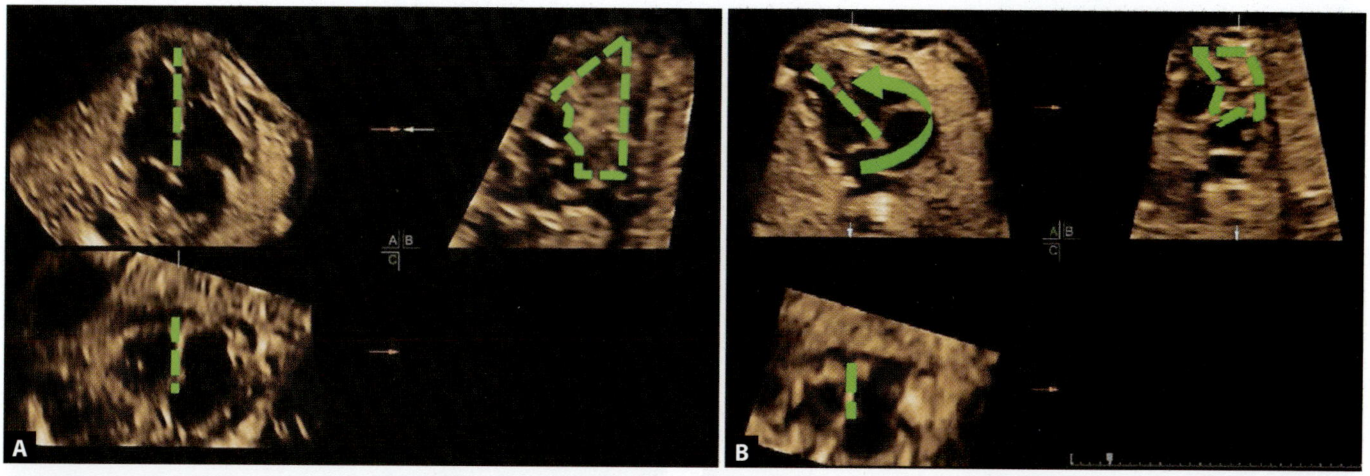

Figs. 16A and B: (A) This picture shows orientation of the volume by using the interventricular septum placed along Y-axis in the A plane, the B plane shows the "IVS in-plane view" and in the C plane the "ventricular short axis view" comes into plane; (B) A Z-axis rotation is the used to again turn the axis of the heart to the left in the A plane.

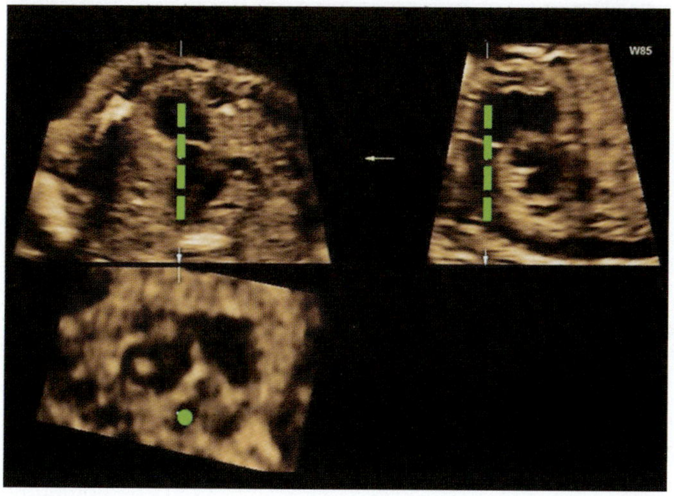

Fig. 17: The ductal arch was aligned vertically along the Y-axis in the A plane.

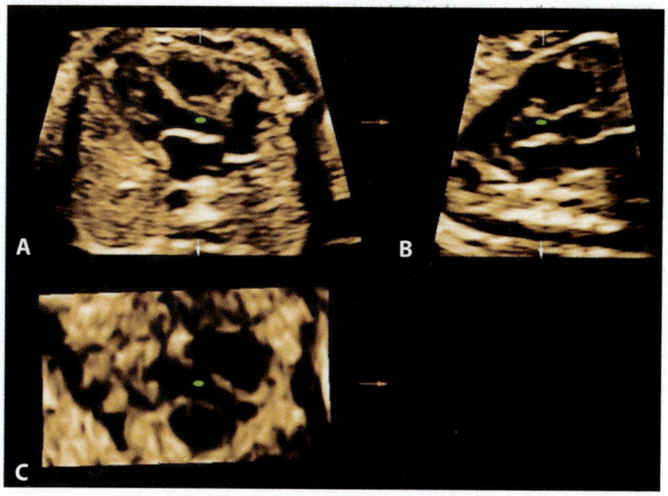

Figs. 18A to C: (A) Multiplanar view showing the pivot point in the aortic root; (B) This same geographic location is represented again by the pivot point in the aortic root, now in a sagittal view; (C) The coronal view of the aortic root is represented again.

STIC Volume Review and the Spectrum of Viewing Options

Once proper orientation of the volume is obtained it is ready for review and interpretation. When the volume is put into motion in the format of a clip, it represents one full heart cycle played over and over again. It is possible to slow down the speed of the clip to about 50%, which creates superb spatial orientation for review. It is also possible to utilize the frame after frame review option. There are many STIC volume three-dimensional viewing options available. These will be discussed below.

Multiplanar view/STIC 2D: Perhaps the most important and most basic of all viewing options is the multiplanar view.[17,18,23-25] In this view 3 planes are shown which are perpendicular to each other **(Figs. 18A to C)**. They have in common one point, the pivot point, which is represented on the screen by a dot. The location of this point in the reference image of plane A, e.g., the root of the aorta, identifies the same structure in the B and C planes. Important tools in the multiplanar view are a parallel shift control, which allows for navigating through the image in a layer after layer manner in any of the 3 planes. Other tools

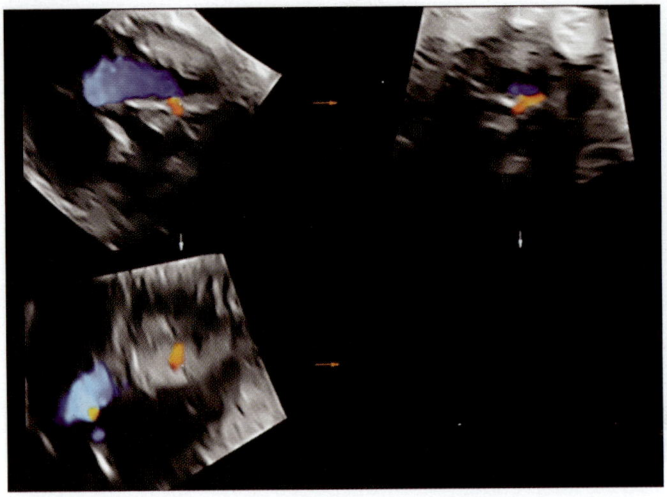

Fig. 19: A muscular ventricular septal defect is show in multiplanar view in all reference images.

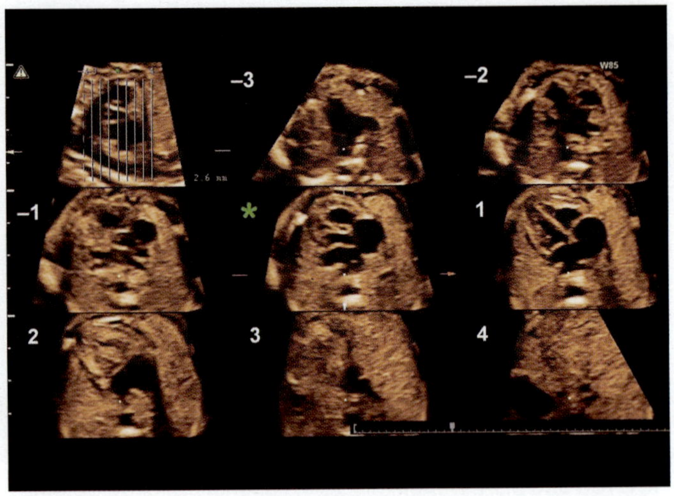

Fig. 21: Ultrasound tomography in systole in a normal heart.

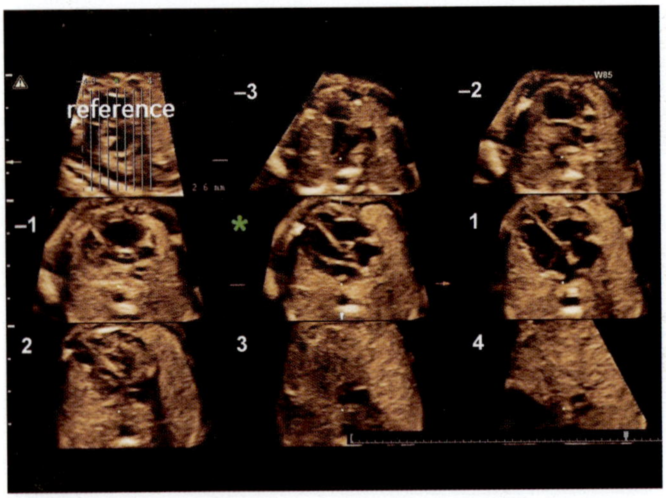

Fig. 20: Tomographic ultrasound imaging in a STIC volume in diastole in a normal heart. In the top left section the overlay image is presented, which is perpendicular to the tomographic layers, demonstrating section levels.

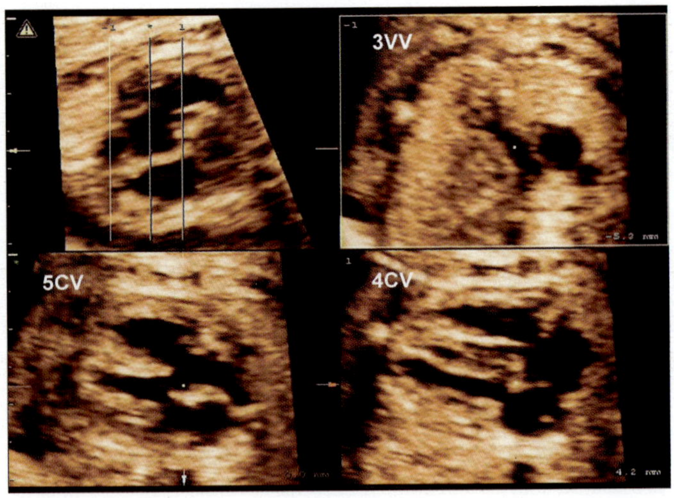

Fig. 22: Tetralogy of Fallot in tomographic ultrasound imaging. Levels of four-chamber view (4CV); five-chamber view (5CV) and three vessel view (3VV) are presented.

are the x, y and z-axis rotational knobs used for volume manipulation.

In **Figure 19** a clinical example of the use of the multiplanar imaging is shown. The anomaly in this case is a ventricular septal defect. The detailed multiplanar evaluation gave the clear picture of this abnormality.

Ultrasound tomography: Another viewing option for a STIC volume is ultrasound tomography (commercial names: Multislice View/Tomographic Ultrasound Imaging/ iSlice). It has many advantages and is utilized often by many examiners.[19,26-28] Tomography allows for the viewing of multiple slices of the same image, by means of **1, 3, 5, 8, 11, or 15** sections on one screen along with a reference image which is perpendicular to the tomographic sections with an overlay of the tomographic lines of slices. The distance between the slices can be set with equal or any distances **(Figs 20 to 23)**. The mid slice is represented on the overlay by an asterisk. Slices to the left of the center line are described by negatives slice numbers and slices to the right of the center line are represented by positive slice numbers. This makes identification of the slices in comparison to the reference image easy. It was proposed

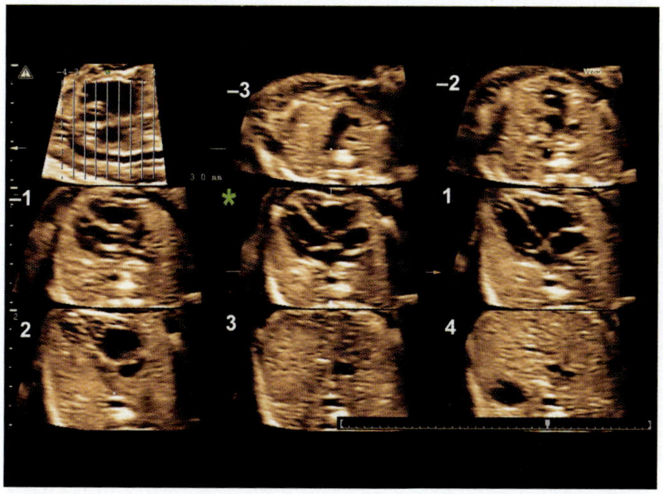

Fig. 23: Presentation of d-transposition of great arteries: Level *shows normal four-chamber view; level 1—two semilunar valves at the same time (five-chamber view); level 2—abnormal arrangement of great arteries (three-vessel view)—aorta pushed anteriorly; and level 3—singular arterial vessel= aortic arch (three-vessel and trachea view).

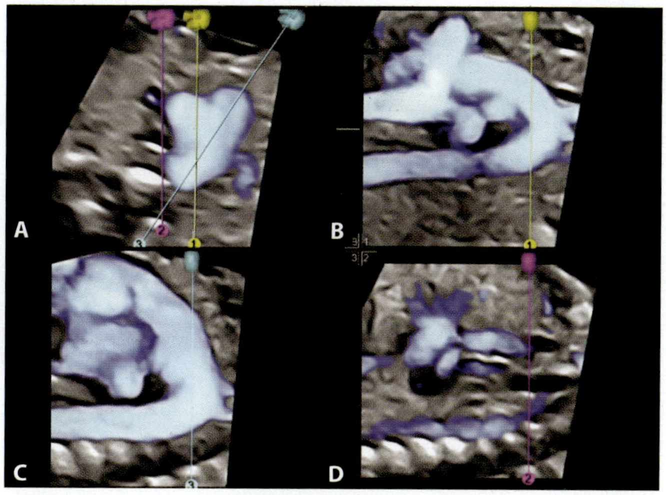

Figs. 24A to D: Omni view imaging in a normal fetal heart: Colored lines are arbitrarily placed on the reference image (A); (B) Represents a perpendicular plane to the yellow line on the reference image (aortic arch view); (C) Represents a perpendicular plane to the blue line on the reference image (the ductal arch view); (D) Represents a perpendicular plane to the purple line on the reference image (the long axis caval view).

the use of 3 standardized tomographic distances, which demonstrate the three cardiac planes in which most of the abnormalities of the heart can be recognized. These 3 planes are the 4-chamber view, the 5-chamber view and the right outflow tract view. In cases of complex defects of the heart ultrasound tomography is an excellent way to illustrate the margins of the defect on one screen. In the pictures below both a normal heart, a heart with tetralogy of Fallot and with d-transposition of great arteries is illustrated with the use of tomographic imaging.

Any plane techniques: Commercially named functionalities Omni View or Oblique View techniques allow for drawing arbitrary straight or curved sections from the reference image and displaying those sections next to the reference image.[29,30] These techniques may simplify fetal heart evaluation in a volume dataset **(Figs. 24A to D)**.

Rendering: A completely different kind of volume viewing option, which can be utilized in STIC is rendering. This is a technique of three-dimensional reconstruction from flat multiplanar images.[18,31,32] Surface rendering gives the impression of depth, causing the final images to resemble autopsy sections. The surface which one wishes to examine can be chosen and applied by the use of a rendering box. Because we are using volumes of information a direction that one wishes to look from can be chosen from any plane. The thickness of the box determines the "depth" of tissue that one wants to see in the rendered image **(Fig. 25)**.

Surface rendering takes place on comparatively narrow thicknesses of the region of interest **(Fig. 26)**.

Most of the rendering directions can be applied in the STIC mode from the volumes obtained by a transverse acquisition technique **(Figs. 27A to D)**.

In surface rendering of the fetal heart the options available for optimization are very important. We have found excellent results with the use of HDlive/Realistic view or *gradient light mode* mixed with *surface* with very low levels of *threshold low* and transparency **(Figs. 28A to D)**.

For the evaluation of the relationships of the great arteries, arches and evaluation of cardiac chambers *minimum transparent mode* or *inversion mode* rendering can be utilized.[35,36] Below is an example of these modes in a case of transposed great arteries. Here the region of interest box has been enlarged so that all of the essential anatomical elements can be seen. The inversion rendering seen on the right image below uses the HDlive/Realistic view mode and an increase of lower threshold and transparency **(Fig. 29)**. This is a particularly good combination utilized with a sagittal acquisition. The visualization rates of inversion mode ranged from 55 to 100%. This method

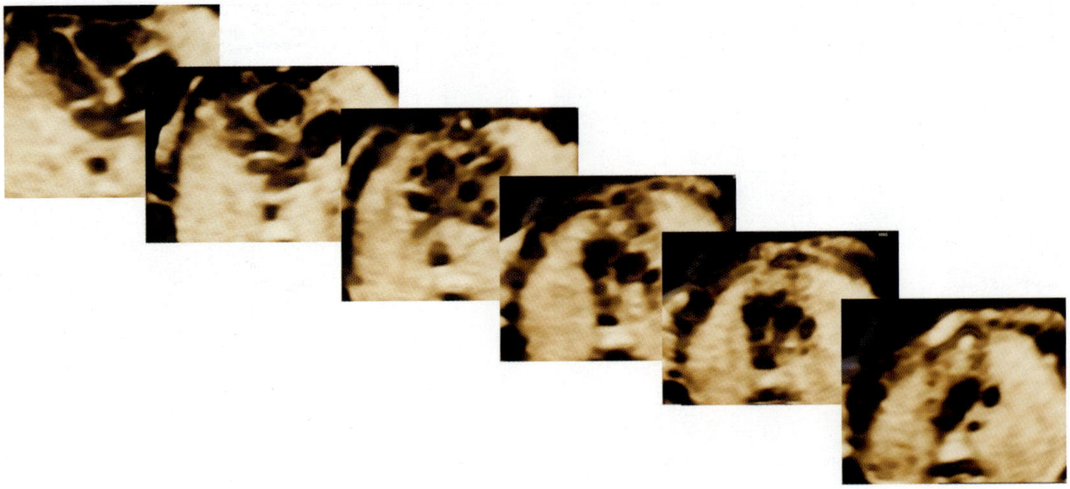

Fig. 25: Surface rendering of the fetal heart from a STIC volume obtained at 21 weeks of gestation. Rendering direction which was applied is front to back. Subsequent cardiac views are represented starting from the four-chamber view through the five-chamber view, the three vessel view, the transverse section through ductal arch, the three vessel and trachea view and the transverse section through aortic arch. In all the presented images the effect of depth is clearly seen.

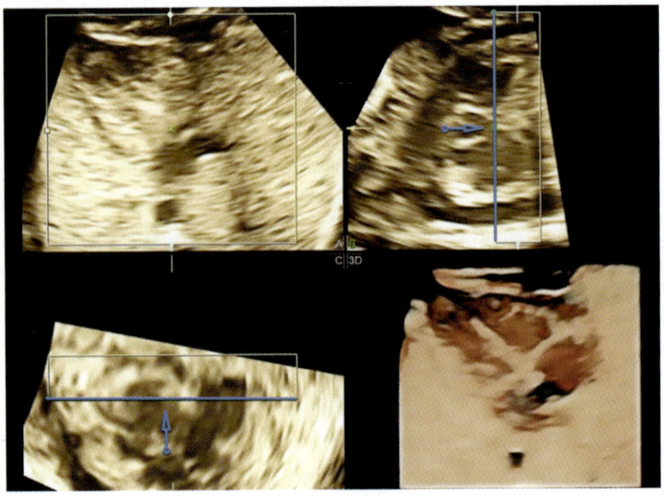

Fig. 26: Multiplanar view of the fetal heart along with 3D rendering. In the B and C reference images a narrow region of interest is chosen which is essential for surface rendering of the heart. Note the blue line representing the direction of rendering.

allows better visualization of complex congenital heart disease and may be considered an addition to 2D fetal echocardiography.[35,36]

In the inversion mode, it is also possible to use a narrow region of interest box, encompassing only the cardiac chambers. This focuses on the relation of the size of ventricles, their contractility, the cross of the heart, the interventricular septum, the composition of the atrioventricular valves, atrial appendages, or the relationship of the outflow tracts **(Figs. 30A and B)**.

For STIC volumes utilizing B-mode information accompanied by color mapping, the same viewing options are accessible as for STIC gray scale datasets.[37,38] A STIC acquisition can be done in gray scale with B-mode alone, or with the addition of color, power, or bidirectional power Doppler mapping (HD flow) **(Figs. 31 and 32)**. These techniques allow for demonstration functional aspects of the fetal heart as well as geometric relation between the ventricles, great arteries and arches.[37] A rendering modality called "glass body" imaging writes the color information on the background of the grayscale information. Below are examples of vascular mapping with STIC.

An option available with STIC imaging is the use of B-flow imaging. B-flow imaging is an exceptionally sensitive form of coding of the blood flow, allowing visualization of extremely small vessels.[41] It is a Doppler independent B-mode option based on the use of the highest frequencies transmitted by the probe allowing for the enhancement of signals representing blood flow while simultaneously ignoring signals from stationary tissue. This allows for the visualization of vascular information independent of tissue information **(Fig. 33)**.

2D and volume measurements in STIC datasets: Measurements can be made from STIC volumes in the same manner as classic two-dimensional measurements. Since 2006 Z-score measurements have been available for use in relating cardiac measurements to gestational age. This method simplifies the expression of measurements providing the examiner with calculations in standard

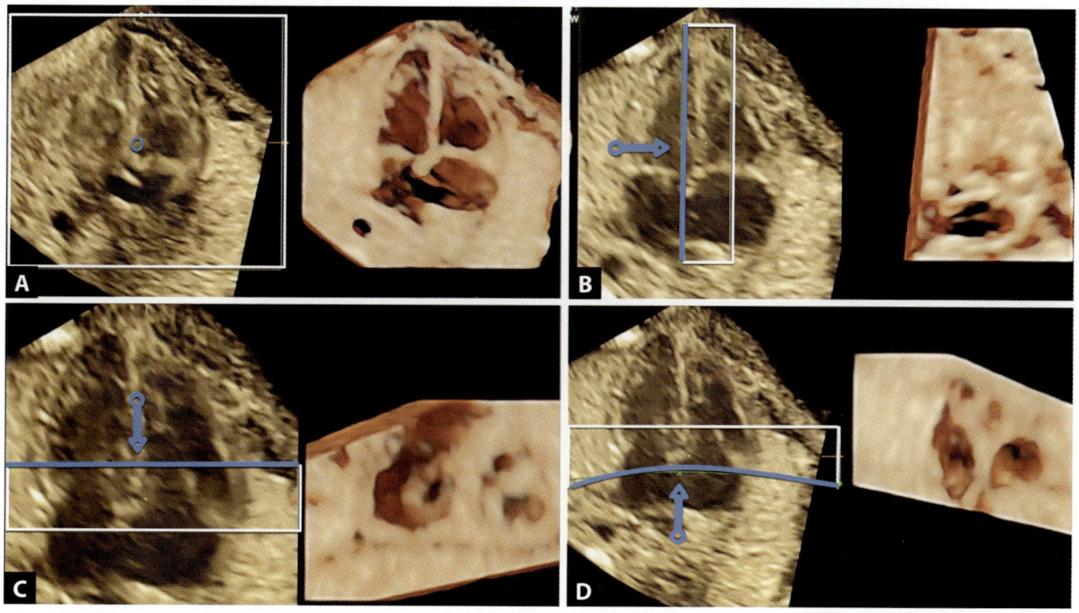

Figs. 27A to D: Rendering directions in surface rendering of the fetal heart shown in the plane A: a 4-chamber rendered view using a front to back render direction (A); in plane view of the interventricular septum (B) left to right direction; atrioventricular valves (C) up to down direction; the base of the heart presenting the relation between the four valves (D) down to up direction.

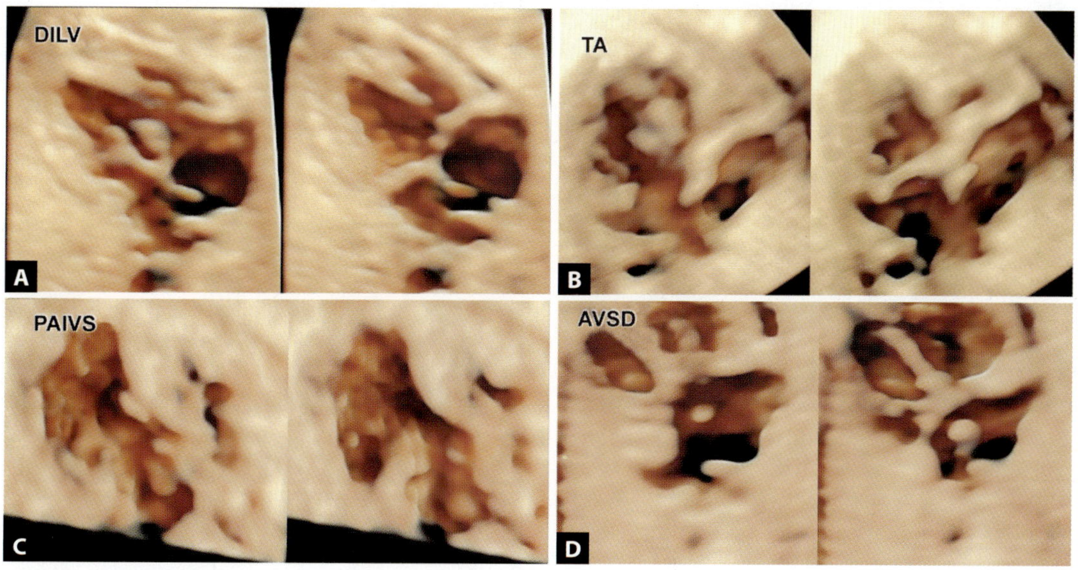

Figs. 28A to D: Surface rendering of four anomalies in diastole and systole at the level of four-chamber view: (A) Double inlet left ventricle (DILV); (B) Tricuspid atresia (TA); (C) Pulmonary atresia with intact interventricular septum (PAIVS); (D) Atrioventricular spetal defect (AVSD).

deviations rather than in millimeters in relation to any given gestational age and measured BPD and FL.[40] It simplifies the precise quantification of the size of fetal cardiac structures. This method of calculation has become a standard in the majority of reference centers nowadays. However, it should be emphasized that there is a risk that in volume datasets of a lower quality, performed measurements would not be in accordance with measurements carried out in 2D.

Because of the capacity of three-dimensional acquisition, STIC datasets allow to calculate typical volume measurements. VOCAL and SonoAVC techniques could be an example.[41,42] The use of the VOCAL method requires mechanical or automated tracing by the examiner

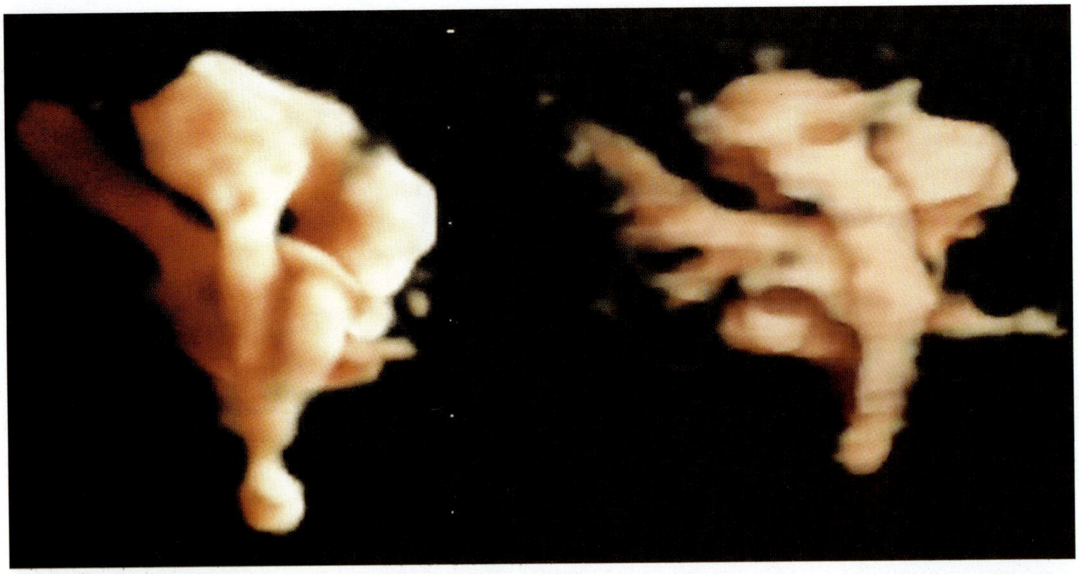

Fig. 29: Normal heart (left) and d-transposition of great arteries in inversion mode rendering. Notice the very different geometry of outflow tracts between these two examples.

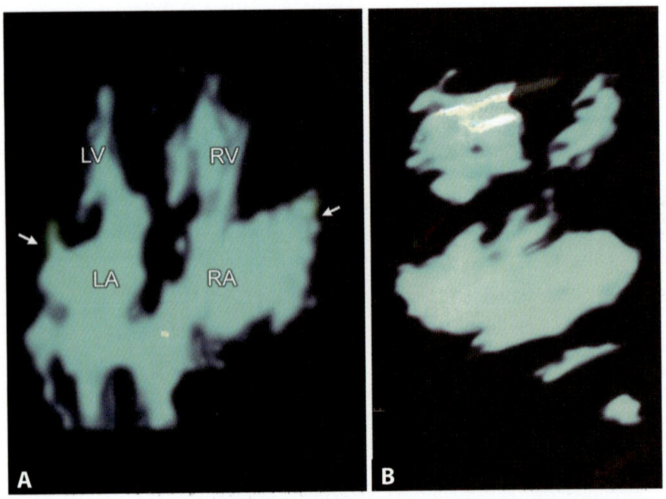

Figs. 30A and B: Inversion mode rendering with the application of a narrow region of interest box focused on the four-chamber view: (A) Shows a normal case; (B) Shows right atrial isomerism with atrioventricular septal defect.

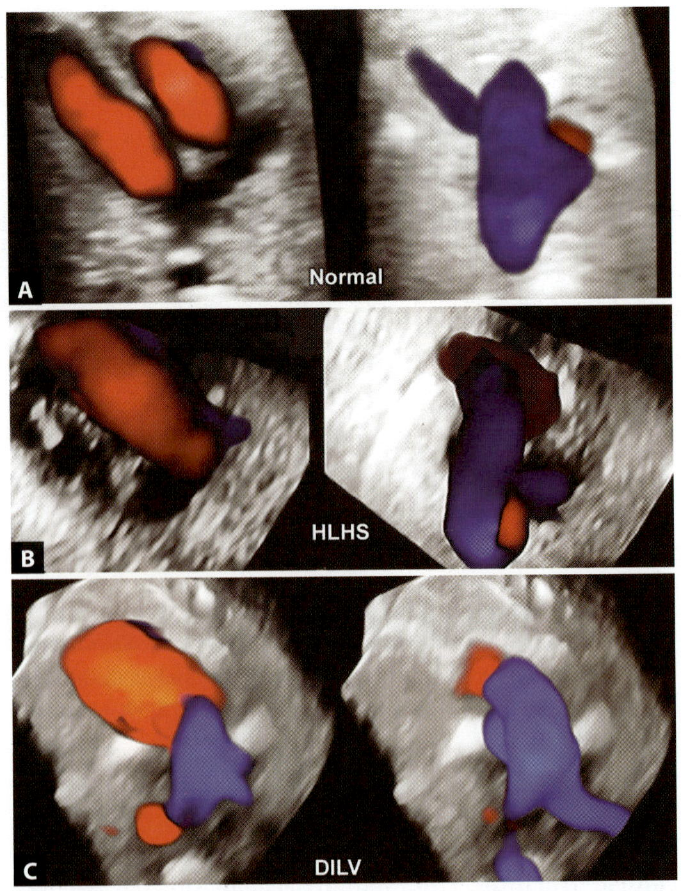

Figs. 31A to C: Glass body rendering in color Doppler mapping using a deep region of interest box in diastole and systole. (A) Normal heart; (B) Hypoplastic left heart (HLHS); (C) Double inlet left ventricle (DILV) with transposed great arteries.

of whatever structure one wishes to perform a volumetric measurement of. SonoAVC is also utilized for volume calculation however it is a machine derived volume, which can only be used for volume measurements of fluid structures. When volumetric measurements are performed in both systole and diastole calculations of cardiac stroke volume can be easily derived. The calculations of these algorithms have been validated on artificial models.[43] An application of this is to assess cardiac chamber volumes

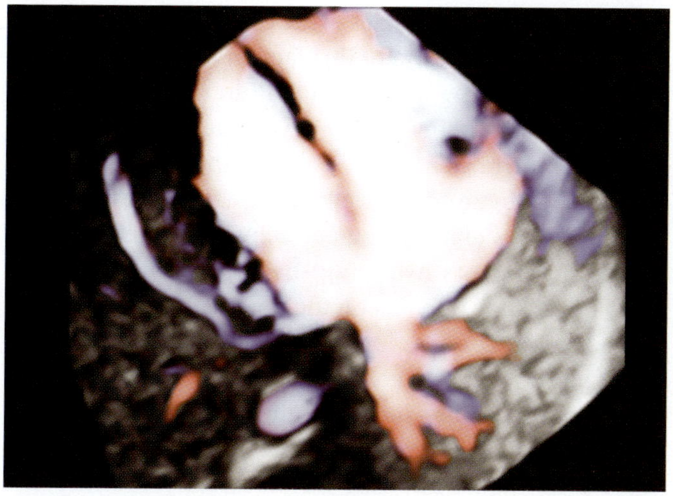

Fig. 32: Glass body rendering in bidirectional Doppler mapping using a shallow region of interest box in diastole in a case of partial anomalous pulmonary venous return (PAPVR). Note the abnormal drainage of pulmonary veins and the small size of the left atrium.

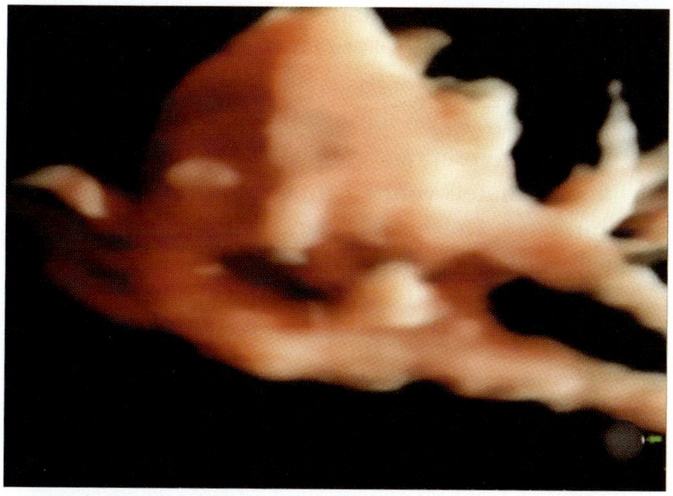

Fig. 33: Surface rendering on the basis of b-flow imaging presenting the aortic arch and brachiocephalic vessels.

in various phases of the cardiac cycle. Due to the contrast between the ventricular walls and cardiac chamber 3D measurements allow for reproducible calculations of ventricular volumes even by the use of automatic contour finder.[44] A good agreement was shown between these two methods for estimating fetal stroke volume and they were even suggested as methods of choice in this area.[45] Basing on 3D measurements normograms for left and right ventricular stroke volumes, ventricular cardiac outputs, and ejection fraction were elaborated with appropriate reproducibility.[46,47] 3D stroke volume readings were compared with 2D Doppler techniques and presented

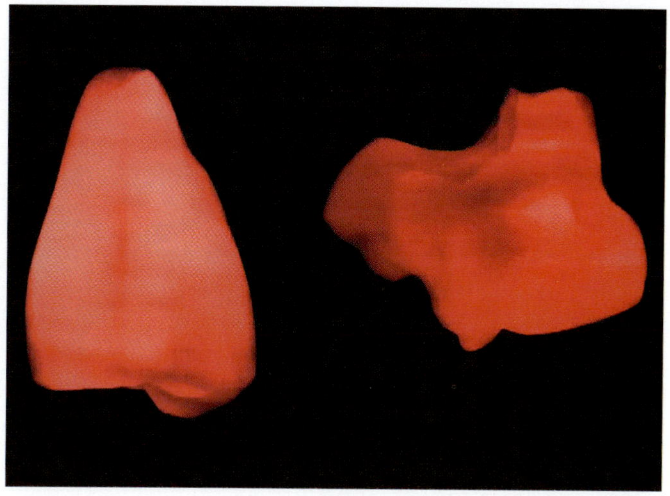

Fig. 34: Volume calculations of cardiac ventricles by the use of vocal technique.

high level of agreement.[48] Thanks to 3D calculations fetal physiology explained similar left and right ventricular stroke volumes and cardiac outputs as a result of larger volume of the fetal right ventricle and a greater ejection fraction of the left ventricle.[59] From diagnostic point of view SonoAVC was also applied for the assessment of atrial appendages in cases of heterotaxy **(Figs. 34 and 35)**.[50]

STIC M-mode: In 2009 STIC M-mode was introduced into clinical practice allowing for the capability of placing arbitrary M-mode lines into the volume dataset allowing for M-mode measurements to be taken from positions that are not available by two dimensional imaging. As an example in 2013 tricuspid annular plane systolic excursion (TAPSE) measurements were described in STIC M-mode.[51] This is an old method of ventricular function assessment that is used in echocardiography of adults in coronary disease. In the fetus it is of importance in the right ventricular function evaluation. For the left ventricle function mitral annular plane systolic excursion (MAPSE) can be applied **(Figs. 36 and 37)**.

Volume automation methods in fetal heart evaluation: A few years after introducing three-dimensional techniques of fetal heart evaluation, examiners began to look for algorithms, which would allow mapping the views of the fetal heart in STIC volume datasets automatically.[13-15] The very first method was volume computer-aided diagnosis (VCAD). This technique was brought into use with fetal heart imaging between 18 and 23 weeks of gestation. In this time period the heart increases in size as the whole

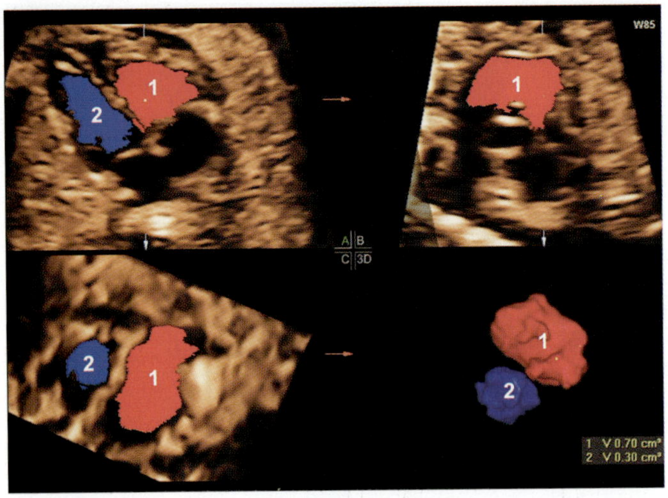

Fig. 35: Volume calculations of cardiac ventricles by the use of SonoAVC.

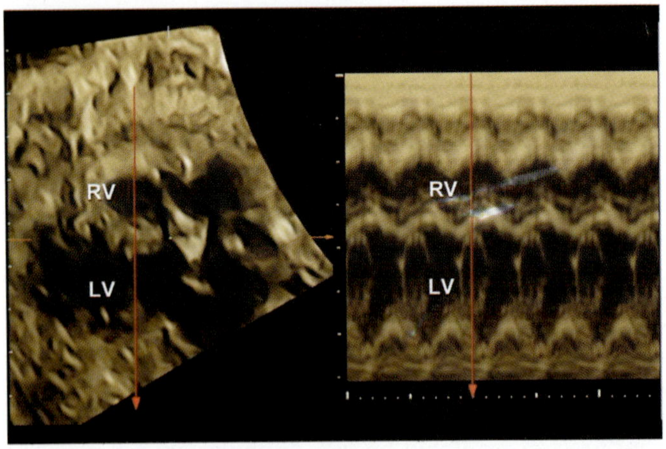

Fig. 36: STIC M-mode technique has the capability of placing arbitrary anatomic lines allowing for M-mode measurements to be taken from positions that are hardly available by two-dimensional imaging. A case of pulmonary atresia with intact interventricular septum (PAIVS)—note the thickening of the right ventricular wall and its small lumen.

but relationships of the sizes of the main cardiac structures remain similar. Because of this fact an automated system can be used during this time to aid in the identification of basic cardiac views. After a volume is achieved the examiner must orient the A plane so that the 4-chamber view is showing and the apex of the heart is to the left. When VCAD is enabled a green template of a heart, ribs and spine appears overlying the A plane image and a green dotted line appears on the B plane representing the sagittal spine. The examiner lines up the volume in the A and B planes with the green templates, which essentially orientates the volume into an optimum position **(Fig. 38)**.

Because the volume is now in a standardized position the VCAD algorithm can automatically identify the following cardiac views: left outflow tract (Cardiac 1); right outflow tract (Cardiac 2); upper abdominal (Cardiac 3); long-axis caval (Cardiac 4); ductal arch (Cardiac 5); and aortic arch (Cardiac 6) **(Fig. 39)**.

In case when the algorithm makes a mistake, assuming, that the examined subject is a normal heart, the examiner can correct the image of particular views owing to the fact that VCAD is based on tomographic ultrasound imaging. It is possible even in case of oblique views, which require partial automated volume rotation such as Cardiac 1 and Cardiac 6. However, in datasets affected by motion artifacts, all sagittal views (Cardiac 4, 5 and 6) will not be shown correctly. The next method, called Fetal Heart Navigation (FHN), was based on automated volume orientation, according to the course of descending aorta and ductal arch. This algorithm does not have limitations resulting from gestational age because after automated orientation is carried out, the examiner himself assigns the levels of representative cardiac views by comparing observed layers with the schematic images presenting

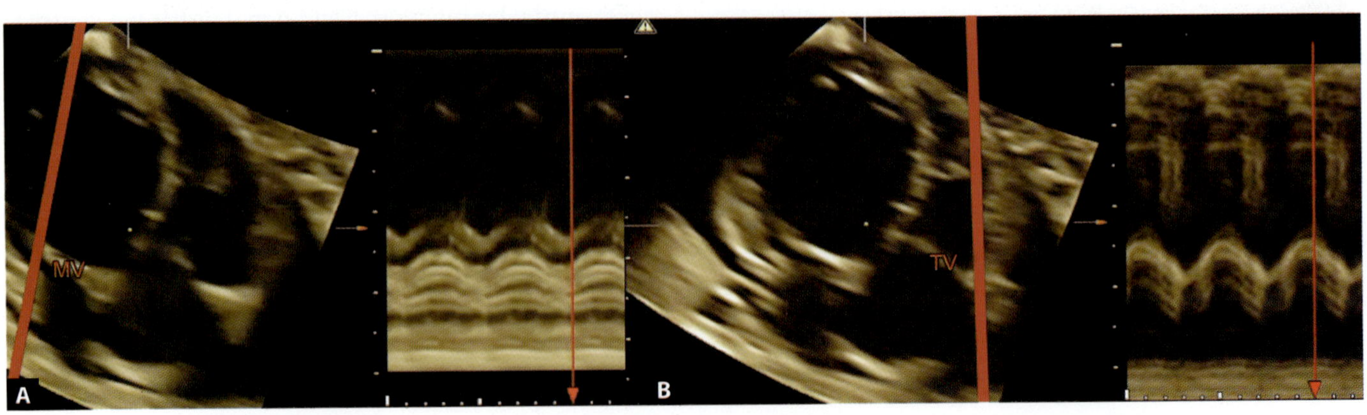

Figs. 37A and B: STIC M-mode technique in a case of critical aortic stenosis. (A) MAPSE; (B) TAPSE.

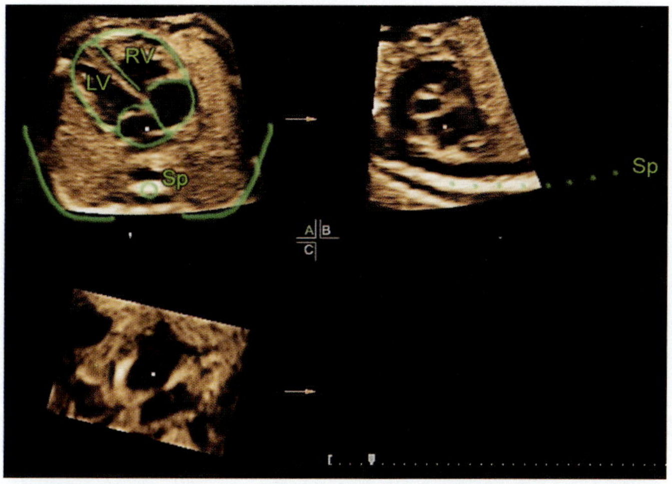

Fig. 38: VCAD modality. Initial stage after simplified orientation according to templates marked with green line (in reference images A and B).

expected views including four-chamber view, left outflow tract, and three-vessel view **(Figs. 40A to D)**.

The newest algorithm is called Fetal Intelligent Navigation Echocardiography (FINE), and is also recognized the under trade name 5D HEART.[13] It is based on geometric landmarks necessary to guide the ultrasound system in identification of 9 cardiac views. After the acquisition, the examiner has to highlight those anatomical points on the screen at particular levels, moving the layers of axial sections through the fetal chest. Those points include: at the level of upper abdominal view: descending aorta, at the level of four chamber view: descending aorta, cardiac crux, interventricular septum and the wall of the right atrium, at the level of three-vessel view: pulmonary valve and superior caval vein, and finally,

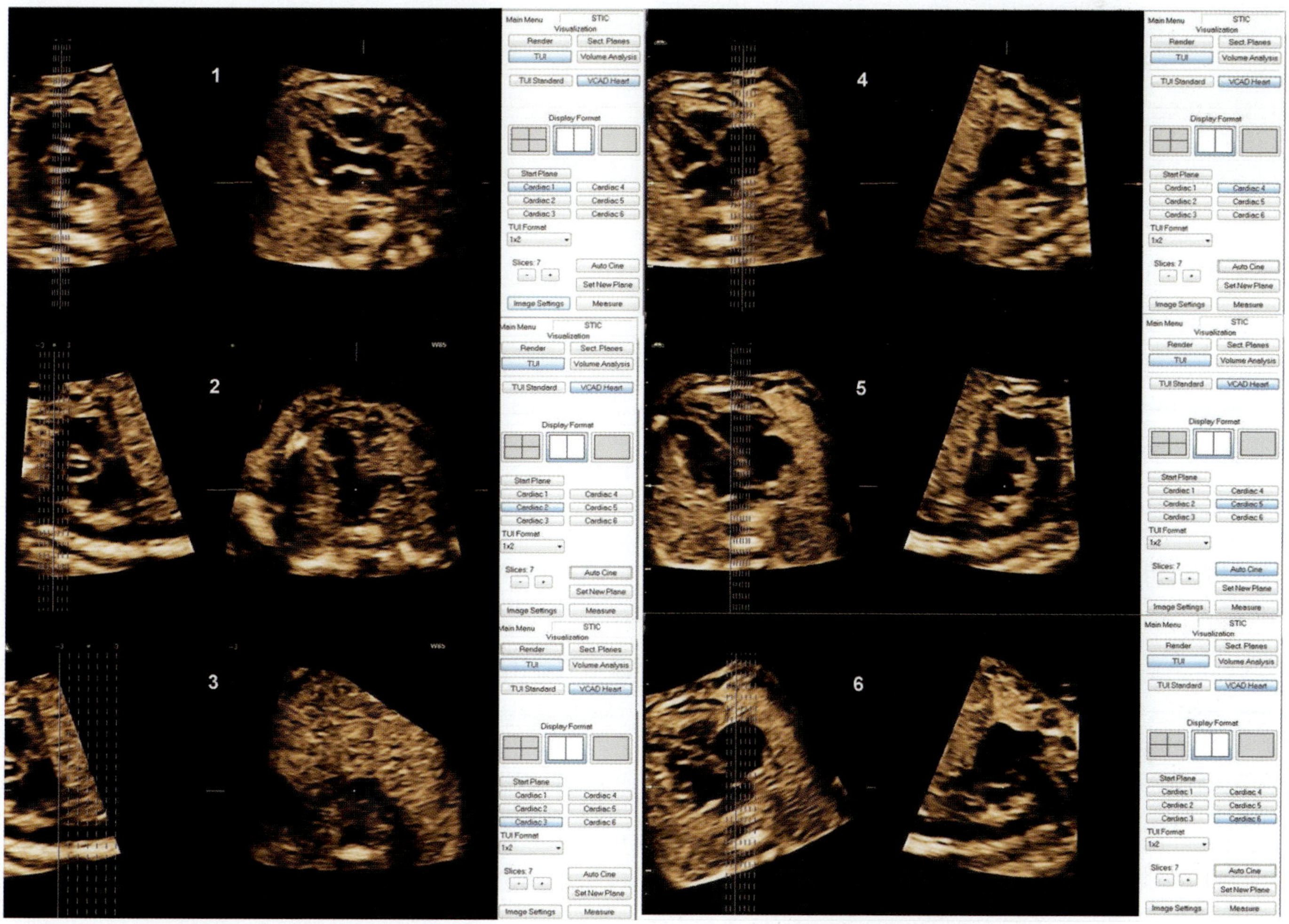

Fig. 39: VCAD modality in the final stage. Automated identification of cardiac views: 1-left outflow tract; 2-right outflow tract; 3-upper abdominal view; 4-long axis caval view; 5-ductal arch; 6-aortic arch.

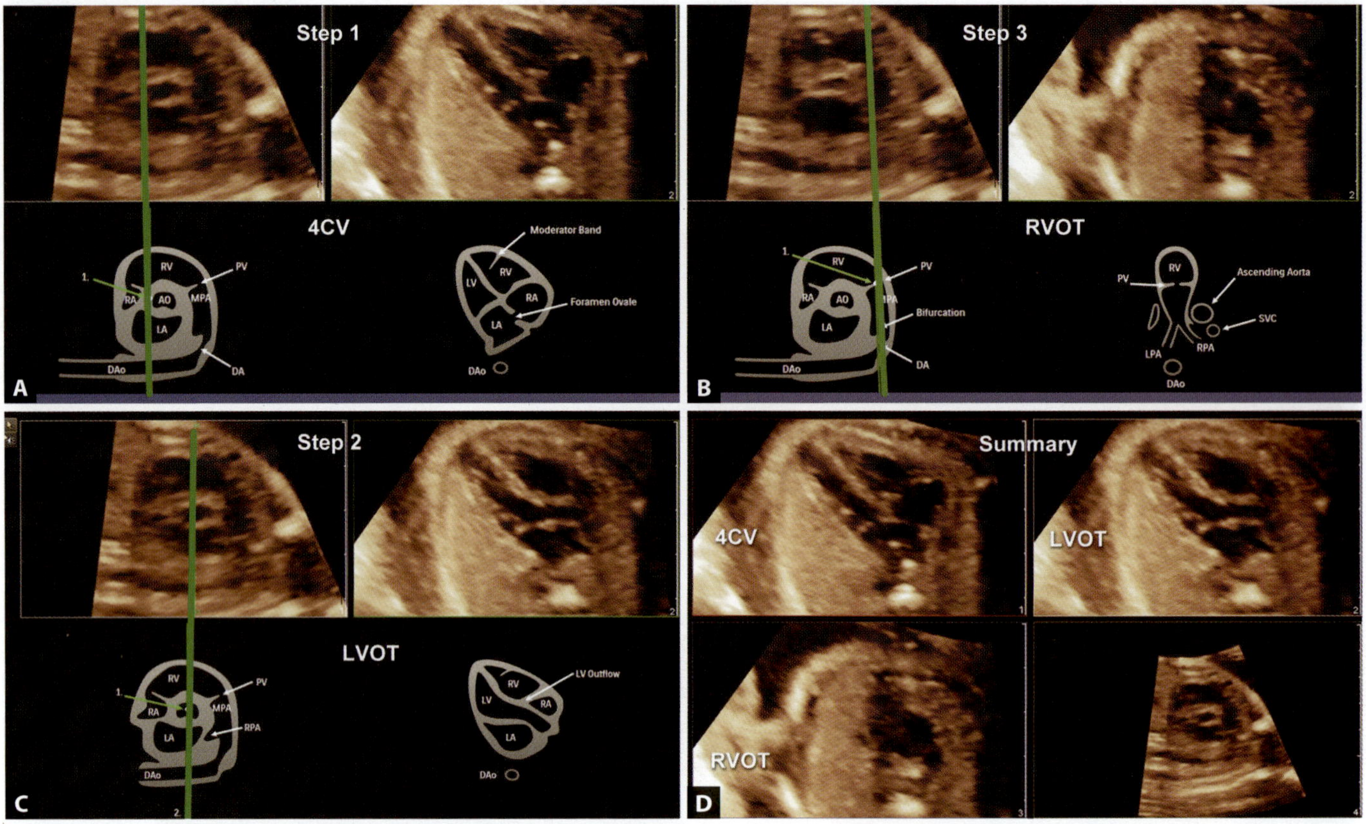

Figs. 40A to D: Fetal heart navigation modality after the arrangement. Identification of cardiac views: Four-chamber view (step 1); left outflow tract (step 2); and right outflow tract view (step 3). After the process is finished all selected cardiac views are summarized (summary).

at the level of transverse aortic arch view: mid-point of the transverse aortic arch **(Fig. 41)**.

After the correct selection, upper abdominal view, four-chamber view, five-chamber view, left outflow tract view, short axis view, three-vessel and trachea view, aortic arch view, ductal arch view and long axis caval view are produced on the screen **(Fig. 42)**.

This method, like the remaining ones, allows analyzing volume datasets, which include information obtained with the use of color mapping.

None of recently introduced methods can identify and align cardiac views correctly in cases of cardiac malformations or mediastinal shift. These algorithms can only provide suspicion of anomaly taking into account that expected cardiac views could not be presented as in a normal fetal heart. In case of congenital heart diseases, the examiner can make a correction manually and assign particular layers of cross-sections to recommended views, e.g., in 5D technique. Nevertheless, it is more difficult and time consuming than a routine 2D sweep, like, for instance, in cases of conotruncal anomalies. It is caused by technical imperfection, which results from basing described algorithms only on the geometry of a normal heart. The geometry of anomalies is unique for most of them, which, in turn, causes technical difficulties in present automated three-dimensional techniques. Therefore, in case of anomalies, 2D evaluation still allows to obtain diagnostic views faster and more efficiently, and as a result, quickly interpret the image.

STIC IN THE FIRST TRIMESTER

The biggest potential obstacle of this method is the first trimester fetal activity that may increase the chance of motion artifacts. Second obstacle is rather suboptimal 2D image resolution for the fetal heart at this stage of gestation. However, first descriptions of the STIC application in the first trimester showed promising results of 71% of success rate in volume acquisitions.[52] It was also presented that first trimester STIC volumes can be applied in teleconsultations.[52] The preferable first trimester STIC viewing

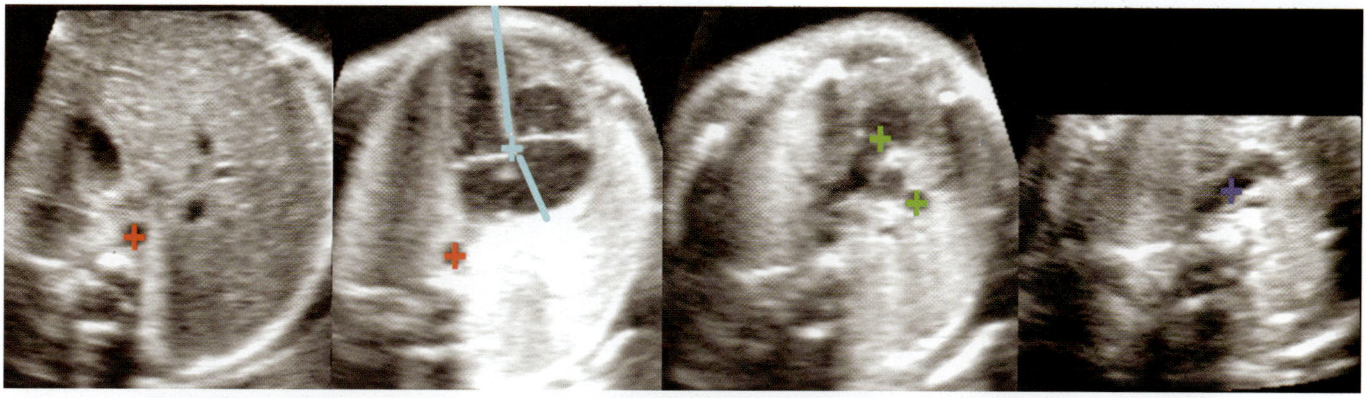

Fig. 41: Fetal intelligent navigation echocardiography (FINE = 5D heart) modality in the early stage. Required anatomical landmarks, which need to be highlighted by the examiner.

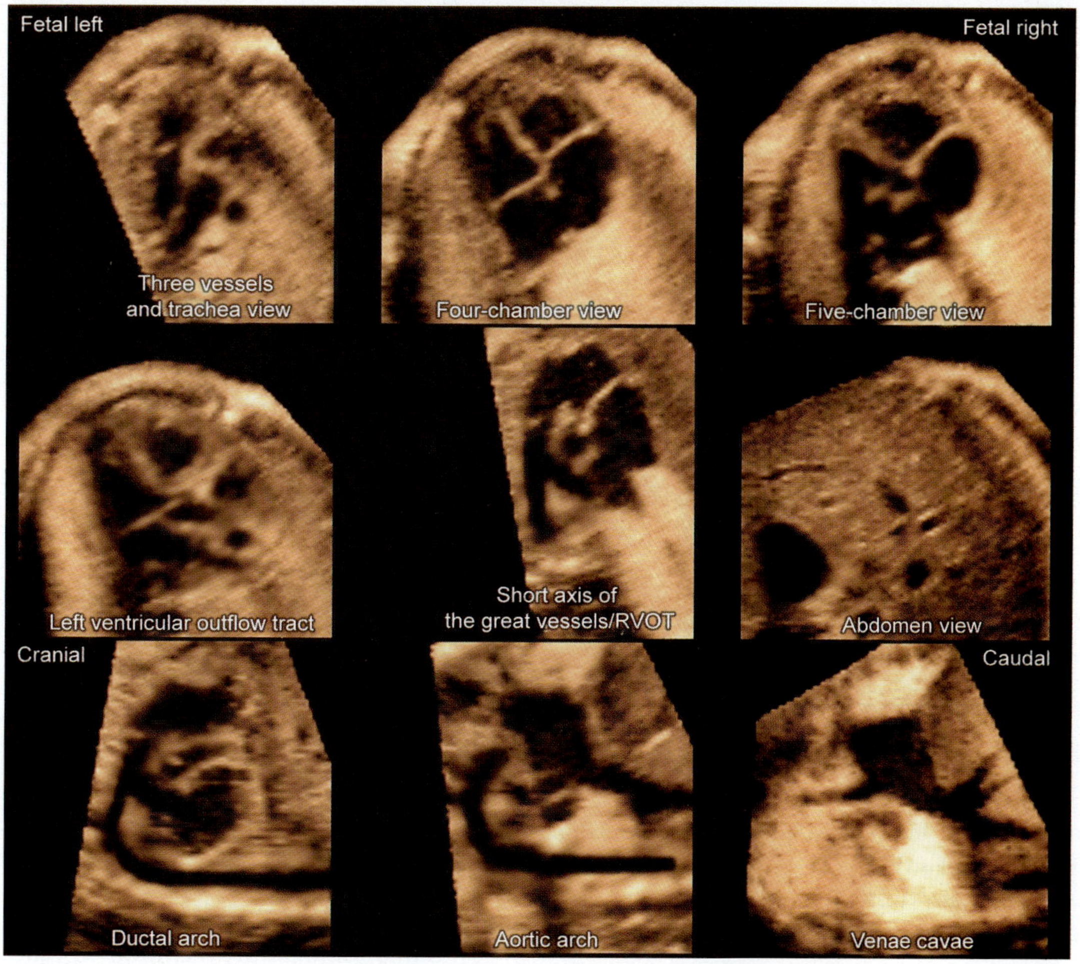

Fig. 42: FINE modality in the final stage. Automated identification of cardiac views.

technique that was raised in literature is ultrasound tomography in color mode **(Fig. 43)**.[53]

But in fact this method shows no more details, which can be presented, in a 2D transversal sweep. This is why 2D remains superior to STIC at 11–14 weeks scan.[54] Optimal imaging of first trimester four-chamber view in STIC 2D pre-acquisition remains crucial for successful volume capture.[55] Other visualization modes are also feasible in

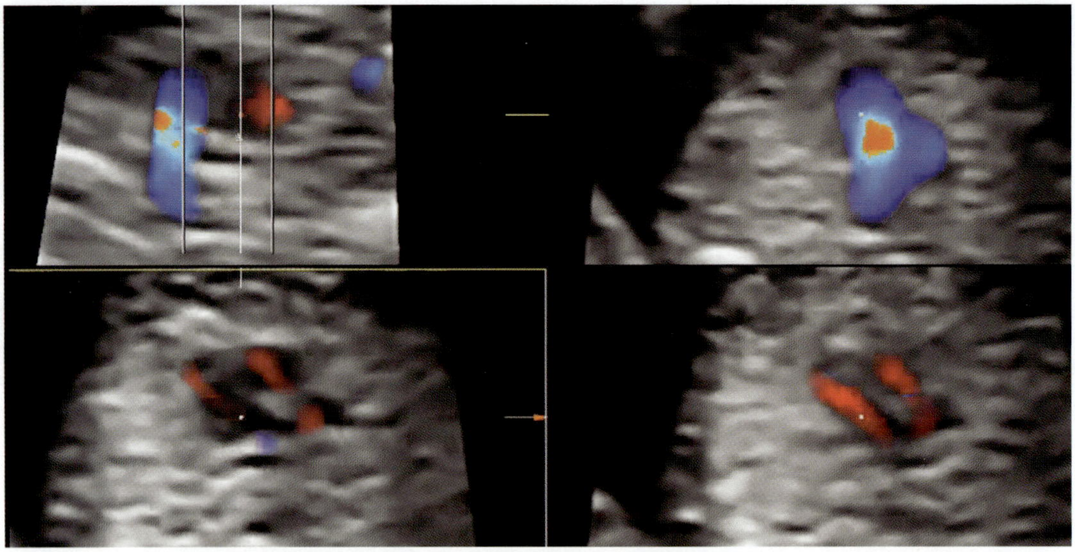

Fig. 43: First trimester STIC ultrasound tomography of a normal heart.

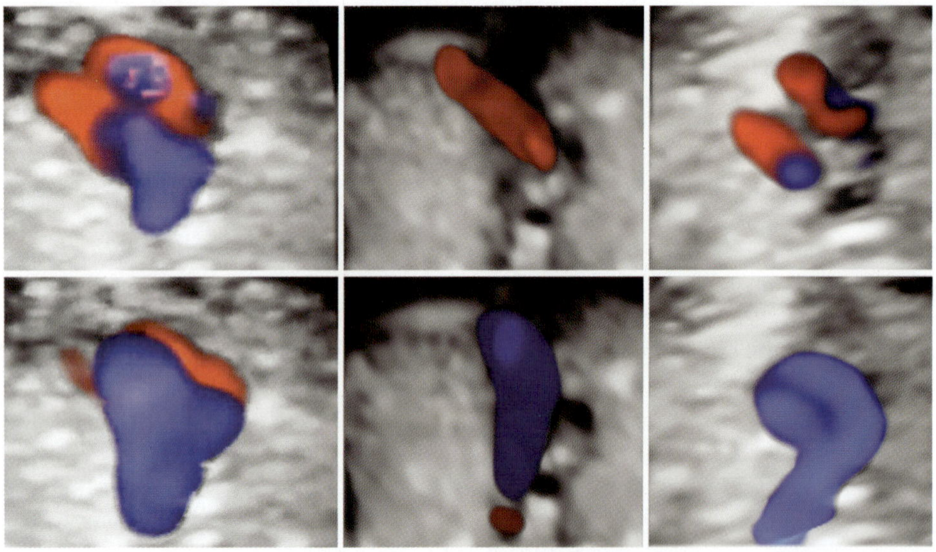

Fig. 44: First trimester STIC color Doppler glass body rendering (four-chamber view-top and three-vessel and trachea view-bottom). Left-normal heart, middle-hypoplastic left heart (HLHS), right- d-transposition of the great arteries (d-TGA).

the first trimester STIC, but they require ideal scanning conditions **(Figs. 44 and 45)**.

In a small-population study the total accuracy of first trimester STIC was 95.3%, with sensitivity, specificity, and positive and negative predictive values of 90.9%, 96.2%, 83.3% and 98.1%. On contrary in this study 2D early fetal echocardiography showed the accuracy of 98.4%, which was better than that of STIC, and presented no false-positive results.[54] In another study also based on a small population accuracy of STIC was 88.7% and of conventional early fetal echocardiography 94.2%.[56]

THREE-DIMENSIONAL PRINTING

The first 3D printouts concerned rare congenital anomalies and were based on views obtained with the use of computed tomography technique.[57] Cardiac surgeons used these printouts in planning of surgery in specific cases. When it comes to the fetal heart, in 2015 the authors of this chapter worked out the first 3D printouts in the world on the basis of STIC volumes **(Figs. 46A to C)**.

According to the authors, they could be significant in education of obstetric and gynecological physicians and

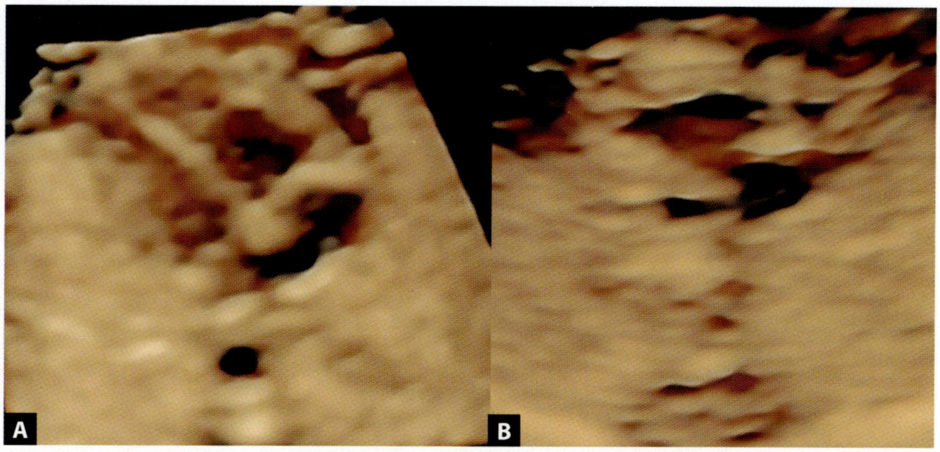

Figs. 45A and B: First trimester STIC surface rendering of the four-chamber view. (A) Normal heart; (B) Hypoplastic left heart.

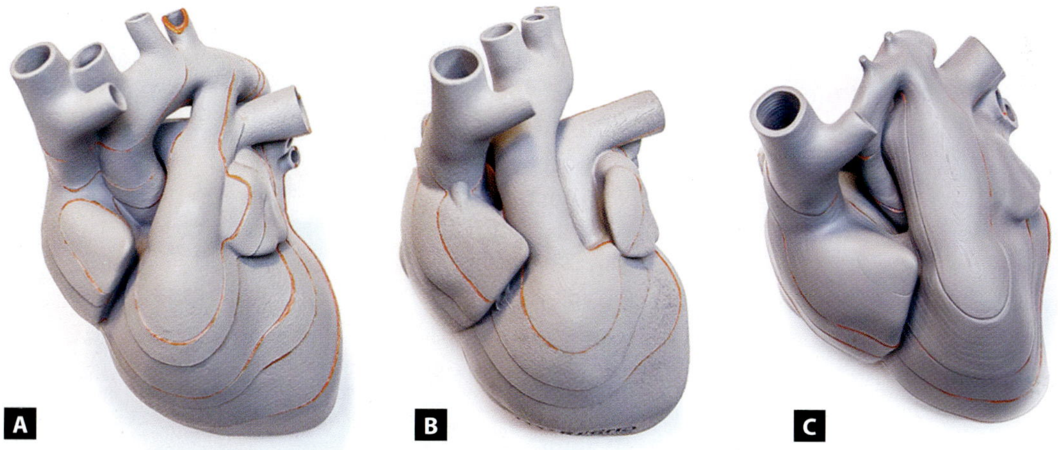

Figs. 46A to C: Fetal heart 3D models as a result of 3D-printing. Left-normal heart, middle- d-transposition of the great arteries (d-TGA), right- hypoplastic left heart (HLHS). Note the very different geometry between cardiac structures in the normal heart and in anomalies.

sonographers learning fetal heart screening and fetal echocardiography. Additionally, 3D printouts of a fetal heart will be used while consulting parents, whose child was prenatally diagnosed with a heart disease.

CONCLUSION

Three-dimensional techniques have had a considerable significance in the development of fetal echocardiography in the recent years.[20] One of the main reasons of this situation was the fact that owing to those methods, advanced fetal heart examination is now open for non-cardiologists. Until the era of 3D ultrasound, only pediatric cardiologists were familiar with geometry of particular congenital heart diseases and their typical patterns, mainly on the basis of cardiac catheterization imaging. This method is not available for the sake of obstetric and gynecological physicians and sonographers' education. However, introducing three-dimensional ultrasound allowed them to understand anatomical differences between a normal fetal heart and particular congenital heart diseases **(Figs. 47A and B)**.

According to the authors, it is the greatest benefit of applying advanced ultrasound imaging techniques in fetal evaluation. However, the routine application of volume fetal echocardiography remains challenging due to the character of fetal ultrasound, which is strongly dependent on the scanning conditions. As an example successful STIC acquisition can be obtained

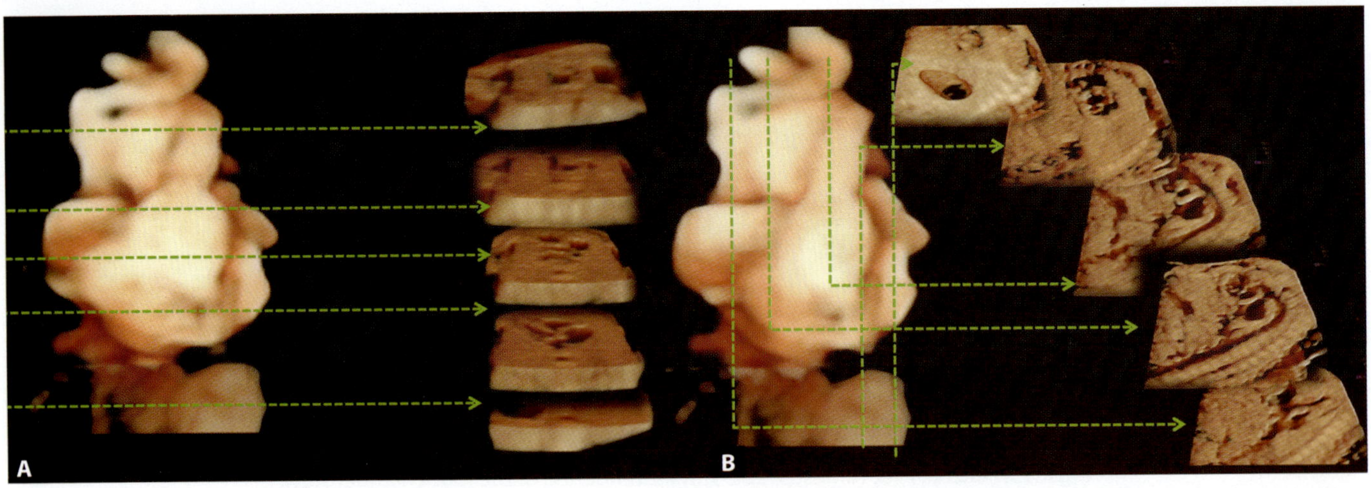

Figs. 47A and B: Better understanding through 3D ultrasound of fetal heart anatomy. From one dataset numerous cross-sections are available [in transversal plane (A) and in sagittal plane (B)].

in approximately 75% of cases. Total time duration dedicated to volume acquisitions of the fetal heart vary between 0.9 to 6 minutes and the interpretation time is significantly longer than the time required for 2D fetal echocardiography.[58] It is also important that the clinical effectiveness of 2D measurements performed in volume datasets showed marginal clinical effectiveness mainly as a result of unsatisfactory STIC acquisitions.[58] On the other hand sonologists with low-to-intermediate expertise in fetal anomaly ultrasound demonstrated reasonably high sensitivity, specificity, positive and negative predictive values at the level of 83%, 87%, 80% and 89%, respectively for outflow tract anomalies in STIC fetal echocardiography.[59] Overall added value of 3D/4D fetal echocardiography was estimated for 6%.[60] As an example it refers to the anomalies of aortic arch and pulmonary veins. In these areas an accurate prenatal 3D imaging shows details to a degree that is conventionally obtainable only by postpartum imaging.[61-63] Also in major anomalies like in atrioventricular septal defect, 3D techniques thanks to the better perception of depth contribute in detailed evaluation of the valvular apparatus.[64] Better spatial understanding translates into the improvement of 2D fetal heart scanning technique in the aspect of obtaining correct symmetric views and the knowledge of layered heart anatomy in every plane. Another example could be the improvement of scanning technique in order to visualize left ventricular outflow tract view, aortic arch view and ductal arch view noted in examiners after training in three-dimensional techniques. Comprehension of the geometry of a heart with a congenital disease gives a chance to make a correct diagnosis on the basis of pattern recognition, what shortens the diagnostic time **(Fig. 48)**.

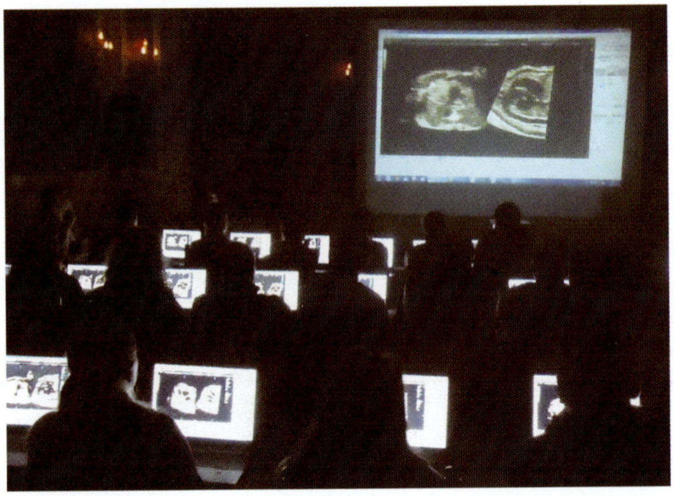

Fig. 48: Teaching session with the use of laptop stations with installed STIC volume dataset review software. A case of d-transposition is discussed—MWU postgraduate School of Ultrasound in Poland.

Some authors believed that 3D ultrasound may reduce operator's dependency in fetal echocardiography.[65] But in fact its application reduced this factor more in 2D than in 3D evaluation by better understanding of fetal heart anatomy. Three-dimensional ultrasound techniques also allow fetal heart models 3D printing, which make the comprehension of the geometry of heart with particular anomalies even easier. Not without significance is also a greater care for image optimization, which examiners gain during three-dimensional ultrasound training. They start realizing the stronger influence of artifacts and shadowing on the quality of 3D and 2D ultrasound images. In order to avoid artifacts, the examiners more carefully utilize larger spectrum of filters correcting the image quality, such as, e.g., compounding, while using 3D as well as 2D. Three-dimensional techniques created new opportunities, not only in tele consulting but also in self-education. They enable the examiner to browse spatial views of fetal heart without the patient's presence with the use of computer 3D volume review software.[65] Owing to this method, tele-consultants or physicians taking part in training are able to analyze saved images without additional stress resulting from the patient's presence. The consultation may take place on the following day after the scan and thorough off-line examination of the volume datasets.

ACKNOWLEDGMENTS

The authors would like to acknowledge Jill Beithon from USA for her valuable input in our manuscripts.

REFERENCES

1. Chaoui R, Heling KS. New developments in fetal heart scanning: Three- and four-dimensional fetal echocardiography. Semin Fetal Neonatal Med. 2005;10: 567-77.
2. Yagel S, Cohen SM, Shapiro I, Valsky DV. 3D and 4D ultrasound in fetal cardiac scanning: a new look at the fetal heart. Ultrasound Obstet Gynecol. 2007;29:81-95.
3. Paladini D. Standardization of on-screen fetal heart orientation prior to storage of spatiotemporal image correlation (STIC) volume datasets. Ultrasound Obstet Gynecol. 2007;29:605-11.
4. Goncalves LF, Lee W, Espinoza J, Romero R. Examination of the fetal heart by four-dimensional (4D) ultrasound with spatio-temporal image correlation (STIC). Ultrasound Obstet Gynecol. 2006;27:336-48.
5. Espinoza J. Contemporary clinical applications of spatio-temporal image correlation in prenatal diagnosis. Current Opinion in Obstetrics and Gynecology. 2011;23:94-102.
6. Espinoza J, Lee W, Comstock C, Romero R, Lami Yeo L, Rizzo G, et al. Collaborative study on 4-dimensional echocardiography for the diagnosis of fetal heart defects. J Ultrasound Med. 2010;29:1573-80.
7. Rizzo G, Capponi A, Pietrolucci ME, Capece G, Cimmino E, Colosi E, et al. Satisfactory Rate of Postprocessing Visualization of Standard Fetal Cardiac Views From 4-Dimensional Cardiac Volumes Acquired During Routine Ultrasound Practice by Experienced Sonographers in Peripheral Centers. J Ultrasound Med. 2011;30:93-9.
8. Xiong Y, Liu T, Wu Y, Xu JF, Ting YH, Leung TY, et al. Comparison of real-time three-dimensional echocardiography and spatiotemporal image correlation in assessment of fetal interventricular septum. The Journal of Maternal-Fetal and Neonatal Medicine. 2012;25:2333-8.
9. Yuan Y, Leung KY, Ouyang YS, Yang F, Tang MHY, Chau AKT, et al. Simultaneous real-time imaging of four-chamber and left ventricular outflow tract views using xPlane imaging capability of a matrix array probe. Ultrasound Obstet Gynecol. 2011;37:302-9.
10. http://www.3dheart.eu
11. Uittenbogaard LB, Haak MC, Spreeuwenberg MD, Van Vugt JMG. A systematic analysis of the feasibility of four-dimensional ultrasound imaging using spatiotemporal image correlation in routine fetal echocardiography. Ultrasound Obstet Gynecol. 2008;31:625-32.
12. Haak MC, Uittenbogaard LB, van Vugt JMG. Spatiotemporal Image Correlation Artifacts in an In Vitro Model. J Ultrasound Med. 2011;30:1411-4.
13. Yeo L, Romero R. Fetal Intelligent Navigation Echocardiography (FINE): a novel method for rapid, simple, and automatic examination of the fetal heart. Ultrasound Obstet Gynecol. 2013;42:268-84.
14. Cohen L, Mangers K, Grobman WA, Gotteiner N, Julien S, Dungan J, et al. Three-Dimensional Fast Acquisition With Sonographically Based Volume Computer-Aided Analysis for Imaging of the Fetal Heart at 18 to 22 Weeks of Gestation. J Ultrasound Med. 2010;29:751-7.
15. Rizzo G, Capponi A, Cavicchioni O, Vendola M, Pietrolucci ME, Arduini D. Application of Automated Sonography on 4-Dimensional Volumes of Fetuses with Transposition of the Great Arteries. J Ultrasound Med. 2008;27:771-6.
16. DeVore GR, Falkensammer P, Sklansky MS, Platt LD. Spatiotemporal image correlation (STIC): new technology for evaluation of the fetal heart. Ultrasound Obstet Gynecol. 2003;22:380-7.
17. Bega G, Kuhlman K, Lev-Toaff A, Kurtz A, Wapner R. Application of Three-dimensional Ultrasonography in the Evaluation of the Fetal Heart. J Ultrasound Med. 2001;20:307-3.
18. Goncalves LF, Lee W, Chaiworapongsa T, Espinoza J, Shoen ML, Falkensammer P, et al. Four-dimensional ultrasonography of the fetal heart with spatiotemporal image correlation. Am J Obstet Gynecol. 2003;189:1792-802.
19. Espinoza J, Romero R, Kusanovic JP, Gotsch F, Lee W, Goncalves LF, et al. Standardized views of the fetal heart using four-dimensional sonograhic and tomographic imaging. Ultrasound Obstet Gynecol. 2008;31:253-42.
20. Paladini D. Standarization of on-screen fetal heart orientation prior to storage of spatio-temporal image correlation (STIC) volume datasets. Ultrasound Obstet Gynecol. 2007;29:605-11.
21. Abuhamad A. Automated Multiplanar Imaging. J Ultrasound Med. 2004;23:573-6.
22. Vinals F, Poblete P, Giuliano A. Spatiotemporal image correlation (STIC): a new tool for the prenatal screening of congenital heart defects. Ultrasound Obstet Gynecol. 2003;22:388-94.

23. Gonçalves LF, Nien JK, Espinoza J, Kusanovic JP, Lee W, Swope B, et al. What Does 2-Dimensional Imaging Add to 3- and 4-Dimensional Obstetric Ultrasonography? J Ultrasound Med. 2006;25:691-9.
24. Goncalves LF, Espinoza J, Romero R, Lee W, Treadwell M, Huang R, et al. Four-dimensional fetal echocardiography with spatiotemporal image correlation (STIC): A systematic study of standard cardiac views assessed by different observers. J Maternal-Fetal Neonatal Med. 2005;17:323-31.
25. DeVore GR, Polanco B, Sklansky MS, Plat LD. The 'spin' technique: a new method for examination of the fetal outflowtracts using three-dimensional ultrasound. Ultrasound Obstet Gynecol. 2004;24:72-82.
26. Paladini D, Vassallo M, Sglavo G, Lapadula C, Martinelli P. The role of spatiotemporal image correlation (STIC) with tomographic ultrasound imaging (TUI) in the sequential analysis of fetal congenital heart disease. Ultrasound Obstet Gynecol. 2006;27:555-61.
27. Rizzo G, Capponi A, Vendola M, Pietrolucci ME, Arduini D. Role of Tomographic Ultrasound Imaging with Spatio-temporal Image Correlation for Identifying Fetal Ventricular Septal Defects. Ultrasound Med. 2008;27:1071-5.
28. Goncalves LF, Espinoza J, Romero R, Kusanovic JP, Swope B, Nien JK, et al. Four-Dimensional Ultrasonography of the Fetal Heart using a Novel Tomographic Ultrasound Imaging Display. J Perinat Med. 2006;34:39-55.
29. Yeo L, Romero R, Jodicke C, Ogge G, Lee W, Kusanovic JP, et al. Four-chamber view and 'swing technique' (FAST) echo: a novel and simple algorithm to visualize standard fetal echocardiographic planes. Ultrasound Obstet Gynecol. 2011;37:423-31.
30. Yeo L, Romero R, Jodicke C, Kim SK, Gonzales JM, Ogge G, et al. Simple targeted arterial rendering (STAR) technique: a novel and simple method to visualize the fetal cardiac outflow tracts. Ultrasound Obstet Gynecol. 2011;37:549-56.
31. Yagel S, Benachi A, Bonnet D, Dumez Y, Hochner-Celiniker D, et al. Rendering in fetal cardiac scanning: the intracardiac septa and the coronal atrioventricular valve planes. Ultrasound Obstet Gynecol. 2006;28:266-74.
32. Vinals F, Pacheto V, Giuliano A. Fetal atrioventricular valve junction in normal fetuses and in fetuses with complete atrioventricular septal defect assessed by 4D volume rendering. Ultrasound Obstet Gynecol. 2006;28:26-31.
33. Goncalves LF, Espinoza J, Lee W, Mazor M, Romero R. Three- and four-dimensional reconstruction of the aortic and ductal arches using inversion mode: a new rendering algorithm for visualization of fluid-filled anatomical structures. Ultrasound Obstet Gynecol. 2004;24:696.
34. Espinoza J, Goncalves LF, Lee W, Chaiworapongsa T, Treadwell M, Stites S, et al. The Use of the Minimum Projection Mode in 4-Dimensional Examination of the Fetal Heart with Spatiotemporal Image Correlation. J Ultrasound Med. 2004;23:1337-48.
35. Qin Y, Zhang Y, Zhou X, Wang Y, Sun W, Chen L, et al. Four-Dimensional Echocardiography with Spatiotemporal Image Correlation and Inversion Mode for detection of Congenital Heart Disease. Ultrasound in Med Biol. 2014;40:1434-41.
36. Gonçalves LF, Espinoza J, Lee W, Nien JK, Hong JS, Santolaya-Forgas J, et al. A new approach to fetal echocardiography digital casts of the fetal cardiac chambers and great vessels for detection of congenital heart disease. J Ultrasound Med. 2005;24:415-24.
37. Chaoui R, Hoffmann J, Heling KS. Three-dimensional (3D) and (4D color Doppler fetal echocardiography using spatio-temporal image correlation (STIC). Ultrasound Obstet Gynecol. 2004;23:535-45.
38. Goncalves LF, Romero R, Espinoza J, Lee W, Treadwell M, Chintala K, et al. Four-Dimensional Ultrasonography of the Fetal Heart Using Color Doppler Spatiotemporal Image Correlation. J Ultrasound Med. 2004;23:473-81.
39. Volpe P, Campobasso G, Stanziano A, De Robertis V, Di Paolo S, Caruso G, et al. Novel application of 4D sonography with B-flow imaging and spatio-temporal image correlation (STIC) in the assessment of the anatomy of pulmonary arteries in fetuses with pulmonary atresia and ventricular septal defect. Ultrasound Obstet Gynecol. 2006;28:40-6.
40. DeVore GR. The use of Z-scores in the analysis of fetal cardiac dimensions. Ultrasound Obstet Gynecol. 2005;26:596-8.
41. Messing B, Cohen SM, Valsky DV, Rosenak D, Hochner-Celnikier D, Savchev S, et al. Fetal cardiac ventricle volumetry in the second half of gestation assessed by 4D ultrasound using STIC combined with inversion mode. Ultrasound Obstet Gynecol. 2007;30:142-51.
42. Tutschek B, Sahn DJ. Semi-automatic segmentation of fetal cardiac cavities: progress towards an automated fetal echocardiogram. Ultrasound Obstet Gynecol. 2008;32:176-80.
43. Uittenbogaard LB, Haak MC, Peters RJH, Van Couwelaar GM, Vanvugt JMG. Validation of volume measurements for fetal echocardiography using four-dimensional ultrasound imaging and spatiotemporal image correlation. Ultrasound Obstet Gynecol. 2010;35:324-31.
44. Hamill N, Romero R, Hassan SS, Lee W, Myers SA, Mittal P, et al. Repeatability and reproducibility of fetal cardiac ventricular volume calculations using spatiotemporal image correlation and virtual organ computer-aided analysis. J Ultrasound Med. 2009;28:1301-11.
45. Rizzo G, Capponi A, Pietrolucci ME, Arduini D. Role of sonographic automatic volume calculation in measuring fetal cardiac ventricular volumes using 4-dimensional sonography. J Ultrasound Med. 2010;29:261-70.
46. Simioni C, Marcondes Machado Nardozza L, Araujo Junior E, Rolo LC, Zamith M, et al. Heart stroke volume, cardiac output, and ejection fraction in 265 normal fetus in the second half of gestation assessed by 4D ultrasound using spatio-temporal image correlation. The Journal of Maternal-Fetal and Neonatal Medicine. 2011;24:1159-67.
47. Uittenbogaard LB, Haak MC, Spreeuwenberg MD, Van Vugt JMG. Fetal cardiac function assessed with four-dimensional ultrasound imaging using spatiotemporal image correlation. Ultrasound Obstet Gynecol. 2009;33:272-81.

48. Rizzo G, Capponi A, Cavicchioni O , Vendola M, Arduini D. Fetal cardiac stroke volume determination by four-dimensional ultrasound with spatio-temporal image correlation compared with two-dimensional and Doppler ultrasonography. Prenat Diagn. 2007;27:1147-50.
49. Hamill N, Yeo L, Romero R, et al. Fetal cardiac ventricular volume, cardiac output, and ejection fraction determined with 4-dimensional ultrasound using spatiotemporal image correlation and virtual organ computer-aided analysis. Am J Obstet Gynecol. 2011;204:76.e1-10.
50. Paladini D, Sglavo G, Masucci A, Pastore G, Nappi C. Role of four-dimensional ultrasound (spatiotemporal image correlation and Sonography-based Automated Volume Count) in prenatal assessment of atrial morphology in cardiosplenic syndromes. Ultrasound Obstet Gynecol. 2011;38:337-43.
51. Messing B, Gilboa Y, Lipschuetz M, Valsky DV, Cohen SM, Yagel S. Fetal tricuspid annular plane systolic excursion (f-TAPSE): evaluation of fetal right heart systolic function with conventional M-mode ultrasound and spatiotemporal image correlation (STIC) M-mode. Ultrasound Obstet Gynecol. 2013;42:182-8.
52. Vinals F, Ascenzo R, Naveas R, Huggon I, Giuliano A. Fetal echocardiography at 11 + 0 to 13 + 6 weeks using four-dimensional spatiotemporal image correlation telemedicine via an Internet link: a pilot study. Ultrasound Obstet Gynecol. 2008;31:633-8.
53. Turan S, Turan OM, Ty-Torredes K, Harman CR, Baschat AA. Standardization of the first-trimester fetal cardiac examination using spatiotemporal image correlation with tomographic ultrasound and color Doppler imaging. Ultrasound Obstet Gynecol. 2009;33:652-6.
54. Bennasar M, Martinez JM, Olivella A, Del Rio M, Gomez O, Figueras F, et al. Feasibility and accuracy of fetal echocardiography using four-dimensional spatiotemporal image correlation technology before 16 weeks of gestation. Ultrasound Obstet Gynecol. 2009;33:645-51.
55. Tudorache S, Cara M, Iliescu DG, Novac, L Cernea N. First trimester two- and four-dimensional cardiac scan: intra- and interobserver agreement, comparison between methods and benefits of color Doppler technique. Ultrasound Obstet Gynecol. 2013;42:659-68.
56. Turan S, Turan OM, Desai A, Harman CR, Baschat AA. First-trimester fetal cardiac examination using spatiotemporal image correlation, tomographic ultrasound and color Doppler imaging for the diagnosis of complex congenital heart disease in high-risk patients. Ultrasound Obstet Gynecol. 2014;44:562-7.
57. http://edition.cnn.com/2015/10/06/health/3d-printed-heart-simulated-organs/
58. Wanitpongpan P, Kanagawa T, Kinugasa Y, Kimura T. Spatiotemporal image correlation (STIC) used by general obstetricians is marginally clinically effective compared to 2D fetal echocardiography scanning by experts. Prenat Diagn. 2008;28:923-8.
59. Paladini D, Sglavo G, Greco E, Nappi C. Cardiac screening by STIC:can sonologists performing the 20-week anomaly scan pick up outflow tract abnormalities by scrolling the A-plane of STIC volumes? Ultrasound Obstet Gynecol. 2008;32: 865-70.
60. Yagel S, Cohen SM, Rosenak D, Messing B, Lipschuetz M, Shen O, et al. Added value of three-/four-dimensional ultrasound in offline analysis and diagnosis of congenital heart disease. Ultrasound Obstet Gynecol. 2011;37: 432-7.
61. Turan S, Turan OM, Maisel P, Gaskin P, Harman CR, Baschat AA. Three-Dimensional Sonography in the Prenatal Diagnosis of Aortic Arch Abnormalities. J Clin Ultrasound. 2009;37:253-7.
62. Volpe P, Tuo G, De Robertis V, Campobasso G, Marasini M, Tempesta A, et al. Fetal interrupted aortic arch: 2D-4D echocardiography, associations and outcome. Ultrasound Obstet Gynecol. 2010;35:302-9.
63. Zhang Y, Ding C, Fan M, Ren W, Guo Y, Sun W, et al. Evaluation of normal fetal pulmonary veins using B-flow imaging with spatiotemporal image correlation and by traditional color Doppler echocardiography. Prenatal Diagnosis. 2012;32:1186-91.
64. Adriaanse BMA, Bartelings MM, Van Vugt JMG, Chaoui R, Gittenberger-De Groot AC, Haak MC. Differential and linear insertion of atrioventricular valves: a useful tool? Ultrasound Obstet Gynecol. 2014;44:568-74.
65. Rizzo G, Capponi A, Muscatello A, Cavicchioni O, Vendola M, Arduini D. Examination of the Fetal Heart by Four-Dimensional Ultrasound with Spatiotemporal Image Correlation during Routine Second-Trimester Examination: The 'Three-Steps Technique'. Fetal Diagn Ther. 2008;24:126-31.

CHAPTER 23

Malformations of the Gastrointestinal System

Vincenzo D'Addario, Grazia Volpe

INTRODUCTION

The ultrasonic appearance of the fetal gastrointestinal system changes according to the different gestational ages and, as regards the gut, to the physiologic peristalsis secondary to fetal swallowing of amniotic fluid. A correct ultrasonic examination of the fetal gastrointestinal tract in the second and third trimesters includes the visualization of the following different segments:

- *Lips and tongue:* The lips are best seen in a coronal view of the face **(Fig. 1A)**; the tongue and the hypopharynx in an axial view of the mouth **(Fig. 1B)**.
- *Esophagus:* In sagittal section of the chest, it appears as a linear echogenic structure made by two parallel lines anterior to the spine **(Fig. 2)**; in apical four chamber view, axial section, this structure however cannot be seen routinely.
- *Diaphragm* **(Fig. 3)**: It appears in the parasagittal section on the thorax and abdomen as a thin anechoic line dividing the lung from the liver.
- *Stomach:* It is best seen in the left side of the upper axial plane of the abdomen, anterior to the spleen **(Fig. 4)**. Its volume changes according to the swallowing of amniotic fluid **(Fig. 5)**.

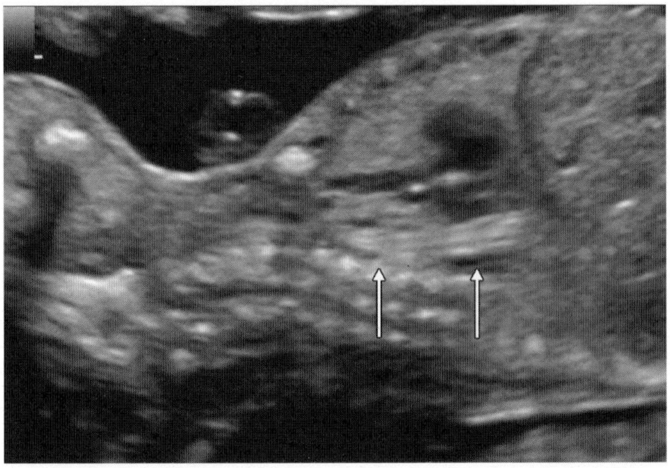

Fig. 2: Sagittal view of the thorax showing the esophagus as a linear echogenic structure anterior to the spine (arrow).

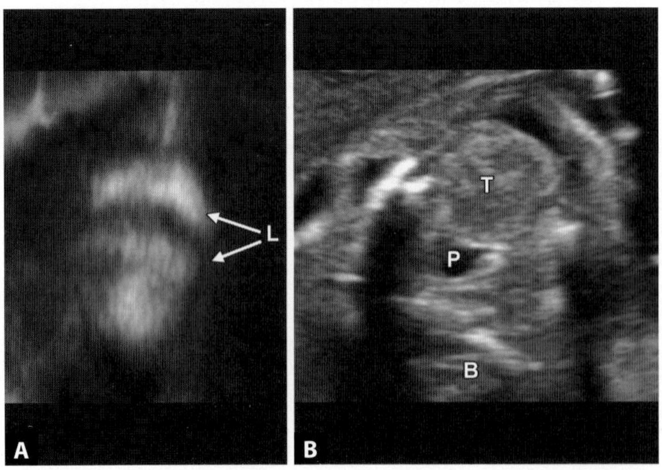

Figs. 1A and B: Coronal view on the lips; (A) Axial view on the mouth; (B) showing the tongue (T) and the hypopharynx (arrows).

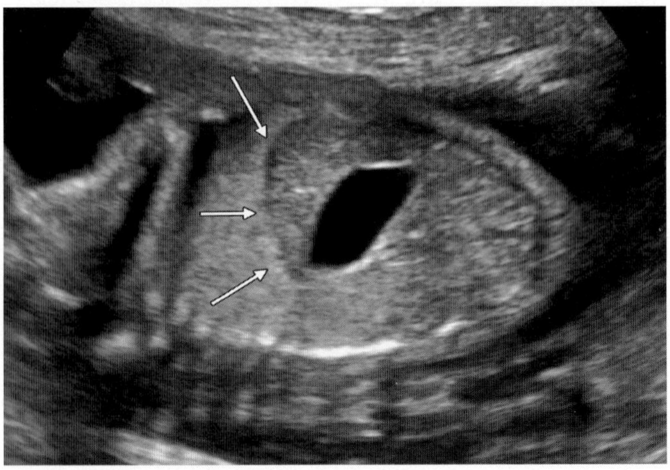

Fig. 3: Parasagittal scan on the fetal chest and abdomen showing the diaphragm (arrows) between the lung and the liver.

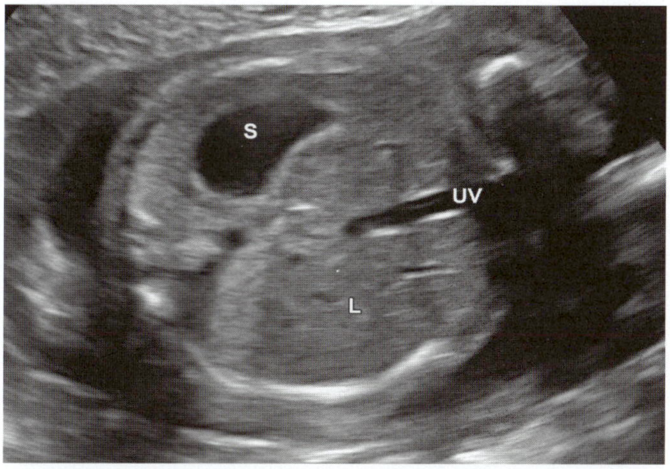

Fig. 4: Axial view of the upper abdomen showing the stomach (S) located on the left side anterior to the spleen, the right lobe of the liver (L), and the intrahepatic portion of the umbilical vein (UV).

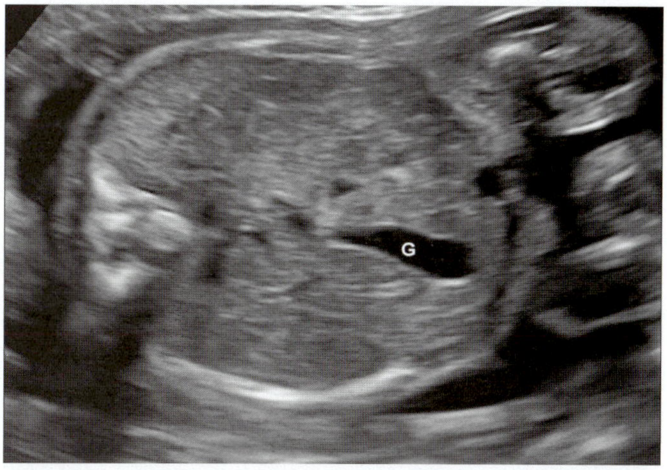

Fig. 6: The gallbladder appears in the right upper axial plane of the abdomen as a pear-shaped anechoic structure below the right hepatic lobe.

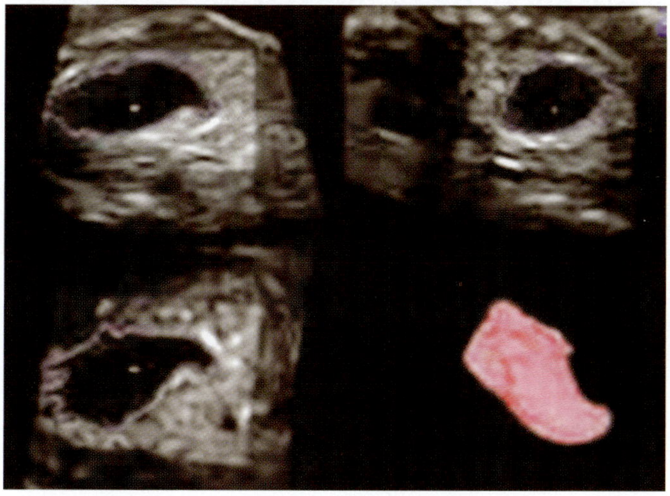

Fig. 5: Stomach volume calculation by 3D US.

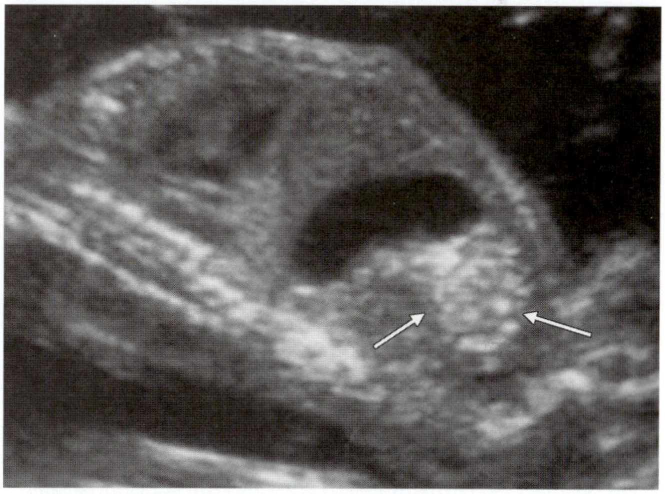

Fig. 7: The echogenic bowel is seen below the stomach.

- *Liver:* In the same upper axial plane of the abdomen, the right lobe of the liver with the intrahepatic portion of the umbilical vein can be visualized **(Fig. 4)**.
- *Gallbladder:* When filled, it appears in the right upper axial plane of the abdomen as a pear-shaped anechoic structure below the right hepatic lobe **(Fig. 6)**.
- *Small bowel (ileum and jejunum):* It appears in the lower axial or in the sagittal scan of the abdomen as an echogenic structure with irregular borders **(Fig. 7)**. Its sonographic appearance changes with the frequency of the ultrasonic beam: high frequencies (6–7 MHz) and the use of second harmonic produce an increased echogenicity.
- *Colon:* It is best seen in the third trimester when it is partially filled by meconium, both in lower axial and in the sagittal planes of the abdomen.
- *Rectum:* It is best seen in the lowest axial scan of the abdomen as an hypoechoic cystic structure posterior to the bladder **(Fig. 8)**.
- *Abdominal wall and the insertion of the umbilical cord:* These are best seen in the midsagittal section of the abdomen **(Fig. 9)**.

The systematic evaluation of the above mentioned structures allows the recognition of several congenital anomalies of the gastrointestinal system. The reported sensitivity of ultrasound in detecting gastrointestinal

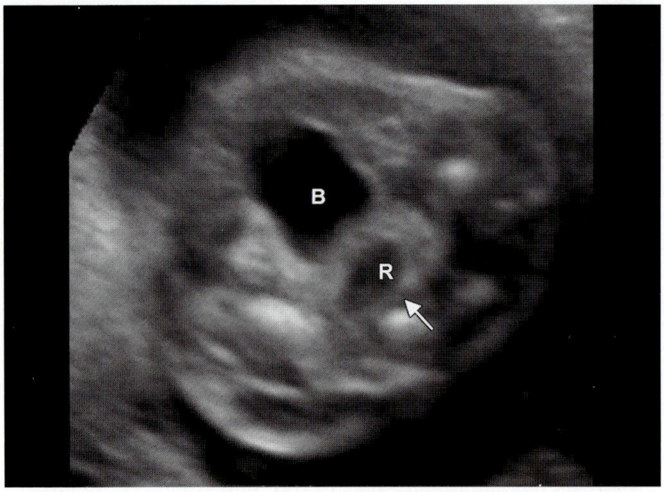

Fig. 8: The rectum appears as a hypoechoic cystic structure (arrow) posterior to the bladder.

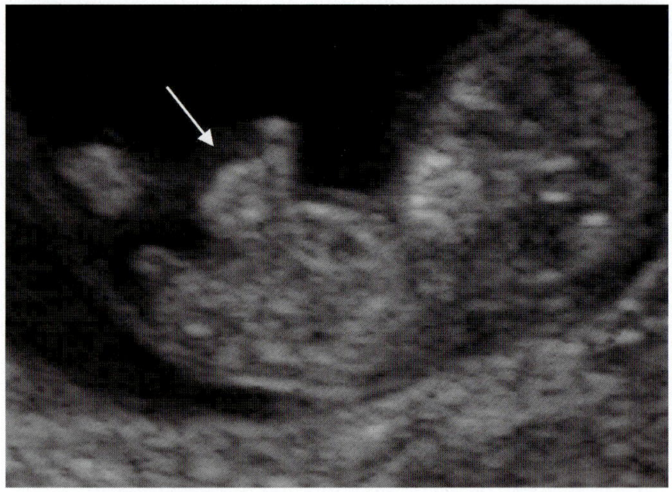

Fig. 10: Physiological herniation of the midgut at 10 weeks of gestation (arrow).

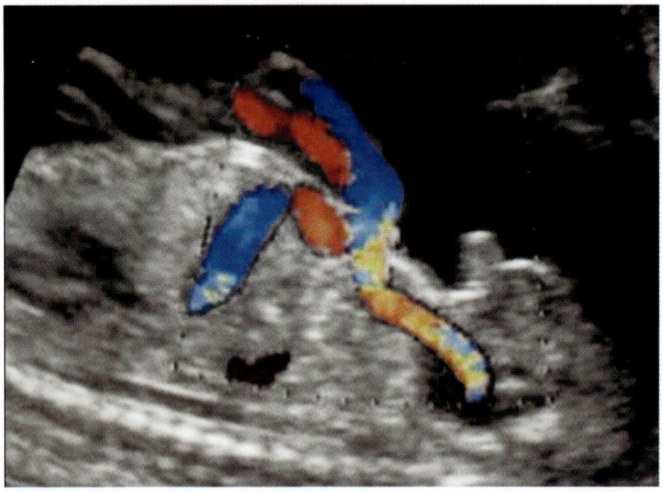

Fig. 9: Insertion of the umbilical cord into the abdominal wall.

malformations varies from 24 to 72%, according to different Authors' results.[1-5] This wide variation is due to the different study designs (mainly the numbers of scans performed during pregnancy), inclusion criteria, levels of examination. Since many gastrointestinal malformations, due to their natural history, appear late in pregnancy, the best results are obtained when the screening design includes a scan also in the third trimester.

The malformations of gastrointestinal tract and abdominal wall can be divided into four groups:

1. Anterior abdominal wall defects
2. Diaphragmatic defects
3. Bowel disorders
4. Non-bowel masses.

ANTERIOR ABDOMINAL WALL DEFECTS

The congenital abdominal wall defects include gastroschisis, omphalocele and body stalk anomaly. The ultrasonic prenatal diagnosis of these defects is relatively simple and possible in the first half of pregnancy. However it must be remembered that there is a physiological herniation of the small intestine outside the abdominal cavity between the 5th and the 11th weeks of gestation **(Fig. 10)** and therefore a prenatal diagnosis of abdominal wall defect cannot be made in the earliest stage of pregnancy.[6,7]

Gastroschisis

Incidence: Rare (1:10.000/15.000 live births)

US diagnosis: Free floating bowels loops in the amniotic fluid

Associated Anomalies: Rare.

Outcome: Good after surgery. Mortality rate ranging from 8 to 28%.

This malformation consists in a paraumbilical full thickness defect of the anterior abdominal wall which is usually located to the right side of the umbilical cord insertion, associated with evisceration of intestinal loops, rarely of the stomach.

The incidence ranges from 1:10.000 to 1:15.000 live births.

Gastroschisis is considered a sporadic event with a multifactorial etiology, but cases of familiar occurrence have been reported. Young maternal age, maternal cigarette use and vasoactive drugs consumption during first trimester are considered as possible etiological factors.

The pathogenesis may be referred to an anomalous regression of the right umbilical vein or to a vascular accident of the omphalomesenteric artery with consequent failed closure of the abdominal wall. The abdominal wall defect is generally small but the amount of bowel protruding from the defect and floating freely in the amniotic fluid may be disproportionately large. The herniated organs include mainly bowel loops, rarely stomach that are not protected by a membrane but usually covered by inflammatory exudates, possibly resulting from chemical irritation by exposure to amniotic fluid.

The ultrasonographic diagnosis of gastroschisis is suggested by the finding of a partly solid, partly cystic mass adjacent to the anterior abdominal wall and freely floating in the amniotic fluid with a typical cauliflower-like appearance **(Figs. 11 and 12)**. Bowel dilatation can be seen both in the herniated and endoabdominal loops as a consequence of the bowel obstruction with associated polyhydramnios. In sever cases, dilatation may disappear as a consequence of ischemia and necrosis of the intestinal walls (vanishing gut).

The differential diagnosis is mainly with omphalocele and is based on the presence of a normal insertion of the umbilical cord, the lateral location of the mass and the absence of a membrane covering the herniated mass.

In contrast to omphalocele, gastroschisis is rarely associated with other malformations and chromosomal anomalies, but additional gastrointestinal abnormalities (malrotation, atresia, volvulus, and infarction) may occur in 20–40% of the cases.[8,9] A high percentage of fetuses with gastroschisis (77%) present intrauterine growth restriction and preterm labor occur in one third of cases. The extent of bowel damage is variable and strictly affects the prognosis. Most of the bowel damage is caused by constriction at the site of the abdominal wall defect: the sonographic evidence of small bowel dilatation and mural thickening correlates with severe intestinal damage and poor clinical outcome.

The mode of delivery of fetuses affected by gastroschisis is still controversial: although there is no striking evidence for CS over vaginal delivery, the former may be preferred in order to avoid trauma and infection of the herniated bowel during the vaginal delivery. Maternal transfer before delivery to a tertiary care center is recommended in order to plan prompt surgical treatment. The mortality rate ranges from about 8 to 28%. The most common causes of the neonatal death are sepsis, prematurity and complications related to the intestinal ischemia.

Gastroschisis requires early surgery after birth, often followed by prolonged neonatal care. However, advances in surgical and postoperative care in the last decade have meant that currently 90% of affected neonates survive, with few long-term problems.[10]

Omphalocele

Incidence: 1:4,000–7,000 live births; higher in utero.

US diagnosis: Mass protruding from the abdomen, covered by a membrane, containing bowels loops or liver; umbilical cord inserted on the protruding mass

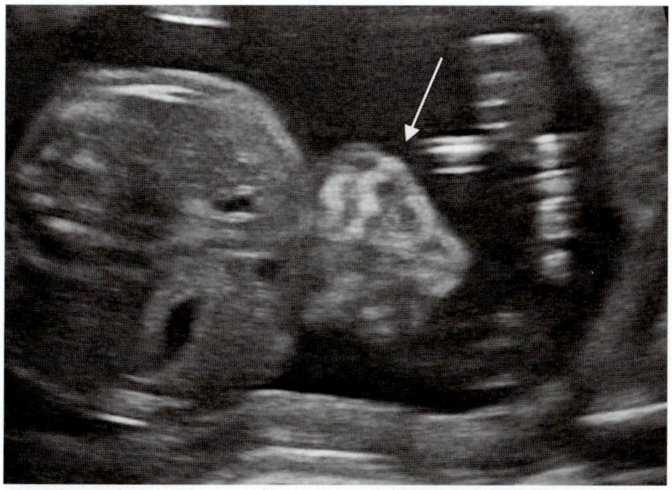

Fig. 11: Gastroschisis: a cauliflower-like mass protrudes from the abdominal cavity into the amniotic fluid (arrow).

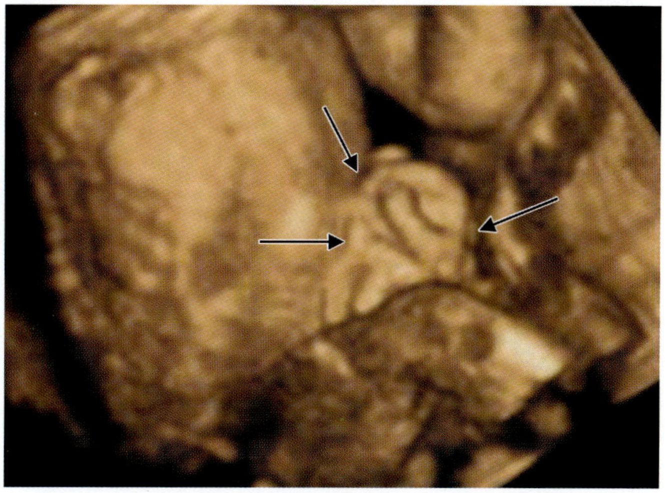

Fig. 12: Gastroschisis: 3D visualization of the intestinal loop protruding from the abdominal wall (arrows).

Associated anomalies: Present in 50–70% of the cases: chromosomopathies in 30% of the cases; present in different syndromes.

Outcome: Good in isolated cases. Poor in the presence of associated anomalies, chromosomopathies and syndromes

Omphalocele is a ventral wall defect characterized by an incomplete development of abdominal muscles, fascia and skin and the herniation of intra-abdominal organs (bowel loops, stomach, liver) into the base of umbilical cord, with a covering amnioperitoneal membrane. The defect is thought to be caused by an abnormality in the process of body infolding. The classic omphalocele is a mid-abdominal defect although there is also a high or epigastric omphalocele (typical of the pentalogy of Cantrell) and a low or hypogastric omphalocele (as seen in bladder or cloacal exstrophy), due respectively to cephalic and caudal folding defects.

The incidence of omphalocele ranges from 1:4.000 to 1:7.000 live births. It is more frequent in older women; most cases are sporadic, although a familial occurrence with a sex-linked or autosomal pattern of inheritance has been reported.

The ultrasonographic appearance of omphalocele varies according to the severity of the defect and to the organs herniated. Small omphalocele contain only omentum and some bowl loops **(Fig. 13)**; in large omphalocele also the liver can be herniated **(Fig. 14)**. 3D sonography may offer a better evaluation of the size of the lesion **(Fig. 15)**. A common finding is the presence of a membrane covering the herniated mass where the insertion of the umbilical cord can be recognized. Sometimes, ascites can be associated. Polyhydramnios is present in one third of the cases as a consequence of bowel obstruction.

The differential diagnosis is mainly with gastroschisis. The presence of a covering amnioperitoneal membrane and the insertion of the umbilical cord on the protruding mass easily allow making the correct diagnosis. However the covering membrane may occasionally disrupt thus making the differential diagnosis with gastroschisis more difficult.

There are different syndromes that include omphalocele, such as pentalogy of Cantrell (midline supraumbilical abdominal defect, lower sternum defect, deficiency of diaphragmatic pericardium, anterior diaphragm defect, cardiac abnormality), Beckwith-Wiedemann syndrome (macroglossia, visceromegaly, omphalocele, diaphragmatic hernia) and OEIS complex

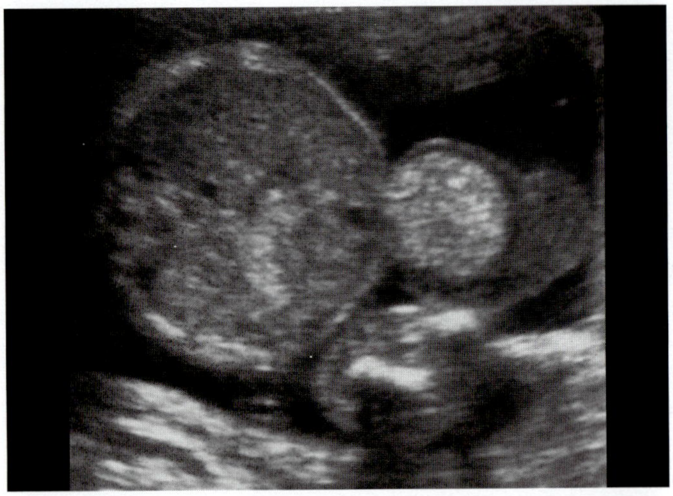

Fig. 13: Omphalocele: an echogenic mass protruding at the level of the cord insertion, covered by an amnioperitoneal membrane.

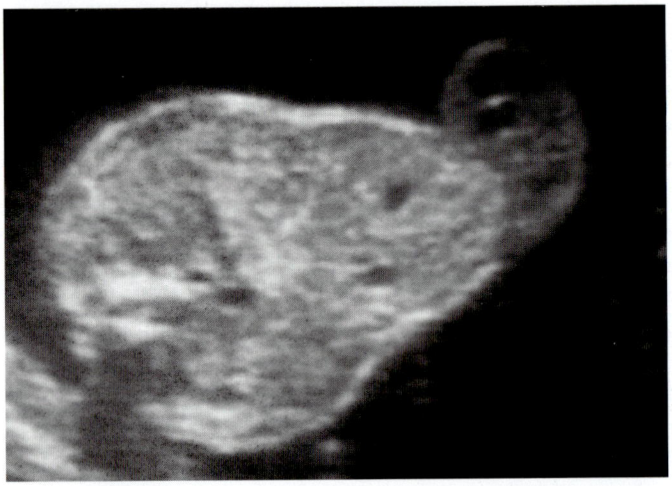

Fig. 14: Large omphalocele containing the liver.

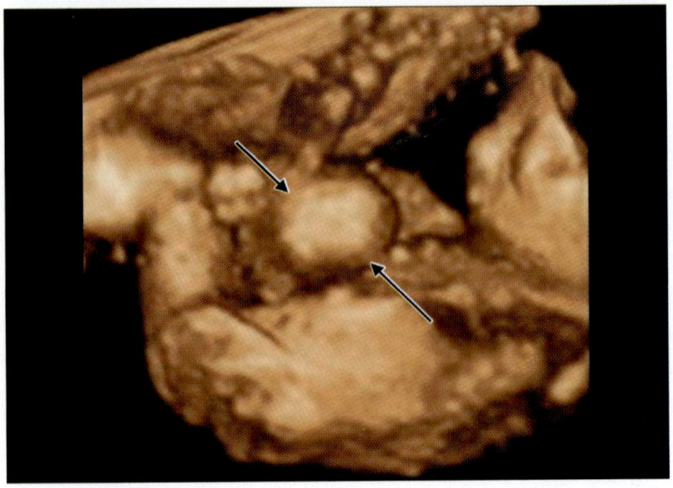

Fig. 15: 3D rendering of a fetus with omphalocele.

(omphalocele, exstrophy of cloaca, imperforate anus, and spinal defect).

Although most cases of omphalocele are sporadic, a familial occurrence of this anomaly with a sex-linked or autosomal pattern of inheritance has been reported.

The most important prognostic variable is the presence of associated malformations (50–70% of cases) or chromosomal abnormalities (30% of cases),[11,12] particularly trisomies 18 and 13 and triploidy.

Some authors have demonstrated that small defects containing only bowel are associated with an increased risk of chromosomal abnormalities, as opposed to large defects that have exposed liver. The main associated malformations are cardiac anomalies (up to 47% of cases), genitourinary abnormalities (40% of cases) and neural tube defects (39% of cases).

The mode of delivery of fetuses with omphalocele has been debated in literature. The goal in the management is to deliver the fetus as close to term as possible in tertiary care centers. Cesarean section may be necessary to avoid dystocia or sac rupture in large omphalocele. In the case of small defects vaginal delivery is recommended. The neonatal mortality after surgery mainly depends from the associated anomalies. In isolated small omphalocele the prognosis is good particularly in small omphalocele. In large omphalocele with herniated liver respiratory distress may be the cause of failure.

Body Stalk Anomaly

Incidence: Rare (1:14.000).

US diagnosis: Large anterior wall defect attaching the fetus to the placenta or uterine wall with absence of umbilical cord.

Associated anomalies: Scoliosis, kyphosis, multiple malformations.

Outcome: Fatal.

The body stalk anomaly is a severe abdominal wall defect caused by the failure of formation of the body stalk; it is characterized by the absence of umbilical cord and umbilicus and the fusion of the placenta to the herniated viscera. The incidence is 1:14.000 births. This malformation is caused by a developmental failure of the cephalic, caudal and lateral embryonic folds.

The ultrasonographic diagnosis is suggested by the finding of a large anterior wall defect attaching the fetus to the placenta or uterine wall, the absence of umbilical cord, and the visualization of abdominal organs in a sac outside the abdominal cavity **(Fig. 16)**.[13] The position of the fetus may lead to scoliosis and kyphosis. Multiple malformations, such as neural tube defects, gastrointestinal and genitourinary anomalies, may be associated. The body stalk anomaly is a uniformly fatal condition.

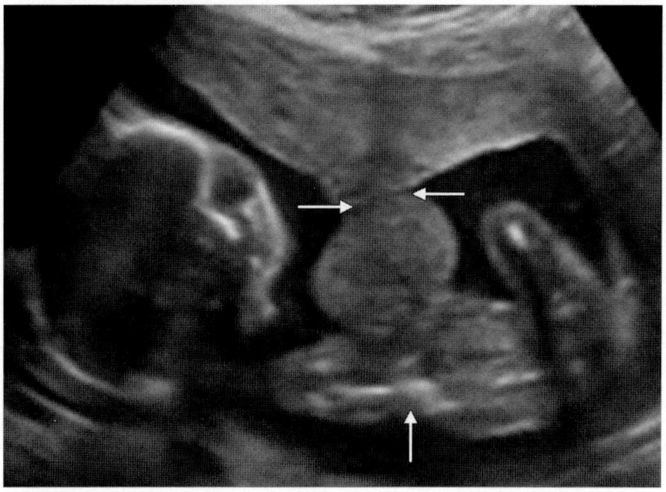

Fig. 16: Body stalk anomaly: a large anterior abdominal wall defect attaches the fetus directly to the placenta (arrows) with subsequent deformity of the spine (thick arrow).

Diaphragmatic Defects

Incidence: 1:3.000 live births.

US diagnosis: Presence of stomach or bowels loops or liver in the thorax with lateral displacement of the heart.

Associated anomalies: Chromosopathies (5–15%); Syndromes (20–30%); other malformations.

Outcome: Poor in syndromic cases; 40–50% survival rate in isolated cases

A diaphragmatic hernia is a defect in the diaphragm, due to failure of the pleuroperitoneal canal to close between 9 and 10 weeks of gestation thus determining the protrusion of the abdominal organs into the thoracic cavity.

The classification of these malformations is based on the location of the diaphragmatic defect:

- Diaphragmatic hernia (Bochdalek and Morgagni types)
- Septum transversum defects (defect of the central tendon)
- Hiatal hernia (congenital large esophageal orifice)
- Eventration of the diaphragm
- Agenesis of the diaphragm.

The incidence of congenital diaphragmatic hernia is 1:3.000 live births.

The most common type of diaphragmatic hernia is the Bochdalek type which is a posterolateral defect mostly located on the left side (80% of cases), less frequently on the right side (15%) and bilateral (5%). Stomach, spleen and colon are the most frequently herniated organs. When the hernia is on the right side, the main organs involved are the liver and the gallbladder.

The Morgagni type is usually a very small hernia which occurs in 1–2% of cases. It is a parasternal defect located in the anterior portion of the diaphragm; it contains liver, which may limit the degree of herniation.

Eventration of the diaphragm consists of an upward displacement of abdominal organs into the thoracic cavity secondary to a congenitally weak diaphragm which has the aspect of an aponeurotic sheet. It occurs in 5% of diaphragmatic defects, and it is more common on the right side.

Diaphragmatic hernia can be either a sporadic or a familiar disorder and although the etiology is unknown this abnormality has been described in association with maternal ingestion of drugs such as thalidomide, quinine and anticonvulsants. There are two hypotheses to explain the mechanism responsible for the origin of a diaphragmatic defect: a delayed fusion of the diaphragm or a primary diaphragmatic defect.

Another classification takes into account the time of onset of the malformation in relation to the lung development:

- Herniation occurring early during bronchial branching causing a severe bilateral pulmonary hypoplasia and lately death.
- Herniation at the stage of distal bronchial branching leading to unilateral hypoplasia, with survival depending on a balance between pulmonary vascular and ductal resistances.
- Late herniation in pregnancy which causes a compression of otherwise normal lung and carries a good prognosis.
- Postnatal herniation without pulmonary pathology and with good chances of viability.

The prenatal sonographic diagnosis of diaphragmatic hernia is mainly based on the visualization of abdominal organs at the same level of the four-chamber view of the heart in the transverse section of the fetal chest. The sonographic signs are different according to the location of the defect. In the most common case (posterolateral left defect) the heart is shifted to the right by the herniated stomach **(Fig. 17)**. Sometimes, only bowel loops and the left lobe of the liver are herniated: in these cases the heart displacement to the right and the irregular echogenicity of the left hemithorax are the signs suggesting the diagnosis. In the sagittal view of the chest and abdomen the stomach may be recognized in the mediastinic cavity **(Fig. 18)**.

Polyhydramnios is common and is secondary to the bowel obstruction.

In the less common cases of right defects the diagnosis is more difficult, since the stomach is not herniated:

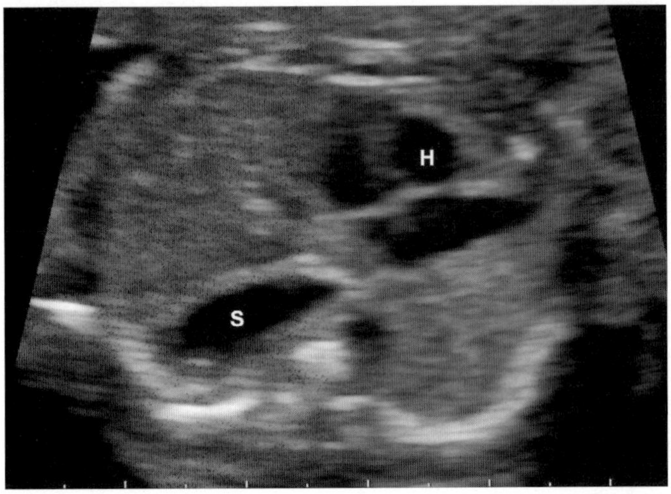

Fig. 17: Transverse section of the fetal chest in a case of posterolateral left diaphragmatic hernia: the heart (H) is displaced to the right side by the presence of the stomach (S) and bowel loops in the thoracic cavity.

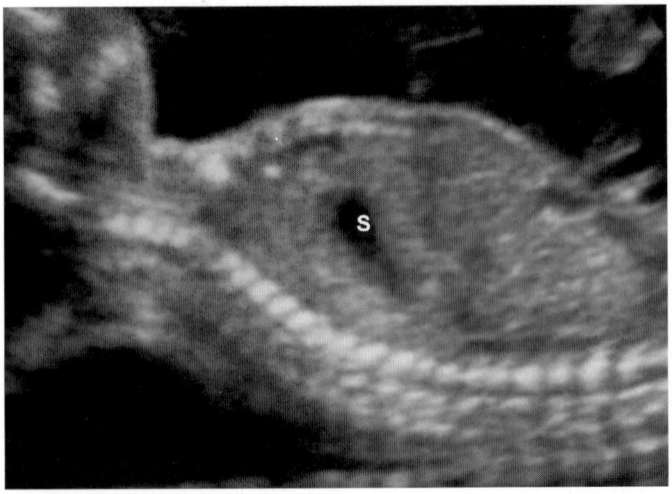

Fig. 18: Longitudinal section of the fetal chest and abdomen in a fetus with diaphragmatic hernia, showing the stomach (S) in the mediastinic cavity.

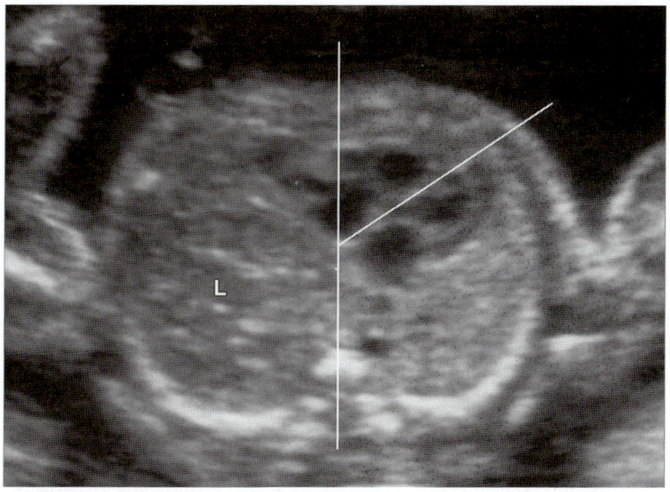

Fig. 19: Right diaphragmatic hernia. The cardiac axis is left rotated by the herniated liver (L).

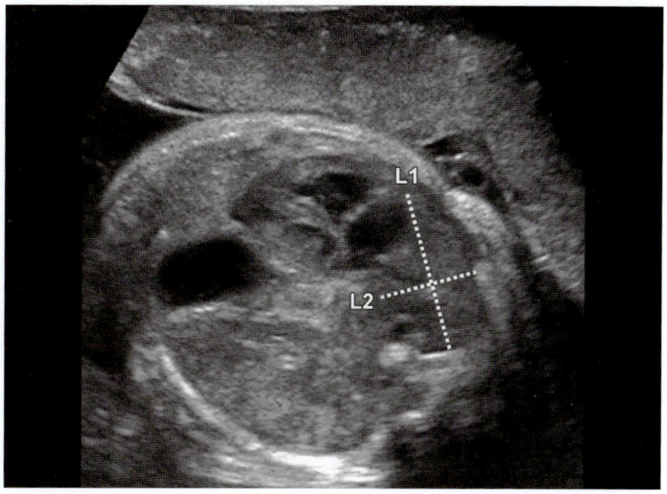

Fig. 21: Technique of measurement of the LHR. The product of the two orthogonal diameters of the collapsed lung, contralateral to the side of herniation, is divided by the head circumference (L1 x L2/HC).

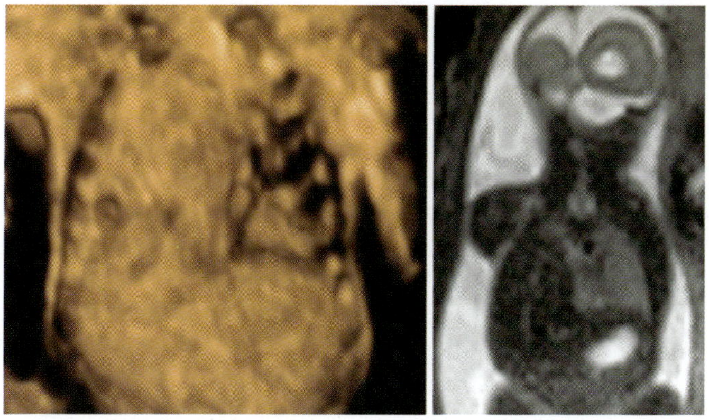

Fig. 20: 3D rendering of the fetal chest in a fetus with right diaphragmatic hernia.

suspicious signs are the left rotation of the cardiac axis and upper displacement of the liver **(Fig. 19)**. In this case the coronal view of the chest is more useful **(Fig. 20)**.

It must be stressed that due to the possible late onset of the herniation, the prenatal diagnosis of diaphragmatic hernia may be missed in up to 40% of the cases.

Recently, 3D ultrasound applications obtained increasingly attention for evaluation of diaphragmatic hernia, particularly the TUI mode that can be useful in case of right-sided hernia to evaluate the liver herniation in the thorax.[14]

The differential diagnosis is with other conditions, such as cystic adenomatoid malformation of the lung, bronchogenic cysts, mediastinal cysts and pulmonary sequestration. The peristalsis of the stomach and bowel is a useful sign to differentiate them from other cystic structure.

The rate of associated anomalies is 25–75% increasing to 95% in stillborns. Such anomalies include central nervous system, cardiac and chromosomal abnormalities, omphalocele and oral cleft.

Furthermore, there are different syndromes that include diaphragmatic hernia: Fryns syndrome (diaphragmatic hernia, central nervous system anomalies and orofacial clefting), Pallister-Killian syndrome (diaphragmatic hernia, facial dysmorphism and micromelia), Beckwith-Wiedemann syndrome (macroglossia, visceromegaly, omphalocele, diaphragmatic hernia).[15,16]

The prognosis for this malformation is still very poor and becomes poorer if other malformations are associated. The poor prognosis mainly depends on the severity of pulmonary hypoplasia-hypertension induced by the prolonged compression of the lungs by the herniated viscera. Different sonographic techniques have been suggested in order to evaluate the risk of lung hypoplasia. The "lung to head ratio" (LHR) is the ratio between the product of the two orthogonal diameters of the collapsed lung, contralateral to the side of herniation, and the head circumference (L1xL2/HC) **(Fig. 21)**. LHR <0, 6 are associated with neonatal death; values >1,35 are associated with good outcome, values between 0,6 and 1,35 have a 60% survival rate.[17] However, a recent meta-analysis demonstrated that the prognostic use of LHR entered in

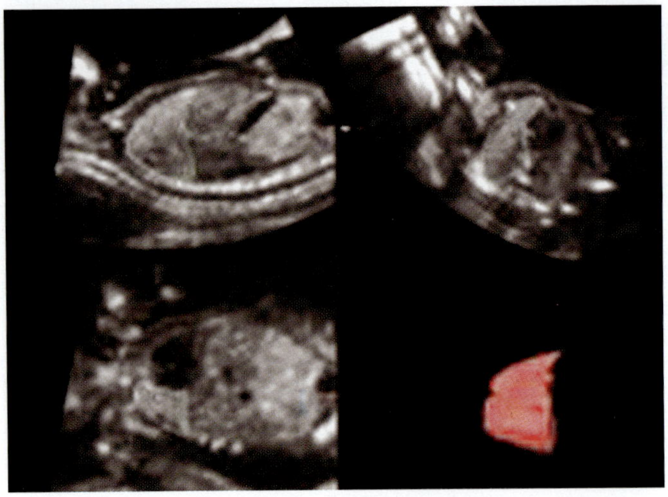

Fig. 22: Technique of the 3D calculation of the lung.

clinical practice prior to publication of important normal data and had not supported by current evidence.[18]

The presence of "liver up" (herniation of the liver in the thorax) reduces the percentage of survival from 93 to 43% and doubles the need of extracorporeal membrane oxygenation (ECMO).[19] The results of these techniques, however, are not uniformly confirmed by different authors;[20] the main limit is the dependency from the gestational age. For this reason alternative techniques have been suggested: one is the ratio between the observed and expected LHR (O/E LHR%), which has the advantage to be independent from the gestational age. Values <15% are indicative of extreme pulmonary hypoplasia, values 15-25% of severe pulmonary hypoplasia, values 25–45% of moderate pulmonary hypoplasia, >45% of mild hypoplasia.[21] 3D evaluation of he lung volumes **(Fig. 22)** and the observed/expected lung volume ratio (O/E LVR%) has also been suggested, but this measurement is technically limited in the third trimester. Better results in the third trimester may be obtained with the use of MRI.[22,23]

Management of fetus with diaphragmatic hernia relies on protecting the controlateral lung hoping that it is normally formed, which depends on the gestational age at diagnosis. If the fetus is less than 24 weeks of gestation, parents may choose to terminate the pregnancy, to continue the pregnancy with postnatal care or even to consider repair of the defect in utero. Between 24 and 32 weeks, parents may choose between conventional postnatal therapy and fetal surgery. Anytime a diaphragmatic defect is diagnosed, prenatal karyotyping and detailed ultrasound examination to detect associated anomalies are recommended. There are no indications for preterm delivery or for caesarean section. The delivery should be planned in a tertiary care center. Prenatal treatment is proposed in highly selected centers with the aim of preventing lung hypoplasia. The first approach was open fetal surgery with hysterotomy during pregnancy, but this technique is carrying several complications. An alternative invasive technique now used is the endotracheal application of a balloon catheter, following the observation that in cases of laryngeal atresia an overgrowth of the lung is observed. The balloon is introduced under endoscopic guidance (FETO = fetal endoscopic tracheal occlusion) and removed at delivery.[24,25]

FETO increased survival rate in severe cases with left-sided diaphragmatic hernia from 24 to 49% and in right-sided cases from 0 to 35%.[26,27]

The prognosis after neonatal surgery mainly depends from the severity of lung hypoplasia-hypertension. In isolated left diaphragmatic hernia the average survival rate is 50–60%. In some surviving infants, however, neurological sequels by brain hypoxia have been reported.

BOWEL DISORDERS

Esophageal Atresia

Incidence: 1:2500/4000 live births.

US diagnosis: Absent stomach bubble, polyhydramnios, dilated esophagus (pouch sign).

Associated anomalies: Frequent association with other malformations, chromosomopathies, syndromes (VACTERL).

Outcome: Depending on the severity of the defect and associated anomalies.

This anomaly consists in the absence of a segment of the esophagus and is often associated with a tracheoesophageal fistula (86–90% of cases). Five types of esophageal atresia may be distinguished, according to the Gross classification:

1. Isolated (type A: 8% of the cases).
2. Associated with a fistula connecting only the proximal part of the esophagus and the trachea (type B: 1% of the cases).
3. Associated with a fistula connecting the lower part of the esophagus and the trachea (type C: 88% of the cases).
4. Associated with proximal and distal fistulas (type D: 1% of the cases).

5. Tracheoesophageal fistula without esophageal atresia (type E: 2% of the cases).

The incidence varies between 1:2500 and 1:4000 live births. The etiology is unknown. The anomaly derives from the failed division at 8 weeks of gestation of the primitive intestine in the ventral tracheobronchial portion and in the dorsal intestinal portion.

The prenatal diagnosis is possible in only 10% of the cases and should be suspected in the presence of polyhydramnios with absent stomach bubble in several and repeated ultrasound examinations; sometimes the dilated proximal tract of the esophagus with absent stomach can also be seen (pouch sign) **(Figs. 23A and B)**;[28-30] the former sign, however, is transient, requires a prolonged examination and usually appears late in gestation. In the remaining 90% of the cases the presence of a tracheoesophageal fistula allows the amniotic fluid to reach and fill the stomach thus making the diagnosis impossible.[31]

The differential diagnosis is with other conditions characterized by failed visualization of the stomach: diaphragmatic hernia, congenital high-way obstruction syndrome (CHAOS), fetal akinesia sequence, anidramnios with consequent failed swallowing of amniotic fluid.

Associated anomalies are present in 50–70% of the cases, including cardiac, genitourinary, chromosomal (trisomy 21), additional gastrointestinal and musculoskeletal anomalies. Characteristic associations are the "VACTERL" (vertebral, anorectal anomalies, cardiac anomalies, tracheoesophageal fistula, esophageal atresia, renal anomalies, limb anomalies) and the "CHARGE" (coloboma of the eye, heart anomaly, choanal atresia, mental retardation, microphallus, ear abnormalities). Fetal karyotyping is suggested. The prognosis depends on the associated malformations and on the severity of polyhydramnios, which can facilitate preterm delivery. The delivery should be planned in a tertiary center for the prompt intensive therapy and surgical treatment.

Duodenal Atresia or Stenosis

Incidence: 1:2500/10.000.

US diagnosis: Double bubble, late polyhydramnios

Associated anomalies: Frequent association to other malformations and chromosomopathies (mainly trisomy 21).

Outcome: Good after neonatal surgery in isolated cases.

The incidence of this malformation is 1:2500/10.000 live births. In most cases the etiology is unknown and its genesis goes back to the 11th week of gestation due to a failure of canalization of the primitive bowel. Another possible cause is focal ischemia with consequent segmental infarction. The obstruction may also be due to external factors, such as intestinal malrotation and volvulus. Atresia is more common than stenosis (70% of cases) and could be associated with chromosomal abnormalities (trisomy 21), skeletal defects and other anomalies.

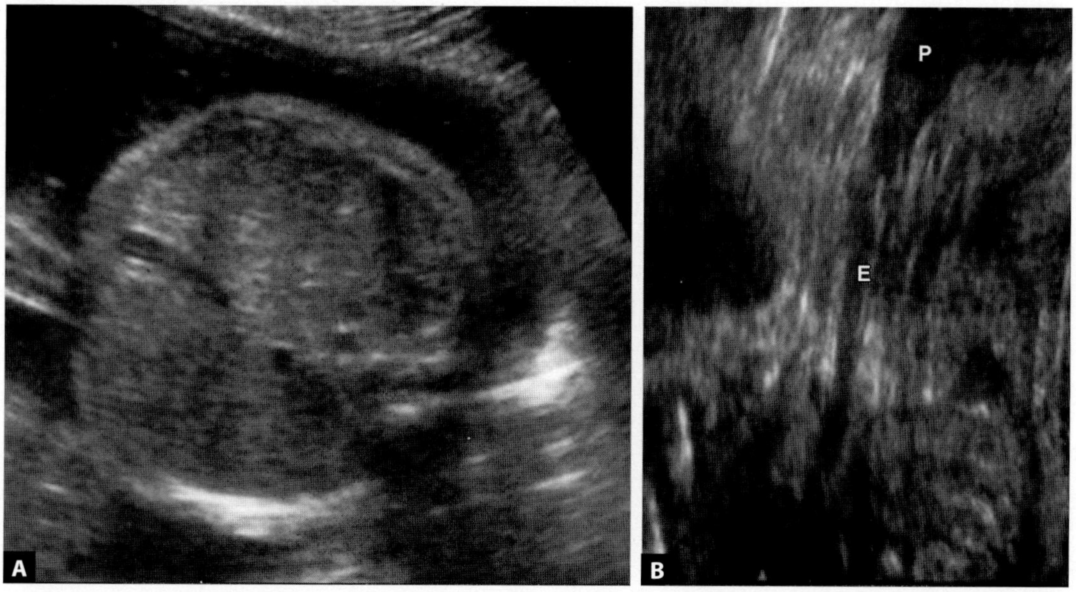

Figs. 23A and B: Esophageal atresia: the diagnosis is suspected by the association of absent stomach (A) and dilatation of the proximal tract of the esophagus in the coronal scan of the neck (B). (P: pharynx; E: esophagus)

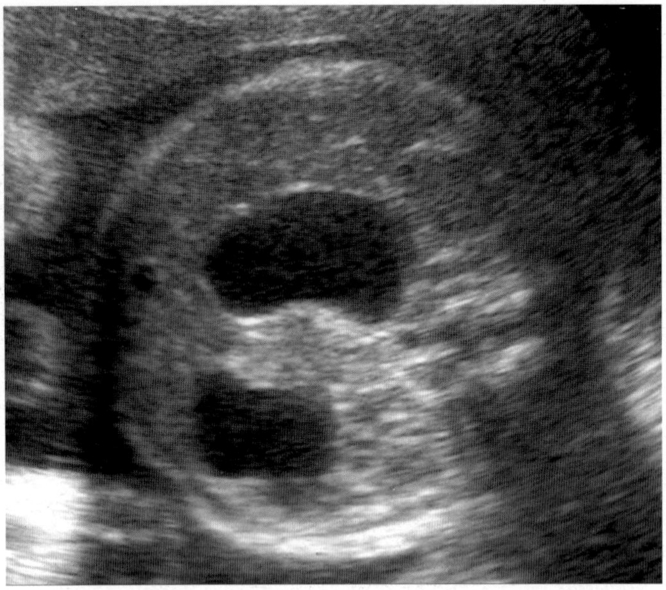

Fig. 24: Duodenal atresia: the dilated stomach and proximal duodenum are clearly recognized with the typical "double bubble" sign.

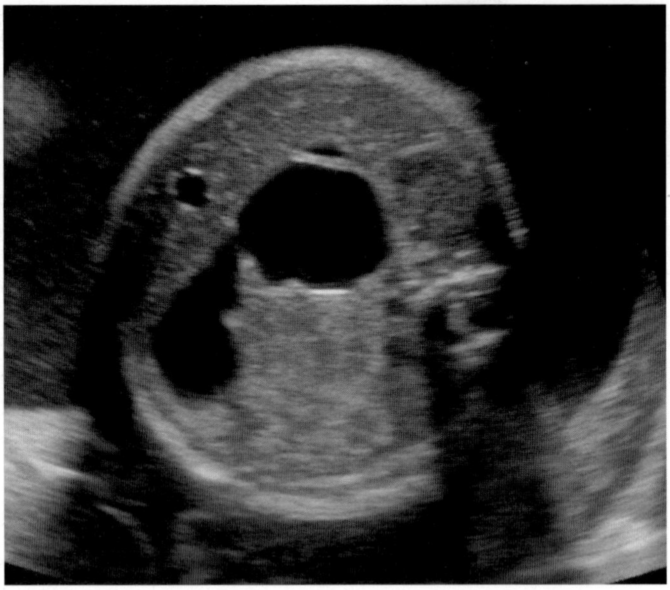

Fig. 25: Duodenal atresia: the continuity of the lumen between the stomach and the duodenum separated by the pylorus can be seen.

The most typical sonographic finding is the characteristic "double bubble" sign caused by the simultaneous dilatation of the stomach and the proximal duodenum **(Fig. 24)**. The diagnosis is usually made in the late second trimester.[32] The differential diagnosis is with other cystic lesions of the upper abdomen, such as duplication cysts, choledochal and hepatic cysts. A useful sign is the visualization of the continuity of the lumen between the stomach and the duodenum **(Fig. 25)**.

Up to half of duodenal atresia cases are complicated by polyhydramnios and this can contribute to preterm labor, but the main cause of death is the associated anomalies. These include gastrointestinal (26–35% of the cases), cardiac (20–30%), genitourinary (5–8%), skeletal (4–8%). In 40–50% of the cases trisomy 21 is associated. Particularly the association of duodenal atresia and atrioventricular canal is highly suspicious for trisomy 21.

The neonatal outcome after surgery is good in 90% of the cases without associated anomalies. Late minor complications, such as megaduodenum and gastric reflux may occur.[33] The delivery should be planned in a tertiary center for the prompt surgical treatment.

Bowel Obstruction

Incidence: 1:2500/5000.

US diagnosis: Multiple dilated bowels loops and late polyhydramnios in ileojejunal atresia; distended sigma-rectum with normal amniotic fluid in anorectal malformations.

Associated anomalies: Rare in ileojejunal atresia; chromosomopathies in anorectal malformations.

Outcome: Usually good in isolated cases.

The incidence of bowel stenosis and atresia is 2–3:10.000 births.

These defects are usually sporadic, although familial cases have been described.

According to the site of the obstruction the defects are divided in: (i) jejunoileal atresia and stenosis, (ii) colonic atresia and (iii) imperforate anus.

In jejunoileal atresia the location of the defect is at proximal jejunum in 31% of the cases, distal jejunum in 20%, proximal ileum in 13% and distal ileum in 36%. In 6% of the cases the atresia interests different intestinal segments. Atresia and stenosis are thought to be a consequence of an ischemic event at the level of the mesenteric artery.

There are four types of jejunoileal atresia:

- *Type I:* Presence of a single or multiple transverse diaphragm of mucosa or submucosa, with regular external intestinal walls and normal mesentery (32%).
- *Type II:* Presence of blind ends of bowel loops connected by fibrous bands with regular mesentery (25%).

- *Type IIIa:* Complete separation of blind ends with a corresponding "V" shaped mesenteric defect (15%).
- *Type IIIb:* "Apple peel" or "christmas-tree" appearance of the blind ended ileum wrapped around the ileocolic artery with loss of the superior mesenteric artery (11%).
- *Type IV:* Multiple atresias of the small intestine (17%).

Colon atresia usually occurs proximal to the splenic flexure with a significant segment of absent colon with distal microcolon.

Anorectal malformations regard the terminal portion of the intestinal lumen and may be divided in high and low level malformations in relation to the elevator ani muscle. The high level anomalies are usually more complex and complicated with genitourinary-perineal fistulas as well as urinary and vertebral malformations. They derive from an anomalous division of the cloaca by the urorectal septum. The low level malformations are more common and less severe and are usually represented by the imperforate anus occasionally associated with perineal fistula.

The sonographic prenatal appearance of the bowel obstruction varies according to the level of the defect. In the case of jejunoileal atresia multiple dilated bowel loops in the fetal abdomen may be seen in association with polyhydramnios **(Fig. 26)**.[33,34] An active peristalsis can be seen.[35] These signs usually appear in the late second or even third trimester. The first sign may be the presence of a single bowel loop with a diameter above 7 mm and with hyperechoic walls **(Fig. 27)**.

In colon atresia the sonographic finding is similar to distal ileal occlusion and the differential diagnosis may not be possible. In cases of distal occlusion dilated intestinal loops with increased peristalsis may be seen as well as intraluminal echogenic material in the distended colon referring to meconium **(Fig. 28)**.[36]

The diagnosis of bowel obstruction is usually made in the third trimester: the lower is the obstruction the later is the appearance of the sonographic signs.

The prognosis of these malformations mainly depends on the level of obstruction (the lower the obstruction, the better the outcome), the length of remaining intestine and birth weight.[37] Other important prognostic factors are the presence of associated malformations (especially gastrointestinal anomalies, including bowel malrotation,

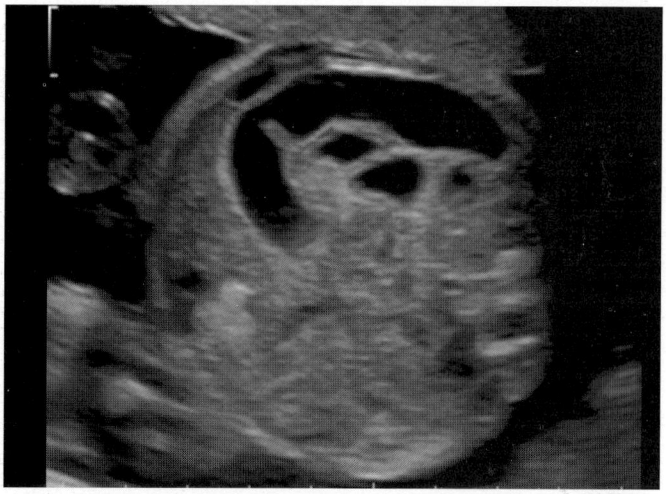

Fig. 27: Early sign of bowel dilatation.

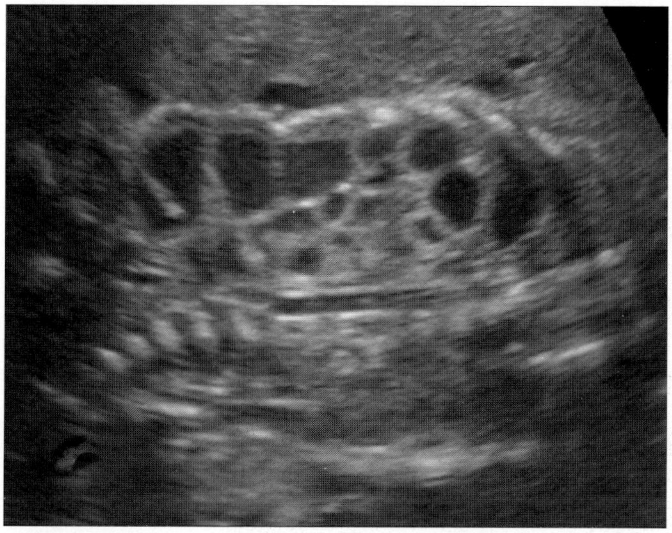

Fig. 26: Jejunal atresia: multiple dilated bowel loops are present in the fetal abdomen.

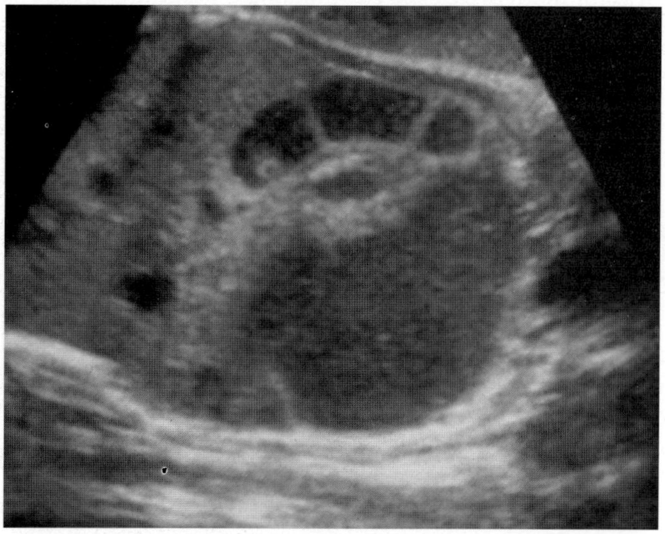

Fig. 28: Colon obstruction in a third trimester fetus: a dilated distal colon is seen containing echogenic material referring to meconium.

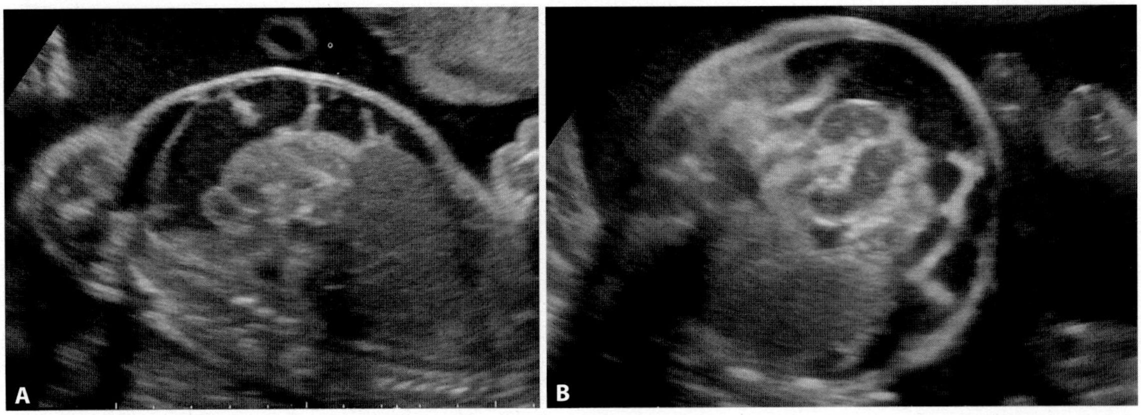

Figs. 29A and B: Meconium peritonitis: fetal ascites caused by exudate and bowel dilatation.

esophageal atresia, microcolon and intestinal duplication), meconium peritonitis and intrauterine growth restriction.

The delivery should be planned in a tertiary center for the prompt neonatal surgery.

Meconium Peritonitis

Incidence: 1:20.000/30.000 live births.

US diagnosis: Intrabdominal diffuse hyperechogenicity, calcifications, ascites, bowel dilatation.

Associated anomalies: Cystic fibrosis frequently associated

Outcome: Usually poor.

This condition is the consequence of in utero perforation of the bowel with spread of meconium into the peritoneal cavity leading to a local sterile chemical peritonitis. The peritonitis may be localized, with the development of a dense calcified mass or fibrous tissue, or diffuse, with a fibrous reaction leading to bowel adhesions and pseudocyst formation. Inflammatory reaction leads to an exudative process and ascites. Its incidence is 1:20.000/30.000 live births. The most common cause of the bowel perforation is cystic fibrosis: in this disease the highly protein meconium causes obstruction, dilatation and subsequent bowel perforation. Other causes of perforation are bowel obstructions.

The prenatal sonographic appearance of meconium peritonitis varies according to the underlying anatomical finding: main signs are intrabdominal diffuse hyperechogenicity and calcifications (85% of cases) and/or fetal ascites caused by exudate and bowel dilatation **(Figs. 29A and B)**.[38]

The prognosis is usually poor since multiple intestinal resections may be required and cystic fibrosis is frequently associated.

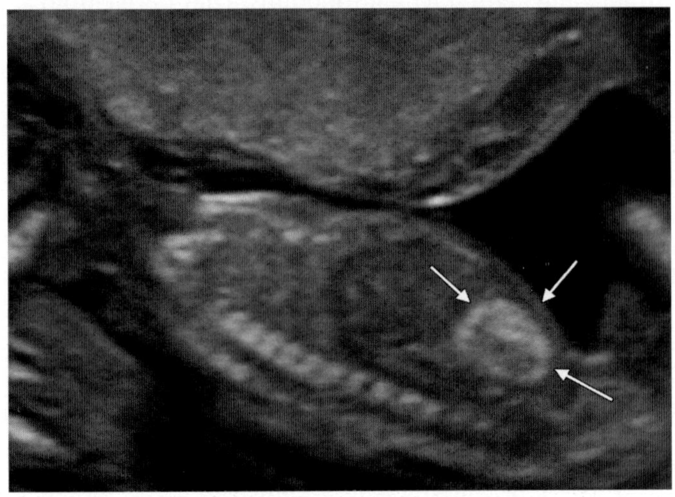

Fig. 30: Echogenic bowel.

Echogenic Bowel

Sonographically, "echogenic bowel" is defined as echogenicity of the bowel loops equal to or greater than the density of the iliac wing **(Fig. 30)**. This feature might depend on a slow or delayed transit of the meconium along the bowel. The reported incidence of "echogenic bowel" in the midtrimester fetuses is 0,2–2%.

In up to 75% of the cases "echogenic bowel" is a normal finding with no pathological significance. It must also be stressed that the use of high frequencies (6–7 MHz) and second harmonic produce an increased echogenicity. In the remaining cases it can be associated to the following pathological conditions:

- Chromosomopathies, mainly trisomy 21, the isolated marker detection rate is 16.7% as reported in a recent meta-analysis [39]

- Congenital infections (mainly CMV,[40] toxoplasmosis, parvovirus B19)
- Cystic fibrosis and meconium ileum
- Intestinal malformations (atresia, volvulus, enteric duplication)
- Fetal growth restriction[41]
- Intra-amniotic bleeding

In the presence of "echogenic bowel" the following management is suggested:[42-44]

- Fetal karyotyping only if additional markers of chromosomopathies are present
- Maternal test for infection
- Parental screening for cystic fibrosis
- Accurate evaluation of fetal growth and well-being
- Rule-out of possible intra-amniotic bleeding (previous bleeding in pregnancy, previous invasive procedures).

In the case of normal results the fetus should be accurately monitored in the third trimester to rule out late onset intestinal anomalies of growth restriction.

NONBOWEL CYSTIC MASSES

Choledocal Cysts

Choledocal cyst is a rare congenital cystic dilatation of the common bile duct. The incidence is about 1:2.000. The cysts can be single or, in rare cases, multiple involving the intrahepatic or extrahepatic portion of the biliary tree. Choledocal cysts are classified into four types:

1. Fusiform dilatation of the common bile duct
2. Diverticular dilatation of the common bile duct
3. Intramural dilatation of the common bile duct
4. Intrahepatic biliary duct dilatation.

The sonographic appearance is that of a cystic structure located in the upper right abdomen with dilated proximal ducts **(Fig. 31)**.[45] Differential diagnosis includes duodenal atresia, hepatic cyst, dilated gallbladder, mesenteric cysts and ovarian cyst. The cystic size and the association with biliary obstruction affect the prognosis.

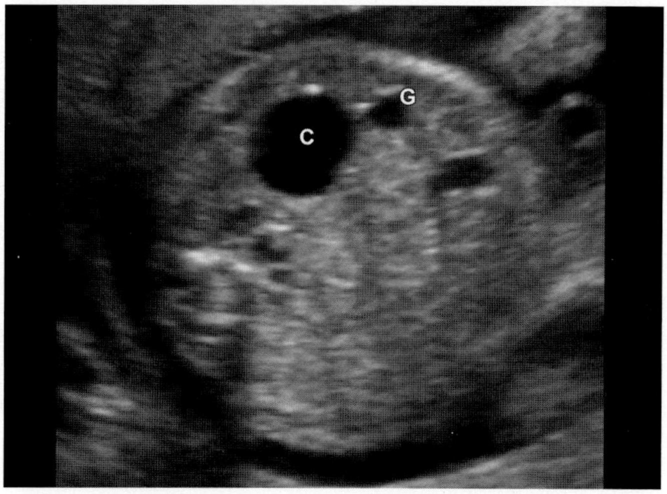

Fig. 31: Choledocal cyst. (C: cyst; G: gallbladder)

Mesenteric and Omental Cyst

These benign malformations consist in cystic structures located in the small or large bowel mesentery or in the omentum filled with serous or chilous fluid. Its sonographic appearance is that of a thin-walled, unilocular or multilocular cystic mass **(Fig. 32)**. It is difficult to make a differential diagnosis with other intrabdominal cystic conditions, such as choledocal, ovarian and hepatic cysts. The prognosis is usually good and no surgical treatment is required in cysts of small size.

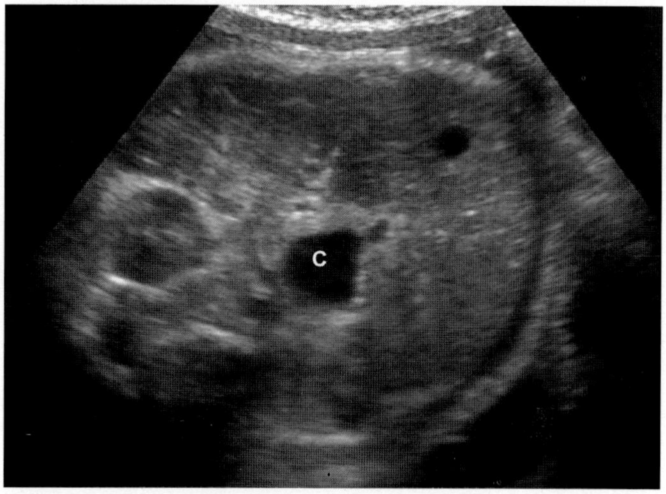

Fig. 32: Mesenteric cyst (C).

Hepatic Masses

Hepatic masses might origin from an obstruction of the hepatic biliary system or might have a tumoral origin (hemangioma, hamartoma, etc...).

Their sonographic appearance changes depending on the origin: cysts are usually isolated and anechoic with regular borders;[46] mesenchymal hamartoma usually appears as irregular hyperechoic areas[47] **(Fig. 33)**, while hemangioma appears hypoechoic, hyperechoic or mixed depending on the degree of fibrosis and stage of involution. Hepatoblastomas and adenomas have a solid appearance.

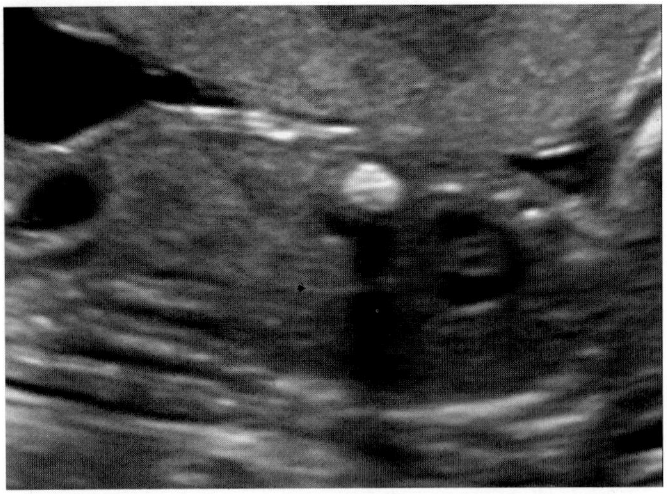

Fig. 33: Hepatic hamartoma appearing as an isolated intrahepatic echogenic area.

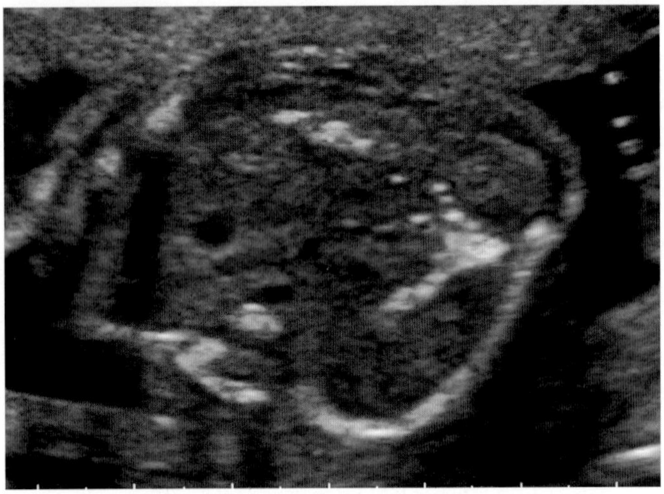

Fig. 34: Multiple hepatic calcifications.

Polyhydramnios may be associated; many cases of reduction in volume or even disappearance in utero have been described.

Multiple intrahepatic calcifications **(Fig. 34)** may be due to congenital infection (CMV, parvovirus B19, herpes, rubella, toxoplasmosis, varicella) or vascular accidents, such as thrombosis or ischemic disorders.

The management is expectant in terms of monitoring the size and evolution of the lesions.

REFERENCES

1. Bernaschek G, Stuempflen I, Deutinger J. The value of sonographic diagnosis of fetal malformations: different results between indication-based and screening-based investigations. Prenat Diagn. 1994;14:807-12.
2. Grandjean H, Larroque D, Levi S. The performance of routine ultrasonographic screening of pregnancies in the Eurofetus Study. Am J Obstet Gynecol. 1999;181:446-54.
3. Luck CA. Value of routine ultrasound scanning at 19 weeks: a four year study of 8849 deliveries. BMJ. 1992;304:1474-8.
4. Queisser-Luft A, Stopfkuchen H, Stolz G, Schlaefer K, Merz E. Prenatal diagnosis of major malformations: quality control of routine ultrasound examinations based on a five-year study of 20,248 newborn fetuses and infants. Prenat Diagn. 1998;18:567-76.
5. Martin RW. Screening for fetal abdominal wall defects. Obstet Gynecol Clin North Am. 1998;25:517-26.
6. Kurkchubasche AG. The fetus with an abdominal wall defect. Med Health R I. 2000;84:159-61.
7. Oguniemy D. Gastroschisis complicated by midgut atresia, absorption of bowel, and closure of the abdominal wall defect. Fetal Diagn Ther. 2001;16:227-30.
8. Brantberg A, Blaas HG, Salvesen KA, Haugen SE, Eik-Nes SH. Surveillance and outcome of fetuses with gastroschisis. Ultrasound Obstet Gynecol. 2004;23:4-13.
9. David AL, Tan A, Curry J. Gastroschisis: sonographic diagnosis, associations, management and outcome. Prenat Diagn. 2008;28(7):633-44.
10. Brantberg A, Blaas HG, Haugen SE, Eik-Nes SH. Characteristics and outcome of 90 cases of fetal omphalocele. Ultrasound Obstet Gynecol. 2005;25:427-37.
11. Blazer S, Zimmer EZ, Gover A, Bronshtein M. Fetal omphalocele detected early in pregnancy: associated anomalies and outcomes. Radiology. 2004;232:191-5.
12. Lakasing L, Cicero S, Davenport M, et al. Current outcome of antenatally diagnosed exomphalos: an 11 years review. J Pediatr Surg. 2006;41:1403-6.
13. Cadkin A, Strom C. Prenatal diagnosis of body stalk anomaly in the first trimester of pregnancy. Ultrasound Obstet Gynecol. 1997;10:419-21.
14. Achiron R, Gindes L, Zalel Y, et al. Three- and four-dimensional ultrasound: new methods for evaluating fetal thoracic anomalies. Ultrasound Obstet Gynecol. 2008;32:36-43.
15. Lyons Jones K. Smith's recognizable patterns of human malformation, 5th edition, Philadelphia: WB Saunders Company; 1996. pp. 176-7.
16. Paladini D, Borghese A, Arienzo M, et al. Prospective ultrasound diagnosis of Pallister- Kilian syndrome in the second trimester of pregnancy: the importance of the fetal facial profile. Prenat Diagn. 2000;20:996-8.
17. Metkus AP, Filly RA, Stringer MD, Harriso MR, Adzick NS Sonographic predictors of survival in fetal diaphragmatic hernia. J Pediatr Surg. 1996;31:148-51.
18. Ba'ath ME, Jesudason EC, Losty PD. How useful is the lung-to-head ratio in predicting outcome in the fetus with congenital diaphragmatic hernia? A systematic review and meta-analysis. Ultrasound Obstet Gynecol. 2007;30:897-90.
19. Geary MP, Chitty LS, Morrison JJ, Wright V, Pierro A, Rodeck CH. Perinatal outcome and prognostic factors in prenatally

diagnosed congenital diphragmatic hernia. Ultrasound Obstet Gynecol. 1998;12:107-11.
20. Heling KS, Wauer RR, Hammer H, Bollmann R, Chaoui R. Reliability of the lung-to-head ratio in predicting outcome and neonatal ventilation parameters in fetuses with congenital diaphragmatic hernia. Ultrasound Obstet Gynecol. 2005;25:112-8.
21. Jani JC, Nicolaides KH. Opinion. Fetal surgery for severe congenital diaphragmatic hernia? Ultrasound Obstet Gynecol. 2012;39:7-9.
22. Cannie M, Jani J, Meersschaert J, Allegaert K, Done E, Marchal G, et al. Prenatal prediction of survival in isolated diaphragmatic hernia using observed to expected total fetal lung volume determined by magnetic resonance imaging based on either gestational age or fetal body volume. Ultrasound Obstet Gynecol. 2008;32:633-63.
23. Jani J, Cannie M, Sonigo P, Roberts Y, Moreno O, Benachi A, et al. Value of prenatal magnetic resonance imaging in the prediction of postnatal outcome in fetuses with diaphragmatic hernia. Ultrasound Obstet Gynecol. 2008;32:793-9.
24. Harrison MR, Keller RL, Hawgood SB, Kitterman JA, Sandberg PL, Farmer DL, et al. A randomized trial of fetal endoscopic tracheal occlusion for severe fetal congenital diaphragmatic hernia. N Engl J Med. 2003;349:1916-24.
25. Deprest J, Jani J, Gratacos E, Vandecruys H, Naulaers G, Delgado J, et al. FETO Task Group. Fetal intervention for congenital diaphragmatic hernia: the European experience. Semin Perinatol. 2005;29:94-103.
26. Done E, Gratacos E, Nicolaides KH, Allegaert K, Valencia C, Castan'on M, et al. Predictors of neonatal morbidity in fetuses with severe isolated congenital diaphragmatic hernia undergoing fetoscopic tracheal occlusion. Ultrasound Obstet Gynecol. 2013;42:77-83.
27. Ruono R, Yoshisaki CT, Da Silva MM, Ceccons MEJ, Grasis MS, Tannuri U, et al. A randomized controlled trial of fetal endoscopic tracheal occlusion versus postnatal management of severe isolated congenital diaphragmatic hernia. Ultrasound Obstet Gynecol. 2012;39:20-7.
28. Centini G, Rosignoli L, Kenanidis A, et al. Prenatal diagnosis of esophageal atresia with the pouch sign. Ultrasound Obstet Gynecol. 2003;21:494-7.
29. Has R, Gunay S, Topuz S. Pouch sign in prenatal diagnosis of esophageal atresia. Ultrasound Obstet Gynecol. 2004;23(5):523-4.
30. Kalache KD, Wauer R, Mau H, et al. Prognostic significance of the pouch sign in fetuses with prenatally diagnosed esophageal atresia. Am J Obstet Gynecol. 2000;182(4):978-81.
31. Shulman A, Mazkereth R, Zalel Y, Kuint J, Lipitz S, Avigad I, et al. Prenatal identification of esophageal atresia: the role of ultrasonography for evaluation of functional anatomy. Prenat Diagn. 2002;22:669-74.
32. Lawrence MJ, Ford WD, Furness ME, Hayward T, Wilson T. Congenital duodenal obstruction: early antenatal ultrasound diagnosis. Pediatr Surg Int. 2000;16:342-5.
33. Shawis R, Antao B. Prenatal bowel dilatation and the subsequent postnatal management. Early Hum Dev. 2006;82:297-303.
34. Haeusler MC, Berghold A, Stoll C, Barisic I, Clementi M; EUROSCAN Study Group Prenatal ultrasonographic detection of gastrointestinal obstruction: results from 18 European congenital anomaly registries. Prenat Diagn 2002;22:616-23.
35. Has R, Gunay S. 'Whirlpool' sign in the prenatal diagnosis of intestinal volvulus. Ultrasound Obstet Gynecol. 2002;20(3):307-8.
36. Chaubal N, Dighe M, Shah M, Chaubal J, Raghavan J. Calcified meconium: an important sign in the prenatal sonographic diagnosis of cloacal malformation. J Ultrasound Med. 2003;22:727-30.
37. Arbell D, Koplewitz BZ, Pinto M, et al. Postpartum sonographic demonstration of "to-and-from" motion in fetal intestinal obstruction: a novel sign formimmediate postnatal surgery. Ultrasound Obstet Gynecol. 2008;32(1): 112-4.
38. Chan KL, Tang MH, Tse HY, Tang RY, Tam PK. Meconium peritonitis: prenatal diagnosis, postnatal management and outcome. Prenat Diagn. 2005;25:676-82.
39. Agathokleous M, Chaveeva P, Poon LC, et al. Meta-analysis of second-trimester markers for trisomy 21. Ultrasound Obstet Gynecol. 2013;41(3):247-61.
40. Goetzinger KR, Cahill A, Macones G. Echogenic Bowel on Second-Trimester Ultrasound: Evaluating the Risk of Adverse Pregnancy Outcome. Obstet Gynecol. 2011;117(6): 1341-8.
41. Zalel Y, Gilboa Y, Berkenshtat M, Yoeli R, Auslander R, Goldberg Y. Secondary cytomegalovirus infection can cause severe fetal sequelae despite maternal preconceptional immunity. Ultrasound Obstet Gynecol. 2008;31(4):417-20.
42. Al-Kouatly HB, Chasen ST, Streltzoff J, Chervenak FA. The clinical significance of fetal echogenic bowel. Am J Obstet Gynecol. 2001;185:1035-8.
43. Berlin BM, Norton ME, Sugarman EA, et al. Cystic fibrosis and chromosome abnormalities associated with echogenic fetal bowel. Obstet Gynecol. 1999;94:135-8.
44. Slotnik RN, Abuhamad AZ. Study of fetal echogenic bowel (FEB) and its implications. J Ultrasound Med. 1999;18:88.
45. Chen CP, Cheng SJ, Chang TY. Prenatal diagnosis of choledochal cyst using ultrasound and magnetic resonance imaging. Ultrasound Obstet Gynecol. 2004;23:93-4.
46. Macken MB, Wright JR Jr, Lau H, Cooper MC, Grantmyre EB, Thompson DL, et al. Prenatal sonographic detection of congenital hepatic cyst in third trimester after normal second-trimester sonographic examination. J Clin Ultrasound. 2000;28:307-10.
47. Laberge JM, Patenaude Y, Desilets V, Cartier L, Khalife S, Jutras L, et al. Large hepatic mesenchymal hamartoma leading to mid-trimester fetal demise. Fetal Diagn Ther. 2005;20:141-5.

24

CHAPTER

Fetal Neck Pathology

Radu Vlădăreanu, Costin Berceanu

INTRODUCTION

Congenital anomalies of the neck are rare or very uncommon conditions, and for this reason their real incidence is practically unknown. Due to the particular anatomical topography, these abnormalities may comprise certain pathophysiological interferences with the base of the fetal skull, mouth, thorax, mediastinum or musculoskeletal structures.

Thus, even with the contribution of new obstetric imaging perspectives, such as fetal MRI, the precise prenatal diagnosis of such anomalies represents a real challenge.

The most important anomalies of the fetal neck, which we present in this chapter, are represented by cystic hygroma, neck teratoma, fetal goiter and fetal thyroid masses, branchial anomalies, vascular neck abnormalities, thyroglossal duct cyst, cervical thymic cyst, other rare anomalies of the fetal neck and congenital high airway obstruction syndrome.

EMBRYOLOGY

Human embryos include four pairs of well-defined pharyngeal arches. The pharyngeal arches form in craniocaudal succession: First arch—day 22nd; second and third arches—sequentially on day 24th; and fourth arch—day 29th.[1,2]

The basic tissues of the head and neck become organized in the branchial apparatus and the origin of many fetal neck abnormalities consist in this embryologic structure.[3]

Pharyngeal arches consist of a mesenchymal core—mesoderm and neural crest cells—that is covered on the outside with ectoderm and lined on the inside with endoderm.[1,2]

Each arch contains: A central cartilaginous skeletal element, striated muscle rudiments, innervated by an arch specific cranial nerve, and an aortic arch artery.[2]

Arterial blood reaches the head via paired vertebral arteries that form from anastomoses among intersegmental arteries and via the common carotid arteries. The common carotid arteries branch to form the internal and external carotid arteries. The common carotids and the roots of the internal carotids are derived from the third arch arteries, whereas distal portions of the internal carotids are derived from the cranial extensions of the paired dorsal aortae. The endothelium of the head vasculature and aortic arch arteries is derived from mesoderm.[1,2]

The external pharyngeal clefts or grooves between the arches remain separated from the apposed, internal pharyngeal pouches by thin pharyngeal membranes. These membranes are initially two-layered, consisting of ectoderm and endoderm, later being infiltrated by mesenchymal cells.[1,2]

All of the pharyngeal pouches give rise to adult structures. These are the tubotympanic recess, the palatine tonsils, the inferior parathyroid glands, and the ultimobranchial body. The parathyroids, thymus primordia, and ultimobranchial bodies separate from the lining of the pharynx and migrate to their definitive locations within the neck and thorax.[2]

The parathyroid glands and the ultimobranchial bodies migrate inferiorly to become embedded in the posterior wall of the thyroid gland. The two parathyroids exchange position as they migrate: Parathyroid III becomes inferior parathyroid, whereas parathyroid IV becomes the superior parathyroid.[1-3]

The thyroid primordium first forms late in the 4th week and appears as a small, solid mass of endoderm proliferating at the apex of the foramen cecum on the developing tongue. The thyroid primordium descends through the tissues of the neck at the end of a slender thyroglossal duct. The thyroglossal duct breaks down by the end of the 5th week, and the isolated thyroid, now consisting of lateral lobes connected by a well-defined isthmus, continues to descend reaching its final position just inferior to the cricoid cartilage by the 7th week.[1,2]

Lymphatic channels arise by vasculogenesis and angiogenesis from venous precursor cells. Lymphangiogenesis begins with the formation of bilateral sprouts from the anterior cardinal veins at about day 42nd of development. These sprouts eventually form a pair of enlargements, the jugular lymphatic sacs, which will collect fluid from the lymphatic vessels of the upper limbs, upper trunk, head, and neck. In the 6th week, four additional lymphatic sacs develop to collect lymph from the trunk and lower extremities: The retroperitoneal lymphatic sac, cisterna chili, and paired posterior lymphatic sacs are associated with the junctions of the external and internal iliac veins.[1,2]

NECK ANOMALIES

Cystic Hygroma

Cystic hygroma (CH) is a congenital lymphatic malformation. It is the most frequently observed fetal neck pathology on prenatal ultrasound (US).[4]

Cystic hygroma refers to the finding of marked skin thickening extending along the entire length of the fetus at early US examination.[5]

Cystic hygroma represents not a tumor, but an anomaly of the lymphatic drainage into the venous system, which leads to the accumulation of lymph in the jugular lymphatic sacs of the cervical region.[1,3,6]

Based on the presence of septations, it can be classified into septated or nonseptated.[1,4]

However, with the improving resolution and the increasing quality of the image offered by the advance of the US machines, it has become clear that all nuchal translucencies (NTs) have visible septations.[1,3,4,7]

Prevalence, Incidence, and Epidemiology

The true incidence of CH remains unknown. It has been reported to be 1:6,000 at birth and 1:750 among spontaneous abortions.[4,8]

Cystic hygroma is normally caused by aberrant development of lymphatic vessels, as a consequence of an abnormal or absent connection with the venous system, leading to lymphatic stasis and enlargement of the jugular sacs.[1,4,9]

Abnormal lymphatic development in the fetal neck could lead to distension of the jugular venous sacs, an accumulation of fluid in the nuchal region, and retrograde increases in venous pressure.[10]

This hypothesis is supported by the observation that reversed or absent ductus venosus flow during atrial contraction is observed in these fetuses. Eventual recanalization or formation of collaterals may explain the transient nature of abnormal ductus venosus waveforms and nuchal edema.[1,10]

Condition, Etiology, and Pathophysiology

Cystic hygroma is seen frequently in the first trimester, affecting about 1 in 300 pregnancies.[5]

Cystic hygroma is also frequently associated with other malformations and chromosomal abnormalities in approximately 75% of the cases **(Table 1)**.[1,3-5,11-17]

TABLE 1: Genetic and structural abnormalities associated with cystic hygroma (CH).

Achondrogenesis	Lethal skeletal dysplasia with extreme hypoplasia of the bones, micromelia, decreased ossification of the bones, and hydrops
Achondroplasia	Autosomal dominant condition with rhizomelic limb shortening, nonlethal, heterozygous type usually is not apparent until late in the second trimester
Arthrogryposis	Sequence of neurologic, muscular, and connective tissue disorders, CH, or thickened nuchal translucency (NT)
Beckwith–Wiedemann syndrome	Gigantism in utero, macroglossia, omphalocele, and renal abnormalities
Cerebrocostomandibular syndrome	Autosomal recessive, micrognathia, vertebral body abnormalities, and CH/nuchal thickening
CHARGE Association	Coloboma of the iris, heart defect, choanal atresia, fetal growth restriction (FGR), genital anomalies, ear anomalies, and CH
Cornelia de Lange syndrome	Facial/limb anomalies, growth restriction, and mental developmental delay

Contd...

Contd…

Cowchock syndrome (CMTX4)	A slowly progressive X-linked recessive disorder with axonal neuropathy, deafness, and cognitive impairment
Cowden disease	Tumor-like growths—hamartomas. Multiple hamartoma syndrome
Cumming syndrome	Autosomal recessive pattern of inheritance, cervical lymphocele (CH), renal-hepatic-pancreatic dysplasia, short gut, polysplenia, generalized lymphedema, short limbs, and bowed limbs (campomelia)
Cri du Chat syndrome (Deletion 5p)	Abnormality of chromosome 5 characterized by microcephaly, hypertelorism, micrognathia, hydrops, FGR, and CH
Ectrodactyly–ectodermal dysplasia–clefting (EEC) syndrome	Autosomal dominant condition, labial clefting, ectrodactyly, genitourinary tract anomalies, and CH
Fraser syndrome	Cryptophthalmos, syndactyly, genital, renal, and tracheal abnormalities
Fryns syndrome	Autosomal recessive condition with diaphragmatic defects, digital and facial abnormalities, and brain anomalies
Hereditary lymphedema	Dysfunction of the lymphatic system. Hypoplasia or aplasia of lymphatic channels. Usually segregating as an autosomal dominant trait
Lymphedema-distichiasis syndrome	Rare genetic multisystem disorder. Lower limb lymphedema and distichiasis. Distichiasis, which may be present at birth, is observed in 94% of affected individuals
Multiple pterygium syndrome	Autosomal recessive condition, multiple contractures and webbing across joints, CH, facial defects
Noonan syndrome	Phenotypically, a Turner-like syndrome, short stature, webbed neck, cardiac abnormalities, and normal karyotype
Oculodentodigital syndrome	Caused by mutations in the *GJA1* gene. Oculodentodigital dysplasia presents with a spectrum of clinical features including craniofacial, ocular, dental, and limb anomalies
Opitz-Frias syndrome	X-linked Opitz G/BBB syndrome (XLOS) is a multiple congenital anomaly disorder, facial anomalies, hypertelorism, prominent forehead, broad nasal bridge, laryngotracheoesophageal defects, and genitourinary abnormalities
Pena–Shokeir syndrome	Autosomal recessive condition, FGR, multiple joint contractures, facial anomalies, and pulmonary hypoplasia
Pentalogy of Cantrell	Ectopia cordis, omphalocele, disruption of the distal sternum, anterior diaphragm, and diaphragmatic pericardium
Perlman syndrome	Autosomal recessive syndrome, fetal overgrowth, macrosomia, bilaterally enlarged kidneys, renal tumors, polyhydramnios, and CH
Polysplenia/asplenia syndrome	Defects in lateralization of normal body asymmetry, severe heart defects, and anomalies of the intrathoracic and intraabdominal viscera
Proteus syndrome	Asymmetric focal overgrowth, subcutaneous tumors, lipomas, hamartomatous, and lymphatic malformations
Roberts syndrome	Severe shortening of the limbs and facial anomalies
Thrombocytopenia-absent radius (TAR) syndrome	Autosomal recessive syndrome, radial aplasia, and thrombocytopenia
Triploidy	Complete extra set of chromosomes, lethal abnormality, early-onset FGR, and multiple anomalies
Williams syndrome	Distinctive facies, congenital cardiovascular malformations, intellectual disabilities, and various other manifestations
Zellweger syndrome	Prototype of peroxisomal disorders characterized by craniofacial dysmorphism and severe neurologic abnormalities, growth restriction, and gastrointestinal malformations

Cystic hygroma has been related to inherited disorders and malformation syndromes in euploid fetuses and to drug intake, including alcohol, aminopterin, and trimethadione.[1,4,18]

There are studies suggesting that septations predict an increased likelihood of aneuploidies.[1,8]

Cystic hygroma in the first trimester has clearly visible septations running transversely between the fetal skin and underlying subcutaneous tissue. It appears that the diagnosis of this finding early in pregnancy represents a completely different entity than the diagnosis of CH in later pregnancy.[5]

The latter condition is typically an isolated structural abnormality of lymphatic drainage and appears to have little or no association with chromosomal abnormality or other malformation.[1,4,5]

The anomaly is visible from the first trimester, and it represents the end of the spectrum of the increased NT.[1]

Recent studies suggest a higher prevalence of Down syndrome on one hand, but on the other hand, Turner syndrome is the most common associated chromosomal abnormality, also affecting approximately 60% of cases.[1,4]

Other chromosomal abnormalities include autosomal trisomies, Klinefelter syndrome, partial trisomies, partial monosomies, translocations, and mosaicisms.[1,4,5,8]

Diagnosis and Imaging Findings

Ultrasound: CH typically develops late in the first trimester and is characterized by the presence of posterior and posterolateral fluid-filled cavities in the fetal neck **(Figs. 1A and B)**. These cavities are quite variable in size. Nuchal hygromas are frequently bilateral, separated by the nuchal ligament, resembling a complex mass with one or more septa in the center[1,4,8,19] **(Fig. 1C)**.

Lymphatic malformations contain dysplastic but mature lymphatic channels.[3] These are multilocular cystic masses with posterior acoustic enhancement and vascular flow limited to the internal septations.[3,8]

The central sonographic criteria for diagnosing CH in the first trimester of pregnancy is the presence of a significantly enlarged NT measurement that extends along the entire length of the fetal back, and in which septations are clearly visible in transverse section through the fetal neck[1,3,5,19] **(Figs. 2A to C)**.

Natural history of CH may be variable. It can resolve spontaneously or progressively affect other fetal structures separate from the neck (pleura, pericardium, and abdomen) leading to hydrops fetalis in 75% of the cases, resulting in fetal demise.[1,4,5,20,21]

Cystic hygroma is associated with other malformations in 60% of cases including cardiac defects, skeletal dysplasias, genitourinary system abnormalities, congenital diaphragmatic hernia, and central nervous system abnormalities.[1,4,22]

The main problem in the diagnosis of CH remains the differential diagnosis in the first trimester, between the enlarged nuchal thickening and when it meets criteria to be termed CH or whether it should be considered a simple increased NT.

Ultrasound imaging: Overdistension of the jugular lymphatic sacs that are located in both sides of the neck results in the formation of a cystic structure that is usually

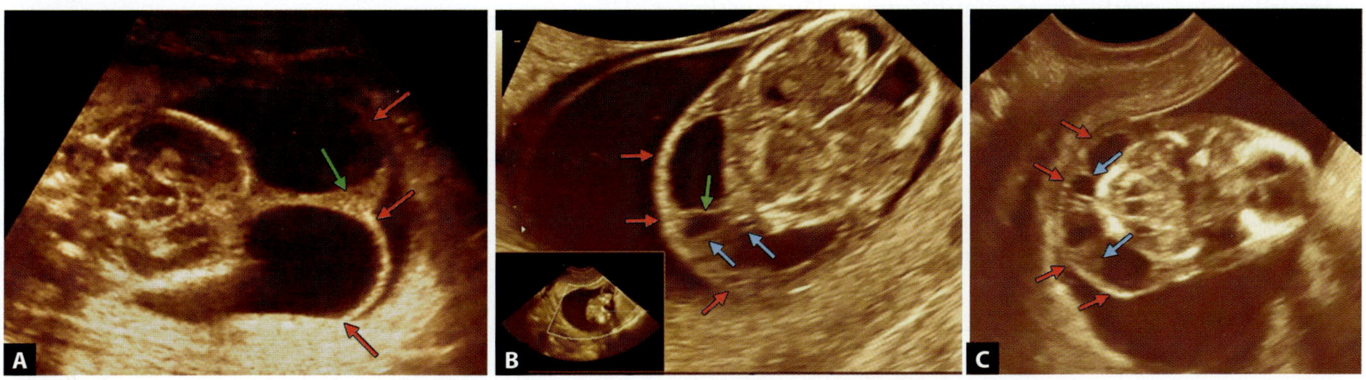

Figs. 1A to C: (A) Axial view of septated cystic hygroma (CH) (red arrows) in early second-trimester ultrasound (US). Two separate fluid accumulations are visible, the nuchal ligament (green arrow) is spotlighted; (B) Axial view of septated CH (red arrows), the nuchal ligament (green arrow), and clearly visible septations (blue arrows); (C) Axial view of septated CH (red arrows), typical honeycomb appearance (blue arrows), and intact calvarial bones.

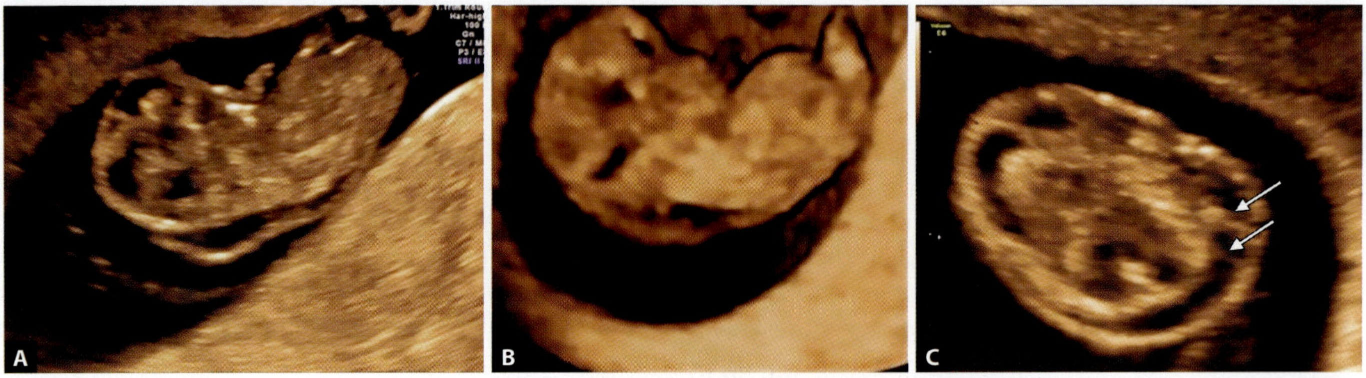

Figs. 2A to C: (A) Sagittal view of cystic hygroma (CH) in the first trimester demonstrating a significantly enlarged nuchal translucency (NT) measurement that extends along the entire length of the fetal back; (B) Three-dimensional surface rendered view of fetus with CH at 9 weeks of gestation. Increased dimensions of the nuchal region extending along the entire length of the fetal back; (C) Axial view of septated CH at 9 weeks of gestation. Septations are clearly visible in transverse section through the fetal neck (arrows).

partitioned by a thick fibrous band corresponding to the nuchal ligament. Within the cystic structure, thinner septa are seen and probably represent fibrous structures of the neck or deposits of fibrin, giving to the lesion a typical honeycomb appearance[1,23] **(Fig. 1C)**.

There is a correlation between increased NT and CH. CH can be regarded as the most severe end of the spectrum of increased NT. Generally, when NT is in excess of 4 mm, septa are seen within it.[23]

Septated CH, using the definition as described above, can be easily identified in the first trimester. If the nuchal thickening does not extend along the entire length of the fetal back, and if transverse septations are not clearly visible, then the term NT should be used[1,5] **(Figs. 3A and B)**.

Magnetic resonance imaging (MRI): MRI demonstrates a multilocular cystic trans-spatial mass. The cystic component is typically isointense to muscle on T1 and hyperintense on T2-weighted images, unless complicated by protein or hemorrhage, in which case there may be fluid-fluid levels.[3]

In late pregnancy, MRI can be useful in prenatal evaluation of airway access and extension of the lymphatic abnormalities to plan an adequate delivery and perinatal management.[4,24]

Differential diagnoses of CH[1,3,4] are spotlighted in **Table 2**.

Management, Outcome, and Recurrence Risk

Cystic hygroma is the most frequently seen fetal neck mass on first trimester US. Overall prognosis is poor with a high

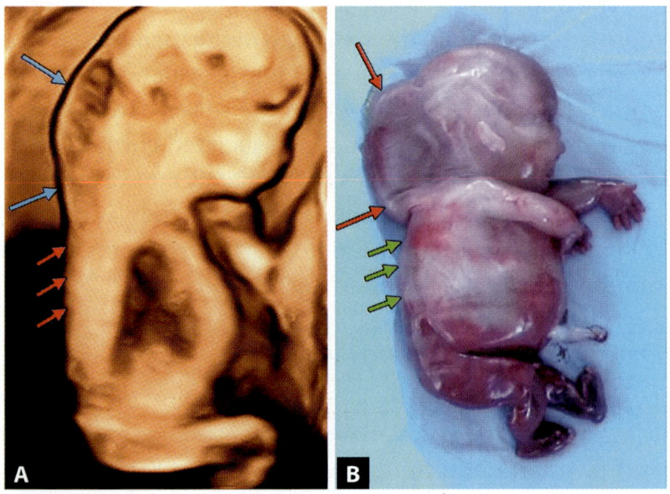

Figs. 3A and B: (A) Three-dimensional surface-rendered view of fetus with cystic hygroma (CH) at 14 weeks of gestation. Increased dimensions of the nuchal region (blue arrows) extending along the entire length of the fetal back (red arrows); (B) Gross image of the postabortum specimen demonstrating CH (red arrows) extending along the fetal back (green arrows) and fetal hydrops.

association with chromosomal and structural defects and progression to hydrops and fetal demise[1,4,5,23] **(Table 3)**.

Recurrence risk for CH associated with fetal aneuploidies should be provided based on the individual chromosomal abnormality. For cases of fetal trisomy, recurrence risk is generally of about 1%, the maternal age-related risk is even higher. For cases with Turner syndrome, there is no significant increased risk of recurrence beyond the general population risk. Similarly, the risk of recurrence in cases with cardiac malformations should be individualized.[4,5,23]

This chapter addresses this lymphatic malformation using the term CH, considering this entity much more widespread in obstetric imaging.

However, the International Society for the Study of Vascular Anomalies, with most recent additions, consider this pathology using the term nuchal macrocystic lymphatic malformation.[25,26]

Neck Teratoma

Cervical teratomas are rare tumors that vary in size and generally consist of a mixture of cystic and solid components, frequently with internal calcifications.[1,23]

Teratomas are the most common histological type of fetal tumors that are rather rare. The neck is the most common location after the sacrococcygeal region for teratomas. The tissues found in fetal and infant teratomas are essentially the same regardless of the site of origin. A neck teratoma may be associated with neonatal mortality in 80–100% of cases if delivery is not managed properly. Ex utero intrapartum treatment (EXIT) and intensive neonatal care are essential to improve outcome.[27]

Fetal cervical teratoma is a normally benign tumor in the neck composed of multiple tissues derived from all three germ layers of the embryonic disk (ectoderm, mesoderm, and endoderm) and are derived from primordial germ cells (PGCc), with a high potential of growing in excess[1,2,27] **(Figs. 4A and B)**.

Some of these tumors may be malignant or may develop malignancies later into adult life.

Cervical teratomas arise from totipotential germ cells or as an end result of a defective twin pregnancy with fetus in fetu.[3,5]

Cervical teratomas are found in about 1:20,000 to 1:40,000 live births, accounting for 3–6% of all neonatal teratomas. The presentation is sporadic, without an apparent relationship to race, maternal age, parity, or fetal sex.[27,28]

TABLE 2: Differential diagnoses of CH.

Increased NT	Main differential diagnosis for CH. Nuchal thickening does not extend along the entire length of the fetal back. Transverse septations are not clearly visible
Occipital encephalocele and meningocele	Defect in the calvaria and the absence of gyral pattern
Hemangioma	Normally irregularly shaped, low-level echoes and color Doppler showing vascularization
Teratoma	Located anteriorly, hyperextension of the fetal neck, and a solid or mixed-solid mass
Goiter	Bilobed mass in the anterior region
Other	Sarcoma, melanoma, brachial cleft cyst, thyroglossal duct cyst, laryngocele, fibroma, lipoma, and metastases

(CH: cystic hygroma; NT: nuchal translucency)

Condition, Etiology, and Pathophysiology

In fetuses, tumors may result from failure of developing tissues to undergo normal cytodifferentiation and maturation.[1,27] Cervical teratomas are mixed cystic and solid lesions arising in the anterior midline neck, being thus constituted of a combination of skin, skin appendages, cartilage, muscle, and respiratory and gastrointestinal epithelium.[3,29]

The pluripotency of teratomas is exhibited by the fact that they can give rise to variety of definitive anatomic structures.[2]

TABLE 3: Management of CH in the first trimester.

Step 1	First trimester diagnosis of CH	Counseling regarding fetal aneuploidy (50%)	Diagnostic testing—CVS
Step 2	CVS—no evidence for aneuploidy	Counseling regarding fetal residual risk of major structural malformation (50%). Most likely malformations are cardiac and skeletal	• Comprehensive fetal US anatomic survey • Fetal echocardiography • Serial assessment of fetal status • 16–20 weeks gestation*
Step 3	Fetal evaluation confirms a structurally normal fetus	Counseling of a 95% likelihood of normal short-term pediatric outcome. A residual risk of 5% for abnormal pediatric outcome should be described	Long-term outcome—minimal data available

*Early fetal anatomic evaluations can be performed using a combined approach, starting with an abdominal survey and assessing details through high-resolution transvaginal ultrasound (US); experienced ultrasonographers can detect many major malformations in the first trimester. Fetal echocardiography may be attempted as early as the first trimester. According to the quality of image and the US findings, fetal heart may be reassessed at 14, 16, 18, or 20 weeks.

(CH: cystic hygroma; CVS: chorionic villus sampling)

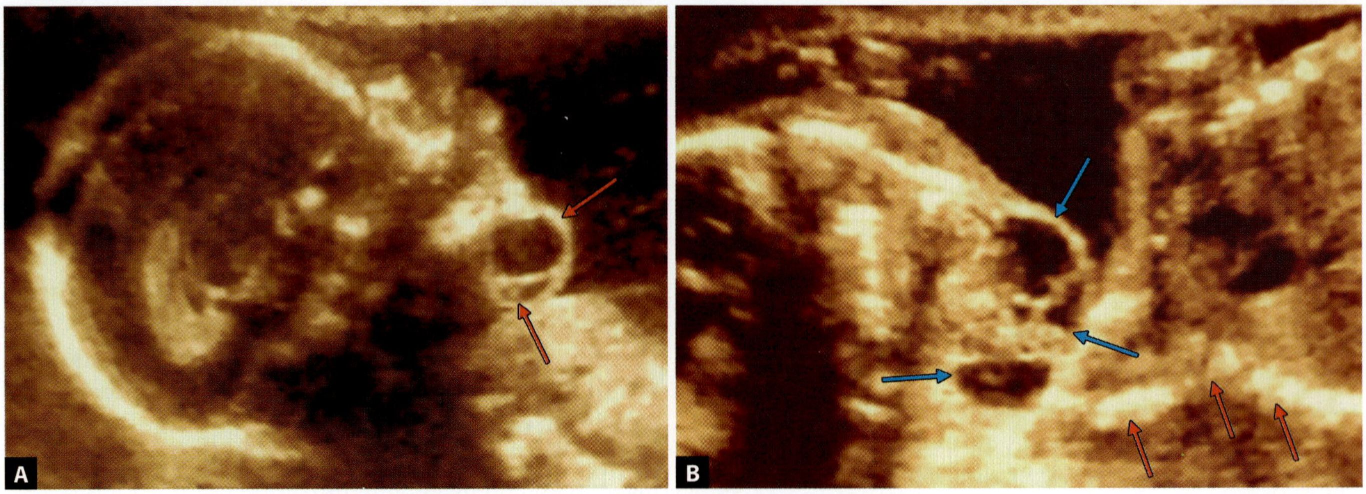

Figs. 4A and B: (A) Sagittal view of a neck teratoma (red arrows), significant distortion in the neck contour, predominantly cystic, well-encapsulated mass; (B) Neck teratoma located in the anterolateral region (blue arrows). The tumor is large and bulky, producing mass effect and extended position of the neck (red arrows).

The development of fetal tumors does not match the same processes as tumors observed in adults. Cervical teratomas may originate from the palate, nasopharynx, or thyrocervical area. They are usually closely thyroid related, and there is also the hypothesis that these masses likely originate in the thyroid gland, based on the presence of a thin pseudocapsule in continuity between the mass and the thyroid.[3,30]

Teratomas are classified into mature and immature types.[2,3] The immature type contains embryonic cells, usually neural, and occur more commonly in the cervical region, compared with other extragonadal teratomas.[3,31]

Mature or immature neuroglial tissues are the most frequent component, but cartilage, respiratory epithelium, and ependymal-lined cysts are common. Malignancy is extremely rare. Immature elements present do not express the biologic behavior.[1,2,27]

Most immature teratomas are not malignant; however, the presence of yolk sac tumor cells carries a higher association with malignancy and recurrence.[3,31,32]

Conventional anatomic US scan, usually in the second trimester, may diagnose the neck teratoma. With large masses, obstruction of the airways and esophagus leads frequently to polyhydramnios. The diagnosis may be as early as the first trimester.

Diagnosis and Imaging Findings

Ultrasound: Targeting the diagnosis as early as the first trimester is not most often possible. However, diagnosis of a teratoma can be made early in pregnancy (15–16 weeks gestation), but the tumor is usually detected on routine second-trimester screening for fetal abnormalities (18–23 weeks gestation) or targeted US scan after initial diagnosis of polyhydramnios **(Figs. 4A and B)**.

The key sign is the distortion in neck contour by the presence of an asymmetric, unilateral, and well-encapsulated mass. The tumor is usually large and bulky (4–12 cm in diameter),[3] with mixed echostructure of cystic and solid components. Echogenic foci of calcifications are present in about half of all cases. The presence of calcifications is fairly specific for the diagnosis of teratoma.[3] Located anterior to the neck, the tumor may produce a mass effect on surrounding tissues from the ear to the jaw or extend into the mediastinum. Large tumors result in severe hyperextension of the fetal head. Polyhydramnios is considered an indication of severity. It is related to tumor size and reflects impaired swallowing by mouth obstruction or esophageal compression[1,3,27,33,34] **(Figs. 5A and B)**.

The differential diagnosis of these anomalies with lymphatic malformations and branchial cleft cysts consists in the first instance, in their location, as cervical teratomas occur anteriorly, while lymphatic malformations are usually located in the posterolateral neck, and branchial cleft cysts are typically lateral.[3,4,27]

The risk of chromosomal anomalies or non-chromosomal syndromes is low, but various associated anomalies have been reported, including trisomy 13, hypoplastic left ventricle, and central nervous system

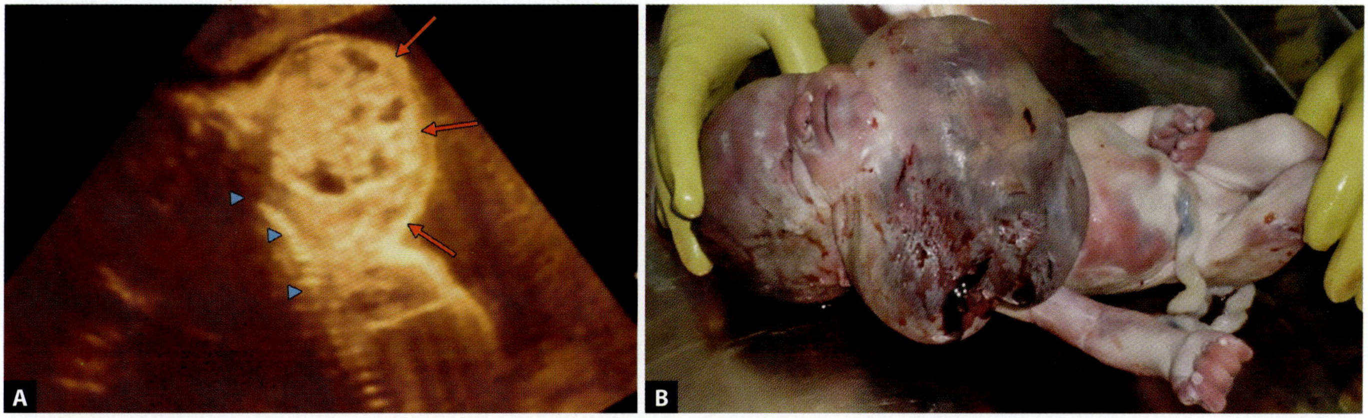

Figs. 5A and B: (A) Two-dimensional sonogram in sagittal view demonstrating a massive neck teratoma (red arrows), severe mass effect, and hyperextended position of the neck (blue arrows), especially with solid component; (B) Macroimage demonstrating the immediate postnatal condition.

TABLE 4: Differential diagnoses of the neck teratoma.

Lymphatic malformations	Large, unilateral, multiloculated, predominantly cystic tumor often with intrathoracic extension, complicated by hydrops
Cystic hygroma (CH)	Posteriorly located, septated cystic tumors, relatively characteristic
Goiter	Homogenous, echogenic, and symmetric mass in the anterior neck
Other neck masses	Amniotic band syndrome, solid thyroid tumors, thyroglossal duct cyst, branchial cleft cyst, laryngocele, parotid tumor, neuroblastoma, hemangioma, hamartoma, lipoma, and fibroma

anomalies. The protocol should include detailed fetal US, echocardiography, neurosonogram, and fetal caryotype.[27,35,36]

Tumor vascularization and characteristics could be assessed by color Doppler, power or high definition modes.

Differential diagnoses of the neck teratoma[1,11,27] are marked out in **Table 4**.

Three-dimensional US may enhance the accuracy of prenatal diagnosis and provide additional detailed information on aspects related with location, extension, and intracranial spread.[1,27]

Magnetic resonance imaging: MRI is valuable in confirming the diagnosis of cervical teratomas[3] and may provide additional information about tumor location calcifications, extension, facial involvement, and intracranial spread.[27]

Magnetic resonance imaging can estimate lung volumes, helpful in predicting the presence of pulmonary hypoplasia complicating fetal cervical teratoma.[37] In these cases, the carina is retracted superiorly, resulting in compression of the lungs in the upper thorax with resultant poor lung development.[3,38]

It can demonstrate the internal architecture and extent of the tumor, showing a well-defined complex mass with multiloculated cystic and solid components. Intratumoral hemorrhage can be seen as dark signal on gradient echo images and bright signal on T1-weighted images.[3]

Magnetic resonance imaging also allows evaluation of the relationship of the mass to the trachea, information of critical importance in planning delivery, normally by EXIT, and postnatal surgery.[1,3,27,39-41]

Fetal MRI performed during the pregnancy for investigation of fetal neck masses detected on US gives compatible results observed in the neonate after birth and maintains adequate findings for follow-up and planning of treatment.[24]

Management, Outcome, and Recurrence Risk

Cervical teratomas are associated with high mortality rates. Prenatal US diagnosis of cervical teratoma can be made at 15–16 weeks of gestation. Tracheal and esophageal obstruction can lead to polyhydramnios or to airway compromise in the newborn. No direct fetal treatment is available, but management often requires amnioreduction secondary to polyhydramnios and risk of preterm labor. Delivery must be planned with EXIT in a tertiary care center to reduce the risk of serious complications, which can occur even in apparently successful resuscitations and include brain damage or death associated with severe pulmonary hypoplasia.[27,42-44]

Early resection is the treatment of choice. Delaying surgery can result in further complications, including retention of secretions, atelectasis, and pneumonia owing to interference with swallowing.[27,45]

Because the thyroid and parathyroid glands may be removed or affected by tumor excision, the risk of permanent hypothyroidism must be considered. Malignancy risk is very low.[1,27,46]

Fetal endoscopic tracheal intubation (FETI) is targeting to ensure extrauterine tracheal permeability.[47]

Fetal endoscopic tracheal intubation is a technique where the fetal airway is secured in utero via intubation by percutaneous endoscopic fetal tracheoscopy under US guidance. FETI has been described in large fetal neck masses with anatomical airway compression as a feasible airway management strategy and a potential alternative to an EXIT procedure in select cases.[48,49]

Neck teratoma is considered to be a spontaneous malformation such that risk for recurrence in subsequent pregnancies would not be anticipated.[50]

Fetal Goiter and Fetal Thyroid Masses

Fetal goiter (FG) or thyromegaly is a diffuse enlargement of the fetal thyroid gland. Goiter in the fetus can occur as part of a hypothyroid, hyperthyroid, or euthyroid state.[1,5]

It is defined on US as a thyroid circumference or diameter greater than the 95th centile for gestational age. It is frequently associated with maternal thyroid dysfunction, generally hypothyroidism.[51,52]

Goiter associated with fetal hypothyroidism can be caused by transplacental passage of antithyroid medications being used by a mother with hyperthyroidism, iodine deficiency or intoxication, transplacental passage of antithyroid antibodies, congenital metabolic disorders of thyroid hormone synthesis, or hypothalamic-pituitary hypothyroidism.[1,5,53]

Prevalence, Incidence, and Epidemiology

Fetal goiter is very rare.[3] The prevalence of goitrous hypothyroidism is 1:30,000 to 1:50,000 live births in Europe and North America.[51] Hypothyroid goiter is more common than hyperthyroid goiter.[1,5] Iodine deficiency is still considered a major health problem worldwide.[52] However, only a small fraction of the estimated prevalence will be diagnosed prenatally with FG.[1,5]

Condition, Etiology, and Pathophysiology

In the euthyroid fetus, the main potential problem associated with goiter is obstruction of trachea or esophagus as the goiter enlarges with pregnancy progression. This may lead to polyhydramnios on one hand, and on the other hand to hyperextension of the fetal neck.[5,54,55]

Congenital goiters are most commonly diagnosed in mothers with known thyroid disease, usually Graves' disease. Graves' disease is a common cause of hyperthyroidism that is present in 0.2% of pregnant.[51,56,57] Fetuses of mothers with thyroid disease are especially susceptible to develop congenital hyperthyroid goiter owing to the passage of antibodies against the thyroid-stimulating hormone (TSH) receptor (TRAb), also called thyroid-stimulating immunoglobulin, found in 1% of children born from mothers with Graves' disease. Fetuses can also develop congenital goitrous hypothyroidism because of the transplacental passage of propylthiouracil, or occasionally inhibitory immunoglobulins.[1,51]

Fetal goiter associated with hyperthyroidism may result in significant fetal changes including: Tachycardia, cardiac hypertrophy, hydrops, FGR, fetal death, intellectual impairment, and preterm birth.[5] Congenital goitrous hyperthyroidism is most frequently caused by maternal antibodies or dyshormonogenesis.[1,51]

When considering all cases of congenital goitrous hypothyroidism, almost 80% are due to thyroid dysgenesis and may be related to somatic mutations in the TSH receptor. Nearly 15% of cases are due to dyshormonogenesis or transplacental passage of TSH receptor blocking antibodies.[1,58] Dyshormonogenesis is the most frequent cause in the absence of maternal thyroid disease or iodine deficiency; it is frequently caused by recessively inherited biochemical defects in one or more steps in the pathway leading to the normal synthesis of thyroid hormones.[1,51]

Fetal goiter secondary to hypothyroidism may result in fetal bradycardia, heart block, or cardiomegaly[1,5,51] **(Table 5)**.

Fetal goiter as a result of the enlarged thyroid gland, progressing to a global thyroid mass, can be detected by a dedicated US evaluation of the fetal neck or by the complications that it may cause.

Exceptionally, FG with hypothyroidism has been associated with other congenital abnormalities, such as Prader–Willi syndrome.[3,59]

Sonographic screening for FG may be difficult because of problems in accurately identifying the fetal thyroid during early gestation.[1,5]

TABLE 5: Fetal complications of the goiter and thyroid masses.

Fetal complications by compression and the mass effect:	
Esophageal obstruction	• Can cause polyhydramnios • Risk of preterm delivery
Tracheal obstruction	• Can cause perinatal asphyxia • Need for intubation • EXIT (ex utero intrapartum treatment)
Neck hyperextension	Consequent fetal dystocia
Fetal complications consequent to thyroid dysfunction:	
Fetal hyperthyroidism	• Fetal growth restriction (FGR) • Tachycardia • Cardiac hypertrophy • Intrauterine death by cardiac failure • Accelerated bone maturation • Thyrotoxicosis • Hepatosplenomegaly • Craniosynostosis with intellectual impairment • Hydrops • Preterm birth
Fetal hypothyroidism or untreated congenital hypothyroidism	• Bradycardia • Heart block • Cardiomegaly • Impaired motor and intellectual development in the later stages of life in some affected infants • The degree of neurologic impairment has been related to the severity of fetal hypothyroidism as assessed by the age at diagnosis, the lower serum thyroxine concentrations, and the delay in postnatal treatment • An early diagnosis should be made • Subsequent treatment should be promptly started before potentially irreversible neurologic damage occurs secondary to insufficient thyroid hormone levels

Diagnosis and Imaging Findings

Ultrasound: FG is diagnosed by US at an average gestational age of 26 weeks.[3,60] The classic US findings of the FG spotlight a homogeneous, echogenic, symmetric mass in the anterior fetal neck, and sometimes with some lobulation.[1,5] The thyroid is symmetrically enlarged with bilobed configuration and varying echogenicity, either homogeneous or heterogeneous with multiple cysts[3] **(Fig. 6A)**.

When FG is suspected, the transverse width and circumference of the thyroid gland should be measured. The diagnosis should be made when these measurements are above the 95th centile based on the nomograms for gestational age. Some US signs can be helpful in determining if the FG is associated with hypothyroidism or hyperthyroidism[1,23,51,56] **(Table 6)**.

The fetal neck is often maintained in a state of hyperextension and the trachea and esophagus may be compressed or displaced by the enlarged gland.[1,3] Later in pregnancy, as swallowing becomes more difficult, polyhydramnios may be induced[1,3] **(Fig. 6C)**.

In fetuses with hyperthyroid goiter, additional US findings include tachycardia, advanced bone age, hydrops, FGR, and hepatosplenomegaly. In those with hypothyroid goiter, US may reveal cardiac dysfunction and delayed bone age[1,3,51,56] **(Table 6)**.

Color Doppler US showing a high-flow pattern confirms the diagnosis of FG but does not imply fetal hyperthyroidism, as hypothyroid FGs may also have increased vascularity. Color Doppler of the thyroid may show peripheral vascularization that reflects a hypertrophic but inactive thyroid gland, more commonly present in hypothyroid goiters.[1]

However, in fetuses with hyperthyroid goiter with high-output cardiac failure, Doppler may show

TABLE 6: Indirect ultrasound (US) signs of fetal thyroid dysfunction.

Bone maturation	• Accelerated bone maturation is defined as the presence of distal femoral ossification before 31 weeks of gestation and is frequently present in hyperthyroidism • Delayed bone maturation is defined as the absence of this center after 33 weeks of gestation and is more frequently present in hypothyroidism
Fetal tachycardia	Fetal tachycardia, defined as a continuous heart rate >160 beats/min, is an indirect sign of hyperthyroidism
Fetal movements	Hypothyroid fetuses showed more frequently increased jerky movements, which were absent in cases of hyperthyroidism
Polyhydramnios	When fetal goiter (FG) is suspected, the amniotic fluid should be always evaluated using the amniotic fluid index because of the potential compression of the fetal esophagus. Polyhydramnios is related to goiter volume rather than etiology. When polyhydramnios is present, cervical length should be measured

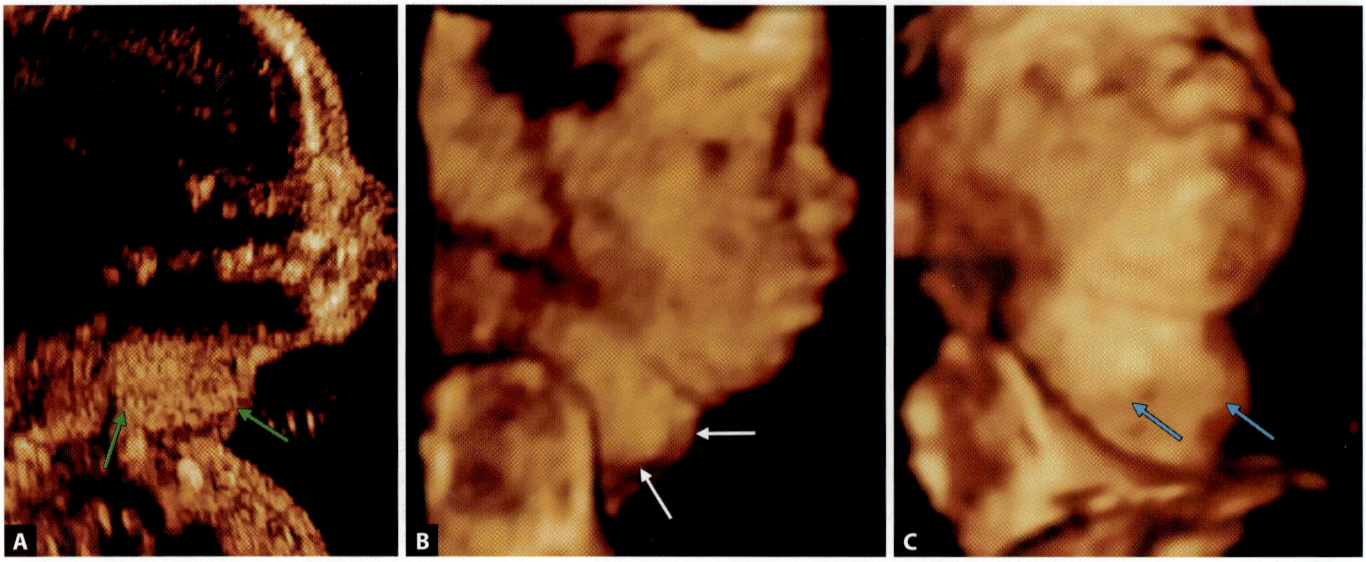

Figs. 6A to C: (A) Fetal goiter (FG) in sagittal view (green arrows). Homogeneous, echogenic mass in the anterior fetal neck; (B and C) Three-dimensional imaging of a FG. Surface rendering demonstrating the appearance of the thyroid mass (white arrows), sometimes with some lobulation (blue arrows).

increased velocities in the common carotid artery and descending aorta, and dilatation of the superior vena cava.[3] Cardiomegaly and pleural effusions have been also reported.[3,61]

The disappearance or reduction of the mass or the Doppler signal may be associated with improvement in fetal thyroid status.[1,51,56]

Enlargement of the thyroid may result in neck hyperextension seen via 2D and 3D US.[3] 3D US in fetal thyroid masses is helpfully **(Figs. 6B and C)** and may facilitate the mother's understanding of the FG, which may obtain better treatment compliance. 3D US could also be useful in assessing the reduction in size and volume of the FG after treatment.[51]

Magnetic resonance imaging: It is a complementary imaging mode to study fetal thyroid masses, and its use has been reported in cases of goitrous hypothyroidism during pregnancy.[1,5,51]

The normal thyroid gland is hyperintense on T1-weighted images and isointense on T2-weighted images, relative to muscle.[3,62]

In FG, there is symmetric thyroid enlargement with increased T1 and intermediate T2 signals.[3,63]

Magnetic resonance imaging of congenital hypothyroid goiters shows a T1 and T2 signal hyperintensity.[1,51] Thyroid enlargement with T2 signal greater than muscle suggests thyroid dysfunction, either hypo- or hyperthyroid state. Intrinsic thyroid T1 hyperintensity persists despite hypo- or hyperthyroid state.[3,64]

Fetal MRI can be beneficial in assessing the compromise and compression of the esophagus and trachea and when neonatal intubation may seem unavoidable.[1,3,5,51]

Differential diagnoses of FG[1,3,5,51] are marked out in **Table 7**.

Management, Outcome, and Recurrence Risk

Fetal goiters are rare. FG is usually self-limited and has good prognosis.[3]

They are associated more frequently with fetal hypothyroidism and less frequently with fetal hyperthyroidism. Prenatal euthyroid goiters can also exist. Screening for FGs should be carried out in pregnancies of mothers with thyroid disease, especially Graves' disease. If an FG is detected, a detailed US examination should be performed looking for signs of either hyperthyroidism or hypothyroidism. If the neck mass is large enough to compress the esophagus, polyhydramnios may be present, and a preterm delivery could occur. If there is tracheal occlusion, there is a risk of neonatal asphyxia, and the need for intubation should be anticipated. When an FG is detected, fetal thyroid function should be assessed, preferentially by cordocentesis. If there is congenital hypothyroidism, intra-amniotic instillation of LT-4 is the preferred treatment option, although the dosage and the

TABLE 7: Differential diagnoses of the fetal goiter and thyroid masses.

Thyroglossal duct cysts	• The most common congenital anomaly of thyroid development • Persistence of the thyroglossal duct • Usually disappears by the 8th week of gestation • Accumulation of fluid can result in a ductal cyst • It can be located anywhere from the base of the tongue to the thyroid isthmus • It can be anechoic, hypoechoic, or complex
Thyroid teratomas	• They can be solid, semicystic, or multiloculated • Derive from the embryonic thyroid anlage • Fetal thyroid teratomas generally are considered benign tumors
Cervical teratomas	• Usually midline • Mixed (cystic and solid) • Rapid growth and greater degree of mass effect upon the airway and esophagus • Faster and more important secondary polyhydramnios when compared with goiter
Ectopic thymus	• Aberrant migration of the thymus causes the ectopic presence of remnants anywhere in the mediastinum, base of the skull, tracheal bifurcation, or cervical region • Ectopic thymus is rarely symptomatic
Lymphatic malformations	• Usually lateral rather than medial • Predominantly cystic
Branchial cleft cysts	• Result from incomplete involution of the branchial apparatus • Lack of any solid elements or septations
Hemangiomas	Characteristically high vessel density and flow
Other conditions	Cystic hygroma (CH), lymphatic malformations or hemangiomas, cervical rhabdomyosarcoma, cervical neuroblastomas, and cervical meningocele

intervals of administration are not standardized. The main objective of intrauterine treatment for FGs is to decrease the mass size and secondarily to normalize thyroid function.[1,23,51,56,65]

Recurrence of FG in subsequent pregnancies is a significant circumstance when a mother has thyroid dysfunction. About 2–12% of all infants of mothers with Graves' disease will have hypo- or hyperthyroidism. Overall, the recurrence risk in such circumstances is 25%.[3,5,23,51,56]

Branchial Anomalies

Branchial anomalies are a consequence of abnormal development of the branchial apparatus during embryogenesis.[66] Prenatal diagnosis of branchial apparatus anomalies is very rare.[3]

Branchial remnants are congenital malformations that arise from incomplete obliteration of the branchial apparatus during embryogenesis.[67]

Condition, Etiology, and Pathophysiology

Up to 95% of branchial cleft cysts are thought to arise from the second branchial arch, with the remaining 5% originating from the first and third arches, and only a few cases of fourth branchial cleft cysts have been reported.[66]

Defects in the embryogenesis of the branchial apparatus include branchial, parathyroid, and thymic anomalies, which may manifest as sinuses, fistulas, or cysts.[3]

The vast majority of branchial cysts originate from the second branchial cleft and pouch, and they are usually located at the anterior border of the sternocleidomastoid muscle, at the junction of its upper and middle thirds.[66]

The pathogenesis seems to emphasize the fact that branchial anomalies have vestigial remnants resulting from incomplete obliteration of the branchial apparatus or buried epithelial cell rests.[3,66,67] Third and fourth branchial apparatus anomalies are rare. These anomalies arise from the piriform sinus and course through the deep spaces of the neck, often descending into the mediastinum along the tracheoesophageal groove.[68]

Diagnosis and Imaging Findings

Ultrasound: Branchial cysts are round or ovoid anechoic or hypoechoic thin-walled cysts. Real-time imaging can demonstrate movement of internal echoes differentiating from a solid lesion.[3]

TABLE 8: Differential diagnoses and associated conditions of the branchial anomalies.

Differential diagnoses (branchial cysts are typically lateral)	• Thymic cyst • Lymphatic malformation • Thyroglossal duct cyst (predominately midline) • Fetal goiter and fetal thyroid masses
Associated anomalies	• Branchio-oto-renal syndrome • Usually isolated

Other US findings can demonstrate a lateral cystic neck mass and communication between the airway and cyst.[68] Doppler imaging can demonstrate the absence of intralesional vascular flow. Real-time imaging can show fluctuation in the size of the cystic lesion with fetal breathing motion.[66-68]

Magnetic resonance imaging: Cysts are hypointense on T1-weighted sequences and hyperintense on T2-weighted sequences.[3] Second trimester T2-weighted fetal MRI can demonstrate unilocular cystic lesion, having tubular shape with a medial beak, with or without mass effect on the airway. Postcontrast T1-weighted image can show communication with the airway.[68]

Differential diagnoses and associated anomalies[3,51,66-68] are marked out in **Table 8**.

Management and Outcome

Surgical excision is considered the definite therapy, and earlier treatment may potentially spare these patients from associated morbidity.[68] Also, surgical resection, and marsupialization of the tract, is curative.[3] Rarely, branchial cleft cyst can cause airway or esophageal obstruction and necessitate EXIT procedure.[3,66-68]

As complications, there can be hemorrhage, infection, and questionable predisposition to cancer.[3] In most cases, the prognosis is excellent following complete resection.[3,66-68]

Vascular Neck Abnormalities

Vascular anomaly is an all-encompassing term that includes both vascular malformations and vascular tumors.[3]

Vascular malformations assume the existence of a combination of anomalous primordial arterial, venous, or lymphatic vessels.[69] They are classified according to hemodynamics into high-flow and low-flow malformations[3,69] **(Table 9)**.

TABLE 9: Vascular malformations classification.

Low-flow malformations	• Often present as mass-like lesions • Consist of pure or combined malformations of capillary, lymphatic, and venous channels • Head and neck—the most common locations • When the lymphatic vascular component is prevalent, lesions are called lymphatic malformations • Predominantly lymphatic lesions are often detected prenatally • Predominantly venous lesions are usually detected later in life
High-flow malformations	Include both arteriovenous malformations and fistulas

Vascular tumors include hemangiomas, which are classified into congenital or infantile types.[3] Vascular tumors are classified as benign, locally aggressive or borderline, and malignant.[69]

As previously stated, although the International Society for the Study of Vascular Anomalies considers the term nuchal macrocystic lymphatic malformation instead of CH, considering the latter's usefulness in the clinical practice of obstetric imaging, it was described separately and will not be discussed in this subsection.

Vascular Neck Tumors

Congenital Neck Hemangioma

Congenital hemangioma is the most frequent vascular tumor of the fetal head and neck.[25,69] Congenital hemangioma is a benign endothelial tumor with increased mitotic activity during the proliferative phase.[69]

Hemangiomas are the result of vascular endothelial proliferation. They can occur anywhere in the skin, mucous membranes, or internal organs. Hemangiomas range in size from a few millimeters to many centimeters in diameter. They may be superficial, deep, or combined.[1]

Congenital hemangiomas are classified according to their postnatal involution patterns[25,69,70] **(Table 10)**.

Diagnosis and imaging findings

Ultrasound: Congenital hemangiomas appear as a large heterogeneous vascular mass originating from the posterolateral neck or head.[1,25,69] Congenital hemangiomas

TABLE 10: Congenital hemangiomas classification.

RICH	• Rapidly involuting congenital hemangioma • Most congenital hemangiomas in the head and neck • Usually achieve complete involution by 14 months of age
NICH	• Noninvoluting congenital hemangioma • Never involutes
PICH	• Partially involuting congenital hemangioma • Usually achieve involution by 14 months of age

TABLE 11: Differential diagnoses and associated conditions of the congenital neck hemangioma.

Differential diagnoses	• Congenital fibrosarcoma • Occipital cephalocele (when located in the posterior neck) • Other perinatal vascular neck tumors
Associated anomalies	• Brain cortical malformations • PHACES* syndrome

*Posterior fossa malformations, Hemangiomas, Arterial anomalies, Cardiac defects and coarctation of the aorta, Eye abnormalities, Sternal defect with or without supraumbilical raphe.

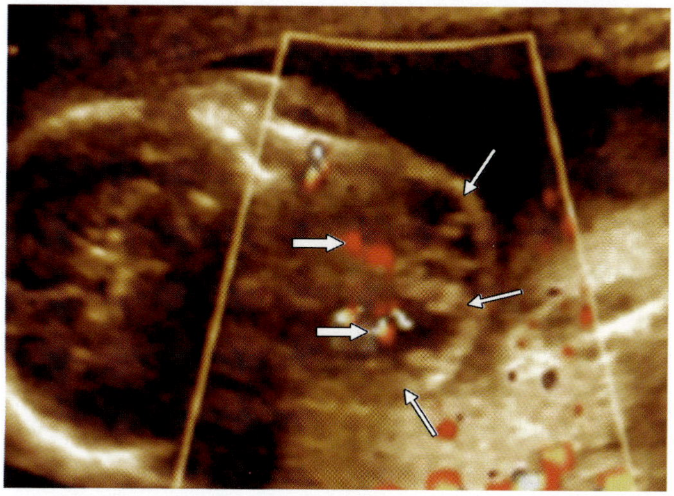

Fig. 7: Axial view of a neck hemangioma (white thin arrows). Mixed heterogeneous, solid and vascular tumor—color Doppler (white thick arrows).

have been diagnosed as early as 12 weeks gestation.[3] There is no apparent imaging differentiation between RICH (rapidly involuting congenital hemangioma) and NICH (noninvoluting congenital hemangioma). They share location, size, and similar imaging features. These tumors are heterogeneous, solid, and vascular masses with high vessel density and high-flow velocity, and low-resistance index and broadening of spectrum on Doppler US[3,25,69,70] **(Fig. 7)**.

Later in pregnancy, hemangiomas may be large size tumors, which makes the prenatal diagnosis easy.[1]

Other possibly associated imaging findings may be polyhydramnios, neck hyperextension, lateral head tilting, or congestive heart failure secondary to arteriovenous shunting.[3,71]

Magnetic resonance imaging: Congenital hemangiomas usually present a very heterogeneous appearance on prenatal MRI.[3,25] It demonstrates a well-defined heterogeneous solid mass in the neck region with intermediate signal intensity on T1-weighted images and increased signal intensity on T2-weighted images. High T2 signal intensity is likely secondary to slow vascular flow through small vascular spaces of the hemangioma. Flow void signal can be seen in high-flow vessels within the mass.[3,25,69]

Differential diagnoses and associated anomalies[3,25,72-74] are marked out in **Table 11**.

Management and outcome: Large RICH may have an impressive presentation at birth with high output heart failure.[69] RICH usually regress by 14 months of age and may leave behind atrophic skin or large veins in the region of prior hemangiomas.[3] Usually, RICH is managed conservatively, although complications based on size and location may prompt surgical excision.[25,69]

Noninvoluting congenital hemangioma may even grow with the child.[69] It usually requires surgical treatment.[3]

Maternal administration of steroid may accelerate involution of the hemangioma, and if there is compression upon the airway, delivery by cesarean section or EXIT procedure to secure the airway should be performed.[3,25,69]

Kaposiform Hemangioendothelioma

Kaposiform hemangioendothelioma (KHE) has been described in both the prenatal and neonatal periods.[25,75] It is a very infrequent locally aggressive vascular tumor.[25,69]

The head and neck location is not typical for KHE.[25,69,75] However, it should be considered in the differential diagnosis of a large fetal vascular mass.[25,69]

Diagnosis and imaging findings: The imaging features are nonspecific and the lesion might present as a vascular mass with ill-defined margins, subcutaneous fat stranding, intralesional calcification, and prominent feeding and draining vessels.[25]

TABLE 12: Vascular malformations spectrum.

Vascular malformations	*Vascular malformations based on flow type*	
	Low-flow	*High-flow*
• Venous malformation (VM) • Lymphatic malformation (LM) • Arterial malformation (AM) • Capillary malformation (CM) • Arteriovenous malformation (AVM) • Arteriovenous fistula (AVF) • Mixed (CLVM, VLM, CLAVM, and CVAVM)	• VM • LM • CM • CLVM • VLM	• AM • AVM • AVF • CLAVM • CVAVM

(CLAVM: capillary lymphatic arteriovenous malformation; CLVM: capillary lymphatic venous malformation; CVAVM: capillary venous arteriovenous malformation; VLM: venolymphatic malformation)

Kaposiform hemangioendothelioma tends to cause bony destruction and can also result in the development of Kasabach–Merritt phenomenon (a form of coagulopathy due to severe thrombocytopenia caused by platelet trapping within the rapidly enlarging vascular tumor and microangiopathic hemolytic anemia).[25,69]

Benign Vasoproliferative Hemangioendothelioma: Not Otherwise Specified

Benign vasoproliferative hemangioendothelioma—not otherwise specified (NOS) is a tumor only recently described as a separate entity. Benign vasoproliferative hemangioendothelioma is a very uncommon perinatal neoplasm that has imaging features similar to those in congenital hemangioma, but it can grow postnatally and might demonstrate intracranial invasion.[25,69]

Vascular Neck Malformations

Vascular malformations are classified as arterial, venous, capillary, lymphatic, or a combination of these (mixed) based on their predominant vascular channels.[76]

Vascular defects that have arterial components associate high-flow malformations, whereas anomalies with capillary, lymphatic, or venous components associate low-flow malformations[3,69,76] **(Table 12)**.

Venolymphatic Malformations

Venolymphatic malformations (VLMs) can significantly range in size and morphology.[25,69] The current classification of these vascular malformations includes a wide spectrum **(Table 12)**, so that this type of anomalies may be purely venous, venolymphatic, or arteriovenous.[3,76] The most common are VLM.[3,25,69]

TABLE 13: Differential diagnoses and associated conditions of the venolymphatic malformation (VLM).

Differential diagnoses	• Lymphatic malformations • Arteriovenous malformation • Hemangioma • Soft tissue sarcoma
Associated anomalies	• Klippel–Trenaunay syndrome[a,*] • Parkes-Weber syndrome[b,*] • Maffucci syndrome[c] • Blue rubber bleb nevus syndrome[d]

[a]Asymmetric limb or trunk enlargement, deep and superficial lymphatic malformations, venous malformations, and cutaneous hemangiomata of the affected limb or body part
[b]Capillary, venous, lymphatic, and arteriovenous malformation, diffuse arteriovenous fistulas and enlargement of the limb
[c]Congenital, nonhereditary condition, multiple enchondromas, and hemangiomas
[d]Extremely rare disorder, multifocal venous malformations
*Overgrowth condition

Venous malformations occur in approximately 1% of the general population, and of these, approximately 40% occur in the head and neck.[3,76] Mixed vascular malformations often are more diffuse than focal abnormalities and can be associated with soft-tissue and skeletal hypertrophy.[76]

Diagnosis and imaging findings: US Doppler is helpful to differentiate venous from other vascular malformations. It can show slow velocity with monophasic to biphasic waveforms. Fluid–fluid levels and acoustic shadowing related to phleboliths may be present.[3]

Venolymphatic malformation presents as a large, trans-spatial, multicystic mass with intervening septa and blood–fluid levels. On the other hand, a small malformation may present as a unilocular cyst. VLMs typically have no or minimal solid components, no increased vascularity, and no calcification. Also, they produce a rather mild mass effect on surrounding structures despite the large size of these anomalies.[3,25,69,76]

Magnetic resonance imaging demonstrates that VLM is typically isointense to muscle on T1- and hyperintense on T2-weighted images, but appears heterogeneous if thrombus or hemorrhage is present.[3,25,69]

Differential diagnoses and associated anomalies[3,76] are marked out in **Table 13**.

TABLE 14: Lymphatic malformations (LMs) classification.

Type I	Transpatial cystic lesions with multiple thin and/or thick internal septations
Type II	Predominantly cystic with no more than three septations
Type III	Purely cystic
Type IV	• Mixed cystic and solid with at least a 30% solid component • Most challenging to diagnose correctly • Complex appearance resembling that of teratoma* • Large structures with solid fields • Calcified phleboliths—can simulate tumoral calcification

*Type IV LM vs. teratoma: Teratoma tends to cause more mass effect and tissue distortion rather than invasion.

Management and outcome: Most venous malformations are treated conservatively, either with elastic compression, sclerotherapy, or surgical excision.[3,69,76,77]

Many VLMs are present at birth, most are small and often go unrecognized on prenatal imaging.[3] Anyway, after birth they tend to grow proportionally to the growth of the child.[3,76,77] On the other hand, some lesions may enlarge suddenly because of hemorrhage, infection, thrombosis, or hormonal changes.[3,76,77]

Lymphatic Malformations

It is recognized that lymphatic malformations (LMs) may have a very complex and atypical appearance.[3,25,69,76,78-80] There is a great variability in the prenatal sonographic appearance of LM.[69,78]

Therefore, there is a new classification of LM that categorizes the lesions by their internal architecture. According to this classification, all LMs may be divided into four distinct types[25,69,78] **(Table 14)**.

Diagnosis and imaging findings: Non-nuchal LM may be cystic masses with posterior acoustic enhancement. Vascular flow is not seen in pure LM (venous flow is present in VLM).[3,25,69]

Magnetic resonance imaging demonstrates a multilocular cystic trans-spatial mass. The cystic component is typically isointense to muscle on T1- and hyperintense on T2-weighted images. Non-nuchal LM may cause airway compromise.[3,69] MRI can assess the deep extent and airway involvement, in order to guide perinatal management, respectively the decision for EXIT procedures.[3,25,69]

TABLE 15: Differential diagnoses and associated conditions of the non-nuchal lymphatic malformation (LM).

Differential diagnoses	• Hemangioma • Venous malformation • Cystic teratoma • Arteriovenous malformation • Soft tissue sarcoma
Associated anomalies	• Klippel–Trenaunay syndrome • Parkes-Weber syndrome

Differential diagnoses and associated anomalies[3,76] are marked out in **Table 15**.

Management and outcome: Management options include observation, pharmacotherapy, sclerotherapy, and surgical procedures.[81]

In the presence of airway obstruction, delivery via the EXIT procedure may be imperative. Surgical resection is the treatment of choice but can be difficult in the presence of neural, vascular, or muscular invasion.[3,81,82] Macrocystic LM are often successfully treated postnatal with sclerotherapy, but other treatment strategies include radiofrequency ablation and laser.[3,81-83]

Large, infiltrating lesions can be difficult to treat fully; however, small focal LMs have excellent prognosis by percutaneous sclerosis and surgical resection.[3,81-83]

The outcome for isolated non-nuchal LM is favorable, depending on the extent and treatment response of the lesion.[3,84,85]

Arteriovenous Fistula and Arteriovenous Malformation

Arteriovenous malformation (AVM) is an interlacement of abnormal thin-walled vessels connecting dilated high-flow arteries to an often enlarged draining vein.[3,86] AVM are fast-flow vascular malformations composed of a complex vessel network directly connecting feeding arteries to draining veins.[87]

It seems that AVM arises in the fetus from failure of regression of arteriovenous channels in the primitive retiform plexus.[3]

Arteriovenous fistulas (AVFs) are similar to AVM, instead these lesions lack the entanglement of dysplastic vessels that are present in AVM.[3]

Arterial malformations are most common in the head and neck.[3,87]

Diagnosis and imaging findings: AVMs are typically described by US as a vascular lesion without soft tissue mass.[3,86,87] However, in the fetus, a soft tissue mass is often seen in conjunction with high-flow images. Also, multiple hypoechoic channels with or without soft tissue mass are observed.[3]

Ultrasound with color and spectral Doppler interrogation can reliably identify arteriovenous (AV) shunting and characterize the flow pattern in AVM and AVF.[87] Doppler demonstrates high systolic, high diastolic flow in the arteries and also arterialized venous waveforms with spectral broadening.[3]

Magnetic resonance imaging allows assessment of the lesion and the adjacent soft tissue. It demonstrates dilated veins without a discrete mass.[87] Also, MRI may show multiple tubular structures with flow void and heterogeneous T2 signal intensity. A single or multiple large vessels can be seen coursing through the mass.[3] Moreover, signal abnormalities may be present in the surrounding tissue representing fibrofatty changes, edema, and disorganized overgrowth. Osseous involvement manifests as overgrowth and lytic changes with diffuse abnormal bone signal.[87] Cardiac failure and hydrops may develop in the presence of high AV shunting.[3]

Differential diagnoses and associated anomalies[3,85,88,89] are marked out in **Table 16**.

Management and outcome: Treatment of AVM is very challenging and requires an interdisciplinary approach.[87] Transarterial embolization or surgery is the option of choice.[3,87] The main goal of AVM therapy is often maximal control of shunting and palliation of the clinical manifestations.[87] Cure is possible in some of the favorable angiographic types and AVF.[3,87] These anomalies are prone to recurrence, and interventions can be associated with serious side effects.[87]

TABLE 16: Differential diagnoses and associated conditions of the AVM and AVF.

Differential diagnoses	• Hemangioma • Venous malformation • Non-nuchal LM
Associated anomalies	• Cowden syndrome[a,*] • Bannayan–Riley–Ruvalcaba syndrome[b,*] • *RASA* (angiogenic) gene mutations • Parkes-Weber syndrome • Hereditary hemorrhagic telangiectasia (HHT)

[a]Rare inherited condition, autosomal dominant manner, multiple hamartomas in a variety of tissues from all three embryonic layers, and a cancer predisposition syndrome

[b]Rare genetic disorder, multiple lipomas, hamartomatous intestinal polyps, macrocephaly, developmental delay, pigmented macules of the penis, and autism spectrum disorder

*PTEN (phosphatase and tensin) homolog gene mutations

(AVF: arteriovenous fistula; AVM: arteriovenous malformation; LM: lymphatic malformation)

Thyroglossal Duct Cyst

Thyroglossal duct cyst (TGDC) is the most common midline cervical anomaly representing 70% of all congenital neck masses.[3] However, prenatal diagnosis of TGDC is rare.[3,90]

Thyroglossal duct cyst is formed by mucus production in an incompletely degenerated thyroglossal duct.[90] The majority of duct remnants are midline or parasagittal, adjacent to the hyoid bone.[3]

Diagnosis and Imaging Findings

The classic appearance by US of TGDC is a thin-walled anechoic unilocular lesion. Sometimes, TGDC may be hypoechoic or has heterogeneous echotexture, appearing pseudo solid and mimicking ectopic tissue, all of which are due to high protein content.[3] US can also demonstrate posterior acoustic enhancement in the majority TGDC, absence of color Doppler flow and a normal thyroid gland.[3,91]

Most TGDCs are typically bright on T1 and T2 sequences on MRI assessment.[3]

Differential diagnoses and associated anomalies[3,91,92] are marked out in **Table 17**.

Management and Outcome

Postnatal therapy is surgical resection with the Sistrunk procedure, which involves excision of cyst, remnant tract, and a portion of the hyoid bone.[3,93] Approximately 30% of patients with TGDC will have subsequent infection. There is a 1% risk of cancer. TGDC can rarely cause airway obstruction and EXIT procedure may be necessary.[3]

TABLE 17: Differential diagnoses and associated conditions of the thyroglossal duct cyst (TGDC).

Differential diagnoses	• Dermoid cyst • Esophageal duplication cyst • Ranula • Branchial cyst • Thymic cysts • Lymphatic malformations • Teratoma
Associated anomalies	Cowden syndrome

Cervical Thymic Cyst

Cervical thymic cysts (CTC) are very rare and infrequently diagnosed in utero.[3] CTC are a rare cause of cervical mass, different studies indicating an incidence of 0.3–1% of all congenital neck masses.[94] CTC are benign lesions of the thymus characterized by thymic tissue within the cyst wall.[95] Thymic cysts may be encountered in the neck, thoracic inlet, or mediastinum because of persistence of the thymopharyngeal tracts.[3]

Cervical thymic cysts usually manifest as a slowly growing asymptomatic mass in the region between the gonial angle of the mandible and the sternum, in proximity of the carotid sheath. They occur mostly on the left side, and there is a slight predominance among males.[94]

Diagnosis and Imaging Findings

Cervical thymic cysts are commonly multilocular, but may be unilocular and vary in size from 1.4 to 8 cm^3. CTC are intimately associated with the carotid space, elongating the carotid artery and jugular vein.[3,96] CTC are anechoic by US, but they may present intracystic echoes (protein fluid content).[3,94]

Magnetic resonance imaging demonstrates that CTC are hypointense on T1-weighted images and hyperintense on T2-weighted images.[3] The signal can be heterogeneous if they are complicated by hemorrhage.[3,97]

Differential diagnoses include branchial cleft cyst, TGDC, lymphatic malformation, or thyroid cyst.[3,94,95,97]

Management and Outcome

Cervical thymic cysts management includes surgical excision of the cyst and residual tract. Spontaneous remission has been also reported.[3,94-97] CTC are usually asymptomatic, or can cause respiratory distress, dysphagia, and vocal cord paralysis.[3,95,97]

Other Rare Anomalies of the Fetal Neck

In this subsection, we have included certain extremely rare pathologies that can affect the fetal neck such as ranula, congenital epulis, dermoid and epidermoid, epignathus, congenital neck neuroblastoma, rhabdomyosarcoma, and congenital infantile fibrosarcoma **(Table 18)**.[3,25,69,98-108]

Apart from the fact that they are very rare, all these entities present certain peculiarities of prenatal diagnosis, sometimes extremely difficult, along with particularities of management through special procedures.

Congenital High Airway Obstruction Syndrome

Congenital high airway obstruction syndrome (CHAOS) involves the partial or complete obstruction of the fetal upper airways, usually caused by atresia or stenosis of the larynx or trachea.[109]

Congenital high airway obstruction syndrome is a rare fetal anomaly that is associated with mortality in about 80–100% of cases. CHAOS is an exceedingly rare condition consisting of complete intrinsic obstruction of the fetal upper airway that can be located at the level of the larynx, trachea, or bronchi. As a result of the obstruction, the fetal lungs are completely expanded secondary to retention of bronchial secretions leading to tracheobronchial dilatation and pulmonary developmental impairment.[1,110]

Congenital high airway obstruction syndrome is a clinical entity manifested by the presence of extremely large echogenic fetal lungs, flattened or inverted diaphragm, dilated tracheobronchial tree, ascites, other manifestations of nonimmune hydrops, and due to complete obstruction of the fetal airway.[1,5,110]

When fetal hydrops and complete airway obstruction are associated, CHAOS is lethal without intervention.

In one-third of the cases, there is a spontaneous perforation of the laryngeal or tracheal atresia, resulting in the resolution of the hydrops.[1,5]

The airway obstruction may be generated by laryngeal atresia, tracheal atresia, or laryngeal cyst and the fetal clinical presentation in quite the same. CHAOS can be bilateral or unilateral (bronchial atresia). The incidence is unknown as the disease is very rare.[1,5,110,111]

Condition, Etiology, and Pathophysiology

Isolated CHAOS is a sporadic fetal malformation with low risk of chromosomal anomalies, but CHAOS can also be present within a syndrome. A significantly high proportion of cases can be associated with Fraser syndrome.[1,110,112]

Other syndromes reported in association with CHAOS are Cri-du-Chat syndrome, short-rib polydactyly syndrome, and velocardiofacial syndrome.[112]

Moreover, other conditions may induce an extrinsic obstruction of the tracheobronchial tree, such as lymphatic congenital malformations, cervical teratoma, or vascular rings, such as double aortic arch or aberrant right subclavian artery.[1,110,113]

Congenital high airway obstruction syndrome is characterized by retention of bronchial and alveolar

TABLE 18: Other rare anomalies of the fetal neck.

Ranula	• Congenital ranula are rare and benign cysts • Sublingual or minor salivary gland retention cyst • Located at the floor of the mouth • Obstruction or rupture of the sublingual gland ducts • Atresia of the salivary gland ducts or ostial adhesion • Histopathology is distinctive—salivary duct epithelium lining the walls of the cyst • Distinct from LM	
	Classification	• Simple—intraoral type • Plunging—oro-cervical type
	Diagnosis and imaging findings	• Prenatal diagnosis is very rare • US—well-defined anechoic or hypoechoic cysts in the floor of the mouth. May extend into the submandibular/cervical region. Usually, no color Doppler is observed • MRI—well-delineated borders. Low T1 and high T2 signals
	Differential diagnoses	• LM • Thyroglossal duct cyst • Dermoid
	Management and outcome	*Management:* Marsupialization, aspiration, and resection of the sublingual salivary gland. No recurrence except for marsupialization *Outcome:* Spontaneous resolution in the neonatal period is possible. Rarely grow to completely fill the oral cavity, possibly obstructing the upper airway at birth. Giant congenital ranula may result in airway obstruction, necessitating EXIT procedure (infrequent)
Congenital epulis	• Benign gingival tumor • Rare, occurring almost exclusively in females • Can cause obstruction of the airway • Arises from the gingival mucosa of the alveolar ridge of the—maxilla and less commonly the mandible • Usually solitary • Few synchronous epulides described	
	Diagnosis and imaging findings	• Well-defined pedunculated mass protruding through the fetal mouth • US—solid mass with internal blood flow with a vascular pedicle from the mouth Fetal swallowing is not affected usually. If the lesion becomes large it may impair fetal swallowing (subsequent polyhydramnios or airway obstruction) • MRI—hypointense on T2-weighted images. The origin from the maxilla or mandibular alveolar ridge can be seen
	Differential diagnoses	• Teratoma • Hemangioma • Epignathus • LM • Oropharyngeal rhabdomyosarcoma • Dermoid cysts
	Management and outcome	Surgical excision is the treatment of choice. No reported recurrence. Small lesions may regress spontaneously
Dermoid and epidermoid	• Aberrant ectodermal tissues during the fetal period cause DC and EC • DC and EC—inclusion of ectodermal tissue during the fusion of the branchial arches • DC—two germ layers (ectoderm and mesoderm) • EC—one germ layer (ectoderm) • 7.0% in the head and neck region	
	Diagnosis and imaging findings	• Prenatal diagnosis is rare • US—well-circumscribed, thin-walled unilocular mass with internal echoes and small posterior echo enhancement • MRI—T1 hyperintense to isointense. T2 hyperintense

Contd...

Contd...

	Differential diagnoses	• Congenital epulis • Ranula
	Associated conditions	Gardner syndrome
	Management and outcome	• Surgical resection—the treatment of choice • DC and EC are at risk for rupture or infection • Approximately 5% may undergo malignant degeneration • May cause airway obstruction • EXIT may be considered
Epignathus	• Extremely rare teratoma in the oral cavity or oropharyngeal region • More common in females • Frequently associated with life-threatening airway obstruction • Components of all three germ layers	
	Diagnosis and imaging findings	• Usually present in the second trimester • Unidirectional or bidirectional masses • US and MRI—similar characteristics with cervical teratomas. Tumors can vary in size
	Differential diagnoses	• Neck teratoma • Other neck masses
	Associated conditions	• Branchial cleft cyst • Agenesis of the corpus callosum • Cleft palate • Congenital heart disease • Duplicated pituitary gland
	Management and outcome	• Surgical excision is the treatment of choice • Prognosis is very poor in cases of intracranial extension • Can rapidly grow • May cause swallowing dysfunction, airway obstruction, or polyhydramnios • EXIT procedures are required to secure the airway
Congenital neck neuroblastoma	• CNNB is a rare occurrence • Primary CNNB—<5% of all cases • Embryonal cancer that may develop at any site of sympathetic nervous system tissue	
	Diagnosis and imaging findings	• US—solid or mixed (solid-cystic) mass in the lateral neck with or without calcification • MRI—mass with low signal intensity on T1 and high signal intensity on T2-weighted images
	Differential diagnoses	• LM • Branchial cleft cyst • Other solid or mixed lateral neck masses
	Associated conditions	Horner's syndrome
	Management and outcome	• Disappearance of the tumor before birth has been reported • CNNB, especially purely cystic, has a better prognosis than those occurring during childhood • Extension to the brain and metastasis are extremely rare • CNNB may cause compression upon the airway and esophagus and neck hyperextension
Rhabdomyosarcoma	• Highly malignant congenital neoplasm • Extremely rare • Exceptionally rare diagnosed prenatally • Often associated with chromosomal translocations • Can occur in the soft tissues of the head and neck, fetal brain, or extremities	

Contd...

Contd...

	Associated conditions	• Robert syndrome • Beckwith–Wiedemann syndrome • Neurofibromatosis
Congenital infantile fibrosarcoma	• Uncommon soft tissue tumor • Can be detected prenatally • May occur in the head and neck (primarily occurs in the extremities) • MRI—similar features with congenital neck hemangioma • More favorable prognosis compared to adult fibrosarcoma	

(CNNB: congenital neck neuroblastoma; DC: dermoid cysts; EC: epidermoid cysts; EXIT: ex utero intrapartum treatment; LM: lymphatic malformation)

secretions, resulting in elevated intratracheal pressure and a significant increment in the amount of fluid within the lungs and tracheobronchial tree leading to severely increased lung volume and tracheal dilatation. The massively enlarged lungs deform the fetal thorax inducing a regression in the diaphragmatic convexity and a mediastinal shift. These findings can be detected on US in the first trimester of pregnancy.[1,110-113]

The diagnosis is usually made on examination of the fetal thorax, which is typically characterized by hyperexpanded and hyperechoic lungs, flattened diaphragms, and dilated airways below the level of the obstruction.[1,110]

Diagnosis and Imaging Findings

Ultrasound: It shows signs related to complete airway obstruction. In a transverse view and at the level of the four-chamber view of the fetal heart, the lungs appear severely enlarged and highly hyperechoic. Secondary to the exceedingly high intrathoracic pressure and the degree of pulmonary expansion, the heart is squeezed into the middle of the fetal mediastinum between the lungs and shows a reduction of the cardiac angle. The sagittal and coronal views of the fetal thorax reveal two pathognomonic signs: Flattening or inversion of the diaphragmatic convexity and greatly dilated airways filled with bronchial secretions with an anechoic appearance, which allows observation of the entire tracheobronchial tree as a bronchogram. The dilated trachea and bronchi are better displayed with a coronal view of the fetal chest.[1,110,113,114]

In addition, absence of flow in the trachea during fetal breathing or swallowing can be shown using color Doppler US. Extrapulmonary signs include nonimmune hydrops fetalis and placentomegaly secondary to cardiac failure or impeding venous return, or both, and polyhydramnios secondary to esophageal compression.[1,110-114]

Magnetic resonance imaging: MRI findings of CHAOS include confirmation of dilated airways below the level of obstruction, increased lung signal intensity, and large lung volumes with flattened or inverted hemidiaphragms. Differential diagnosis between unilateral CHAOS and congenital cystic adenomatoid malformation (CCAM) can be challenging by US, and MRI can be useful in differentiating among congenital lung lesions. MRI may also help to exclude additional congenital malformations and other conditions associated with extrinsic compression of the tracheobronchial tree, such as adjacent tumors. MRI may play an important role in better identification of the level of obstruction, particularly in unilateral cases.[1,5,110,114,115]

Differential diagnosis of CHAOS: The main diagnosis mistaken for CHAOS is CCAM. CCAM is usually lobar, not involving the entire lung, and very few of the cases are bilateral. CHAOS may be a part or a morbid association to Fraser syndrome.[1,5,110-115]

Management, Outcome, and Recurrence Risk

Congenital high airway obstruction syndrome is usually a lethal abnormality, especially in the presence of hydrops. Fetuses with suspected CHAOS should be referred to a fetal medicine center with teams able to perform EXIT delivery. Perinatal mortality is 100% without intervention. Preliminary studies reported that fetuses with CHAOS could benefit from in utero fetal therapy, as EXIT is associated with increased maternal morbidity.[1,110,114-116]

However, even if there are some published cases with encouraging results,[116-118] fetoscopic methods require future studies.[1,110-115]

Most cases of CHAOS occur sporadically, isolated malformations without a known risk of recurrence. When Fraser syndrome is associated, there is a 25% risk of recurrence.[1,5,110]

CONCLUSIONS

- Congenital anomalies of the neck are uncommon and their real incidence is unknown.
- CH is the most frequently seen fetal neck mass on first trimester US, and the overall prognosis is poor.
- Cervical teratomas are associated with high mortality rates and the risk for recurrence in subsequent pregnancies could not be anticipated.
- FG is rare and usually self-limited, having a good prognosis.
- Branchial cleft cyst can cause airway or esophageal obstruction and surgical excision is the definite therapy.
- Vascular neck abnormalities include both vascular malformations and vascular tumors.
- TGDC is the most common midline cervical anomaly and the postnatal therapy is surgical resection.
- CTC are very rare diagnosed in utero and management includes surgical excision.
- Ranula, congenital epulis, dermoid and epidermoid, epignathus, congenital neck neuroblastoma, rhabdomyosarcoma, congenital infantile fibrosarcoma are extremely rare abnormalities of the fetal neck.
- CHAOS is usually a lethal abnormality, and suspected fetuses should be referred to a fetal medicine center able to perform EXIT delivery.

REFERENCES

1. Vladareanu R, Vladareanu S, Berceanu C. Neck. Donald School J Ultrasound Obstet Gynecol. 2016;10(3):256-70.
2. Schoenwolf GC, Bleyl SB, Brauer PR, et al. (Eds). Larsen's Human Embryology, 5th edition. Philadelphia: Churchill Livingstone; 2015. pp. 440-2.
3. Meyers ML, Dannull KA. Neck. In: Kline-Fath BM, Bulas DI, Bahado-Singh R (Eds). Fundamental and Advanced Fetal Imaging: Ultrasound and MRI. Wolters Kluwer Health; 2015. pp. 491-507.
4. Arigita M, Bennasar M, Bienvenido P. Cystic hygroma. In: Copel JA, D'Alton ME, Gratacos E, et al. (Eds). Obstetric Imaging. Philadelphia: Elsevier Saunders; 2012. pp. 370-2.
5. Bianchi DW, Crombleholme TM, D'Alton ME, et al. Fetology-Diagnosis and Management of the Fetal Patient, 2nd edition. McGraw-Hill Medical; 2010. pp. 237-41.
6. Sherer DM, Hsieh V, Soyemi S, et al. First-trimester septated cystic hygroma, marked non-immune fetal hydrops, 45,X and coarctation of the aorta with neonatal survival. J Clin Ultrasound. 2023;51(6):1024-6.
7. Pashaj S, Merz E. First trimester screening: Increased nuchal translucency or cystic hygroma? Ultraschall Med. 2022;43(2):111-4.
8. Chen YN, Chen CP, Lin CJ, et al. Prenatal Ultrasound Evaluation and Outcome of Pregnancy with Fetal Cystic Hygromas and Lymphangiomas. J Med Ultrasound. 2017;25(1):12-5.
9. Grapsa D, Mavrigiannaki P, Kleanthis C, et al. Autopsy findings in fetuses with cystic hygroma: a literature review and our center's experience. Clin Exp Obstet Gynecol. 2012;39(3):369-73.
10. Haak MC, Twisk JW, Bartelings MM, et al. Ductus venosus flow velocities in relation to the cardiac defects in first-trimester fetuses with enlarged nuchal translucency. Am J Obstet Gynecol. 2003;188(3):727-33.
11. Benacerraf B. Ultrasound of Fetal Syndromes, 2nd edition. Churchill Livingstone: Elsevier; 2008. pp. 50-2.
12. Uller W, Fishman SJ, Alomari AI. Overgrowth syndromes with complex vascular anomalies. Semin Pediatr Surg. 2014;23(4):208-15.
13. Boudon E, Levy Y, Abossolo T, et al. Antenatal presentation of hereditary lymphedema type I. Eur J Med Genet. 2015;58(6-7):329-31.
14. Cheng YKY, Huang J, Law KM, et al. Prenatal diagnosis of maternally inherited X-linked Opitz G/BBB syndrome by chromosomal microarray in a fetus with complex congenital heart disease. Clin Chim Acta. 2014;436:140-2.
15. Herwegen JV. Williams syndrome and its cognitive profile: the importance of eye movements. Psychol Res Behav Manag. 2015;8:143-51.
16. Ueda K, Yamada J, Takemoto O, et al. Eight patients with Williams syndrome and craniosynostosis. Eur J Med Genet. 2015;58(6-7):355-7.
17. Aydemir O, Kavurt S, Esin S, et al. Fetal echogenic bowel in association with Zellweger syndrome. J Obstet Gynaecol Res. 2014;40(6):1799-802.
18. Mastromoro G, Guadagnolo D, Hashemian NK, et al. A Pain in the Neck: Lessons Learnt from Genetic Testing in Fetuses Detected with Nuchal Fluid Collections, Increased Nuchal Translucency versus Cystic Hygroma-Systematic Review of the Literature, Meta-Analysis and Case Series. Diagnostics (Basel). 2022;13(1):48.
19. Chen M, Lee CP, Lin SM, et al. Cystic hygroma detected in the first trimester scan in Hong Kong. J Matern Fetal Neonatal Med. 2014;27(4):342-5.
20. Kagan KO, Sonek J, Kozlowski P. Antenatal screening for chromosomal abnormalities. Arch Gynecol Obstet. 2022;305(4):825-35.
21. Edwards L, Hui L. First and second trimester screening for fetal structural anomalies. Semin Fetal Neonatal Med. 2018;23(2):102-11.
22. Nicolaides KH. First-trimester screening for chromosomal abnormalities. Semin Perinatol. 2005;29(4):190-4.
23. Pilu G, Segata M, Perolo A. Ultrasound evaluation of the fetal face and neck. In: Callen PW (Ed). Ultrasonography in Obstetrics and Gynecology, 5th Edition. Philadelphia: Saunders Elsevier; 2008. pp. 392-418.

24. Doğer E, Ceylan Y, Çakıroğlu AY, et al. Prenatal diagnosis and management of a fetal neck mass. J Turk Ger Gynecol Assoc. 2015;16(2):118-20.
25. Feygin T, Bilaniuk LT. Fetal head and neck tumors. Pediatr Radiol. 2020;50(13):1999-2008.
26. Merrow AC, Gupta A, Patel MN, et al. 2014 Revised Classification of Vascular Lesions from the International Society for the Study of Vascular Anomalies: Radiologic-Pathologic Update. Radiographics. 2016;36(5):1494-516.
27. Puerto B, Eixarch E, Sanz-Cortéz M. Neck teratoma. In: Copel JA, D'Alton ME, Gratacos E, et al. (Eds). Obstetric Imaging. Philadelphia: Elsevier Saunders; 2012. pp. 373-8.
28. Sheikh F, Akinkuotu A, Olutoye OO, et al. Prenatally diagnosed neck masses: Long-term outcomes and quality of life. J Pediatr Surg. 2015;50(7):1210-3.
29. Tonni G, De Felice C, Centini G, et al. Cervical and oral teratoma in the fetus: A systematic review of etiology, pathology, diagnosis, treatment and prognosis. Arch Gynecol Obstet. 2010;282(4):355-61.
30. Riedlinger WF, Lack EE, Robson CD, et al. Primary thyroid teratomas in children: a report of 11 cases with a proposal of criteria for their diagnosis. Am J Surg Pathol. 2005;29(5):700-6.
31. Bianchi B, Ferri A, Silini EM, et al. Congenital cervical teratoma: A case report. J Oral Maxillofac Surg. 2010;68(3):667-70.
32. Isaacs H Jr. Perinatal (fetal and neonatal) germ cell tumors. J Pediatr Surg. 2004;39(7):1003-13.
33. Walz PC, Schroeder JW Jr. Prenatal diagnosis of obstructive head and neck masses and perinatal airway management: The ex utero intrapartum treatment procedure. Otolaryngol Clin North Am. 2015;48(1):191-207.
34. Ng TW, Xi Y, Schindel D, et al. Fetal Head and Neck Masses: MRI Prediction of Significant Morbidity. AJR Am J Roentgenol. 2019;212(1):215-21.
35. Goldstein I, Drugan A. Congenital cervical teratoma, associated with agenesis of corpus callosum and a subarachnoid cyst. Prenat Diagn. 2005;25(6):439-41.
36. Köchling J, Karbasiyan M, Reis A. Spectrum of mutations and genotype-phenotype analysis in Currarino syndrome. Eur J Hum Genet. 2001;9(8):599-605.
37. Wolfe K, Lewis D, Witte D, et al. Fetal cervical teratoma: What is the role of fetal MRI in predicting pulmonary hypoplasia? Fetal Diagn Ther. 2013;33(4):252-6.
38. Liechty KW, Hedrick HL, Hubbard AM, et al. Severe pulmonary hypoplasia associated with giant cervical teratomas. J Pediatr Surg. 2006;41(1):230-3.
39. Knox EM, Muamar B, Thompson PJ, et al. The use of high resolution magnetic resonance imaging in the prenatal diagnosis of fetal nuchal tumors. Ultrasound Obstet Gynecol. 2005;26(6):672-5.
40. Lazar DA, Olutoye OO, Moise KJ Jr, et al. Ex-utero intrapartum treatment procedure for giant neck masses-fetal and maternal outcomes. J Pediatr Surg. 2011;46(5):817-22.
41. Bahado-Singh RO, Goncalves LF. Techniques, terminology, and indications for MRI in pregnancy. Semin Perinatol. 2013;37(5):334-9.
42. Kamil D, Tepelmann J, Berg C, et al. Spectrum and outcome of prenatally diagnosed fetal tumors. Ultrasound Obstet Gynecol. 2008;31(3):296-302.
43. Sichel JY, Eliashar R, Yatsiv I, et al. A multidisciplinary team approach for management of a giant congenital cervical teratoma. Int J Pediatr Otorhinolaryngol. 2002;65(3):241-7.
44. Preciado DA, Rutter MJ, Greenberg JM, et al. Intrapartum management of severe fetal airway obstruction. J Otolaryngol. 2004;33(5):283-8.
45. Azizkhan RG. Perinatal tumors. In: Carachi R, Grosfeld J, Azmy AF (Eds). The surgery of childhood tumors, 2nd edition. Berlin: Springer-Verlag; 2008. pp. 155-6.
46. Martino F, Avila LF, Encinas JL, et al. Teratomas of the neck and mediastinum in children. Pediatr Surg Int. 2006;22(8):627-34.
47. Cruz-Martinez R, Moreno-Alvarez O, Garcia M, et al. Fetal Endoscopic Tracheal Intubation: A New Fetoscopic Procedure to Ensure Extrauterine Tracheal Permeability in a Case with Congenital Cervical Teratoma. Fetal Diagn Ther. 2015;38(2):154-8.
48. Mendoza HF, Campisi P, Deshpande P, et al. Fetal Endoscopic Tracheal Intubation: Modification of the Fetal Endoscopic Tracheal Intubation Procedure to Establish an Airway in a Fetus with a Congenital Cervical Teratoma. Fetal Diagn Ther. 2022;49(11-12):496-501.
49. Chmait RH, Chon AH, Anselmo D, et al. In utero Fetal Intubation for a Large Neck Mass: A Minimally Invasive EXIT Option. Fetal Diagn Ther. 2019;45(4):275-80.
50. Johnson MP, Mann S. Fetal tumors. In: Rodeck CH, Whittle MJ (Eds). Fetal Medicine - Basic Science and Clinical Practice, 2nd edition. UK: Elsevier Health; 2009. pp. 528-37.
51. Sanz-Cortéz M, Fernández S, Puerto B. Fetal thyroid Masses and Fetal Goiter. In: Copel JA, D'Alton ME, Gratacos E, et al. (Eds). Obstetric Imaging. Philadelphia: Elsevier Saunders; 2012. pp. 378-86.
52. Polak M, Van Vliet G. Therapeutic approach of fetal thyroid disorders. Horm Res Paediatr. 2010;74(1):1-5.
53. Rosner G, Shahar SB, Yaron Y, et al. Treatable fetal endocrine and metabolic disorders. In: Rodeck CH, Whittle MJ (Eds). Fetal Medicine - Basic Science and Clinical Practice, 2nd edition. Churchill Livingstone: Elsevier; 2009. pp. 592-601.
54. Polak M, Luton D. Fetal thyroidology. Best Pract Res Clin Endocrinol Metab. 2014;28(2):161-73.
55. Mastrolia SA, Mandola A, Mazor M, et al. Antenatal diagnosis and treatment of hypothyroid fetal goiter in an euthyroid mother: a case report and review of literature. J Matern Fetal Neonatal Med. 2015;28(18):2214-20.
56. Huel C, Guibourdenche J, Vuillard E, et al. Use of ultrasound to distinguish between fetal hyperthyroidism and hypothyroidism on discovery of a goiter. Ultrasound Obstet Gynecol. 2009;33(4):412-20.

57. Fujishima A, Sato A, Miura H, et al. Fetal goiter identified in a pregnant woman with triiodothyronine-predominant graves' disease: a case report. BMC Pregnancy Childbirth. 2020;20(1):344.
58. Munoz JL. Fetal thyroid disorders: Pathophysiology, diagnosis and therapeutic approaches. J Gynecol Obstet Hum Reprod. 2019;48(4):231-3.
59. Insoft RM, Hurvitz J, Estrella E, et al. Prader-Willi syndrome associated with fetal goiter: a case report. Am J Perinatol. 1999;16(1):29-31.
60. Agrawal P, Ogilvy-Stuart A, Lees C. Intrauterine diagnosis and management of congenital goitrous hypothyroidism. Ultrasound Obstet Gynecol. 2002;19(5):501-5.
61. Didier-Mathon H, Bouchghoul H, Senat MV, et al. Prenatal management of fetal goiter alternating between hypothyroidism and hyperthyroidism in a mother with Graves' disease. Clin Case Rep. 2021;9(4):2281-4.
62. Rubio EI. Imaging of the fetal oral cavity, airway and neck. Pediatr Radiol. 2021;51(7):1122-33.
63. Karabulut N, Martin DR, Yang M, et al. MR imaging findings in fetal goiter caused by maternal graves disease. J Comput Assist Tomogr. 2002;26(4):538-40.
64. Kondoh M, Miyazaki O, Imanishi Y, et al. Neonatal goiter with congenital thyroid dysfunction in two infants diagnosed by MRI. Pediatr Radiol. 2004;34(7):570-3.
65. Delay F, Dochez V, Biquard F, et al. Management of fetal goiters: 6-year retrospective observational study in three prenatal diagnosis and treatment centers of the Pays De Loire Perinatal Network. J Matern Fetal Neonatal Med. 2020;33(15):2561-9.
66. Misawa K, Imai A, Sugiyama K, et al. A right-sided fourth branchial cleft cyst: a case report. Int J Pediatr Otorhinolaryngol. 2011;75(3):438-40.
67. Lind RC, Hulscher JB, van der Wal JE, et al. A very rare case of a giant third branchial pouch remnant discovered in utero. Eur J Pediatr Surg. 2010;20(5):349-51.
68. Li Y, Mashhood A, Mamlouk MD, et al. Prenatal Diagnosis of Third and Fourth Branchial Apparatus Anomalies: Case Series and Comparison with Lymphatic Malformation. AJNR Am J Neuroradiol. 2021;42(11):2094-100.
69. Feygin T, Khalek N, Moldenhauer JS. Fetal brain, head, and neck tumors: Prenatal imaging and management. Prenat Diagn. 2020;40(10):1203-19.
70. Fadell MF, Jones BV, Adams DM. Prenatal diagnosis and postnatal follow-up of rapidly involuting congenital hemangioma (RICH). Pediatr Radiol. 2011;41(8):1057-60.
71. Alamo L, Beck-Popovic M, Gudinchet F, et al. Congenital tumors: imaging when life just begins. Insights Imaging. 2011;2(3):297-308.
72. Miyakoshi K, Tanaka M, Matsumoto T, et al. Occipital scalp hemangioma: Prenatal sonographic and magnetic resonance images. J Obstet Gynaecol Res. 2008;34(4 Pt 2):666-9.
73. Proisy M, Powell J, McCuaig C, et al. PHACES Syndrome and Associated Anomalies: Risk Associated With Small and Large Facial Hemangiomas. AJR Am J Roentgenol. 2021;217(2):507-14.
74. Sepulveda W, Sepulveda F. Fetal neuroimaging findings in PHACE syndrome: case report and review of the literature. J Matern Fetal Neonatal Med. 2022;35(14):2751-8.
75. Martinez AE, Robinson MJ, Alexis JB. Kaposiform hemangioendothelioma associated with nonimmune fetal hydrops. Arch Pathol Lab Med. 2004;128(6):678-81.
76. Calvo-Garcia MA, Kline-Fath BM, Adams DM, et al. Imaging evaluation of fetal vascular anomalies. Pediatr Radiol. 2015;45(8):1218-29.
77. Dubois J, Alison M. Vascular anomalies: What a radiologist needs to know. Pediatr Radiol. 2010;40(6):895-905.
78. Oliver ER, Coleman BG, DeBari SE, et al. Fetal Lymphatic Malformations: More Variable Than We Think? J Ultrasound Med. 2017;36(5):1051-8.
79. Rogerson D, Alkelai A, Giordano J, et al. Investigation into the genetics of fetal congenital lymphatic anomalies. Prenat Diagn. 2023;43(6):703-16.
80. Crivelli L, Millischer AE, Sonigo P, et al. Contribution of magnetic resonance imaging to the prenatal diagnosis of common congenital vascular anomalies. Pediatr Radiol. 2021;51(9):1626-36.
81. Kulungowski AM, Patel M. Lymphatic malformations. Semin Pediatr Surg. 2020;29(5):150971.
82. Oosthuizen JC, Burns P, Russell JD. Lymphatic malformations: A proposed management algorithm. Int J Pediatr Otorhinolaryngol. 2010;74(4):398-403.
83. Greene AK, Perlyn CA, Alomari AI. Management of lymphatic malformations. Clin Plast Surg. 2011;38(1):75-82.
84. Hathaway BA, Radu S, Wilson J, et al. Lymphatic and Mixed Malformations. Lymphat Res Biol. 2021;19(1):41-50.
85. Fordham LA, Chung CJ, Donnelly LF. Imaging of congenital vascular and lymphatic anomalies of the head and neck. Neuroimaging Clin N Am. 2000;10(1):117-36, viii.
86. Schimmel K, Ali MK, Tan SY, et al. Arteriovenous Malformations-Current Understanding of the Pathogenesis with Implications for Treatment. Int J Mol Sci. 2021; 22(16):9037.
87. Uller W, Alomari AI, Richter GT. Arteriovenous malformations. Semin Pediatr Surg. 2014;23(4):203-7.
88. Abdel Razek AAK, Elmokadem AH, Soliman M, et al. MR Imaging of Vascular Malformations and Tumors of Head and Neck. Magn Reson Imaging Clin N Am. 2022;30(1):199-213.
89. Fernández-Alvarez V, Suárez C, de Bree R, et al. Management of extracranial arteriovenous malformations of the head and neck. Auris Nasus Larynx. 2020;47(2):181-90.
90. Fang N, Angula LN, Cui Y, et al. Large thyroglossal duct cyst of the neck mimicking cervical cystic lymphangioma in a neonate: A case report. J Int Med Res. 2021;49(4):300060521999765.
91. Keizer AL, Deurloo KL, van Vugt JM, et al. A prenatal diagnosis of a thyroglossal duct cyst in the fetal anterior neck. Prenat Diagn. 2011;31(13):1311-2.

92. Zheng W, Gai S, Qin J, et al. Role of prenatal imaging in the diagnosis and management of fetal facio-cervical masses. Sci Rep. 2021;11(1):1385.
93. Kartini D, Panigoro SS, Harahap AS. Sistrunk Procedure on Malignant Thyroglossal Duct Cyst. Case Rep Oncol Med. 2020;2020:6985746.
94. Betti M, Hoseini NH, Martin A, et al. Cervical thymic cyst in childhood: A case report. Fetal Pediatr Pathol. 2015;34(1):65-9.
95. Joshi J, Ganguly A, Ventakataramana CG, et al. Cervical Thymic Cyst - A Rare Diagnosis. J Indian Assoc Pediatr Surg. 2022;27(6):753-5.
96. Cigliano B, Baltogiannis N, De Marco M, et al. Cervical thymic cysts. Pediatr Surg Int. 2007;23(12):1219-25.
97. Prosser JD, Myer CM 3rd. Branchial cleft anomalies and thymic cysts. Otolaryngol Clin North Am. 2015;48(1):1-14.
98. Rao AR, Parakh H, Rao PMM, et al. Unusual Presentation of a Congenital Ranula Cyst in a Newborn. Cureus. 2023;15(5):e38749.
99. Regaieg C, Triki M, Charfi M, et al. Congenital Epulis Diagnosed Antenatally. Fetal Pediatr Pathol. 2023; 42(4):675-8.
100. López de Lacalle JM, Aguirre I, Irizabal JC, et al. Congenital epulis: Prenatal diagnosis by ultrasound. Pediatr Radiol. 2001;31(6):453-4.
101. Suga K, Muramatsu K, Uchiyama T, et al. Congenital epidermoid cyst arising in soft palate near uvula: a case report. Bull Tokyo Dent Coll. 2010;51(4):207-11.
102. Goto S, Nakazawa A, Yoshizawa T, et al. Case Report: a Giant Epignathus with a Well-Developed Skeleton of Head and Neck. Int J Surg Pathol. 2022:10668969221133739.
103. Runggaldier D, Reinehr M, Friedrich H, et al. Case report and review of the literature: rare fetus-in-fetu presenting as oropharyngeal epignathus. Front Surg. 2023;10:1122327.
104. Lele Mutombo F, Nzanzu Kikuhe J, Kasereka Mwanamolo N, et al. Congenital epignathus associated with a cleft palate: A case report. J Med Case Rep. 2021;15(1):422.
105. Zafeiriou DI, Economou M, Koliouskas D, et al. Congenital Horner's syndrome associated with cervical neuroblastoma. Eur J Paediatr Neurol. 2006;10(2):90-2.
106. Hoellen F, Noack F, Ribbat J, et al. Foetal rhabdomyosarcoma with massive cardiac and placental infiltration associated with intrauterine foetal death. Z Geburtshilfe Neonatol. 2010;214(4):167-9.
107. Yoshino K, Takeuchi M, Nakayama M, et al. Congenital cervical rhabdomyosarcoma arising in one fetus of a twin pregnancy. Fetal Diagn Ther. 2005;20(4):291-5.
108. AbouZeid AA, Mohammad SA, Aly NH, et al. Differential diagnostic features between congenital haemangioma, KHE, and congenital fibrosarcoma: A single-centre experience. Eur J Pediatr. 2021;180(8):2581-9.
109. Werner H, Lopes J, Ribeiro G, et al. Congenital High Airway Obstruction Syndrome (CHAOS): Virtual Navigation in the Fetal Airways After Intrauterine Endoscopic Treatment. J Obstet Gynaecol Can. 2021;43(7):879-83.
110. Cruz-Martinez R, Puerto B. Congenital High Airway Obstruction Syndrome and Bronchial Atresia. In: Copel JA, D'Alton ME, Gratacos E, et al. (Eds). Philadelphia: Elsevier Saunders; 2012. pp. 386-9.
111. D'Eufemia MD, Cianci S, Di Meglio F, et al. Congenital high airway obstruction syndrome (CHAOS): Discussing the role and limits of prenatal diagnosis starting from a single-center case series. J Prenat Med. 2016;10(1-2):4-7.
112. Ashraf A, Abdelrahman AM, Senna A, et al. Congenital High Airway Obstruction Syndrome (CHAOS): No Intervention, No Survival-A Case Report and Literature Review. Case Rep Radiol. 2020;2020:1036073.
113. Ravikanth R, Khanapure VP. Prenatal Diagnosis of Congenital High Airway Obstruction Syndrome due to Laryngeal Atresia. J Med Ultrasound. 2020;29(4):298-9.
114. Afzal S, Fatima K, Ambareen M. Antenatal Ultrasound Diagnosis of Congenital High Airway Obstruction Syndrome: A Case Report and Review of Literature. Cureus. 2019;11(5):e4772.
115. Courtier J, Poder L, Wang ZJ, et al. Fetal tracheolaryngeal airway obstruction: prenatal evaluation by sonography and MRI. Pediatr Radiol. 2010;40(11):1800-5.
116. King A, Bedwell JR, Mehta DK, et al. Fetoscopic Balloon Dilation and Stent Placement of Congenital High Airway Obstruction Syndrome Leading to Successful Cesarean Delivery. Fetal Diagn Ther. 2022;49(1-2):29-35.
117. Sabra R, Gheorghe CP, Monson MA, et al. In utero Treatment of Congenital High Airway Obstruction Syndrome via Fetal Laryngoscopy and EXIT Procedure. Fetal Diagn Ther. 2022;49(9-10):385-93.
118. Peiro JL, Nolan HR, Alhajjat A, et al. A Technical Look at Fetoscopic Laser Ablation for Fetal Laryngeal Surgical Recanalization in Congenital High Airway Obstruction Syndrome. J Laparoendosc Adv Surg Tech A. 2020; 30(6):695-700.

25

CHAPTER

Diagnostic Sonography of Fetal Urinary Tract Anomalies

Zoltán Tóth, Zoltán Papp

INTRODUCTION

Over the course of embryogenesis, fetal kidneys and the urinary tract develop from the intermediate mesoderm. Following the formation of the pronephros, the mesonephric (or Wolffian) duct gives rise to the ureteric bud, which grows into the tissue of the metanephros, induced by the transiently developing and then regrediating mesonephros, and after 15 division generations gives rise to the ureter, the renal pelvis, the minor and major calyces and the collecting ducts. Until gestational week 15, the formation of the collecting ducts takes place fast; thereafter, it is somewhat slower. By week 20, however, nearly all ducts are present. The collecting ducts induce the arising of nephrons, juxtamedullar glomeruli and the definitive kidney from the metanephric blastema. Development of nephrons is intensive during the first 15 weeks, but at that time, merely one-third of nephrons have developed, whereas the final nephron number is reached by week 32. The kinetics of nephrogenesis is also marked by the changing amount of amniotic fluid. Agenesis of the pronephros, the mesonephric duct or the ureteric bud as well as disorders of the interactions between the ureteric bud and the metanephric blastema lead to a totally or partially absent permanent kidney.[1,2]

The urorectal septum divides the cloaca into two sinuses: (i) the urogenital and (ii) the anorectal sinus. The distal segment of the mesonephric duct forms part of the wall of the urogenital sinus called the trigone. The upper, wider part of the urogenital sinus gives rise to the urinary bladder, the middle segment forms the prostatic and membranous urethra, the lower part forms the definitive urogenital sinus (phallic portion). The hydrostatic pressure of the urine produced results in the opening of the membrane between the ureter and the urinary bladder at week 9, if this step does not take place ureterovesical obstruction or ureterocele develops. At week 9, the membrane of the urigenital sinus is absorbed, from then on, urine is excreted into the amniotic space. Problems with this step lead to obstruction or valve of the urethra.[3]

Over the course of embryogenesis transient pronephros does not produce any urine, the mesonephros produces more or less, whereas the permanent kidney developed from the metanephros produces real urine. Following the conjoining of the ureter and the bladder, urinary bladder filling begins at week 9. With the development of the urethral orifice at week 10, urine is excreted into the amniotic fluid, thus from that time on, the amount and composition of the amniotic fluid is also determined by the urine produced by the active kidney. Oligohydramnios due to abnormal kidney function and absence of urine excretion can be visualized from gestational week 15. Elimination of fetal waste products and maintenance of fetal electrolyte balance are primarily carried out by the placenta. After birth, maintaining homeostasis becomes a role of the kidneys, and the 15% glomerular filtration rate at birth is doubled in the first 2 weeks of life, and reaches the adult rate at 1–2 years of age. This process starts from a smaller value in case of premature babies.[4,5] During ultrasound imaging, malformations of the fetal kidney and urinary tract can be recognized based on differences in comparison with the normal image. The importance of recognizing these malformations is that some of these malformations is severe and incompatible with life, in these cases continuing pregnancy may be pointless, in certain cases the further damage of the kidneys can be prevented by the intrauterine diversion of the accumulated urine, while other malformations can be asymptomatic in 80% of newborns, thus absence of prenatal recognition makes early and successful treatment, aimed at saving the kidney, impossible.

ULTRASOUND IMAGING OF NORMAL FETAL KIDNEYS AND URINARY TRACT

Fetal kidneys can be recognized sonographically using a transvaginal probe from gestational week 11 **(Fig. 1)**, and transabdominally from gestational week 12 **(Fig. 2)**, aided by their characteristic shape and the echogenic appearance of medullary pyramids and the renal cortex. In the parasagittal plane, kidneys appear next to the lumbar spinal column as elliptic, whereas in the horizontal plane as oval paraspinal organs. The central echogenic pyelon–calyx complex composed of fat, connective tissue and hilar blood vessels is surrounded by the less echogenic parenchyma, and around that there is the echogenic perirenal capsule **(Fig. 3)**. There is less than 5 mm of fluid in the pyelon, later the less echogenic medullar and the more echogenic cortical structure can also be differentiated **(Fig. 4)**. The size (length, width and depth) of the kidneys keep growing constantly during pregnancy. Their circumference, the renal circumference/abdominal circumference ratio is constant during pregnancy with a value between 0.27 and 0.30. The normal length of a fetal kidney equals the height of 4–5 vertebrae, and the renal volume can also be determined using 3D ultrasound technique **(Fig. 5)**.

Adrenal glands initially appear as suprarenal hyperechogenic organs and after 30 weeks gestation they

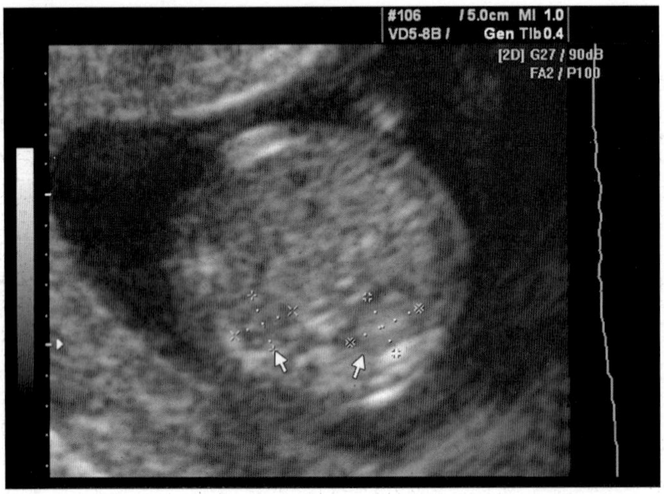

Fig. 1: Transvaginal sonographic view of fetal kidneys at gestational week 11.

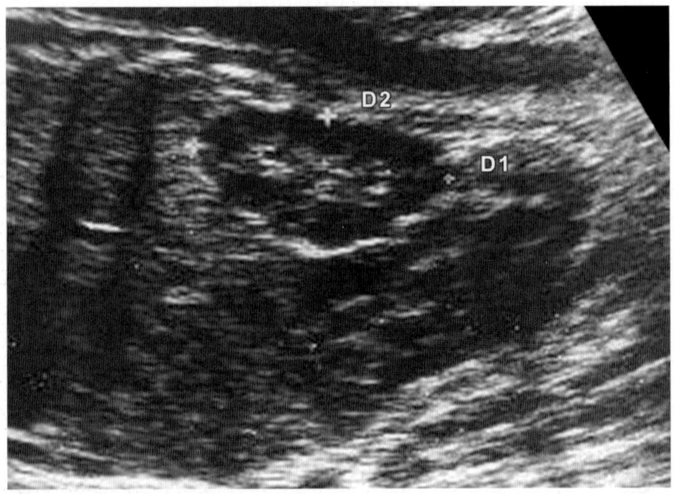

Fig. 3: The perirenal capsule of the fetal kidney is more echogenic, the medulla is less echogenic, the central echo complex is more echogenic.

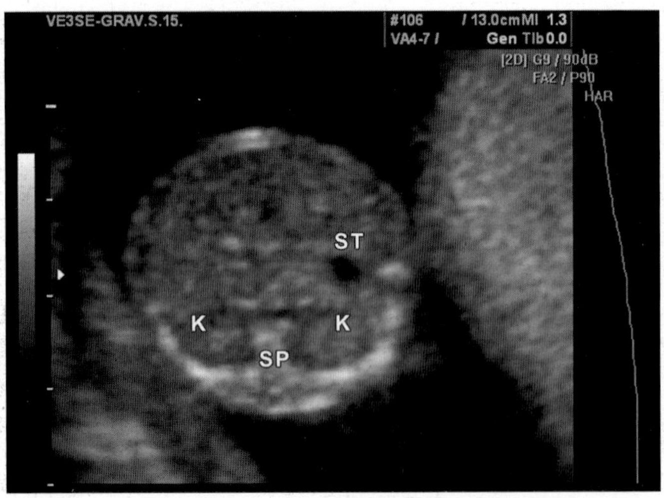

Fig. 2: Transabdominal sonographic view of fetal kidneys at gestational week 14.

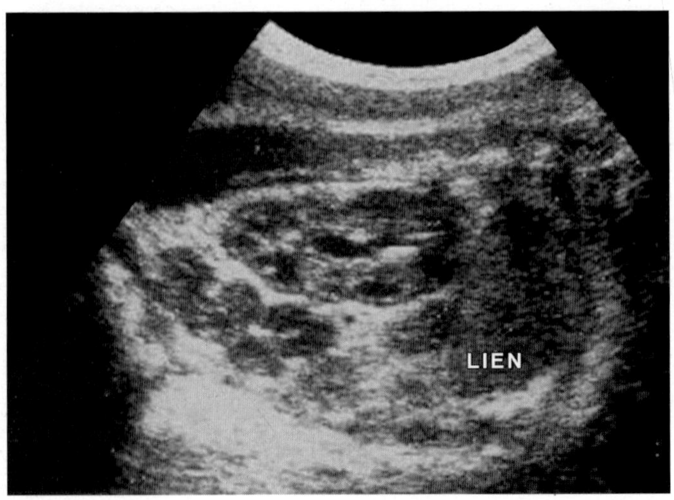

Fig. 4: Less than 5 mm fluid in the pyelon.

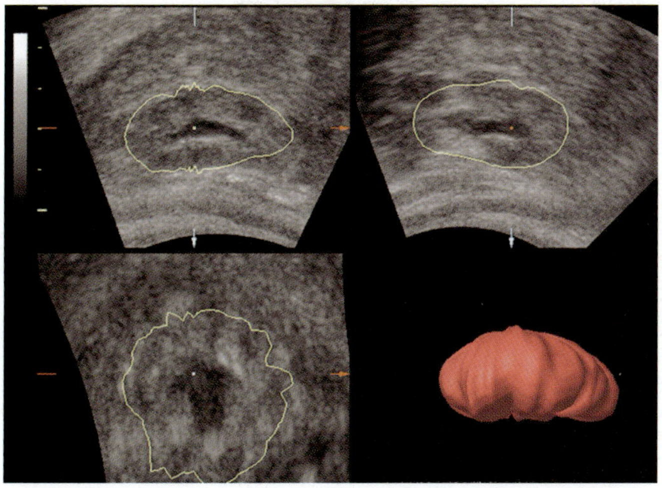

Fig. 5: Imaging the renal volume using 3D technique.

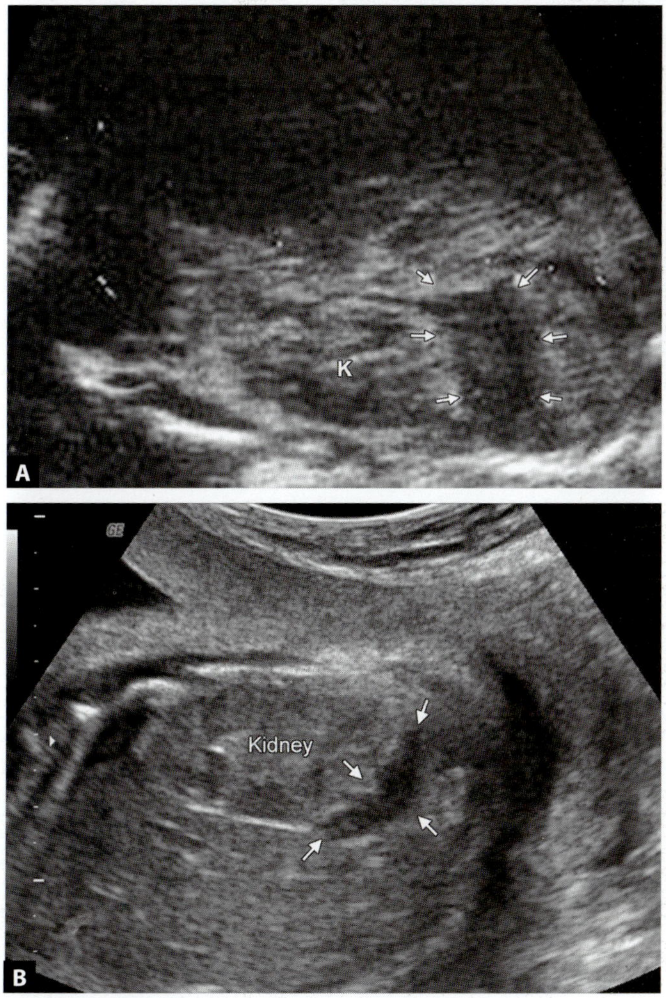

Figs. 6A and B: The fetal adrenal gland is less echogenic.

can be imaged as less echogenic discoid-shaped organs of a size equaling one third of that of the kidneys **(Figs. 6A and B)**. Normally developing ureters cannot be imaged by ultrasound.

The fetal urinary bladder appears as an sonolucent spherical organ between the ischial and iliac ossification centers in the lesser pelvis. Its size changes constantly over 20 to 30-minute intervals due to urination **(Figs. 7 and 8)**. On the two sides of the bladder, the intra-abdominal segments of the umbilical arteries can be easily demonstrated using the color-Doppler technique **(Fig. 9)**.

Anomalies of the renal kidneys and urinary tract can be diagnosed prenatally by detecting the abnormal amount of amniotic fluid (oligohydramnios, polyhydramnios) and

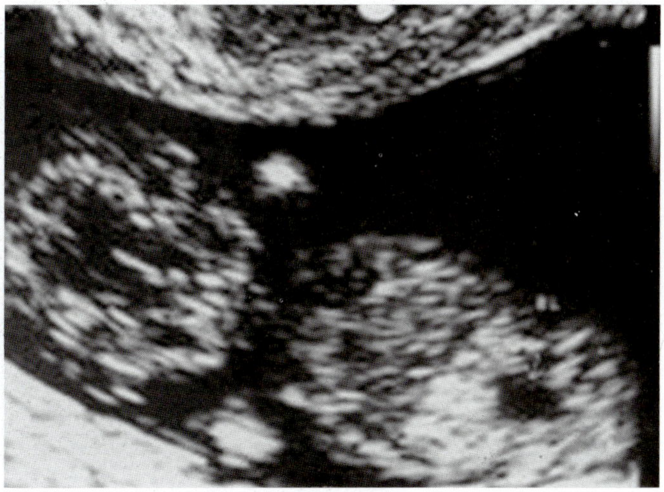

Fig. 7: The unechogenic region of the bladder in the pelvis minor.

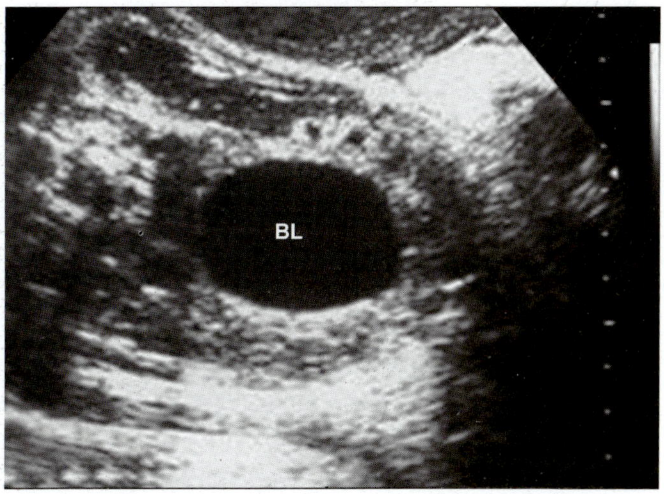

Fig. 8: The full bladder appears as a round unechogenic organ.

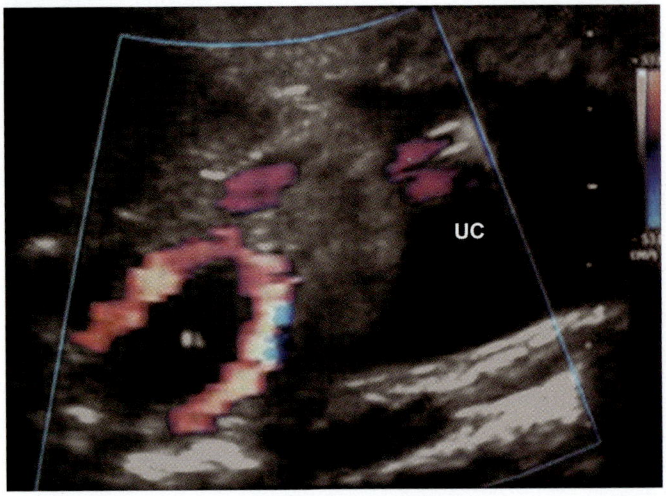

Fig. 9: The umbilical arteries can be detected next to the wall of the bladder.

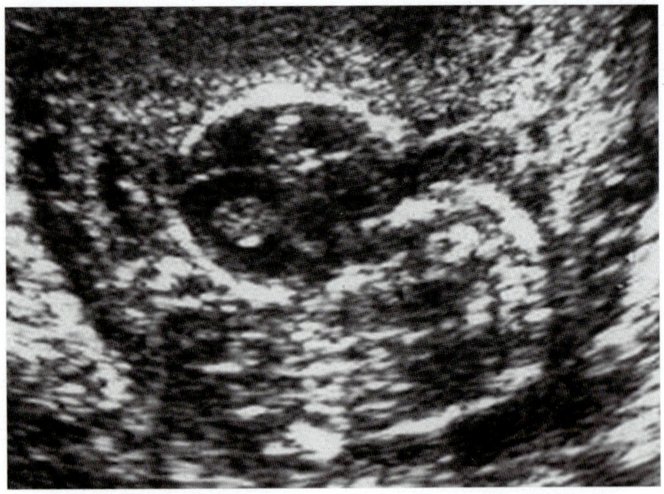

Fig. 10: Forced position of the fetus due to renal agenesia.

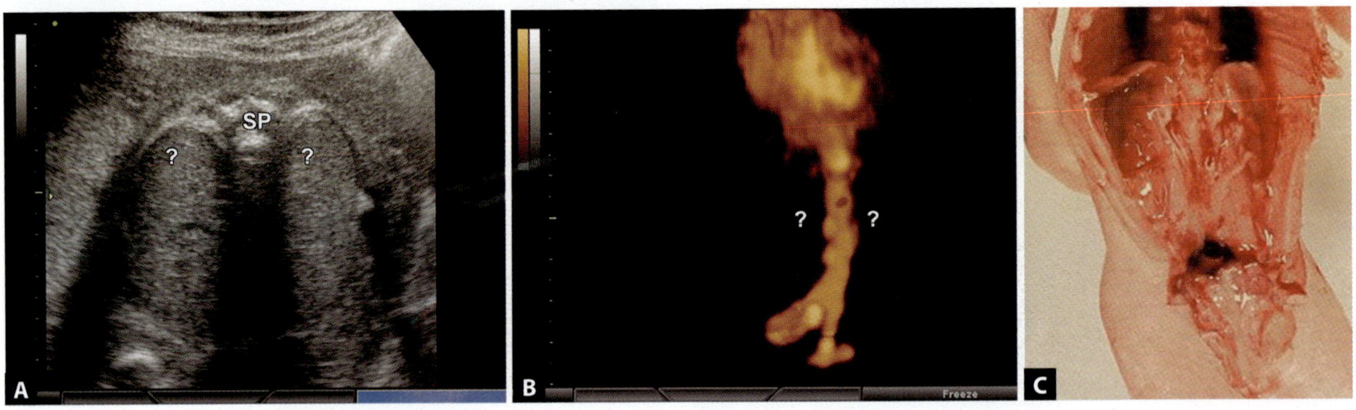

Figs. 11A to C: Bilateral renal agenesia: (A) No kidneys; (B and C) No renal arteries.

fetal urine, analysis of their components, the absence of the regular filling and emptying of the urinary bladder, the uni- or bilateral dilation of the urinary tract (urethra, urinary bladder, ureters, pyelons, calyces), and the alteration of the size and structure of the kidneys (hyperechogenic, cystic).[6-18]

RENAL AGENESIS

This bilateral abnormality appears almost exclusively in males, its incidence is 1/4,000-10,000. It is incompatible with life. Its autosomal dominant form has incomplete penetrance with unilateral agenesis and hypoplasia, but it can also be autosomal recessive or of multifactorial origin. As a consequence of the resulting oligohydramnios, facial and limb deformities, pulmonary hypoplasia, retardation appear, called Potter syndrome. Deformities resulting from oligohydramnios of any origin are called Potter sequence or oligohydramnios deformation sequence. In the case of bilateral agenesis, ultrasonography reveals severe oligohydramnios, arthrogryposis **(Fig. 10)**, growth restriction, the absence of kidneys and absent bladder filling, whereas color-Doppler fails to detect the renal arteries **(Figs. 11 and 12)**. The accompanying central nervous system, cardiovascular, musculoskeletal and gastrointestinal malformations can hardly be imaged due to the decreased amount of amniotic fluid. Adrenal glands that are one third of the kidneys in size can be misleading, especially in the case of the unilateral form of renal agenesis that is 4–20 times more common and is characterized by a urinary bladder of normal volume and a normal amount of amniotic fluid.[6-9,12-16,19]

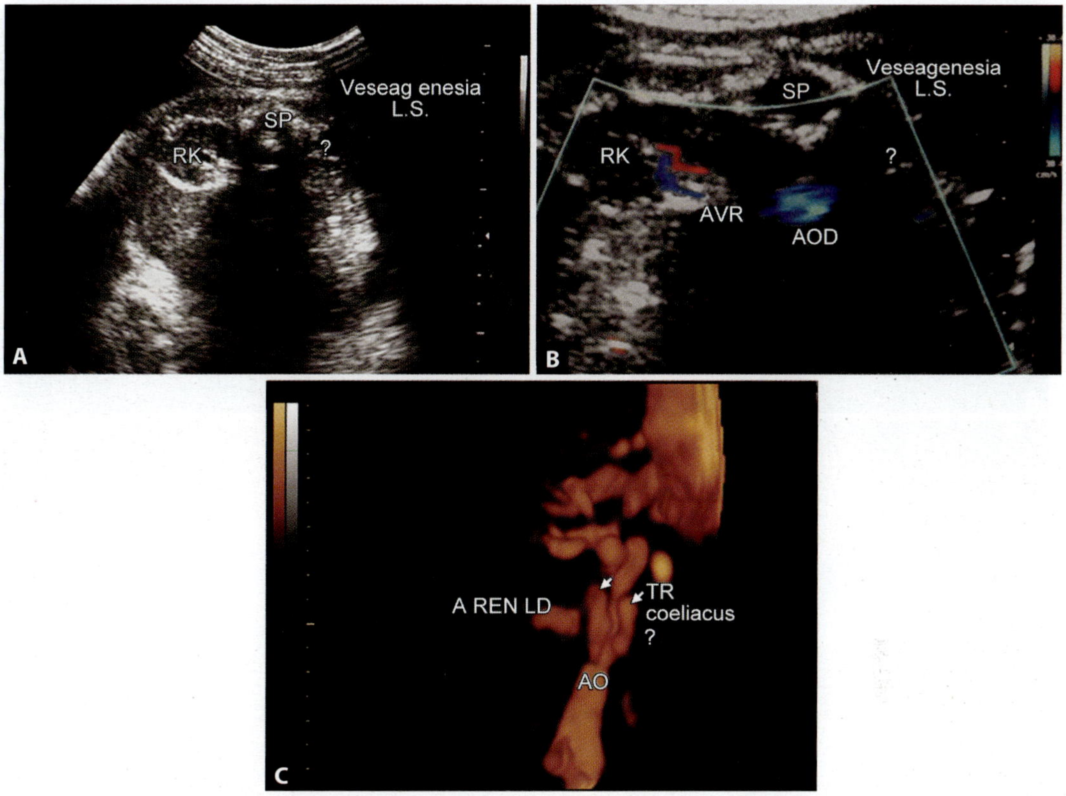

Figs. 12A to C: (A) Unilateral renal agenesia—only one normal kidney; (B and C) One renal artery.

■ CYSTIC RENAL DYSPLASIA

Cystic renal dysplasia refers to a group of congenital renal parenchymal malformations of different origins. Their etiology, manifestation and clinical course cover a wide range.

Autosomal Recessive (Infantile) Polycystic Renal Dysplasia

The incidence of the disease is 1/40,000, the recurrence risk is 25%, the localization of the gene responsible for the disease is as yet unknown. The development of ureters, pyelons, calyces, papillas is regular, the number of nephrons is normal, but in the medulla collecting ducts form 1–2 mm small cysts, which causes the kidneys to be enlarged and lobular **(Figs. 13A to D)**. The affected kidneys do not produce urine, thus the bilateral disease results in oligohydramnios and anuria. The liver is also cystically degenerated accompanied by periportal and intralobular fibrosis, and bile duct proliferation (biliary dysgenesis) and polycystic pulmonary malformation also appear. Based on the different degree of involvement of the kidneys and the liver and based on the course of the disease, fetal, neonatal, infantile, and juvenile types are differentiated. The fetal and neonatal forms lead to death after birth due to the absence of renal function.

The small (1–2 mm) cysts cannot be detected separately during sonography. At the beginning, kidneys appear moderately, later significantly enlarged and as a result of reverberation of echos the medullary segment appears hyperechogenic, the central echo complex cannot be differentiated. Later as the pregnancy progresses, the cortex appears less echogenic. As urine production is missing, urinary bladder filling cannot be detected, the oligohydramnios forces the fetus in an arthrogrypotic position. Calculating the renal/abdominal circumference ratio can help detect the enlargement of the kidneys at an early stage. Depending on the extent of the abnormality of the kidney, the characteristic ultrasonographic image might be recognized only in the second trimester. The prenatally diagnosed autosomal recessive polycystic kidney disease is incompatible with life and thus the pregnancy can be terminated upon request of the parents.[6-9,12-15,20]

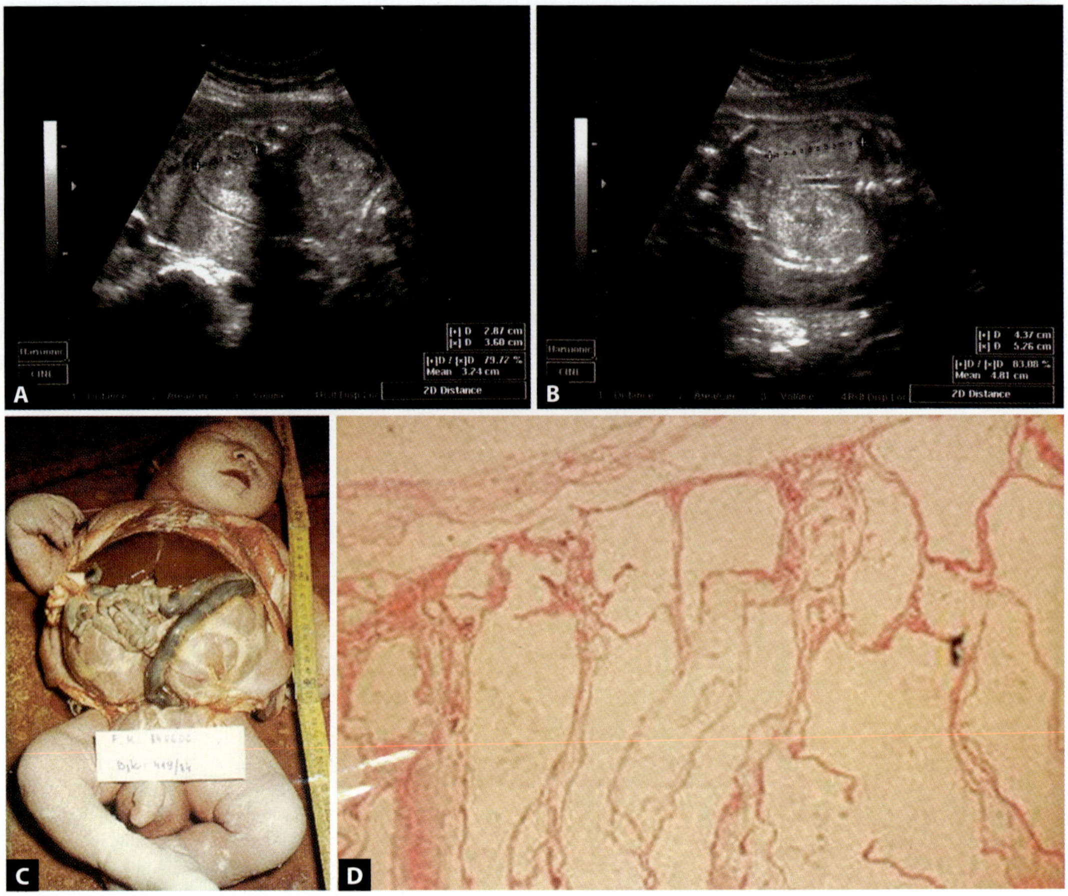

Figs. 13A to D: (A and B) Infantile polycystic renal dysplasia, enlarged kidneys in horizontal and longitudinal planes; (C) At autopsy typically enlarged, lobular kidneys are seen; (D) The histologic section shows small cysts only.

Autosomal Dominant (Adult) Polycystic Renal Dysplasia

The incidence of the disease is 1/15,000. Its recurrence is 50%, the gene responsible for the disease is localized on the short arm of chromosome 16. The expressivity of the disease is variable, it manifests in feti, infants or young children, but occasionally, it causes no symptoms until around 40 years of age, when hypertensive disease, hematuria and constantly deteriorating renal function reveal it. Some nephrons and loops of Henle turn into cysts with thin walls, collecting ducts form thick-walled cysts, but normally functioning tubules and nephrons are also present; therefore, renal dysfunction is less severe. Cysts can also be present in the liver, pancreas and lungs, but hepatic fibrosis and dysfunction are not common. The bilateral manifestation of the disease does not lead to the inability to produce urine, thus urinary bladder filling is present, and it does not result in an oligohydramnios.

In case of adult polycystic renal dysplasia manifesting in fetal life ultrasonography reveals hyperechogenic, more or less enlarged kidneys, macrocysts can be seen only in severe cases, but the central echo complex can be recognized **(Figs. 14A to C)**. As urine is produced, urinary bladder filling is present and oligohydramnios complicates some severe cases only. Following the sonographic imaging of the fetus, it is also necessary to examine the kidneys of the parents as well, with respect to the hereditary nature of the disease. In uncertain situations, molecular genetic examination of the family members may be helpful in differentiating between the autosomal recessive and autosomal dominant forms of the disease.[6-9,12-15,20,21]

Multicystic Renal Dysplasia

The incidence of the disease is 1/10,000, it is more common in males, and its etiology is unclear. The activity of the ampules at the end of the collecting tubules is inhibited,

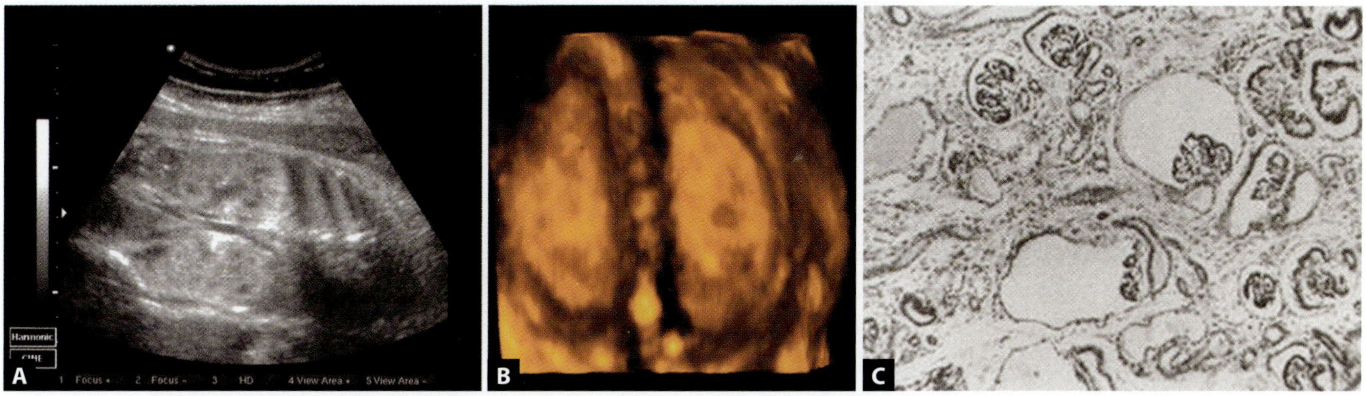

Figs. 14A to C: (A and B) Enlarged adult polycystic kidneys with central echo complex; (C) Histology—small cysts between glomeruli.

the branching of the collecting tubules decreases, the induction of nephrons is reduced. Collecting tubules form cysts with thick walls, nephrons turn into thin-walled cysts, in between which loose connective tissue is present. The kidney is enlarged, normal renal parenchyma and urine production are missing. In 2/3 of the cases, the abnormality is unilateral, in 1/3 it is bilateral, and rarely, it is segmental. Unilateral multicystic renal dysplasia is often accompanied by other urogenitary or chromosomal aberrations. Bilateral multicystic renal dysplasia is not accompanied by the cystic dysplasia of other organs, it causes Potter sequence and is incompatible with life. In its isolated form it cannot be inherited, but as part of a syndrome, such as Meckel-Gruber syndrome or Zellweger syndrome, it shows autosomal recessive inheritance.

Ultrasonographic imaging reveals cysts of diverse size in the expected position of the kidneys, but renal parenchyma or central echo complex cannot be identified **(Figs. 15A to E)**. If the disease is unilateral, urinary bladder filling can not be detected, oligohydramnios is present. In unilaterally manifesting cases, normal bladder filling and amniotic fluid amount is seen. Sometimes, even the compensatory hypertrophy of the contralateral kidney and a resulting moderate polyhydramnios can be detected. It is important to differentiate it from dilated, tortuous ureters caused by ureterovesical obstruction and dilated calyces seen in mild hydronephrosis.[6-9,12-15,20-24]

Obstructive Cystic Renal Dysplasia

Obstruction of the urinary tract at any level (ureteropelvical, ureterovesical, urethral) will cause cystic dysplasia due to increased intraluminar pressure. Morphology depends on the place and time of obstruction during nephrogenesis.

Early obstruction causes cystic dysplasia at the end of the primitive mesonephric duct and the ampulles of the collecting tubules leading to multicystic kidney disease.

Increased pressure beginning later in development will be transferred to the collecting tubules and causes parenchymal disorganization, cystic dilation of the capsule of Bowman, forming of subcapsular cysts[25] and fibrosis at the other end of the collecting ducts.

Starting even later, increased pressure will lead to the degeneration of the parenchyma and as a result, a hydronephrotic kidney appears.

Early obstruction at the upper segment of the ureter results in the appearance of a multicystic kidney. Obstruction at lower parts of the ureter during the second trimester, as well as obstruction at the level of the urethra lead to increased urinary tract pressure later, causing formation of subcapsular cysts and hydronephrosis. Early deviation of urine decreases the intraluminal pressure and thus cystic dysplasia can be prevented.

Ultrasound imaging after gestational week 20 shows the dilation of the pyelon and calyces of the affected kidney, the increased echogenity due to the small subcapsular cysts, and later the growing subcapsular cysts **(Fig. 16)**.[6-9,12-15,20]

OBSTRUCTIVE UROPATHY

Strictures and blockages at different levels of the urinary tract cause urinary retention and increased intraluminal pressure and thus lead to dilation of different degree not only in the renal parenchyma but also in the urinary tract. Depending on the place and duration of the blockage, the upper segment of the urethra, the bladder, the ureter, the pyelon and the calyces can be dilated **(Figs. 17A to D)**. The final result can be hydronephrosis with the

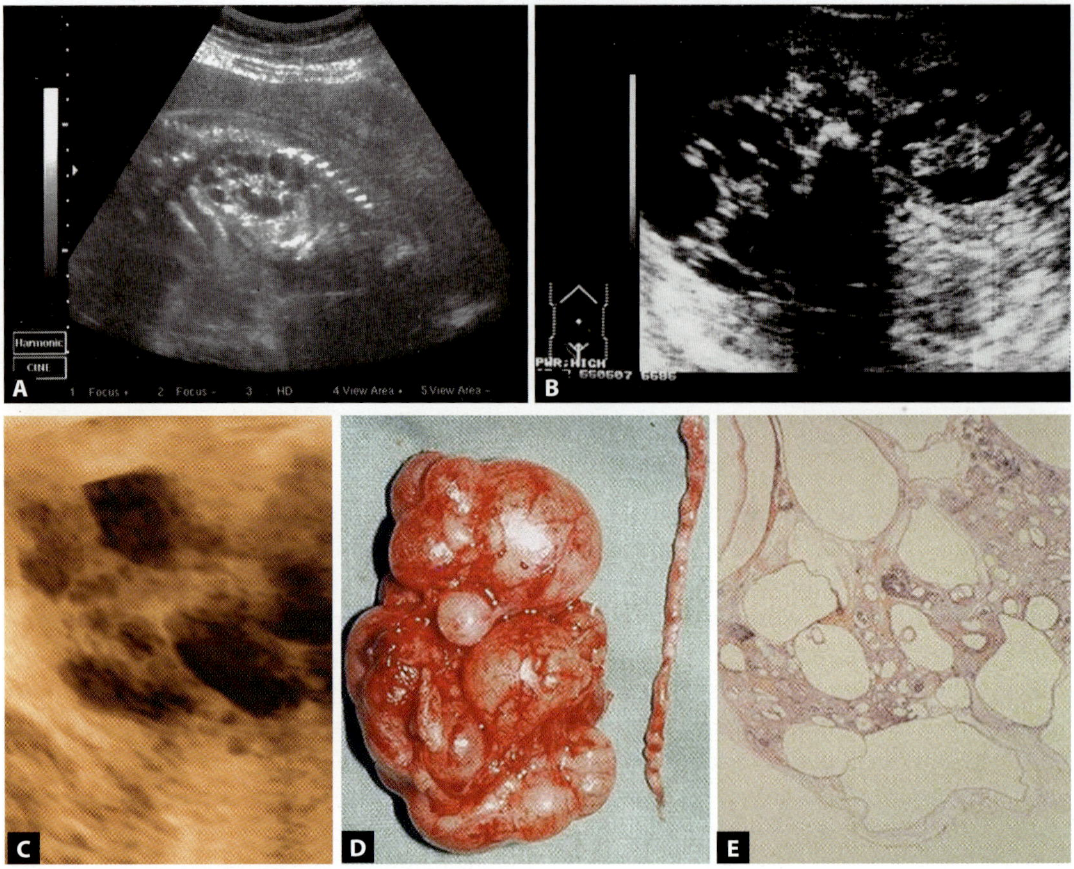

Figs. 15A to E: Multicystic renal dysplasia: there are 10–20 mm cysts in the kidneys, no central echo complex is present. (A) Unilateral; (B and C) Bilateral; (D) The kidney is made up of various size cysts; (E) Histology—cysts with thin and thick walls.

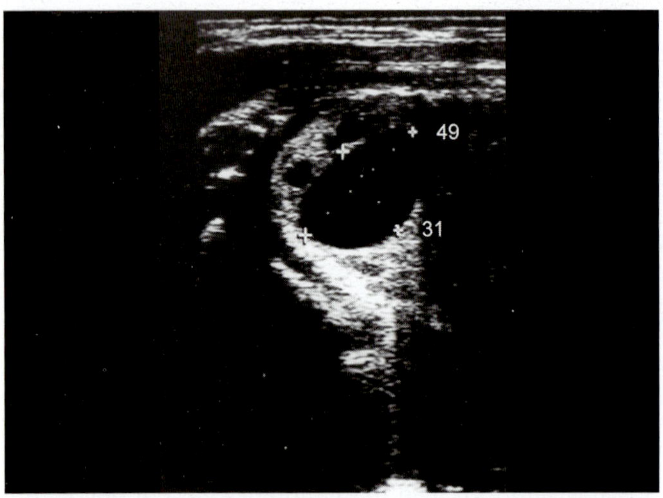

Fig. 16: Subcapsular cyst in a hydronephrotic kidney.

degeneration of renal parenchyma. Anteroposterior dilation of the renal pelvis can have five degrees. Dilation above 10 mm or exceeding 50% of the anteroposterior size of the kidney is considered hydronephrosis.[6,7,13,14,17,26-34]

Obstruction of the Ureteropelvic Junction

Urine passage can be blocked by the abnormal shape of the pyeloureteral junction, adhesion of the lumen, folding of the mucosa, ureteral valve or absence of longitudinal muscle fibers, leading to hydronephrosis. It is twice as common in males as in females, it is sporadic and inheritance is uncommon. In 70% of the cases, it is unilateral with a left side predominance, but in these cases the abnormality of the other kidney (renal agenesis, multicystic dysplasia, ectopic kidney) can also be detected. In the bilateral manifestation (30% of cases), the extent of renal damage on the two sides is different. It is rare that is accompanied by abnormalities of other organs. 80% of the cases will cause no symptoms after delivery, 10% will regress spontaneously, and in 90% conservative or surgical treatment becomes necessary.

Ultrasonography shows a certain degree of pyelectasia in the affected kidney **(Figs. 18A to C)** and at the ureteropelvic junction the renal cortex becomes thinner.

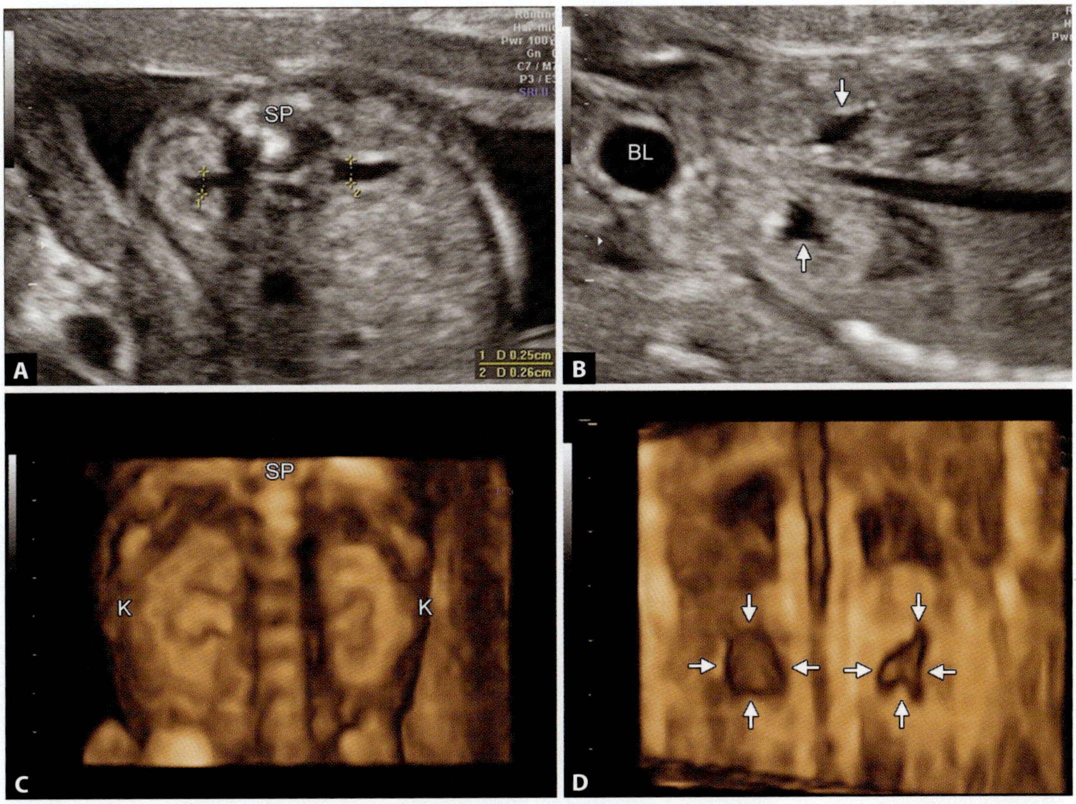

Figs. 17A to D: The pyelon and calyces are dilated.

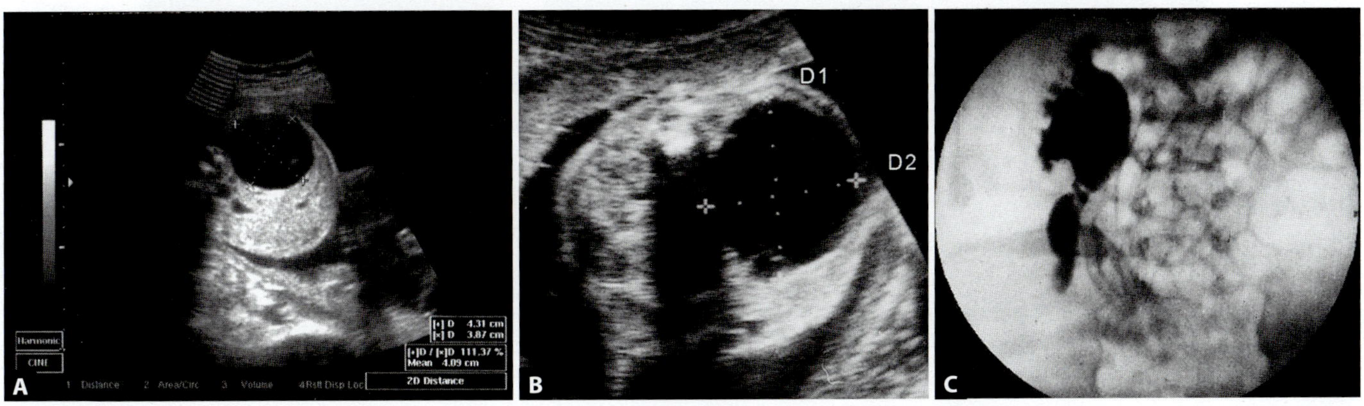

Figs. 18A to C: (A and B) Extremely dilated hydronephrotic kidney; (C) X-ray image.

Below the block, ureters are not dilated and thus are invisible. If the disease is unilateral, bladder filling is present and the amount of the amniotic fluid is normal, but when an incomplete manifestation is encountered, polyhydramnios can also be found. If the kidney is severely damaged and the contralateral kidney does not function either, bladder filling is missing and the amount of the amniotic fluid is minimal.[6,7,14]

Stricture or Valve of the Ureter

A circular or semicircular mucosal fold or valve containing muscle bands can appear at any level of the ureter and may lead to blockage of urine flow.

Sonography shows the segment of the ureter above the valve as being dilated and having active peristalsis, whereas the segment below the blockage cannot be visualized.

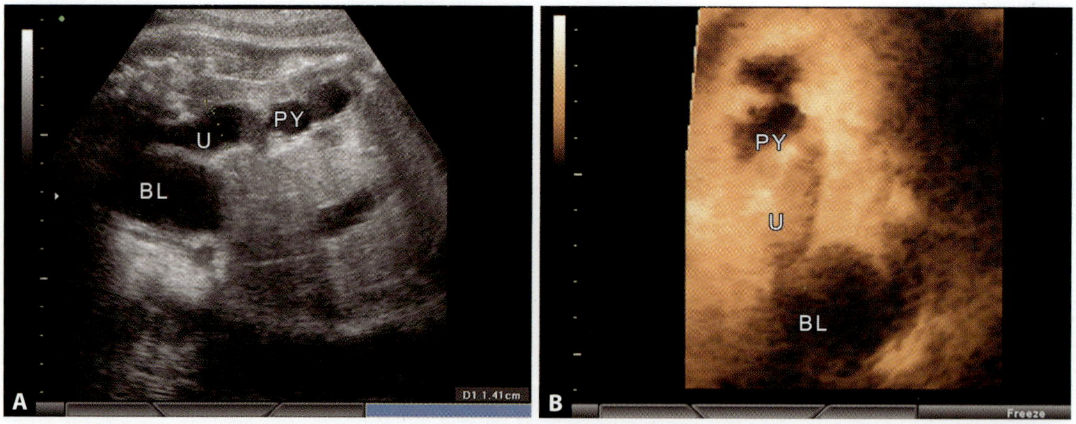

Figs. 19A and B: (A) Behind the bladder (BL), dilated ureter (U) and dilated pyelon (PY) in (A) 2D and (B) 3D image.

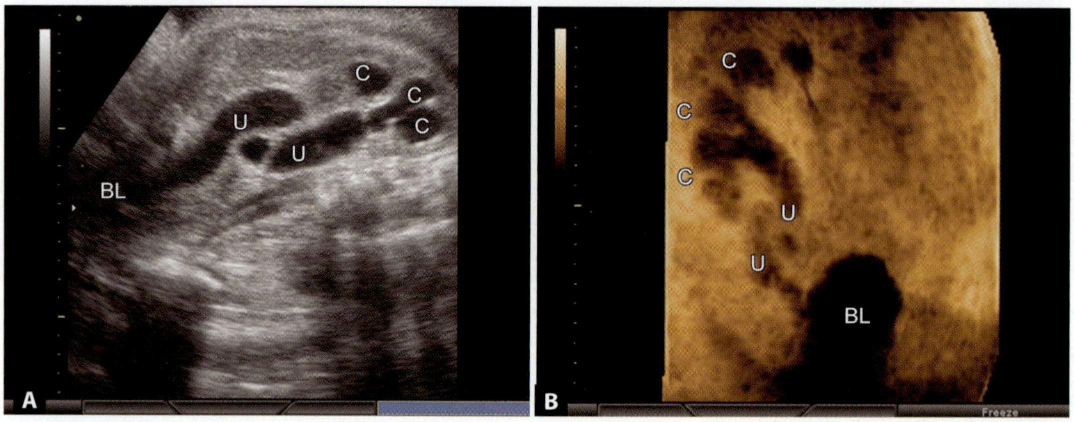

Figs. 20A and B: Double kidney and ureter, with a ureter connected to the dilated lower pole of the kidney.

Obstruction of the Ureterovesical Junction: Megaureter

Pathologic dilation of the ureter is 4 times more common in males, 2–3 times more frequent on the left side, and in 20% of the cases it can be bilateral. It is sporadic, but inherited forms have also been reported. Stenosis, fibrosis, abnormal muscular layer, segmental absence of peristalsis or absence of the antireflux mechanism at the ureterovesical junction leads to primary megaureter and consecutive hydronephrosis. Blockage at a lower segment of the urinary bladder and consecutive reflux leads to secondary megaureter. Megaureter can be accompanied by renal agenesis, incomplete or complete duplication, contralateral cystic renal dysplasia or Hirschsprung's disease.

Ultrasonography reveals pyelectasia and a dilated (sometimes even 1–2 cm wide), sonolucent, peristaltic, tortuous ureter that can be followed down to the bladder **(Figs. 19A and B)**. Double renal pelvis and dilation of the upper part can indicate ureter duplex with the dilation of only one of the two ureters.[6,7,13,14,35,36]

Vesicoureteral Reflux

The ureterovesical junction is positioned higher and more laterally, therefore the submucosal part of the ureter is shorter, thus urine can regurgitate from the bladder into the ureter more easily.[37] The abnormality can be uni- or bilateral, if there is double ureter present, it belongs to the lower one and leads to mild or moderate hydronephrosis **(Figs. 20A and B)**. It is considered to be a multifactorial disease, but autosomal recessive and sex chromosome linked cases have also been reported.

Ultrasonography reveals mild, nonprogressive, sometimes only intermittently appearing hydronephrosis, a dilated ureter showing no peristalsis and normal amount of amniotic fluid.[6,7,38,39]

Ureterocele

It is 4 times more common in males, usually it appears on the left side, in 15% of the cases it is bilateral. Simple ureterocele means that the thin membrane of the lower segment of the ureter fails to disappear, it appears in the urinary bladder as a cyst with a thin wall. It hinders urinary flow and leads to hydroureter and hydronephrosis. If ureteral duplication is present,[39] the ectopic ureterovesical junction can result in ectopic ureterocele. The ectopic junction can be at the neck of the bladder or even the urethra, and the ureterocele may block the ipsilateral or contralateral ureteral orifice or the neck of the bladder. The renal segment connected to the ectopic ureterocele is often found to be abnormal (hypoplasia, dysplasia, hydronephrotic atrophy) with deteriorated function.

Ultrasonography shows the ureterocele as a cyst with a thin wall inside the bladder and the dilated hydroureter.[7,15] In two cases we managed to fenestrate the membrane of the ureterocele by transabdominal ultrasound-guided punctures and let the urine excrete into the bladder, and managed to relieve the bilateral hydroureter and hydronephrosis and prevent the kidneys from damage. Under close observation after birth, there was no need for surgical intervention, the function of the kidneys is normal and there is no urinary tract obstruction (**Figs. 21A to H**).

Megacystis, Microcolon and Intestinal Hypoperistalsis Syndrome

The disease is most probably of multifactorial origin, more common in females, and sometimes seems to be hereditary. The affected organs display neurodysplasia, indicating some innervation disorder, which leads to the dilation of the bladder without obstruction (megacystis), small intestines are shorter and dilated, the colon is narrower (microcolon), and intestinal peristalsis is weak or missing. Unable to empty, the distended bladder pushes the abdominal wall forward, the increased pressure affects the ureters and the kidneys, too, resulting in dilation. Intestinal dysfunction leads to polyhydramnios.

Ultrasonography reveals polyhydramnios, an extremely dilated (**Fig. 22**) bladder with a thin wall, megaureter and hydronephrosis.[13,14]

Urethral Obstruction

The incidence of the disease at birth is between 1/35,000 and 1/50,000. It has a multifactorial etiology, sometimes it is hereditary. The partial or complete blockage of the urethra leads to urine retention, bladder dilation, bilateral hydroureter, hydronephrosis, cystic renal dysplasia, consecutive oligohydramnios, pulmonary hypoplasia, facial and limb deformity (urethral obstruction sequence), cryptorchism in males, rectus diastasis of the abdominal wall and a dilated abdominal wall (prune-belly syndrome).[7,40] The posterior urethral valve is found almost exclusively in males, whereas the rare urethra agenesis is seen in females. The ejaculatory duct evolving from the distal part of the mesonephric duct has an abnormal junction formation, resulting in the appearance of the posterior urethral valve and the dilation of the urinary tract. Increased intraluminal pressure may also lead to a subcortical perinephric urinoma, and in case it ruptures, urine ascites can result (**Fig. 23**). The disease is accompanied by other urogenital or other organ or chromosomal (chromosomes 13 and 18) abnormalities.

Ultrasonography reveals oligohydramnios (in 50% of the cases), dilated bladder with a thick wall, the funnel-shaped dilation of the neck of the bladder and the first part of the urethra (**Figs. 24 and 25**), bilateral hydroureter, bilateral hydronephrosis, the damaged renal parenchyma, subcapsular cysts or sometimes urinomas.[6,7,14,41-43]

Persistent Cloaca

If the urorectal septum fails to develop, a persistent cloaca is the result. This sand-glass-shaped sinus is the terminal collecting cavity of the urogenitary and the gastrointestinal tracts. This common sinus surrounded by the abdominal wall is filled with urine and bowel content, the increased pressure leads to the dilation of the ureters and pyelons. Because of the intact cloaca membrane, urine will not pass into the amniotic space, therefore oligohydramnios will be present.

Ultrasonography shows oligohydramnios, the fetal abdomen is pushed forward and inside of it an unusually shaped cystic region can be seen, sometimes containing septa (**Figs. 26A and B**). In the horizontal plane, this region extends into the space next to the spinal column.[3,6,7]

Cloaca Exstrophy

The incidence of the malformation is 1/200,000 and can be seen in both sexes. During embryogenesis, the urorectal septum dividing the cloaca fails to reach the cloaca membrane, the fusion of the mesodermal crests that normally leads to the closure of the abdominal wall as well as the caudal retraction of the membrane do not take place, and after the membrane dissolves, the bladder

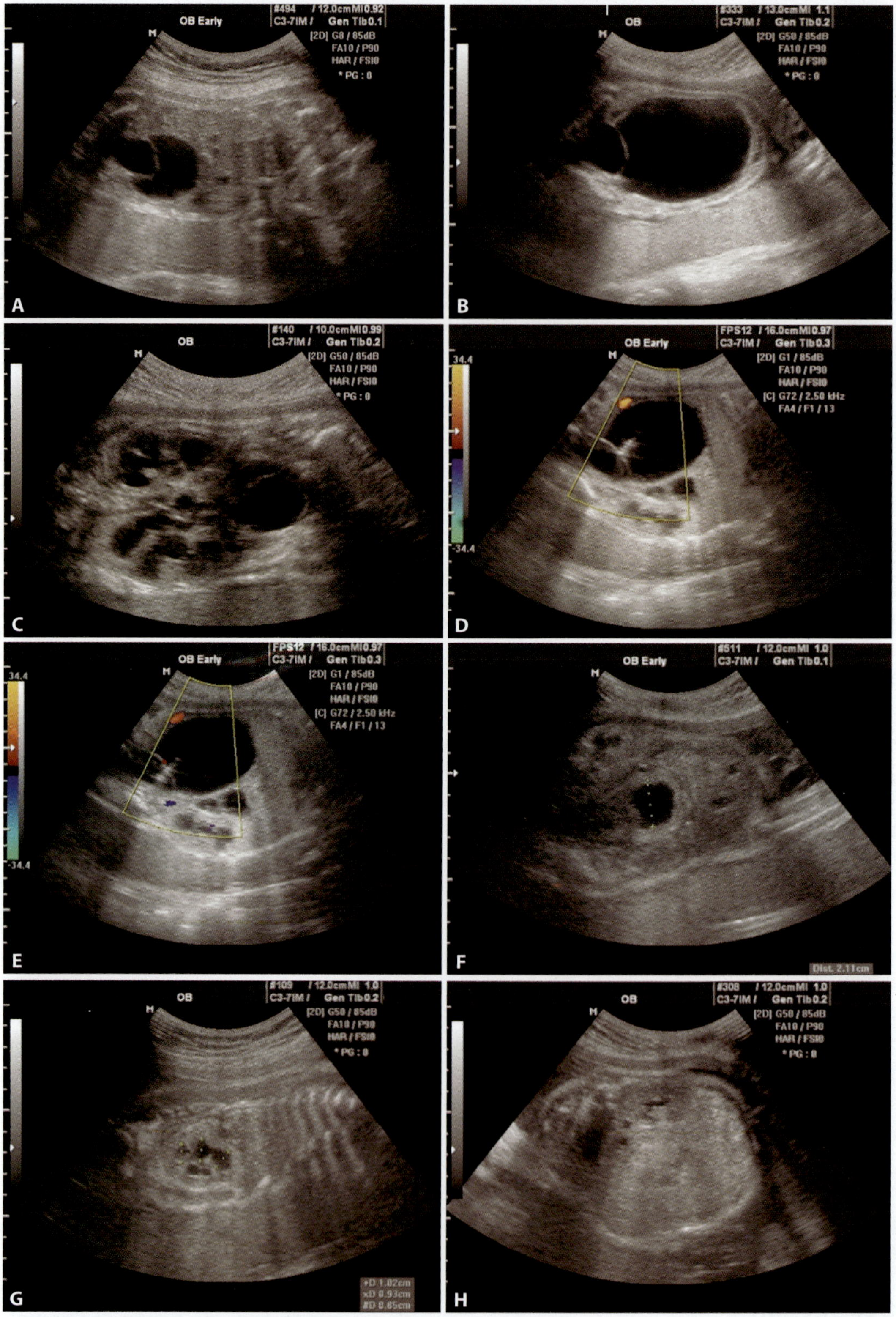

Figs. 21A to H: (A) Unilateral cystic protrusion of the ureterocele into the bladder at 26 weeks of gestation; (B) Ureterocele and hyperextended bladder at 29 weeks of gestation; (C) Bilateral severe hydronephrosis at 29 weeks of gestation; (D) Intrauterine vesicocentesis at 29 weeks of gestation; (E) Intrauterine fenestration of the ureterocele at 29 weeks of gestation; (F) Moderate dilatation of the urinary bladder after the fenestration of the ureterocele; (G) Moderate dilatation of the calycies on the affected side; (H) Normal kidney on the contralateral side after the fenestration.

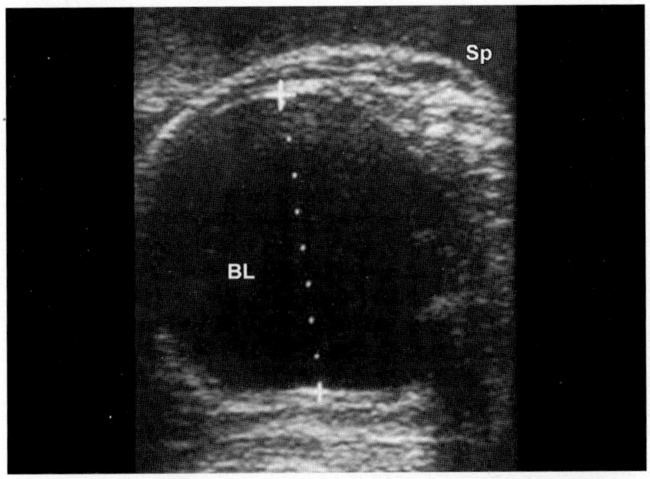

Fig. 22: Megacystis-microcolon-intestinal hypoperistalsis syndrome—the wall of the dilated bladder (BL) is thin.

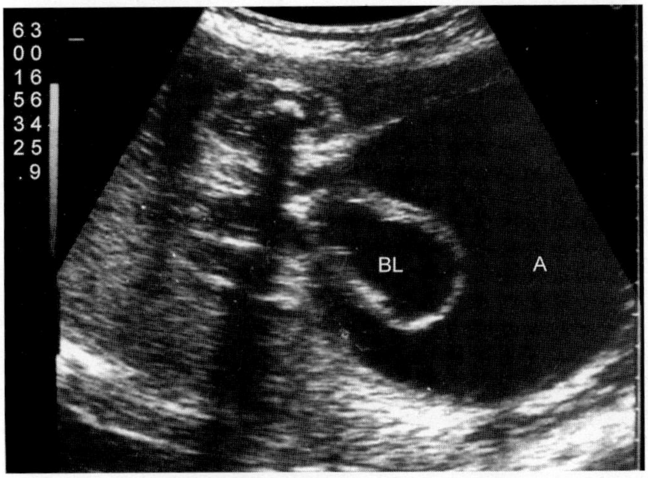

Fig. 23: Urine ascites—dilated bladder with thick wall (BL) appears in the ascites (A).

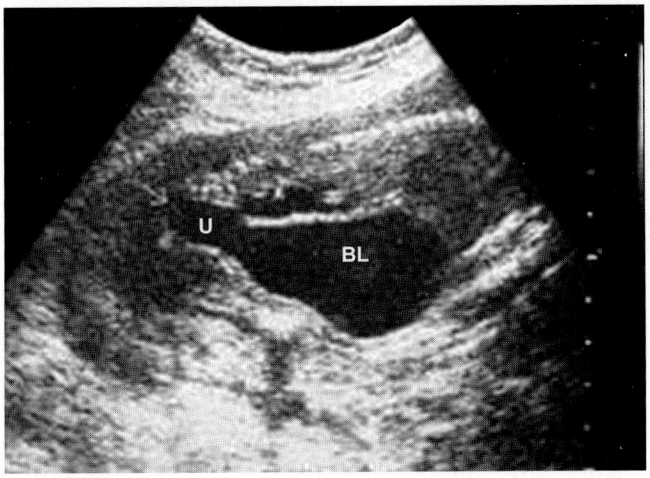

Fig. 24: Urethral obstruction—the first part of the urethra and the neck of the bladder show funnel-shaped dilation.

and the rectum is placed externally, resulting in cloaca exstrophy.[3]

Urinary Bladder Exstrophy

The incidence of the malformation is 1/40,000 births, and it is more common in males. The cloaca is divided by the cloaca membrane, but the retraction of the cloaca membrane is abnormal and the posterior wall of the bladder is externalized. The defect of the lower abdominal wall and the absence of the anterior wall of the bladder results in the extra-abdominal position of the bladder. In a mild case, the divergence of the rectus abdominis muscle and the symphysis is minimal. In the common moderate case, beside bladder exstrophy, the abdominal wall and the symphysis joint is split. In the most severe situation, all the above mentioned abnormalities are present, accompanied by umbilical and inguinal hernia, a ventrally positioned anus with a relaxed sphincter and intermittent rectal prolapse.

Ultrasonography reveals absence of bladder filling. At the abdominal wall below the umbilicus, sometimes cystic structure or extra soft tissue can be demonstrated. The umbilical arteries can be visualized using color-Doppler outside the abdominal wall **(Figs. 27A to D)**. Deformity of the pubic bone can be suspected only in severe cases. Accompanying genital or renal malformations can hardly be visualized due to the oligohydramnios.[44]

RENAL TUMORS

Mesoblastic Nephroma

It is a leiomyomatous renal hamartoma containing connective, adipose, smooth muscle tissue, and tubular epithelial cells. Clinically, it is a benign tumor, histologically dominated by the presence of mesenchymal tissue.

Ultrasonography shows a large, mainly solid bulk in the region of one of the kidneys, it can have cystically degenerated parts, the renal capsule is blurred. The other kidney has a normal structure. It almost always produces polyhydramnios.[7,45]

Wilms' Tumor

It is a multifocal, often bilateral tumor, composed mainly of epithelial tissues. It has a more malignant clinical course.

Prenatal ultrasonography shows a bilateral solid bulk, indicating Wilms' tumor. This, however, does not allow to determine the exact diagnosis, but it gives information to arrange the necessary postnatal examinations and treatment.

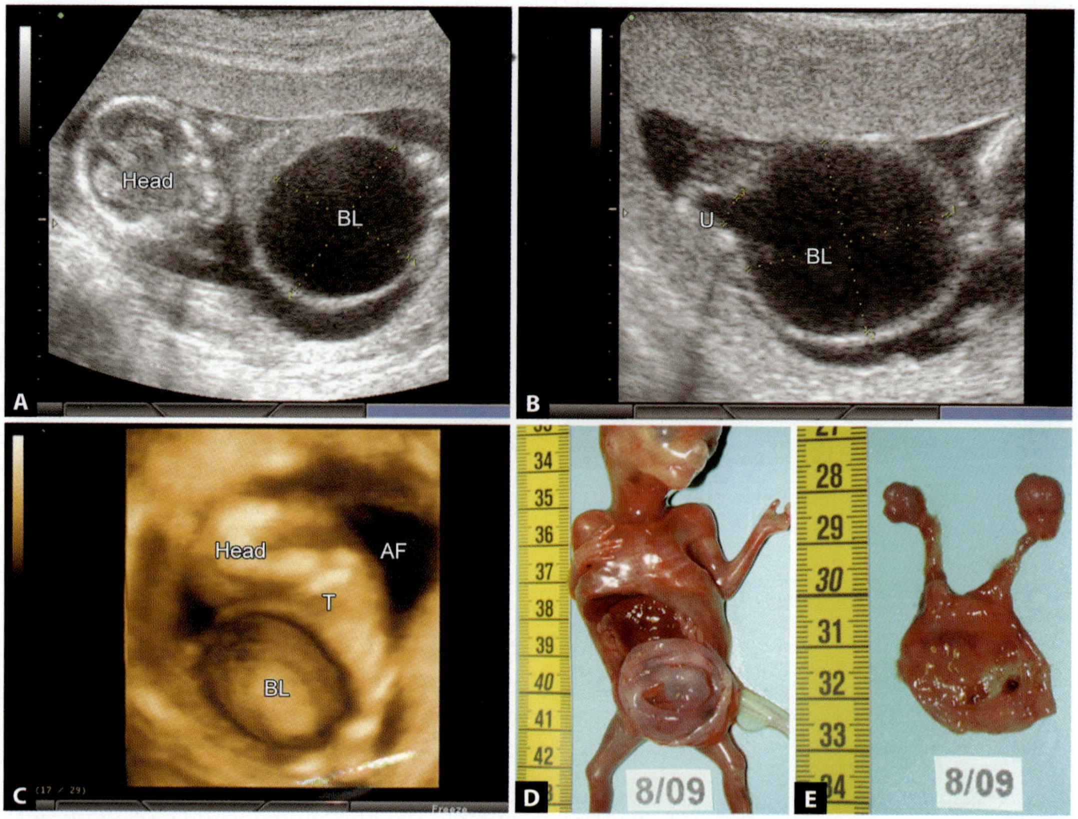

Figs. 25A to E: Urethra obstruction diagnosed at gestational period of 14 weeks. (A and B) 2D sonographic images; (C) 3D sonographic image; (D and E) Autopsy photographs.

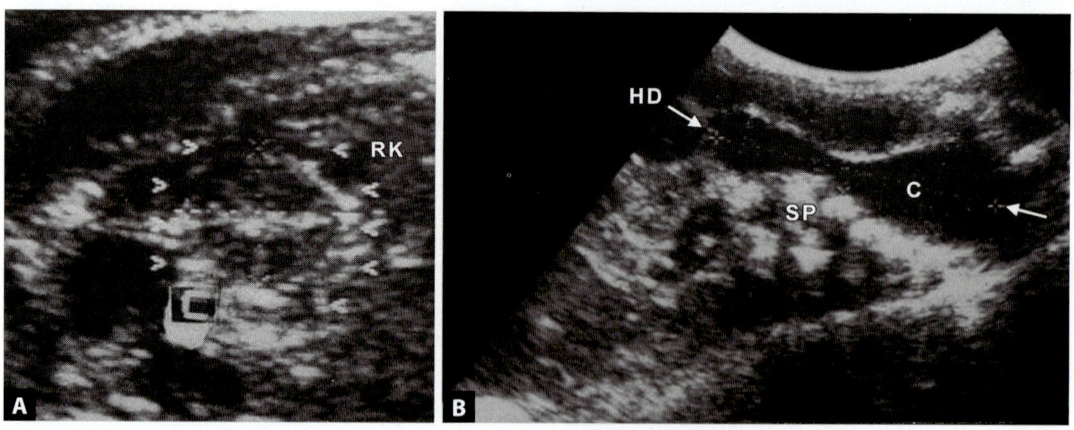

Figs. 26A and B: Ultrasound image of persistent cloaca, appearing as an unusual cystic region in the abdomen. (A) Prenatal; (B) Postnatal.

DETERMINATION OF FETAL RENAL FUNCTION

Following the prenatal diagnosis of kidney and urinary tract malformations, it is important to determine renal function of the fetus. Following points need to be taken care of in determining the renal function of the fetus:

- The amount of amniotic fluid is an indirect indicator of renal function. Early oligohydramnios indicates renal agenesis or severe problems with renal function. Normal or excessive amount of amniotic fluid requires at least one functioning kidney.[46-48]

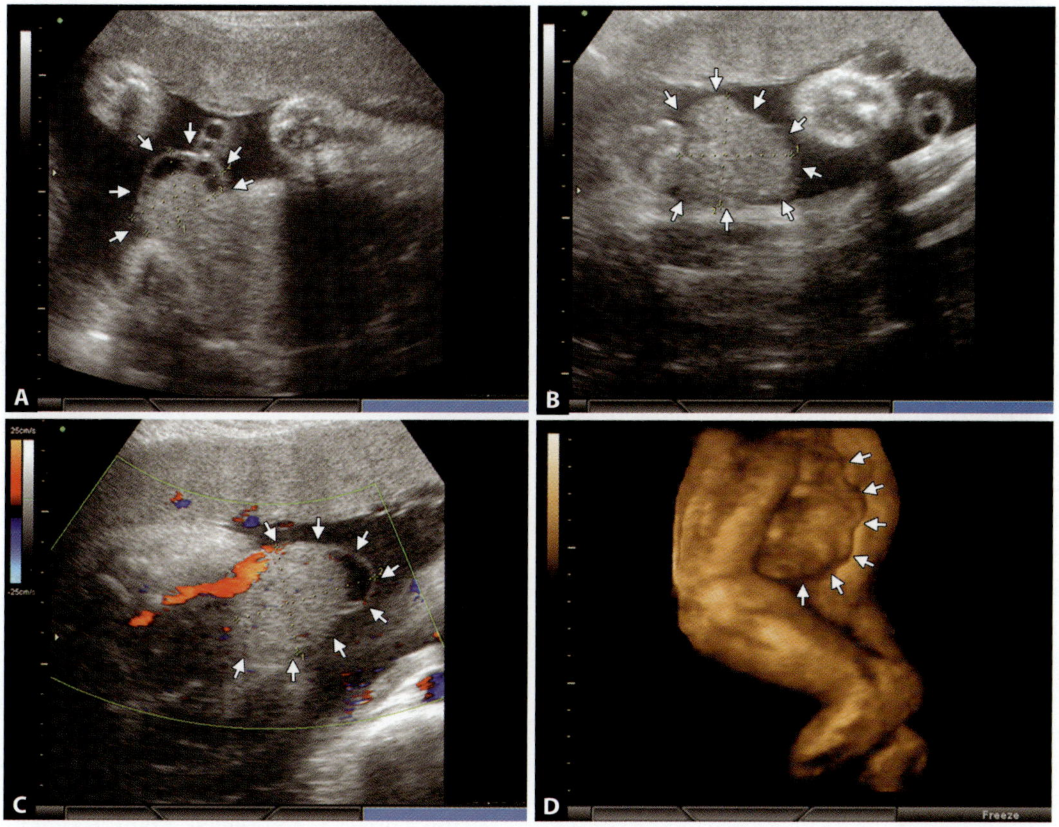

Figs. 27A to D: (A and B) Urinary bladder exstrophy—in the subumbilical region of the abdominal wall, small, protruding, cystic tissue or; (C) Soft tissue surplus is seen; (D) Umbilical arteries are found outside the abdominal wall using color-Doppler imaging.

- Urinary bladder filling indicates at least one functioning kidney. Absence of filling raises the possibility of renal agenesis, bilateral ureteral obstruction or kidney damage. Distension of the bladder indicates conduction problems at the level of the urethra.
- Ureteral dilation can be observed due to obstruction of the lower segments. There is only a weak correlation between the severity of the dilation and renal impairment.
- Echogenicity of the renal parenchyma and visualization of subcapsular cysts are not suitable for determining precise renal function.[7,26]
- Examination of the circulation of renal arteries can prove to be a useful tool which helps determine kidney functional impairment in case retrograde pressure increases.[15]
- Biochemical analysis of fetal urine consists of examination of urine acquired from the dilated urinary bladder or the dilated calyces through transabdominal puncture. Urinary Na^+ <100 mmol/L, Cl^- <90 mmol/L, osmolarity <210 mOsmol/L and creatinine <150 umol/L indicate good prognosis. Elevated levels and the appearance of proteins smaller than 70,000 dalton molecular weight indicate probable renal functional impairment.[6,7,15]

TREATMENT OF PRENATALLY DIAGNOSED RENAL AND URINARY TRACT ANOMALIES

In cases of bilateral, severe renal impairment incompatible with postnatal life (renal agenesis, infant polycystic kidney, multicystic renal dysplasia, hydronephrotic kidneys, unilateral multicystic and contralateral nonfunctioning kidney, early abnormalities with severe oligohydramnios and pulmonal hypoplasia) termination of pregnancy can be offered to the parents.

In cases of a unilateral, severe anomaly (agenesis, multicysticrenaldysplasia, severehydronephrosis) accompanied by other severe concomitant malformation(s), termination of the pregnancy can be offered before week 24. Unilateral malformations without severe concomitant abnormalities and a normal amount of amniotic fluid require regular control and multidisciplinary (obstetrical, neonatological, surgical, urological) counseling.[49]

Urethric obstruction can be solved by a vesicoamnial shunt prepared before week 24. So far open fetal surgical techniques have been carried out with poor outcomes.

Dilation of the renal pelvis requires follow-up by repeated ultrasound examinations. Prenatally diagnosed pyelectasy, hydronephrosis is best controlled at day 3–7 after birth, after physiologic postnatal dehydration passes. Cases showing spontaneous regression should be examined by ultrasound again two weeks later. In case of an abnormal finding, a detailed examination of the neonate is necessary (IV urography, voiding cystography, nuclear renography, laboratory examinations).

Early prenatal diagnosis, timely interventions and thorough postnatal examinations create the possibility to significantly decrease the morbidity and mortality of fetuses and neonates suffering [50,51] from kidney and urinary tract anomalies, and to minimize the number of future dialyses.

ACKNOWLEDGMENTS

We should like to express our sincere gratitude to Dr András Tankó for his permission to insert some sonographic pictures from his collection and for his helpful comments on the manuscript.

REFERENCES

1. Potter EL. Normal and abnormal development of the kidney, Medical Publishers, Chicago; 1972.
2. Gersh I. The correlation of structure and function in the developing mesonephros and metanephros Contrib Embryol. 1937;26:35-9.
3. Tank ES. Urologic complications of imperforate anus and cloacal dysgenesis. In: Cambell S (Ed). Urology. 4th edition. WB Saunders Co, Philadelphia; 1986. pp. 1889-2000.
4. McCrory WW. Embryonic development and prenatal maturation of the kidney. In: Edelmann CM (Ed). Pediatric kidney disease, Boston, Little Brown; 1978. pp. 3-25.
5. McCrory WW. Developmental nephrology, Cambridge, Harward University Press; 1972.
6. Callen PW (Ed). Ultrasonography in obstetrics and gynecology. 4th edition, WB Saunders Company, Philadelphia, London, New York, St Louis, Sydney Tokyo; 2000.
7. Filly RA, Feldstein VA. Fetal genitourinary tract. In: Callen PW (Ed). WB Saunders Company. Ultrasonography in obstetrics and gynecology. 4th edition, Philadelphia, London, New York, St Louis, Sydney Tokyo; 2000. pp. 517-50.
8. Grannum PA. The genitourinary tract. In: Nyberg DA, Mahony BS, Pretorius DH (Eds). Diagnostic ultrasound of fetal anomalies: Text and atlas. Mosby Year Book, St Louis; 1990. pp. 433-91.
9. Kurjak A, Chervenak FA (Eds). Donald School Textbook of ultrasound in obstetrics and gynecology. Jaypee Brothers Medical Publishers (P) Ltd, New Delhi; 2004.
10. Kurjak A, Kupesic S. Color Doppler and 3D ultrasound in gynecology, infertility and obstetrics. Jaypee Brothers Medical Publishers (P) Ltd, New Delhi; 2003.
11. Khurana A, Dahiya N. 3D and 4D ultrasound. A text and atlas. Anshan Ltd, Tunbridge Wells, Kent, UK; 2004.
12. Latin V, Kos M, Marton U. Urinary tract malformations. In: Textbook of perinatal medicine. In: Kurjak A (Ed). Parthenon Publishing, London, New York; 1998. pp. 325-34.
13. Sanders RC. Ultrasonic assessment of genitourinary anomalies in utero. In: Sanders RC, James AE (Eds). The principles and practice of ultrasonography in obstetrics and gynecology. 3rd edition. Appleton Century Crofts, Norwalk, Connecticut; 1985. pp. 195-209.
14. Papp Z (Ed). Atlas of Fetal Diagnosis. Elsevier, Amsterdam, London, New York, Tokyo; 1992.
15. Luque JMT, Rodriguez MTC. Fetal geniotourinary tract: Prenatal diagnosis and assessment of nephrouropathies. In: Kurjak A, Chervenak Frank E (Eds). Donald school textbook of ultrasound in obstetrics and gynecology. Jaypee Brothers Medical Publishers (P) Ltd, New Delhi; 2004. pp. 298-319.
16. Isaksen CV, Eik-Nes SH, Blaas H-G, et al. Fetuses and infants with congenital urinary system anomalies: correlation between prenatal ultrasound and postmortem findings. Ultrasound Obstet Gynecol. 2000;15:177-85.
17. Grignon A, Filion R, Filiatrault D, et al. Urinary tract dilatation in utero: Classification and clinical applications. Radiology. 1986;160:645-7.
18. Roume J, Ville Y. Prenatal diagnosis of genetic renal diseases: breaking the code. Ultrasound Obstet Gynecol. 2004;24:10-8.
19. Kovács T, Csécsei K, Tóth Z, et al. Familial occurrence of bilateral renal agenesis. Acta Paediat Hung. 1991;31:13-21.
20. Tóth Z, Török O, Csécsei K, et al. Cystic kidney diseases diagnosed prenatally by ultrasound. In: Tankó A, Berbik I, Petri E (Eds). Practical Aspects of Gynaecourology. Akadémiai Kiadó, Budapest; 1986. pp. 439-46.
21. Brun M, Maugey-Laulom B, Eurin D, et al. Prenatal sonographic patterns in autosomal dominant polycystic kidney disease: a multicenter study. Ultrasound Obstet Gyneco. 2004;24:55-61.
22. van Eijk L, Cohen-Overbeek TE, den Hollander NS, et al. Unilateral multicystic dysplastic kidney: a combined pre- and postnatal assessment. Ultrasound Obstet Gynecol, 2002;19:180-3.

23. Csécsei K, Szeifert GT, Tóth Z, et al. Prenatal detection and morphology of dysplastic kidneys in Meckel syndrome. In: Tankó A, Berbik I, Petri E (Eds). Practical Aspects of Gynaecourology. Akadémiai Kiadó, Budapest; 1986. pp. 425-30.
24. Damen-Elias HAM, De Jong TPVM, Stigter RH, et al. Congenital renal tract anomalies: outcome and follow-up of 402 cases detected antenatally between 1986 and 2001. Ultrasound Obstet Gynecol. 2005;25:134-43.
25. Gorincour G, Rypens F, Toiviainen-Salo S, et al. Fetal urinoma: two new cases and a review of the literature. Ultrasound Obstet Gynecol. 2006;28:848-52.
26. Chaumoitre K, Brun M, Cassart M, et al. Differential diagnosis of fetal hyperechogenic cystic kidneys unrelated to renal tract anomalies: a multicenter study. Ultrasound Obstet Gynecol. 2006;28:911-7.
27. Török O, Tóth Z, Csécsei K, et al. Obstructive uropathies diagnosed prenatally by ultrasound. In: Tankó A, Berbik I, Petri E (Eds). Practical Aspects of Gynaecourology. Akadémiai Kiadó, Budapest; 1986. pp. 431-7.
28. Bronshtein M, Yoffe N, Brandes JM, et al. 1st and early 2nd trimester diagnosis of fetal urinary tract anomalies using transvaginal sonography. Prenat Diagn. 1990;10:653-66.
29. Bouzada MCF, Oliveira EA, Pereira AK, et al. Diagnostic accuracy of fetal renal pelvis anteroposterior diameter as a predictor of uropathy: a prospective study. Ultrasound Obstet Gynecol. 2004;24:745-9.
30. Chudleigh TM, Chitty LS. The postnatal significance of mild fetal pyelectasis. Ultrasound Obstet Gynecol. 2001;18:F63.
31. Cohen-Overbeek TE, Wijngaard-Boom P, Ursem NTC, et al. Mild renal pyelectasis in the second trimester: determination of cut-off levels for postnatal referral. Ultrasound Obstet Gynecol. 2005;25:378-83.
32. Kilby MD, Somerset DA, Khan KS. Potential for correction of fetal obstructive uropathy: time for a randomized, controlled trial? Ultrasound Obstet Gynecol. 2004;23:527-30.
33. Sairam S, Al-Habib A, Sasson S, et al. Natural history of fetal hydronephrosis diagnosed on mid-trimester ultrasound. Ultrasound Obstet Gynecol. 2001;17:191-6.
34. Wollenberg A, Neubaus TJ, Willi UV, et al. Outcome of fetal renal pelvic dilatation diagnosed during the third trimester. Ultrasound Obstet Gynecol. 2005;25:483-8.
35. Abuhamad AZ, Horton CE Jr, Horton SH, et al. Renal duplication anomalies in the fetus: clues for prenatal diagnosis. Ultrasound Obstet Gynecol. 1996;7:174-7.
36. Yang JM, Yang SH, Hsu HC, et al. Transvaginal sonography in the morphological and functional assessment of segmental dilation of the distal ureter. Ultrasound Obstet Gynecol. 2006;27:449-51.
37. Chen CP, Liu YP, Huang JP, et al. Prenatal evaluation with magnetic resonance imaging of a giant blind ectopic ureter associated with a duplex kidney. Ultrasound Obstet Gynecol. 2008;31:360-2.
38. van Eerde AM, Meutgeert MH, de Jong TPVM, et al. Vesicoureteral reflux in children with prenatally detected hydronephrosis: a systematic review. Ultrasound Obstet Gynecol. 2007;29:463-9.
39. Whitten SM, McHoney M, Wilcox DT, et al. Accuracy of antenatal fetal ultrasound in the diagnosis of duplex kidneys. Ultrasound Obstet Gynecol. 2003;21:342-6.
40. Hoshino T, Ihara Y, Shirane H, et al. Prenatal diagnosis of prune belly syndrome at 12 weeks of pregnancy: case report and review of the literature. Ultrasound Obstet Gynecol. 1998;12:362-6.
41. Carroll SGM, Soothill PW, Tizard J, et al. Vesicocentesis at 10–14 weeks of gestation for treatment of fetal megacystis. Ultrasound Obstet Gynecol. 2001;18:366-70.
42. Kim SK, Won HS, Shim JY, et al. Successful vesicoamniotic shunting of posterior urethral valves in the first trimester of pregnancy. Ultrasound Obstet Gynecol. 2005;26:666-8.
43. Rohyr R, Benachi A, Daikha-Dahmane F, et al. Correlation between ultrasound and anatomical findings in fetus with lower urinary tract obstruction in the first half of pregnancy. Ultrasound Obstet Gynecol. 2005;25:478-82.
44. Lee EH, Shim JY. New sonographic finding for the prenatal diagnosis of bladder exstrophy: a case report. Ultrasound Obstet Gynecol. 2005;21:498-500.
45. Schwärzler P, Bernard JP, Senat MV, et al. Prenatal diagnosis of fetal adrenal masses: differentiation between hemorrhage and solid tumor by color Doppler sonography. Ultrasound Obstet Gynecol. 1999;13:351-5.
46. Gramellini D, Delle Chiaie L, Piantelli G, et al. Sonographic assessment of amniotic fluid volume between 11 and 24 weeks of gestation: construction of reference intervals related to gestational age. Ultrasound Obstet Gynecol. 2001;17:410-5.
47. Lee SM, Jun JK, Lee EJ, et al. Measurement of fetal urine production to differentiate causes of increased amniotic fluid volume. Ultrasound Obstet Gynecol. 2010;36:191-5.
48. Lee SM, Park SK, Shim SS, et al. Measurement of fetal urine production by three-dimensional ultrasonography in normal pregnancy. Ultrasound Obstet Gynecol. 2007;30:281-6.
49. Bhide A, Sairam S, Farrugia M-K, et al. The sensitivity of antenatal ultrasound for predicting renal tract surgery in early childhood. Ultrasound Obstet Gynecol. 2005;25:489-92.
50. Carrera JM, Torrents M, Mortera C, et al. Routine prenatal ultrasound screening for fetal abnormalities: 22 years' experience. Ultrasound Obstet Gynecol. 1995;5:174-9.
51. Papp Z, Tóth-Pál E, Papp CS, et al. Impact of prenatal mid-trimester screening on the prevalence of fetal structural anomalies: a prospective epidemiological study. Ultrasound Obstet Gynecol. 1995;6:320-6.

CHAPTER 26

Fetal Musculoskeletal System

Anna Maroto, Carlota Rodó, Elena Carreras

INTRODUCTION

Fetal Musculoskeletal Abnormalities

- *Osteochondrodysplasias*:
  - Thanatophoric dysplasia
  - Osteogenesis imperfecta
  - Achondroplasia
  - Achondrogenesis
  - Others
- *Reductional defects*:
  - Terminal defects
  - Constriction band sequence
  - Phocomelia
  - Proximal femoral focal deficiency (PFFD)
  - Split-hand and split-foot malformation (SHFM), ectrodactyly
  - Hand and foot deformities
- Polydactyly
- Syndactyly
- Hemivertebrae
- Fetal akinesia deformation syndrome (FADS)
- *Other skeletal defects:* Patellar anterior luxation; teratogenic effects: Misoprostol.

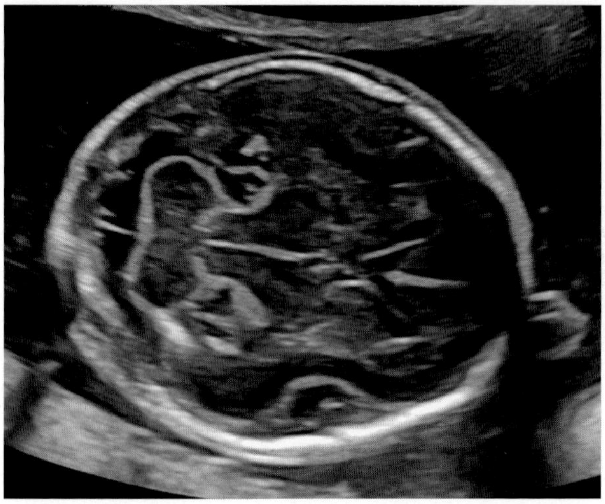

Fig. 1: Assessment of normal ossification of the skull at 20 weeks of gestation. The exploration of the upper hemisphere is limited because of the acoustic shadow of the skull.

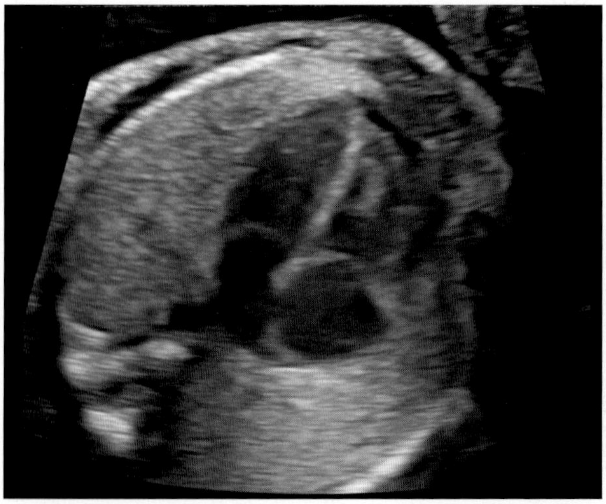

Fig. 2: Axial view of a normal fetal thorax. The thoracic shape is correct and there is no thoracic hypoplasia, therefore, it is not expected to have respiratory compromise at birth.

NORMAL ULTRASOUND APPEARANCE OF FETAL SKELETON

A systematic fetal musculoskeletal evaluation requires the inspection of all four extremities. Fetal head, thorax **(Figs. 1 and 2)**, and spine must also be assessed.

A standardized approach to sonographic evaluation must include:

- All three portions of the limb (proximal, middle, and distal) **(Figs. 3 to 11)**
- Bone characteristics [long bone measurements, degree of mineralization **(Fig. 12)**, and presence of

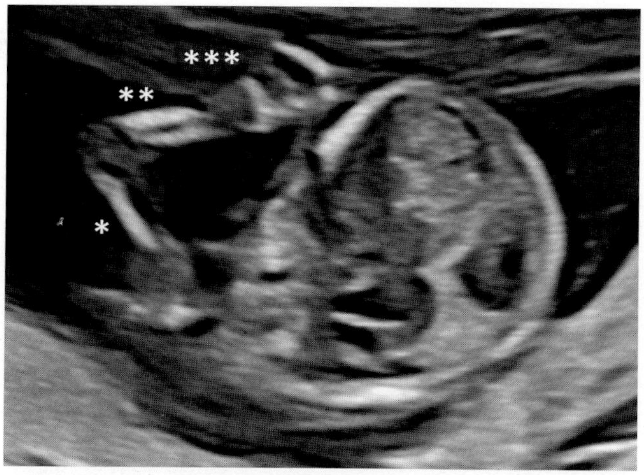

Fig. 3: A 12-week embryo. All three portions of the upper limb must be distinguished (proximal humerus*), middle (ulna and radius**) and distal (hand***), with five fingers.

bone fractures and bowing] are helpful in categorizing skeletal dysplasias.[1,2]

- Fetal posture and movement
- Hand (metacarpals and phalanges) **(Figs. 13 to 15)** and foot (metatarsals and phalanges) configuration **(Figs. 16 to 18)**.

Fetal head, spine, and thorax **(Figs. 19A and B)** should be evaluated for abnormal configuration and echogenicity or degree of mineralization. Many of the skeletal disorders may have a familial component, so it is important to ask the parents about the findings and relate to them if it is possible.

Some sonographic features of serious skeletal dysplasias are already present in the first trimester, which may allow early diagnosis, mainly in cases with a known family history.[3]

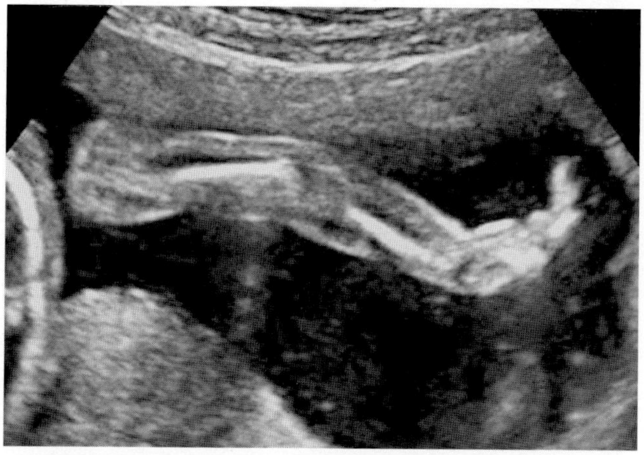

Fig. 4: Upper limb. For a correct ultrasonographic assessment, all three portions of fetal limbs must be visualized (proximal, middle, and distal) aligned following the same axis. Fetal posture and shoulder, elbow, and wrist movement must be assessed.

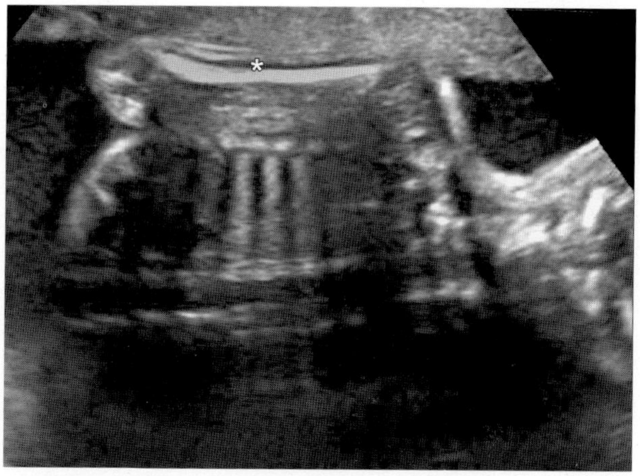

Fig. 5: Humerus (*). Long bone length is the measurement of the ossification center of bone diaphysis.

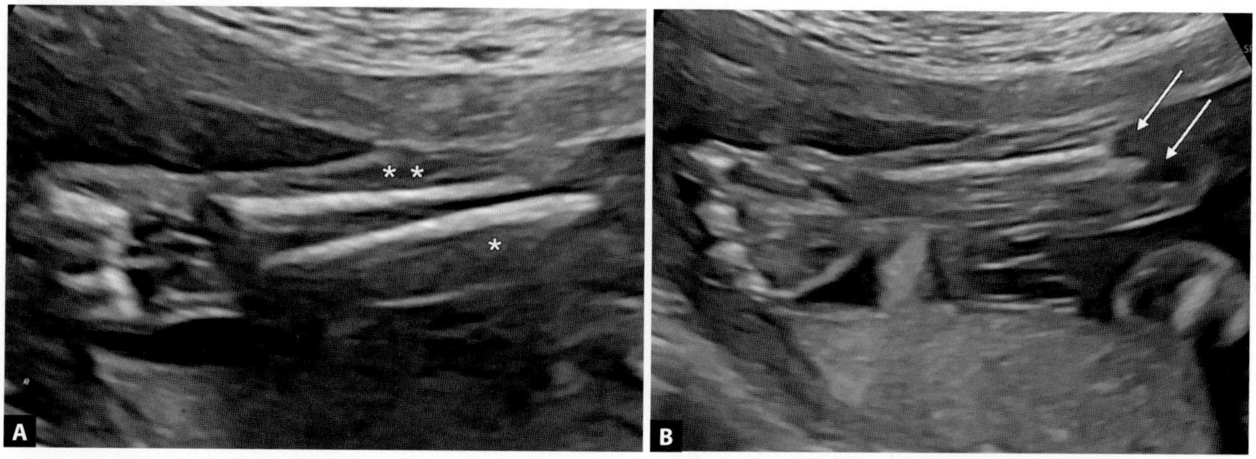

Figs. 6A and B: Ulna (*) and radius (**). Ulnar diaphysis is longer than radial one. Proximal noncalcified epiphyses may be assessed, as round anechogenic structures (arrows).

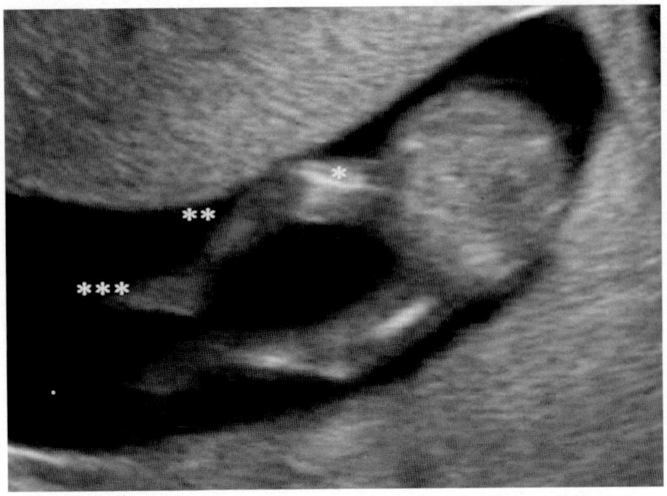

Fig. 7: A 12-week embryo. All three portions of the lower limb must be distinguished: Proximal (femur*), middle (tibia and fibula**), and distal (foot***).

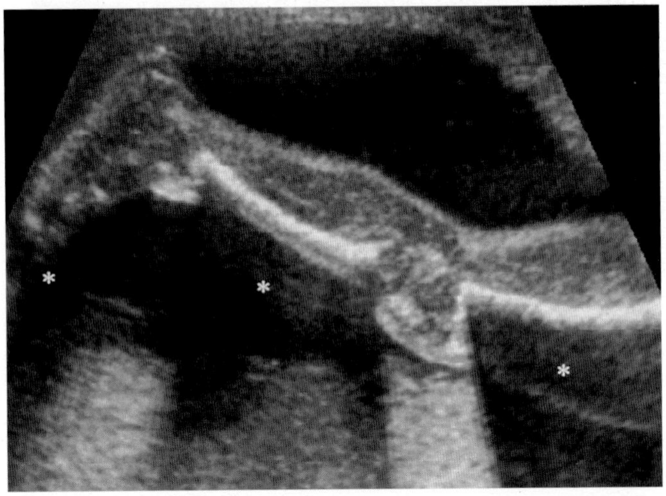

Fig. 8: Lower limb showing all three portions. All of them responsible of a posterior shadow effect (*). One must assess the femur, tibia, and foot normally aligned and the hip, knees, and elbows motility.

OSTEOCHONDRODYSPLASIAS

Osteochondrodysplasias or skeletal dysplasias **(Figs. 20A and B)** are a genetically heterogeneous group of disorders that involves the growth and development of bones and cartilage. More than 500 conditions have been described.[4] They are traditionally classified in terms of which portions of the limbs[5] are shortened:

- *Rhizomelia* denotes shortening of the proximal limb—humerus and femur

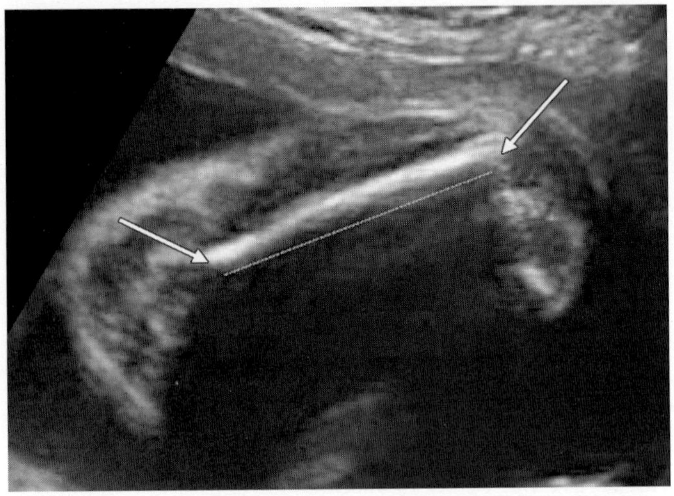

Fig. 9: Femoral diaphysis. A normal degree of mineralization is indirectly assessed by the appearance of a posterior shadow (arrows) that enables a clear visualization of all diaphyseal thickness (discontinued line). For this reason, bone appears thinner than soft tissues that surround it.

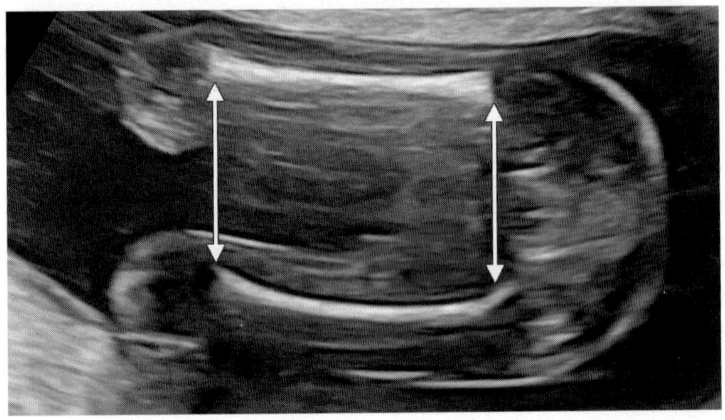

Fig. 10: Even if you only measure one of them, it is important to assess that both femurs have the same length (arrows).

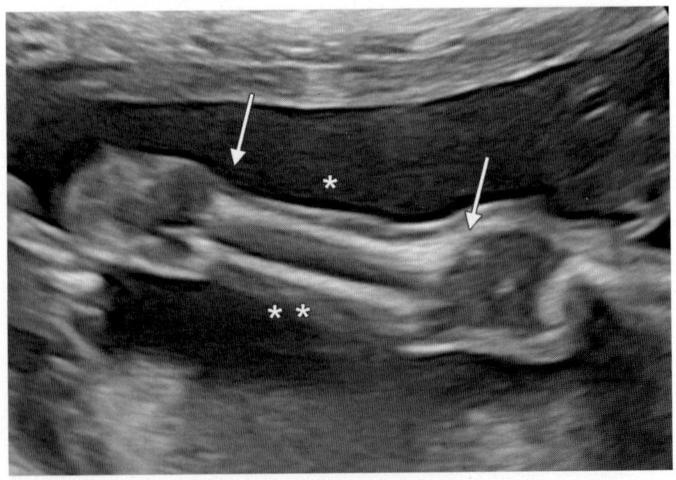

Fig. 11: Tibia (*) and fibula (**). Tibial diaphysis is longer and thicker than fibular diaphysis. Nonmineralized fibular epiphysis (arrows).

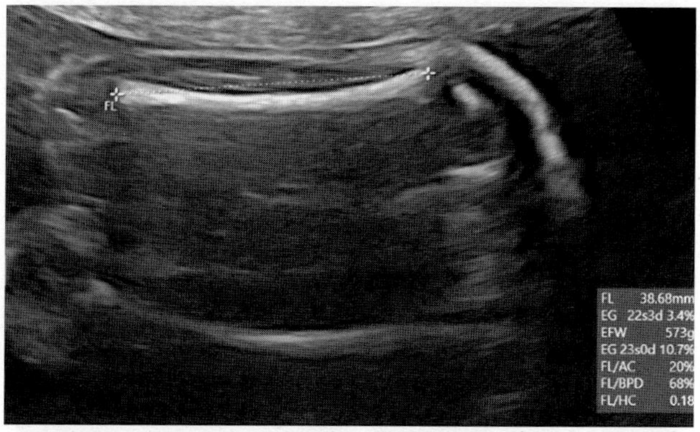

Fig. 12: Shortened femoral length (FL) with correct degree of mineralization, no angulations or fractures.

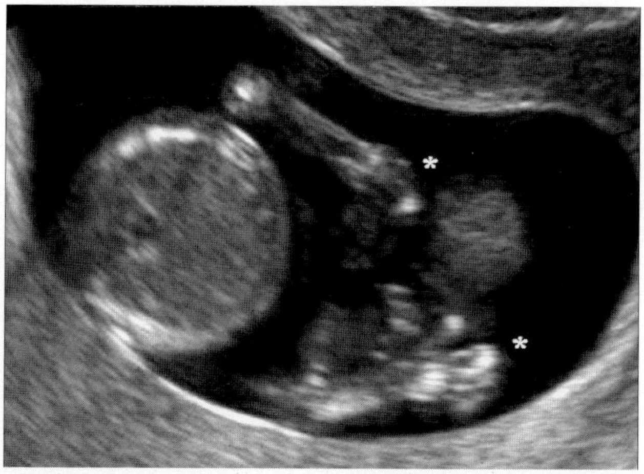

Fig. 13: A 12-week embryo. Both upper limbs can be assessed simultaneously (*). A common pitfall is to assess the same limb twice. To avoid this one should try to visualize simultaneously both hands. It is the ideal gestational age to perform this.

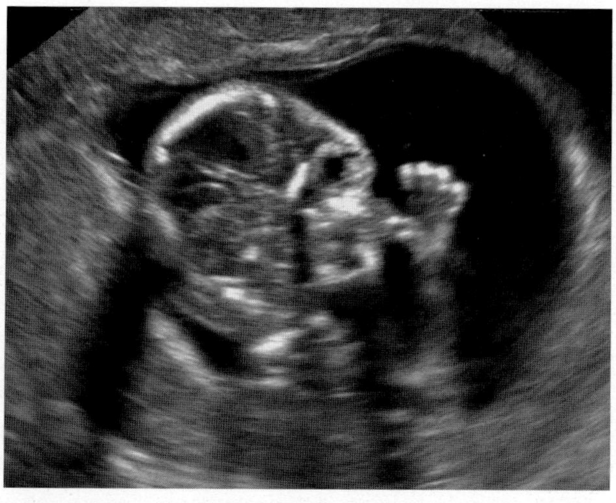

Fig. 14: A 12-week embryo. Hands are best assessed when they are opened so one can confirm the integrity of all the phalanges and the normal separation of fingers.

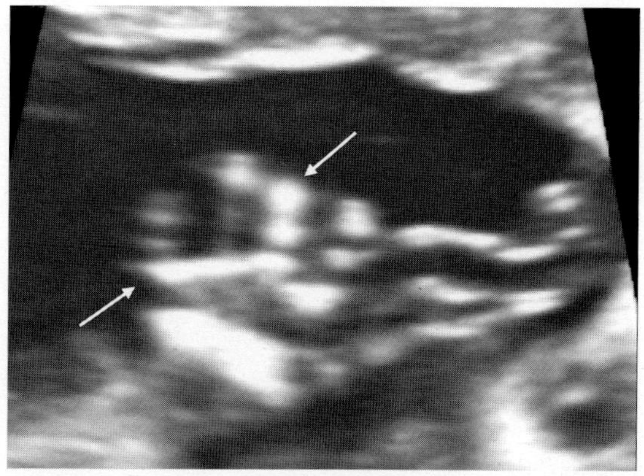

Fig. 15: A 15-week fetal hand. Arrows showing phalanges and metacarpals.

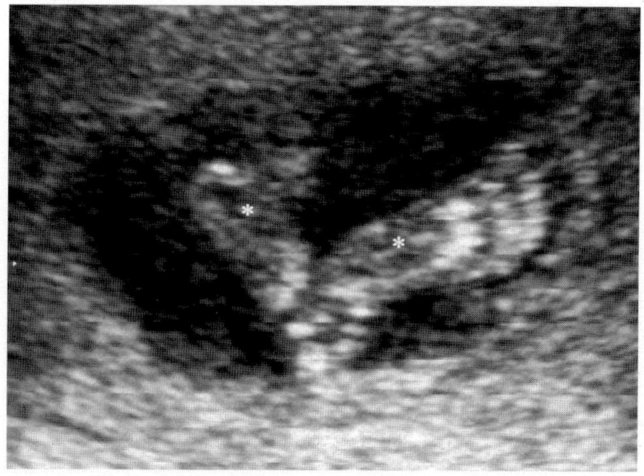

Fig. 16: A 12-week embryo. Both feet are simultaneously assessed (*) in order to avoid exploring the same limb twice.

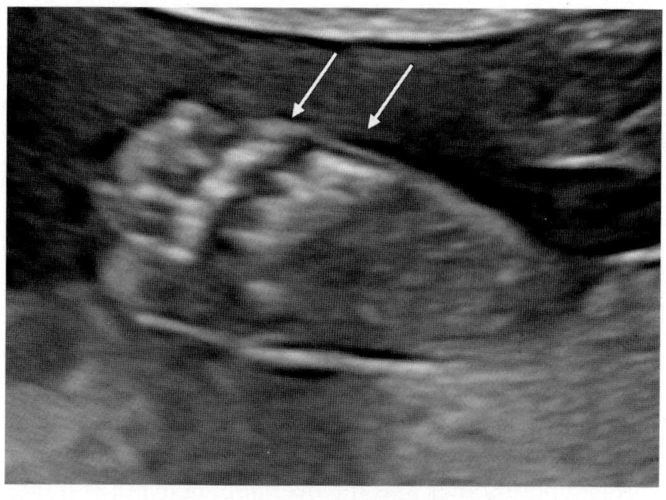

Fig. 17: Forefoot. Arrows showing metatarsal and phalanges. Fetal tarsus completes its calcification process at 26 weeks of gestation.

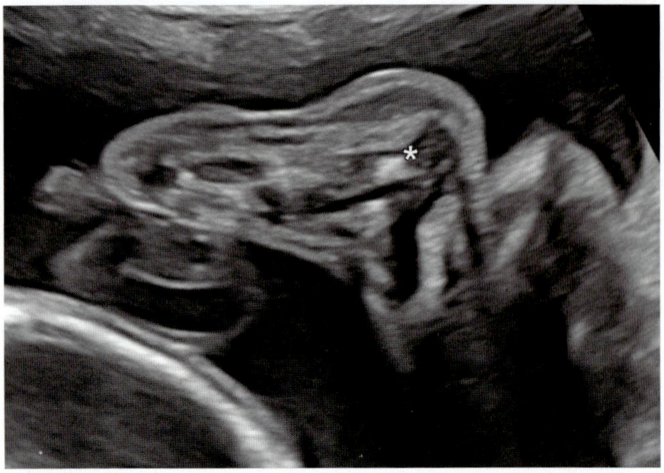

Fig. 18: Foot in a 28-week fetus. By 26 weeks, one can visualize the tarsal ossification centers (*) showing a posterior shadow.

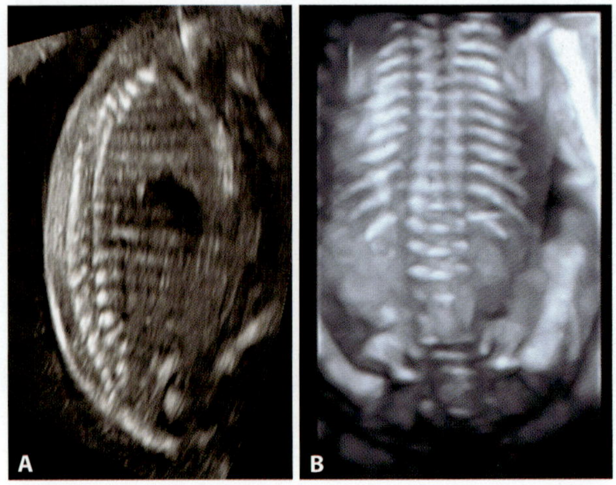

Figs. 19A and B: Normal appearance of fetal spine at 20 weeks by 2D and 3D ultrasound.

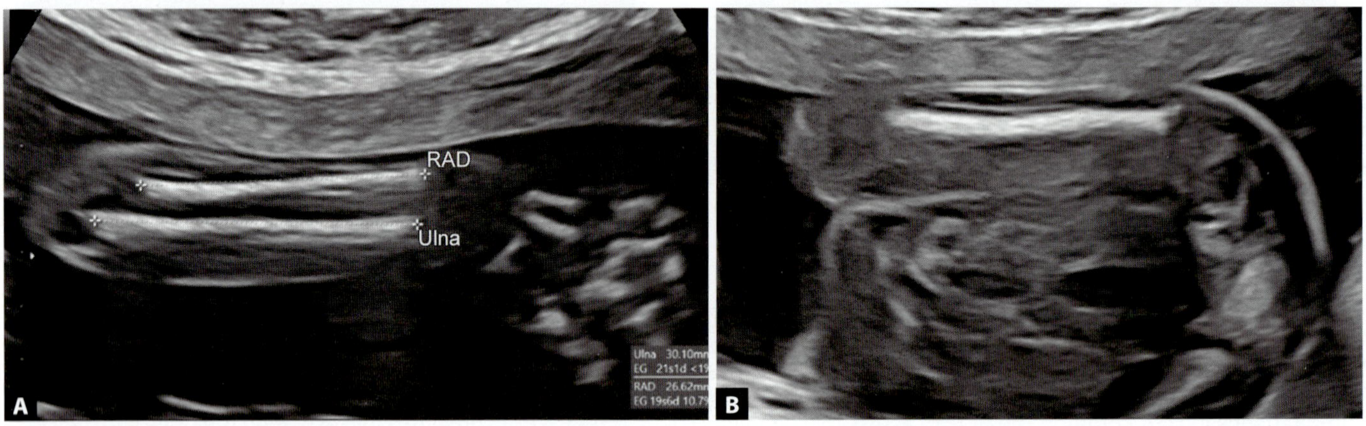

Figs. 20A and B: A 23-week fetus with correct configuration but shortened long bones. It may represent an osteochondrodysplasia, but also intrauterine growth restriction or a normal variant. Parental phenotype must be assessed. When the diagnosis is not achieved prenatally, in postnatal period the growing pattern must be followed up. (RAD: radius)

- *Mesomelia* indicates shortening of the middle portion of the limb—forearm or lower leg bone
- *Acromelia* refers to shortening of the distal portion of the limb—hand and foot
- *Micromelia* technically means severe shortening of all portions of a limb, but the term is also used to indicate shortening of a limb without a specific reference of the particular portion that is shortened **(Figs. 21 to 27)**.

Many of the skeletal dysplasias can be assessed by ultrasound.[5] However, the variability in expression of ultrasound findings and the overlapping features hinder prenatal diagnosis for even the most common skeletal dyplasias.[5-9]

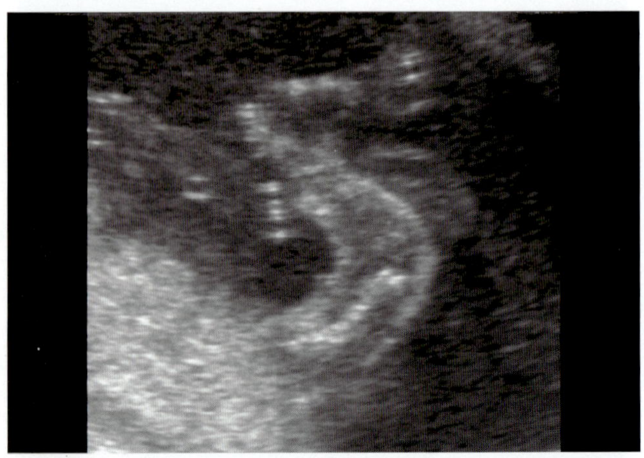

Fig. 21: Upper limb showing all three portions. They are uniformly shortened, well aligned on their axes, without angulations, or fractures.

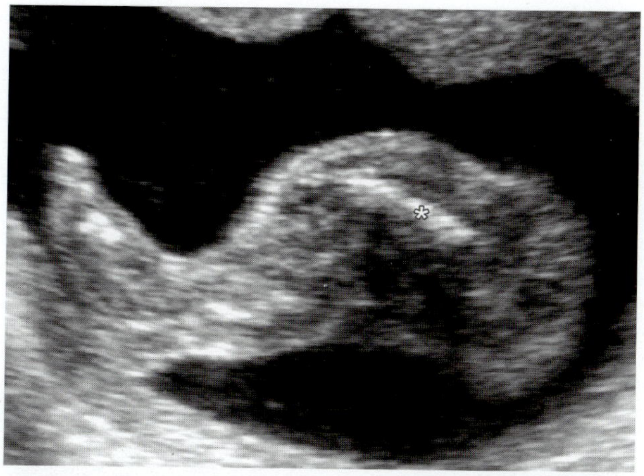

Fig. 22: Three portions of a lower extremity. The limb is much shortened (micromelia). One can compare femur (*) and foot length.

The osteochondrodysplasias most commonly assessed by ultrasound[9] are:

- Thanatophoric dysplasia
- Osteogenesis imperfecta
- Achondroplasia
- Achondrogenesis
- Campomelic dysplasia **(Fig. 28)**
- Spondylothoracic dysplasia
- Atelosteogenesis
- Others

The prevalence of skeletal dysplasias **(Figs. 29A to C)** in newborn is 3–4/10,000 and the frequency of them among perinatal deaths is about 9/1,000. Skeletal dysplasias have a variety of phenotypic expressions. In the last years, 3D ultrasound, fetal magnetic resonance

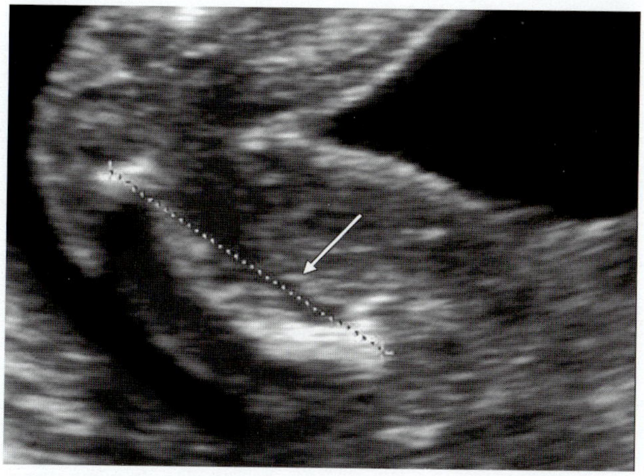

Fig. 23: Very short lower limbs (micromelia) but without axial deviation of the three portions. A curved femur showing the classical "telephone receiver" configuration (arrow). There are no fractures, and the degree of bone mineralization is normal.

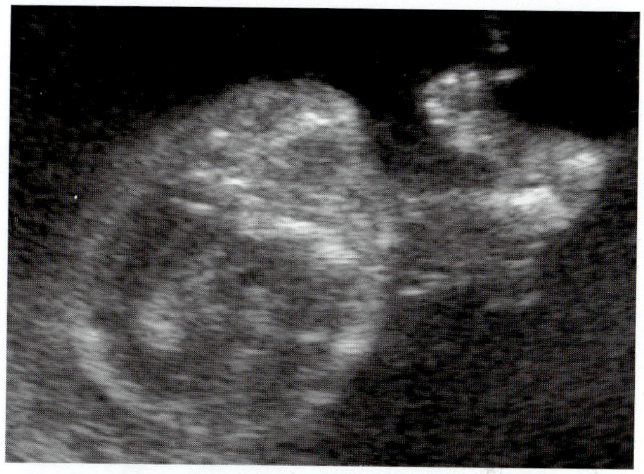

Fig. 24: Extremely short upper limb (micromelia) showing all three portions.

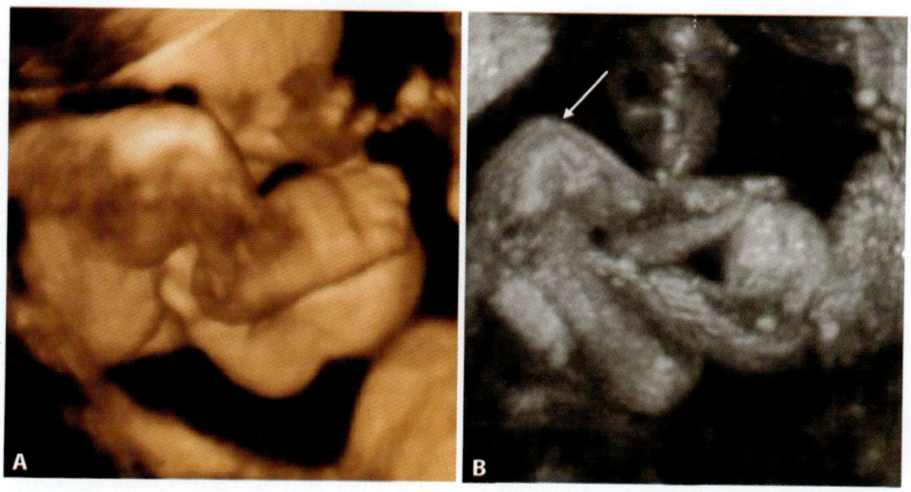

Figs. 25A and B: 3D view of extremely short lower limb (micromelia). The arrow shows multiple irregularities in tibial diaphysis secondary to postfracture callous tissue formation.

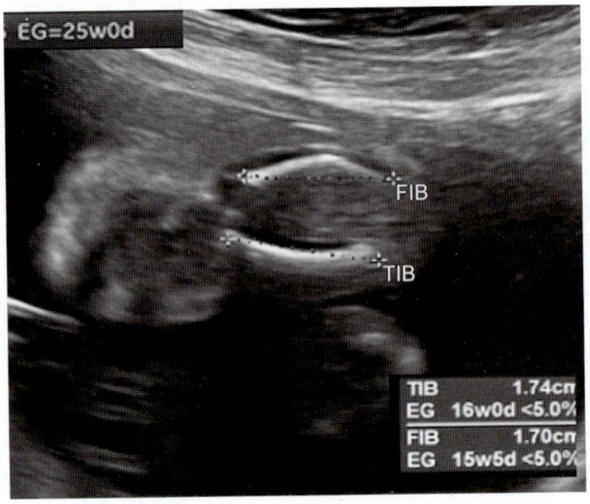

Fig. 26: Sonogram demonstrating severe micromelia at 25 weeks of gestation, showing a good degree of mineralization. The measurements of the tibia (TIB) and fibula (FIB) are showed.

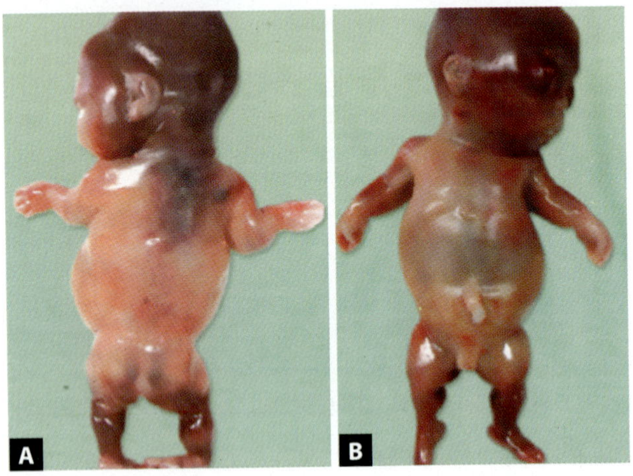

Figs. 27A and B: Hydropic fetus showing extremely short extremities (severe micromelia). Macrocrania. Very shortened long bones.

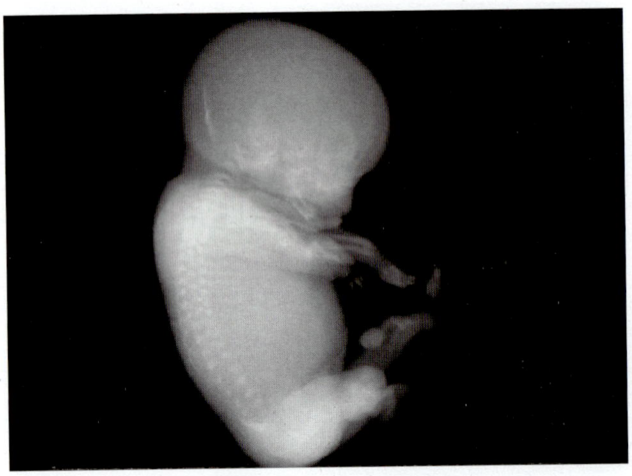

Fig. 28: Campomelic dysplasia. Postmortem fetography showing short neck and evident long bones anterior bowing.

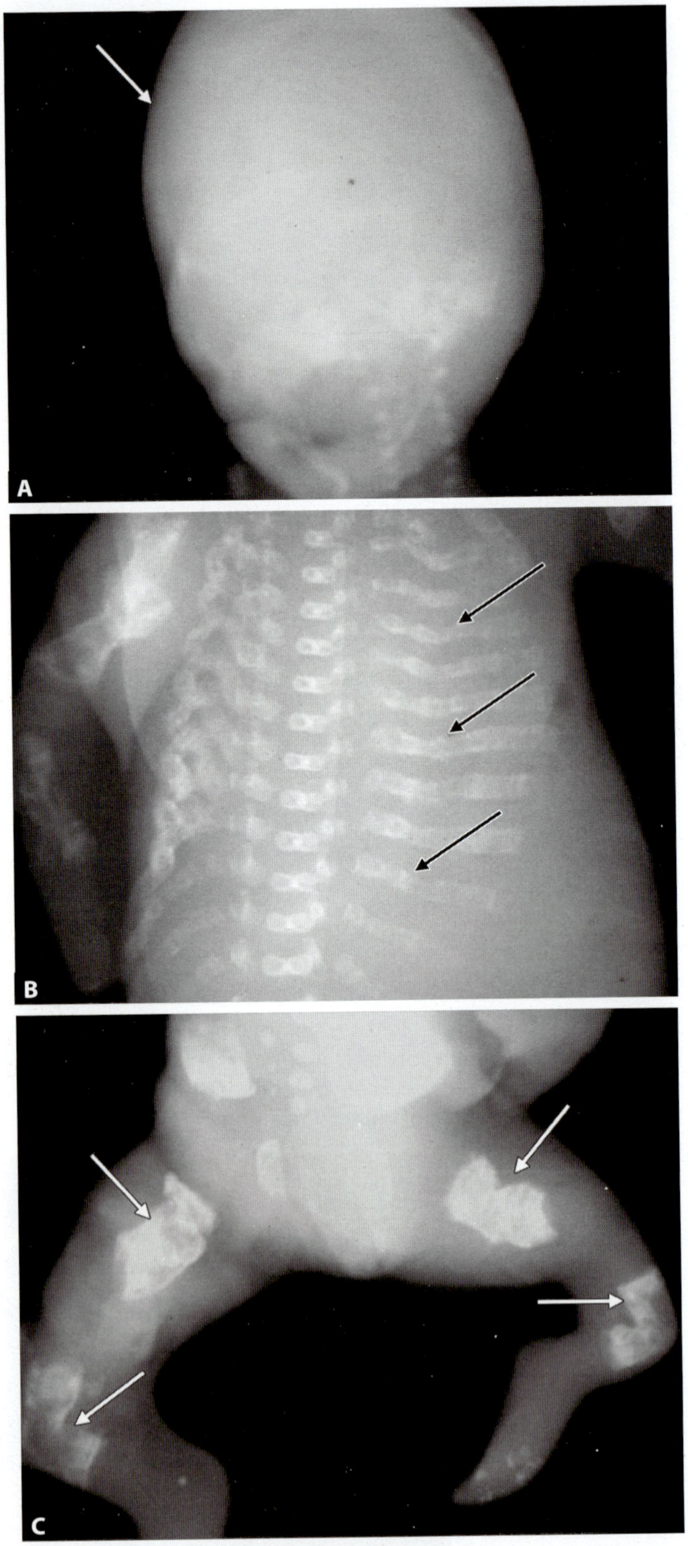

Figs. 29A to C: *Postmortem fetographies:* (A) Demineralization of the fetal skull (arrow); (B) Narrow chest caused by multiple fractures of the ribs (arrows); (C) Long bone shortening and angulation due to multiple fractures (arrows).

imaging and fetal CT have been introduced in order to improve diagnostic accuracy.[2] However, the existence of overlapping signs makes it difficult to establish a specific diagnosis. Other disorders may mimic skeletal dysplasias including dysmorphic syndromes and intrauterine growth restriction (IUGR) **(Fig. 30)**. A systematic evaluation of the long bones, thorax, hands **(Figs. 31A and B)** and feet, skull **(Figs. 32 to 35)**, spine **(Figs. 36A to C)**, and pelvis is required to obtain detailed information of the abnormality. Other relevant information about the skeletal disorders can be obtained from anatomopathological study, assessing the characteristics of enchondral ossification **(Figs. 37 to 41)** line. The development of advanced genomic study techniques has increased the diagnostic yield of fetal structural abnormalities. Currently, whole exome or genome sequencing has considerably increased the detection of diagnostic genetic variants in skeletal anomalies.[8]

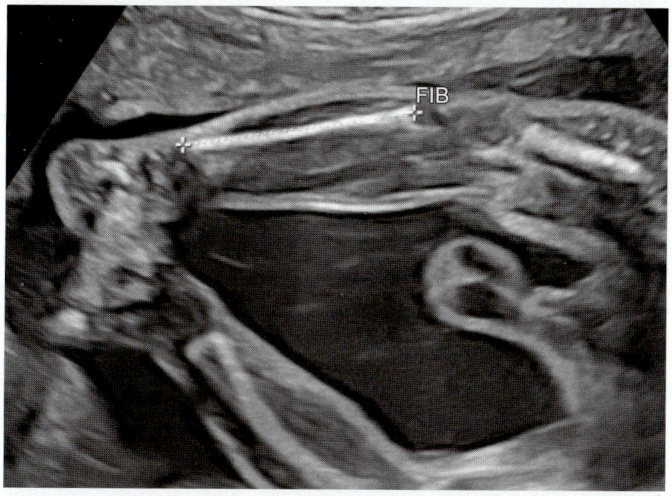

Fig. 30: Assessment of all fetal biometrics. In some cases of fetal growth delay, the long bones are found below normality but with normal shape and mineralization. The image shows the measurement of the fibula in a fetus with early IUGR (FIB).

Although it is not always possible to reach the diagnosis, being able to differentiate lethal from nonlethal disorders, providing differential diagnoses before delivery and determining postpartum management may improve patients care and postnatal counseling for future pregnancies.[6,9]

Thanatophoric Dysplasia

Thanatophoric dysplasia is the most common lethal skeletal dysplasia.[10-12] The name is derived from the Greek word *thanatophoras* meaning "death bearing" because of the uniformly lethal outcome of this dysplasia in the perinatal period, mainly due to pulmonary hypoplasia secondary to thoracic hypoplasia.[6] Two types have been described, both caused by *FGFR3* gene pathogenic variants with an autosomal dominant inheritance. Thanatophoric dysplasia is characterized by a severe micromelia [affecting all portions of a limb **(Figs. 42A and B)**] with bowing bones **(Figs. 43 to 45)**. The extremities are very short while the chest length is normal **(Fig. 46)**. Bones are well mineralized without fractures in long bones. The thorax is bell shaped and the ribs are shortened **(Figs. 47 to 50)**. The platyspondyly (flattened vertebral shape) of the spine is a typical finding **(Figs. 51 and 52)**.

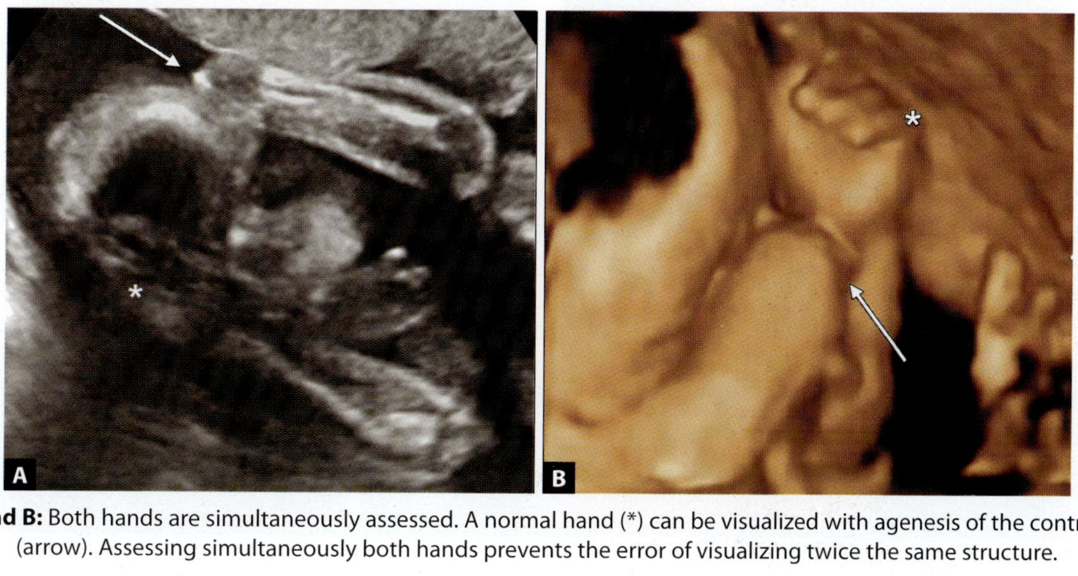

Figs. 31A and B: Both hands are simultaneously assessed. A normal hand (*) can be visualized with agenesis of the contralateral one (arrow). Assessing simultaneously both hands prevents the error of visualizing twice the same structure.

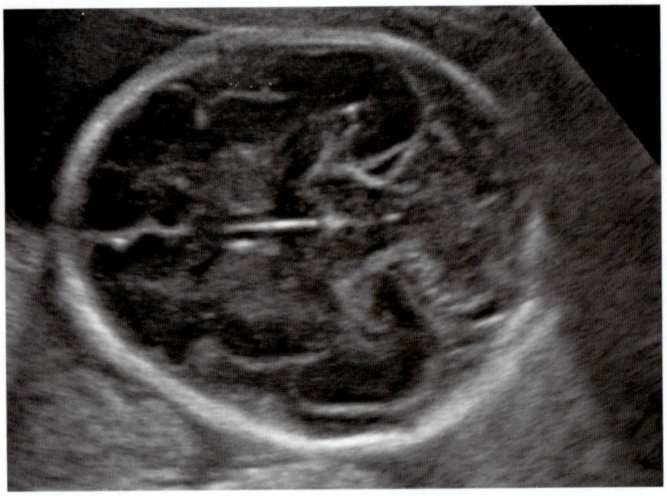

Fig. 32: The skull demonstrates markedly decreased echogenicity. Normally, the distal cortical is shadowed out by the proximal but not in the severe demineralization of osteogenesis imperfecta. It permits an easy visualization of intracranial structures.

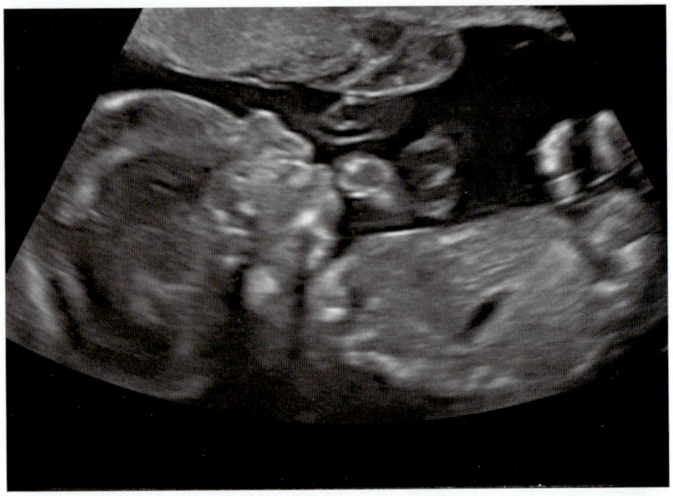

Fig. 34: Middle sagittal section of the fetal profile assessing the skull demineralization.

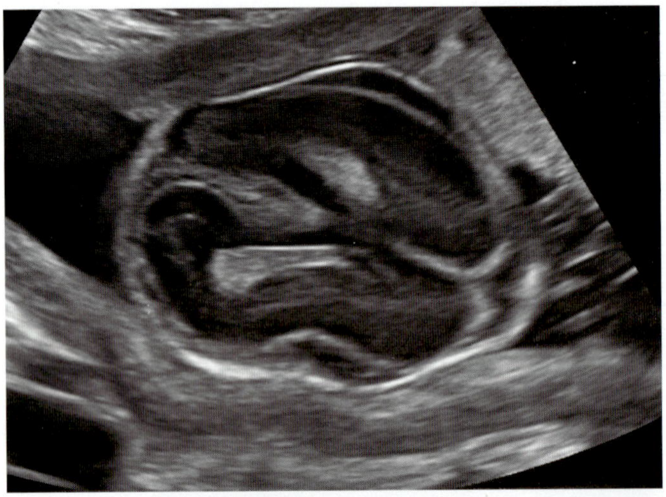

Fig. 33: Due to the markedly decreased skull mineralization the encephalic structures may seem abnormal. Note that atrial shape and measure is normal. The weight of the ultrasound (US) probe may deform the head.

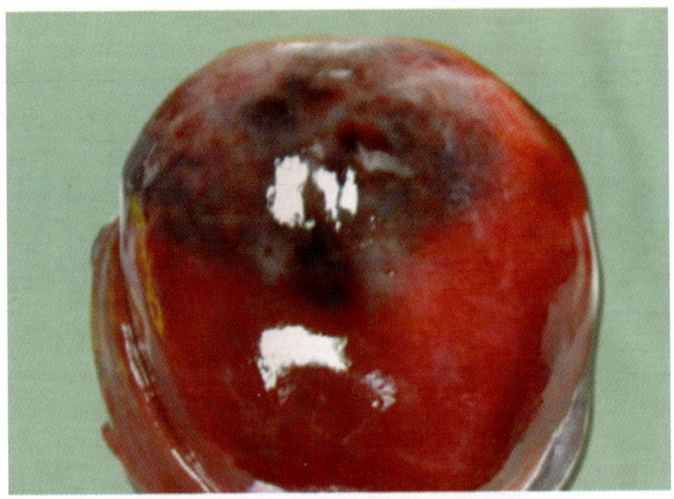

Fig. 35: Demineralized fetal skull. Encephalic tissues can be assessed through the dura mater.

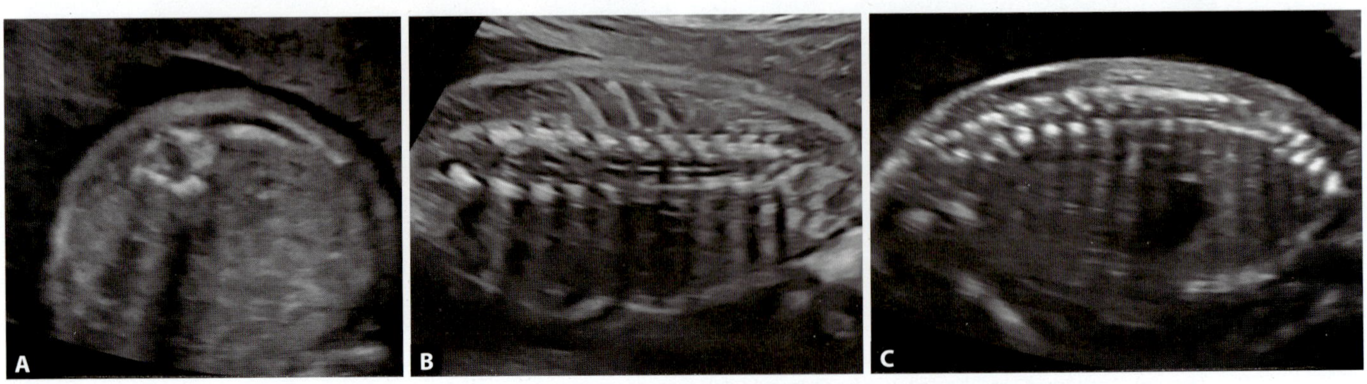

Figs. 36A to C: Axial, coronal, and sagittal planes of a normal fetal spine at 20 weeks.

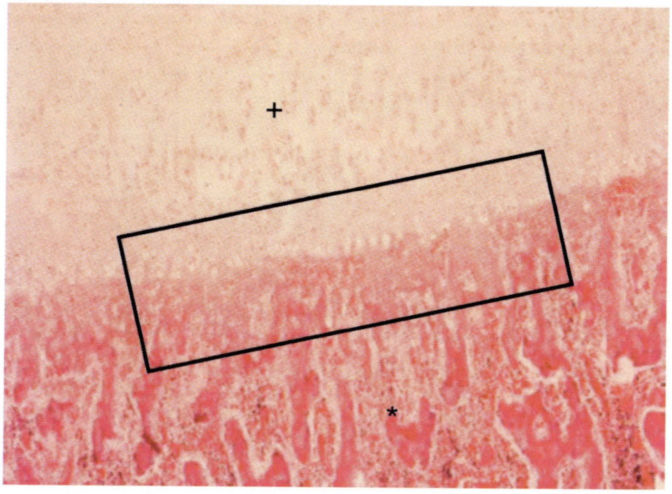

Fig. 37: Normal enchondral ossification line. Metaphyseal growing region shows a regular aspect (box). One can distinguish the cartilaginous epiphyseal portion (+) and the trabecular bone diaphyseal portion (*).

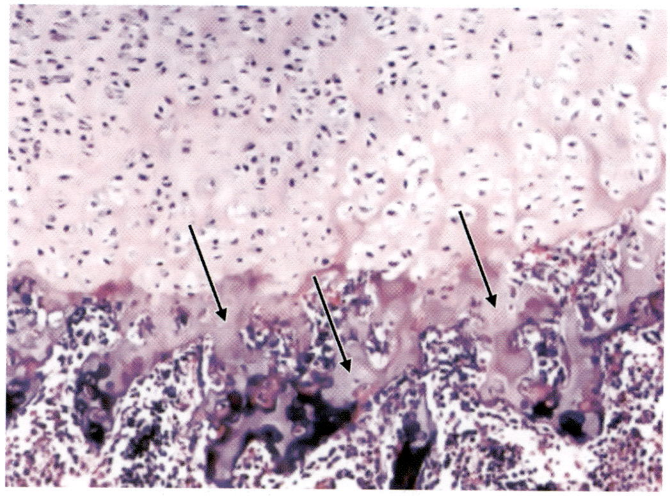

Fig. 39: Enchondral ossification line of long bones metaphysis showing thick osseous trabeculae that run parallel to the line (arrows).

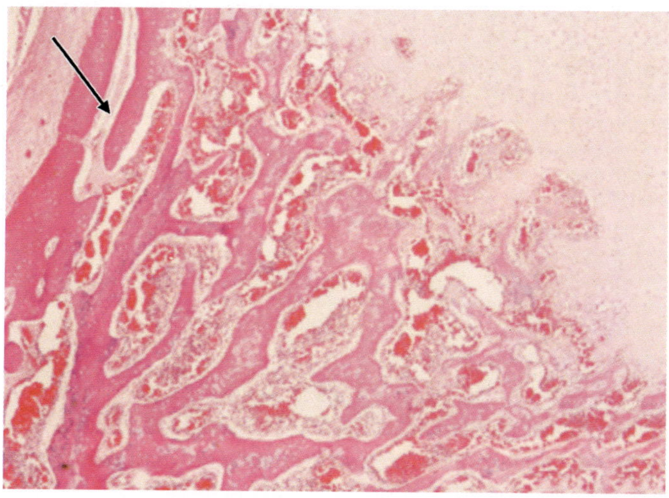

Fig. 38: Long bones enchondral ossification line showing a severe disruption secondary to vascular invasion (arrow) extending from the metaphyseal ossification zone to the chondrocitary region.

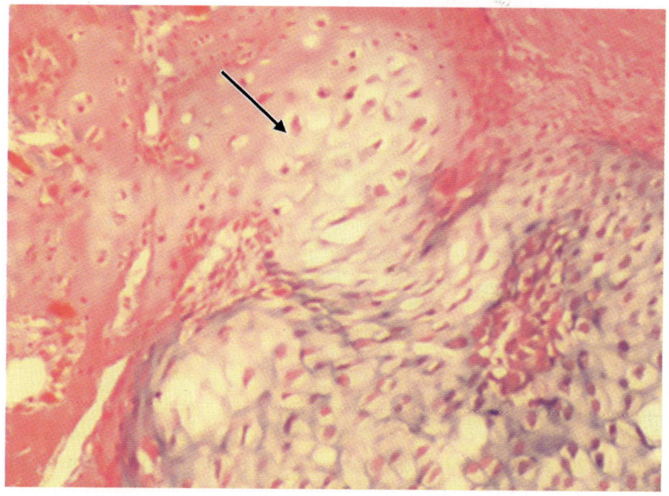

Fig. 40: Detail of the box contain in **Figure 37**. Note the severe distortion of the enchondral ossification line showing giant anomalous chondrocytes disposed concentrically (arrow).

Usually, there is macrocrania **(Fig. 53)**, frontal bossing, and a depressed nasal bridge **(Fig. 54)**. Approximately 15% of all cases are type II in which the skull is markedly cloverleaf in configuration **(Fig. 55)**, with a trilobed appearance in the coronal view, due to the premature closure of cranial sutures. It may associate renal, heart, and central nervous system anomalies **(Fig. 56)**. Polyhydramnios occurs in almost 50% of cases.[6]

OSTEOGENESIS IMPERFECTA

Osteogenesis imperfecta is a heterogeneous group of genetic disorders[4,9-13] that affect the type I collagen. It is characterized by severe bone fragility, blue sclera, and prenatal growth deficiency. It is due to mutations in the genes related to collagen formation: COL1A, COL1A2, CRTAP, and P3H1. In most cases, the inheritance pattern is dominant; however, autosomal recessive and X-linked

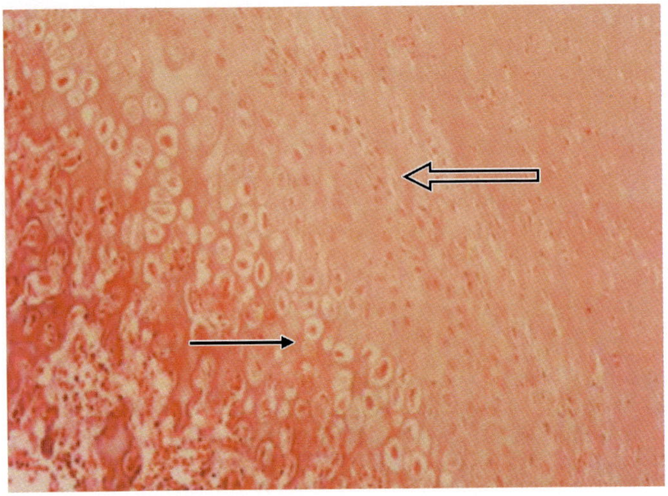

Fig. 41: Regular enchondral ossification line (arrow). Note the incurvation of epiphyseal region chondrocytes (opened arrow).

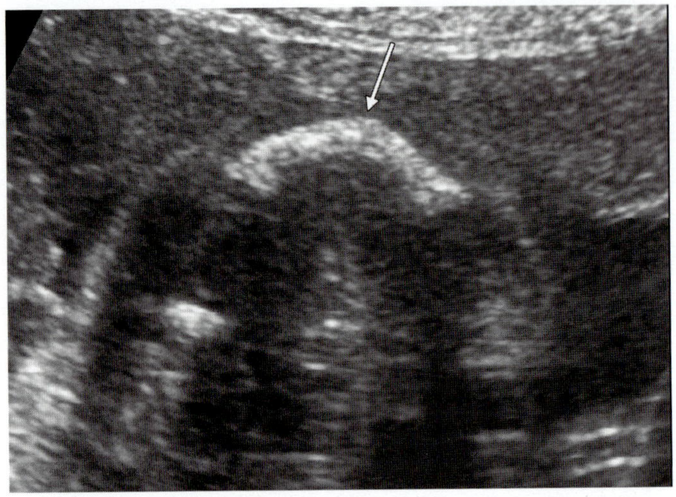

Fig. 43: Characteristic bowing of the femur (arrow). The classical "bent" bone on ultrasound may mimic a fracture because of the acute angulation.

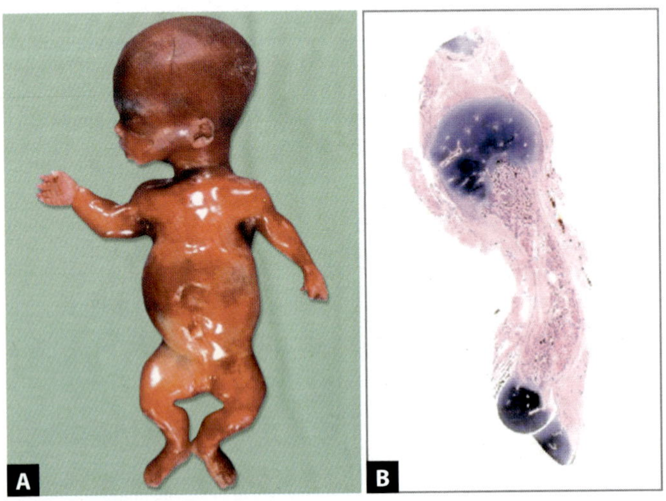

Figs. 42A and B: (A) *Thanatophoric dysplasia:* Prominent skull, hypoplastic thorax, and severe micromelia. Short and curved thighs; (B) Femur showing the classical telephone receiver configuration, short and curved.

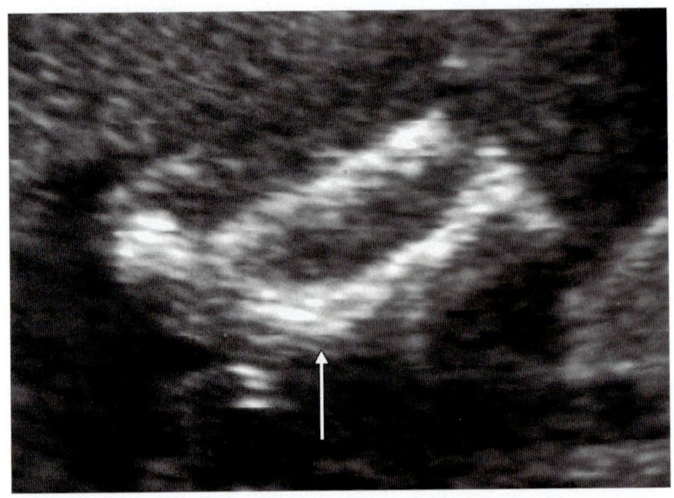

Fig. 44: Middle portion of lower extremity showing long bone bowing (arrow) without fractures.

cases or de novo mutations have also been described. Currently, eight types have been described but only type II and III can be detected prenatally. Type II is the most severe form and the most frequently diagnosed by antenatal ultrasonography. Osteogenesis imperfecta type II is a severe global osteochondrodysplasia affecting all segments (micromelic type). It is characterized by severe bone fragility, leading to abnormal ossification **(Fig. 57)** and multiple fractures **(Fig. 58)** and bone angulations **(Figs. 59A and B)**. There are no associated visceral malformations and fetal movements may be reduced. Type II is lethal and the most frequent causes are respiratory failure due to pulmonary hypoplasia secondary to thoracic hypoplasia as a consequence of multiple rib fractures **(Figs. 60 and 61)** and cerebral hemorrhage.

ACHONDROPLASIA

Achondroplasia is an osteochondrodysplasia characterized by a rhizomelia (short humerus and femur) **(Fig. 62)**. Bone mineralization is normal and the long

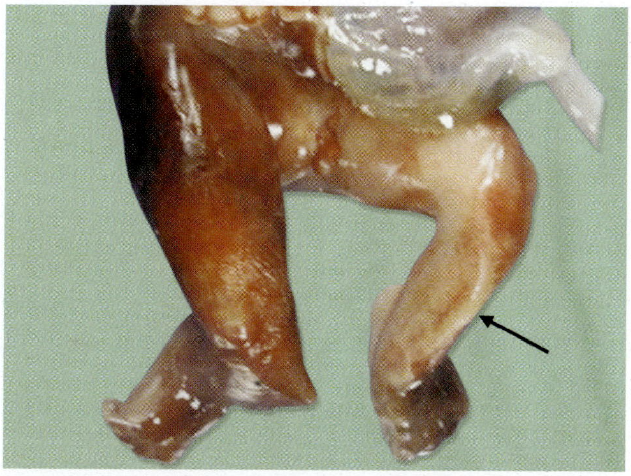

Fig. 45: Flattened aspect of the lower limbs with tibial bowing (arrow).

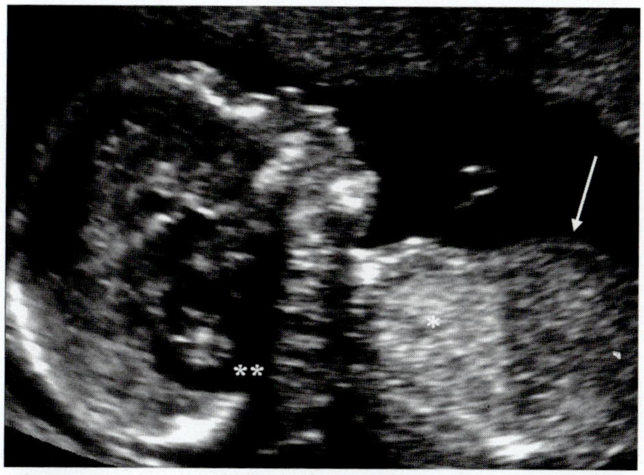

Fig. 46: Sagittal view of the trunk. A normal abdomen that appears falsely protuberant (arrow) compared to the hypoplastic thorax (*). Bones show a correct mineralization as demonstrated by the posterior shadow behind the jaw (**).

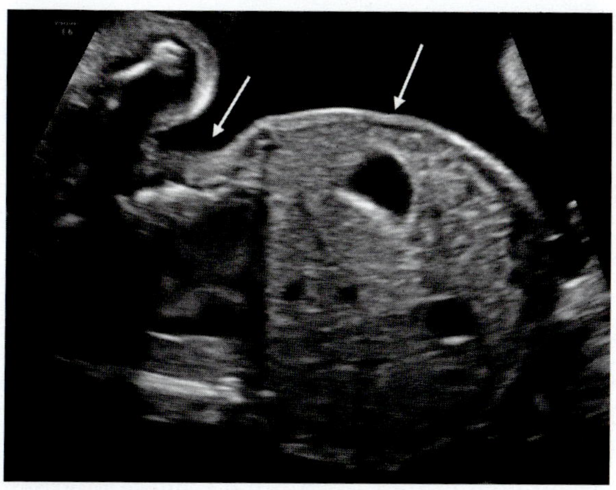

Fig. 47: Coronal view of the trunk. The thorax is bell shaped, and the ribs are shortened (but normally mineralized). A normal abdomen appears protuberant compared to the small thorax (arrows).

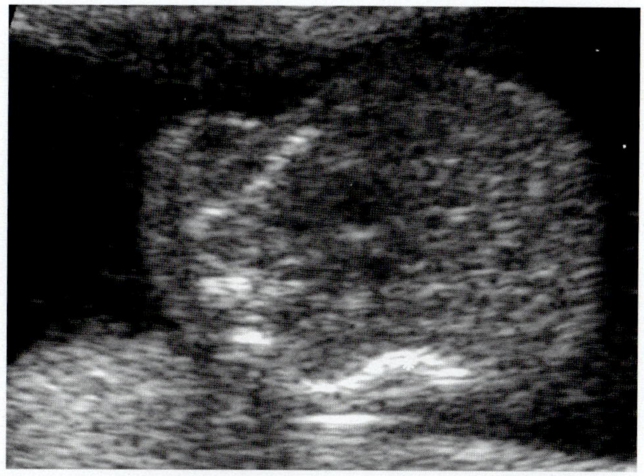

Fig. 48: Axial section of the fetal thorax. A narrow and bell-shaped thorax can be assessed. Note the anomalous appearance of the ribs.

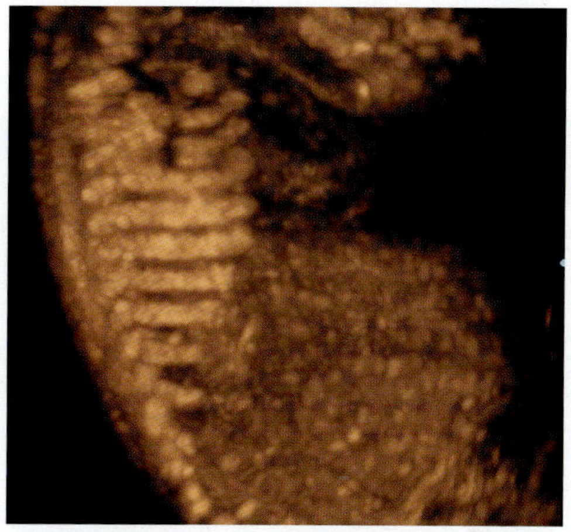

Fig. 49: Fetal thorax with rib shortening.

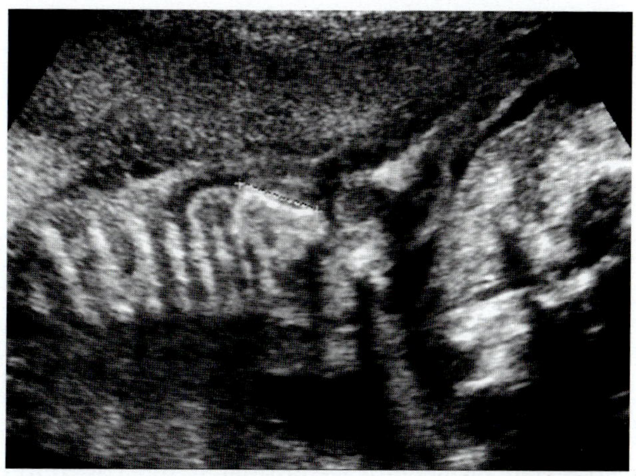

Fig. 50: Oblique view of fetal thorax. Note the absence of posterior shadow effect behind the scapulae (crosses). Short and bell-shaped thorax.

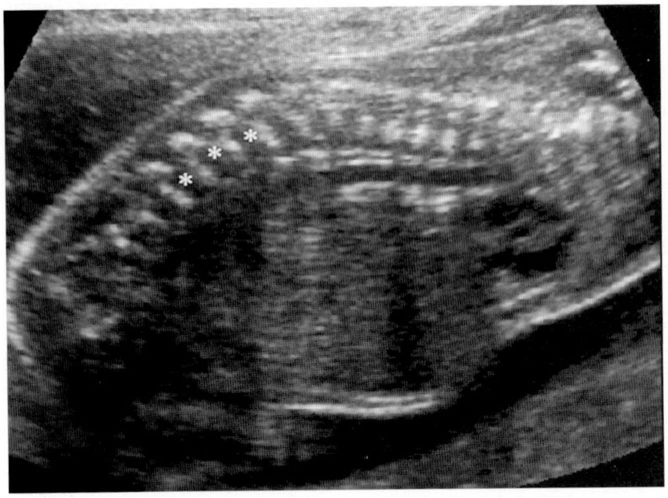

Fig. 51: Sagittal section of the trunk. Platyspondyly (*) is severe; the vertebral ratio is the smallest of the skeletal dysplasias.

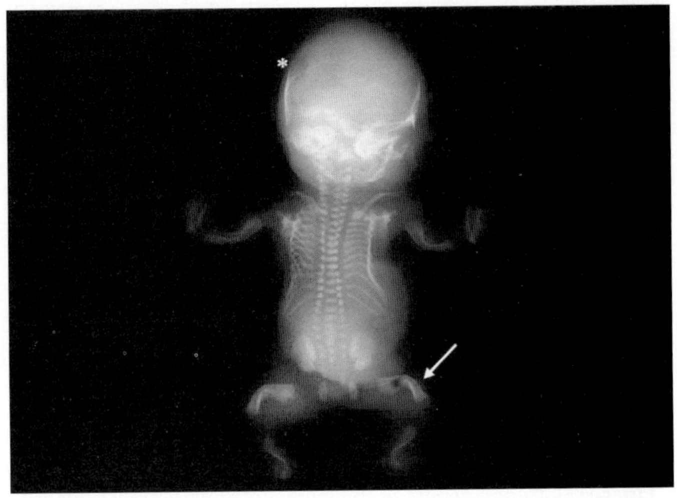

Fig. 53: Postmortem fetography of a fetus with thanatophoric dysplasia. Macrocrania, normal skull mineralization (*), hypoplastic thorax, and micromelic limbs. Femur showing the classical telephone receiver configuration (arrow).

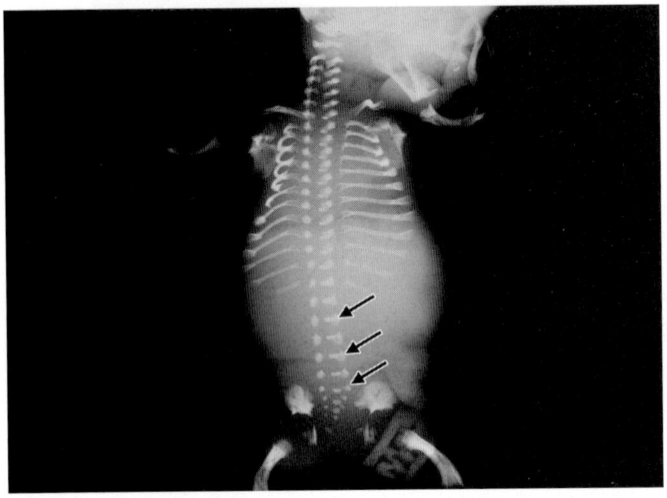

Fig. 52: Severe platyspondyly (arrows) by postmortem fetography.

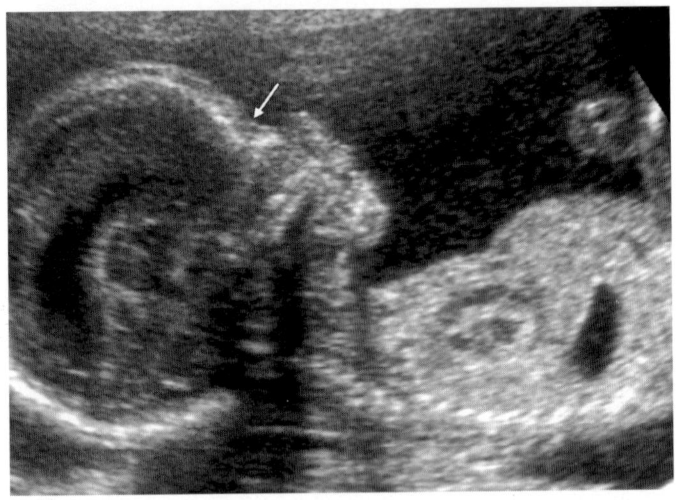

Fig. 54: Sagittal view. Macrocrania, frontal bossing, and depressed nasal bridge (arrow). The thorax is hypoplastic and responsible of the classical pulmonary hypoplasia that determines its ominous prognosis. There are no associated visceral anomalies.

bones are not bowed. Thoracic shape is also normal. Phenotypically, macrocrania, frontal bossing, and depressed nasal bridge **(Figs. 63 and 64)** can also be recognized. The trident hand (an increased interspace between the third and fourth digit) or the lack of widening of the lumbar canal can also be identified by ultrasound **(Figs. 65A to C)**. Prenatal detection is usually established at late second or third trimester because, in most cases, osseous **(Fig. 66)** lengths are normal up to 25 or 26 weeks of gestation, at this moment the growing pattern reaches a plateau. Homozygous achondroplasia is uniformly lethal but the most frequent form, the heterozygous type, has a good global and intellectual prognosis. The genomic cause is also a mutation in *FGFR3* gene.[4,6]

ACHONDROGENESIS

Achondrogenesis is rare group of lethal osteochondrodysplasias characterized by a severe demineralization of intramembranous and endochondral bone resulting in marked global limb shortening (severe micromelia) associated with severe pulmonary hypoplasia because of very narrow barrel-shaped thorax.[7] There is a poor

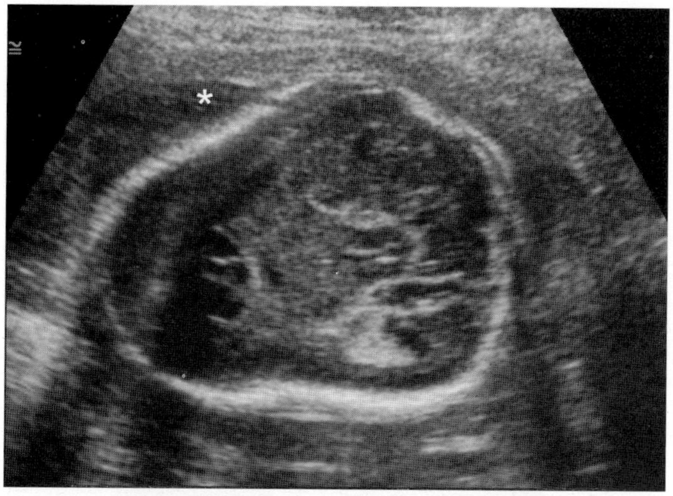

Fig. 55: Transverse view of fetal skull. Initial form of a cloverleaf skull (*). This sign in association with a severe micromelia is pathognomonic of thanatophoric dysplasia. The encephalic structures are usually normal. Other abnormalities that may be seen include gyration disorders.

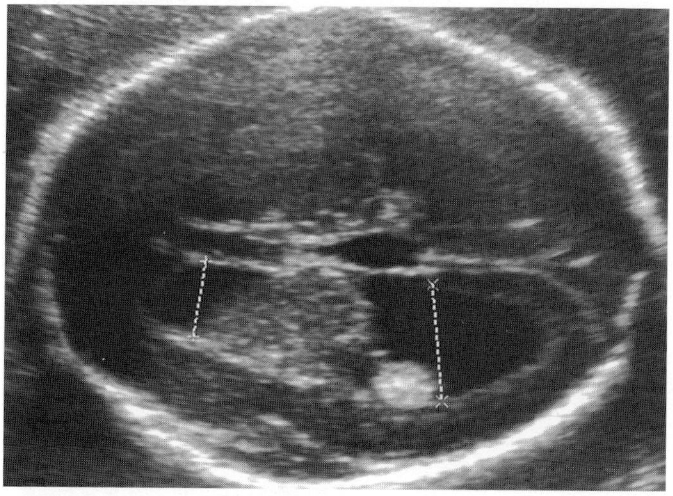

Fig. 56: Ventriculomegaly (between calipers) secondary to a reduced magnum foramen.

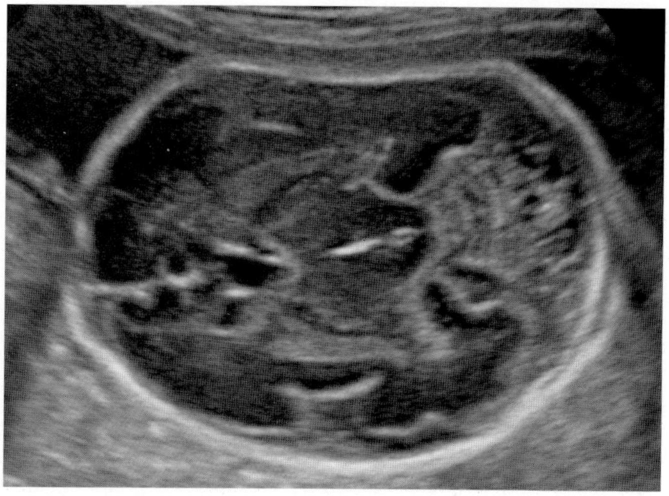

Fig. 57: Transverse view. Abnormal ossification of the fetal skull, as shown by the absence of posterior shadowing and the deformation caused by the pressure of the transducer.

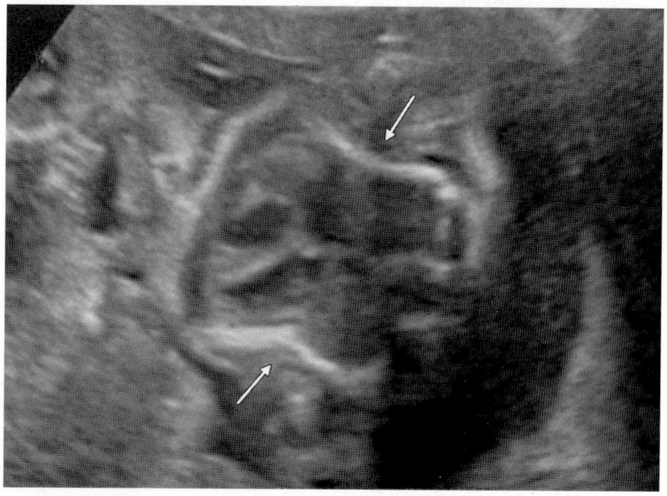

Fig. 58: The four-chamber view. Narrow chest caused by fractures of the ribs and wrinkling of the surface of the bones due to multiple fractures (arrows).

skull and vertebral ossification and bone fractures. Other possible associations are gastrointestinal abnormalities with polyhydramnios and marked redundancy of the subcutaneous tissue (pseudohydrops) with generalized subcutaneous edema due to lymphatic ectasia **(Fig. 67)**. Three types have been described with different radiological, histological, and inheritance patterns:

- Types IA and IB (autosomal recessive) involve a lack of ossification of the skull and the spine, with short bones and rib fractures, pseudohydrops, short neck and trunk, narrow thorax, and severe micromelia.
- Type II (autosomal dominant) is characterized by severe micromelia; skull ossification is relatively normal, small thorax without rib fractures. The outcome is fatal, although type II may survive for short periods in the neonatal period.

CAMPOMELIC DYSPLASIA

Campomelic dysplasia is a congenital disorder characterized by development of abnormal curvatures of long bones, particularly from lower extremities such as femur and tibia **(Fig. 68)**. Other sonographic features that are commonly present include bell-shaped narrow chest, eleven pairs of ribs, and hypoplasia of the mid-thoracic vertebral bodies, fibula, and scapula **(Fig. 69)**. Even if karyotypic sex ratio is approximately M2:F13, the vast majority shows a female phenotype with ambiguous genitalia. It may associate heart anomalies, hydronephrosis, and hydrocephalus. Almost all result in neonatal or infant death due to respiratory complications secondary to tracheobronchomalacia. The cause is a mutation in *SOX9* gene, which promotes the reproductive and skeletal development.[4-6]

SPONDYLOTHORACIC DYSPLASIA (JARCHO–LEVIN SYNDROME)

The spondylothoracic dysplasia is a group of disorders,[4] characterized by delayed ossification of spine and ribs and defects of vertebral segmentation **(Fig. 70)**. The prognosis is variable, with some lethal forms and some types that can reach the adult life. It is important to establish the differential diagnosis with other osteochondrodysplasias, such as asphyxiating thoracic dysplasia (Jeune thoracic dystrophy) and short rib polydactyly syndrome.

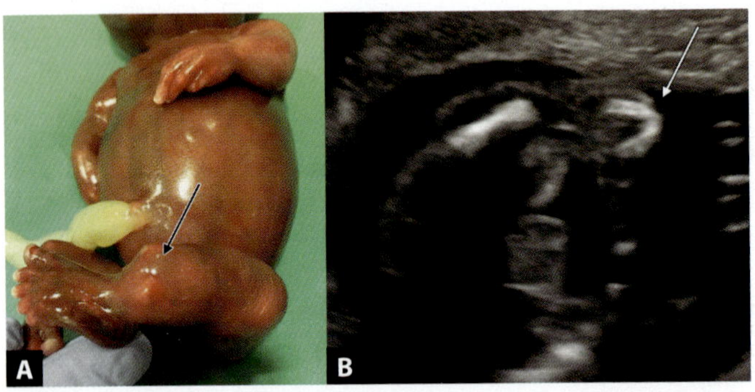

Figs. 59A and B: Osteogenesis imperfecta type II. Long bone shortening and angulation due to multiple fractures (arrows).

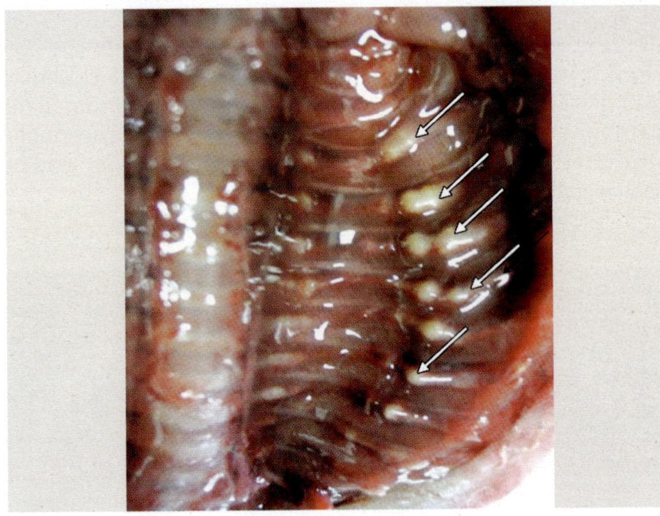

Fig. 60: Osteogenesis imperfecta type II. Multiple fractures of the ribs. The callous formation may be assessed during necropsy (arrows).

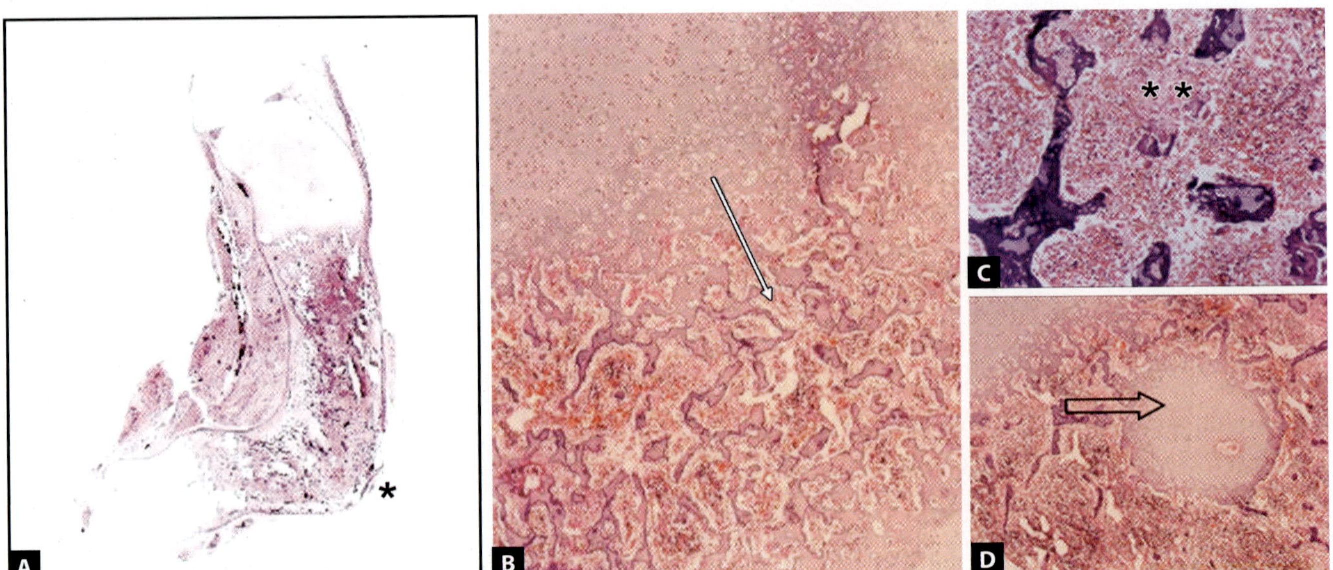

Figs. 61A to D: Short and angulated long bones due to multiple intrauterine fractures (*) at metaphyseal level conditioning bone shortness (arrow) at diaphyseal level (**) responsible of trabecular destruction and callus formation (open arrow) and pseudoarticulation creation.

ATELOSTEOGENESIS

Atelosteogenesis is also known as spondylo-humero-femoral dysplasia. It is characterized by a "bent" tibia **(Fig. 71)** showing a "boomerang" configuration **(Figs. 72 and 73)** and the absence of fibula, with shortened long bones.

OTHER OSTEOCHONDRODYSPLASIAS

In occasions long bones have a normal appearance, but they are shortened **(Fig. 74)**. The differential diagnosis between some conditions, such as an authentic osteochondrodysplasia, a normal variant or an IUGR **(Fig. 75)**, must be considered and sometimes it can be a big challenge. The molecular study, the monitoring of fetal growth, and the growth of long bones and the Doppler study can provide the key for the differential diagnosis. Postnatally, the newborn and child must be strictly followed-up.

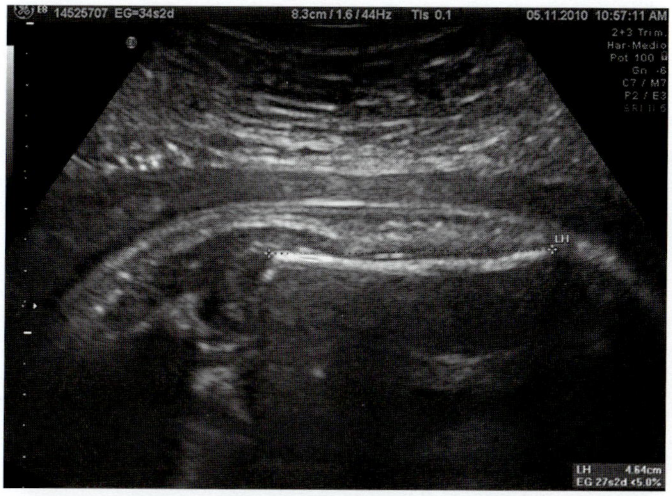

Fig. 62: Short femur at third trimester in fetus affected with achondroplasia.

REDUCTIONAL DEFECTS

Reductional defects are heterogeneous group of diseases characterized by the absence of any portion of a limb. Currently, the term amputation **(Fig. 76)** has been substituted, because in the vast majority of cases the defect is due to an abnormal development[13-15] **(Fig. 77)**. It includes:

- Terminal defects
- Phocomelia
- Proximal focal femoral deficiency
- Split-hand and split-foot syndromes

They are often (50% of cases) isolated defects and usually affect only one extremity. 25% may affect more than one limb and 25% may be associated with other structural defects or are features of a genetic syndrome **(Fig. 78)**. The outcome depends on the degree of compromise and the possibility of a correct postnatal orthopedic surgical repair. The term *amelia* means the complete absence of the limb and *meromelia* is used when there is a partial absence of a limb **(Fig. 79)**.

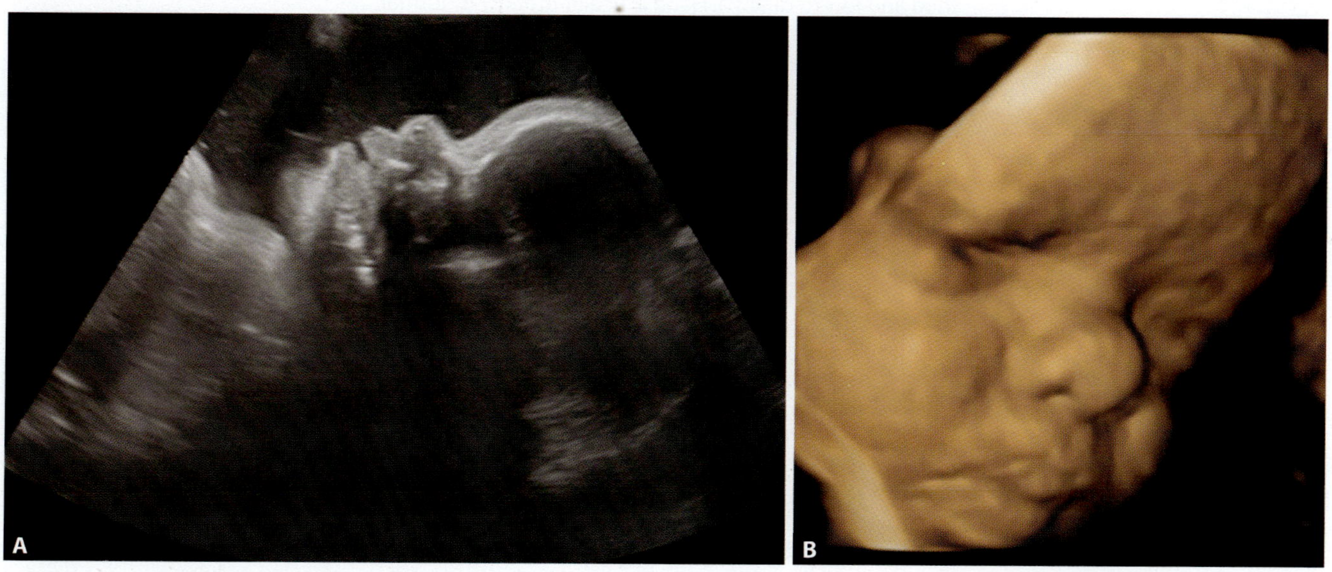

Figs. 63A and B: Fetal profile by 2D and 3D ultrasound. Frontal bossing and depressed nasal bridge.

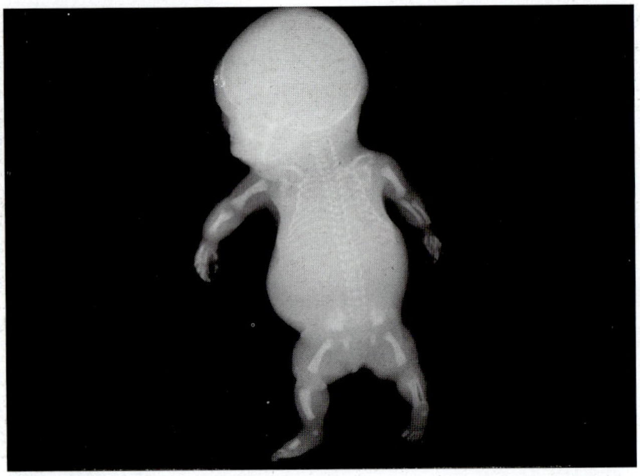

Fig. 64: Postmortem photography of an achondroplasic fetus showing frontal bossing, depressed nasal bridge, and rhizomelia.

TRANSVERSE TERMINAL DEFECTS

Transverse terminal defects are defects of the distal part of the limb with the proximal portion preserved. These defects can affect any long bone, however 75% of cases affect the distal portion of the left upper limb **(Figs. 80, 81 and 31)**. They may be associated with other structural defects such as esophageal atresia, heart malformations, kidney dysgenesis, hypospadias, microretrognathia or abdominal wall defects as part of genetic syndromes.[13-15] As a differential diagnosis of transverse terminal defects, it is important to consider the amniotic band sequence.

CONSTRICTION BAND SEQUENCE

Constriction band sequence or amniotic band syndrome sporadic is characterized by the presence of multiple

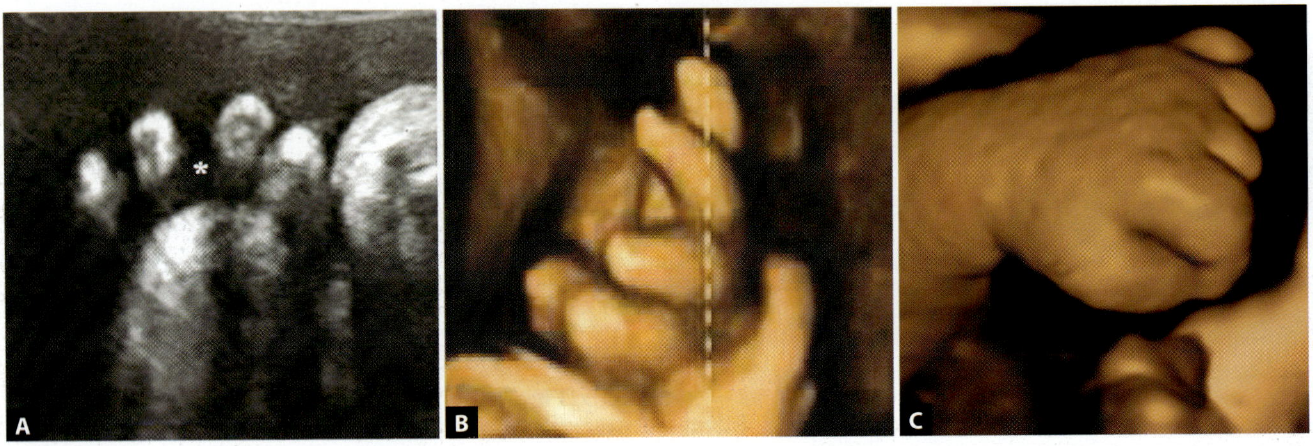

Figs. 65A to C: 2D and 3D views. A trident hand. The four fingers have the same length. Note the increased interspaces between the third and fourth digit (*). Hand articular motility is normal.

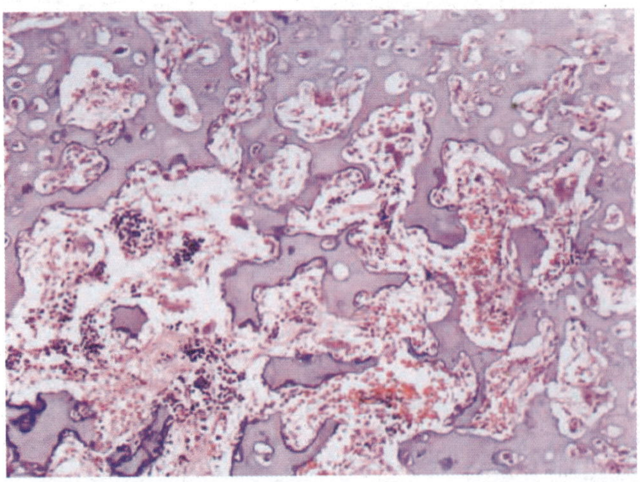

Fig. 66: Chondrocostal ossification abnormality showing a reduced chondrocytary component. Thick and disorganized osseous trabeculae.

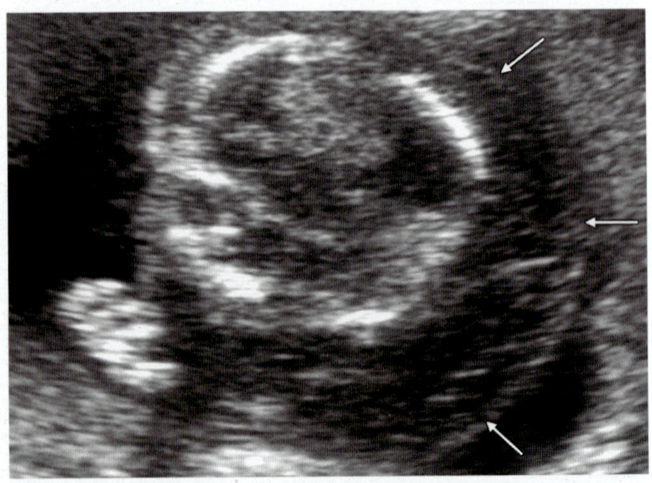

Fig. 67: View of the head of fetus affected by achondrogenesis. Note the double contour of the skull (arrows) that suggests a generalized lymphatic drainage defect.

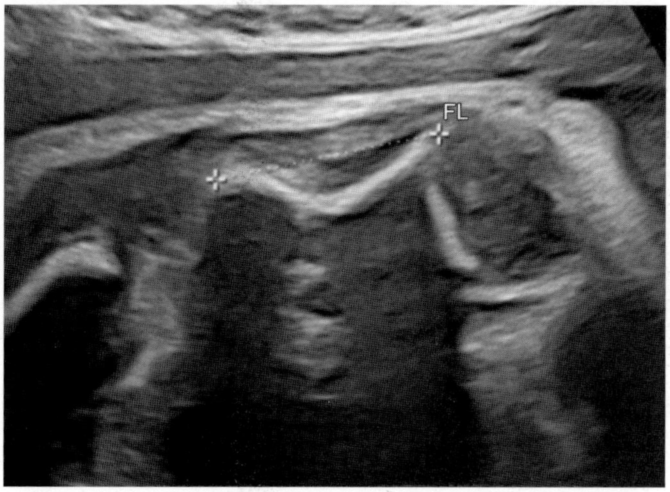

Fig. 68: Longitudinal view of short bowed femur. The image shows the femur length (FL).

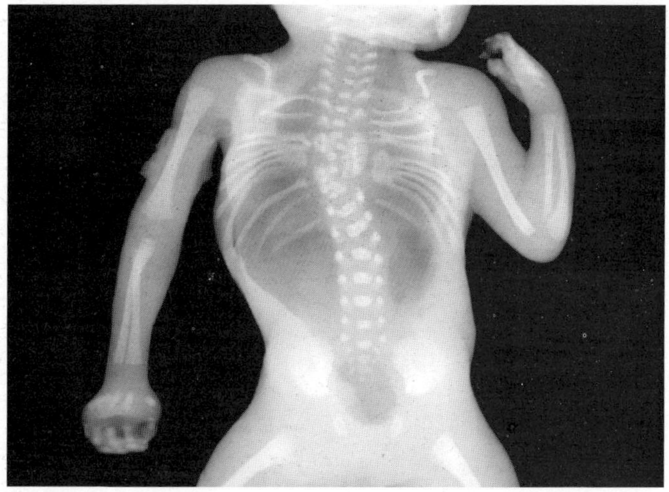

Fig. 70: Postmortem fetography of a fetus with spondylothoracic dysplasia type Jarcho–Levin, showing hemivertebrae and vertebral fusion. Fused dorsal vertebrae and ribs.

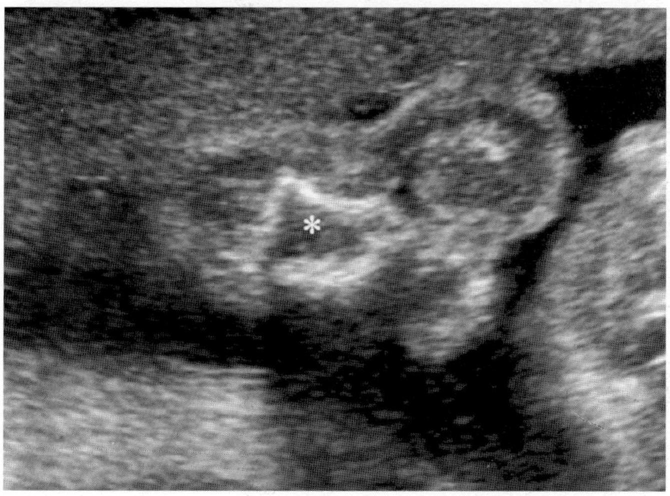

Fig. 69: Coronal view of hypoplastic scapula (*).

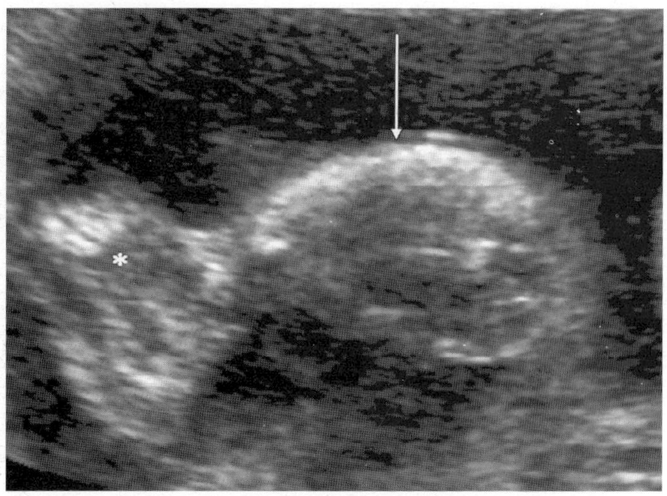

Fig. 71: Tibia is "bent". Similar length of tibia (arrow) and foot (*).

loose amniotic bands that adhere to the fetus and cause constriction, vascular compromise, and amputation of the limbs[16] **(Figs. 82 to 88)**. They must be distinguished from placental septation that is a septum that crosses the uterine cavity **(Fig. 89)** without affecting the fetus.

PHOCOMELIA

The name is derived from the "seal" aspect of the fetuses **(Figs. 90A and B)**. The terminal and middle portion of the limbs are aplastic or hypoplastic. Feet and hands are directly articulated to the ankle or shoulder and they may be normal or abnormal. Phocomelia can occur sporadically (e.g., related to thalidomide drug) although it can be seen in many genetic syndromes and conditions such as Holt-Oram syndrome, thrombocytopenia absent radius (TAR) syndrome **(Fig. 91),** and Robert's syndrome (characterized by tetraphocomelia and midface anomalies with microcephaly and growth restriction) **(Figs. 90A and B)**.[13-15]

PROXIMAL FEMORAL FOCAL DEFICIENCY

Proximal femoral focal deficiency is a rare anomaly varying in severity from a marginally short femur **(Fig. 92)** to a complete absence of femur **(Figs. 93 to 95)**. It may be a

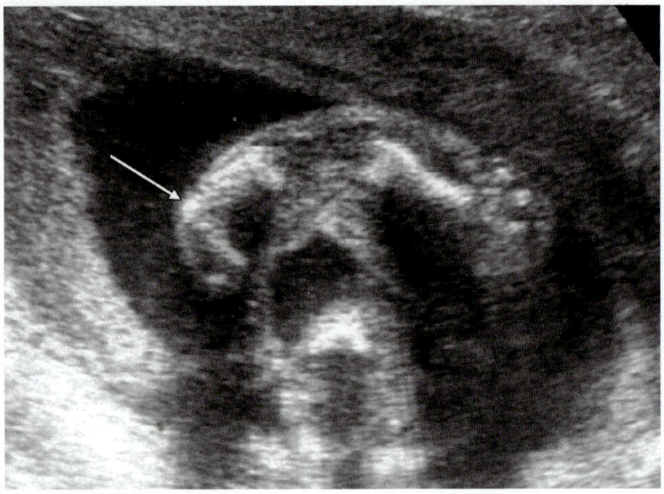

Fig. 72: Bowing tibia showing the "boomerang" configuration (arrow). The fibula cannot be assessed.

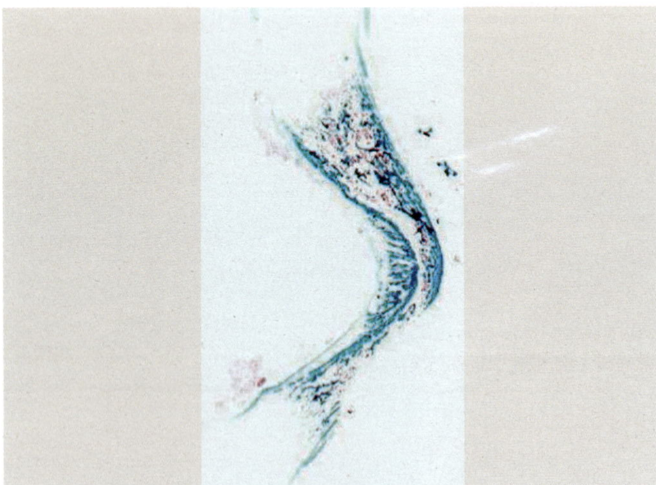

Fig. 73: Bowing tibial diaphysis by microscopy showing the classical "boomerang" configuration.

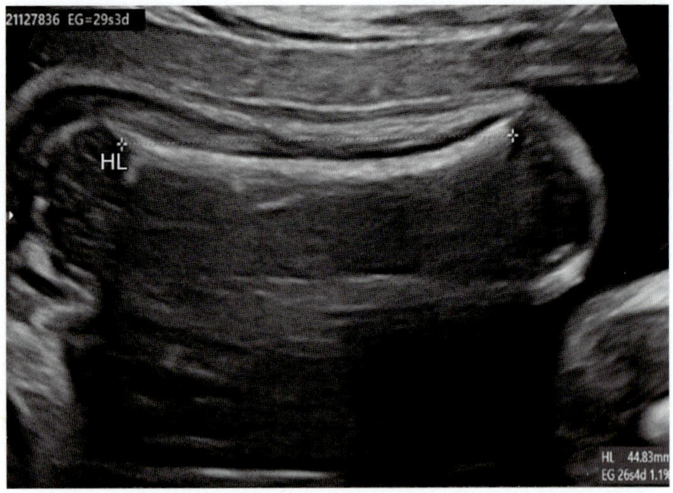

Fig. 74: Longitudinal view of shortened humerus with normal appearance at 26 weeks of gestation.

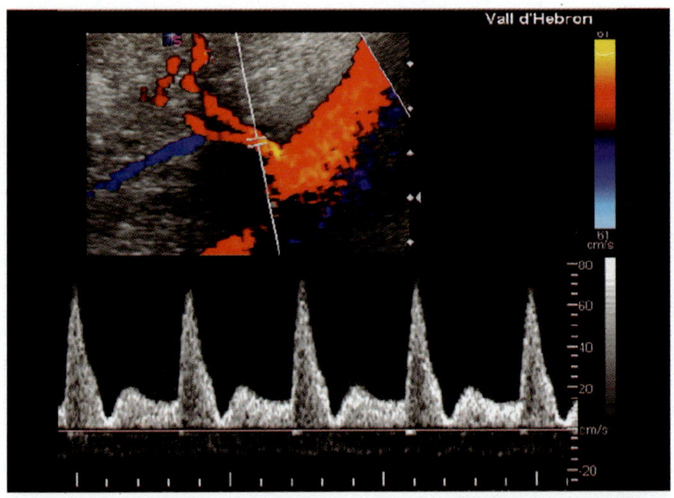

Fig. 75: Pathological uterine artery Doppler waveform suggesting an intrauterine growth restriction (IUGR) as the most likely cause of short femur.

unilateral defect (usually right sided) or bilateral in 10–15% of cases. PFFD is almost always an isolated occurrence except for associated ipsilateral fibular hemimelia (sporadic) or ulnar hemimelia (genetic).[13-15]

SPLIT-HAND AND SPLIT-FOOT MALFORMATION (ECTRODACTYLY)

Split-hand and split-foot malformation is a limb anomaly[17] **(Fig. 96)** involving the central rays of the autopod (the distal division of the limb such as hands or feet), syndactyly, median clefts of the hands and feet, and aplasia and/or hypoplasia of the phalanges, metacarpals, and metatarsals. Currently, 12 different mutations have been identified in SHFM phenotype. There are several classifications based on phenotype or molecular genetic alterations. The two typical manifestations are:

1. *Type 1 isolated SHFM:* Classical cleft affecting all four limbs with aplasia of one or more central digits in a "V" configuration **(Figs. 97 to 102)**
2. *Type 2 with long bone deficiency:* More severe form with aplasia of central and preaxial rays of the autopod (monodactyly) **(Figs. 103 and 104)**

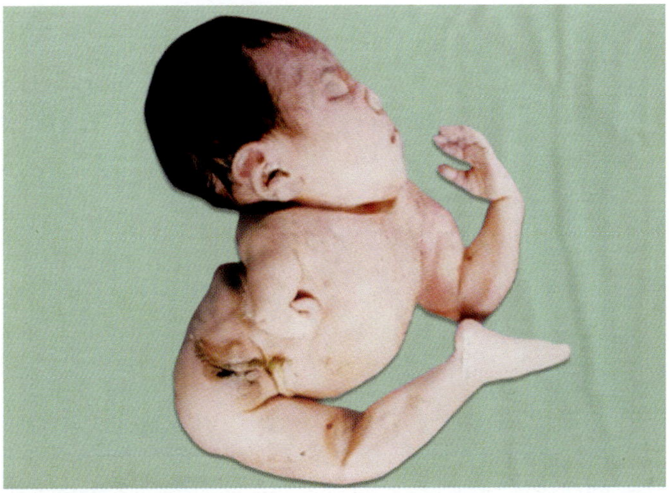

Fig. 76: Limb reductional defects secondary to constriction in a right lower limb. Amputation of the forearm and hand probably secondary to constriction of the developing limb during fetal life.

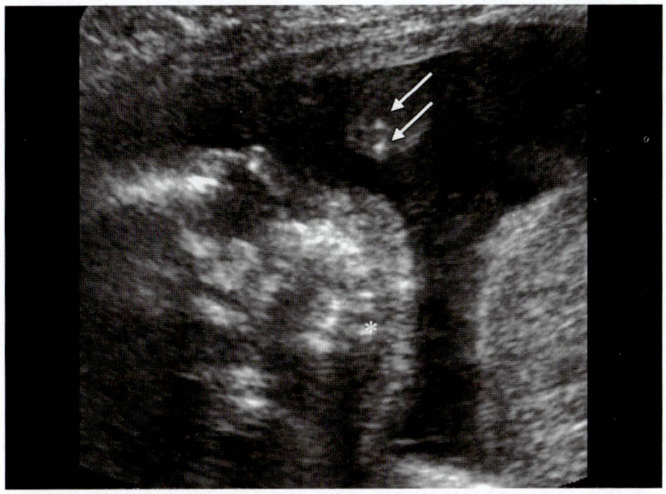

Fig. 78: Arrows showing hypoplastic ulna and radius as typically seen in reductional defect cases. One must assess facial structures (*) in order to find cleft lips, tongue defects, or microretrognathia that may be associated with constituting a genetic syndrome.

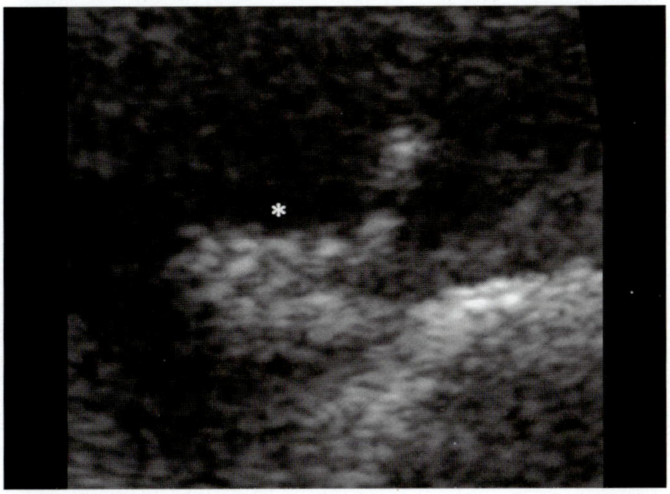

Fig. 77: Fetal hand showing a reductional defect. Oligodactyly. Absent phalanges of third, fourth, and fifth digits (*). To evaluate fetal phalanges, the hand must be opened. A closed hand must not be misinterpreted as an adactyly.

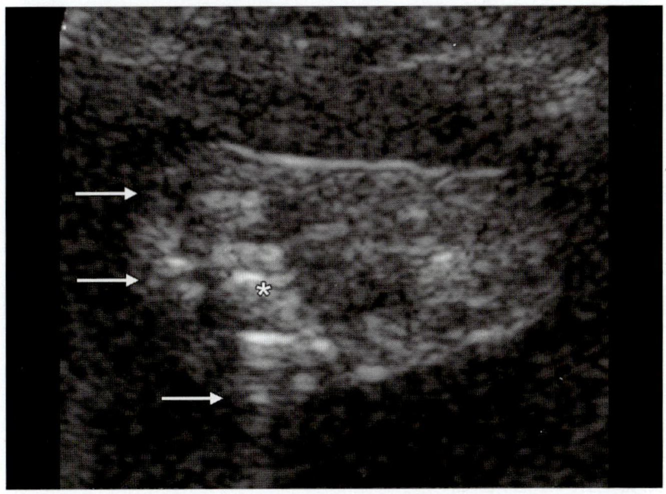

Fig. 79: Fetal forefoot view showing a reductional defect of toes. Normal metatarsal (*) with hypoplastic digits and without distal osseous component (arrows).

The most common pattern of inheritance for SHFM is an autosomal dominant with reduced penetrance. Autosomal recessive and X-linked inheritance have also been described. SHFM may be associated with other structural defects, such as cleft lip/palate, ectodermal dysplasia, or developmental delay. There are some syndromes related to ectrodactyly (cleft hand and absent tibia syndrome or absent ulna syndrome, ectrodactyly-ectodermal dysplasia-cleft palate, etc.).

HAND AND FOOT DEFORMITIES

Clubhands[18]

Malposition of the hands is much less common than feet malposition. They are classified according to the side of the deviation:

- *Ulnar clubhands are* rare and usually isolated **(Fig. 105)**.
- *Radial clubhands* include a spectrum of anomalies with absent, hypoplastic **(Figs. 106 to 108)**, or triphalangeal

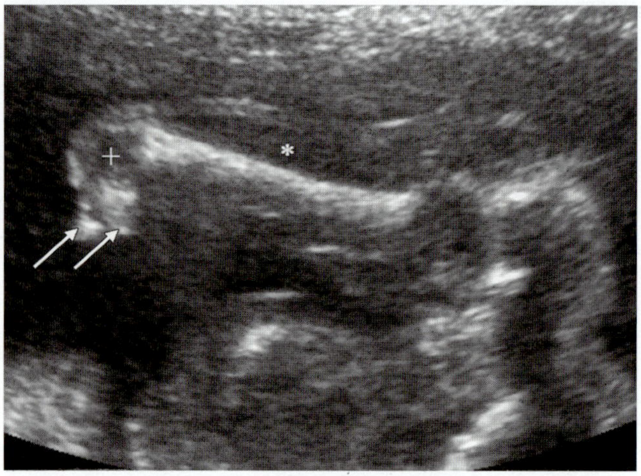

Fig. 80: Upper extremity view showing a terminal defect. Normal humerus (*) with a hypoplastic radius and ulna (arrows) and absence of almost all forearm and hand. The articulation below the humerus usually remains unaffected (+).

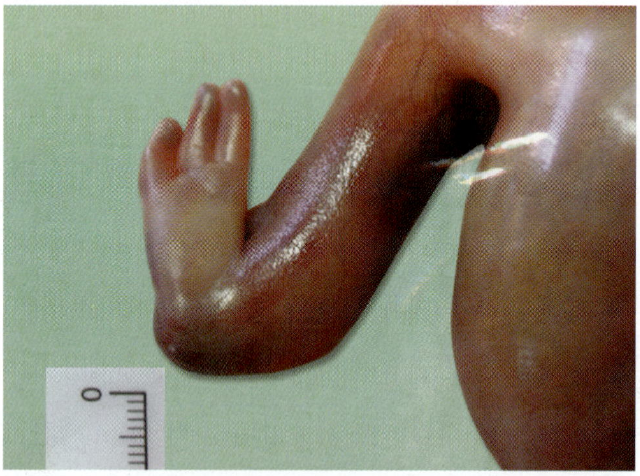

Fig. 81: Upper extremity showing a terminal defect. Normal humerus with a hypoplastic ulna and radius and absence of almost all forearm and hand.

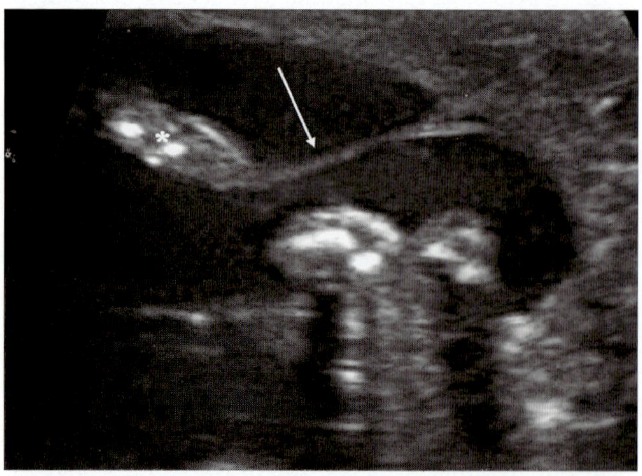

Fig. 82: Amniotic band (arrow) connecting amnios and hand (*).

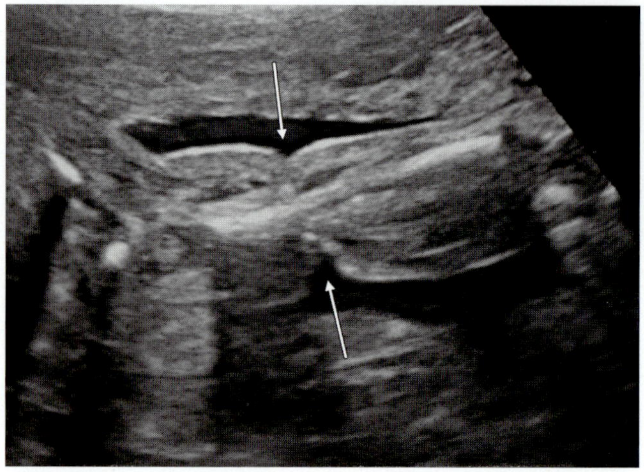

Fig. 83: Constriction band in a low extremity (arrows). Note the lymphedema secondary to vascular constriction.

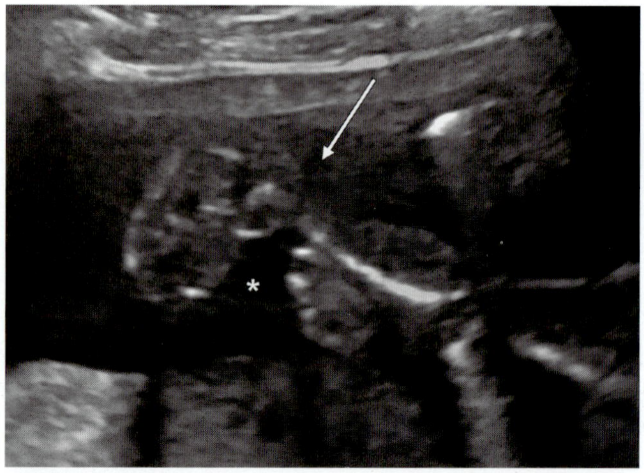

Fig. 84: Longitudinal view of the lower limb. Constriction band attached at malleolar level (arrows) with distal edema (*).

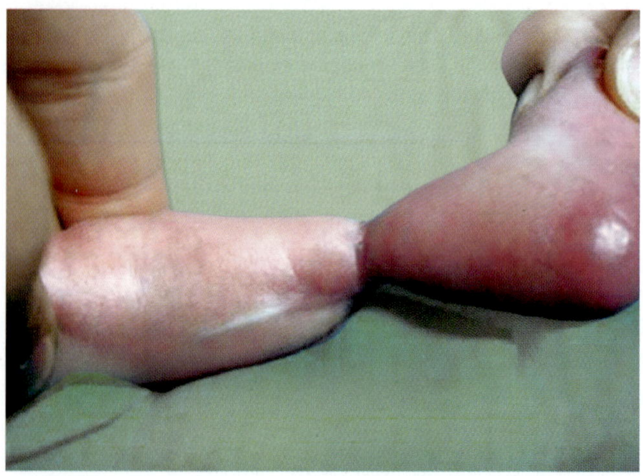

Fig. 85: A 28-week newborn with a constriction band in a low extremity.

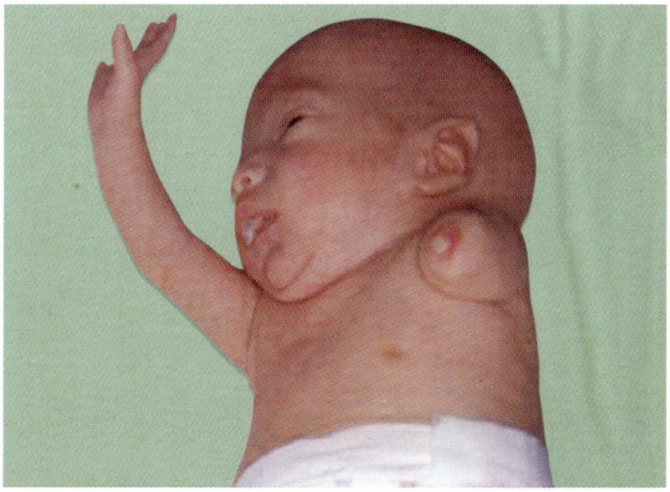

Fig. 86: Newborn with a reductional defect due to an amniotic band. The articulation remains unaffected. Contralateral upper extremity showing a normal appearance.

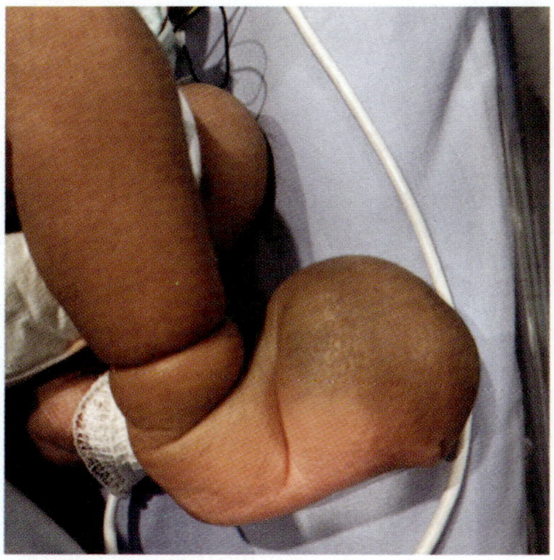

Fig. 87: Forefoot edema due to a vascular compromise secondary to amniotic band syndrome.

thumb and radial aplasia or hypoplasia. Radial deformity is usually associated to genetic syndromes and in 50% of cases is bilateral. The most common associations are chromosome anomalies (trisomy 18), hematological disorder (Fanconi pancytopenia and thrombocytopenia-absent radius) **(Fig. 109)**, cardiac disorders (Holt–Oram syndrome) **(Figs. 110A and B)**, or scoliosis.

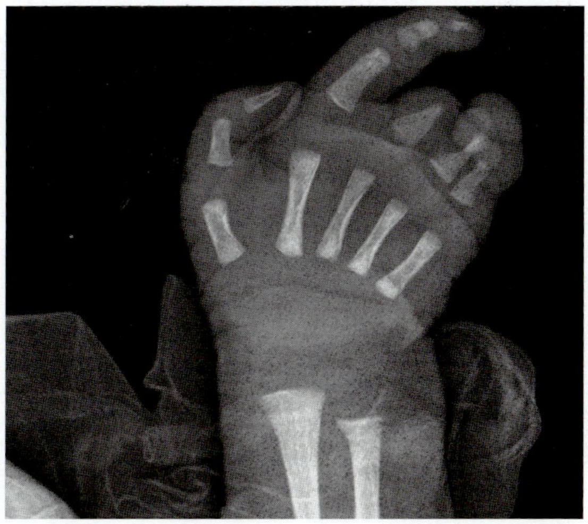

Fig. 88: Reductional defects of the distal part of the fingers due to amniotic band syndrome. In this case, the contralateral hand was normal. In 50% of cases, the compromise is isolated and the contralateral limb is unaffected. The ultrasound (US) assessment of fetal extremities must be meticulous and must include visualization of both extremities independently.

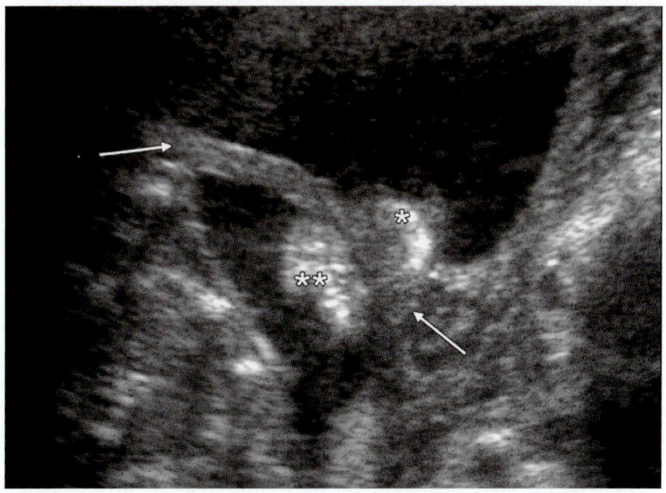

Fig. 89: Placental septation that does not affect the fetus. It crosses the uterine cavity. Arrows show its myometrial insertions. Fetus with his opened mouth is surrounding the septation (upper maxilla*, lower maxilla**). Finding a placental septation is relatively frequent and does not require a special follow-up.

Clubfeet[19,20]

Clubfeet or talipes equinovarus are one of the most common congenital defects and affect four components of the feet: (1) Cavus, (2) forefoot adductus, (3) hindfoot varus, and (4) ankle equinus. The majority of cases are isolated with a certain familial predisposition. However, to date, the responsible genes have not been identified.

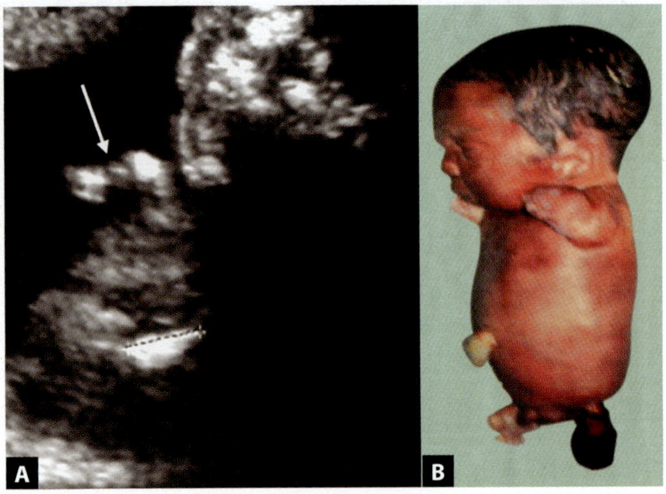

Figs. 90A and B: *Ultrasound image of phocomelia of upper limbs:* (A) Anomalous hand (between callipers) directly inserted in the trunk without evidence of middle or proximal portions of the upper limb (arrow); (B) Macroscopic image of tetraphocomelia due to a Robert's syndrome.

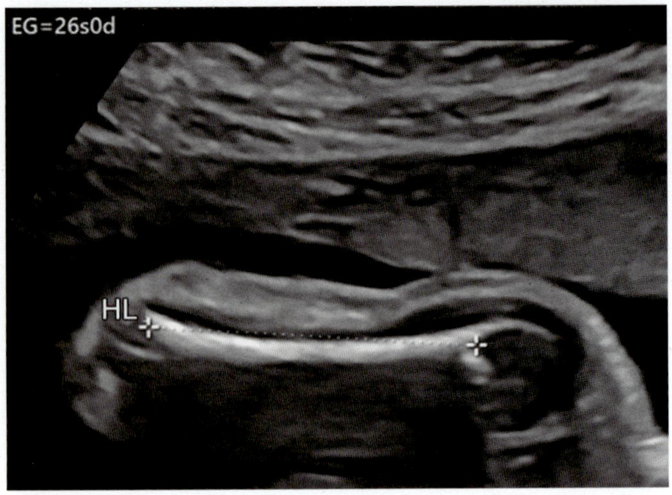

Fig. 92: Sonogram of a fetal femur that shows a normal configuration but extremely shortened (<1 percentile). Note the difference between the real gestational age (EG) and the corresponding to the femur measurement on the legend of the picture.

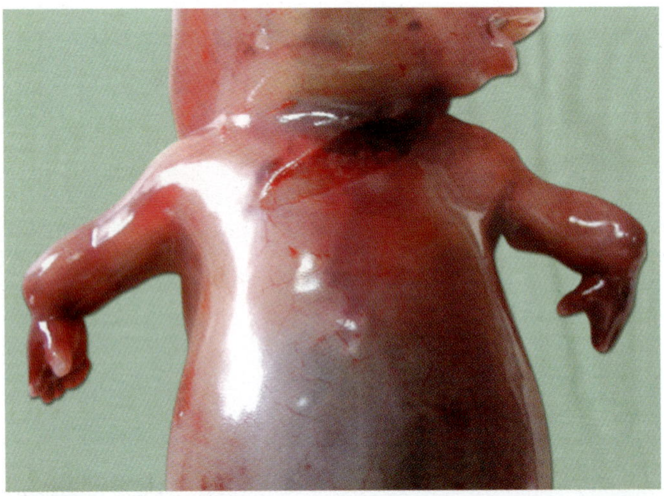

Fig. 91: Thrombocytopenia-absent radius (TAR) syndrome. Note that fetal thumbs are present.

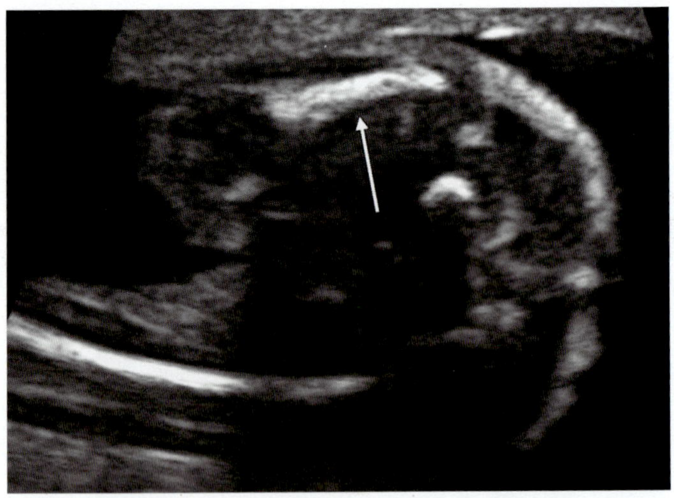

Fig. 93: The femur appears shorter than the contralateral one (arrow). Even if one measure only one femur diaphysis both bones must be visualized in order to exclude any long bone asymmetry.

Clubfeet can also be associated with chromosome defects (trisomy 18) and skeletal dysplasias. Fetal clubfeet are shown in **Figures 111 to 124**. When clubfeet are isolated (unilateral or bilateral) the prognosis is good, and most of the cases can be treated postnatally with conservative management.

POLYDACTYLY

Polydactyly is the most common hand anomaly. Prenatal detection is made by finding more than the normal number of digits in the fetal hand, foot, or both **(Figs. 125 to 132)**. It may be a unilateral or bilateral defect. Extra digits may consist solely of soft tissue elements or may contain bone.

They may be isolated defects (showing dominant inheritance pattern) or may occur with a number of associations.

There are three types depending on the location:

1. Preaxial polydactyly involves the radial aspect of the hand or foot **(Figs. 125 and 126)**.

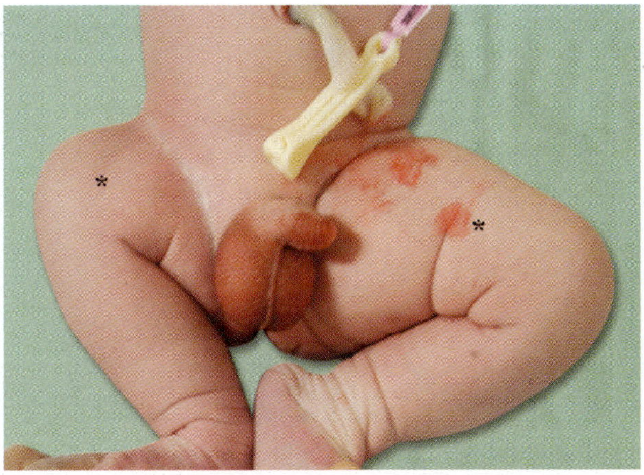

Fig. 94: Femoral focal deficiency in a newborn. Note the significant difference on the length between the proximal part of the low extremities (*).

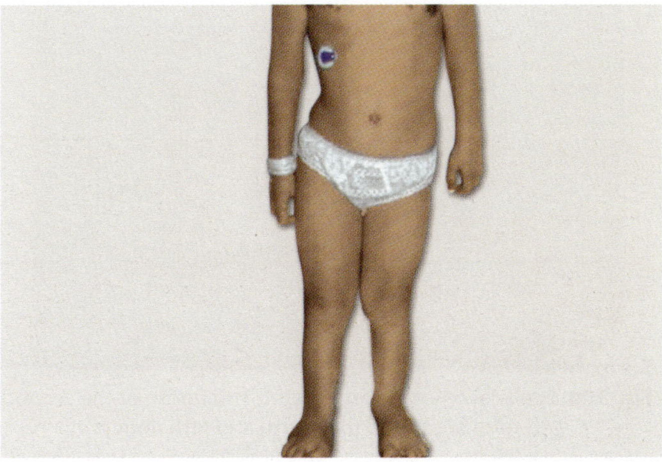

Fig. 95: Proximal femoral focal deficiency. Asymmetrical shortening of lower extremities.

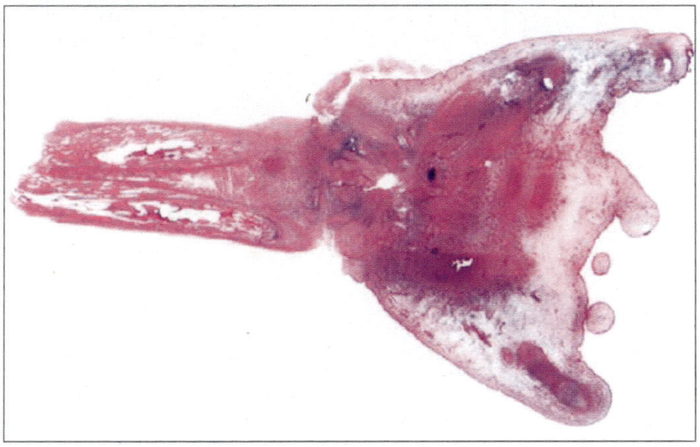

Fig. 96: Macro-microscopic image (histological specimen) of a characteristic ectrodactyly.

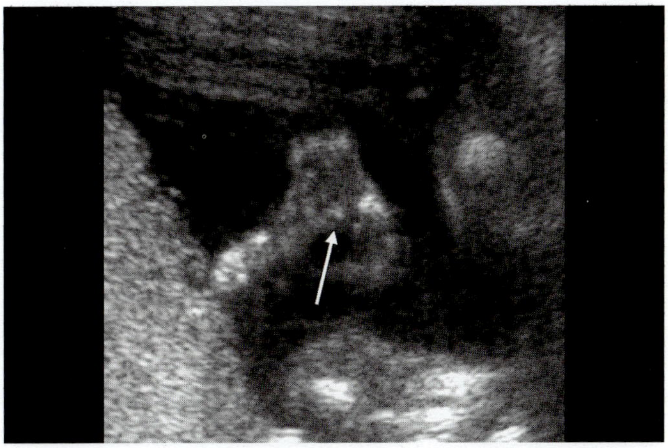

Fig. 97: Deep fetal hand cleft showing a "V" configuration (arrow). Absence of differentiation of metacarpals and phalanges.

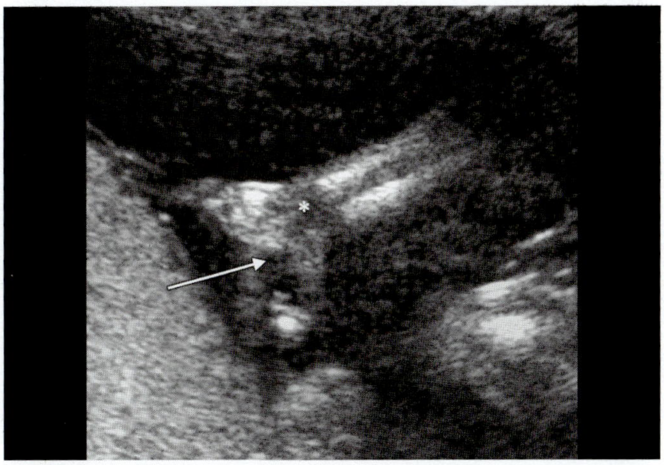

Fig. 98: Deep cleft in fetal hand, demonstrating a "V" configuration (arrow). The ulna, radius, and wrist joint show a normal aspect.

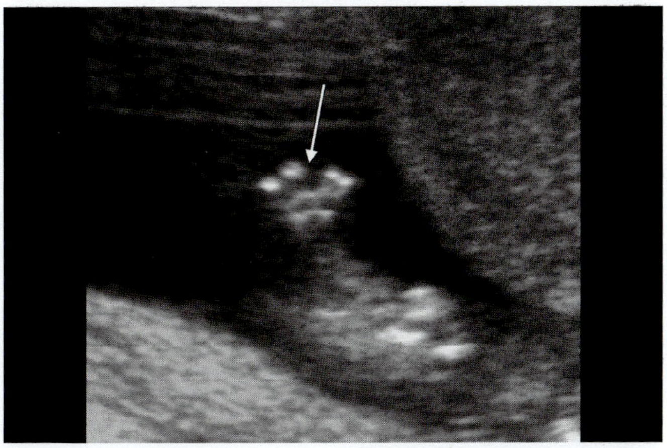

Fig. 99: A 12-week fetal ultrasound showing a "V" configuration hand cleft. Both hands must be assessed in the first trimester sonographic examination.

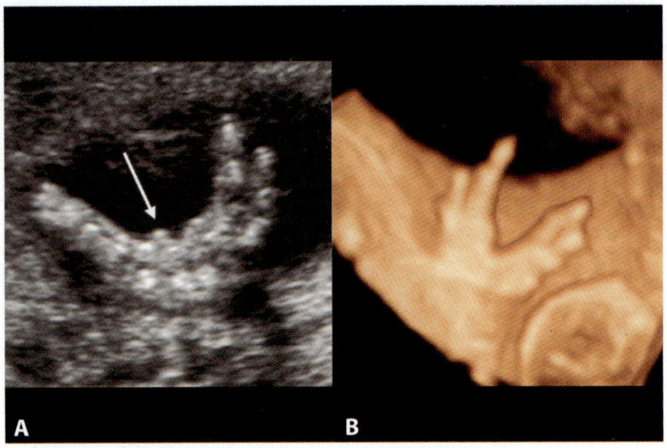

Figs. 100A and B: Split hand (arrow). Only three and four digits can be identified showing a normal differentiation of metacarpals and phalanges.

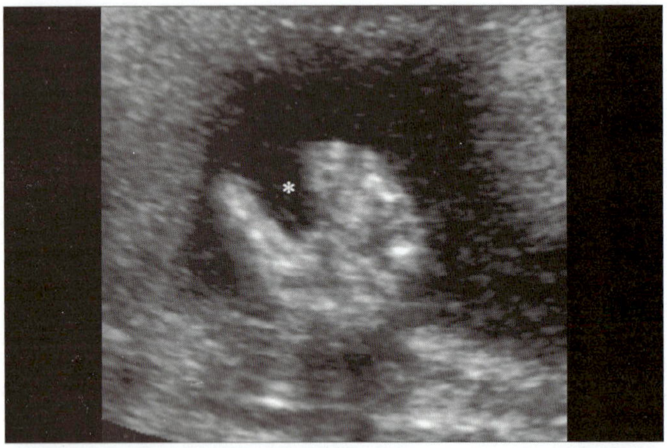

Fig. 101: Split hand (*) demonstrating poorly differentiated fingers (syndactyly).

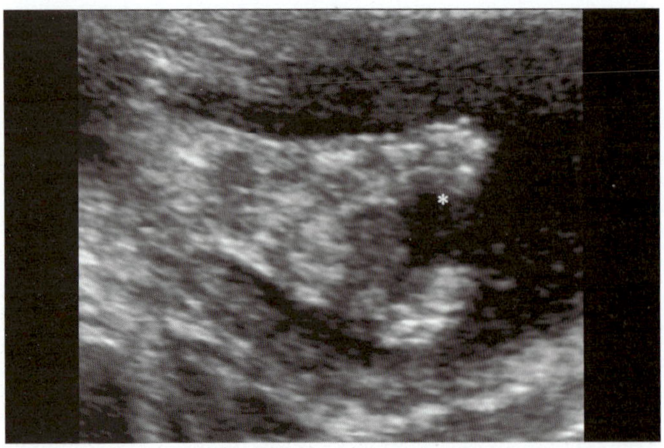

Fig. 102: Ultrasound view of the foot showing a deep central cleft (*) and syndactyly.

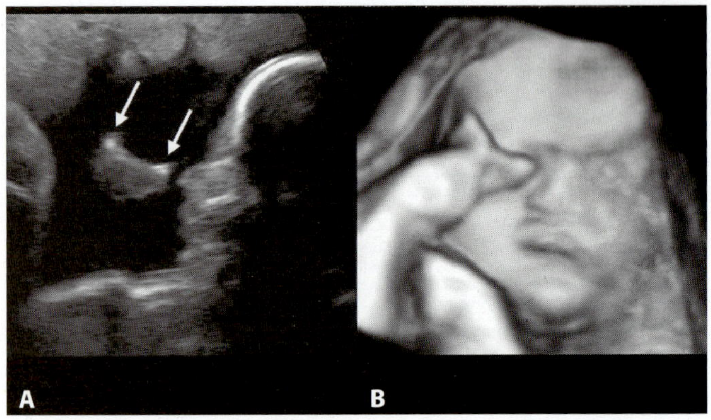

Figs. 103A and B: Ectrodactyly. Split "V" shaped hand. The arrows show the two fingers ("lobster-claw" anomaly). If it is isolated, the prognosis is good.

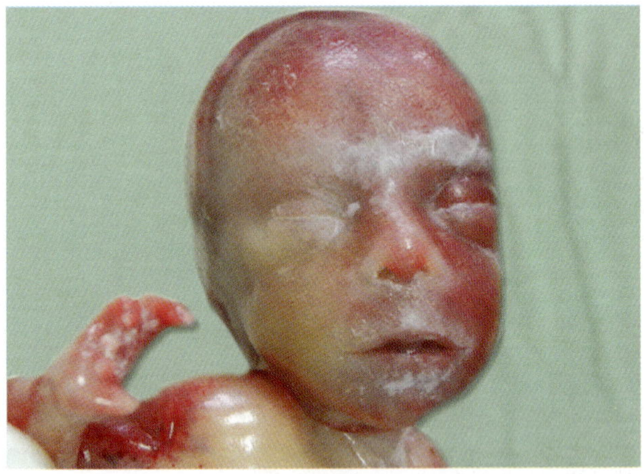

Fig. 104: Ectrodactyly with central cleft and fusion of the second and third digits and the fourth and fifth fingers.

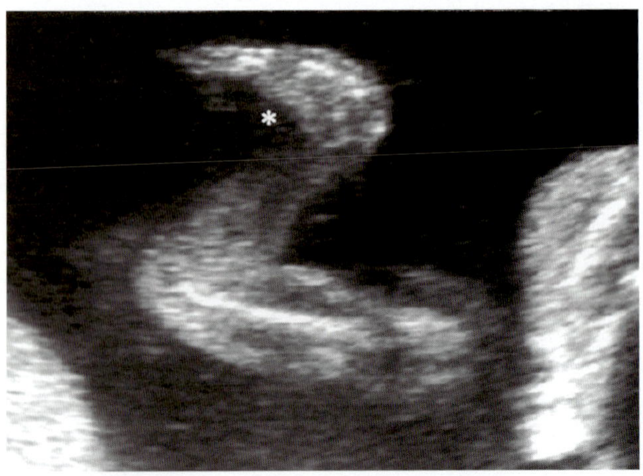

Fig. 105: The hand is malpositioned, describing a 90° angle with the forearm (*). The ulnar deviation was sustained even when articular movements of shoulder and elbow are normal. A transient cubital or radial deviation is considered normal, but if it is fixed, a postural defect must be suspected.

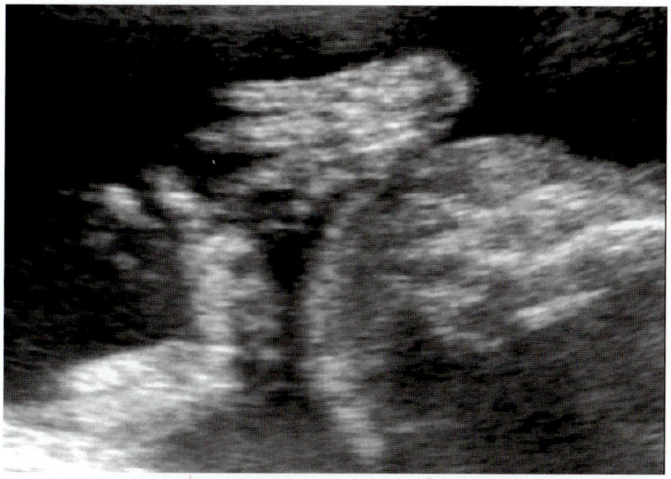

Fig. 106: Bilateral radial deviation of fetal hands. The thumb is present.

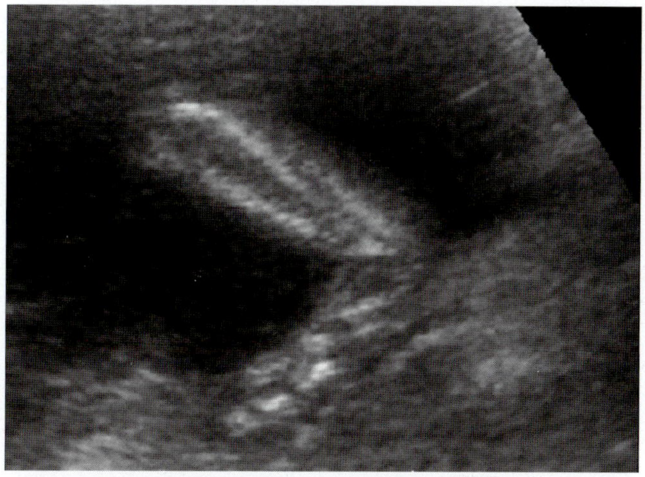

Fig. 108: Clubhand with radial hypoplasia.

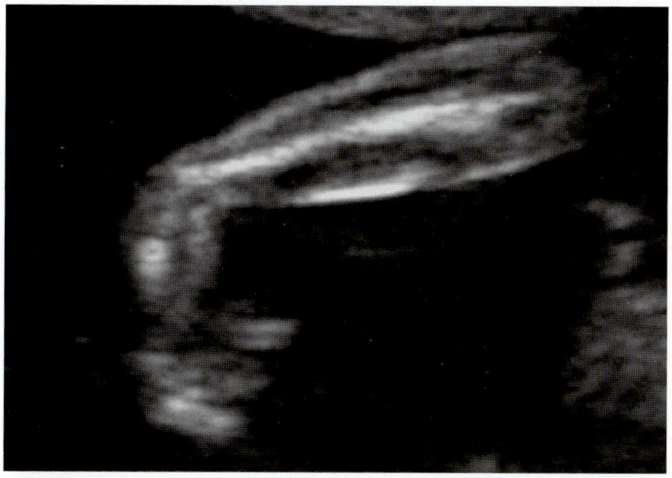

Fig. 107: Clubhand. The hand persisted in a fixed malposition throughout the exploration.

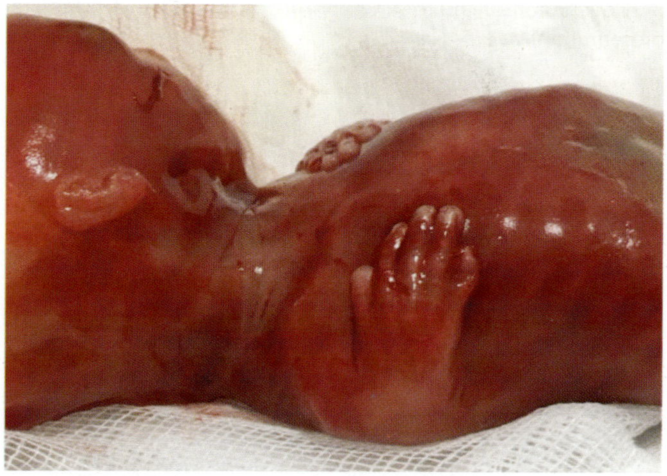

Fig. 109: Severe form of thrombocytopenia-absent radius (TAR) syndrome (phocomelia). The affectation is typically bilateral and symmetric with normal thumbs.

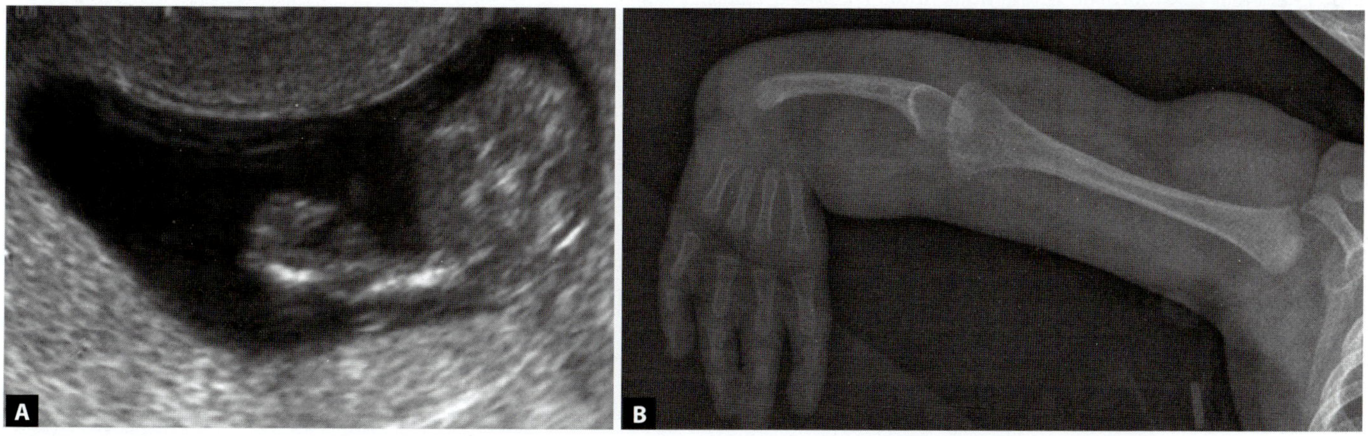

Figs. 110A and B: Hand deformity with radial aplasia and absent thumb in (A) a 12-week ultrasound due to Holt–Oram syndrome; (B) Postnatal X-ray.

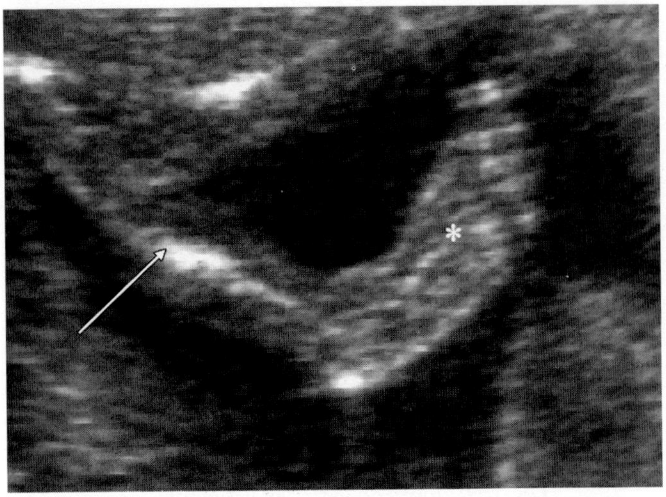

Fig. 111: Foot deformity (*). Fetal leg showing a single bone (arrow), probably the fibula. This defect may be isolated or part of the femur-tibia-radius complex (classically with familial presentation).

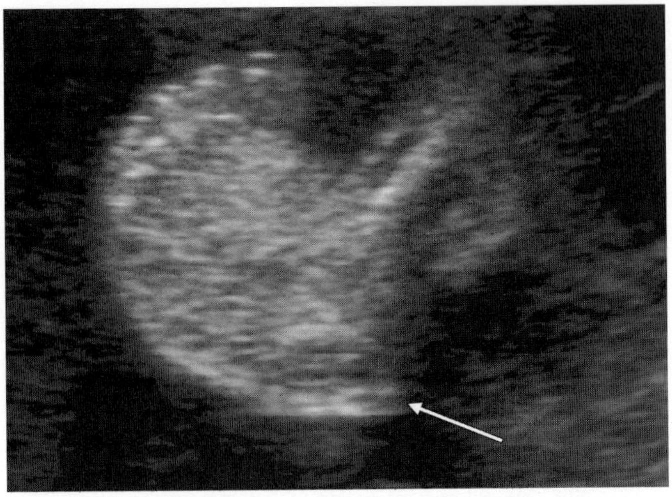

Fig. 113: Talipes equinovarus foot. The heel cannot be assessed. Forefoot is oriented in the same plane as the lower leg with loss of heel angle (arrow). Even if the knee joint movement is normal, the foot joint is fixed and the foot is permanently malpositioned.

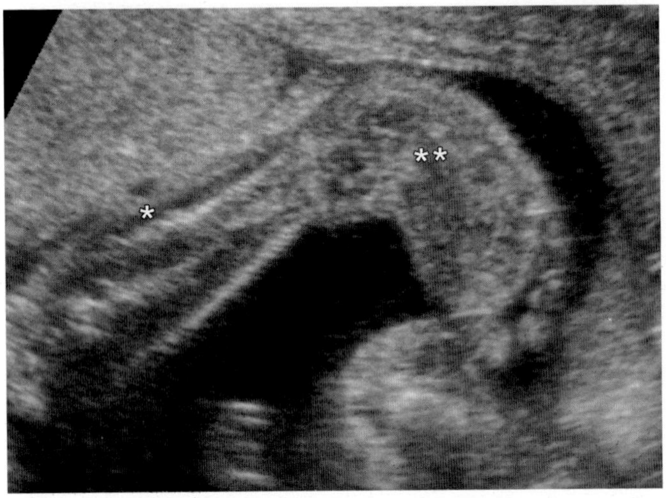

Fig. 112: Fetal clubfoot. The whole tibia, fibula (*), and the sole of the foot (**) can be assessed in the same plane. In normal conditions, in a sagittal view, the foot is visualized in profile.

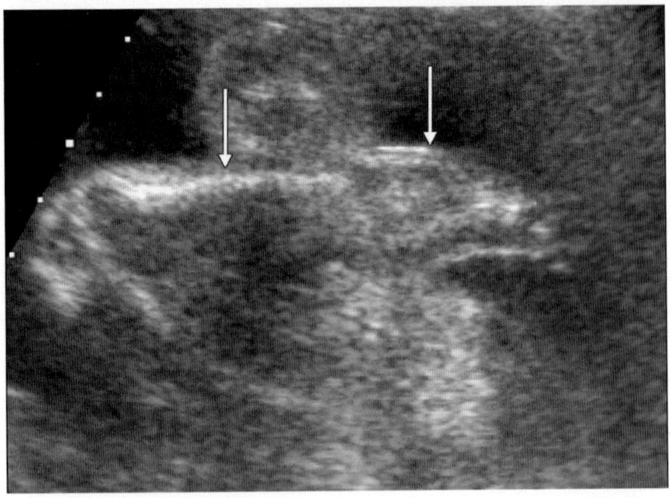

Fig. 114: Talipes equinovarus with a marked equinus component (permanent plantar flexion). The lower leg's bone is practically aligned with the hindfoot (arrows).

2. Postaxial polydactyly involves the ulnar aspect of fetal hand or foot **(Figs. 127 to 132)**.
3. Central polydactyly, when the three central digits are affected.

Postaxial polydactyly is the most frequent form, and it is normally isolated; however, it can also be associated to some syndromes. Preaxial and central polydactyly usually involve a syndromic association.

The most common syndromes that need to be considered are Meckel-Gruber syndrome (with encephalocele and multicystic kidneys), Bardet-Biedl syndrome (with syndactyly and big hyperechogenic kidneys), Pallister-Hall syndrome (with facial abnormalities and cleft palate), and Ellis-Van Crevelt syndrome (narrow chest, short limbs, and heart defects).

SYNDACTYLY

Syndactyly is an abnormal fusion between digits. This fusion can involve only soft tissues (simple) or include bones (complex). The complex syndactyly is easier

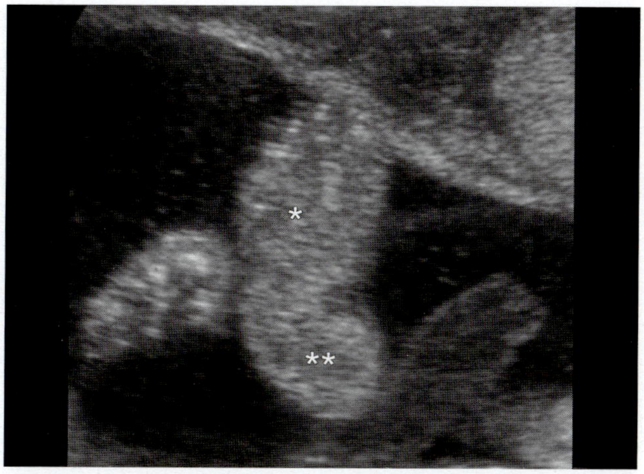

Fig. 115: Talipes equinovarus with marked varus component. Note the prominent metatarsal adduction (*) respect to heel (**).

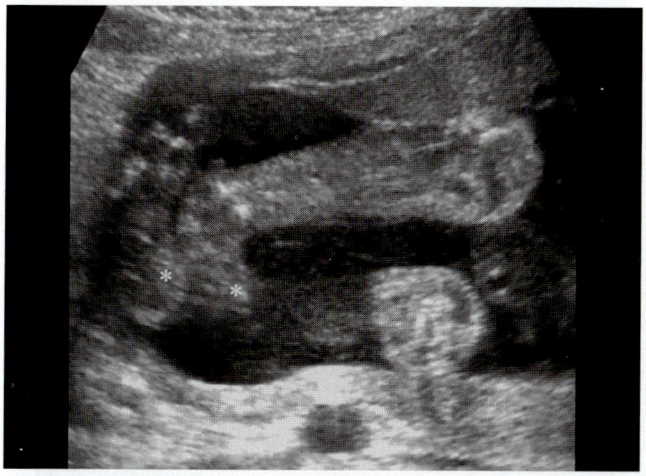

Fig. 116: Bilateral clubfeet (*). Forefeet are oriented in the same plane as the lower leg with loss of calcaneus angulation.

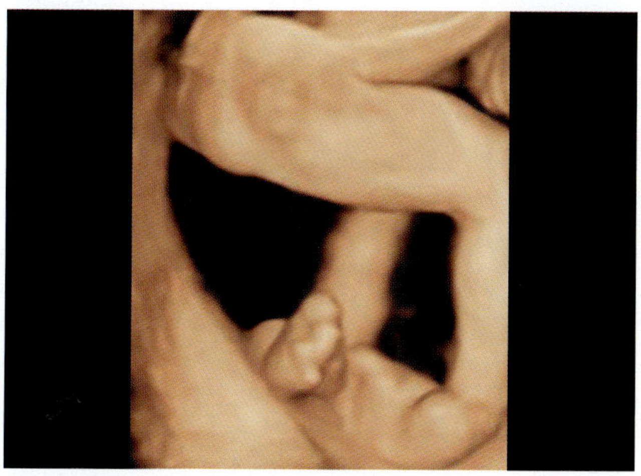

Fig. 117: 3D view of bilateral clubfeet.

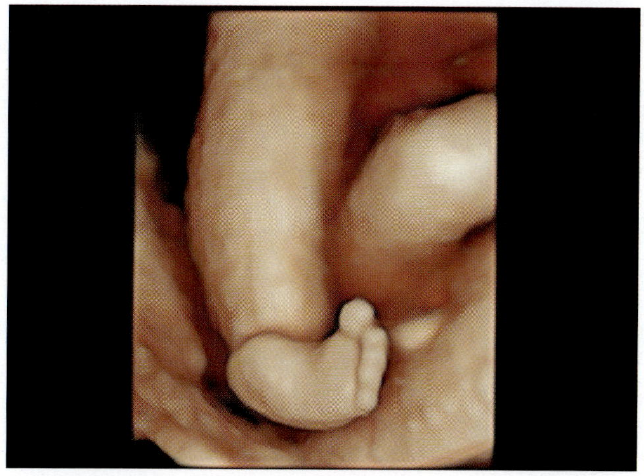

Fig. 118: 3D ultrasound of unilateral fetal clubfoot.

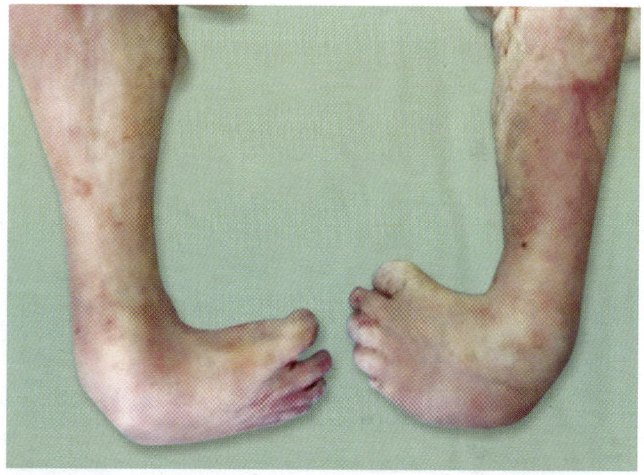

Fig. 119: Neonatal photograph demonstrating that the angle formed by the lower leg and hindfoot may be rounded laterally in talipes equinovarus deformity.

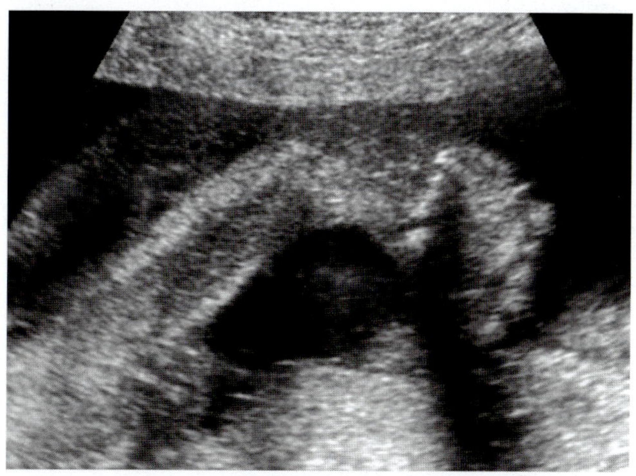

Fig. 120: Fetal foot showing a 90° angle with the forefoot. The foot was in a fixed position throughout the duration of the sonographic examination.

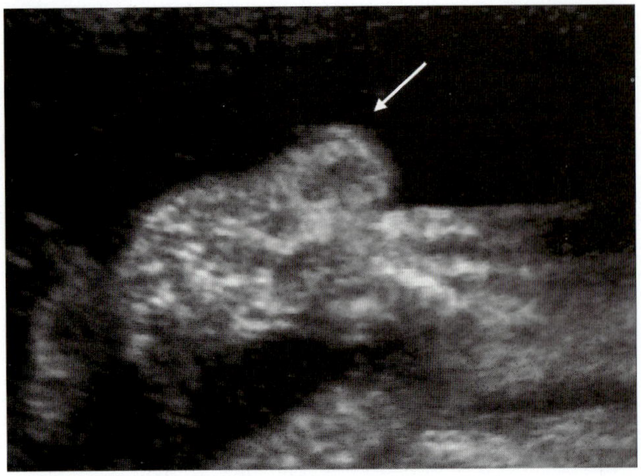

Fig. 121: Malpositioned calcaneus valgus foot. Prominent calcaneus (arrow). As in talipes equinovarus, the forefoot is oriented in the same plane as the lower leg.

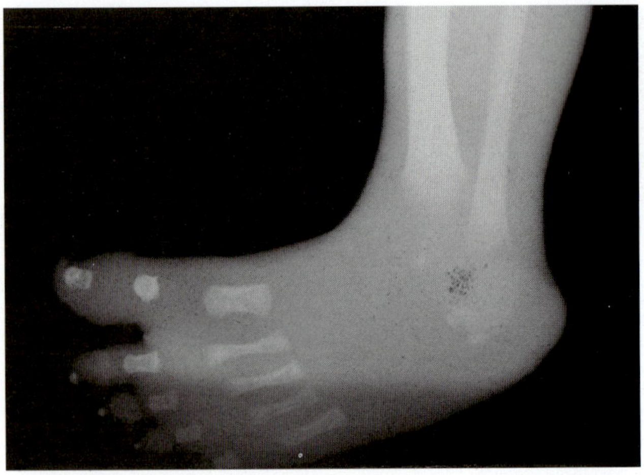

Fig. 122: Postmortem fetography showing a prominent calcaneus typical of the calcaneus valgus deformity.

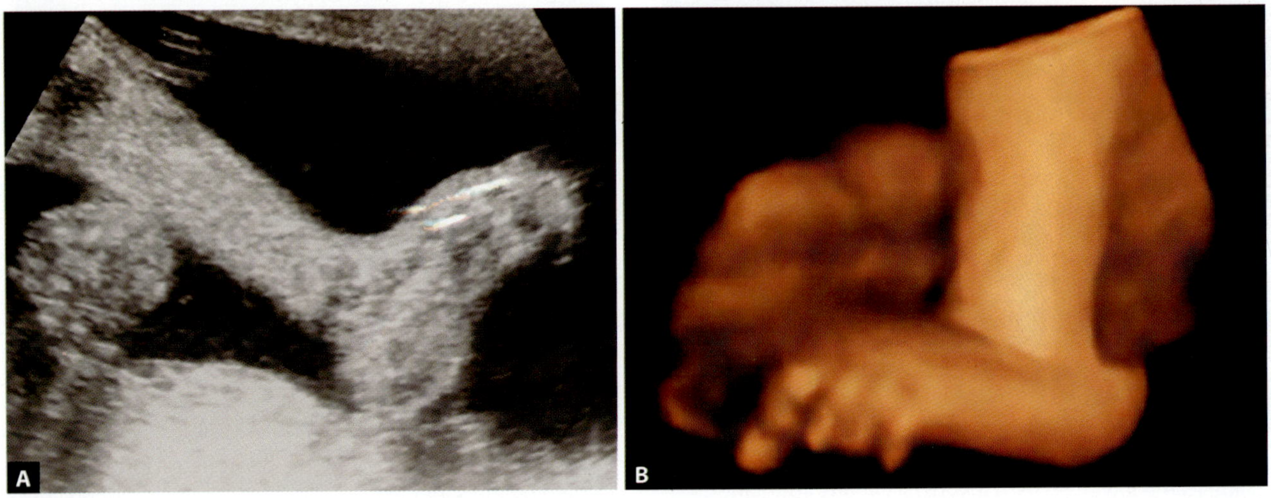

Figs. 123A and B: Malpositioned fetal foot. The foot is in a fixed position throughout the duration of the sonographic examination.

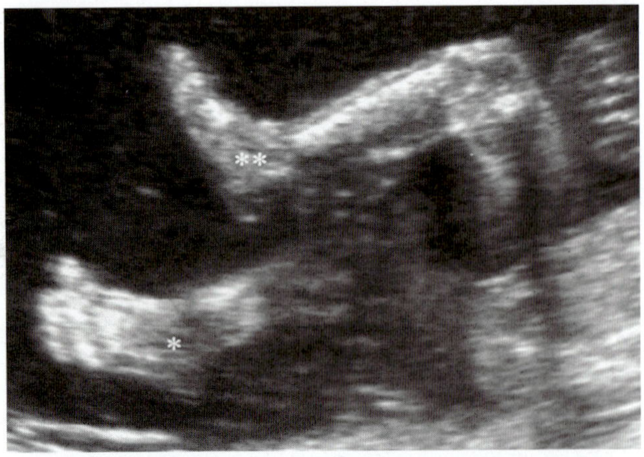

Fig. 124: Normal fetal foot can achieve startling degrees of dorsiflexion (**) or plantar flexion (*). Fetal movements and transient correction of the suspected malposition can be assessed.

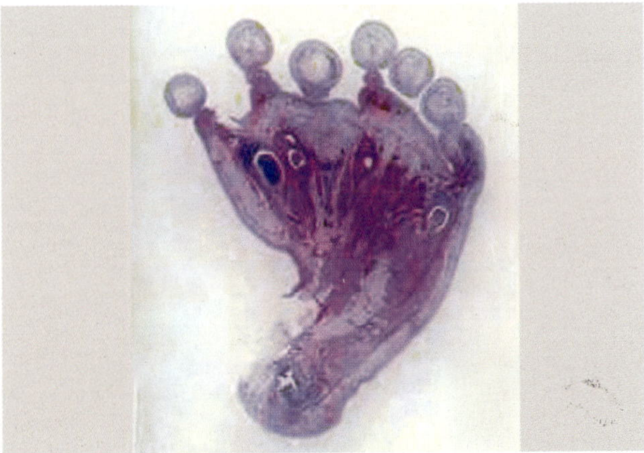

Fig. 125: Macro-micro examination (histological specimen) of a foot preaxial polydactyly.

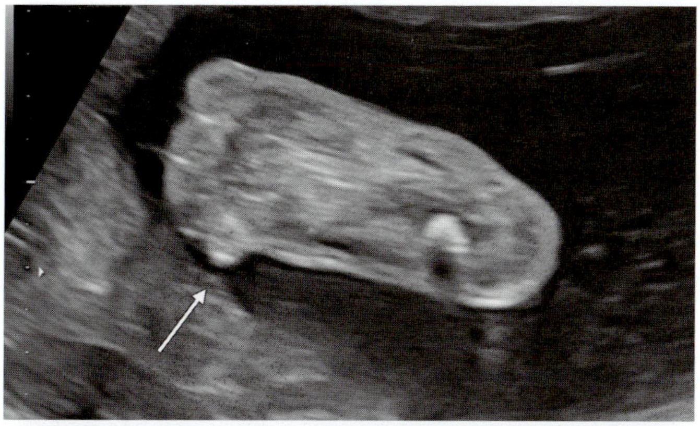

Fig. 126: View of the sole of the foot. Fetal foot preaxial polydactyly (arrow). The accessory digit contains solely soft tissue elements.

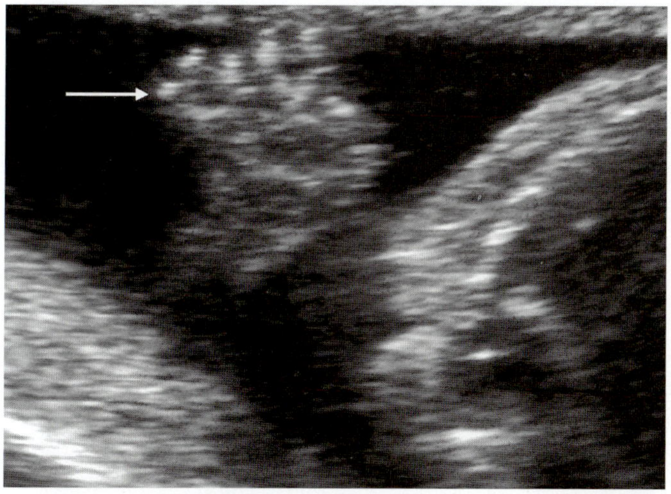

Fig. 127: Sometimes the first sign of polydactyly is a thicker than normal hand. With ultrasound examination a postaxial polydactyly can be detected (arrow).

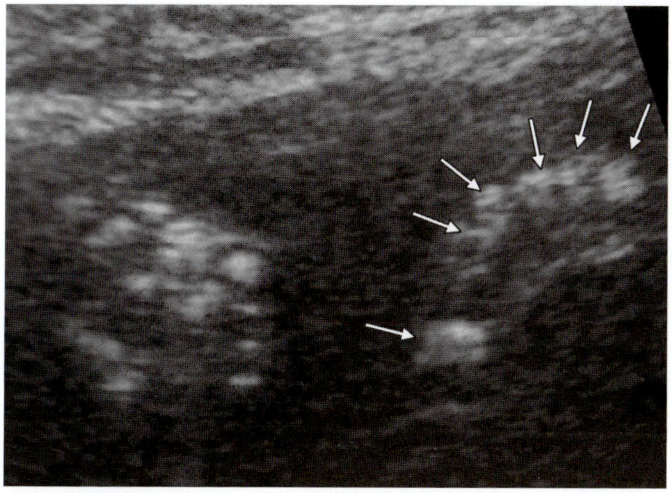

Fig. 128: Polydactyly is better assessed in the opened hand. Nevertheless sometimes can also be identified in a closed hand (arrows).

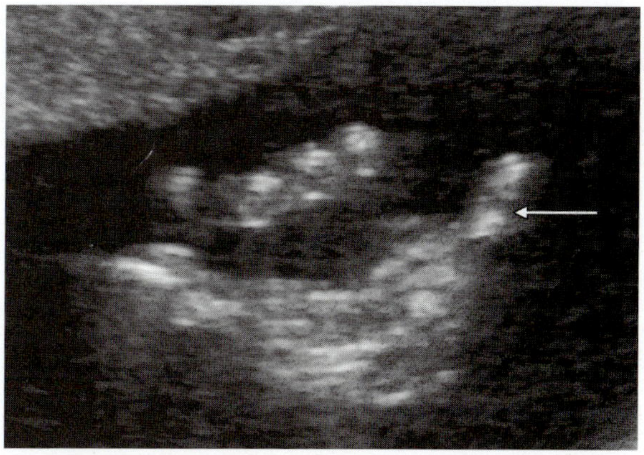

Fig. 129: Fetal hand with postaxial polydactyly. The accessory digit contains bone (arrow).

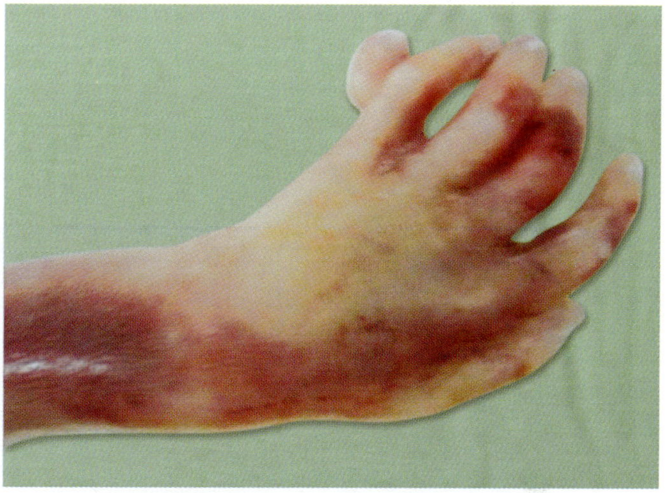

Fig. 130: Postaxial polydactyly of the left hand.

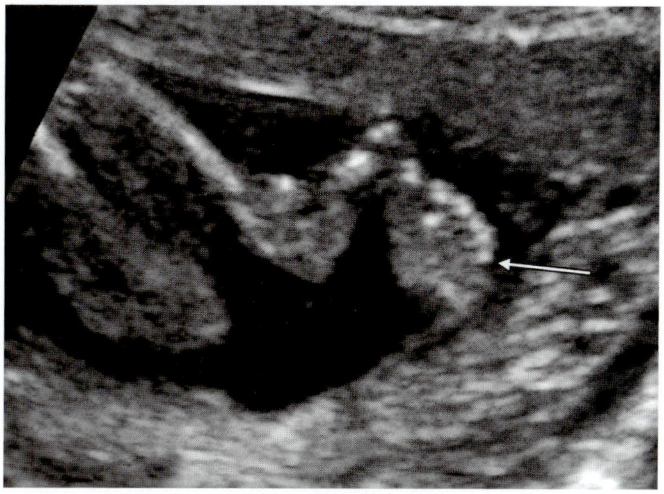

Fig. 131: Fetal foot postaxial polydactyly (arrow). The accessory digit contains bone.

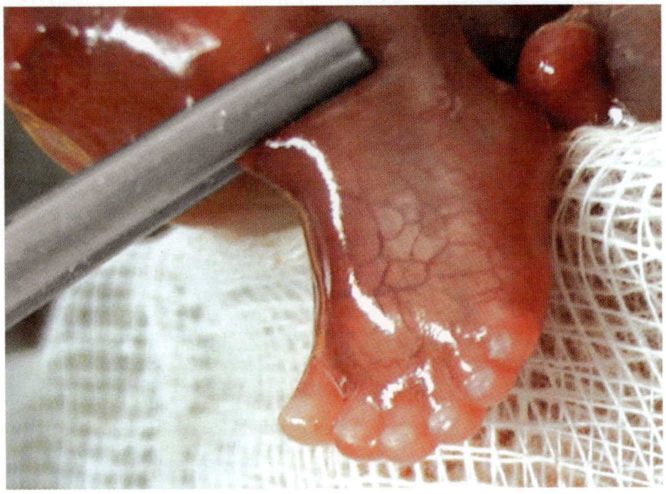

Fig. 132: Postaxial polydactyly of the left foot.

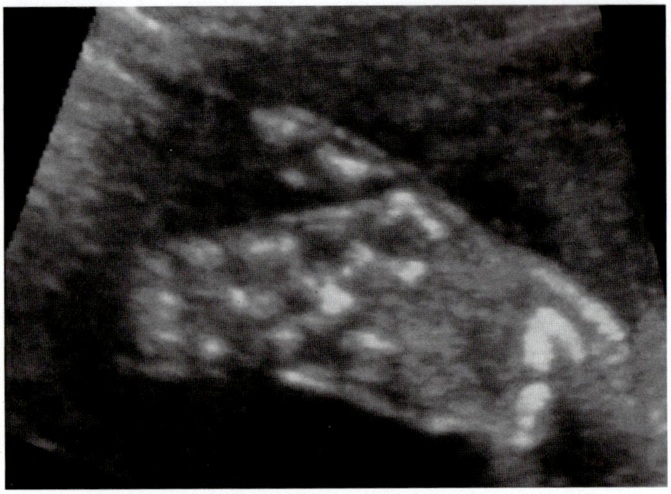

Fig. 133: Fetal hand syndactyly. 3D ultrasound.

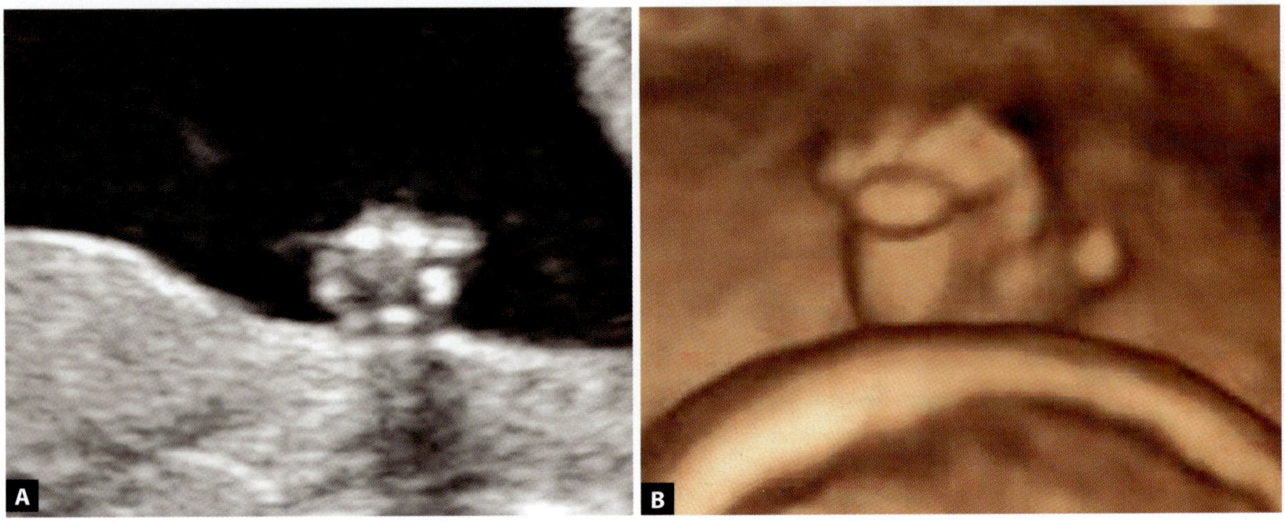

Figs. 134A and B: Fetal hand syndactyly. 2D and 3D views.

to diagnose in utero, because the affected fingers are deformed. Syndactyly **(Figs. 133 and 134)** can be complete (involving the hole digit) or incomplete (when spares the distal part).

Any number of fingers can be linked. When more than two fingers are involved, the hand takes a strange appearance (spoon hand or mitten hand). It can be sporadic with a familial tendency, or associated with other anomalies (syndromes or constriction band sequence).

HEMIVERTEBRAE

Abnormal curvature of the spine is due to a failure in formation of vertebral bodies, resulting in triangular shaped vertebrae (hemivertebrae) **(Figs. 135 and 136)** or due to a failure in vertebral segmentation (block vertebrae) **(Figs. 137 and 138)**. Any segment of the spine may be involved; the thoracolumbar is the most frequent and it has the worst prognosis. Mild spinal curvature may be an isolated finding. However, the association with other structural abnormalities or syndromes is common **(Fig. 139)** (such as Klippel-Feil, characterized by fusion of cervical vertebrae with short neck aspect or Jarcho-Levin).

FETAL AKINESIA DEFORMATION SEQUENCE

Deformative sequence secondary to fetal akinesia **(Figs. 140 and 141)** due to two or more intrauterine joint contractures. It is not a specific diagnosis; it refers

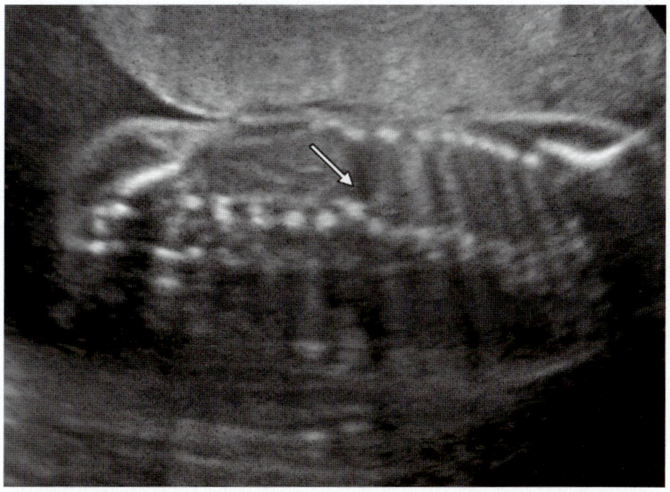

Fig. 135: Coronal view of fetal spine. Lumbar hemivertebrae (arrow).

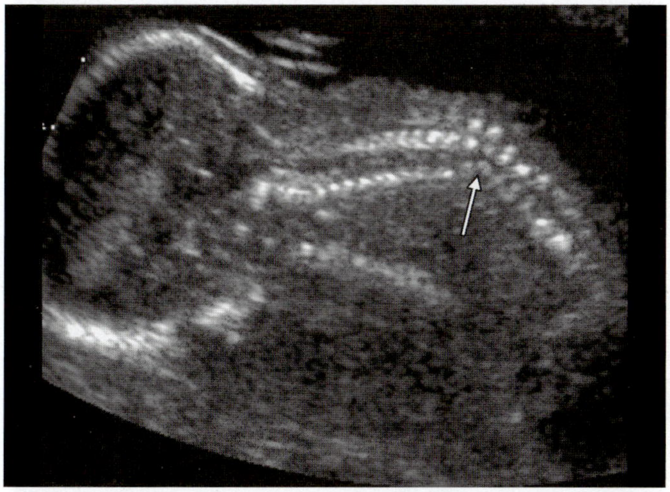

Fig. 136: Severe fetal scoliosis. Longitudinal view of the spine demonstrating a persistent angulation of the spine. The paired neural arch ossification centers appear disordered or mismatched (arrow). It was not associated with a neural tube defect.

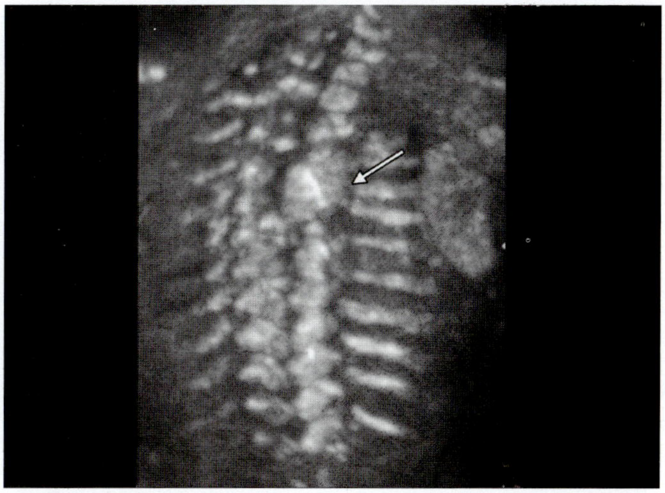

Fig. 137: 3D view of fetal spine. One can assess multiple vertebral fusion (arrow), without any visible intervertebral space.

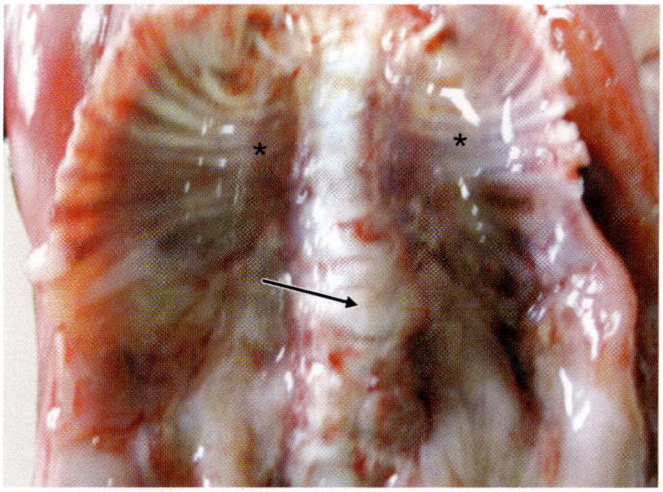

Fig. 138: Radial disposition of ribs (*) and protrusion of vertebral bodies (arrow).

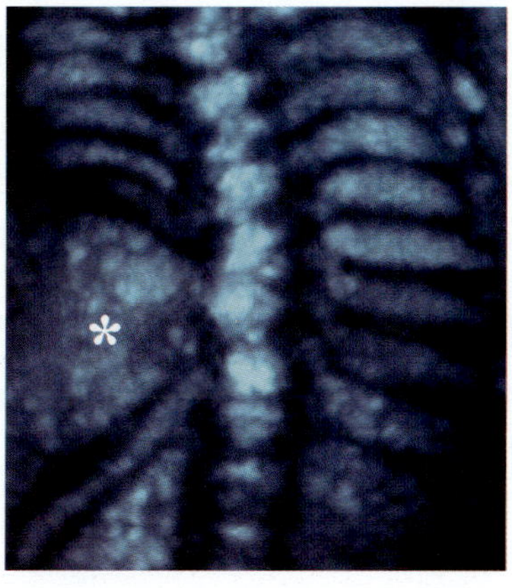

Fig. 139: 3D ultrasound of a fetal spine. There is a scoliosis due to the presence of multiple hemivertebrae associated with absence of some ribs (*).

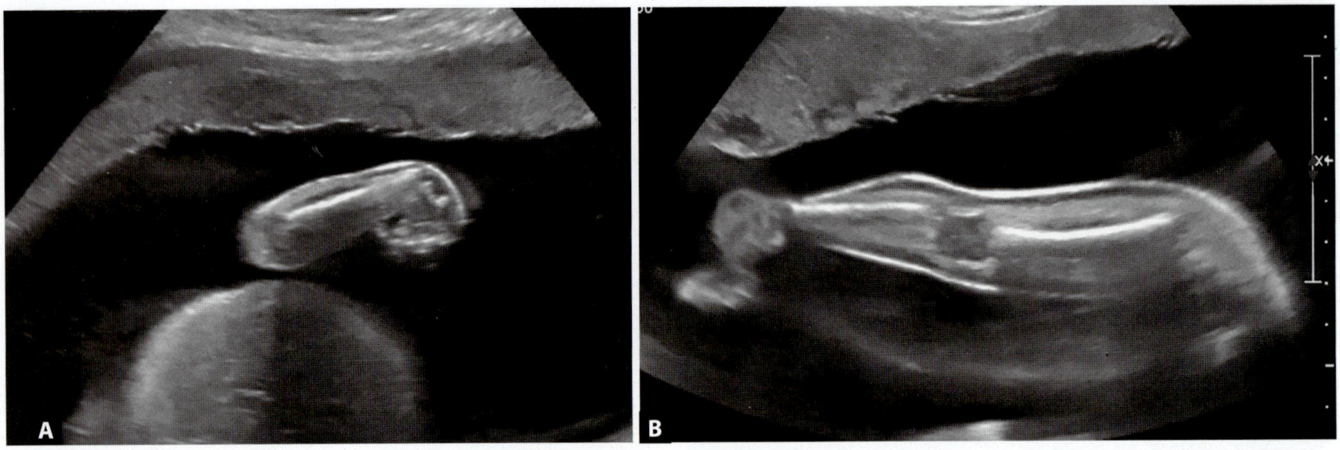

Figs. 140A and B: Fetus with fetal akinesia deformation syndrome (FADS). Rigid hyperextension lower limbs can be observed together with wrist contracture and polyhydramnios.

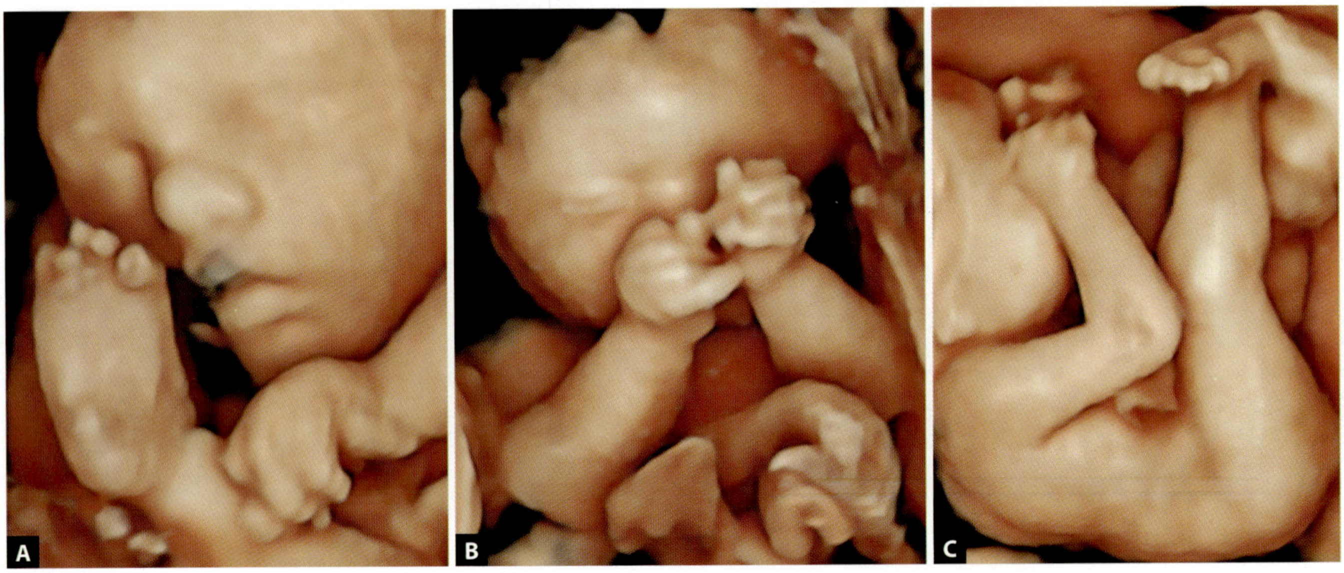

Figs. 141A to C: 3D images of fetuses with fetal akinesia deformation syndrome (FADS). Contractures in upper and lower limbs and fetal akinesia can be assessed.

to more than 400 entities with neurological, muscular, connective, skeletal, or mechanical origin. Typical features include bilateral feet malposition, heel, knee, and elbow deformities (in flexion or extension). The compromise is usually symmetric, sometimes progressive, affecting all the extremities. Sometimes, at the first trimester, a thick nuchal translucency can be observed. It may be found in association with polyhydramnios due to jaw contractures, thoracic hypoplasia, micrognathia, fetal growth restriction, palate disorders, and slightly shortened long bones (Pena-Shokeir phenotype). Some features may be present in other syndromes such as multiple lethal arthrogryposis and multiple pterygium **(Figs. 142 to 145)** syndrome. About 30% of cases are associated with genetic anomalies. Some infections and mechanical compression due to oligohydramnios are other possible origins.[21]

OTHER SKELETAL DEFECTS[13-15]

Patellar Anterior Luxation

Patellar anterior luxation is an anterior flexion of the knee joint. It is secondary to a patellar abnormality **(Figs. 146 to 148)**.

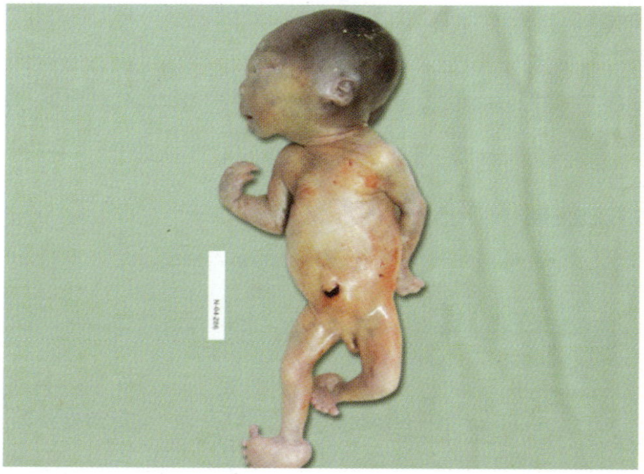

Fig. 142: Malpositioned fetal extremities with deformation and hyperflexion secondary to fetal akinesia.

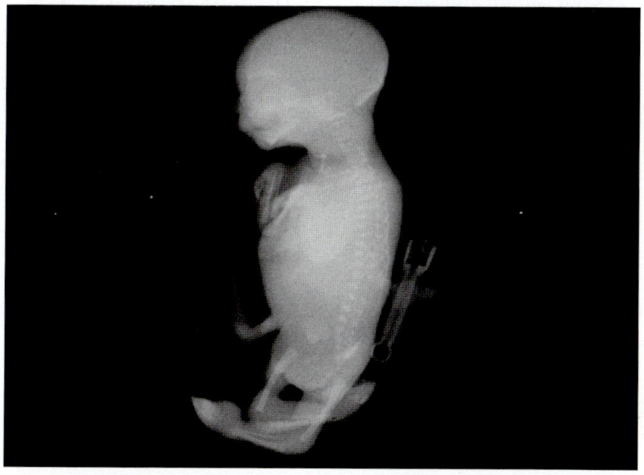

Fig. 143: Fetography of a fetus with fetal akinesia deformation sequence.

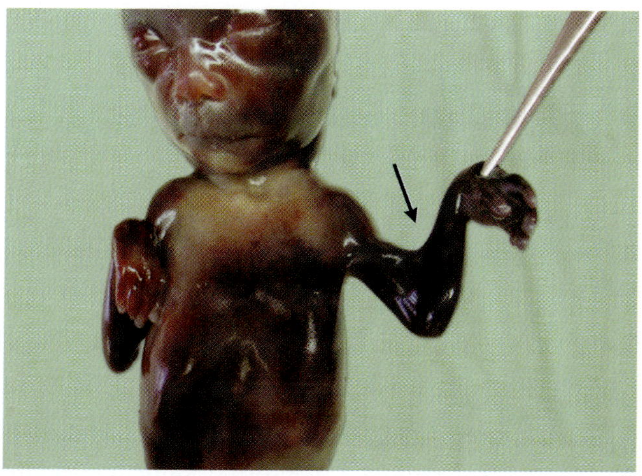

Fig. 144: Pterygium multiple. Cutaneous membrane joining the forearm and hand (arrow).

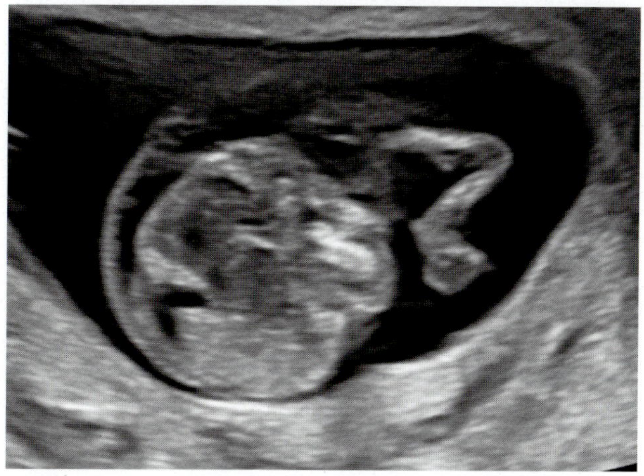

Fig. 145: Ultrasound image of pterygium multiple at 12 weeks of gestation. Increased nuchal translucency can be assessed.

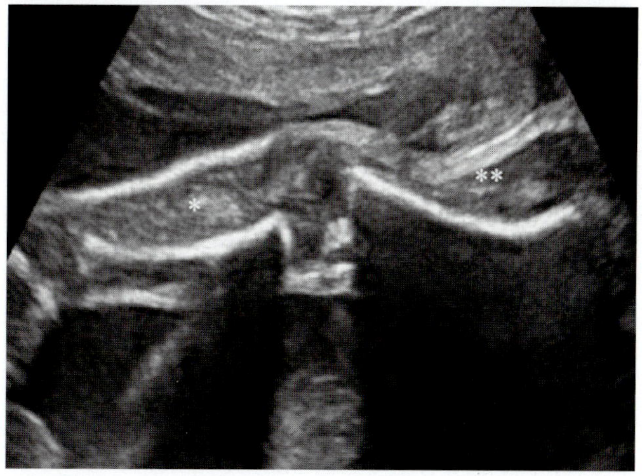

Fig. 146: Congenital patellar luxation. The middle portion of lower extremity is malpositioned (*) compared to the proximal portion of the extremity (**).

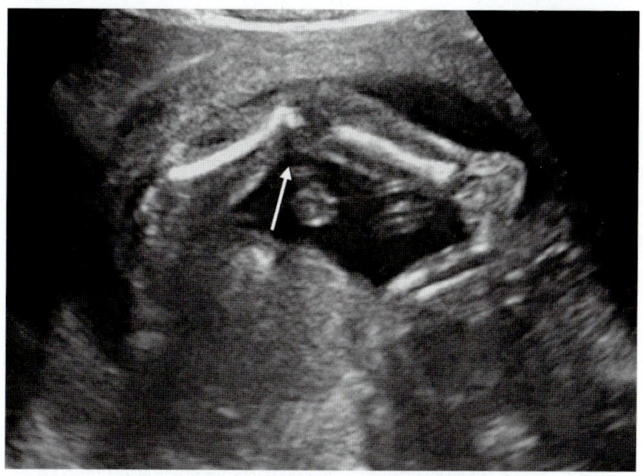

Fig. 147: Congenital patellar luxation. Anterior knee flexion (arrow) due to a patellar anomaly. Other fetal joints seem normal.

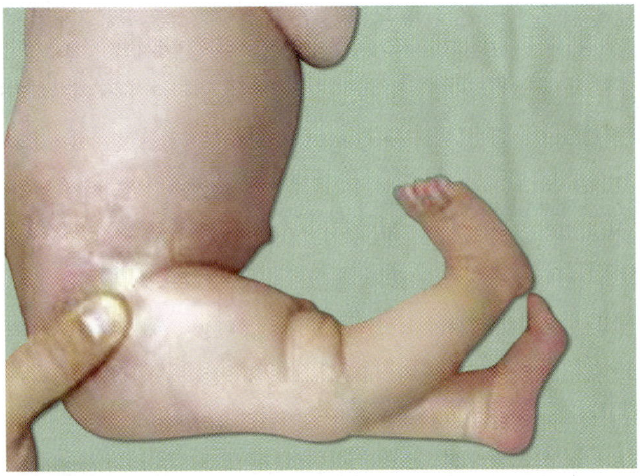

Fig. 148: Newborn demonstrating a congenital knee luxation.

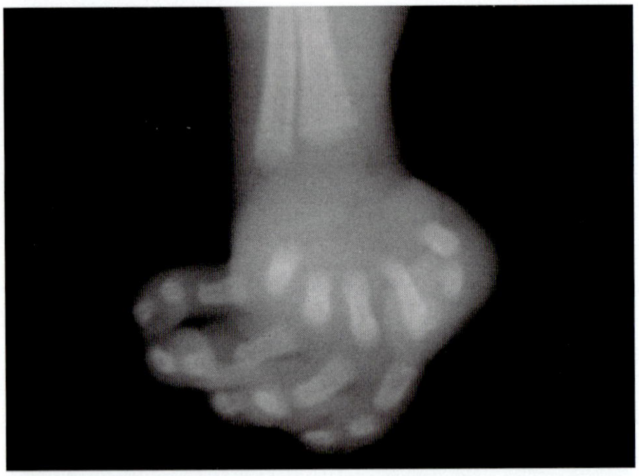

Fig. 149: Fetography showing malpositioned, disorganized phalanges due to cutaneous compression probably secondary to misoprostol use.

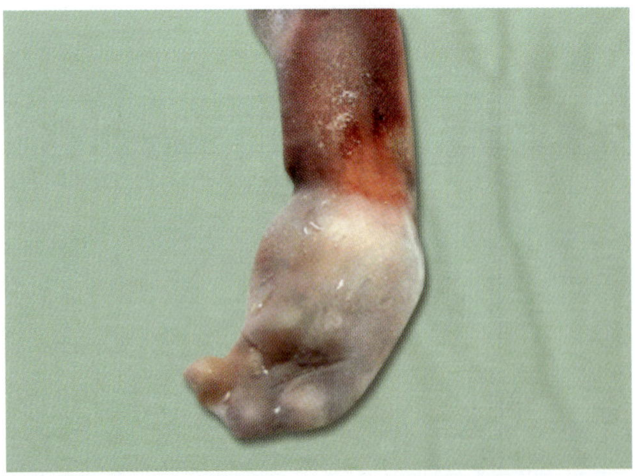

Fig. 150: Photograph of a dysmorphic hand. Digits are fused and disorganized. It may be associated with misoprostol use.

Teratogenic Effects: Misoprostol

The use of misoprostol in the first trimester of pregnancy has been associated with limb distal anomalies **(Figs. 149 and 150)**.

REFERENCES

1. Salomon LJ, Alfirevic Z, Berghella V, et al. ISUOG Practice Guidelines (updated): Performance of the routine mid-trimester fetal ultrasound scan. Ultrasound Obstet Gynecol. 2022;59(6):840-56.
2. Ruano R, Molho M, Roume J, et al. Prenatal diagnosis of fetal skeletal dysplasias by combining two-dimensional and three-dimensional ultrasound and intrauterine three-dimensional helical computer tomography. Ultrasound Obstet Gynecol. 2004;24(2):134-40.
3. Khalil A, Pajkrt E, Chitty LS. Early prenatal diagnosis of skeletal anomalies. Prenat Diagn. 2011;31(1):115-24.
4. Unger S, Ferreira CR, Mortier GR, et al. Nosology of genetic skeletal disorders: 2023 revision. Am J Med Genet A. 2023;191(5):1164-209.
5. Kos M, Hafner T, Funduk-Kurjak B, et al. Limb deformities and three-dimensional ultrasound. J Perinat Med. 2002;30(1):40-7.
6. Krakow D. Skeletal dysplasias. Clinical Perinatol. 2015;42:301-19.
7. Schramm T, Gloning KP, Minderer S, et al. Prenatal sonographic diagnosis of skeletal dysplasias. Ultrasound Obstet Gynecol. 2009;34(2):160-70.
8. Lord J, McMullan DJ, Eberhardt RY, et al. Prenatal exome sequencing analysis in fetal structural anomalies detected by ultrasonography (PAGE): Cohort study. Lancet. 2019;393(10173):747-57.
9. Milks KS, Hill LM, Hosseinzadeh K. Evaluating skeletal dysplasias on prenatal ultrasound: An emphasis on predicting lethality. Pediatr Radiol. 2017;47(2):134-45.
10. Yeh P, Saeed F, Paramasivam G, et al. Accuracy of prenatal diagnosis and prediction of lethality for fetal skeletal dysplasias. Prenal Diagn. 2011;31(5):515-8.
11. Cassart M. Suspected fetal skeletal malformations or bone diseases: How to explore. Pediatr Radiol. 2010;40:1046-51.
12. Carreras E, Toran N (Eds). Atlas de Malformaciones Fetales Congénitas. S.A: Ediciones Mayo; 2000.
13. Lowry RB, Bedard T. Congenital limb deficiency classification and nomenclature: The need for consensus. Am J Med Genet A. 2016;170(6):1400-4.
14. Vij N, Goncalves LF, Llanes A, et al. Prenatal radiographic evaluation of congenital transverse limb deficiencies: a scoping review. World J Orthop. 2023;14(3):155-65.
15. Rosano A, Botto LD, Olney RS, et al. Limb defects associated with major congenital anomalies: clinical and epidemiological study from the International

Clearinghouse for birth defects monitoring systems. Am J Med Genet. 2000;93(2):110-6.

16. López-Muñoz E, Becerra-Solano LE. An update on amniotic bands sequence. Arch Argent Pediatr. 2018;116(3):e409-e420.
17. Sowinska-Seidler A, Socha M, Jamsheer A. Split-hand/foot malformation - molecular cause and implications in genetic counseling. J Appl Genet. 2014;55(1):105-15.
18. Rypens F, Dubois J, Garel L, et al. Obstetric US: Watch the fetal hands. Radiographics. 2006;26:811-32.
19. Werler MM, Yazdy MM, Mitchell AA, et al. Descriptive epidemiology of idiopathic clubfoot. Am J Med Genet A. 2013;161A(7):1569-78.
20. Di Mascio D, Buca D, Khalil A, et al. Outcomes of isolated fetal talipes: A systematic review and meta-analysis. Acta Obstet Gyneocol Scand. 2019;98(11):1367-77.
21. Rac MWF, McKinney J, Gandhi M; Society for Maternal-Fetal Medicine. Arthrogryposis. Am J Obstet Gynecol. 2019;221(6):B7-9.

27

CHAPTER

Sonographic Assessment of the Umbilical Cord

Edoardo Di Naro, Luigi Raio, Antonella Cromi, Alessandra Giocolano

INTRODUCTION

For several decades, the morphological and morphometric aspects of the umbilical cord have been studied and retrospectively correlated with the perinatal outcome by pathologists after delivery. The advent of ultrasound has increased our knowledge and added a dynamic form of information in particular on the development of the fetus and its supporting structures such as the placenta and the umbilical cord. However, at the beginning, the umbilical cord has received only little interest mainly due to the limited resolution of the initial ultrasound machines. Indeed, the prenatal sonographic morphologic investigation of the umbilical cord has for long time been limited to the assessment of the number of vessels and later to the evaluation of the impedance to blood flow by Doppler waveform analysis.

However, an increasing body of clinical and experimental evidences show that both prenatal morphology and morphometry of the umbilical cord and its vessels may help in understanding the physiology of development as well as adaptive processes of the fetoplacental unit to pathologic insults. Moreover, studying the umbilical cord may in some circumstances help in the prediction of adverse pregnancy outcome. In the last decade, a considerable amount of scientific work has been published on this topic. We have learned that the umbilical cord is not an inert structure which is suspended between the fetus and placenta but is actively involved in important processes such as fetal growth restriction, preeclampsia, diabetes, stillbirth and chromosomal defect or genetic syndromes.[1-5] The aim of this chapter is to evaluate the role of the sonographic assessment of the umbilical cord during fetal life.

MORPHOLOGY

A normal umbilical cord at term is about 50–60 cm long and its surface is covered by a single layer of amniotic epithelium. The ground substance, in which three vessels—two arteries and one vein—are embedded, is called Wharton's jelly. The characteristic structure of the umbilical cord is determined by the helical course of the arteries around the vein. Between the fetal umbilical ring and the placental insertion, the vessels fulfill usually 10–11 coils. This structure is very dynamic, as its morphology is influenced by a number of factors including gestational age, amount of amniotic fluid and its composition, fetoplacental hemodynamics as well as maternal complications during pregnancy. The evaluation of the umbilical cord can be accomplished either from the long-axis view or from a cross-sectional view. Probably the latter method is more appropriate because it allows quantification not only of the umbilical vessels' size but also of the amount of the Wharton's jelly.

What can be observed in an umbilical cord? How can we read each sign?

Basically, the morphology and morphometry of the umbilical cord is influenced by external factors and/or by factors which are inherent to the cord itself. Nomograms for the diameter of the umbilical vessels have been reported by Weissman and Raio,[6,7] showing that the diameter of the umbilical arteries increases from 1.2 ± 0.4 mm at 16 weeks to 4.2 ± 0.4 mm at term of gestation and the umbilical vein diameter varies from 2.0 ± 0.6 mm at 16 weeks of gestation to 8.2 ± 0.8 mm at the term of gestation. These nomograms have showed that the diameter increases as a function of gestational age, progressively up to 32 weeks of gestation followed then by a plateau towards the end of the pregnancy due to a reduction of water content of the Wharton's jelly. Moreover, a significant relationship between umbilical cord diameter and cross-sectional area and fetal anthropometric parameters (biparietal diameter, femur length, abdominal circumference) has been described. Experimental and clinical evidence suggest that

Wharton's jelly plays a metabolically active role throughout pregnancy; Vizza et al.[8] reported that the collagen fibrillar network of the Wharton's jelly, studied by scanning electron microscopy, shows the presence of a wide system of interconnected cavities consisting of canalicular-like structures as well as cavernous and perivascular spaces. Considering that the Wharton's jelly lack of a proper vasculature, this system of cavities may have an important role facilitating a bidirectional transfer of water and metabolites between amniotic fluid and umbilical cord vessels through the Wharton's jelly. Moreover, Wharton's jelly cushions umbilical blood vessels, preventing disruption of flow due to compression or bending caused by fetal movements and uterine contraction, i.e. at delivery. Modifications in the amount and composition of Wharton's jelly of three-vessel cords have been described in a number of pathological conditions, usually associated with a modification of the amniotic fluid volume and composition, occurring in pregnancy (i.e. hypertensive disorders, gestational diabetes). The reduction of the amount of Wharton's jelly may be the consequence of either an extracellular dehydration or a reduction in extracellular matrix component.

The sonographic cross-sectional area of Wharton's jelly can be computed by subtracting the vessels area from the cross-sectional area of umbilical cord. The umbilical vein and arteries areas are to be computed at the maximal magnification using the software of the ultrasound machine. A reference range for the total vascular area has been generated by Weissman and colleagues.[6]

The umbilical cord can be defined as:

- LEAN, if it's sonographic cross-sectional area is below the 10th percentile for gestational age **(Fig. 1)**, and
- LARGE if it's sonographic cross-sectional area is above the 90th percentile for gestational age.

"LEAN" UMBILICAL CORD

Just over 40 years ago, observing two cases of macroscopically thin umbilical cord (UC) associated with stillbirth and fetal distress, Hall stated that "*The thin cord is a dangerous cord, and a fat cord is a safe cord, all other factors being equal*".[9]

Pathologic studies and case reports demonstrated that a lean umbilical cord is associated with adverse pregnancy outcome, oligohydramnios and fetal distress.[10,11] Raio et al. found an association between the presence of a "lean" umbilical cord and the delivery of a small-for-gestational-age infant. Patients with a "lean" UC after 20 weeks of gestation had a 4.4-fold higher risk (95% confidence interval, 2.16–8.85) of having an SGA infant than those with a normal umbilical cord. Wharton's jelly appears to serve the function of adventitia, which the UC lacks, binding and encasing the umbilical vessels. It has been speculated that the cells of Wharton's jelly appear to possess contractility comparable to that of smooth muscle cells and participate in the regulation of umbilical blood flow and that, at least in some cases, the reduction in fetal growth could be the consequence of Wharton's jelly decrease leading to hypoplasia of the umbilical vessels. In fact, a reduction of wall thickness of umbilical cord arteries and vein has been found in intrauterine growth retardation (IUGR) infants with abnormal umbilical artery flow when compared to IUGR infants without increased umbilical artery resistance. Cumulative evidence suggests that an umbilical cord less than 10th centile for gestational age is a simple and early marker SGA infant and the occurrence of intrapartum complication.[11-14] Moreover, a lean UC is frequently associated with signs of fetal distress at the time of delivery (oligohydramnios, low Apgar score and meconium-stained amniotic fluid).

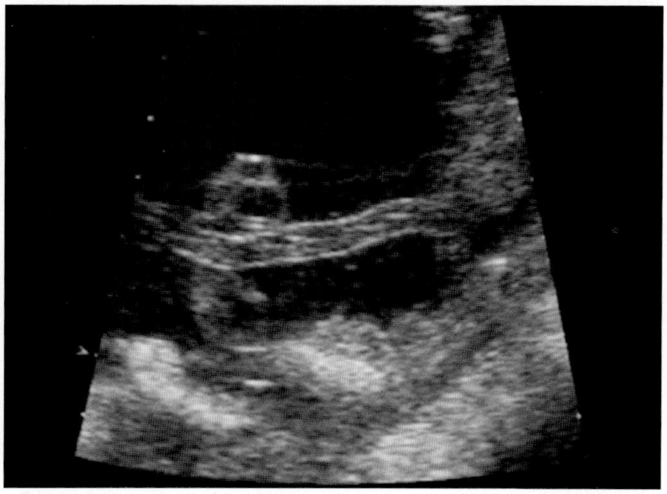

Fig. 1: Lean cord.

LARGE UMBILICAL CORD

Several reports in the literature have described a large UC associated with other fetal structural anomalies such as umbilical cord tumor, urachal cysts, umbilical cord mucoid degeneration and omphalomesenteric cyst.[15-17] Generally, in these conditions, the morphology is altered in a limited portion of the umbilical cord **(Figs. 2A and B)**.

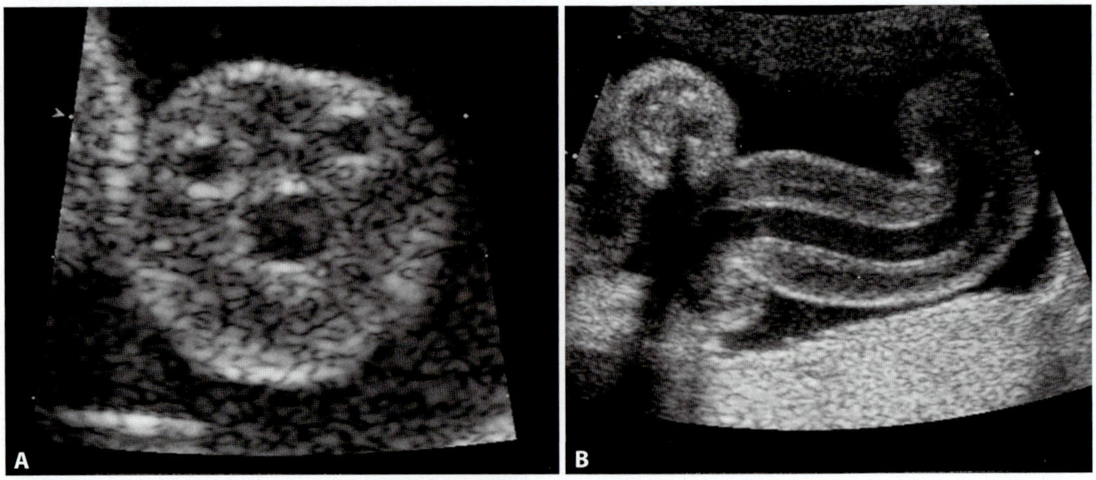

Figs. 2A and B: Giant umbilical cord.

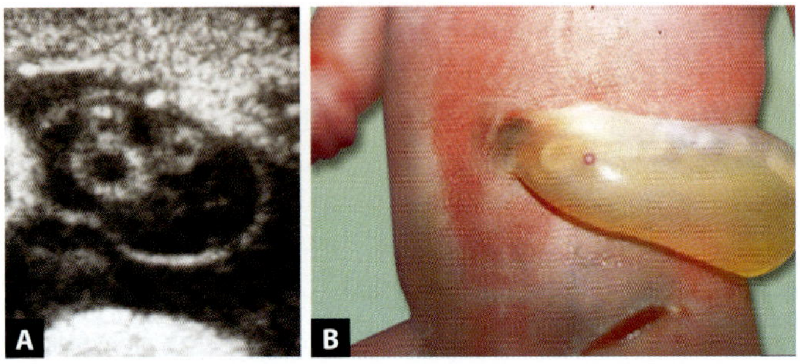

Figs. 3A and B: Hydropic Wharton's jelly in a syndromic fetus.

However, a consistent association between an ultrasonographic large UC and the presence of a gestational diabetes mellitus has been reported. A large UC can be considered as an additional parameter useful to identify fetuses of a mother with some kind of glucose intolerance during pregnancy. Fetuses of patients with gestational diabetes have a larger UC and this is mainly due to a higher content of Wharton's jelly. Weissman and Jakobi found an alteration in the distribution of Wharton's jelly fibers with large empty spaces among them and speculated that this could be caused by an abnormal accumulation of fluid and plasma proteins within the Wharton's jelly, resulting in an increased surface area and in an increased permeability and hemorrhages due to an increased oncotic pressure in the interstitial spaces of the Wharton's jelly[18,19] **(Figs. 3A and B)**. This modification can be observed at 24 gestational weeks, suggesting that the involvement of the umbilical cord in fetuses of diabetic mothers is a phenomenon that occurs early in pregnancy.

In addition, it has been shown that sonographic assessment of umbilical cord area may improve the prediction of fetal macrosomia; although ultrasound remains imprecise in the recognition of fetal macrosomia, obstetrician should not shun the use of biometric methodology to assist in the management of suspected macrosomia, but rather should look forward to further improvements that will enhance its accuracy as a diagnostic tool. Umbilical cord area is an easily obtained sonographic measurement, with highly reliable intraobserver and interobserver reproducibility. The time required to obtain an adequate and satisfactory image of cross-section of UC is about 2 minutes. A large cross-sectional area of the UC performs poorly by itself as a predictor of fetal macrosomia. A sonographic large UC can be used in addition to estimated fetal weight (EFW) as a further marker that may facilitate the detection of fetal overgrowth, potentially improving the performance of ultrasound-based policies for the management of suspected macrosomia.[5]

DISCORDANT UMBILICAL ARTERY

Discordance between the umbilical arteries is considered to be present when the difference between the diameter of the two arteries is at least 1 mm in three different portions of the UC in both transverse and longitudinal section[20,21] **(Figs. 4A to D)**.

Moreover, these arteries are also characterized by differences in the impedance to blood flow measured by Doppler flow methods with usually a higher resistance index measured in the smaller artery.[21]

Therefore, the information provided by Doppler velocimetry of the smaller umbilical artery should be taken with caution, because the significance of high-resistance patterns observed in other populations seems to represent a more benign condition in patients with discordant umbilical arteries. Therefore, from a clinical point of view, the presence of discordant umbilical artery seems to be a benign condition that does not affect the development of the fetus.

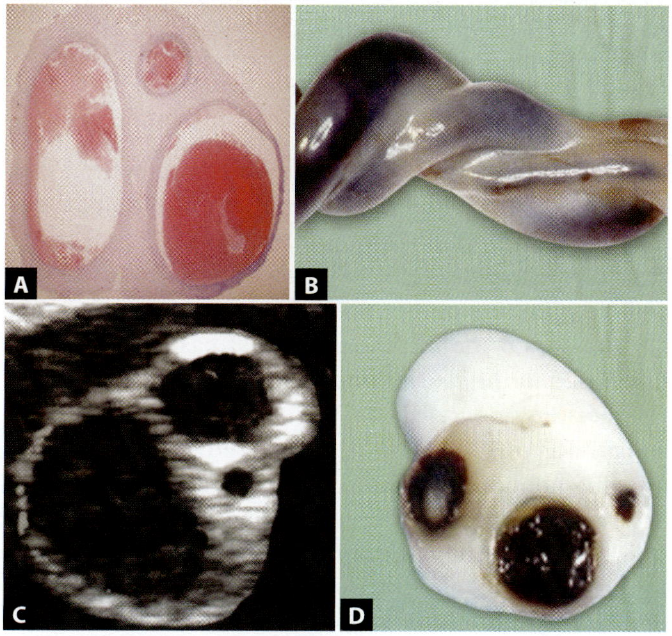

Figs. 4A to D: Discordant umbilical arteries.

However, cases with discordant arteries are associated with a higher incidence of morphologic placental alterations (placenta bipartite, placenta succenturiata, absence of Hyrtl anastomosis) and anomalous placental insertion (marginal, velamentous). These placental anomalies are similar to those frequently seen in cases of single umbilical artery (SUA) supporting the theory that the presence of a single artery represents the greatest expression of umbilical artery discordance.[22,23] The presence of the Hyrtl anastomosis is a common feature of the vascular system in the human placenta, present in at least 95% of all placentae. This anastomosis is the only vessel that connects the umbilical arteries or their branches on the placental surface, close to the site of cord insertion, playing an active role in equalizing the blood pressure between the territories supplied by each umbilical artery; in fact, although the areas supplied by each of the umbilical arteries may show great discrepancy, the corresponding UC arteries are usually of equal caliber **(Fig. 5)**. This equalizing effect might be of utmost importance in particular during uterine contractions when the blood pressure and resistance in the corresponding portion of the intervillous space and cotyledons may differ in different part of the placenta **(Figs. 6 and 7)**.

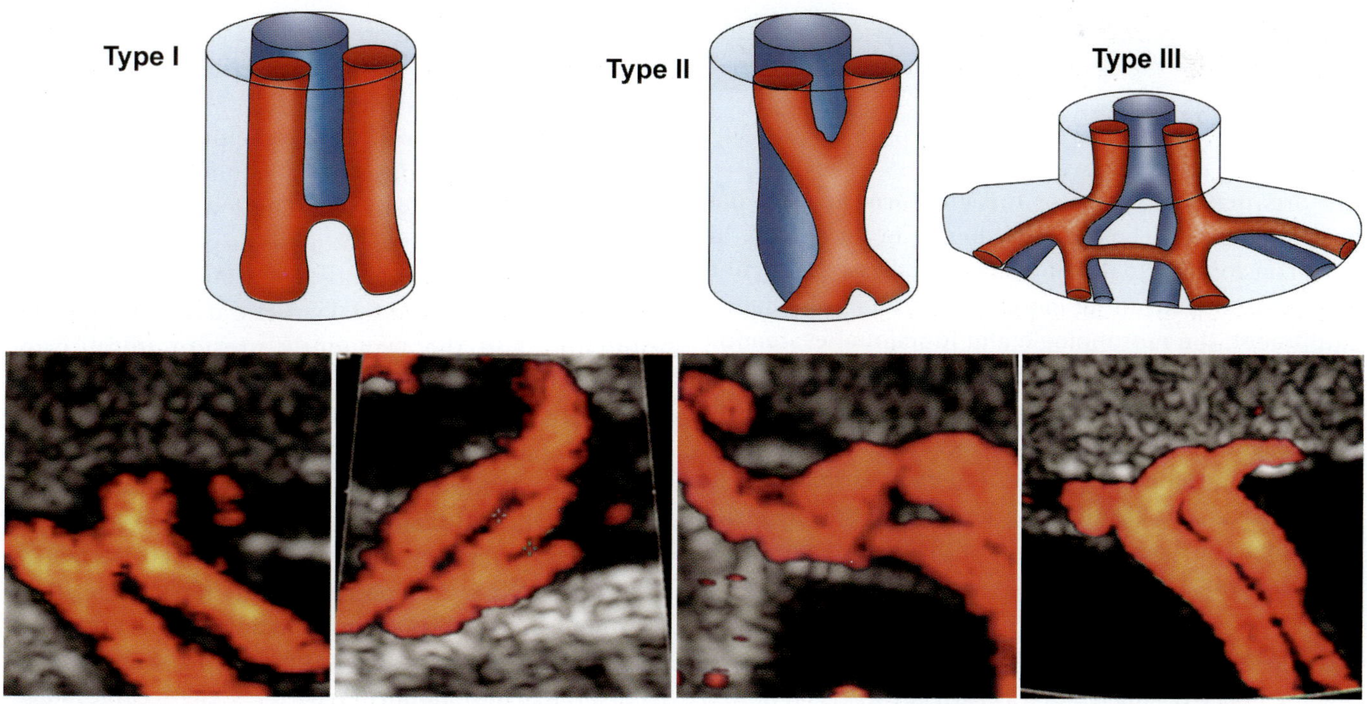

Fig. 5: Doppler ultrasound demonstration of Hyrtl anastomosis.

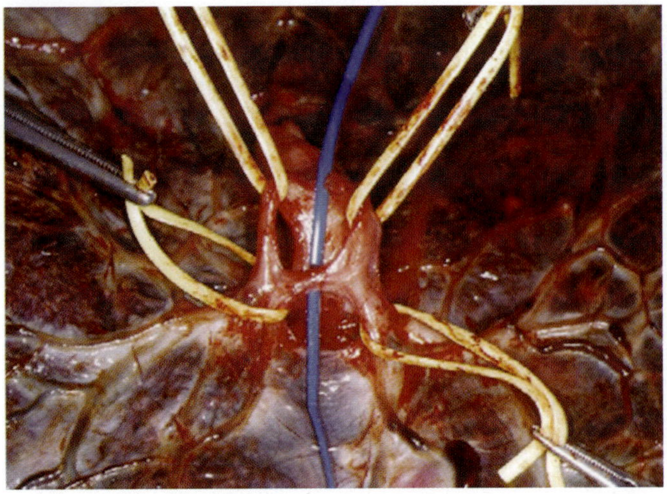

Fig. 6: Hyrtl anastomosis.

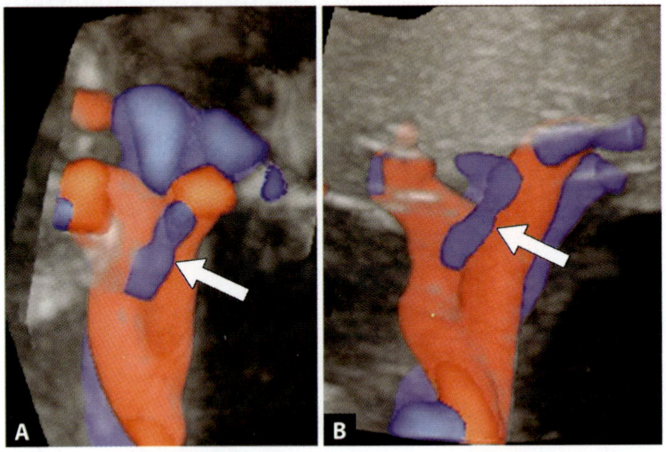

Figs. 7A and B: 3D view of Hyrtl anastomosis.

Discordance in calibers of the umbilical arteries has been postulated to be the consequence of a failure of the Hyrtl anastomosis to develop anatomically or to function fully. With the advent of more sophisticated ultrasound equipment, the morphologic and functional evaluation of this vessel has now become possible. The absence of a Hyrtl anastomosis has recently been associated with the presence of discordant umbilical arteries; similarly, abnormal umbilical cord insertion such as marginal or velamentous cord insertion has also been associated with a missing Hyrtl anastomosis and discordant umbilical cord arteries.[24,25]

SINGLE UMBILICAL ARTERY

The incidence of single umbilical artery (SUA) is reported to be 0.5–2.5% in uncomplicated neonates, but is higher in aborted (1.5–7%) and aneuploid fetuses (9–11%). Multiple gestations have a three to seven-fold increased risk of SUA. Fetuses whose umbilical cord has a single artery are at increased risk of intrauterine and intrapartum death, regardless of the presence or not of congenital or chromosomal malformations. Most cases of SUA are diagnosed in the late second trimester **(Figs. 8A and B)**. Despite the apparently easy recognition of SUA, a low sensitivity of ultrasound is reported. Color Doppler imaging allows earlier and more confident diagnosis of SUA, but its apparent efficacy has to be proven. The patent artery is usually larger than normal and it may approximate to the vein diameter. It has been estimated that the risk of anomalies is seven times greater than in infant with three-vessels cord. The list of anomalies identified to be associated with SUA is long. Persutte and Hobbins[22] divided the reported abnormalities into three groups:

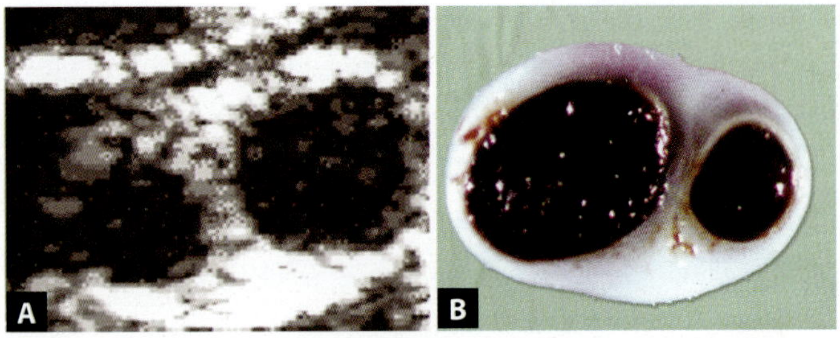

Figs. 8A and B: Single umbilical arteries

1. To be identified with prenatal ultrasonography
2. To be difficult to be identified prenatally
3. To be unidentifiable prenatally.

Using these criteria, they conclude that prenatal ultrasonography can consistently identify only 37% of fetal anomalies associated with SUA. This low accuracy should well be kept in mind when counseling a patient with a fetus affected by SUA. The prognosis of SUA infants is mainly related to be associated fetal structural or chromosomal anomalies and the frequently present intrauterine growth retardation. The lower amount of Wharton's jelly present in two-vessels cord could be responsible of a higher vulnerability of the UC during the third trimester of pregnancy and during labor. The elevated incidence of stillbirth at the end of pregnancy in patients with a SUA may be in part explained by the cumulative effect of the relative Wharton's jelly reduction that occurs physiologically in the third trimester of pregnancy, acting on a constitutional deficiency of jelly in umbilical cord with a single artery.[26] It is likely that the amount of Wharton's jelly at earlier stages of pregnancy exerts a sufficient protection to the vessels

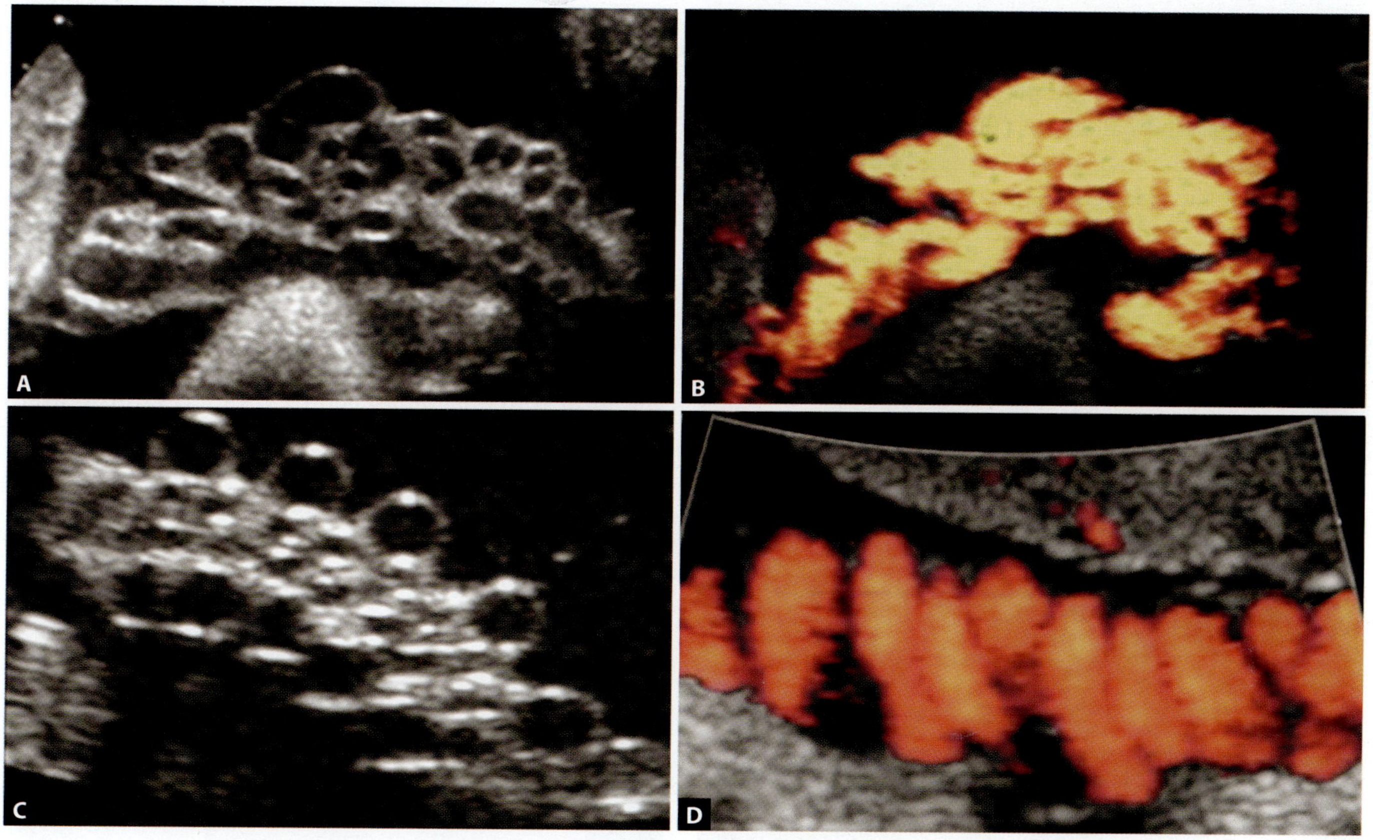

Figs. 9A to D: Atypical coiling. (A and B) Uncoordinated coiling; (C and D) Supercoiling.

without affecting blood flow and therefore fetal growth. The SUA fetuses have a lack of the safety warranted by the presence of Hyrtl's anastomosis, a safety valve and this fact partially explains the increased rate of unexplained intrauterine fetal demise in the third trimester of gestation and during labor.

UMBILICAL CORD ANGIOARCHITECTURE

Although, the origin and significance of the umbilical cord angioarchitecure has been the subject of extensive research, the developmental process and functional importance of this vascular coiling are not fully understood.

Regardless of its origin, data from both pathologic and ultrasonographic investigations suggest that umbilical coiling is well-established as early as 8 weeks of gestation, and the total number of coils at the end of the first trimester is similar to that observed in fully term cords. Moreover, the direction of twist is not randomly determined, since several investigators have found a clear prevalence of left-twisted umbilical cords.

Color flow mapping could be used to enhance the definition of the umbilical cord vascular architecture. The sonographic assessment of the coiling pattern is performed in different UC segments in order to exclude segmental morphologic anomalies (i.e. false knots, varices). The length of one complete umbilical vascular coil (distance between the right outer surface of consecutive arterial coils) is measured in a longitudinal midsection of the UC and a mean of three measurements is used for analysis. The sonographic umbilical coiling index (UCI) is defined as the reciprocal value of that measurement and it represents the number of vascular coils in a given cord. According to the umbilical coiling pattern the UC can be classified as:

- Normal
- Uncoiled (two straight umbilical arteries with an umbilical coiling angle equal to zero)
- Hypocoiled, if the UCI is below the 10th percentile for gestational age
- Hypercoiled, if the UCI is above the 90th percentile for gestational age
- Atypical Coiling (**Figs. 9A to D**):
    - *Uncoordinated coiling or bizarre, or aperiodic coiling pattern*, if there is an atypical coiling, in

which the absence of a repetitive pattern doesn't allow the measurement of the UCI
- *Supercoiling*, in the presence of a spring spatial configuration of the UC **(Figs. 10 to 12)**.

The only reference in the pathologic literature on anomalous helical patterns dates back to Hyrtl and Malpas and Symonds,[27,28] which described in their postnatal series some "complicated" cords with different directions of twists, occurring in different segments or a combination of coiled and uncoiled portions.

Compelling evidence has demonstrated a correlation between abnormal umbilical coiling pattern and suboptimal pregnancy outcome in singleton pregnancy. The mechanisms leading to the coiling of the UC are largely unknown and whether it represents a genetically determined or an acquired phenomenon is still the subject of debate. Since the etiology of the vascular coil in normal UC is still an enigma, it is even more intriguing to find a plausible pathophysiologic explanation for an abnormal umbilical cord angioarchitecture. A variety of hypotheses have been advanced to explain the origin of umbilical vascular coiling, including fetal movements,[29] unequal umbilical vascular growth rate (Roach), fetal hemodynamic forces, umbilical vascular wall mechanism and genetics factors. Since, the helical course of umbilical vessels is

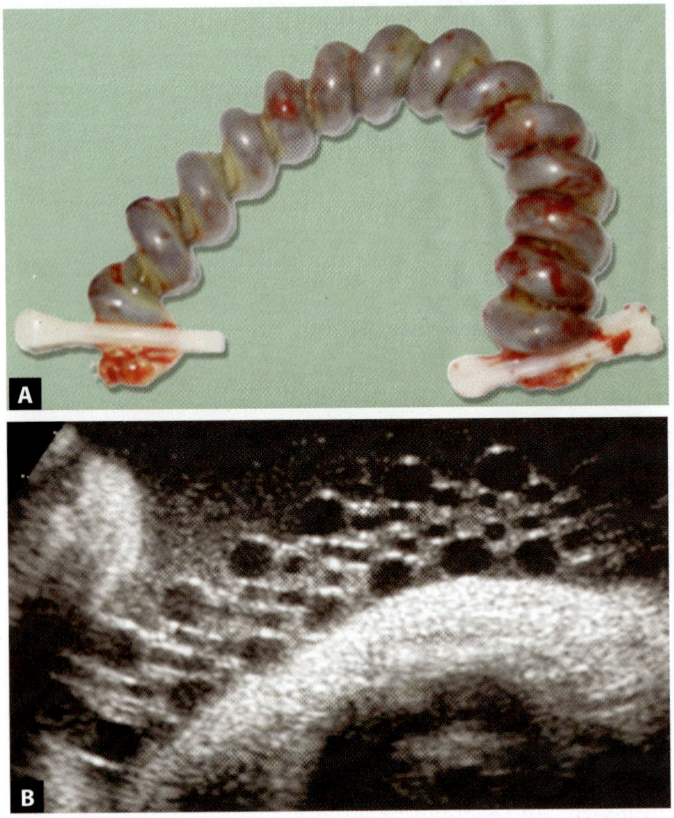

Figs. 10A and B: Supercoiling postnatal vs. ultrasound aspect.

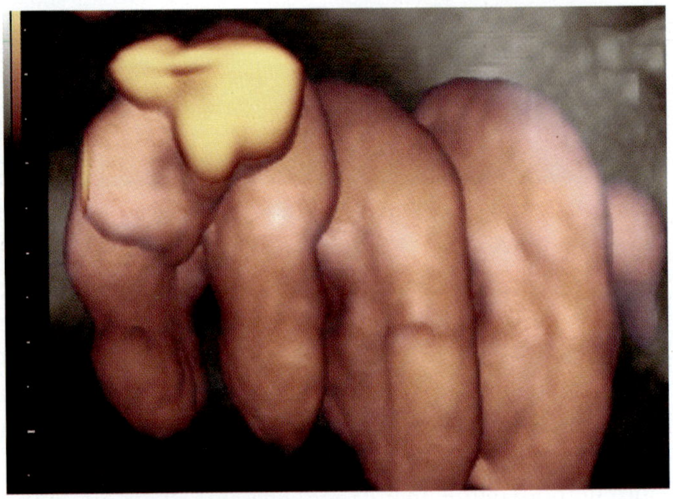

Fig. 11: Supercoiling cord 3D power flow view.

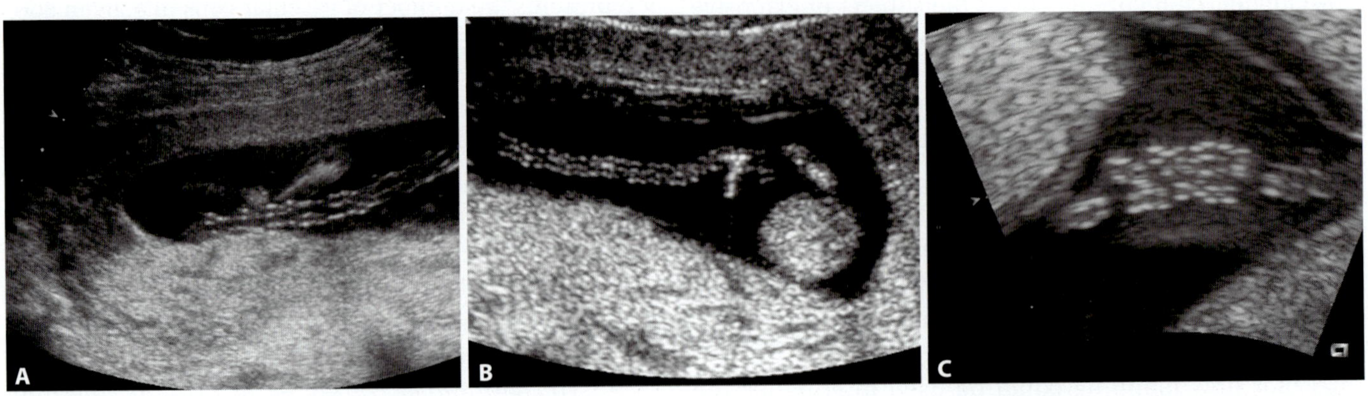

Figs. 12A to C: First trimester (A) normal; (B) hypercoiled and (C) supercoiled cord.

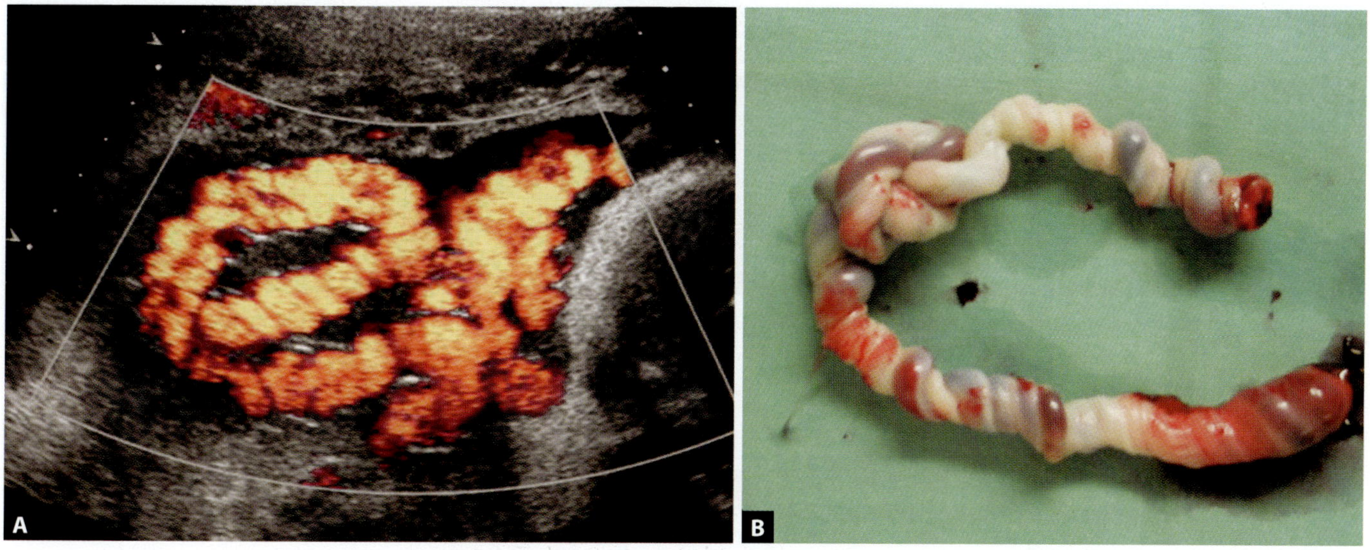

Figs. 13A and B: Hypercoiling in SUA with UC knot.

established by 9 weeks of gestation, a hemodynamic imbalance leading to unequal cord morphology is supposed to occur very early in gestation. As this typical repetitive vascular pattern of the umbilical cord is fully established at the end of the first trimester, uncoordinated coiling may be the result of an abnormal coiling process, which takes place during early pregnancy **(Figs. 13A and B)**. It has been postulated that coiling is determined by an interaction between the intrinsic properties of the fibers in the umbilical cord vessels wall and hemodynamic forces acting on it during development.

Data from clinical and experimental studies show that the umbilical cord is a dynamic structure where both hemodynamic factors and gestational age influence the vascular umbilical cord pattern.[30-32] Before the fetal kidneys start the excretion of significant amount of urine, fetal membranes are involved in fetal fluid accumulation and regulation by transmembranous mechanism.[33] In early gestation, the fluid exchange between umbilical vessels and amniotic fluid is facilitated by the limited amount of Wharton's jelly wrapped around the umbilical cord vessels.

Reynolds et al. postulated that the UC is a pistonless pulsometer pumping system acting as a cardiac assist pump to sustain the venous return from the placenta.[34] The fetal blood flows through the umbilical vein pumped by slight but definite decreases and increases in venous pressure that are generated from the force of the rising limb of the arterial pressure pulse. The presence of arterial coils that surround the vein along the length of the cord provide multiple variations in an additive fashion; the presence of vascular coils plays a central role in determining the blood flow from the placenta to the fetus. This mechanism is of utmost importance in early gestation when the placental resistance to blood flow is particularly elevated. Therefore, a reduced number of coils in lean umbilical cords could be responsible for a reduced umbilical blood flow which in turn leads to a fetal growth impairment.

Reynolds' hypothesis, according to which the umbilical coils serve as a peristaltic pump mechanism enhancing the venous return to the fetus, has been advocated by several authors to explain how an abnormal coiling could influence the perinatal outcome.

Alterations in morphology and ultrastructure of UC components have been described in pregnancy complications that affect fetoplacental hemodynamics **(Figs. 14A to D)**. In particular, a high frequency of uncoiled and hypocoiled cords has been reported in intrauterine growth restriction and maternal hypertensive disorders. According to Poiseuille's law, the three factors that might influence blood flow are the caliber of the vessel, the blood flow velocity and the viscosity of the blood. Di Naro stated that the vein blood flow is lower in fetuses with an umbilical cord cross-sectional area below the 10th centile than in those with an umbilical cord of normal caliber and the risk to have an IUGR is very high. The alterations of vein blood flow can be detected earlier than arteries. The umbilical vein area and the umbilical vein blood

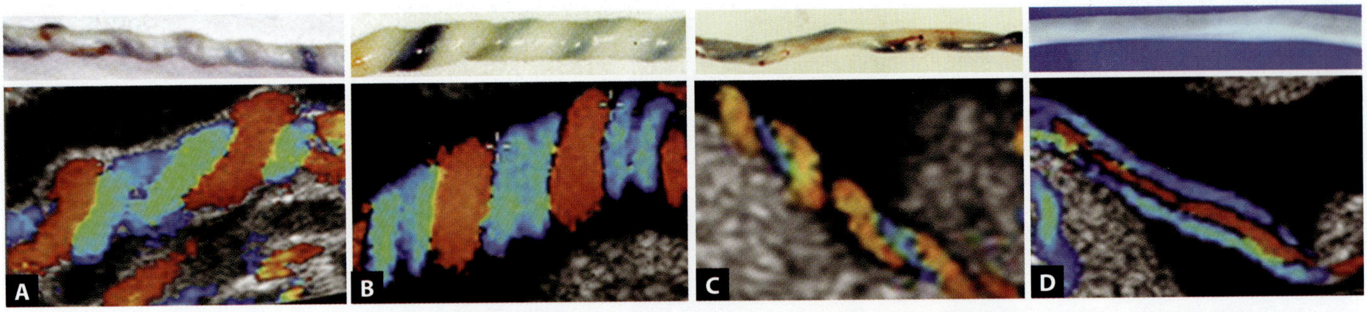

Figs. 14A to D: Adverse perinatal outcome and coiling. (A) Normal cord; (B) Hypercoiling; (C) Hypocoiling; (D) Uncoiled cord.

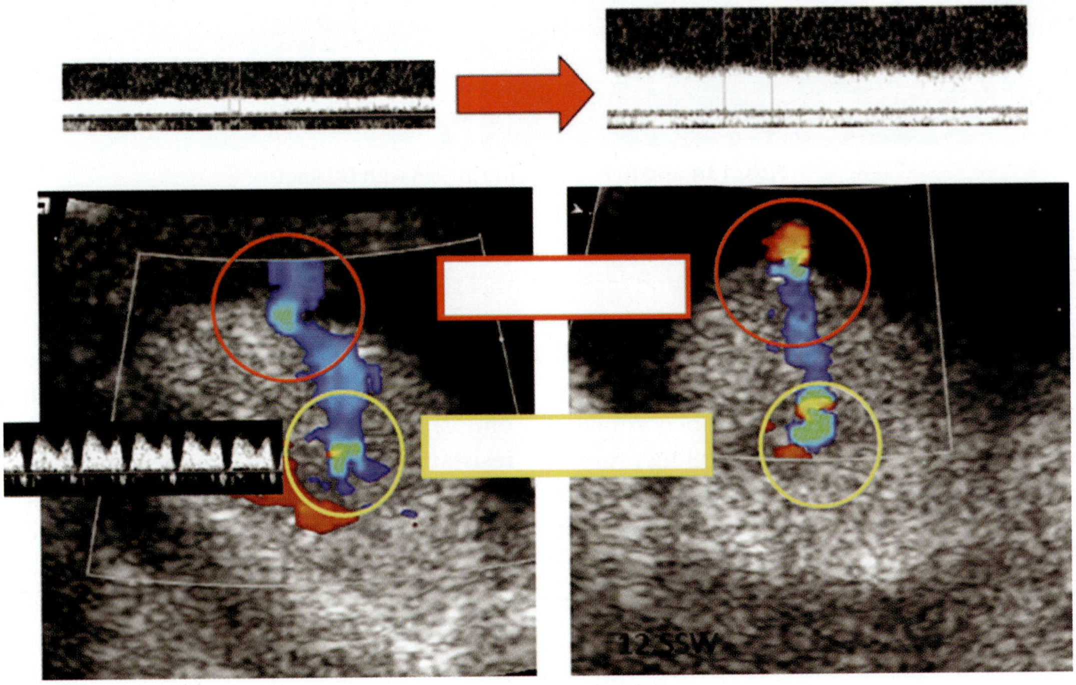

Fig. 15: Umbilical ring.

flow are significantly reduced in growth restricted fetuses compared to normally grown fetuses.[35] The discrepancy in the umbilical vein size might represent an adaptive response to venous overload on the one hand and chronic hypovolemia on the other hand.[36] Supercoiling can be associated with pathologic fetal intra-abdominal process and may be explained by a relative increase in resistance at the level of the umbilical ring, which in turn induces a venous congestion of the extra-abdominal umbilical vein **(Fig. 15).** Kilavuz and Skulstad[37,38] were able to show that blood velocity in the umbilical vein at the abdominal wall is higher than that in the extra-abdominal portion of the umbilical cord and that this increase in velocity is due to a progressive tightening of the fetal umbilical ring starting after that the physiologic midgut herniation is completed at 12 weeks of gestation.

Thereafter, umbilical vein constriction is a common finding and does not change during the second half of gestation. As Skulstad stated, the exact role of the fetal umbilical ring remains to be elucidated, and whether extreme degrees of constriction could affect placental circulation and are associated with any type of pregnancy complication is unknown.

UMBILICAL CORD AND ANEUPLOIDIES

A number of studies have reported a higher incidence of umbilical cords with decreased coiling index or even absence of coils in fetuses with aneuploidy.[39-41] The UC extracellular matrix is a tissue composed by a high amount of glycosaminoglycans. The Wharton's jelly is composed of an insoluble fibrillar network of different collagen types within which soluble open-coil polysaccharides are held. Hyaluronan, the most represented glycosaminoglycan in the Wharton's Jelly, is known to influence cell behavior and to play a crucial role in angiogenesis, morphogenesis and tissue remodeling especially during embryogenesis. Hyaluronic acid can entrap large amount of water. A smaller part of the Wharton's jelly extracellular matrix is formed by sulfated glycosaminoglycans, which, in turn, are linked to proteins to form proteoglycans.[42] An alteration of the extracellular matrix has been indicated as one of the possible causes of increased nuchal translucency in trisomy 21 human fetuses. The variation in the amount of hyaluronan found in the skin of trisomy 21 fetuses may be present in the extracellular matrix of umbilical cords influencing their macroscopic appearance. There is evidence that fibroblast synthesis of hyaluronic acid is not different between healthy and trisomy 21 fetuses. Fibroblast of fetuses with trisomy 21 overexpress collagen type VI and experimental evidence has been provided that an inverse correlation exists between collagen synthesis and hyaluronan degradation.[43,44] An increase in collagen type VI may contribute to hyaluronan accumulation. There is evidence that a reduced turnover of hyaluronan could also influence the growth of the umbilical cord vessels and coiling formation.

CONCLUSION

The antenatal measurement of umbilical cord area is probably a better parameter than determination of umbilical cord diameter to identify fetuses at risk of being small for gestational age at delivery or of having distress in labor, or to identify macrosomic fetuses born diabetic mothers. Since, the UC area is easy to measure and nomograms are available, its measurement should be part of a routine scan and should prompt a careful and thorough evaluation whenever there is a discrepancy between the observed and the normal values.

REFERENCES

1. Raio L, Ghezzi F, Di Naro E, et al. Sonographic measurement of the umbilical cord and fetal anthropometric parameters. J Obstet Gynecol Reprod Biol. 1999;83(2):131-5.
2. Di Naro E, Ghezzi F, Raio L, et al. Umbilical cord morphology and pregnancy outcome. Eur J Obstet Gynecol Reprod Biol. 2001;96(2):150-7.
3. Todros T, Adamson SL, Guiot C, et al. Umbilical cord and fetal growth—a workshop report. Placenta. 2002;23 (Suppl) A: S130-2.
4. Raio L, Ghezzi F, Di Naro E, et al. Altered sonographic umbilical cord morphometry in early-onset preeclampsia. Obstet Gynecol. 2002;100(2):311-6.
5. Cromi A, Ghezzi F, Di Naro E, Siesto G, Bergamini V, Raio L. Large cross-sectional area of the umbilical cord as a predictor of fetal macrosomia.Ultrasound Obstet Gynecol. 2007;30(6):861-6.
6. Weissman A, Jakobi P, Bronshtein H, et al. Sonographic measurements of the umbilical cord and vessels during normal pregnancies. J Ultrasound Med. 1994;13(1):11-4.
7. Raio L, Ghezzi F, Di Naro E, et al. Sonographic measurement of the umbilical cord and fetal anthropometric parameters. Eur J Obstet Gynecol Reprod Biol. 1999;83(2):131-5.
8. Vizza E, Correr S, Goranova V, et al. The collagen skeleton of the human umbilical cord at term. A scanning electron microscopy study after 2N-NaOH maceration. Reprod Fertil Dev. 1996;8(5):885-94.
9. Hall SP. The thin cord syndrome. A review with a report of two cases. Obstet Gynecol. 1961;18:507-9.
10. Raio L, Ghezzi F, Di Naro E, et al. Prenatal diagnosis of a lean umbilical cord: a simple marker for the fetus at risk of being small for gestational age at birth. Ultrasound Obstet Gynecol. 1999;13(3):176-80.
11. Silver RK, Dooley SL,Tamura RK, et al. Umbilical cord size and amniotic fluid volume in prolonged pregnancy. Am J Obstet Gynecol. 1987;157(3):716-20.
12. Bruch JF, Sibony O, Benali K, et al. Computerized microscope morphometry of umbilical vessels from pregnancies with intrauterine growth retardation and abnormal umbilical artery Doppler. Hum Pathol. 1997;28(10):1139-45.
13. Ghezzi F, Raio L, Günter Duwe D, et al. Sonographic umbilical vessel morphometry and perinatal outcome of fetuses with a lean umbilical cord. J Clin Ultrasound. 2005;33(1):18-23.
14. Goodlin RC. Fetal dysmaturity, "lean cord," and fetal distress. Am J Obstet Gynecol. 1987;156(5):1357.
15. Benirschke K, Kaufmann P. Pathology of the human placenta. 3rd edition. New York: Springer; 1995.
16. Chantler C, Baum JD, Wigglesworth JS, et al. Giant umbilical cord associated with a patent urachus and fused umbilical arteries. J Obstet Gynaecol Br Commonw. 1969;76(3):273-4.
17. Iaccarino M, Baldi F, Persico O, et al. Ultrasonographic and pathologic study of mucoid degeneration of umbilical cord. J Clin Ultrasound. 1986;14(2):127-9.
18. Weissman A, Jakobi P. Sonographic measurements of the umbilical cord in pregnancies complicated by gestational diabetes. J Ultrasound Med. 1997;16(10):691-4.
19. Singh SD. Gestational diabetes and its effect on the umbilical cord. Early Hum Dev. 1986;14(2):89-98.
20. Dolkart LA, Reimers FT, Kuonen CA. Discordant umbilical arteries: ultrasonographic and Doppler analysis. Obstet Gynecol. 1992;79(1):59-63.

21. Raio L, Ghezzi F, Di Naro E, et al. The clinical significance of antenatal detection of discordant umbilical arteries. Obstet Gynecol. 1998;91(1):86-91.
22. Persutte WH, Hobbins J. Single umbilical artery: a clinical enigma in modern prenatal diagnosis. Ultrasound Obstet Gynecol. 1995;6(3):216-29.
23. Heifetz SA. Single umbilical artery. A statistical analysis of 237 autopsy cases and review of the literature. Perspect Pediatr Pathol. 1984;8(4):345-78.
24. Raio L, Ghezzi F, Di Naro E, et al. Prenatal assessment of the Hyrtl anastomosis and evaluation of its function: case report. Hum Reprod. 1999;14(7):1890-3.
25. Raio L, Ghezzi F, di Naro E, et al. In-utero characterization of the blood flow in the Hyrtl anastomosis. Placenta. 2001;22(6):597-600.
26. Raio L, Ghezzi F, Di Naro E, et al. Prenatal assessment of Wharton's jelly in umbilical cords with single artery. Ultrasound Obstet Gynecol. 1999;14(1):42-6.
27. Hyrtl J. Die Blutgefasse der menshlichen nachgeburt in normalen und abnormen Veuhatmissen. Wien: Wilhelem Beamüller; 1870.
28. Malpas P, Symonds EM. Observations on the structures of the human umbilical cord. Surg Gynecol Obstet. 1966;123(4): 746-50.
29. Lacro RV, Jones KL, Benirschke K. The umbilical cord twist: origin, direction, and relevance. Am J Obstet Gynecol. 1987;157(4 Pt 1):833-8.
30. Di Naro E, Ghezzi F, Raio L, et al. Umbilical vein blood flow in fetuses with normal and lean umbilical cord. Ultrasound Obstet Gynecol. 2001;17(3):224-8.
31. Degani S, Lewinsky RM, Berger H, et al. Sonographic estimation of umbilical coiling index and correlation with Doppler flow characteristics. Obstet Gynecol. 1995;86(6):990-3.
32. Langille BL. Remodeling of developing and mature arteries: endothelium, smooth muscle, and matrix. J Cardiovasc Pharmacol. 1993;21(Suppl 1):S11-7.
33. Gilbert WM, Brace RA. Amniotic fluid volume and normal flows to and from the amniotic cavity. Semin Perinatol. 1993;17(3):150-7.
34. Reynolds RR. Mechanisms of placentofetal blood flow. Ostet Gynecol. 1978;51(2):245-9.
35. Di Naro E, Ghezzi F, Raio L, et al. Umbilical vein blood flow in fetuses with normal and lean umbilical cord. Ultrasound Obstet Gynecol. 2001:17:224-8.
36. Di Naro E, Raio L, Ghezzi F, et al. Longitudinal umbilical vein blood flow changes in normal and growth-retarded fetuses. Acta Obstet Gynecol Scand. 2002;81(6):527-33.
37. Kilavuz O, Vetter K. The umbilical ring—the first rapid in the fetoplacental venous system. J Perinat Med. 1998;26(2): 120-2.
38. Skulstad SM, Rasmussen S, Iversen OE, et al. The development of high venous velocity at the fetal umbilical ring during gestational weeks 11-19. BJOG. 2001;108(3):248-53.
39. Strong TH, Elliott JP, Radin TG. Non-coiled umbilical blood vessels: a new marker for the fetus at risk. Obstet Gynecol. 1993;81(3):409-11.
40. Qin Y, Lau TK, Rogers MS. Second-trimester ultrasonographic assessment of the umbilical coiling index. Ultrasound Obstet Gynecol. 2002;20(5):458-63.
41. Ghezzi F, Raio L, Di Naro E, et al. First-trimester sonographic umbilical cord diameter and the growth of the human embryo. Ultrasound Obstet Gynecol. 2001;18(4):348-51.
42. Sobolewski K, Bańkowski E, Chyczewski L, et al. Collagen and glycosaminoglycans of Wharton's jelly. Biol Neonate. 1997;71(1):11-21.
43. von Kaisenberg CS, Brand-Saberi B, Christ B, et al. Collagen type VI gene expression in the skin of trisomy 21 fetuses. Obstet Gynecol. 1998;91(3):319-23.
44. Rooney P, Kumar S. Inverse relationship between hyaluronan and collagens in development and angiogenesis. Differentiation. 1993;54(1):1-9.

CHAPTER 28

Placenta: From Basic Facts to Highly Sophisticated Placenta Accreta Story

Giuseppe Calì, Gabriella Minneci

INTRODUCTION

The study of the placenta is a fundamental aspect of pregnancy management since the first to the third trimester. In the last years, the increased ultrasound technology has given us new possibilities of diagnosis, often with great importance in the clinical practice. This chapter discusses the most known placental diseases, but highlights the importance of some emerging pathological entities, whose early diagnosis or suspect may significantly improve maternofetal outcomes.

ANATOMOPATHOLOGICAL ASPECTS OF PLACENTA

A normal pregnancy depends on the harmonious balance of three biologic systems: Mother, fetus, and placenta. The last one permits the transfer from woman to fetus of the elements it needs to grow up. O_2, active metabolites, hormones, and growth factors reach the fetus through the umbilical vein.

Gaseous and metabolic exchanges between mother and fetus take place in a vascular microenvironment, which is composed of intervillous space (where maternal blood flows, oxygenated and full of nutrients), villus venous capillary (where fetal blood flows, deoxygenated and full of metabolic waste) and vasculosyncytial membrane consisting of basal membrane, trophoblast, and villus capillary endothelium.

The anatomical elementary unit of placenta is the lobule, whose function (fetal oxygenation and nutrition) depends on the presence and integrity of vasculosyncytial membrane. The lobule includes the villus tree (the vascular ramification of the trophoblast) and the intervillous space. Around 5/10 placental lobules together form the placental cotyledon.

At the end of its morphological development [33 weeks of gestation (GW)], the villus tree of placental lobule consists of stem villi, immature intermediate villi, mature intermediate villi, and terminal villi, developing between 13 and 41 GW, 8 and 24 GW, 25 and 32 GW, after 33 GW, respectively.

The progressive ramification of villi ensures both greater ease in gaseous and metabolic maternal–fetal exchanges and greater extension of exchange surface. The reduction of villi thickness implicates the approach of villus capillary to the intervillous space, with the formation of the vasculosyncytial membrane.

Placental lobule inlet is constituted by uterine-placental arteries, which derive from the remodeling of spiral arteries of decidua basalis. Blood returns to maternal circulation via drain-like uterine veins.

Placental oxygenation depends on an adequate perfusion of the intervillous vascular space by oxygenated maternal blood flowing through uterine–placental arteries.

After 3–4 weeks of implantation, the invasive intermediate trophoblast commences to progressively invade maternal spiral arteries.[1] This invasion results in disruption of extracellular matrix and replacement of maternal endothelium by cells of trophoblastic origin leading to the development of a low impedance and large capacitance vascular bed that will cater to the increased requirement of blood flow in pregnancy.[2]

There is the progressive passage from a "low flow and high resistance circle" (spiral arteries) to a "high flow and low resistance circle" (uterine-placental arteries).

The physiologic remodeling of spiral arteries can be hindered by a broad range of anomalies, such as atherosis, persistence of tunica media, fibrinoid necrosis, lymphocytic vasculitis, etc. The lack of remodeling leads to the reduction of uterine-placental arteries and the consequent inadequate supply of oxygen and active metabolites to intervillous space.

The complete cessation of maternal vascular perfusion of the intervillous space induces placental infarct, acute and chronic. Small infarcts in a terminal placenta can have not clinical significance, while big or multiple small infarcts involving a great part of the placenta (>10% of its surface) are functionally devastating and important markers of maternal vascular disease, in particular hypertension. Decidual vasculopathy, fast maturation of villi, and placental infarct have been observed in pregnancies complicated by preeclampsia and gestational hypertension, systemic lupus erythematosus, lupus anticoagulant, and antiphospholipid antibody syndrome.[3,4]

Shape and Dimension

Sonographically, the placenta can be identified since 8 GW. It appears evenly isoechoic till 20 GW and its thickness is not >3 cm. After this age, we can observe the appearance of calcifications and hyperechoic areas and placental thickness reaches about 4–5 cm. At term of pregnancy, placental diameter usually is 15–20 mm. However, during the course of ultrasound examination, assessment of the size of the placenta is often subjective.[5]

According to many authors, placental shape and dimension are mirror of fetal well-being.[6] A thin placenta can be index of intrauterine growth restriction (IUGR). The excessive increase of placental thickness in the second/third trimester can be associated to negative perinatal outcome. A homogeneous thickening can be related to diabetes mellitus, anemia, hydrops, infections **(Table 1)**. A heterogeneous thickening can be caused by a previous intraplacental hemorrhage.

Placental calcifications are usually present during pregnancy. They generally are considered signs of maturation/aging of placenta. According to their frequency and distribution Grannum et al.[7] created a system of ultrasound evaluation (placental grading) (**Figs. 1A to D**):

- *Grade 0:* Homogeneous placenta
- *Grade 1:* Lobulations of the surface are evident. Chorionic indentations do not extend to the basilar plate. Cotyledons are not delineated and no hyperechogenicities or calcification are evident.
- *Grade 2:* There are chorionic indentations extending to the basilar plate and echogenic marginal delineation of placental cotyledons. No calcification is evident.
- *Grade 3:* Extensive calcification is evident.

TABLE 1: Diseases associated with increase of placental thickness or placentomegaly.

• Uteroplacental insufficiency	• Intrauterine infection
• Diabetes mellitus	• Congenital neoplasia
• Maternal anemia	• Beckwith–Wiedemann syndrome
• Fetal anemia	• Chromosomal abnormalities
• Fetal hydrops	• Placental mosaicism
• Placental hemorrhage	

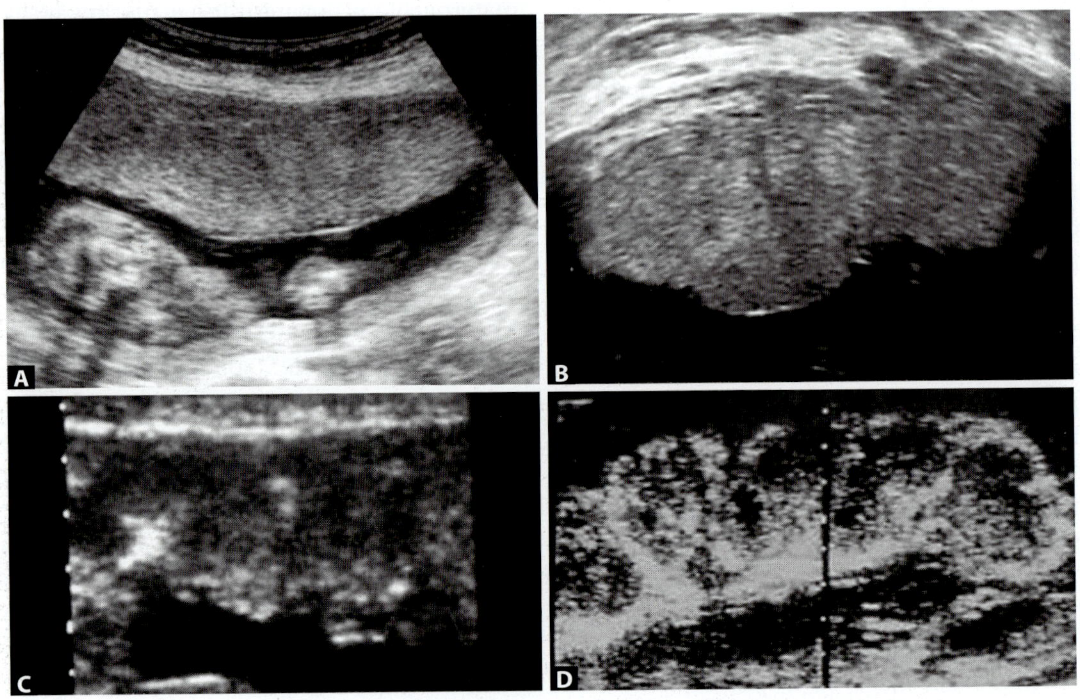

Figs. 1A to D: Grannum scale: (A) Grade 0; (B) Grade 1; (C) Grade 2; (D) Grade 3.

Widespread calcification may be favored by various factors (hypertension, diabetes, IUGR, and smoking).

Aging signs can be seen very well with a macroscopic examination of the placenta. An eventual vascular injury causes thrombosis and consequential infarct areas. In case of arterial occlusion, these areas are generally whitish, while they are prevalently cyanotic in case of venous obliteration. However, infarcts are not evident on an ultrasound examination.

Succenturiate Placenta

This is a morphologic anomaly characterized by a smaller accessory placental lobe that is not part of the main disc of the placenta but is linked to it by blood vessels. There can be >1 succenturiate lobe. It can work normally but can be associated to complications such as placenta previa or vasa previa.

Succenturiate placenta is similar to bilobate placenta and the difference between these two entities is not clear. Some authors use the term "bilobate" when the placental segments have almost the same dimension, while "succenturiate" when there is a greater difference between them.[8]

The incidence is of 3–6%. At the basis of its development, there is the tendency of trophoblast to grow where decidua is richly vascularized (concept of placental trophotropism). Instead, in the areas of insufficient vascularization, placenta is atrophic.[9,10]

On ultrasound, we can see two separated portions of placenta: the main one (which presents the insertion of umbilical cord) and the succenturiate lobe **(Fig. 2)**.

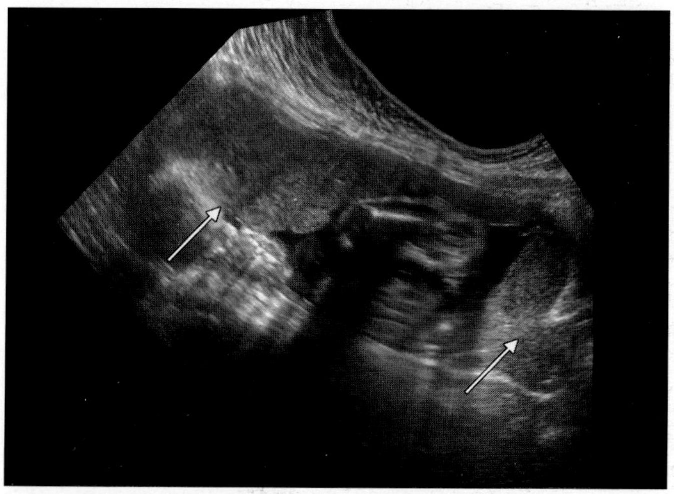

Fig. 2: Succenturiate placenta. Note the main disc (left arrow) and the succenturiate lobe (right arrow). In this case, the accessory lobe covers the internal uterine orifice (IUO).

It is important not to confuse this image with the normal placental extension across the uterus; in this case, there is a flap of placental tissue that links the two parts. When succenturiate placenta is diagnosed, we have to evaluate the insertion of the umbilical cord and the communicating vessels in order to identify eventual vasa previa.

The succenturiate lobe must be distinguished from subchorionic hematoma, myoma, or myometrial contracture. In this last condition, there is not any connection between the two parts and the image disappears within 30 minutes or less.

The retention of the succenturiate lobe can cause postpartum hemorrhage or infections, which can manifest days or weeks after the delivery. Rarely, there is the rupture of communicating vessels, with fetal hemorrhage.

Placenta Membranacea

It is a rare anomaly. All or the main part of fetal membranes remains covered by chorial villi. This anomaly is caused by nondifferentiation of chorion leave and chorion frondosus.[11] The frequency is 0.25–0.5/10,000.[12]

Ultrasound examination shows placenta covering the main part or the whole uterine wall.

Placenta is very thin and deeply adherent, often it presents areas of acretism requiring manual removal. The risk of metrorrhagia must be taken into consideration.

Circumvallate/Circummarginate Placenta

Circumvallate placenta is a variant with the evidence of a relieved ring of membranous tissue on the fetal surface of the placenta, variably distant from umbilical cord insertion. It is determined by a double crease of chorion and amnios, with decidual degeneration and fibrin in the middle. Circummarginate placenta is a similar variant, but the ring of membranous tissue is thinner. It can be found in 20% of placentas, while circumvallate placenta has a minor incidence (1–2%). Both have not clinical significance.

They are the result of the discrepancy between the dimensions of the chorial plate, which is smaller, and the basal plate. This causes the growth of extrachorial placental tissue. The ring can involve the whole placental circumference or just a part of it. The portion of placenta which is not covered by the chorion is called extrachorial.

Ultrasound image is characterized by the fold of fetal membranes, associated to hyperechoic tissue in correspondence of the placental edge **(Fig. 3)**.

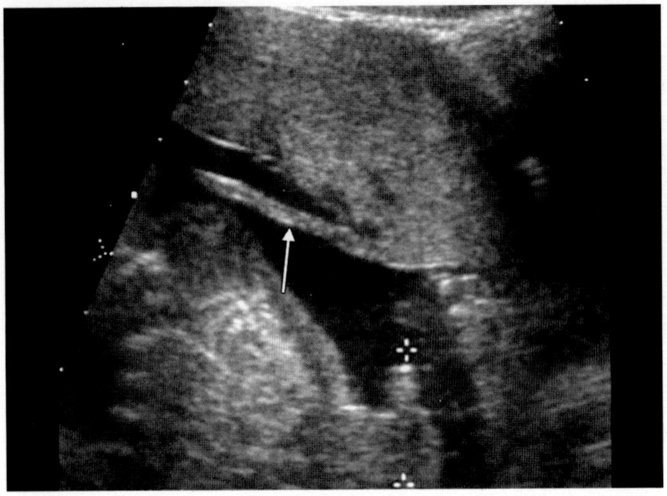

Fig. 3: Circumvallate placenta. Note the fold (arrow) of membranes in correspondence of the placental edge.
Courtesy: Dr Francesco Labate.

Ultrasound accuracy is small. Differential diagnosis is done with intrauterine synechiae and subchorionic hemorrhage.

Circumvallate placenta increases the risks of metrorrhagia for placental abruption and IUGR. However, to find it does not change the management.[13,14]

Abruptio Placentae

It is a complex clinic syndrome determined by the detachment of the placenta before fetal birth. It is a particularly dangerous condition, with high maternal and fetal morbidity and mortality.

Placental abruption is frequently associated with preterm delivery and high perinatal mortality (15–25%) for anoxia, prematurity, and exsanguination fetalis.

Detachment extension can widely vary from minor forms having very little effect on outcomes to major forms, which are associated with fetal death and unfavorable maternal outcomes.

Placental abruption can be total or partial, and it occurs in the 0.4–1% of pregnancies.[15]

Etiology and pathogenesis are not clear yet. They appear complex and multifactorial, with interaction between genetic and environmental factors. The most important risk factors are smoking, preeclampsia, and previous placental abruption. Other risk factors are old maternal age, hypertension, IUGR, anomalous fetal presentation, polyhydramnios, oligohydramnios, multiparity, low body mass index, intrauterine infections, premature rupture of membranes, chorioamnionitis, twin pregnancies, thrombophilia (in association with hyperhomocysteinemia), diabetes mellitus, anemia, uterine anomalies, abdominal traumas, and use of alcohol or drugs. An abdominal trauma can cause the detachment since 6–48 hours to a maximum of 5 days after. A previous cesarean section (CS) increases the risk of about 40% more than spontaneous delivery.[16]

About pathogenesis, abruptio placentae is the result of a bleeding between decidua and placenta, determining their separation and the consequent functional exclusion of the involved placental area. The detachment can also derive from contrasting forces in the decidua-placental interface after abdominal traumas or after the sudden decompression of a overextended uterus (e.g., after rupture of membranes in case of polyhydramnios or twin pregnancy).

The diagnosis is mainly clinic and based on vaginal bleeding, abdominal pain, and eventual cardiotocographic anomalies. It is confirmed by the inspection of the placenta after delivery.

Clinical presentation can be extremely variable, with a range from asymptomatic forms to forms with vaginal hemorrhage.

In the most severe forms, the uterus appears tense and hypertonic at palpation, there are signs of fetal distress and the possibility of maternal shock with the insurgence of consumptive coagulopathy. The quantity of vaginal bleeding is not indicative of the amount of abruption. In 10% of the cases, the hemorrhage is hidden, and there is not any vaginal bleeding.

Ultrasound can be an auxiliary instrument even if not always decisive for diagnosis. In the evaluation of the placenta, scrupulous attention should be given to its localization, dimension, anatomy, morphology, and implantation, excluding the presence of placenta previa.

The placenta usually appears like a homogeneous hyperechoic mass, when compared to the myometrium. In the third trimester, it is more heterogeneous for the presence of calcification and vascular lacunae (anechoic region in the intervillous spaces).

The echogenicity of hemorrhage depends on the time interval between the onset of symptoms to the ultrasound examination. Acute hemorrhaging appears hyperechoic/isoechoic when its echogenicity is greater than the placenta or equal. So, it can be distinguished hardly. Not always it is possible to evaluate the hemorrhage extension in the first scans.

In a week, with resolution, the hemorrhage area becomes hypoechoic, so less echoic than the placenta and similar to myometrium. In 2 weeks, this area becomes anechoic, so similar to amniotic fluid.

The volume of hemorrhage is estimated by the measurement of the three perpendicular diameters (D), on the basis of the formula: 0,52 × (D1 D2 D3).

The localization of hemorrhage is defined on the basis of the mainly involved region and is classified as:

- Subchorial (between myometrium and placental membranes)
- Retroplacental (between myometrium and placenta)
- Preplacental (between placenta and amniotic cavity).

In subchorial forms, the hemorrhage can be limited and hidden. The hematoma can remain confined under membranes or the blood can make its way between membranes and reach the cervix appearing outside. Subchorial hemorrhage is the most common location (67% of cases) of placental hemorrhage observed by ultrasound after 20 GW. Generally, it starts from marginal disconnection between membranes and myometrium and not always it is associated to placental abruption.

In retroplacental forms, the hematoma under the placenta increases and can penetrate the myometrium, determining hemorrhage (uterine-placental apoplexy). Retroplacental hemorrhage (29% of cases) on ultrasound is characterized by placental thickening and sometimes by the view of retroplacental clots (**Figs. 4A and B**).

Preplacental forms can be characterized by rupture of membranes near the placental detachment and the blood reaches the amniotic cavity. Subamniotic hematoma (4% of cases) appears like a hemorrhage along the amniotic surface of placenta.[17,18]

Ultrasound sensibility in the diagnosis of placental abruption is low. As the blood not always forms a hematoma, a negative ultrasound examination cannot exclude the diagnosis of abruption placentae. Ultrasound does not recognize three-fourths of the cases.

Nuclear magnetic resonance (NMR) acquired an important role in the diagnosis of abruption placentae. It has a greater sensibility than ultrasound (100% vs. 53%). It is not conditioned by placenta localization and can distinguish blood from other fluid collections. Between disadvantages of NMR, there are costs, time, and the lack of experts in the evaluation of the examination.

Gestational Trophoblastic Disease

Gestational trophoblastic diseases are a heterogeneous group of pathologies, all originating from the abnormal proliferation of gestational trophoblast. On the basis of anatomical and pathological characteristics and clinic evolution, they are classified as follows in **Table 2**.[19]

TABLE 2: Classification of the gestational trophoblastic diseases.

Hydatidiform mole	*Trophoblastic tumors*
• Complete • Partial	• Invasive mole • Choriocarcinoma • Placental site trophoblastic tumor • Epithelioid trophoblastic tumor

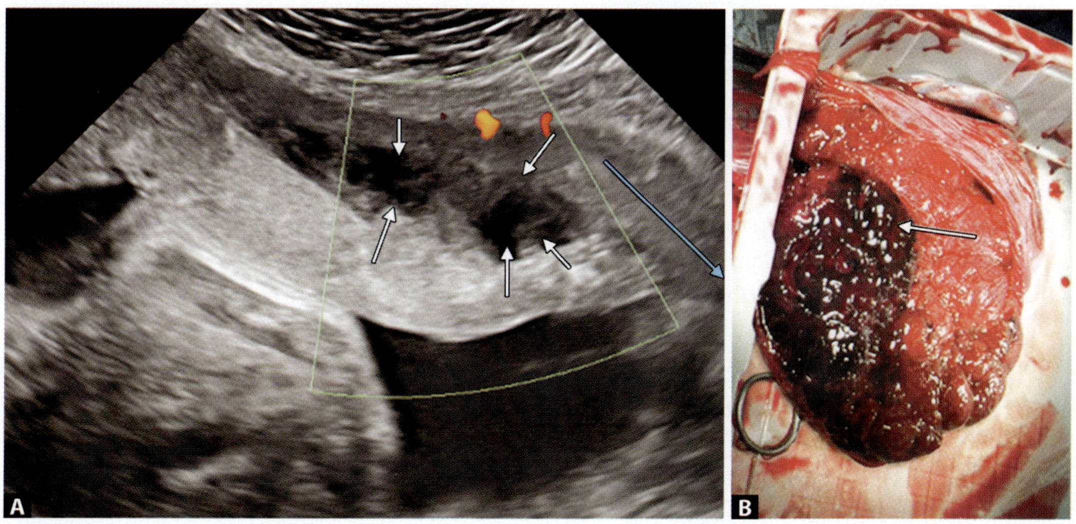

Figs. 4A and B: (A) Image of retroplacental hematoma (arrows), which appears hypoanechoic; (B) Surgical specimen.

The most frequent gestational trophoblastic disease is the hydatidiform mole. It derives from a wrong process of fertilization, with consequent abnormal proliferation and degeneration of the gestational trophoblast.

Partial moles are due to a fertilization error in which a normal ovum is fertilized by two spermatozoa or by one spermatozoon which duplicates. The result is a triploid karyotype (69,XXY) or, rarely, tetraploid (92,XXXY).

About 90% of complete moles derive from the fecundation of an ovum without nucleus (so without maternal chromosomes), by an haploid spermatozoon 23,X, which duplicates its chromosomes giving origin to a homozygous 46,XX androgen diploid entity (entirely paternally derived).[20]

The invasive mole often is the degeneration of a hydatidiform mole. It locally invades the myometrium but does not metastasize.

The choriocarcinoma is a highly malignant epithelial tumor. It metastasizes above all to the lung and pelvic organs.

The placental site tumor is the most rare trophoblastic disease. It origins from the placenta implantation site after pregnancy at term or abortion, rarely after molar pregnancy.

The diagnosis of gestational trophoblastic disease is mainly based on symptomatology, ultrasound image, and plasmatic beta-human chorionic gonadotropin (hCG) values. The clinic aspect of all the forms of trophoblastic disease is the presence of abnormal vaginal bleeding, from minimal to severe hemorrhage.

Beta-hCG concentration is higher than normal.

Ultrasound is the gold standard in the evaluation of a suspected molar pregnancy. It generally appears like an echoic endometrial complex mass containing many small cysts with a diameter of 2–3 mm. This is the classical snowstorm appearance which uniformly involves the whole mass **(Fig. 5)**.[21]

In case of partial mole, an ultrasound shows a bigger placenta than normal, with multiple hypoanechoic cystic areas. It is often associated to an embryo without heart activity or to a malformed fetus and/or with severe growth restriction.

In >30% of cases of complete mole on ultrasound, we can find the presence of multiple ovarian cysts, secondary to the high level of beta-hCG.

Invasive mole, choriocarcinoma, and placental site trophoblastic tumors have a similar aspect, and it is difficult to distinguish them from not invasive molar disease by ultrasound. The most common image is that of an irregular echoic mass invading the myometrium, which appears inhomogeneous for the presence of multiple areas of necrosis and hemorrhage (**Figs. 6A to D**). Color Doppler can be useful to demonstrate an accentuated vascularization at the level of the uterine spiral arteries.[21] In case of suspect of invasive forms, it is opportune to evaluate with ultrasound also the pelvis and the liver, which are frequent sites of metastasis.

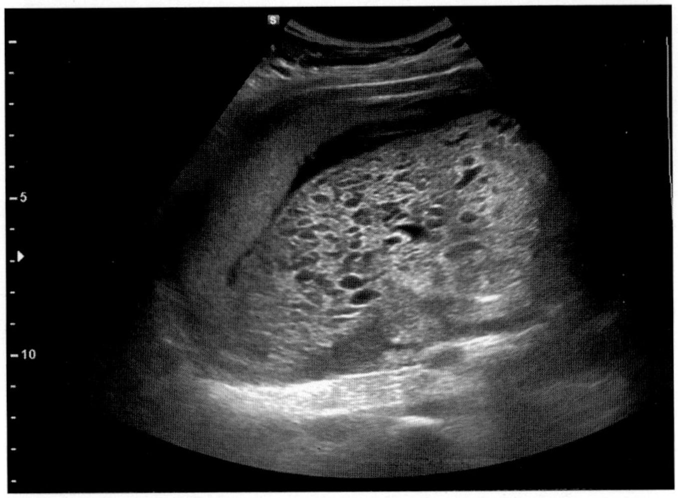

Fig. 5: Complete molar pregnancy, with the classical "snowstorm" appearance. Note the multiple hypoanechoic cystic areas.

There is a high percentage of false-positives and false-negatives on an ultrasound examination. So, the histological examination is fundamental, because the misdiagnosis of gestational trophoblastic disease increases the morbidity and the consequent necessity of chemotherapeutic and surgery treatments.

Chorioangioma

It is a nontrophoblastic benign tumor deriving from an excessive proliferation of small vessels in chorial villous stroma, with variable association of stromal solid areas. Chorioangioma can be singular or multifocal.

Small chorioangiomas are present in 1% of examined placentas, while tumors reaching clinically evident dimensions are relatively uncommon (incidence between 1/3,500 and 1/9,000 pregnancies).[22] Actually, the real incidence of chorioangioma is not exactly identifiable, because the study of placental structure is not included between the criteria of ultrasound screening of the second trimester. Moreover, its identification can be conditioned by the gestational age, because chorioangioma

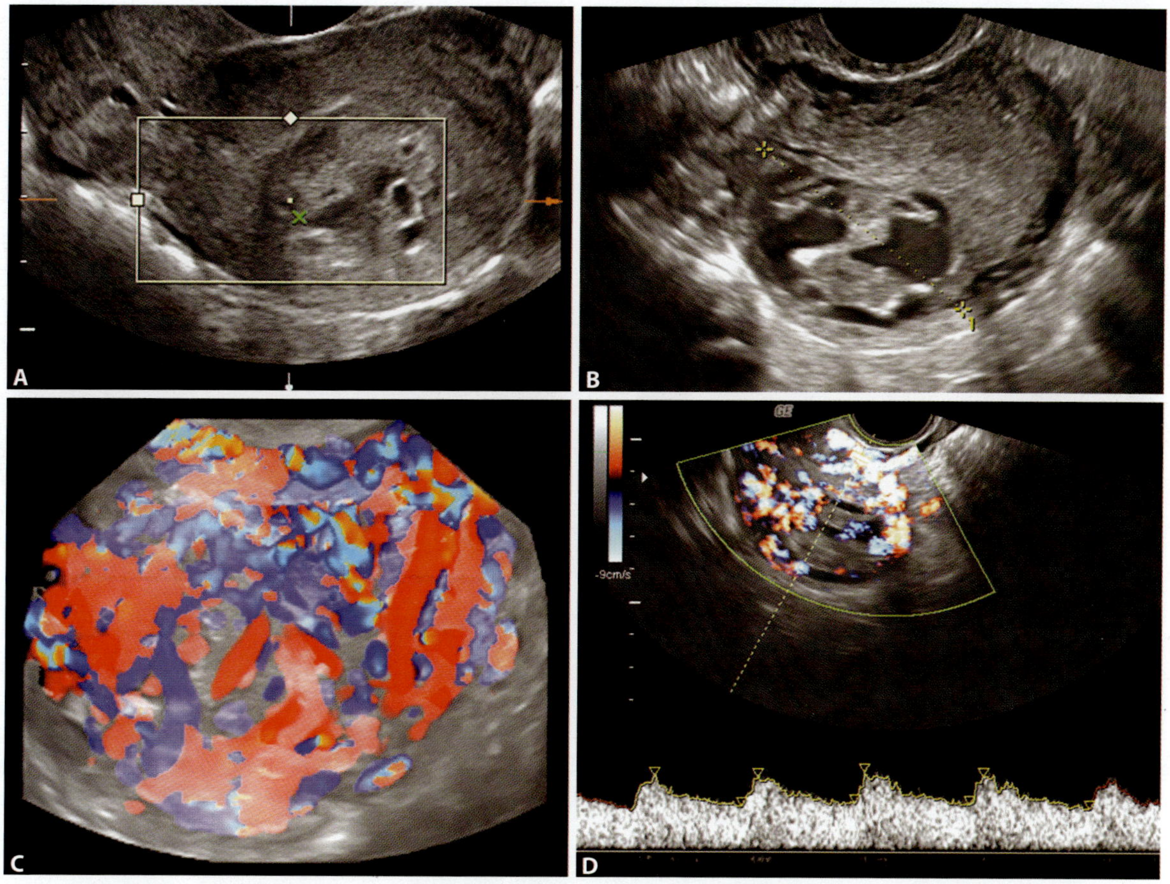

Figs. 6A to D: (A to C) Poorly marginated, heteroechoic, intensely vascular myometrial lesion, compatible with the diagnosis of choriocarcinoma; (D) The lesion is characterized by low resistance flow.

is more easily diagnosable during the third trimester of gestation.

Its pathogenesis is not well defined, yet. Histologically, chorioangioma is made of a group of big and dilated villi, which are not demarked by a fibrous capsule but are surrounded by villous tissue.

The ultrasound image is that of a confined solid formation with hyperechoic or hypoechoic echostructure, sometimes complex, protruding from the placental surface and presenting hypervascularity (**Figs. 7A to C**). It is often localized in proximity of the umbilical cord insertion.[23] To identify intraplacental chorioangiomas is difficult if they are small. Chorioangiomas bigger than 5 cm of diameter are defined as "giant".

Chorioangioma must be distinguished from hematoma, placental lacunae,[24] placental teratomas, partial hydatidiform mole, maternal metastases to placenta,[25] and vascular aneurysms.[26]

It is usually asymptomatic. However, when it is big, it can cause unfavorable fetal outcomes, such as nonimmune fetal hydrops, cardiomegaly, heart failure, anemia, thrombocytopenia, coagulopathy, preterm delivery, severe IUGR, sudden fetal death, and mirror syndrome.[27]

Placental Mesenchymal Dysplasia

Placental mesenchymal dysplasia (PMD) is a rare placental vascular anomaly.[28]

True incidence is not known, but it has been estimated at 0.02%. The underlying cause of PMD is unclear. Some genetic anomalies are considered as etiology of PMD.[29]

It is characterized on ultrasound by an enlarged, hydropic placenta, depicting multiple cysts and tangles of intestine-like chorionic vessels on gross examination (**Figs. 8A to D**).[30] Placentomegaly is mostly >90th percentile.

The differential diagnosis of PMD is broad and includes partial molar pregnancy, complete mole with coexisting normal fetus, chorioangioma, subchorionic hematoma, confined placental mosaicism, and spontaneous abortion with hydropic changes.[31]

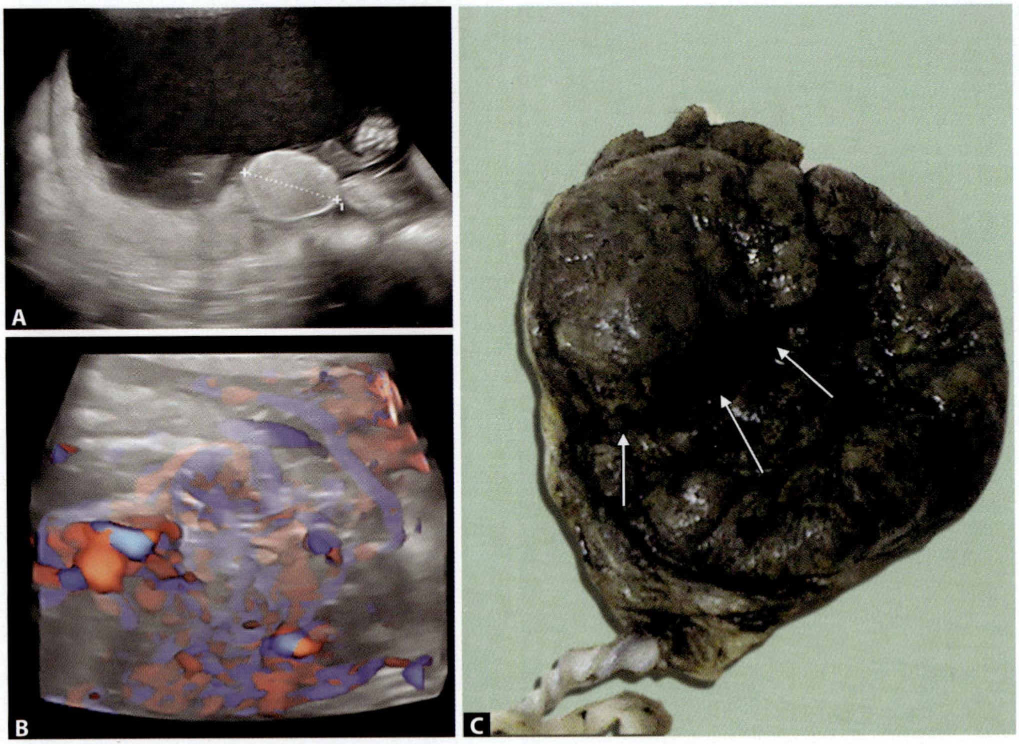

Figs. 7A to C: Chorioangioma: (A) Confined solid formation with hyperechoic structure, protruding from placental surface; (B) 3D color power Doppler image showing hypervascularity; (C) Surgical specimen.

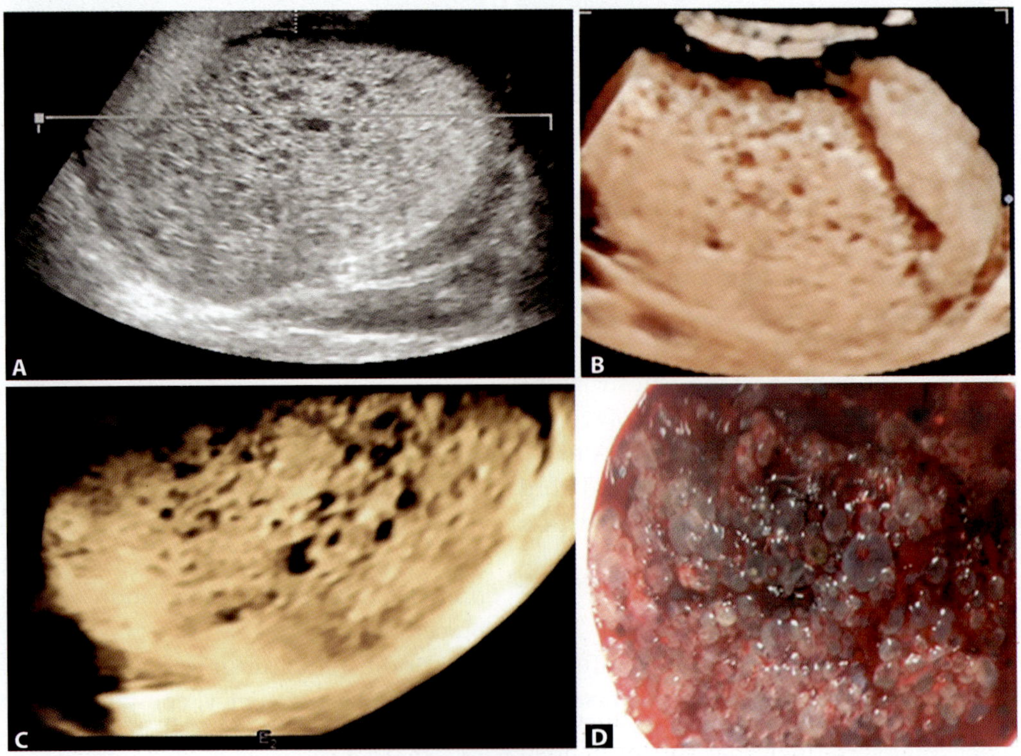

Figs. 8A to D: (A to C) Placental mesenchymal dysplasia. Enlarged, hydropic placenta depicting multiple cysts and dilated chorionic vessels; (D) Surgical specimen.

In the placental parenchyma, multiple vesicles are seen especially in the first and second trimesters. These vesicular changes grossly and ultrasonographically resemble partial mole measuring 0.3–2.5 cm.[32]

On a histologic level, however, both conditions can be clearly distinguished. A partial mole is characterized by trophoblastic proliferation, which is completely absent in PMD. The characteristic changes of the latter are essentially vascular abnormalities: enlarged stem villi with dilated vessels, a focal cistern-like formation, and possibly chorangiomatoid changes. Cytogenetically, both conditions are also distinctly different: partial moles are triploid (usually diandric), whereas aneuploidy is uncommon in PMD, but it is sometimes associated with rare genetic syndromes; the best known association is with Beckwith–Wiedemann syndrome (BWS). PMD is associated with raised maternal serum alfa-fetoprotein (AFP) levels but normal or mildly elevated beta-hCG levels.

Placental mesenchymal dysplasia is usually associated with normal fetus; unlike hydatidiform mole, the pregnancy extends to the third trimester.[33-35]

The fetus usually has normal karyotype with female predominance, but PMD is associated with intrauterine growth retardation, stillbirth, prematurity, and BWS.[28,36-38]

Beckwith–Wiedemann syndrome is present in 25% of cases and is characterized by macrosomia, visceromegaly, hemihyperplasia, macroglossia, omphalocele, and increased childhood tumors.

Diagnosis should be considered with specific sonographic findings, including enlarged, cystic placenta with dilated chorionic vessels. Abnormal levels of biochemical analytes, identified as part of aneuploidy screening, especially elevated msAFP, further support the diagnosis. Karyotype should be obtained to exclude partial molar pregnancy, as this is the most common misdiagnosis of PMD, and termination of pregnancy is recommended in this situation. A detailed anatomical survey should be performed to rule out fetal anomalies, especially abnormalities consistent with BWS.

The anatomical ultrasound should include a thorough evaluation of the fetal abdomen to rule out hepatic tumors. The placenta should be sent for pathological evaluation after delivery for confirmation of PMD.

Pregnancy outcomes range from healthy, uncomplicated pregnancies to adverse maternal and/or neonatal complications.

DIAGNOSIS OF PLACENTA ACCRETA SPECTRUM

Introduction

The study of the placenta is one of the most important aspects of pregnancy management since the first trimester. In this period, ultrasonography allows the diagnosis of possible subchorionic hematomas, gestational trophoblastic disease, and twin chorionicity.

In the last years, because of the increase of CSs and the improvement of imaging techniques, we have observed a rising incidence of scar pregnancies and morbidly adherent placenta in the first trimester.

In the second and third trimesters, the study of placental insertion is fundamental. Above all, it enables to select cases with risk of acretism.

The anomalies in placental insertion and invasion, such as placenta previa and the various forms of acretism [placenta accreta (PA), increta, and percreta], are today a rising obstetric pathology.

In the past, PA was a catastrophic but extremely rare event, while in the last decades its incidence gradually and steady increased. According to epidemiological data, it occurs in 2 cases out of 1,000 pregnancies. It is important to underline the existence of known risk factors, first of all a previous CS. Also, placenta previa is a condition associated with placenta accreta spectrum (PAS) disorders and its frequency is correlated to CS too.[39-44]

In the United States, the rate of CS increased from 5% to 32.9% in 2009.[45] Similar or even higher rates of CSs are reported elsewhere in the world with countries such as Brazil (45%), Mexico (44%), China (42%), and Italy (38%).[46]

In consideration of the epidemiologic emergency, the great maternofetal morbidity and mortality and the possible medicolegal implications, the prenatal diagnosis of acretism is extremely important above all for a correct management.[47]

Placenta Previa

Placenta is defined *previa* when it is implanted on the lower segment of the uterus. We distinguish it into the following:

- *Placenta previa major*, when it completely covers the internal uterine orifice (IUO) (**Figs. 9A and B**)
- *Placenta previa minor*, when the IUO is not covered but placenta is far <2 cm from it (**Figs. 10A and B**)
- *Placenta low-lying*, when placenta is far >2 cm but <3.5 cm from the IUO

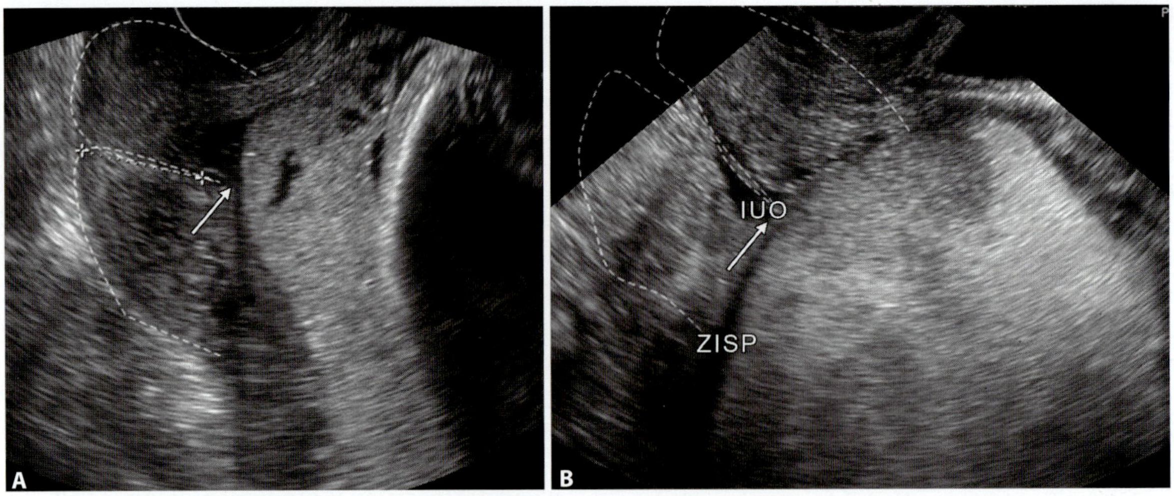

Figs. 9A and B: Placenta previa major. The placenta completely covers the IUO (arrows).

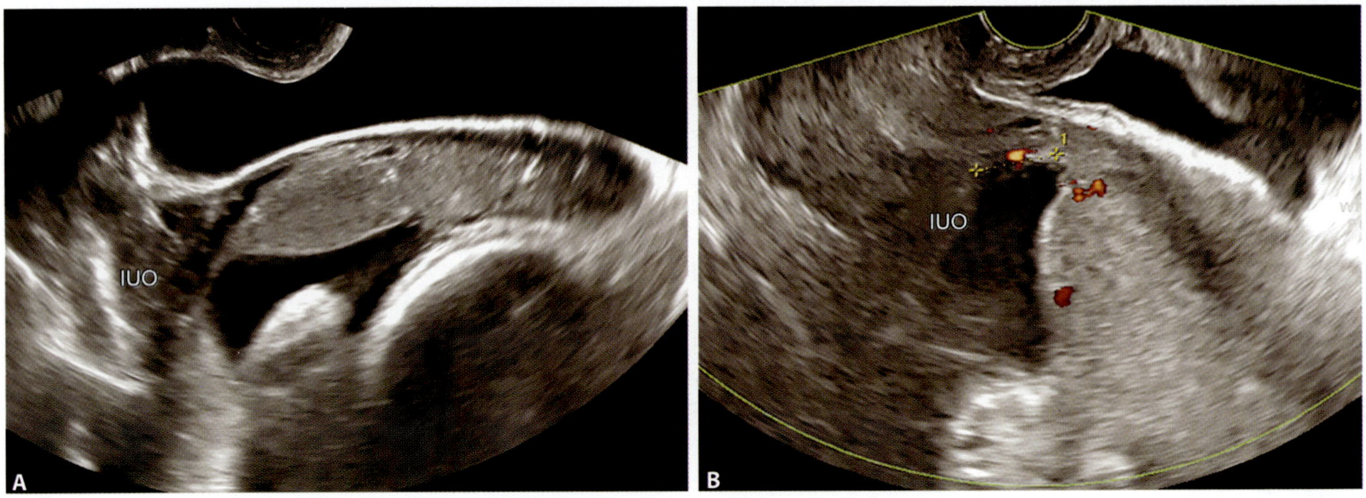

Figs. 10A and B: Placenta previa minor. The IUO is not coverd by the placenta.

Recently placenta previa has been more easily classified in:

- *Placenta previa,* when it covers the IUO
- *Placenta low-lying,* when the IUO is not covered, but the placenta is far <2 cm from it
- *Placenta normal,* if its edge is at least 2 cm far from the IUO.

The best imaging modality to evaluate a placenta implanting on the lower uterine segment is transvaginal ultrasound (TVU), which shows with good precision the topographic relation and the distance between the placenta and IUO.[48]

Furthermore, TVU allows to overcome the possible limits about bladder filling, scant echogenicity, and/or fat.

The incidence of placenta previa is different in relation to the gestational age, with a range from 5% in the second trimester to 0.5% at the end of pregnancy.[49] In fact, in diagnosis of placenta previa, it has to be considered the phenomenon of "placental migration", that is to say the physiologic moving of the placenta to the fundus of uterus.

This event is linked to the progressive development of the uterine lower segment[50] and to the lower vascularization of cervicoisthmic region.[51] The migration is more evident during the second trimester and continues, but in a smaller scale, in the third trimester.[52] Oppenheimer et al.[53] highlighted that, since the 26th week of gestation, if the placental edge is >2 cm distant from the IUO, the following migration cancels the risk of placenta previa at the end of pregnancy. On the contrary, when the placental edge covers the IUO for >20 mm, placenta remains previa.

The Royal College of Obstetricians & Gynaecologists (RCOG) guidelines (2011) suggest a careful ultrasound follow-up since the 20th week of gestation when the placenta is implanted on the lower uterine segment involving completely or marginally the IUO. Through this follow-up we can monitor the process of placental migration and exclude the evolution to acretism in patients at risk (with previous CS).

Placenta Accreta (Increta, Percreta)

Placenta accreta is an abnormal adherence of the placenta to the uterine wall. It occurs when chorionic villi have an excessive capacity of infiltration or when the decidual reaction is inadequate in containing villi penetration. The Nitabuch fibrinoid layer is a layer of fibrin between the endometrium and cytotrophoblast. When this membrane is compromised, the placenta will attach itself deeply into the uterine wall between the myometrial fibers.

Placenta accreta spectrum disorders include three forms of abnormal placentation:

1. PA (or adherent), when the villi adhere to the myometrium without invasion
2. Placenta increta, when the villi invade the myometrium
3. Placenta percreta, when villi invade the full thickness of the myometrium including the uterine serosa and sometimes adjacent pelvic organs.

According to the lateral extension of the myometrial invasion and the number of cotyledons involved, PAS disorders can also be divided into focal, partial, or total.

There is not a specific clinical symptomatology of PAS, and in many forms of acretism there is no bleeding during the gestation. So, we have to suspect its presence if the patient has risk factors. Placenta previa, previous curettage, multiparity, maternal age >35 years, hysterotomy scars, and above all previous CS are linked to a high risk of PAS. In fact, the increasing rate of these events correlates with the rising incidence of PAS in western countries.

At delivery, this condition exposes to a big risk of severe hemorrhage with possible necessity of hysterectomy. So, an accurate prenatal diagnosis (or at least a suspect) is required to reduce the risk of maternal/fetal morbidity and mortality.[54]

Prenatal diagnosis allows to plan the availability of compatible blood to consider the various therapeutic options and to ensure the presence of a multidisciplinary team with adequate experience. Furthermore, if the patient shows a strong desire of preserving fertility, a prompt diagnosis could permit the planning of a conservative treatment.[55]

In the past, the diagnosis of PA was made intrapartum often with catastrophic consequences for the woman because of the attempts of instrumental removing of placenta.

Therefore, in order to have a diagnosis of placental acretism as early as possible, in the last years, many authors have studied the validity of various ultrasound criteria.[56-59]

The generally used criteria are:

- Loss or irregularity of hypoechoic area between placenta and myometrium (*clear space*)
- Placental vascular *lacunae*
- Thinning or interruption of the hyperechoic interface between uterine serosa and bladder wall (*bladder line*)
- Papillar extroversion of placental-like tissue on the uterine serosa and/or into the bladder
- The reduction of myometrial thickness.

Clear space: It is the hypoechoic area between the placenta and myometrium (**Fig. 11A**). It coincides with the vessels of the basalis decidua.[60] Even if it is evident since the 12th GW, sometimes the clear space is not well viewable also in cases of placenta not accreta, especially if it is implanted on the anterior wall of the uterus.[61] There is a clear correlation between PAS and the absence or irregularity of clear space, related to the insufficient presence of basalis decidua (**Fig. 11B**).[62]

Other authors studied the efficacy of clear space as single diagnostic criterion, highlighting a high rate of false positives.[63,64]

In 2004, Comstock suggested that an altered representation of the clear space, above all in case of anterior placenta, could depend on the pressure employed on the probe during the examination.[58] However, the high negative predictive value (NPV) and sensitivity legitimize the use of this criterion in the ultrasound diagnosis of acretism, in association with other criteria.[65,66]

Placental vascular lacunae: Number and small dimension of lacunae relate with the diagnosis of PAS **(Fig. 12)**.

In case of PAS lacunae present a flow with high speed and low resistance (**Figs. 13A and B**).[24]

The exact histogenetic course is not totally clear; however, it seems that in case of acretism the increasing vascularization and the abnormal placental insertion could represent mechanical causes of intraplacental disruption with consequent formation of lacunae.[67] In 1992, Findberg and Williams proposed a grading for placental lacunae: grade 0 when no lacuna is present (low risk of acretism);

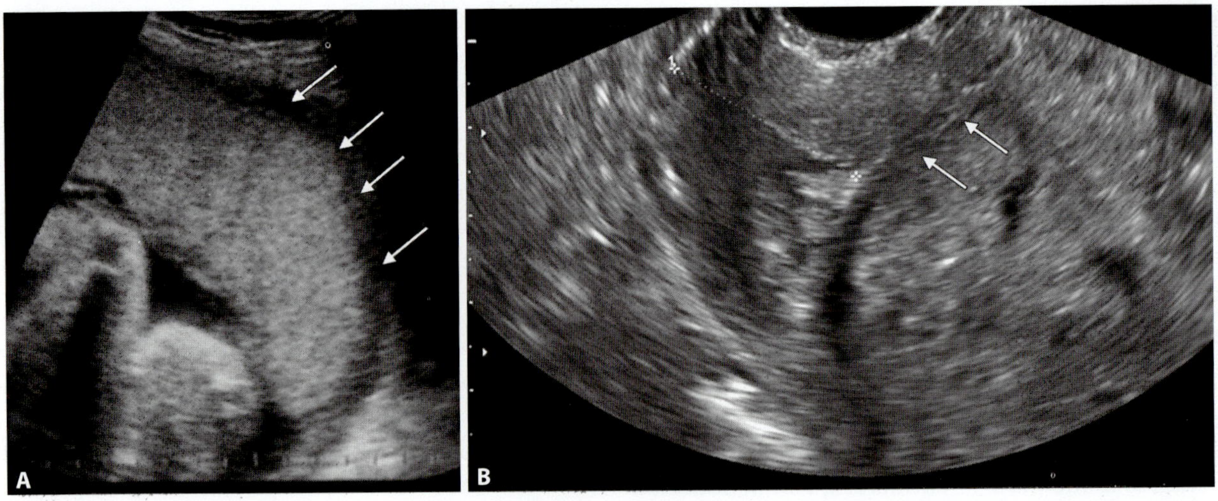

Figs. 11A and B: Clear space: (A) Normal clear space: Hypoechoic area between placenta and myometrium. It coincides with the vessels of the basal decidua; (B) Partial absence and irregularity of clear space between myometrium and placenta (arrows).

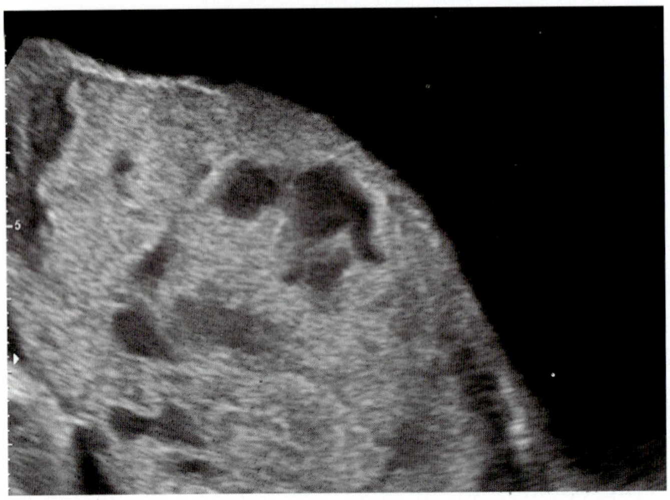

Fig. 12: Intraparenchymal placental lacunae (vascular spaces).

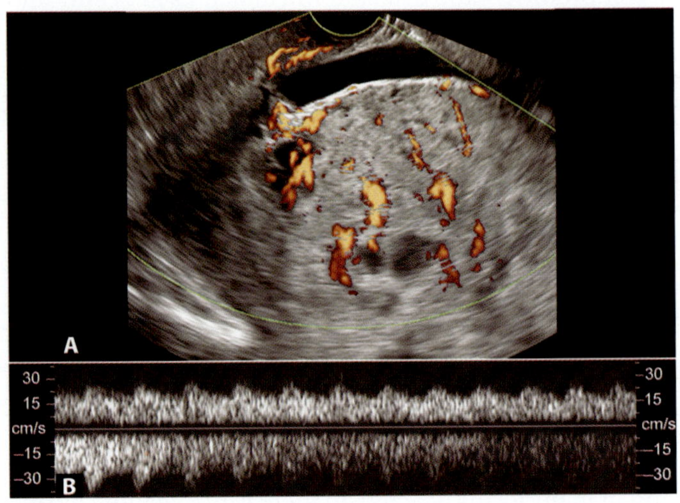

Figs. 13A and B: (A) Placental lacunae characterized by turbulent flow; (B) High velocity flow of lacunae.

grade 1+ in presence of 1–3 lacunae; grade 2+ if there are 4–6 lacunae; grade 3+ in presence of many lacunae with irregular shape affecting most of placental parenchyma (high risk of acretism).[63]

Figure 14 shows placental vascular lacunae displayed by color Doppler.

In 2004, Comstock et al. observed that placental vascular lacunae showed 93% of sensitivity in women at ≥20 GW.[58] D'Antonio et al. obtained 77.43% of sensitivity and 95.02% of specificity.[66]

Bladder line: It is a hyperechoic line corresponding to the interface between bladder and myometrium, better viewable when the bladder is partly filled and the probe is positioned at 90° respect to its wall **(Fig. 15)**.[67] The thinning or interruption of the bladder line depends on the development of blood vessels in the space between the myometrium and bladder. In case of PAS, they can reach the bladder wall **(Figs. 16 and 17)**. This sign can be present also in absence of acretism, above all in patients with >1 previous CS, because they develop neovascularization on the vesicouterine fold.[59]

In an already mentioned meta-analysis of 2013, authors found that the interruption of the bladder line presented sensitivity of 49.66% and specificity of 99.75%.[66] Calì et al. proved that sensitivity of bladder line interruption was 70% with gray-scale ultrasound, but it reaches 90% with color Doppler ultrasound **(Fig. 18)**.[24]

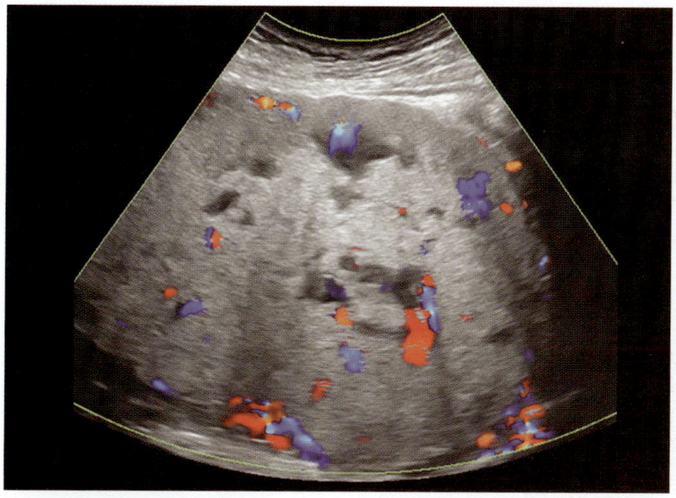

Fig. 14: Color power Doppler image of intraparenchymal placental lacunae.

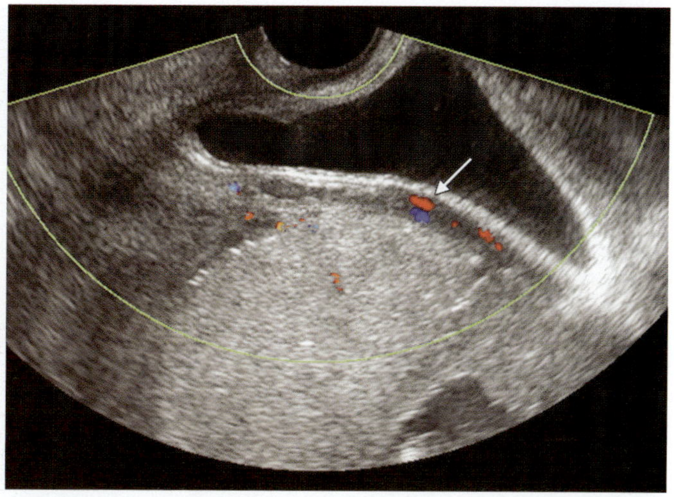

Fig. 15: Normal bladder line: Hyperechoic line corresponding to the interface between bladder and myometrium.

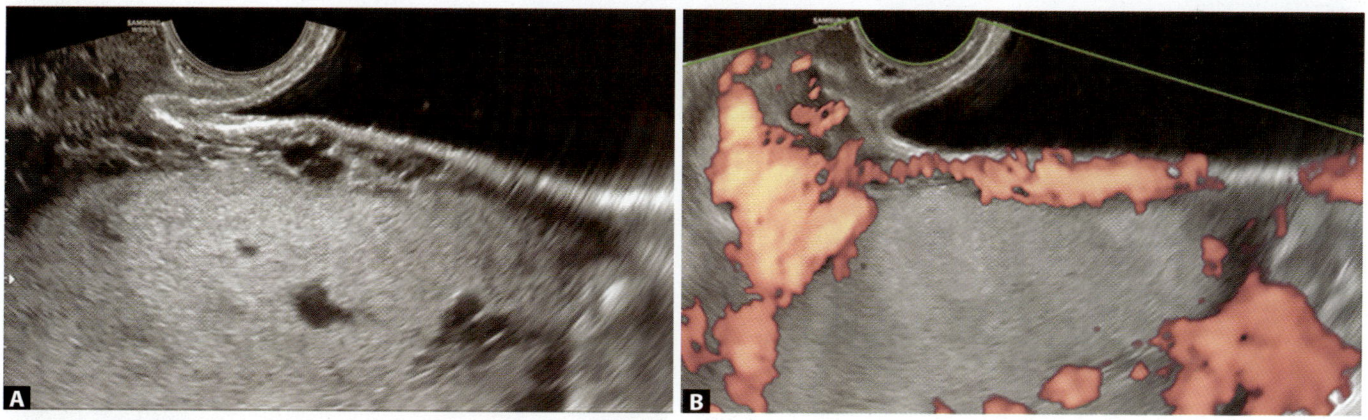

Figs. 16A and B: (A) Thin and interrupted bladder line in a case of placenta percreta; (B) Interruption and thinning of the interface between uterine serosa and bladder wall are caused by its hypervascularization.

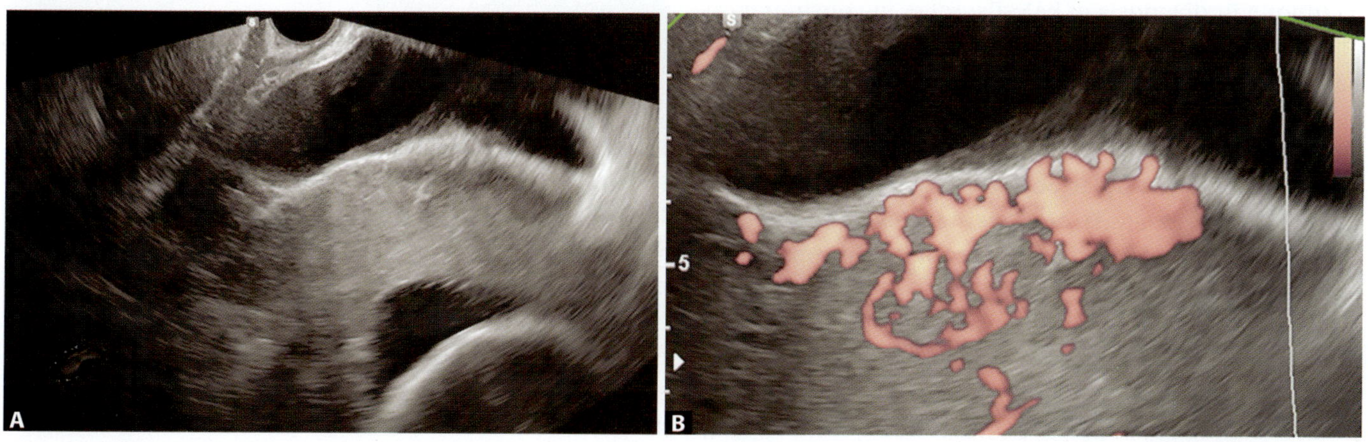

Figs. 17A and B: (A) An other case of placenta percreta, showing irregularity and interruption of the bladder line; (B) Blood vessels reach the bladder wall.

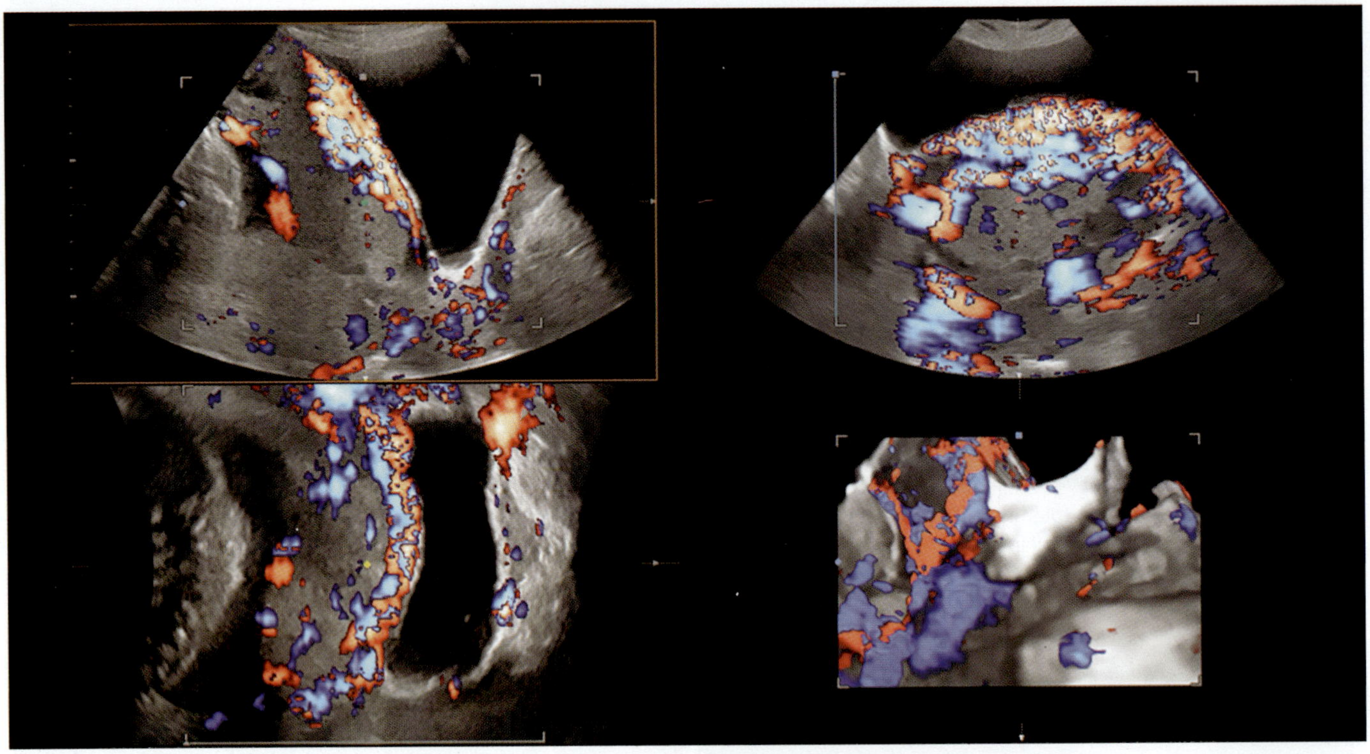

Fig. 18: Color power Doppler images showing the hypervascularization of the bladder line.

The presence of a chaotic vascularization with confluent and tortuous vessels seems to represent the best single diagnostic criterion, with sensitivity and sensibility of 97% and 92%, respectively.[65] However, to date, there is not a single diagnostic criterion that has high confidence in order to diagnose or exclude placental acretism.

3D Power Doppler

Although bidimensional ultrasound is the standard technique in diagnosis of PAS disorders in consideration of the important maternofetal implications of this pathology, it is useful to employ all the available diagnostic techniques, such as 3D ultrasound and 3D power Doppler.

A 3D power Doppler became an instrument of frequent use in the study of placental development and vascularization, allowing not just qualitative but also a quantitative evaluation.

This instrument has the capability of obtaining multiplanar images on axial, coronal, and sagittal planes, and with rotational technique permits to visualize placenta-bladder interface more accurately. So, it allows a better study of the degree of bladder invasion.[68] This information, obviously, is very important for counseling and following management. Many studies in the literature support the employment of 2D ultrasound and color Doppler in the diagnosis of placental acretism,[57,63,69] but until recently, there was no evidence in literature about the possibility of differential diagnosis between PA, increta, or percreta **(Fig. 19)**.

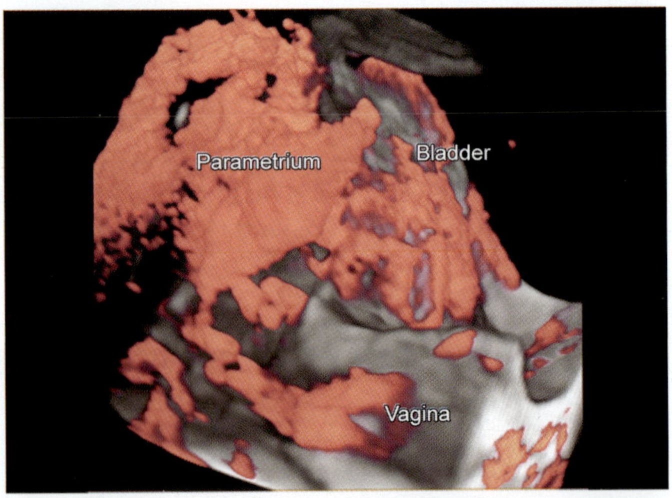

Fig. 19: 3D power Doppler image. Extensive and chaotic hypervascularization involving the whole placental parenchyma in placenta percreta. Note the parametrial vascular invasion.

According to the RCOG guidelines published in 2011, 3D power Doppler diagnostic criteria are as follows:[70]

- Presence of vessels (linear, confluent) involving the uterine-bladder interface in basal images
- Placental hypervascularization in lateral images
- Inadequate distinction between intervillous and cotyledonoid circulation, tortuous vessels, and chaotic ramifications in lateral images.

Calì et al., using 3D color power Doppler, demonstrated that the hypervascularization observed at the uterine-bladder interface was extended from side to side in all cases of placenta percreta they examined, with sensitivity, specificity, NPV, and positive predictive value (PPV) of 90, 100, 100, and 97%, respectively.[24]

Combination of 2D and 3D Power Doppler Ultrasound Criteria

Diagnostic accuracy increases using more ultrasound criteria. Calì et al. used three bidimensional signs (clear space, lacunae, and bladder line interruption) and two tridimensional power Doppler signs (chaotic vascularization with confluent and tortuous vessels in the whole placental parenchyma and hypervascularization of serosa-bladder interface) and observed that all women in examination with 5 positive criteria had placenta percreta. On the contrary, no woman with normal placental insertion showed >1 ultrasound criterion.[24] On the basis of ultrasound criteria evidenced in 2D ultrasound, Comstock et al. found that using ≥2 criteria, the sensitivity was 80% and the PPV was 86%.[58]

An important contribute in the comparison of 3D power Doppler and gray scale has been given by a study by Shih et al.; the results demonstrated that the use of 3D power Doppler increases the diagnostic information we can obtain with bidimensional, both in terms of PPV than NPV.[65] The hypervascularization of serosa-bladder interface observed by 3D power Doppler presents PPV of 100% and, in case of percretism, is always associated to an abnormal intraparenchymal vascularization (3D power Doppler) similar to an aneurysmatic formation.[24] In this study, the bladder line, evaluated with TVU 3D power Doppler and with standard bladder filling of 300 mL, can predict placental acretism with high accuracy; furthermore, the spatial reconstruction of neovascularization of bladder-myometrium interface with a 3D ultrasound gives more effective results than a 2D technique in the differentiation between acretism/incretism and percretism.

An additional contribute to definition of percretism is given by the publication by Calì et al. about the utilization of "virtual cystoscopy";[71] in the diagnostic workup of patients with PAS, 3D-HD-flow TVU was used to analyze the vascular topography of uterine-bladder interface. Using bladder filling of 300 mL, the authors obtained information about bladder posterior wall, which was adjacent to the abnormal placental invasion. In particular, they obtained information about the amount of vascularization under the bladder mucosa **(Figs. 20 and 21)**. The technique allows to highlight the final stages of placental invasion before the perforation of bladder mucosa.

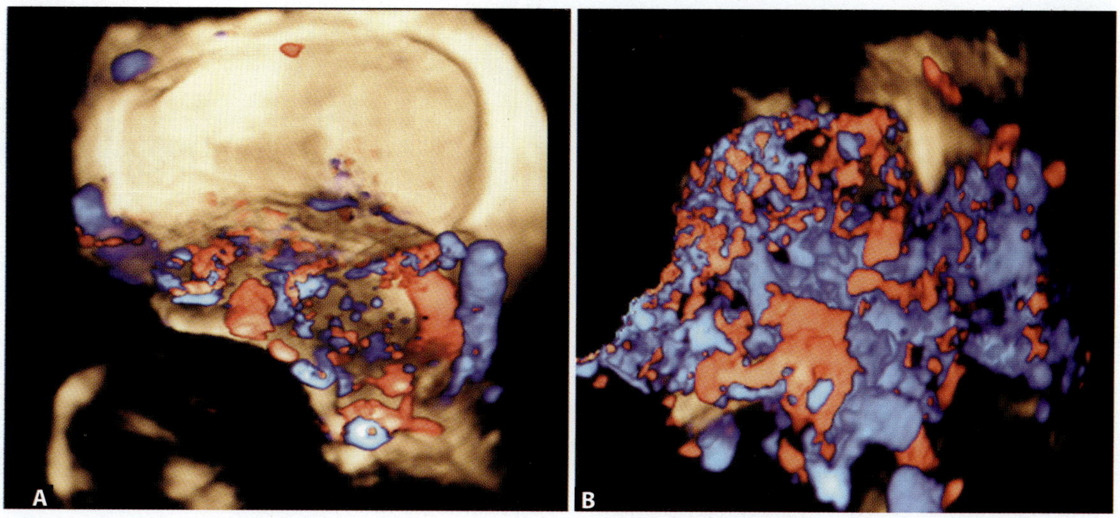

Figs. 20A and B: Virtual cystoscopy images in a case of placenta percreta. The hypervascularity is extended below the bladder urothelium.

Virtual cystoscopy, worthy of further confirmation on big data, could permit the identification of the cases of PA/placenta increta, which tend to evolve into percretism. This kind of diagnosis would justify an intensive monitoring and the planning of delivery through CS also at an early gestational age.

Nuclear Magnetic Resonance

Even if an ultrasound remains the main diagnostic technique in the study of placental implantation, in the last years, the interest on the utilization of NMR has increased.

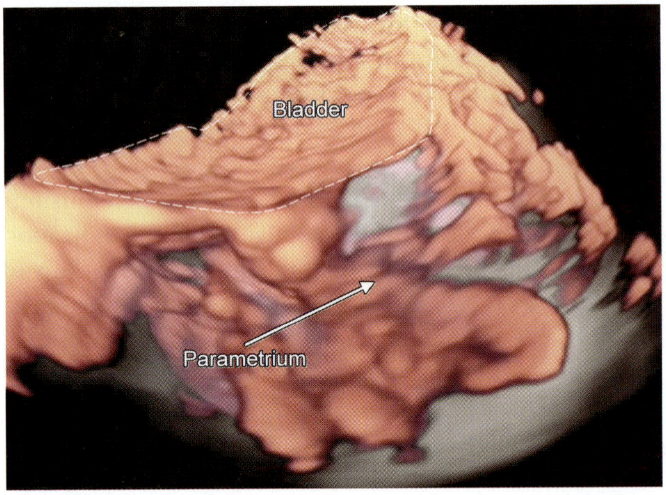

Fig. 21: An other case of placenta percreta on virtual cystoscopy. The image shows the hypervascularization of the uterine serosa-bladder interface. Note the extreme development of neovascularization with confluent vessels involving also the parametrium.

Nuclear magnetic resonance seems to give more information in the diagnosis of acretism when an ultrasound examination is ambiguous or in presence of posterior placental insertion.[69,72] Actually, its employment in clinical management of patients with the risk of PA is to date subject of debate.[70]

In a review of literature, there are almost never big differences in terms of sensitivity and specificity between ultrasound and NMR in the diagnosis of PA.

Nuclear magnetic resonance seems more useful to better define placental acretism degree, selecting cases of placenta increta and percreta. Anyway, few studies confirmed this result, and they are all small case series or case reports.[73,74]

In most cases, magnetic resonance imaging (MRI) does not seem to give more information, compared to ultrasound.[75]

In 2013, Calì et al.'s study on patients with placenta previa and previous CS, ultrasound accuracy was so satisfactory that NMR was not necessary for choosing pre- and intrapartum management **(Figs. 22 and 23)**.[24]

Anyway, in literature, there are no data collection sufficiently large for a comparison between 3D power Doppler ultrasound and NMR.

The individual experience of an obstetrician and radiologist is fundamental; these techniques are strictly operator-dependent in this specific situation.

The guidelines published in 2021 by the Italian Society of obstetric and gynecological ultrasound recommend employing NMR in the study of placenta accreta spectrum,

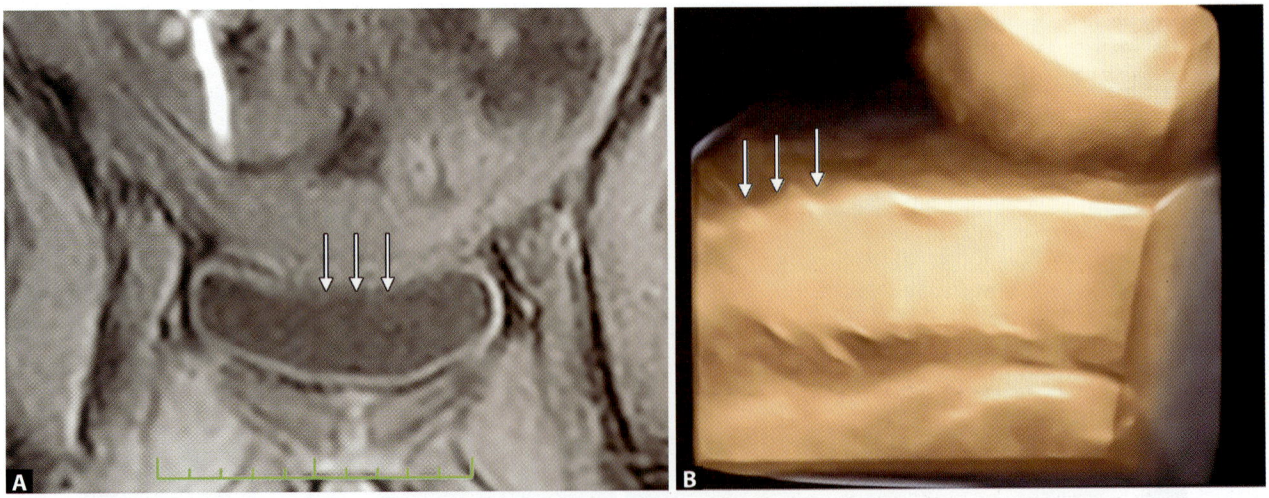

Figs. 22A and B: Comparison between (A) nuclear magnetic resonance (NMR) and (B) 3D ultrasound in the evaluation of bladder invasion in case of placenta percreta. The arrows show the interruption of the bladder line.

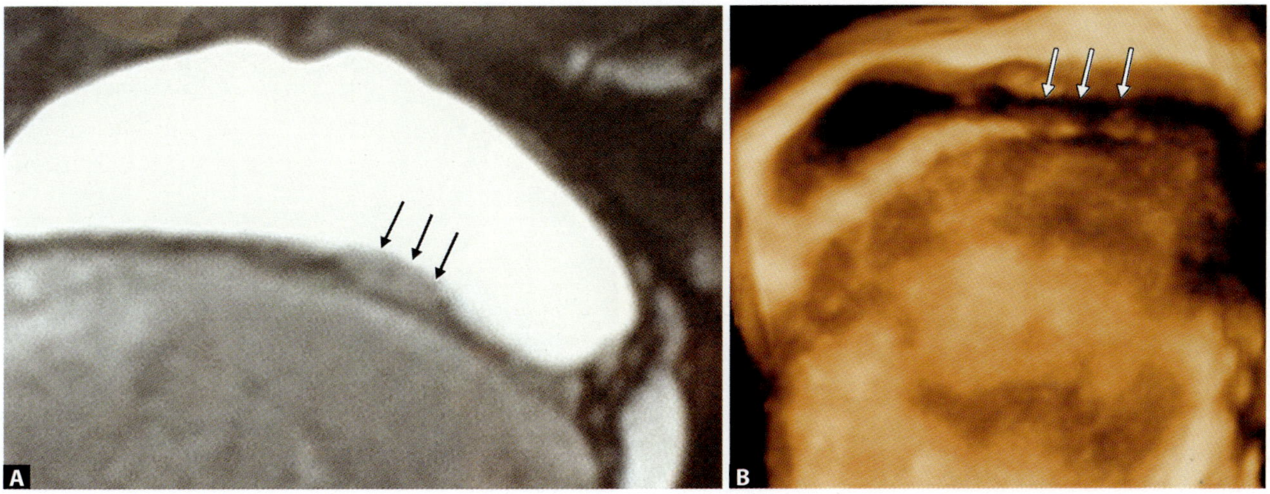

Figs. 23A and B: Other images of comparison between (A) nuclear magnetic resonance (NMR) and (B) 3D ultrasound in diagnosis of placenta percreta.

although not always NMR allows to reach conclusive data.[76]

The most recent literature shows that in a selected population, the diagnostic accuracy of NMR is high. So, we can affirm that it can be a useful diagnostic instrument for a second step, when the ultrasound examination is confounding or in case of posterior placenta.[59,77,78]

In consideration of the importance of diagnosis and the possible severe consequences in case of misdiagnosis, it is appropriate that all suspected cases are subjected to a careful diagnostic study in referral centers, where it is possible to benefit from a more advanced technology and operators with higher experience.[76,79]

Cesarean Scar Pregnancy

Cesarean scar pregnancy (CSP) is a serious consequence of a previous CS: pregnancy with implantation of the gestational sac in the area of the scar of a previous CS. The steadily mounting rate of CS mirrors the increasing number of CSP as well as those of MAP.[80-82]

The true incidence of CSP is unknown. It is estimated in a the range from 1/1,800 to 1/2,500 of all CS performed.[83-85] Previous uterine surgery leads to thin or absent decidua basalis in scarred areas of the lower uterine segment. A low oxygen tension seems to be an important prerequisite for the invading trophoblast.[86,87]

The scar tissue into which the placenta implants may provide the exact environment of low oxygen tension stimulating the cytotrophoblast to deeply invade the scarred area.[88]

Cesarean scar pregnancy is the result of the implantation of blastocyst on the uterine scar or inside the "niche" (dehiscence) left after the healing process of the uterine wall. The mechanism is similar to implantations after uterine surgery (myomectomy, curettage, endometrial ablation, and manual removal of placenta or any intrauterine surgical manipulation).

The niche is usually larger than it appears with a TVU on a sagittal section of the uterus; so, a transverse/coronal section may reveal the real size of the defect. This can be seen on a 3D ultrasound image of the uterus.

Vaginal bleeding may be the first clinical sign of a CSP, which usually is diagnosed before 12–13 weeks. The amount of blood may range from minimal to severe hemorrhage. Pain is usually not the first symptom and some patients may be asymptomatic.

The initial ultrasound examination is critical since many CSPs are misdiagnosed as threatened abortion or simply intrauterine pregnancies.[89]

Such misdiagnoses may lead to a curettage for a presumed failed pregnancy resulting in profuse bleeding and emergency surgical interventions, at times ending with hysterectomy.[90-92]

Every woman in the first trimester with a history of a previous CS and a low, anterior gestational sac with or without heart activity should be considered at risk of CSP until proven otherwise.

The best imaging modality to diagnose a CSP is TVU. Sonographic criteria for CSP identification are as follows **(Fig. 24)**:[93,94]

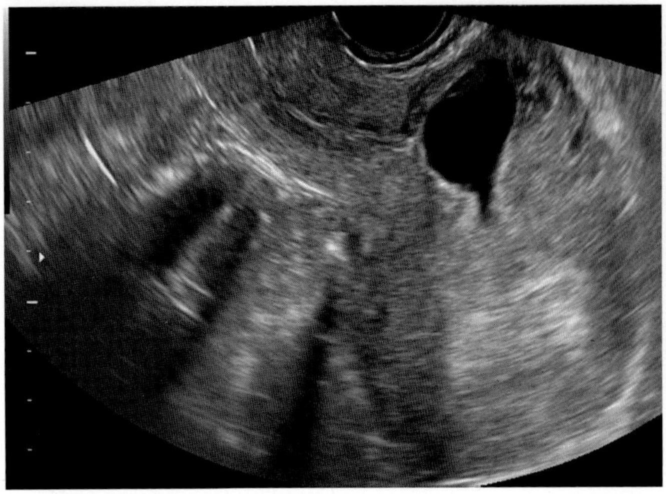

Fig. 24: Cesarean scar pregnancy. The gestational sac is implanted in the niche.

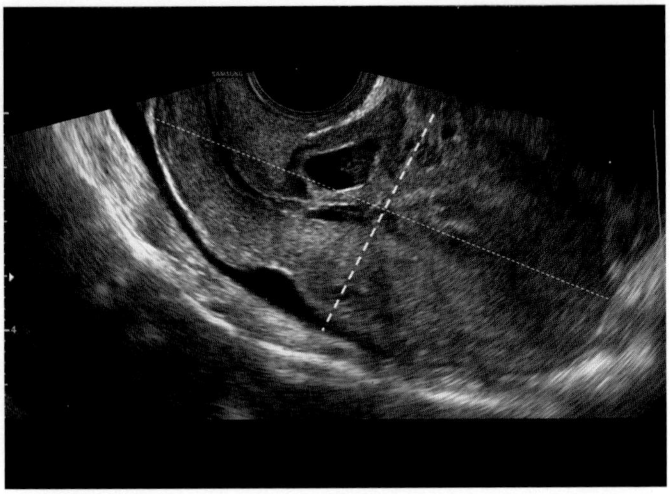

Fig. 25: Cesarean scar pregnancy. The gestational sac is below an imaginary line, which divides the uterus in half.

- An empty uterine cavity and closed empty endocervical canal
- Detection of an early gestational sac and/or placenta in close proximity of the hysterotomy scar/niche with fetal or embryonic pole and/or yolk sac with or without heartbeat. Before the age of 7 GW, the gestational sac may assume the shape of the niche
- An absent or thin appearing myometrial layer between the gestational sac and the bladder wall
- Abundant blood flow around the gestational sac determined by Doppler examination.

The diagnosis of a CSP can easily be made very early by its location in the uterus. The location of the center of the gestational sac relative to the midpoint axis of the uterus can be used as an easy, noninvasive "point-of-service" method for sonographic differentiation of intrauterine pregnancies and CSPs between 5 and 10 completed GW.[95] Dividing the uterus in half by an imaginary line on a longitudinal sagittal scan, we can determine the location of the gestational sac:

- If the gestational sac is above the line, mostly the implantation is normal
- If the gestational sac is below it, we can suspect a CSP or a cervical pregnancy **(Fig. 25)**.

A CSP has differential diagnosis with a cervical pregnancy and a miscarriage in progress in transition, close to the IUO or the cervical canal. Cervical pregnancies are rare and usually do not occur in patients with previous CS.[96]

Miscarriages do not present heart activity. Pressure on the uterus with the vaginal probe at the level of the distorted gestational sac results in a sliding of the sac toward the cervical canal and back when the pressure is released. Instead, a true CSP does not move away.

If in the second trimester, a low, anterior placenta or previa is diagnosed in a patient with a previous CS, the examination of a first-trimester ultrasound image is indicated for a retroactive application of the sonographic criteria of CSP.

CONCLUSIONS

The study of placenta is a fundamental step in the management of pregnancy. Many placental pathologies can occur since the first to the third trimester of gestation, sometimes with severe complications. Prenatal detection of these conditions can significantly improve maternofetal outcomes.

With the increasing incidence of cesarean delivery in the last decades, anomalies of placental implantation and invasion have become an emerging pathology that clinicians must consider with great attention. Prenatal diagnosis plays a fundamental role in identifying patients at risk who must be directed to second level investigations in referral Centers.

REFERENCES

1. Kliman HJ. Trophoblast infiltration. Reprod Med Rev. 1994;3(2):137-57.
2. Kliman HJ. The placenta revealed. Am J Pathol. 1993; 143(2):332-6.
3. Sebire NJ, Sepulveda W. Correlation of placental pathology with prenatal ultrasound findings. Clin Pathol. 2008; 61(12):1276-84.

4. Fox H. The development and structure of the placenta. In: Fox H (Ed). Pathology of the Placenta. Philadelphia: WB Saunders; 1997. pp. 1-16.
5. Abramowicz JS, Sheiner E. Ultrasound of the placenta: a systematic approach. Part I: Imaging. Placenta. 2008;29(3): 225-40.
6. Harris RD, Alexander RD. Ultrasound of the placenta and umbilical cord. In: Callen PW (Ed). Ultrasonography in Obstetrics and Gynecology, 4th edition. Philadelphia: WB Saunders Co; 2000. pp. 597-625.
7. Grannum PA, Berkowitz RL, Hobbins JC. The ultrasonic changes in the maturing placenta and their relation to fetal pulmonic maturity. Am J Obstet Gynecol. 1979;133(8): 915-22.
8. Angtuaco TL, Boyd CM, Marks SR, Quirk JG, Galwas B. Sonographic diagnosis of the bilobate placenta. J Ultrasound Med. 1986;5(11):672-4.
9. Finberg HJ. Umbilical cord and amniotic membranes. In: McGahan JP, Goldberg BB (Eds). Diagnostic ultrasound—a logical approach, 1st edition. Philadelphia: Lippincott-Raven Publishers; 1998. pp. 201-29.
10. Predanic M, Perni SC, Baergen RN, Chasen ST. A sonographic assessment of different patterns of placenta previa "migration" in the third trimester of pregnancy. J Ultrasound Med. 2005;24(6):773-80.
11. Ekoukou D, Ng Wing Tin L, Nere MB, Bourdet O, Elalaoui Y, Bazin C. Placenta membranacea. Review of the literature, a case report. J Gynecol Obstet Biol Reprod (Paris). 1995;24(2):189-93.
12. Greenberg JA, Sorem KA, Shifren JL, Riley LE. Placenta membranacea with placenta increta: a case report and literature review. Obstet Gynecol. 1991;78(3 Pt 2):512-4.
13. McCarthy J, Thurmond AS, Jones MK, Sistrom C, Scanlan RM, Jacobson SL, et al. Circumvallate placenta: sonographic diagnosis. J Ultrasound Med. 1995;14(1):21-6.
14. Harris RD, Wells WA, Black WC, Chertoff JD, Poplack SP, Sargent SK, et al. Accuracy of prenatal sonography for detecting circumvallate placenta. AJR Am J Roentgenol. 1997;168(6):1603-8.
15. Tikkanen M. Placental abruption: epidemiology, risk factors and consequences. Acta Obstet Gynecol Scand. 2011;90(2):140-9.
16. Tikkanen M. Etiology, clinical manifestations, and prediction of placental abruption. Acta Obstet Gynecol Scand. 2010;89(6):732-40.
17. Nyberg DA, Mc Gahan JP, Pretorius DH, Pilu G. The placenta Umbilical Cord and Membranes—Placental Hemorrhage/ Abruption. In: "Diagnostic Imaging of fetal Anomalies". Lippincot: Williams & Wilkins; 2003. pp. 99-102.
18. Nyberg DA, Cyr DR, Mack LA, Wilson DA, Shuman WP. Sonographic spectrum of placental abruption. AJR Am J Roentgenol. 1987;148(1):161-4.
19. FIGO Oncology Committee. FIGO staging for gestational trophoblastic neoplasia 2000. FIGO Oncology Committee. Int J Gynaecol Obstet. 2002;77(3):285-7.
20. Palmer JE, Macdonald M, Wells M, Hancock BW, Tidy JA. Epithelioid trophoblastic tumor: a review of the literature. J Reprod Med. 2008;53(7):465-75.
21. Nguyen D, Nguyen C, Yacobozzi M, Bsat F, Rakita D. Imaging of the placenta with pathologic correlation. Semin Ultrasound CT MRI. 2012;33(1):65-77.
22. Guschmann M, Henrich W, Entezami M, Dudenhausen JW. Chorioangioma—new insights into a well-known problem. I. Results of a clinical and morphological study of 136 cases. J Perinat Med. 2003;31(2):163-9.
23. Abramowicz JS, Sheiner E. In utero imaging of the placenta: importance for diseases of pregnancy. Placenta. 2007;28 Suppl A:S14-22.
24. Calì G, Giambanco L, Puccio G, Forlani F. Morbidly adherent placenta: an evaluation of ultrasound diagnostic criteria and an attempt to differentiate placenta accreta from percreta. Ultrasound Obstet Gynecol. 2013;41(4):406-12.
25. Wolfe BK, Wallace JHK. Pitfall to avoid: chorioangioma of the placenta simulating fetal tumor. J Clin Ultrasound. 1987;15(6):405-8.
26. Reinhart RD, Wells WA, Harris RD. Focal aneurysmal dilatation of subchorionic vessels simulating chorioangioma. Ultrasound Obstet Gynecol. 1999;13(2):147-9.
27. Braun T, Brauer M, Fuchs I, Czernik C, Dudenhausen JW, Henrich W, et al. Mirror syndrome: a systematic review of fetal associated conditions, maternal presentation and perinatal outcome. Fetal Diagn Ther. 2010;27(4):191-203.
28. Moscoso G, Jauniaux E, Hustin J. Placental vascular anomaly with diffuse mesenchymal stem villous hyperplasia. A new clinicopathological entity? Pathol Res Pract. 1991;187(2-3):324-8.
29. Arizawa M, Nakayama M. Suspected involvement of the X chromosome in placental mesenchymal dysplasia. Congenital Anomalies. 2002;42(4):309-17.
30. Nayeri UA, West AB, Grossetta Nardini HK, Copel JA, Sfakianaki AK. Systematic review of sonographic findings of placental mesenchymal dysplasia and subsequent pregnancy outcome. Ultrasound Obstet Gynecol. 2013; 41(4):366-74.
31. Robertson M, Geerts LT, de Jong G, Wainwright H. Mesenchymal dysplasia in a monochorionic diamniotic twin pregnancy with review of the differential diagnosis of cystic changes in the placenta. J Ultrasound Med. 2007;26(5):689-93.
32. Gizzo S, Gangi SD, Patrelli TS, Saccardi C, Antona D, Nardelli GB. Placental mesenchymal dysplasia: can early diagnosis ensure a good materno-fetal outcome? A case report. Arch Gynecol Obstet. 2012;286(1):15-7.
33. Parveen Z, Tongson-Ignacio JE, Fraser CR, Killeen JL, Thompson KS. Placental mesenchymal dysplasia. Arch Pathol Lab Med. 2007;131(1):131-7.
34. Umazume T, Kataoka S, Kamamuta K, Tanuma F, Sumie A, Shirogane T, et al. Placental mesenchymal dysplasia: a case of intrauterine sudden death of fetus with rupture

of cirsoid periumbilical chorionic vessels. Diagn Pathol. 2011;6:38.
35. Gibson BR, Padilla JM, Champeaux A, Suarez ES. Mesenchymal dysplasia of the placenta. Placenta. 2004; 25(7):671-2.
36. Pham T, Steele J, Stayboldt C, Chan L, Benirschke K. Placental mesenchymal dysplasia is associated with high rates of intrauterine growth restriction and fetal demise. Am J Clin Pathol. 2006;126(1):67-78.
37. Paradinas FJ, Sebire NJ, Fisher RA, Rees HC, Foskett M, Seckl MJ, et al. Pseudo-partial moles: placental stem vessel hydrops and the association with Beckwith-Wiedemann syndrome and complete moles. Histopathology. 2001; 39(5):447-54.
38. Heazell AEP, Sahasrabudhe N, Grossmith AK, Martindale EA, Bhatia K. A case of intrauterine growth restriction in association with placental mesenchymal dysplasia with abnormal placental lymphatic development. Placenta. 2009;30(7):654-7.
39. Committee on Obstetric Practice ACOG Committee opinion. Placenta accrete. No 266, January 2002. Int J Obstet Gynecol. 2002;77(1):77-8.
40. Izabela UW, Krzysztof N, Ryszard P, Aneta P. Placenta previa increta with caesarean section scar invasion. Ginekol Pol. 2011;82(6):471-3.
41. Miller DA, Chollet JA, Goodwin TM. Clinical risk factors for placenta previa-placenta accrete. Am J Obstet Gynecol. 1997;177(1):210-4.
42. Esakoff TF, Sparks TN, Kaimal AJ, Kim LH, Feldstein VA, Goldstein RB, et al. Diagnosis and morbidity of placenta accreta. Ultrasound Obstet Gynecol. 2011;37(3):324-7.
43. Gielchinsky Y, Rojansky N, Fasouliotis SJ, Ezra Y. Placenta accrete—summary of 10 years: a survey of 310 cases. Placenta. 2002;23(2-3):210-4.
44. Clark SL, Koonings PP, Phelan JP. Placenta previa/accrete and prior caesarean section. Obstet Gynecol. 1985;66(1): 89-92.
45. Spong CY, Berghella V, Wenstrom KD, Mercer BM, Saade GR. Preventing the first cesarean delivery: summary of a joint Eunice Kennedy Shriver National Institute of Child Health and Human Development, Society for Maternal-Fetal Medicine, and American College of Obstetricians and Gynecologists Workshop. Obstet Gynecol. 2012;120(5):1181-93.
46. Arnold J. (2012). World Cesarean Rates: OECD Countries. Available from: https://www.cesareanrates.org/ [Last accessed June, 2024].
47. Calì G, Giambanco L. Abnormal placental adherence: An obstetrical arising complication. A proposal of early diagnostic work-up. Ital J Gynaecol Obstet. 2011;23(1):9-18.
48. Leerentveld RA, Gilberts ECAM, Arnold KJCW, Wladimiroff JW. Accuracy and safety of transvaginal sonographic placental localization. Obstet Gynecol. 1990;76(5 Pt 1):759-62.
49. Cho JY, Lee YH, Moon MH, Lee JH. Difference in migration of placenta according to the location and type of placenta previa. J Clin Ultrasound. 2008;36(2):79-84.
50. Morrison J. The development of the lower uterine segment. Aust NZ J Obstet Gynaecol. 1982;12(3):182-5.
51. Benirschke K, Kaufmann P. The pathology of the human placenta. New York: Springer-Verlag; 1990. pp. 202-4.
52. Lauria MR, Smith RS, Treadwell MC, Comstock CH, Kirk JS, Lee W, et al. The use of second-trimester transvaginal sonography to predict placenta previa. Ultrasound Obstet Gynecol. 1996;8(5):337-40.
53. Oppenheimer L, Holmes P, Simpson N, Dabrowsky A. Diagnosis of low-lying placenta: can migration in the third trimester predictor outcome? Ultrasound Obstet Gynecol. 2001;18(2):100-2.
54. Calì G. Prevention of postpartum hemorrhage and hysterectomy in patients with morbidly adherent placenta: A cohort study comparing outcomes before and after introduction of the Triple-P procedure. V Teixidor Viñas, AM Belli, S Arulkumaran and E Chandraharan. Ultrasound Obstet Gynecol 2015;46:350-355. Ultrasound Obstet Gynecol. 2015;46(3):265.
55. D'Antonio F, Palacios-Jaraquemada J, Lim PS, Forlani F, Lanzone A, Timor-Tritsch I, et al. Counseling in fetal medicine: evidence-based answers to clinical questions on morbidly adherent placenta. Ultrasound Obstet Gynecol. 2016;47(3):290-301.
56. Lerner JP, Deane S, Timor-Tritsch IE. Characterization of placenta accreta using transvaginal sonography and color Doppler imaging. Ultrasound Obstet Gynecol. 1995;5(3):198-201.
57. Chou MM, Ho ES, Lee YH. Prenatal diagnosis of placenta previa accreta by transabdominal color Doppler ultrasound. Ultrasound Obstet Gynecol. 2000;15(1):28-35.
58. Comstock CH, Love JJ Jr, Bronsteen RA, Lee W, Vettraino IM, Huang RR, et al. Sonographic detection of placenta accreta in the second and third trimesters of pregnancy. Am J Obstet Gynecol. 2004;190(4):1135-40.
59. Comstock CH. Antenatal diagnosis of placenta accreta: a review. Ultrasound Obstet Gynecol. 2005;26(1):89-96.
60. Callan PW, Filly RA. The placental-subplacental complex: a specific indicator of placental position on ultrasound. J Clin Ultrasound. 1980;8(1):21-6.
61. McGahan JP, Phillips HE, Reid MH. The anechoic retroplacental area: a pitfall in diagnosis of placental-endometrial abnormalities during pregnancy. Radiology. 1980;134(2):475-8.
62. Pasto ME, Kurtz AB, Rifkin MD, Cole-Beuglet C, Wapner RJ, Goldberg BB. Ultrasonographic findings in placenta increta. J Ultrasound Med. 1983;2(4):155-9.
63. Finberg HJ, Williams JW. Placenta accreta: prospective sonographic diagnosis in patients with placenta previa and prior cesarean section. J Ultrasound Med. 1992;11(7):333-43.

64. Wong HS, Cheung YK, Zuccollo J, Tait J, Pringle KC. Evaluation of sonographic diagnostic criteria for placenta accreta. J Clin Ultrasound. 2008;36(9):551-9.
65. Shih JC, Palacios Jaraquemada JM, Su YN, Shyu MK, Lin CH, Lin SY, et al. Role of three-dimensional power Doppler in the antenatal diagnosis of placenta accreta: comparison with gray-scale and color Doppler techniques. Ultrasound Obstet Gynecol. 2009;33(2):193-203.
66. D'Antonio F, Iacovella C, Bhide A. Prenatal identification of invasive placentation using ultrasound: systematic review and meta-analysis. Ultrasound Obstet Gynecol. 2013;42(5):509-17.
67. Comstock CH. The antenatal diagnosis of placental attachment disorders. Curr Opin Obstet Gynecol. 2011; 23(2):117-22.
68. Chou MM, Chen W, Tseng J, Chen Y, Yeh T, Chu E. Prenatal detection of bladder wall involvement in invasive placentation with sequential two-dimensional and adjunctive three- dimensional ultrasonography. Taiwan J Obstet Gynecol. 2009;48(1):38-45.
69. Levine D, Hulka CA, Ludmir J, Li W, Edelman RR. Placenta accreta: evaluation with color Doppler US, Power Doppler US, and MR imaging. Radiology. 1997;205(3):773-6.
70. Royal College of Obstetricians & Gynaecologists. (2011). Placenta praevia, placenta praevia accreta and vasa praevia: diagnosis and management. RCOG Green-top Guideline No. 27. Available from: https://www.rcog.org.uk/guidance/browse-all-guidance/green-top-guidelines/placenta-praevia-placenta-praevia-accreta-and-vasa-praevia-diagnosis-and-management-green-top-guideline-no-27/ [Last accessed June, 2024].
71. Calì G, Forlani F. Three-dimensional sonographic virtual cystoscopy in a case of placenta percreta. Ultrasound Obstet Gynecol. 2014;43(4):481-2.
72. Palacios-Jaraquemada JM. Diagnosis and management of placenta accreta. Best Pract Res Clin Obstet Gynaecol. 2008;22(6):1133-48.
73. DeFriend DE, Dubbins PA, Hughes PM. Sacculation of the uterus and placenta accreta: MRI appearances. Br J Radiol. 2000;73(876):1323-5.
74. Maldjian C, Adam R, Pelosi M, Pelosi M 3rd, Rudelli RD, Maldjian J. MRI appearance of placenta percreta and placenta accreta. Mag Reson Imaging. 1999;17(7):965-71.
75. Ito T, Katagiri C, Ikeno S, Takahashi H, Nagata N, Terakawa N. Placenta previa increta penetrating the entire thickness of the uterine myometrium: ultrasonographic and magnetic resonance imaging findings. J Obstet Gynaecol Res. 1999; 25(5):303-7.
76. Società Italiana di Ecografia Ostetrico Ginecologicae Metodologie Biofisiche. Linee guida per ecografia ostetrica e ginecologica 2021. Editeam. Available from: https://www.sieog.it/wp-content/uploads/2021/11/LINEE-GUIDA-MINISTERIALI-SIEOG-2021-compresso.pdf
77. Warshak CR, Eskander R, Hull AD, Scioscia AL, Mattrey RF, Benirschke K, et al. Accuracy of ultrasonography and magnetic resonance imaging in the diagnosis of placenta accreta. Obstet Gynecol. 2006;108(3 Pt 1):573-81.
78. Palacios-Jaraquemada JM. Efficacy of surgical tecniques to control obstetric hemorrhage: analysis of 539 cases. Acta Obstet Gynecol Scand. 2011;90(9):1036-42.
79. Calì G, Giambanco L, Vallone M, Fundarò G, Buonasorte R, Amico ML, et al. Placenta accreta: multidisciplinary management improves maternal outcome. Int J Gynaecol Obstet. 2012;119(S3):S357-S358.
80. Timor-Tritsch IE, Monteagudo A, Cali G, Palacios-Jaraquemada JM, Maymon R, Arslan AA, et al. Cesarean scar pregnancy and early placenta accreta share common histology. Ultrasound Obstet Gynecol. 2014;43(4):383-95.
81. Timor-Tritsch IE, Monteagudo A, Cali G, Vintzileos A, Viscarello R, Al-Khan A, et al. Cesarean scar pregnancy is a precursor of morbidly adherent placenta. Ultrasound Obstet Gynecol. 2014;44(3):346-53.
82. Timor-Tritsch IE, Monteagudo A, Calì G, Viscarello R, Mayberry P, Vintzileos A, et al. Sonographically-proven caesarean scar pregnancies (CSP) can result in a live offspring and morbidly adherent placenta (MAP). Ultrasound Obstet Gynecol. 2014;44(S1):178.
83. Jurkovic D, Hillaby K, Woelfer B, Lawrence A, Salim R, Elson CJ. Cesarean scar pregnancy. Ultrasound Obstet Gynecol. 2003;21(3):310.
84. Jurkovic D, Hillaby K, Woelfer B, Lawrence A, Salim R, Elson CJ. First-trimester diagnosis and management of pregnancies implanted into the lower uterine segment Cesarean section scar. Ultrasound Obstet Gynecol. 2003;21(3):220-7.
85. Rotas MA, Haberman S, Levgur M. Cesarean scar ectopic pregnancies: etiology, diagnosis, and management. Obstet Gynecol. 2006;107(6):1373-81.
86. Rosen T. Placenta accreta and cesarean scar pregnancy: overlooked costs of the rising cesarean section rate. Clin Perinatol. 2008;35(3):519-29, x.
87. Norwitz ER. Defective implantation and placentation: laying the blueprint for pregnancy complications. Reprod Biomed Online. 2006;13(4):591-9.
88. Kliman HJ, Feinberg RF, Haimowitz JE. Human trophoblast- endometrial interactions in an in vitro suspension culture system. Placenta. 1990;11(4):349-67.
89. Giambanco L, Doveri T, Amico ML, Forlani F, Incandela D, Alio L, et al. Scar pregnancies: early diagnosis allows conservative non surgical management. Supplement to Int J Gynecol Obstet. 2012;119(3):261-530.
90. Timor-Tritsch IE, Calì G, Monteagudo A, Ramos J, Berg RE, Forlani F. The use of a Foley balloon catheter as an adjuvant in treating caesarean scar (CSP) and cervical pregnancies (CxP). Ultrasound Obstet Gynecol. 2014; 44(S1):308.

91. Timor-Tritsch IE, Calì G, Monteagudo A, Khatib N, Berg RE, Forlani Fet al. Foley balloon catheter to prevent or manage bleeding during treatment for cervical and cesarean scar pregnancy. Ultrasound Obstet Gynecol. 2014;46(1): 118-23.
92. Timor-Tritsch IE, Calì G, Monteagudo A, Berg R, Forlani F. The adjuvant, hemostatic use of a Foley balloon catheter in the treatment of cesarean scar and cervical pregnancies. Ultrasound Med Biol. 2015;41(4):S59.
93. Timor-Tritsch IE, Monteagudo A. Unforeseen consequences of the increasing rate of cesarean deliveries: early placenta accreta and cesarean scar pregnancy. A review. Am J Obstet Gynecol. 2012;207(1):14-29.
94. Timor-Tritsch IE, Monteagudo A, Santos R, Tsymbal T, Pineda G, Arslan AA. The diagnosis, treatment, and follow-up of cesarean scar pregnancy. Am J Obstet Gynecol. 2012;207(1):44e1-e13.
95. Timor-Tritsch IE, Monteagudo A, Calì G, El Refaey H, Arslan AA. How to avoid misdiagnosis of cesarean scar pregnancy: an easy and reliable method for sonographic differentiation of the 5–10 completed weeks intrauterine and cesarean scar pregnancies. (in press).
96. Alio L, Giambanco L, Alio W, Doveri T, Incandela D, Calì G. Cervical pregnancy in a nulliparous woman: case report. Int J Gynecol Obstet. 2012;119:S275.

CHAPTER 29

Measurement of Cervical Length

Oliver Vasilj, Berivoj Miskovic

INTRODUCTION

Preterm birth (PB) is one of the greatest challenges in modern perinatal medicine. Despite the improvements in perinatal management over the last two decades the rate of PB has not declined and it is still a major cause of perinatal morbidity and mortality.[1] One of the reasons behind this is the fact that the complex underlying ethiopathogenic causes of PB are not fully understood yet. The role of uterine cervix in PB is undisputed.

GENERAL FACTS ABOUT UTERINE CERVIX

The uterine cervix is a unique organ composed predominately of extracellular matrix, proteins, collagen, elastin and glycosaminoglycans. Among all biological processes, the phenomenal connective tissue remodeling that occurs in the cervix during and after parturition is unparalleled in scope and magnitude. During the pregnancy cervix undergoes changes that have to be understood prior to transvaginal ultrasonography (TVU) assessment. It changes from a closed, rigid structure before pregnancy to a soft, distensible organ proximate to parturition. Cervical remodeling begins soon after conception and continues throughout pregnancy and the puerperium. It consists of four overlapping phases:

1. Softening alone
2. Ripening (softening with effacement, dilation and change in position)
3. Dilation in response to contractions and
4. Postpartum repair.[2]

Dynamic changes and shortening of the cervix during pregnancy differs from one pregnant woman to another. Mean reduction in cervical length in mid second trimester of pregnancy is around 1.1 mm, but it may be as high as 2.7 mm weekly.[3] This data may be used only for primiparous patients as multiparous patients have different dynamic of cervical shortening.[3,4] According to studies the 50th percentiles for cervical length before 20 weeks of gestation is 40 mm and at 22 to 32 weeks of gestation is 35 mm.[5]

What is Cervical Insufficiency?

Cervical insufficiency (CI) is defined as asymptomatic cervical dilatation in second and third trimester of pregnancy.[6] Causes of CI may be congenital or acquired. The congenital causes include biological variations in cervical length and collagen or uterine anomalies, all of these can affect the way the cervix functions during pregnancy. [7] Acquired factors that are most commonly attributed to CI are different mechanical or operative procedures on cervix (pregnancy termination with dilatation, hysteroscopy, cervical biopsy, laser ablation, loop excision or cold knife conization).[7] It is unclear whether the increase is due to procedure-related structural injury leading to CI, adverse effects of the underlying cervical disease on cervical function or another mechanism such as subclinical upper genital tract infection.[7] It has been shown that processes that lead to both term and preterm spontaneous labor resemble an inflammatory reaction. Up regulation of inflammatory cytokines and prostaglandins that occurs over a period of several weeks leads to cervical ripening and membrane rupture.[1] This will again lead to myometrial contractility and labor.[1] The cervix acts as a barrier to this stimulus maintaining the distance from the vagina and retaining the cervical mucus plug as an additional barrier. Women with a short cervix or CI will be at much greater risk of this cervical barrier being breached.

Diagnosis of Cervical Insufficiency

Detection of CI in the first pregnancy is difficult because the symptoms are usually dismissed as normal pregnancy effects, so that cervical effacement and dilation often progress to a clinical presentation of a bulging amniotic sac or ruptured membranes. The diagnosis of CI is based on a combination of past and present pregnancy history, physical examination and ultrasound findings.

The main goal of physical examination is digital palpation and visualization of the cervix using a speculum. The physical examination is a subjective method and is not ideal for assessment and prediction of PB. This was clearly shown in our study, where the physical examination was compared with ultrasonographic examination of the cervix in the low-risk population regarding the prediction of PB.[6]

Transvaginal ultrasonography is the gold standard for assessment of cervix in pregnancy. Transabdominal and transperineal ultrasound of the cervix can be used but are more difficult and less precise than TVU.[8] If screening of cervical changes in pregnancy is employed to predict PB, this should be done with TVU and not with physical exam or a different ultrasound technique. The TVU cervical measurement is a well-described method with intra and interobserver variations that are acceptable for clinical use.[9]

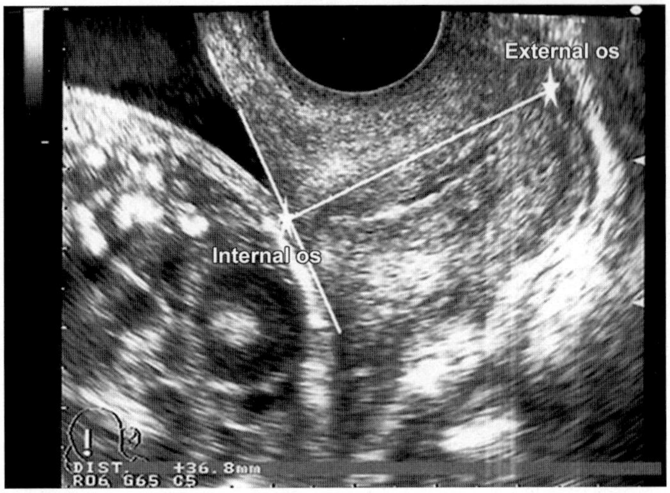

Fig. 1: The ultrasound assessment of the cervix in pregnancy. Normal "T" shape of the cervix. The linear measurement of cervical length between internal and external os is presented.

Transvaginal Ultrasonographic Cervical Assessment and Recommendations for Clinical Application

Measurement of cervical length by TVU examination is a technique that can be learnt rapidly. About 23 supervised ultrasound scans appear necessary for an operator with no experience in TVU.[10] Substantially fewer are required for an operator already familiar with this approach for other indications.[10] For an adequate exam the maternal bladder has to be emptied. Ultrasound gel is placed on a transvaginal probe before covering it with a condom or specialized cover and then more ultrasound gel is placed on the cover. If the membranes are ruptured sterile materials should be used. The transducer should be placed in the anterior fornix until the cervix is visualized. The image is enlarged to fill at least one-half of the ultrasound screen. The appropriate sagittal view for measuring cervical length includes the V-shaped notch at the internal os, the triangular area of echo density at the external os, and the endocervical canal, which appears as a faint line of echo density or echolucency between the two. Cervical length is the linear distance between calipers placed at the internal and external os and should only be determined from images when the anterior and posterior lips of the cervix are of equal thickness **(Fig. 1)**. When three measurements have been obtained that satisfy measurement criteria the shortest is chosen and recorded as the "shortest best." If the cervix is curved there is no need to measure it in several points or by using a tracer since in these cases the cervical length is usually very long and no additional clinical information is obtained by these procedures.

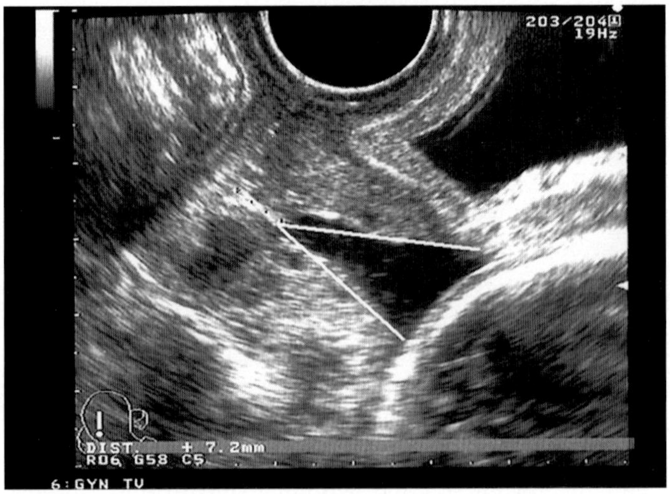

Fig. 2: "V" shape of the cervix.

Two ultrasound based criteria are found to be related to CI. These are the length of the closed part of the cervical canal and the shape of the internal cervical os ("T" **Fig. 1**, "V" **Fig. 2**, "Y" **Fig. 3**, "U" so called "funneling" **Fig. 4**).[11] Funneling is defined in percentages according to the ratio of the funnel length to the total cervical length (funnel length + remaining closed cervix). The presence or absence of a funnel and its length should be recorded

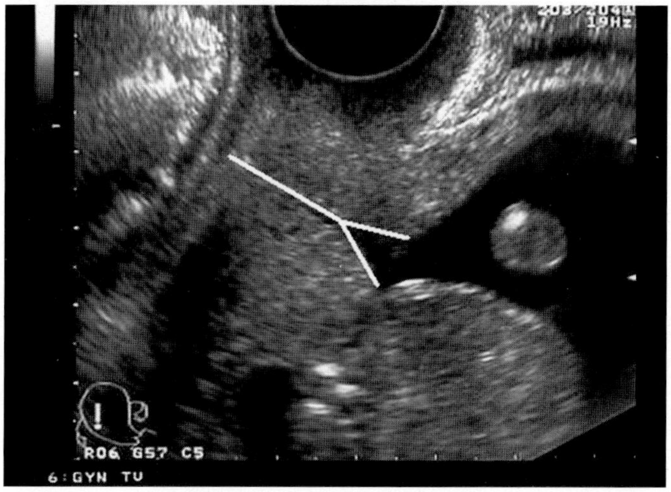

Fig. 3: "Y" shape of the cervix.

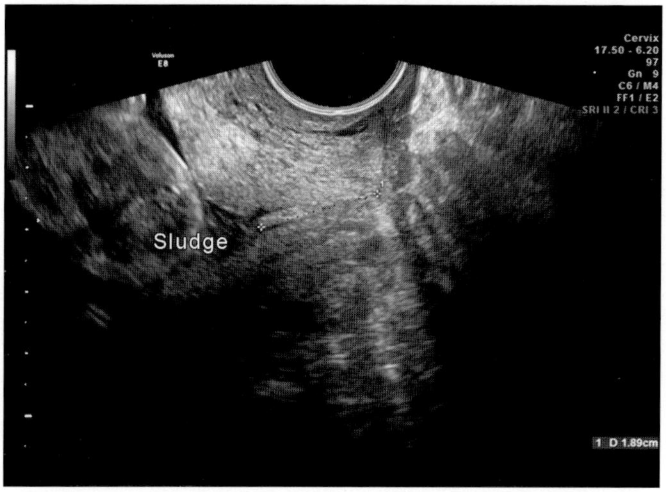

Fig. 5: Cervical sludge at the level of internal cervical os.

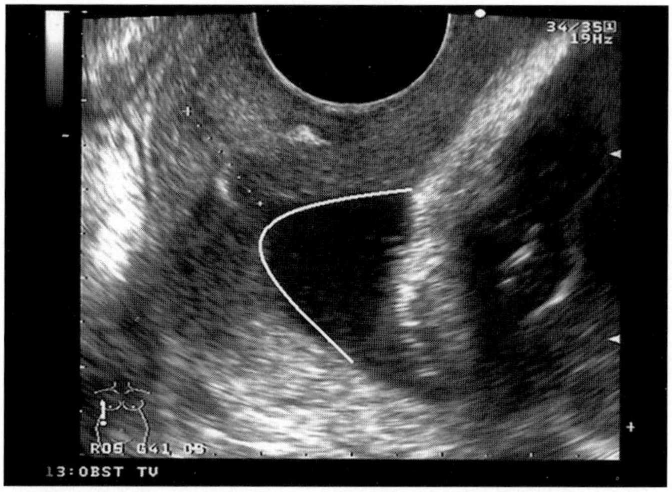

Fig. 4: Funneling or "U" shape cervix suspicious of cervical insufficiency.

but it is believed that funneling is not clinically important. If funneling is present, the length of the residual closed portion of the cervix is recorded as the true length of the cervix. The length of the funnel is often uncertain because landmarks, such as the shoulder of the internal os, may not be distinct. Dynamic spontaneous funneling seen occasionally above a normal length cervix has little prognostic value.[12]

Intraamniotic debris ('sludge') refers to the sonographic finding of hyperechoic matter in the amniotic fluid close to the internal cervical os. The composition of the debris is unclear; it may be blood clot, meconium, vernix, or cellular material related to infection/inflammation. Some studies, but not all, have reported an association between the presence of intra-amniotic debris and preterm delivery and other pregnancy complications **(Fig. 5)**.[13,14]

The most common mistake during TVU of the cervix is the excess pressure on the anterior cervical lip with the artificial elongation of cervical canal. This can be avoided by withdrawing the probe when the internal and external os are visualized until slight blurring occurs, and then the probe is inserted slightly until a clear image returns.

With well-known cervical length and shape in recent years, a new ultrasound based parameter of CI was presented. The presence of cervical glands and cervical mucus were introduced as additional parameters used in order to define CI.[15,16] The hypoechogenic translucency of cervical mucus area in the middle of the endocervical canal was measured by area trace.[16] Hypo- or hyperechogenic translucencies surrounding the canal that probably corresponds to the histological cervical gland area was measured under a 90° angle from the endocervical canal, as the linear distance from the outer boundary of the deepest invasion of cervical glands.[16] Sonographic images of cervical glands and cervical mucus are presented in **Figures 6 and 7**. In our study it was shown that absence or diminishment of glandular area of the cervix could be one of the early signs of PB.[16] We defined a new term Qualitative Glandular Cervical Score (GQCS).[16] As a potential screening test for PB low QGCS had sensitivity 83.3% (≤34 weeks) and 55.5% (34–37 weeks) with positive predictive value (PPV) 31.2% (≤34 and 34–37 weeks). Shortened CL had sensitivity 66.6% (≤ 34 weeks) and 22.2% (34–37 weeks) with PPV 23.5% (≤34 weeks) and

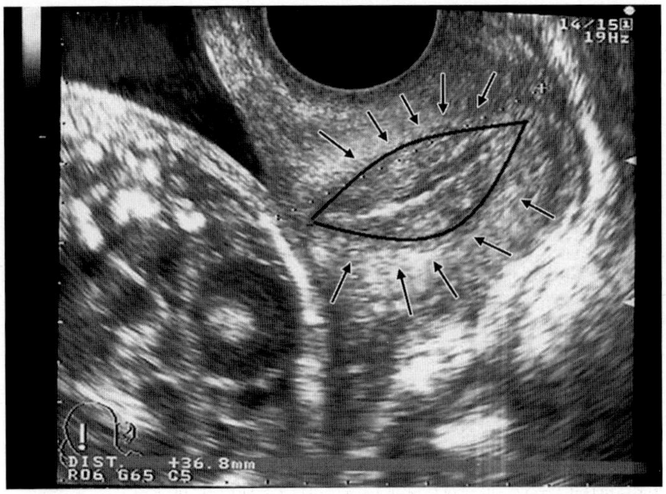

Fig. 6: The presence of cervical glands as a normal finding.

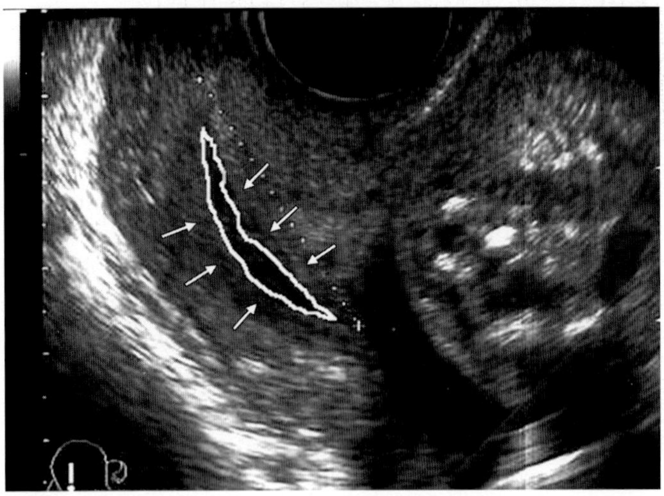

Fig. 7: Cervical mucus anechoic translucency inside the cervical canal measured with area trace.

11.7% (34–37 weeks).[20] The diagnostic accuracy of this test in predication of risk for PB was the same if not better than the sole measurement of the closed part of the cervical canal.[16]

In recent years three-dimensional ultrasound was introduced in the screening program for detection of CI. It was not found to be significantly better regarding the measurements of the cervical length but it introduced the new term of cervical volumetry that may be of help in the further assessment programs.[17]

Numerous studies evaluating the use of TVU cervical measurement for prediction of PB in asymptomatic and symptomatic high-risk and low-risk women were performed. The following is a summary of recommendations for the use of TVU cervical assessment in prediction of PB:

- Transvaginal ultrasound does not differentiate between CI and other causes of short cervix. It identifies women who are at higher risk of PB regardless of the etiology, and one of those etiologies may be CI. The risk of PB is highest for cervical length below the 10th percentile (about 25 mm between 22 and 30 weeks of gestation), there is no threshold value and not all patients with a short cervix will have PB.[18]
- In asymptomatic women with a history of spontaneous PB measurement of cervical length in the second trimester predicted risk of recurrence.[1]
- The low sensitivity and low PPV of cervical length screening limit the usefulness of this test in low-risk asymptomatic obstetric populations. Thus the use of sonographic measurement of cervical length to screen low-risk populations to determine risk of PB is not recommended.[19]
- In symptomatic women the use of TVU may be useful for distinguishing women with false preterm labor. A high negative predictive value was shown for a 30 mm threshold, but there is no threshold of cervical length that establishes diagnosis.[20]

Is Cerclage Needed?

Cochrane database of systematic reviews included a total of 12 randomized controlled studies involving 3,328 pregnant women at high-risk of pregnancy loss. When cerclage was compared with no treatment (nine trials), there was no clear difference in the number of babies dying before (as a result of miscarriages, stillbirths) or around the time of birth or neonatal illness, despite a clear reduction in the number of preterm births. Compared with no treatment, cervical cerclage reduces the incidence of preterm birth in women at risk of recurrent preterm birth without statistically significant reduction in perinatal mortality or neonatal morbidity and uncertain long-term impact on the baby. Cesarean section is more likely in women who had cervical suture inserted during pregnancy.

The authors conclusion on how best to minimize the risk of recurrent preterm birth in women at risk, either because of poor history of a short or dilated cervix, should be 'personalized', based on the clinical circumstances, the skill and expertise of the clinical team and, most importantly, woman's informed choice.[21]

What the Future Might Bring?

The limitation of cervicometry is in the fact that it assesses only the cervical length. The consistency of cervix is a very important factor as well. Recently, a novel approach to this problem has been described. The main focus behind this new approach is based on biochemical and biophysical changes associated with cervical ripening.[22] Changes in collagen organization, water content, as well as concentration of proteoglycans in the extracellular matrix are considered to be the basis for the modifications in biomechanical properties that make a cervix soft or hard.[23] Elastography measures the percentage of tissue deformation that occurs when oscillatory compression is applied.[24] The degree of tissue deformation can be expressed as strain where increased strain reflects increased deformation (softer tissue), while decreasing strain reflects reduced deformation (stiffer tissue).[25] Standardized protocol for obtaining cervical strain measurements in pregnancy has been describe with estimated strain values differed across anatomical planes and regions of interest. Cervical strain values differed even further by patient characteristics including parity and prior preterm delivery, gestational age at examination, and cervical length.[26] The risk of spontaneous preterm delivery was significantly lower in women with low strain (stiffer tissue) values obtained in the internal cervical os. The authors conclude that ultrasound elastography may have a role in the assessment of risk for preterm delivery.[27]

REFERENCES

1. Conde-Agudelo A, Romero R. Predictive accuracy of changes in transvaginal sonographic cervical length over time for preterm birth: a systematic review and metaanalysis. Am J Obstet Gynecol. 2015;213(6):789-801.
2. Word RA, Li XH, Hnat M, Carrick K. Dynamics of cervical remodeling during pregnancy and parturition: mechanisms and current concepts. Semin Reprod Med. 2007;25:69.
3. Bergelin I, Valentin L. Patterns of normal change in cervical length and width during pregnancy in nulliparous women: a prospective, longitudinal ultrasound study: Ultrasound Obstet Gynecol. 2001;18:217-22.
4. Bergelin I, Valentin L. Normal cervical changes in parous women during the second half of pregnancy—a prospective, longitudinal ultrasound study. Acta Obstet Gynecol Scand. 2002;81:31-8.
5. Hibbard JU, Tart M, Moawad, AH. Cervical length at 16-22 weeks' gestation and risk for preterm delivery. Obstet Gynecol. 2000;96:972.
6. Matijevic R, Grgc O, Vasilj O. Is sonograpic assessment of the cervical length better than digital examination in screening for preterm delivery in a low risk population? Acta Obstet Gynecol Scand. 2006;85(11):1342-7.
7. Vyas NA, Vink JS, Ghidini A, et al. Risk factors for cervical insufficiency after term delivery. Am J Obstet Gynecol. 2006;195:787.
8. Meijer-Hoogeveen M, Stoutenbeek P, Visser GHA. Transperineal versus transvaginal sonographic cervical length measurement in second- and third-trimester pregnancies. Ultrasound Obstet Gynecol. 2008;32:657-62.
9. Valentin L Bergelin I. Intra- and interobserver reproducibility of ultrasound measurements of cervical length and width in the second and third trimesters of pregnancy. Ultrasound Obstet Gynecol. 2002;20:256-62.
10. Vayssière C, Morinière C, Camus E, Le Strat Y, Poty L, Fermanian J, et al. Measuring cervical length with ultrasound: evaluation of the procedures and duration of a learning method Ultrasound Obstet Gynecol. 2002;20:575-9.
11. Rozenberg P, Gillet A, Ville Y. Transvaginal sonographic examination of the cervix in asymptomatic pregnant women: review of the literature. Ultrasound Obstet Gynecol. 2002;19:302-11.
12. Crane JMG. Hutchens D. and Transvaginal sonographic measurement of cervical length to predict preterm birth in asymptomatic women at increased risk: a systematic review. Ultrasound Obstet Gynecol. 2008;31:579-87.
13. Hatanaka AR, Mattar R, Kawanami TE, et al Amniotic fluid "sludge" is an independent risk factor for preterm delivery. J Matern Fetal Neonatal Med. 2016;29(1):120-5.
14. Fuchs F, Boucoiran I, Picard A, et al Impact of amniotic fluid "sludge" on the risk of preterm delivery. J Matern Fetal Neonatal Med. 2015;28(10):1176-80.
15. Yoshimatsu K, Sekiya T, Ishihara K, Fukami T, Otabe T, Araki T. Detection of the cervical gland area in threatened preterm labor using transvaginal sonography in the assessment of cervical maturation and the outcome of pregnancy. Gynecol Obstet Invest. 2002;53:149-56.
16. Grgic O, Matijevic R, Vasilj O. Qualitative glandular cervical score as a potential new sonomorphological parameter in screening for preterm delivery. Ultrasound Med Bio. 2006;32(3):333-8.
17. Severi FM, Bocchi C, Florio P, Picciolini E, D'Aniello G, Petraglia F. Comparison of two-dimensional and three-dimensional ultrasound in the assessment of the cervix to predict preterm delivery. Ultrasound Med Biol. 2003;29(9):1261-5.
18. Iams JD, Goldenberg RL, Mercer BM, et al. The Preterm Prediction Study: Can low-risk women destined for spontaneous preterm birth be identified?. Am J Obstet Gynecol. 2001;184:652.
19. ACOG Practice Bulletin. Cervical insufficiency. Obstet Gynecol 2003;102:1091.

20. Sotiriadis A, Papatheodorou S, Kavvadias A, Makrydimas G. Transvaginal cervical length measurement for prediction of preterm birth in women with threatened preterm labor: a meta-analysis. Ultrasound Obstet Gynecol. 2010;35:54.
21. Alfirevic Z, Stampalija T, Roberts D, Jorgensen AL. Cervical stitch (cerclage) for preventing preterm birth in singleton pregnancy. Cochrane Database Syst Rev. 2012; 18;4:CD008991.
22. Gonzalez JM, Romero R, Girardi G. Comparison of the mechanisms responsible for cervical remodeling in preterm and term labor. J Reprod Immunol. 2013;97:112-9.
23. Winkler M, Rath W. Changes in the cervical extracellular matrix during pregnancy and parturition. J Perinat Med. 1999;27:45-60.
24. Parker KJ, Doyley MM, Rubens DJ. Imaging the elastic properties of tissue: the 20 year perspective. Phus Med Biol. 2011;56:R1-R29.
25. Garra BS. Elastography: current status, future prospects, and making it work for you. Ultrasound Q. 2011;27:177-86.
26. Hernandez-Andrade E, Hassan SS, Ahn H, Korzeniewski SJ, Yeo L, Chaiworapongsa T, et al. Evaluation of cervical stiffness during pregnancy using semiquantitative ultrasound elastography. Ultrasound Obstet Gynecol. 2013;41:152-61.
27. Hernandez-Andrade E, Romero R, Korzeniewski SJ, et al. Cervical strain determined by ultrasound elastography and its association with spontaneous preterm delivery. J Perinat Med. 2014;42(2):159-69.

30

CHAPTER

Monochorionicity: Unveiling the Black Box

Alexandra Matias, Miguel Pereira-Macedo, Nuno Montenegro

INTRODUCTION

Multiple pregnancy represents about 1.2% of all pregnancies. About 30% of these pregnancies are iatrogenic. In fact, an "epidemic" of multiple pregnancies is being observed in the world, as a consequence of both the increase in the reproductive age of pregnant women[1] and the widespread use of ovulation induction and assisted reproduction techniques (ARTs).[2-4]

The contribution of ART toward the increase in the rate of twins is well known. Namely in the USA, an increase of 30% in the prevalence of twins was observed since the beginning of the 1990s. ART techniques show a twin rate 20 times higher than that of spontaneous conceptions, and a dizygotic twin rate higher than the monozygotic (MZ) twin rate (10:1). However, the rate of MZ twinning as a consequence of ART seems to be increased as well,[5-8] mainly associated with the transfer of blastocysts (when compared with the transfer of embryos on the third day), and seems not to be affected by the manipulation of the zona pellucida. In a study that included 15.644 cycles and the transfer of a single embryo in 7,832 cases of in vitro fertilization (IVF), the monozygosity rate was 2.3%, a figure six times higher than the 0.4% described in the literature.[7] In contrast, the frequency of MZ twins recorded after ovulation induction (6.4%) was 14 times higher than the rate of spontaneous twins, and more than twice the rate of MZ twins after IVF.

The growing concern with multiple pregnancies is mainly related to the higher mortality and greater incidence of adverse perinatal outcomes when compared to singleton pregnancies.[9,10] There is a duplication of risk for structural defects[11-13] and a higher risk of chromosomal anomalies.[14] Though multiple pregnancies represent 1.2% of the population, they heavily contribute toward perinatal mortality representing 12.6% of deaths. In the case of monochorionic (MC) twin pregnancies, the known perinatal morbidity and mortality are even more dramatic.[15] This should encourage more differentiated and specialized surveillance.[9,16]

THE MONOZYGOSITY PHENOMENON

The human female was programmed by evolution to ovulate only once in every menstrual cycle, leading to monofetal pregnancies and to the nurturing of only one infant at a time. Therefore, in about 99% of spontaneous pregnancies, a unique fetus derives from a single zygote. As a consequence of a *reproductive disorder,* which occurs in 0,8% of spontaneous conceptions, more than an oocyte is produced and fertilized in each cycle, resulting in polyzygotic multiple pregnancies. In another 0.4% of spontaneous pregnancies, as a result of a *reproductive anomaly*, a single ovum normally destined to produce a single embryo, splits to form MZ multiples.

The MZ twinning is a form of "vegetative" reproduction whereby more than one individual results from a single zygote. MZ twins, at birth, weigh somewhat less than twice the birth weight of singletons of corresponding gestational age. Hence, a single fertilized egg is capable of producing much more somatic and placental mass than a singleton pregnancy, though the mechanisms of overgrowth in MZ twinning are not fully understood. We can consider the existence of extramitotic cycles and/or reduced apoptosis, but it is a tribute to the plasticity of early embryogenesis that anatomically and well-grown normal MZ twins, triplets, or higher-order multiples, can be produced from a single fertilized egg.

The prevalence of MZ twinning is fairly constant worldwide, strongly suggesting that MZ twinning derives from an intrinsic "anomalous" property of human zygotes. Based on this stability, Weinberg's law was established and allows the accurate prediction of zygosity based on the frequency assessment of twin pairs of different sexes. In spontaneous conceptions, the rate of MZ twins represents about a third of all twin pregnancies, that is, about 4:1,000 births, and about two-thirds of MZ twin pregnancies will develop an MC placentation, that is, 2–3:1,000 births. In iatrogenic pregnancies, the ratio is altered and MZ twin pregnancies are more prevalent (1:15–20 instead of 1:3). In certain cases, a familial tendency to MZ twinning was disclosed, probably due to molecular mechanisms that cause postzygotic cells to disaggregate more easily than usual, forming two or more internal masses.

It is awkward to consider MZ twins "genetically identical," based on an equal number of multipotential "founder" cells exposed to the same intrauterine milieu. These assumptions seem untrue, and they are more inaccurate in some fetuses than in others.[17,18] The complexity and variety of the initial development of MZ twins lend a degree of sophistication and fascination toward the understanding of MZ twinning, introducing biases in twin studies. A lot of them do not take into consideration the possibility of discordance at birth that can exist caused by the different environmental, genetic, postzygotic, and epigenetic factors of prenatal occurrence.

Why does the division of a single zygote occur? Though scientific evidence does not exist, different hypotheses have been proposed but all are at present merely speculative. Presently, four theories are available to explain the mechanism of zygotic splitting: The so-called *repulsion hypothesis*[19]—cells in the developing zygote express genetic differences that translate into repulsive forces that lead to the splitting of the zygote; the existence of codominant axes[12]—the continuous *presence of a codominant axis* will cause the zygote to split; *depressed calcium levels* in the early embryo,[20] and the *blastomere herniation* hypothesis—the integrity of the zona pellucida is breached during embryonic development, thereby losing its sequestering and protective role and permitting herniation of pluripotent cells through a gap in the zona pellucida.[21,22] All these theories are, however, not convincingly clear in explaining the origin of MZ triplets and quadruplets, and do not elucidate the higher rate of MZ twins related to ART techniques (with or without manipulation of the zona pellucida). This particular difficulty is due to the inexistence of animal models of monozygosity, in which, with the exception of the human race and the armadillo (*Dasypus novemcinctus*), in no other mammals is this process expected to occur. More recently the hypothesis that human fertilized oocytes more splitting-prone are able to undergo one or two successive binary fissions, or various combinations offered by subsequent secondary fissions, just as the case for the nine-banded armadillo, and give rise to a variety of combinations of MZ pregnancies has been proposed (zona pellucida-assisted binary fission theory).[23] This latter theory would be able to explain MZ triplets and quadruplets, as well as "mirror-image" characteristics[24] and some midline asymmetries in MZ twins.[25]

The true frequency of zygotic division is not exactly known but inferred by the number of fetuses that exceed the number of transferred embryos. Clearly, this estimation is not reliable. If we consider that after the transfer of two embryos, one is lost and the other originates an MZ pregnancy with dichorionic placentation, no excess of fetuses would be found. Moreover, it is not clinically possible to differentiate between dichorionic dizygotic twins of the same sex from MZ twins with dichorionic placentation. Finally, Weinberg's law is based on proportions observed in spontaneous conceptions that are not necessarily reproducible in ART pregnancies.

In a hypothetical model, we can calculate the risk of iatrogenic twins per 1,000 births: Natural conceptions comprise 1.2% twins including 0.4% MZs; whereas, ART conceptions comprise 25% twins, of which 2.5% are MZs. In a department with 10% deliveries after ART, six MZ twins are predictable for every 1,000 deliveries as compared with four MZs after spontaneous conception. An increase of 1% in iatrogenic conceptions will translate into an increase of monozygosity by 6.25% compared to a 50% increase when 10% of the conceptions are iatrogenic. It can be concluded that the number of MZs increases as a linear function of iatrogenic pregnancies and the overall increase in iatrogenic multiples will significantly increase the total number of MZs in any given population.[8]

Still addressing the issue of iatrogenic pregnancies, it was noticed that the early spontaneous embryonic/fetal loss was slightly superior in the pregnancies resulting from ART than in spontaneous pregnancies. Nevertheless, whenever the end result of ART was a twin pregnancy, this early loss rate appeared importantly reduced. Thus, multiple pregnancies may be seen as a marker of reproductive advantage.[26,27] A sensible explanation for this advantage of twins over singletons would be that the higher levels of placental hormones produced by a larger placental mass in twin gestations would improve the implantation capacity of the egg. Several studies support this evidence,[26-32] showing loss rates of 24% in singleton pregnancies versus 3–11% in twin pregnancies. The early fetal loss rate associated with ART is two to five times higher in singleton pregnancies.

Time Matters in Monozygosity: Sharing Levels and a Model of Placentation

The timing of MZ twinning events can be inferred from the type of placentation, X chromosome-inactivation in female MZ twins, asymmetric language function in the cerebral hemispheres, and asymmetric dermatoglyphics.

The *dizygotic* twins, fraternal or nonidentical, result from the fertilization of two ova by different spermatozoids, possessing therefore different genetic content. The type of placenta resulting from this process of fertilization, in which the trophoblast formation precedes the egg implantation, has two chorions and two amniotic sacs, defining a dichorionic diamniotic pregnancy.

Monozygotic twins result from the early division of a single egg (originating from the fertilization of an oocyte and a single spermatozoid) in two identical cell masses, that contain the same genotype (exception—heterokaryotypic monozygotes). This cleavage will occur between the fertilization and the gastrulation period. Individual variations are the result of postzygotic mutations and arbitrary division of mitochondrial deoxyribonucleic acid (DNA). The placentation inherent to these twins is more complex, depending on the very moment in which the separation occurs.

Dichorionic Diamniotic

Dichorionic diamniotic (DC-DA) MZ twins (18–36%) have separate membranes and placentas and result from abnormal splitting at the two-cell stage to morula (day 0–3). Consequently, each twin receives trophoblastic and somatic stem cells into their cell masses. Therefore, twinning must have happened before the differentiation and physical separation of somatic and trophoblastic cells into the outer and inner cell masses, respectively, in the cavitated blastocyst at about 3 days postconception. Dichorionic diamniotic placentas are derived from the splitting of about eight blastomeres.

Splitting at any time thereafter, results in a single MC placenta that continues as such even in the face of subsequent MZ twinning in the inner cell mass.

Monochorionic Diamniotic

Monochorionic diamniotic (MC-DA) twins (~80%) separate at the inner cell mass, after the chorion has formed (day 4–7). Consequently, two fetuses will develop with the same genome, a single placenta, and two amniotic cavities, as the amniotic cavity will only be formed after the eighth day after conception. The sharing of a single placenta is an anomaly, creating unequal vascular territories for each twin and a more common eccentric location of the umbilical cords.[33,34] Eventually 5–15% will develop a twin-to-twin transfusion syndrome (TTTS), and a late discrepancy in fetal growth can be a frequent finding.

If the division occurs between the 9th and 12th day, at the late blastocyst stage, a single placenta and a unique amniotic cavity will be formed, that is, all placental structures will be shared, resulting in a *monochorionic monoamniotic* (MC-MA) twin pregnancy (1%).

The highest level of sharing occurs very rarely when the division happens circa the 13th day, resulting in the incomplete division of the embryonic disc, originating *conjoined twins* (estimated prevalence of 1 in 100,000). After that time, the undivided egg will maintain the expected course to produce a singleton pregnancy.

If MZ twinning events would take place at a constant rate during the first 12 days postconception, proportions of DC, MC-DA, and MC-MA twins would vary from those observed. The underrepresentation at birth of MC-MA and conjoined twins is explained by the higher intrauterine lethality. The relative excess of DC-MZ twins may be the result of their having less placental complications. Considering the level of sharing, it is inversely proportional to the incidence of twins that result from this sharing (the incidence of MZ twins is about 1:250, and the incidence of MC twins is two-thirds of the MZ pregnancies (1:350–400 births). The incidence of MC monoamniotic twins is 1:2,500 liveborn, and the one from conjoined twins is <1:40,000 liveborn). On the other hand, perinatal mortality and morbidity are related directly with the level of sharing, that is, the greater the level of sharing the greater the risk of pregnancy adverse outcomes. Whereas MZ with dichorionic placentation and dizygotic twins present pregnancies with similar risks, those with MC placentation have an important increase in worse outcomes, mainly if the shared circulation is unbalanced or if we are dealing with monoamniotic or conjoined twins.

How Identical are Monozygotic Twins?—Phenomena of Genetic and Epigenetic Discordance

Unexpectedly MZ twins may be of a different chromosomal composition (heterokaryotypic twins).[35] Heterokaryotypic twins may be explained by two mechanisms: (1) When the mitotic error occurs *before* the twinning event, the mosaic will be present in both fetuses with different distribution of the two cell lines between the twins and (2) when the mitotic error occurs *after* the twining event, the mosaic will be present in only one twin.[36,37] All possible combinations of karyotypes observed in twins can be attributed to the unequal allocation of the abnormal cells to each twin: abnormal/normal, mosaic/mosaic, abnormal/mosaic, and normal/mosaic.[38]

Adding to the complexity of the situation, we must consider the timing of the event (responsible for the presence of the mitotic error in somatic regions of one twin) and the placental status of the chromosomes.

Monozygotic twins with chromosomal anomalies and discordant phenotypes have been reported, including discordant sex phenotype with mosaicism 46XY/45X, Turner's syndrome in female twins with mosaicism 46XX/45X,[36,39,40] trisomy 21,[39] and trisomy 13.[41] There are a few case reports of MZ twins with discordant phenotype and rare partial chromosomal anomalies including 22q11 deletion (Lu et al., 2001),[42] 7q syndrome,[43] monosomy 21,[44] and partial trisomy 1.[43] Trisomy 11p have already been reported[38] either associated with a nonspecific clinical pattern or with the Beckwith–Wiedemann syndrome (BWS) when the additional region causes paternal disomy.[38] MZ pairs discordant for 45X emerging from 47XXY, 47XXX, 46XY, and 46XX zygotes have been reported (Machin, 1996).[45]

Therefore, various postzygotic events determine a discordant phenotype for MZ twins, that are not so identical as would be expected.[46]

Concordant or Reciprocal X Chromosome Inactivation

X-inactivation (or lyonization) refers to the inactivation of one of the X chromosomes in females to achieve dosage compensation of X-linked genes with males.

Several studies link random inactivation of the X chromosome of maternal or paternal inheritance to subtypes and timing of MZ twins and indicate that the allocation of cells to the twins is not always equal.[47] Despite the female excess in MC twinning, it is not clear that X-inactivation is a major stimulus to MZ twinning *per se*. The discordance in the inactivated X may justify the phenotypic discordance for aspects linked to chromosome X, such as Duchenne muscular dystrophy. This inactivation precedes the MC placentation and confirms that the production of a monoamniotic sac is a late event in the MC placentation.

An excess of females over males has been observed in surviving MZ twins, mainly with MC placentation, suggesting a relationship with the time of twinning. Discordance for several X-linked recessive conditions have been reported in MZ twins, suggesting, and often demonstrating non-random X-inactivation.[21]

Finally, the highly similar patterns of X chromosome inactivation among MC twins may indicate that X chromosome inactivation occurs before the twinning event in this subgroup of MZ twins.

Chromosomal Mosaicism

The presence of two or more cell lines derived from the same zygote having different chromosomal constitutions (secondary to postzygotic events) is well recognized in aneuploid singletons. Depending on the relative timing of the twinning and chromosomal events, two or more cell lines may be distributed largely or exclusively in the somatic cells of one twin or the other. Blood mosaicism might also be present in normal twins, as a result of interfetal anastomoses, and therefore, karyotyping in MZ twins that are discordant for some fetal abnormality should be performed in amniocytes rather than in fetal blood.[36]

This mosaicism is particularly problematic for those fetuses initially 46,XY with loss of a Y chromosome, which will result in a male fetus and a mosaic 46,XY/45,XO reared as a female. This female fetus may suffer masculinization due to the fetal passage of testosterone produced by the 46,XY cotwin through the vascular anastomoses. Whether derived from a 46,XX or 46,XY zygote, the MZ twin with a predominant or total 45,XO constitution is likely to develop fetal jugulolymphatic obstruction, endangering the life of the cotwin.

Imprinted Genes

Genomic imprinting is a phenomenon in which one of two alleles, from maternal or paternal origin, is inactivated by DNA methylation.[48]

Imprinting is initiated during gametogenesis and transmitted to embryos via mature male and female gametes. Appropriate imprinting of the two gametes is critical and implicated in prenatal growth, development and differentiation, behavior, and human disease.[49]

Discordance between MZ twins has been reported for several diseases where genomic imprinting is suspected or implicated, such as BWS. BWS has a higher prevalence than expected between monozygotic female (MZF) twins and they are mostly discordant.[21,48] These parent-of-origin effects, together with the finding of paternal uniparental disomy of chromosome 11p15 in 20% of BWS cases, suggest that abnormal genomic imprinting might play an important role in the etiology of BWS. Discordance for hyperinsulinemic hypoglycemia[50] and Russell–Silver syndrome[51] has also been reported and although these are likely to be heterogeneous conditions, it is possible that imprinted genes play nonetheless an important role.[21]

Discordance in MZ twin pairs is well recognized for diseases thought to result from abnormal imprinting of genes. Beckwith–Wiedemann syndrome is caused by abnormal *imprinting* of one or more of a cluster of genes in the p15 region chromosome 11. It is not clear however how the abnormal imprinting relates to the MZ twinning process, through unequal splitting, postzygotic chromosomal rearrangements, or abnormal imprinting at the crucial moment of twinning.

Trinucleotide Repeat Sequence

Several progressive neurological disorders are characterized by phenotypic expression only when a threshold of trinucleotide repeat sequence number is exceeded, such as fragile X syndrome. Discordance has been found in some MZ twin pairs. A more severely affected twin had a complete mutation, whereas his less severely affected sibling had a "mosaic" for premutation and full mutation. Therefore, there may be some difficulty in offering predictive tests for these kinds of diseases to MZ twins.

Epigenetics

Epigenetic phenomena are characterized by "modifications in gene expressions that are controlled by heritable but potentially reversible changes in DNA methylation and/or chromatin structure."[52,53] Epigenetic modifications consist of methylation of cytosines, as well as modifications of histones by methylation, acetylation, phosphorylation, and ubiquitination.[54]

Deoxyribonucleic acid methylation may occur more frequently in MZ twins and may influence susceptibility to bipolar disorder and schizophrenia. MZ twins discordant for schizophrenia have been more frequently reported. Different DNA methylation patterns have been implicated in the discordance of schizophrenia in relation to specific schizophrenia candidate genes. Other studies also focused on the role of epigenetics in twin discordance, implying different methylation patterns in age-related diseases, risk-taking behavior, and caudal duplication anomaly.[54-56]

More recently, Bianchi et al. (2010)[57] as well as Liao et al. (2017),[58] Leonard and Martin (2020),[59] and Caroto et al (2020),[60] pointed out in different meta-analyses to alternative methods for evaluating in vivo genetic differences in MZ twins, such as cell-free fetal DNA [free fetal deoxyribonucleic acid (ffDNA)] in maternal blood, messenger ribonucleic acid (mRNA) in amniotic fluid and RNA single nucleotide polymorphism (SNP) allelic ratio analysis. Therefore, prenatal gene expression investigation in vivo may open a new field for prenatal twin research.

Phenotypic Discordance for a Single Gene Mutation

It would be expected that MZ twins affected by an autosomal dominant disorder such as type 1 neurofibromatosis might show different somatic patterns of distribution of discrete lesions because of somatic mosaicism. However, major somatic differences may be attributed to a postzygotic discordance for the causative point mutation.

Phenotypic Discordance with Same Genetic Predisposition

Monozygotic twins are usually discordant for the extent and severity of congenital heart diseases when they have microdeletion 22q1.1. probably due to a second epigenetic effect on the phenotype.

Discordance for Major Malformation

The prevalence of structural defects in a dizygotic twin pregnancy is the same as in a singleton pregnancy whereas in MZ twins, it will be two to three times higher.[12,13] The concordant defects (both fetuses are affected) are rare, occurring in 10% of DC twin pregnancies and 20% of MC twin pregnancies.[61]

The discordance in DZ twins is due to a genetic predisposition. In the MZ pregnancy this discordance is more prevalent and may be explained by:

- Variable gene expression (postzygotic mutation and asymmetrical X inactivation)
- Asymmetric splitting of the cellular mass
- Splitting after laterality gradients have been established (midline defects and cardiac)
- Hemodynamic factors, in MC gestations with TTTS (putatively responsible for disruptions).

Monozygotic are usually discordant for malformations such as cardiac and urinary tract defects, omphalocele, and neural tube defects, but on the contrary, are usually concordant for malformations such as cloacal dysgenesis and omphalocele-exstrophy-imperforate anus-spinal defects syndrome.

Pseudoconcordance of malformations may occur in MZ twins. Though they are frequently discordant for thyroid dysgenesis, both may only be mildly ill. Due to interfetal connections, the affected fetus may be protected from hypothyroidism by the transplacental transfusion of thyroxin from the thyroid of the unaffected cotwin and present at birth with almost normal thyroxin levels.

Another example of pseudoconcordance of phenotype exists for monoamniotic twins with urinary tract malformations, in which the anuric fetus is protected from pulmonary hypoplasia and deformities by the urine output from the other fetus.

Disruptions in MZ twins including limb reduction defects, hemifacial microsomia, and amyoplasia, may be the result of shared placental circulation leading to secondary disruptions and sometimes to single intrauterine fetal death.

Finally, clubfeet, dislocated hips, and cranial synostosis are deformations associated with spatial constraint and intrauterine crowding, which are apparently related to limited space in utero for the bearing of two fetuses.

"Mirroring" in Monozygotic Twins

In about 25% of MZ twins, the development of normal lateralization may be impaired by the twinning process itself in such a way that for some of the asymmetrical features, the resulting twins would not be duplicated, but mirror-images.[62]

The concept of mirror-image MZ twins is based on inverse laterality. This may suggest that the event that originated the twins began after the cells of the embryonic plate were beginning to lateralize but before the formation of the primitive streak. Later MZ twinning could occur when the molecular determinants of left/right asymmetry are beginning to be expressed with lateral discordance. Opposite-handedness is more prevalent among both DZ and MZ twin pairs.

"Fine-Tuning": Detailed Peripheral Patterning

MZ twins are not concordant for dermatoglyphics, this being one of the examples by which MZ twins are not "identical." The extent of discordance in dermatoglyphic patterns varies with chorionicity and MC twins show more within-pair variability than DC-MZ twins. There is also evidence of an effect from placental crowding: MZ twins with DC placentation show greater variability than those with MC placentas. This effect was also noted in like-sexed DC twin pairs.

Unequal Placental Territoriality

The unequal allocation of stem cells/blastomers to the twins can determine the existence of unequal placental masses or the differential sharing of placental territory in MZ twins. As a consequence, discrepant fetal growth and different phenotypes can occur in MZ twins.[63]

Limits of Zygosity Testing: Postnatal Importance

The estimation of MZ twins is frequently based on the number of MC twins observed in obstetric ultrasound. Though all MC placentas correspond to MZ twins, and all twin pairs of different sexes are DZ, the majority of like-sexed twins with dichorionic placentation are blind to their zygosity. The recognition of zygosity in dichorionic MZ twins is based on physical similarities but even the most experienced practitioner may misclassify zygosity in about 6% of cases.[19,64] In liked-sex dichorionic twins, we are blind to zygosity in about 44% of the cases. Despite observations of DZ MC twins, the so-called "gold standard" defining monozygosity is that all MC twins are MZ. Biochemical characteristics such as blood type, enzyme polymorphisms, and HLA types have also been used to classify zygosity. However, the "gold standard" for the determination of zygosity should be based on several genetic markers (including "DNA fingerprinting") in buccal swabs or blood sampling, applied to like-sexed dichorionic twin pregnancies. Though this determination would have been more scientific than clinically justified, in particular cases it can be lifesaving as in solid organ transplantation. This may be, however, a somewhat misleading approach as all MZ twins share vascular placental connections and might have exchanged DNA (chimerism).

In reality, the final diagnosis of zygosity cannot be accomplished in about 43% of cases without DNA evaluation.[65] In daily practice, the estimation of MZ twins is based roughly on chorionicity and fetal sex, disregarding about one-third of MZ twins. Therefore, whatever the method used it will underestimate the real incidence of MZ twins.

Considering the data from the East Flanders Prospective Twin Survey, in which zygosity was studied in all like-sexed dichorionic twins, the frequency of MZ twins after ART was 4.5% (10× superior to the 0.45% MZ rate found in twins after spontaneous conception). The frequency of MZ twins after IVF was 2.6% (6× the rate of spontaneous conceptions).[65]

Chorionicity: A (Re)definition of Perinatal Prognosis

Clearly, it is chorionicity rather than zygosity that determines several aspects of antenatal management and perinatal outcome. Thus, the routine assignment of chorionicity and the earliest possible diagnosis of MC twinning is highly desirable, though seldom achieved in practice.

Zygosity refers to the type of conception whereas chorionicity reflects the type of placentation. The type of placentation depends on the time of splitting of the fertilized ova. One study suggests the possibility of determining zygosity, by means of ultrasound, at the beginning of the first trimester by counting the number of yolk sacs;[66] however, a unique placental mass and the same fetal sex suggest but do not prove monozygosity. It is not possible to determine zygosity in about 45% of the cases because dizygotic twins of the same sex (about half of the dizygotic twins) and MZ dichorionic twins (a one-third of all MZ twins) cannot be differentiated unless molecular tests are used.

Caution should be taken when using the number of chorionic sacs and the number of yolk sacs alone to determine the number of embryos. Shortly after the sixth postmenstrual week, embryonic heartbeats are visible, and one can confidently count the number of embryos by the number of beating hearts. By that time, to determine the number of amnions in an MC twin pregnancy, in which two embryos are seen within the chorionic sac, it is wise to wait until the eighth postmenstrual week to ascertain amnionicity. The amniotic membrane is so thin that it may remain inconspicuous until 8–9 weeks, leading to the incorrect consideration of an MC-monoamniotic gestation.

After that gestational age, it becomes clear that no amniotic membrane is present between the embryos and only one yolk sac is visualized. When two embryos or fetuses assume a parallel, head-to-head position, conjoined twins should be suspected. A jerk with the probe should be inflicted to induce movement between the two fetuses, away from each other or close together when conjoined twins are in question. From then on it is important to look for sonographic signs of cord entanglement, potentially depicted as early as 12 weeks, with the help of color Doppler.

At 10–14 weeks, the gold standard "window" for chorionicity definition, the chorion frondosum is sufficiently thick to be identified between the two layers of amnion. We can see with ultrasound a wedge-shaped structure in a dichorionic twin pregnancy (not obligatorily a dizygotic twin pregnancy), yielding the fully diagnostic "twin peak" or "lambda" or "delta" sign[67-69] **(Figs. 1A and B)**. However, the number of "twin-peak" signs is no secure indication of how many chorionic sacs exist within a given pregnancy. If two fused layers of amnion, without any chorion interposed, are found in the scan creating a T-shaped "take-off" (T sign), showing a very thin membrane with strictly two layers, an MC twin pregnancy can be diagnosed with a 100% certainty[69,70] **(Figs. 1A and B)**.

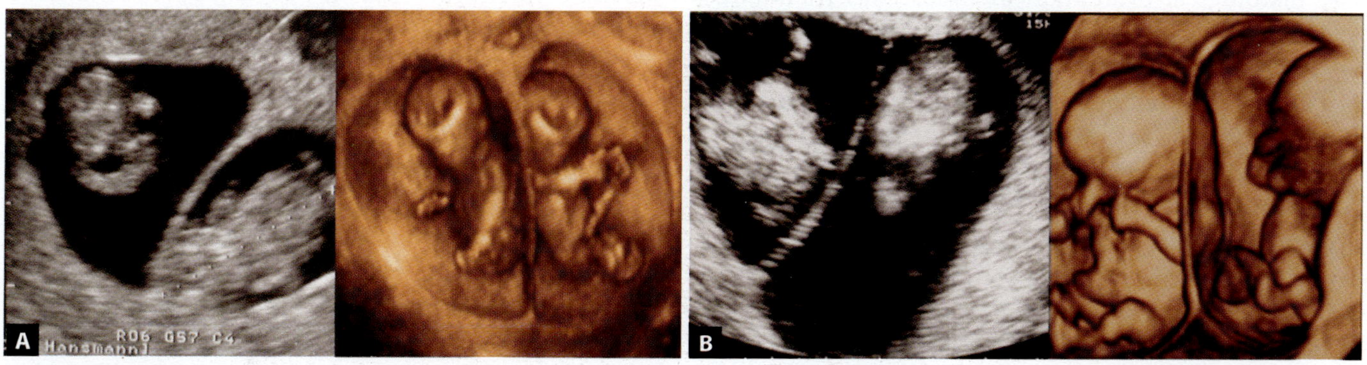

Figs. 1A and B: Diagnosis of chorionicity by ultrasound. (A) Lambda sign (dichorionic placentation); (B) T-sign (monochorionic placentation) at 10–14 weeks of gestation.

After 16 weeks physiologically the chorion frondosum regresses and chorionicity becomes a more confounding issue (in the second trimester a false characterization of chorionicity can occur in about 10% of cases).[68,71] The delta sign disappears[72,73] and, if sexes are alike, monochorionicity can be wrongly inferred. It is the conjugation of several sonographic criteria that approaches the correct diagnosis of chorionicity, the ultimate determinant of perinatal prognosis. Therefore, an adequate first-trimester scan of a multifetal pregnancy makes the subsequent second and third-trimester evaluation more meaningful, simpler, and faster.

If one finds two separate placentas of different locations, or two fetuses of a different sex, or a thick interfetal membrane >2 mm with more than two layers, dichorionicity is strongly suggested. Note that to identify the interfetal membranes, a right-angled orientation of the probe in relation to the membranes should be obtained to take advantage of the axial over the lateral resolution. In order to count the number of layers one must "zoom in." In contrast, a membrane placed parallel to the ultrasonic beam will appear thinner and poorly imaged, rendering it impossible to be sure about the number of layers of the intertwin membrane.

The confirmation of an MC placentation by the detailed examination of the placenta is the most reliable proof of monozygosity. Not only is it possible to identify the pathological aspects that interfere with placental function but also the relationship between the chorion and fetal membranes (chorionicity), and the pattern and the type of anastomoses of the chorionic vessels. This exam includes the careful macroscopic examination of the placenta with consideration of aspects such as the fusion of the chorion and amnion, thickness and translucency of the septum, and the vascular pattern of the fetal surface. The histological evaluation includes cord fragments, membranes and placental parenchyma, and fragments of the transitional zone. To study vascular anastomoses, the placenta should not be fixed, and the amnion should be removed.

When chorionicity is established, stratification of risk is possible, anticipating the characteristic complications of each type of placenta. In fact, complications of MC twin pregnancies are by far more common, such as preterm delivery (in Portugal, out of 7,551 newborns of very low birth weight born between 1996 and 2003, 25.6% resulted from multiple gestations), fetal malformations, TTTS, intrauterine death of one fetus, and cerebral palsy. Recently an update on the management of twin pregnancies was published, discussing the peculiarities of MC twins' clinical orientation.[74]

Prenatal Screening and Diagnosis: Pathology Unique to Twins

Twins present unique issues in prenatal diagnosis. The performance of screening tests designed for singleton pregnancies is altered. Having correctly established the chorionicity, specific aspects of prenatal screening and diagnosis can be adequately programmed. Chromosomal abnormalities in twin pregnancies give rise to serious clinical, ethical, and moral problems that need to be addressed:[75]

- Effective methods of screening, such as maternal serum biochemistry, are not applicable and have lower detection rates
- In the presence of a "screen-positive" result, there is no feature to suggest which fetus may be affected
- *Noninvasive prenatal test (NIPT) is prone to quality issues in case of multiple gestations*: The minimum total amount of cell-free fetal DNA must be higher to reach a comparable sensitivity and vanishing twins may cause results that do not represent the genetics of the living sibling.[59,76]
- Invasive testing techniques are more demanding in twins and it may be difficult to ensure that fetal tissue is obtained from each fetus.
- Increased risk of miscarriage of an invasive test in twins.
- Which invasive test to offer
- The paucity of data in abnormally affected pregnancies when the fetuses are either concordant or discordant for an abnormality.
- The difficulties of clinical management of fetal reduction and the potential increased risk to the unaffected cotwin.

The overall probability that a multiple gestation contains an aneuploid fetus is directly related to its zygosity. In *dizygotic* pregnancies, each fetus has an independent risk of aneuploidy, thus, the maternal age-related risk for chromosomal abnormalities for each twin may be the same as in singleton pregnancies, but the chance that at least one fetus will be affected by a chromosomal defect is twice as high as in singleton pregnancies[77] **(Figs. 2A to D)**. This means that for dizygotic twin pregnancies, the pregnancy-specific risk is calculated by adding the

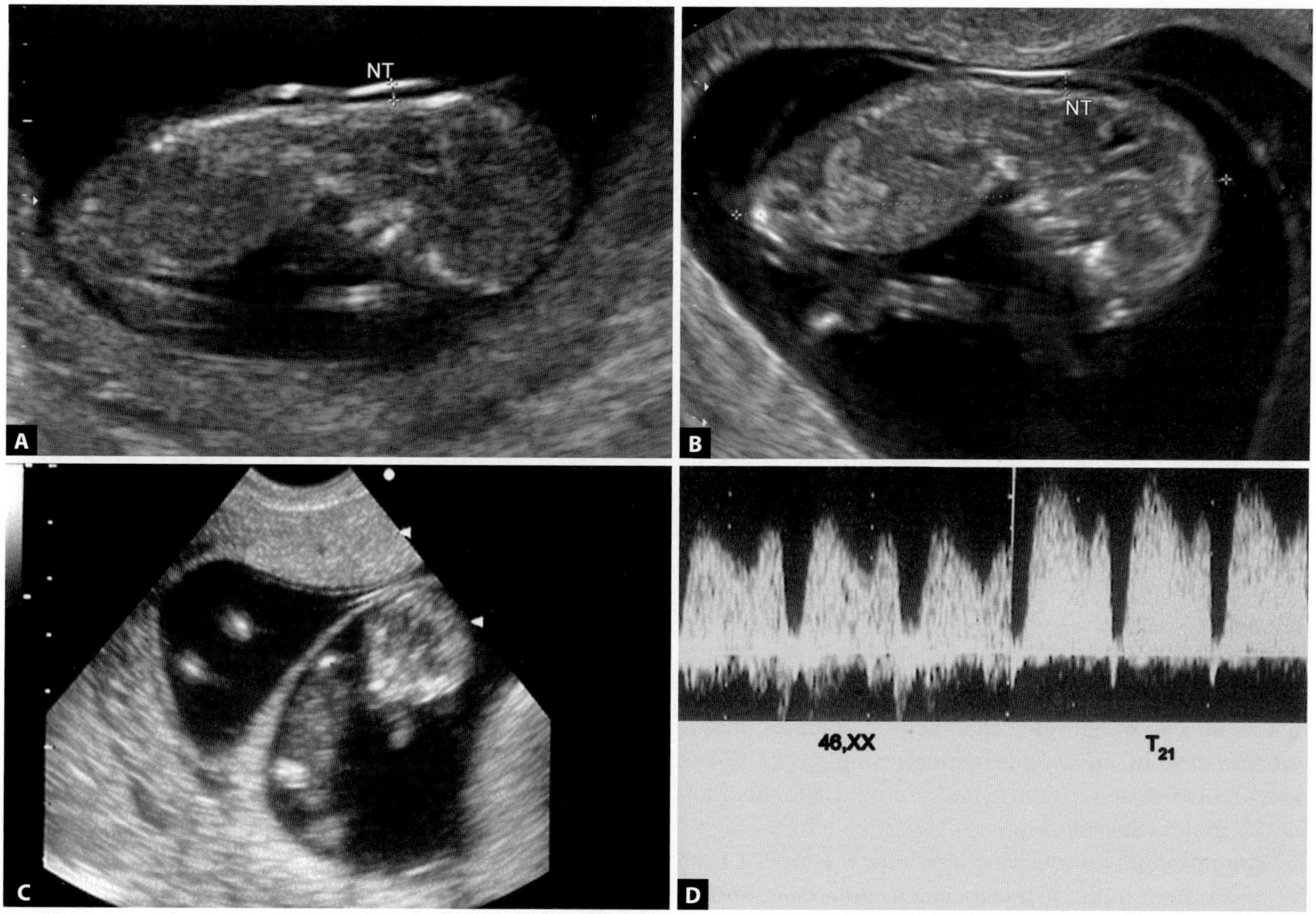

Figs. 2A to D: Screening for trisomy 21 in dichorionic twins (summing method)—the lambda sign is evident at 10–14 weeks. We can observe discrepant nuchal translucencies (NTs) = 1.1 and 5.7 mm. Ductus venosus Doppler blood flow is abnormal in the fetus with increased NT that eventually revealed to be a fetus affected by trisomy 21.

individual risk estimates for each fetus. Furthermore, since the rate of dizygotic twinning increases with maternal age, the proportion of twin pregnancies with chromosomal defects is higher than in singleton pregnancies. The 10% of dichorionic twin pregnancies that are MZ will incorrectly have their risks calculated by addition rather than the averaging method. However, the ultimate effect on screening performance and clinical meaning will be a negligible one.

In MZ twins, the risk of an affected fetus is similar to the maternal age risk of a singleton pregnancy and, in the vast majority of cases, the risk for one fetus is the same as the risk for the other.[75,78] There is no reason to attribute different risks to the two fetuses because, presumably, both will be affected or both will be unaffected. The most reliable and reproducible method of screening is nuchal translucency (NT), and it is, therefore, appropriate to take the average of the two NT measurements so that a single risk estimate can be calculated (averaging method).

This ignores the small possibility of heterokaryotypic MZ twins resulting from a mitotic nondisjunction after the zygote splits. There are occasional reports of MZ twins discordant for abnormalities of autosomes or sex chromosomes, most commonly with one fetus presenting a Turner syndrome and other either a normal male or female phenotype, but usually with a mosaic karyotype, or a Klinefelter syndrome.

The relative proportion of spontaneous dizygotic to MZ is about 2:1 and; therefore, the prevalence of chromosomal abnormalities affecting at least one fetus in a twin pregnancy would be expected to be about 1.6 times that of singletons.

If zygosity is unknown the risk of at least one aneuploid fetus can be approximated as five-thirds that of the singleton risk. This is based on the assumption that a third of all twin pairs are MZ.[14] Counseling based on chorionicity, clinically more feasible than zygosity, means that in MC twins both fetuses can be affected equally. If the pregnancy is dichorionic, then the parents should be counseled that the risk of discordance for a chromosomal abnormality is about twice that in singleton pregnancies, whereas the risk that both fetuses are affected is a much rarer event, corresponding to the singleton risk squared. However, with higher risk conditions, such as autosomal recessive disorders, this could be as high as one in 16. In a dizygotic twin pregnancy, the risk that one fetus would be affected would be 1 in 50 (1 in 100 plus 1 in 100), whereas the risk that both fetuses would be affected is 1 in 10,000 (1 in 100 × 1 in 100). This is, however, an oversimplification since, unlike all MC pregnancies that are always MZ, only about 90% of dichorionic pregnancies are dizygotic.

When calculating the risk of higher-order multiples, estimates can be made by multiplying the singleton risk by the number of fetuses.[79] This method assumes unique chorionicity for each fetus, though monozygosity can occur more frequently than usually thought at higher rates in ART multiple gestations.[5,6]

The possibility of deriving a risk for trisomy 21 from NT assessment in the first trimester of pregnancy shifted the consideration of a pregnancy-specific risk to a fetus-specific risk (Sebire et al., 1996).[80] This assumption was based on the observation that the distribution of NT measurements in twin fetuses with trisomy 21 was similar to that in singletons (Sebire et al., 1996a).[81-83] The higher rate of false positives for NT among MC twins (8.4%) should be ascribed to the possibility of early hemodynamic imbalance (the risk of developing TTTS if NT is increased is augmented 3–5-fold).[84-86]

Though assessing nasal bones in multiple pregnancies can be more demanding due to the more difficult acquisition of adequate fetal face planes, whenever they are assessed, they can be combined with NT and biochemical screening for calculating first-trimester risks. With the addition of nasal bone evaluation, sensitivity for trisomy 21 screening increased from 79 to 89%, for the same false positive rate of 5%.[87,88]

In contrast, though biochemical screening in twins was the first alternative to age-derived risk it can still be a source of confusion and clearly has a lower detection rate for fetal aneuploidies (50%) and higher rates of false positives. (Spencer et al., 2010).[89-91] This kind of screening only allows the calculation of a pregnancy and not a fetus-specific risk. In twin pregnancies, the levels of maternal serum markers are, on average, expected to be about twice as high in unaffected twin pregnancies as in unaffected singleton pregnancies,[92] that is, proportional to the number of fetoplacental units. However, as biochemical screening in twins is still investigational and far less powerful than in singletons, it should not be recommended in general practice without extensive counseling.[93,94]

MONOCHORIONIC PREGNANCY AS A HIGH-RISK PREGNANCY: TWIN-TO-TWIN TRANSFUSION SYNDROME AS A PARADIGM TO TREAT

Over the last decade, perinatal mortality in singleton pregnancies has fallen due to advances in fetal medicine and improvements in perinatal care. A similar reduction has not been observed in multiple pregnancies in which perinatal loss remains six times higher than in singleton pregnancies. Even more striking is the perinatal mortality of MC twins (260/1,000) which remains three to five-fold higher than in dichorionic pregnancies (90/1,000): The rate of perinatal loss before 24 weeks in MC compared with dichorionic pregnancies is 12.2% versus 1.8% (Sebire et al., 1997b).[95]

The MC twin placenta is designed and built for a singleton fetus; hence, attempts to cater to the needs of twin fetuses can often be suboptimal. Twin fetal circulations are seldom separate and several intertwin vascular communications of various kinds may be present and quite often there is an unequal sharing of placental parenchyma. An example of a complication almost unique to MZ twinning is TTTS. By way of intertwin vascular connections, blood is transfused from the *donor*, who becomes growth-restricted and develops high output cardiac insufficiency and oligohydramnios (depleted-donor twin), to the recipient, who develops circulatory overload with congestive heart failure and polyhydramnios (volume and an overfilled recipient twin). Therefore, TTTS reflects primarily a pathological form of circulatory imbalance that develops chronically between hemodynamically connected MC twin fetuses.

Twin-to-twin transfusion syndrome affects about 5–15% of MC twin pregnancies (1:400 pregnancies) and thus occurs in 1 in 1,600 deliveries. This syndrome accounts for 17% of perinatal mortality, nearly 12% of neonatal deaths, and 8.4% of infant deaths in twins. This is 3–10 times higher than that attributed to singletons. This syndrome was always recognized as a devastating complication of "identical" twins, but it took roughly 400 years to understand the way it works. Though clinically identifiable, this condition is still far from being effectively anticipated and treated. Twin-to-twin transfusion syndrome presents unique characteristics and the greatest therapeutic challenges in perinatal medicine:

- It affects *two* fetuses, not one.
- It affects *structurally normal* fetuses.
- Its basis resides in the *placenta*, not in the fetus.
- It is associated with important *perinatal morbidity* and *mortality*.
- It is amenable to *curative* therapy.

Vascular anastomoses are found invariably in almost all MC placentas. Thus, interfetal transfusion is a normal event in MC twin pregnancies. When intertwin transfusion in MC twins is balanced, clinical manifestations of TTTS are not expected to occur.

More than a century ago, Schatz et al. (1890)[96] suggested that TTTS is due to discordant hemodynamics secondary to transfusional imbalance. Later Bajoria et al. (1995)[97] related TTTS with unbalanced intertwin transfusion mediated by one or more arteriovenous (AV) anastomoses in association with absent bidirectional superficial anastomoses: Those affected by TTTS had fewer arterioarterial (AA) anastomoses present in 24% versus 84% of MC twins without TTTS.[98] For about 78% of MC pregnancies in this series with one or more AV anastomoses and no AA anastomoses developed TTTS.[98] When an AA anastomosis is found, the risk of developing TTTS is reduced ninefold.

Therefore, due to a particular vascular anatomy of the placenta, some MC twins are unable to compensate for the unidirectional flow in a "causative" AV anastomosis. MC twins have a continuous spectrum of severity in the imbalance between their fetoplacental circulations, depending on an angioarchitectural basis, hemodynamic, and hormonal factors. The progressive nature of TTTS in utero is thought to be due to one twin (the donor) slowly pumping blood to the other (the recipient) through these anastomoses.

The net result of transfusion between twins depends on:

- *Vascular anastomoses*: Combination of type of connections (number, type, and diameter) and direction of connections. In some cases, the normal transfusion from the donor's arterial to the recipient's venous circulation is not adequately compensated by oppositely directed flow by other deep or superficial anastomoses.[97]
- *Placental sharing*: Unequal placental sharing, both by the discrepant size of the placental territory or by velamentous insertion of the umbilical cord, may further impair growth in TTTS fetuses.[99]
- *Asymmetry* in the progressive reduction of an initially large number of bidirectional AV connections formed during the embryonic unification of placental and fetal vessels.
- *Unbalanced renin-angiotensin system* (RAS): Upregulation of RAS (donor) and downregulation of RAS (recipient) with the transfer of angiotensin II may cause or contribute to the development of TTTS.[100]
- *Incomplete remodeling* and defective trophoblastic invasion of maternal spiral arteries.

The pathophysiology of TTTS is poorly understood, and, although transfusion has been confirmed in vivo, the pathophysiology of TTTS includes more than shunting of blood from donor to recipient. A vicious cycle of hypervolemia-polyuria-hyperosmolality is established, leading in about one-third of the cases to the development of acute polyhydramnios/oligohydramnios sequence in the second trimester of pregnancy.

Diagnosis of Twin-to-Twin Transfusion Syndrome

In the past, diagnosis of the syndrome was made only after delivery of the affected twin pair and careful examination of the placenta. The standard neonatal criteria comprised:

- A difference in *cord hemoglobin* concentrations of 5 g/dL or more (false positives should be considered whenever there is untimely umbilical cord clamping of either donor or recipient or reversed intrapartum shunts).
- A difference in *birth weights* of 20% or more (this criterion is not necessarily present in the acute form of fetofetal transfusion syndrome that occurs in labor, and hydroptic fetuses may obscure the real intertwin size disparity).

Danskin and Neilson (1989),[101] revisiting the neonatal criteria for diagnosis of TTTS, found that an intertwin hemoglobin disparity of 5 g/dL or more and birth weight differences of >20% were found in both in MC and dichorionic twins at similar rates. Wenstrom et al. (1992)[102]

concordantly found that weight and hemoglobin level discordance were relatively common among MC twins. Therefore, a definitive diagnosis of TTTS solely based on neonatal criteria seemed insufficient.

Considering the many pitfalls of neonatal findings in TTTS and the more consistent sonographic antenatal criteria,[103-105] the emphasis on screening and diagnosis of TTTS is being pushed backward in pregnancy. In the early 1980s, the contribution of antenatal ultrasound for redefining the diagnostic criteria of TTTS was recognized by Wittmann and Brennan. Wittmann et al. proposed as discriminating findings in TTTS the discrepancy in the sizes of twins and the polyhydramnios surrounding the larger twin. Brennan et al. added to the former criteria, the disparity in the size of the vessels in the umbilical cords, same-sex, single placenta showing different echogenicity of the cotyledons supplying the two cords, and evidence of hydrops in either twin or congestive heart failure in the recipient. More recently, more useful sonographic criteria have been adopted, which are discussed further.

Discordance in Amniotic Fluid Volume (Oligohydramnios Sequence)

In 1988, Chescheir and Seeds disclosed a powerful clue based on the fact that six out of seven twin pregnancies with MC placentas and TTTS had concurrent polyhydramnios and oligohydramnios. This is not surprising when we understand TTTS as a manifestation of a hemodynamic imbalance.[106] Fetal renal perfusion is asymmetric—the congestive heart failure in the recipient will overperfuse the kidneys with consequent polyuria and excess of amniotic fluid; hypovolemia in the donor causes inadequate perfusion of the kidneys with a decrease in urinary output and oligohydramnios.

More uniform criteria for the oligohydramnios sequence have been proposed for a quantitative definition—deepest vertical pool in the donor sac <2 cm and >8 cm in the recipient's sac. Not infrequently anhydramnios in the donor sac results in it becoming "stuck," shrouded by the intertwin membrane, while the recipient's sac becomes severely polyhydramniotic.

One should bear in mind that sonographic pitfalls may exist in the presence of discordant anomalies in twins that imply differences in amniotic fluid volume, such as one twin with esophageal atresia and consequent polyhydramnios, or with renal agenesis, with consequent oligohydramnios/anhydramnios.

Other related confirmatory features include a small or nonvisible bladder due to hypovolemia and renal hypoperfusion in the donor, along with a distended urinary bladder with resulting excessive micturition in the recipient.

Discordance in Fetal Size

Discordant growth is a common complication of twin pregnancies. The need for stricter sonographic criteria to define growth has changed gold standards over time. Abdominal circumference rather than head measurements of twins was proposed as the most reproducible and meaningful one. Besides, considering that fetal weight estimations based on singleton growth charts may be inadequate for twins, the abdominal circumference criterion should be definitely used for the sonographic diagnosis of divergent twin growth. A cut-off value of 20 mm for the difference in abdominal circumference between twins indicated growth discordance of >20%.

Abnormal Doppler Findings

Alterations in cardiac hemodynamics are indirectly put on evidence by alterations in venous blood flow waveforms. The receptor presents with pulsatility in the umbilical vein and absent or reverse flow in the ductus venosus[107] as signs of congestive heart failure due to hypervolemia and increased preload from placental vascular anastomotic transfusion.

Fetal Echocardiography

Both donor and recipient twins have dynamic changes in volume/pressure loading during cardiovascular development constituting a hostile intrauterine environment. Considering the hemodynamic imbalance between the circulations of the twins involving some excess of blood flowing from the donor to the recipient fetus, cardiac involvement is logically expected. Echocardiography is a well-established tool for antenatal assessment of structural and functional heart disease, turning it possible in TTTS to assess cardiovascular adaptation to intertwin transfusion, early recognition of deterioration, and evaluation of antenatal management.

Zosmer et al. (1994)[108] showed that some surviving twins of TTTS had a persistent right ventricular hypertrophic cardiomyopathy and proposed that cardiac dysfunction could be induced in utero by sustained strain upon the heart by TTTS, predominantly affecting the right ventricle.

The right ventricle is stiffer and more afterload-sensitive than the left ventricle, mostly due to the redistribution of blood in the cerebral arteries which decreases the left ventricular afterload. Additionally, recipients remain at increased risk of pulmonary artery stenosis and maintain a slightly reduced early diastolic ventricular filling as compared to donors (diastolic dysfunction).[109]

In contrast, the significant reduction of blood flow velocity in the umbilical artery recorded in the "donor" is consistent with hypovolemia and increased placental resistance, increasing cardiac afterload, and decreasing umbilical venous return. This is in good agreement with some studies, which show that the donor twin has a trend toward a lower Tei-index than in the normal population. Finally, there have been speculations about an increased incidence of aortic coarctation in donors due to a lower venous return from the placenta and hence a decreased loading of the left ventricular outflow tract (Wohlmuth et al., 2011).[109]

In the study from Fesslova et al. (1998),[110] all recipient fetuses showed cardiac hypertrophy and dilatation, well-known compensatory mechanisms of blood volume overload, and high cardiac output (Frank–Starling mechanism).

After birth about half of the recipients showed biventricular hypertrophy, with prevalent left ventricular hypertrophic cardiomyopathy.[108,110,111] A smaller subgroup will develop right ventricular tract obstruction (functional pulmonary stenosis) and pulmonary hypertension in the neonatal period, which may be aggravated by systolic right ventricular dysfunction. Recently diastolic abnormalities were described in the right ventricle, with abnormal filling patterns, prolonged isovolumic relaxation time, and abnormal flow patterns in the inferior vena cava and ductus venosus. In addition to hemodynamic remodeling, it is well recognized the role of increased endothelin-1 in the recipient, mainly in the hydropic recipient, as a mitogenic factor to smooth muscle cells in systemic and pulmonary vasculature and for ventricular myocyte proliferation.

More recently, abnormalities of vascular distensibility were described in survivors of TTTS in infancy.[111] The donor fetus shows evidence of chronic hypovolemia resulting in activation of the RAS. This upregulation initially attempts to correct volume depletion, and transfusion of increased concentrations of angiotensin II will probably cause increased vascular stiffness in the surviving donor in childhood.

Signs of Hydrops in the Recipient Twin

In an advanced stage of TTTS the recipient twin affected by congestive heart failure may present signs of serosa effusions, such as ascites, pleural effusion, and subcutaneous edema.

Other Ultrasonographic Findings

- *Identification of cord insertion:* Velamentous insertion of the cord is a frequent finding.
- *Funipuncture*: Theoretically it may allow the antenatal assessment of intertwin hemoglobin difference, the degree of fetal anemia in the donor twin, and the twin's zygosity through blood group studies. However, the possible benefit of this procedure seems to be very poor on clinical grounds and the risks importantly outweigh the informative gain.
- *Difference in the color of the placentas*: Due to blood transfusion from one twin to the other, the placenta of the donor twin tends to be whitish ("pale"), and the placenta of the recipient, of a denser color (excess of blood).

Treatment of Twin-to-Twin Transfusion Syndrome

Fetoscopic laser coagulation of inter-twin vascular anastomoses on the MC placenta is the preferred treatment for TTTS. Severe postoperative complications can occur when intertwin vascular anastomoses remain patent including twin-anemia polycythemia sequence or recurrent TTTS. To minimize the occurrence of residual anastomoses, a modified laser surgery technique, the Solomon technique, was developed in which the entire vascular equator is coagulated. This technique was associated with a significant reduction in short-term complications (twin-anemia polycythemia sequence and recurrence of TTTS) when compared with the standard laser surgery technique. No differences in survival or neurodevelopmental impairment between both techniques were found.[112]

Prediction of Twin-to-Twin Transfusion Syndrome

While accounting for only 1.2% of the population, twins are responsible for 12.6% of the perinatal mortality. In the particular case of MC twinning the fetal loss rate is even more relevant and there is an increased risk of adverse perinatal outcome. Therefore, targeted surveillance of MC twins at earlier stages of gestation could anticipate and provide timely management of the pregnancies at risk of one of the most devastating type-specific complications including TTTS.

Nuchal Translucency

Data gathered from the literature show that increased NT thickness at 10–14 weeks of gestation was found twice as much as in MC than in singleton pregnancies, and the likelihood ratio of developing TTTS in those twins with increased NT was 3.5.[95,113] Considering that MC pregnancies do not show a higher prevalence of chromosomal abnormalities, the higher prevalence of increased NT in those twins could be ascribed to cardiac dysfunction. With advancing gestation, this transient heart failure eventually resolves with increased diuresis and ventricular compliance. More recently, it was observed that whenever the discrepancy of NT values was above 20%, the detection rate for early fetal death was 63% and for severe TTTS of 52%.[114] In a study by Lewi et al. (2008)[115] showed that significant predictors in the first trimester were the difference in crown–rump length (CRL) [odds ratio (OR) = 11] and discordant amniotic fluid (OR = 10). Later in pregnancy, at 16 weeks, significant predictors were the difference in abdominal circumference (OR = 29), discordant amniotic fluid (OR = 7), and discordant cord insertions (OR = 3). Risk assessment in the first trimester and at 16 weeks detected 29% and 48% of cases with a complicated fetal outcome, respectively, with a false-positive rate of 3 and 6%, respectively. Combined first-trimester and 16-week assessments identified 58% of fetal complications, with a false-positive rate of 8%.[115]

Ductus Venosus Flowmetry

Can the characteristic circulatory imbalance of TTTS, fully expressed later in pregnancy, disclose indirect signs of cardiac dysfunction in earlier stages of gestation? In studies of vascular hemodynamics in fetuses with increased NT at 10–14 weeks, the abnormal flow in DV more frequently recorded in fetuses with chromosomopathies, with or without cardiac defects, was related to heart strain.[116-119] These findings are in good agreement with the overt hemodynamic alterations found in TTTS later in pregnancy. Therefore, strong evidence suggests that increased NT along with abnormal flow in the DV, even in the presence of a normal karyotype, may be early signs of cardiac impairment or defect.

In a study from our Unit,[77] in which nuchal translucency and Doppler blood flow waveforms in the DV were recorded in both twins between 11 and 14 weeks of gestation, TTTS was recorded in those fetuses with combined increased NT and abnormal flow in the DV. Whenever NT was discrepant but with the normal flow in the DV, no cases of TTTS were found [78,120] **(Figs. 3A and B)**.

More recently, in a more inclusive study, we showed that discrepant values for NT over 0.6 mm had a sensitivity of 45.5% and a specificity of 86.9%. The presence of at least one abnormal blood flow waveform in the DV translated into a relative risk for developing TTTS of 11.86 (3.05–57.45) with a sensitivity of 72.7% and a specificity of 91.7%. The combination of abnormal DV blood flow with discrepant NT >0.6 mm, yielded a relative risk for the development of TTTS 21 times higher [confidence interval (CI): 95% 5.47–98.33].[86]

In those uncomplicated MC twin pregnancies, in which abnormal DV flow was found in at least one of the fetuses, a higher discordance in birth weight was recorded in the third trimester of pregnancy when compared to those with the normal flow in both fetuses.[121]

Therefore, both increased NT and abnormal flow in the ductus venosus in MC twins may translate into early manifestations of hemodynamic imbalance between donor and recipient. In these pregnancies, in addition to NT measurement at 11–14 weeks, the Doppler assessment of DV blood flow increases relevantly the performance of screening for those at risk of developing TTTS.

More recently, Stagnati et al. (2017)[122] published a systematic review and a metanalysis to evaluate the performance of each ultrasonographic early marker (intertwin NT discrepancy, NT >95th percentile, intertwin CRL discrepancy >10% or abnormal DV flow) in the prediction of TTTS in the 1st trimester of pregnancy. An increased risk of TTTS was associated with: intertwin NT discrepancy [positive likelihood ratio (LR+), 1.92 (95% CI: 1.25–2.96); negative likelihood ratio (LR–), 0.65 (95% CI, 0.50–0.84); NT >95th percentile [LR+, 2.63 (95% CI: 1.51–4.58); LR–, 0.85 (95% CI: 0.75–0.96)]; CRL discrepancy >10% (LR+, 1.80 (95% CI: 1.05–3.07); LR–, 0.92 (95% CI: 0.81–1.05)); abnormal DV flow [LR+, 4.77 (95% CI: 1.33–17.04; LR–, 0.49 (95% CI: 0.17–1.41)]. The highest sensitivities were observed for intertwin NT discrepancy [52.8% (95% CI: 43.8–61.7%)] and abnormal DV flow [50.0% (95% CI: 33.4–66.6%)].[122]

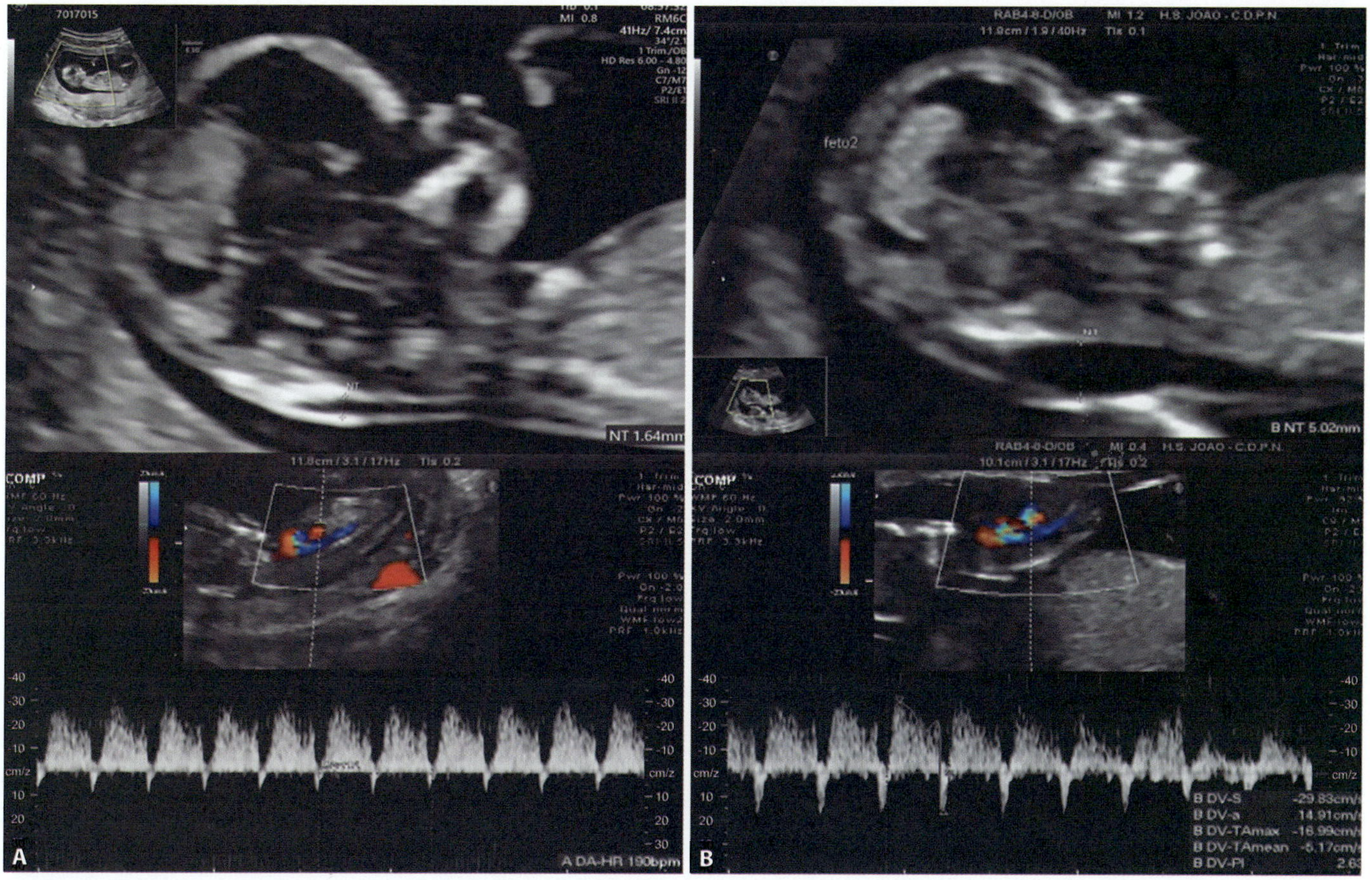

Figs. 3A and B: Screening for trisomy 21 in monochorionic twins (averaging method). We can observe discrepant nuchal translucencies (NTs) = 1.25 and 5.02 mm. Ductus venosus Doppler blood flow is abnormal in the fetus with increased NT. This pair of twins was chromosomally normal and developed a twin-to-twin transfusion syndrome at 16 weeks.

Arterioarterial Anastomoses

The search of AA anastomoses in the placental plate of MC placentas by color Doppler has until now mainly provided a negative value: only 5% of MC twins will develop TTTS if AA anastomoses are present; if absent, 58% will develop TTTS. In the studies of Taylor et al., the sensitivity and positive predictive value for absent AA anastomoses in predicting TTTS were 74% and 61%, respectively.[123] The major limitation to the use of absent AA anastomoses in predicting TTTS is the difficulty in being sure that an AA anastomosis is really absent or simply not yet seen, as it frequently happens before 18 weeks.

Intertwin Membrane Folding

At 15–17 weeks of gestation, the disparity in amniotic fluid volume between the two amniotic sacs seems to cause membrane folding: if present, 28% of cases developed severe TTTS and 72% developed mild TTTS. If membrane folding was absent, no cases of TTTS were recorded.

DISCORDANCE OF FETAL GROWTH: WHAT IS ADAPTATION, PROMOTION, AND GROWTH RESTRICTION IN MULTIPLES?

The restriction of intrauterine fetal growth is more frequently found in multiple pregnancies: about 52% of twins and 92% of triplets present low birth weight (<2,500 g) compared to 6% of singletons, whereas 10% of twins and 32% of triplets are born with very low birth weight (<1,000 g) when compared to 1% of singletons. This has not been scrutinized in depth because of three limitations including (1) when we define fetal growth restriction (FGR) growth curves of fetuses with comparable growth potentials twin curves should be adopted. At present, it is believed that multiples do not have the same growth potential as singletons and there are serious doubts concerning the appropriateness of singleton standards for multiples. Second, the growth pattern of late pregnancy is practically unknown because preterm birth (by singleton standards) is the rule rather than the exception in multiple gestations (before 37 weeks, about 50% of twins and 91% of triplets were already born in comparison with 9% of singletons). Finally, there are few longitudinal studies and most of our knowledge is derived from birth weight by gestational age relationships (growth curves).

Grande et al. (2015)[124] demonstrated that early discordant twin pregnancies were at significant higher risk of chromosomal (OR: 11.42; 95% CI: 2.78–46.94), structural anomalies (OR: 5.91; 95% CI: 2.25–15.54), spontaneous fetal loss (OR: 4.23; 95% CI: 1.79–10.01), birthweight discordance (OR: 2.8; 95% CI: 1.48–5.65) and small for gestational age (SGA) (OR: 3.48; 95% CI: 1.78–6.79). In fact, CRL discordance (≥10%) presented with higher rates of structural anomalies, stillbirth, birthweight discordance, and small newborns. Fetal anomalies and growth restriction increased in severe CRL discordance (≥16%).[124] More recently, Curado et al. (2019)[125] and Litwinska et al. (2019)[126] demonstrated that a large discordance in CRL is associated with a high risk for fetal loss and ominous perinatal outcome.

If we monitor fetal growth in multiple pregnancies by singleton standards, >50% of triplets are considered (SGA) at 35 weeks, and more than 50% of twins are considered SGA at 38 weeks. Though many authors classify twin infants as IUGR by using a gender, and a gestational age-specific birth weight below the 10th centile,[127,128] the truth is that a biological phenomenon with a frequency of over 50% reluctantly will be considered a pathological event. The reevaluation of the median birth weight centile of twins and triplets compared to the 10th centile for singletons showed that the average multiple is not "SGA" and weighs more than the 10th birth weight percentile for singletons until 35 weeks in triplets and 38 weeks in twins.[129]

The common growth curves show that deviations from singleton standards occur after 28 weeks.[129] The uterine milieu, comprising uteroplacental, maternal, and fetal components, limits physiologically the growth potential of the individual fetus in a multiple pregnancy. This concept implies that most multiples delivered after 28 weeks are growth-restricted compared to singletons, as a result of an adaptative process. The total twin and total triplet birth weights exceed that of the 90th birth weight centile for singletons as early as 25 weeks gestation (data derived from 3.6 million singletons from the Matria database). The uterine potential adaptation to multiple pregnancies is also appreciated by realizing that the average singleton birth weight at 40 weeks is reached as early as 32 weeks in twins and as early as 29 weeks in triplets.

Consequently, the individual multiple is relatively growth-restricted compared to singletons whereas the entire pregnancy is growth promoted.[130] This physiological restriction (reduction in fetal size) is a way to promote a more advanced gestation as long as possible, to overcome the tremendous increase in volume, uterine overdistention, and the higher frequency of preterm delivery in multiples.[129] The variables that most strongly influence uterine adaptation are parity (less in nulliparous), maternal age, maternal height, and weight gain.

Discordant growth is another potential way to reduce uterine volume in order to promote an advanced gestational age at birth. The problem is to distinguish between natural variation and pathological growth restriction. Differences as large as 15% may be normal; whereas, 15–25% discordance may denote adaptation, and differences of >25% reveal the inability to maintain growth.[8] This latter group presents the best correlation with adverse outcomes, namely neonatal mortality and morbidity and intensive care admission (Blickstein e Keith, 2004b).[131]

The risk of occurring a fetal growth restriction in a multiple pregnancy is 10 times greater than in a singleton pregnancy,[132] being even greater in an MC (34%) compared to a dichorionic pregnancy (23%) (Sebire et al., 1997c).[133] More recently, our group put in evidence that in uncomplicated MC twin pregnancies, abnormal DV flow in at least one of the fetuses seems to be associated with a higher discordance in birth weight than in those with normal flow in both fetuses.[121] In fact, in pregnancies with abnormal DV flow in at least one of the fetuses the median discordance in birth weight was higher than in those with normal DV flow in both twins (13.2% vs. 7.8%, $P = 0.006$).

Hence, the meaning of *fetal growth discordance* in multiples depends on chorionicity. The abdominal circumference is the most reliable sonographic criterion for the establishment of growth discrepancy. A difference of 20 mm translates into a birth weight discrepancy of 20% or more. In a dichorionic twin pregnancy (dizygotic in 90%) may be ascribed to a different genetic constitution of the twins or to an unequal placental function. In an

MC pregnancy, as the genetic content is the same, the growth discordance may be due to an unequal division of the cellular mass (unequal sharing of the placenta), velamentous insertion (VCI) of the cord, vasa previa or to the unbalanced transfusion of blood through the vascular anastomoses. Our group demonstrated that VCI is not associated with the development of TTTS but increases the risk of adverse outcomes. Both VCI and TTTS independently increased the prevalence of intrauterine fetal death and lower gestational age at birth in a similar way, showing that VCI is an important indicator of adverse perinatal outcomes in MC twins.[33,34]

By using data from the Matched Multiple Birth Data Set from the National Centre for Health Statistics it was noticed that 10.683 pairs showed a discordance >25% (8.2% of the entire population of twins). This population was subdivided into three groups according to the birth weight of the smaller twin (<10th centile, 10–50th centile, or >50th centile). These subgroups correspond to severely discordant twin pairs that are growth restricted, growth adapted, or growth promoted, respectively. The frequencies of each subgroup were unaltered through the third trimester: 6,668 (62.4%), 3,514 (32.9%), and 501 (4.7%) severely discordant sets (Blickstein & Keith, 2004).[134] Neonatal mortality was significantly higher (29.1%) when the smaller twin weighed <10th centile for gestational age compared with other subgroups (11.2 and 11%). The data proves that even among severely discordant pairs, 40% are appropriately grown twins, of which 6% are, in fact, growth promoted.

Importantly this growth restriction among twins, mainly the MC subgroup has well-known ominous consequences in fetal neurodevelopment. What is new is that this issue has a negative impact on all three areas of development including cognition, language, and motor skills.[135]

MULTIPLES AND CEREBRAL PALSY: THE EFFECT OF PREMATURITY OR MORE?

In 1897, Sigmund Freud suggested that multiple pregnancy was the most important cause of cerebral palsy more relevant than perinatal asphyxia or preterm birth. A century later, this postulate remains valid:[136-140] We know that the risk of one of the fetuses being affected by cerebral palsy is 1.5% in twins, 8% in triplets, and 43% in quadruplets.[141] In reality, there is an exponential relationship between the number of fetuses in a pregnancy and the rate of cerebral palsy. There is a higher prevalence of brain damage in MC and like-sex twins than in dichorionic pregnancies, namely when the death of the cotwin occurs: the incidence of the lesions of the white matter after the death of the cotwin in an MC pregnancy is 25% in contrast with 3% in the survivor of a dichorionic twin pregnancy.[142] Prematurity and low birth weight are the most relevant risk factors for long-term neurological morbidity. Factors such as zygosity, intrauterine growth restriction, fetal weight discordance, and type of birth are less powerfully correlated with the risk of cerebral palsy in multiple pregnancies.[143]

In a population-based retrospective cohort study comparing neurological problems in Swedish children born after IVF with matched controls, the former was 70% more likely to need rehabilitation. The risk of cerebral palsy was four-fold increased in children born after IVF. The data confirm a model that suggested a significantly lower estimated cerebral palsy rate (2.7/1,000 neonates) after spontaneous pregnancies as compared with transfer of three embryos (OR = 6.3), two embryos (OR = 3.3), and transfer of three embryos in which all triplets have been reduced to twins (OR = 3.8). Similar estimations suggested that iatrogenic multiples contribute 8% to the annual number of cerebral palsy cases in the USA.

In the specific case of TTTS, Lopriore, et al. (2003)[144] presented important data concerning the psychomotor development of survivors from TTTS evaluated until school entry. From a total of 29 children affected in utero by TTTS and evaluated for 8 years, 41% presented cerebral anomalies disclosed by ultrasound and about 21% had cerebral palsy.[144] This figure rose to 50% in the cases of TTTS complicated by intrauterine fetal demise of the cotwin whereas rates of 14% of cerebral palsy were found in the cases in which both twins survived.

To anticipate the neurologic risk in cases of TTTS complicated with the death of the cotwin, Senat et al. (2003)[145] proposed the sequential evaluation of the fetal middle cerebral artery peak systolic velocity to predict fetal anemia within 24 hours of the death of one MC twin and to monitor hemoglobin concentration in the surviving fetus at risk for acute anemia.[145] This method was found to be a reliable non-invasive diagnostic tool and may be helpful in counseling and planning invasive testing.

CONCLUSION

In clinical terms, the assignment of chorionicity is more relevant than zygosity determination and will dramatically influence the perinatal outcome. In fact, about 30% of MC twin pregnancies are complicated by TTTS, isolated discordant growth, twin anemia-polycythemia sequence, congenital defects, or intrauterine demise. About 15% will be eligible for invasive fetal therapy. Combining several sonographic markers, ultrasound examination in the first and early second trimester can differentiate MC twins at high risk for adverse outcomes from those likely to be uneventful, useful information for patient counseling and planning of care.

REFERENCES

1. Tromp M, Ravelli AC, Reitsma JB, et al. Increasing maternal age at first pregnancy planning: health outcomes and associated costs. J Epidemiol Community Health. 2010;65(12):1083-90.
2. Blickstein I. The worldwide impact of iatrogenic pregnancy. Int J Gynecol Obstet. 2003;82(3):307-17.
3. Blickstein I. Estimation of iatrogenic monozygotic twinning rate following assisted reproduction: pitfalls and caveats. Am J Obstet Gynecol. 2005;192(2):365-8.
4. de Mouzon J, Goossens V, Bhattacharya S, et al. Assisted reproductive technology in Europe, 2006: results generated from European registers by ESHRE. Hum Reprod. 2010;25(8):1851-62.
5. Wenstrom KD, Syrop CH, Hammitt DG, et al. Increased risk of monochorionic twinning associated with assisted reproduction. Fert Steril. 1993;60(3):510-4.
6. Blickstein I, Verhoeven HC, Keith LG. Zygotic splitting after assisted reproduction. N Eng J Med. 1999;340(9):738-9.
7. Blickstein I, Jones C, Keith LG. Zygotic-splitting rates after single-embryo transfers in in vitro fertilization. N Eng J Med. 2003;348(23):2366-7.
8. Blickstein I. Growth aberration in multiple pregnancy. Obstet Gynecol Clin North Am. 2005;32(1):39-54,viii.
9. Blickstein I, Arabin B, Lewi L, et al. A template for defining the perinatal care of monochorionic twins: the Istanbul international ad hoc committee. J Perinat Med. 2010;38(2):107-10.
10. Marleen S, Dias C, Nandasena R, et al. Association between chorionicity and preterm birth in twin pregnancies: a systematic review involving 29 864 twin pregnancies. BJOG. 2021;128(5):788-96.
11. Myrianthopoulos NC. Congenital malformations: the contribution of twin studies. Birth Defects Orig Artic Ser. 1978;14(6A):151-65.
12. Baldwin VJ. Anomalous development of twins. In: Baldwin VJ (Ed). Pathology of Multiple Pregnancy. New York: Springer-Verlag; 1994. pp. 169-97.
13. Casati D, Faiola S, Lanna M. Major discordant anomalies in MZ twins: management and outcome. In: Alexandra Matias, Isaac Blickstein (Eds). Developmental and fetal origins of differences in monozygotic twins: from Genetics to Environmental factors. Amsterdam: Elsevier Inc; 2020. pp. 181-96.
14. Rodis JF, Egan JF, Craffey A, et al. Calculated risk of chromosomal abnormalities in twin gestations. Obstet Gynecol. 1990;76(6):1037-41.
15. Hack KE, Derks JB, Elias SG, et al. Increased perinatal mortality and morbidity in monochorionic versus dichorionic twin pregnancies: clinical implications of a large Dutch Cohort Study. BJOG. 2008;115(1):58-67.
16. Buca D, Di Mascio D, Khalil A, et al. Neonatal Morbidity of Monoamniotic Twin Pregnancies: A Systematic Review and Meta-analysis. Am J Perinatol. 2022;39(3):243-51.
17. Silva S, Martins Y, Matias A, et al. Why are monozygotic twins different? J Perinat Med. 2011;39(2):195-202.
18. Matias A, Blickstein I. In: Alexandra Matias, Isaac Blickstein (Eds). Developmental and fetal origins of differences in monozygotic twins: from Genetics to Environmental factors. Amsterdam: Elsevier Inc.; 2020.
19. Hall JG. Twinning: mechanisms and genetic implications. Curr Opin Genet Dev. 1996;6(3):343-7.
20. Steinman G, Valderrama E. Mechanisms of twinning. III. Placentation, calcium reduction and modified compaction. J Reprod Med. 2001;46(11):995-1002.
21. Hall JG. Twinning. Lancet. 2003;62(9385):735-43.
22. Blickstein I, Keith LG. The decreased rates of triplet births: temporal trends and biologic speculations. Am J Obstet Gynecol. 2005;193(2):327-31.
23. Blickstein I, Keith LG. On the possible cause of monozygotic twinning: lessons from the 9-banded armadillo and from assisted reproduction. Twin Res Hum Genetics. 2007;10(2):394-9.
24. Teplica D, Peekna K. The mirror phenomenon in monozygotic twins. In: Blickstein I, Keith LG (Eds). Multiple pregnancy, 2nd edition. London, UK: CRC Press; 2005. pp. 277-88.
25. Blokage CE. Embryogenesis of chimeras, twins and anterior midline asymmetries. Human Reprod. 2006;21(3):579-91.
26. Matias A, Montenegro N, Blickstein I. Sonographic evaluation of multiple pregnancies. In: Kurjak A, Chevernak F (Eds). Textbook of Perinatal Medicine, 2nd edition. London, UK: CRC Press; 2006. pp. 1591-603.
27. Matias A, La Sala G, Blickstein I. Early loss rates of entire pregnancies after assisted reproduction are lower in twin than in singleton pregnancies. Fert Steril. 2007;88(5):1452-4.
28. Oliviennes F. Avoiding multiple pregnancies in ART. Double trouble: yes a twin pregnancy is an adverse outcome. Hum Reprod. 2000;15(8):1663-5.
29. Tummers P, De Sutter P, Dhont M. Risk of spontaneous abortion in singleton and twin pregnancies after IVF/ICSI. Hum Reprod. 2003;18(8):1720-3.
30. Zegers-Hochschild F, Bravo M, Fernandez E, et al. Multiple gestation as a marker of reproductive efficacy: learning from assisted reproductive technologies. Reprod Biomed Online. 2003;8(1):125-9.
31. La Sala GB, Nicoli A, Villani MT, et al. Spontaneous embryonic loss rates in twin and singleton pregnancies after transfer of top- versus intermediate-quality embryos. Fertil Steril. 2005;84(6):1602-5.

32. Lambers MJ, Mager E, Goutbeek J, et al. Factors determining early pregnancy loss in singleton and multiple implantations. Hum Reprod. 2006;22(1):275-9.
33. Costa-Castro T, De Villiers S, Montenegro N, et al. Velamentous cord insertion in monochorionic twins with or without twin-twin transfusion syndrome: Does it matter? Placenta. 2013;34(11):1053-8.
34. Costa-Castro T, DP Zhao, Lipa M, et al. Lopriore. Velamentous cord insertion in dichorionic and monochorionic twin pregnancies - Does it make a difference? Placenta. 2016;42:87-92.
35. Lewi L, Couck I, Deprest J. Twin-reversed arterial perfusion sequence: different identical twins. In: Alexandra Matias, Isaac Blickstein (Eds). Developmental and fetal origins of differences in monozygotic twins: from Genetics to Environmental factors. Amsterdam: Elsevier Inc.; 2020. pp. 169-78.
36. Schmid O, Trautmann U, Ashour H, et al. Prenatal diagnosis of heterokaryotypic mosaic twins discordant for fetal sex. Prenat Diagn. 2000;20(12):999-1003.
37. Jonsson H, Magnusdottir E, Eggertsson HP, et al. Differences between germline genomes of monozygotic twins. Nat Genet. 2021;53(1):27-34.
38. Bourthoumieu S, Yardin C, Terro F, et al. Monozygotic twins concordant for blood karyotype, but phenotypically discordant: a case of "mosaic chimerism". Am J Med Genet A. 2005;135(2):190-4.
39. Nieuwint A, Van Zalen-Sprock R, Hummel P, et al. 'Identical' twins with discordant karyotypes. Prenat Diagn. 1999;19(1):72-6.
40. Zech NH, Wisser J, Natalucci G, et al. Monochorionic-diamniotic twins discordant in gender from a naturally conceived pregnancy through postzygotic sex chromosome loss in a 47,XXY zygote. Prenat Diagn. 2008;28(8):759-63.
41. Heydanus R, Santema JG, Stewart PA, et al. Preterm delivery rate and fetal outcome in structurally affected twin pregnancies: a retrospective matched control study. Prenat Diagn. 1993;13(3):155-62.
42. Lu, JH, Chung MY, Hwang B, Chien HP. Monozygotic twins with chromosome 22q11 microdeletion and discordant phenotypes in cardiovascular patterning. Pediatr Cardiol. 2001;22(3):260-3.
43. Tsukamoto H, Inui K, Taniike M, et al. Different clinical features in monozygotic twins: a case of 7q--syndrome. Clin Genet. 1993;43(3):139-42.
44. Cheng PJ, Shaw SW, Shih JC, et al. Monozygotic twins discordant for monosomy 21 detected by first-trimester nuchal translucency screening. Obstet Gynecol. 2006;107(2 Pt 2):538-41.
45. Machin GA. Some causes of genotypic and phenotypic discordance in monozygotic twin pairs. Am J Med Genet. 1996;61(3):216-28.
46. Matias A, Pereira-Macedo M, Montenegro N. Spotting the differences in the first trimester of pregnancy in monozygotic twins: the issue of aneuploidies and TTTS screening. In: Alexandra Matias, Isaac Blickstein (Eds). Developmental and fetal origins of differences in monozygotic twins: from Genetics to Environmental factors. Amsterdam: Elsevier Inc.; 2020. pp. 215-26.
47. Zito A, Roberts AL, Visconti A, et al. Escape from X-inactivation in twins exhibits intra- and inter-individual variability across tissues and is heritable. PLoS Genet. 2023; 19(2):e1010556.
48. Kato T, Iwamoto K, Kakiuchi C, et al. Genetic or epigenetic difference causing discordance between monozygotic twins as a clue to molecular basis of mental disorders. Mol Psychiatry. 2005;10(7):622-30.
49. Singh SM, Murphy B, O'Reilly R. Epigenetic contributors to the discordance of monozygotic twins. Clin Genet. 2002;62(2):97-103.
50. Santer R, Hoffmann H, Suttorp M, et al. Discordance for hyperinsulinemic hypoglycemia in monozygotic twins. J Pediatr. 1995;126(6):1017.
51. Blakely EL, He L, Taylor RW, et al. Mitochondrial DNA deletion in "identical" twin brothers. J Med Genet. 2004;41(2):e19.
52. Haque FN, Gottesman, II, Wong AH. Not really identical: epigenetic differences in monozygotic twins and implications for twin studies in psychiatry. Am J Med Genet C Semin Med Genet. 2009;151C(2):136-41.
53. Homfray T. Genetics and epigenetics differences in monozygotic twins: the vision of the geneticist. In: Alexandra Matias, Isaac Blickstein (Eds). Developmental and fetal origins of differences in monozygotic twins: from Genetics to Environmental factors. Amsterdam: Elsevier Inc; 2020. pp. 95-110.
54. Kaminsky Z, Petronis A, Wang SC, et al. Epigenetics of personality traits: an illustrative study of identical twins discordant for risk-taking behavior. Twin Res Hum Genet. 2008;11(1):1-11.
55. Oates NA, van Vliet J, Duffy DL, et al. Increased DNA methylation at the AXIN1 gene in a monozygotic twin from a pair discordant for a caudal duplication anomaly. Am J Hum Genet. 2006;79(1):155-62.
56. Poulsen P, Esteller M, Vaag A, et al. The epigenetic basis of twin discordance in age-related diseases. Pediatr Res. 2007;61(5 Pt 2):38R-42R.
57. Ferguson-Smith MA, Bianchi DW. Prenatal Diagnosis: past, present, and future. Prenat Diagn. 2010;30(7):601-4.
58. Liao H, Liu S, Wang H. Performance of non-invasive prenatal screening for fetal aneuploidy in twin pregnancies: a meta-analysis. Prenat Diagn. 2017;37(9):874-82.
59. Leonard S, Martin K. Noninvasive prenatal screening in twin pregnancies. In: Alexandra Matias, Isaac Blickstein (Eds). Developmental and fetal origins of differences in monozygotic twins: from Genetics to Environmental factors. Amsterdam: Elsevier Inc.; 2020. pp. 229-42.
60. Caroto T, Santos V, Matias A. Accuracy of NIPT for detection of trisomy 21, trisomy 18 and trisomy 13 in twin pregnancies: a systematic review. Obstet Gynecol. 2021 (submitted).
61. Machado AP, Ramalho C, Portugal R, et al. Concordance for bilateral congenital diaphragmatic hernia in a monozygotic

dichorionic twin pair - first clinical report. Fetal Diagn Ther. 2010;27(2):106-9.
62. Sommer IE, Ramsey NF, Bouma A, et al. Cerebral mirror-imaging in a monozygotic twin. Lancet. 1999;354(9188):1445-6.
63. Benassar M, Gratacos E. Differences in growth: selective intrauterine growth restriction in monochorionic twins. In: Alexandra Matias, Isaac Blickstein (Eds). Developmental and fetal origins of differences in monozygotic twins: from Genetics to Environmental factors. Amsterdam: Elsevier Inc.; 2020. pp. 135-44.
64. Gringras P, Chen W. Mechanisms for differences in monozygous twins. Early Hum Dev. 2001;64(2):105-17.
65. Derom C, Derom R. The East Flanders Prospective Twin Survey. In: Blickstein I, Keith LG (Eds). Multiple Pregnancy, 2nd edition. London, UK: Taylor & Francis; 2005. pp. 39-47.
66. Tong S, Vollenhoven B, Meagher S. Determining zygosity in early pregnancy by ultrasound. Ultrasound Obstet Gynecol. 2004;23(1):36-7.
67. Sepulveda W, Sebire N, Hughes K, et al. The lambda sign at 10-14 weeks of gestation as a predictor of chorionicity in twin pregnancies. Ultrasound Obstet Gynecol. 1996;7(6):421-3.
68. Wood SL, St Onge R, Connors G, et al. Evaluation of the twin peak or lambda sign in determining chorionicity in multiple pregnancy. Obstet Gynecol. 1996;88(1):6-9.
69. Maruotti GM, Saccone G, Morlando M, et al. First-trimester ultrasound determination of chorionicity in twin gestations using the lambda sign: a systematic review and meta-analysis. Eur J Obstet Gynecol Reprod Biol. 2016;202:66-70.
70. Bennett PR, Overton TG, Lighten AD, et al. Lancet. 1995;345(8950):661-2.
71. Pretorious D, Budorick N, Sciosia A, et al. Twin pregnancies in the second trimester in women in an alpha-fetoprotein screening program: sonographic evaluation and outcome. Am J Roentgenol. 1993;161(5):1007-13.
72. Blickstein I. The twin-twin transfusion syndrome. Obstet Gynecol. 1990;76(4):714-22.
73. Sepulveda W, Sebire N, Hughes K, et al. Evolution of the lambda or twin-chorionic peak sign in dichorionic twin pregnancies. Obstet Gynecol. 1997;89(3):439-41.
74. Khalil A, Rodgers M, Baschat A, et al. ISUOG Practice Guidelines: role of ultrasound in twin pregnancy. Ultrasound Obstet Gynecol. 2016;47(2):247-63.
75. Matias A, Silva S, Blickstein I. Mechanisms of discordance in MZ twins: why and when? In: Alexandra Matias, Isaac Blickstein (Eds). Developmental and fetal origins of differences in monozygotic twins: from Genetics to Environmental factors. Amsterdam: Elsevier Inc.; 2020. pp. 61-77.
76. Grömminger S, Yagmur E, Erkan S, et al. Fetal Aneuploidy Detection by Cell-Free DNA Sequencing for Multiple Pregnancies and Quality Issues with Vanishing Twins. J Clin Med. 2014;3(3):679-92.
77. Matias A, Montenegro N. Down syndrome screening in multiple pregnancies. Obst Gynecol Clin North Am. 2005;32(1):81-96.
78. Matias A, Ramalho C, Montenegro N. Search for hemodynamic compromise at 11-14 weeks in monochorionic twin pregnancy: is abnormal flow in the ductus venosus predictive of twin-twin transfusion syndrome? J Matern Fetal Neonatal Med. 2005;18(2):79-86.
79. Jenkins TM, Wapner RJ. The challenge of prenatal diagnosis in twin pregnancies. Curr Opin Obstet Gynecol. 2000;12(2):87-92.
80. Sebire NJ, Snijders RJ, Hughes K, Sepulveda W, Nicolaides KH. Screening for trisomy 21 in twin pregnancies by maternal age and fetal nuchal translucency thickness at 10-14 weeks of gestation. Br J Obstet Gynaecol. 1996; 103(10):999-1003.
81. Pandya PP, Snijders RJ, Johnson SP, et al. Screening for fetal trisomies by maternal age and fetal nuchal translucency thickness at 10 to 14 weeks of gestation. Br J Obstet Gynaecol. 1995;102(12):957-62.
82. Sebire NJ, Snijders RJ, Johnson S, Noble PL, Nicolaides KH. First-trimester ultrasound screening for chromosomal defects. Ultrasound Obstet Gynecol. 1996;7(3):216-26.
83. Sebire NJ, D' Ercole C, Hughes K, Carvalho M, Nicolaides KH. Increased nuchal translucency thickness at 10–14 weeks of gestation as predictor of severe twin-to-twin transfusion syndrome. Ultrasound Obstet Gynecol 1997a; 10:86-9.
84. Sebire NJ, D' Ercole C, Hughes K, et al. Increased nuchal translucency thickness at 10-14 weeks of gestation as a predictor of severe twin-to-twin transfusion syndrome. Ultrasound Obstet Gynecol. 1997;10(2):86-9.
85. Cheng PJ, Huang SY, Shaw SW, et al. Difference in nuchal translucency between monozygotic and dizygotic spontaneously conceived twins. Prenat Diagn. 2010;30(3):247-50.
86. Matias A, Montenegro N, Loureiro T, et al. Screening for twin-twin transfusion syndrome at 11-14 weeks of pregnancy: the key role of ductus venosus blood flow assessment. Ultrasound Obstet Gynecol. 2010;35(2):142-8.
87. Cleary-Goldman J, Rebarber A, Krantz D, et al. First-trimester screening with nasal bone in twins. Am J Obstet Gynecol. 2008;199(3):283.e1-3.
88. Sepulveda W, Wong AE, Casasbuenas A. Nuchal translucency and nasal bone in first-trimester ultrasound screening for aneuploidy in multiple pregnancies. Ultrasound Obstet Gynecol. 2009;33(2):152-6.
89. Spencer K, Salonen R, Muller F. Down's syndrome screening in multiple pregnancies using alpha-fetoprotein and free beta hCG. Prenat Diagn. 1994;14(7):537-42.
90. Spencer K, Kagan KO, Nicolaides KH. Screening for trisomy 21 in twin pregnancies in the first trimester: an update of the impact of chorionicity on maternal serum markers. Prenat Diagn. 2008;28(1):49-52.
91. Spencer K, Staboulidou I, Nicolaides KH. First trimester aneuploidy screening in the presence of a vanishing twin: implications for maternal serum markers. Prenat Diagn 2010;30(3):235-40.

92. Cuckle H. Down's syndrome screening in twins. J Med Screen. 1998;5(1):3-4.
93. Nicolaides KH, Spencer K, Avgidou K, et al. Multicenter study of first-trimester screening for trisomy 21 in 75 821 pregnancies: results and estimation of the potential impact of individual risk-orientated two-stage first-trimester screening. Ultrasound Obstet Gynecol. 2005;25(3):221-6.
94. Madsen H, Ball S, Wright D, et al. A reassessment of biochemical marker distributions in trisomy 21-affected and unaffected twin pregnancies in the first trimester. Ultrasound Obstet Gynecol. 2010;37(1):38-47.
95. Sebire NJ, Snijders RJM, Hughes K, Sepulveda W, Nicolaides KH. The hidden mortality of monochorionic twin pregnancies. Br J Obstet Gynecol. 1997;104:1203-7.
96. Schatz F. Clinical for the physiology of the fetus. Berlin: Hirschwald; 1890.
97. Bajoria R, Wigglesworth J, Fish NM. Angioarchitecture of monochorionic placentas in relation to the twin-twin transfusion syndrome. Am J Obstet Gynecol. 1995;172(3): 856-63.
98. Denbow ML, Cox P, Taylor M, et al. Placental angioarchitecture in monochorionic twin pregnancies: relationship to fetal growth, fetofetal transfusion syndrome, and pregnancy outcome. Am J Obstet Gynecol. 2000;182(2):417-26.
99. Lewi L, Cannie M, Blickstein I, et al. Placental sharing, birthweight discordance, and vascular anastomoses in monochorionic diamniotic twin placentas. Am J Obstet Gynecol. 2007;197(6):587e.1-8.
100. Mahieu-Caputo D, Muller F, Joly D, et al. Pathogenesis of twin-twin transfusion syndrome: the renin-angiotensin system hypothesis. Fetal Diagn Ther. 2001;16(4):241-4.
101. Danskin FH, Neilson JP. Twin-to-twin transfusion syndrome: what are appropriate diagnostic criteria? Am J Obstet Gynecol. 1989;161(2):365-9
102. Wenstrom KD, Tessen JA, Zlatnik FJ, et al. Frequency, distribution, and theoretical mechanisms of hematologic and weight discordance in monochorionic twins. Obstet Gynecol. 1992;80(2):257-61.
103. Wittmann BK, Baldwin VJ, Nichold B. Antenatal diagnosis of twin transfusion syndrome by ultrasound. Obstet Gynecol. 1981;58(1):123-7.
104. Brennan JN, Diwan RV, Rosen MG, et al. Fetofetal transfusion syndrome: prenatal ultrasonographic diagnosis. Radiology. 1982;143(2):535-6.
105. Storlazzi E, Vintzileos AM, Campbell WA, et al. Ultrasonic diagnosis of discordant fetal growth in twin gestations. Obstet Gynecol. 1987;69(3 Pt 1):363-7.
106. Sá R, Nassar Carvalho P, Moreira de Ávila L. Differences in amniotic fluid in MZ twins. In: Alexandra Matias, Isaac Blickstein (Eds). Developmental and fetal origins of differences in monozygotic twins: from Genetics to Environmental factors. Amsterdam: Elsevier Inc.; 2020. pp. 157-67.
107. Hecher K, Ville Y, Snijders R, Nicolaides KH. Doppler studies of the fetal circulation in twin-twin transfusion syndrome. Ultrasound Obstet Gynecol. 1995;5(5):318-24.
108. Zosmer N, Bajoria R, Weiner E, et al. Clinical and echographic features of in utero cardiac dysfunction in the recipient twin in twin-twin transfusion syndrome. Br Heart J. 1994;72(1):74-9.
109. Wohlmuth C, Gardiner HM, Diehl W, Hecher K. Fetal cardiovascular hemodynamics in twin-twin transfusion syndrome. Acta Obstet Gynecol Scand. 2016;95(6):664-71.
110. Fesslova V, Villa L, Nava S, et al. Fetal and neonatal echocardiographic findings in twin-twin transfusion syndrome. Am J Obstet Gynecol. 1998;179(4):1056-62.
111. Gardiner HM, Taylor MJ, Karatza A, et al. Twin-twin transfusion syndrome: the influence of intrauterine laser photocoagulation on arterial distensibility in childhood. Circulation. 2003;107(14):1906-11.
112. van Klink JM, Slaghekke F, Balestriero MA, et al. Neurodevelopmental outcome at 2 years in twin-twin transfusion syndrome survivors randomized for the Solomon trial. Am J Obstet Gynecol. 2016;214(1):113.e1-7
113. Sebire NJ, Souka A, Skentou H, et al. Early prediction of severe twin-to-twin transfusion syndrome. Human Reprod. 2000;15(9):2008-10.
114. Kagan O, Gazzoni A, Sepulveda-Gonzalez G, et al. Discordance in nuchal translucency thickness in the prediction of severe twin-to-twin transfusion syndrome. Ultrsound Obstet Gynecol. 2007;29(5):527-32.
115. Lewi L, Lewi P, Diemert A, et al. The role of ultrasound examination in the first trimester and at 16 weeks' gestation to predict fetal complications in monochorionic diamniotic twin pregnancies. Am J Obstet Gynecol. 2008;199(5):493.e1-7.
116. Montenegro N, Matias A, Areias JC, et al. Increased nuchal translucency: possible involvement of early cardiac failure. Ultrasound Obstet Gynecol. 1997;10(4):265-8.
117. Matias A, Montenegro N, Areias JC, et al. Anomalous fetal venous return associated with major chromosomopathies in the late first trimester of pregnancy. Ultrasound Obstet Gynecol. 1998;11(3):209-13.
118. Matias A, Gomes C, Flack N, et al. Screening of chromosomal defects at 11-14 weeks: the role of ductus venosus blood flow. Ultrasound Obstet Gynecol. 1998;12(6):380-4.
119. Matias A, Huggon I, Areias JC, et al. Cardiac defects in chromosomally normal fetuses with abnormal ductus venosus blood flow at 10-14 weeks. Ultrasound Obstet Gynecol. 1999;14(5):307-10.
120. Matias A, Montenegro N, Areias JC. Anticipating twin-twin transfusion syndrome in monochorionic twin pregnancy. Is there a role for nuchal translucency and ductus venosus blood flow evaluation at 11-14 weeks? Twin Res. 2000;3(2):65-70.
121. Matias A, Maiz N, Montenegro N, et al. Ductus venosus flow at 11-13 weeks in the prediction of birth weight discordance in monochorionic twins. J Perinat Med. 2011;39(4):467-70.

122. Stagnati V, Zanardini C, Fichera A, et al. Early prediction of twin-to-twin transfusion syndrome: systematic review and meta-analysis. Ultrasound Obstet Gynecol. 2017;49(5):573-82.
123. Taylor MJ, Denbow ML, Tanawattanacharoen S, et al. Doppler detection of arterio-arterial anastomoses in monochorionic twins: feasibility and clinical application. Hum Reprod. 2000;15(7):1632-6.
124. Grande M, Goncé A, Stergiotou I, et al. Intertwin crown-rump length discordance in the prediction of fetal anomalies, fetal loss and adverse perinatal outcome. J Matern Fetal Neonatal Med. 2015;29(17):2883-8.
125. Curado J, Sileo F, Bhide A, et al. Early- and late-onset selective fetal growth restriction in monochorionic diamniotic twin pregnancy: natural history and diagnostic criteria. Ultrasound Obstet Gynecol. 2020;55(5):661-6.
126. Litwinska E, Syngelaki A, Cimpoca B, et al. Intertwin discordance in fetal size at 11-13 weeks' gestation and pregnancy outcome. Ultrasound Obstet Gynecol. 2020;55(2):189-97.
127. Luke B, Minogue J, Witter FR. The role of fetal growth restriction and gestational age on length of hospital stay in twin infants. Obstet Gynecol. 1993;81(6):949-53.
128. Fraser D, Picard R, Picard E, et al. Birth weight discordance, intrauterine growth retardation and perinatal outcomes in twins. J Reprod Med. 1994;39(7):504-8.
129. Blickstein I. Normal and abnormal growth of multiples. Semin Neonatol. 2002;7(3):177-85.
130. Blickstein I. Is it normal for multiples to be smaller than singletons? Best Pract Res Clin Obstet Gynecol. 2004;18(4):613-23.
131. Blickstein I, Keith LG. Neonatal mortality rates among growth-discordant twins, classified according to the birth weight of the smaller twin. Am J Obstet Gynecol. 2004;190(1):170-4.
132. Luke B, Keith LG. The contribution of singletons, twins and triplets to low birth weight, infant mortality and handicap in the United States. J Reprod Med. 1992;37(8):661-6.
133. Sebire NJ, D'Ercole C, Hughes K, Rennie J, Nicolaides KH.Dichorionic twins discordant for intrauterine growth retardation. Arch Dis Child Fetal Neonatal Ed. 1997c;77(3): F235-6.
134. Blickstein I, Keith LG. Neonatal mortality rates among growth-discordant twins, classified according to the birth weight of the smaller twin. Am J Obstet Gynecol 2004;190: 170-4.
135. Halling C, Malone FD, Breathnach FM, et al. Neuro-developmental outcome of a large cohort of growth discordant twins. Eur J Pediatr. 2016;175(3):381-9.
136. Pharoah P. Neurological outcome in twins. Semin Neonatol. 2002;7(3):223-30.
137. Pharoah P. Risk of cerebral palsy in multiple pregnancies. Clin Perinatol. 2006;33(2):301-13.
138. Pharoah P. Twins and locomotor disorder in children. J Bone Joint Surg Br. 2006;88(3):295-7.
139. Blickstein I. Do multiple gestations raise the risk of cerebral palsy? Clin Perinatol. 2004;31(3):395-408.
140. Topp M, Huusom LD, Langhoff-Roos J, et al. Multiple birth and cerebral palsy in Europe: a multicenter study. Acta Obstet Gynecol Scand. 2004;83(6):548-53.
141. Yokoyama Y, Shimizu T, Haykawa K. Prevalence of cerebral palsy in twins, triplets and quadruplets. Int J Epidemiol. 1995;24(5):943-8.
142. Bejar R, Vigliocco G, Gramajo H, et al. Antenatal origin of neurologic damage in newborn infants. II. Multiple gestations. Am J Obstet Gynecol. 1990;162(5):1230-6.
143. Malone FD. Monochorionic pregnancy—Where have we been? Where are we going? Am J Obstet Gynecol. 2003;189(5):1308-9.
144. Lopriore E, Nagel HT, Vandenbussche FP, et al. Long-term neurodevelopmental outcome in twin-to-twin transfusion syndrome. Am J Obstet Gynecol. 2003;189(5):1313-8.
145. Senat MV, Loizeau S, Cooudere S, et al. The value of middle cerebral artery peak systolic velocity in the diagnosis of fetal anemia after intrauterine death of one monochorionic twin. Am J Obstet Gynecol. 2003;189(5):1319-23.
146. Bush MC, Malone FD. Down syndrome screening in twins. Clin Perinatol. 2005;32(2):373-86.
147. Chescheir NC, Seeds JW. Polyhydramnios and olygohydramnios in twin gestations. Obstet Gynecol. 1988;71(6 Pt 1):882-4.
148. Gjerris AC, Loft A, Pinborg A, et al. The effect of a 'vanishing twin' on biochemical and ultrasound first trimester screening markers for Down's syndrome in pregnancies conceived by assisted reproductive technology. Hum Reprod. 2009;24(1):55-62.
149. Goncé A, Borrell A, Fortuny A, et al. First-trimester screening for trisomy 21 in twin pregnancy: does the addition of biochemistry make an improvement? Prenat Diagn. 2005;25(12):1156-61.
150. Hamasaki S, Shirabe S, Tsuda R, et al. Discordant Gerstmann-Sträussler-Scheinker disease in monozygotic twins. Lancet. 1998;352(9137):1358-9.
151. Linskens IH, Spreeuwenberg MD, Blankenstein MA, et al. Early first-trimester free beta-hCG and PAPP-A serum distributions in monochorionic and dichorionic twins. Prenat Diagn. 2009;29(1):74-8.
152. Saunders NJ, Snijders RJ, Nicolaides KH. Therapeutic amniocentesis in twin-twin transfusion syndrome appearing in the second trimester of pregnancy. Am J Obstet Gynecol. 1992;166(3):820-4.
153. Van Mieghem T, Lewi L, Gucciardo L, et al. The Fetal Heart in Twin-to-Twin Transfusion Syndrome. 2010; 2010:379792.
154. Valsky DV, Eixarch E, Martinez-Crespo JM, et al. Fetoscopic laser surgery for twin-to-twin transfusion syndrome after 26 weeks of gestation. Fetal Diagn Ther. 2012;31(1):30-4.
155. Wald NJ, Rish S, Hackshaw AK. Combining nuchal translucency and serum markers in prenatal screening for Down syndrome in twin pregnancies. Prenat Diagn. 2003;23(7):588-92.

31

CHAPTER

Ultrasonography and Birth Defects

Narendra Malhotra, Neharika Malhotra Bora, Jaideep Malhotra

INTRODUCTION

"Care is Absolute, Prevention is ideal"

What is a birth defect?

A birth defect (congenital anomaly) is a health problem or an abnormal physical change that is present when a baby is born.

What are the common visible birth defects?

More than 4,000 different kinds of birth defects are reported, which range from minor defects that need no treatment to serious defects that cause disabilities or require medical or surgical treatment. Of these defects in the development of the brain or spinal cord, cleft lip and palate and clubfoot are most common.

How common are the common birth defects?

Birth defects constitute the fifth largest cause of death in the newborn babies in our country. Globally, congenital anomalies affect 2–3% of births. In India too, 1–3 out of 100 babies are born with birth defects accounting for 27 million babies being born with birth defects each year.

Birth defects are a global problem. Birth defect is one of the leading causes of perinatal mortality and morbidity, accounting for 2–3% of all live-births.[1]

Presence of anomalies and their undesirable consequences for the affected neonate, family, and medical fraternity is a very convincing argument by many experts on universal screening.

Regardless whether a woman is in low-risk (majority cases) or high-risk category (genetic, diabetes, etc.), the risk of fetal malformation is always there and because there are no symptoms and these pregnancies may be uneventful.

It is estimated that every year 7.9 million children are born with a serious birth defect of genetic or partly genetic origin. A further 1 million are born with serious birth defects of postconception origin, which result from environmental teratogens such as alcohol, rubella, syphilis, and iodine deficiency, which can either cause death or lifelong disability.[2]

Whilst this problem has been addressed in the West, it is yet to be addressed in developing countries where 94% of those born with birth defects reside and where 95% of the children who die from birth defects are born.[2]

The prevalence of fetal malformations is 65%, though only 2–2.5% are potentially life-threatening, lethal, or represent a major cosmetic defect **(Fig. 1)**.[1] It is seen that the incidence of aneuploidy (trisomy 21) increases with maternal age **(Fig. 2)**.

Ultrasound routine screening is a very valuable tool for detecting birth defects.[3,4]

In India, due to its high birth rate, population, and consanguinity in certain communities, the burden of birth defects is significant [The Federation of Obstetric and Gynecological Societies of India (FOGSI) Birth Defects Registry unpublished data].

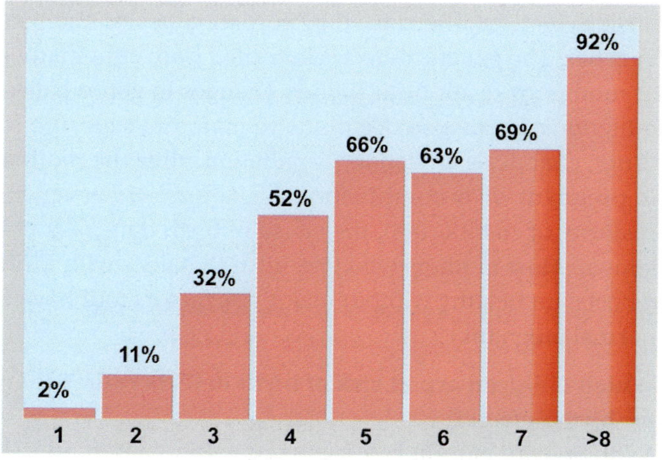

Fig. 1: Frequency of aneuploidies versus number of anomalies.

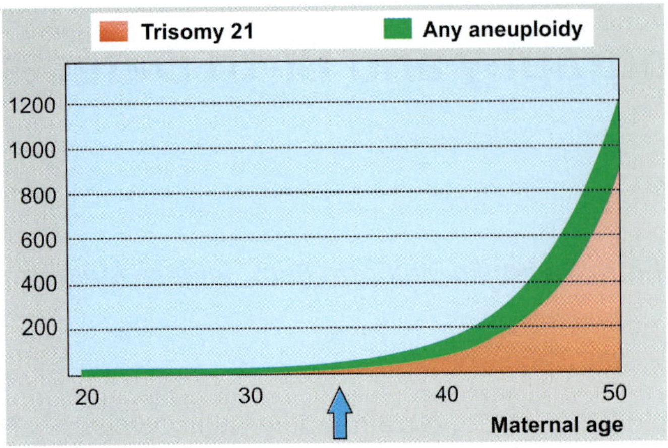

Fig. 2: Incidence of aneuploidy (Trisomy 21) screen with maternal age.

India has the highest number of children with birth defects. They affect approximately 1 in 33 infants and result in approximately 3.2 million birth defect-related disabilities every year. The prevalence of high-risk pregnancies in India is about 15% with only about 4% being diagnosed before delivery.

An estimated prevalence of 495,000 infants are born with congenital malformations every year.[5] In addition, 21,400 with Down syndrome; 9,000 with thalassemia; 5,200 with sickle cell anemia; 390,000 with glucose-6-phosphate dehydrogenase (G6PD) deficiency; and 9,760 with amino acid disorders are born every year.[6]

Diagnosis is generally late or ineffective and the infrastructure for management and rehabilitation of the families is not easily accessible. This makes the burden of genetic diseases and birth defects particularly severe as compared to the western countries.

What causes the birth defects?

Birth defects can be caused by certain genes or changes in genes. The genetic defect is inherited from either father or mother or result from sudden changes in genes called mutations. It can also occur due to maternal exposure to drugs, chemicals, infection, or radiation while the mother is pregnant or a combination of factors. However, in majority of cases (70%), the cause of birth defects is not known. Most mothers who give birth to babies with birth defects are healthy without major risk factors and have a normal pregnancy.

Which children are at risk of birth defects rather than for birth defects?

Mothers with certain risk factors are at an increased risk of having a baby with a birth defect. These include older age (beyond 35 years), previous baby with birth defect, presence of a family or personal history of birth defects, medical conditions such as poorly controlled diabetes, use of medications around the time, and she conceives the baby or in the first few months of becoming pregnant. Mothers who use recreational drugs such as cocaine, marijuana, or drink alcohol during pregnancy are also at higher risk. The risk for certain mutation in genes and thus the risk of birth defects is higher among certain ethnic communities and when parents are related by blood (consanguinity).[1]

The International Statistical Classification of Diseases and Related Health Problems, tenth revision (ICD-10), includes birth defects in Chapter XVII: Congenital malformations, deformations and chromosomal abnormalities. Birth defects such as inborn errors of metabolism and blood disorders of prenatal origin appear in other chapters. Birth defects can be defined as structural or functional abnormalities, including metabolic disorders, which are present from birth. The term congenital disorder is considered to have the same definition; the two terms are used interchangeably. The eleventh revision of the classification provides an opportunity for a review of the current entry.

Congenital disorders are a common condition. The World Health Organization (WHO) estimates that some 260,000 deaths worldwide (about 7% of all neonatal deaths) were caused by congenital anomalies in 2004. They are most prominent as a cause of death in settings where overall mortality rates are lower, e.g., in the European Region, where as many as 25% of neonatal deaths are due to congenital anomalies.

There are currently no sound estimates of the number of children born with a serious congenital disorder attributable to genetic or environmental causes. The most common serious congenital disorders are congenital heart defects, neural tube defects (NTDs), and Down syndrome. Hemoglobinopathies (including thalassemia and sickle cell disease) and G6PD deficiency, which are not covered by the ICD-10 definition of congenital anomalies, account for 6% of all congenital disorders.

Considerable uncertainties remain as to the incidence of and mortality attributable to congenital disorders, especially in countries that lack adequate registration of deaths. However, existing figures indicate that work on reducing the incidence of and mortality associated with congenital anomalies needs to be linked to efforts to achieve the Millennium Development Goal 4 target of a two-thirds reduction in the mortality rate of children under 5 years of age between 1990 and 2015.[5]

Ultrasound has revolutionized obstetric practice world over, there is no doubt about this. With good resolution machines, color Doppler and 3D and 4D scanning, it is now possible to make a prenatal diagnosis of many structural anomalies, which are lethal, life-threatening, and debilitation.

All pregnancies are at risk of producing fetal malformations or birth defects. Some pregnant women are at a greater risk. The world consensus on whether all pregnancies should be screened by ultrasound for anomalies and when, is still divided.

As per the National Family Health Survey (NFHS)-3 data, ultrasound was performed in only 24% of pregnancies. Out of these, only 4% women in the lowest socioeconomic quintile had an ultrasound test compared with 62% among the highest wealth quintile.

Social stigma, discrimination, lost hopes, and lack of opportunities add to the emotional and financial burdens. To reduce the impact of birth defects, National Health Policy makers need to first recognize the prevalence, disability, and burden of the disease.

Most of developed countries have guidelines for ultrasonography (USG) during pregnancy. The European and Canadian guidelines recommend two USGs as a part of standard prenatal care, first for dating at 8–14 weeks and second to detect fetal abnormalities at 18–20 weeks. A recent workshop of joint committee of American association of fetal imaging held in 2014 gave recommendations that in the absence of specific indications for a first-trimester ultrasound, a single USG should be performed at 18–20 weeks of gestation. At present, in India, there are no set standards for the number of ultrasounds to be done in pregnancy, their interpretation, and reporting. In view of the above evidence, the Government of India (GOI) constituted an expert group to deliberate on use of USG in pregnancy in detail and formulate guidelines for India. The present guidelines have been prepared based on the recommendations of the experts and available national/international evidences. The GOI has introduced Pradhan Mantri Surakshit Matritva Abhiyan (PMSMA) from June 2016 onward, where on 9th of every month pregnant women (in 2nd/3rd trimesters of pregnancy) will receive all essential antenatal care (ANC) services by Medical Officer and OB-GYN specialist including USG services. So these guidelines will also give states more clarity for implementing PMSMA program.

CAUSES

The incidence of birth defects in USA is 1 out of 33 and may be much more in developing countries and countries where no formal and structured registry exists.

There are three major categories of causes:

1. Genetic
2. Environmental
3. Complex genetic/unknown.

Genetic Causes

Chromosomal or single-gene disorders are known to account for about 25–30% of all birth defects. Chromosomal abnormalities are seen in about 0.5% of live newborns. Recently, use of "telomeric probes" has increased this incidence further as about 5–7% of mentally challenged children have a cryptic translocation that cannot be detected by traditional cytogenetic methods. A "mutation" in the genetic locus can give rise of "single gene disorder". Not all mutant genes manifest at birth or lead to structural problems.

Some birth defects are caused by errors in *genes* or *chromosomes*. Those caused by genes can be inherited—passed by parents to their children. Some inherited disorders are more common in certain ethnic groups, such as *sickle cell disease*, *cystic fibrosis*, and *Tay-Sachs disease*.

Chromosomal defects are caused by missing, damaged, or extra chromosomes. These defects are often the result of an error that occurred when the egg and sperm were joining. Common chromosomal disorders are *Down syndrome* and *trisomy 18*. Generally, the risk of having a baby with Down syndrome, trisomy 18, and other chromosomal disorders increases as a woman ages.[6]

Environmental Causes

These account to 5–10% of causes of birth defects. These include nutritional deficiencies, maternal illnesses, teratogenic drugs, or radiation and infectious agents. However, the extent of the damage depends upon the timing of exposure and the individual's genetic susceptibility.

Other birth defects result from the *fetus* being exposed to harmful agents, such as medications, chemicals, and infections. Whether a woman or her baby is harmed depends on how much of the agent they have been exposed to, when during her pregnancy a woman is exposed to the agent, and for how long.

Complex Genetic/Unknown Causes

These comprise about 65–70% of birth defects. This may be caused by defects in more than one gene or a complex interaction of the environment and genes.

Sometimes, a mixture of factors is the cause. For many birth defects, the exact cause is not known.

SCREENING METHODS AND TESTS

Maternal and Fetal Screening Tests

Noninvasive and Invasive

There are many screening tests conducted on the mother or directly on the fetus/pregnancy products, which may be invasive or noninvasive. These tests vary in their effectiveness, that is, the detection rate or the sensitivity and specificity of the test. The best way to assess which is the best screening test would be to fix the false-positive rate and compare the detection rate of various tests.

Noninvasive tests: These tests are performed on maternal blood (serum screening) and by an ultrasound scan. Detection of any abnormal level of hormones in maternal blood or abnormal measurement of fetal parameters increases the relative risk for the fetus to have a chromosomal defect. The "detection rate" of any test depends upon following the highest standards of practice, in both, scanning and in the laboratories. Hence, the "efficacy" of the test largely depends upon the laboratory performing the blood tests and the operator performing the fetal scan.

Invasive tests: These tests are largely done to confirm a suspected diagnosis of genetic disease and in a few cases for fetal infections. Test samples are taken from the placenta [chorionic villous sampling (CVS)], amniotic fluid (amniocentesis), or fetal blood (cordocentesis). These tests involve inserting a needle into the pregnancy sac to retrieve the sample. This requires expertise as it carries a risk of miscarriage of the entire pregnancy, which largely depends upon the operator skills.

Screening Tests Versus Diagnostic Tests

It is important to understand the difference between a screening test and a diagnostic test:

- Screening tests help to evaluate the risk for certain birth defects, but they cannot diagnose a birth defect. Screening tests are noninvasive and pose no risk to mother or baby.
- Diagnostic tests, such as CVS, are highly accurate at diagnosing or ruling out a birth defect. However, these tests are invasive and may pose a very small risk of miscarriage.

Application of Various Maternal and Fetal Screening Tests to Pregnant Women

Screening tests such as ultrasound can be performed at any stage of the pregnancy. However, most screening tests, particularly blood tests, are not performed after 22 weeks, firstly because the efficacy of the tests declines steeply after that and secondly in most countries late termination of pregnancy is restricted. The best detection rate for the tests can be obtained when performed in the particular window period of gestations. The following tests are the most widely performed.

Ultrasound Screening

Through screening of all pregnant patients is impossible in the current scenario. But we can and should offer ultrasound to all possible pregnant women as a prenatal diagnostic test.[7]

Most of the birth defects can be identified and diagnosed in utero. A careful history, proper biochemical screening, and ultrasound added with invasive testing where required can pick up structural, chromosomal, and metabolic abnormalities in the unborn. An early diagnosis leads to good counseling and informed choice to the parents with option of termination.

Clinically high-risk groups for a detailed anomalies scan are shown in **Box 1**.

Sonographic findings that are indications for a detailed anomalies scan are listed in **Boxes 2 and 3**.

Nonsonographic laboratory investigations that can warrant a detailed anomalies scan are listed in **Box 4**.

Technical guidelines for use of USG in pregnancy: Technical aspects will focus on the following:

- Number of ultrasounds in pregnancy
- Timing of obstetric ultrasound

BOX 1: Clinical markers of high-risk pregnancy.

- Advanced maternal age
- Previous birth of a malformed fetus
- Family history of a malformed fetus
- Consanguinity
- Exposure to drugs/radiation
- Maternal diabetes mellitus
- Bad obstetric history
- Bleeding in early pregnancy

BOX 2: Sonographic findings: First trimester.

- Oligoamniotic sac
- Embryonic bradycardia
- Abnormal yolk sac
- Increased nuchal translucency
- One identified anomaly
- Dates size discrepancy at 9–12 weeks

BOX 3: Sonographic findings: Second and third trimester.

- Increased nuchal translucency
- Symmetric intrauterine growth restriction (IUGR)
- Polyhydramnios
- Oligohydramnios
- Breech presentation
- Twins
- One identified anomaly

BOX 4: Nonsonographic findings.

- Abnormal results from a chorionic villus sampling (CVS)/ amniocentesis
- Abnormal immunoglobulin profile
- Abnormal triple test/increased alfa-fetoprotein/abnormal pregnancy-associated plasma protein (PAPP)
- Abnormal first trimester dual marker test

- Who will perform obstetric ultrasound?
- Purpose/indication of obstetric ultrasound
- Components of the routine obstetric ultrasound scan
- Equipment and maintenance
- Consent forms and reporting formats
- Follow-up action

Components of the routine obstetric ultrasound scan: The following systems are examined to assess for any congenital anomalies and screen for high-risk pregnancy:

- Fetal number, multiple gestations—chorionicity, amnionicity, comparison of fetal sizes, estimation of amniotic fluid volume (increased, decreased, or normal) in each gestational sac
- Qualitative or semiquantitative estimate of amniotic fluid
- Placental location, appearance, and relationship to the internal cervical Os
- Umbilical cord—number of vessels in the cord and placental cord insertion site
- *Measurements:* Biparietal diameter (BPD), head circumference, abdominal circumference, and femoral diaphysis length
- Fetal anatomic survey:
    - Head, face, and neck
    - Lateral cerebral ventricles, choroid plexus, midline falx, cavum septi pellucidi, cerebellum, cistern magna, upper lip
    - *Chest:* Shape/size of chest and lungs
    - *Heart:* Four-chamber view, left ventricular outflow tract, right ventricular outflow tract
    - *Abdomen:* Stomach (visualization, size, and sites), kidneys, and urinary bladder
    - Umbilical cord insertion site into the fetal abdomen
    - *Spine:* Cervical, thoracic, lumbar, and sacral spine
    - *Extremities:* Legs and arms
    - *Maternal anatomy:* Evaluation of the uterus, adnexal structures, and cervix should be performed when appropriate.

ULTRASOUND FOR CHROMOSOMAL ABNORMALITIES AND CONGENITAL DEFECTS

First Trimester Scan (NT/NB Scan)

Nuchal Translucency Scan

All major chromosomal abnormalities and congenital heart diseases are mostly associated with increased nuchal translucency (NT). It is the sonographical appearance of subcutaneous accumulation of fluid behind the fetal neck. Babies with abnormalities tend to accumulate more fluid at the back of their neck during the first trimester, causing this clear space to be larger than average.

Principles of NT measurement (Fetal Medicine Foundation guidelines):

- The period of gestation should be 11–14 weeks and the fetal crown–rump length (CRL) should be 45–84 mm.
- The fetus should be in the neutral position.
- A midsagittal section of the fetus should be obtained.
- Only the fetal head and upper thorax should be included in the image.
- The magnification should be as large as possible and always such that each slight movement of the calipers produces only a 0.1 mm change in the measurement.
- The maximum thickness of the subcutaneous translucency between the skin and the soft tissue overlying the cervical spine should be measured.
- The calipers should be placed on the lines that define the NT thickness—the crossbar of the caliper should be such that it is hardly visible as it merges with the white line of the border and not in the nuchal fluid.
- More than one measurement must be taken and the maximum one should be recorded.

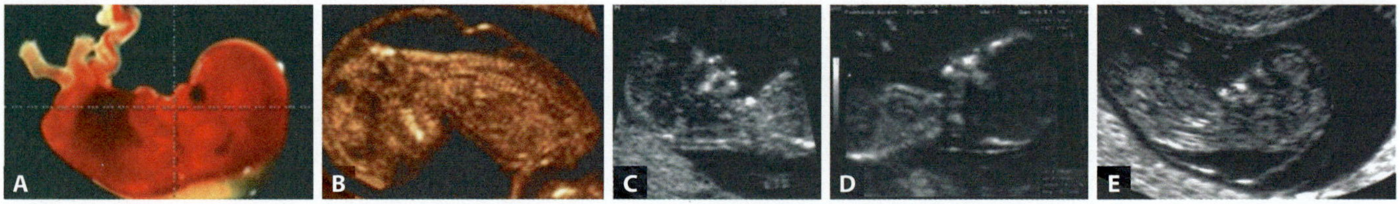

Figs. 3A to E: Measurement of nuchal translucency in the first trimester.

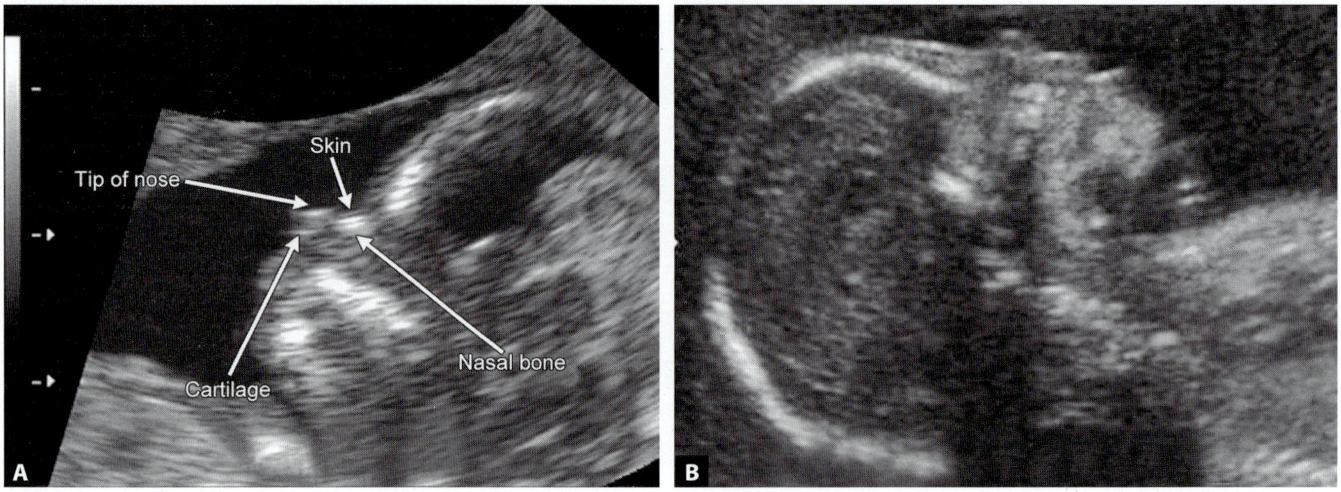

Figs. 4A and B: (A) Nasal bone; (B) Absent nasal bone.

Pitfalls in measuring the NT include the presence of an encephalocele, a nuchal cord, an amniotic band, or a loose amnion that can be mistaken for the nuchal skin edge.[8] It is therefore imperative to magnify the image **(Figs. 3A to E)**.

In trisomies 21, 18, and 13, the average NT is about 2.5 mm above the normal median for CRL. In Turner syndrome, the median NT is about 8 mm above the normal median.

Nasal Bone

The fetal nasal bone (NB) can be seen by USG at 11–14 weeks of gestation.[9] If NB is present, then there should be three distinct lines. The topmost line represents the skin and the bottom more echogenic represents the NB. A third line in continuity with the skin, present at a higher level, represents tip of the nose.

Several studies have demonstrated a high association between absent NB at 11–14 weeks and trisomy 21, as well as other chromosomal abnormalities.[10] It is absent in 60–70% of cases with trisomy 21, 50% of trisomy 18, and 30% of trisomy 13 **(Figs. 4A and B)**.

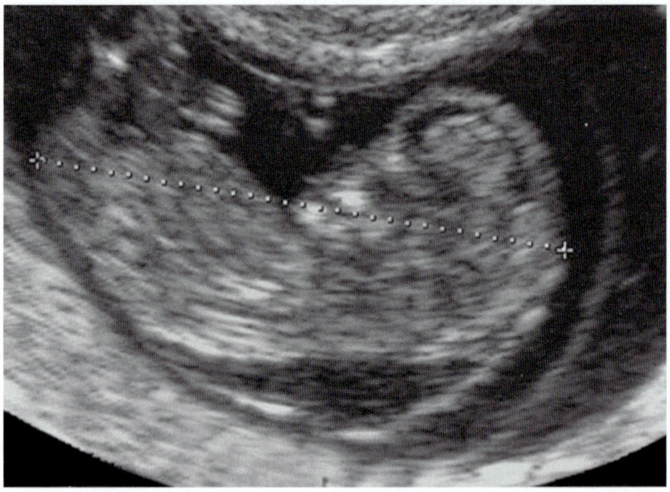

Fig. 5: Measurement of crown–rump length.

Other First Trimester Signs of Aneuploidy

Crown-rump length: Growth patterns of the CRL have been evaluated to determine whether growth abnormalities could be utilized as signs of aneuploidy.[11] Growth rates are significantly reduced among fetuses with trisomies 13 and 18 and with triploidy **(Fig. 5)**.

Fetal heart rate: At 11–14 weeks, trisomy 13 and Turner syndrome are associated with tachycardia, whereas in trisomy 18 and triploidy there is fetal bradycardia.[12] Fetal heart rate (FHR) measurement in the first trimester is unlikely to improve screening for trisomy 21, but it is a useful in detecting trisomy 13.

Doppler in the ductus venosus: At 11–14 weeks, abnormal ductal flow is associated with chromosomal defects, cardiac abnormalities and adverse pregnancy outcome.[13]

Abnormal flow in the ductus venosus is seen in about 80% of trisomy 21 fetuses and in about 5% of chromosomally normal fetuses.[10]

Other sonographic methods for detecting aneuploid fetus includes abnormal fetal heart rate at 10–14 weeks: Absent NB, faciomaxillary angle, intracranial translucency (IT), umbilical cord thickness, and wide iliac angle.

By combining maternal age, NT, and heart rate, 83% fetuses with trisomy 21 were detected.[14]

Second Trimester

The checklist for the anomalies scan can be a combination of the following recommendations:

Components of the standard fetal examination at 18–20 weeks of gestation:

- *Fetal cardiac activity, fetal number, and presentation should be documented:*
  - An abnormal heart rate and/or rhythm should be documented.
  - Multiple gestations require the documentation of additional information—chorionicity, amnionicity, comparison of fetal sizes, estimation of amniotic fluid volume (increased, decreased, or normal) in each gestational sac, and fetal genitalia (when visualized).
- A qualitative or semiquantitative estimate of amniotic fluid volume should be documented.
- Placental location, appearance, and relationship to the internal cervical os should be documented. The umbilical cord should be imaged and the number of vessels in the cord documented. The placental cord insertion site should be documented when technically possible.
- *Measurements:* BPD, head circumference, abdominal circumference, and femoral diaphysis length
- *Fetal anatomic survey:*
  - Head, face, and neck:
    - Lateral cerebral ventricles
    - Choroid plexus
    - Midline falx
    - Cavum septi pellucidi
    - Cerebellum
    - Cistern magna
    - Upper lip
    - Nuchal fold measurement may be helpful during a specific age interval to assess the risk of aneuploidy.
  - *Chest—Heart:*
    - Four-chamber view
    - Left ventricular outflow tract
    - Right ventricular outflow tract
    - Three-vessel view
  - *Abdomen:*
    - Stomach (presence, size, and situs)
    - Kidneys
    - Urinary bladder
    - Umbilical cord insertion site into the fetal abdomen
    - Umbilical cord vessel number
  - *Spine:* Cervical, thoracic, lumbar, and sacral spine
  - *Extremities:* Legs and arms
  - *Gender: Only* in circumstances permitted under the Pre-Conception and Pre-Natal Diagnostic Techniques (PCPNDT) Act
- *Maternal anatomy: Evaluation of the uterus, adnexal structures, and cervix should be performed when appropriate.*

Nuchal Fold

Excessive soft tissue in the back of the neck is known to be a feature of newborns with Down syndrome. Callen et al.[7] described the use of thickened nuchal fold as a sonographic marker for Down syndrome in 1985, they showed that 2/6 fetuses with Down syndrome had a nuchal thickness of ≥6 mm. This measurement is done using the transverse section of the fetal head angled posteriorly to include the cerebellum and the occipital bone. The measurement is made outside the occipital bone to the outer skin edge. This measurement has remained the most sensitive and specific single marker for the midtrimester detection of Down syndrome.

Major Anomalies

Infants with trisomy 21 have a 50% incidence of heart defects, most commonly ventricular septal defects and common atrioventricular canal.

Other major anomalies include ventriculomegaly, cerebellar hypoplasia, duodenal atresia, hydrops, omphalocele, and limb anomalies.[15]

Femur Length

Individuals with trisomy 21 have short stature, small femur, and humerus.[15]

Pyelectasis (Fig. 6)

Mild fetal pyelectasis was associated with an increased risk of Down syndrome. Crane and Gray defined pyelectasis as an anteroposterior diameter of the renal pelvis ≥4 mm.[16]

Hyperechoic Bowel (Fig. 7)

Nyberg et al.[17] were the first to demonstrate that hyperehoic bowel is associated with Down syndrome. There is also an increased risk of cystic fibrosis among fetuses with this sonographic finding, and parental allele testing for cystic fibrosis carrier status is recommended to evaluate this risk.

Echogenic Intracardiac Focus (Fig. 8)

The echogenic intracardiac focus (EIF) has been seen among normal fetuses for many years and was considered a normal variant till 1994. Brown, Roberts, and Miller in a case report showed that mineralization of the papillary muscle was associated with trisomy 21 in one of three fetuses.[18]

Lehman et al.[19] were the first to report the association of EIF with trisomy 13.

Several investigators have suggested that the association between an EIF and chromosomal abnormalities is low enough that, in the absence of other findings in an otherwise low-risk patient, fetal karyotyping is unwarranted.

Minor Markers/Soft Markers

Anomalies of the pelvic bones, particularly the iliac wings, are associated with Down syndrome. Children with Down syndrome have a wider lateral span of the iliac wing than do normal children.

It is known among pediatricians and geneticists that infants with Down syndrome have brachycephaly and frontal lobe shortening. An attempt is made to evaluate the use of this feature in detecting second trimester fetuses with Down syndrome.

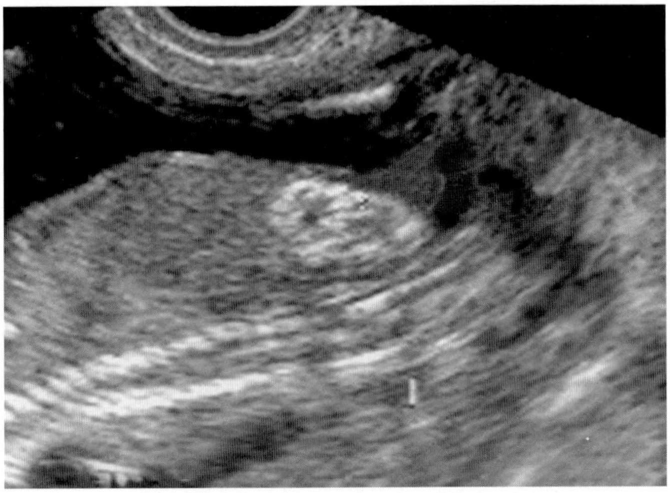

Fig. 7: Echogenic mass in the small bowel.

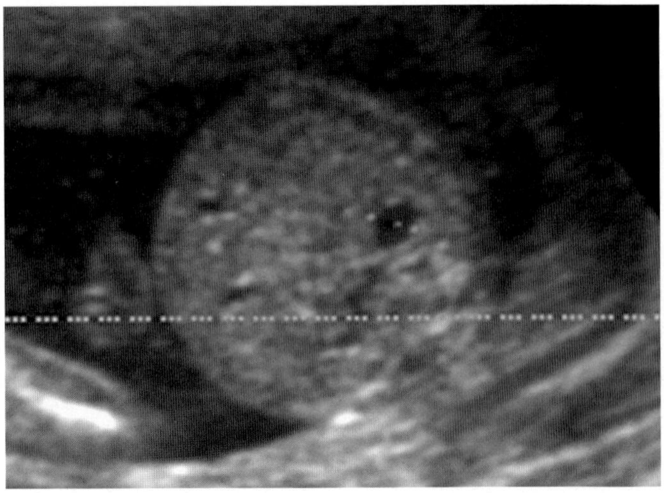

Fig. 6: Fetal pyelectasis crease of the palm.

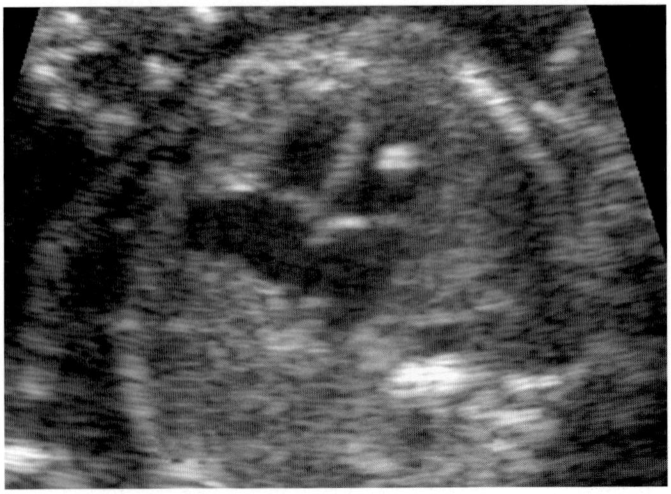

Fig. 8: Echogenic intracardiac focus.

The transverse cerebellar diameter was evaluated as a possible marker for Down syndrome.

Other possible markers for the prenatal detection of Down syndrome have been put forth, including abnormal fetal heart rate patterns, abnormally shortened ear length, flat facies, clinodactyly, sandal gap great toe, and the simian.

TRISOMY 13 (PATAU SYNDROME)

The incidence of trisomy 13 is 1/5,000 births, and it is the most severe of the three autosomal trisomies that can lead to live-born infants. The fetal anomalies most commonly seen with these fetuses include abnormalities of the brain, face, extremities, and heart. In particular, holoprosencephaly is a common finding that is invariably associated with severe midline facial defects, including hypotelorism, cyclopia, midline clefts, microphthalmia, and absence of the nose. Other intracranial anomalies that can be seen with trisomy 13 include microcephaly, abnormal posterior fossa, agenesis of corpus callosum, and ventriculomegaly. In addition, approximately 40% fetuses with trisomy 13 have echogenic intracardiac focus. More than 90% of these fetuses have cardiac defects. Abnormalities of the limbs include polydactyly and radial aplasia. Other major defects include NTDs and anterior abdominal wall defects. 30% of affected fetuses have enlarged echogenic kidneys, similar to polycystic kidneys. Placental anomalies such as partial mole also have been described with trisomy 13.[19,20]

TRIPLOIDY

Triploidy is a syndrome that results from three sets of chromosomes yielding 69 chromosomes. Most triploid conceptions end in spontaneous abortion. When the extra set of chromosome arises from the maternal side, the placenta is small and senescent, and there is severe early IUGR. When the extra set of chromosome arises from the paternal side, the placenta is large, full of echolucency, and often associated with a partial mole.[21]

Usually fetuses with triploidy have multiple congenital abnormalities of particularly every organ system. Characteristically, they also have the first trimester onset IUGR. They also give rise to the unusual appearance of a very thin body with an almost normal-sized head.

Fetal malformations associated with triploidy include early-onset IUGR, facial anomalies such as hypertelorism, micrognathia, and microphthalmia, brain anomalies such as ventriculomegaly, Dandy–Walker malformation, agenesis of corpus callosum, holoprosencephaly, and meningomyelocele. Affected fetuses also have thickened NT/cystic hygroma, heart defects, renal anomalies, clubbed feet, single umbilical artery, and oligohydramnios. Most helpful of all in the specific diagnosis of triploidy is the syndactyly of the third and fourth digits of the hand, recognizable sonographically.

TURNER SYNDROME

Turner syndrome is a chromosomal anomaly due to the loss of one sex chromosome, resulting in a 45X karyotype. The missing chromosome is usually paternal. And the syndrome is not related with maternal age. In most cases, conceptions with Turner syndrome are spontaneously aborted, some fetuses may persist into the second trimester with severe lymphatic abnormalities. These fetuses have large cystic hygromas that are typically septate but clear.

Hydrops, pleural effusion, ascites, and edema of all body parts is seen.

Mosaicism for Turner syndrome is more likely to result in live births, and these individuals are often not diagnosed until puberty. They suffer from sexual infantilism and short stature.

In general, half of the fetuses with Turner syndrome have cardiac anomalies and 19% have renal anomalies.[22]

TRISOMY 18 (EDWARDS SYNDROME)

Trisomy 18 have an incidence of 3/10,000 live births and is associated with multiple severe structural abnormalities that mostly involve the heart, extremities, face, and brain. Affected fetuses are often miscarried or die in utero.[23]

Structural abnormalities associated with trisomy 18 involve abnormal cisterna magna and Dandy–Walker syndrome. Affected fetuses can also have myelomeningoceles and ventriculomegaly. Limb abnormalities include preaxial upper limb reduction and clenched hands with overlapping index fingers. Second trimester fetuses with trisomy 18 tend to have strawberry-shaped skull, cerebellar deviation beyond two standard deviation below the mean, rocker-bottom feet, clubbed feet, single umbilical artery, and renal anomalies such as hydronephrosis. Gastrointestinal tract anomalies include omphalocele and diaphragmatic hernia. The triad of polyhydramnios, growth restriction, and abnormal hand posturing is highly predictive of trisomy 18 in the third trimester.

Umbilical cord cysts have also been associated with an increased incidence of trisomy 18.

Choroid plexus cysts are present in approximately one-third of fetuses with trisomy 18.

NEURAL TUBE DEFECTS

It is one of the most common malformations with a worldwide prevalence of 1–3/1,000 live births.

The most common types of NTDs are anencephaly and spina bifida, which are caused by failure of closure of cranial pore and spinal part of neural tube, respectively.

First Trimester Ultrasound Findings

First trimester diagnosis of NTDs is possible at around 11–14 weeks of gestation with transvaginal USG 2D or 3D **(Figs. 9A to D)**.

- Reduced or absent IT
- Brainstem thickening
- Shortening of the distance between the brainstem and occipital bone
- Increase in the ratio of brainstem diameter to brainstem-occipital bone distance to >1 (N<0.9)
- Posterior shift of the midbrain with parallelism of the cerebral peduncles
- Decreased BPD (<10th centile)

Second Trimester Ultrasound Findings (Fig. 10)

Society of Fetal Medicine Protocol for the Second Trimester Anomalies Scan

The second trimester scan includes three components. These are a detailed anatomical evaluation of the fetus, fetal biometry, and an evaluation of the fetal environment.

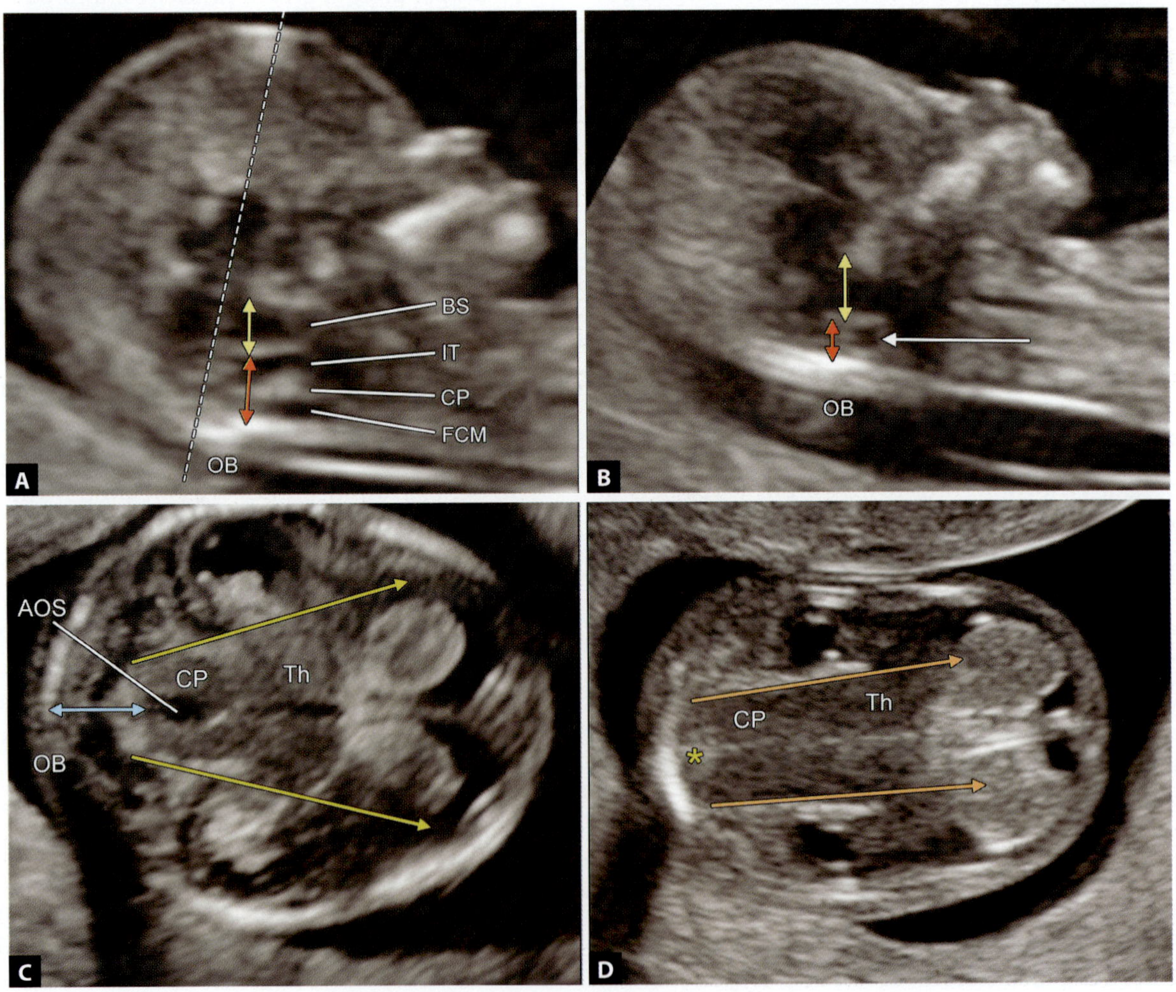

Figs. 9A to D: First trimester ultrasound findings. (AOS: aqueduct of Sylvius; BS: brainstem; CP: choroid plexus; FCM: future cisterna magna; IT: intracranial translucency; OB: occipital bone; Th: thalami)

The use of high frequency transducers, transvaginal scanning, color and power Doppler studies, and three dimensional and real-time 3D scans enhances accuracy in several situations and is encouraged but not mandatory.

The study should document the following:

- Fetal number
- Chorionicity and amnionicity in case of multiple gestations
- Fetal cardiac activity
- Fetal biometry as recommended in the following section
- Estimation of fetal weight

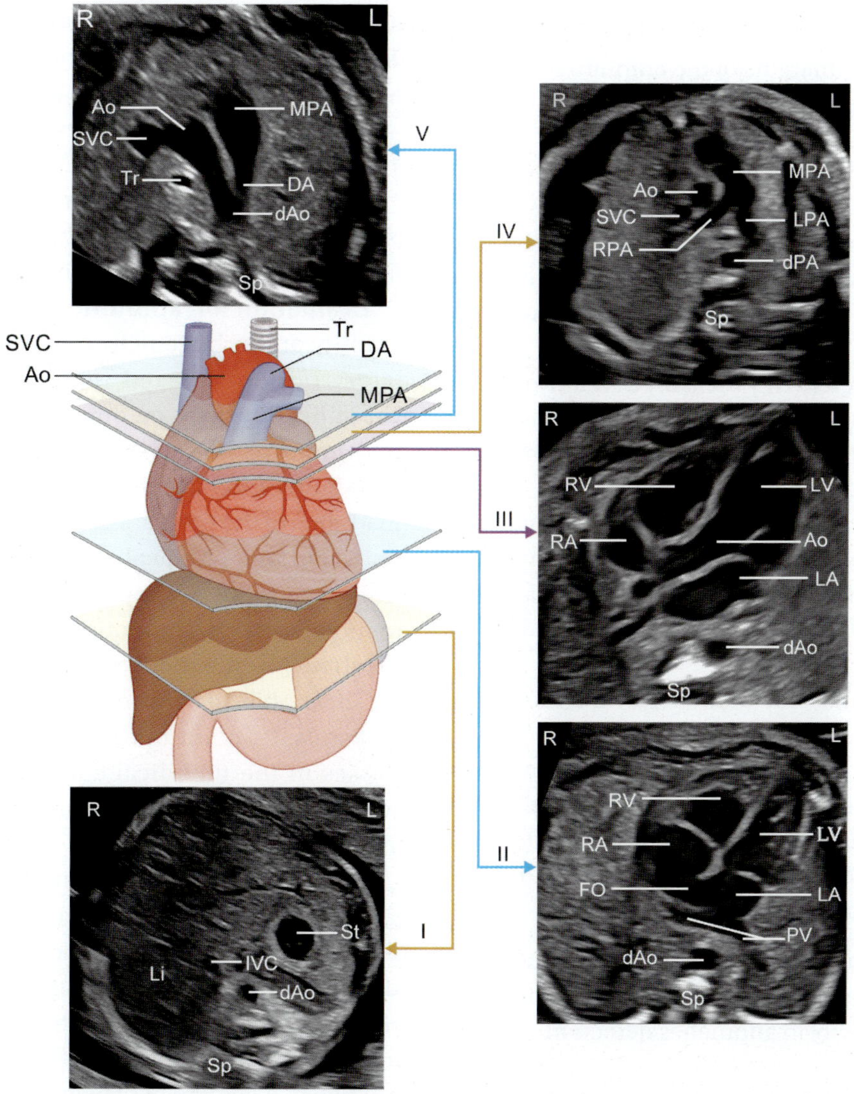

Fig. 10: Fetal cardiac evaluation. Five axial views for optimal fetal heart screening, corresponding to planes shown in figure. Diagram shows the trachea, heart and great vessels, liver, and stomach, with five planes of insonation indicated by polygons, corresponding to grayscale images, as indicated. Most caudal plane, showing fetal stomach (St), cross-section of descending aorta (dAo) and inferior vena cava (IVC), spine (Sp), and liver (Li). (II) Four-chamber view of the fetal heart, showing right and left ventricles (RV and LV) and atria (RA and LA), foramen ovale (FO), and pulmonary veins (PV) to right and left of dAo. (III) Left ventricular outflow tract view, showing proximal ascending aorta (Ao), LV, RV, LA, and RA and cross-section of dAo. (IV) Slightly more cephalad view (right ventricular outflow tract view) showing main pulmonary artery (MPA) and bifurcation into right (RPA) and left (LPA) pulmonary arteries and cross-sections of Ao and dAo. (V) Three-vessel-and-trachea view, showing superior vena cava (SVC), MPA, ductus arteriosus (DA), transverse aortic arch (from proximal Ao to dAo), and trachea (Tr). L, left, R, right.

Source: Modified from Yagel et al. with permission.

- A detailed fetal anatomic survey as recommended in the following sections
- Evaluation of the fetal environment including the placenta, amniotic fluid, umbilical cord and maternal uterus, cervix and adnexa, as recommended in the following sections.

Fetal biometry should include the following measurements:

- BPD measured from the leading edge to the leading edge of the osseous margins of the cranium in an axial section that includes the cavum septum pellucidum and the thalami
- Head perimeter (HP) at the same level as the BPD, traced at the outer margin of the osseous skull vault
- Occipitofrontal distance at the same level as the BPD from the anterior edge of the osseous surface to the posterior edge of the osseous surface on the outer aspect
- Abdominal perimeter (AP) measured in a transverse view of the abdomen at the level of the junction of the umbilical vein and portal vein anteriorly and the spine in a true transverse section posteriorly
- Femur length includes the shaft only; vertical orientation of the bone is inappropriate. Measurements are to be taken end to end, and, if both femora are seen in the same plane, the bone in the near field is to be measured
- The cerebellar transverse diameter at the maximum axial extent of the cerebellum.

Every effort must be made to obtain ideal planes for measurement. If these are not possible, several of the suboptimal planes described in literature may be used. However, the compromise on an ideal view should be mentioned in the report.

The following measurements are not mandatory but encouraged in appropriate clinical situations and serve the purpose of objectivity in anomalies detection:

- Humeral length
- Radial length, ulnar length, tibial length, fibular length, foot length, and clavicular length
- Depth of the cisterna magna
- Width of the atrium of the lateral ventricle
- Nasal bone length
- Binocular distance, interocular distance, and orbital diameter
- Lung length
- Kidney length

The nuchal skin fold should be necessarily measured. This is ideally measured in an axial section showing the fold and including the cerebellum and cavum septum pellucidum.

Fetal weight estimates should be deprived from customized charts, or in case these are not available, from standard charts. The chart used should be quoted in the report/report table. Measurements should include cranial measurements, abdominal perimeter, and femoral length. Deviation of measurements from norm has traditionally been reported as equivalents in weeks and days. There is a recent trend of reporting deviations as centiles and this is encouraged.

Evaluation of the fetal environment includes assessment of the amniotic fluid, the umbilical cord, the placenta, the cervix, and the myometrium and adnexa.

Evaluation of amniotic fluid includes assessing quantity and echogenicity. Measurements are not mandatory but encouraged to facilitate serial evaluation. Quantification may be done by assessing the amniotic fluid index or the maximum vertical pocket. The index is the sum of the deepest fluid pocket in each of the four quadrants of the uterus. The pockets should be free of fetal limbs and the umbilical cord. In multifetal pregnancies, the maximum vertical pocket should be measured in each amniotic sac. If the amniotic fluid is excessively echogenic, this should be mentioned in the report.

The umbilical cord should be assessed for the number of vessels, its point of origin, and its point of insertion. Masses in the umbilical cord, if any, should be noted. Cord length is unreliable to assess but a short cord if noted should be documented.

Placental evaluation should include location, echogenicity, thickness, and the retroplacental area. Accessory lobes should be looked for and noted if present. Location includes a measurement of the distance of the inferior margin of the placenta from the internal os. Focal areas of altered echogenicity should be characterized if possible and noted. Assessment of placental thickness is subjective. Abnormally thin or thick placentas should be documented and maximum thickness should be measured in these situations. Although the sensitivity of ultrasound for assessing abnormal invasion of the myometrium by the placenta is poor, an attempt should be made to assess this.

The myometrium should be assessed for fibroids and any thinning of previous scars. Any maternal adnexal mass should be noted and characterized if possible.

The cervix should be assessed for its length and for a closed internal os. Emerging evidence suggests that a transvaginal scan is more accurate for this assessment and future direction is awaited.

The anomalies survey is the most significant component of the second trimester fetal study. A systematic and meticulous approach is necessary. This should not be limited by time constraints. Low-end equipment with its lower resolution is often inadequate for an adequate study. At the same time, very high-end technology is not necessary but encouraged.

The cranium should be assessed for shape, ossification, and bony defects. The intracranial anatomic survey should include a subjective assessment of symmetry, the falx, cavum septum pellucidum, thalami, cerebellum, cisterna magna, the third ventricle, lateral ventricles, and early sulcation of the cerebrum. Any focal abnormalities in the cerebrum should be noted. Deviations from norm should be reported.

The nuchal skin fold should be measured from the outer margin of skin to the surface of the occipital bone.

The anatomic survey of the face should include an assessment of the slope of the forehead, the orbit, eyelids, lens, NB, nasal configuration, upper lip, lower lip, maxilla, mandible, cheek, and chin. Location and configuration of the external ear is required only in specific clinical scenarios and does not form part of routine anomalies evaluation

The neck should be assessed for anterior, posterior, or lateral masses.

The spine including the osseous components, soft tissues, and skin should be assessed in longitudinal, coronal, and axial sections.

The thorax should be systematically assessed for the chest wall, lungs, heart, mediastinum, and diaphragm. The chest wall should include the ribs, scapula, and clavicles. The cardiac survey should include cardiac situs, size, axis, rate, rhythm, four-chamber view, outflows, and the three vessel/three-vessel trachea view (3VTV). The lungs should be assessed for extent and echogenicity. The mediastinum should be evaluated for masses and displacements. The diaphragm and interruptions should be looked for.

Anatomical assessment of the abdomen should include observing visceral situs, the anterior and posterior abdominal wall, filling and emptying of the stomach, bowel echogenicity, size and echogenicity of the liver and spleen, abnormal masses if any, kidney location, contour and echogenicity, urinary dilatation if any, and the urinary bladder in a full and empty phase.

Evaluation of the fetal genitalia should be considered only in the perspective of sex-related disorders and in the context of local legislation.

The extremities should be assessed for the presence of bones and soft tissues in the proximal, middle, and distal segments of both upper limbs and both lower limbs. Counting of the digits does not form part of the anomalies protocol. Clinodactyly and sandal-gap deformity should be looked for. Movements should be surveyed.

- Spinal lesion variably involving the skin, subcutaneous tissue, muscular or neural elements
- Lemon sign
- Banana sign
- Ventriculomegaly
- Clubfeet
- Associated abnormalities of the urinary bladder or lower limbs

ROLE OF FETAL ECHOCARDIOGRAPHY IN FIRST AND SECOND TRIMESTER

Cardiac defects are one of the most common congenital abnormalities found. Most of these can be missed during routine USG at 18–22 weeks and can only be detected by specialist fetal echocardiography at same gestation or earlier by 14 weeks. A major screening study examining the sensitivity of the four-chamber view at 16–22 weeks during a routine scan reported identification of only 26% of major cardiac defects.[24]

A retrospective screening study has found that >50% of cardiac defects can be found in fetuses with an increased NT at 10–14 weeks.[25] Hence, increased NT at 11–14 weeks is an indication for fetal echocardiography.

Congenital heart disease (CHD) has a prevalence of 8.2 per 1,000 live births and is a leading cause of infant morbidity and mortality. Prenatal diagnosis can improve birth outcome prior to intervention,[7] particularly for certain types of cardiac lesion. Prenatal awareness of CHD and parental education allow preparation for the birth of a neonate that will require specialized care and services. The impact of prenatal diagnosis may also be relevant to long-term neurodevelopmental outcome and it maximizes options for the family. However, prenatal detection rates vary widely in different geographic regions and for various types of CHD, with fewer than one half of cardiac anomalies being identified before birth. Some variation can be attributed to differences in examiner ability, transducer frequency, patient body habitus, abdominal scars, gestational age, amniotic fluid volume, and fetal position. Continuous feedback-based training of healthcare professionals, a low threshold for echocardiography referrals, use of standardized ultrasound protocols, and easy access to fetal-heart specialists can improve the performance of a screening program.

EARLY FETAL CARDIAC SCREENING

Screening for CHD in the first trimester has been shown to be effective in low-risk populations. However, it is neither performed routinely nor considered mandatory. In countries or centers in which this is possible, early screening can be carried out at the time of the NT scan. Minimum requirements for early screening include visualization of the heart within the chest and ascertainment of regular rhythm. It should be borne in mind that due to the small size of the fetal heart in early gestation, the success rate of visualization of the cardiac structures on detailed anatomic survey is significantly higher after 12 + 3 gestational weeks.

Though transvaginal transducers may be used, the recommended methodology includes use of high-frequency transabdominal transducers, owing to their higher resolution, and use of color and/or high-quality power Doppler (bidirectional flow mapping) in addition to grayscale imaging. Color and power Doppler ultrasound should be adjusted to prioritize the color signal over the grayscale to enhance visualization of the blood flow across the small structures in the first-trimester fetal heart. Doppler should be used primarily for screening the four-chamber view and the 3VTV for safety reasons. The most recent ISUOG safety statement suggests that the various Doppler modalities may be used routinely between 11 + 0 and 13 + 6 weeks for certain clinical indications, including screening for cardiac anomalies. Nevertheless, it is important to observe the displayed thermal index, which should be ≤1.0, and the exposure time should be kept as short as possible (usually no longer than 5–10 minutes). The following components are recommended as part of a detailed early cardiac screening examination (GOOD PRACTICE POINT):

- Situs, determined on grayscale imaging, to ascertain the normal position of the stomach and heart, both of which should be on the left side of the fetus. It is also important to assess the cardiac axis, as this is a useful marker for CHD.
- Four-chamber view, displayed using grayscale and color and/or bidirectional power Doppler imaging. Ideally, the spine is visualized posteriorly for adequate demonstration of biventricular filling.
- 3VTV, displayed using color and/or bidirectional power Doppler ultrasound, to demonstrate the left-sided aortic and ductal arches.

Visualization of left and right outflow tracts at this early gestational age is often challenging and prone to both false-negative and false-positive diagnosis. Hence, if early cardiac screening is performed at the time of the NT scan, this should be based mainly on determining situs and obtaining the four-chamber view and 3VTV. Should any suspicion of CHD be raised at this scan, the patient should be referred for early fetal echocardiography.

The four-chamber view along with origin and crossing of the great blood vessels can be seen in the majority of cases at 11–14 weeks. In suspected cases, fetal echo at 14 weeks can effectively reassure most of the patients regarding cardiac defects. Follow-up scan can be done at 18–20 weeks.[27]

Indications for Fetal Echocardiography

- Exomphalos
- Diaphragmatic hernia
- Growth retardation
- Hydrops
- Increased nuchal translucency
- Family history
- Maternal diabetes mellitus

ULTRASONOGRAPHY FOR EXTRA FETAL EVALUATION

Liquor Amnii

Quantity

The measurement of the amniotic fluid can be done either by a single pocket measurement or the four-quadrant approach [amniotic fluid index (AFI)]. The AFI is easily reproducible and more accurate **(Figs. 11 and 12)**.

Fetal swallowing and urinary flow are the primary regulators of amniotic fluid. So abnormalities of these systems cause oligohydramnios (decreased liquor amnii) **(Fig. 13)** or polyhydramnios (increased liquor amnii) **(Fig. 14)**, which can be indirect, signs for detecting anomalies.

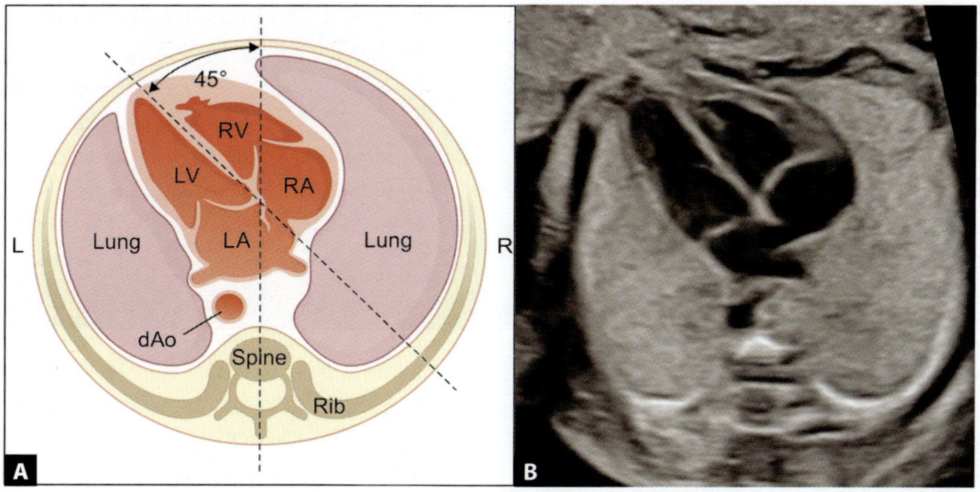

Figs. 11A and B: Determination of cardiac position and axis, shown in schematic diagram (A) and corresponding grayscale ultrasound image (B). Imaginary line drawn from spine posteriorly to sternum anteriorly divides thorax into two equal parts, left (L) and right (R). Normal fetal heart lies mainly on left, with cardiac apex pointing to left at an angle of 45°–20° in relation to anteroposterior axis of the chest. (dAo: descending aorta; LA: left atrium; LV: left ventricle; RA: right atrium; RV: right ventricle)

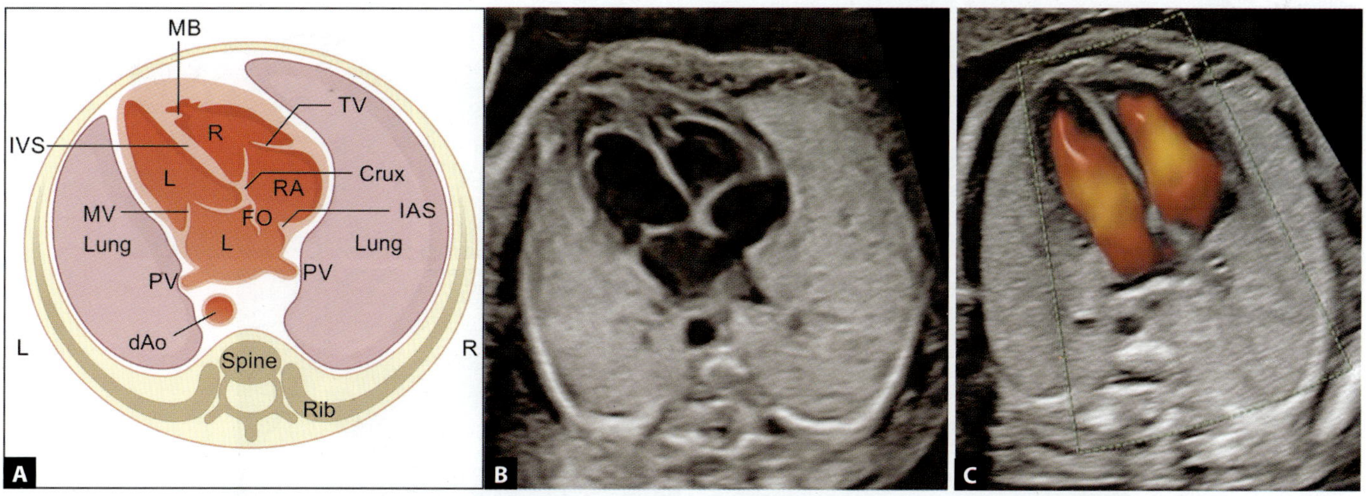

Figs. 12A to C: Schematic drawing (A) and corresponding grayscale (B) and color Doppler (C) ultrasound images of the four-chamber view. Key elements of normal second-trimester four-chamber view include heart area no more than one-third of the chest area, right- and left-sided structures approximately equal (in chamber size and wall thickness), patent foramen ovale (FO) with valve in left atrium (LA), intact cardiac "crux" with normal offset of the two atrioventricular valves and intact interventricular septum (IVS). In (A) and (B), morphological right ventricle (RV) is identified by the presence of moderator band (MB) and tricuspid valve (TV), with septal leaflet inserting in septum more apically compared with insertion of mitral valve (MV) (normal offset). Pulmonary veins (PV) are also seen to enter LA. On color Doppler (C), two separate blood inflows into the ventricles can be seen during diastole. (dAo: descending aorta; IAS: interatrial septum; L: left; LV: left ventricle; R: right; RA: right atrium)
Source: Adopted from Carvalho JS, et al.[26]

Amniotic Bands

Whenever one sees amniotic bands in the uterine cavity traversing the gestational sac, be careful of evaluating whether any fetal part is impinged upon by these bands causing limb reduction defects or any other external anomaly of the cranium, face, anterior abdominal wall or spine **(Fig. 15)**.

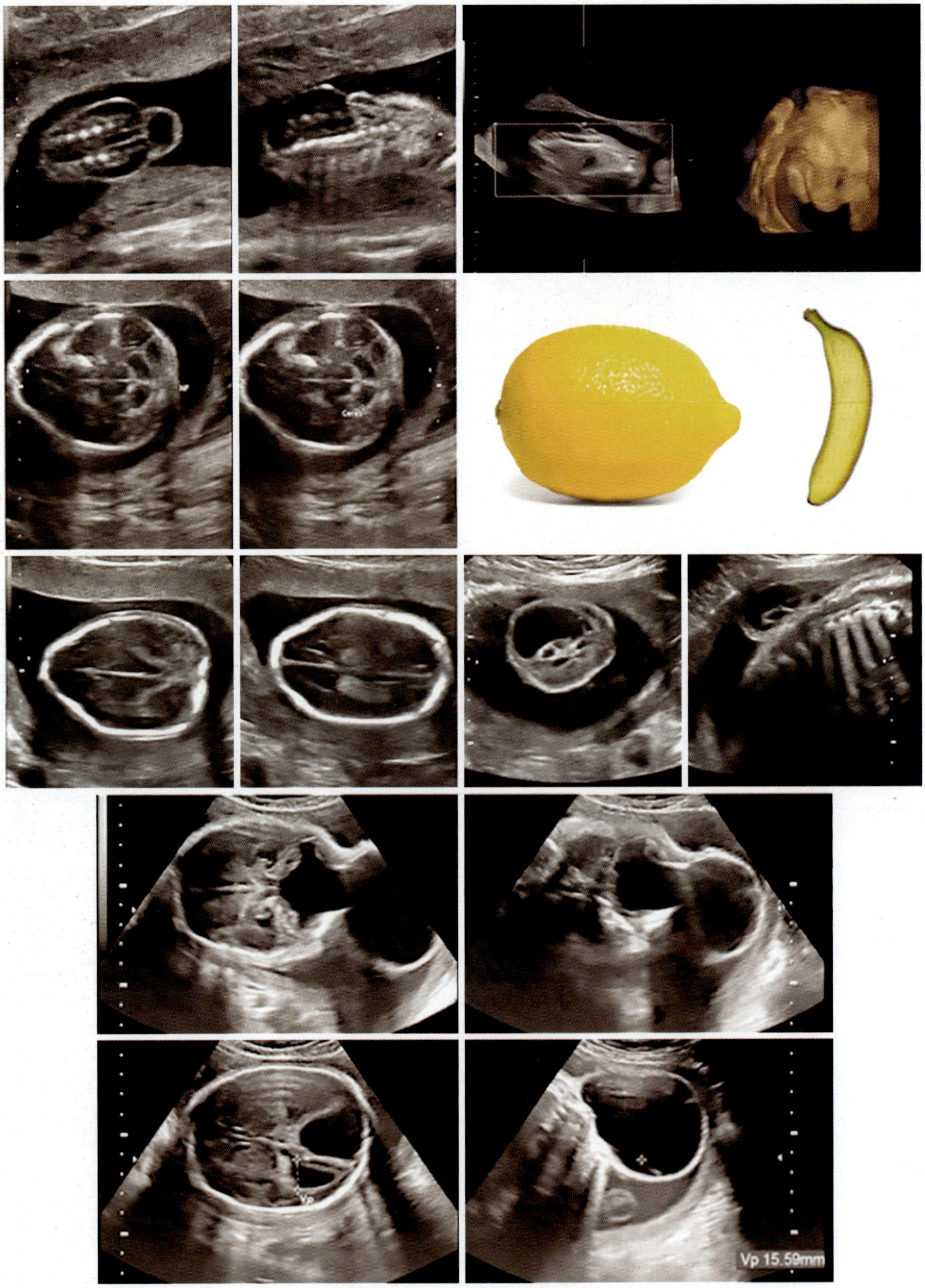

Fig. 13: Second trimester ultrasound findings.

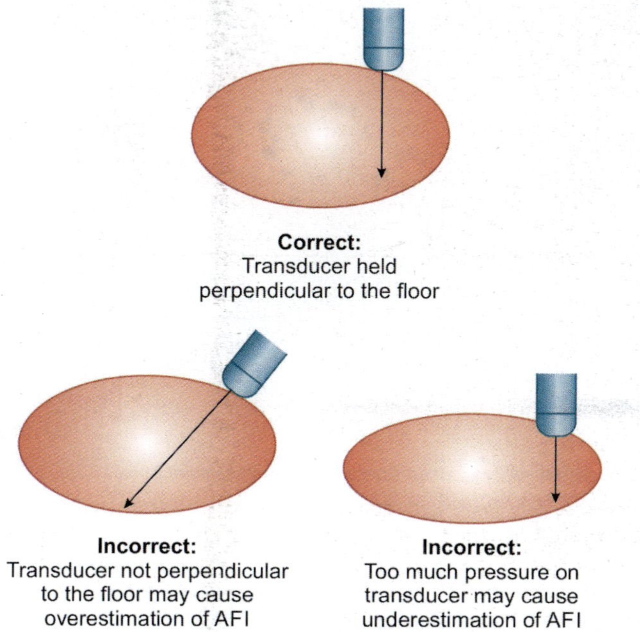

Fig. 14: Amniotic fluid index (AFI) measurement technique.

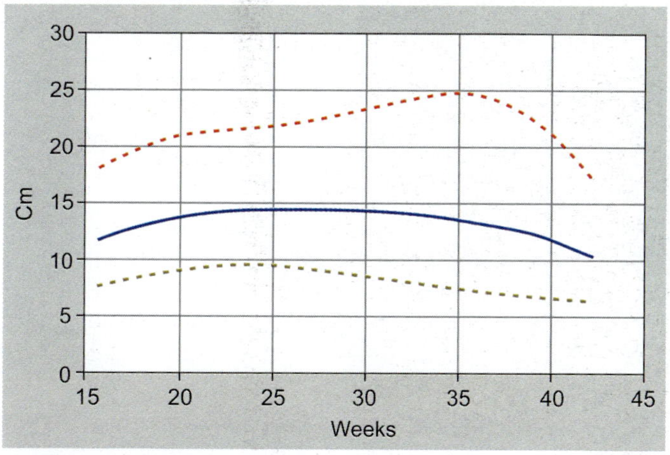

Fig. 15: Amniotic fluid index (AFI) in normal singleton pregnancy.

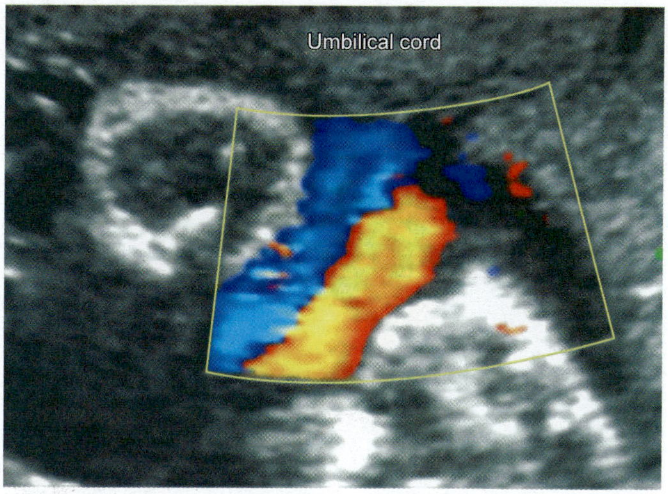

Fig. 16: Two vessel cord as seen on color flow mapping. Single umbilical artery (red) and single umbilical vein (blue) can be seen.

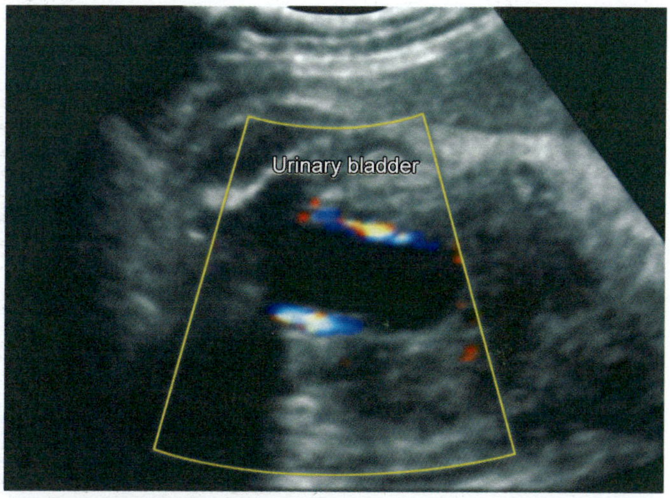

Fig. 17: Hypogastric arteries seen adjacent to the urinary bladder on both sides confirming a three vessel cord.

Umbilical Cord

Number of Vessels (Fig. 16)

- There should be two arteries and one vein in the umbilical cord **(Fig. 17)**.
- Whenever a single umbilical artery is diagnosed, a careful search for anomalies should be done especially chromosomal abnormalities, major cardiac defects, holoprosencephaly, anterior abdominal wall defects, and skeletal deformities. With no other anomaly detected, continuation of pregnancy can be thought of.
- In a 2D ultrasound, look for the rail-track appearance **(Fig. 18)** to assess for number of vessels.
- On color flow mapping, it is easy to see for two arteries and one vein **(Figs. 19 and 20)**, but whenever in doubt always look for the hypogastric arteries adjacent to the urinary bladder **(Figs. 21 and 22)** to evaluate whether there are two arteries or not.

Origin and Insertion

Origin in respect to anomalies is important to differentiate between omphalocele and gastroschisis.

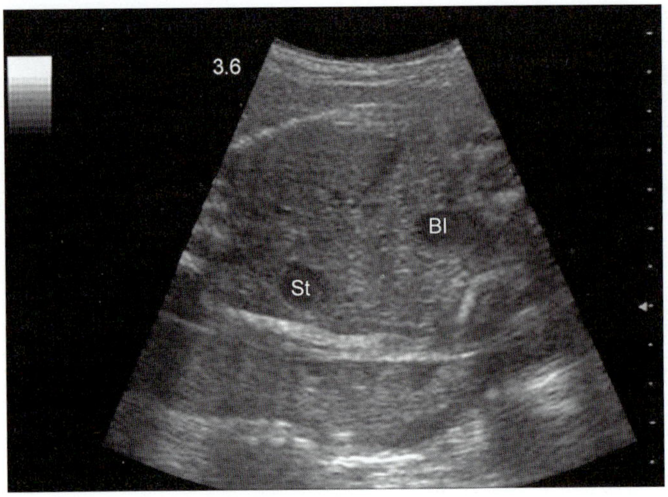

Fig. 18: Oligohydramnios.
(St: stomach; Bl: urinary bladder)

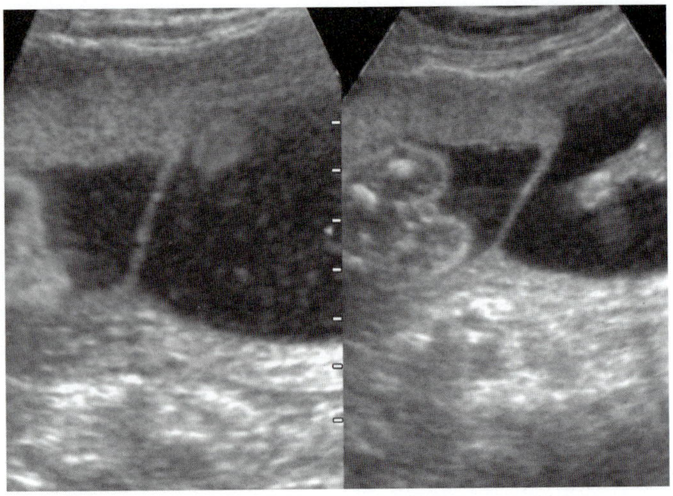

Fig. 20: Amniotic fold/band seen traversing the uterine cavity. Be careful to check for any limb or digit reduction/constriction defects, external anomalies of the face (cleft lip and palate and nasal abnormalities), cranium (anencephaly or encephalocele), anterior abdominal wall defects, and abnormal curvature of the spine.

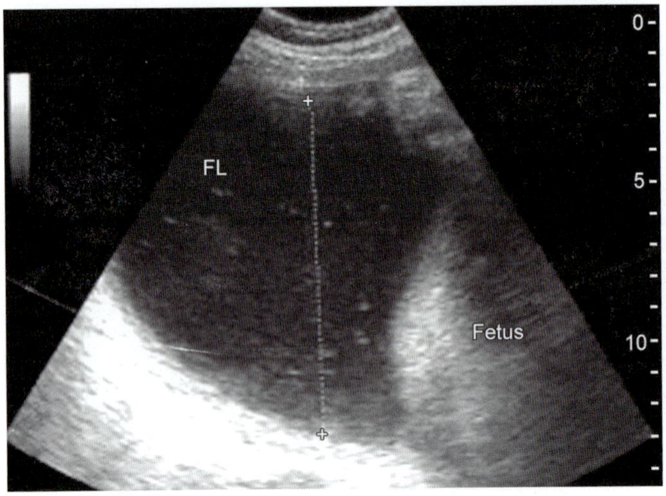

Fig. 19: Polyhydramnios.

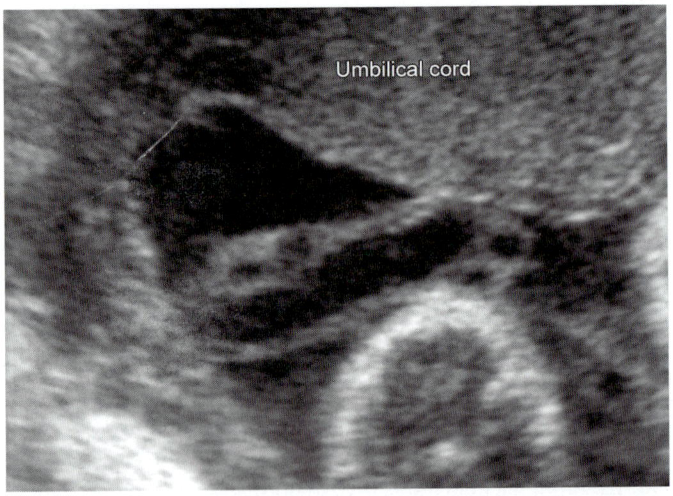

Fig. 21: Three vessel cord as seen on 2D ultrasound. The single umbilical vein and two umbilical arteries are seen as a rail-track appearance.

ULTRASONOGRAPHY FOR FETAL MORPHOLOGY EVALUATION

Choroid Plexii (Fig. 23)

- Cysts
- Hydrocephalus
- Isolated ventricular dilatation
- Tumors

Cerebellum

- Cerebellar transverse diameter
- Superior and inferior cerebellar vermis
- Communication between fourth ventricle and cisterna magna

Cisterna Magna

- Posterior fossa cyst
- Depth

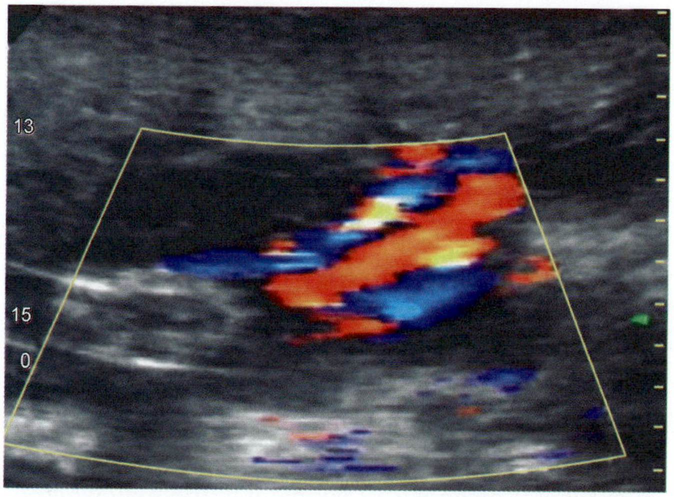

Fig. 22: Three vessel cord as seen on color flow mapping. Two umbilical arteries (blue) and single umbilical vein (red) can be easily demonstrated. On color flow mapping the red and blue to not specify arteries and veins but flow toward the transducer or away from it.

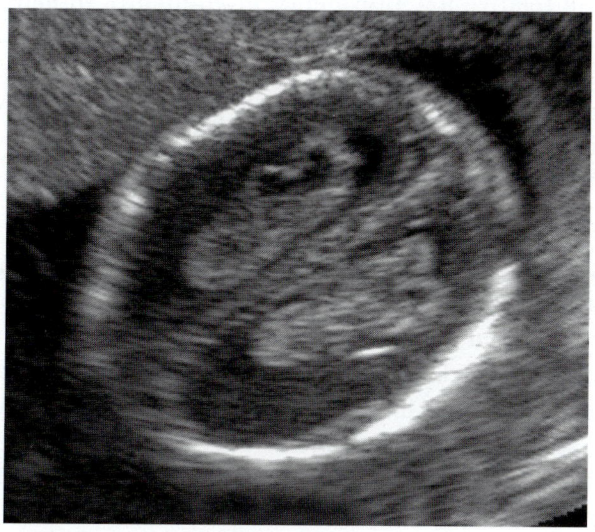

Fig. 23: Choroid plexii.

Nuchal Skin

- Thickness
- Septation
- Generalized hydrops

Fetal Orbits and Face

- Hypo- or hypertelorism
- Lens
- Lips
- Nostrils
- Ears

Fetal Spine

- Soft tissues
- Longitudinal
- Coronal
- Axial
- Ossification centers

Fetal Thorax

- Ribs
- Diaphragm
- Echotexture of lung
- Lung length
- Masses
- Cardiothoracic ratio

Fetal Heart

- Situs
- Size
- Rate
- Rhythm
- Configuration
- Connections
- Tumors

Fetal Abdomen

- Gastrointestinal
  - Stomach
  - Duodenum
  - Small bowel
  - Large bowel
  - Omentum
  - Mesentery
- Pancreas
- Spleen
- Hepatobiliary
  - Liver
  - Gallbladder
- Genitourinary
  - Kidneys
  - Urinary bladder
  - Genitalia

Fetal Skeleton

- Cranium
- Mandible

- Clavicle
- Spine
- Extremities

Fetal Biometry

- Biparietal diameter
- Occipitofrontal distance
- Head perimeter
- Abdominal perimeter
- Femoral length
- Humeral length
- Nuchal skin
- Cerebellar transverse diameter
- Cisterna magna depth
- Width of body of lateral ventricle
- Ocular diameter
- Interocular distance
- Binocular distance
- Foot length

FREQUENTLY ASKED QUESTIONS ABOUT ULTRASOUND

Is routine screening justified?

Screening to be justified should fulfill many criteria; the procedure should be safe, reliable, reproducible, easily available, and cost effective. For an "at risk" population, an ultrasound scan is justified but in developing countries such as India where still almost half our pregnant women have no access to a proper antenatal care. A routine ultrasound currently may not be practically feasible test for screening even though its utility and efficacy are beyond doubt.[3]

Is incidence of fetal malformation high enough to merit screening?

According to Heinonen 1977, approximately 150,000 children are born with malformations annually in USA where almost 100% pregnant women have antenatal care and institutional deliveries.[2] In developing countries, the incidence is higher due to inability for detection, screening, and more exposure to teratogens.

Is outcome of undetected congenital malformations detrimental enough to warrant a routine screening?

Out of an incidence of around 6% congenital malformations, almost half (2.5%) are lethal, life-threatening, and have a major cosmetic defect.[28]

Major congenital defect mostly manifest in fetal intrauterine life (ultrasound detectable), sometimes in fetal life (ultrasound suspicion), and occasionally in childhood (ultrasound undetectable); for this reason, some experts question the need of routine prenatal ultrasound screening.[29] Fetal medicine is still not advanced to treat potential life-threatening conditions such as open NTDs and cardiac defects where death is the expected outcome after delivery, occasionally these defective babies survive and are severely handicapped. Diagnosis of such conditions during pregnancy can give the couple an option of termination.

Current technology enables detection of >60% fetal malformations.[30,31]

Can prenatal diagnosis of anomalies ease emotional pain?

An antenatal diagnosis of congenital anomaly whether lethal, life-threatening, or even lesser serious anomaly can still help couples and doctors prepare themselves to the challenge to come.[32] There is a definite benefit of screening for both patients and physicians. A normal ultrasound scan is usually a good news to the parents to be because of the relative low prevalence of anomalies in general population and relative low incidence of false-positive results by ultrasound.[33]

If the ultrasound screening is positive for anomaly, then counseling and discussion of all options can be done and choice left open to the parents to be.[34]

Is ultrasound prenatal screening cost effective?

It is difficult to assess cost effectiveness of screening, and there are only a few studies on this. Certain costs such as purchase, maintenance of equipment, and salary of well-trained technicians and doctors can be assessed and is expensive.[35] Emotional costs of family disorganization and suffering cannot be calculated. Because of the many options for handling anomalies available from termination to plastic major surgery, it is again difficult to assess whether it is cost effective to detect an anomaly. Helsinki ultrasound trial (1996)[36] has shown that second-trimester screening for anomalies by ultrasound is cost effective.

How does prenatal anomaly scan for screening influence infant health?

Ultrasound screening is not a primary prevention because it cannot prevent the anomaly, it can detect the problem, and if the anomaly is lethal, it gives the parents "to be" an option to terminate pregnancy—secondary prevention. Also, in many cases severe but curable defects (cardiac) can be managed by treating newborn without delay if the pediatric surgery unit is prepared. Expertly performed prenatal ultrasound screening and autopsy reports correlate and provide accurate information.[37]

What are the options after diagnosis of congenital malformations?

The options for managing congenital malformation pregnancy have to be discussed with the parents "to be" and the final choice lies with the parents. A team of specialists should provide all information and counseling. This team should consist of obstetrician, sonologist, geneticist, neonatologist, pediatric surgeon, and a psychologist.

Options depend on severity of the anomaly and can be as follows:

- Termination of pregnancy
- Intrauterine treatment
- Maternal transport to tertiary care center
- Premature delivery
- Immediate specialized neonatal care
- Additional diagnostic tests
- Extensive monitoring.

Alternatives or adjuncts to ultrasound?

There are various blood tests such as maternal serum alpha-fetoprotein (MSAFP), triple test, quadruple tests, and many interventional procedures such as CVS and amniocentesis, cordocentesis, and fetal biopsy, which can help to directly karyotype and chromosomally analyze the fetus, but these are expensive, not easily available, and carry a procedure-related risk of miscarriage.

Noninvasive magnetic resonance imaging (MRI) is definitely not a cost-effective method for screening.

Ultrasound advances have made this technology for screening an ideal test because it is:

- Relatively low in cost
- Ease to perform
- Real-time display
- Acceptable to all
- Widely available
- Accurate
- Safe
- Reproducible
- Available as office investigation
- Can now be applied from late first trimester also.[38]

How long does it take?

A primary screening ultrasound examination is a systemic analysis of fetal growth and fetal morphology is system-wise and will take 10–20 minutes to scan. The screening will stop if everything appears normal in all significant organs and structures.

Depending on image quality, maternal obesity, gestational age, type of anomaly, color Doppler, or 3D scan, still the total scan duration rarely exceeds 30 minutes. For subtle defects or solitary markers or inexperienced sonologists, a second opinion scan might be required by an expert, which will take another 30 minutes.

What does a prenatal ultrasound scan show?

Depending on the gestational age, the defects can be seen and identified, e.g., NT in the first trimester and duodenal atresia, gastrointestinal defects, NTDs, and some cardiac defects in the second trimester.[39]

When we do not see the expected image of the fetus, we suspect a defect. Sometimes, we have to look for soft markers and signs of chromosomal anomalies, e.g., banana sign, lemon sign, etc.

Ultrasound can also pick up functional abnormalities and abnormal fetal biophysical profile and abnormal fetal behaviors.

- Abnormal fetal activity
- Rapid uncoordinated fetal movements
- Fetal arrhythmia
- Fetal vomiting
- Fetal gastrointestinal stenosis.

When should a screening prenatal scan be done?

Nicolaides has suggested a 11–14 weeks scan for screening for chromosomal anomalies, trisomy 21 by looking at the NT and NB ossification.[39] Other workers have suggested addition of biochemical markers.[40] The detection rate for trisomies varies from 80 to 89% with a false-positive rate of 5% by using multiple markers study in the first trimester scan (11–14 weeks).

A second trimester anomaly scan should be done between 18 and 22 weeks and a detailed fetal echocardiography and color Doppler uterine artery and ductus venosus should be done.

Third trimester screening should not be delayed more than 32 weeks of gestation and is mainly done for growth and color Doppler studies for hypoxia detection. Late anomaly screening for gastrointestinal and urinary tract anomaly is usually done at 32 weeks.

Ideal time for ultrasound screening for each and every gravida should be a monthly ultrasound, but as this is not practical and feasible at least each pregnancy should have two scans, one 11–14 weeks scan and one second trimester scan.[41,42]

Ultrasound: How sensitive it is for malformation detection?

In a major study on 500,000 cases, 11,000 (2.2%) were found to be malformed fetus with a range of sensitivity from 14 to 80% (mean 45.5%).

In another study on 170,000 pregnant women, 4,000 malformed fetus were detected with a sensitivity of 61%.[42]

What counts as success in genetic counseling?

Whenever anomaly is detected, for some people abortion and termination of pregnancy is a matter of course response and no ethical dilemma arises; however, among certain religious groups objections to termination pose an ethical dilemma.

Advances in fetal surgery?

This option is still a research tool and there is an ethical aspect that many of these fetal surgical procedures are still experimental and of uncertain value and to give or not to give this option to couples carrying a malformed pregnancy is a dilemma.

3D and 4D scans for screening are they useful or gimmick?

There is now an increasing availability 3D ultrasound. The benefits of 3D/4D scans are now a matter of debate. The 3D and 4D scans help in maternal fetal bondage and also help for recognition and better confirmation of certain anomalies such as cleft lips, polydactyly, micrognathia, malformed ears, clubfoot, vertebral malformations, and other exterior surface anomalies. The development of transvaginal scan (TVS) 3D probes have further enhanced its value in early diagnosis of malformations.

Reassurance scans—how reassuring?

Proposed by Professor Stuart Campbell, a 3D routine scan to reassure the parents and to rule out anomalies. But criticized as entertainment scans and consumerized for unprecedented profit marketing particularly after 4D ultrasound.

CONCLUSION

- With improved technology, in particular, the development of high frequency transvaginal ultrasound probes and its increased acceptance with the patients, it has become possible to examine the detailed fetal anatomy even in the late first trimester and early second trimester.
- The new panorama of normal embryological development is possible with 3D ultrasound and with computers handling the pre- and postprocessing of the ultrasound images give us a future insight into the future of technology being applied to achieve a better understanding of early human developments and its errors.

ACKNOWLEDGMENTS

The authors are grateful to Dr Jaideep Malhotra, Dr Shipra Singla, Dr JP Rao, Dr Asim Kurjak, Dr JP Shah, Dr Ashok Khurana, Dr Kuldeep Singh, and Dr P Radhakrishan for their inputs.

REFERENCES

1. Indian Academy of Pediatrics. (2021). Guidelines for Parents "Birth Defects". Available from: https://iapindia.org/pdf/Ch-054BirthDefectsIAPParentalGuidelines.pdf [Last accessed May, 2024].
2. Heinonen OP, Sloane D, Shapiro S. Birth defects and drugs in pregnancy. Littleton, MA: PSG Publishing; 1977.
3. Hill LM, Breckle R, Gehrking WC. The prenatal detection of congenital malformations by ultrasonography. Mayo Clin Proc. 1983;58(12):805-26.
4. American College of Radiology. ACR-ACOG-AIUM-SRU Practice Guideline for the Performance of Obstetrical Ultrasound. Revised 2013 (Resolution 17).
5. World Health Organization. (2010). Sixty-Third World Health Assembly. Available from: https://apps.who.int/gb/ebwha/pdf_files/WHA63-REC1/WHA63_REC1-en.pdf [Last accessed May, 2024].
6. Benacerraf, Beryl R. Ultrasound of Fetal Syndromes. Philadelphia, Churchill Livingston; 1998.
7. Callen PW (Ed). Ultrasonography in Obstetrics and Gynecology, 4th edition, Philadelphia, PA: WB Saunders; 2000.
8. Pandya PP, Santiago C, Snijders RJ, Nicolaides KH. First trimester fetal nuchal translucency. Curr Opin Obstet Gynecol. 1995;7(2):95-102.
9. Cicero S, Curcio P, Papageorghiou A, Sonek J, Nicolaides KH. Absence of nasal bone in fetuses with trisomy 21 at 11–14 weeks of gestation: an observational study. Lancet. 2001;358(9294):1665-7.
10. Nicolaides KH. Nuchal translucency and other first-trimester sonographic markers of chromosomal abnormalities. Am J Obstet Gynecol. 2004;191(1):45-67.
11. Schemmer G, Wapener RJ, Johnson A, Schemmer M, Norton HJ, Anderson WE. First trimester growth patterns of aneuploid fetuses. Prenat Diag. 1997;17(2):155.
12. Liao AW, Snijders R, Geerts L, Spencer K, Nicolaides KH. Fetal heart rate in chromosomally abnormal fetuses. Ultrasound Obstet Gynecol. 2000;16(7):610-3.
13. Borrell A, Martinez JM, Seres A, Borobio V, Cararach V, Fortuny A. Ductus venosus assessment at the time of

nuchal translucency measurement in the detection of fetal aneuploidy. Prenat Diagn. 2003;23(11):921-6.
14. Hyett JA, Noble PL, Snijders RJ, Montenegro N, Nicolaides KH. Fetal heart rate in trisomy 21 and other chromosomal abnormalities at 10-14 weeks of gestation. Ultrasound Obstet Gynecol. 1996;7(4):239-44.
15. Rotmensch S, Liberati M, Bronshtein M, Schoenfeld-Dimaio M, Shalev J, Ben-Rafael Z, et al. Prenatal sonographic findings in 187 fetuses with Down syndrome. Prenat Diagn. 1997;17(11):1001-9.
16. Rotmensch S, Mandell J, Estroff JA. Fetal Pyelectasis: a possible association with Down syndrome. Obstet Gynecol. 1992;76:770.
17. Nyberg DA, Resta RG, Mahony BS, Dubinsky T, Luthy DA, Hickok DE, et al. Fetal hyperechogenic bowel and Down's syndrome. Ultrasound Obstet Gynecol. 1993;3(5):330-3.
18. Brown DL, Roberts DJ, Miller WA. Left ventricular echogenic focus in the fetal heart. Pathologic correlation. J Ultrasound Med. 1994;13(8):613-6.
19. Lehman CD, Nyberg DA, Winter TC 3rd, Kapur RP, Resta RG, Luthy DA. Trisomy 13 syndrome: prenatal US findings in a review of 33 cases. Radiology. 1995;194(1):217-22.
20. Jones KL. Smith's Recognizable Patterns of Human Malformations. Philadelphia: WB Saunders; 1997.
21. Rubenstein JB, Swayne LC, Dise CA, Gersen SL, Schwartz JR, Risk A. Placental changes in fetal triploidy syndrome. J Ultrasound Med. 1986;5(10):545-50.
22. Sherard J, Bean C, Bove B, DelDuca V Jr, Esterly KL, Karcsh HJ, et al. Long survival in a 69,XXY triploid male. Am J Med Genet. 1986;25(2):307-12.
23. Droste S, FitzSimmons J, Pascoe-Mason J, Shepard TH. Growth of linear parameters in trisomy 18 fetuses. Am J Obstet Gynecol. 1990;163(1 Pt 1):158-61.
24. Tegnander E, Eik-Nes SH, Johansen OJ, Linker DT. Prenatal detection of heart defects at the routine fetal examination at 18 weeks of gestation in a non-selected population. Ultrasound Obstet Gynecol. 1995;5(6):372-80.
25. Hyett J, Perdu M, Sharland GK, Snijders RJM, Nicolaides KH. Using fetal nuchal translucency to screen for major cardiac defects at 10–14 weeks of gestation. Population base cohort study. BMJ. 1999;318(7176):81-5.
26. Carvalho JS, Axt-Fliedner R, Chaoui R, Copel JA, Cuneo BF, Goff D, et al. ISUOG Practice Guidelines (updated): fetal cardiac screening. Ultrasound Obstet Gynecol 2023;61:788-803.
27. Gembruch U, Knopfle G, Bald R, Hansmann M. Early diagnosis of fetal congenital heart disease by transvaginal echocardiography. Ultrasound Obstet Gynecol. 1993; 3(5):310-7.
28. Snijders RJM, Nicolaides KH. Ultrasound markers for fetal chromosomal defects. New York, NY: Parthenon Publishing Group; 1996.
29. Grandjean H, Larroque D, Levi S. The performance of routine ultrasonographic screening of pregnancies in the Eurofetus study. Am J Obstet Gynecol. 1999;181(2):446-54.
30. Levi S. Cost effectiveness of antenatal screening for fetal malformation by ultrasound: an evaluation of antenatal mass screening by ultrasound for the diagnosis of birth defects (1990–1993). Report to the European Commission, European Union, contract MR4*-0225-B; 1995.
31. McNeil TF, Torstensson G, Nimby G. Psychological aspects of screening. In: Kurjak S (Ed). Textbook of Perinatal Medicine. London, England: Parthenon Publishing; 1998. pp. 717-29.
32. Levi S. Screening for congenital malformations by ultrasound. In: Kurjak S (Ed). Textbook of Perinatal Medicine. London, England: Parthenon Publishing; 1998. pp. 587-609.
33. Reed KL. Why (not) do obstetric ultrasound? An observation on uncertainty. Ultrasound Obstet Gynecol. 1996;8(1):1-2.
34. Leivo T, Tuominen R, Saari-Kemppainen A, Ylöstalo P, Karjalainen O, Heinonen OP. Cost-effectiveness of one-stage ultrasound screening in pregnancy: a report from the Helsinki ultrasound trial. Ultrasound Obstet Gynecol. 1996;7(5):309-14.
35. Cheschiery NC, Reitnauer PJ. A comparative study of prenatal diagnosis and perinatal autopsy. J Ultrasound Med. 1994;13(6):451-56.
36. Salvesen KA, Eik-Nes SH. Is ultrasound unsound? A review of epidemiological studies of human exposure to ultrasound. Ultrasound Obstet Gynecol. 1995;6(4):293-98.
37. Rosendahl H, Kivinen S. Antenatal detection of congenital malformations by routine ultrasonography. Obstet Gynecol. 1989;73(6):947-51.
38. Nicolaides KH, Azar G, Byrne D, Mansur C, Marks K. Fetal nuchal translucency: ultrasound screening for chromosomal defects in first trimester of pregnancy. BMJ. 1992;304(6831):867-9.
39. Spencer K, Souter V, Tul N, Snijders R, Nicolaides KH. A screening program for trisomy 21 at 10-14 weeks using fetal nuchal translucency, maternal serum free beta-human chorionic gonadotropin and pregnancy-associated plasma protein-A. Ultrasound Obstet Gynecol. 1999;13(4):231-7.
40. Levi S, Montenegro N. Eurofetus: an evaluation of routine ultrasound screening for the detection of fetal defects: aims and method. In: Chervenak F, Levi S (Eds). Ann NY Acad Sci. 1998;847:103-17.
41. Clarke A. What counts as success in genetic counselling. J Med Ethics. 1993;19(1):47-9.
42. Langham MR Jr, E Reiger KM. Advances in fetal surgery. Surg Annu. 1994;26:193-226.

32

CHAPTER

Postpartum Ultrasound

Ajlana Mulic-Lutvica

INTRODUCTION

Postpartum period usually includes six subsequent weeks during which normal pregnancy involution occurs and the uterus returns to the nonpregnant state. Our knowledge about postpartum changes in the uterus has mainly been based on clinical examinations as well as from histological studies from the end of the 19th century and the early part of the 20th century when maternal mortality was high.[1] The involution of the uterus, as a main characteristic of the puerperium was previously assessed by palpation of the fundal height.

Since the introduction of ultrasound (US) in clinical practice by Ian Donald et al.[2] in 1958 the uterus became one of the first organs to be examined.[3-7] However, few studies have focused on US investigations during the puerperium and results of published studies are not unambiguous.[1-16] In published studies concerning the involution process, the length[4, 6-9,11,12,14,] width,[8,9,12] AP-diameter,[3,4,6,7,11-13,16] area,[9] thickness of the uterine wall[10] and volume of the uterus and the uterine cavity,[15] have been used as a measure of uterine involution. Majority of the studies described pathological conditions without knowledge about normal findings[4,5,8,] they were restricted to the early puerperium and designs were cross-sectional.[3-7,12] A few studies concerning uterine cavity during normal puerperium have been published.[13-16]

Postpartum complications involving the uterus occur in about 8–10% of cases. Immediate and late postpartum hemorrhage, puerperal sepsis, and septic pelvic thromboembolism are still potentially life-threatening conditions. Abnormal placentation (placenta accreta, increta or percreta) is a rare cause of postpartum hemorrhage that may continue postpartum. Several studies investigated antenatal ultrasound diagnosis of this condition[17-23] but a few papers have focused on postpartum ultrasound monitoring of retained placenta accreta.[24] Ultrasound can help to diagnose vascular lesions, congenital or acquired,[25-31] placental site tumor[32] and choriocarcinoma, which can also cause severe postpartum hemorrhage.

Thus, whenever puerperal complication occurs, the obstetricians should not hesitate to switch on ultrasound machine.

NORMAL PUERPERIUM

A description of normal ultrasound changes of the uterus and uterine cavity during puerperium is a prerequisite for ultrasound diagnosis of pathological conditions. We can follow the physiological involution of the uterus weighing more than 1 kg soon after delivery to an organ weighing about 80 grams at the end of the puerperium by means of ultrasound. The involution changes concerning the size, shape, position, and texture of the uterus have been relatively well examined by ultrasound.[3-16] The influence on the involution process of parity,[7,9,11,13,15,16] route of delivery,[11] oxytocin administration during labor[7] breast-feeding[6,7,9,11-13,15,16] or the infant's weight[11-13] have been studied. Previously published studies involving sonographic examination of uterine cavity are not unambiguous.[6,11,13-16]

In the early and middle puerperium (in the first 2 weeks) the transabdominal approach is to be recommended. A relatively short focal length of the vaginal probe limits its use during the early postpartum period when the uterus is too large and lies near to abdominal wall. In contrast, during the late postpartum period (>2 weeks) a high frequency transvaginal probe, which better distinguishes minor details, should be used. At that time the uterus is considerably decreased in size and it lies in the true pelvis. The postpartum uterus should be examined in three standard sections: sagittal, transverse and coronal **(Figs. 1 and 2)**. Urinary bladder should be moderately filled.

Gentle compression with the probe should be used in order to avoid uterine distortion.

We can differentiate three typical ultrasound images during normal puerperium: in the early, middle and late puerperium **(Figs. 3 and 4)**. The involution of the uterus is a dynamic process that has no parallel in normal adult life.[1] There are two physiological lifesaving processes occurring soon after placenta delivery: myotamponade (compression of the vessels by myometrial contraction) and thrombotamponade (enhanced blood clotting activity).

The appearance of ultrasound finding in the early postpartum period reflects these physiological changes. The uterus has an angulated form **(Fig. 4A)**. It lies in a slightly retroflected position and arches over the sacral promontory. Wachsberg et al.[12] pointed out the impact of uterine angulation on the measurement of uterine length and recommended segmental measurement. This angulated form of the early puerperal uterus is typical only in early puerperium and it is artificial. An extremely great degree of uterine deformability is caused by a heavy uterine corpus, a hypotonic lower uterine segment and supine position of the examined woman. Lifesaving uterine contraction approaches anterior and posterior uterine walls and just a virtual cavity appears. The uterine cavity is empty and decidua appears as a thin white line from the fundus to the level of the internal cervical os **(Fig. 4A)**. Sometimes, this line can be irregular and thicker, which probably depends on the amount of retained decidua **(Fig. 5A)**. The separation of the placenta and membranes generally, occurs in the spongy layer; however, the level varies. Already in the 1931 Williams wrote concerning the line of separation of the placenta and membranes: "While separation generally occurs in the spongy layer, the line is very irregular so that in places a thick layer of decidua is retained, in others only a few layers of cells remain, while in still others the muscularis is practically bare".[33] The variation in sonographic appearance of the cavity could be seen as a demonstration of these physiological variations in retained decidua. The white thin line seen on ultrasound might possibly represent cases in which only the basal decidual layer is retained or if the muscularis is practically bare **(Fig. 4A)**. Whereas the thicker and more irregular lines might represent cases with retention of more amount of spongy decidual layer, and perhaps fragments of membranes **(Fig. 5A)**.

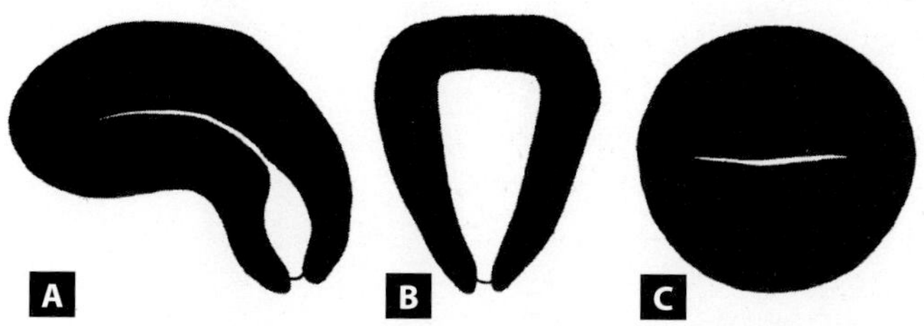

Figs. 1A to C: Three standard ultrasound sections of the puerperal uterus. (A) Longitudinal; (B) Coronal; (C) Transverse.

Fluid or echogenic mass is not common finding in the cavity in the early postpartum period.[13] Small echogenic or echolucent dots in the cavity are harmless physiological findings.[13,34] A heterogeneous mass with fluid and solid components can be seen in the cervical area.[13,14,34,35] This finding has no clinical significance and the mass is usually expelled spontaneously. It probably reflects a collection of blood, blood clots and parts of membranes. On the posterior wall of the uterus the prominent uterine vascular channels are regularly seen.[11] They usually disappear during the 2nd and 3rd postpartum weeks as a result of involution process, which decreases both the size and the amount of uterine vessels. Gas in the cavity is not common finding in the early postpartum period although it can be

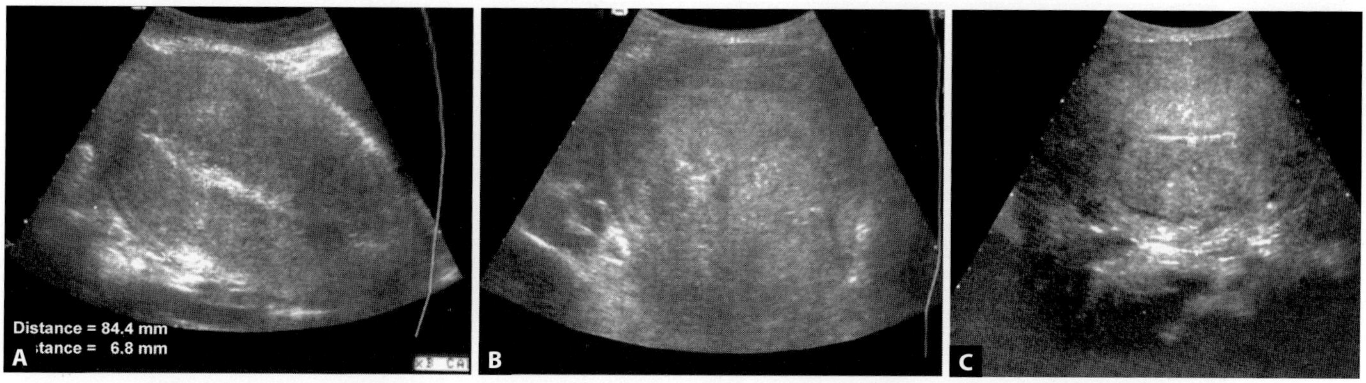

Figs. 2A to C: Transabdominal ultrasound scans of a normal puerperal uterus on day 1. (A) Longitudinal scan; (B) Coronal scan; (C) Transverse scan.

occasionally seen.[13] Wachsberg detected gas in 19% of normal population during the early postpartum period.[36]

In the middle part of the puerperium (1-2 weeks postpartum): The uterus is diminished, the shape of the uterus is oval. It rotates along its internal cervical os towards an anteflected position probably due to forming a firm isthmus.[13] The vascular channels are not so prominent. Either pure fluid or mixed echo with fluid and solid components can be seen in the whole cavity not only in the cervical area **(Figs. 4B and 5B andC)**. This finding reflects

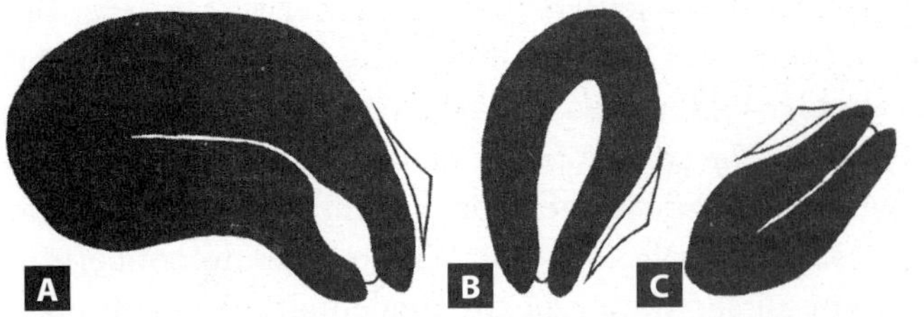

Figs. 3A to C: The normal ultrasound appearance of the uterus and uterine cavity during the puerperium. (A) Transabdominal approach during the early puerperium; (B) During the middle part of the puerperium; (C) Transvaginal approach during the late puerperium.

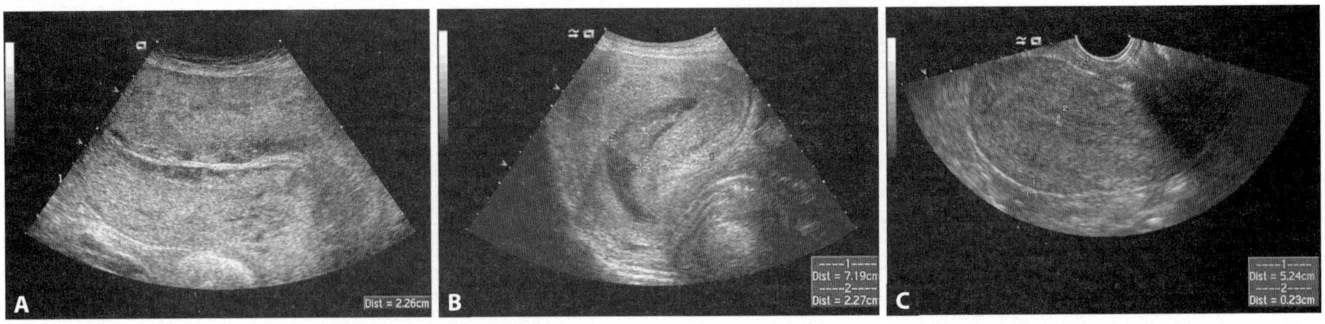

Figs. 4A to C: Three typical USG images during normal puerperium. (A) In the early puerperium: uterus is retroverted. The cavity is seen as a thin white line; (B) In the middle puerperium: uterus is anteverted. An abundant fluid or mixed echo pattern with echogenic and echo-free area is seen in the whole cavity; (C) In the late puerperium: uterus is considerably decreased in size; the cavity is empty and appears as a thin white line.

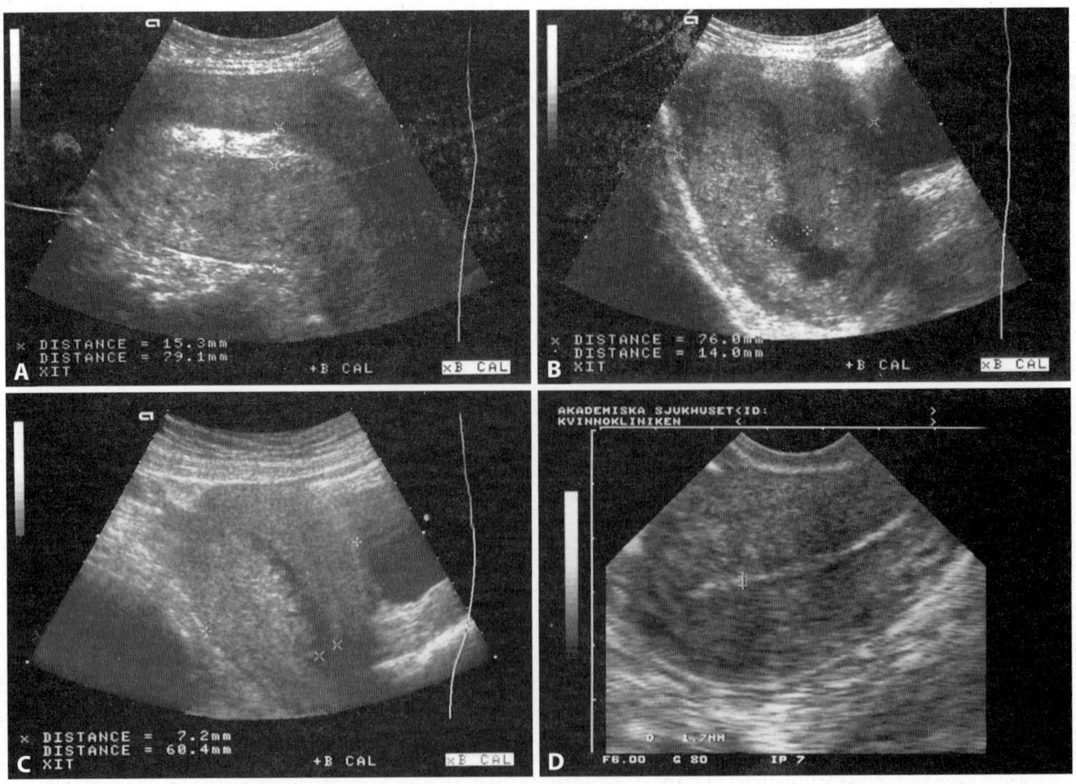

Figs. 5A to D: Transabdominal, longitudinal scans of the uterus from an uncomplicated puerperium. (A) On day 1; (B) On day 7; (C) On day 14; (D) On day 28.

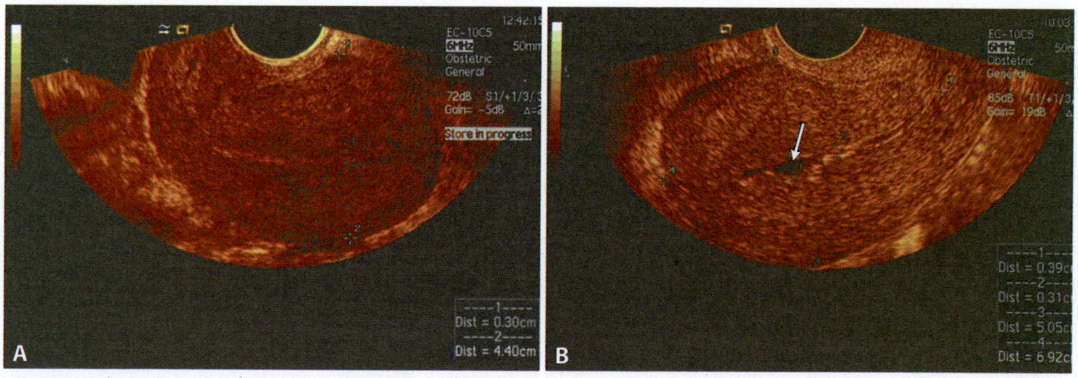

Figs. 6A and B: (A) Transvaginal ultrasound image of the uterus on day 28 postpartum shows a retroverted uterus on day 28 postpartum; (B) Transvaginal ultrasound image of the uterus on day 28 postpartum shows a small amount of fluid with echogenic foci in the cavity (white arrow).

a normal healing process of the placental site inside uterine cavity, necrotic changes of retained decidua and an abundant shedding of lochia. Echogenic mass or gas is not common finding during middle part of the puerperium. In contrast Edwards et al.[15] found an echogenic mass in a great proportion of normal puerperal women.

During late puerperium (>2 weeks postpartum): The uterus is considerably diminished **(Figs. 4C and 5D)**. It lies in an anteflected position in 88% of cases.[13] In 12% of cases the uterus has a retroflected position corresponding well to normal prevalence of retroversion of the uterus in general population **(Fig. 6A)**. The uterine cavity is again empty. Decidua and necrotic vessel ends are exfoliated, the placental site is recovered, and a new endometrium is regenerated from the basal layer of the decidua adjacent to the myometrium. Ultrasonically, the cavity in the late puerperium appears as a thin white line **(Figs. 4C and 5D)**. This corresponds to an inactive endometrium and reflects the hypo estrogenic state of the puerperium ("the physiologic menopause"). Sometimes, a small amount of fluid or echogenic dots can be seen (arrow) **(Fig. 6B)**.

In 1953 Sharman performed endometrium biopsies and identified fully restored endometrium from the 16th postpartum day.[37] In contrast a study published in 1986 by Oppenheimer[38] showed that duration of puerperal lochia may be up to 60 days in 13% of women. Similarly, in a recently published study[39] on the duration of postpartum bleeding among 477 breastfeeding, women it was reported that the median duration of lochia was 27 days with a range from 5–90 days. Only 15% of the women reported that their lochia had stopped within 2 weeks postpartum. They also pointed to the fact that bleeding associated with the postpartum healing process commonly stops and starts again. So, the normal physiological time span for the placental site to recover is probably 4–6 and not 2 weeks as previously considered.

Doppler Ultrasound during Normal Puerperium

Besides conventional ultrasound, Doppler technology is used to study hemodynamic events occurring during the puerperium. Normal pregnancy requires the growth of many new vessels. Consequently, during puerperium dramatically regressive changes must occur. The physiological involution of the uterus involves not only muscle cells and decidua but also the arteries. From histological studies we know that normal involute placental bed is characterized by a disappearance of trophoblasts and completely thrombosed spiral arteries.[40-42] High diastolic flow velocities in combination with a disappearance of the early diastolic notch are the main characteristics of the uterine artery Doppler flow pattern from gestational week 20–26 and they reflect the physiological conversion from high (nonpregnant) to low (pregnant) resistance state.[43,44] How fast these physiological changes return to the nonpregnant state is a controversial issue.[45-48] Tekay and Jouppila[14] assessed the peripheral vascular resistance of the uterine arteries in 42 postpartum women and found that the pulsatility index (PI) increased significantly in early puerperium compared to pregnancy, remained unchanged during the next 6 weeks and then gradually started to increase again. However, nonpregnant values were not reached even 3 months after delivery. Jaffa et al.[46] on the other hand, described that PI decreased in the 2nd and remained relatively low until the 4th postpartum week. Similar differences regarding the reappearance of

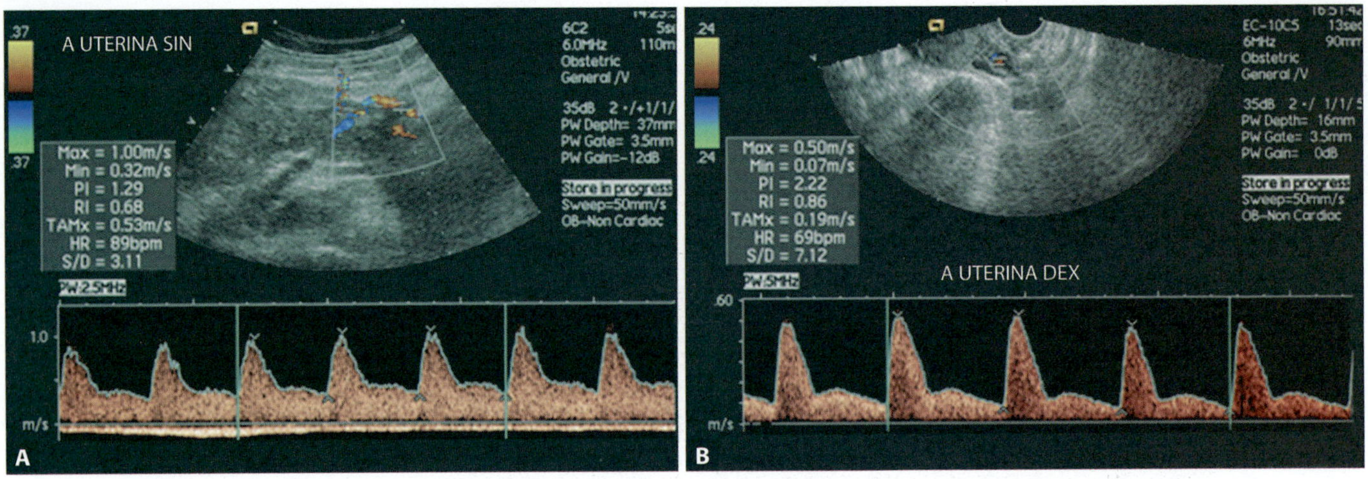

Figs. 7A and B: (A) Normal flow velocity waveforms of the uterine artery on day 1 (Transabdominal approach) and; (B) 56 (Transvaginal approach) postpartum.

the early diastolic notch have been reported. Tekay and Jouppila[14] noted a reappearance of the early diastolic notch already in early puerperium in 40 of 42 women, while Jaffa et al.[46] found that the early diastolic notch had reappeared in only 1 of 60 women five weeks postpartum.

According to our findings,[48] in early puerperium the means of Doppler flow resistance indices are higher than those reported in late pregnancy. Thereafter they do not change markedly until day 28 postpartum. On day 56 postpartum they are still lower compared to the values reported for non-pregnant women, which speaks for longer duration of physiological vascular return from a pregnant to a nonpregnant state. We observed a diastolic notch in 13% of women on day 1 and in 90.6% of women on day 56 postpartum **(Figs. 7A and B)**.

Color and Power Doppler ultrasound may detect a localized area of increased vascularity within the myometrium. It may be a common transient ultrasound finding if asymptomatic and it does not require treatment.[47]

Three-dimensional (3D) Ultrasound Postpartum

Although the volume of the uterus and uterine cavity were previously measured using 2D ultrasound,[15] the volumes assessed by 3D ultrasound may provide more accurate measurements than does the conventional ultrasound. 3D ultrasound using VOCAL program (virtual organ computer-aided analysis) has recently been used to measure the volumes of the uterus and the uterine cavity after normal delivery and in cases with suspicion of retained placental tissue[49-51] **(Figs. 8A to F)**.

3D power Doppler angiography is a new unexplored method for quantifying noninvasively the vascular network of the uterus **(Fig. 8C)**.

RETAINED PLACENTAL TISSUE

Both ultrasound diagnosis of retained placental tissue (RPT) and appropriate management for Secondary postpartum hemorrhage (SPH) is still controversial issue. An SPH is defined as any abnormal bleeding from the uterus occurring between 24 hours and 12 weeks postpartum[52] and occurs in 1–2% of deliveries.[52,53] In developed countries, half of postpartum women who are admitted to hospital with this condition undergo uterine surgical evacuation.[52-56] In developing countries, it is a major contributor to maternal death.[52] The most common causes of SPH are abnormal involution of the placental site in the uterine cavity that may be idiopathic[42] or it can be caused by RPT[56] or by endometritis.[54] Subinvolution of the placental bed in the absence of RPT or endometritis is a distinctive entity, characterized by widely distended spiral arteries, only partly occluded by thrombi of various ages and invested with extravillous trophoblasts.[40,42] The diagnosis, however, requires histological examination and clinically it is a diagnosis of exclusion. Moreover, placental vascular subinvolution is often under recognized by general surgical pathologists.[42] Carlan et al.[57] performed manual exploration of the cavity on 131 asymptomatic women 5 min after placental delivery and within 2 minutes after an ultrasound examination. They found that 24 of 131(18.8%) women had documented evidence of RPT. This is a surprisingly higher figure compared to Jones et al.[58]

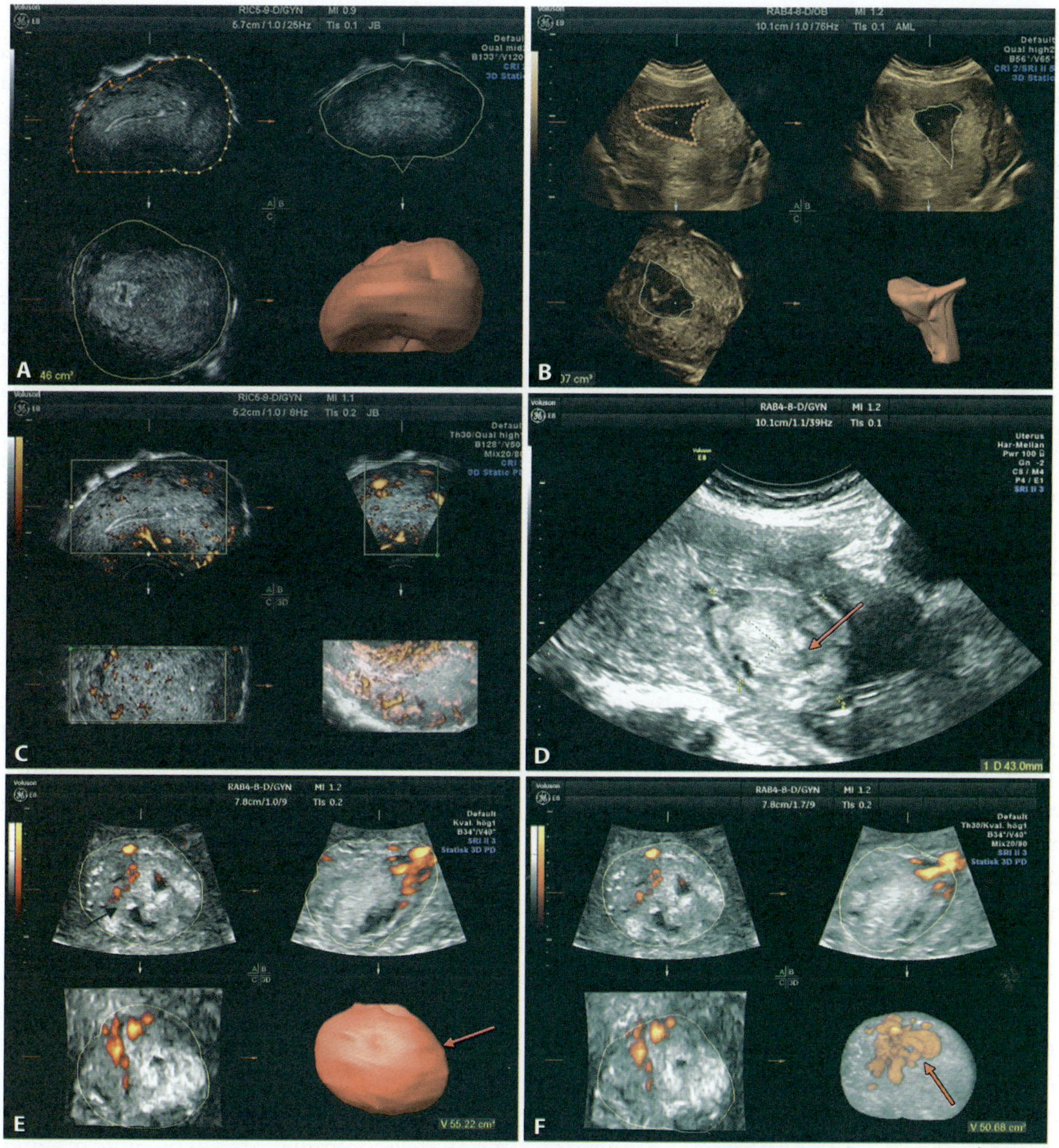

Figs. 8A to F: (A) Three-dimensional USG of the volume of the uterus on day 28 and; (B) Uterine cavity on day 7 after normal delivery; (C) With 3D power Doppler a localized area of increased vascularity within the myometrium is seen; (D) Transabdominal longitudinal scan of the uterus on day 17 postpartum. Suspected retained placental tissue seen as an echogenic mass in the uterine cavity (red arrow); (E) 3D USG shows the volume of the suspected retained placental tissue; (F) Power Doppler angiography, glass body mode shows vessels in the placental tissue (red arrow).

who performed manual intrauterine explorations routinely after 1000 births and removed placental fragments or bits of membranes in only 2.4% of cases. Defective decidua, which can be scanty or completely absent in some patients, is a predisposing factor for abnormal attachment of the placenta and for partially RPT.[40] Vascular abnormalities of the uterus have recently been described as possibly more common causes of severe SPH than previously thought.[25-31]

In a Cochrane Review, Alexander et al.[52] identified 45 papers about the management of SPH and concluded that little information is available from randomized trials to guide clinicians in the management of this condition. Since the causes of SPH may be various the best treatment options should be chosen according to the underlying cause of bleeding. However, an essential problem is that the underlying cause of SPH often is unknown and that clinical or ultrasound diagnosis of RPT, which is the indication for surgical treatment, is still a controversial issue.[59-75] There is a few number of published guidelines for management of secondary postpartum hemorrhage (DSOG), as the evidence is sparce. It is the best for diagnostic, and very sparce for the treatment and for the prevention of the complications. The decision whether to perform uterine evacuation for RPT depends on both, clinical finding and the ability to visualize retained placenta by ultrasound.[58-69] In contrast to Hoveyda who reported that uterine evacuation was more frequent for women who underwent ultrasound examination than for those who did not, Dossou et al.[74] found that the use of ultrasound did not influence of the rate of surgical interventions. Although prompt curettage seems to be necessary in many cases it usually does not remove identifiable placental tissue.[74] Moreover, it is more likely to traumatise the implantation site and incite more bleeding. Consequently, the complications rate is high. Hoveyda et al. reported in his review regarding secondary postpartum hemorrhage that the frequency of perforation of the uterus was 3% and hysterectomy about 1%.[56] Similar results are reported from an Audit of 200 cases concerning puerperal curettage.[76] They showed that 8.5% of patients experienced major morbidity and 7% required a repeat procedure with further morbidity. In addition to immediate complications, late sequelae related to surgical treatment for SPH may influence the reproductive health of women. If curettage damages stratum basalis of the endometrium one to four weeks postpartum during the hypoestrogen status of the puerperium, the endometrium may fail to regenerate, leading to Asherman's syndrome.[77] Asherman's syndrome is characterized by intrauterine synechia, hypo- or amenorrhea and infertility. During subsequent pregnancy, an abnormal placental implantation may occur. Westendorp et al.[78] prospectively examined 50 women undergoing either a repeat removal of placental remnants after delivery or a repeat curettage for incomplete abortion. At a later hysteroscopy, 20 out of 50 (40%) women had intrauterine adhesions. The prevalence of Asherman's syndrome is 2% after manual evacuation of the placenta but 37.5% after postpartum curettage.[76-78] More recently, an update on intrauterine adhesions has been published and the importance of prevention has been emphasized.[79] First studies concerning RPT performed with old ultrasound equipment showed high rate of false-positive diagnosis.[4,5,8] Similar results have been obtained by modern ultrasound equipment.[58-68] Published studies have demonstrated a variable sensitivity (42–94%) and specificity (62–92%) for ultrasound diagnosis of RPT.[59-71] On the other side ultrasound appears as a valuable tool to confirm an empty cavity. Lee and Mandrazzo[8] found empty cavity in 20 of 27 patients with late puerperal bleeding. In only one case RPT was confirmed. The same authors reported that histological confirmation was obtained in eight of nine patients with ultrasound suspected RPT. Although ultrasound technology becomes considerably improved the diagnosis of RPT is still difficult. Ultrasound finding of RPT may vary depending on many different factors. We cannot expect the same ultrasound image during early **(Figs. 5A and B)** and late period of the puerperium **(Figs. 5C and D)**. The presence of blood, blood clots, necrotic decidua, membranes or gas can give various ultrasound images and a proper diagnosis is sometimes difficult. Nevertheless, the most common ultrasound finding associated with RPT is an echogenic mass[8,34,35,57,59-70] **(Figs. 8D to F; 9A to F; 10 and 11; and 12A)**. In contrast, Edwards et al.[15] found in his study an echogenic mass on day 7 in 51% of normal cases, in 21% on day 14 and in 6% on day 21. He questioned ultrasound finding of an echogenic mass in uterine cavity as a sign of RPT. However, the definition of an echogenic mass was not specified and we may hypothesise that other investigators would probably classify many of their "echogenic mass" as "heterogeneous patterns". A heterogeneous pattern is a common and insignificant finding of the involuting uterus[13] **(Figs. 4B, and 5C and D)**. It is located in the cervical area in the early puerperium, in the whole uterine cavity in the middle part of the puerperium and it is not common during late postpartum period.[13] Sokol et al.[16] used the same classification and found "echogenic material" in 40% of women 48 hours after a normal delivery. However, 14 of the 16 cases demonstrated echogenic material in the lower uterine segment while only two had such findings in the fundus. It is unclear if "echogenic material" is the same as an "echogenic mass" or if it might be a mixed echo pattern. If dysfunctional postpartum bleeding persists for a long time, RPT is highly suspected. Hertzberg et al.[34] described so-called "Stippled pattern" of scattered hyperechogenic foci that later on became increasingly generalized echogenic, reflected secondary regressive changes in RPT **(Fig. 11A)**.

Two studies[63,64] compared the diagnostic accuracy of clinical assessment with transabdominal US in the management of SPH and concluded that both methods were of limited value. In contrast, recently published studies that assessed diagnostic accuracy of combined

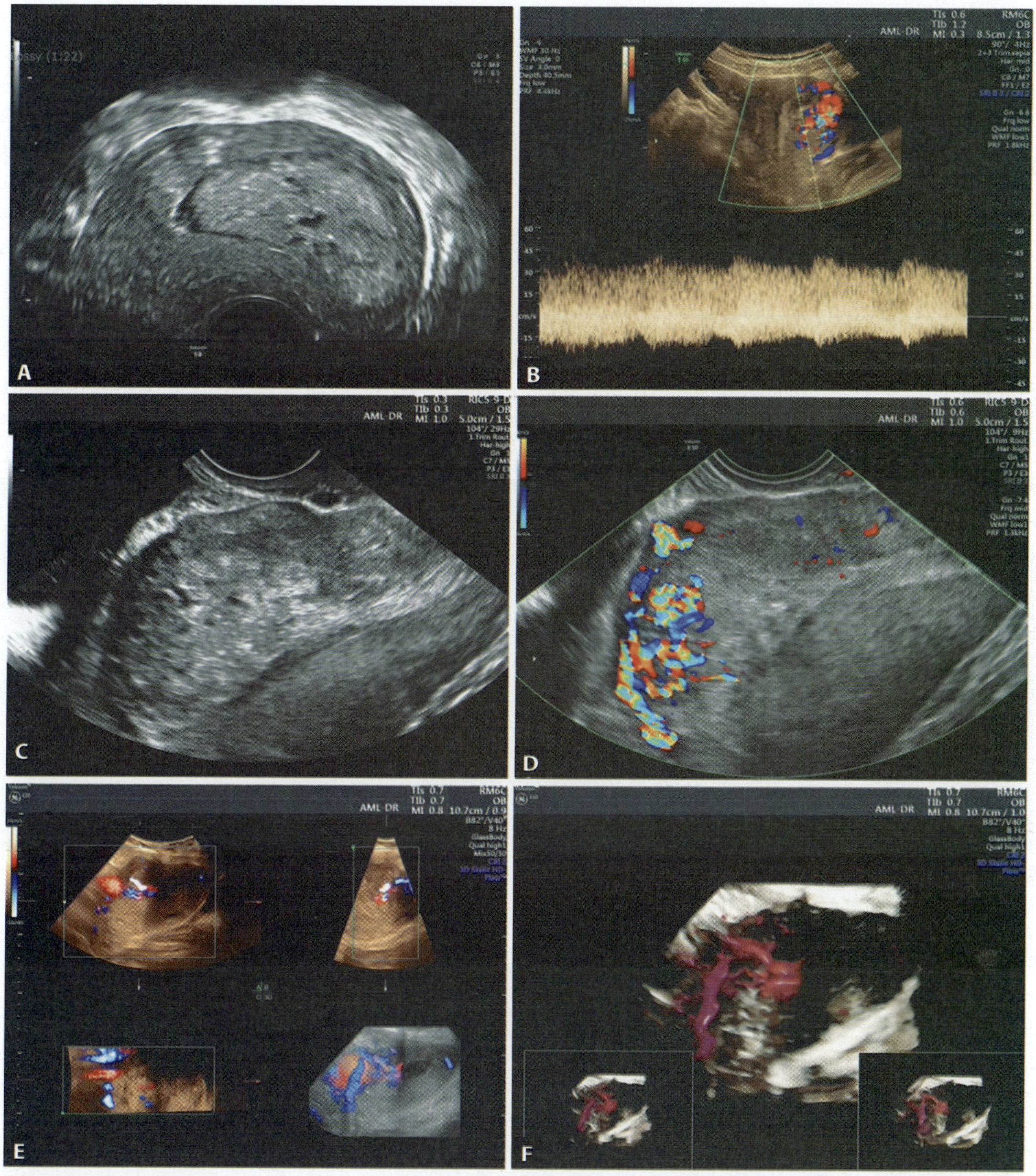

Figs. 9A to F: Puerperal abnormalities revealed by ultrasound: (A) Retained placental tissue 5 weeks postpartum; (B) Blood flow in relation to retained placental tissue 2 weeks postpartum; (C) A huge retained placental tissue 2 weeks after preterm delivery in pregnancy week 22; (D) The same image with abundant blood flow in the top of the uterine myometrium; (E) 3D glass body modality shows a retained placental tissue one week postpartum; (F) The same retained placental tissue visualised in 3D HD live modality.

clinical and sonographic protocol, concluded that the combined approach was accurate and highly sensitive tool for the diagnosis of retained placental tissue.[68-71]

There are many reasons for discrepancies in the published reports. Factors that might explain the low sensitivity and high false-positive rate include a vague definition of the US diagnosis of RPT,[60-64] retrospective study design[34,62,66,67] and mixed study populations including women with bleeding after an abortion and women with postpartum hemorrhage.[8,62,66-68] Three studies often cited in the published literature evaluated asymptomatic women.[57,60] The accuracy of postpartum US for detection of RPT was calculated either from a small proportion of women who underwent curettage, assuming that women who had an uneventful puerperal course after conservative treatments had no RPT,[34,62-64] or from histological findings

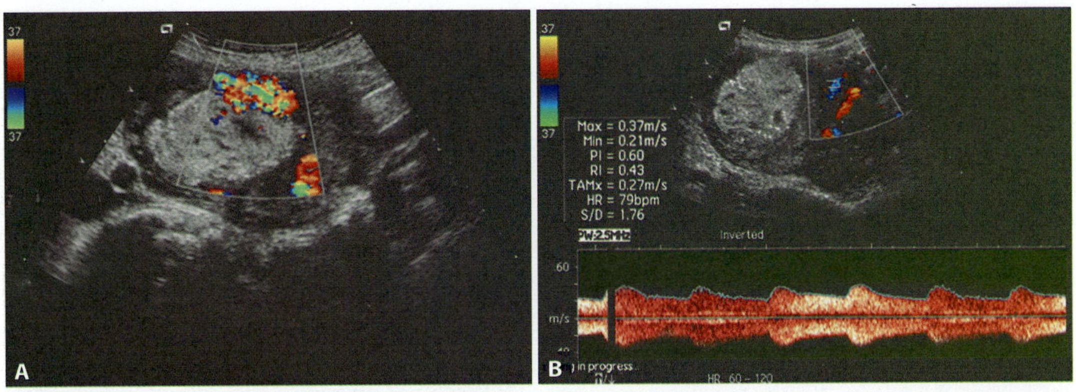

Figs. 10A and B: Puerperal abnormalities revealed by ultrasound. (A) Transabdominal transverse scan, 9 days postpartum, shows retained placental tissue seen as an echogenic mass; (B) A low resistance blood flow is seen on one side of the echogenic mass.

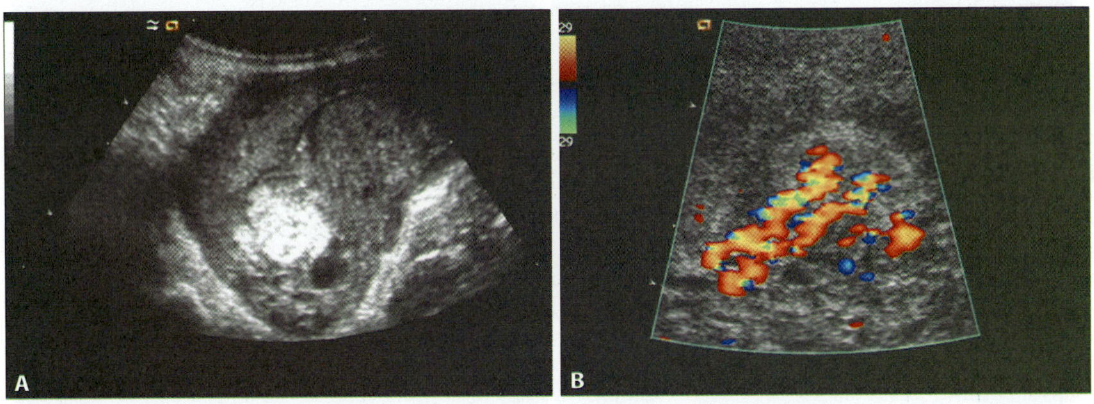

Figs. 11A and B: (A) Transvaginal longitudinal scan shows retained placental tissue 6 weeks postpartum; (B) By color Doppler, feeding vessels are seen inside the echogenic mass.

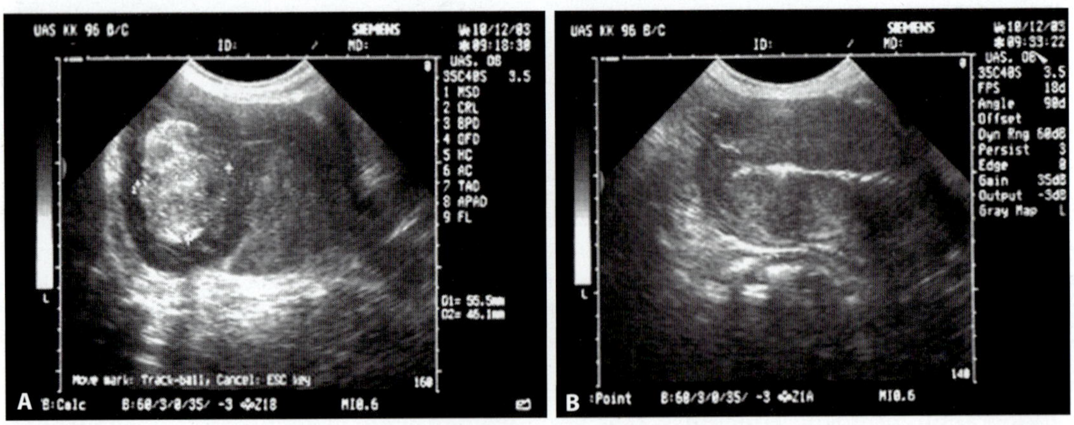

Figs. 12A and B: (A) Transabdominal scan, 11 days postpartum, shows retained placental tissue seen as an echogenic mass; (B) A thin echogenic endometrium is visible soon after curettage.

among asymptomatic women.[57,60] Finally, the patients and clinicians have not been blinded to the sonographic results in any of the published studies. If ultrasound finding shows an empty cavity with thin white decidua/endometrium during early **(Figs. 2A and 4A)** or late puerperium **(Figs. 4C, 5D and 6A)**, pure fluid/heterogeneous content in the cavity during the middle part of the puerperium **(Figs. 4B and 5B and C)**, or only small echolucent or hyperechogenic dots throughout whole postpartum period, a clinically significant amount of retained placental tissue is unlikely.[13,34] Transvaginal ultrasound with high frequency probe as well as transvaginal sonohysterography may better differentiate intrauterine puerperal pathology.[80-83] If in doubt we recommend to use medical treatment initially, as a first-line treatment, reserving surgical management for patients when the first treatment fails.

Doppler Ultrasound during Pathological Puerperium

A few studies investigated pulsed and color Doppler during puerperium in order to improve diagnostic accuracy of ultrasound regarding RPT.[62,80,81,89] Some investigators observed low resistance blood flow around intracavitary contents[81-86] **(Figs 9B and 9D to F)**. Ashiron et al.[74] measured resistance index (RI) in relation to RPT and found that diagnosis is highly suspected if RI is below 0.35 **(Fig. 9B)**. These patients are suitable for invasive treatment. RI above 0.45 should exclude diagnosis. Values between 0.35 and 0.45 form a "gray zone" Conservative treatment and repeated ultrasound examinations should be performed.

Power Doppler seems to be a new unexplored modality that could improve our abilities to diagnose clinically significant RPT. Retained placental tissue in the uterine cavity might cause a delay in the normal involution of uterine vessels.[40,41] By colour Doppler ultrasound, a localized area of increased vascularity within the myometrium may be detected.[47,84-88] The presence of a hypervascular area in the myometrium, within or close to the echogenic mass, has previously been interpreted alternatively as a common physiological finding,[47] as a finding associated with the presence of RPT[60,80,81,89,90] or with arteriovenous (AV) malformations.[25,84,85] Pulsed Doppler usually demonstrates a low resistance turbulent flow with high systolic velocity, resembling AV malformations. It has recently been suggested that curettage should not be performed on patients who present with SPH and a color Doppler image of a hypervascular area within the myometrium.[84,85] Van den Bosch[86] examined 385 consecutive postpartum women and reported that a hypervascular area in the uterus was relatively common (8.3%) and disappeared either spontaneously or after removal of placental remnants. Mungen[87] has drawn attention to a tendency to overdiagnose true AV malformations. He pointed out that a majority of hypervascular areas in the myometrium probably represented normal "perivillous flow" in the spiral arteries. The regression period may be prolonged in the presence of RPT. Only in very rare instances do they represent true arteriovenous malformations. In our recent work on angiographic embolization for treatment of major postpartum hemorrhage, no true AV malformation was diagnosed among 20 patients but 4 cases had pseudoaneurysm **(Figs. 13A and B)**.[90]

Summary of recommendations
(Adapted from danish guideline on retained placental tissue dsog 2014[72]).

Statements	*Evidence level*
Combination of clinical and ultrasound suspicion of retained placental tissue in cases of secondary postpartum hemorrhage (SPH), gives the highest rate of histologic confirmation of placental tissue	IIB
Ultrasound examination of the uterus in cases of postpartum bleeding is an effective diagnostic method with high sensitivity (88.8%–99.9%)	IIB
Specificity of ultrasound diagnosis increases with using of Colour Doppler technology (52.2%–82.4%)	IIB
Hydrosonography increases sensitivity and specificity to 100% but it implies a high risk for complications (fever and infection)	IIB
In cases of Ultrasound image of an intrauterine focal echogenic mass the probability of retained placental tissue is high	IIB
A temporarily found ultrasound image of thickened uterine cavity, or mixed echo pattern, without a focal intrauterine mass and without significant clinical symptoms, is not an indication for surgical treatment as these findings are associated with ultrasound image of normal uterus within the first three weeks postpartum	IIB

Clinical recommendations	***Grades of recommendations A-D***
In cases of secondary postpartum hemorrhage should Ultrasound examination always be a part of patient's examination	B
Color Doppler examination should be used as a complement to 2D imaging	B
Ultrasound image of an intrauterine focal echogenic mass and clinical symptoms of SPH are associated with retained placental tissue	B

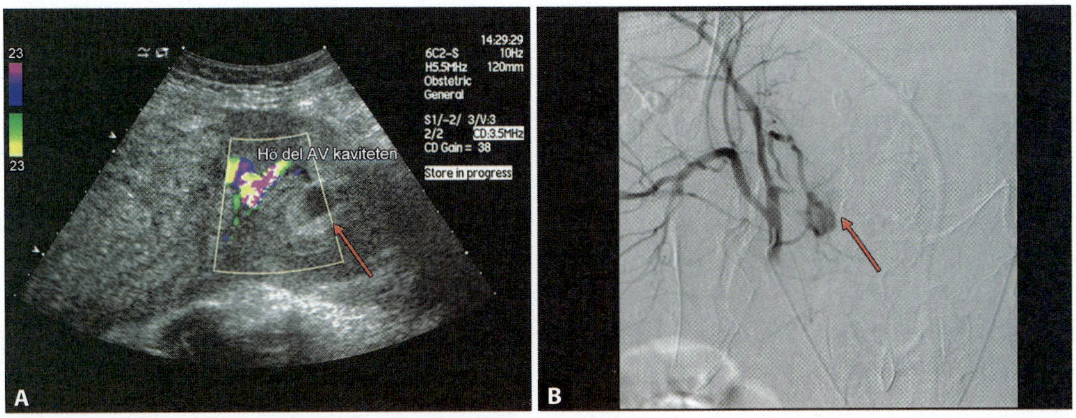

Figs. 13A and B: (A) Transabdominal scan of the uterus on day 8 postpartum shows a huge defect in the uterus forming a pseudoaneurysm (arrow). Color Doppler reveals a feeding damaged uterine artery; (B) Angiography confirmed the ultrasound finding.

Our knowledge on uterine artery flow in women with RPT is sparse. It could be that RPT prevents the physiological changes in uterine blood flow during the puerperium. The results of our small study8 showed the resistance flow indices in uterine artery below the 10th percentile for 8 of 20 (40.0%) women of which 7 had histological confirmation of RPT and 1 did not. There was, however, considerable overlap. No patient had resistance indices above the 90th percentile. In 12 of 20 (60.0%) patients an early diastolic notch was absent. Early diastolic notches appeared relatively late compared to the findings in normal population. Only one woman had a notch before postpartum day 28. Colour Doppler showed a hypervascular area close to the echogenic mass in 12 of 20 (60%) patients, all with histologically confirmed RPT. This figure is slightly higher than that reported by Durfee et al.[62] (55%) and by Zalel et al. (46%).[83] A hypervascular area was absent in 8 patients (40%) of which six had an echogenic mass that was histologically confirmed RPT. Our findings that the absence of blood flow does not exclude RPT are in concordance with previously reported results.[62,83] Kamaya et al.[67] *tried to classify color Doppler (CD) mapping in an assumed retained placental tissue:*

0: No CD signal in the RPT
1: CD signal in the RPT is lower than in the adjacent myometrium.
2: CD signal in the RPT has the same level as the adjacent myometrial vessels.
3: CD signal in the RPT is stronger than in the adjacent myometrium.

POSTPARTUM ENDOMETRITIS

Postpartum endometritis is a fairly common clinical condition, affecting 2–5% women following delivery.[92,93] Caesarean section (CS) is the leading predisposing factor.[94] It has been considered that the typical ultrasound finding in cases of endometritis is the presence of gas in the uterine cavity.[10] Madrazo found gas in uterine cavity in 15% of patients with puerperal endometritis.[10] Nowadays infections caused by gas-forming organisms *C. perfringens* are very rare and large gas-bubbles are almost never seen. Moreover, Wachsberg and Kurtz[36] detected gas in about 19% of normal cases, which is in accordance with results of a computed tomographic study performed within 24 hours of uncomplicated vaginal delivery (21%). Ultrasound appearance of gas is seen as an intensively hyperechogenic focus equivalent on echogenicity to bowel gas with clean and dirty shadowing or a reverberation artifact.[95] According to our experience gas is mostly observed following intrauterine manipulations[96] **(Fig. 12B)** although it is occasionally observed after normal vaginal delivery.[13] The detection of gas within the uterine cavity may be a normal finding during the puerperium and does not necessarily indicate the presence of endometritis or RPT.[13,36] After CS or intrauterine manipulations highly echogenic foci can obscure an existing mass in the uterine cavity or be mistaken for retained placental tissue.[34,96] Thus whenever highly echogenic foci are present in the uterine cavity the physician who interprets ultrasound finding must be aware of recent uterine manipulations. Gas usually disappears within 1–2 weeks after instrumentation **(Figs. 14A and B)**.[96] Furthermore, it has been claimed that ultrasound image of RPT and endometritis overlap.[8,54] Results from published

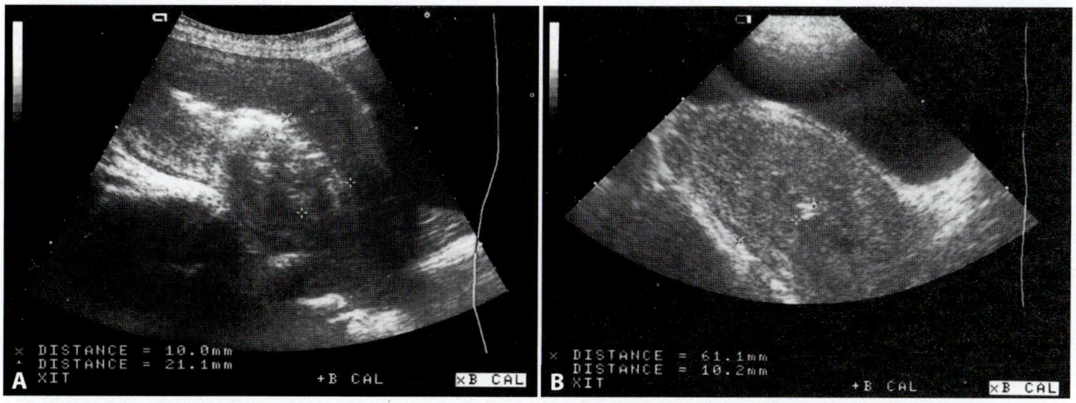

Figs. 14A and B: (A) Gas in uterine cavity one-day post-curettage; (B) Six days post curettage.

studies on this issue are inconsistent.[8,41, 54,55,64,76,96] Pelage et al.[97] described 14 cases with uncontrollable SPH undergoing selective angiographic embolization. Six of 14 patients had clinical and ultrasound signs of endometritis with RPT. In 4 cases histological confirmation was obtained. Two patients had pure endometritis. Conversely, Kong et al.[41] pointed out that endometritis appeared to be an overstated cause of SPH. He found that less than 5% of cases could be ascribed to endometritis. Ben-Ami et al.[64] found that a majority of the patients presenting with fever ≥38°C postpartum were falsely diagnosed by ultrasound as having suspected RPT.

The presence of RPT may result in intrauterine infection and in these cases, ultrasound examination can help us to select patients suitable for invasive treatment. In the vast majority of cases of isolated endometritis, ultrasound findings are normal and have no pathognomonic ultrasound image.[35,96] Kirkinen et al.[45] found that blood flow to the infected uterus could be different from normal. Deutchman and Hartman described postpartum pyometra as a lucent area within the uterus.[98] They also advocated the usage of Ultrasound to assist in guiding a drainage procedure. Septic pelvic thrombophlebitis, well known as an "enigmatic puerperal fever" is another uncommon complication of the puerperium. It most commonly presents in early postpartum period and antibiotic treatment is usually unsuccessful. Rudoff et al.[99] suggests ultrasound examination in case of clinical suspicion of pelvic thrombophlebitis. Although ultrasound diagnosis of ovarian vein thrombophlebitis is well described,[100-102] the diagnosis is still difficult and an ultrasound expertise is needed. Asymmetric dilatation of the ovarian or other pelvic vein may sometimes be observed.[101] Furthermore,

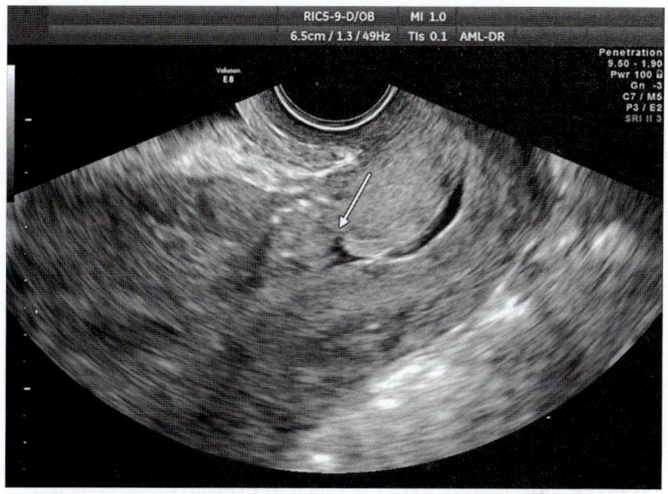

Fig. 15: Transvaginal, longitudinal view of the lower uterine segment 8 weeks postpartum shows an irregular utero-bladder junction with the defect in the myometrium in the cesarean scar area (arrow).

a complex or hypoechoic mass near the lower pole of the kidney particularly in clinical setting of an "enigmatic puerperal fever" should suggest thrombophlebitis. An echogenic intracaval mass is considered diagnostic and anticoagulation treatment should be added.[102]

CESAREAN SECTION

Nowadays when CS rates are continuously rising, higher incidence of all puerperal complications can be expected.[94] The ultrasound image of the uterus following CS usually shows three distinctive patterns: (i) gas in the cavity, (ii) a small rounded area at the incision site that reflects tissue reaction due to localized edema, and (iii) several echogenic dots at the incision site, which is related to the type of closure and the suture material used **(Fig. 15)**.[88,96,103]

All these characteristics are normal findings and no correlation with pathological conditions is found. The involution rate of the uterus following CS is not markedly different from the involution rate after vaginal delivery.[96,104-106] We observed a few morphological differences between the women delivered by CS and the women who had a vaginal delivery, such as the less common anteverted position of the uterus and the less common the empty uterine cavity in early puerperium, which might reflect slightly delayed uterine involution process.[96] The significant infectious morbidity is associated with CS.[94] Ultrasound may be useful in postpartum women with clinical suspicion of a postoperative complication like phlegmona,[107] abscess, pyometra, hematometra, wound infection, subfascial hematoma or intra-abdominal postoperative hemorrhage. Baker et al. described bladder flap hematoma after a low uterine transverse CS.[108] A solid or complex mass between the posterior bladder wall and the anterior uterine wall may be observed by ultrasound. An abscess appears as a cystic structure with internal debris surrounded by thicker irregular walls. An infected hematoma initially has similar ultrasound appearance. During the resolution process, it may change and appears more solid. However, the physician must be aware that ultrasound diagnosis is just a complement and clinical condition of the patient should guide the therapeutic approach.

UNCOMMON BUT POTENTIALLY LIFE-THREATENING CAUSES OF POSTPARTUM BLEEDING

There are a few uncommon but potentially life-threatening causes of postpartum bleeding which contribute significantly to maternal mortality and morbidity. These are placenta accreta/increta/percreta,[17-23] vessel's lesions (true AV malformations,[25] pseudoaneurysm[26-31]), placental site tumor[32] and choriocarcinoma.

PLACENTA ACCRETA/INCRETA/PERCRETA

The incidence of abnormal placentation, placenta accreta/increta/percreta, has increased in recent years, particularly due to the increasing rates of cesarean section. It is the most common factor for uncontrolled postpartum hemorrhage leading to emergency postpartum hysterectomy, which is associated with significant maternal morbidity and mortality.[17] Antenatal diagnosis of severe invasive placentation is feasible with ultrasound. Both, conventional 2D and 3D ultrasound have been used and several reports have been recently published.[18-24]

Diagnostic criterion by 2D ultrasound:

1. Retroplacental sonolucent zone: irregular/absent **(Fig. 16B)**.
2. Hyperechoic bladder mucosa: thinning/interruption **(Fig. 16B)**.
3. Hypervascularity of uterine serosa-bladder wall interface **(Fig. 16B)**.
4. Placental lacunae: appearance "moth-eaten" lacunae with/without high-peak systolic velocity (PSV) and low resistance turbulent flow by color Doppler mapping.

Diagnostic criterion by 3D ultrasound:

1. Irregular intraplacental vascularization with tortuous confluent vessels crossing placental width and with chaotic branching **(Fig. 16A)**.
2. Hypervascularity of uterine serosa-bladder wall interface **(Fig. 16A)**.

Optimal management strategies for placenta accreta is highly dependent on accurate antenatal diagnosis and it is also associated with decreased maternal morbidity.[109,110]

According to our experience a high corporal incision and placenta left in situ, followed by hysterectomy, is the most beneficial treatment option with the lowest complication rate, for both the mother and her child **(Figs. 16E and F)**.

Placenta accreta may be left in situ, as the whole or just partly[109] and ultrasound may be of help monitor spontaneous resorption of the retained tissue. However, the reports about ultrasound findings in these cases are sparse[24] **(Figs. 16A to D)**.

Uterine Arteriovenous Lesions (True Av Malformations, Acquired Av Malformations/Pseudoaneurysm)

True arteriovenous malformations (AV) are a rare errors of morphogenesis, which do not regress spontaneously and they are extremely rare causes of SPH.[25,87] In contrast, acquired AV abnormalities of the uterus are associated with trauma after previous intrauterine procedures, RPT, infection or malignancy and are more common.[26-31] The difference between normal peri-villous blood flow increased myometrial flow related to RPT and AV malformations seems to be difficult.[25,47,87] Three typical ultrasound signs of pseudoaneurysm include: a pulsating hypoechoic area connected to feeding artery by a narrow neck on gray-scale ultrasound, a turbulent flow inside the

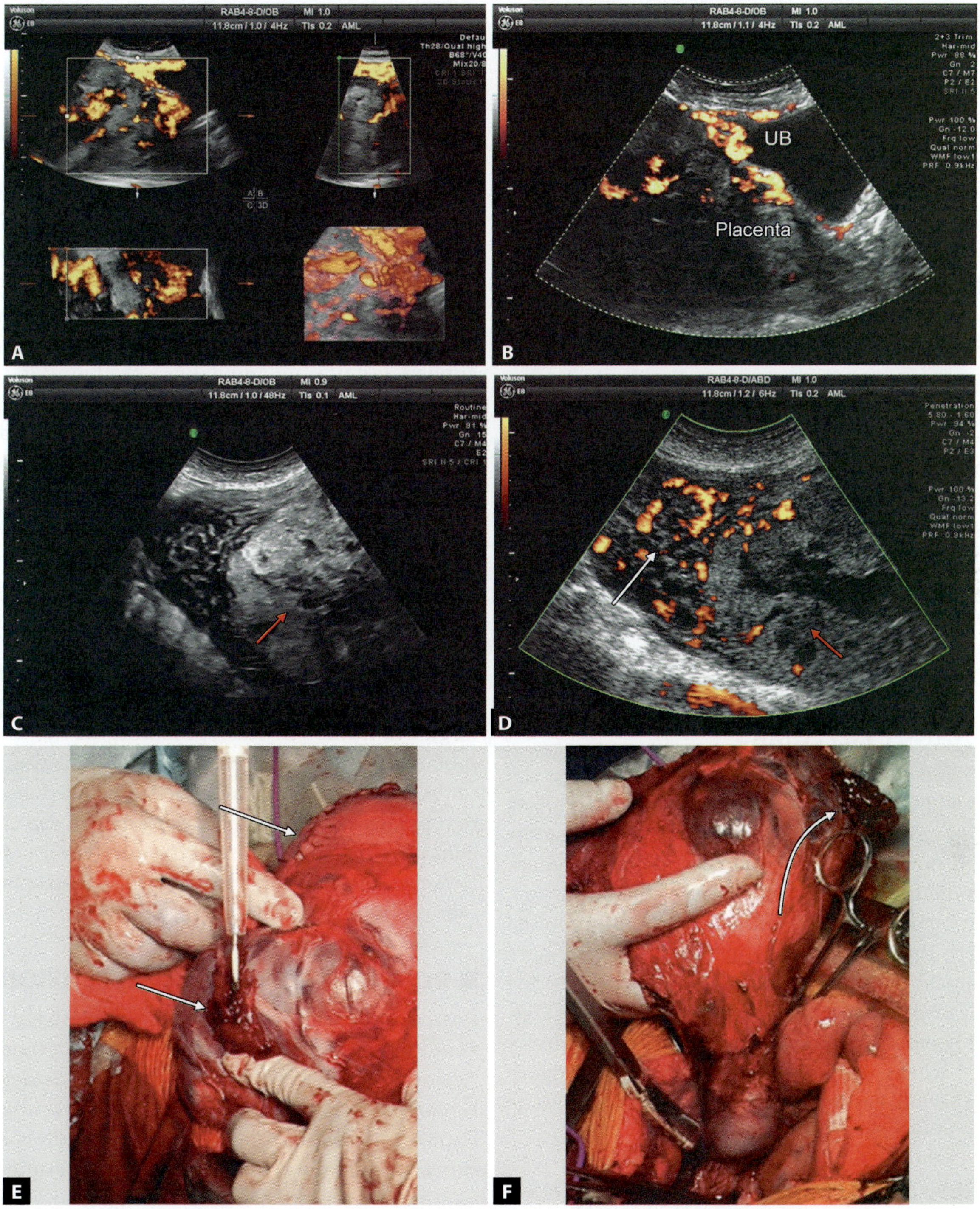

Figs. 16A to F: (A to D) Ultrasound image of placenta praevia perccreta left in situ. (A) Color Doppler and; (B) Power Doppler show the interface between the uterus and urinary bladder 7 days after cesarean section; (C) Retained placenta occupies the most part of the uterine cavity (arrow); (D) Power Doppler shows increased myometrial vascularity behind the retained placenta (arrow); (E and F) The uterus together with placenta percreta extirpated by total hysterectomy: (E) A high corporal section is seen (upper white arrow); (F) Lower uterine segment with placental tissue growing throughout the whole myometrium is seen (lower white arrow).

pseudoaneurysm on color Doppler and a reversed flow on the neck of the pseudoaneurysm on Pulse Doppler. During systole blood enters the pseudoaneurysm and during diastole it reverses into the uterine artery because of the pressure gradient between the pseudoaneurysm and the feeding artery **(Figs. 13A and B)**. Curettage should not be performed on patients who present with severe postpartum bleeding and a pseudoaneurysm is suspected on colour Doppler scan. Further investigation with pelvic angiography or MRI should be performed.

Placental Site Tumor and Choriocarcinoma

These are rare forms of gestational trophoblastic disease and ultrasound image is difficult to distinguish them from each other as well as from retained placenta accreta and from acquired arteriovenous lesions. MRI findings are more sensitive but not specific. Thus the appropriate diagnosis may be delayed.

Placental site tumor[32] and choriocarcinoma may appear as an irregular mass with both cystic and hyperechoic components in the cavity often involving myometrium **(Fig. 17A)**. With colour Doppler low-resistance flow may be seen **(Fig. 17B)**.

PREGNANCY LUTEOMAS

Pregnancy luteomas are bilateral benign neoplasms of the ovary caused by the hormonal effects of pregnancy. They are most commonly asymptomatic, but they often grow throughout pregnancy and they may mimic malignant tumors. Sometimes luteomas may cause ovarian torsion, which can lead to rupture and severe intra-abdominal bleeding.[116] However, most pregnancy luteomas are incidentally detected on ultrasound examination during pregnancy or postpartum or at caesarean section **(Figs. 17A to F)**. Luteomas usualy decrease in size after delivery within 2–3 weeks. Differential diagnosis is androgen-producing Sertoli–Leydig cell tumors, which in contrast do not regress in size after delivery.

CONGENITAL UTERINE MALFORMATIONS

The prevalence of the congenital uterine malformations in general population is largely unknown. Failed fusion of the two Mullerian ducts to form the genital organs may cause reproductive, fetal and maternal hazards (infertility, premature labor, abnormal fetal presentations, retained placental tissue and postpartum hemorrhage). It is well known that uterine anomalies may remain undiscovered except when they are associated with reproductive or obstetric problems. Already in 1976 Bennett suggested puerperal ultrasonic hysterography as a screening procedure prior to radiological examination in women whose reproductive performance suggests a diagnosis of congenital malformation of the uterus.[111] Since that a few studies concerning the issue were published. Szoke and Kiss[112] examined in 1977 patients where manual examination revealed a uterus differing in shape from normal, the patient had a breech presentation in her previous or present pregnancy and the involution of the uterus was slow. The ultrasound echo technique was applied and uterine anomalies were found in five cases postpartum.[112] In 1984 Land et al. performed ultrasonic hysterography in 104 patients between the 2nd and 5th postpartum day. An unexpectedly high number of women (16%) showed an abnormal uterine configuration.[113]

The coronal section seems to be the most appropriate section in order to reveal uterine cavity anatomy **(Figs. 18A to C)**.[13,82] It is difficult to obtain the coronal section by abdominal examination in nonpregnant patients. However, the puerperium when the uterus is extremely large makes an exception. The ultrasound examination should perform in the early puerperium because a large uterus lies in near proximity to the ultrasound probe and highly echogenic decidua outlines well the shape of the cavity Puerperal ultrasound might detect uterine developmental abnormality, providing an explanation for complications in labour and the puerperium **(Fig. 18C)**. However, the best way to assess the coronal plane of the uterus is by 3D VCI-C rendering **(Fig. 8B)**.

POSTPARTUM URINARY RETENTION

Postpartum urinary retention is a relatively common condition and incidence ranges between 1% and 18%.[114] According to the International Continence Society, 100 mL is considered as the upper limit of residual urine. Ultrasound is the method of choice when assessing urinary bladder and residual urine postpartum. Invasive catheterization with the discomfort and the risk of infection can be avoided. Conventional bladder scanner is not to be recommended during the puerperium. Large uterus may content fluid and thus, a misinterpretation may be done. Many different techniques for bladder volume measurement are used and the accuracy of the method varies widely. We prefer a method where the longest distance of the maternal bladder (d1) is measured

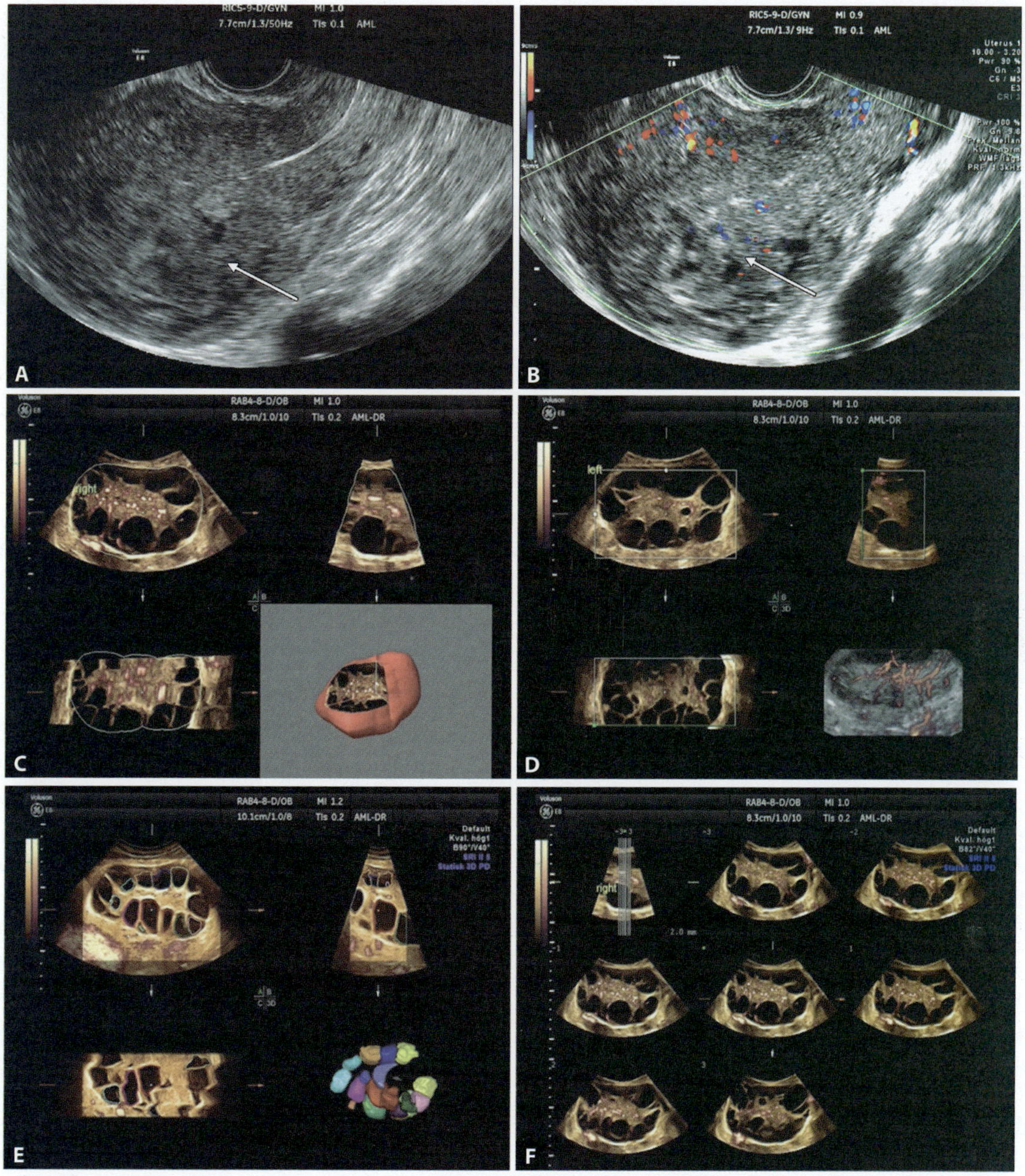

Figs. 17A to F: (A and B) Pregnancy luteomas: 2D view of the bilateral huge ovaries detected incidentally postpartum. (A) Color Doppler in the periphery of the right ovary; (B) Power Doppler in the periphery of the left ovary; (C to F) Pregnancy luteomas: Various 3D modalities used to assess ovarian luteomas. (C) 3D volumetry, (D) 3D power Doppler angiography glassbody, (E) 3D niche volumetry; (F) Tomographic ultrasound imaging.

in a longitudinal section, and then two perpendicular diameters (d2 and d3) are measured in the transverse section **(Fig. 19)**. The estimated amount of residual urine can be calculated using the formula for approximation of the ellipsoid:

Volume (mL) = (d1 × d2 × d3)/2 **(Fig. 20A to D)**.

PUERPERAL MASTITIS AND BREAST ABSCESS

Puerperal mastitis is a common complication in lactating women, particularly in primiparous women. Reported incidence varies from 1% to 24%.[115] If treatment with antibiotics is delayed or inadequate it can progress to more

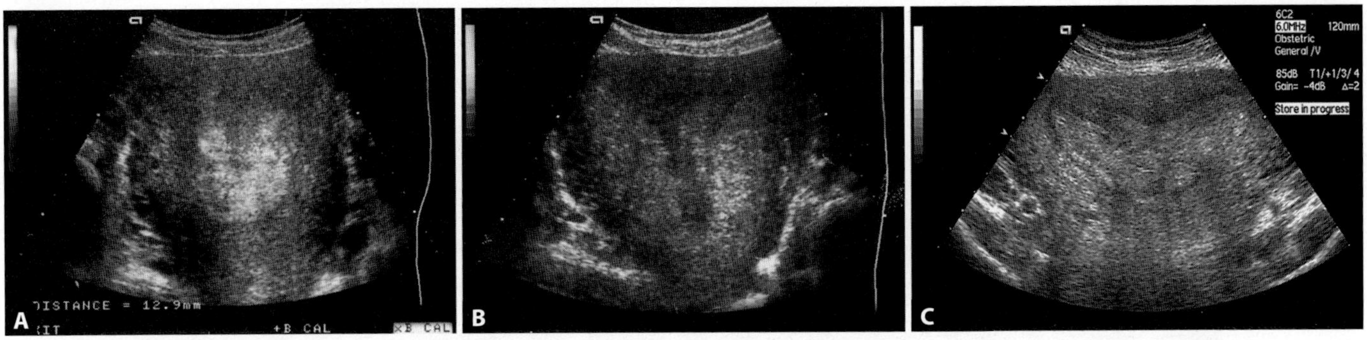

Figs. 18A to C: (A) A coronal section shows a subseptate uterus one day after manual evacuation of the placenta; (B) The uterus of the same patient 8 days later; (C) A coronal section on day three postpartum shows uterus arcuatus in a woman who had twice breach position and preterm delivery.

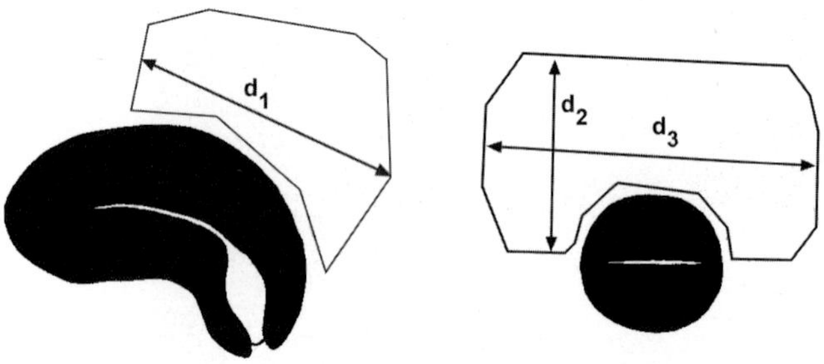

Fig. 19: Residual urine volume measurement

serious complication, breast abscess. Breast tenderness limits clinical assessment and clinical diagnosis may be difficult, particularly if the abscess lies deeply in the breast or if it is too small. Ultrasound with a 7.5–12 MHz probes is being used to differentiate abscess from puerperal mastitis.[115] Ultrasound findings of mastitis are increased parenchyma/fat echogenicity, skin thickening and increased vascularity by colour Doppler. Ultrasound diagnosis of breast abscess, in contrast, is made when a round/oval or irregular hypoechogenic lesion is detected **(Fig. 21A)**. Color Doppler detects any vessels. The traditional treatment of breast abscess by surgical incision and drainage requires general anesthesia, major duct may be damaged and it usually makes a poor cosmetic result due to scar formation. More recently US-guided needle aspiration of breast abscess or catheter placement was used instead of surgical treatment. Ulitzsch et al.[115] reported ultrasound treatment of 56 breast abscesses among 43 breastfeeding women and the treatment was successful in all but one woman. In 52% of cases repeat needle aspirations were required. The authors recommended a 21-gauge needle aspiration alone if the abscess diameter <3 cm. In contrast an abscess ≥3 cm should treat with placement of pigtail catheter **(Fig. 21B)** which should be removed when ultrasound shows no residual fluid and when only minimal saline can be irrigated into the residual cavity. Breastfeeding is not contraindicated. However, in cases of recurrence, lactation stop with dopamine agonist is to be required.

CONCLUSION

Present ultrasound technology with high image resolution has made ultrasound a valuable diagnostic tool for assessing numerous postpartum clinical conditions. Suspicion of retained placental tissue, unknown cause of the puerperal sepsis, surgical complications or acute abdominal pain is some of the possible reasons to switch on ultrasound machine. Not only the involution changes of the uterus or pathological changes in uterine cavity but also the other organs like kidneys, urinary bladder, gallbladder, ovaries and abdominal cavity can be easily examined by ultrasound during postpartum period.

Sonohysterography may better differentiate intrauterine pathology by injecting saline under sonographic control and so, improve the accuracy of the diagnosis of puerperal pathology.

Color, pulsed and power Doppler have improved our ability to study for the first time the vascular changes of the uterine involution noninvasively. With 3D ultrasound the possibility to measure volumes of the uterus and the cavity postpartum has been introduced. Uterine vascular network can also be investigated by 3D PD angiography more extensively.

More studies are required in this important area and all these new modalities need further evaluation. Moreover, the knowledge obtained through ultrasound examinations can help us to better understand both the physiology

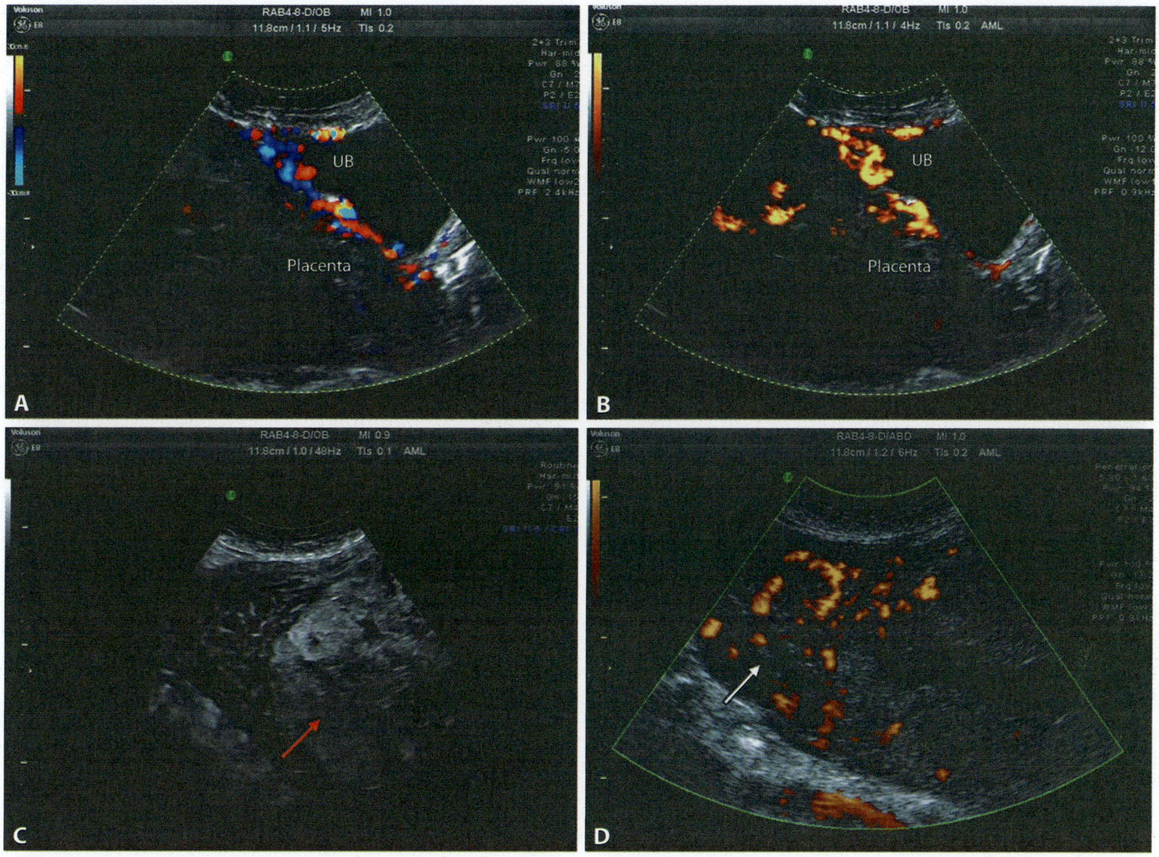

Figs. 20A to D: (A) 3D Power Doppler image of placenta praevia percreta just before surgery; (B) Power Doppler of placenta praevia percreta left in situ shows the interface between the uterus and urinary bladder 7 days after cesarean section. (C) Retained placenta occupies the most part of the uterine cavity (red arrow), (D) Power Doppler shows increased myometrial vascularity behind the retained placenta (white arrow).

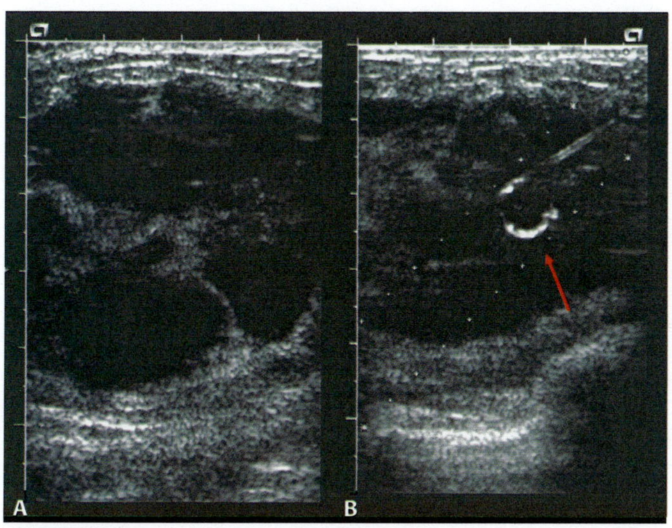

Figs. 21A and B: (A) Ultrasound image of breast abscess before drainage with pigtail catheter; (B) After drainage with pigtail catheter (arrow) .

and pathophysiology of the puerperium. The usefulness of ultrasound examinations during puerperium is not questioned any more, but ultrasound has become the first imaging modality used whenever puerperal complications are suspected.

Summary of recommendations (adapted from guideline on retained placental tissue DSOG 2014).[72]

REFERENCES

1. Hytten F. The Clinical Physiology of the Puerperium. London, UK: Farrand Press; 1996.
2. Donald I, MacVicar J, Brown TC. Investigation of abdominal masses by pulsed ultrasound. Lancet. 1958;1:1188.
3. Robinson HP. Sonar in the puerperium. Scott Med J. 1972; 17:364.
4. Szoke B, Kiss D. The use of the ultrasonic echo technique in examining the normal and pathological involution in the puerperium. Int J Gynaecol Obstet. 1976;14:513-6.

5. Malvern J, Campbell S. Ultrasonic scanning of the puerperal uterus following postpartum haemorrhage. J Obstet Gynaecol Br Commonw. 1973;80:320-4.
6. Rodeck CH, Newton JR. Study of the uterine cavity by ultrasound in the early puerperium. Br J Obstet Gynaecol 1976;83:795-801.
7. Defoort P, Benijts G, Thiery M, et al. Ultrasound assessment of puerperal uterine involution. Eur J Obstet Gynaecol. 1978;8:95-7.
8. Lee CY, Madrazo B, Drukker BH. Ultrasonic evaluation of the postpartum uterus in the management of postpartum bleeding. Obstet Gynaecol. 1981;58:227-32.
9. VanRees D, Bernstine RL, Crawford W. Involution of the postpartum uterus. An ultrasonic study. J Clin Ultrasound 1981;9:55.
10. Madrazo BL. Postpartum Sonography. The principle and Practice of Ultrasonography in Obstetrics and Gynecology, 3rd edn. East Norwalk: Appleton-Century-Crofts; 1985. pp. 449-56.
11. Lavery JP, Shaw LA. Sonography of the postpartum uterus. J Ultrasound Med. 1989;8:481-6.
12. Wachsberg RH, Kurtz AB, Levine CD, et al. Real-time ultrasonographic analysis of the normal postpartum uterus: technique, variability and measurements. J Ultrasound Med. 1994;13:215-21.
13. Mulic-Lutvica A, Bekuretzion M, Axelsson O, et al. Ultrasonic evaluation of the uterus and uterine cavity after normal, vaginal delivery. Ultrasound Obstet Gynecol. 2001;18:491-8.
14. Tekay A, Jouppila P. A longitudinal Doppler ultrasonographic assessment of the alterations in peripheral vascular resistance of uterine arteries and ultrasonographic findings of the involuting uterus during the puerperium. Am J Obstet Gynecol. 1993;168:190-7.
15. Edwards A, Ellwood DA. Ultrasonographic evaluation of the postpartum uterus. Ultrasound Obstet Gynecol. 2000;16:640-3.
16. Sokol ER, Casele H, Haney EI. Ultrasound examination of the postpartum uterus what is normal? J Maternal Fetal Neonat Med. 2004;15:95-9.
17. Rossi AC, Lee RH, Chmait RH. Emergency Postpartum Hysterectomy for Uncontrolled Postpartum Bleeding A systematic Review, Obstetrics 6 Gynecology 2010;115(3): 637-44.
18. Chou MM, Ho ESC, Lee YH. Prenatal diagnosis of placenta previa accreta by transabdominal color Doppler ultrasound. Ultrasound Obstet Gynecol. 2000;15:28-35.
19. Yang JI, Lim YK, Kim HS, Chang KH, Lee JP, Ryu HS. Sonographic findings of placental lacunae and the prediction of adhaerent placenta in women with placenta previa totalis and prior Cesarean section. Ultrasound Obstet Gynecol. 2006;28:178-82.
20. Japaraj RP, Mimin TS, Mukudan K. Antenatal diagnosis of placenta previa ccreta in patients with previous cesarean scar. J Obstet Gynaecol Ress. 2007;33(4):431-7.
21. Bauer ST, Bonanno C. Abnormal placentation. Semin Perinatol. 2009;33:88-96.
22. Shin JC, Jaraquemada JMP, Su YN, SHYU MK, Lin CH, Lin SY, et al. Role of three-dimensional power Doppler in the antenatal diagnosis of placenta accreta: comparison with gray-scale and color Doppler technique. Ultrasound Obstet Gynecol. 2009;33:193-203.
23. Chou MM, Chen WC, Tseng JJ, Chen Ya-F, Yeh TT, Ho E.S-C Prenatal detection of bladder wall involvement in invasive placentation with sequential two-dimensional and adjunctive three-dimensional ultrasonography. Taiwan J Obstet Gynecol. 2009;48(1):38-45.
24. Shapiro JL, Sherer DM, Hurley JT, et al. Postpartum ultrasonographic findings associated with placenta accreta. Am J Obstet Gynecol. 1992;167:601-2.
25. Kelly SM, Belli AM, Campbell S. Arteriovenous malformation of the uterus associated with secondary postpartum hemorrhage. Ultrasound Obstet Gynecol. 2003;21:602-5.
26. Henrich W, Fuchs I, Luttkus A, et al. Pseudoaneurysm of the uterine artery after cesarean delivery: sonographic diagnosis and treatment. J Ultrasound Med. 2002;21:1431.
27. Cooper BC, Hocking-Brown M, Sorosky JI, Hansen WF. Pseudoaneurysm of the Uterine Artery Requiring Bilateral Uterine Artery Embolization. J Perinat. 2004;24:560-2.
28. Eason DE, Tank Avoidable Morbidity in a Patient with Pseudoaneurysm of the Uterine Artery after Cesarean Section. J of Clin Ultrasound. 2006;34(8)407-11.
29. Mammen T, Shanthakumari H, Gopi K, Lionel J, Ayyappan AP, Kekre A. Iatrogenic secondary post-partum haemorrhage: Apropos of two uncommon cases. Australian Radiology. 2006;50:392-4.
30. McGonegle SJ, Scott Dziedzic T, Thomas J, Hertzberg BS. Pseudoaneurysm of the Uterine Artery After an Uncomplicated Spontaneous Vaginal Delivery. J Ultrasound Med. 2006;25:1593-7.
31. Marnela K, Saarelainen S, Palomäki O, Kirkinen P. Sonographic diagnosis of postpartum pseudoaneurysms of the uterine artery: a report of 2 cases. J Clin Ultrasound. 2010;38(4):205-8.
32. Vaswani K, Vitellas KM, Bennet WF et al. Sonography case o the day. Am J Roentgenol.2000;175:895-901.
33. Williams JW. Regeneration of the uterine mucosa after delivery with special reference to the placental site. Am J Obstet Gynecol. 1931;22:640-64.
34. Hertzberg BS, Bowie JD. Ultrasound of the postpartum uterus, prediction of retained placental tissue. J Ultrasound Med. 1991;10:451-6.
35. Sakki A, Kirkinen P. Ultrasonography of the uterus at early puerperium. Eur J Ultrasound. 1996;4:99-105.
36. Wachsberg RH, Kurtz AB. Gas within the endometrial cavity at postpartum US. A normal finding after spontaneous vaginal delivery. Radiology. 1992;183:431-3.
37. Sharman A. Reproductive Physiology of the Post-Partum Period. Livingston: Edinburgh E.& S; 1966.

38. Oppenheimer LW, Sherriff EA, Goodman JDS, Shah D, James CE. The duration of lochia. Br J Obstet Gynaecol. 1986;93:754-7.
39. Visness CM, Kennedy KI, Ramos R. The Duration and Character of Postpartum Bleeding Among Breastfeeding Women. Obstet Gynecol. 1997;89:159-63.
40. Andrew AC, Bulmer JN, Wells M, Morrison L, Buckley CH. Subinvolution of the uteroplacental arteries in the human placental bed. Histopathology. 1989;15(4):395-405.
41. Khong TY, Khong TK. Delayed postpartum hemorrhage: a morphologic study of causes and their relation to other pregnancy disorders. Obstet Gynecol. 1993;82(1):17-22.
42. Weydert JA, Benda JA. Subinvolution of the Placental Site as an Anatomic Cause of Postpartum Uterine Bleeding. A Review. Arch Pathol Lab Med. 2006,130;1538-42.
43. Campbell S, Diaz-Recasen J, Griffin D, Cohen-Overbeek TE, et al. New Doppler technique for assessing uteroplacental blood flow. Lancet. 1983;1:675-7.
44. Bernstein IM, Ziegler WF, Leavitt T, Badger GJ. Uterine Artery Hemodynamic Adaptations Through the Menstrual Cycle Into Early Pregnancy. Obstet Gynecol. 2002;99:620-4.
45. Kirkinen P, Dudenhausen J, Baumann H, et al. Postpartum blood flow velocity waveforms of the uterine arteries. J Reprod Med. 1988;33:745-8.
46. Jaffa AJ, Wolman I, Har-Toov J, et al. MR. Changes in uterine artery resistance to blood flow during puerperium–a longitudinal study. J Matern-Fetal Invest 1996;6:27-30.
47. Van Schoubroeck D, Van den Bosch T, Scharpe K, Lu C, Van Huffel S, Timmerman D. Prospective evaluation of blood flow in the myometrium and uterine arteries in the puerperium. Ultrasound Obstet Gynecol. 2004;23:378-81.
48. Mulic-Lutvica A, Eurenius K, Axelsson O. Longitudinal study of Doppler flow resistance indices of uterine artery after normal vaginal delivery. Acta Obstet Gynecol Scand. 2007;86:1207-14.
49. Belachew J, Mulic-Lutvica A, Eurenius K. Three-dimensional ultrasound of the uterus postpartum. Abstract, Presented as an oral poster at 20th World Congress on ultrasound in Obst and Gynecol in Prag 10-14 October. 2010.
50. Belachew J, Axelsson O, Mulic-Lutvica A, Eurenius K. Longitudinal study of the uterine body and cavity with three-dimensional ultrasonography in the puerperium. Acta Obstet Gynecol Scand. 2012;91:1184-90.
51. Belachew J, Axelsson O, Eurenius K, Mulic-Lutvica A. Three-dimensional ultrasound does not improve diagnosis of retained placental tissue compared to two-dimensional ultrasound. Acta Obstet Gynecol Scand. 2015;94:112-6.
52. Alexander J, Thomas P, Sanhghera J. Treatments for secondary postpartum haemorrhage. The Cochrane Library, Issue 4: 2002.
53. Dewhurst C. Secondary postpartum hemorrhage. J Obstet Gynaecol Br Commonwealth. 1966;73:53-8.
54. Rome RM. Secondary postpartum haemorrhage. Br J Obstet Gynaecol. 1975;82(4):289-92.
55. King PA, Duthie SJ, Dong ZG, et al. Secondary postpartum haemorrhage. Aust NZ Obstet Gynaecol 1989;29(4):394-8.
56. Hoveyda F, MacKenzie IZ. Secondary postpartum haemorrhage: incidence, morbidity and current management. Br J Obstet Gynaecol. 2001;108:927-30.
57. Carlan SJ, Scott WT, Pollack R, et al. Appearance of the uterus by ultrasound immediately after placental delivery with pathologic correlation. J Clin Ultrasound. 1997;25(6):301-8.
58. Jones RF, Warren BL, Thorton WN. Planned postpartum exploration of uterus, cervix and vagina. Obstet Gynecol 1996;27:699-702.
59. Shalev J, Royburt M, Fite G, Mashiach R, Schoenfeld A, Bar J, Ben-Rafael Z, Meizner I. Sonographic evaluation of the puerperal uterus: correlation with manual examination. Gynecol Obstet Invest. 2002;53(1):38-41.
60. Shen O, Rabinowitz R, Eisenberg VH, Samueloff A. Transabdominal sonography before uterine exploration as a predictor of retained placental fragments. J Ultrasound Med. 2003;22(6):561-64.
61. Sadan O, Golan A, Girtler O, Lurie S, Debby A, Sagiv R, Evron S, Glezerman M. Role of sonography in the diagnosis of retained products of conception. J Ultrasound Med. 2004;23(3):371-4.
62. Durfee SM, Frates MC, Luong A, Benson CB. The Sonographic and Color Doppler Features of Retained Products of Conception. J Ultrasound Med. 2005;24:1181-6.
63. Neill AMC, Nixon RM, Thornton S. A comparison of clinical assessment with ultrasound in the management of secondary postpartum haemorrhage. Eur J Obstet Gynecol Reprod Biol. 2002;104:113-5.
64. Ben-Ami I, Schneider D, Maymon R, Vaknin Z, Herman A, Halperin R. Sonographic versus clinical evaluation as predictors of residual trophoblastic tissue. Hum Reprod. 2005; 20(4):1107-1111.
65. Mulic-Lutvica A, Axelsson O. Ultrasound finding of an echogenic mass in women with secondary postpartum hemorrhage is associated with retained placental tissue. Ultrasound Obstet Gynecol. 2006;28(3):312-9.
66. Rufener SL, Adusumilli S, Weadock WJ, Caoili E. Sonography of Uterine Abnormalities in Postpartum and postabortion Patients. A Potential Pitfall of Interpretation. J Ultrasound Med. 2008;27:343-48.
67. Kamaya A, Petrovitch I, Chen B, et al. Retained Products of Conception. Spectrum of Color Doppler Findings. J Ultrasound Med. 2009;28:1031-41.
68. Van den Bosch T, Daemen A, Van Schoubroeck D, Pochet N, De Moor B, Timmerman D. Occurrence and Outcome of Residual Trophoblastic Tissue. J Ultrasound Med. 2008;27:357-61.
69. Matijevic R, Knezevic M, Grgic O, et al. Diagnostic accuracy of sonographic and clinical parameters in the prediction of retained products of conception. J Ultrasound Med. 2009;28(3):295-9.

70. Wolman I, Altman E, Faith G, Har-Toov J, Amster R, Gull I, Jaffa A. Combined clinical and ultrasonographic work -up for the diagnosis of retained products of conception. Fertil Steril. 2009;92:1162-4.
71. Wolman I, Altman E, Faith G, Har-Toov J, Amster R, Gull I, et al. Evaluating retained products of conception in the setting of an ultrasound unit. Fertil Steril, 2009;91(4):1586-8.
72. Retineret-vaev efter födsei, Sandbjerg, DSOG Guideline; 2014 (www.dsog.dk).
73. Steinkeler J, Coldwell BJ, Warner MA. Ultrasound of the Postpartum Uterus, Review Article. Ultrasound Quarterly. 2012;28:97-103.
74. Dossou M, Debost-Legrand A, Déchelotte P, Severe Secondary Postpartum Hemorrhage A Historical Cohort, BIRTH. 2005;42:2.
75. Lousqui R, Morel O, Soyer P, Malartic C, Gayat E, Barranger E. Routine use of abdominopelvic ultrasonography in severe postpartum haemorrhage: retrospective evaluation in 125 patients. Am J Obstet Gynecol. 2011;204:232.e1-6.
76. Pather S, Ford M, Reid R, Sykes P. Postpartum curettage: an audit of 200 cases. Aust N Z J Obstet Gynaecol. 2005; 45(5):368-71.
77. Jensen PA and Stromme WB. Amenorrhhea secondary to puerperal curettage (Asherman's Syndrom) Am J Obstet Gynecol. 1972;113:150-7.
78. Westendorp IC, Ankum WM, Mol BW, et al. Prevalence of Asherman's syndrome after secondary removal of placental remnants or a repeat curettage for incomplete abortion. Hum Reprod. 1998;13(12):3347-50.
79. Al-Inany H. Intrauterine adhesions. An update. Acta Obstet Gynecol Scand. 2001;80:986-93.
80. Achiron R, Goldenberg M, Lipitz S, et al. Transvaginal duplex Doppler Ultrasonography in bleeding patients suspected of having residual trophoblastic tissue. Obstet Gynecol. 1993;81:507-11.
81. Alcazar JL, Lopez-Garcia G, Zornoza A. A role of color velocity imaging and pulsed Doppler sonography to detect retained trophoblastic tissue. Ultrasound Obstet Gynecol. 1996;8(Suppl 1):41.
82. Wolman I, Hartoov J, Amster R, et al. Transvaginal sonohysterography for the early detection of residual trophoblastic tissue. Ultrasound Obstet Gynecol. 1986;8:37.
83. Zalel Y, Gamzu R, Lidor A, Goldenberg M, Achiron R. Color Doppler imaging in the sonohysterographic diagnosis of residual trophoblastic tissue. J Clin Ultrasound. 2002;30: 222-5.
84. Timmerman D, Van Den Bosch T, Peeraer K, Debrouwere E, Van Schoubroeck D, Stockx L, et al. Vascular malformations in the uterus: ultrasonographic diagnosis and conservative management. Eur J Obstet Gynecol Reprod Biol. 2000; 92:171-8.
85. Timmerman D, Wauters J, Van Calenbergh S, Van Schoubroeck D, Maleux G, Van Den Bosch T, et al. Color Doppler imaging is a valuable tool for the diagnosis and management of uterine vascular malformations. Ultrasound Obstet Gynecol. 2003;21:570-7.
86. Van den Bosch T, Van Schoubroeck D, De Brabanter J, et al. Color Doppler and gray- scale ultrasound evaluation of the postpartum uterus. Ultrasound Obstet Gynecol. 2002; 20:586-91.
87. Müngen E. Vascular abnormalities of the uterus: have we recently over-diagnosed them? Opinion. Ultrasound Obstet Gynecol. 2003;21:529-31.
88. Mulic-Lutvica A, Axelsson O. The chapter "Labor and Puerperium" in the section" Ultrasound in perinatal medicine in the Textbook of Perinatal Medicine, July 2001.
89. Mulic-Lutvica Ajlana, Eurenius K, Axelsson O. Uterine artery Doppler ultrasound in postpartum women with retained placental tissue. Acta Obstet Gynecol Scand. 2009;88:724-8.
90. Kido A, Togashi K, Koyama Y, Ito H, Tatsumi K, Fujii S, et al. Retained products of conception masquerading as acquired arteriovenous malformation. J Comput Assist Tomogr 2003;27:88-92.
91. Eriksson LG, Mulic-Lutvica A, Jangland L, et al. Massive postpartum hemorrhage treated with transcatheter arterial embolization: long-term effects, implication on fertility and technical considerations. Acta Radiologica. 2007;48:63-42.
92. Stovall TG, Ambrose SE, Ling FW, et al. Short-term course antibiotic therapy for the treatment of chorioamnionitis and postpartum endomyometritis. Am J Obstet Gynaecol. 1998;159(2):404-7.
93. Calhoun BC, Brost B. Emergency management of sudden puerperal fever. Obstetrics and Gynecology Clinics North Am. 1995;22(2):357-7.
94. Zelop C.Heffner Lj. The downside of caesarean delivery; short-and long-term complications. Clin Obstet Gynecol. 2004;47:386-93.
95. Carson PL. Clean and dirty shadowing at US: a reappraisal. Radiology. 1991;181:231-6.
96. Mulic-Lutvica A, Axelsson O. Postpartum ultrasound in women with postpartum endometritis, after cesarean section and after manual evacuation of the placenta. Acta Obstet Gynecol Scand. 2007;86:210-7.
97. Pelage JP, Soyer P, Repiquet D, Herbreteau D, Le Dref O. Houdart E. et al. Secondary Postpartum Hemorrhage: Treatment with Selective Arterial Embolization. Radiology. 1999;212:385-9.
98. Deutchman ME, Hartmann KJ. Postpartum pyometra: a case report. J Fam Pract 1993;36:449-52.
99. Rudoff JM, Astranskas LJ, Rudoff JC, et al. Ultrasonographic Diagnosis of Septic Pelvic Thrombophlebitis. J Ultrasound Med 1988;7:287-91.
100. Warhit JM, Fagelman D, Goldman MA, et al. Ovarian vein thrombophlebitis: diagnosis by ultrasound and CT. J Clin Ultrasound 1984;12:301.
101. Wilson PC, Lerner RM. Diagnosis of ovarian vein thrombophlebitis by ultrasonography. J Ultrasound Med 1983;2:187.

102. Sherer DM, Fern S, Mester J, et al. Postpartum ultrasonographic diagnosis of inferior vena cava thrombus associated with ovarian vein thrombosis. Am J Obstet Gynecol. 1997;177(2):474-5.
103. Burger NF, Dararas B, Boes EGM. An echogenic evaluation during the early puerperium of the uterine wound after caesarean section. J Ultrasound Med. 1983;2:18.
104. Meyenburg M, Schulze-Hagen K, Schaller G. Involution of the uterus following vaginal or abdominal delivery. Z Geburtshilfe Perinatol. 1983;187(4):200-2.
105. Negishi H, Kishida T, Yamada H, Hirayama E, Mikuni M, Fujimoto S. Changes in uterine size after vaginal delivery and caesarean section determined by vaginal sonography in the puerperium. Arch Gynecol Obstet. 1999;263(1-2): 13-6.
106. Koskas M, Nizard J, Salomon LJ, Ville Y. Abdominal and pelvic ultrasound findings within 24 hours following uneventful cesarean section. Ultrasound Obstet Gynecol. 2008;32(4):520-6.
107. Lavery JP, Howell RS, Shaw L. Ultrasonic demonstration of a phlegmona following Caesarean section - case report. J Clin Ultrasound. 1985;13:134-6.
108. Baker ME, Bowie JD, Killan AP. Sonography of postcaesarean-section bladder-flap hematoma. Am J Roentgenol. 1984;144:757-9.
109. Sentilhes L, Ambroselli C, Kayem G, Provansal M, et al. Maternal Outcome After Conservative Treatment of Placenta Accreta. Obstetrics & Gynecology, 2010;115(3):526-39.
110. Warshak CR, Ramos GA, Eskander R, Benirschke K, Saenz CC, Kelly TF, et al. Effect of Predelivery Diagnosis in 99 Consecutive Cases of Placenta accreta. Obstetrics & Gynecology. 2010;115(1):65-9.
111. Bennett MJ. Puerperal ultrasonic hysterography in the diagnosis of congenital uterine malformations. Br J Obstet Gynaecol. 1976;83(5):389-92.
112. Szoke B, Kiss D. The use of ultrasonic echo technique in the diagnosis of developmental anomalies of the uterus. Ann Chir Gynecol. 1977;66(1):59-61.
113. Land JA, Stoot JE, Evers JL. Puerperal ultrasonic hysterography. Gynecol Obstet Invest. 1984;18(3):165-8.
114. Weissman A, Grisarn D, Shenhav M, et al. Postpartum Surveillance of urinary retention by ultrasonography: the effect of epidural analgesia. Ultrasound obstet Gynecol 1995;6:130-4.
115. Ulitzsch D, Nyman MKG, Carlson RA. Breast Abscess in Lactating Women: US-guided Treatment, Radiology. 2004;232(3):904-9.
116. Masarie K, Katz V, Balderston K. Pregnancy luteomas Clinical Presentations and Management Strategies. Obstet & Gynecol Survey. 2010; 65(9):575-82.

33

CHAPTER

Three-dimensional Sonoembryology

Ritsuko K Pooh, Kohei Shiota, Asim Kurjak

INTRODUCTION

Owing to recent reproductive revolution, the beginning of human life has been marvelously elucidated. Furthermore, in a field of embryology, advanced technologies of experimental magnetic resonance (MR) microscopy of embryos[1,2] and computer graphic[3] have contributed to comprehensive early human development. "Sonoembryology" was first described in 1990[4] after introduction of high-frequency transvaginal transducer in obstetrical field. Combination of transvaginal approach and three-dimensional (3D) ultrasound has been establishing "3D sonoembryology", producing more objective and accurate information of early embyonal and fetal development and natural history of fetal abnormalities.[5] Although 3D sonoembryology has been approaching modern high-tech embryology, it still cannot demonstrate internal organs of embryos as clearly as by embryonal MR microscopy. However, a great advantage in sonoembryology, which human embryology cannot possess, is "demonstration of living embryos with circulation in vivo". Human embryology is based on dead embryos which had been well preserved. 3D sonoembryology has a remarkable potential to discover new findings of living embryos and fetuses in utero. In this chapter, we introduce up-date embryology and 3D sonoembryology. The staging and aging of embryos are different in embryology from in obstetrics. Although "gestational age" usually used in obstetrical field based on menstrual period or crown lump length, has been criticized in the embryological point of view,[6] it is used in this chapter on description of sonograms.

MODERN EMBRYOLOGY BY MAGNETIC RESONANCE MICROSCOPY AND COMPUTER GRAPHICS

Carnegie stages **(Fig. 1)**, well-known embryonal staging system till 8 weeks after conception, was named after the famous institute which began collecting and classifying embryos in the early 1900s. An embryo is assigned a Carnegie stage (numbered from 1 to 23) based on its external morphological features. Age and size proves a poor way to organize embryos. It is very difficult to accurately age an embryo, and it could shrink a full 50% in the preserving fluids. Therefore, this staging system is not dependent on the chronological age nor the size of the embryo. The stages, are in a sense, arbitrary levels of maturity based on multiple physical features. Embryos that might have different ages or sizes can be assigned the same Carnegie stage based on their external appearance because of the natural variation which occurs between individuals. **Table 1** shows the Carnegie stages from stage 1 to 23.

The recent advance in magnetic resonance (MR) microscopic technology has made it possible to scan and visualize relatively small samples, including mammalian embryos.[1] MR microscopy demonstrates tomographic imaging of small objects, and the digitized data can be manipulated to achieve 3D reconstruction of the samples.[1] Although the resolution and long imaging speed were initial problems in MR microscopy, those have been solved by invention of a super-parallel MR microscope.[2] Additionally, recent advanced computer graphics techniques combined MR microscopy have produced detailed 3D images of human embryos. Yamada, et al.[3] successfully constructed a series of 3D images of human embryos, based on the MR microscopy data of human embryo specimens in the Kyoto Collection (**Figs. 2A to C**), with the aid of CG techniques, to illustrate 3D structures and morphogenetic movements in human embryos **(Figs. 3 and 4)**. In addition, they produced movies using these 3D images (Supplementary Movies, which can be viewed at http://www.interscience.wiley.com/jpages/1058-8388/suppmat) to show the entire process of morphogenesis in human embryos from fertilization to the completion of organogenesis.[3]

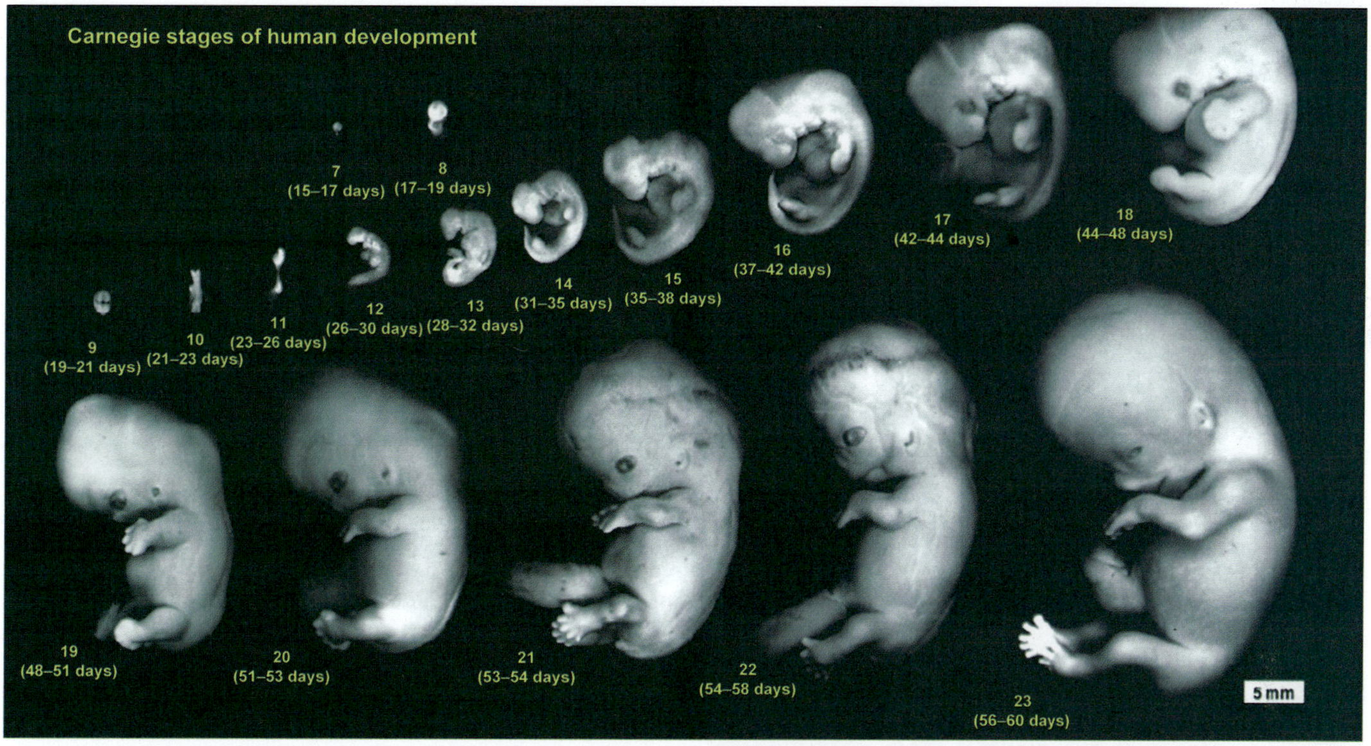

Fig. 1: Development of human embryos at 4–8 weeks after conception (Kyoto collection of human embryos).

TABLE 1: Carnegie stages table.

Stage	*Days after conception (approx)*	*Size (mm)*	*Events*
1	1 (week 1)	0.1–0.15	Fertilized oocyte, pronuclei
2	2–3	0.1–0.2	Cell division with reduction in cytoplasmic volume, formation of inner and outer cell mass
3	4–5	0.1–0.2	Loss of zona pellucida, free blastocyst
4	5–6	0.1–0.2	Attaching blastocyst
5	7–12 (week 2)	0.1–0.2	Implantation
6	13–15	0.2	Extraembryonic mesoderm, primitive streak
7	15–17 (week 3)	0.4	Gastrulation, notochordal process
8	17–19	1.0–1.5	Primitive pit, notochordal canal
9	19–21	1.5–2.5	Somite Number 1–3: Neural folds, cardiac primordium, head fold
10	22–23 (week 4)	2–3.5	Somite Number 4–12: Neural fold fuses
11	23–26	2.5–4.5	Somite Number 13–20: Rostral neuropore closes
12	26–30	3–5	Somite Number 21–29: Caudal neuropore closes
13	28–32 (week 5)	4–6	Somite Number 30: Leg buds, lens placode, pharyngeal arches
14	31–35	5–7	Lens pit, optic cup
15	35–38	7–9	Lens vesicle, nasal pit, hand plate
16	37–42 (week 6)	8–11	Nasal pits moved ventrally, auricular hillocks, foot plate
17	42–44	11–14	Finger rays
18	44–48 (week 7)	13–17	Ossification commences
19	48–51	16–18	Straightening of trunk
20	51–53 (week 8)	18–22	Upper limbs longer and bent at elbow
21	53–54	22–24	Hands and feet turned inward
22	54–56	23–28	Eyelids, external ears
23	56–60	27–31	Rounded head, body and limbs

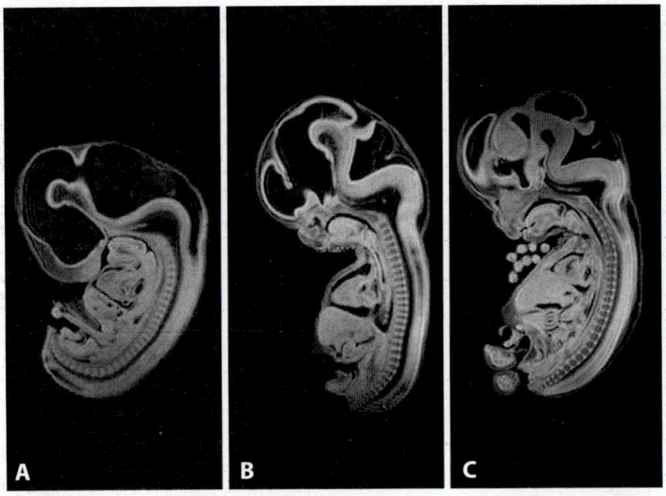

Figs. 2A to C: Magnetic resonance images of 2D cross sections selected from 3D data sets of fixed human embryos: (A) Carnegie stage (CS)18; (B) CS20; (C) CS23.

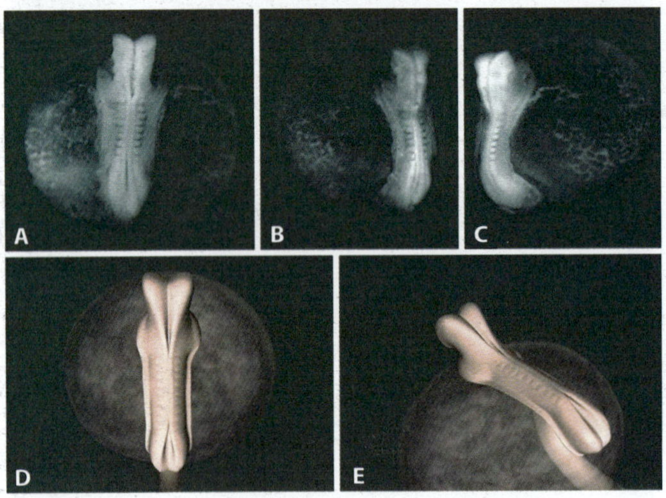

Figs. 3A to E: A neurulating human embryo [Carnegie stage (CS) 10] and its three-dimensional (3D) computer graphics model. (A to C) Photographs of a CS10 embryo with the closing neural tube. Ten pairs of somites are recognizable. The round ball-like structure on the ventral side of the embryo is the yolk sac; (D and E) A 3D computer graphics model of the embryo shown in A to C. This model was reconstructed based on its gross pictures and histological sections.

NORMAL EMBRYO VISUALIZATION BY THREE-DIMENSIONAL SONOEMBRYOLOGY

Since the introduction of high frequency transvaginal transducer, ultrasonographic visualization of embryos and fetuses in early stage has been remarkably progressed and sonoembryology[4] has been established. In addition, recent introduction of three-dimensional and four-dimensional ultrasounds combined with the transvaginal approach has produced more objective and accurate information on

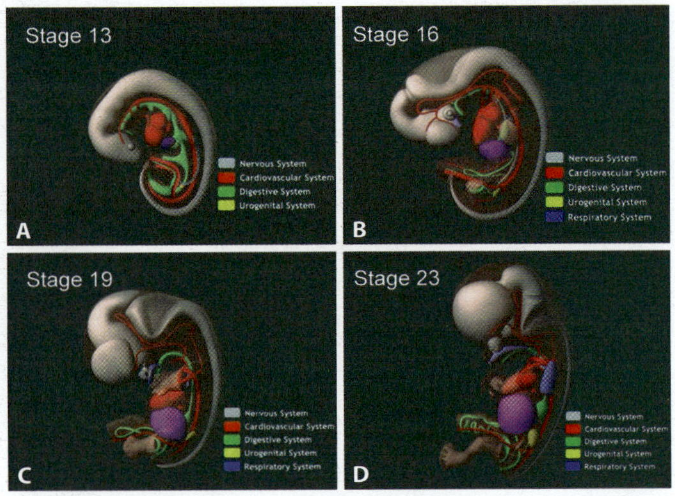

Figs. 4A to D: Computer graphics model of human embryos showing major internal organs overlapped with the surface contour. The internal organs were reconstructed according to magnetic resonance images, histological sections, and textbook illustrations: (A) Carnegie stage (CS) 13; (B) CS16; (C) CS19; (D) CS23.

embryonal and early fetal development.[5,7] **Figures 5A and B** show a gestational sac at 4 weeks of gestation and **Figures 6A and B** demonstrate the yolk sac visualization at 5 weeks of gestation. Although it has been difficult to demonstrate small embryos less than 10 mm of greatest length by ultrasound, **Figures 7 and 8** show 5.5 mm-long-embryo with yolk sac at 6 weeks of gestation and 18.3 mm-CRL-embryo at 8 weeks of gestation respectively, depicted by using 3D equipment with high-frequency transvaginal transducer (Voluson® E8 with 12 MHz/256 element vaginal probe, GE Healthcare, Milwaukee, USA). Early neural tube and premature spinal cord are successfully demonstrated in a small embryo. **Figures 9A and B** is macrographic images of an aborted specimen taken just after abortion. Premature spinal cord is visualized on the back, which is compatible with 3D image on **Figure 8**. **Figure 10** shows the development of spinal cord in embryonal size of 5.5 mm, 18.3 mm and 26.3 mm.[7] Thereafter, the vertebral bony structure can be visualized from 11 weeks of gestation and gradual closure of bilateral laminae caudally from the cervical region **(Fig. 11)**. Recent 3D technology of HDlive imaging demonstrates the fetal structure with more reality **(Figs. 12 and 13)**.

The development of the embryonic circulation became visualized by 3D power Doppler imaging technology.[8] **Figures 14A and B** illustrates the vascular network of an embryo at 7 weeks of gestation. In 1993 and 1994, color Doppler detection and assessment of brain vessels in the early fetus using a transvaginal approach was reported.[9,10] Clear visualization by transvaginal power Doppler of the

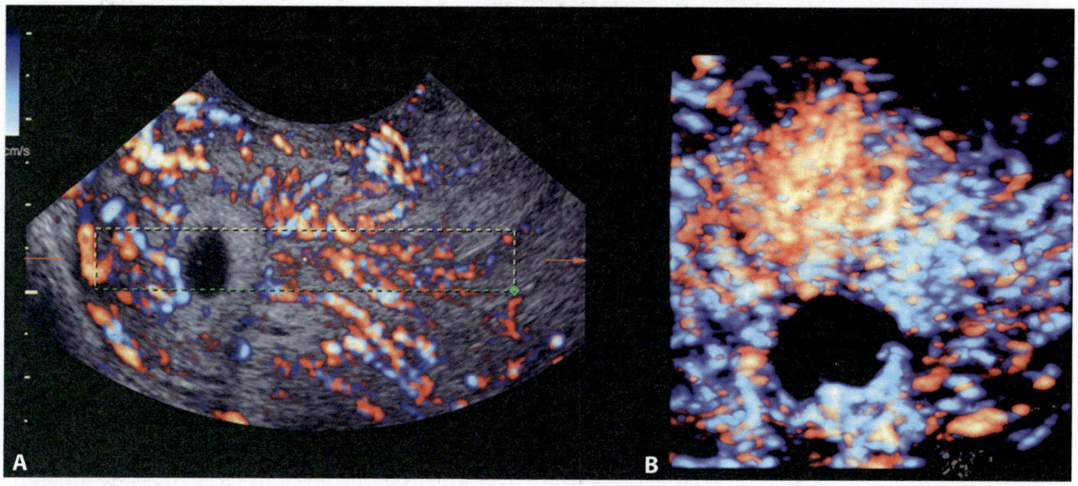

Figs. 5A and B: Gestational sac with uterine hypervascularity: (A) Bidirectional power Doppler 2D image; (B) 3D HD reconstructed image.

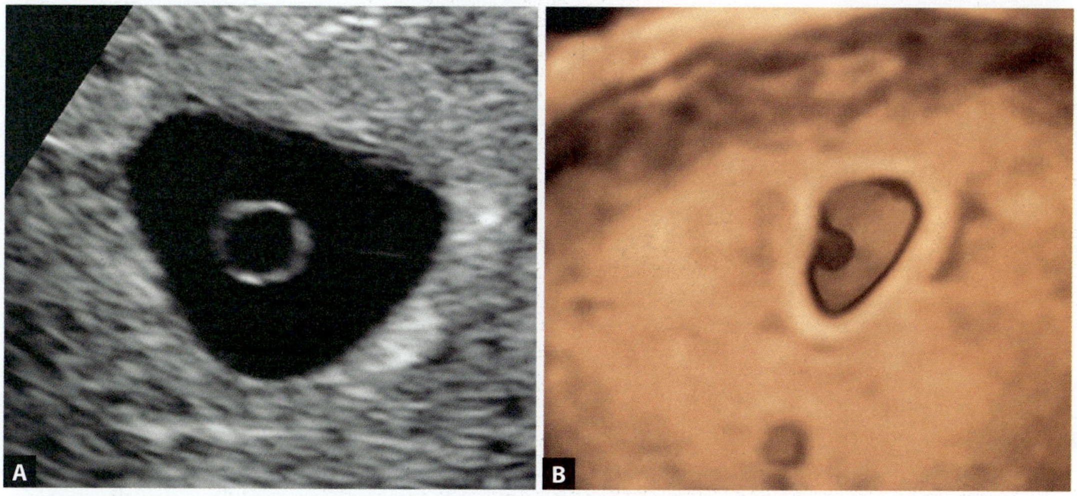

Figs. 6A and B: Yolk sac at the beginning of 5 weeks: (A) 2D image; (B) 3D reconstructed image.

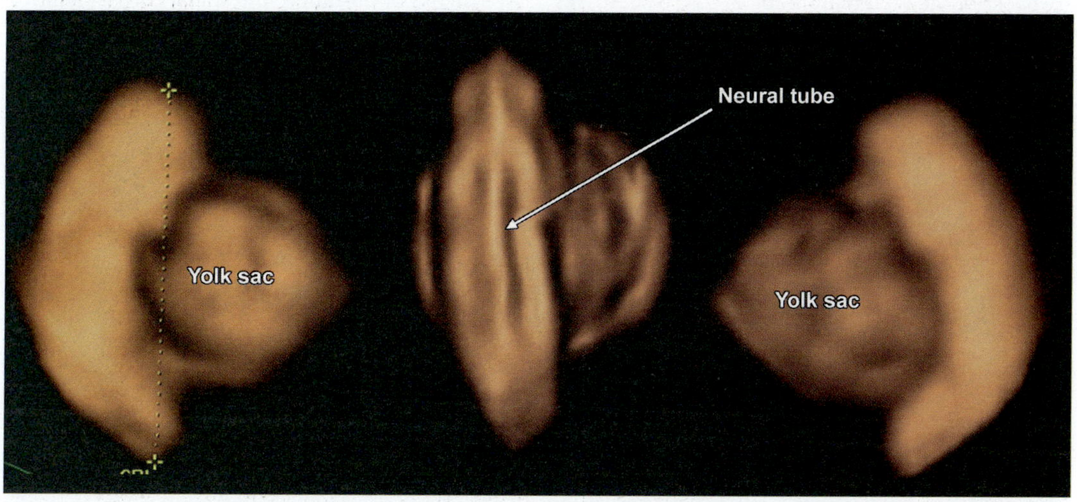

Fig. 7: 3D reconstructed image of the yolk sac and 5.5 mm-CRL-embryo (6 weeks of gestation); normal 6-week-embryo (CRL 5.5 mm) and yolk sac. Occipital view shows the neural tube on the embryonal back.

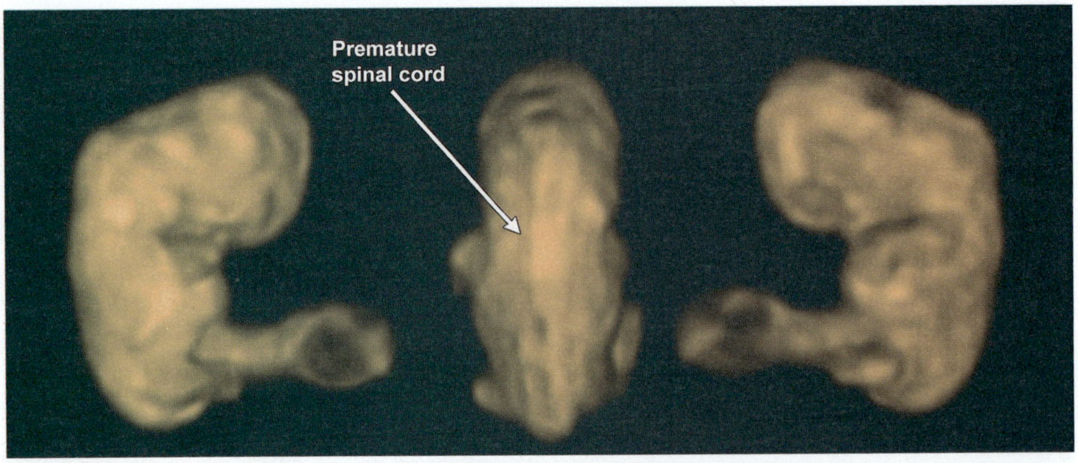

Fig. 8: 3D reconstructed image of the embryo (8 weeks of gestation); normal 8-week-embryo. Occipital view shows the premature spinal cord which is seen in the **Figure 4** (right).

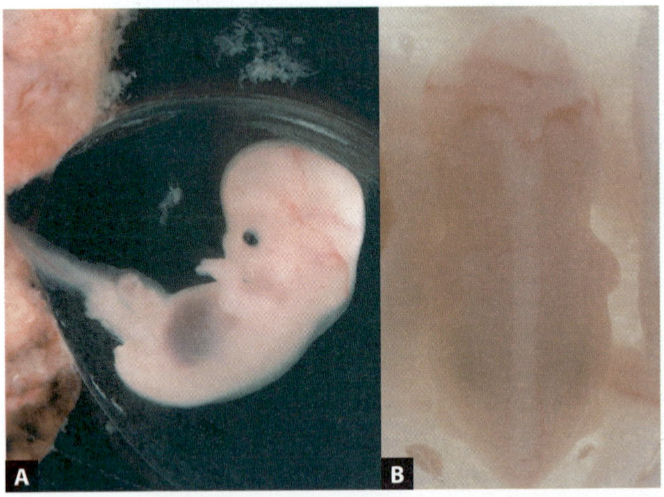

Figs. 9A and B: Lateral and back view of aborted embryo at 8 weeks of gestation: (A) Lateral view. Physiological umbilical hernia is seen; (B) Backside view. Premature spinal cord is seen. This photo was taken just after abortion before preserving in formalin.

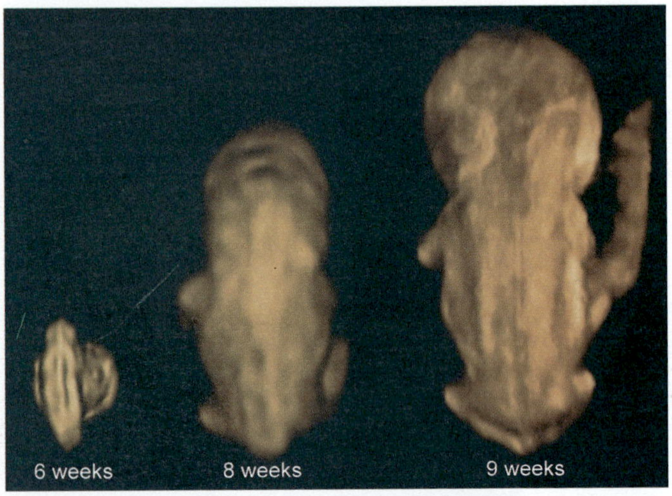

Fig. 10: 3D reconstructed image of the embryo (6–9 weeks of gestation); embryonal sizes are 5.5 mm, 18.3 mm and 26.3 mm. At 9 weeks of gestation, the spinal cord is demonstrated as a thin line, compared with that at 8 weeks of gestation.

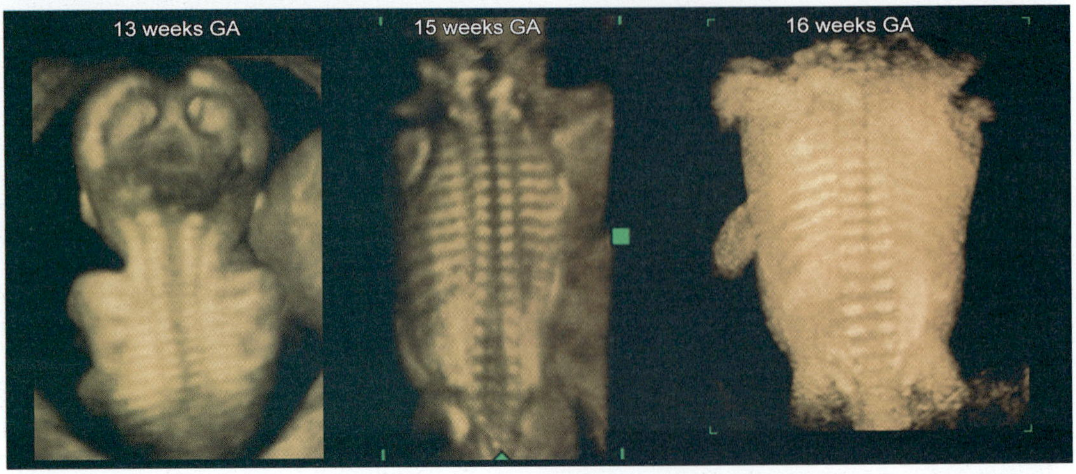

Fig. 11: 3D reconstructed image of fetal vertebral development between 13 and 16 weeks of gestation.

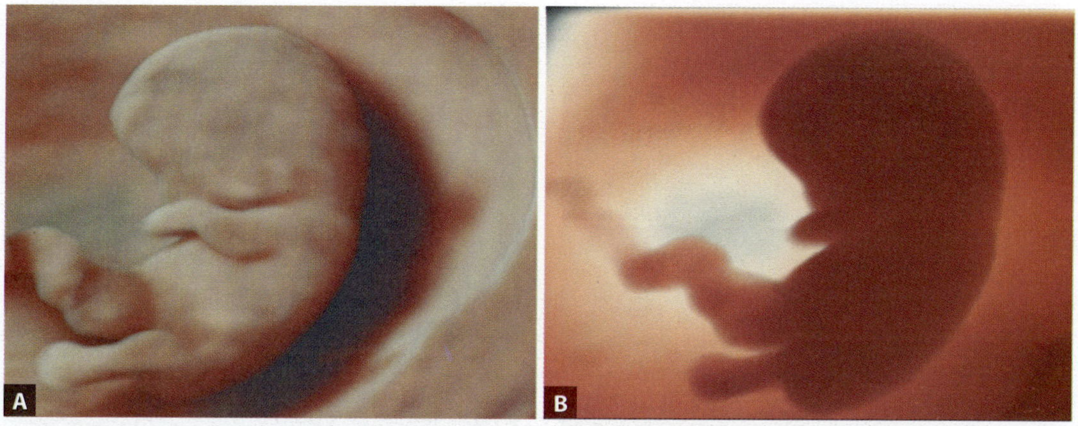

Figs. 12A and B: HDlive images of 9-weeker fetus. At this stage, physiological omphalocele is visible in all of normal fetuses. Two pictures are exactly the same 3D image with different shadowing.

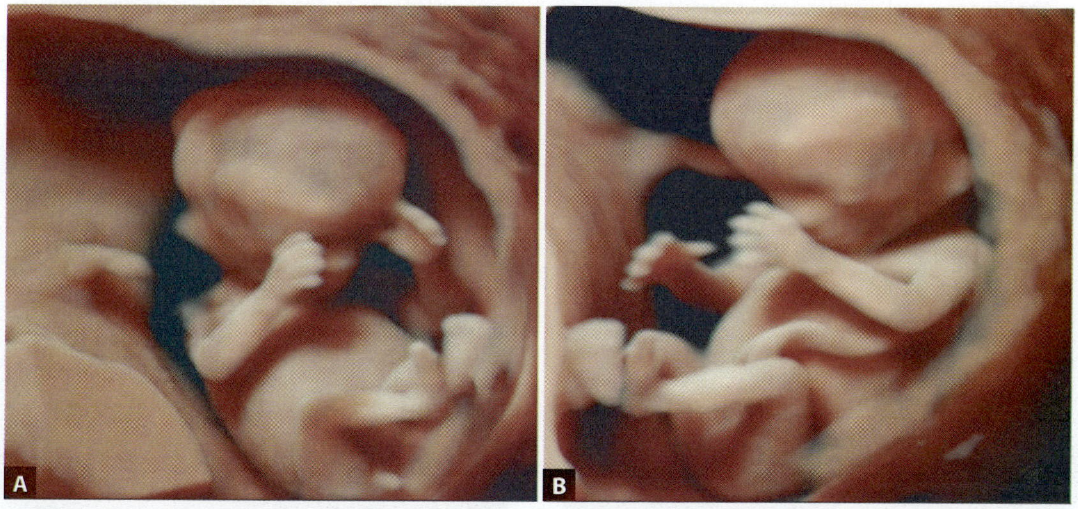

Figs. 13A and B: HDlive images of 12-weeker fetus. At this stage, detailed surface structure including fingers and face is well demonstrated.

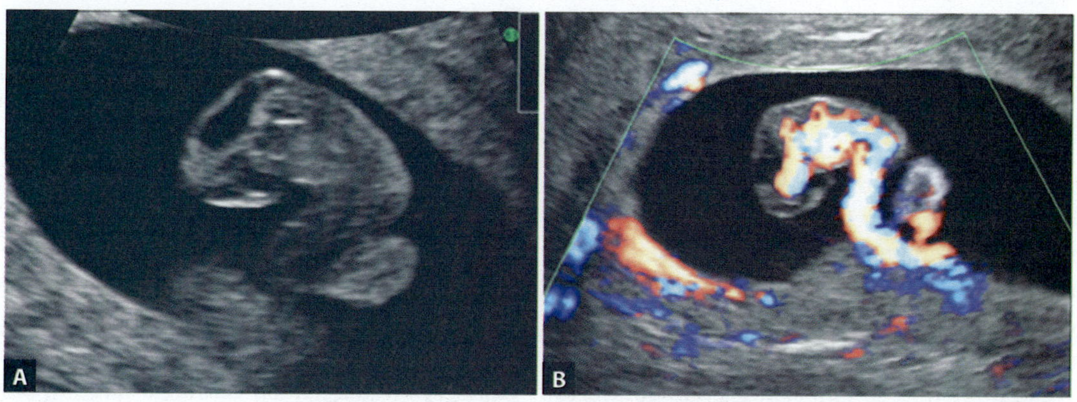

Figs. 14A and B: Early vascular system at 7 weeks of gestation: (A) 2D gray mode; (B) Power Doppler image.

common carotid arteries, internal and external carotid arteries, middle cerebral arteries at 12 weeks of gestation was reported in 1996.[11] By using 3D power Doppler technology, the vascular anatomy can now be imaged clearly by identification of the anterior and middle cerebral arteries and its branches (**Figs. 15A and B**).

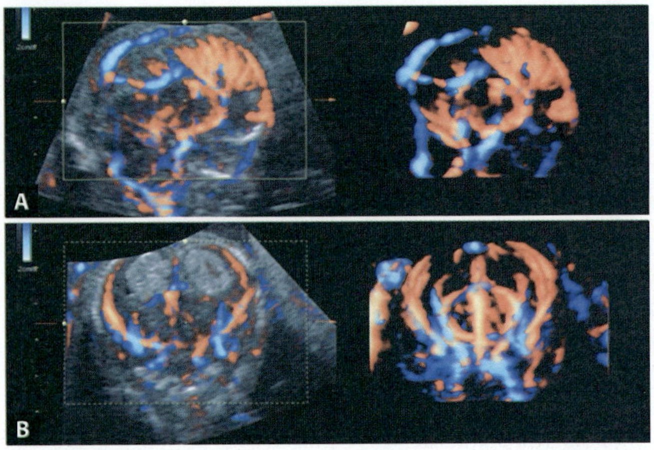

Figs. 15A and B: Premature vascularity of normal 12 weeks brain: (A) 2D power Doppler image and 3D reconstructed image in the sagittal section. Anterior cerebral arteries and its branches are well demonstrated; (B) 2D power Doppler image and 3D reconstructed image in the coronal section. Middle cerebral arteries and its branches are well demonstrated.

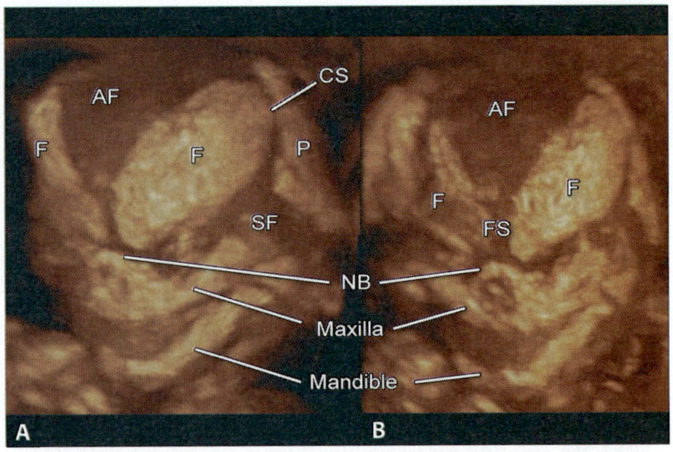

Figs. 17A and B: 3D maximum mode image of normal craniofacial structure at 14 weeks of gestation: (A) Oblique view; (B) Frontal view. Anterior fontanelle (AF), sphenoidal fontanelle (SF), frontal suture (FS), coronal suture (CS), nasal bone (NB), maxilla and mandible are gradually formed according to cranial bony development.

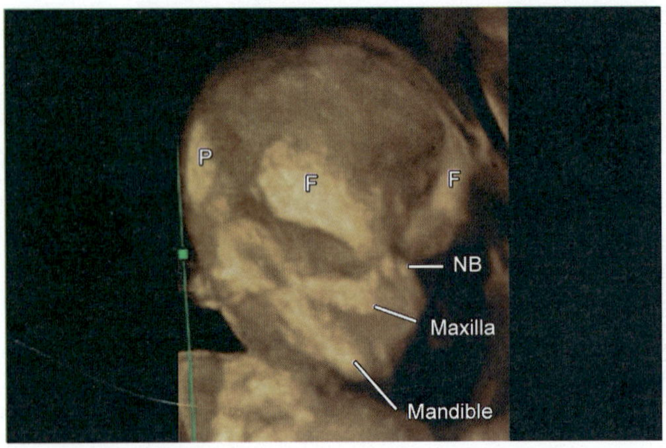

Fig. 16: 3D maximum mode image of normal craniofacial structure at 11 weeks of gestation. Premature bony structure of frontal bone (F), parietal bone (P), nasal bone (NB), maxilla and mandible are recognizable.

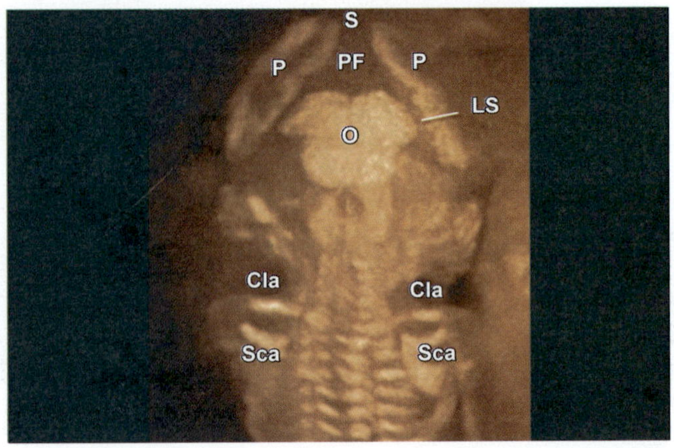

Fig. 18: 3D maximum mode image of occipital view at 13 weeks of gestation. Note the premature occipital bone appearance. Midline crack is demonstrated. (S: sagittal suture; P: parietal bone; PF: posterior fontanelle; O: occipital bone; Cla: clavicula; Sca: scapula; LS: lambdoid suture)

The utilization of post-processing algorithms such as maximum mode can be used to demonstrate the fetal skeleton. Chaoui et al.[12] reported clear 3D images for the identification of an abnormally wide metopic suture in the second trimester of pregnancy. However, rapid ossification of the craniofacial bones occurs during the first trimester of pregnancy. We demonstrate in this chapter the identification of the craniofacial skeleton from 10 weeks of gestation onwards. **Figures 16 and 17** show early fetal craniofacial bony structures at 11 and 14 weeks, respectively, using the maximum mode algorithm. The difference of frontal bone morphology between 11 and 14 weeks demonstrates membranous ossification of the cranium at this stage. **Figure 18** demonstrates the structure of the skull in the occipital region at 13 weeks of gestation.

During the early embryonic period, the central nervous system anatomy rapidly changes in appearance. MR images (*see* **Fig. 2**) shows remarkable change of CNS appearance in a short period between Carnegie stage 18 and 23. Detailed cerebrospinal structure at Carnegie stage 23 is visualized in **Figure 19**.

3D sonography using transvaginal sonography with high-resolution probes allows imaging of early structures in the embryonic brain. Fetal brain detailed morphology at the beginning of 8th week is shown in **Figures 20 to 22** and this can be accomplished by tomographic ultrasound imaging **(Figs. 20A and B)**, multiplanar imaging **(Fig. 21)** and thick-slice 3D reconstructed imaging **(Fig. 22)**. Serial examinations allow obtaining exact the same sections of the fetal brain at different stages of development. **Figures 23 and 24** show 10th and 12th week brain respectively. Thus, it is possible to document the changes in CNS development between 8th and 12th week as demonstrated in **Figure 25**. Reports published on embryonal ventricular development from 6th or 7th week by use of 3D inversion-rendering mode, have made sonoembryology more sophisticated and objective.[13,14] It is possible that by

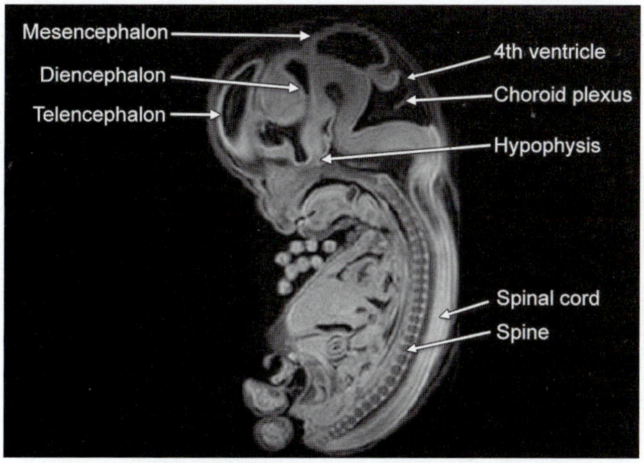

Fig. 19: Embryo structures visualized by MR image (Carnegie stage 23).

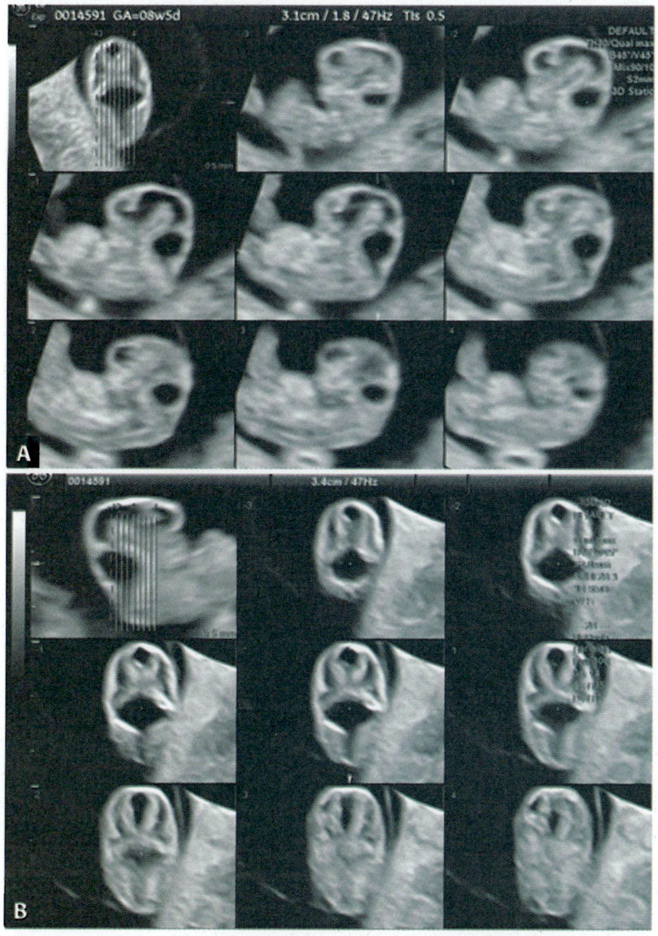

Figs. 20A and B: Tomographic sagittal image (A) and coronal image (B) of normal fetus at the beginning of 8 weeks of gestation.

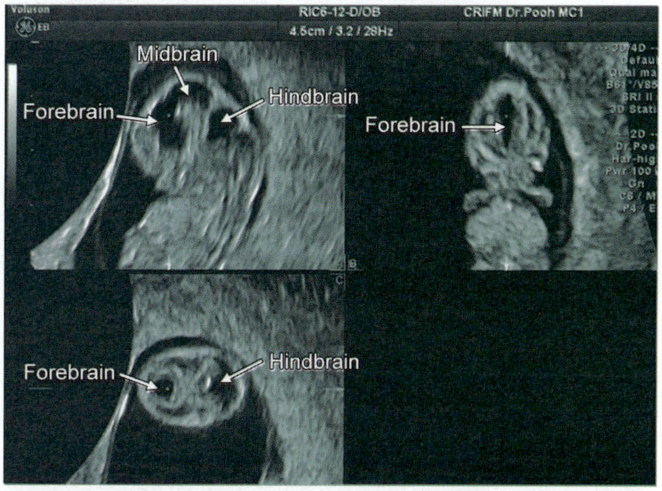

Fig. 21: Three orthogonal image of normal brain at the end of 8 weeks of gestation. The development of premature ventricular system is seen. Note the different appearance from the beginning of 8 weeks of gestation **(Figure 17)**.

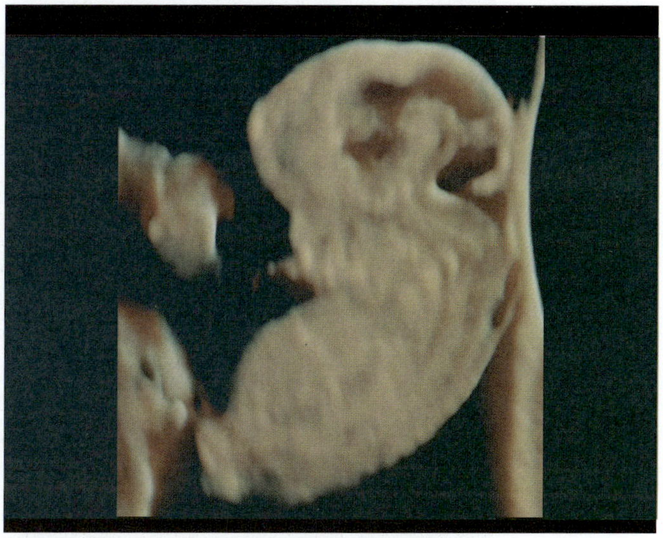

Fig. 22: Thick slice 3D reconstructed image of the brain in the mid-sagittal cutting section at the end of 8 weeks of gestation.

developing 3D neurosonoembryology imaging in-utero, current fetal staging (which uses gestational age based on last menstrual period or crown-rump length measurement) may change into a "morphological staging system," such as the Carnegie staging system, which has been central to embryology.[7]

Thoracoabdominal structures can also be imaged in the first trimester. For example, **Figure 26** shows tomographic ultrasound imaging of fetal chest and abdomen at 13 weeks of gestation. Clear visualization of the lung-liver interface can be of value in the early diagnosis of thoracoabdominal abnormalities, such as a diaphragmatic hernia.

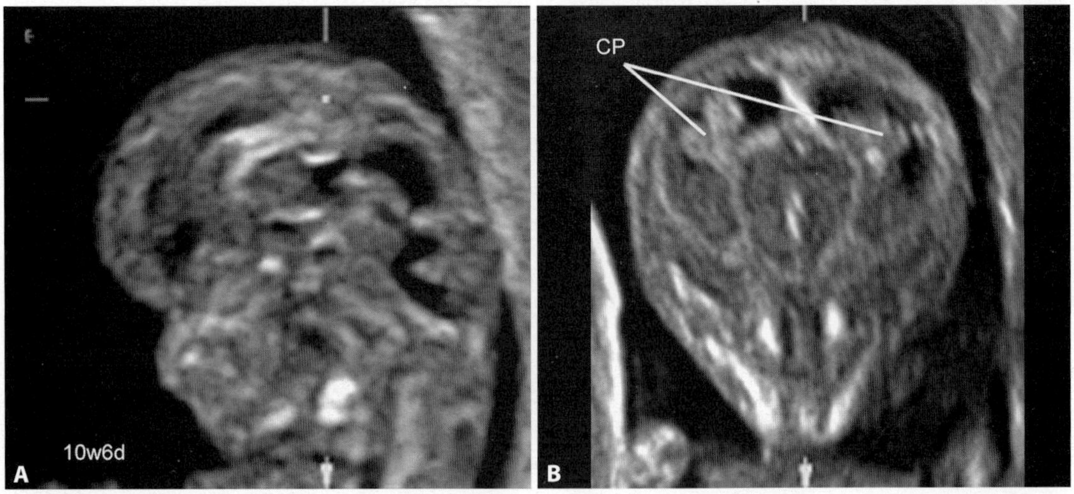

Figs. 23A and B: Sagittal section and coronal sections of 10-week-fetus. (CP: Choroid plexus of the lateral ventricles)

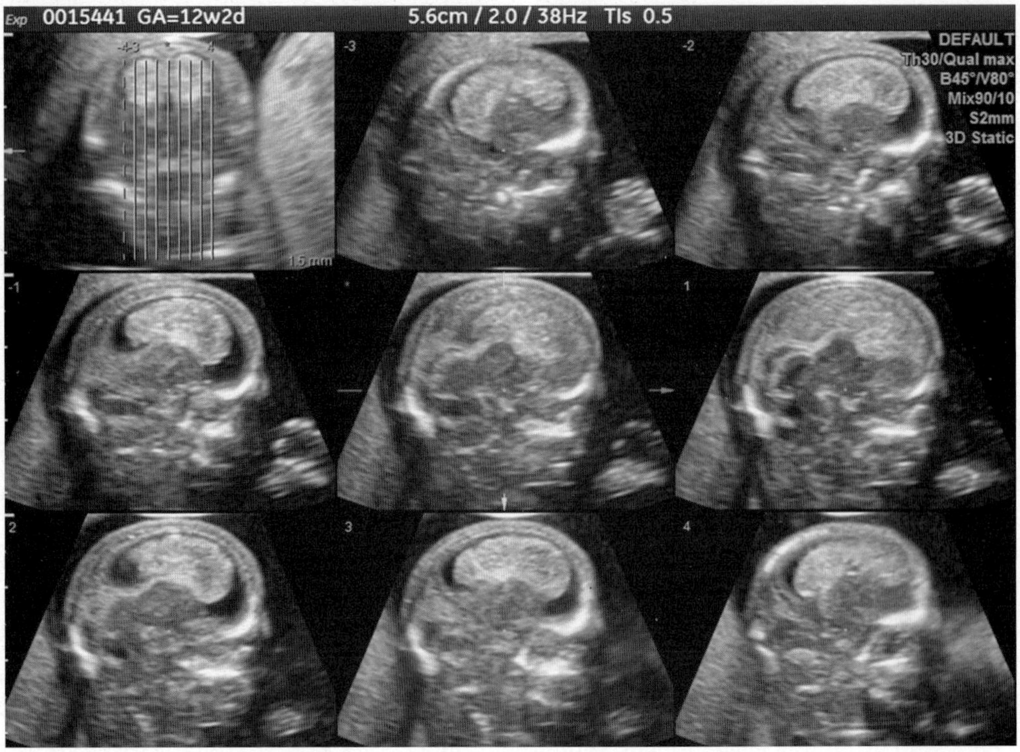

Fig. 24: Normal sagittal TUI image of fetal brain at 12 weeks. Hyperechogenic choroid plexus occupies most of lateral ventricle.

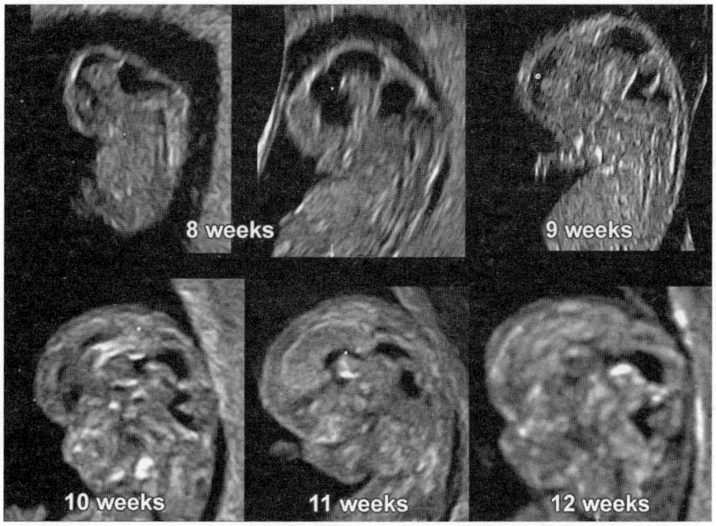

Fig. 25: Normal brain development by mid-sagittal 3D US section between 8 and 12 weeks of gestation.

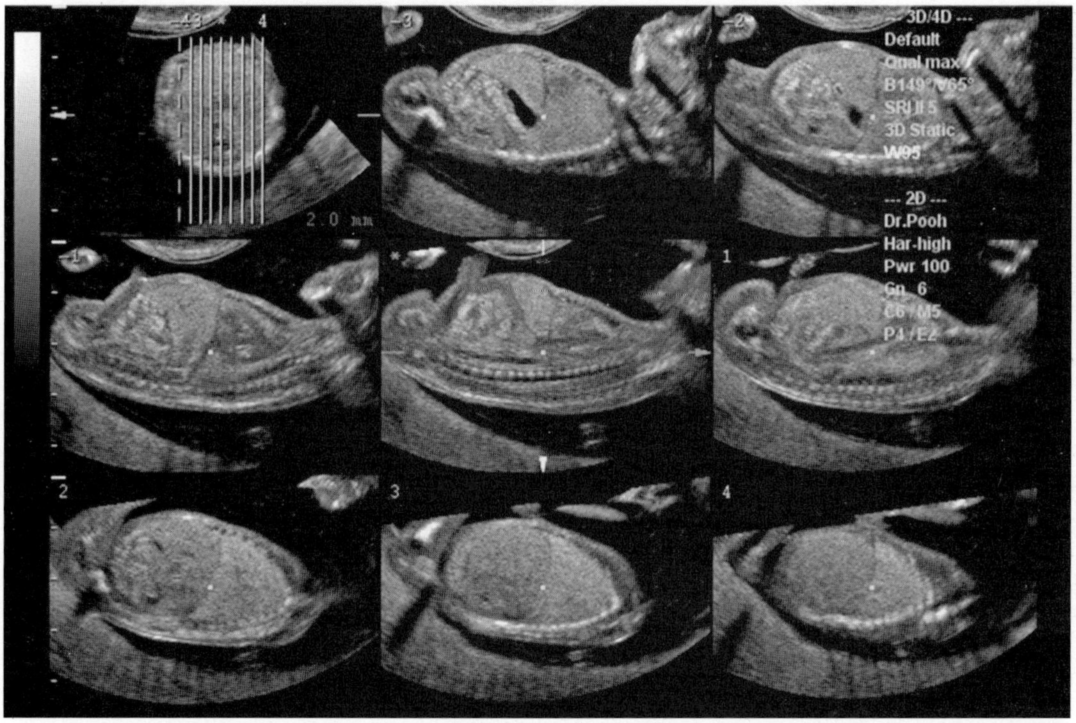

Fig. 26: Tomographic ultrasound imaging of normal thoracoabdominal structure at 13 weeks of gestation. Parallel sagittal sections are shown. Lung-liver border and intra-abdominal organs are clearly visualized.

The sagittal and axial cutting sections shown in **Figure 27** provide us clinically significant information. In the first trimester, genetic and morphological screening is important role. Especially nuchal translucency (NT) shown in **Figures 28 and 29** is well-known as a significant ultrasound marker for genetic screening as well as morphological screening for congenital heart abnormality or skeletal disorder. In the same cutting section, brain structure including midbrain, medulla oblongata, intracranial translucency (IVth ventricle), cisterna magna are well demonstrated.

The external ear position goes higher with advance of gestational age as shown in **Figure 30** and 3D images demonstrate precisely changing position of the external ear **(Figs. 31A and B)**.

The number of umbilical arteries is clearly depicted by bidirectional power Doppler **(Figs. 32A and B)** or color Doppler, and placental vasculature is quite comprehensively demonstrated by 3D reconstructed power Doppler images as shown in **Figures 33 and 34**.

FETAL ABNORMALITIES IN EARLY GESTATION

Yolk Sac

The yolk sac plays an important role in embryonal hemopoiesis and fetomaternal transportation

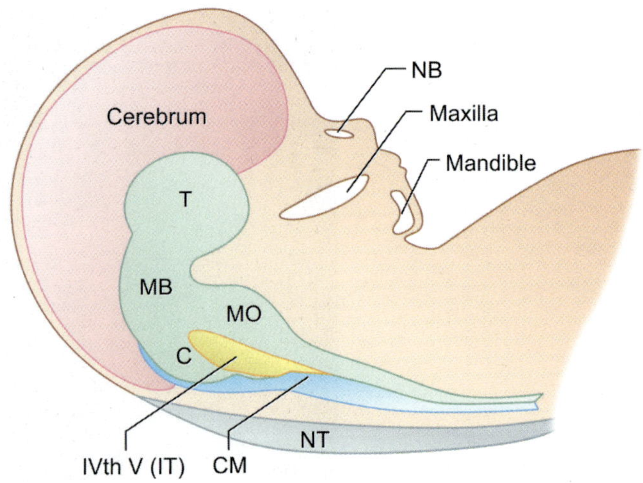

Fig. 28: Schematic picture of mid-sagittal section of the face in the first trimester. (NB: nasal bone; T: thalamus; MB: midbrain; C: cerebellum; IVth V: fourth ventricle; IT: intracranial translucency; MO: medulla oblongata; CM: cisterna magna; NT: nuchal translucency)

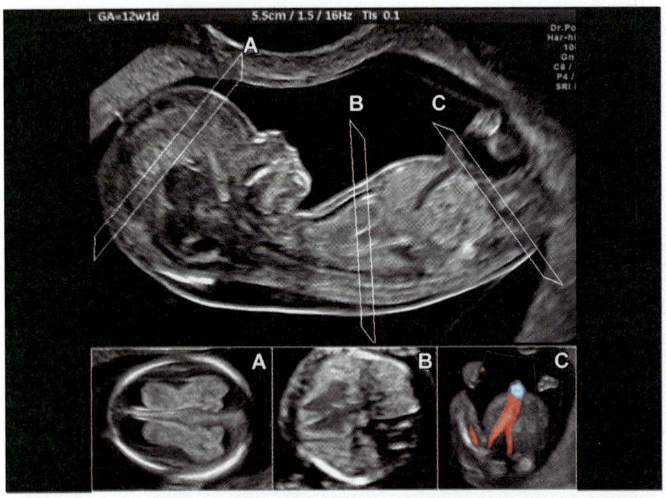

Fig. 27: Normal mid-sagittal and axial sections of 12-weeker fetus. Mid-sagittal section shows profile, mid-cutting section of the brain, nuchal area, and lung-liver border and genitalia. 90-degree-rotation of transducer leads to axial section (A, B, C) from mid-sagittal section.

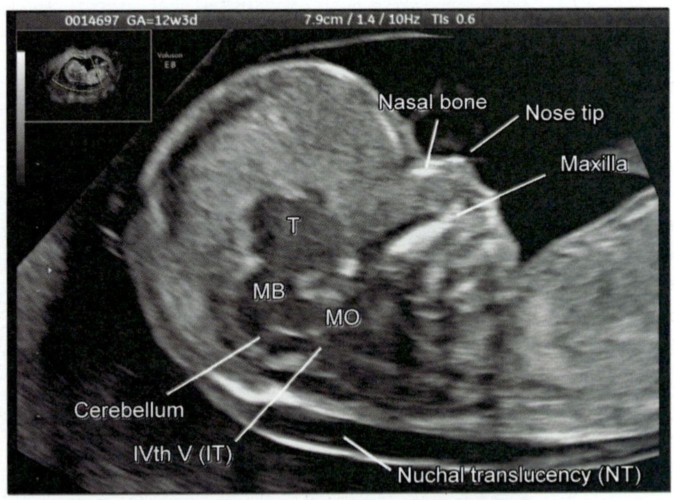

Fig. 29: Normal profile image at the beginning of 12 weeks. Note the nasal bone, maxilla, diencephalon and nuchal translucency. (T: thalamus; MB: midbrain; IVth V: fourth ventricle; IT: intracranial translucency; MO: medulla oblongata).

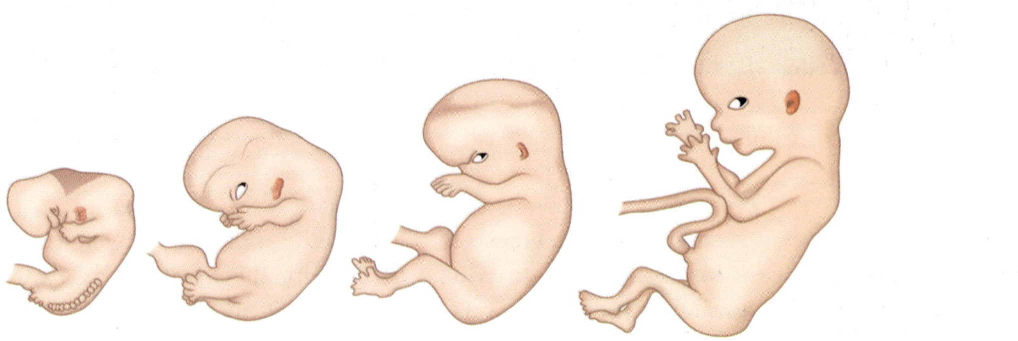

Fig. 30: External ear development in early pregnancy. External ear is located on the neck but gradually the position goes higher with gestational age.

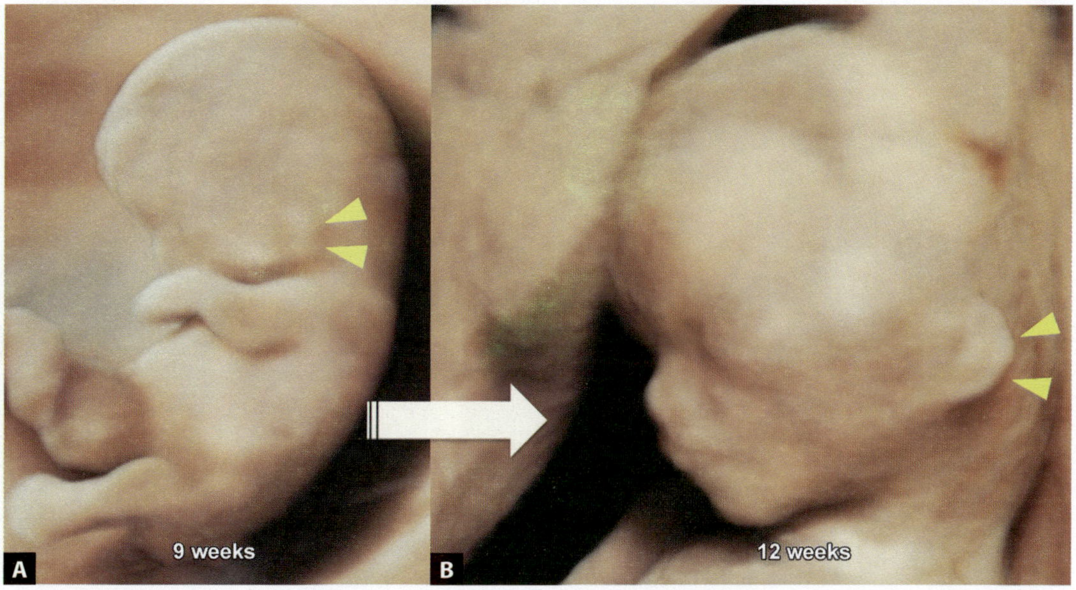

Figs. 31A and B: External ear position change between 9 and 12 weeks of gestation in normal fetus. External ear position is low at 9 weeks (A, arrowheads) but normal positioned ear is demonstrated at 12 weeks (B, arrowheads).

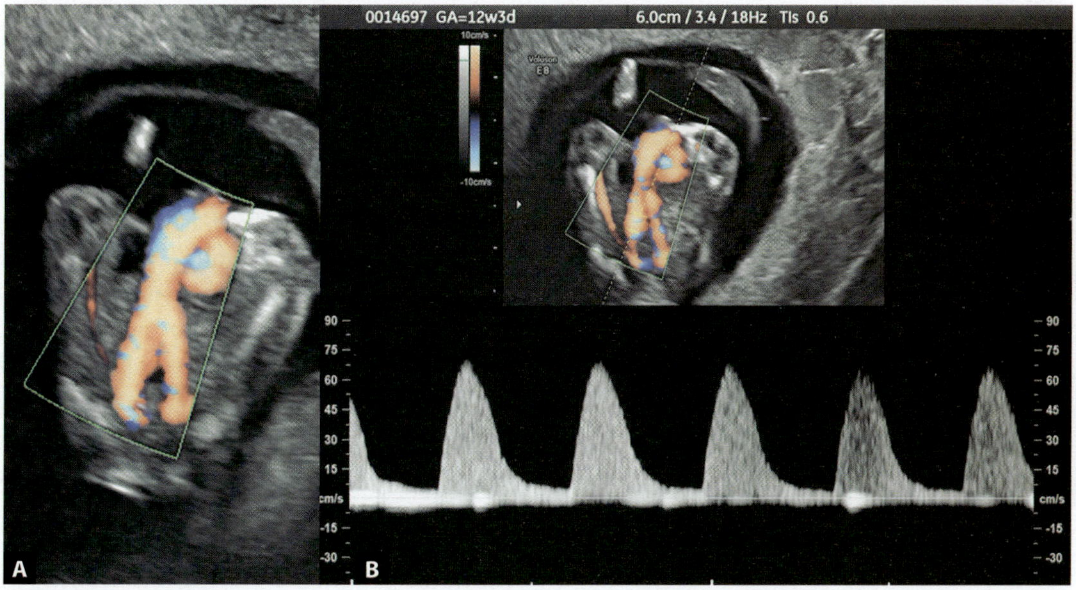

Figs. 32A and B: Normal two umbilical arteries and its blood flow: (A) Two arteries are along with bladder wall; (B) Normal umbilical artery blood flow. In most of cases in the first trimester, umbilical artery diastolic blood flow velocity is positive with low velocity or absent.

of nutritive properties before establishment of fetoplacental circulation. The primary yolk sac forms at around 3rd weeks of the menstrual age, then following the formation of the extraembryonic coelom, and the secondary yolk sac is formed. From the 5th weeks of gestation, it appears as a spherical and cystic structure covered by numerous superficial small vessels merging at the basis of the vitelline duct. This connects the yolk sac to the ventral part of the embryo, the gut and main blood circulation. During the 10th week of gestation, the yolk sac begins to degenerate and rapidly ceases to function.[15]

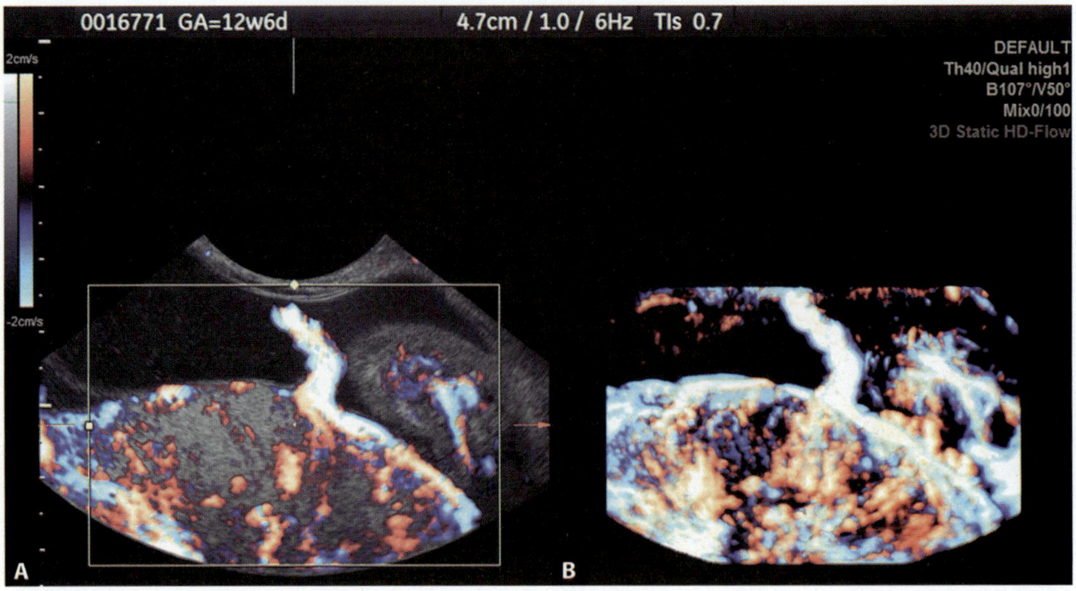

Figs. 33A and B: Placental circulation and umbilical cord at 12 weeks of gestation: (A; 2D HD power Doppler image; (B) 3D reconstructed bidirectional PD image. Rich vascularity inside placenta is visible.

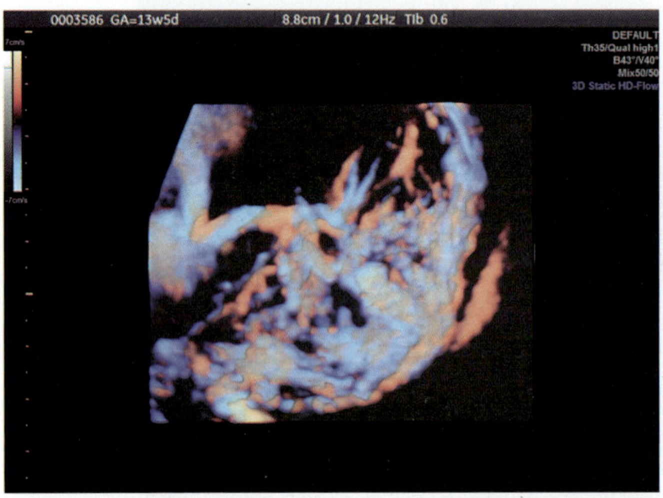

Fig. 34: Normal placenta—umbilical cord vascularity at 13 weeks.

It has been reported that abnormal size and/or shape of yolk sac may be associated with ominous pregnant outcome.[16] Large yolk sac is defined more than two standard deviations above the mean, which indicates over 5.6 mm of diameter at less than 10 weeks menstrual age.[16,17] Large yolk sac is associated with chromosomal aberration of autosomal trisomy **(Figs. 35 to 37)**. Echogenic yolk sac **(Figs. 38A and B)** is also related to adverse pregnant outcome with autosomal trisomy.

Prenatal Diagnosis of Anatomical Congenital Anomalies in the Human Embryo

The prenatal diagnosis of congenital anomalies with ultrasound is based upon identification of a substantial departure of normal anatomy. This has been possible in the second and third trimester of pregnancy, and this achievement has made the diagnosis of congenital anomalies one of the objectives of modern prenatal care. The definition of the "normal anatomy" of the human embryo provides the basis for the identification of congenital anomalies at the earliest stages of human development. This goes beyond the mere identification of nuchal translucency, because it is now possible to identify anomalies even in the absence of an abnormal nuchal translucency. Therefore, the scope of prenatal diagnosis during embryonic life has been widened by sonoembryology with three-dimensional ultrasound.[7]

Conjoined Twin

Conjoined twins are defined as monochorionic-monoamniotic twins fused at any portion of their body as a result of an incomplete division of the embryonic disk after the 13th day of conception. Pathogenesis of the condition is considered as the result from failure of complete separation. Careful observation in the first trimester can reveal this condition from the early pregnancy. **Figure 39A and B** demonstrate conjoined twin at 9 weeks of gestation. Three-dimensional ultrasound can objectively depict this rare abnormality.

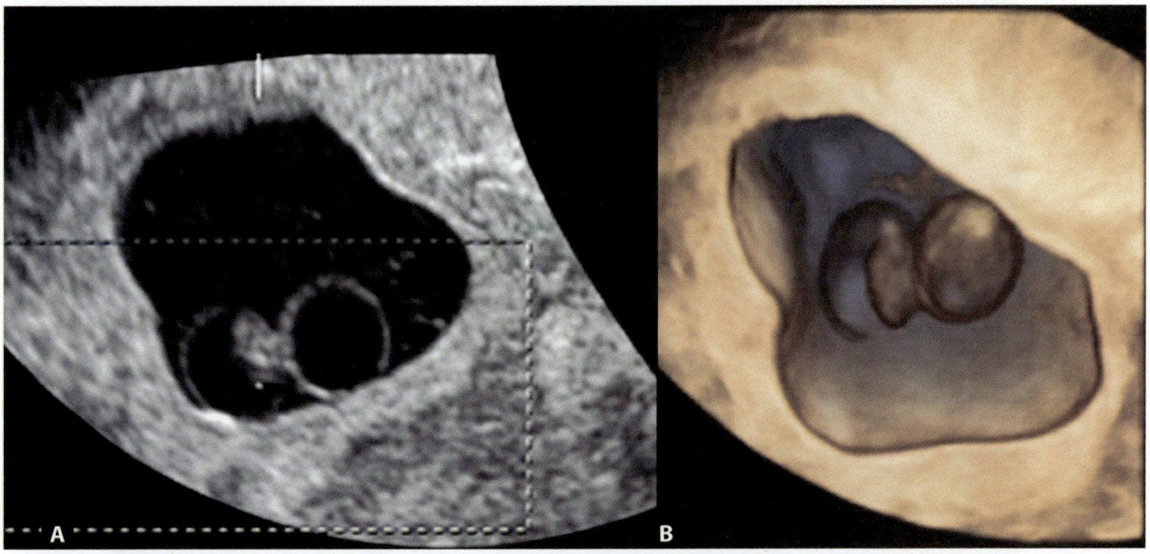

Figs. 35A and B: Large yolk sac: (A) 2D image; (B) 3D HDlive image. Large yolk sac is one of ominous signs of fetal loss.

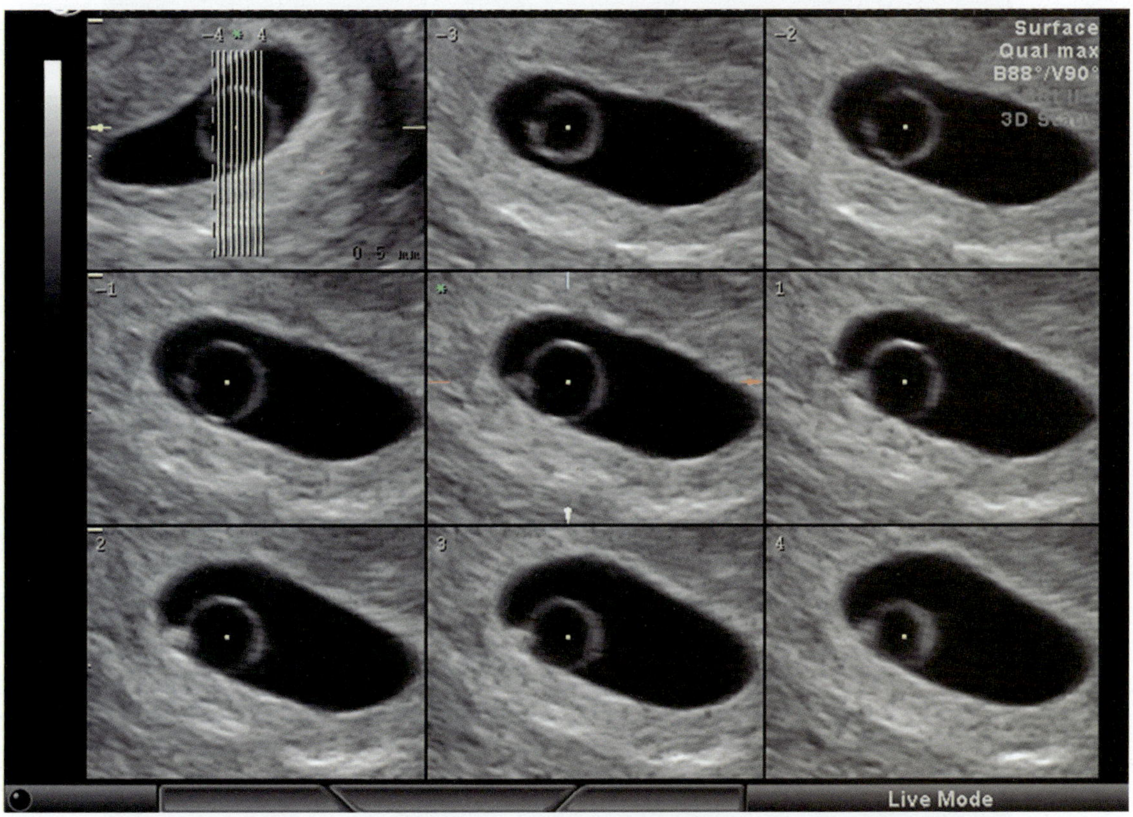

Fig. 36: Tomographic imaging of large yolk sac at 6 weeks of gestation. Large yolk sac with normal fetal heart beat was observed. Fetal demise was confirmed at 8 weeks. Villous chromosome exam resulted in 47,XY, +22.

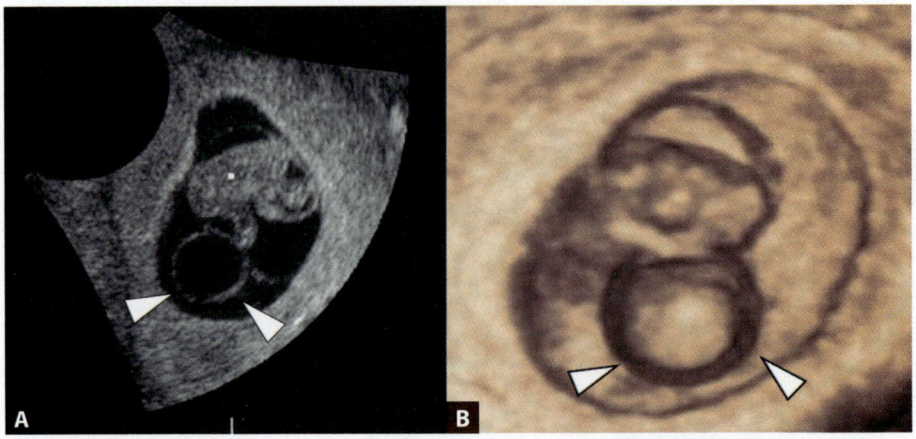

Figs. 37A and B: Large yolk sac (arrowheads) at 8 weeks of gestation. (A) 2D sagittal section of the fetus. Normal appearance of 8-week-fetus and amniotic membrane are visible, but large yolk sac with 12 mm of diameter is demonstrated; (B) 3D image. Intrauterine fetal demise was confirmed 30 hours later. Villous chromosome exam resulted in doubled trisomy of 48,XY, +15, +21.

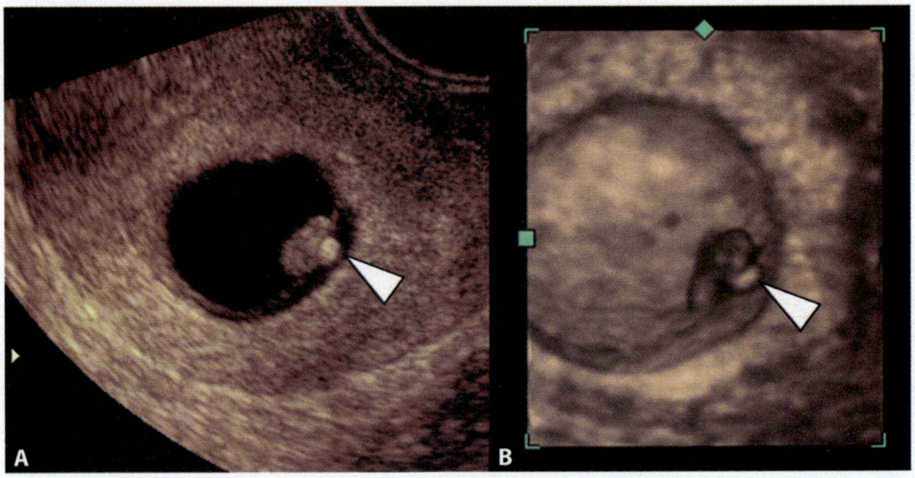

Figs. 38A and B: High echogenic yolk sac: (A) 2D ultrasound image of yolk sac (arrowhead) at 9 weeks and 1 day. Small embryo compatible with 7-week-embryo was visible with regular heart beats in the abnormally large amniotic sac; (B) 3D ultrasound image. Intrauterine fetal demise was confirmed 3 days later and villous chromosome was trisomy 15.

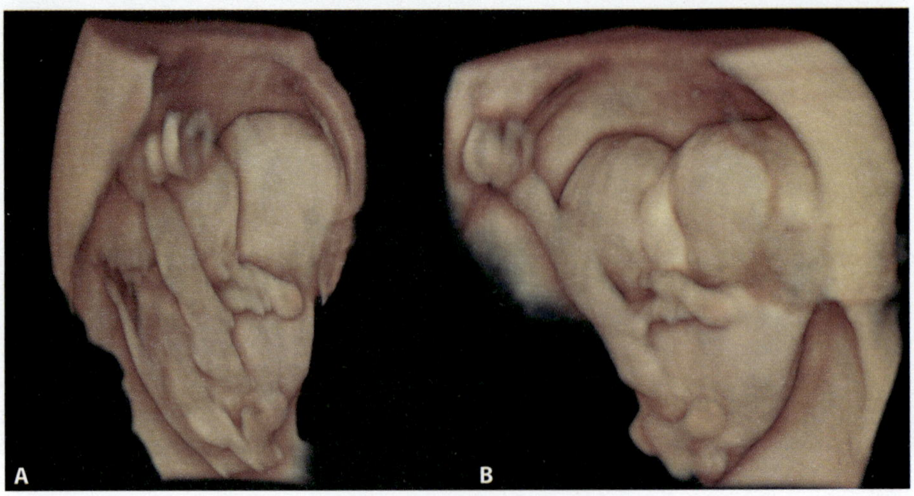

Figs. 39A and B: Conjoined at 9 weeks of gestation.

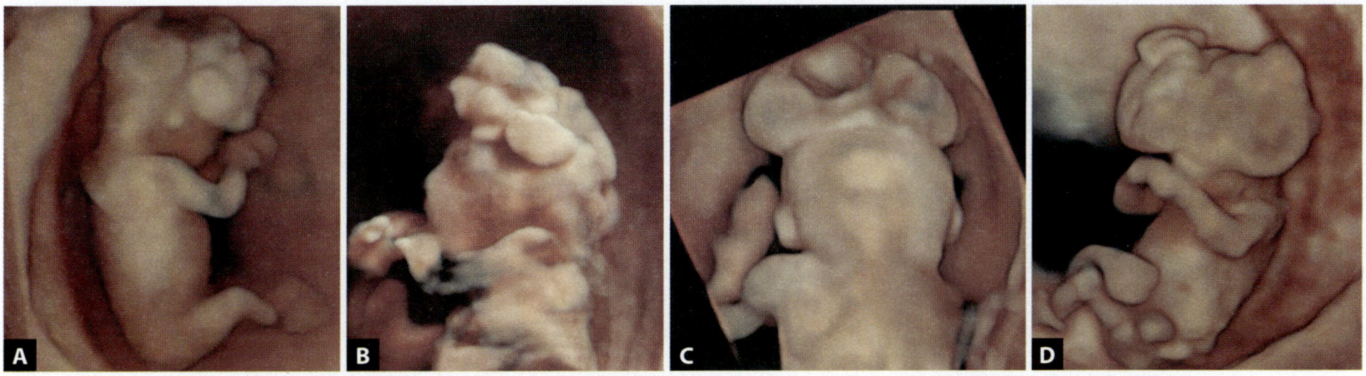

Figs. 40A to D: 3D images of various types of exencephaly in acranial cases between 10 and 12 weeks.

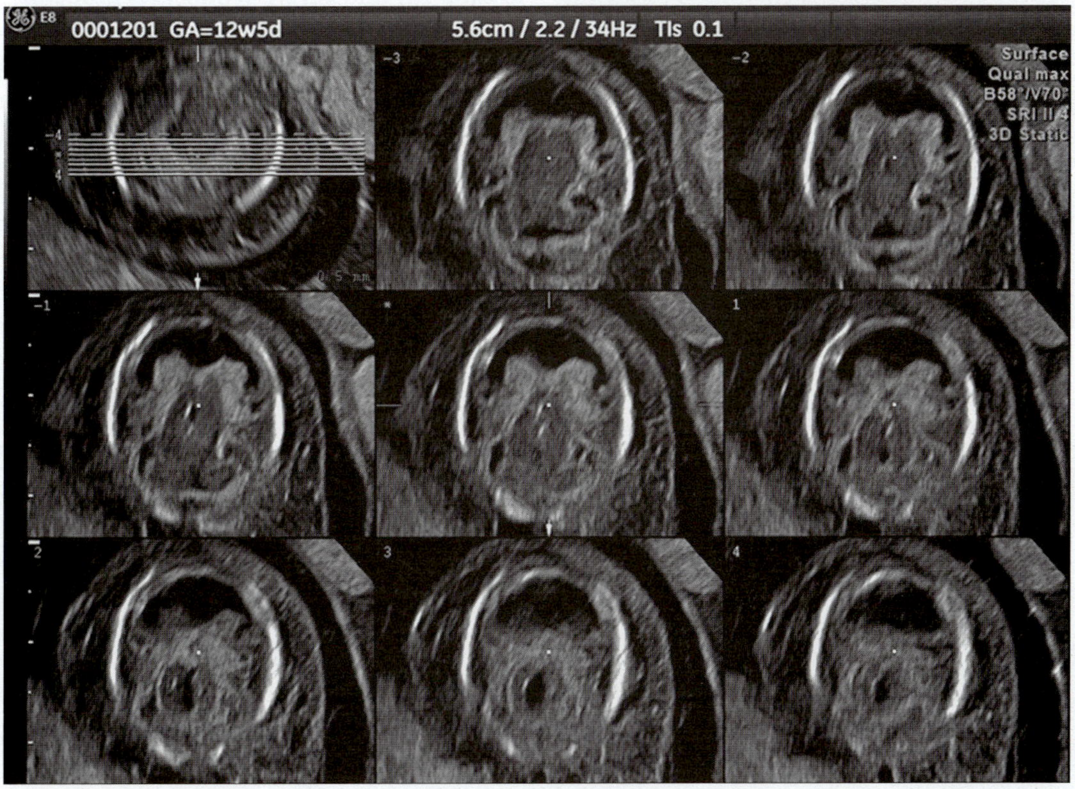

Fig. 41: Holoprosencephaly at 12 weeks of gestation. Tomographic ultrasound imaging shows a single ventricle due to non-separated hemispheres.

Central Nervous System (Cranium, Brain, Vertebra and Spinal Cord) Anomalies

Acrania, frequently found by early ultrasound scan, is characterized by a partial or complete absence of the cranium. The cranial shape and appearance vary, according to the extent of brain destruction. **Figures 40A to D** show various exencephalic appearances of acrania demonstrated by 3D reconstructed imaging. Holoprosencephaly can be detectable by careful observation of the midline and choroid plexus appearance **(Figs. 41 and 42)**. Occasionally, cephalocele is detectable as shown in **Figures 43A and B**.

Spina bifida is the most common congenital spinal cord anomaly. It is often detected during the second and third trimesters. However, the fundamental basis for this anomaly is a failure of the neural tube to close during early embryonic age. Most reports of the diagnosis of spina bifida in utero have occurred after 12 weeks of gestation. Blaas et al.[18] reported an early diagnosis using 2D and 3D ultrasound before 10 weeks of gestation. **Figures 44A and B** show the early diagnosis of spina bifida in a case of OEIS complex (omphalocele, bladder exstrophy, imperforate anus, spina bifida) at 9 weeks of gestation. 3D surface rendering image shown in **Figure 45A** is not enough for differentiating myelomeningocele from meningocele. A close observation in the sagittal section **(Fig. 45B)** is quite helpful because the spinal cord from spinal canal to the surface of myelomeningocele is clearly demonstrated. In the sagittal section of the head, absence of the intracranial translucency is a good ultrasound marker for suspecting spina bifida as shown in **Figures 46A and B**.

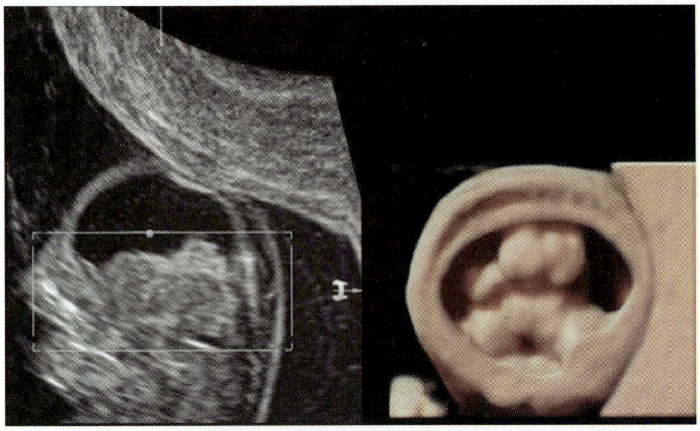

Fig. 42: Holoprosencephaly alobar type at 11 weeks of gestation.

Iniencephaly is a rare neural tube defect that combines extreme retroflexion (backward bending) of the head with severe defects of the spine, associated with acrania, anencephaly and encephalocele. The prognosis for those with iniencephaly is extremely poor. Early detection of iniencephaly is possible **(Figs. 47A and B)**. Scoliosis is often associated with limb body-wall complex **(Figs. 48 and 49)** and rarely scoliosis is associated with early vertebral fusion as shown in **Figures 50A to C**. Extreme hyper-dorsiflexion (backward bending) is a rare finding with unknown clinical significance. **Figures 51A to C** demonstrate extreme hyper-dorsiflexion seen in a case of trisomy 21.

Facial Abnormalities

A facial anomaly can be associated with a central nervous system anomaly (e.g., holoprosencephaly as shown in **Figures 52A to C**), be an isolated finding,

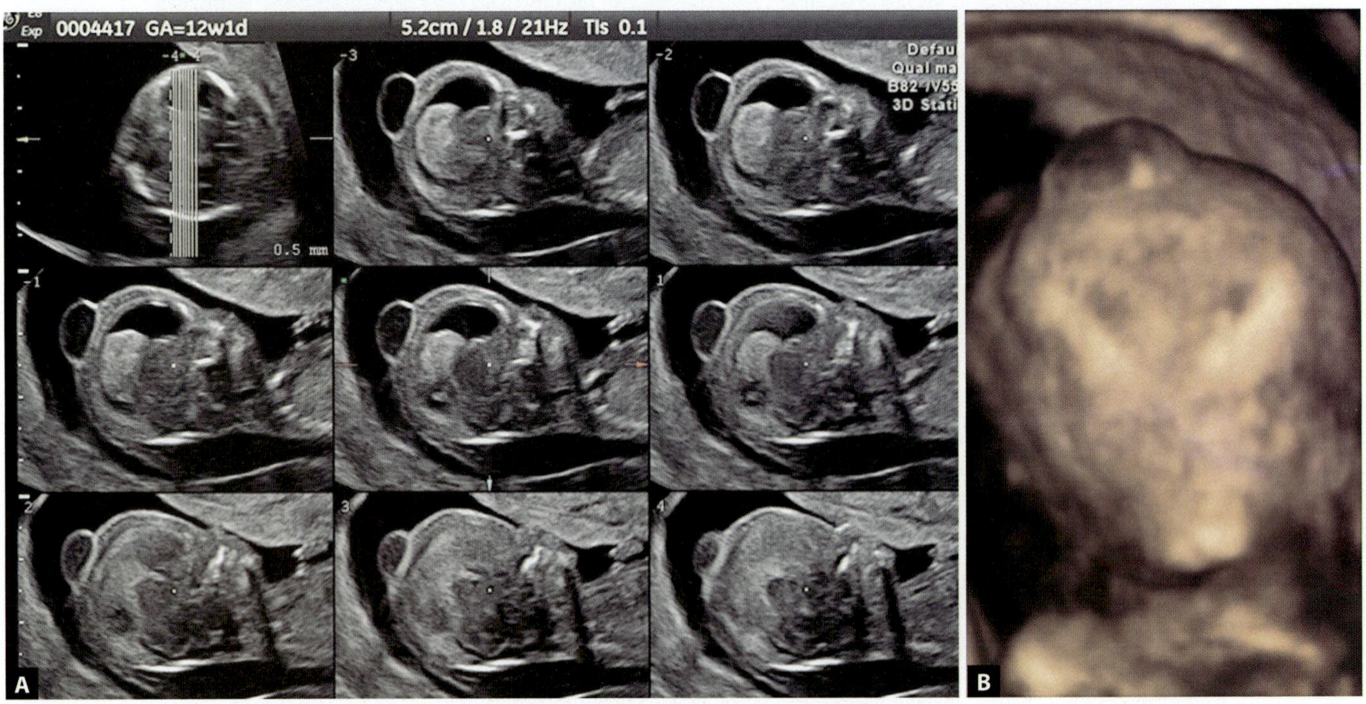

Figs. 43A and B: Cephalocele at 12 weeks of gestation. Cephalocele containing translucent fluid is seen on the parietal right side of the head. This cyst disappeared 2 weeks later.

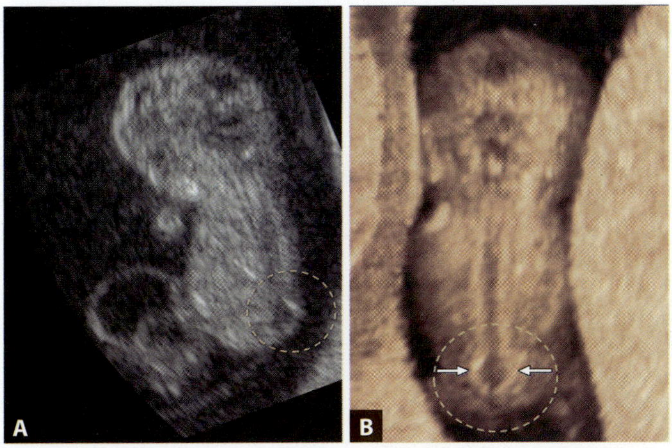

Figs. 44A and B: Spina bifida at 9 weeks of gestation: (A) 2D sagittal image. Cystic formation was seen (white circle) at lumbar part; (B) 3D image of neural tube. Clear dilatation of the neural tube is demonstrated (arrows).

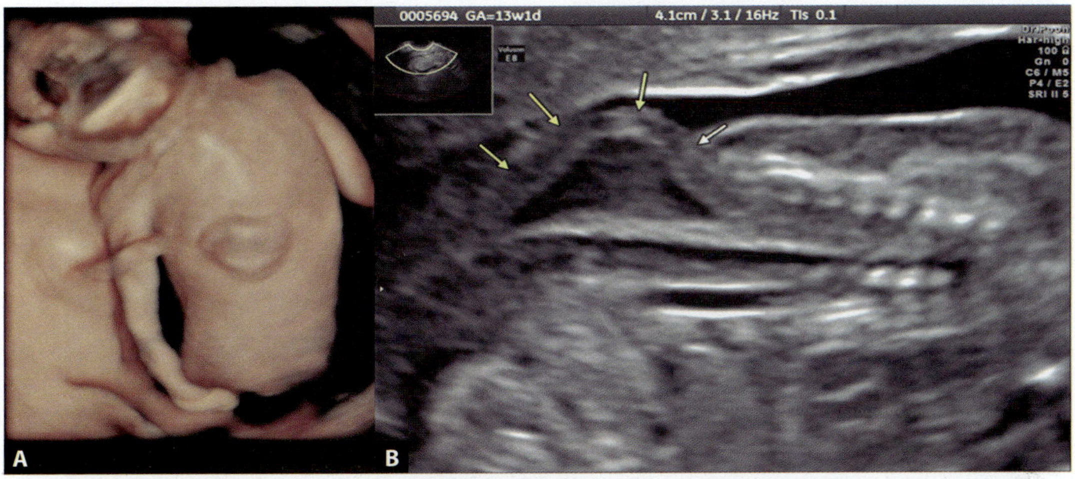

Figs. 45A and B: Myelomeningocele at 13 weeks of gestation: (A) 3D reconstructed image of fetal back; (B) 2D sagittal image. Ectopic spinal cord (arrows) is obvious.

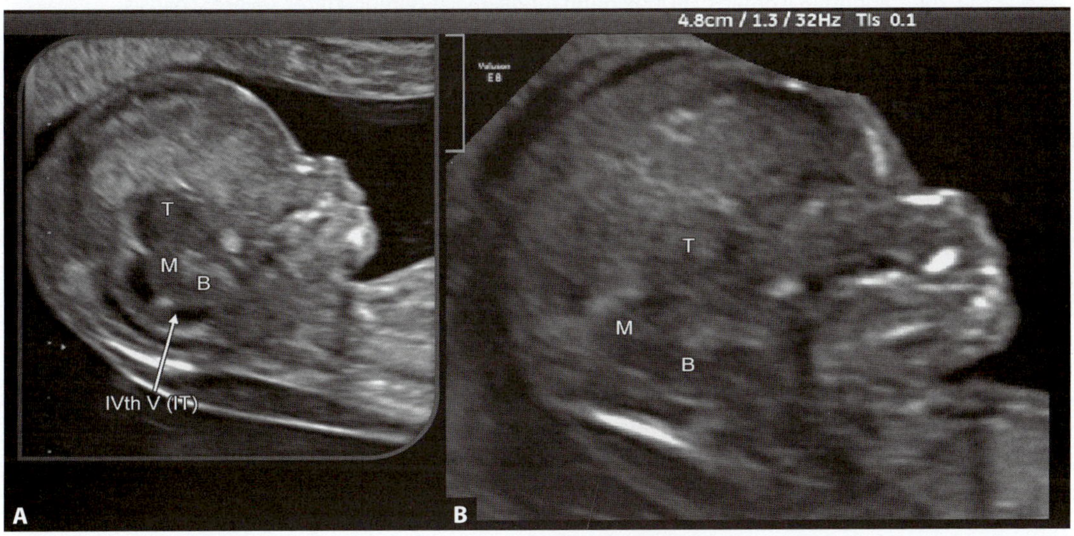

Figs. 46A and B: Disappearance of intracranial translucency (IT) in a case of spina bifida at 12 weeks: (A) Normal median structure; (B) Absence of IT.

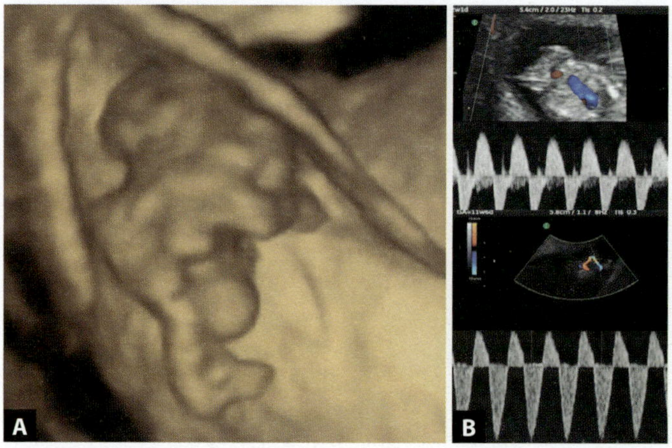

Figs. 47A and B: Iniencephaly at 12 weeks of gestation. (A) 3D reconstructed image. Acrania, short body with dorsiflexion are well demonstrated; (B) This fetus had reverse flows of descending aorta (upper) and umbilical artery (lower) and intrauterine fetal demise was confirmed 1 week later.

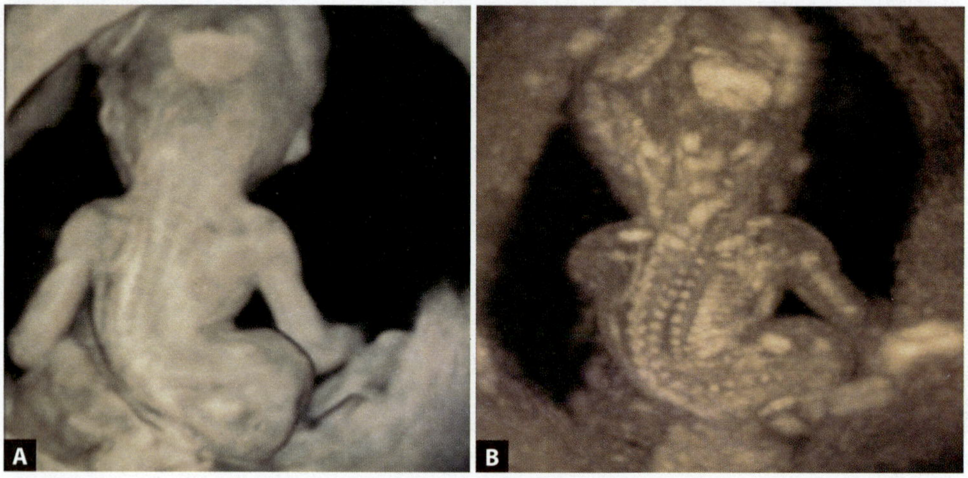

Figs. 48A and B: Body stalk anomaly with severe scoliosis at 13 weeks: (A) Conventional 3D surface image showing scoliosis with ectopic abdominal organs; (B) Maximum mode image demonstrates severe scoliosis.

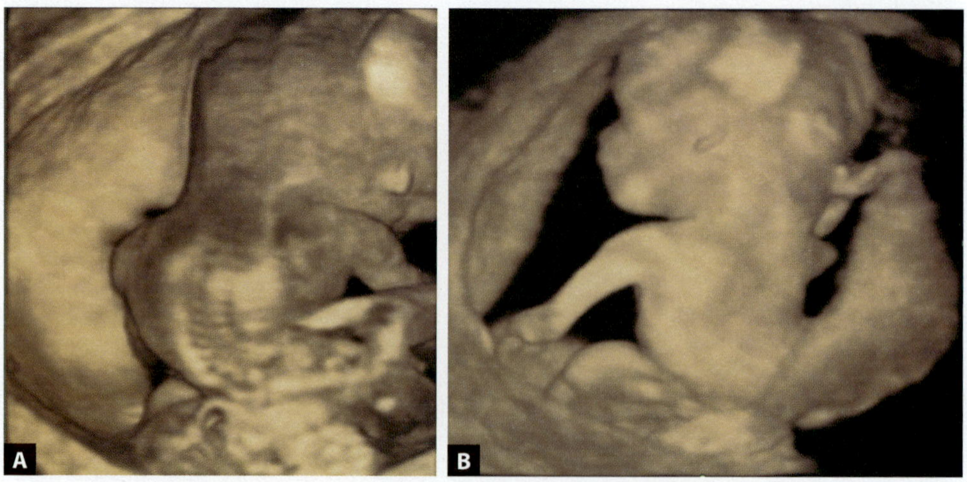

Figs. 49A and B: Body stalk anomaly with severe scoliosis at 13 weeks: (A) Maximum mode image demonstrates severe scoliosis with ectopic abdominal organs; (B) Conventional 3D surface image showing scoliosis.

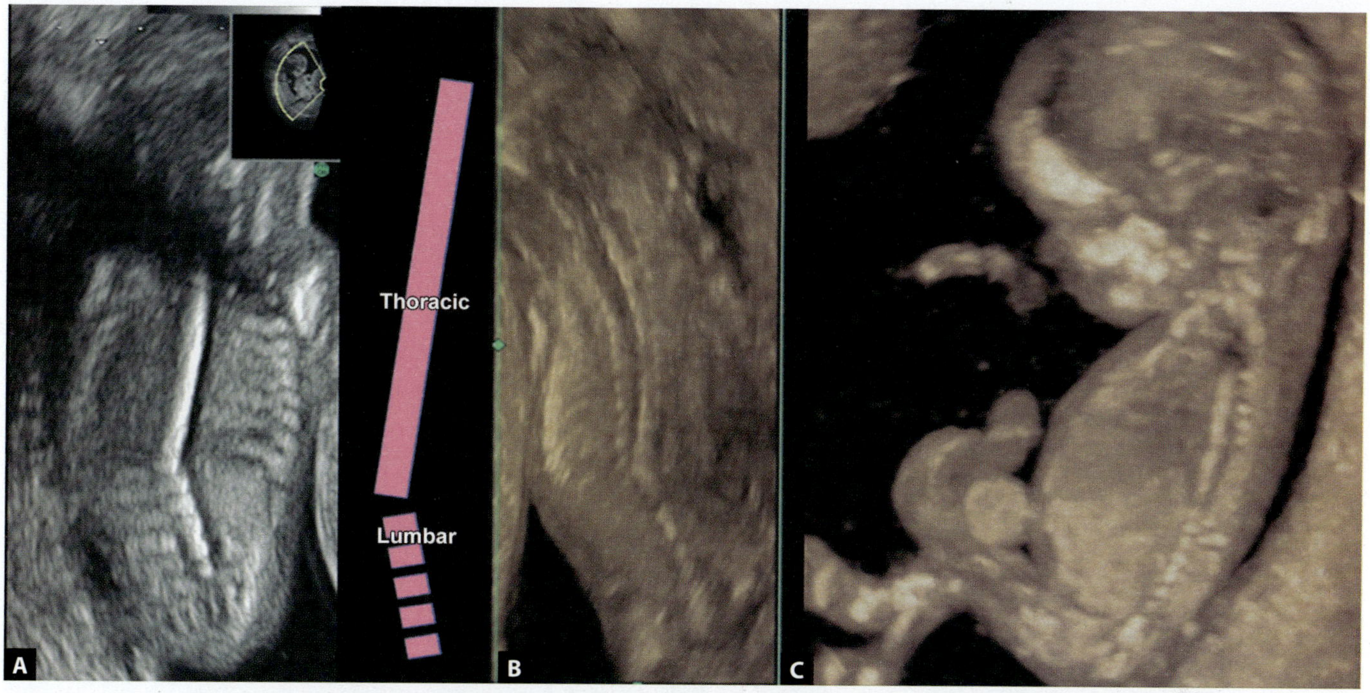

Figs. 50A to C: Fused thoracic vertebral body with scoliosis at 13 weeks of gestation: (A) 2D sagittal image. Thoracic vertebral body is completely fused while lumbar vertebral bodies are apart; (B) 3D maximum mode of dorsal view; (C) 3D maximum mode of lateral view.

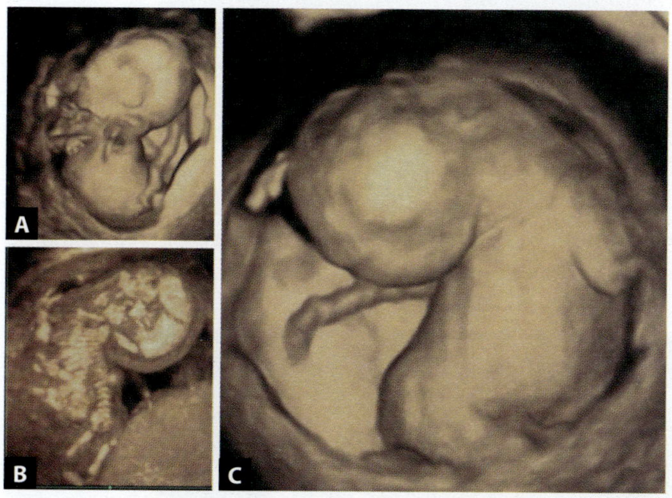

Figs. 51A to C: Extreme hyper-dorsiflexion seen in a case of trisomy 21 at 14 weeks of gestation: (A and C) 3D reconstructed oblique anterior and lateral views of the fetus; (B) 3D maximum mode demonstrating bony structure.

or part of a syndrome. Detection of the presence or absence of a nasal bone has been found to be of value in the assessment of aneuploidy in the first trimester of pregnancy (risk assessment for trisomy 21).[19-23] Cicero et al. reported that the nasal bone was absent in 113 (0.6%) of the 20,165 chromosomally or phenotypically normal fetuses and in 87 (62.1%) of the 140 fetuses with trisomy 21.[23] 3D sonography allows a mid-sagittal section of the fetal face to be obtained by utilizing the three orthogonal planes, and avoids the pitfall of obtaining a parasagittal view, which could lead to false-negative results. Tomographic ultrasound imaging also allows demonstration of facial midline structures in detail, by examining close parallel sections **(Figs. 53A and B)**. It is important to be aware that the quality of the orthogonal planes or tomographic imaging **(Fig. 54)** is strongly dependent upon the original plane of acquisition. Rembouskos et al.[24] described that routine application of 3D scanning for the nasal bone in screening for trisomy 21 is likely to be associated with a very high false-positive rate due to the possible limits of 3D technology. Benoit and Chaoui[25] described the diagnosis of bilateral or unilateral absence or hypoplasia of nasal bones in second trimester screening for Down syndrome by using 3D sonography with maximal mode rendering. **Figures 55A to C** show the midsagittal section of fetal face and craniofacial bony reconstructed image of normal fetus and trisomy 21 fetuses in the first trimester.

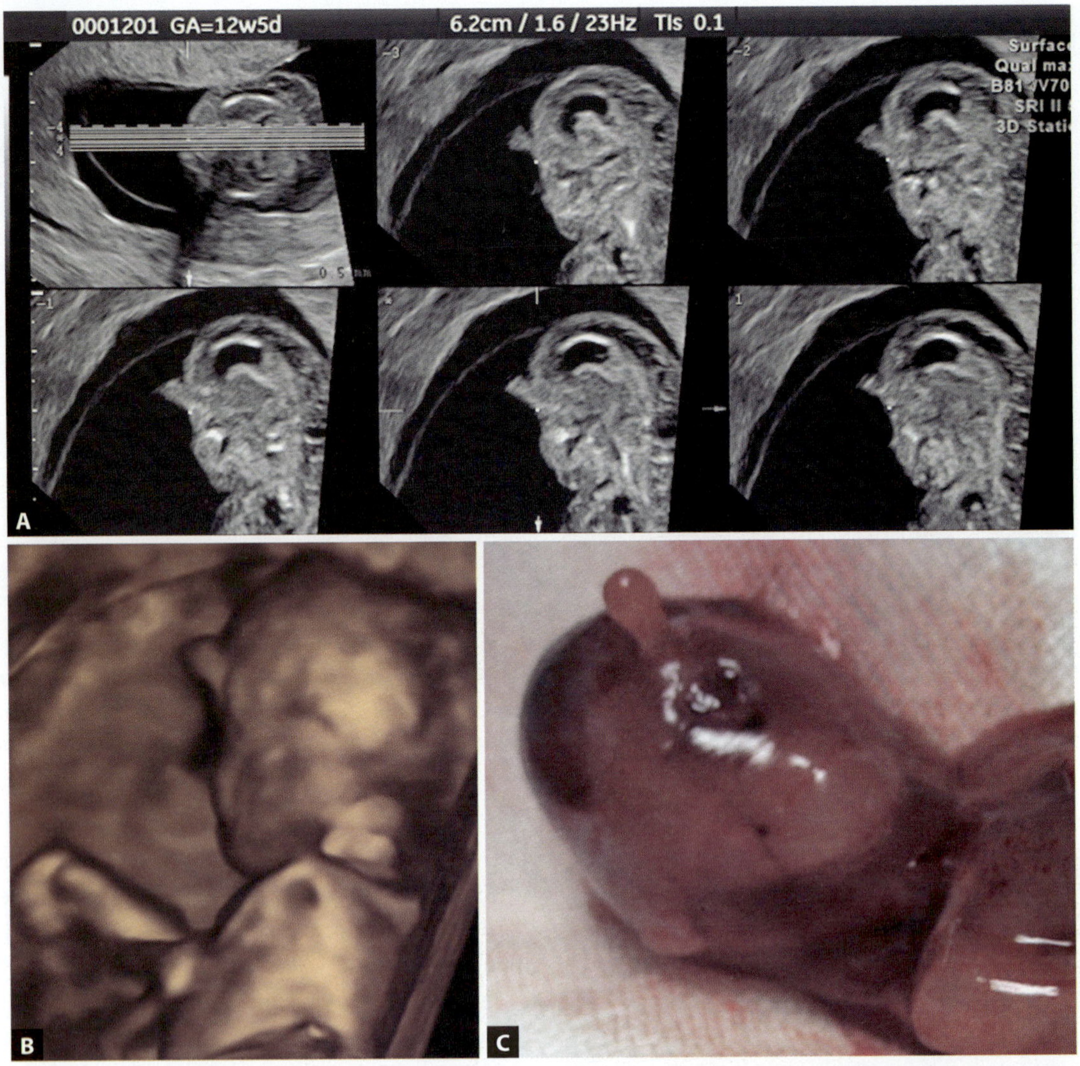

Figs. 52A to C: Proboscis associated with holoprosencephaly at 12 weeks of gestation: (A) Tomographic facial sagittal imaging of holoprosencephalic fetus; (B) 3D reconstructed image of fetal face, lateral view; (C) Macroscopic picture after termination of pregnancy.

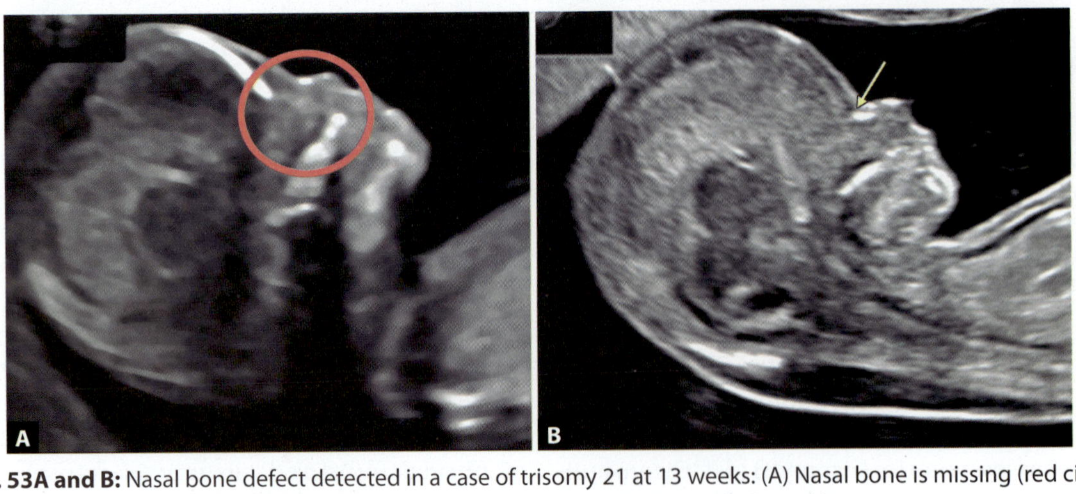

Figs. 53A and B: Nasal bone defect detected in a case of trisomy 21 at 13 weeks: (A) Nasal bone is missing (red circle); (B) Normal case for comparison. Arrow indicates normal nasal bone.

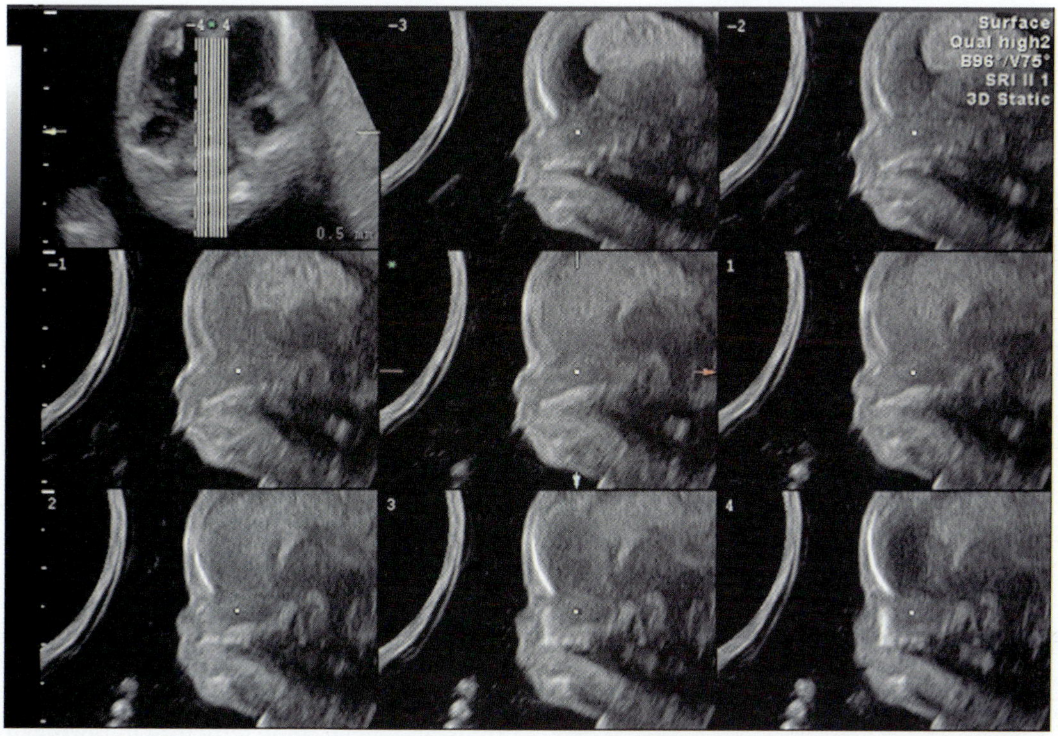

Fig. 54: Tomographic ultrasound image of fetal profile with hypoplastic nasal bone at the end of 13 weeks of gestation. Thinly sliced parallel cutting section of mid-sagittal plane shows fetal profile in detail and hypoplastic nasal bone. Trisomy 21 was confirmed by CVS.

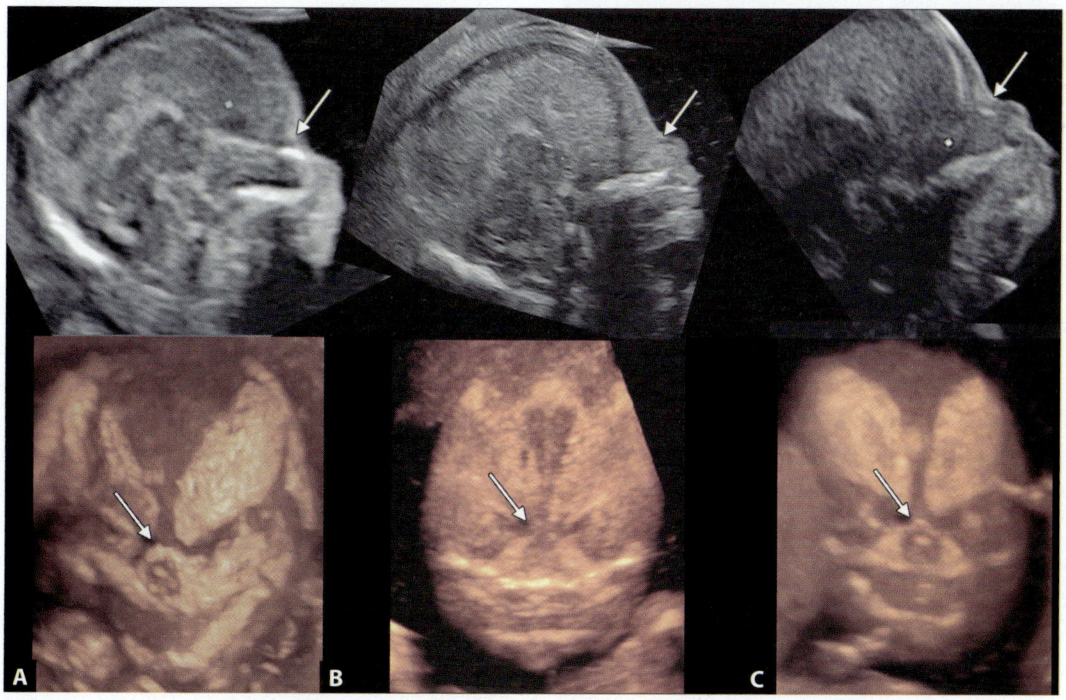

Figs. 55A to C: Mid-sagittal 2D image of fetal profile and craniofacial bony reconstructed image of normal fetus (A) and trisomy 21 fetuses (B and C) at 13–14 weeks of gestation. (A) Normal fetus. Nasal bone is clearly visualized in both 2D and 3D images (arrows); (B) Nasal bone defect in a case of trisomy 21. Nasal bone is completely missing in both 2D and 3D; (C) Nasal bone hypoplasia in a case of trisomy 21. Small nasal bone is visualized in both 2D and 3D.

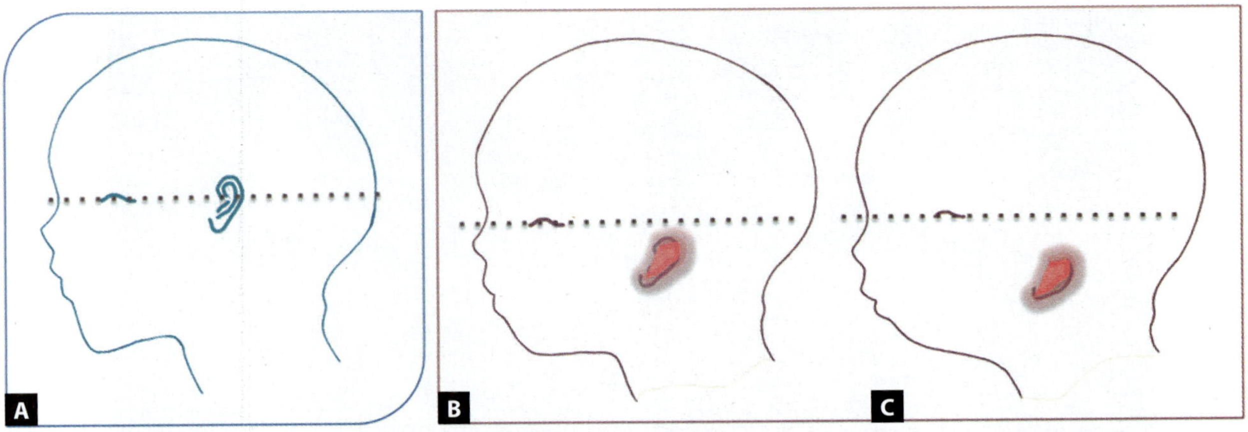

Figs. 56A to C: Schematic picture of low-set ear associated with micrognathia; (A) Normal ear position with normal jaw development after 11 weeks of gestation; (B) Low-set ear with micrognathia; (C) Shows more premature type of low-set ear and micrognathia. Micrognathia is often associated with low-set ears. If the line is drawn from the outer canthus of the eye straight back to the occiput (blue dot lines), a low-set ear will fall completely below the line.

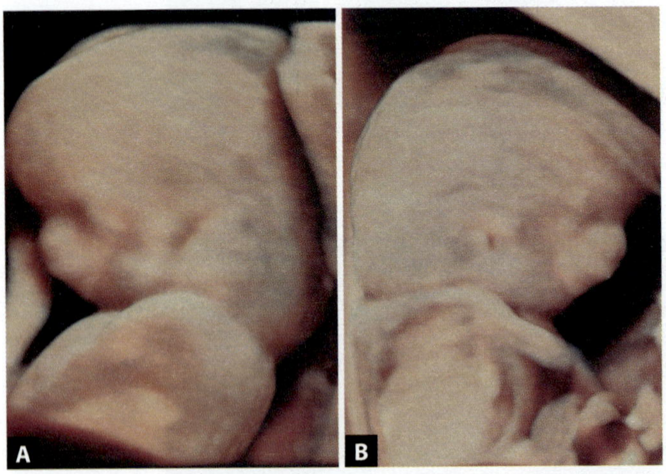

Figs. 57A and B: Low-set ear and micrognathia in cases of trisomy 18 at 12 weeks of gestation. HDlive images demonstrating typical trisomy 18 facial appearance.

A short maxillary length has been associated with trisomy 21.[26] Micrognathia can be detected as an isolated structural anomaly, as one of the features of a chromosomal abnormality, or a syndrome.[27] Congenital micrognathia and lowest ears are frequently detected together as shown in **Figures 56 to 59**, in cases with chromosomal aberrations and other syndromic diseases, because mandibula and ears arises from the first pharyngeal (branchial) arch. However, bilateral ear development is not always symmetrical and occasionally asymmetrical ear development is seen as demonstrated in **Figures 60A and B**. Assessment of the facial features, chin development and mandibular size by 3D ultrasound in the second and third trimesters has been reported.[28] By using the surface mode and maximum mode (**Figs. 61A to D**), the fetal profile and facial bone structure in normal and abnormal fetuses can be described in the first trimester.

Cleft lip and palate is usually demonstrated and diagnosed in the second and third trimesters. However, 3D imaging has provided accurate and informative diagnostic images of cleft lip (**Figs. 62 and 63**). Furthermore, 3D tomographic ultrasound imaging can provide the precise demonstration of palate shown in **Figures 63 and 64**. In the 2D mid-sagittal cutting section without 3D technology, the maxilla bone appearance may be helpful for suspecting the presence of cleft palate (**Figs. 65A and B**).

Eye abnormality is often associated with holoprosencephaly (**Figs. 66A and B**). Eyeballs and lenses are detectable by ultrasound from the late first trimester. Cataract is defined by the presence of any lens opacity. The incidence of congenital cataract ranges from 1 to 6 newborn infants out of 10,000 births.[29] Cataract development is strongly linked to the embryonic ocular development. The lens differentiates from the surface ectoderm before the 6th week of gestation, explaining the absence of cataract in case of late first-trimester fetal infection.[30,31] A genetic cause is responsible for 30% of unilateral cataracts and 50% of bilateral cataracts. Prenatal diagnosis of fetal cataract was reported in the late second and third pregnancy.[32-36] **Figures 67A and B** show fetal bilateral cataract with microphthalmia as early as 14 weeks of gestation.

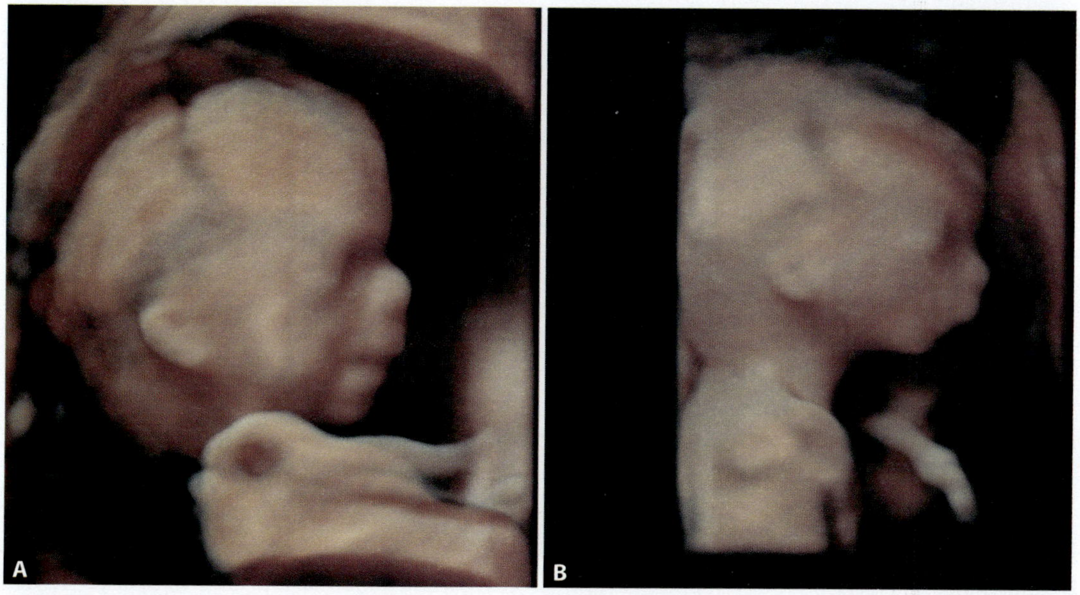

Figs. 58A and B: Low-set ear associated with micrognathia by 3D ultrasound images. Two cases with low-set ear and micrognathia. Micrognathia is often associated with low-set ears. If the line is drawn from the outer canthus of the eye straight back to the occiput, a low-set ear will fall completely below the line. Low-set ear cannot be detected by conventional 2D ultrasound technique. Only 3D ultrasound can detect low-set ears. Recent advanced technology demonstrates low-set ear in the first trimester.

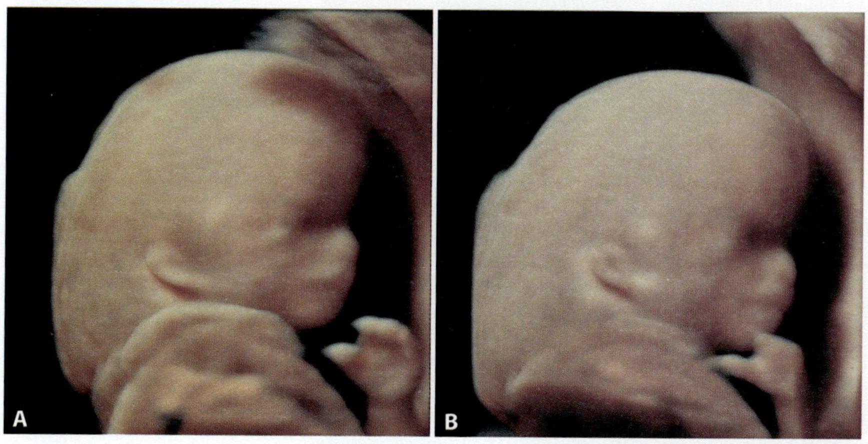

Figs. 59A and B: Micrognathia and low-set ears at 12 weeks of gestation. Both images are from the same fetus. Micrognathia and low set ears are clearly demonstrated by 3D reconstructed images.

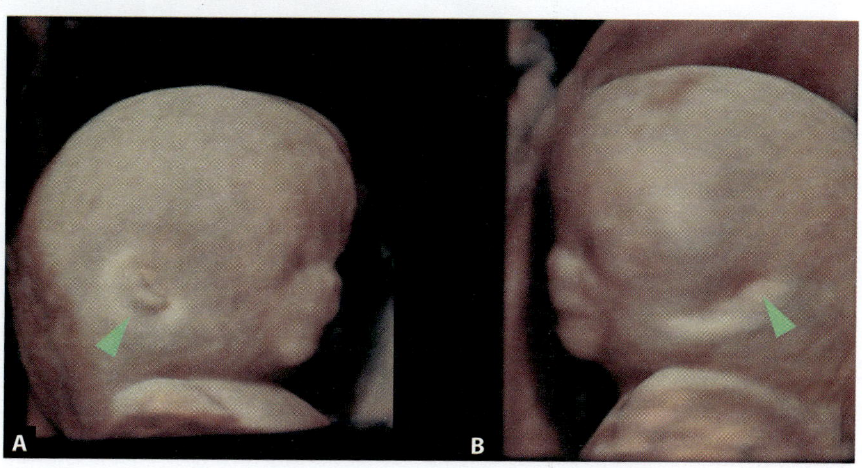

Figs. 60A and B: Asymmetrical ear development. (A) Low-set ear of the right ear; (B) Low-set and hypoplastic ear of the left ear in the same fetus.

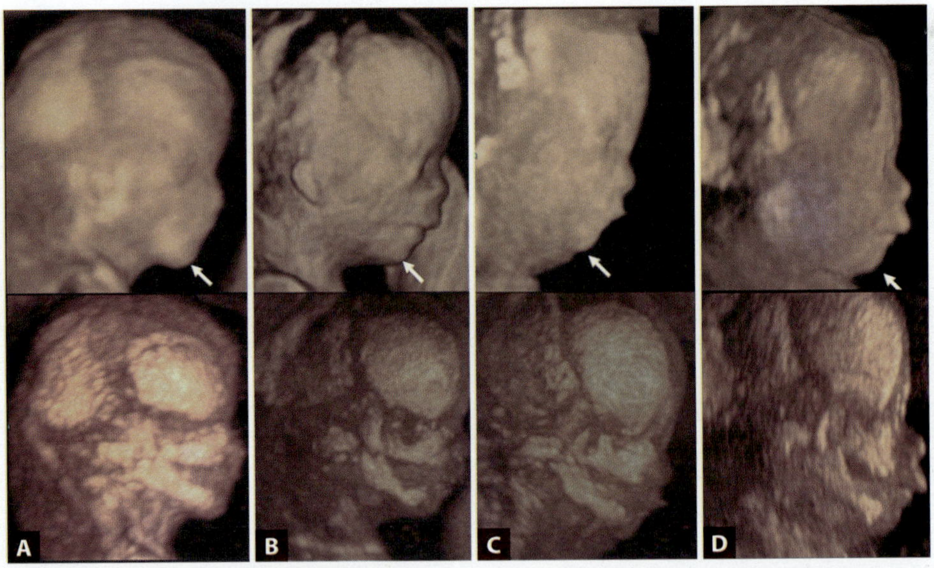

Figs. 61A to D: Fetal profile and facial bone development in normal fetus (A) and abnormal fetuses (B to D) at 12–13 weeks of gestation. (A) Normal fetus; (B) Trisomy 21 fetus; (C) Trisomy 18 fetus; (D) Mild micrognathia with normal chromosome. Lateral views of fetal profile (upper Figures) show the difference of chin-angle. Maximum mode images (lower Figures) indicate the hypoplastic maxilla and mandible in B to D.

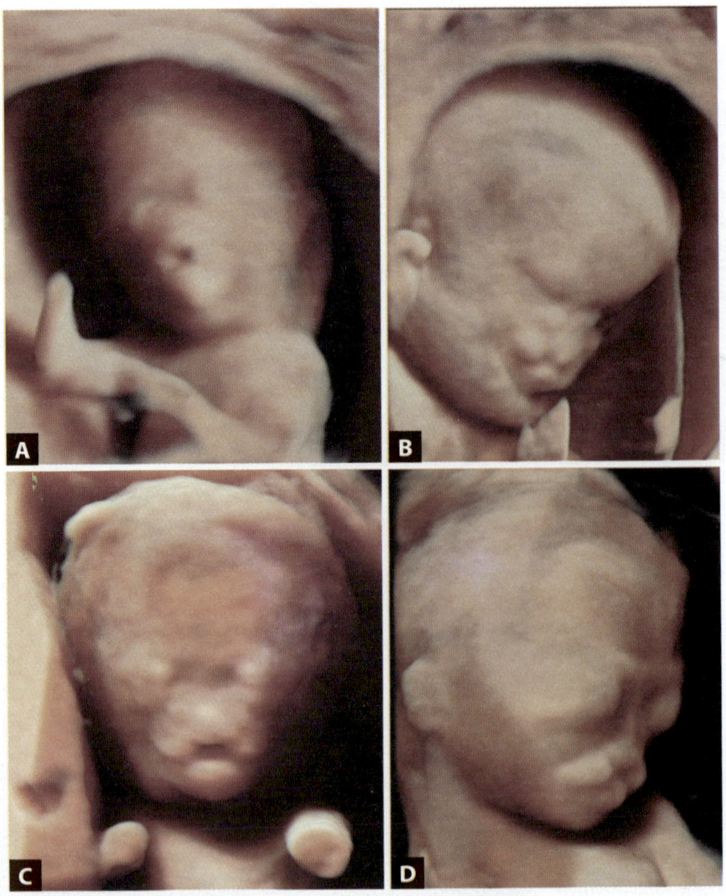

Figs. 62A to D: HDlive images of fetal face with bilateral or middle cleft lip in 4 cases of trisomy 13 with holoprosencephaly at 12–13 weeks.

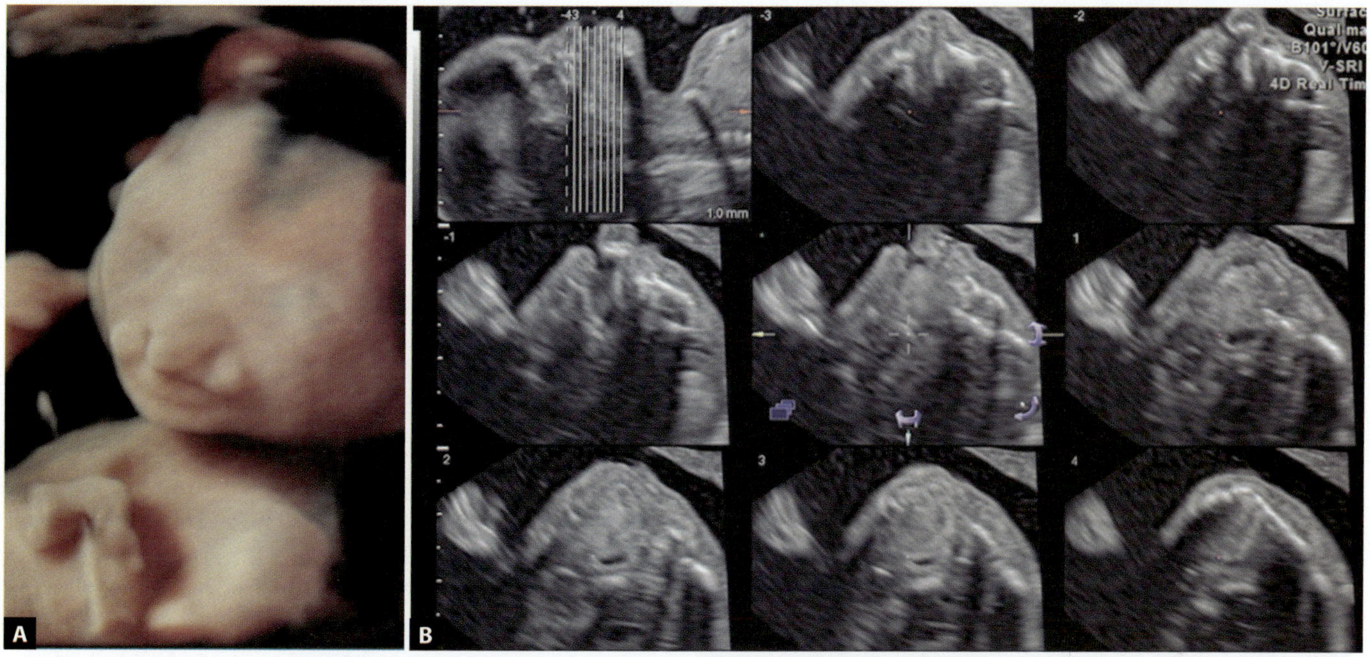

Figs. 63A and B: Bilateral cleft lip/palate seen in a case with multiple anomalies: (A) 3D HDlive image of bilateral cleft lip; (B) TUI demonstrates hypoplastic palate. Cardiac anomaly (common AV canal) and ectrodactyly were found in this case with normal karyotype.

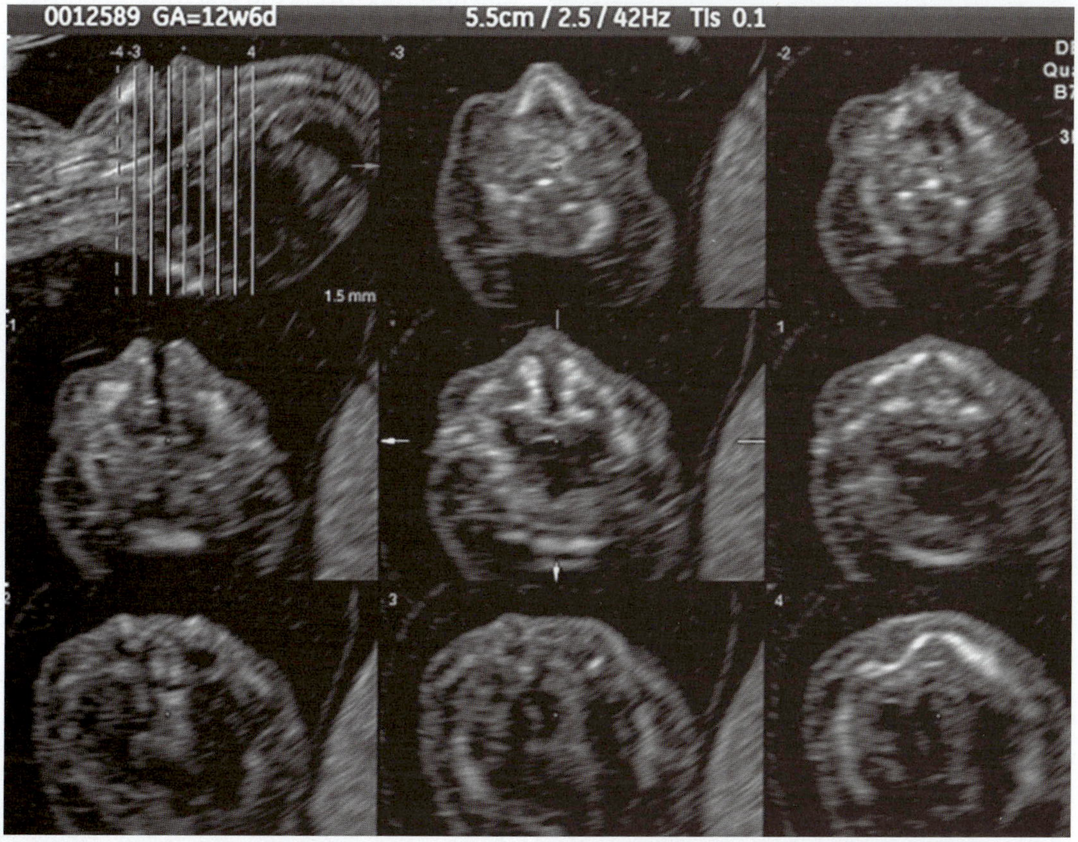

Fig. 64: Cleft lip/palate seen in a case of holoprosencephaly at 12 weeks. TUI demonstrates a central wide defect of maxilla bone (arrow) indicating cleft palate.

Limb Abnormalities

Limb abnormalities can occur as isolated findings or as one component of a syndrome or sequence. However, only 5% of congenital hand anomalies occur as part of a recognized syndrome.[37] Overlapping fingers, wrist contracture (**Figs. 68A and B**) and forearm deformities are often associated with a chromosomal abnormality such as trisomy 18. Most skeletal anomalies are recognizable in the second trimester. However, several reports on congenital skeletal abnormalities (such as sirenomelia and others) in the first trimester have been documented.[38-42] Short limb abnormality in the first trimester was shown in **Figures 69 and 70**. **Figures 71A to C** show an 11 weeks fetus with elbow joint abnormality of the bilateral upper limbs and normal lower extremities. Clubfoot as shown in **Figures 72A to D** is not common in the first trimester. Finger and toe abnormalities such as polydactyly, oligodactyly and syndactyly, are detectable by 3D ultrasound (**Figs. 73 and 74**).

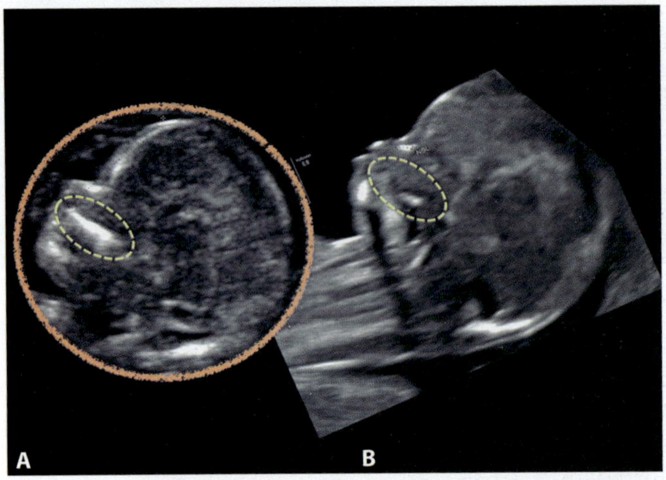

Figs. 65A and B: 2D profile showing cleft palate at 12 weeks of gestation. (A) Normal maxilla bone in a normal case; (B) No maxilla bone is detected in the mid-sagittal section due to the central part of cleft palate.

Thoracoabdominal Abnormalities

Congenital diaphragmatic hernia (CDH) occurs in 1 of every 2,000–4,000 live births and accounts for 8% of all major congenital anomalies.[43] There are three types of CDH; posterolateral or Bochdalek hernia (occurring at approximately 6 weeks of gestation), the anterior Morgagni hernia, and a hiatus hernia. The left-sided Bochdalek hernia occurs in approximately 90% of cases. Left-sided hernias allow herniation of both small and large bowel as well as intra-abdominal solid organs into the thoracic cavity. Early diagnosis of CDH in the first trimester has been reported.[44] **Figures 75A and B** show the thoracoabdominal area of a fetus with a congenital diaphragmatic defect where the lung-liver borderline acutely changes its angle from 13 to 15 weeks, due to progressive liver upward movement into the chest. Early diagnosis of this defect is important.[44]

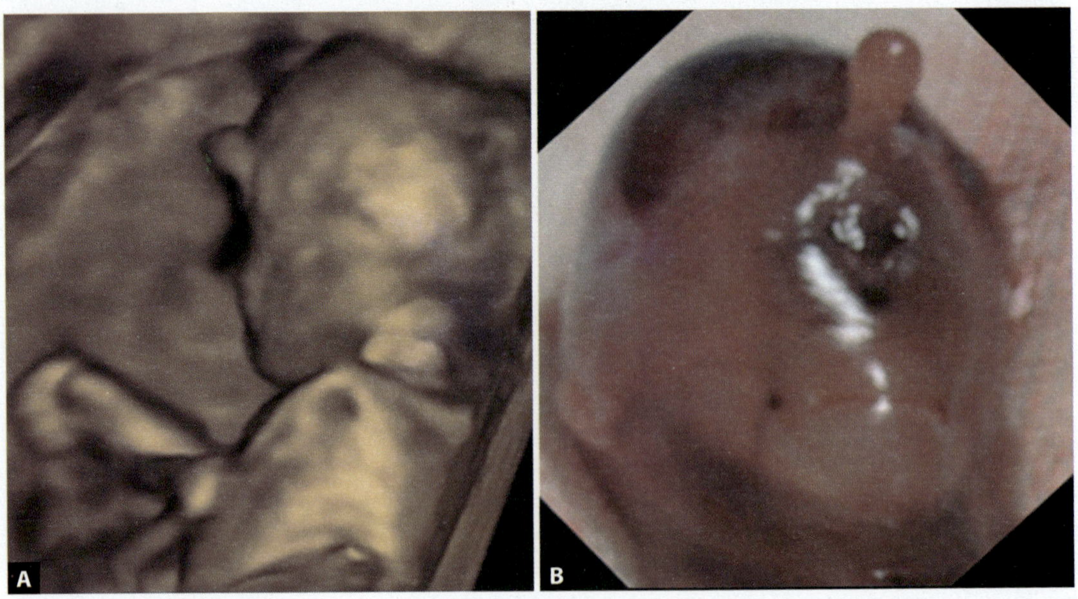

Figs. 66A and B: Cyclops and proboscis seen in a case of holoprosencephaly at 11 weeks. 3D image (A) and aborted fetus (B).

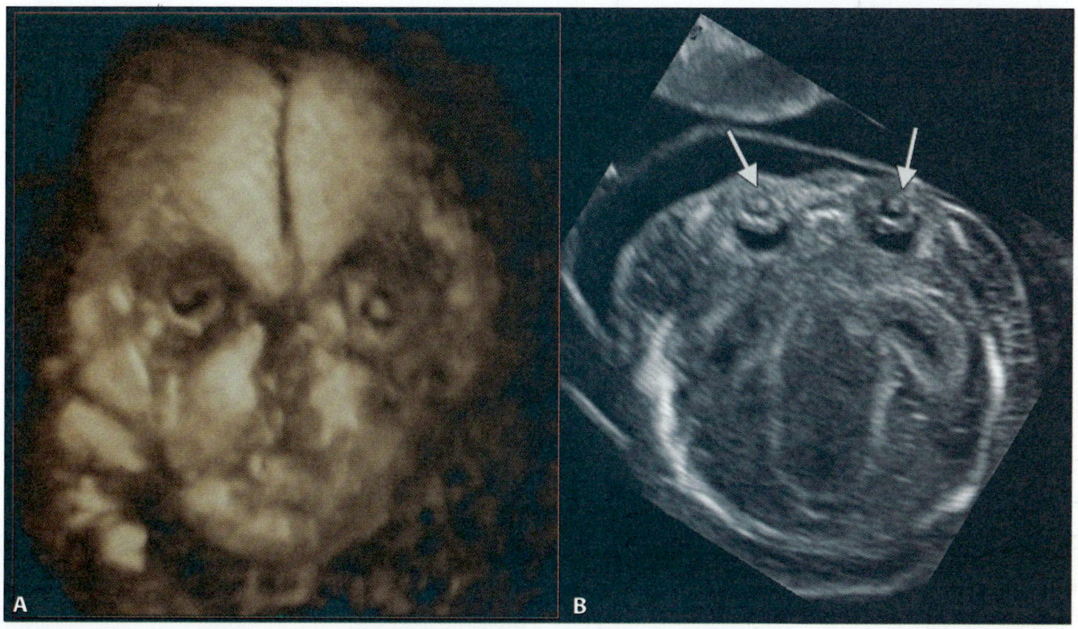

Figs. 67A and B: Congenital cataract at 14 weeks of gestation. Bilateral congenital cataract with microphthalmia is demonstrated as lens opacity (arrows) in 3D (A) and 2D (B) images.

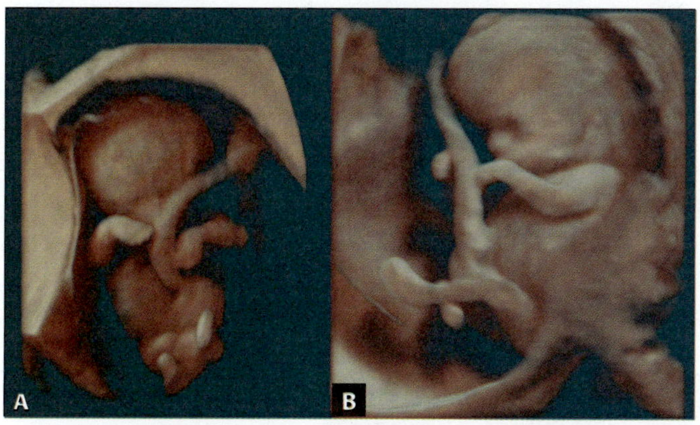

Figs. 68A and B: Mild-to-moderate wrist contracture seen in cases of trisomy 18 at 12–13 weeks of gestation.

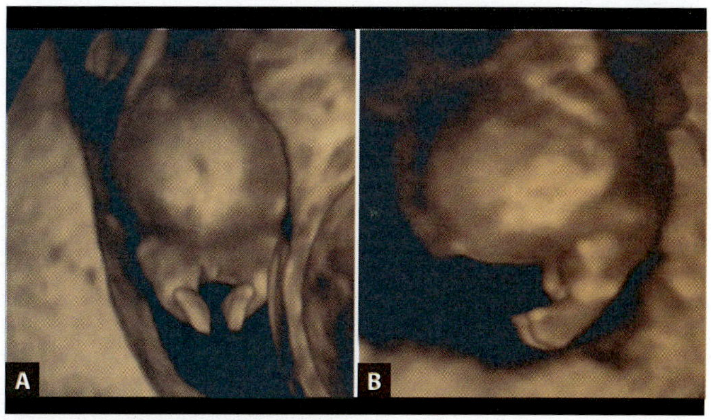

Figs. 69A and B: Short limb abnormality at 13 weeks of gestation. Short lower extremities with large abdomen is clearly demonstrated in the frontal (A) and lateral (B) views.

Omphalocele is often seen from the first trimester. Physiological umbilical hernia is usually observed around 8–10 weeks of gestation, however, umbilical hernia seen after the beginning of 12 weeks is definitely pathological **(Figs. 76 and 77)**. Ectopic abdominal organs outside of amniotic cavity is often associated with short umbilical cord, abnormal limbs and this condition is called as short umbilical cord complex, limb body-wall complex or body-stalk anomaly as shown in **Figures 78 to 81**, different from amniotic band syndrome.

Urinary Tract Abnormality

Bladder exstrophy **(Figs. 82A and B)** is a rare abnormality, which may be associated with cloaca malformation or the OEIS (omphalocele, bladder exstrophy, imperforate anus, spine defect) complex. Prune-Belly syndrome **(Figs. 83 to 85)** describes the triad of dilation of the urinary tract, a deficiency of the abdominal wall musculature, and failure of testicular descent. Hydronephrosis is the most common pathologic finding in the urinary tract on

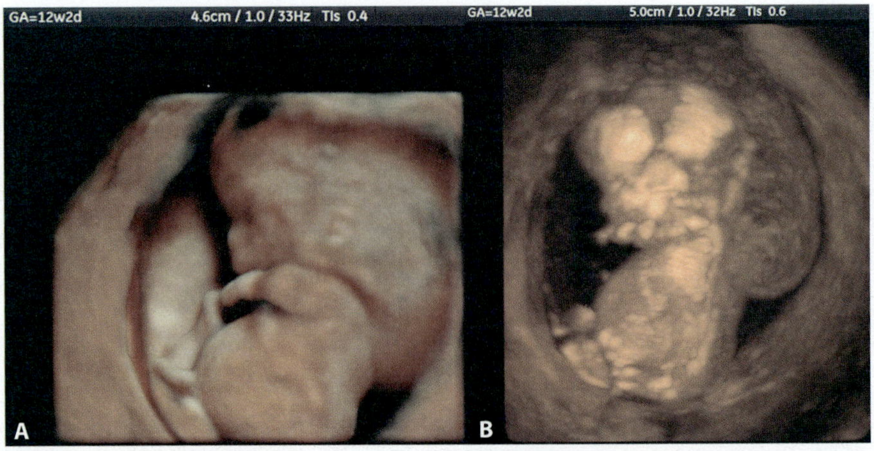

Figs. 70A and B: Short limbs at 12 weeks of gestation. Extremely short arms in early pregnancy.

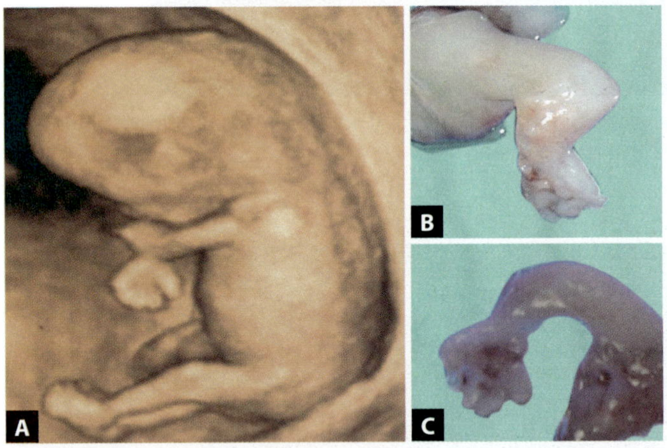

Figs. 71A to C: Upper limb abnormality at 11 weeks of gestation. (A) 3D ultrasound revealed contracted elbow joint abnormality; (B and C) Show macroscopic appearance of upper limbs of aborted fetus.

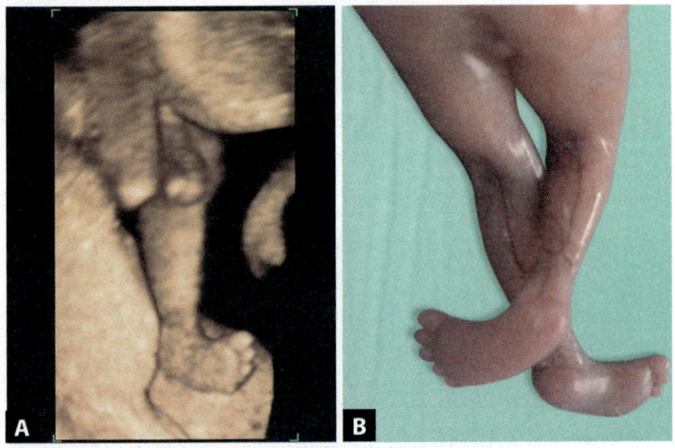

Figs. 72A and B: Fetal clubfoot at 13 weeks of gestation (A) 3D image of fetal leg; (B) Legs of aborted fetus. This case was associated with chromosomal aberration.

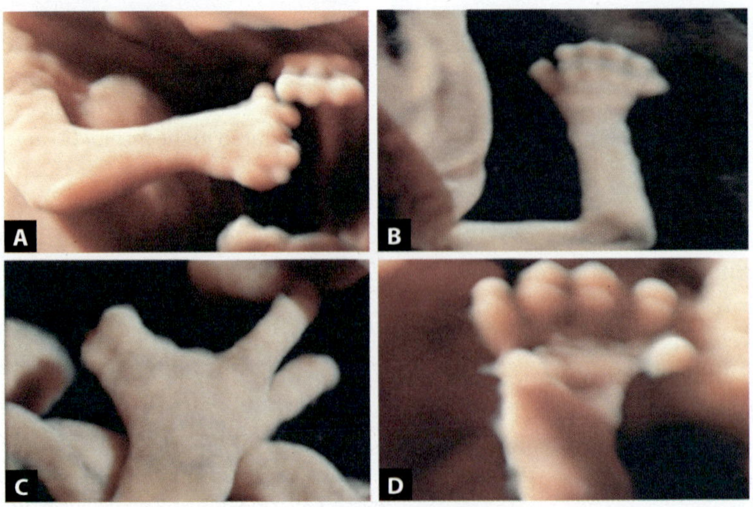

Figs. 73A to D: 3D HDlive images of finger abnormality at 12–14 weeks of gestation. (A) Hypoplastic fingers; (B) Polydactyly; (C) Oligodactyly with syndactyly; (D) Polydactyly.

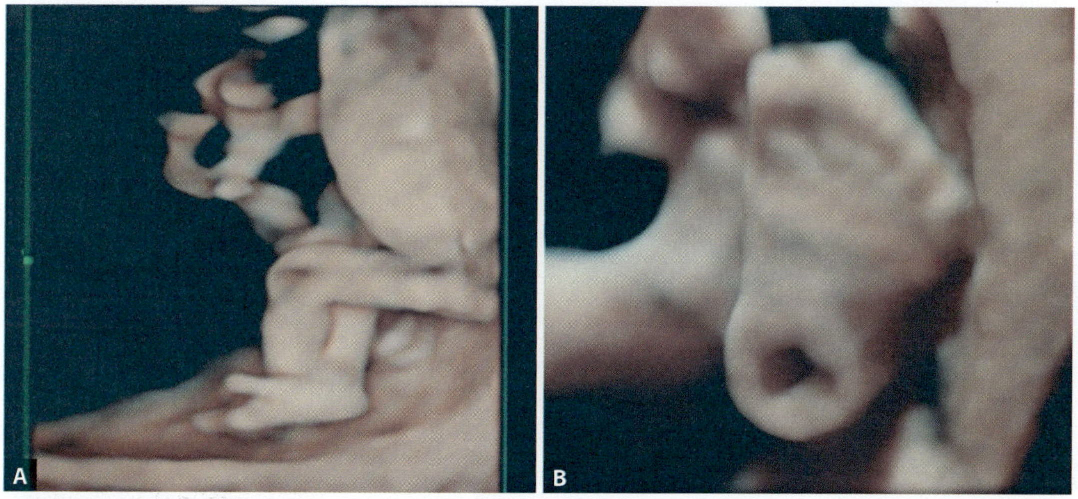

Figs. 74A and B: 3D HDlive images of toe abnormality at 12–14 weeks of gestation: (A) Split toe; (B) Polydactyly.

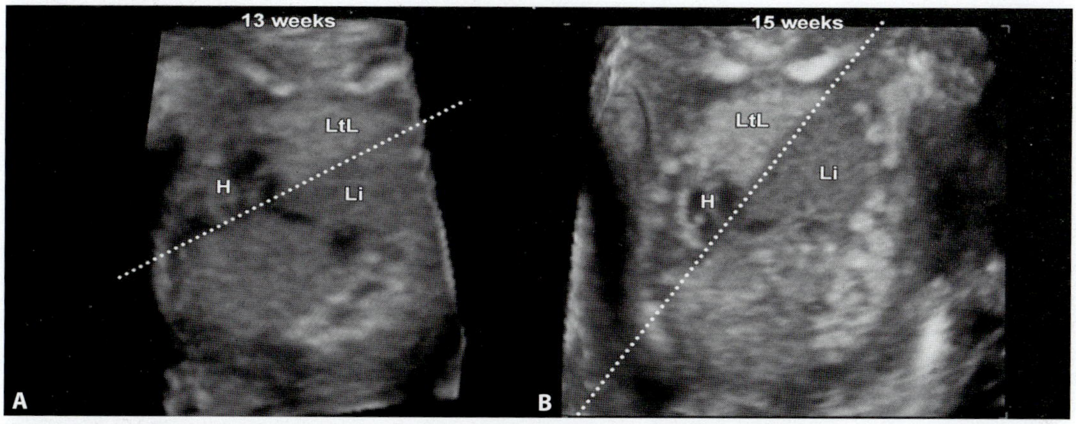

Figs. 75A and B: Congenital diaphragmatic defect at 13 and 15 weeks of gestation. Referral case due to nuchal translucency of 3 mm at 11 weeks of gestation: (A) Frontal view at 13 weeks. Dextrocardia (H), liver-up (Li) and oppressed left lung (Lt L) are demonstrated; (B) Frontal view at 15 weeks. The line of lung-liver border indicates acute angle changing in a short period due to progressive liver-up.

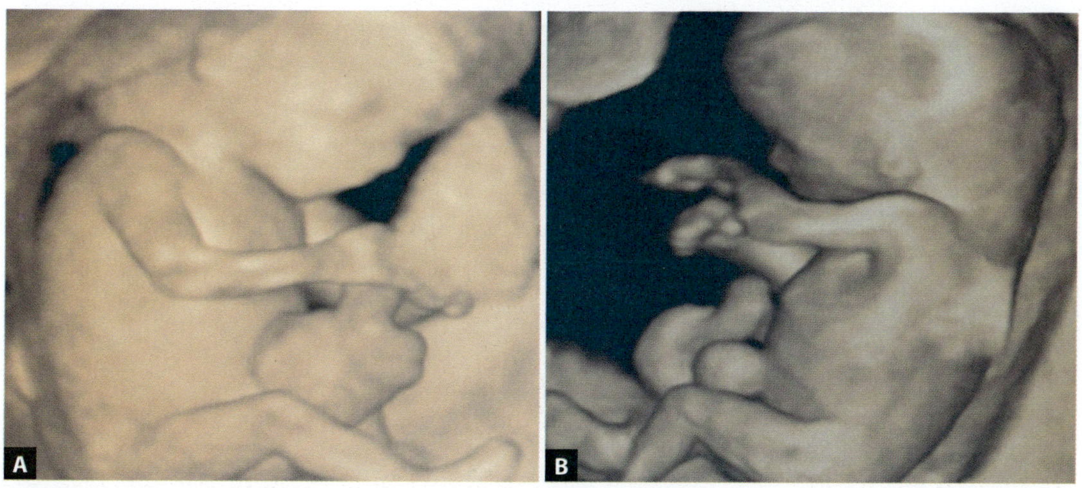

Figs. 76A and B: Omphalocele at 12 and 13 weeks of gestation 3D reconstructed ultrasound images clearly demonstrates omphalocele. Trisomy 18 was confirmed by chorionic villi sampling in both cases.

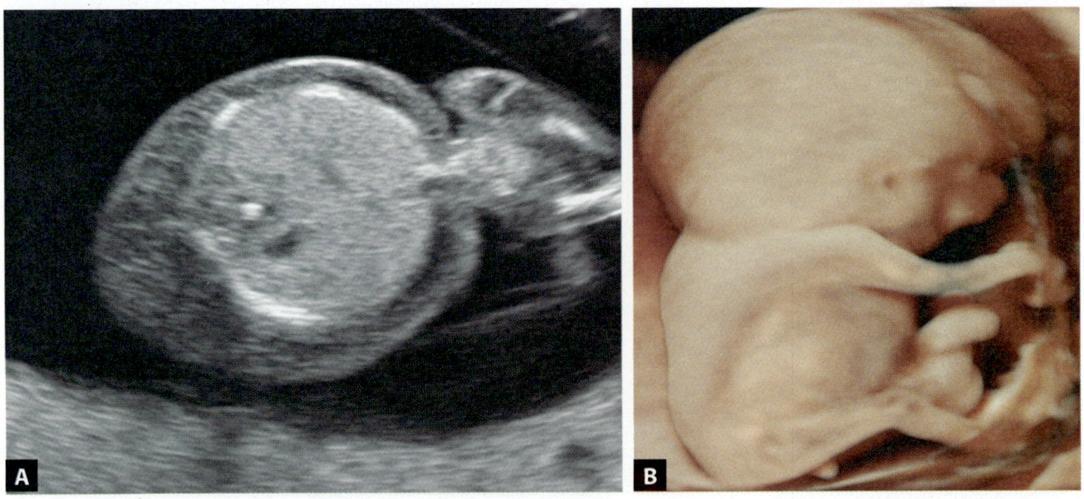

Figs. 77A and B: Omphalocele, low-set hypoplastic ear and micrognathia in a case of trisomy 18 at 13 weeks of gestation. (A) 2D axial abdomen showing small omphalocele containing with bowels; (B) HDlive image demonstrating low-set and hypoplastic ear with micrognathia.

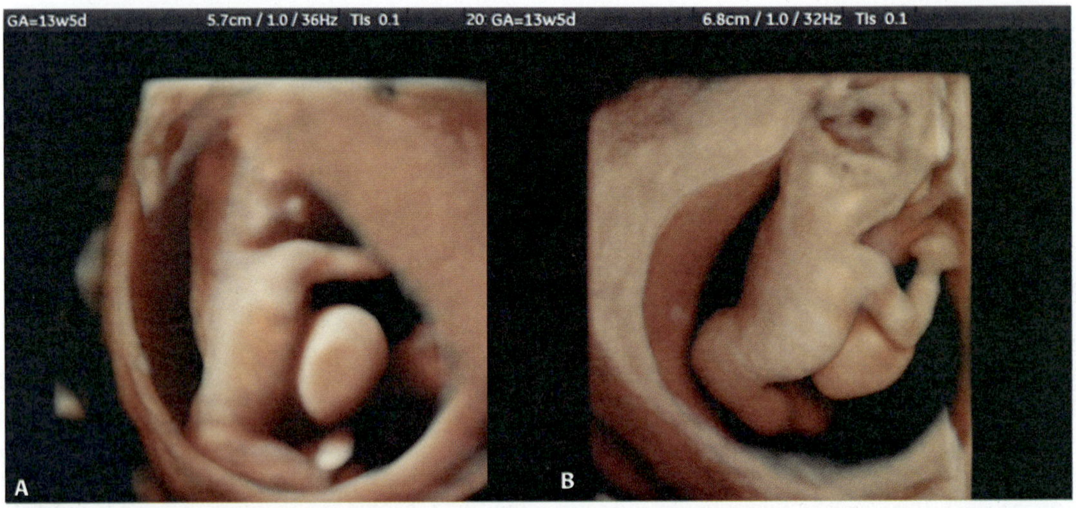

Figs. 78A and B: Omphalocele with scoliosis (body stalk anomaly) at 13 weeks of gestation. HDlive images shows ectopic liver and scoliosis. This is the mild type of body stalk anomaly.

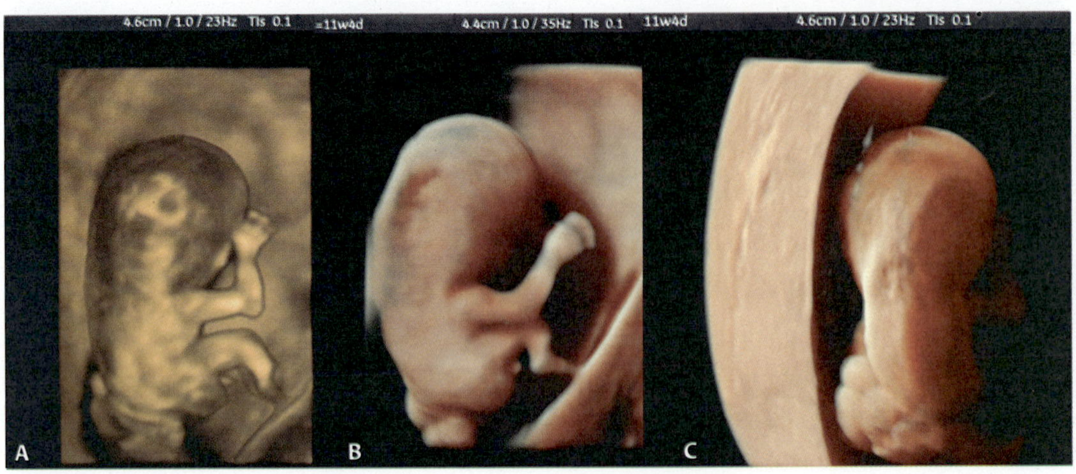

Figs. 79A to C: Body stalk anomaly with severe scoliosis at 11 weeks. (A) Conventional 3D image showing scoliosis with ectopic abdominal organs; (B) 3D HDlive image; (C) HDlive image objectively demonstrates the contents of ectopic organs.

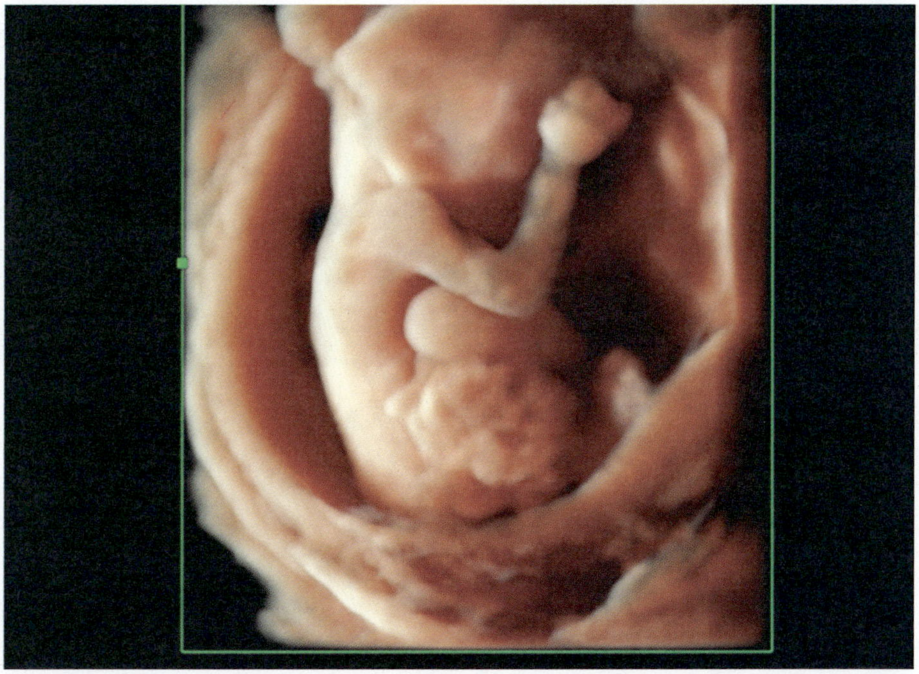

Fig. 80: Ectopic abdominal organs containing liver and bowels in a case of body stalk anomaly at 13 weeks of gestation. HDlive image shows clearly contents of ectopic organs.

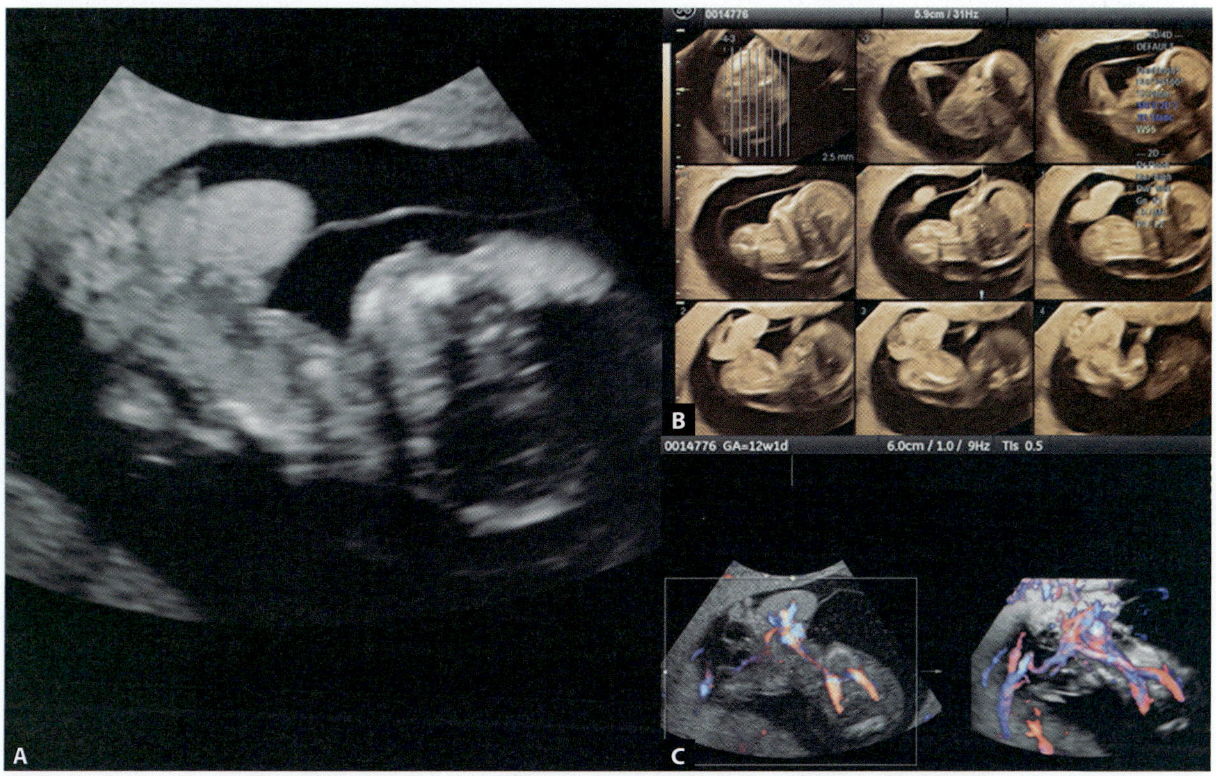

Figs. 81A to C: Body stalk anomaly at 12 weeks of gestation. (A) 3D VCI image. Liver and bowels are ectopic out of amniotic membrane; (B) TUI image; (C) 3D power Doppler image showing vascularity of cord and ectopic organs.

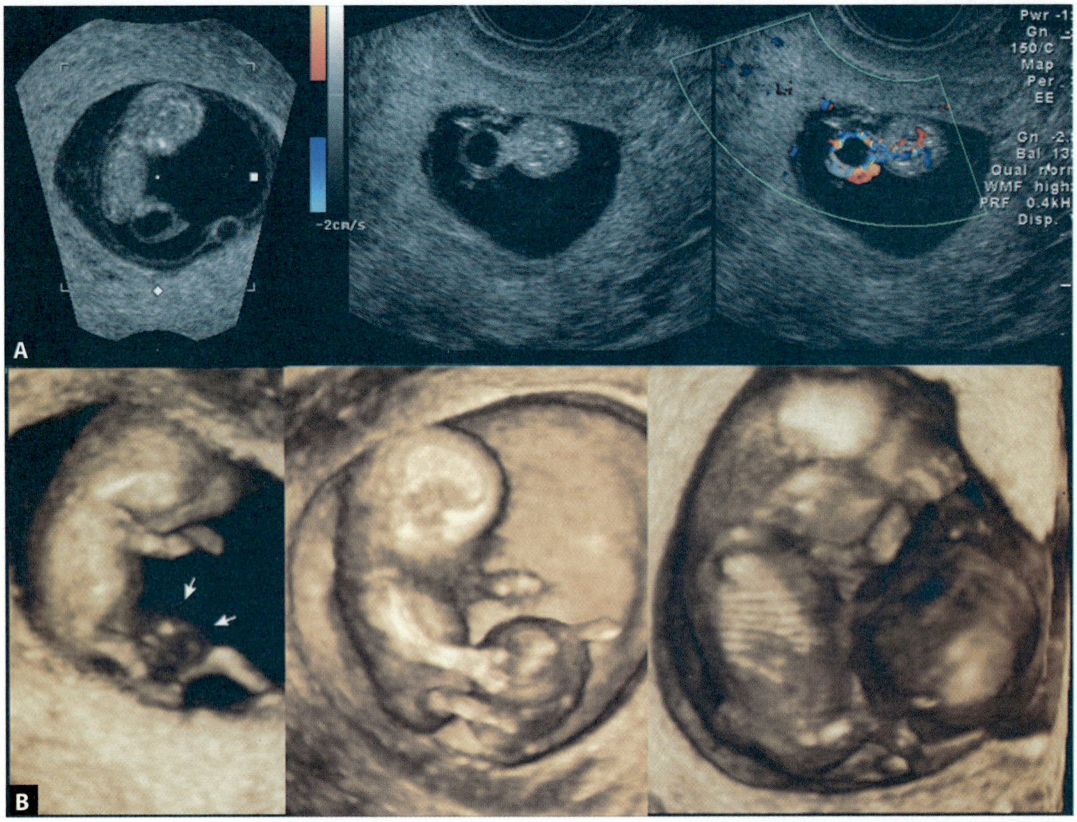

Figs. 82A and B: Bladder exstrophy in the first trimester. (A) Cystic formation between bilateral umbilical arteries. No bladder is visible inside of the fetus; (B) 3D US images at 10, 11 and 12 weeks from the left. Rapid increase in size of external bladder is clearly demonstrated.

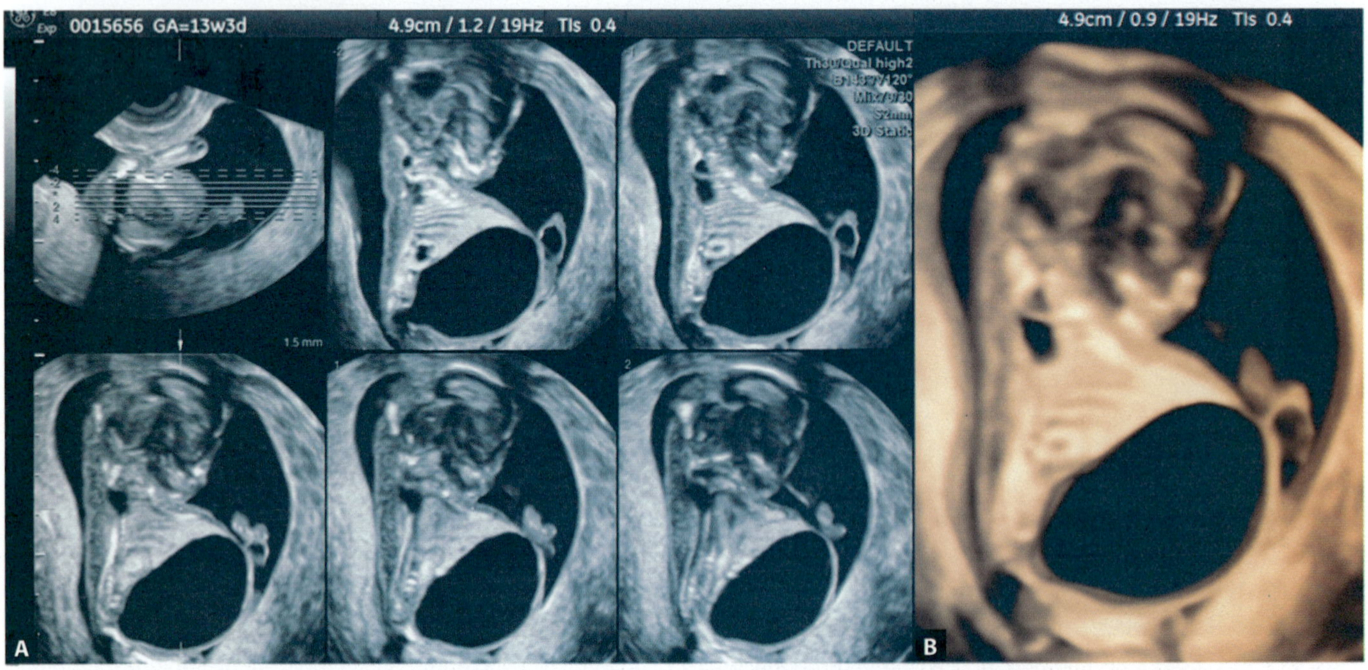

Figs. 83A and B: Prune belly syndrome at 13 weeks of gestation. (A) TUI sagittal image; (B) 3D reconstructed image.

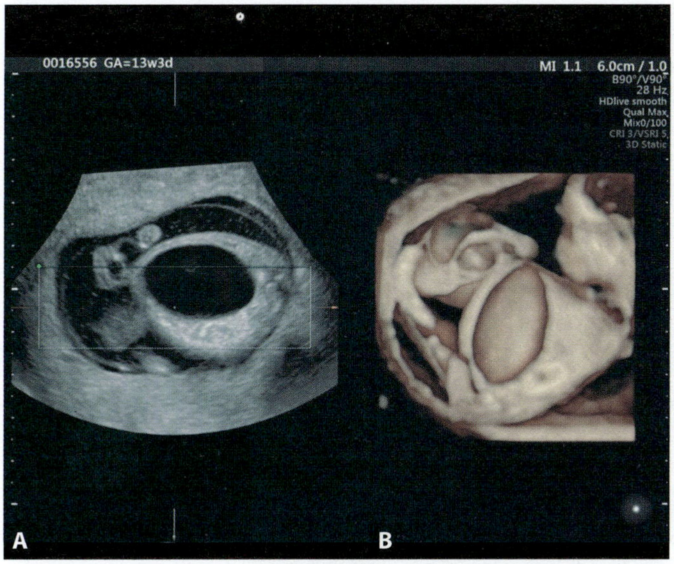

Figs. 84A and B: Prune belly syndrome at 13 weeks of gestation. (A) 2D image; (B) 3D reconstructed image.

prenatal screening by ultrasonography and renal multiple cysts can be observed even in the first trimester **(Fig. 86)**. Fetal obstructive uropathy has become detectable earlier and fetal therapy of vesicoamniotic shunting (VAS) is the accepted procedure in well-defined cases. It has been reported that the long-term outcomes indicate that VAS at 18–30 weeks may not change the prognosis of renal function and that fetal surgery for obstructive uropathy should be performed only for the carefully selected patient who has severe oligohydramnios and "normal"-appearing kidneys.[45] To preserve renal function, however, earlier VAS may be preferable **(Fig. 87)**. Amniotic membranes are well demonstrated by 3D ultrasound and recent HDlive imaging can depict amniotic membranes covering the fetus, amniotic band, constriction ring in a case of amniotic band syndrome from as early as 12 weeks of gestation **(Fig. 88)**.

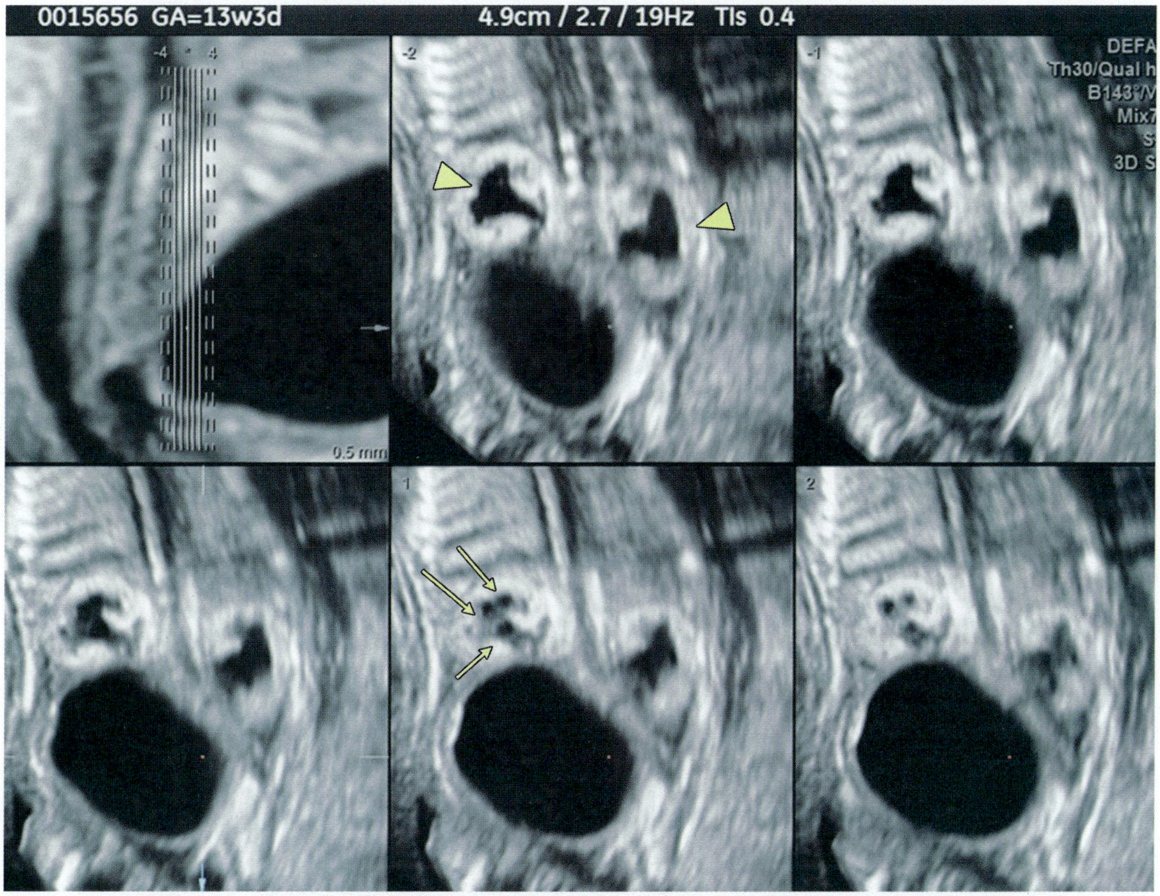

Fig. 85: Renal abnormality associated with Prune belly syndrome TUI image. Bylateral hydronephrosis is obvious (arrowheads) and in addition small multiple cysts are seen (arrows).

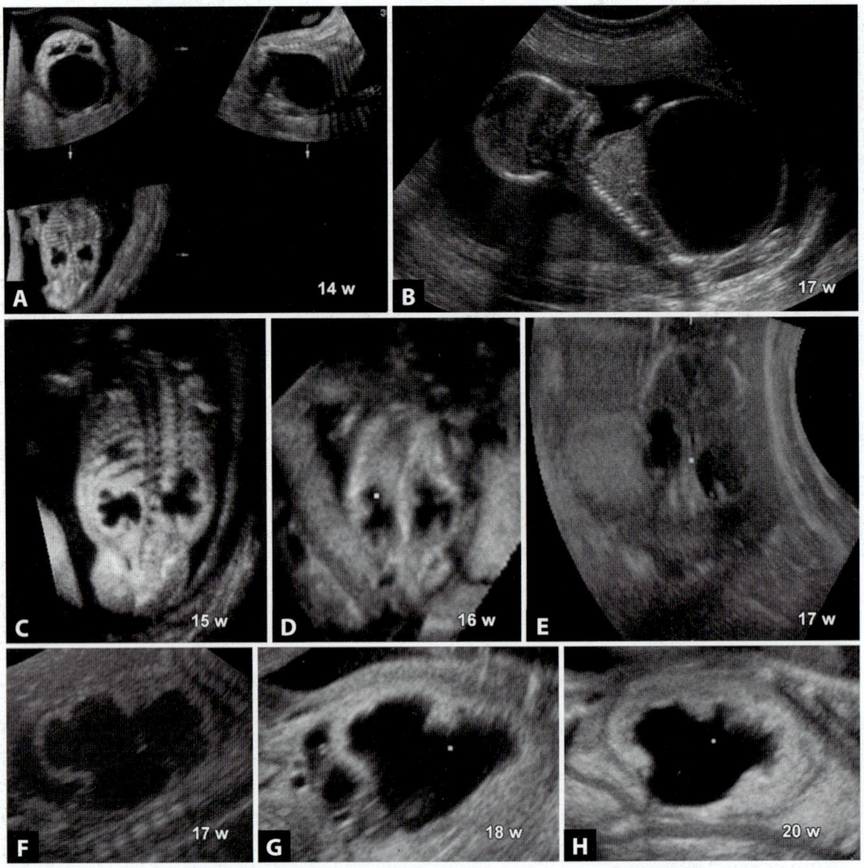

Figs. 86A to H: Huge bladder before and after vesicoamniotic shunt (VAS) operation. (A) 3D orthogonal view at 14 weeks of gestation. Huge bladder and bilateral hydronephrosis are demonstrated. Abdominal wall is not fragile like prune-berry syndrome; (B) Sagittal image at 17 weeks before VAS. Bladder volume is 137.7 mL; (C to E) Changing appearance of kidneys at 15, 16 and 17 weeks from the left. Rapid thinning of renal parenchyma with progressive hydronephrosis is clearly demonstrated; (F to H) Changing appearance of renal parenchyma (17, 18 and 20 weeks from the left) after VAS operation performed at 17 weeks. Renal parenchyma thickness was rapidly recovered after VAS procedure, with improvement of hydronephrosis.

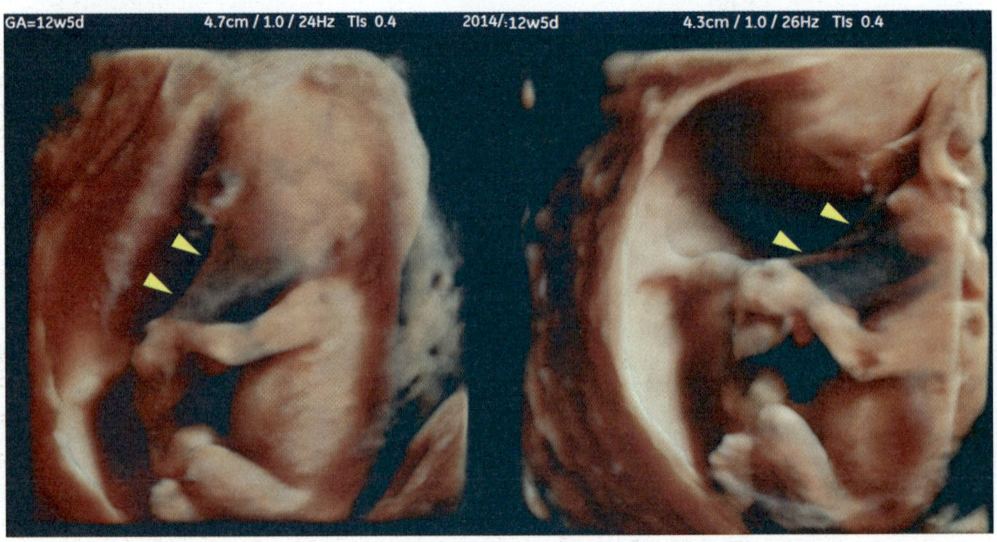

Fig. 87: Amniotic band syndrome at 12 weeks 3D HDlive images clearly demonstrated amniotic membranes (arrowheads) clinging to the fetus.

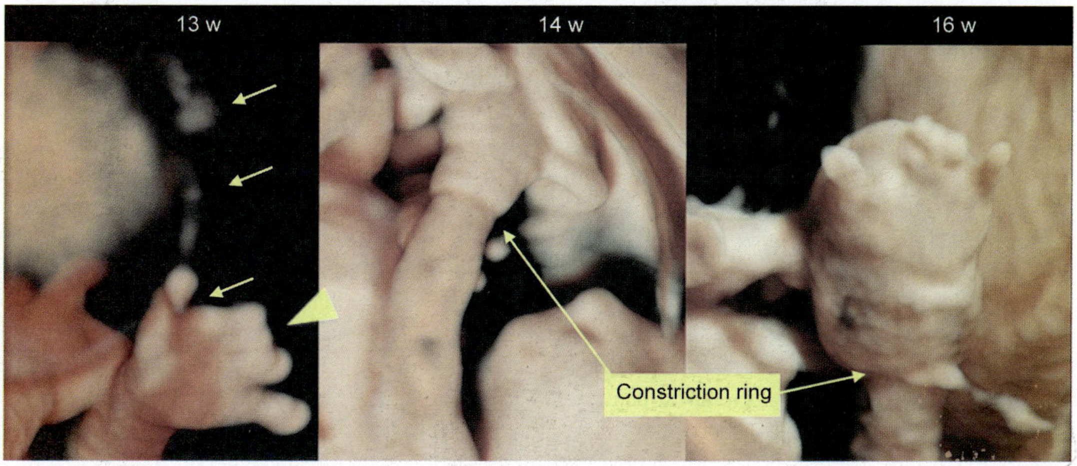

Fig. 88: Amputation of fingers and gradual hand edema with constriction ring in a case of amniotic band syndrome between 13 and 16 weeks (continued from **Figure 87**). 3D HDlive images clearly demonstrated amniotic band (arrows) and amputation of fingers (arrowheads). Note the non-edematous left hand at 13 weeks. At 14 weeks, constriction ring was seen and edematous left hand is seen at 16 weeks.

CONCLUSION

Recent advances of imaging technologies and computerized technologies have greatly contributed to the fields of both embryology and sonoembryology. There has been an immense acceleration in understanding early human development. The anatomy and physiology of embryonic development is a field where medicine exerts its greatest impact on early pregnancy at present, and it opens fascinating aspects of embryonic differentiation. Clinical assessment of those stages of growth relies heavily on 3D/4D HDlive, one of the most promising forms of noninvasive diagnostics and embryological phenomena, once matters for textbooks, are now routinely recorded with outstanding clarity.[46-48] In near future, further new findings will be discovered. We must recognize "the embryo as a patient" as well as "the fetus as a patient".

ACKNOWLEDGMENTS

The authors are grateful to the members of the Academic Center for Computing and Media Studies, Kyoto University, for their collaboration in making computer graphics images. We greatly thank Prof Katsumi Kose of the University of Tsukuba for his contributions to MR imaging of human embryo specimens. We also thank members of Global Ultrasound & IT and Women's Healthcare & Specialty in GE Healthcare (Milwaukee, USA) for their technical support and collaboration.

REFERENCES

1. Smith BR, Huff DS, Johnson GA. Magnetic resonance imaging of embryos: an internet resource for the study of embryonic development. Comput Med Imaging Graph. 1999;23(1):33-40.
2. Matsuda Y, Utsuzawa S, Kurimoto T, Haishi T, Yamazaki Y, et al. Super-parallel MR microscope. Magn Reson Med. 2003;50(1):183-9.
3. Yamada S, Uwabe C, Nakatsu-Komatsu T, Minekura Y, Iwakura M, Motoki T, et al. Graphic and movie illustrations of human prenatal development and their application to embryological education based on the human embryo specimens in the Kyoto collection. Dev Dyn. 2006;235(2): 468-77.
4. Timor-Tritsch IE, Peisner DB, Raju S. Sonoembryology: an organ-oriented approach using a high-frequency vaginal probe. J Clin Ultrasound. 1990;18(4):286-98.
5. Benoit B, Hafner T, Kurjak A, Kupesic S, Bekavac I, Bozek T. Three-dimensional sonoembryology. J Perinat Med. 2002;30(1):63-73.
6. O'Rahilly R, Muller F. Prenatal ages and stages—measures and errors. Teratology. 2000;61(5):382-4.
7. Pooh RK, Shiota K, Kurjak A. Imaging of the human embryo with magnetic resonance imaging microscopy and high-resolution transvaginal three-dimensional sonography: human embryology in the 21st century. Am J Obstet Gynecol. 2011;204(1):77.e1-77.e16. Epub 2010 Oct 25.
8. Kurjak A, Pooh RK, Merce LT, Carrera JM, Salihagic-Kadic A, Andonotopo W. Structural and functional early human development assessed by three-dimensional and four-dimensional sonography. Fertil Steril. 2005;84(5):1285-99.

9. Kurjak A, Zudenigo D, Predanic M, Kupesic S. Recent advances in the Doppler study of early fetomaternal circulation. J Perinat Med. 1993;21:419-39.
10. Kurjak A, Schulman H, Predanic A, Predanic M, Kupesic S, Zalud I. Fetal choroid plexus vascularization assessed by color flow ultrasonography. J Ultrasound Med. 1994;13:841-4.
11. Pooh RK, Aono T. Transvaginal power Doppler angiography of the fetal brain. Ultrasound Obstet Gynecol. 1996;8:417-21.
12. Chaoui R, Levaillant JM, Benoit B, Faro C, Wegrzyn P, Nicolaides KH. Three-dimensional sonographic description of abnormal metopic suture in second- and third-trimester fetuses. Ultrasound Obstet Gynecol. 2005;26:761-4.
13. Kim MS, Jeanty P, Turner C, Benoit B. Three-dimensional sonographic evaluations of embryonic brain development. J Ultrasound Med. 2008;27:119-24.
14. Hata T, Dai SY, Kanenishi K, Tanaka H. Three-dimensional volume-rendered imaging of embryonic brain vesicles using inversion mode. J Obstet Gynaecol Res. 2009;35:2:258-61.
15. Jaumiaux E, Gulbis B, Burton GJ. The Human First Trimester Gestational Sac Limits Rather than Facilitates Oxygen Transfer to the Foetus—A Review. Placenta. 2003;24(17):S86-S93.
16. Kucuk T, Duru NK, Yenen MC, Dede M, Ergűn A, Başer İ. Yolk sac size and shape as predictors of poor pregnancy outcome. J Perinat Med. 1999;27:316-20.
17. Lindsay DJ, Lovett IS, Lyons EA, Levi CS, Zheng XH, Holt SC, et al. Yolk Sac Diameter and Shape at Endovaginal US: Predictors of Pregnancy Outcome in the First Trimester. Radiology. 1992;183:115-8.
18. Blaas HG, Eik-Nes SH, Isaksen CV. The detection of spina bifida before 10 gestational weeks using two- and three-dimensional ultrasound. Ultrasound Obstet Gynecol. 2000;16(1):25-9.
19. Nicolaides KH. Nuchal translucency and other first-trimester sonographic markers of chromosomal abnormalities. Am J Obstet Gynecol. 2004;191:45-67.
20. Cicero S, Curcio P, Papageorghiou A, Sonek J, Nicolaides K. Absence of nasal bone in fetuses with trisomy 21 at 11–14 weeks of gestation: an observational study. Lancet. 2001;358:1665-7.
21. Zoppi MA, Ibba RM, Axiana C, Floris M, Manca F, Monni G. Absence of fetal nasal bone and aneuploidies at first-trimester nuchal translucency screening in unselected pregnancies. Prenat Diagn. 2003;23:496-500.
22. Cicero S, Rembouskos G, Vandecruys H, Hogg M, Nicolaides KH. Likelihood ratio for trisomy 21 in fetuses with absent nasal bone at the 11–14-week scan. Ultrasound Obstet Gynecol. 2004;23:218-23.
23. Cicero S, Avgidou K, Rembouskos G, Kagan KO, Nicolaides KH. Nasal bone in first-trimester screening for trisomy 21. Am J Obstet Gynecol. 2006;195:109-14.
24. Rembouskos G, Cicero S, Longo D, Vandecruys H, Nicolaides KH. Assessment of the fetal nasal bone at 11–14 weeks of gestation by three-dimensional ultrasound. Ultrasound Obstet Gynecol. 2004;23:232-6.
25. Benoit B, Chaoui R. Three-dimensional ultrasound with maximal mode rendering: a novel technique for the diagnosis of bilateral or unilateral absence or hypoplasia of nasal bones in second-trimester screening for Down syndrome. Ultrasound Obstet Gynecol. 2005;25:19-24.
26. Cicero S, Curcio P, Rembouskos G, Sonek J, Nicolaides KH. Maxillary length at 11–14 weeks of gestation in fetuses with trisomy 21. Ultrasound Obstet Gynecol. 2004;24:19-22.
27. Teoh M, Meagher S. First-trimester diagnosis of micrognathia as a presentation of Pierre Robin syndrome. Ultrasound Obstet Gynecol. 2003;21:616-8.
28. Tsai MY, Lan KC, Ou CY, Chen JH, Chang SY, Hsu TY. Assessment of the facial features and chin development of fetuses with use of serial three-dimensional sonography and the mandibular size monogram in a Chinese population. AmJ Obstet Gynecol. 2004;190:541-6.
29. Francis PJ, Berry V, Bhattacharya SS, Moore AT. The genetics of childhood cataract. J Med Genet. 2000;37: 481-8.
30. Thut CJ, Rountree RB, Hwa M, Kingsley DM. A large-scale in situ screen provides molecular evidence for the induction of eye anterior segment structures by the developing lens. Dev Biol. 2001;231:63-76.
31. Karkinen-Jääskeläinen M, Saxen L, Vaheri A, Leinikki P. Rubella cataract in vitro: sensitive period of the developing human lens. J Exp Med. 1975;141:1238-48.
32. Romain M, Awoust J, Dugauquier C, Van Maldergem L. Prenatal ultrasound detection of congenital cataract in trisomy 21. Prenat Diagn. 1999;19(8):780-2.
33. Pedreira DA, Diniz EM, Schultz R, Faro LB, Zugaib M. Fetal cataract in congenital toxoplasmosis. Ultrasound Obstet Gynecol. 1999;13(4):266-7.
34. Daskalakis G, Anastasakis E, Lyberopoulos E, Antsaklis A. Prenatal detection of congenital cataract in a fetus with Lowe syndrome. J Obstet Gynaecol. 2010;30(4):409-10.
35. Reches A, Yaron Y, Burdon K, Crystal-Shalit O, Kidron D, Malcov M, et al. Prenatal detection of congenital bilateral cataract leading to the diagnosis of Nance-Horan syndrome in the extended family. Prenat Diagn. 2007;27(7):662-4.
36. Léonard A, Bernard P, Hiel AL, Hubinont C. Prenatal diagnosis of fetal cataract: case report and review of the literature. Fetal Diagn Ther. 2009;26(2):61-7. Epub 2009 Sep 11.
37. Bolitho DG. Hand, Congenital hand deformities. emedicine 2006. http://www.emedicine.com/plastic/TOPIC298.HTM.
38. Carbillon L, Seince N, Largillière C, Bucourt M, Uzan M. First-trimester diagnosis of sirenomelia. A case report. Fetal Diagn Ther. 2001;16(5):284-8.

39. Monteagudo A, Mayberry P, Rebarber A, Paidas M, Timor-Tritsch IE. Sirenomelia sequence: first-trimester diagnosis with both two- and three-dimensional sonography. J Ultrasound Med. 2002;21:915-20.
40. Schiesser M, Holzgreve W, Lapaire O, Willi N, Lüthi H, Lopez R, et al. Sirenomelia, the mermaid syndrome—detection in the first trimester. Prenat Diagn. 2003;23:493-5.
41. Dugoff L, Thieme G, Hobbins JC. First trimester prenatal diagnosis of chondroectodermal dysplasia (Ellis-van Creveld syndrome) with ultrasound. Ultrasound Obstet Gynecol. 2001;17:86-8.
42. Percin EF, Guvenal T, Cetin A, Percin S, Goze F, Arici S. First-trimester diagnosis of Robinow syndrome. Fetal Diagn Ther. 2001;16:308-11.
43. Doyle NM, Lally KP. The CDH Study Group and advances in the clinical care of the patient with congenital diaphragmatic hernia. Semin Perinatol. 2004;28:174-84.
44. Daskalakis G, Anastasakis E, Souka A, Manoli A, Koumpis C, Antsaklis A. First trimester ultrasound diagnosis of congenital diaphragmatic hernia. J Obstet Gynaecol Res. 2007;33:870-2.
45. Holmes N, Harrison MR, Baskin LS. Fetal Surgery for Posterior Urethral Valves: Long-Term Postnatal Outcomes. Pediatrics. 2001;108:1-7.
46. Pooh RK, Kurjak A. Donald School Atlas of Advanced Ultrasound in Obstetrics and Gyneacology. Jaypee Brothers Medical Publishers, India; 2015.
47. Wataganara T, Pooh RK, Kurjak A. Donald School Textbook of PowerPoint Presentation on Advanced Ultrasound in Obstetrics & Gynecology. Jaypee Brothers Medical Publishers, India; 2015.
48. Pooh RK, Kurjak A. Novel application of three-dimensional HDlive imaging in prenatal diagnosis from the first trimester. Journal of Perinatal Medicine. 2015;43(2):147-58.

34

CHAPTER

Three-dimensional Ultrasound in the Visualization of Fetal Anatomy in the Three Trimesters of Pregnancy

Giovanni Centini, Lucia Rosignoli

INTRODUCTION

Biophysical Monitoring of Pregnancy

Embryo–Fetal Anatomical Study by 3–4D Ultrasound

During the 1970s, the use of ultrasound in obstetric diagnostics was a driving force for the study of the fetus, revolutionizing the concept of prenatal monitoring. The development of increasingly sophisticated techniques such as high frequency, real-time, echo-Doppler flow imaging, color and power Doppler and the second harmonic, was followed in the 90s by a period of relative immobility for ultrasound upgrading. However, since the turn of the millennium, volumetric probes that store volume samples, acquiring up to 25 images per second (and multiples of this figure are already in view), have transformed the classical concept of two-dimensional ultrasound, generating enormous interest and a great spurt of research which still has to be translated into scientific knowledge. So, it is now widely considered that three- and four-dimensional (3–4D), namely 3D with a fourth dimension, time, offer too many possibilities to be ignored.[1-3] Acquisition of a volume or region of interest is the great novelty of 3D technique and just as exciting is the possibility of studying it in movement during ultrasound examination or afterwards, also by other operators and in an infinite number of section planes that can all be perfectly reproduced. Moreover, the many systems of representing acquired volumes make this technique very similar to computed-axial tomography (CAT) and nuclear magnetic resonance (NMR) imaging:

- *Multiplanar scan:* The image can be visualized and studied in the three classical scan planes: coronal, sagittal and transverse
- *Minimum rendering:* This is the classical 3D image of external embryofetal or other anatomical morphology
- *Maximum rendering:* This highlights deep echoes to visualize skeletal details
- *Glass body:* This highlights blood vessels in an anatomical part which is rendered transparent like glass
- *Vocal:* Enabling volumes to be calculated with great accuracy
- *Invert:* Transformation of liquid into solid parts
- *STIC (spatiotemporal imaging correlation):* Storage of a moving volume over a time interval with the possibility of representing and studying it later in slow motion and in different planes
- *Tomography ultrasound imaging (TUI) or multislices:* A field is sectioned in up to 27 scans at predefined distances and in real time (like NMR)
- *4D:* 3D represented in time
- *VCI–c-plane:* Improved tissue contrast resolution in real time (4D), coronal plane imaging (orthogonal plane of the scan plane)
- *B-flow:* The direct visualization of blood reflectors has made B-mode flow imaging (B-flow) possible without the limitations of Doppler technology, angle independent
- *Omni-view:* To study the same volume by VCI–c-plane multiple sections. It is possible shape the box of observation (linear, curve, etc.) to region of interest (ROI). This possibility is very important because the human anatomy usually has a curve or round shape. By omni-view we can realize pictures more detailed.[4]
- *SonoAVC (sono-automated volume calculation):* The possibility to detect areas by different color and to calculate the volume of these areas
- *HDlive (high-definition live source or real-time US):* A new ultrasound software, combines a movable virtual adjustable light source in a software that calculates the proportion of light reflecting through surface

structures, depending on light direction. The light source can be manually positioned to illuminate the desired area of interest. The ultrasound technician can control light intensity to create shadows that enhance image quality. HDlive is an innovation that will render even more realistic images of fetal anatomy and gynecologic lesions.[5] Three-dimensional HDlive further "humanizes" the fetus, enables detailed observation of the fetal face in the first trimester. HDlive is one the most promising forms of noninvasive diagnostic and embryological phenomena, once matters for textbooks are now routinely recorded with outstanding clarity. New advances deserve the adjective "breathtaking", including 4D parallel study of the structural and functional early human development.[6,7]

- Silhouette or transparency, a new advanced tool of HDlive to evidence the shape of embryo-fetal body and internal cavity of brain and body. Silhouette is a good ultrasound tool to study the embryo-fetal head in the first trimester[8] **(Figs. 1 to 12)**.

Other possibilities are the electronic scalpel to eliminate parts not of interest and rotation about orthogonal axes or cine calc to present the volume in different kinds.

Today ultrasound research is so active that new applications have probably been found as these words are being written. One new advance is already available, namely the electronic matrix probe. The possibilities of electronic rather than volumetric probes that combine electronic scans with mechanical movement to cover the area of interest, will provide even more sophisticated images and the possibility of obtaining volume samples from hitherto unthinkable angles and perspectives, especially useful in cardiology.[9] These innovations, however, require relatively long development periods before they are applied.

The above raises the question whether 3-4D offers greater certainty in embryo study and detection of fetal and ovarian pathology.[10-12] The scientific community seems unanimous in considering that we cannot yet fully answer this question, but 10 years after the finalization of volumetric probe were acquired many experiences that can make a real contribution to define the role and importance of 3-4D in the study of various embryo-fetal's organs and systems.

However, there are already very many papers comparing 2D and 3D, and their results define the use of 3-4D complementary to 2D, with the exception for the neurosonology and fetal cardiology, where can offer better possibility to explore physiological and pathological fetal anatomy. This technique has unique applications but it is commonly considered that 3-4D offers an improvement and completion of 2D, of such interest that it cannot be forgone once tried. Hence, there are specific situations in which 3D is indispensable, such as when a coronal scan is needed (visualization of the corpus callosum or a fetal profile in anterior occipital position) though a good instrument in the hands of an experienced sonographer can meet all the needs of ultrasound monitoring in pregnancy. Those with long experience with 2D, and subsequently with 3-4D, know the pleasure of working better and obtaining images superior to those obtained by 2D. The possibility of saving a volume and studying it

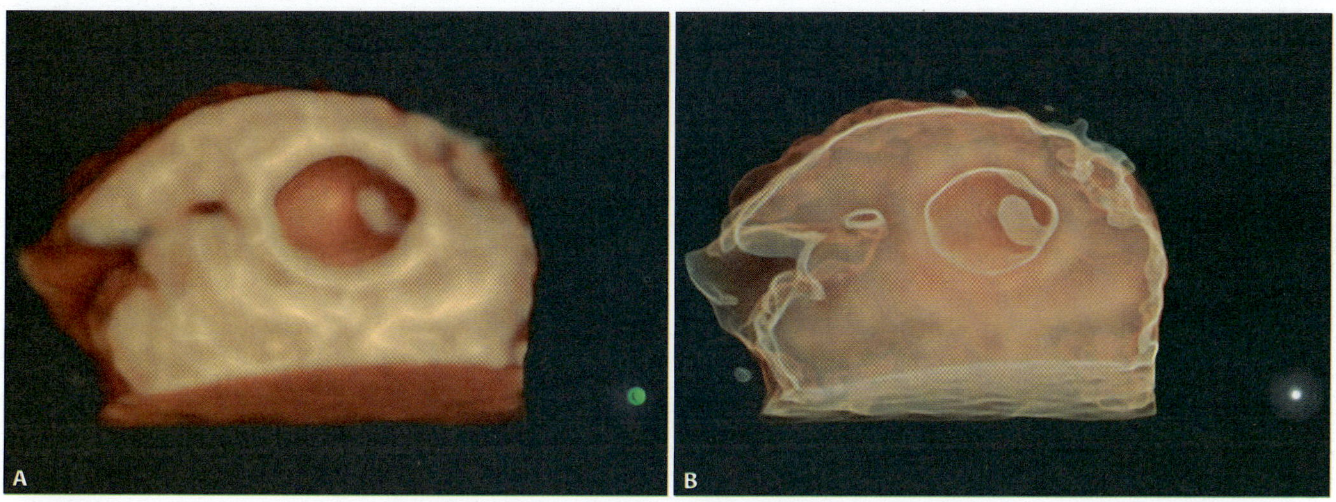

Figs. 1A and B: Weeks 5+5d: (A) HDlive of gestational sac and embryo with front light; (B) The same picture with silhouette. The shape of embryo's cerebral ventricles are highlighted.

later, discussing it with other operators and visualizing it in an infinite number of planes, superior to those obtained with 2D and perfectly reproducible, is as close as one can imagine to CAT or NMR scans, with the advantage of speed, easy repetition and much lower costs. The old recorded cassette to transmit images of a malformation, for example, cannot compare with volumetric acquisition. It seems certain that in the near future nearly all instruments will be equipped with 3-4D, even if not all sonographers know how to exploit it fully. It is therefore necessary to begin to train experts who think and work directly in 3D without having to make the often difficult transition from 2D. Sonographers of tomorrow (today) will certainly obtain better results than those who began with 2D because they will already have in mind the field of interest to explore in 3D.

The aim of this atlas is to provide pictorial documentation of pregnancy monitoring with 3D images, sometimes with the corresponding 2D image, so readers can begin to habituate themselves and hopefully acquire a different and personal key to the 3D image.

FIRST TRIMESTER OF PREGNANCY

From Conception to Week 10

The sophistication achieved by ultrasound instruments associated with clinical and ultrasound knowledge and know-how unthinkable only ten years ago, enables us to monitor pregnancy from before conception. For fertility control, 2D ultrasound with power or color Doppler makes it possible to determine with sufficient certainty the following aspects on day 12:

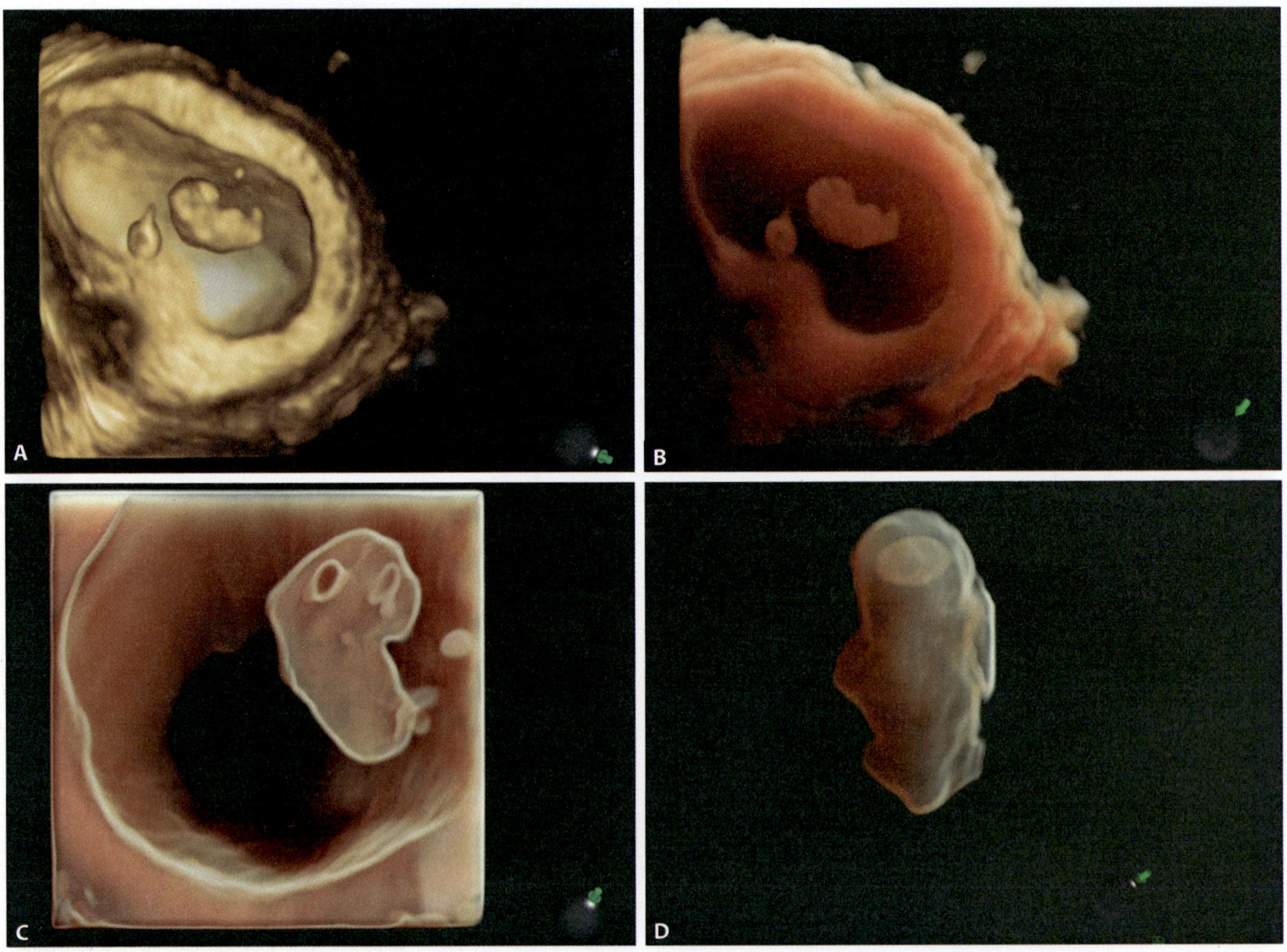

Figs. 2A to D: Weeks 8+4d; (A) HDlive with lateral light; (B) With behind light; (C) Silhouette to evidence the cerebral ventricles; (D)Silhouette, retrovision of embryo with lateral light; the evidence of rhomboencephalon.

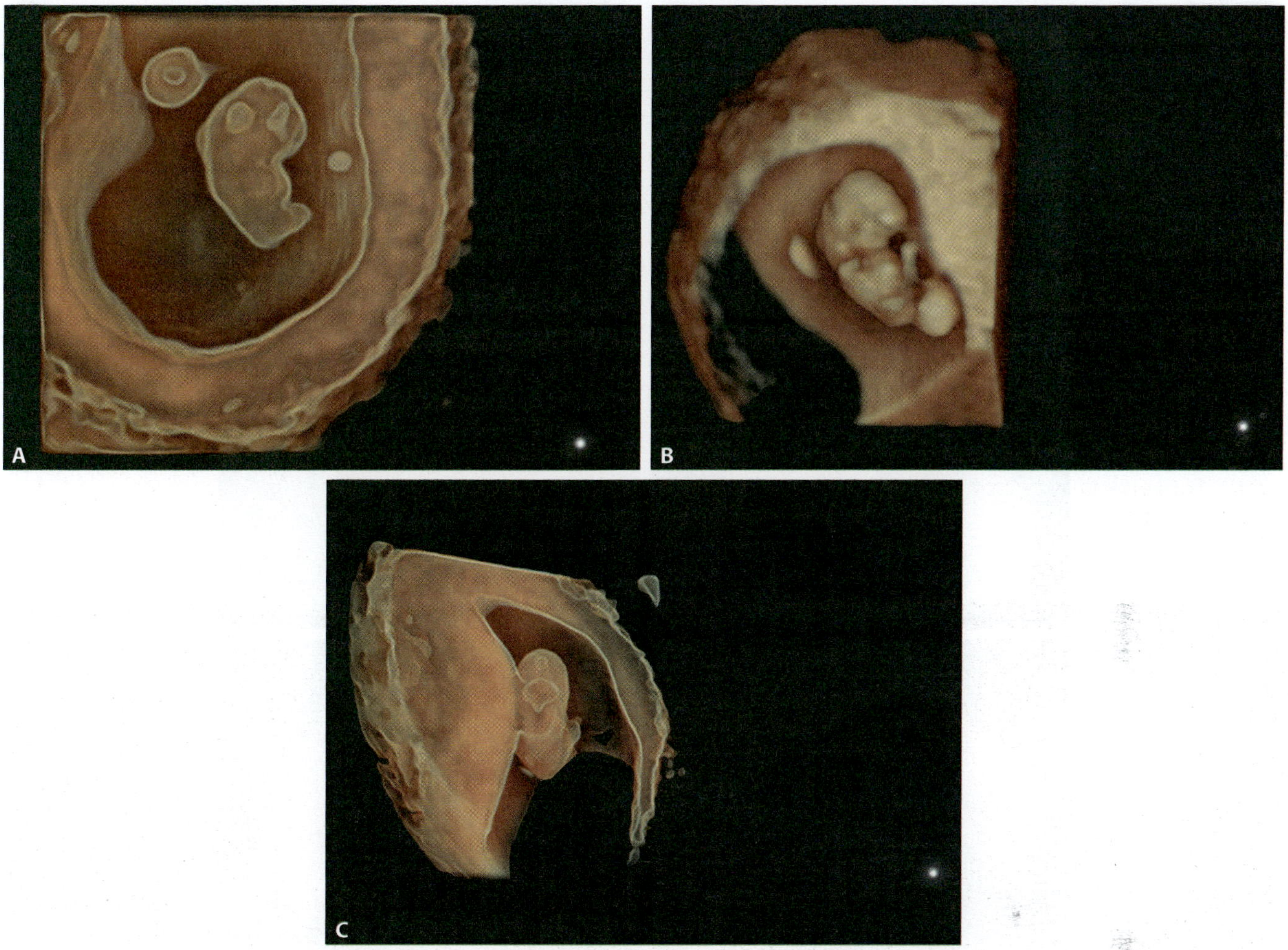

Figs. 3A to C: Weeks 8+5d: (A) HDlive with lateral light to see cerebral ventricles and yolk sac's cavity; (B) HDlive; (C) Silhouette with frontal light; by posterior vision of embryo, it is possible evidence the prosencephalon and rhombencephalon.

- Uterine morphology and myometrial structure; the tridimensional scan in coronal section is a good instrument comparable to ISG-RNM to explore the uterine cavity and find the anatomical uterine malformation which represent 3–5%: arcuate uterus, bidelfus and bicornuate
- Endometrial echostructure and morphology by detecting a three-line image characteristic of the ovulatory period and myometrial vascularization
- Uterine artery flow values which should not have a pulsatility index of less than 3
- The dominant follicle measuring 16–18 mm with peak systolic velocity (PSV) of 5–10 cm/sec in neighboring vessels;
- 4–5 antral follicles per ovary with PSV of 6–12 cm/sec in stromal vessels **(Figs. 13 to 15)**.

By means of 3-4D or better the 4D VCI-c-plane system it is possible to obtain a correct view of the uterine cavity[13,14] **(Fig. 14)**. This means that with only one examination, the existence of anatomical-functional conditions for pregnancy can be ascertained. Once conception has occurred, ultrasound monitoring of pregnancy should not necessarily begin in the first weeks of gestation. This type of protocol is usually used for medically assisted conception, however it is possible to follow the progress of pregnancy week by week, acquiring important information on physiological or pathological evolution by monitoring embryo-fetal growth and studying embryo-fetal anatomy. At the present time, 3-4D volumetric acquisition provides superior images in terms of definition and visual impact, but only slight improvements in diagnostic capacity with respect to 2D.

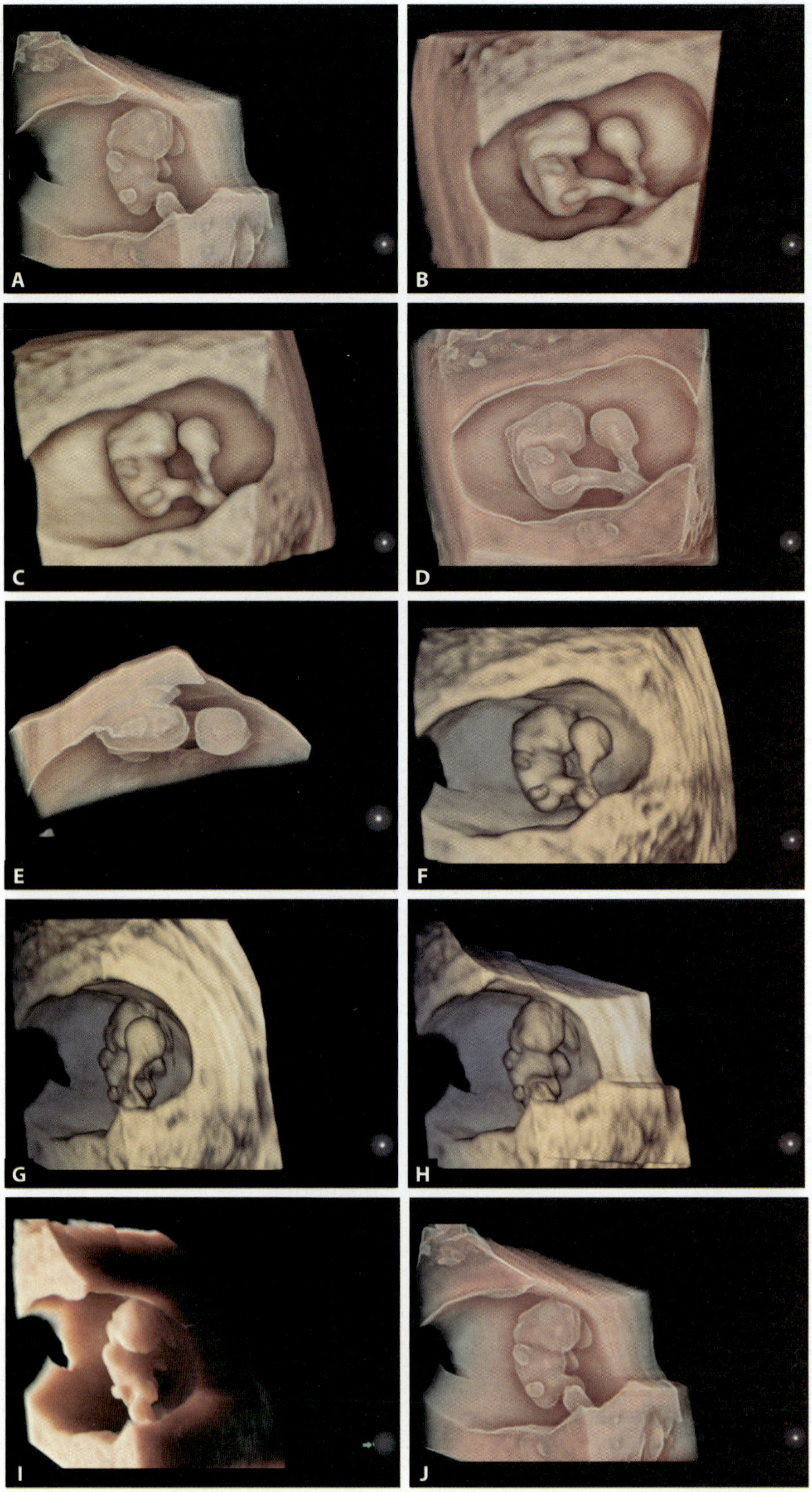

Figs. 4A to J: Weeks 8+6d: A different point of view of the embryo on HDlive and silhouette.

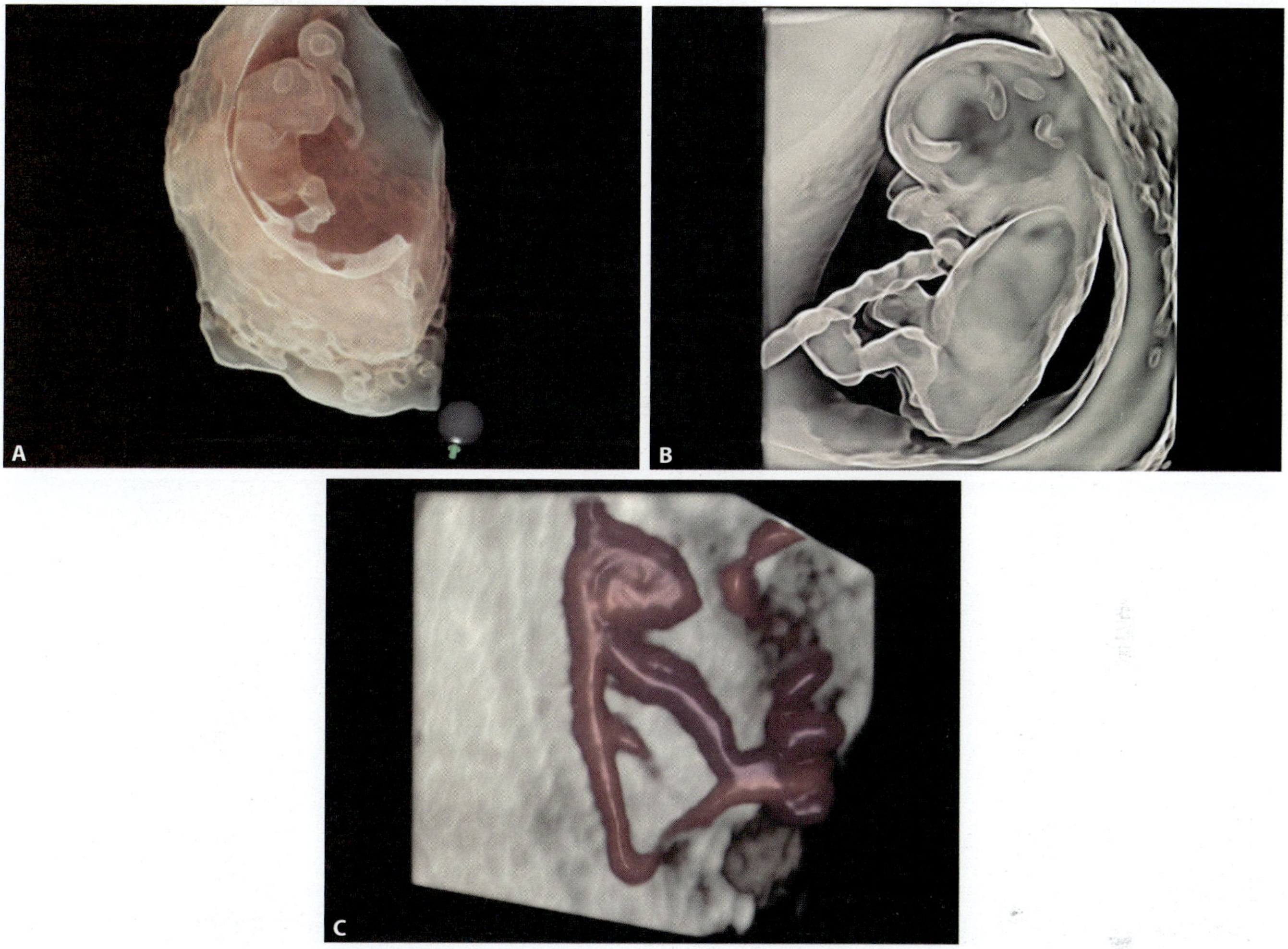

Figs. 5A to C: Weeks 10+0 d: (A and B) Silhouette of the embryo; (C) HDlive of vascular circulation.

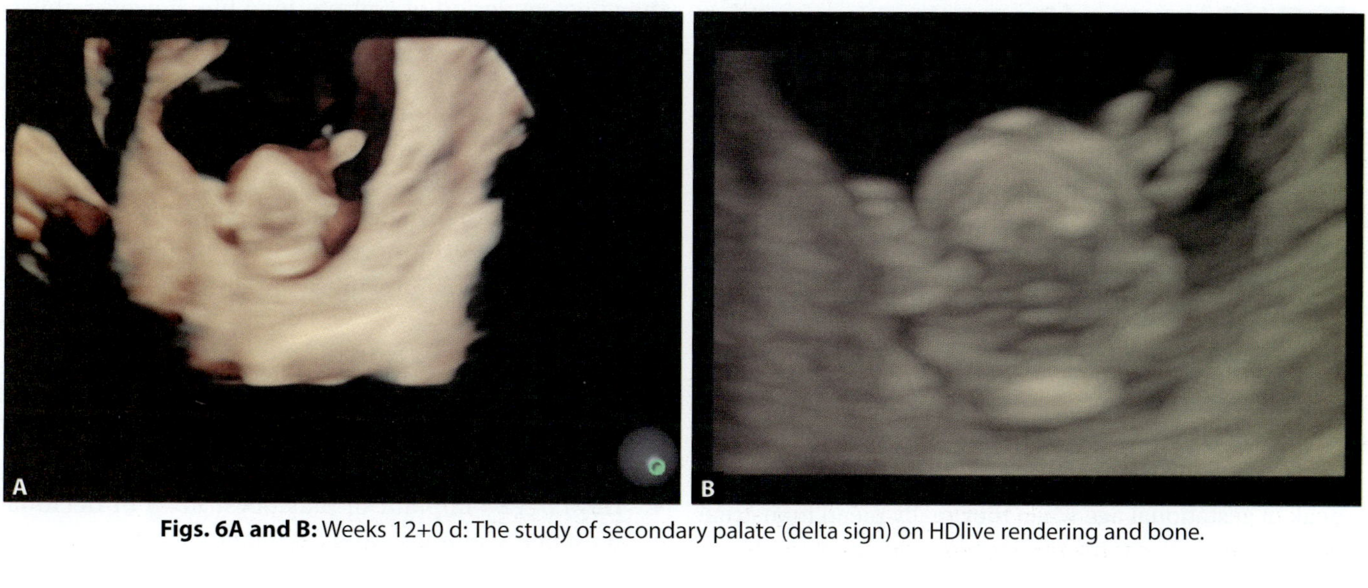

Figs. 6A and B: Weeks 12+0 d: The study of secondary palate (delta sign) on HDlive rendering and bone.

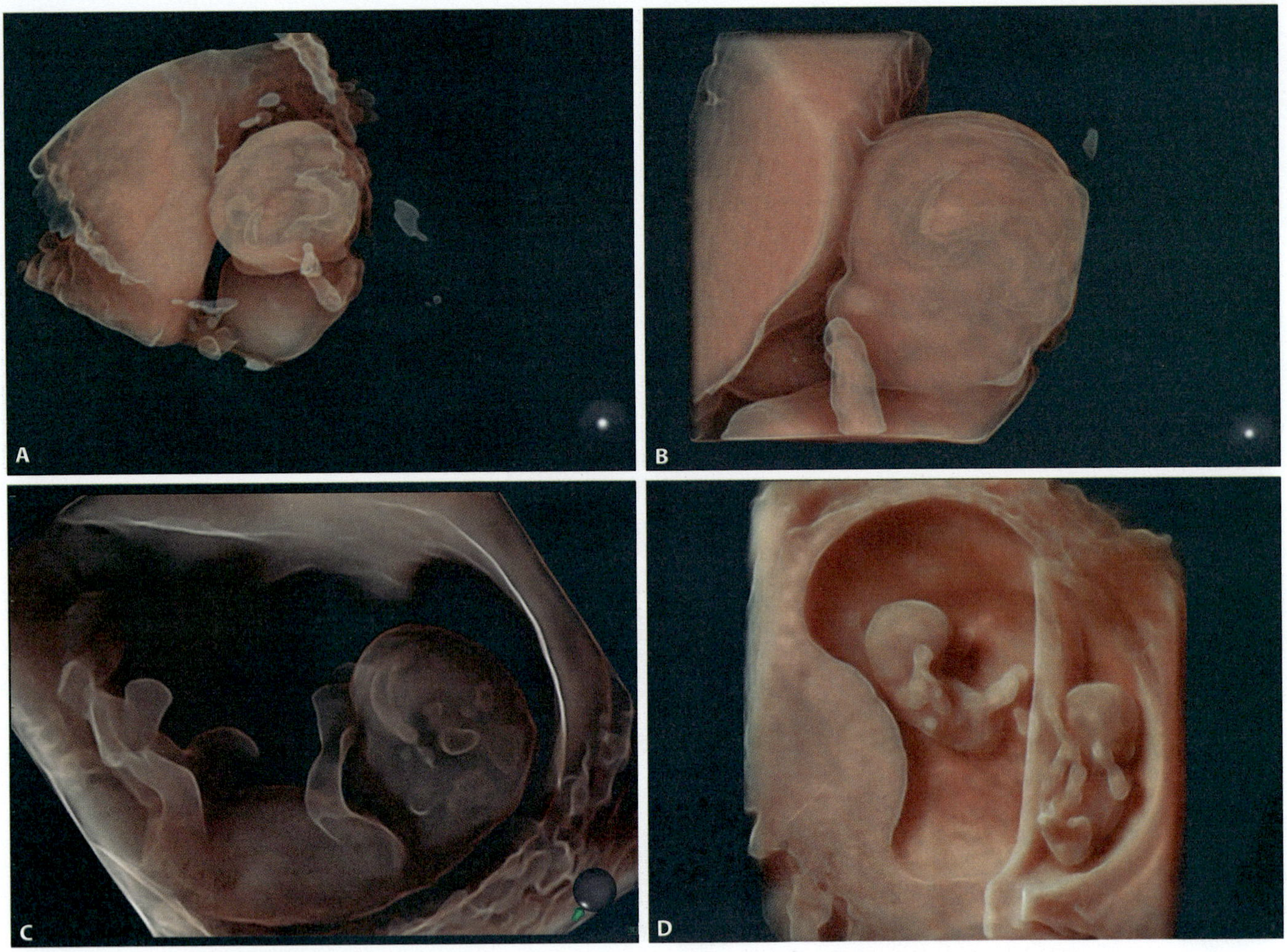

Figs. 7A to D: Weeks 12+0d: (A to C) Silhouette: the vision of right ventricles; (D) Silhouette of twin.

An Ultrasound View of the First Trimester of Pregnancy

In indicating the period of embryo-fetal development, it is correct to distinguish between menstrual age and true gestational age. Menstrual age is counted from the last menstrual period and is unreliable. About 40% of pregnant women, or one in two, have ovulation's problems for various reasons. Moreover, even in women with physiological ovulation's patterns, conception may occur between day 11 and day 17 of the menstrual cycle. It is therefore essential to date pregnancy by means of ultrasound parameters during the first trimester. Gestational age is counted from when the gametes fuse and is on average 14 days less than the menstrual age used by embryologists.[15] Internationally, in fact, obstetricians now speak of gestational age when they really mean menstrual age. A compromise is the term *ultrasound age*, namely age established by ultrasound. When it is desired to indicate the effective period of embryo-fetal life; however, this is usually specified.

In order to better understand ultrasound images, especially for early detection of anatomical structures and embryo-fetal morphology, it is useful to refer to embryology, though naturally the anatomical age is earlier. In practice, it is important to be clear about the terms used.

The first trimester of pregnancy is divided into three periods: pre-embryonic, embryonic and fetal.

Pre-embryonic Period

Embryology: Days 4–19

- Day 4—morula
- Days 4–7—implant of avillous morula in the uterus
- Days 8–12—implant of blastocyst deep in decidua; presence of amniotic and celomatic cavities

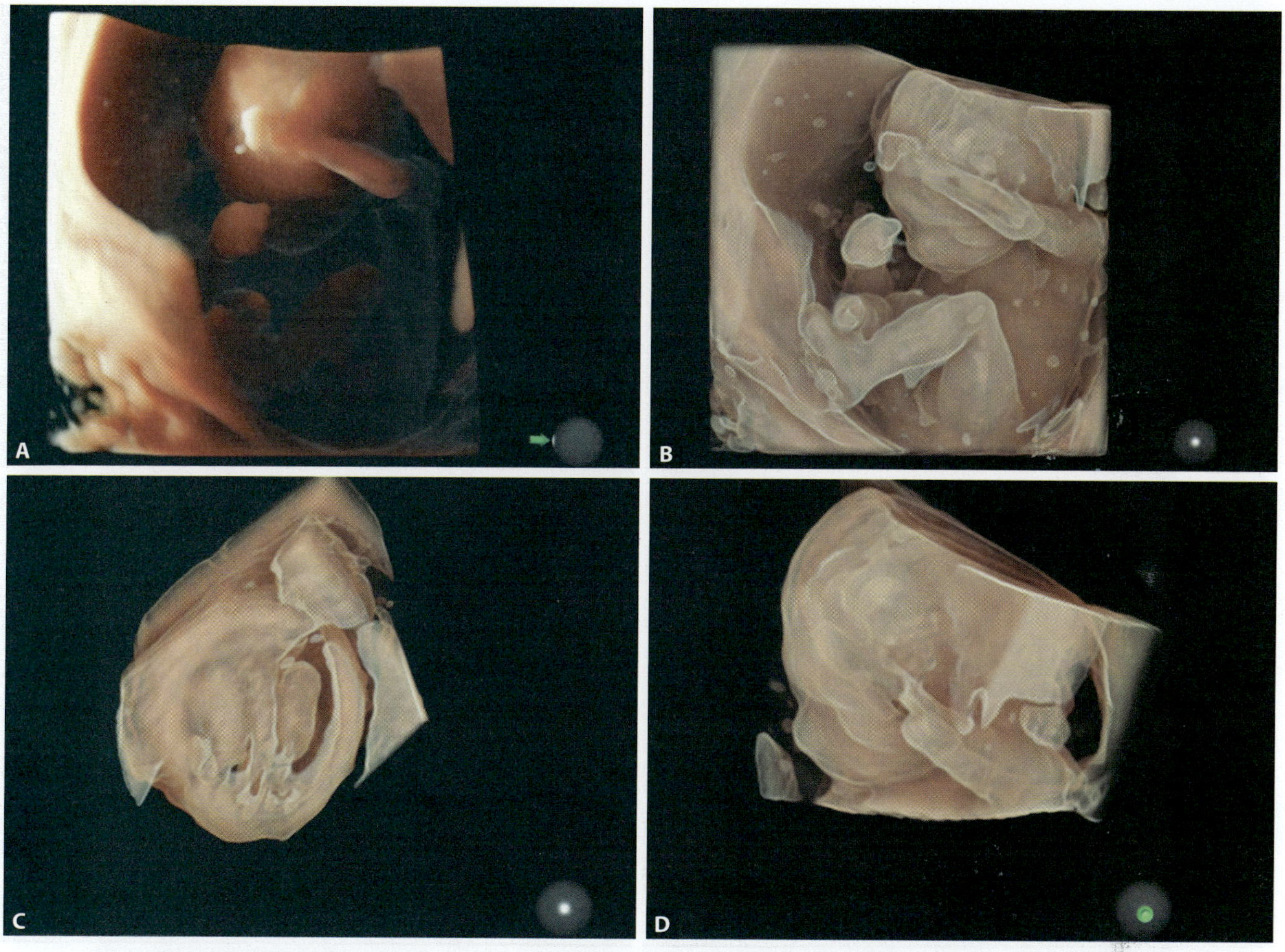

Figs. 8A to D: Weeks 14+0 d: The fetus by HDlive and by silhouette with different point of view light.

- Days 13–19—presence of chorionic villi, yolk sac (YS) and neural plate.

Ultrasonography (Weeks 3 and 4 of Gestation)

Ultrasound detects decidualization of the endometrium and the luteal body but cannot confirm pregnancy. Endometrial flow can be assessed and when absent suggests lack of implantation **(Figs. 16A to E)**.

Embryonic Period

Embryology: days 17–49 (seven full weeks)

Ultrasonography: weeks 5–9 inclusive (up to day 63).

Comparison of tissue, organ and system formation detected and studied anatomically during the embryonic period demonstrates the capacities and limits of ultrasound for monitoring the product of conception. Another small distinction between embryology and ultrasound is that in the former case reference is made to exact parameters such as crown rump length (CRL) or the presence of tissues, organs and systems, whereas in the latter gestational age is usually indicated in weeks (the definition of which we have already discussed), with considerable limitations.

Embryology: Days 20–23

CRL = 1.5–2.0 mm; cloacal membranes and posterior cerebral vesicle (rhombencephalon).

Week 5 (Ultrasonographic)

From 4 weeks + 0 days to 4 weeks + 6 days from the last menstrual period

Week 5 of gestation: It is possible to identify the gestation chamber (GC) from 4 weeks + 2–3 days in pregnancies with regular menstrual cycles, and by the end of week 5 this is

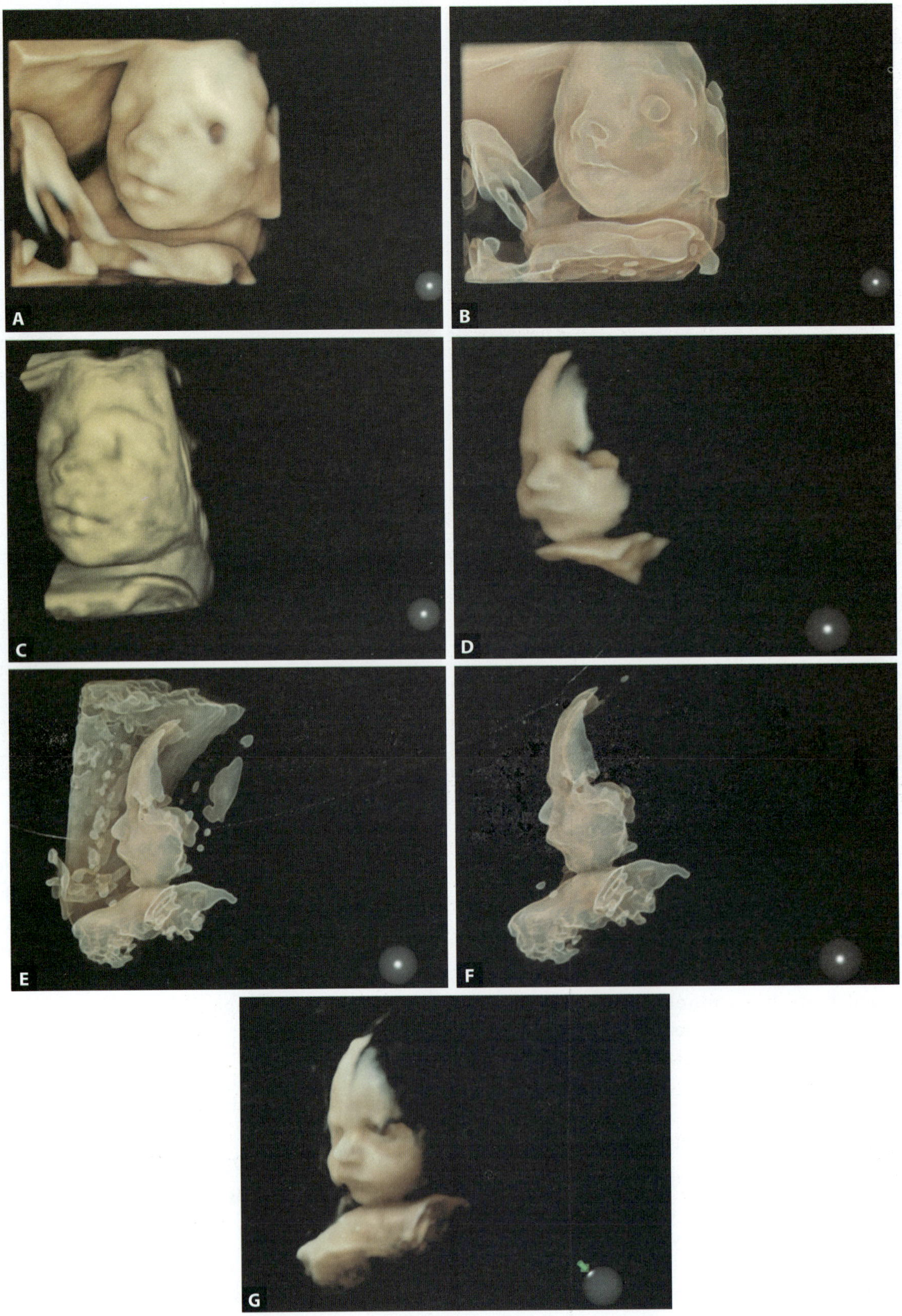

Figs. 9A to G: Weeks 22+0d: "Humanization" of the face by HDlive and silhouette.

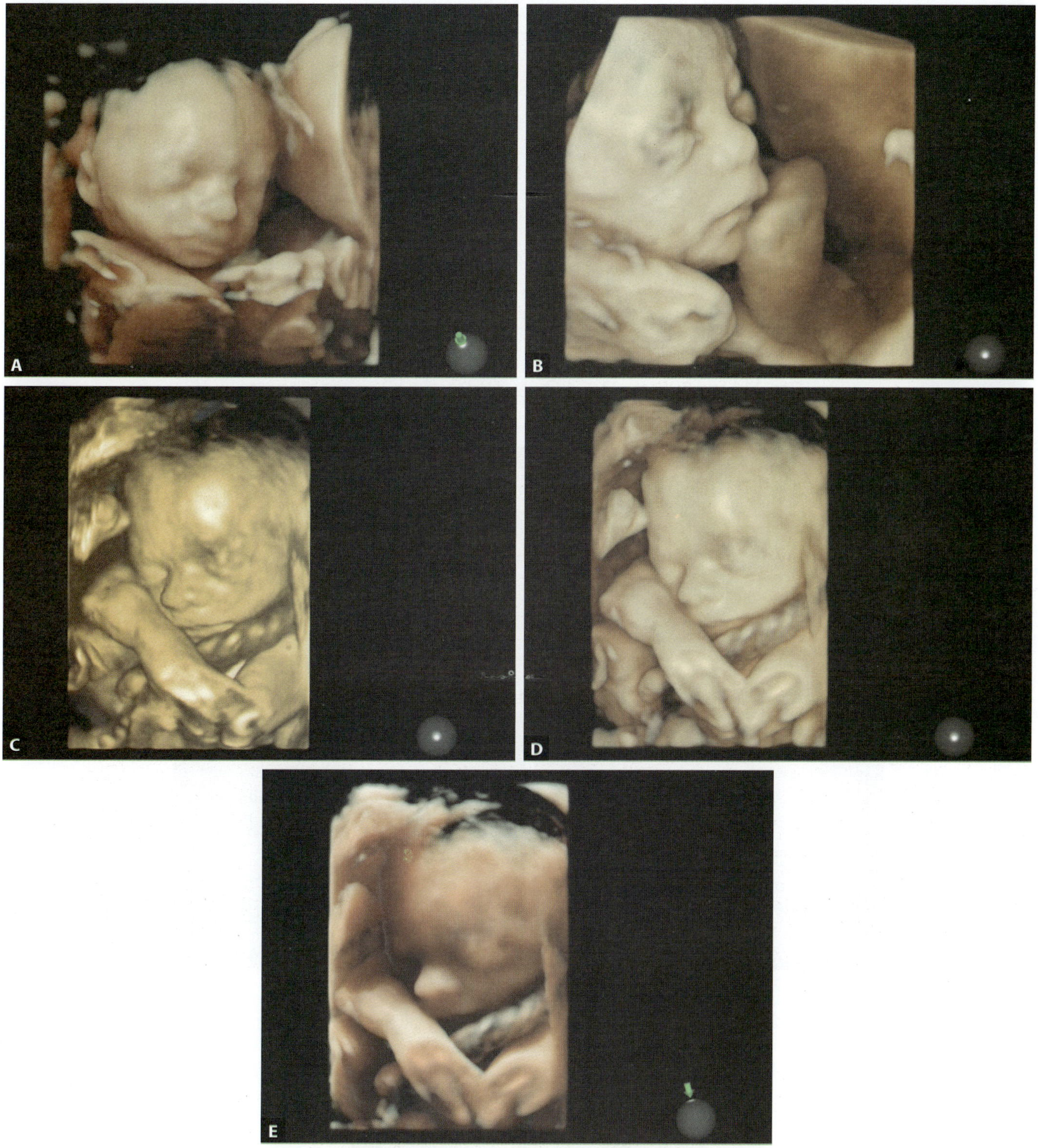

Figs. 10A to E: Weeks 23+0 d: Evidence of the umbilical cord by different use of the light on HDlive.

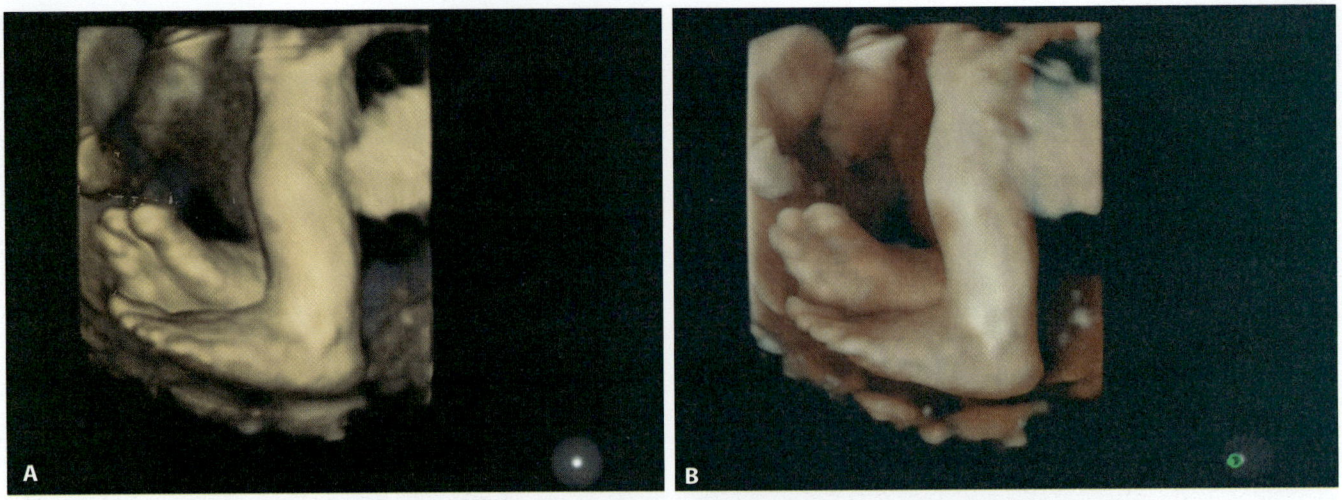

Figs. 11A and B: Weeks 23+0 d: Study of the feet by HDlive and silhouette.

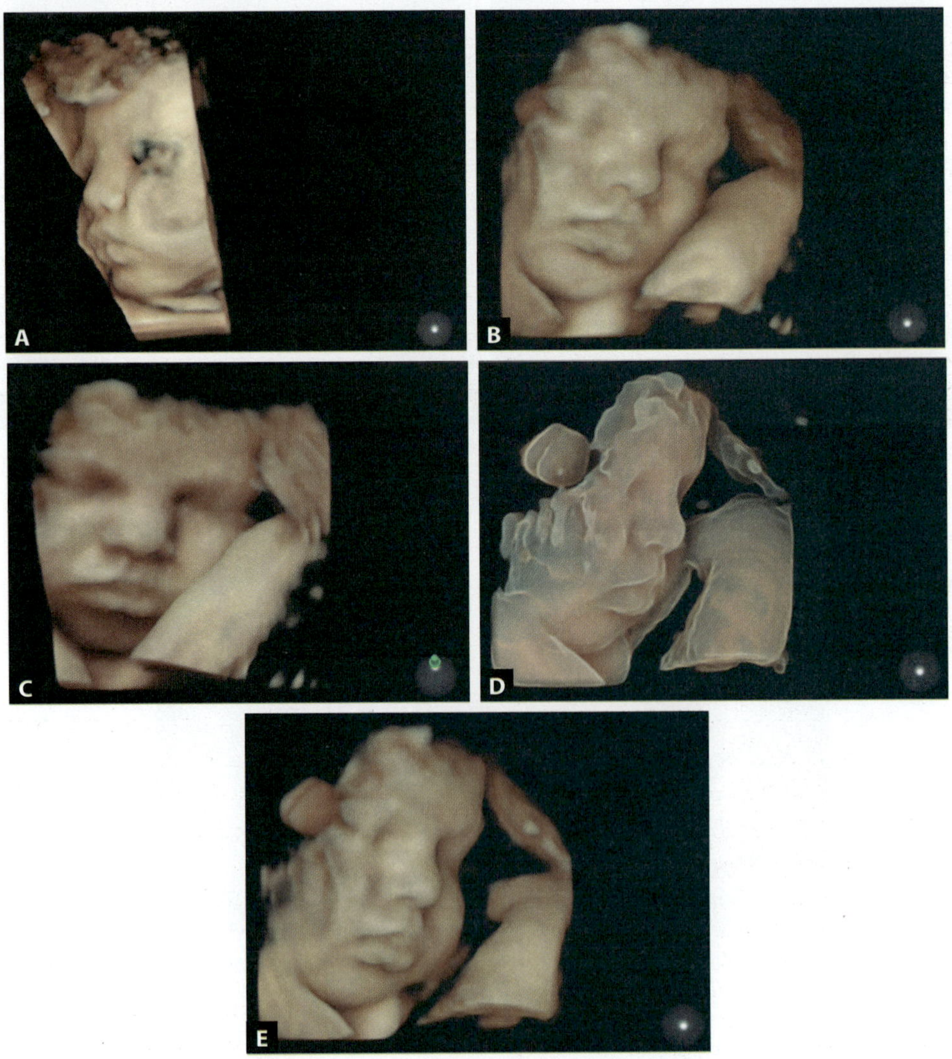

Figs. 12A to E: Weeks 37+0 d: Humanization of the face by HDlive and silhouette.

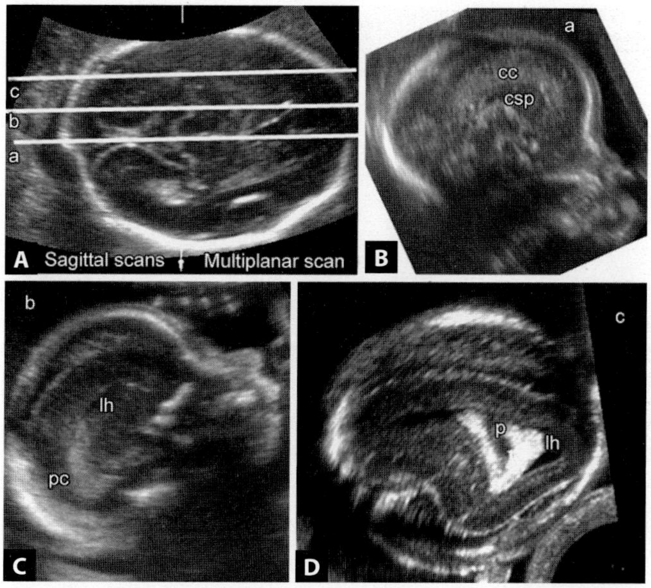

Figs. 13A to D: Sagittal scans. Image *a* shows the corpus callosum and cavum septi pellucidi perfectly. This section is very difficult to obtain by 2D, but easy by 3D multiplanar scan. The parasagittal scan offers a good view of the lateral horn and the anterior, posterior and subtemporal horns. (cc: corpus callosum; csp: cavum septi pellucidi; lh: lateral horn; p, choroid plexus).

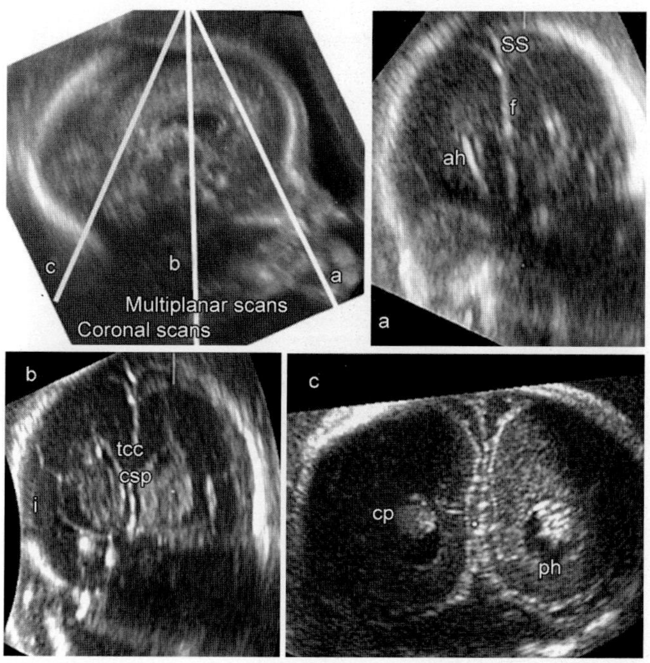

Fig. 14: Coronal scans. Section *a* is known as ox head because the anterior horns resemble those of an ox; section *b* shows a good view of the corpus callosum, cavum septi pellucidi and lateral ventricles; section *c* is known as owl eyes because of the contrast between the posterior horn and the white nervous system with eye-like choroid plexi (ah: anterior horn; csp: cavum septi pellucidi; f: falx; i: insula; cp: choroid plexus; ph: posterior horn).

possible in almost 100% of pregnancies. The number of GCs can also be determined. Spiral circulation around the GC can be detected from week 4; using multiplanar 3D with surface rendering it is easier to see the yolk sac (YS). Detection of the GC in uterus is an essential condition for excluding ectopic pregnancy and its eccentric position with respect to the uterine cavity, the presence of chorionic villi and consequent peripheral vascularisation,[16] combined with hCG monitoring, leave progressively less room for diagnostic uncertainty. It is also possible to visualize vascularization of the myometrium and decidua and check their homogeneous vasculogenesis, though these observation do not yet have clinical implications.

Detection of a GC measuring 2–4 mm in week 5 enables exact dating of pregnancy with an error of only 2–3 days. Visualization of the YS may be possible in the same week and is the first ultrasound-detectable embryonic structure; 2–4 days later, it is possible to see the embryo as a double bubble. In the following days and in practice from week 6, the yolk sac moves away from the embryo and the amnios is seen to divide the celomatic from the amniotic cavity. The yolk sac appears as a transonic ring above the cephalic pole of the embryo, growing slowly until weeks 8–9 without exceeding a diameter of 5 mm and then reducing progressively to disappear between weeks 12 and 14. An absent yolk sac or a large, nonspherical, hyperechogenic one with echo-rich internal structure is a condition associated with a poor prognosis for the pregnancy. A GC of mean diameter greater or equal to 20 mm, of lower than expected volume for gestational age, bounded by a thin trophoblast towards the periphery and devoid of embryo suggests blighted ovum syndrome. In such cases, it is advisable to repeat ultrasound examination a week later (for diagnosis at week 7).

Embryology: Days 24–27

CRL = 4.0 mm, head and body distinguishable; formation of prosencephalic cerebral vesicles or anterior brain, mesencephalon or middle brain and rhombencephalon or posterior brain, which subsequently give rise to:

- Prosencephalon
- Median vesicle (diencephalon) that gives rise to third ventricle
- Two lateral vesicles (telencephalon) that give rise to the hemispheres and lateral ventricles
- Formation of optical vesicles
- Formation of falx cerebri

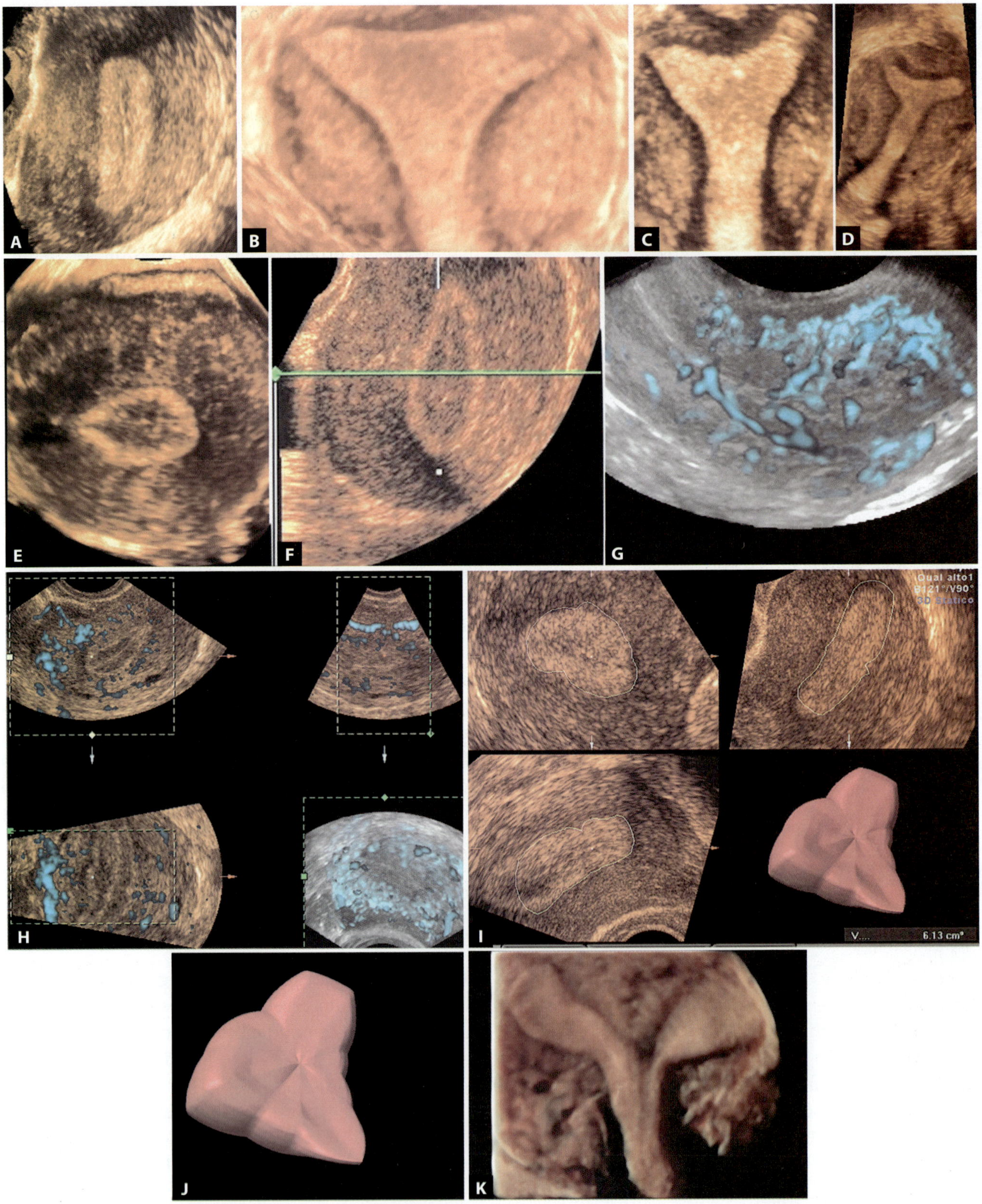

Figs. 15A to K: Different kinds of physiological endometrium at 12 days, a zoom of the three lines and myometrial vascularization and volume by VOCAL. (A) Multiplanar; (B to D) Surface rendering normal uterine shape; (E to H) Luteal phase; (I and J) Vocal; (K) HDlive of bicornuate uterus.

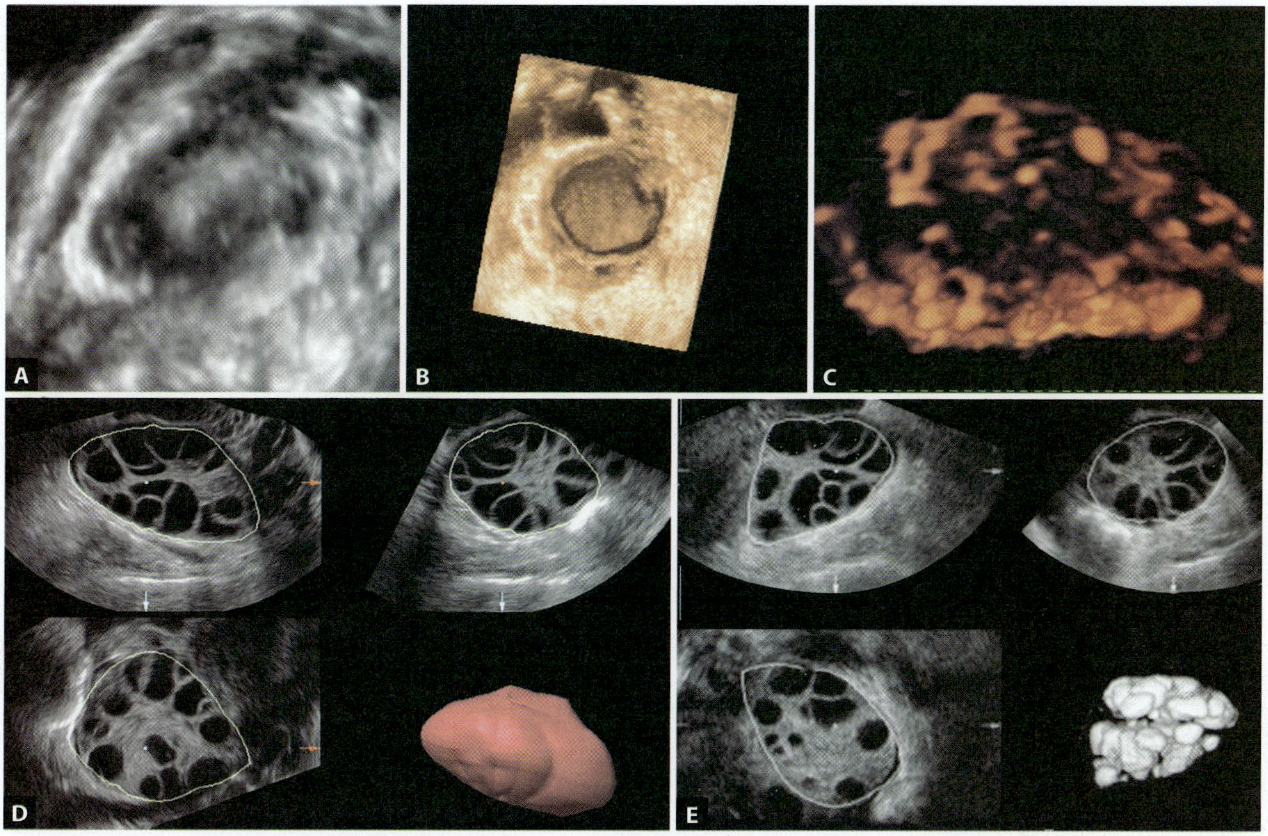

Figs. 16A to E: The number of follicles is easier to determine by 3D in the first part of the cycle (preferably by Vocal and Invert during hyperstimulation) and the morphology and vascularization of the Graafian follicle are more realistic.

- Formation of limbs, liver, pancreas, lungs, thyroid and mesonephrium tubes.

Fusion of two cardiac tubes along the median line and initiation of heart activity **(Figs. 17A to G)**.

Week 6 (Ultrasonographic)

From 5 weeks + 0 days to 5 weeks + 6 days

The GC should still be visible; if not, hCG should be assayed and repeated a week later to determine the possibility of delayed conception or ectopic pregnancy. Bi-, tri-, ..., chorionic multiple pregnancy is readily detected. The YS is detected in almost 100% of cases towards the end of the week and the double bubble image is increasingly frequent with a percentage detection of the embryo of about 20–40%. CRL is 1.5–4.0 mm at the end of week 6 and embryo heart beat (93–106 bpm) is visible. From now until week 12, CRL is the most reliable biometric value for dating pregnancy; mean error in expert hands is ± 2–3 days.

Embryology: 28–35 days

CRL = 6–9 mm;

- Slow heart beat evident through chest wall
- The hemispheres increase
- Budding of limbs
- Primitive intestine present
- First movements of embryo **(Figs. 18A and B)**.

Week 7 (Ultrasonographic)

From 6 weeks + 0 days to 6 weeks + 6 days

The amnios is still distinct from the chorion; the yolk sac is increasingly distant from the embryo, sometimes already compressed between the two membranes; prosencephalon and rhombencephalon detectable; budding of limbs; first movements of embryo.

Embryology: 36–42 days

CRL = 11–20 mm;

- Formation of olfactory and auditory systems.
- Separation of aortic-pulmonary trunk and of right and left atrioventricular canals.
- Herniation of midgut in umbilical cord.
- Formation of limb extremities (fingers and toes).
- Spine detectable (in more detail with 3D) **(Figs. 19A to J)**.

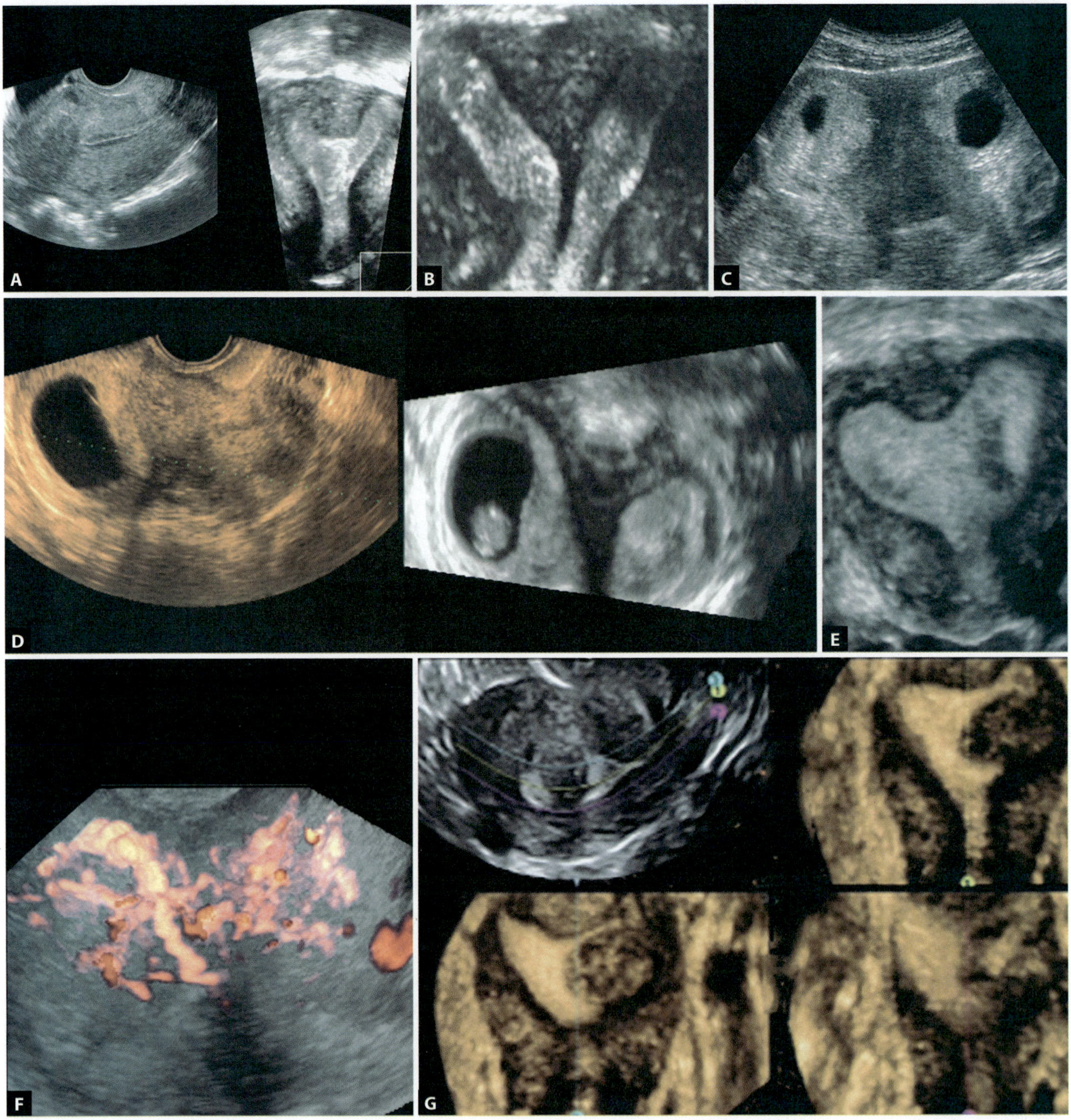

Figs. 17A to G: 3–4D offers a good view of the endometrium and can enable diagnosis of different kinds of uterine malformation. In early pregnancy (8th week) detection is easier, but for correct diagnosis it is important to see vascularization of two cornua. (A and B) Utero didelfo; (C and D) Bicornuate uterus with pregnancy at 6th and 8th week; (E and F) Didelfo uterus with vessels; (G) By multiplanar and surface it is easier to define the position of myoma.

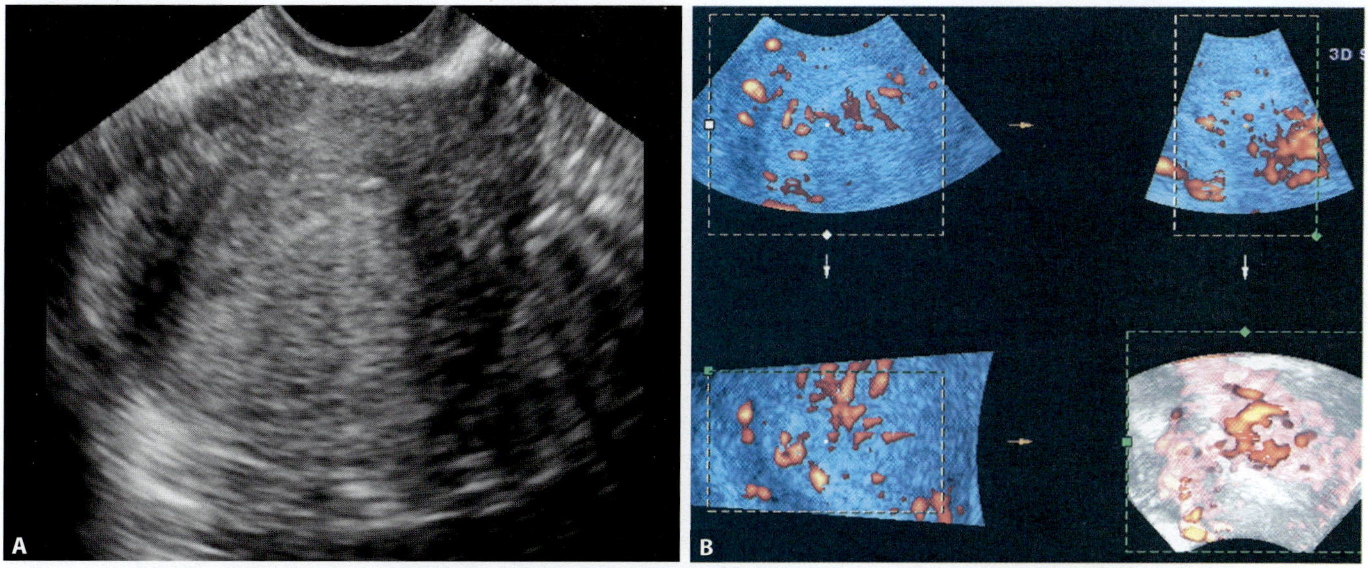

Figs. 18A and B: Until the end of week 4, it is usually possible to observe transformation of the endometrium into decidua and its vascularization.

Week 8 (Ultrasonographic)

From 7 weeks + 0 days to 7 weeks + 6 days

The amnion is still distinct from the chorion; the two membranes constrain and envelop the YS, making it disappear when they fuse, which usually occurs at 14–16 weeks; choroid plexuses present; herniated intestine in umbilical cord which should resume its intra-abdominal position by week 12 (omphalocele differentiation); embryo tachycardia >110 bpm; evident movements of embryo; facial features detectable; extremities detectable.

Embryology: 43–49 days

CRL = 22–30 mm;

- Legs form circle with knees turned out and feet in contact (frog attitude)
- Formation of eyebrows and external ear **(Figs. 20A to I)**.

Week 9 (Ultrasonographic)

From 8 weeks + 0 days to 8 weeks + 6 days

The embryo is clearly visible through vaginal and abdominal windows and begins to appear human. Its movements are often jumpy and abrupt. More articulated and refined movements are not seen until development of the neopallium in months 6–7. The face is clearly delineated, especially by 3D volumetric scans. In the brain, the hemispheres and ventricles with their posterior (choroid plexuses) and anterior horns are observed developing from the two vesicles of the telencephalon. The brainstem is sometimes detectable. The rhombencephalon persists and is dividing to form the fourth ventricle (metencephalon) and the spinal cord (myelencephalon). The spine and ribs are clearly visible. Differentiation of chorion laeve and chorion frondosum.

The embryonic period comes to an end after week 9, ushering in the fetal period with its rapid longitudinal (hyperplastic) growth that continues until week 20, with further differentiation and organization of organs and tissues formed in the embryonic period and with acquisition of specific functions **(Figs. 21A to D)**.

Fetal Period

Anatomy: From day 50–84 (8–12 full weeks).

Ultrasonography: Until Day 98 (10–14 Full Weeks)

Until week 10, the transvaginal route is universally recognized as the acoustic window for embryo study. After week 10, the transabdominal route may also be used with good ultrasound instruments in women with normal fat distribution. By week 10, CRL is no longer precise for dating pregnancy, acquiring an error of ± 5 days (due to fetal flexion and extension). From week 11, biparietal diameter (BPD) is therefore preferred, though CRL is still important, for example in measuring nuchal translucence (NT).

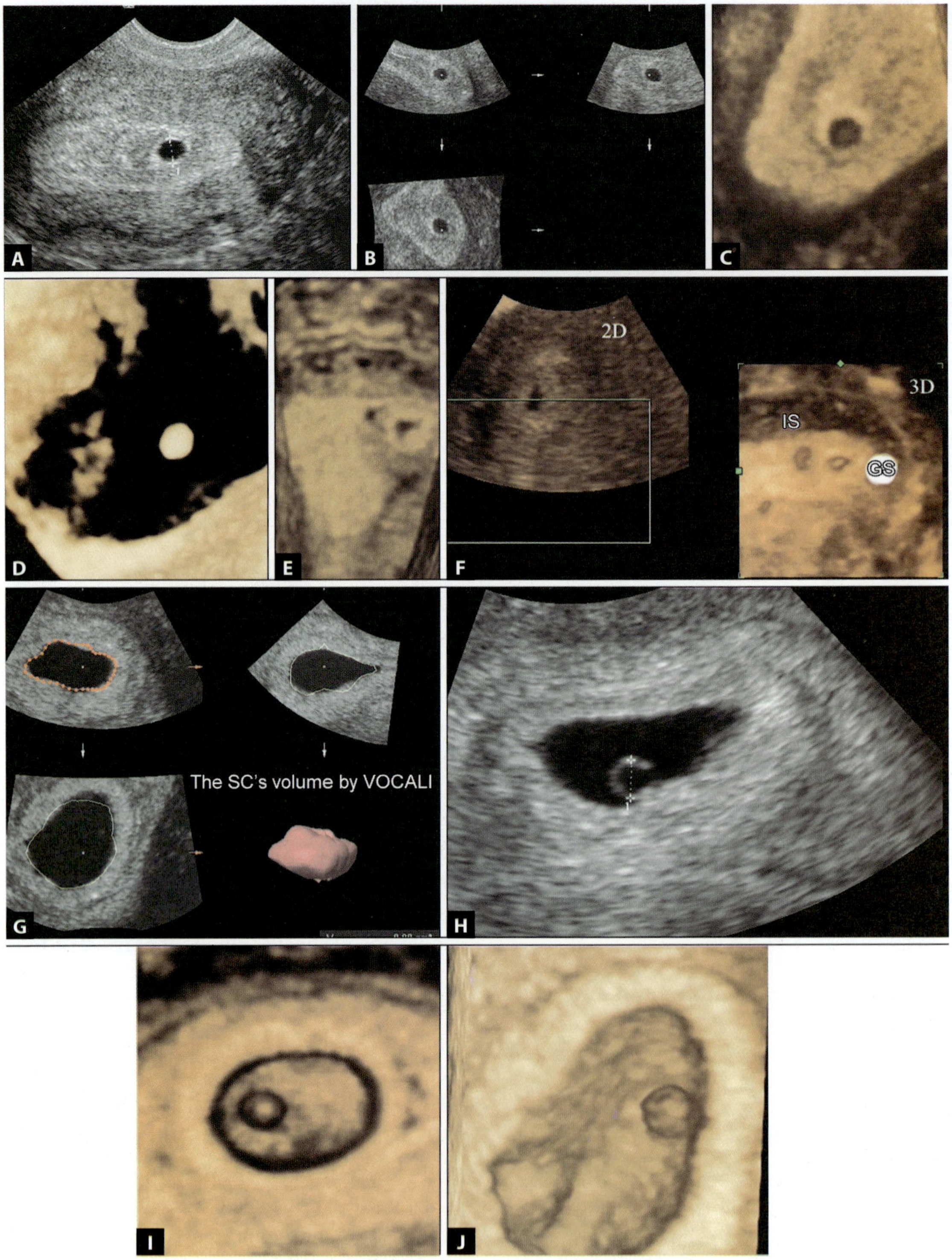

Figs. 19A to J: Week 5: From gestational sac (GS) to yolk sac. The gestational sac is more evident by 3D, and it is possible to see the external wall of the GS, making it easier to distinguish the GS from the interdecidual space (IS).

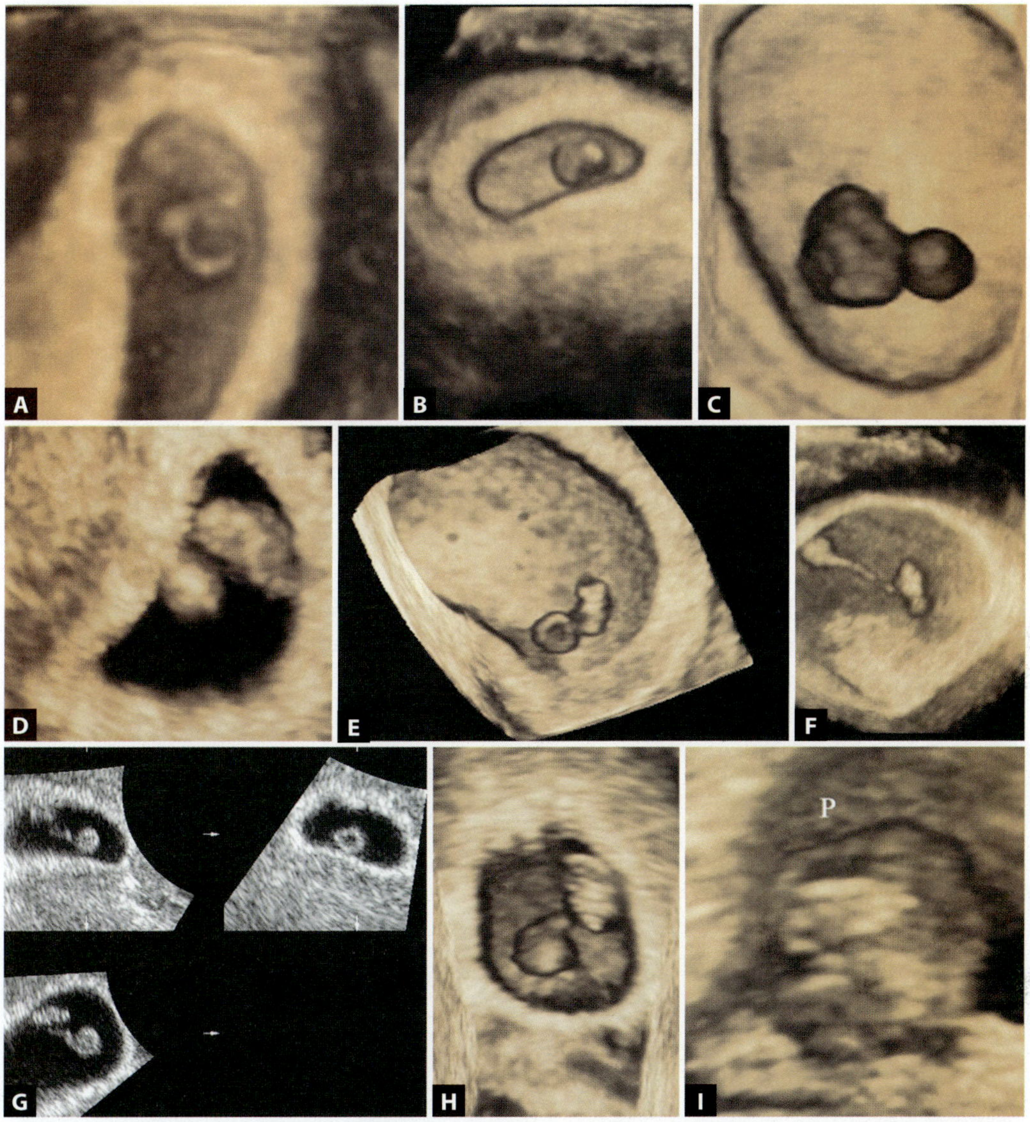

Figs. 20A to I: (A to H) Week 6: The embryo appears and the double bubble becomes more evident during the week. The embryo moves away from the yolk sac, which remains near the uterine wall and disappears in weeks 12–14; (I) Zoom of embryo head showing prosencephalon (P).

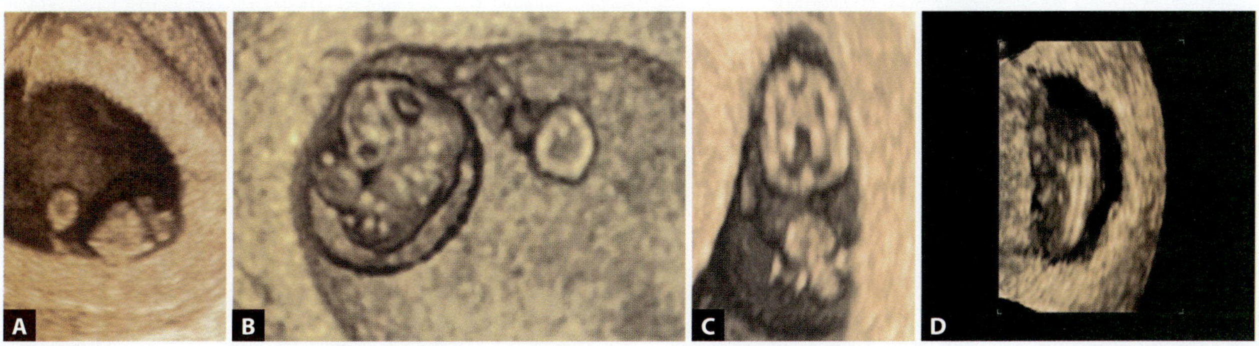

Figs. 21A to D: Week 7 (6–12 mm): Embryo anatomy is more complex: note promesorhomboencephalon and first image of face. Arms and legs are present, as are the queue and the vertebral column. The amniotic membrane is well formed and divides the amniotic cavity from the celomatic cavity; the yolk sac lies between the amniotic and chorionic membranes.

By week 10, the foetus acquires definite anatomical characteristics that will persist for the rest of gestation, albeit with changes in size and function. By week 12, umbilical hernia disappears and by week 14 the YS is hardly visible and the two membranes fuse. In the brain, the choroid plexuses that almost filled the cranial cavity, are relegated to the posterior horns; the brainstem is increasingly evident and the posterior cranial fossa is readily detected by week 14.[17] Although the corpus callosum ceases its formation later and is detectable by ultrasound by weeks 20–22, the cavity of the septum pellucidum can be detected. The heart with its four chambers becomes visible from week 12 transvaginally, however not in all cases.[18] The detection percentage increases dramatically by week 14 and indeed more and more centres are delaying transvaginal screening for cardiopathy until weeks 14–16. The fetal face is increasingly human and offers striking images by 3–4D. By week 12, BPD is the most reliable biometric value for dating pregnancy, having a mean error of ± 1 week **(Figs. 22 to 24).**

Embryo–Fetal Pathology Detectable by Ultrasound in the First Trimester

The acoustic window of the first trimester of pregnancy (until week 14) offers the possibility of suspecting or diagnosing embryo-fetal malformations, chromosome anomalies and perinatal outcome. The possibilities in the first trimester have been described by Nikolaides et al. who concentrated their research on the fetus from week 11–14, documenting the many chromosome pathologies and malformations that can be detected. The fact that ultrasonographic diagnosis is becoming possible increasingly early in pregnancy partly attenuates the psychological problem of the mother and her partner when the painful question of whether or not to interrupt pregnancy arises.[19] There have been many examples illustrating the significance of the first trimester for detecting chromosome and/or structural anomalies or at least for selecting populations at risk, whereas the

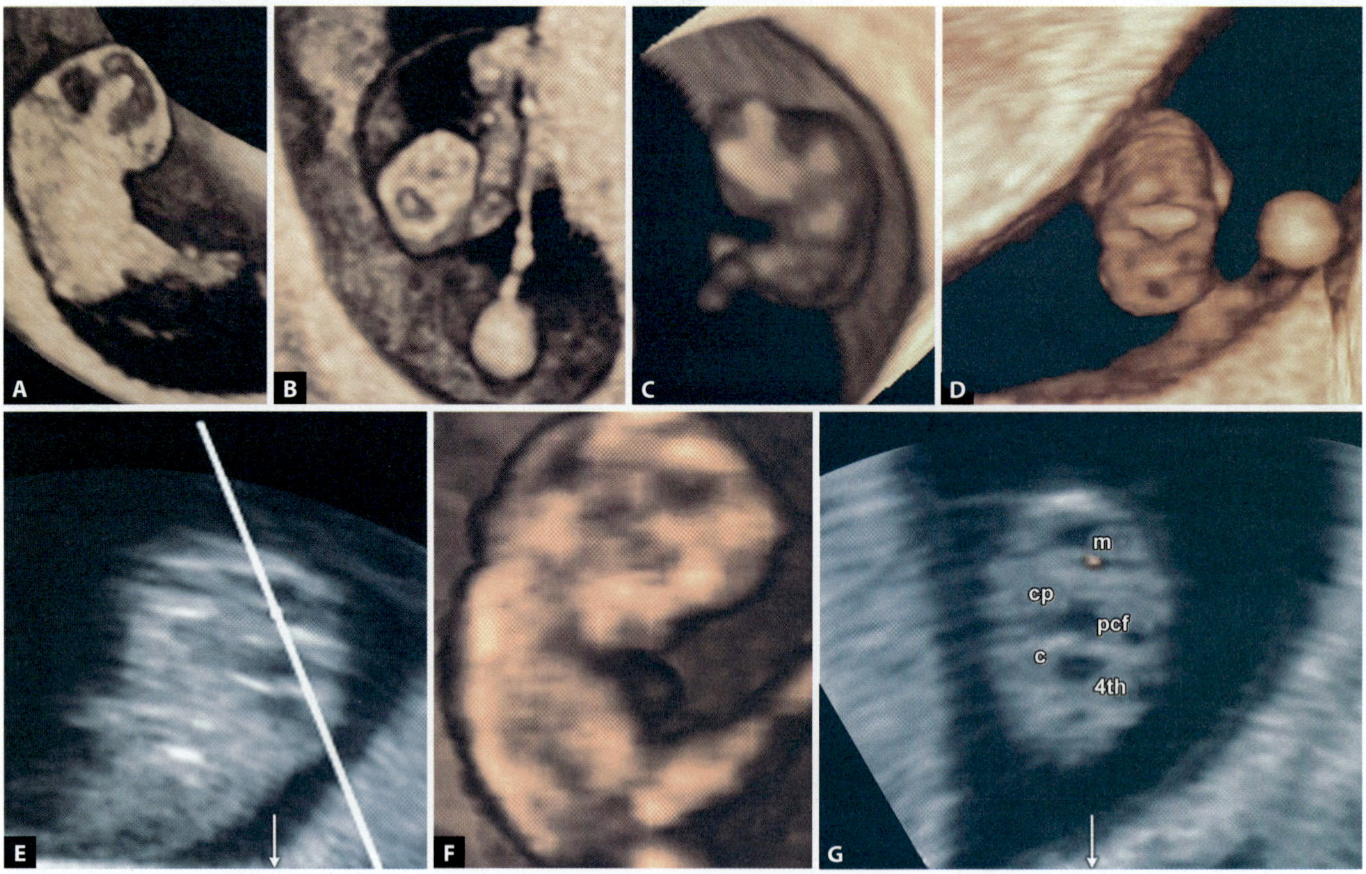

Figs. 22A to G: Week 8 (22 mm): Head structures are better defined. (4th: fourth ventricle; c: cerebellum; pcf: posterior cranial fossa; cp: choroid plexus; m: mesencephalon).

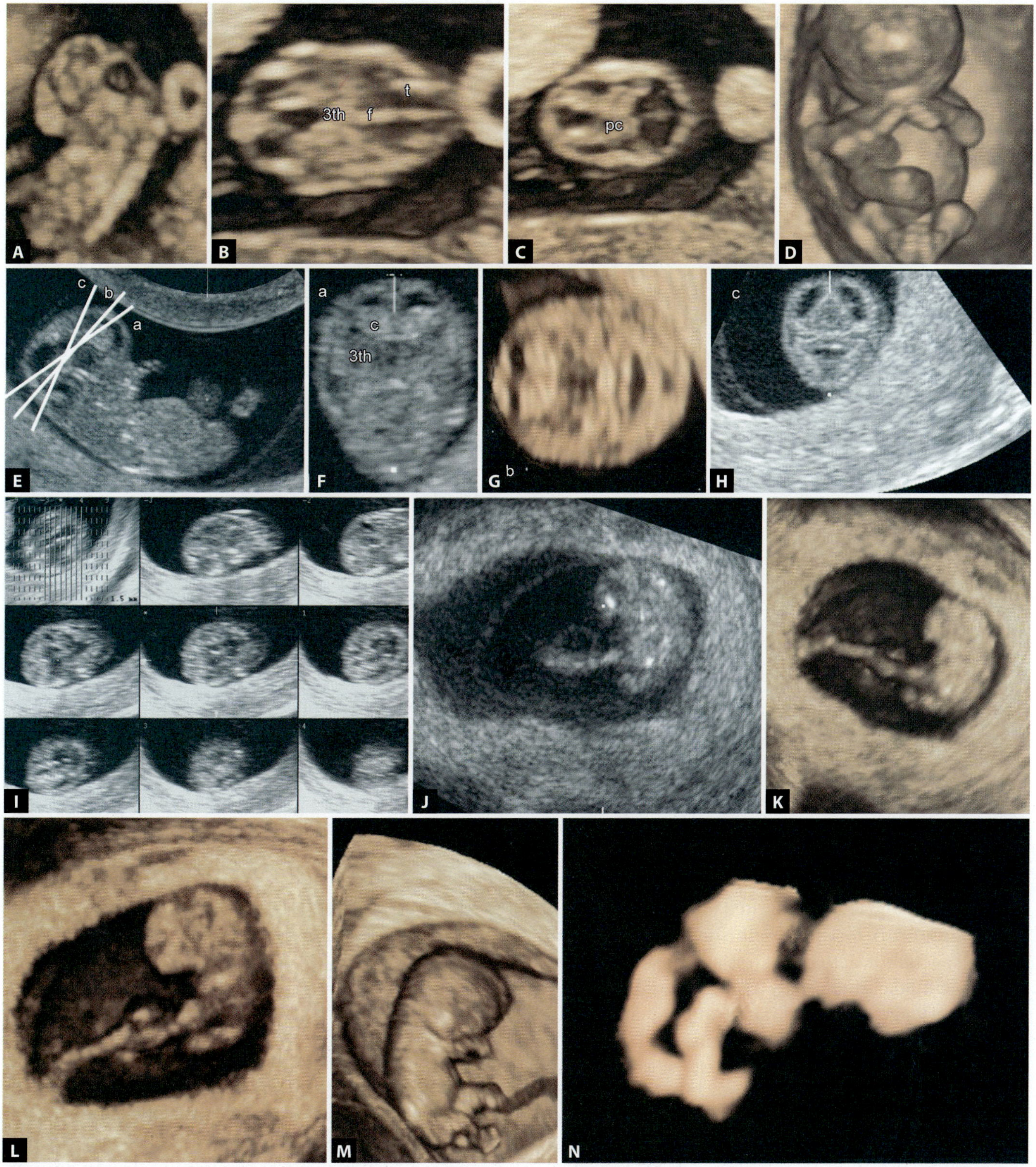

Figs. 23A to N: Week 9 (29 mm): (A to M) Embryo acquires human features and external morphology is now fixed. Detection of physiological umbilical hernia. Complete view of brain clearer with tomography ultrasound imaging which makes ultrasonography similar to NMR (the image can be cut in real time up to 18 times at predetermined distances); (N) Invert mode shows spatial extent of ventricles.

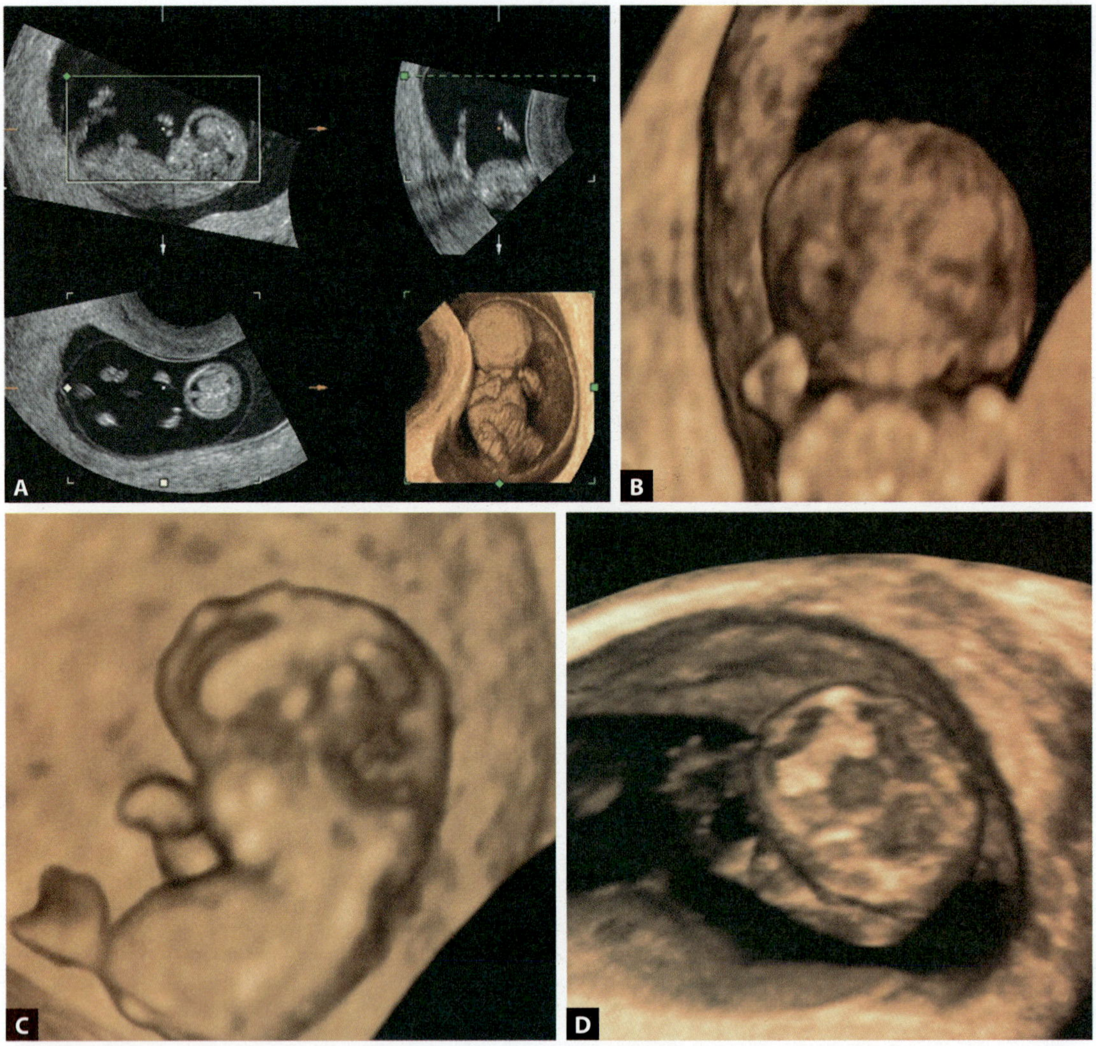

Figs. 24A to D: Week 10: Beginning of fetal period. Body organs have formed and will grow, and acquire organ functions. Multiplanar view of 34 mm fetus, showing face, ventricles and cerebellum.

second trimester is more indicated for malformations, for example the heart (for which there is ample documentation that suspected or actual diagnosis is possible in week, 14), spina bifida[20] and Dandy-Walker syndrome.[21] In any case, knowledge of the natural history of malformations is fundamental for understanding missed diagnoses. For example, partial or total agenesis of the corpus callosum cannot be diagnosed until week 22-24, when the corpus callosum completes its formation. First trimester ultrasonography (weeks 11–14) is increasingly viewed as a time for morphological and structural checkup, similar if not better than second trimester scans, hence increasing use of the term first trimester sonoembryology, meaning the whole of the first trimester **(Figs. 25 to 30)**.

SIGNS PREDICTIVE OF ANEUPLOIDY AND STRUCTURAL EMBRYO-FETAL ALTERATIONS IN THE FIRST TRIMESTER

It is common practice to obtain verbal or written informed consent before determining nuchal translucency. It also seems reasonable to make a similar contract (implying correct counseling and specific request) for predictive markers of aneuploidy in the first trimester, as is customary in the second trimester (so-called "genetic" ultrasonography). In my opinion, consent to scan for structural alterations, the only therapy for which would be interruption of pregnancy, is also advisable. Today, ultrasonography in pregnancy is a powerful instrument for serenity, but may also create gratuitous anguish. Before carrying it out, it is important to discuss it with the woman, not only specifying the limits of the method and of the operator, but also asking clearly what the women expects and wants from the scan.

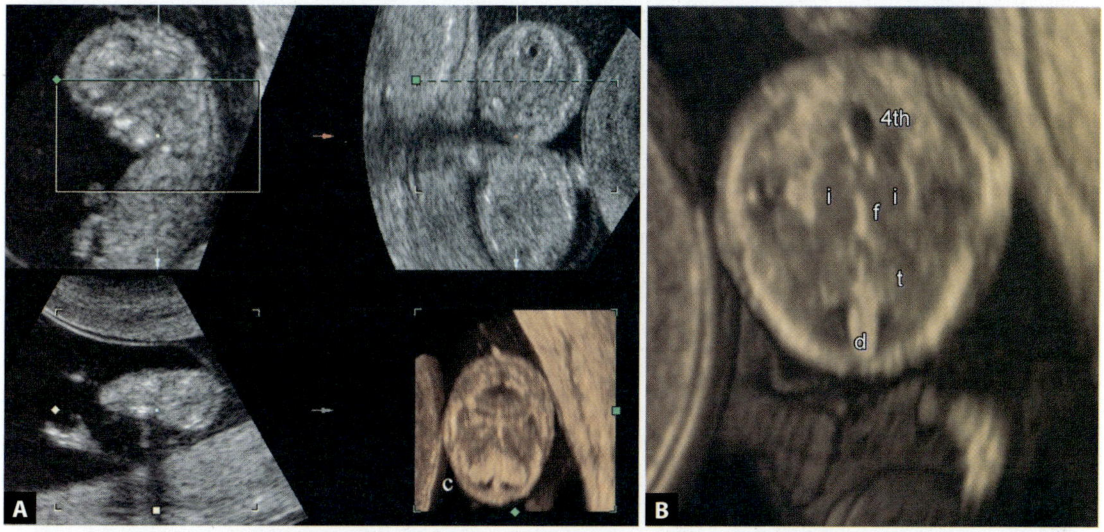

Figs. 25A and B: Weeks 11–12: Multiplanar view showing brain (4th: fourth ventricle; f: falx; d: diencephalon; t: telencephalon).

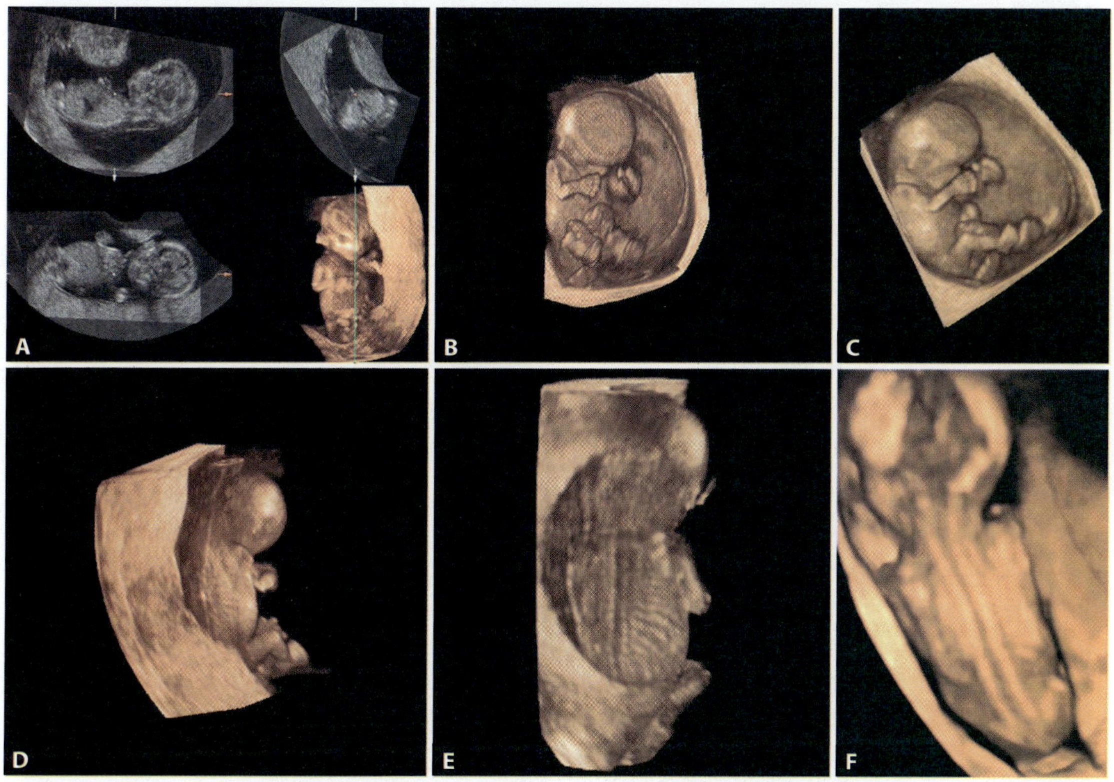

Figs. 26A to F: Weeks 13–14: Fetal morphology is clear; note details of face, limbs, fingers, toes and neck. Detailed study of spine is possible.

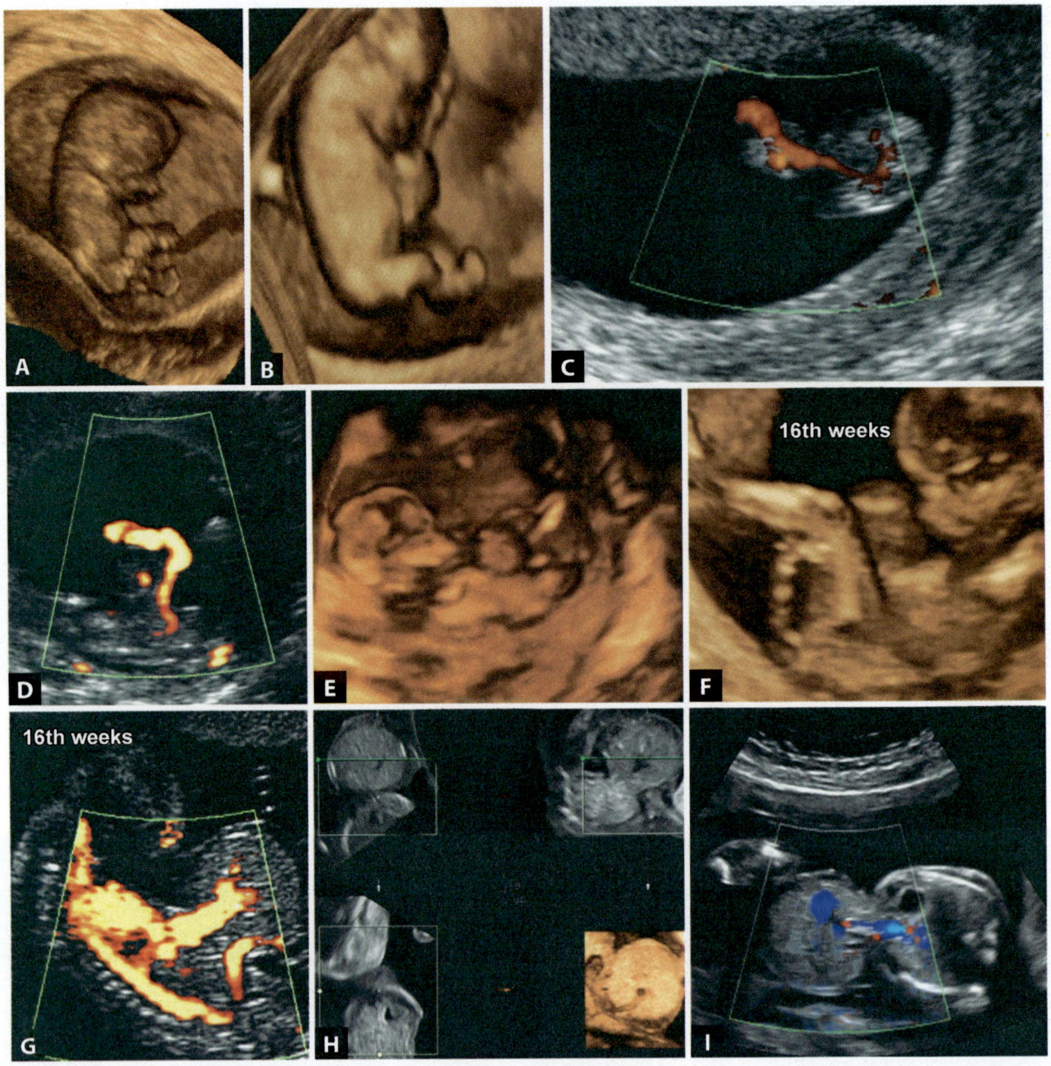

Figs. 27A to I: Omphalocele at weeks 13, 16 and 18. Note difference between normal and abnormal hernia in A and B: umbilical artery starts from top of hernia (color and power glass body mode). Week 16 and 18 images show homogeneous echogenicity of small intestine and stomach.

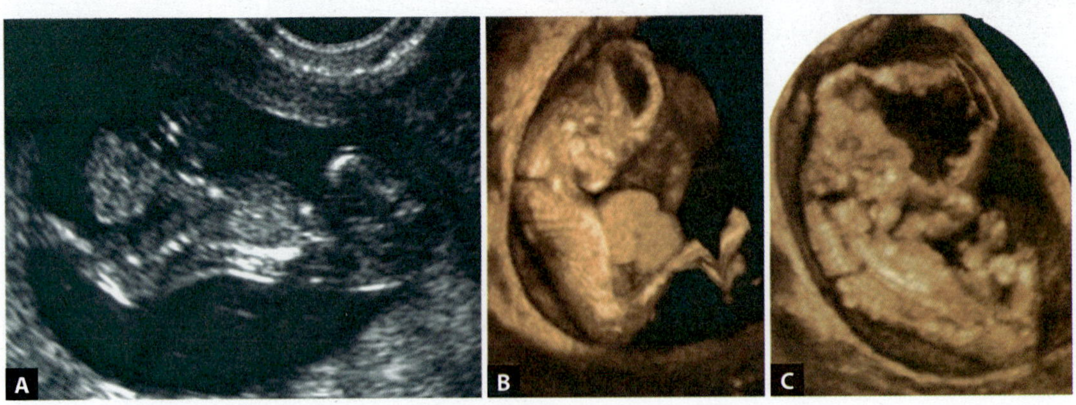

Figs. 28A to C: Alobar holoprosencephaly associated with omphalocele in a 46,XX fetus at week 12. The 3D provides more information than 2D.

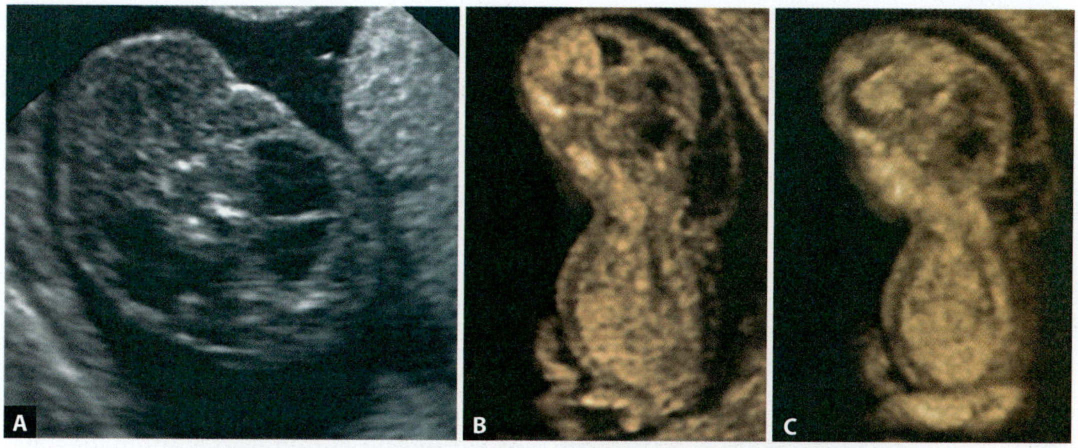

Figs. 29A to C: Septate cystic hygroma at week 13 as shown by 3D and 2D.

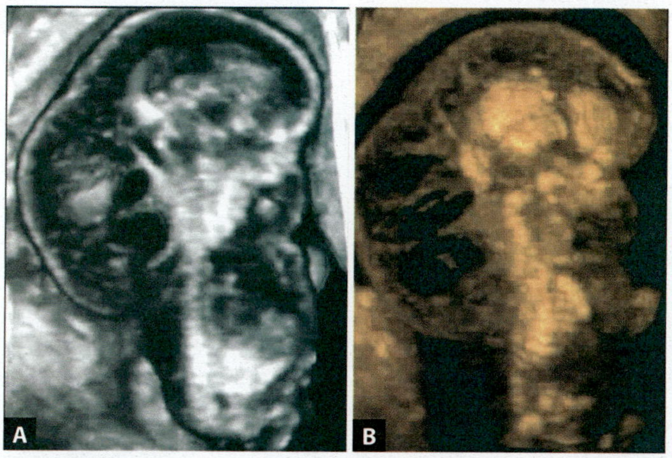

Figs. 30A and B: Hygroma and fetal hydrops at 16 weeks. The hygroma plurisepimentato extends back to the fetus.

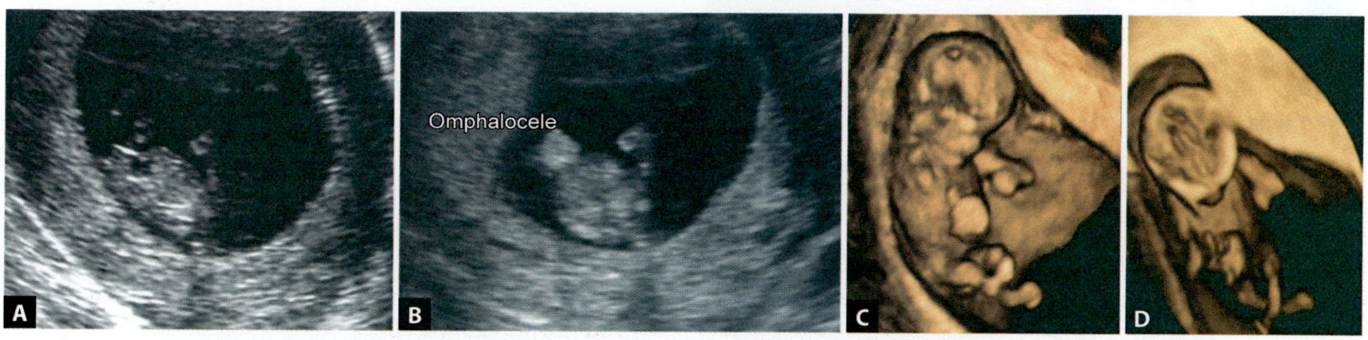

Figs. 31A to D: Radius-ulnar agenesis with omphalocele in fetus with trisomy 18 at week 10.

Transitory Signs

Nuchal Translucency

The problem with screening tests in which nuchal translucency (NT) is a constant component is too complex to discuss in an atlas; however, the detection of this transient sign is easier and quicker with multiplanar than with classical 2D **(Figs. 31 and 32)**. The current scientific findings have shown that it can detect even an intracranial translucency (fourth ventricle) that seems to offer a sensitivity and specificity of nearly 100% in the early detection of spina bifida[22,23] **(refer to Fig. 16)**.

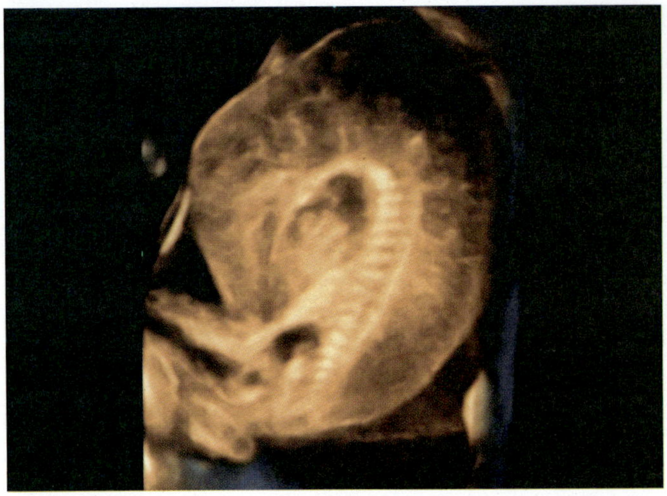

Fig. 32: Twin reversed arterial perfusion syndrome (TRAP). (A) Acardius acephalus (13 weeks) is characterized by amorphous shape of the cephalic pole, the upper limbs are absent; the lower limbs are present and the intrathoracic and abdominal organs are rudimentary, with diffuse subcutaneous edema.

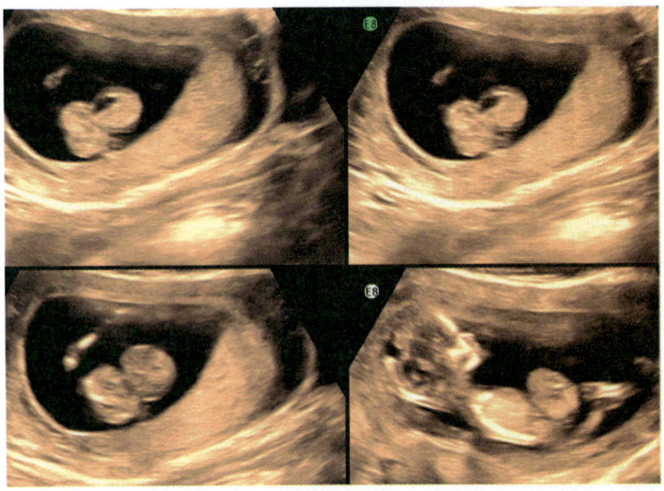

Fig. 33: Omphalocele at 12 weeks.

At 11–13 weeks of gestation, during the first trimester screening of chromosomal abnormalities in the mid-sagittal view of the fetal face, we can to obtain the nuchal translucency thickness and the nasal bone view; in this view is visible the fourth ventricle. In the normal fetuses the fourth ventricle was always visible and the median anteroposterior diameter increased from 1.5 mm at a crown-rump length (CRL) of 45 mm to 2.5 mm at a CRL of 84 mm. In the fetuses with spina bifida the fourth ventricle space was compressed and no could be seen, we can also be used for early detection of open spina bifida.[24]

Pending clinical confirmations is important to be able, during a 11–14 week scan, to detect these markers that can be considered as an alarm bell to identifying cases at risk Assessment of intracranial translucency (IT) in the detection of spina bifida at the 11–13-week scan (**Fig. 23** bis).

Ductus Venosus

Measurement of NT in the first trimester has become a consolidated method for identifying fetuses at risk for chromosomal abnormality. The high percentage of heart defects in fetuses with increased NT, whether isolated or caused by chromosome anomalies, has stimulated considerable interest. The association, together with echo-Doppler modifications of the ductus venosus (DV) in fetuses with increased NT, suggests that altered heart function could play a role in determining an increase in NT.[25,26]

In particular, inverted flow in the DV during heart's contraction (A wave) has been associated with increased NT. The DV is a communicating vessel that carries well oxygenated blood of the umbilical vein into the right atrium, through the oval foramen. This vessel is important for assessing the presence of heart function anomalies. Blood flow in the DV is characterized by high velocity during ventricular systole (S wave) and diastole (D wave) and also by forward flow during atrial contraction (A wave). In heart dysfunction due to heart defects, the A wave is absent or negative.

Assessment of flow in the DV could play a role in secondary screening, permitting further reduction in the percentage of false-positives in screening for chromosome anomalies in the first trimester.[27,28] A major association has been demonstrated between chromosome anomalies and abnormal blood flow in the DV at 11–14 weeks of pregnancy in high risk pregnancies.[29,30] DV flow anomaly associated with heart defects and adverse outcome of pregnancy has also been observed. Some authors suggest that the DV can be an important prognostic factor in fetuses with increased NT and normal karyotype.

In fetuses with chromosome anomalies, whose parents decided to continue the pregnancy, heart dysfunction has been found to be a temporary condition: transitory anomalous flow in the DV, detected by color Doppler, manifested as "reversed flow" during contraction. This marker is detected early, around week 13, and usually disappears by week 20. The dysfunction that caused it aggravates retronuchal edema and may culminate in fetal

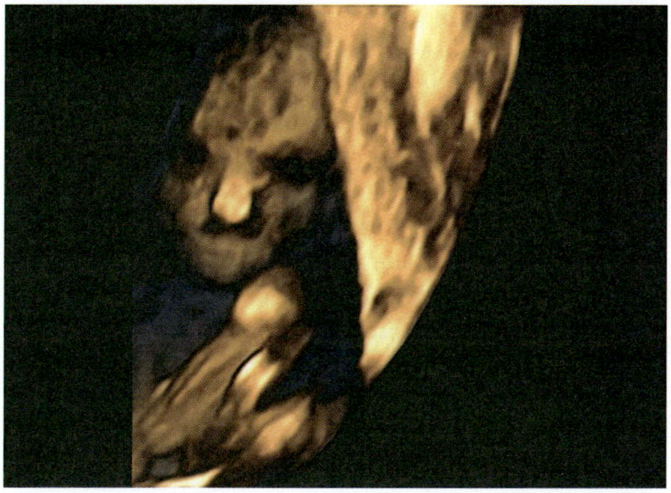

Fig. 34: Frontal holoprosencephaly. Elephant fetus at 11 weeks.

hydrops, which could explain some cases of intrauterine fetal death. At 10–13 weeks + 6 days the duct anomaly is therefore associated with aneuploidy (80% of Down fetuses versus 5% of euploid fetuses), heart malformations and unfavorable outcome of pregnancy. To study the DV, 3-4D does not offer particular advantages, whereas 2D is fundamental and exclusive for correct detection **(Fig. 34)**.

Nuchal Edema, Cystic Hygroma and Nonimmune Hydrops

Subcutaneous edema detected sonographically in the forms of nuchal edema, cystic hygroma, or nonimmune hydrops may be a sign of chromosomal abnormalities.[31]

Cystic hygroma is a congenital malformation of the lymphatic system characterized by a thin walled cystic structure full of liquid. It is usually situated in the nuchal region, extending from the superior occipital bone, caudally and medially to the sternocleidomastoid muscle. It consists of two symmetrical cavities completely separated by a median nuchal ligament and is distinguished from other craniocervical masses, such as encephalocele, meningocele, teratoma, hemangioma and retronuchal edema.[32,33]

At about 40 days of embryo development, the jugular lymphatic sac forms a connection between the jugular duct and the internal jugular veins which become the terminal portions of the lymphatic and thoracic ducts. According to the theory of obstruction of the jugular lymphatic sac, the connection between the jugular lymphatic sac and the jugular veins does not form in the case of cystic hygroma and the lymph builds up in tissues around the neck, causing the sac to swell. Cystic hygroma is often detected by prenatal ultrasound, though some cases develop in the postnatal period, with an incidence of about 1%. The defect may regress spontaneously during pregnancy, leaving extra-skin in the neck region, or progress dramatically towards a form of generalized fetal hydrops.[34]

Fetal cystic hygroma was usually readily diagnosed by transabdominal ultrasound in the second trimester of pregnancy. Today transvaginal ultrasound has increased the percentage of diagnoses in the first trimester.[35] Ultrasound diagnosis of cystic hygroma is based on visualization of a prominent anechogenic or hypoechogenic area (more than 3 mm thick) in the occipital, nuchal or upper thoracic regions, bilaterally. On the other hand, physiological build-up of fluid or the nuchal bleb is generally considered normal when it is less than 3 mm thick: these build-ups seem to occur in 40% of embryos before week 10 and disappear at week 11.

Cystic hygroma may be single or consist of multiple cysts and is classified as septate and non septate. Though confused for years by various authors, this distinction is important for prognosis, because septate cystic hygroma is strongly associated with aneuploidies.[36]

The presence of cystic hygroma in the first trimester is associated with increased risk of fetal chromosome anomalies: about 50% of fetuses with ultrasound diagnosis of cystic hygroma in the first trimester also have a chromosome anomaly. A high percentage of the cases undergoing cytogenetic analysis show Turner syndrome, often associated with trisomy 21, 18, 13 or other structural anomalies. The risk of this transient anomaly increases with increasing maternal age.

As yet there are no ultrasonographic elements for distinguishing cystic lesions that may regress from those that persist. However, when the nuchal cyst is small and non septate and karyotype is normal, it usually resolves spontaneously with good fetal outcome. When septate cystic hygroma is diagnosed early in pregnancy, the risk of chromosome aberrations is much greater and the outcome is therefore worse, also because septate hygroma is often larger and frequently develops into fetal hydrops. Spontaneous regression of cystic hygroma has been reported in chromosomally normal fetuses and in Down, Turner and Robert syndrome fetuses.

Fetuses diagnosed with nonseptate and septate forms, with or without associated malformations, are at high risk of chromosome aneuploidies. The mothers need correct counseling to assess the possibility of cytogenetic tests to determine fetal karyotype, to program subsequent ultrasound monitoring to exclude morphological anomalies, particularly of the heart and circulatory system, and to evaluate any worsening of edema or its resolution. Fetuses with normal karyotype are usually free of hygroma by weeks 16–17 and many have normal phenotypes at birth. Ultrasound parameters such as hygroma size and the time of its disappearance associated with fetal echocardiography may be useful to identify pregnancies at risk for dysmorphic conditions such as Noonan syndrome **(refer to Fig. 27)**.

Persistent Signs

Nasal Bone

In 1866, Langdon Down noticed that subjects with trisomy 21 had a small nose. An anthropometric study on 105 Down patients confirmed that the nasal bone (NB) was smaller than normal in 49.5% of cases. Recent radiological and ultrasound studies have shown that nasal hypoplasia is already present in the uterus.[37,38] A study of 105 fetuses with trisomy 21, aborted at weeks 12–25, showed lack of ossification of the NB in 32.4% of cases and hypoplasia in 21.4%. The correlation between absence of NB at weeks 11–14 and increased risk of trisomy 21 was reported for the first time in 2001. Indeed, about 65% of Down fetuses lack, or have a small, NB.

The nasal bone can be seen by scan from week 11.[39] Many recent studies show a strong association between absence of NB at this gestational age and trisomy 21 and other chromosome anomalies.[40,41] We can therefore say that at 11–13 weeks + 6 days, fetal profile can be examined correctly in more than 95% of cases and that the NB is absent in about 70% of fetuses with trisomy 21 and in about 55% of fetuses with trisomy 13. The incidence of absence of NB in euploid fetuses is less than 1%. Absence of NB is therefore a major marker of trisomy 21. There are some limiting factors in the ultrasonographic assessment of NB.[42,43] Between weeks 11 and 14 from the last menstrual cycle, the probability of visualizing the NB increases with increasing gestational age. The presence of NB is not independent of fetal nuchal thickness, since the possibility of visualizing it seems to decrease with increasing NT. Finally, ultrasound detection of NB at 11–14 weeks requires much technical skill of the operator, unlike later in pregnancy.[44]

Absence of NB has a higher incidence in fetuses of African origin than in Caucasians and decreases with CRL. In calculating individual patient-specific risk of Down syndrome, it is necessary to consider these demographic and ultrasonographic aspects.

If examination of fetal profile to detect NB is associated with NT and maternal serum proteins (free β hCG and PAPP-A) during first trimester screening for trisomy 21, the detection rate can increase substantially and the false positive rate decrease. For a false-positive rate of about 5%, the detection rate increases from about 75% [NT] and 90% [NB + maternal serum proteins] to 93% [NT+NB] and 97% [NT+NB+ maternal serum proteins]. For a false-positive rate of 1%, the detection rate could be about 57% for NT, 86% for NT + NB and 93% for NT, NB and maternal serum proteins.

In conclusion, the absence of NB or small NB are more common in fetuses with chromosome anomalies. It is therefore clear that NB is becoming a major marker in the prenatal diagnosis of aneuploidies.

There is a statistically significant difference between detection of NB by 2D and 3D techniques. Traditional scan is about 20% less reliable in detecting presence/absence of NB and also for the number of bones detected. This difference can be as high as 40% when 2D is performed with mediosagittal scan of the fetal face, since detection of the NB requires a longitudinal fetal scan as for detection of NT, but in the case of NB the section is 1–2 mm from the sagittal median. Further studies seem to suggest greater reliability in the second trimester, with a cutoff of 2.5 mm for NB and the presence of both nasal bones; in the second trimester, 3D plays an important role, making detection of the bones simpler and more reliable[45] **(Fig. 35)**.

Palate

It is possible investigate the normality of the secondary palate better than the primary palate, because it is very difficult define a normality of the lips in the first trimester (foto 14 settimane). We can detect the secondary palate by two methods: by the evidence of the retronasal angle with a 100% confidence by the authors) using 2D or 3D multiplanar or omni-view and by the Faure method with a coronal/sagittal 3D scan of the foetus's profile and rotation of the picture avoiding the maxillary shadow and maximum or minimum rendering of the palate by axial section (delta sign) **(Fig. 35)**.

Jaw Bone

In a series 89 Down fetuses compared with a population of 900 euploid fetuses, Cicero (2004) found jaw bones shorter

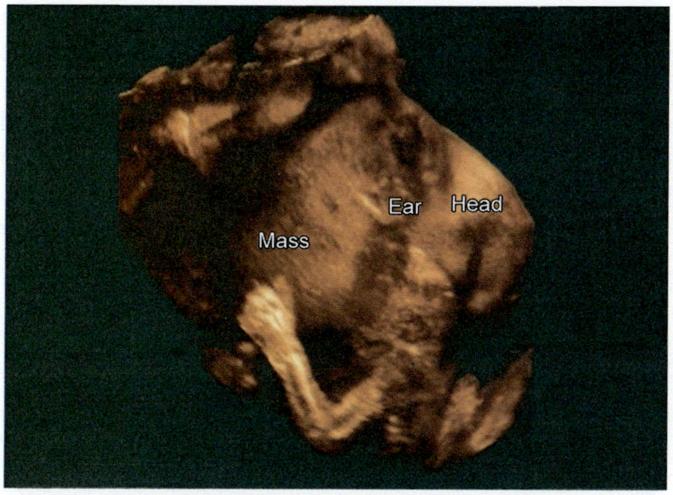

Fig. 35: Epicanto at 14 weeks. The mass distance morphology of the face.

by about 0.7 mm (with variations in growth from 4.8 - 8.3 mm from 11–14 weeks) in fetuses with NB and 0.5 mm in fetuses without NB.[46] This characteristic is specific to trisomy 21 and not detectable in other aneuploidies. It is important to assess the jaw correctly by sagittal scan taking the mandibular condyle as reference point.

Single Umbilical Artery

A single umbilical artery in the first trimester of pregnancy is associated with trisomy 21 and especially trisomy 18. Nikolaides et al. showed that an umbilical artery is missing in 77% of cases of trisomy 18[47] **(Fig. 33)**.

The screening tests for Down syndrome in the first trimester with the use of NT and other marker (nasal bone, ductus venosus....) have focused the investigator's attention to the first trimester 11–14 week and today it is possible to diagnose about the 50% of structural foetal malformation that we can detect in the second trimester[43] **(Figs. 26 to 29)**.

SECOND AND THIRD TRIMESTERS

The scan performed in the second trimester, usually around week 20 (range week 18–23, depending on the protocol), is used to study foetal anatomy and detect fetal malformations, as well as to evaluate foetal growth by means of biometric parameters.[49] Despite the high expectations of pregnant women about the diagnostic capacity of ultrasound (presumably due to incorrect information in the media and often also from specialists), the various studies on detection of fetal malformations by standard ultrasound in the second trimester show rates that do not exceed 40-60% of all malformations detected at birth, with a homogeneous mean prevalence of 2.5%. The Eurocat report,[50] for example, documents a diagnostic capacity of 62% for 11 major pathologies among 4,366 malformations in 1,198,519 babies born in 17 European regions in the period 1995–1999. Variability was high, ranging from 25% in Croatia to 88% in Paris, with enormous regional differences. Moreover, about 30–40% of cases were diagnosed after week 24, for various reasons, not least of which the natural history of malformations. No malformation was diagnosed in all carriers; for example, anencephaly was diagnosed in 94% of cases. It is therefore necessary to be precise and careful when informing women about the intrinsic limits of general ultrasound, as well as individual limits determined by the type of equipment and operator experience. As mentioned for ultrasound in the first trimester, the sophistication of instruments and operator experience also make very accurate and difficult diagnoses possible in the second trimester. Indeed, today the study of fetal anatomy can be much more detailed than in the 1990s. Thus greater experience, attention to districts, such as the face, heart and circulatory system, should improve the sensitivity of diagnosis of malformations, though this quite reasonable claim has not yet been demonstrated. Specialists in prenatal diagnosis can also achieve great morphological detail with the aid of sophisticated new instruments with 3-4D technology.[51] For specific use of these instruments, we consider the various systems and organs.

The Head

The head offers the possibility of detailed examination of a series of morphological signs by 3-4D.[52-54] The face is accessible, and it is relatively easy to exclude or diagnose cleft lip in this period.[55] Note that 3D technology includes 2D as base, so the capacity to visualize the fetal face by 3-4D in the second trimester is certainly much better than with 2D, with due enhancement and limitation related to fetal position, maternal abdominal fat, the placenta and quantity of amniotic fluid.[56] Given time (and perhaps more than one session) it is possible to obtain a good image of the foetal face in almost all cases in the period 19–23 weeks in 85–90% of cases (our personal percentage for 3,540 pregnancies is 92%). In the next period of pregnancy, the possibility of exploring the foetal face decreases as pregnancy proceeds. Indeed, in the third trimester, after week 35, the face can only be visualized in 30–50% of cases

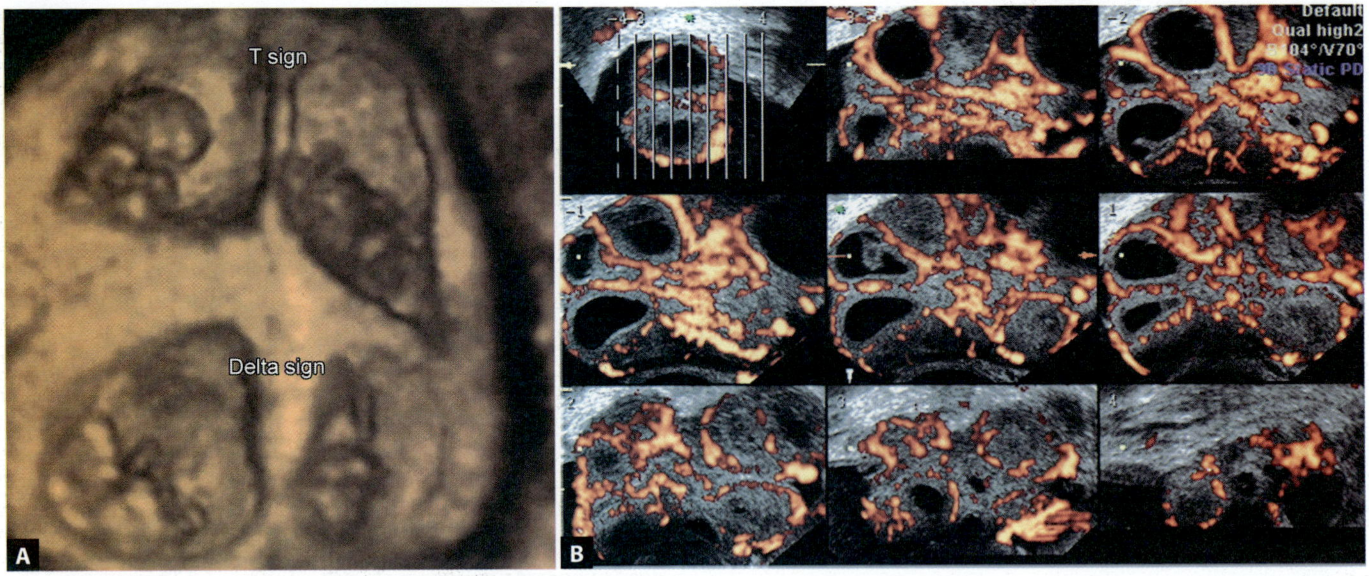

Figs. 36A and B: Unusual scan of quadrigeminal pregnancy arising from FIVET of three oocytes: two twins are clearly bichorionic-biamniotic (delta sign) and two monochorionic-monoamniotic (T sign) and a distribution of vessels in multiple pregnancy in the first trimester.

and sometimes requires two or three sessions in the case of suspected diagnosis **(Figs. 36A and B)**.

Operator experience is critical. After initial successes, considerable difficulty is often encountered in analyzing a saved volume: to obtain good images, 3D takes time and application as well as interest and predisposition. 3–4D is much less instinctive than 2D, which gratifies the operator with interpretable images after a few hours of practice (for example, measurement of BPD). The first impression of a face naturally cannot have scientific value, though many facial dysmorphisms depend on genetic syndromes and aneuploidies. Hyper- and hypotelorism, a weak chin and low ear position are easily and immediately detectable by 3D and this prompts us to consider the fetus as if it were a newborn. Moreover, with 4D we can observe sucking movements and attitudes, yawning, extraflexion of the tongue and movements of the hands, arms and legs, all characteristic of fetal wellbeing.[57] Maximum mode rendering enables exact views of bones,[58] detailed study of cranial bones and sutures, as well as measurement and counting of nasal bones making easier a diagnosis of craniosynostosis.[59-61] Minimum mode surface rendering can show details, such as ear lobes which are markers of urinary system pathology. The study of the fetal face is now the less important and significant field of the 3D study of the cephalic extreme. The so called "granny" effect that is achieve pleasing images of the fetal face to take home is the playful part of the use of ultrasound that has always existed,

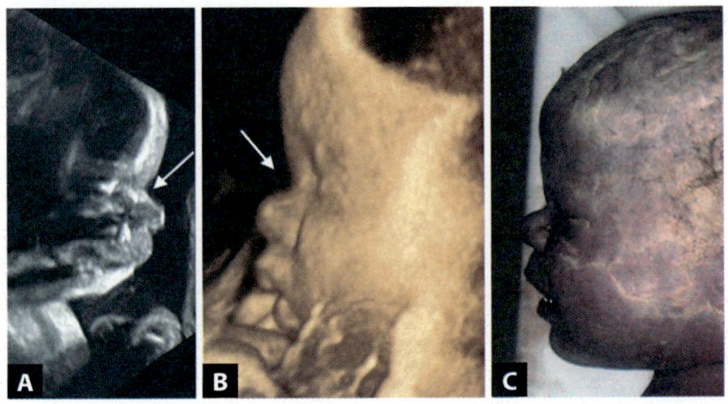

Figs. 37A to C: Typical face of achondroplasia.

even when we were only able to hear the heartbeat. The facial dimorphisms are relevant in certain diseases such as achondroplasia **(Figs. 37A to C)** and in many syndromes (holoprosencephaly, elephant man) where the face is often one of many markers, though often very impressive. Finally, today the 3D have bought or better earned its place as a complement or as a significant contribution to the 2D ultrasound diagnostic of malformations.

Internal structures of the brain can be explored in more detail. A correct view of the corpus callosum and pellucid fossa can be obtained in real time by 3–4D with volume contrast imaging in the C-plane. The posterior horns and the vermis can also be explored and their volume calculated.[62,63] The optic chiasma is easily detected and is an important prognostic factor in cases of anterior brain anomalies. Brain vascularization provides much material for future study. The Willis circle and the pericallosa and marginal arteries are easily detected in glass-body mode and angio-mode of power or color Doppler from the first trimester **(Figs. 38 to 40)**.

Detailed study of the jaw and oral cavity is another aspect of the head. We have extensively studied the ears, their size, morphology and position (normal or low), prompted by observations of neonatologists who attribute importance to the anatomy of the external ear **(Figs. 36 and 41 to 51)**. Neurosonology represents the area in which the three-dimensional really makes the difference enabling the operator to browse inside the brain structures using multiplanar method; the study of the corpus callosum has become a reality in almost all cases, with the ability to detect the partial agenesis, while both ventricles and posterior fossa are now easier to explore.

Inside the cranium is now possible to highlight structure otherwise unimaginable as the optic chiasm or sphenoid bone **(Figs. 43H to I)**, although currently there is a lack of clinical utility, but it is representative to signify the depth anatomical study allowed by 3–4D. Finally, the study of the palate which today represents a new barrier demolished by ultrasound with a great contribution of the 3D **(Figs. 42 to 51)**.

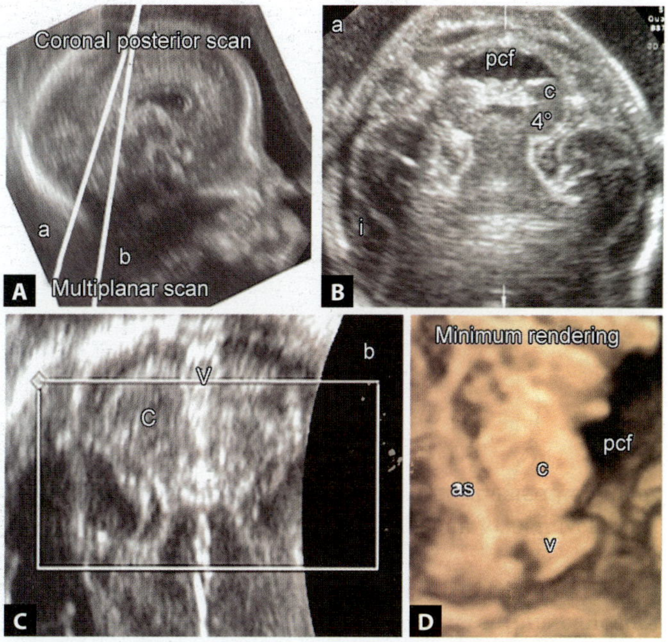

Figs. 38A to D: Posterior coronal scan. By 3D multiplanar and minimum rendering we can obtain a view of the cerebellum, fourth ventricle, acqueductus silvii and vermis that is difficult to obtain by 2D. (as: aqueductus silviani; c: cerebellum; pcf: posterior cranial fossa; i: insula; v: vermis; 4: fourth ventricle).

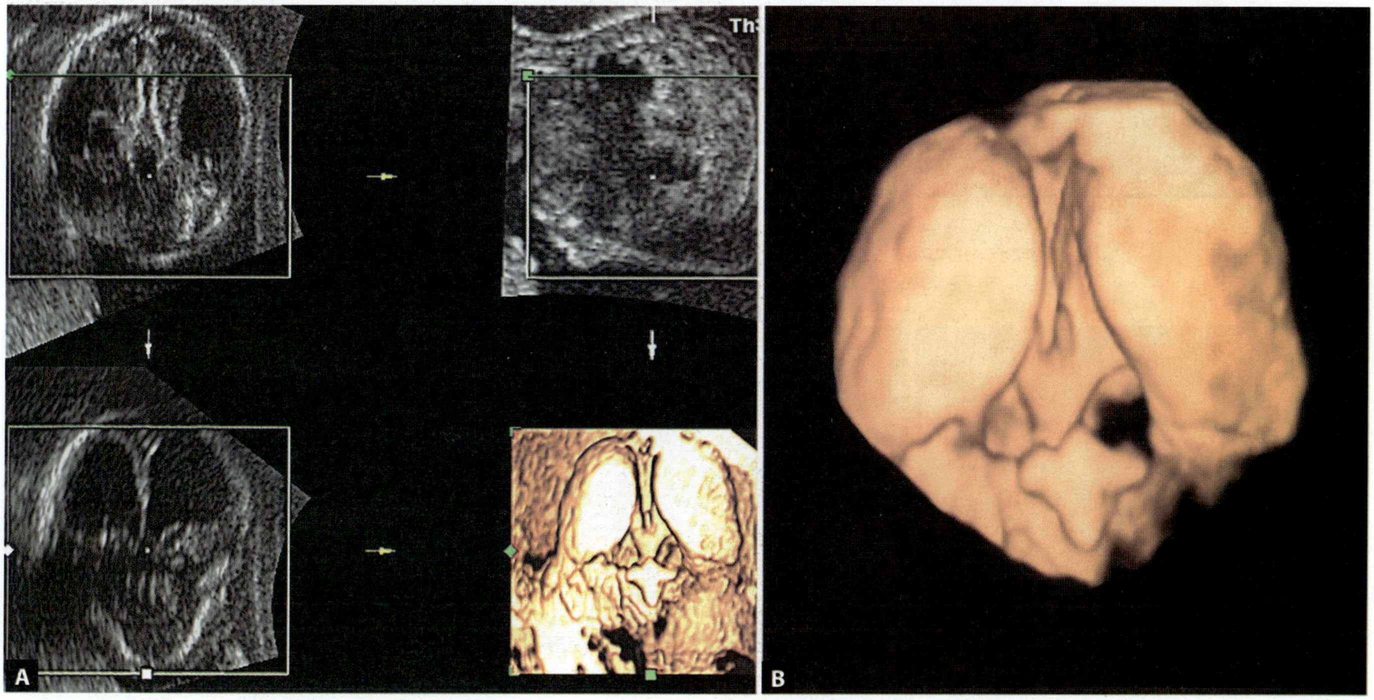

Figs. 39A and B: Invert and vocal modes are suitable for determining hydrocephaly.

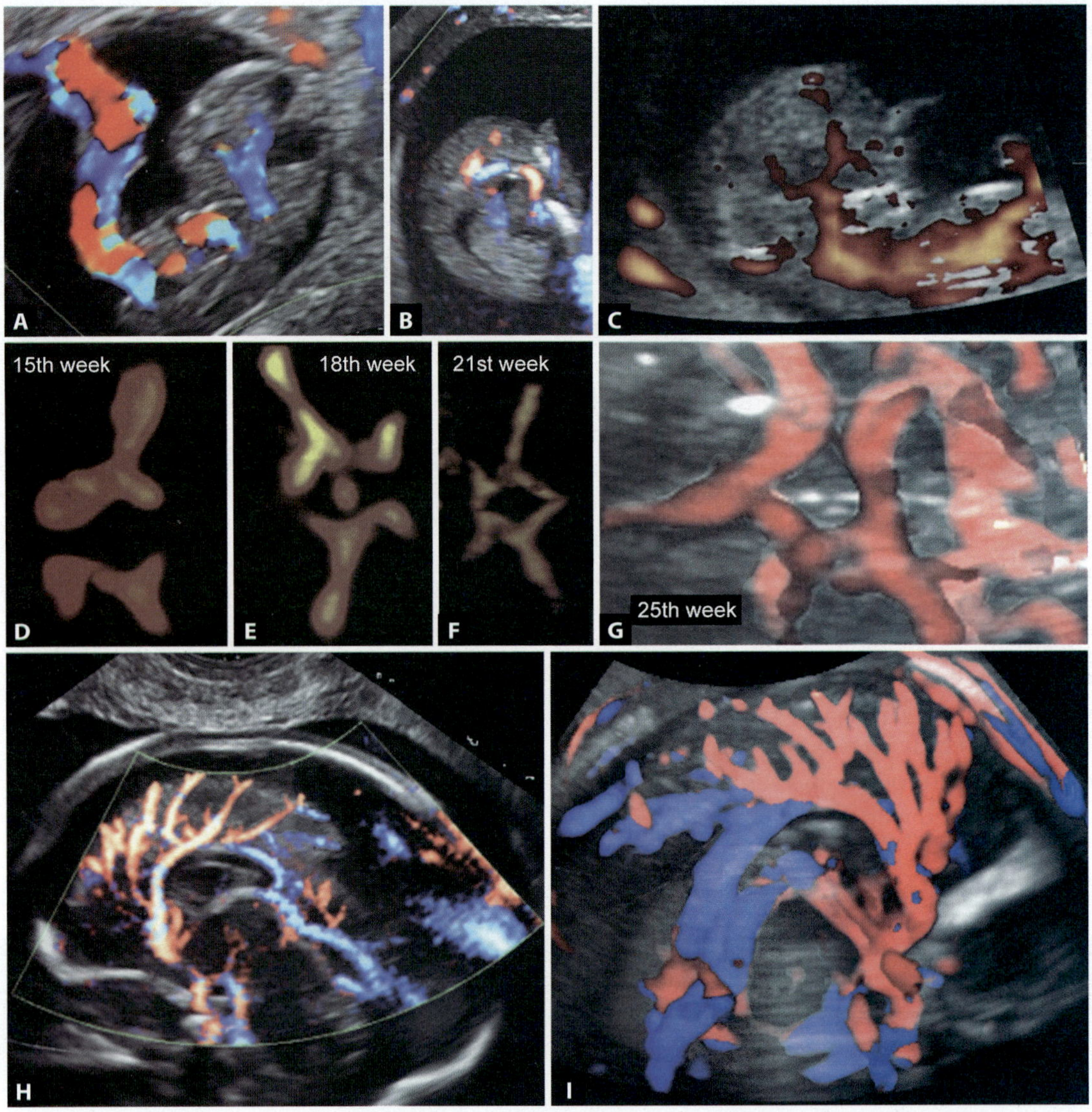

Figs. 40A to I: Brain circulation starts in the first trimester of pregnancy. The Willis circle and pericallosa artery are readily viewed by power or color glass–body mode.

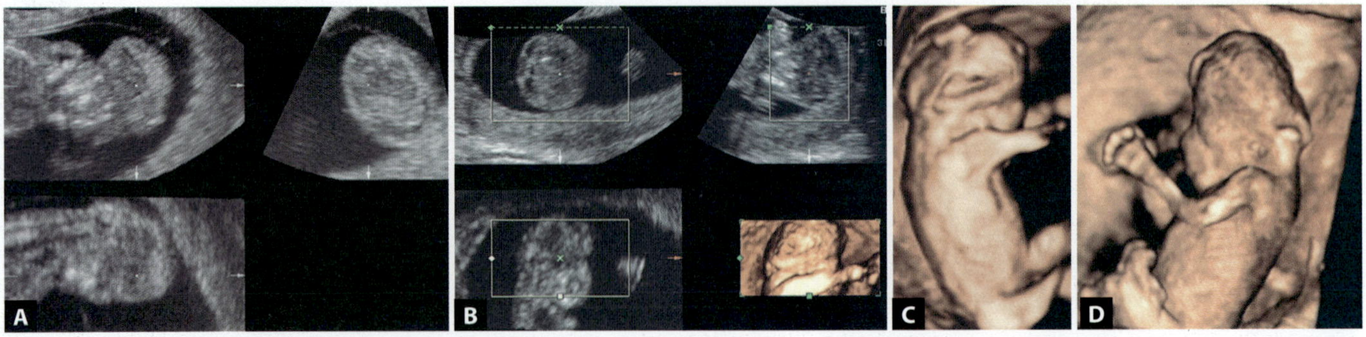

Figs. 41A to D: Anencephaly at week 11. The image shows the typical face and the absent skull.

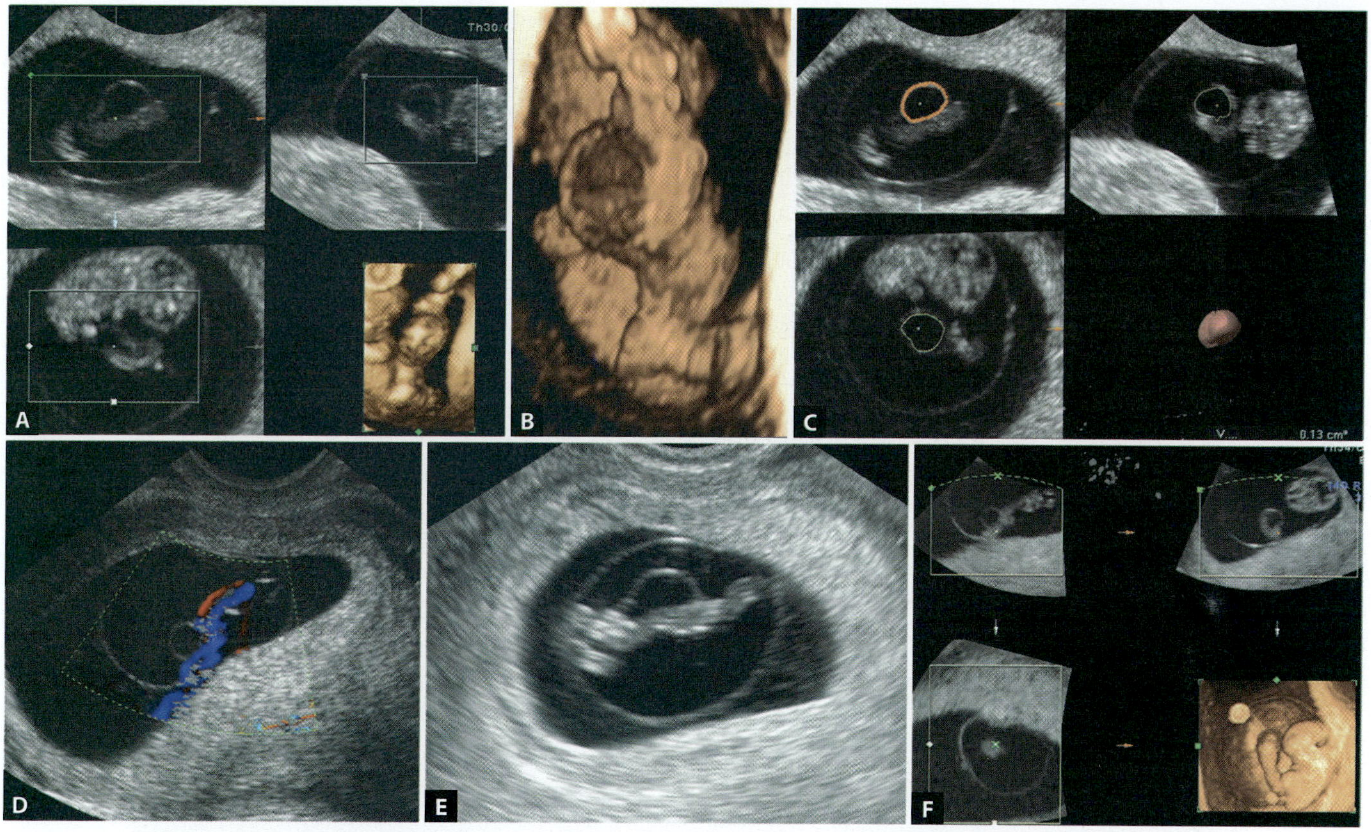

Figs. 42A to F: Umbilical cord cyst at week 9. This is a transient soft marker of aneuploidy (about 25% sensitivity—present in about 5% of pregnancies).

Renewed interest in the study of primary and secondary palatal morphology has arisen with new ultrasound diagnostic methods in 3-4D[64-66] and the fact that facial cleft accounts for 13% of all congenital malformations.[67] Malformation of the lip and palate may be isolated, associated with other malformations and/or sequences of malformations, associated with chromosome anomalies or with manifestations of a syndrome. Typical facial cleft, including cleft lip, cleft lip/cleft palate and cleft palate, have a prevalence of 9.1/10,000 and 6.4/10,000 births, respectively. Cleft lip accounts for 36% of all lip and palate malformations and the birth prevalence of isolated orofacial clefts accounts for 61.67% of total facial clef.[68] The prevalence is high (about one/1000) and in about two thirds of cases not only involves the lips but also the palate. Unfortunately in 45–47% of cases the defect affects the palate only.[69] From an epidemiological viewpoint, isolated malformations of the palate are associated with other malformations in about 18% of cases and with syndromes in 27.2%.[70] Cleft lip-cleft palate is isolated in 70–79% of cases and in the other 21–29% it is part of a syndrome or associated with other malformations.[71-73] Chmait 2006[74] reports 45 cases of cleft lip-cleft palate diagnosed by 2D and 3-4D scan, among which 21.6% of forms diagnosed as isolated revealed malformations not detected by ultrasound at follow-up. The report EUROSCAN 2000[75] documents a total ultrasound sensitivity of 27% for cleft lip-cleft palate, a sensitivity of 17% for isolated forms and 7% for isolated cleft palate. Other reports indicate a detection rate of up to 73% for cleft lip by 2D scan performed after week 20 of pregnancy ultrasound but there are papers which report sensibility for isolated cleft of palate about 0%.[76] The prevalence of this malformation and especially the high incidence of associations with other anatomic and genetic malformations has prompted research to improve ultrasound definition of the secondary palate. Usually the amniocentesis for caryotype should be offered in all cases of cleft lip/palate because of the risk of aneuploidy; also the patients should be counseled that ultrasound occult additional anatomic abnormalities might be present with all clefts.[77,78]

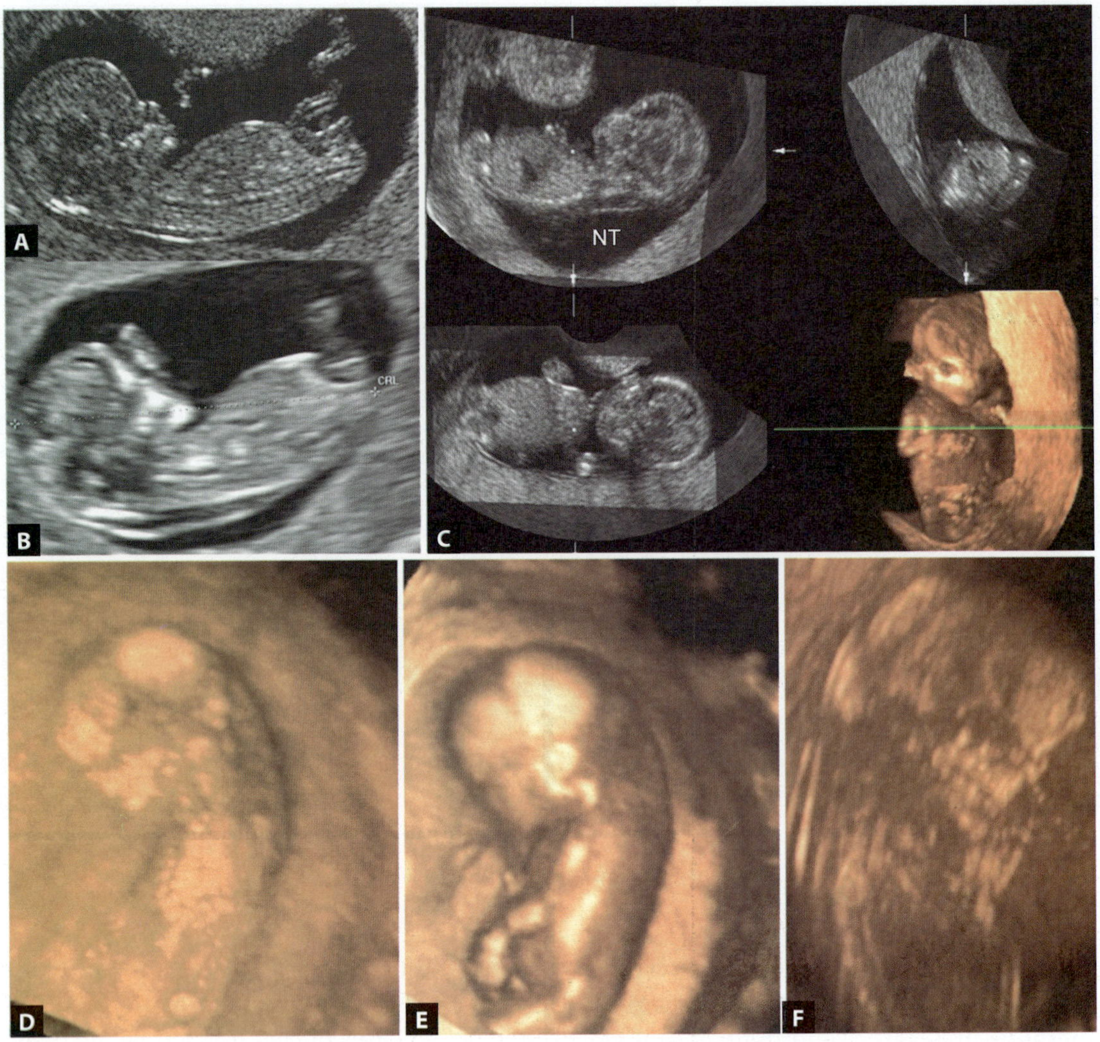

Figs. 43A to F: The difference between 2D and 3D for detection of nuchal translucency (NT) is usual minor: 2D is better for routine scan; 3D sometimes has advantages when the fetus is in an inappropriate position.

Ultrasonographic Detection of the Palate

The primary palate includes the lips and jaw bone to the nose root and is the most easily detected part of the anatomy by 2D scan **(Figs. 52 and 53)**. Indeed, many sustain that it is worthwhile visualizing the lips, jaw bone and nose root with an oblique coronal scan, scrolling upwards during the routine second trimester scan, and it is evident to users of 3D that this suggestion is almost superfluous when a scan of the fetal face is part of the routine **(Figs. 54A to C)**. The secondary palate consists of a hard palate, which runs posterior and horizontal to the incisive foramen and soft palate or velum, which curves downwards and backwards from the posterior aspect of the hard palate and ends in the uvula. In the fetus the hard/soft palate is 2.1 and the soft palate has the similar thickness **(Figs. 15 to 22)**. Usually the cleft of the secondary palate is always midline and results from failure of the palatine processes to elevate and grow **(Figs. 16 to 18 and 20)**. Cleft of the secondary palate starts from uvula and soft palate, but it is possible the cleft of soft palate with an intact hard palate[79] **(Fig. 19)**. The severe shadowing of the maxilla made difficult but not impossible the visualization and the diagnosis of clefts of the secondary palate. Sherer et al.[80] says that visualization of the secondary palate is not difficult by axial plane 2D scan, but he does not report any cases of defects of secondary palate. In this case the new volumetric probe 3D multiplanar and surface rendering offers greater possibilities of study of the normality and

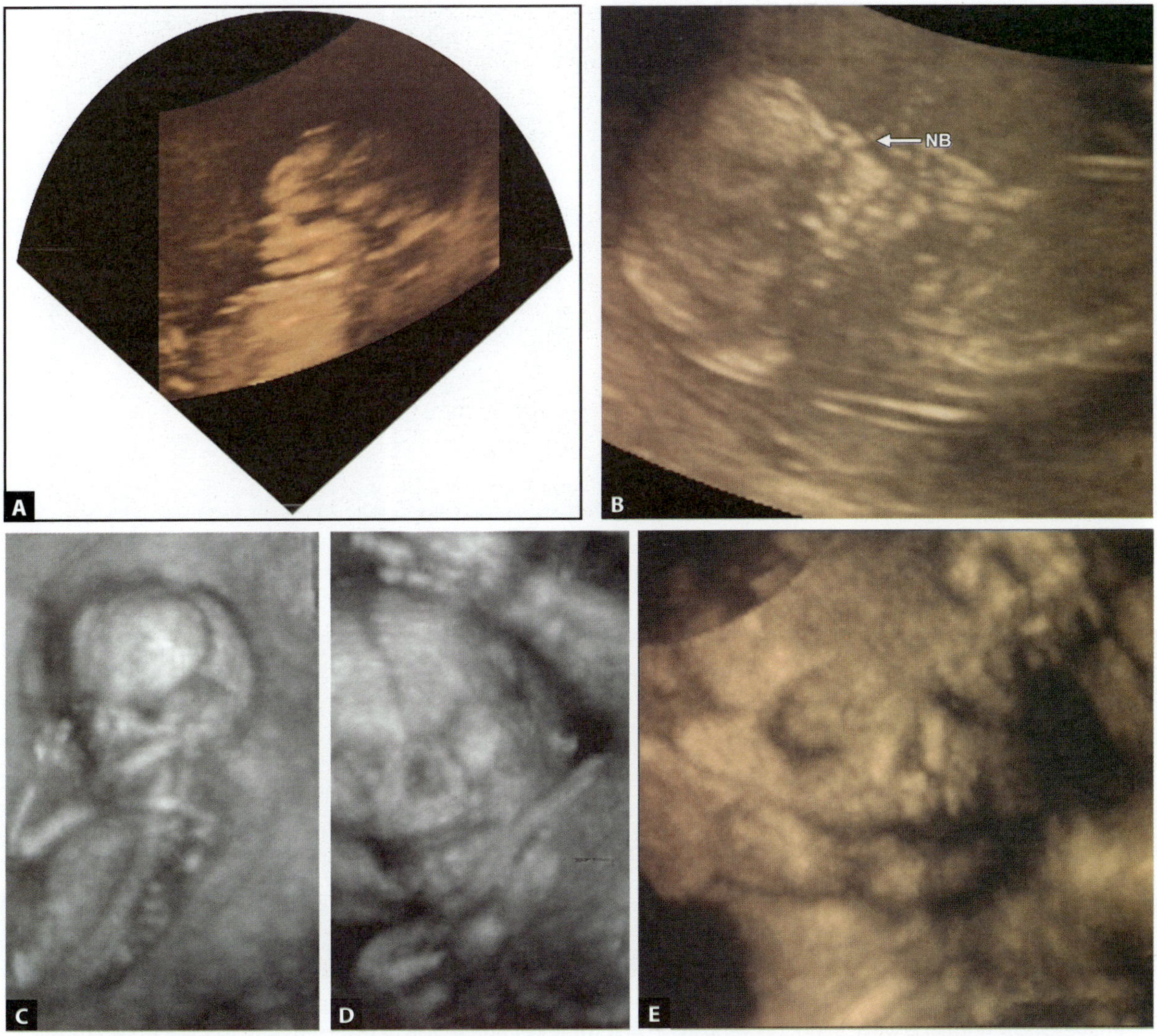

Figs. 44A to E: Weeks 13 and 20. It is easy to find the nasal bone (NB) and to detect both bones by 3D in the first and second trimesters; it is more difficult by 2D. The pictures are at 13th and 20th weeks. *(*nb: nasal bone).

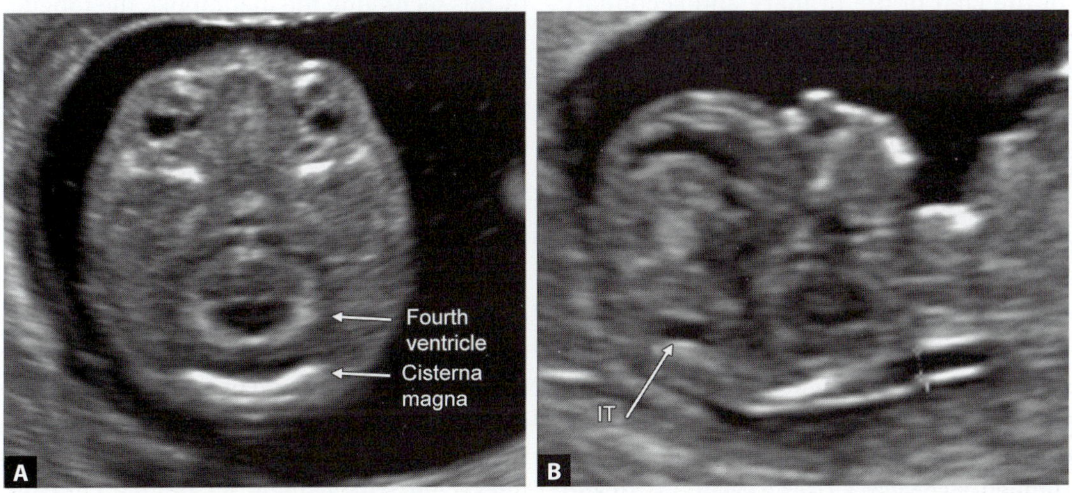

Figs. 45A and B: Intracranial translucency (IT) 2D and 3D. It is easy with a correct scan to find the IT between two hyperechoic lines.

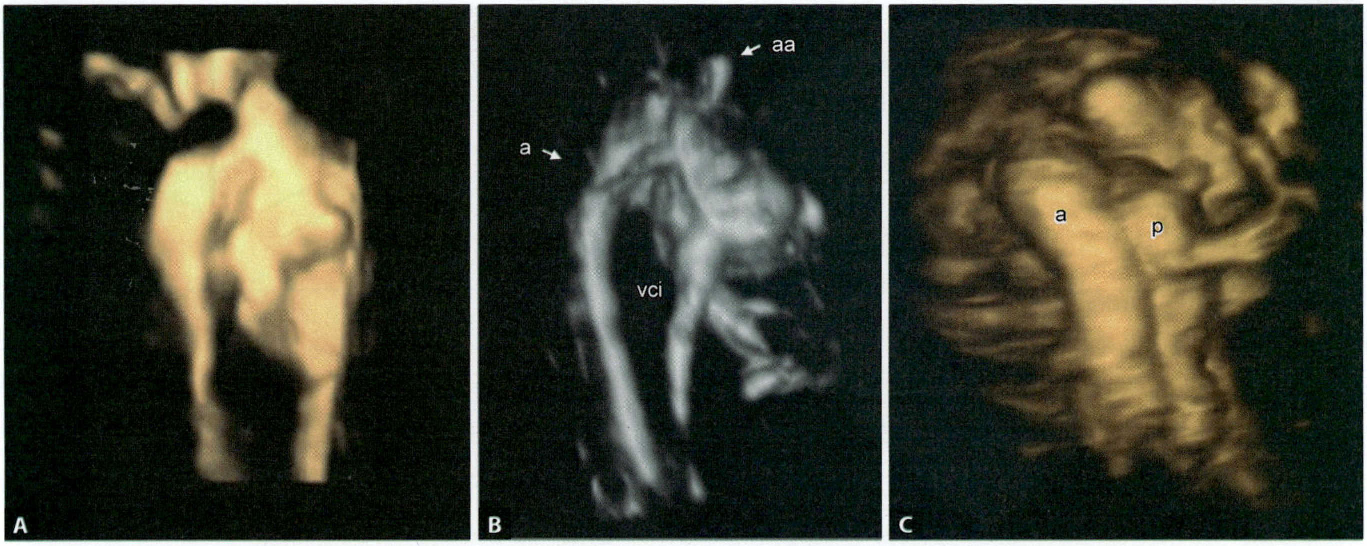

Figs. 46A to C: An example of great vessels transposition. The b-flow is not an easy technique but improves the heart defects about pulmonary veins. (a: aorta; p: pulmonary artery; vci: inferior vena cava; aa: anonymous artery).

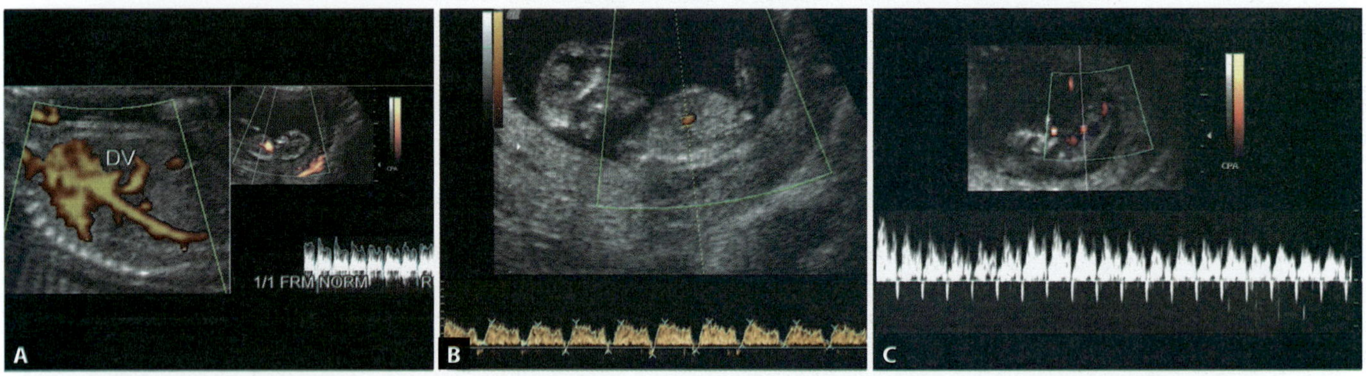

Figs. 47A to C: Ultrasound flow imaging of the ductus venosus is only feasible by 2D, but 3D provides good images of the vessel. The images show normal A wave in ductus venosus in first trimester and a case of reversed flow. (DV; ductus venosus).

of diagnosis of the cleft of the primary and secondary palate[81-83] By 3D, it is possible to see the alveolus and maxilla by axial scan and secondary palate by coronal scan by scrolling front-to-back in coronal plane. But with this method, there is the problem of the maxillary shadow. Campbell[84] overcame this problem by rotating the face through 180° and scrolling from back-to-front. This technique, described as 'reverse face view' eliminate the shadowing of the maxilla, but it offers the possibility to have a good vision of the hard palate but not of the soft palate. Platt et al.[85] found a different technique to see also the soft palate by axial 3D plane (multiplanar and surface rendering) with inverted picture to avoid the shadowing of the maxilla and using a little acoustic box scrolling from chin to nose (flipped-face view'). Uses a sagittal scan and by this technique the mandibula, the tongue, the maxilla, the alveolar ridge, the secondary complete palate are systematically seen and offers a good mode to diagnosis the clefts of the primary and secondary palate. Faure et al.[86] propose the same technique of Platt by coronal scan, because were able to obtain the view of the palate in all 100 low-risk cases, all with normal anatomy after delivery, from 17 to 23 wks. Pilu and Segata[87] describe a new multiplanar approach to study the secondary palate using tomography ultrasound imaging (TUI); to avoid the shadowing of the alveolar ridge the authors used a scan with an angle of 45° and obtained a satisfactory view in 10 of 15 cases between 19 and 28 wks. Now, then, we have many possibility to study systematically the primary and the secondary palate by 2D, but with greater possibilities

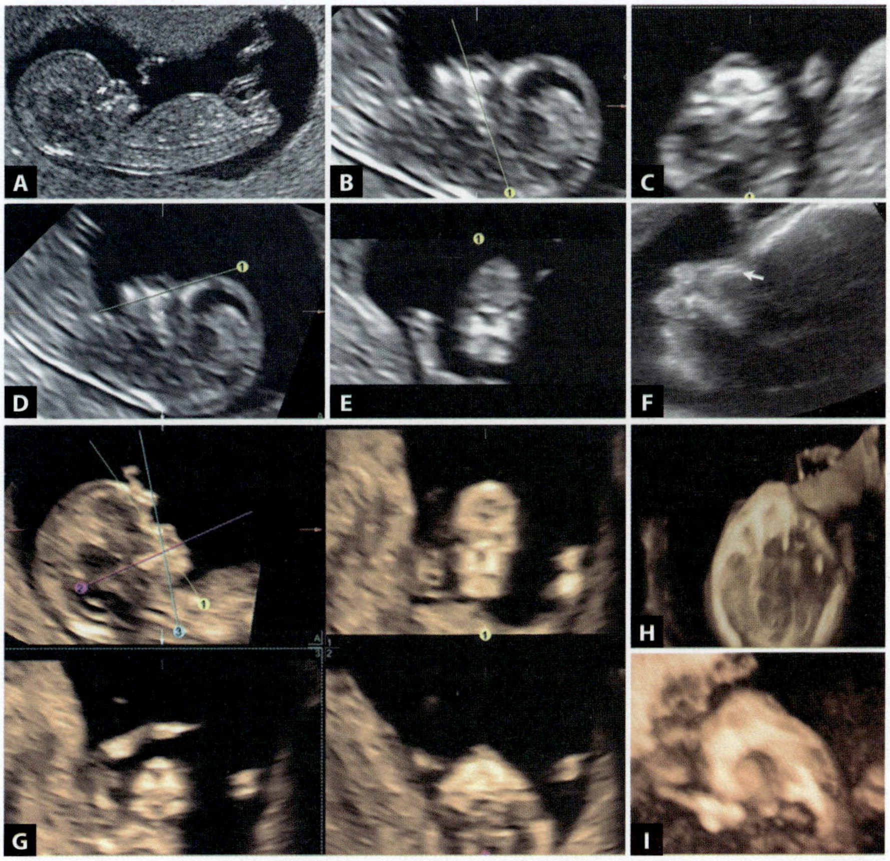

Figs. 48A to I: It is possible to control the normal secondary palate in the first trimester of pregnancy by Faure technique 3D (delta sign (D and E) by rendering surface or (C) by omniview) or by retronasal triangle (A to C) by 2D or by omniview).

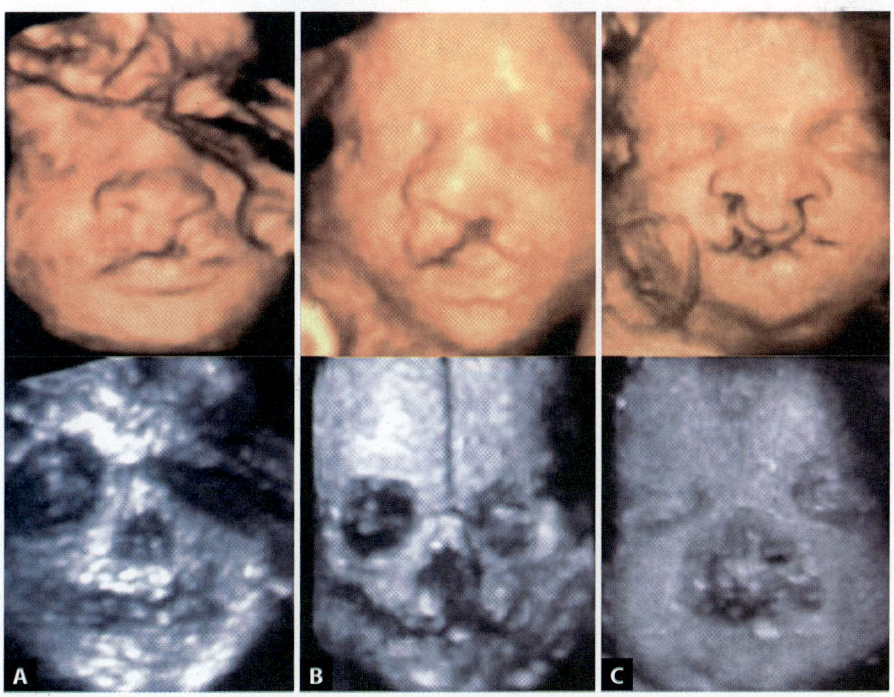

Figs. 49A to C: Maximum and minimum rendering in three cases of l-p cleft. It is easy to understand the extension of the cleft.

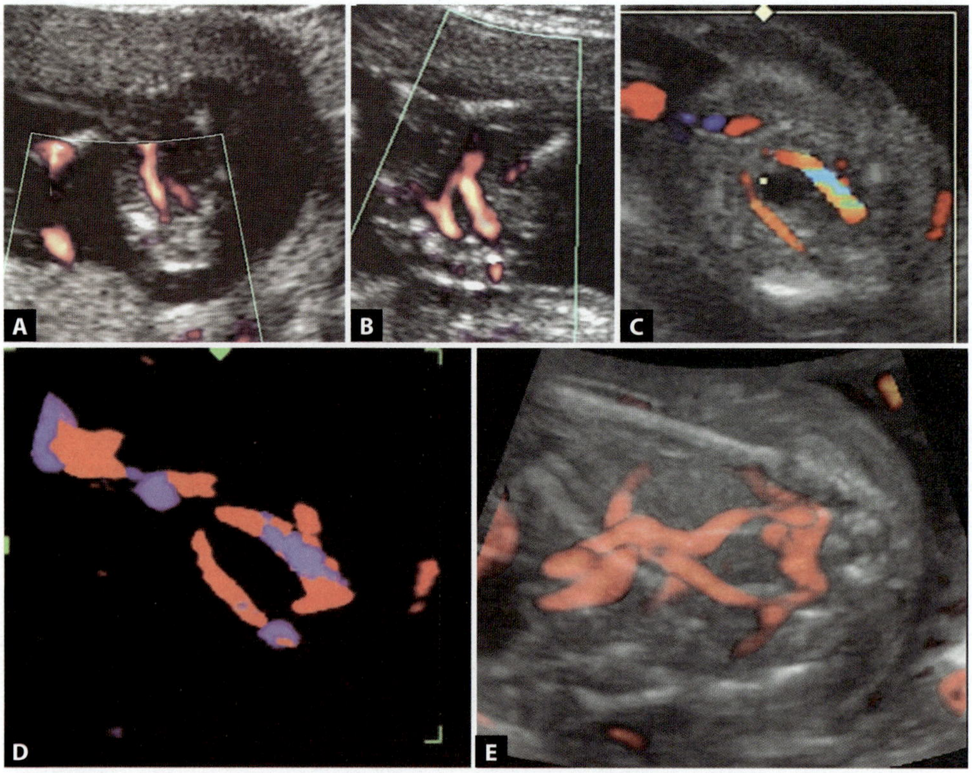

Figs. 50A to E: In the first and second trimesters, it is easy to find both umbilical arteries at bladder level; 3D color, power and glass body modes provide more realistic images.

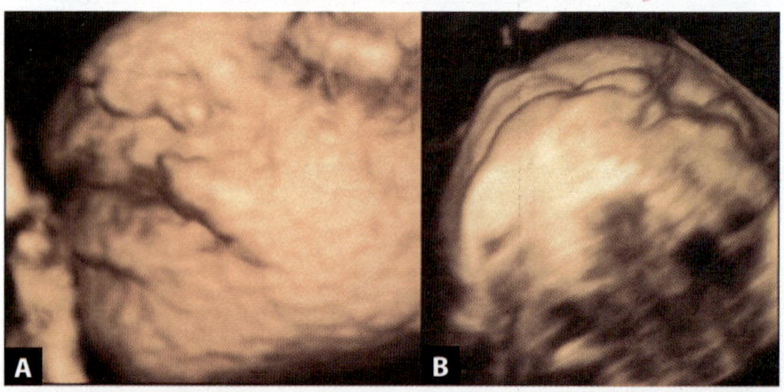

Figs. 51A and B: Cleft-lip and cleft alveolar ridge by surface rendering front face

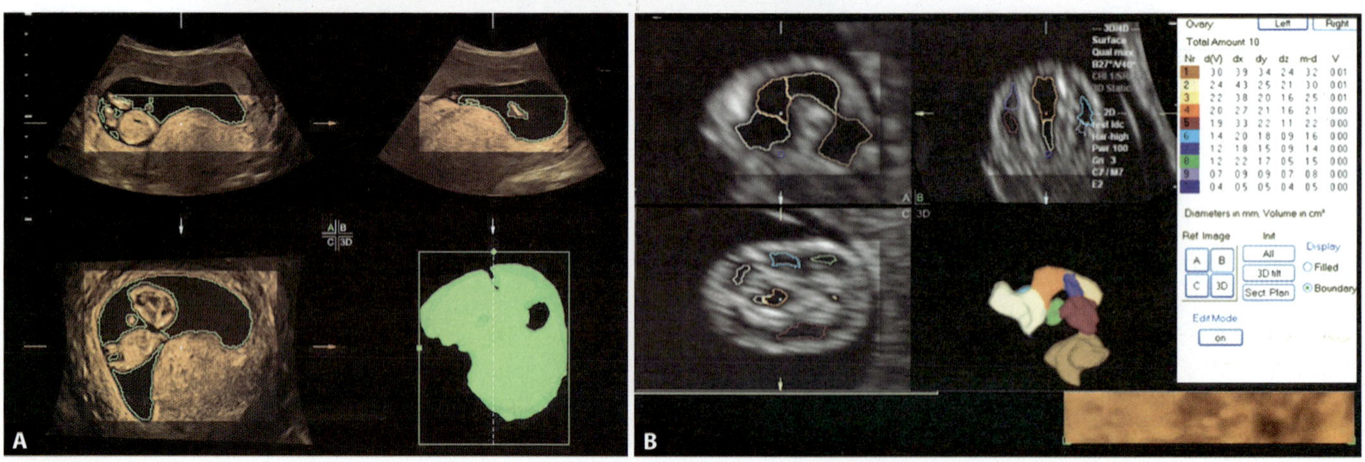

Figs. 52A and B: The control of volume of amniotic fluid in the first trimester or the dimension of ventricles is possible by sonoAVC.

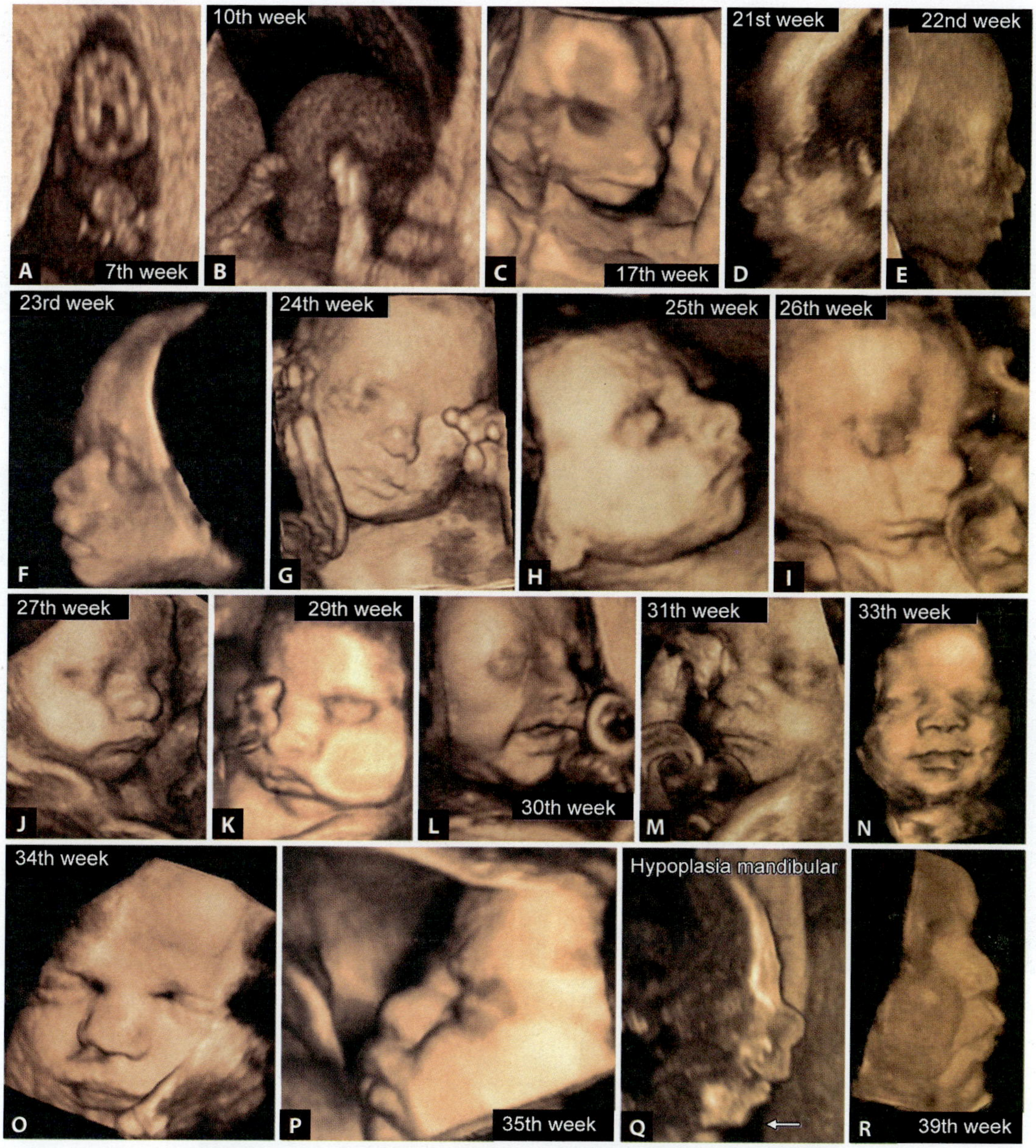

Figs. 53A to R: The fetal face acquires human features during gestation. The face of the embryo is quite unattractive; whereas in the second trimester, it becomes softer and more pleasant and remains thus into the postnatal period. Facial modeling is related to the formation of facial musculature, fat and the thick consistency of skin due to soaking. 3–4D provides completely realistic images, especially with high quality instruments and experienced operators. It is therefore relatively easy to assess facial symmetry and reliably recognize facial dysmorphisms (e.g. mandibular hypoplasia), which may be of genetic disorders and to diagnose cleft lip or palate.

by 3D;[88] it is reasonable says that gold standard is to have experience with all techniques, above all in cases of doubt or of diagnosis of facial cleft to define exactly the limit of lesion. By axial 3D plane (sagittal or coronal scan) Campbell[89] propose a screening of secondary palate in the first trimester; in fact, it is easy from 11–14 weeks to see the secondary palate (delta sign) but, if the screening is effective in diagnosing orofacial clefting will require further study, (delta sign)(**Figs. 55 and 56**). The scan in the second trimester, week 19-22, is associated with a greater possibility of detecting the primary and secondary palate and of diagnosis of facial clefts (**Figs. 57 to 61**).

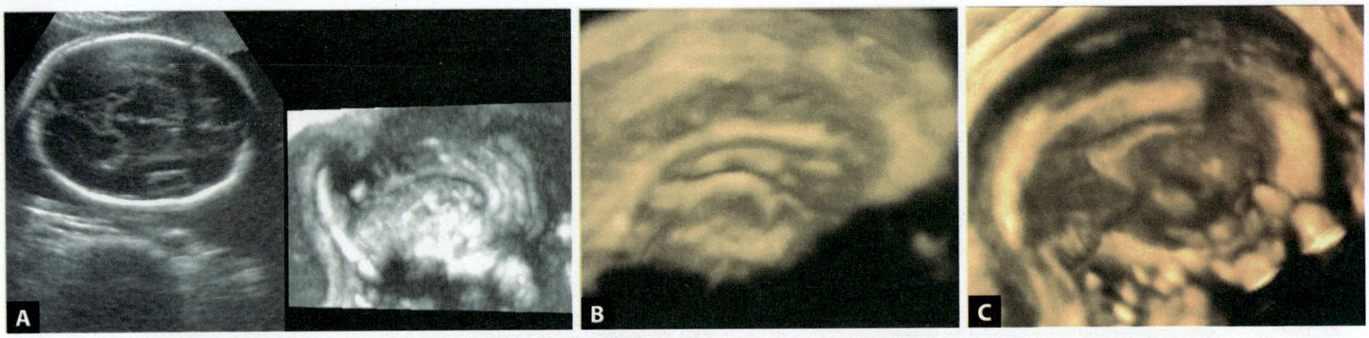

Figs. 54A to C: Examination of the corpus callosum is easy and quick by 3D and volume contrast imaging in c-plane; by 2D it is very difficult.

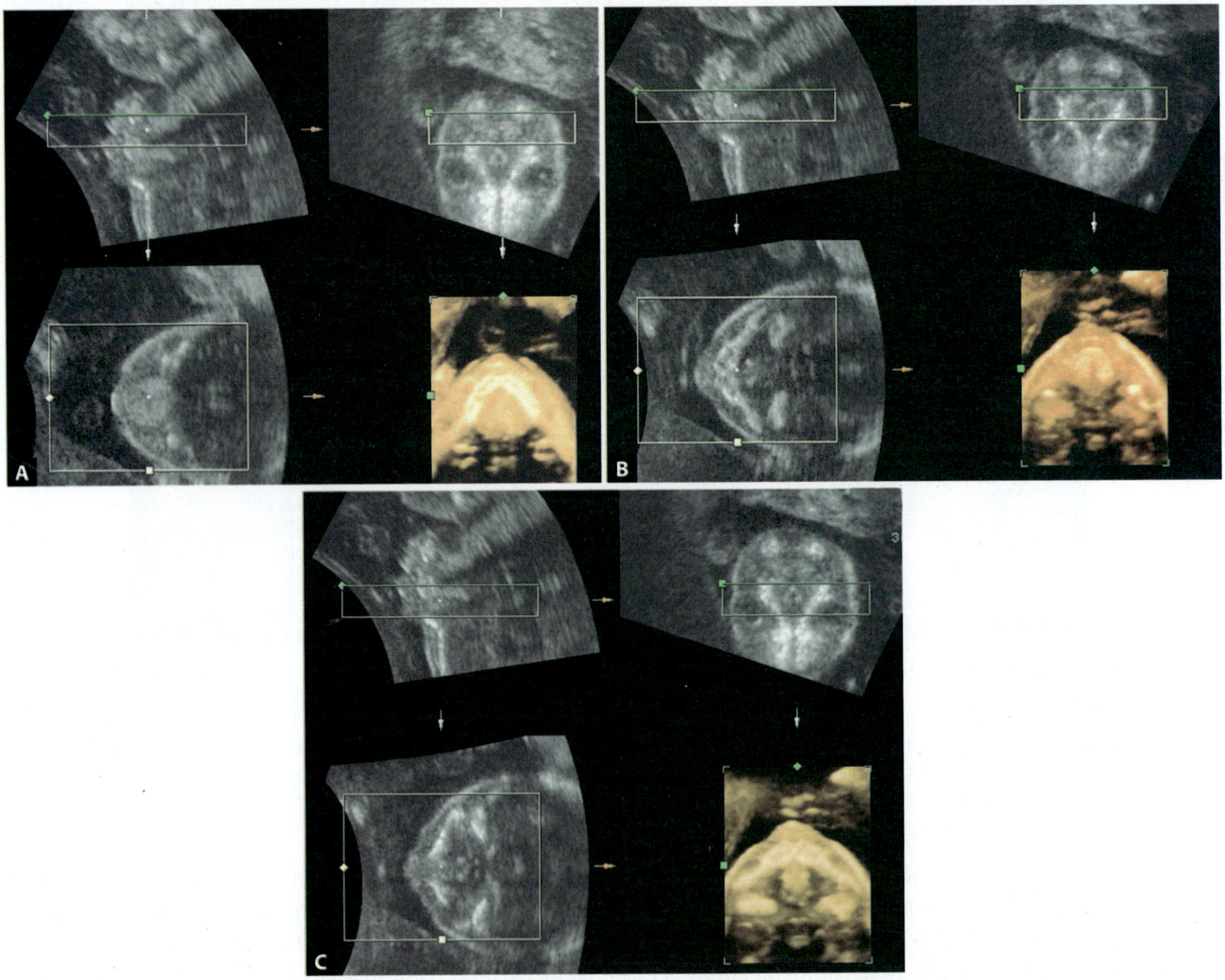

Figs. 55A to C: Secondary palate by 3D multiplanar and surface rendering; axial plane (flipped view face) with sagittal inverted (to avoid the maxillary shadow) scan; scrolling up-down: (A) The mandibula; (B) The tongue; (C) The maxilla.

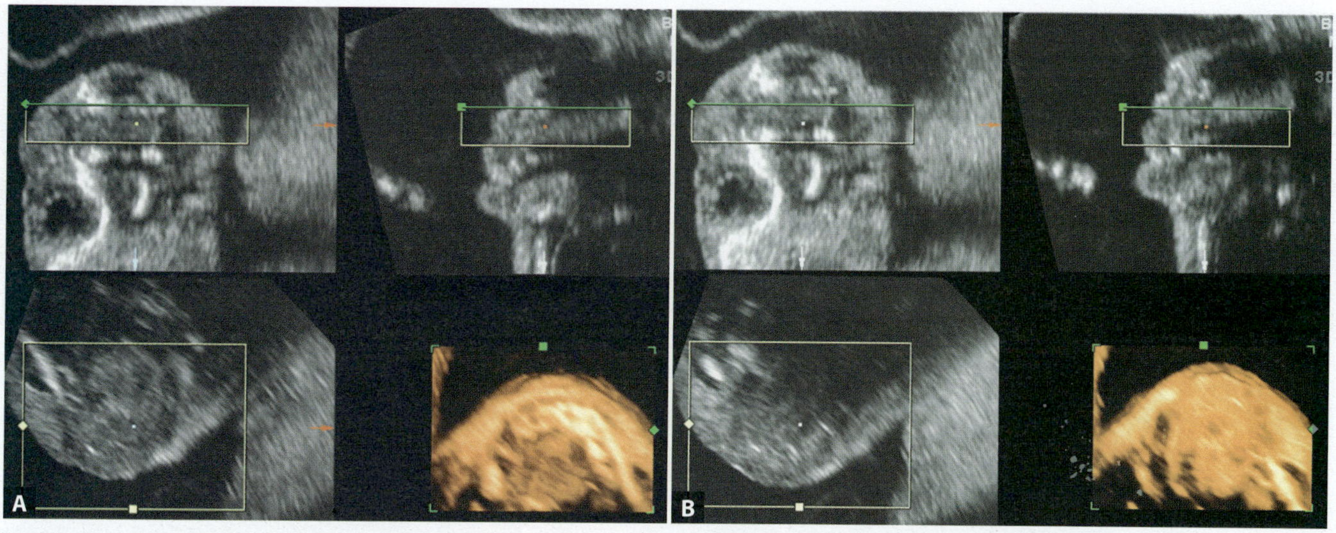

Figs. 56A and B: Secondary palate by 3D multiplanar and surface rendering: axial plane with coronal inverted (to avoid the maxillary shadow) scan; scrolling up-down: (A) Mandibula; (B) Tongue and maxillary bone.

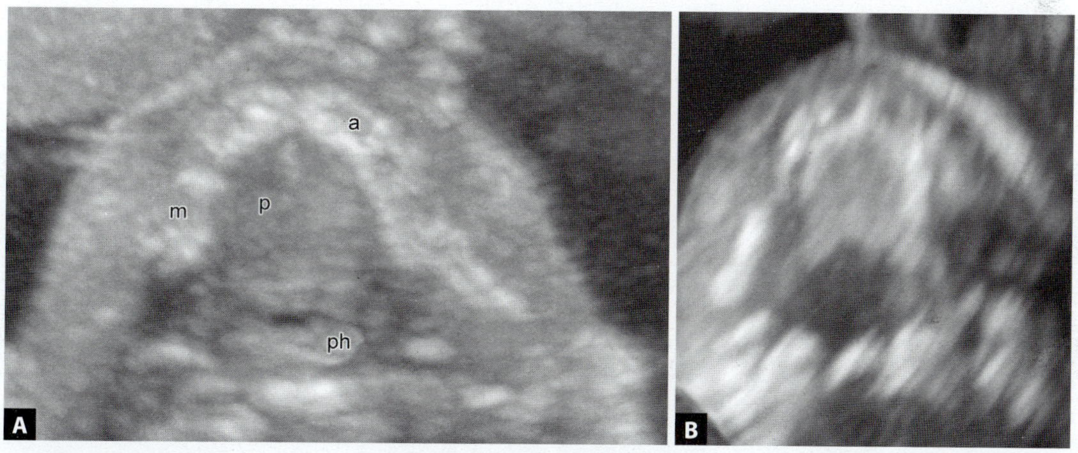

Figs. 57A and B: Secondary palate by axial 3D plane (A) Maximum mode and (B) Minimum mode.

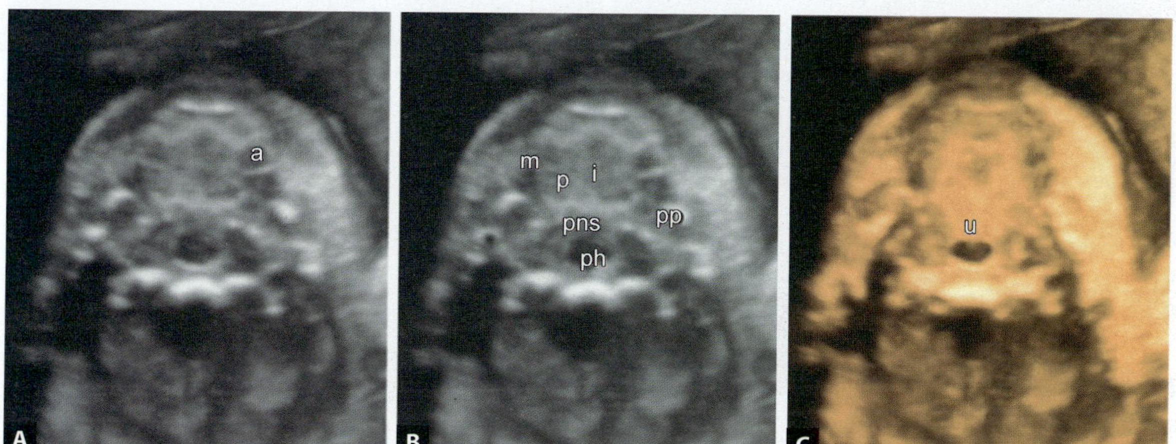

Figs. 58A to C: Secondary palate by 3D plane minimum mode without and with captions. (a: alveolar ridge; m: maxilla; i: interpalatal suture; p: palatine process; pns: posterior nasal spine; pp: pterygoid process; u, uvula).

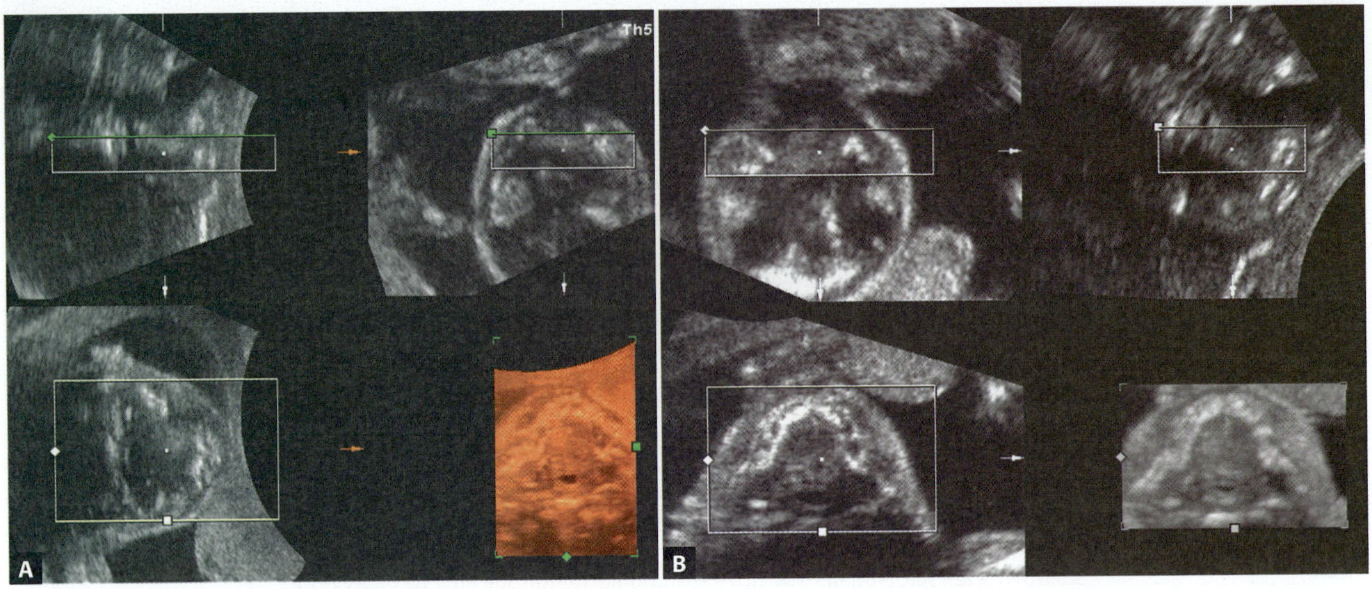

Figs. 59A and B: By axial 3D plane, there is no difference between (A) sagittal and (B) coronal scan to see the secondary palate.

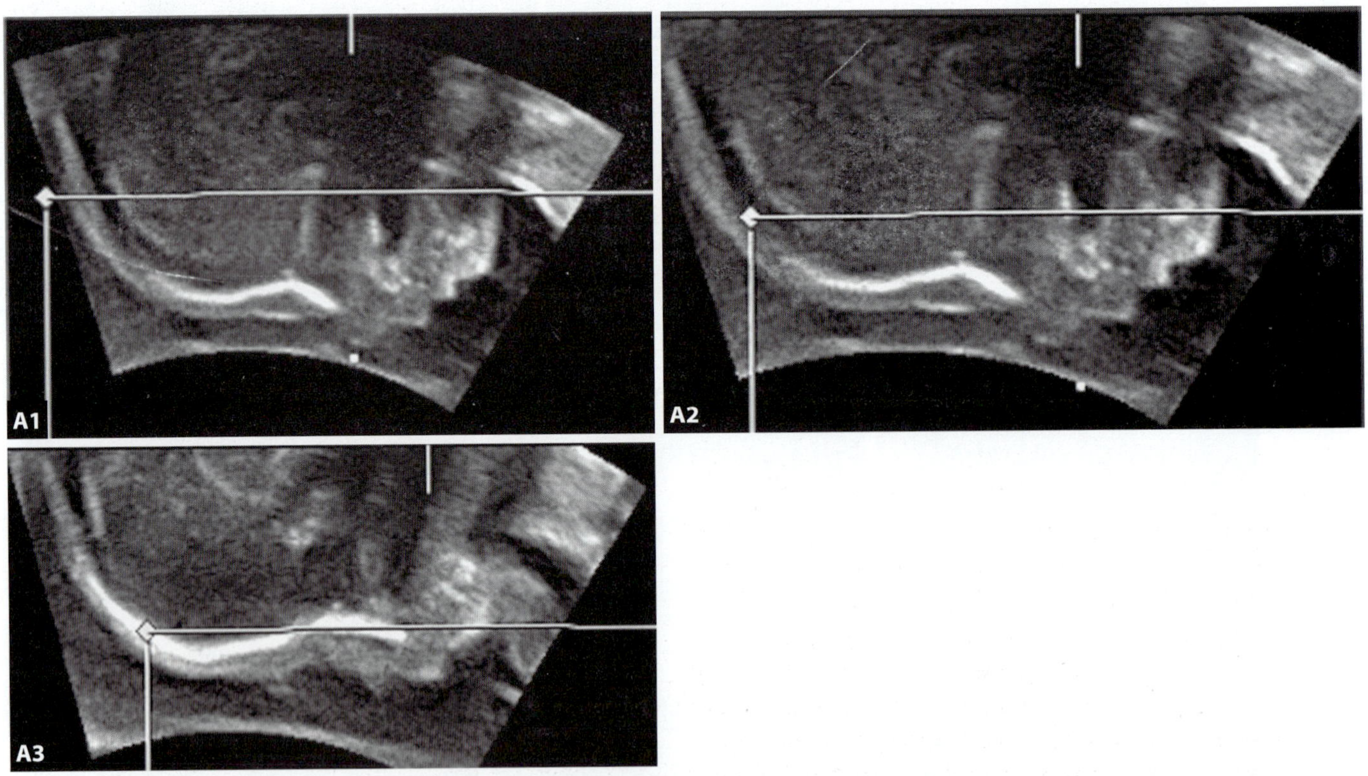

Figs. 60 A1 to A3: Secondary palate by coronal 3D plane multiplanar and surface rendering; scrolling forwards (reverse face); A1-B1; A2-B2; A3-B3. The arrow points at hard palate.

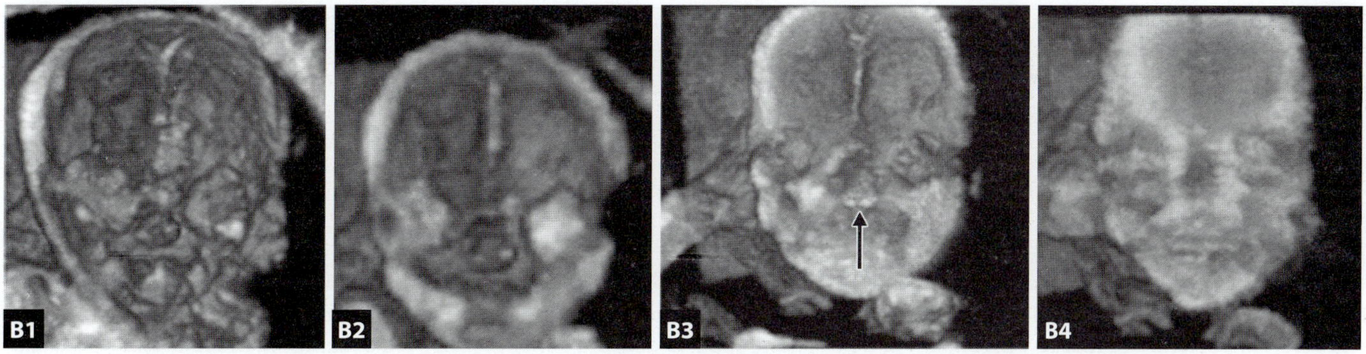

Figs. 61 B1 to B4: Secondary palate by coronal 3D plane multiplanar and surface rendering; scrolling forwards (reverse face); A1-B1; A2-B2; A3-B3; A4-B4. The arrow points at hard palate.

Secondary Palate

The scheme of Berkowitz **(Figs. 62A to D)** illustrates that the uvula is always involved in cleft palate and could simplify detection; but in practice, it is difficult to detect this small anatomical part with 2D and 3–4D.

2D

Two-dimensional scans can be used to study the hard and soft parts of the secondary palate and detect the uvula **(Fig. 20)**. However it is necessary that the fetal head be in a favorable position, possibly with the lips slightly apart. Today (2010 Whilhelm) a new marker "the equal sign" offers a new easy possibility to detect or suspect an isolated palate cleft. In axial scan (better than coronal, inusual and difficult),with the same scan to messure the BPD with a little inclination, is relatively easy find the farinx like an anechoic round area with a double signs of the uvula foto. In case of the bifidus uvula it is important to study the secondary palate and the 3D (min-max rendering, Faure method or others, omniview) became a beautiful tool to investigate.

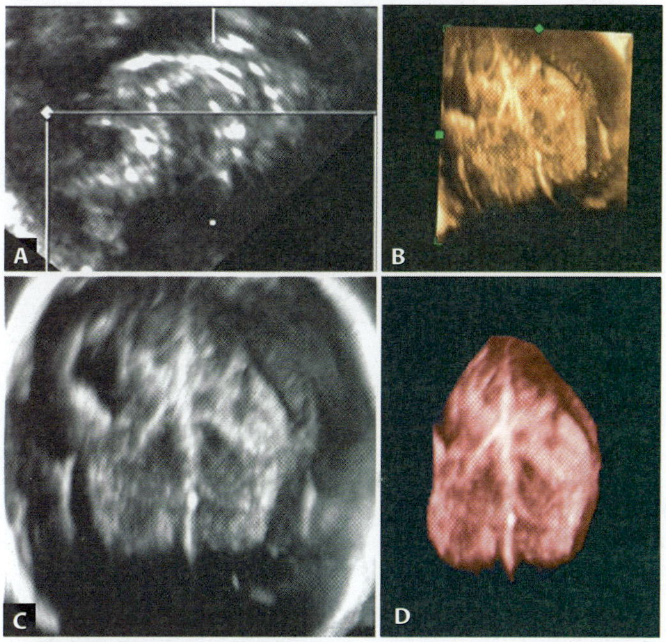

Figs. 62A to D: Exploration of the brain by 3D multiplanar mode offers a splendid view of the optic chiasma, important in cases of partial agenesis of the corpus callosum.

3–4D

Three-dimensional scans have greater possibilities because a volume can be saved and examined later in an infinite number of scanning planes. Various methods have been proposed: axial surface rendering plane with a small box ("flipped-face view") and inverted scan to avoid maxillary shadow (scrolling upwards) by sagittal or coronal scan **(Figs. 55 to 61 and 63 to 70)** coronal surface rendering plane, reverse-face (scrolling forwards) or front face (scrolling backwards) scan **(Figs. 68 and 69).**

TUI tomography ultrasound imaging sagittal scan with angle of 45° **(Fig. 70)**.

Ultrasound technicians will be increasingly called upon to check the integrity of the secondary palate due to the high prevalence of facial defects at birth and the high percentage of malformations, syndromes and chromosome anomalies, associated especially with cleft palate. Three-dimensional techniques offer ways of achieving this. Among those described above, the 3D axial plane is the fastest and easiest to apply, and has been reported to detect the secondary palate in almost all cases in 2–3 minutes when echographic conditions do not pose an impediment. Variable fetal position in relation to maternal fat is the only

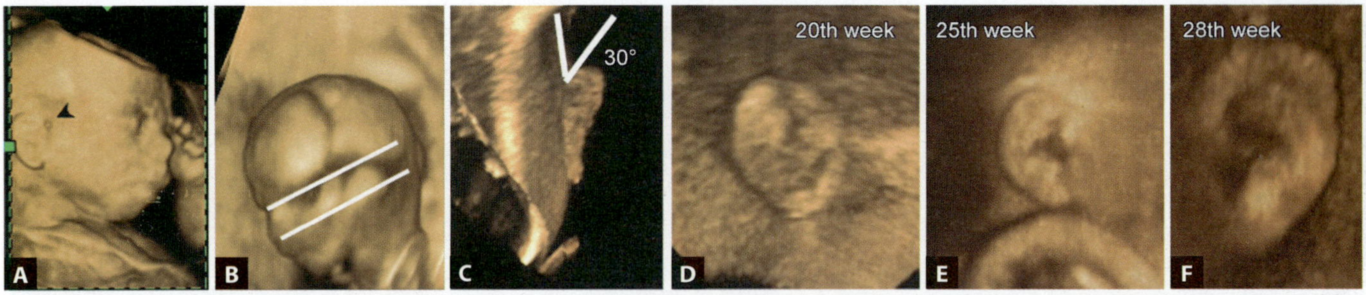

Figs. 63A to F: By 3D it is possible to detect very small appendix auricularis (an important marker for many other malformations); ear position is important, because low placement or a helix more than 30 degrees out of the skull are a marker of aneuploidy. External ear morphology changes during gestation: until week 20 it is a ring; final morphology is only achieved at about week 29.

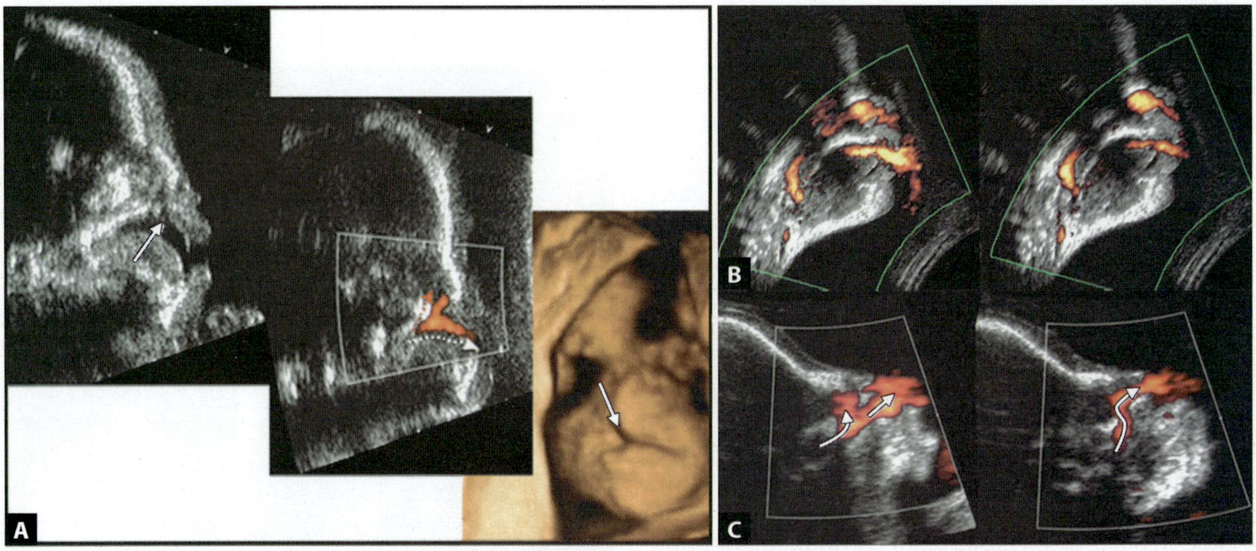

Figs. 64A to C: (A) The use of 2D, 3D and color Doppler offers a good possibility to diagnose the l-p cleft. It is suggestive of the passage of amniotic fluid directly from oral to nasal choana; (B) Sagittal scan power-color to demonstrate the normality of secondary palate during swallowing; (C) The amniotic fluid crosses through the palate.

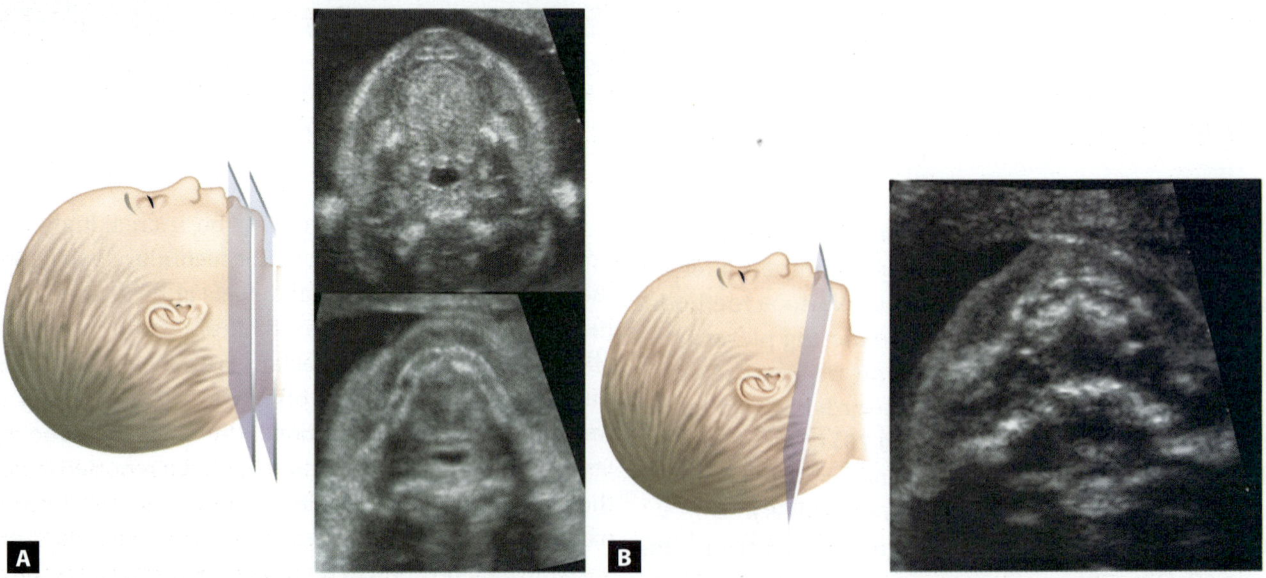

Figs. 65A and B: Different planes of axial 2D scan for the jaw and the tongue. (A) The maxilla; (B) The proximal part of the maxilla and the eyes.

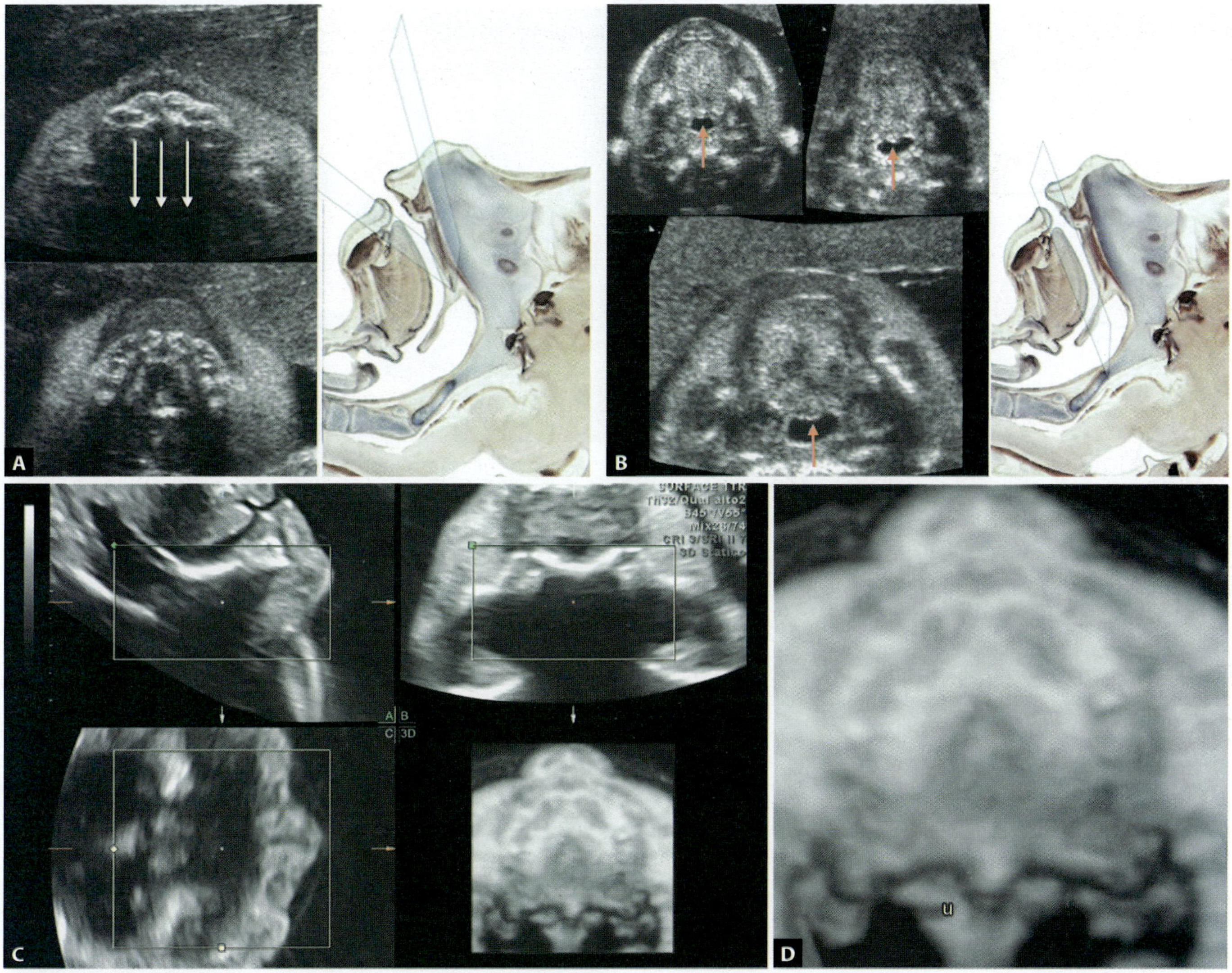

Figs. 66A to D: (A) A correct axial 2D scan for the maxillary bone; (B) The tongue and the uvula; (C) The secondary palate with the uvula by 3D flipped-face view multiplanar; (D) Surface rendering.

serious obstacle to its correct detection. Today it would seem reasonable to propose study of the hard and soft palate only in cases with suspected or confirmed diagnosis of facial clefting and in cases with a positive family history or after non visualization of the "equals sign" in 2D **(Figs. 71 to 76)**.[90]

Chest

The chest contains the heart, an organ fundamental for human life. Study of the heart, efflux and the circulatory system[91] has exploited 3-4D technology and STIC mode (spatio-temporal imaging correlation), which being in four dimensions, cannot be illustrated in an atlas. However, fixed, invert, power, color and Doppler 3D images and study in real time by TUI are striking, interesting, and considerably improve diagnostic capacity. At this time the b-flow is the alone possibility to study the vein efflux with low flow and can also became complementary to STIC in heart pathology; but it is not easy to learn the b-flow. Lung volume can be measured by the VOCAL system,[92,93] improving the prognosis and outcome of fetuses with diaphragm hernia, and is expected to replace thickness as an indication for therapy in utero. With special experience it is possible to correctly visualize the course and morphology of the esophagus. The volume of the thymus, an important fetal organ, can be assessed. The diaphragm

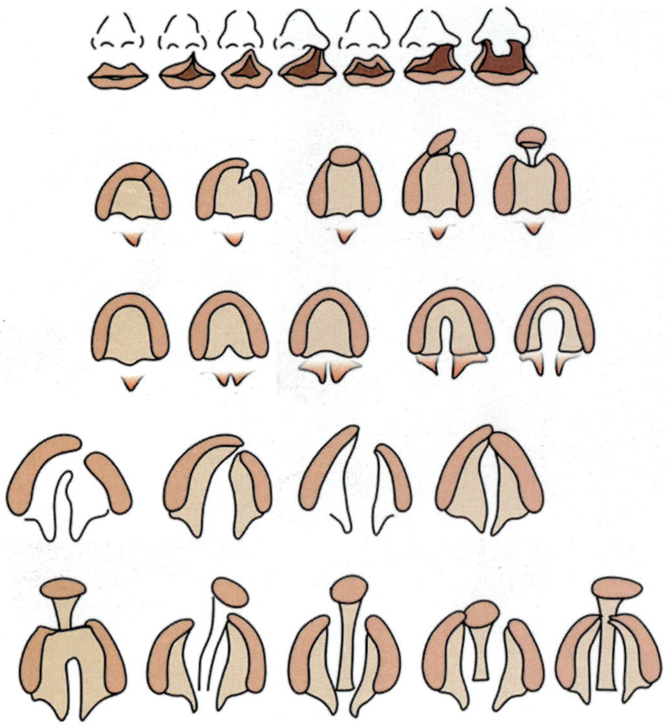

Fig. 67: Picture of Berkowitz (2006) shows the different possibilities of facial cleft. It is important to note that the palate-cleft starts from the uvula until the primary palate.

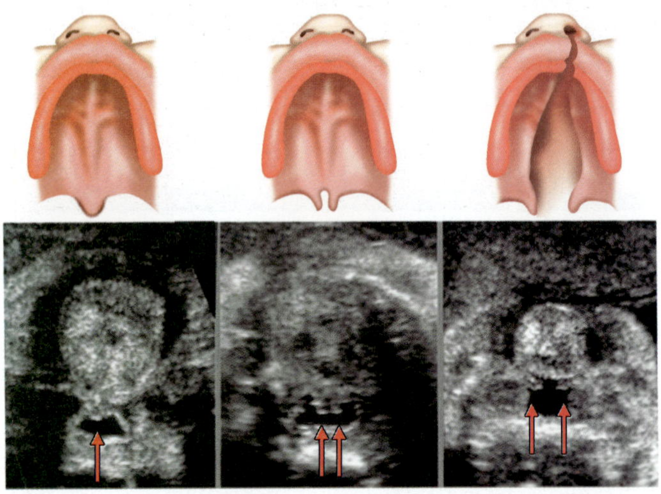

Fig. 68: Beautiful 2D pictures of uvula-cleft; the uvula-cleft is always associated with palate-cleft.

is quite evident, reducing diagnostic doubts about hernia. The gallbladder is also easily visualized **(Figs. 77 and 78)**.

Abdomen

Visualization of the viscera and stomach are less exciting than the face, though the vascularization of the liver is

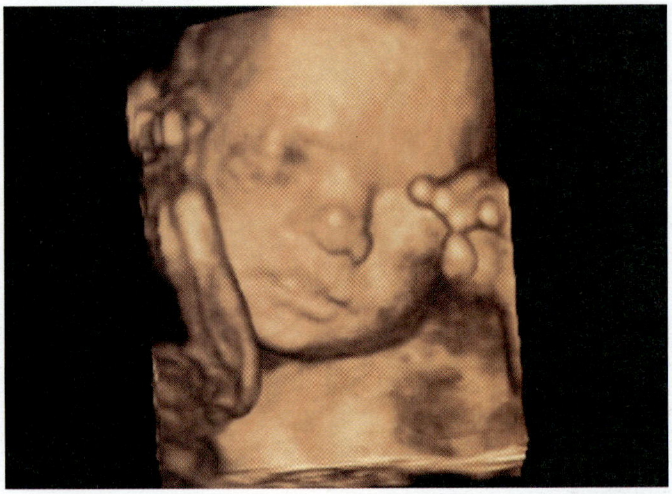

Fig. 69: The study of the nose and the lips is very easy in the second trimester of pregnancy by 3D.

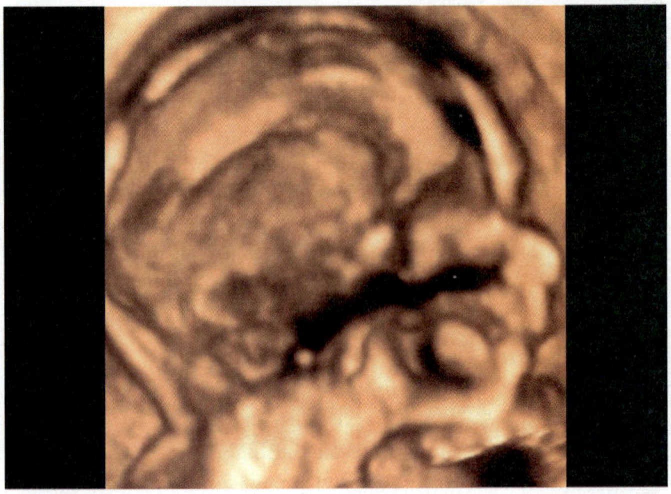

Fig. 70: The sagittal section of secondary palate shows the two portions of hard and soft palate with the uvula.

striking.[94] Regarding the urinary system, it is easier to study the renal arteries and parenchyma vessels, and kidney volume is a better index of development than traditional biometry.

Neural Tube and Limbs

Volume acquisition is one of the most important technological achievements of the last decade in diagnostic ultrasound and offers a good possibility to study the spine. In particular, there is the multiplanar which gives the possibility to navigate within a volumetric space through infinite reproducible imaging planes (including the crown), in real time. There is also rendering which

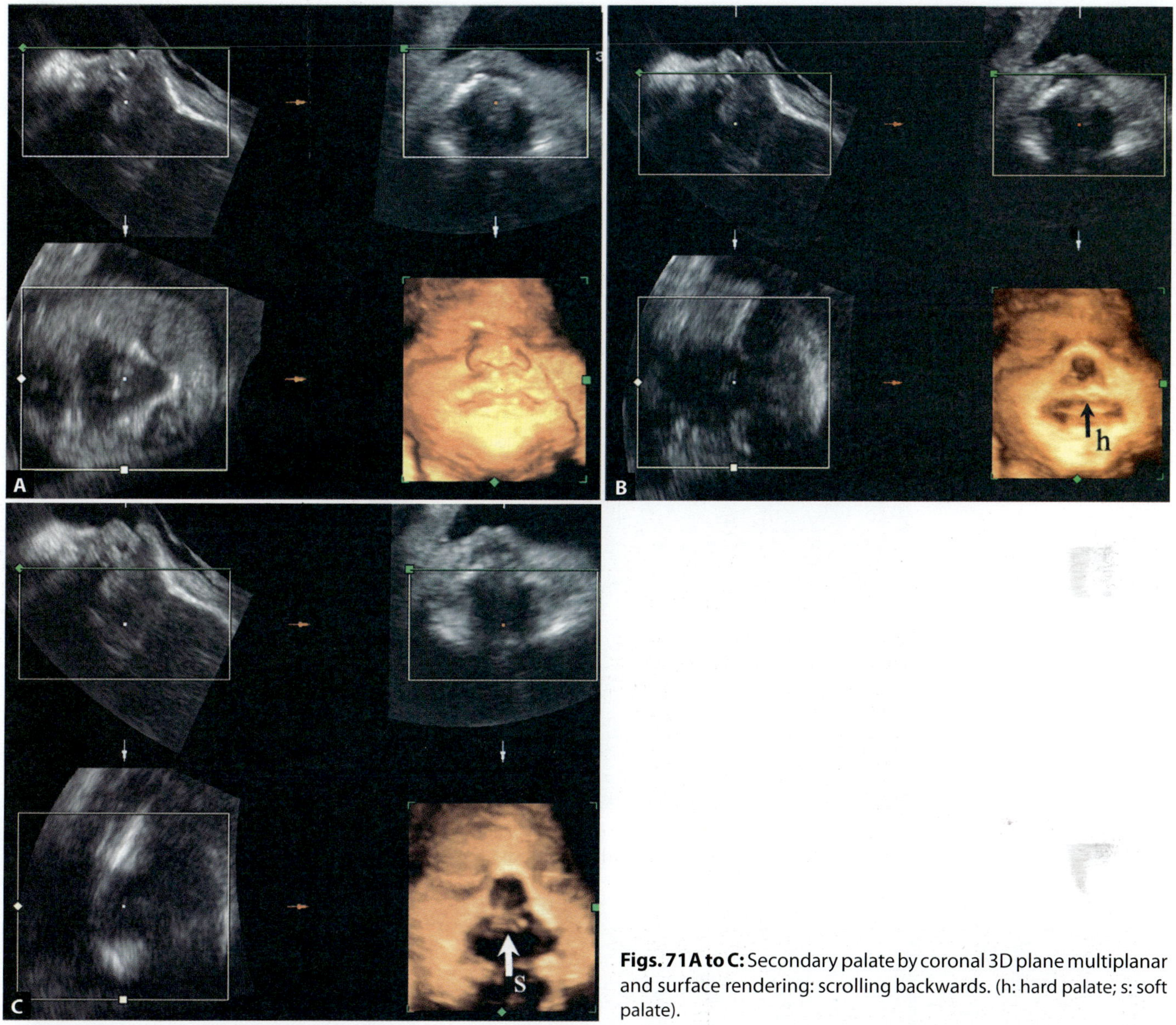

Figs. 71A to C: Secondary palate by coronal 3D plane multiplanar and surface rendering: scrolling backwards. (h: hard palate; s: soft palate).

has the ability to represent surfaces, as well as the VCI–c-plane that makes it possible to dissect an orthogonal plane with ultrasound scanning by integrating multiplanar and rendering.[95] A further step forward is the VCI-OmniView, which has the ability to model the source of 3D insonation by adapting to the structures of the fetal body that are normally represented by curved and straight lines (also the median line at the bottom is an artifact ultrasound).[96] This technique allows direct and relatively simple scans which adapt to the adjustable thickness of the structures corpus studied (20 mm spine). There is no doubt that with a 3D-4D instrument equipped with VCI–c-plane adapted to insonation, can produce virtually overlaping results in terms of detecting anatomical structures in almost all three trimesters, also if with significantly reduced times using the omni-view in the second trimester. The VCI-OmniView, sharing the latest technological achievements, allows one to specify the anatomical study of the fetus by choosing the ideal section plane. Regarding the multiple planes, that being in 3D and 4D in the same volume, it can better yet follow the natural curves and angles of the structures, while rotating like a real scanner box that can focus on very small points, which would otherwise be very difficult to explore.

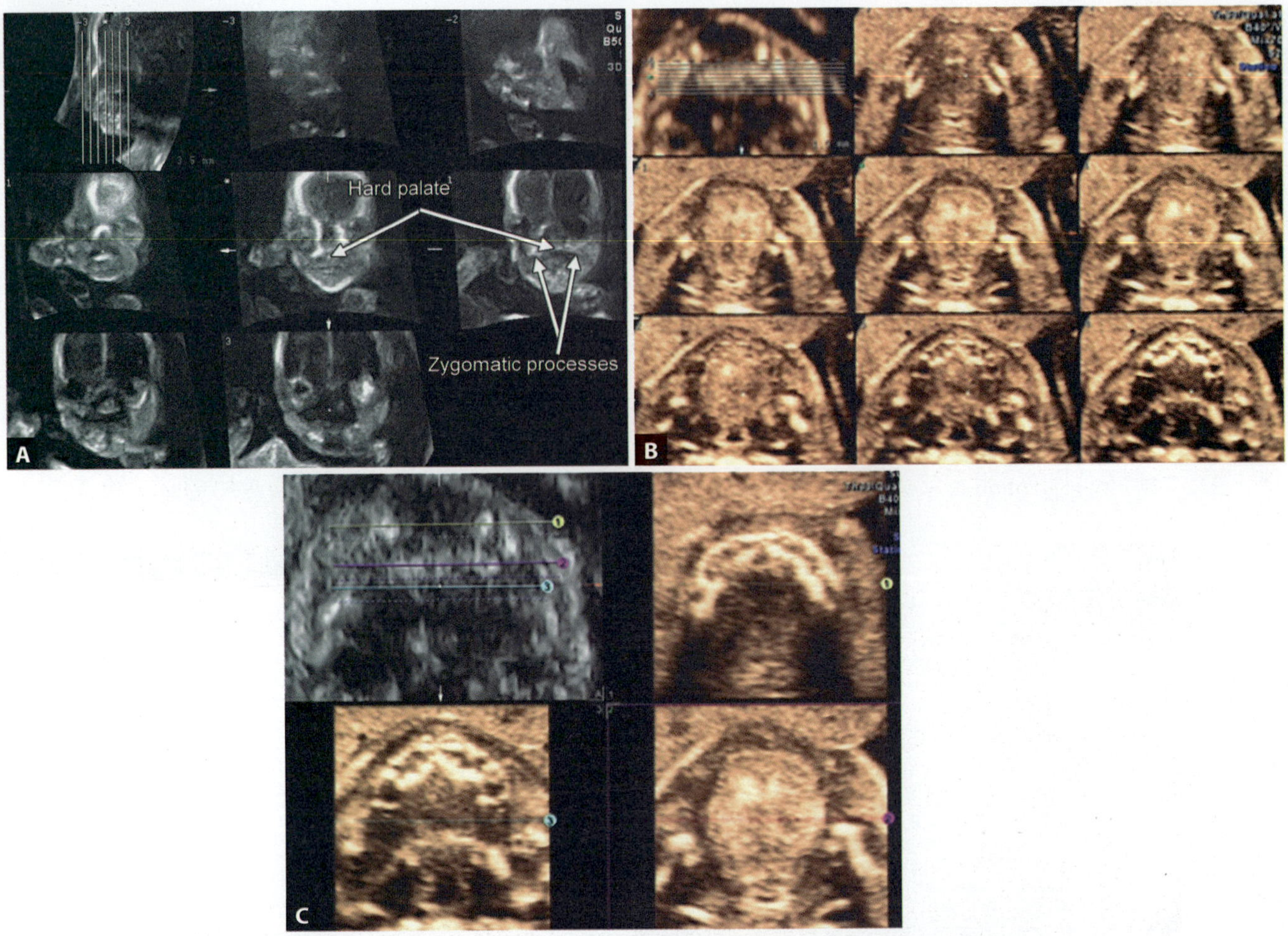

Figs. 72A to C: (A) Tomographic ultrasound imaging (TUI) of the secondary palate in the coronal plane; (B) TUI of the secondary palate in the axial plane; (C) Omniview of the secondary palate in the axial plane.

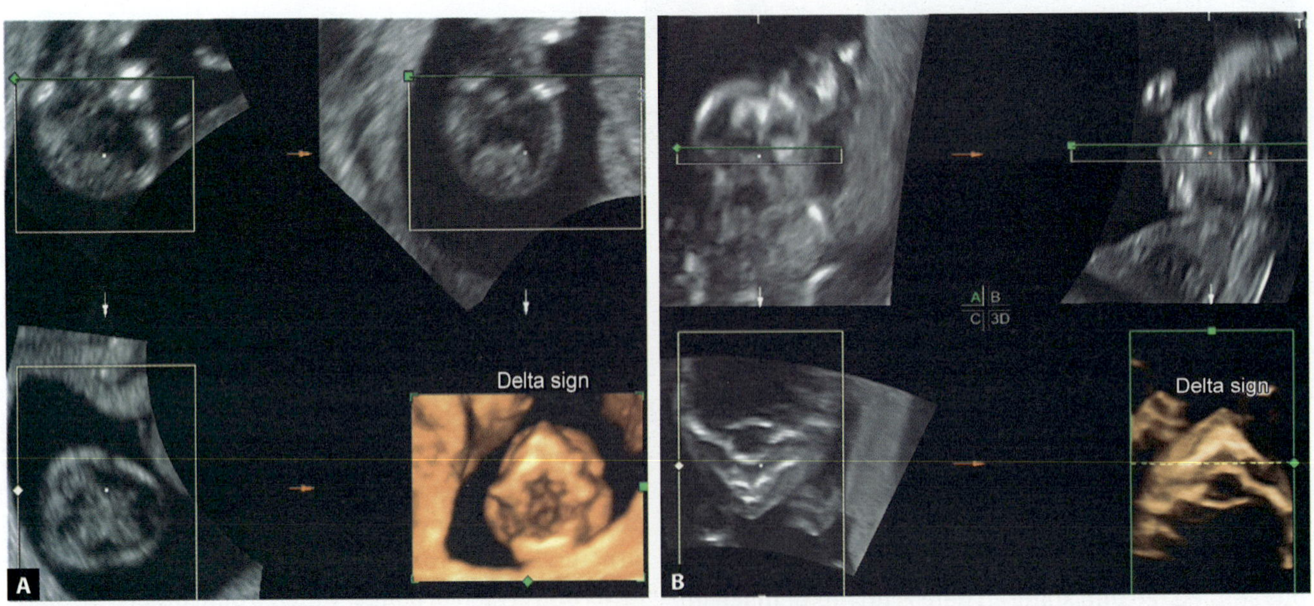

Figs. 73A and B: Axial 3D plane multiplanar and surface rendering (flipped view) to see the maxilla (delta sign) and hard palate at 12 weeks by (A) sagittal and (B) coronal scan.

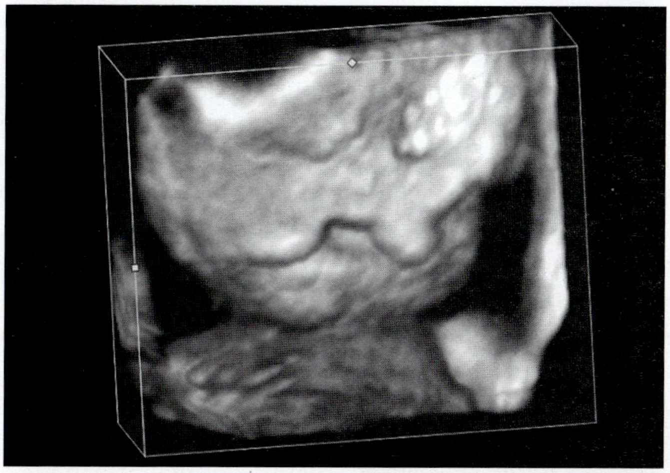

Fig. 74: A diagnosis at 14 weeks of cleft lip associated to holoprosencephaly by 3D vaginal probe 9–12 MHz (E8 GE).

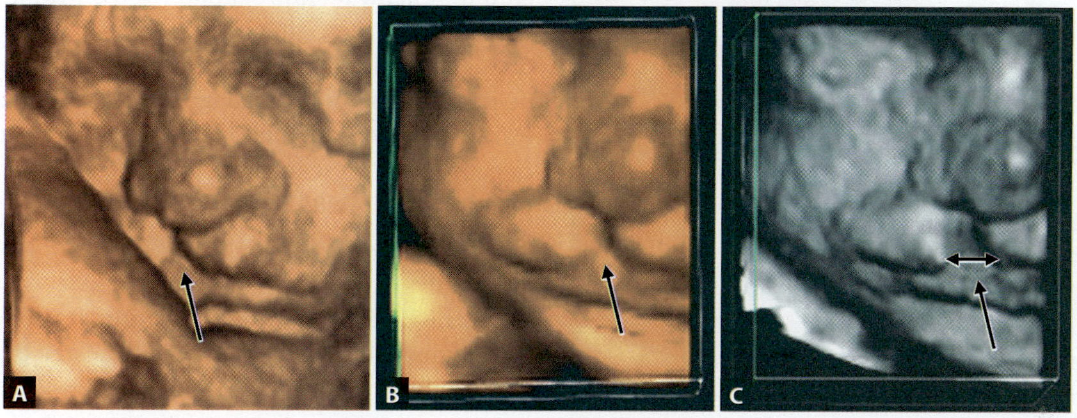

Figs. 75A to C: Three images of cleft lip.

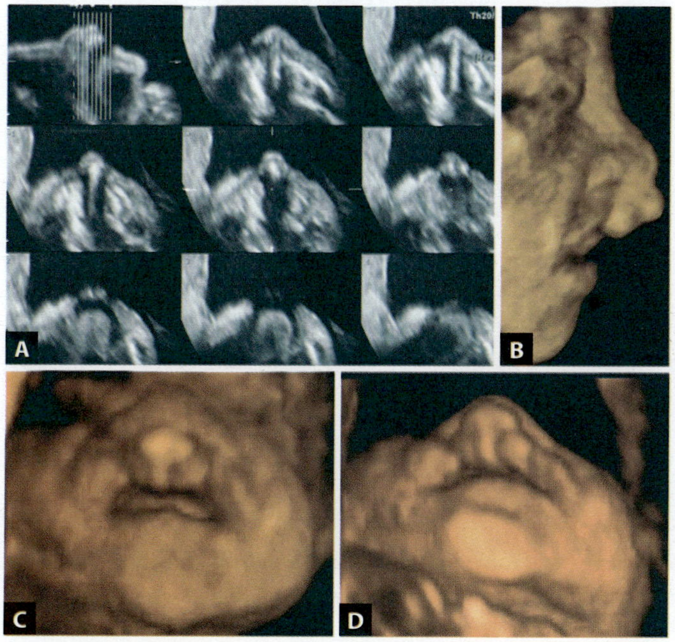

Figs. 76A to D: Bilateral l-p cleft with TUI and rendering surface.

The detailed study is therefore quite superior since it can easily and quickly visualize the structures, that with 3D–4D can be sometimes detectable only under particular conditions.

Study of the vertebral column and possible anomalies is much more convenient with 3–4D maximum mode which provides easy visualization of all bones, including the phalanges, as well as faster identification of any anomalies (platyspondyly, hemivertebrae, kyphosis, scoliosis such as absence (agenesis) or extraelements **(Figs. 52 and 79).** The ostechondrodysplasia have a prevalence of approximately 2.4 per 10,000 births and are rappresenatate in about 70% of four conditions: thanatophoric dysplasia, achrondroplasia, achondrogenesis, osteogeneis imperfecta **(Figs. 80A to C)**.

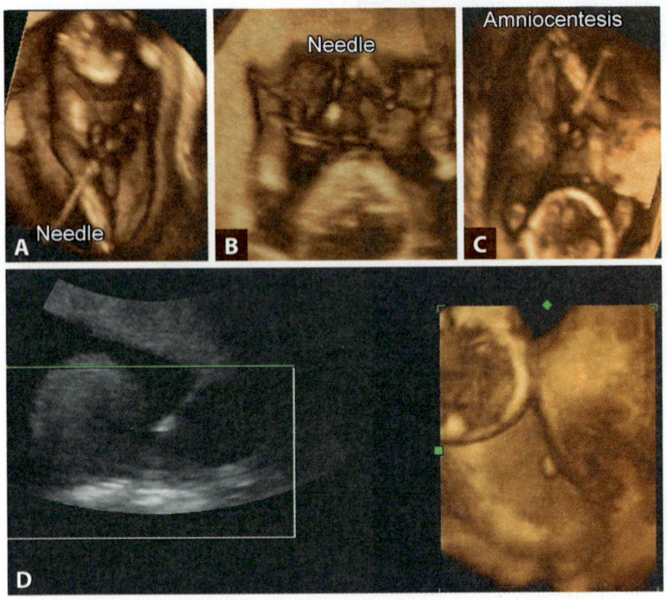

Figs. 77A to D: (A to C) 3D images of amniocentesis; (D) Gives a good idea of the difference between 2D and 3D.

The use of 3D does not offer a better condition to study the long bones, even if it is a good tool to store a volume and to explore by infinitive planes; but the study of dimension of the long bones, for instance the femur and the humerus for the suspicious of Down syndrome is the same by 2D or 3D. Instead the control of the extremity is a good field of exploration for 3D scan. The club foot varus or valgus meet 415 syndromes in London Medical Databases; it is an important malformation because is often associated with other malformations or in about 2% with aneuploid malformation and in the last decade the detection rate of club foot achieve approximately 80% with about 15% of false positive rate.[97] It is reasonable to think that the use of 3–4D, by tools maximum mode and omni-view, will be possible improve the diagnosis of malformation of the extremity (feet and hands) and decrease the false-positive rate, because 3D scan is better in the study of anatomical detail **(Figs. 81 to 85)**.

Genitals

The genitals are a new field of study. It is relatively easy to diagnose sex in the second trimester by 2D and to determine descent of the testicles at 26–28 weeks (third trimester), however diagnosis of pathology of the external genitalia, such as hypospadia, is much easier with 3D (tulip sign)[98] **(Figs. 86A to L)**.

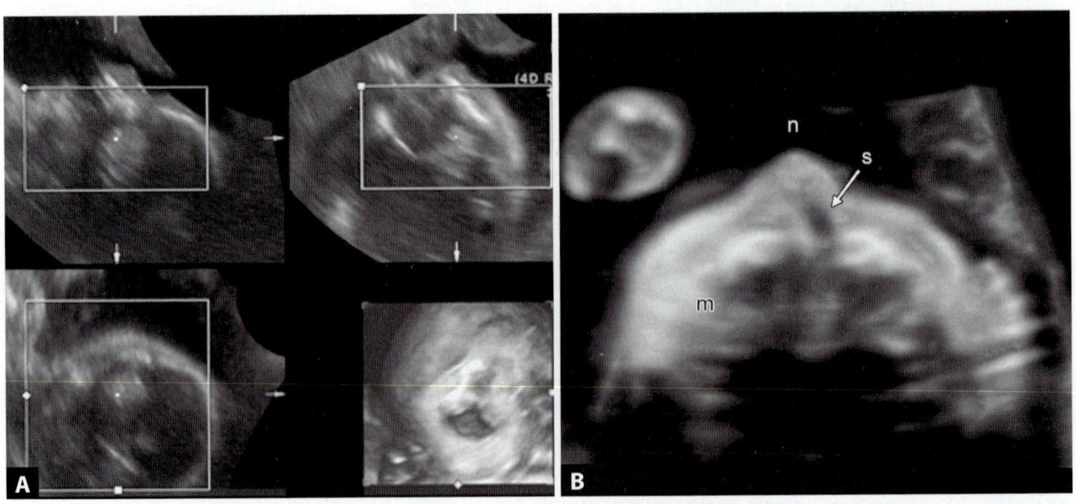

Figs. 78A and B: The axial 3D plane by multiplanar and surface rendering "flipped view face" to see a cleft-lip cleft alveolar ridge.

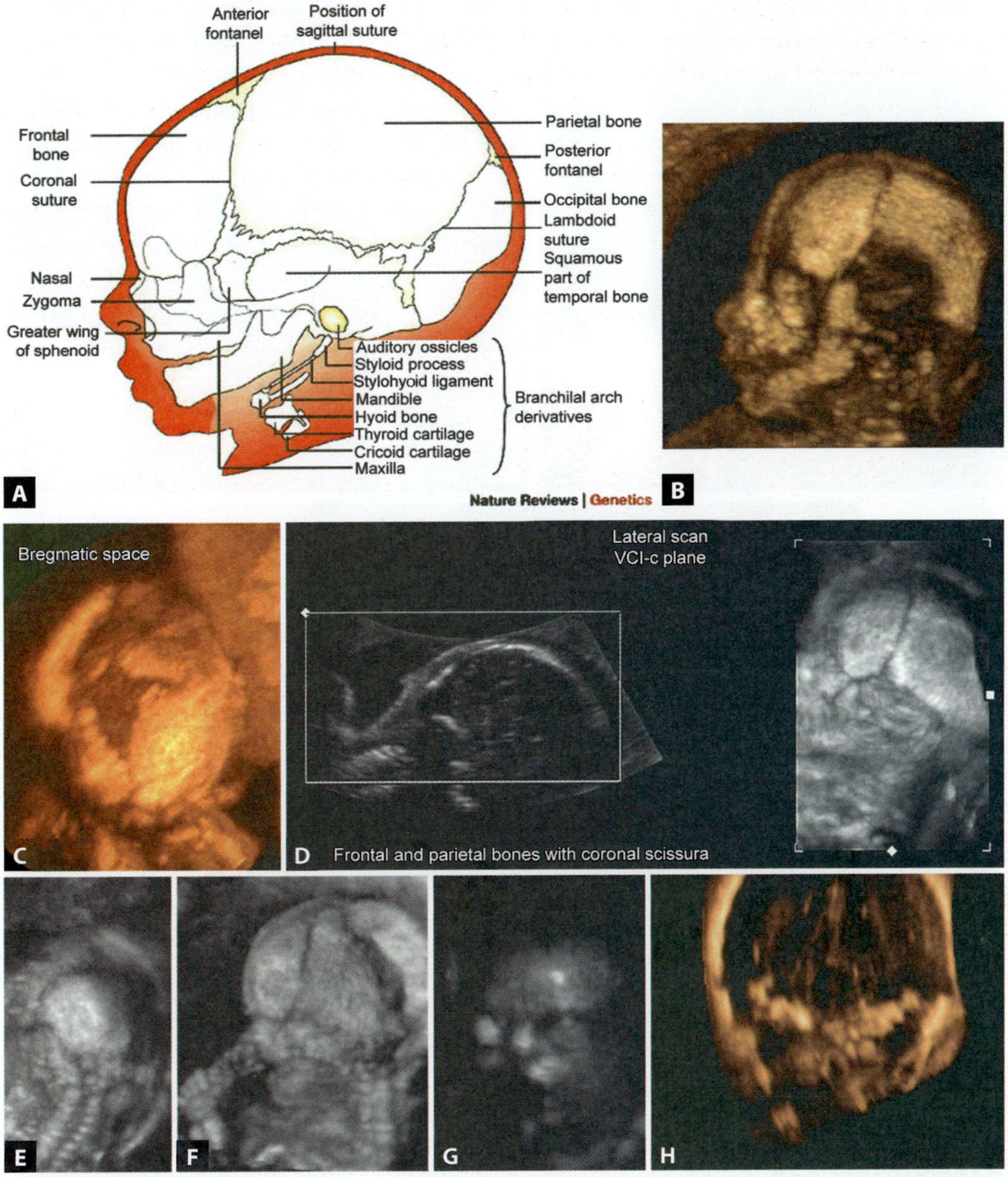

Figs. 79A to H: (A to C) The maximum mode imaging can detect so many features of the skull than it is possible to compare the image with a design; (D to G) Examination of the skull can detect many malformations: cranial bones and fissures are detectable by 3D, pathology of the bones like craniosynostosis at 20th week detected by maximum mode, or (H) Sphenoid bone.

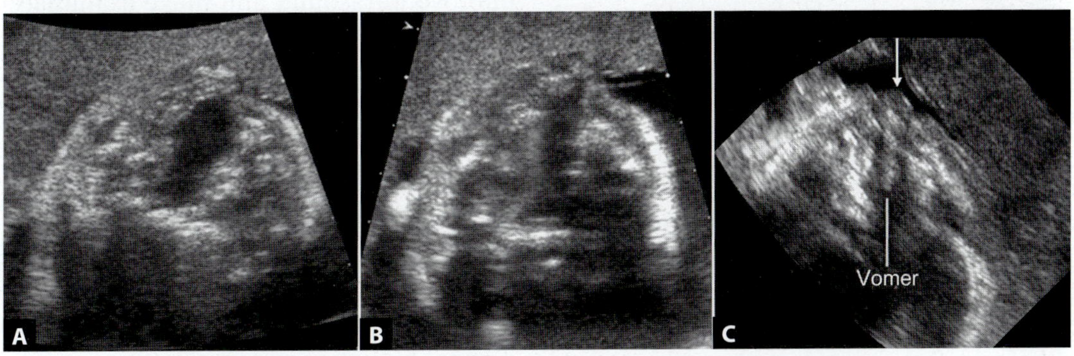

Figs. 80A to C: Monolateral cleft-lip and cleft-palate by axial 2D scan.

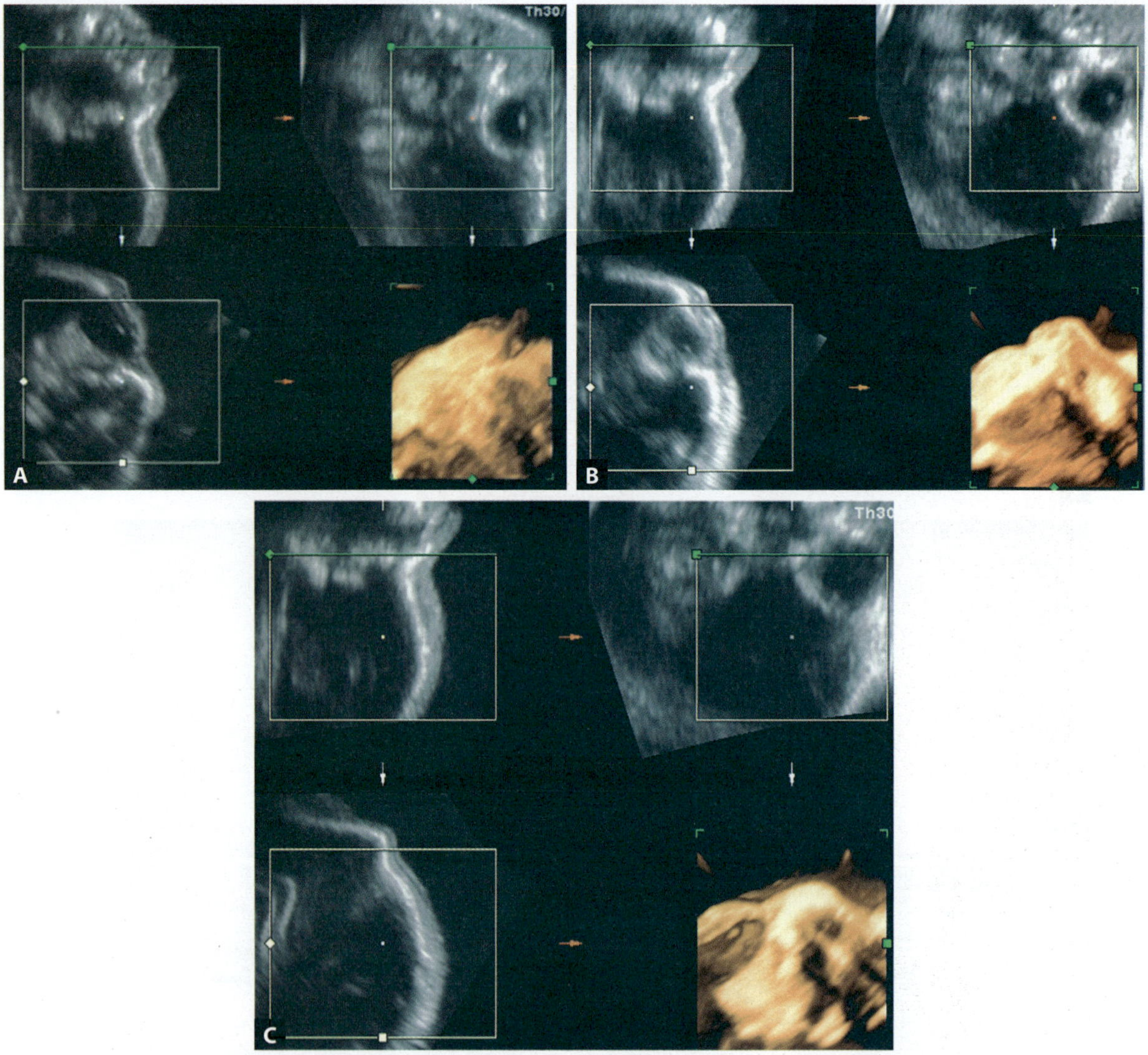

Figs. 81A to C: Axial 3D plane, inverted image, "flipped view face", sagittal scan: (A) Cleft lip; (B) Cleft alveolar ridge; (C) Cleft palate.

Placenta and Umbilical Cord

Detection of cord pathology (such as cysts), retrocervical position and number of twists is especially easy and reliable with power color glass-body mode **(Figs. 87A and B)**. Also the study of position and vascularity of the placenta is easier by 3-4D[99,100] **(Figs. 88A to H)**.

The above is not intended as a scientific evaluation of the merits of 3-4D with respect to 2D; however, almost all researchers report improved sensitivity and a better detection rate using 3-4D to measure volumes, determine orientation and definition of vessels and more precise definition of malformation, study coronal planes and the fetal face, diagnose heart malformations (by STIC), visualize limbs and fingers and study embryo-fetal anatomy (especially neurosonology). All this does not establish a "need" for 3D for the structural study of the foetus, but certainly indicates that 3D instruments can improve ultrasound and make examination easier and more pleasant.

Motor Activity and Facial Expression

The structure of the fetal brain is in the process of development, and in each phase of intrauterine life it has a maximum functional level. The first regions to mature are those necessary for life, such as sucking, swallowing and breathing. A first growth spurt is recognized between 10 weeks of gestation and 18 months of neonatal life, with synapse formation and myelination.

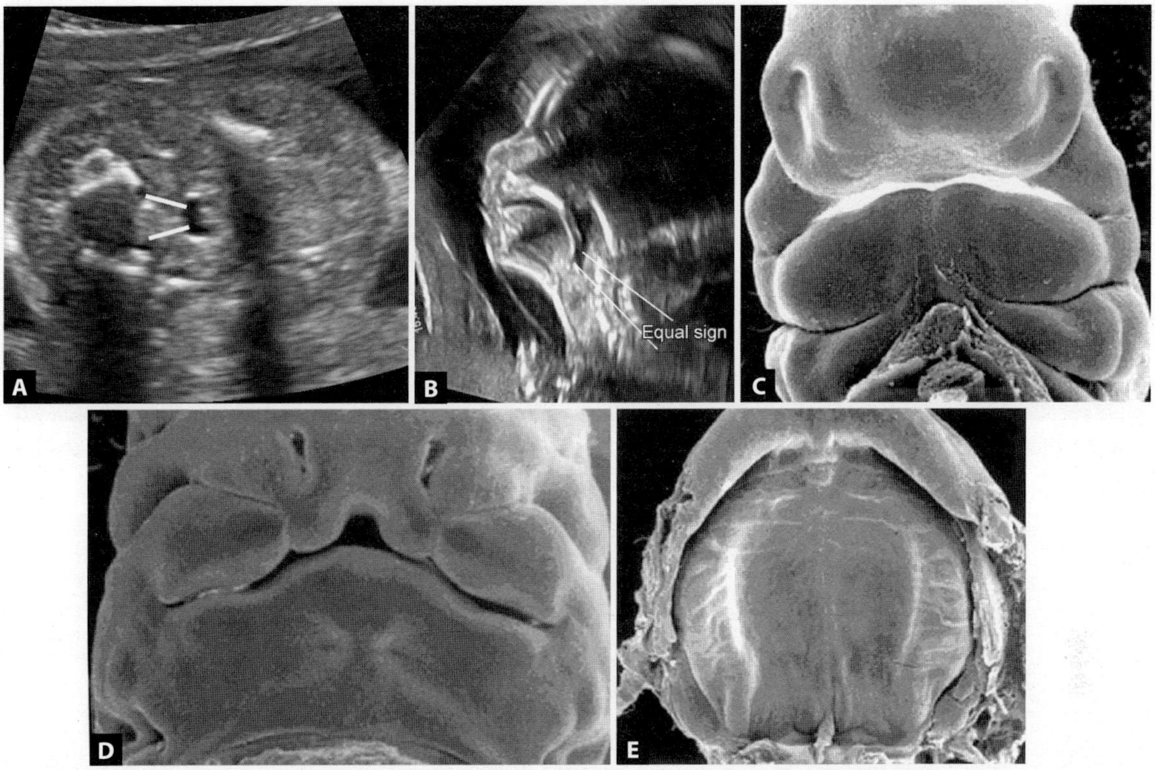

Figs. 82A to E: (A and B) Sagittal and axial scan offer a good possibility to see the "equal sign". The arrows indicate the two signs; (C) 6-weeks-old embryo: maxillary swellings fuse with medial nasal swellings, which merge with each other. The upper lip is still incompletely formed; (D) 53-day-old embryo: secondary palate: the fusion with primary palate has occurred; (E) 59-days-old embryo: complete fusion of the secondary palate has occurred.
Courtesy: K Sulik, Chapel Hill, North Carolina

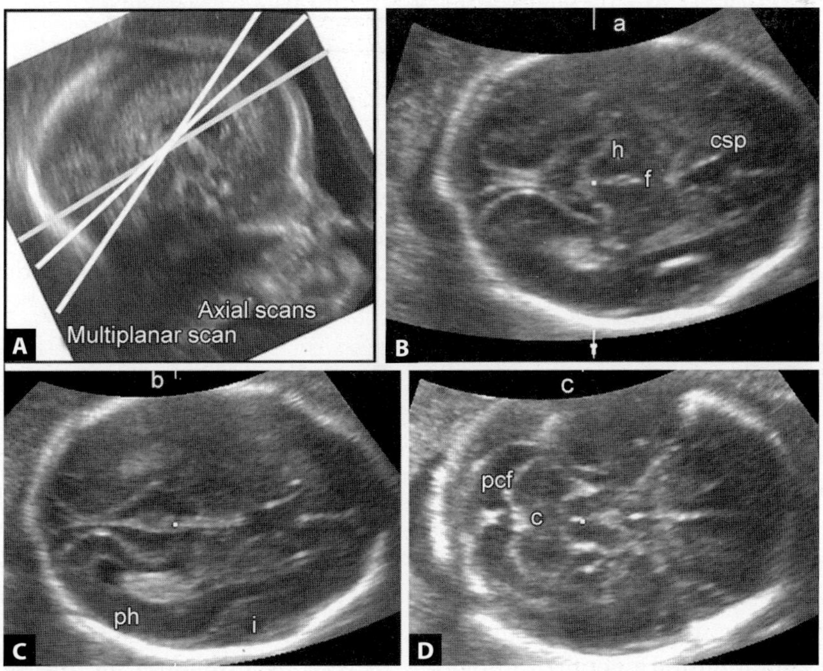

Figs. 83A to D: Axial scans of fetal head. The three scans are the usual sections to measure BPD, to see the posterior horns and to measure the cerebellum. (c: cerebellum; csp: cavum septi pellucidi; f: falx; pcf: posterior cranial fossa; ph: posterior horn; h: hypothalamus).

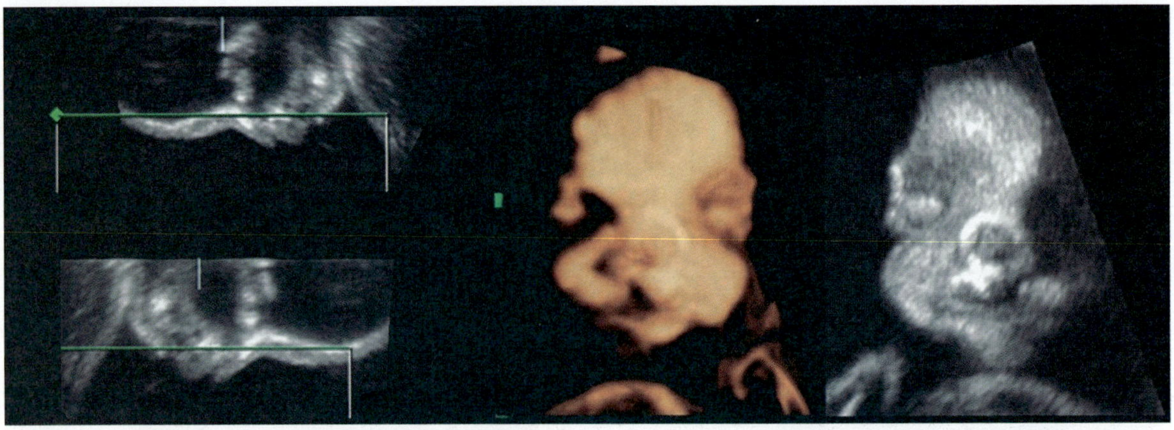

Fig. 84: Cleft-lip by "reverse face" mode and "front face" in the same case, of course change the position of the cleft.

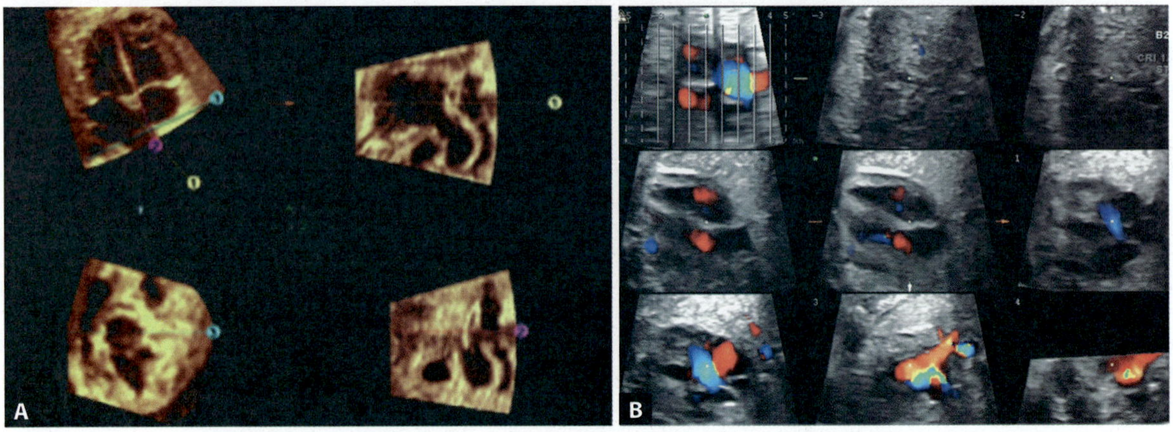

Figs. 85A and B: The omniview and STIC are good tools to explore the heart.

Fetal movements can be divided into primary motor patterns and primary automatisms. The former are present in the first half of pregnancy and are genetically determined, whereas the latter depend on interaction of the fetus with its environment and occur from week 10 of gestation into the first years of exstrauterina life. Active fetal movements increase with maturation of the nervous system, reaching a maximum at 32 weeks (after which they begin to decline);[101] in the term fetus, movements are similar to neonatal movements. Fetal circadian rhythm and fetal behavioral states, such as quiet sleep, active sleep, quite waking state, active waking state and crying, are recognized. Alternation of these fetal behaviors in the 24-hour period is a sign of neurological maturation. Ultrasound can assess a foetal biophysical profile composed of fetal movements, muscle tone, respiratory movements, placental maturation and amount of amniotic fluid.

Doppler flow imaging plays a fundamental role in assessing foetal wellbeing, by evaluating alterations in blood flow in the placenta, fetus and mother. Robles de Medina, et al. sustain that male and female fetuses do not show behavioral differences.[102] Dynamic 3D scan (4D) can be useful together with 2D to study foetal behavior in the second trimester of pregnancy.[103]

Brain Function

Though up to a few years ago the study of fetal brain function and hence motor activity, attitudes, posture and facial expression were of little interest, now, with 4D techniques that enable more accurate visualization in real time of everything the fetus can do in utero, studies of fetal activity have become increasingly numerous. These studies are concerned with activity from the point of view of physiology as well as brain pathology.[104] We now know much about fetal cognitive and emotional

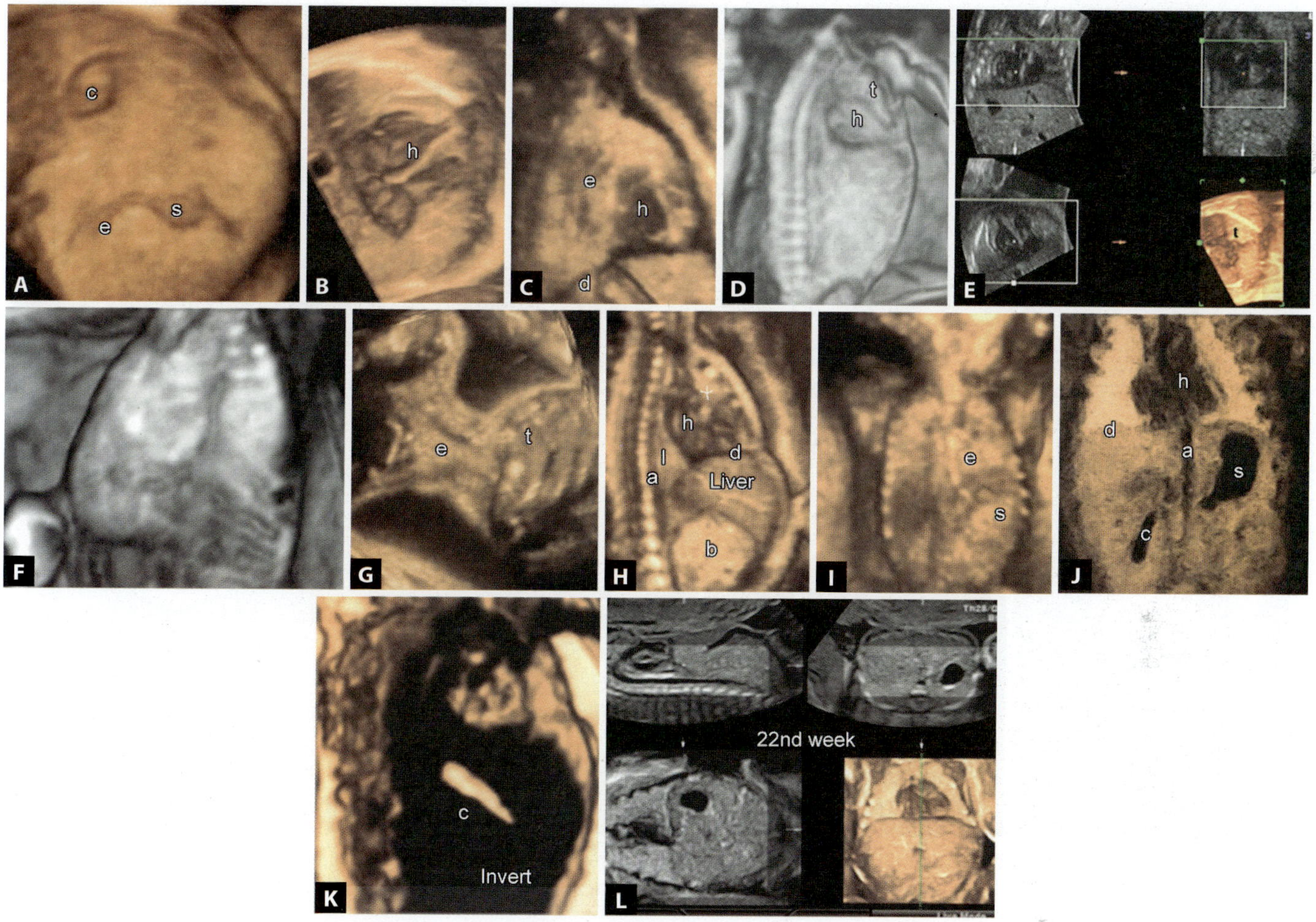

Figs. 86A to L: The chest and abdomen from the oral cavity to the esophagus are conveniently examined by 3-4D. The esophagus can be viewed from the oral cavity to the stomach by 3D, aiding diagnosis of stenosis-agenesis. All organs (lung, diaphragm, heart, thymus and bowel) are realistically represented by 3D. (a: aorta; b: bowel; c: gallbladder; d: diaphragm; e: esophagus; h: heart; t: thymus).

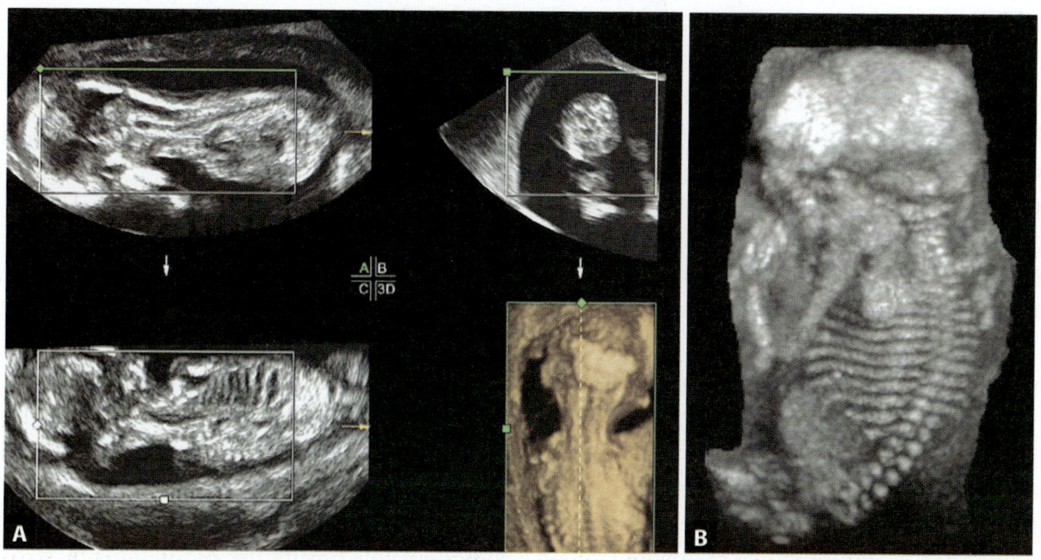

Figs. 87A and B: It is possible in the first trimester to study the bones of the skull. (A) Occipital bone at 12 week or the total skeleton with the spina; (B) The skeleton at 12th weeks by maximum mode.

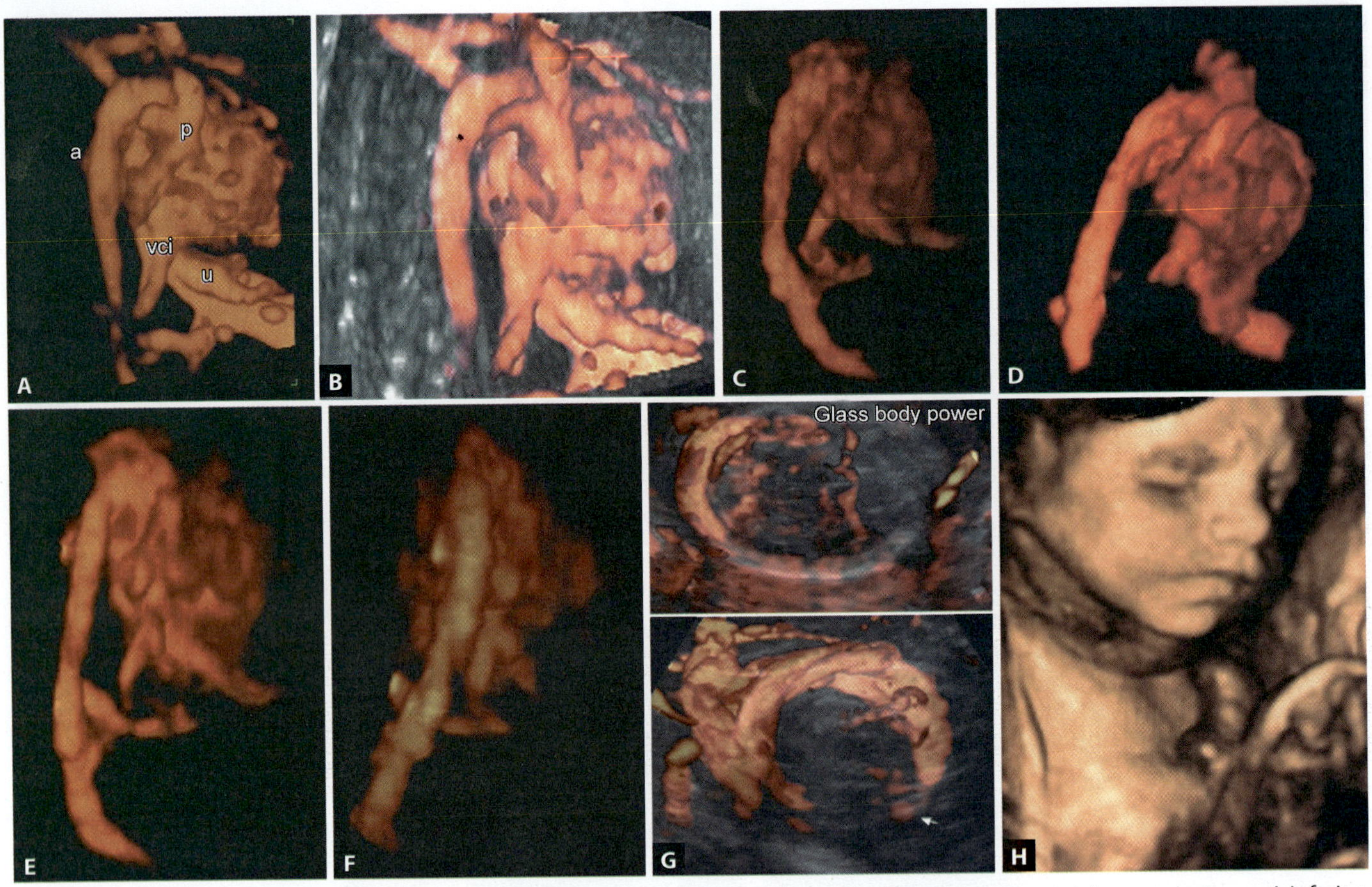

Figs. 88A to H: The glass body tool enhance the fetal circulation and thoracic conformation. (a: aorta; p: pulmonary artery; vci: inferior vena cava; u: umbilical artery).

development from observation of premature babies who now survive from as early as 22–23 weeks of gestation. Clearly, extrauterine life involves stressors that force the premature baby along the path of brain development, often with irremediable delays due to anoxia. Observation of premature babies therefore cannot be taken as validation of the physiological evolutionary milestones of the fetal brain. Renewed interest in this field has been spearheaded by Kurjak, who foresees major clinical benefits for 4D study of fetal behavior. We personally have studied the moment when laterality, the predominance of one hemisphere over the other, is established. Laterality has been the same all over the world for thousands of years. No scientific explanation of the predominance of the left over the right hemisphere has yet been found, if not an ancestral genetic mutation. Today, there have been many papers, especially from Scandinavia, associating predominance of the right hemisphere, and hence predominant use of the left side of the body, with a significant increase in mental disorders. 4D scan enabled us to determine laterality in about 90% of fetuses between weeks 10 and 11.

Behavior, Senses and Response to Stimulation in the Second and Third Trimesters

As mentioned, much is now known about fetal behavior at various gestational ages from the study of premature babies. However, the possibility of observing the fetus in its natural habitat in real time by 3–4D has led much research that may help us to assess fetal wellbeing and specifically, the degree of neurological development in physiological situations and in the presence of CNS pathology. It is fairly easy to detect a fetus who yawns, puts out its tongue, touches itself and its surroundings, developing its sense of touch, pulls faces after ingesting amniotic fluid (taste), opens its eyes (attempts at seeing?), responds to sounds (hearing), responds to manual stimulation (many sustain that parental stimulation of the fetus by stroking or patting the maternal abdomen leads to faster and more intense development of neuronal function), starts (from weeks 11–12 the fetus can be observed reacting whenever its fingers and toes touch the wall of the uterus), hiccups, smiles, grimaces, frowns and expresses pain or serenity. The fetus therefore sends us many messages through its behavior. Though much progress has been made, no scientifically demonstrated clinical applications of behavior have yet been developed. It is certainly fascinating for parents and specialists to observe a fetus by 4D, and it reinforces the hedonistic aspect of ultrasound examination in pregnancy.

ACKNOWLEDGMENT

The autors wish to thank Dr Mario Lituania, Chief Prenatal Diagnosis, Galliera Hospital,Genova, Italy for collaboration.

REFERENCES

1. Dyson RL, Pretorius DH, Budorick NE, Johnson DD, Sklansky MS, Cantrell CJ, et al. Three-dimensional ultrasound in the evaluation of fetal anomalies. Ultrasound Obstet Gynecol. 2000;16(4):321-8.
2. Merz E, Bahlmann F, Weber G, et al. Three-dimensional ultrasonography in prenatal diagnosis. J Perinat Med. 1995; 23(3):213-22.
3. Merz E, Welter C. 2D and 3D Ultrasound in the evaluation of normal and abnormal fetal anatomy in the second and third trimesters in a level III center. Ultraschall Med. 2005; 26(1):9-16.
4. GL Pilu, T Ghi. Preliminary experience with advanced volume contrast imaging (VCI) and OmniView obstetric and gynecologist ultrasound. GE Healthcare; 2010.
5. Bonilla-Musoles F, Raga F, Osborne NG, Bonilla F Jr; Caballero O, Climent MT, et al. Multimodality 3-dimensional volumetric ultrasound in obstetrics and gynecology with an emphasis in HDlive technique. Ultrasound Q. 2013;29(3): 189-201.
6. Pooh RH, Kurjak A. Novel application of three-dimensional HDlive imaging in prenatal diagnosis from the first trimester. J Perinat Med. 2015;43(2):147-58.
7. Grigore M, Mares A. The role of HDlive technology in improving the quality of obstetrical images. Med Ultraso. 2013;15(3):209-14.
8. AboEllail MA1, Tanaka H1, Mori N1, et al. HDlive silhouette mode in antenatal diagnosis of jejunal atresia. Ultrasound Obstet Gynecol. 2015; doi: 10.1002/uog.15737. [Epub ahead of print]
9. Forsberg F, Berghella V, Merton DA, Rychlak K, Meiers J, Goldberg BB. Comparing image processing techniques for improved 3-dimensional ultrasound imaging. J Ultrasound Med. 2010;29(4):615-9.
10. Michailidis GD, Papageorgiou P, Economides DL. Assessment of fetal anatomy in the first trimester using two- and three-dimensional ultrasound. Br J Radiol. 2002;75(891):215-9.
11. Xu HX, Zhang QP, Lu MD, et al. Comparison of two-dimensional and three-dimensional sonography in evaluating fetal malformations. J Clin Ultrasound. 2002; 30(9):515-25.
12. Downey DB, Fenster A, Williams JC. Clinical utility of three-dimensional US. Radiographics. 2000;20(2):559-71.
13. Campbell S. Doppler and 3D ultrasound in infertility - do they alter the outcome for the patient? Ultrasound Ostet Gynecol. 2003; 23(1):24.
14. Rosignoli L, Periti E. Centini G. 3D Omniview sonography in the pre-assisted reproductive medicine programme. Ultrasound Obstet Gynecol. 2010;36 (Suppl.1):52-167.
15. Timor-Tritsch IE, Fuchs KM, Monteagudo A, D'alton ME. Performing a fetal anatomy scan at the time of first-trimester screening. Obstet Gynecol. 2009;113:402-7.
16. Hafner E, Metzenbauer M, Stümpflen I, Waldhör T, Philipp K. First trimester placental and myometrial blood perfusion measured by 3D power Doppler in normal and unfavourable outcome pregnancies. Placenta. 2010; 31(9):756-63.
17. Souka AP, Pilalis A, Kavalakis Y, Kosmas Y, Antsaklis P, Antsaklis A. Assessment of fetal anatomy at the 11-14-week ultrasound examination. Ultrasound Obstet Gynecol. 2004;24:730-4.
18. Tonni G. Centini G, Taddei F. Can 3D uktrasound and doppler angiography arteries be included in second trimester ecocrdiograpphic examination? A prospective study on low-risk pregnancy population. Echocardiography. 2009;26(7):815-22.
19. Centini G, Sollazzi S, Rosignoli L, Ciani V, Imperatore A, Petraglia F, et al. Capacità diagnostica ecografica dei processi mal formativi nel primo trimestre di gravidanza: è proponibile l'ecografia morfologica dalla 11a alla 14a settimana? Il Ginecologo. 2010;5(1-2):22-9.
20. Merz E. Spina bifida aperta—detection of a shallow defect of the spine by 3D sonography. Ultraschall Med. 2007;28(3):246-7.
21. Tonni G, Centini G. Three dimensional first-trimester diagnosis of alobar holoprosencephaly associated with onphalocele in a 46,xx fetus. Am J Perinat. 2006.
22. Chaoui R, Nicolaides KH. From nuchal translucency to intracranial translucency: towards the early detection of spina bifida. Ultrasound Obstet Gynecol. 2010;35(2):133-8.
23. Chaoui R, Benoit B, Mitkowska-Wozniak H, et al. Ultrasound Obstet Gynecol. 2009;34(3):249-52.
24. Schramm T, Gloning KP, Minderer S, Tutschek B. 3D ultrasound in fetal spina bifida. Ultraschall Med. 2008;29(5):289-90.
25. Bilardo CM, Muller MA, Zikulnig L, Schipper M, Hecher K. Ductus venosus studies in fetuses at high risk for

chromosomal or heart abnormalities: relationship with nuchal translucency measurement and fetal outcome. Ultrasound Obstet Gynecol. 2001;17:288-94.
26. Nicolaides KH. Nuchal translucency and other first-trimester sonographic markers of chromosomal abnormalities. Am J Obstet Gynecol. 2004;191(1):45.
27. Matias A, Gones C, Flack N, et al. Screening for chromosomal abnormalities at 10-14 weeks: the role of ductus venosus blood flow. Ultrasound Obstet Gynecol. 1998;12:380-4.
28. Borrell A, Martinez JM, Serès A, Borobio V, Cararach V, Fortuny A. Ductus venosus assessment at the time of nuchal translucency measurement in the detection of fetal aneuploidy. Prenat Diagn. 2003;23:921-6.
29. Matias A, Montenegro N. Ductus venosus blood flow in chromosomally abnormal fetuses at 11 to 14 weeks of gestation. Seminars in Perinatology. 2001;25:32-7.
30. Toyama JM, Brizot ML, Liao AW, Lopes LM, Nomura RMY, Saldanha FAT, Zugaib M. Ductus venosus blood flow assesment at 11 to 14 weeks of gestation and fetal outcome. Ultrasound Obstet Gynecol. 2004;23:341-5.
31. Gezer C, Echin A, Gezer NS, Ertas IE, Avuc ME, Uyar I, et al. Prenatal karyotype results of fetuses with nuchal edema, cystic hygroma, and non-immune hydrops. Clin Exp Obstet Gynecol. 2015;42(5):586-9.
32. Chevernak FA, Isaacson G, Blakemore KJ, Breg WR, Hobbins JC, Berkowitz RL, Tortora M, Mayden K, Mahoney MJ. Fetal cystic hygroma: cause and natural history. N Engl J Med. 1983;309:822.
33. Mathias B, Forrester BS, Ruth D. Merz MS. Descriptive epidemiology of cystic hygroma: Hawaii, 1986 to 1999. Southern Medical Journal. 2004;97:631-6.
34. Bernstein HS, Filly RA, Goldberg JD, Golbus MS. Prognosis of fetuses with a cystic hygroma. Prenat Diagn. 1991;11:349-55.
35. Podobnik M, Singer Z, Podobnik-Sarkanji S, Bulic M. First trimestre diagnosis of cystic hygromata using transvaginal ultrasound and cytogenetic evaluation. J Perinat Med. 1995;23:283-91.
36. Rosati P, Guariglia L. Transvaginal ultrasound detection of septated and non-septated cystic hygroma in early pregnancy. Fetal Diagn Ther. 1997;12:132-5.
37. Farkas LG, Katic MJ, Forrest CR, Litsas L. Surface anatomy of the face in Down's syndrome: linear and angular measurements in the craniofacial regions. J Craniofac Surg. 2001;12:373-9.
38. Stempfle N, Huten Y, Fredouille C, Brisse H, Nessman C. Skeletal abnormalities in fetuses with Down's syndrome: a radiographic post-mortem study. Pediatr Radiol 1999;29: 682-8.
39. Rosignoli L. An early diagnosis of trisomy 18 by 2-3-4D at 10th week. Ultrasound Obstet Gynecol. London 3-7 September 2006.
40. Sonek J, Nicolaides KH. Prenatal ultrasonographic diagnosis of nasal bone abnormalities in three fetuses with Down syndrome. Am J Obstet Gynecol. 2002;186:139-41.
41. Cicero S, Rembouskos G, Vandecruys H, Hogg M, Nicolaides KH. Likelihood ratio for trisomy 21 in fetuses with absent nasal bone at the 11-14 weeks scan. Ultrasound Obstet Gynecol. 2004;23:218-23.
42. Kelekci S, Yazicioglu HF, Oguz S, Inan I, Yilmaz B, Sommez S. Nasal bone measurement during the first trimester: Is it useful? Gynecol Obstet Invest. 2004;58:91-5.
43. Peralta CF, Falcon O, Wesrzyn P, Faro C, Nicolaides KH. Assessment of the gap between the fetal nasal bone at 11 to 13+6 weeks of gestation by three-dimensional ultrasound. Ultrasound Obstet Gynecol. 2005;25(5):464-7.
44. Cicero S, Binda R, Rembouskos G, Spencer K, Nicolaides. KH Integrated ultrasound and biochemical screening for trisomy 21 at 11 to 14 weeks. Prenat Diagn. 2003;23(4): 306-10.
45. Benoit B, Chaoui R. Three dimensional ultrasound with maximal mode rendering: a novel technique for the diagnosis of bilateral or unilateral absence or hypoplasia of nasal bones in second-trimester screening for Down syndrome. Ultrasound Obstet Gynecol. 2005;25(1):19-24.
46. Cicero S, Curcio P, Rembouskos G, Sonek J, Nikolaides KH. Maxillary length at 11-14 weeks gestation in fetuses with trisomy 21. Ultrasound Obstet Gynecol. 2004;24(1):19-22.
47. Rembouskos G, Cicero S, Sacchini C, Nikolaides KH. Single umbilical artery at 11-14 weeks of gestation: relation to chromosomal defects. Ultrasound Obstet Gynecol. 2003; 22(6):567-70.
48. Sollazzi S, Centini G, Ciani V, Lmperatore A, Servillo R, Rosignoli L. First trimester ultrasonography in detection of fetal anomalies. Ultrasound Obstet and Gynecology. 36(1):119.
49. Guidelines SIEOG, Editeam, Cento, Italy, 2010. ISBN: 88-6135-124-7;978-88-6135-124-0.
50. Eurocat Group. Prenatal diagnosis of severe structural congenital malformations in Europe. Ultrasound Obstet Gynecol. 2005;25:6-11.
51. Rosignoli L, Tonni G, Centini G. Cranial development in the first trimester: the use of 3D in the study of complex structures. Imaging Med. 2010;2(3):251-7.
52. Rotten D, Levaillant JM. Two- and three-dimensional sonographic assessment of the fetal face. 1. A systematic analysis of the normal face. Ultrasound Obstet Gynecol. 2004;23(3):224-31.
53. Rotten D, Levaillant JM. Two- and three-dimensional sonographic assessment of the fetal face. 2. Analysis of cleft lip, alveolus and palate. Ultrasound Obstet Gynecol. 2004; 24(4):402-11.
54. Tonni G, De Felice C, Centini G, Gianneschi G. Cervical and oral teratome in the fetus: a systematic review of etiology, pathology, diagnosis, treatment and prognosis. Arch Gynecol Obstet. 2010.
55. Lee W, Kirk JS, Shaheen KW, Romero R, Hodges AN, Comstock CH. Fetal cleft lip and palate detection by three-dimensional ultrasonography. Ultrasound Obstet Gynecol. 2000;16(4):299-301.

56. Hata T, Kenenishi K, Akiyama M, Tanaka H, Kimura K. Real-time 3-D sonographic observation of fetal facial expression. J Obstet Gynecol Res. 2005;31(4):337-40.
57. Kurjak A, Stanojevic M, Azumendi G, Carrera JM. The potential of four-dimensional (4D) ultrasonography in the assessment of fetal awareness. J Perinat Med. 2005;33(1):46-53.
58. Yanagihara T, Hata T. Three-dimensional sonographic visualization of fetal skeleton in the second trimester of pregnancy. Gynecol Obstet Invest. 2000;49(1):12-6.
59. Dikkeboom CM, Roelfsema NM, Van Adrichem LN, Wladimiroff JW. The role of three-dimensional ultrasound in visualizing the fetal cranial sutures and fontanels during the second half of pregnancy. Ultrasound Obstet Gynecol. 2004; 24(4):412-6.
60. Faro C, Benoit B, Wegrzyn P, Chaoui R, Nicolaides KH. Three-dimensional sonographic description of the fetal frontal bones and metopic suture. Ultrasound Obstet Gynecol. 2005;26(6):618-21.
61. Chaoui R, Levaillant JM, Benoit B, Faro C, Wegrzyn P, Nicolaides KH. Three-dimensional sonographic description of abnormal metopic suture in second-and third-trimester fetuses. Ultrasound Obstet Gynecol. 2005;26(7):761-4.
62. Vinals F, Munoz M, Naveas R, Shalper J, Giuliano A. The fetal cerebellar vermis: anatomy and biometric assessment using volume contrast imaging in the C-plane(VCI-C). Ultrasound Obstet Gynecol. 2005; 26(6):622-7.
63. Chang CH, Chang FM, Yu CH, Ko HC, Chen HY. Assessment of fetal cerebellar volume using three dimensional ultrasound. Ultrasound Med Biol. 2000;26(6):981-8.
64. Benacerraf, BR, Sadow PM. Barnewolt CE. Estroff JA. Benson C. Cleft of the secondary palate without cleft lip diagnosed with three-dimensional ultrasound and magnetic resonance imaging in a fetus with Fryns' syndrome. Ultrasound Obstet Gynecol. 2006; 27(5):566-70.
65. Tonni G, Panteghini M, Pattacini P, De Felice C, Centini G, Ventura A. Integrating 3D sonography with targeted MRI in the prenatal diagnosis of posterior cleft lip. Journal of Diagnostic Medical Sonography. 2006;22:367-71.
66. Tonni G, Centini G, Rosignoli L. Prenatal screening for fetal face and clefting in a prospective study on low-risk population: can 3-4dimensional ultrasound enhance visualization and detection rate? Oral Pathology, Oral Radiology and Endodontics. 2005;100:420-6.
67. Gorlin RJ, Cervenka J. Pruzansky S. Facial clefting and its syndromes. Birth Defects Orig Artic Ser. 1971;7(7):3-49.
68. Calzolari E., Pierini A, Astolfi G, et al. Associated anomalies in multi-malformed infants with cleft lip and palate: An epidemiologic study of nearly 6 million births in 23 EUROCAT registries. Am J Med Genet A. 2007;143(6):528-37.
69. Stoll C, Alembik Y, Dott B, et al. Associated malformations in cases with oral clefts. Cleft Palate Craniofac J. 2000;37(1):41-7.
70. Calzolari E. Bianchi F, Rubini M, Ritvanen A et al. Epidemiology of cleft palate in Europe: implications for genetic research. Cleft Palate Craniofac J. 2004;41(3):244-9.
71. Milerad J, Larson O, Ph DD, et al. Associated malformations in infants with cleft lip and palate: a prospective, population-based study. Pediatrics. 1997:100(2 Pt 1):180-6.
72. Walker SJ, Ball RH, Babcook CJ, et al. prevalence of aneuploidy and additional anatomic abnormalities in fetuses and neonates with cleft lip with or without cleft palate: a population-based study in Utah. J Ultrasound Med. 2001;20(11):1175-80.
73. Ghi T, Tani G, Savelli L, Colleoni GG, Pilu G, Bovicelli L. Prenatal imaging of facial clefts by magnetic resonance imaging with emphasis on the posterior palate. Prenat Diagn. 2003;23(12):970-5.
74. Chmait R, Pretorius D, Moore T, et al. Prenatal detection of associated anomalies in fetuses diagnosed with cleft lip with or without cleft palate in utero. Ultrasound Obstet Gynecol. 2006;27(2):173-6.
75. Clementi M, Tenconi R, Bianchi F, et al. Evaluation of prenatal diagnosis of cleft lip with or without cleft palate and cleft palate by ultrasound: experience from 20 European registries. EUROSCAN study group. Prenat Diagn. 2000;20(11):870-5.
76. Hanikeri M, Savundra J, Gillett D, et al. Antenatal transabdominal ultrasound detection of cleft lip and palate in Western Australia from 1996 to 2003. Cleft Palate Craniofac J. 2006;43(1):61-6.
77. Walker SJ, Ball RH, Babcook CJ, et al. Prevalence of aneuploidy and additional anatomic abnormalities in fetuses and neonates with cleft lip with or without cleft palate. L Ultrasound Med. 2001;20:1175-80.
78. Mulliken, JB, Benacerraf BR. Prenatal diagnosis of cleft lip: what the sonologist needs to tell the surgeon. J Ultrasound Med. 2001:20(11):1159-64.
79. Berkowitz S. Cleft lip and palate: Diagnosis and management. Berlin: Springer-Verlag; 2006.
80. Sherer DM, Sokolovski M, Santoso PG, et al. Nomograms of sonographic measurements throughout gestation of the fetal hard palate width, length and area. Ultrasound Obstet Gynecol. 2004;24:35-41.
81. Shipp TD, Mulliken JB, Bromley B, et al. Three-dimensional prenatal diagnosis of frontonasal malformation and unilateral cleft lip/palate. Ultrasound Obstet Gynecol. 2002;20:290-3.
82. Centini G, Rosignoli L, Faldini E, et al. Comparison between three different methods of scan to visualize the secondary foetal palate by thre-dimensional ultrasonography.17th World Congress on Ultrasound in Obstetrics and Gynecology. Florence. ISUOG. 2007.
83. Centini G, Rosignoli L, Faldini E. L'ecografia del primo e secondo trimestre in 3D: Diagnosi Prenatale Ed Paletto; 2006;82-104.
84. Campbell S, Lees C, Moscoso G, et al. Ultrasound antenatal diagnosis of cleft palate by a new technique: the 3D "reverse face" view. Ultrasound Obstet Gynecol. 200;25(1):12-8.
85. Platt LD, Devore GR, Pretorius DH. Improving cleft palate/cleft lip antenatal diagnosis by 3-dimensional sonography: the "flipped face" view. J Ultrasound Med. 2006;25:1423-30.

86. Faure JM, Captier G, Baumler M, et al. Sonographic assessment of normal fetal palate using three-dimensional imaging: a new technique. Ultrasound Obstet Gynecol. 2007;29(2):159-65.
87. Segata M, Pilu G. A novel technique for visualization of the normal and cleft fetal secondary palate: angled insonation and three-dimensional ultrasound. Ultrasound Obstet Gynecol. 2007;29(2):166-9.
88. Tonni G, Centini G, Inaudi P, Rosignoli L, Ginanneschi C, De Felice C. Prenatal diagnosis of severe epignathus in a twin: case report and review of the literature. Cleft Palate Craniofac J. 2010;47(4):421-5.
89. Campbell S. Prenatal ultrasound examination of the secondary palate. Ultrasound Obstet Gynecol. 2007;29(2): 124-7.
90. Wilhelm L, Borgers H. The 'equals sign': a novel marker in the diagnosis of fetal isolated cleft palate. Ultrasound Obstet Gynecol. 2010;36(4):439-44.
91. Cohen L, Mangers K, Grobman WA, Gotteiner N, Julien S, Dungan J, et al. Three-dimensional fast acquisition with sonographically based volume computer-aided analysis for imaging of the fetal heart at 18 to 22 weeks' gestation. J Ultrasound Med. 2010;29(5):751-7.
92. Ruano R, Martinovic J, Dommergues M, Aubry MC, Dumez Y, Benachi A. Accuracy of fetal lung volume assessed by three-dimensional sonography. Ultrasound Obstet Gynecol. 2005;26(7):725-30.
93. Ruano R, Benachi A, Joubin L, Aubry MC, Thalabard JC, Dumez Y, et al. Three dimensional ultrasonographic assessment of fetal lung volume as prognostic factor in isolated congenital diaphragmatic hernia. Br J Ostet Gynaecol. 2004;111(5):423-9.
94. Chang CH, Yu CH, Chang FM, et al. The assessment of normal fetal liver volume by three-dimensional ultrasound. Ultrasound Med Biol. 2003;29(8):1123-9.
95. Rosignoli L, Periti E, Tonni G, et al. VCI-Omniview e studio della colonna vertebrale. XVII Congresso Nazionale Società Italiana Ecografia Ostetrica-Ginecologica (SIEOG). Ottobre Sorrento. 2010;17-20
96. Pilu GL, Ghi T. Preliminary experience with advanced volume contrast imaging (VCI) and OmniView obetric and gynecologist ultrasound. GE Heltcare 2010 White book.
97. Lauson S, Alvarez C, Patel MS, Langlois S. Outcome of prenatally diagnosed isolated clubfoot. Ultrasound Obstet Gynecol. 2010;35(6):708-14.
98. Cafici D, Iglesias A. Prenatal diagnosis of severe hypospadias with two-and three-dimensional sonography. J Ultrasound Med. 2002;21(12):1423-6.
99. Costa J, Rice H, Cardwell C, et al. An assessment of vascularity and flow intensity of the placenta in normal pregnancy and pre-eclampsia using three-dimensional ultrasound. J Matern Fetal Neonatal Med. 2010;23(8):894-9.
100. Huster KM, Haas K, Schoenborn J, et al. Reproducibility of placental volume and vasculature indices obtained by 3-dimensional power Doppler sonography. Ultrasound Med. 2010;29(6):911-6.
101. D'Elia A, Pighetti M, Moccia G, et al. Spontaneous motor activity in normal fetuses. Early Hum Dev. 2001;65(2):139-47.
102. Robles de Medina PG, Visser GH, Huizink AC, et al. Fetal behaviour does not differ between boys and girls. Early Hum Dev. 2003;73(1-2):17-26.
103. Kuno A, Akiyama M, Yamashiro C, Tanaka H, Yanagihara T, Hata T. Three-dimensional sonographic assessment of fetal behaviour in the early second trimester of pregnancy. J Ultrasound Med. 2001;20(12):1271-5.
104. Blaas HG, Eik-Nes SH. Sonoembryology and early prenatal diagnosis of neural anomalies. Prenat Diagn. 2009;29(4): 312-25.

35

CHAPTER

Three-dimensional Ultrasound in Detection of Fetal Anomalies

Ritsuko K Pooh, Asim Kurjak

INTRODUCTION

Recent Advances of 3D Ultrasonography

Recent advances of 3D/4D sonography have assessed not only structural but also functional early human development.[1] 3D images of embryos were generated using the high-frequency transducer. Demonstration of an embryo of less than 10 mm (greatest length) has been difficult in the past and not visualized in detail[2–4] (See the Chapter of Three Dimensional Sonoembryology). 3D/4D sonography moved prenatal diagnosis of fetal anomalies from the second to the first trimester of pregnancy.[5] In the second and third trimesters, 3D ultrasound imaging provides us the detailed superficial structure such as external ear and hair as shown in **Figure 1**. The detailed structure of small parts, for instance the lenses of eyeballs **(Fig. 2)** can be visualized by 3D orthogonal view. 3D ultrasound technology will contribute to demonstration of in-utero pathological changes of congenital diseases arising in-utero. This can be accomplished through the use of not only surface rendered imaging but also three orthogonal planes, and tomographic ultrasound imaging. Serial examinations allow obtaining exactly the same cutting section at different stages of fetal development. Therefore, it is possible to document the changes of development from early embryonic period.

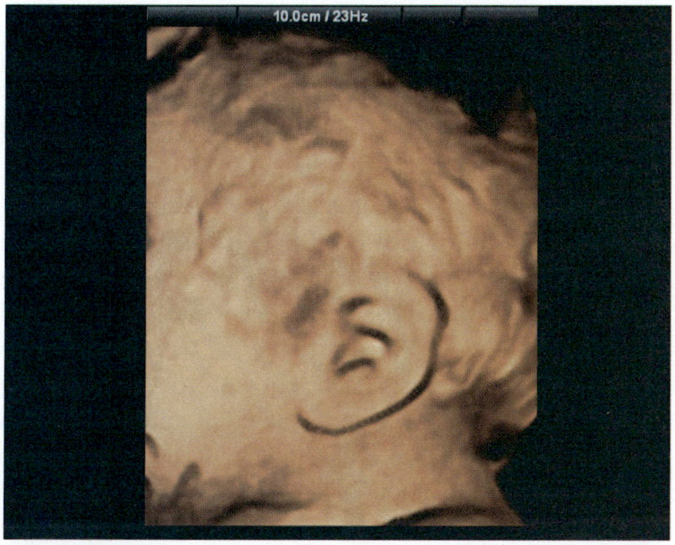

Fig. 1: Normal ear and hair at 35 weeks of gestation by 3D surface rendering.

In the history of 3D/4D ultrasound technology, the great achievement was HD (high definition) live technology.[6] This technology is a novel ultrasound technique that improves the 3D/4D images. HDlive ultrasound has resulted in remarkable progress in visualization of early embryos and fetuses and in the development of sonoembryology.[7] HDlive uses an adjustable light source and software that calculates the propagation of light through surface structures in relation to the light direction.[8] The virtual light source produces selective illumination, and the respective shadows are created by the structures where the light is reflected. This combination of light and shadows increases depth perception and produces remarkable images that are more natural than those obtained with classic 3D ultrasound. The virtual light can be placed in the front, back, or lateral sides, where viewing is desired until the best image is achieved. A great advantage is that the soft can be applied to all images stored in the machine's memory[7]. With HDlive ultrasound, both structural and functional developments can be assessed from early pregnancy more objectively and reliably and indeed, the new technology has moved embryology from postmortem studies to the in vivo environment. Practically in obstetrical ultrasound, HDlive could be used during all three trimesters of pregnancy. As shown in **Figures 3 and 4**, HDlive image of the fetus is more clearly demonstrated by shadowing with virtual light than classic 3D image.

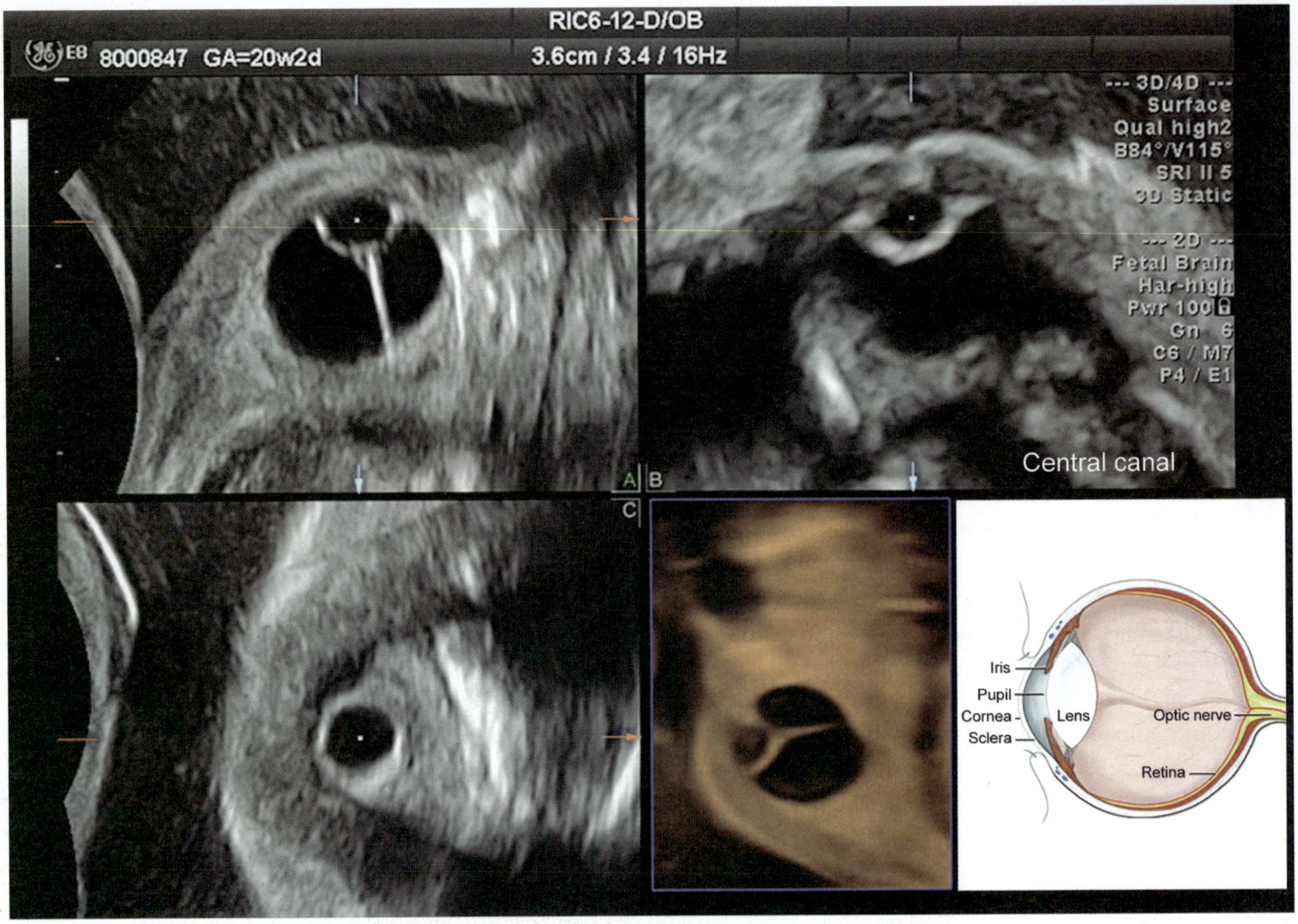

Fig. 2: Eyeball structure at 20 weeks: Three orthogonal view and reconstruction image of the eyeball. Lens and central canal are clearly demonstrated.

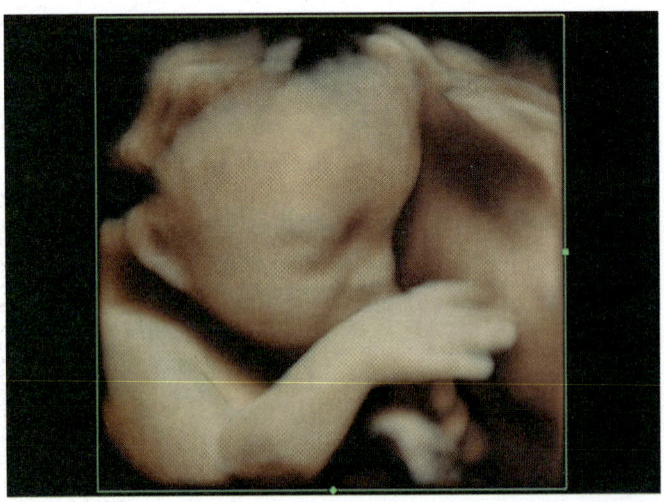

Fig. 3: Normal fetal face and hand at 30 weeks of gestation by 3D HDlive imaging.

There have been several reports on HDlive demonstration of fetal surface.[9-12] Three-dimensional HDlive further "humanizes" the fetus, enables detailed observation of detailed facial appearance even in the first trimester, and reveals that a small fetus is not a fetus but a "person" with its personality from the first trimester.[11] Detailed structural abnormalities of face, fingers, toes and even amniotic membranes in the first trimester could be well demonstrated by HDlive technique.[11,12] New applications of HDlive silhouette and HDlive flow were released at the end of 2014. The algorithm of HDlive silhouette creates a gradient at organ boundaries, fluid filled cavity and vessels walls, where an abrupt change of the acoustic impedance exists within tissues.[13,14] By HDlive silhouette mode, an inner cystic structure with fluid collection can be depicted through the outer surface structure of the body and it

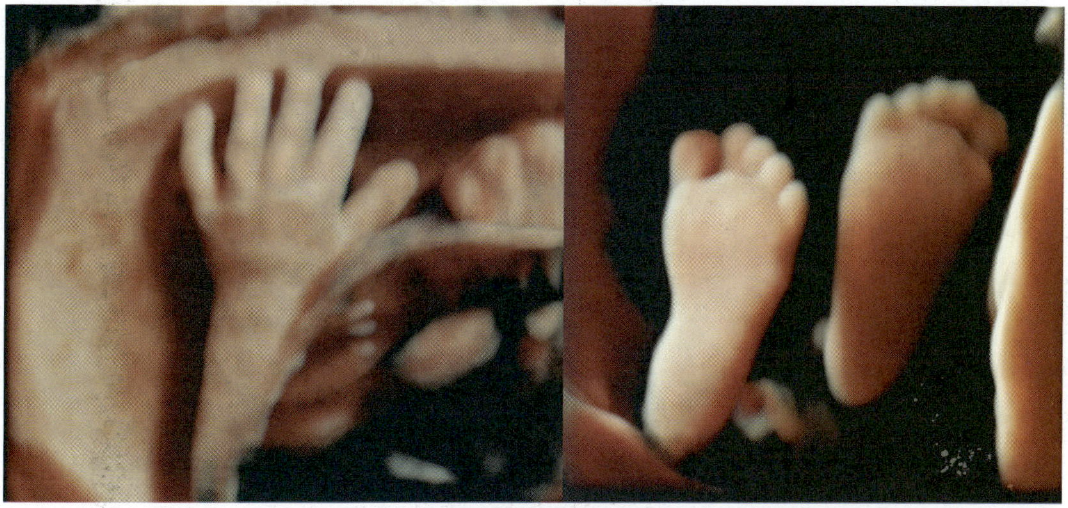

Fig. 4: Normal fetal limbs at 19 weeks of gestation by 3D HDlive imaging.

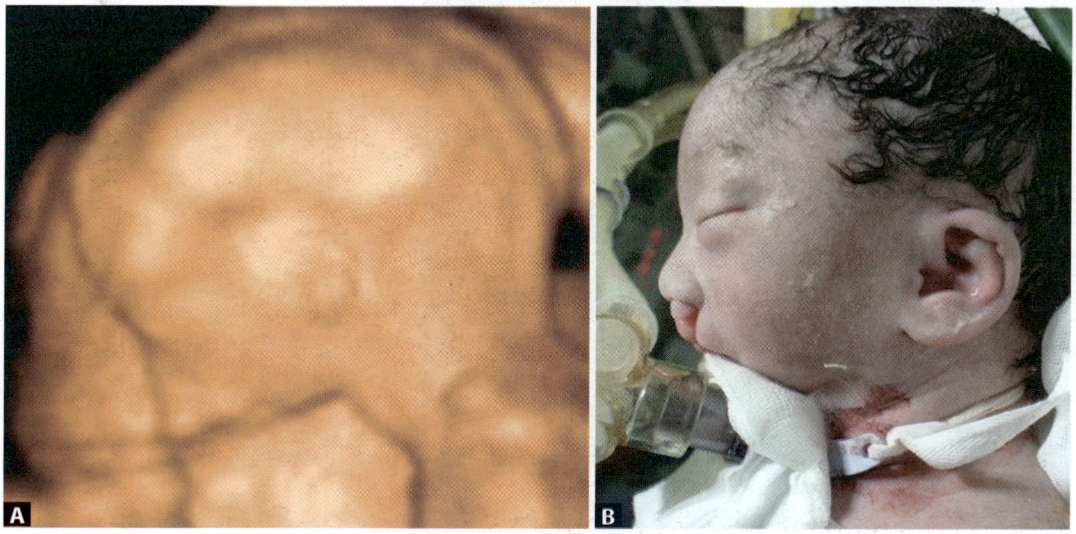

Figs. 5A and B: Agnathia with cleft lip at 19 weeks: (A) 3D reconstructed lateral image of the fetal face at 19 weeks; (B) Postnatal facial appearance.

can be appropriately named as 'see-through fashion'.[13] (see the Chapter of "HDlive Silhouette and HDlive Flow—New Application of 3D Ultrasound in Prenatal Diagnosis").

PRENATAL DIAGNOSIS OF ANATOMICAL CONGENITAL ANOMAILES

The prenatal diagnosis of congenital anomalies with ultrasound is based upon identification of a substantial departure of normal anatomy. This has been possible in the second and third trimester of pregnancy, and this achievement has made the diagnosis of congenital anomalies one of the objectives of modern prenatal care.

Facial Anomalies

A facial anomaly can be associated with a central nervous system anomaly, be an isolated finding, or part of a syndrome. Micrognathia **(Figs. 5A and B)** can be detected as an isolated structural anomaly, as one of the features of a chromosomal abnormality, or a syndrome[15] **(Figs. 6A to C)** demonstrates the slow jaw development during pregnancy in a case of Pierre Robin sequence, detected by serial 3D ultrasound scans. Congenital micrognathia and lowest ears are frequently detected together as shown in **Figures 7A to C**, in cases with chromosomal aberrations and other syndromic diseases, because mandibule and

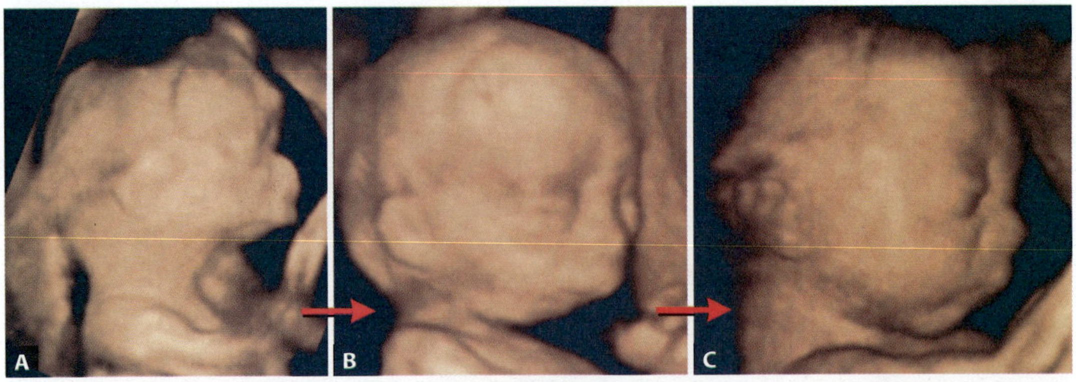

Figs. 6A to C: Slow jaw development in a case of Pierre Robin sequence during pregnancy: (A) Serial 3D scan clearly reveals slow jaw development at 17 weeks (A); 20 weeks (B) and 29 weeks (C) associated with Pierre Robin sequence.

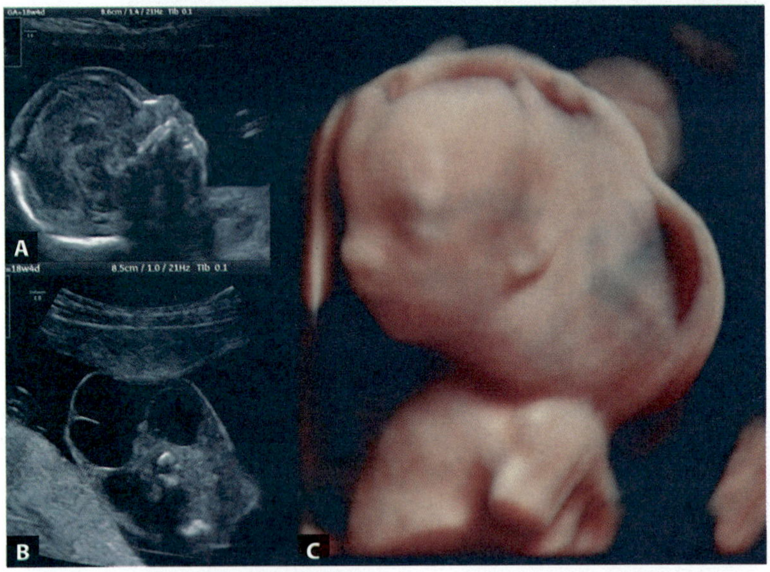

Figs. 7A to C: Low-set ear with micrognathia in a case of cystic hygroma at 18 weeks: (A) 2D profile image. Micrognathia is demonstrated; (B) 2D image showing cystic hygroma around the neck; (C) HDlive image. Low-set ear with micrognathia and dilated neck due to cystic hygroma are demonstrated.

ears arises from the first pharyngeal (branchial) arch. Assessment of the facial features, chin development and mandibular size by 3D ultrasound in the second and third trimesters has been reported.[16] Facial abnormalities are often associated with maldevelopmental brain **(Figs. 8A and B)** or craniosynostosis **(Figs. 9A to E)** due to deformed cranial structure. Cleft lip and palate is one of common congenital facial anomalies. Cleft lip occurs unilaterally **(Figs. 10A to C)** or bilaterally **(Figs. 11 and 12)**. Recent 3D tomographic ultrasound can demonstrate anterior maxillary structure, indicating the evidence of alveolar cleft presence shown in the **Figures 10 and 12**. A single nostril is occasionally seen as demonstrated in **Figures 13A and B**, associated with holoprosencephaly. Maldevelopment of eyes is often associated with brain abnormalities. **Figure 14** shows the holoprosencephalic fetus with cyclops. 3D ultrasound proved the presence of two eye lenses inside. Exophthalmos and microphthalmia are well-demonstrated in **Figures 15 and 16** respectively.

Brain Anomalies

The brain structure should be understood as three-dimensional structure.[17,18] 3D sonographic assessment of premature brain in the early pregnancy was reported from 1995.[19,20] From 2000, fetal brain assessment in the second and third trimesters by 3D ultrasound was reported.[17,18,21-30] Recent advanced 3D ultrasound has enabled to assess detailed brain structure as an understandable organ. 3D ultrasound abilities, such as tomographic ultrasound imaging and three orthogonal view, greatly contribute

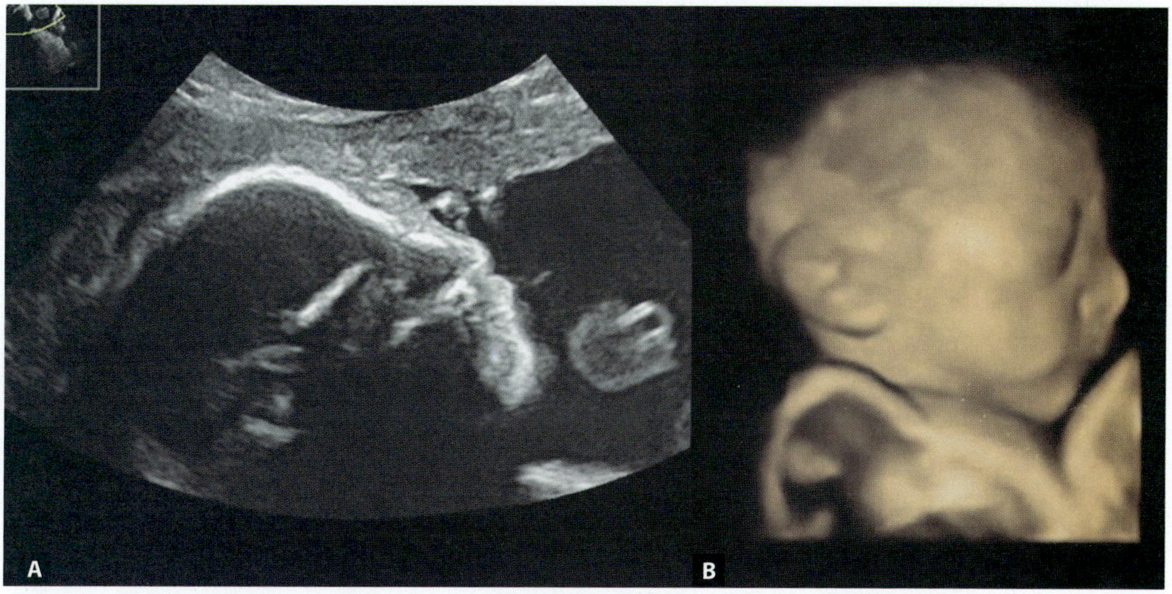

Figs. 8A and B: Face of microcephalic fetus at 23 weeks of gestation: (A) 2D image showing flat face; (B) 3D image.

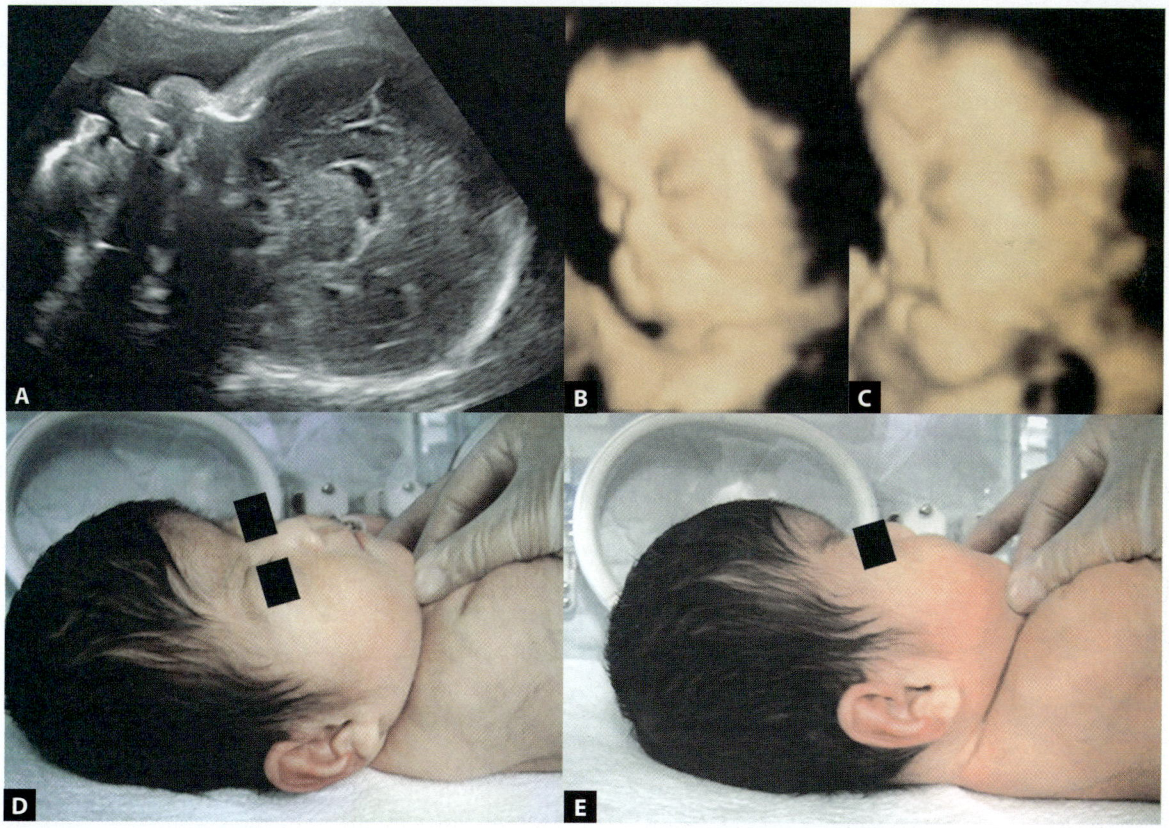

Figs. 9A to E: Facial abnormality associated with Apert syndrome at 31 weeks: (A) 2D sagittal image of the fetal face. Note the marked frontal bossing and low nasal bridge. (B and C) 3D reconstructed images of fetal face. Exophthalmos is clearly visualized. This facial appearance occurs due to craniosynostosis of coronal sutures seen in a case of Apert syndrome. (D and E) Postnatal facial appearance of the same baby.

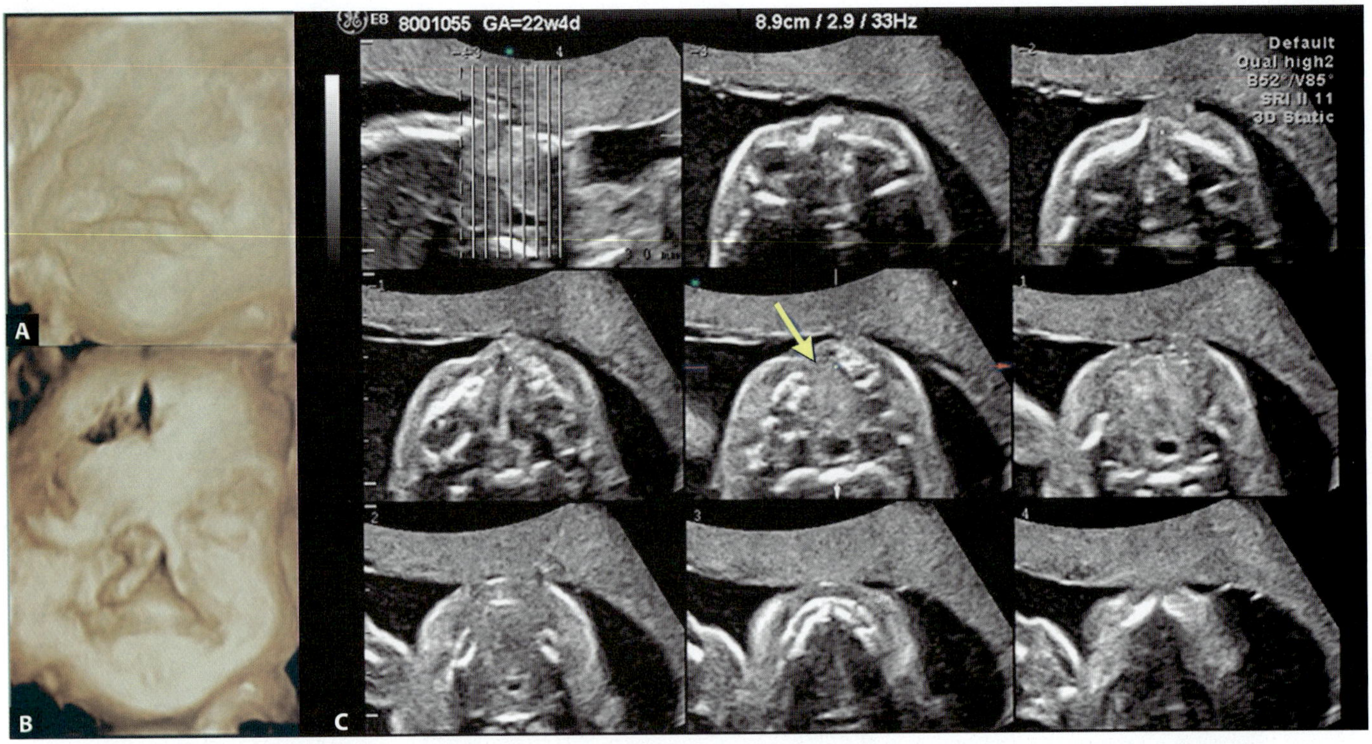

Figs. 10A to C: Cleft lip and palate at 22 weeks: (A) Surface image of the fetal face. Left sided cleft lip and deformed nasal structure is clearly demonstrated. (B) 3D reconstructed image inside the oral cavity. Cleft palate is visualized. (C) Tomographic ultrasound image of the anterior maxillary structure, indicating the evidence of alveolar cleft presence (arrow).

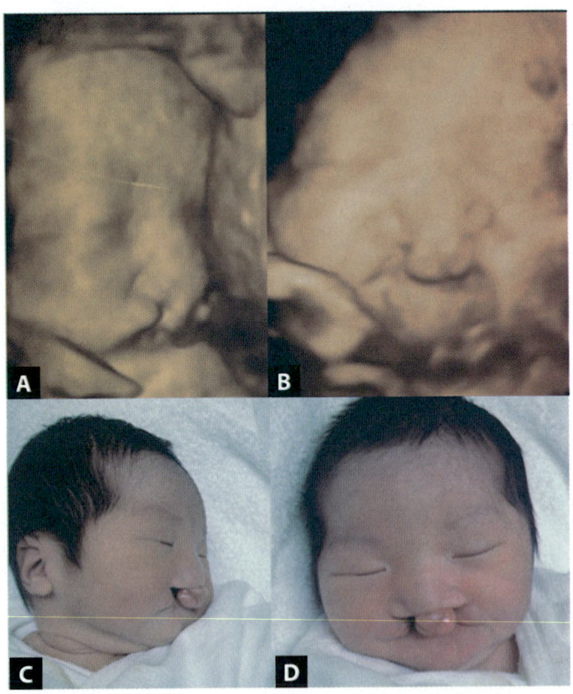

Figs. 11A to C: Bilateral cleft lip at 35 weeks: Bilateral cleft lip is often overlooked because of its symmetrical facial structure. (A and B) 3D ultrasound shows the clear visualization of the bilateral cleft lip. (C) Postnatal facial appearance of the same baby.

to evaluation of fetal brain morphology.[29,30] **Figures 17A to C** shows transvaginal 3D tomographic coronal, sagittal and axial ultrasound views of intracranial structure in a case of ventriculomegaly at 20 weeks of gestation. Thus, accurate assessment of brain pathology can be done by 3D ultrasound. Furthermore, ventricular appearance can be demonstrated comprehensively by inversion mode, as shown in **Figures 18A to C**. Cortical development of fetal brain can also be visualized by 3D surface imaging, demonstrating gyral and sulcal development and migration disorder **(Figs. 19A and B)** which had been difficult to be detected during pregnancy, can be depicted by 3D ultrasound.[31] **Figures 13A and B** demonstrate the asymmetrical cortical development due to migration disorder by 2D ultrasound and 3D surface imaging. The 3D volume contrast imaging demonstrated the cortical development **(Fig. 20)**. Thus, 3D ultrasound surface imaging is useful in objective assessment of brain surface. The cranial bone abnormality, seen in a case of encephalocele, can be also visualized by 3D ultrasound maximum mode imaging as shown in **Figures 21A and B**.

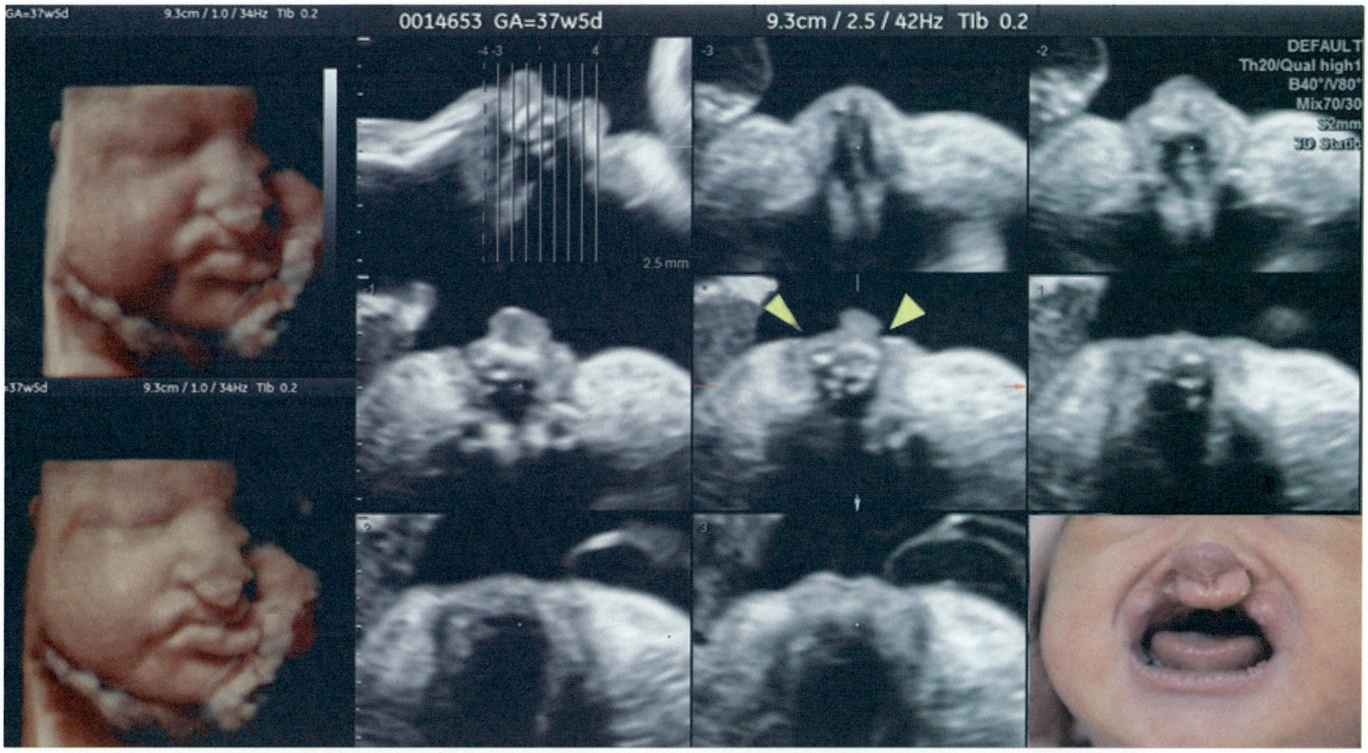

Fig. 12: Bilateral cleft lip/palater at 37 weeks of gestation: Left; HDlive images of fetal face. Cleft is very thin and difficult to be detected by surface rendering mode. Right; TUI of lip, alveolus and palate. By tomographic images, narrow cleft lines are bilaterally visible (arrowheads). Right lower; Neonatal cleft lip.
Courtesy: Dr Shimaoka, Shimaoka Clinic, Kyoto, Japan.

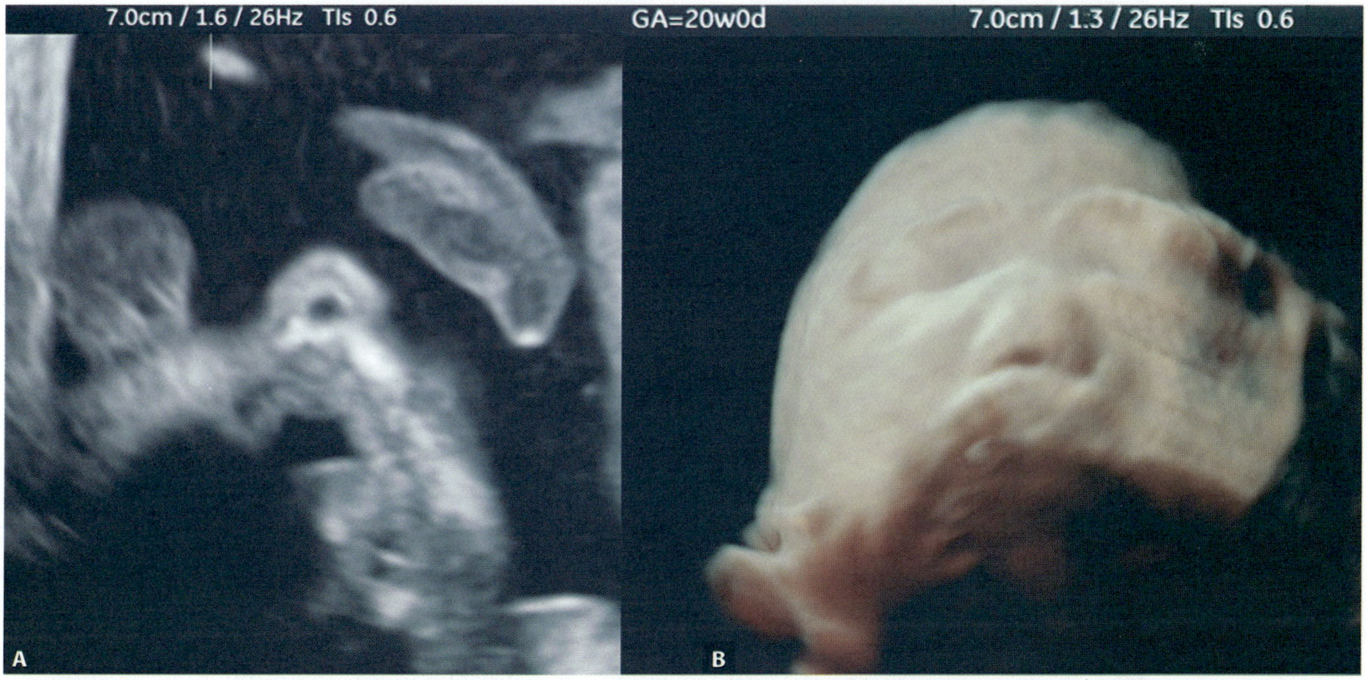

Figs. 13A and B: Single nostril at 20 weeks of gestation in a case of holoprosencephaly: (A) 2D image; (B) 3D HDlive image.

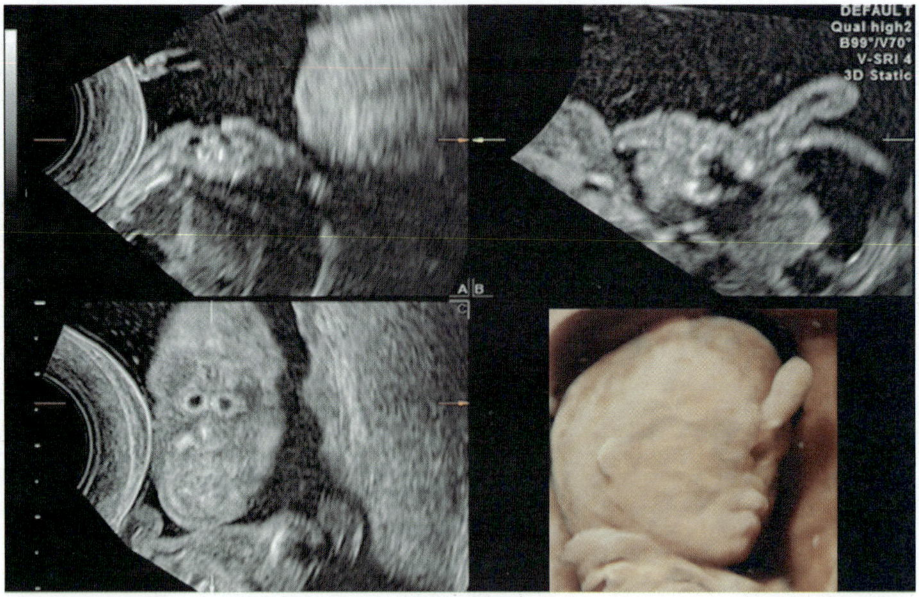

Fig. 14: Two eye lenses seen in a cycloptic eye: Three orthogonal view demonstrates the two eye lenses inside, despite 3D view demonstrates cyclops.

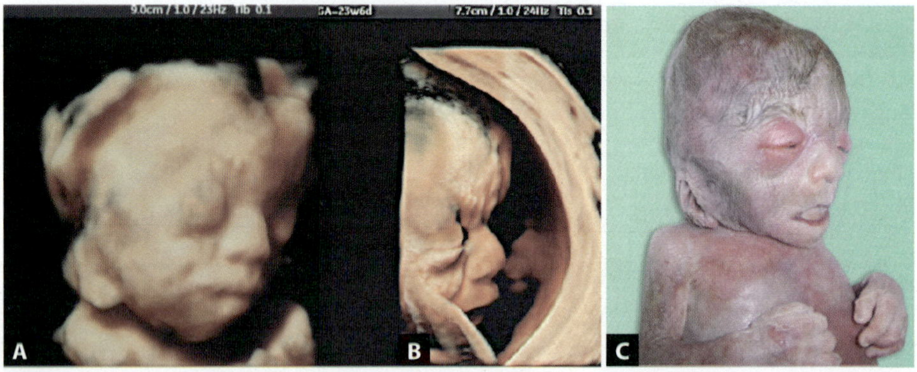

Figs. 15A to C: Exophthalmia, low-set ear and micrognathia at 23 weeks in a case of multiple anomalies: (A and B) HDlive images showing exophthalmia, low-set ear and micrognathia; (C) Stillbirth baby. Normal karyotype and the cause was unknown.

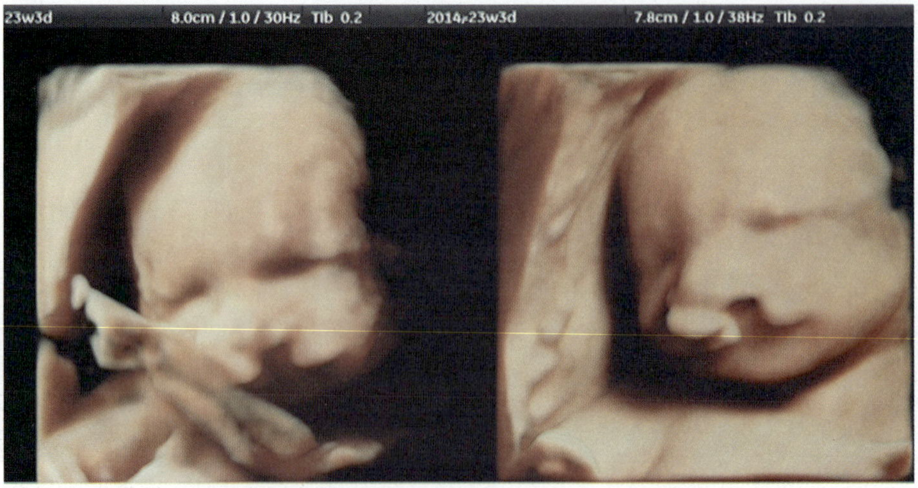

Fig. 16: Microphthalmos and cleft lip seen in a case of trisomy 13.

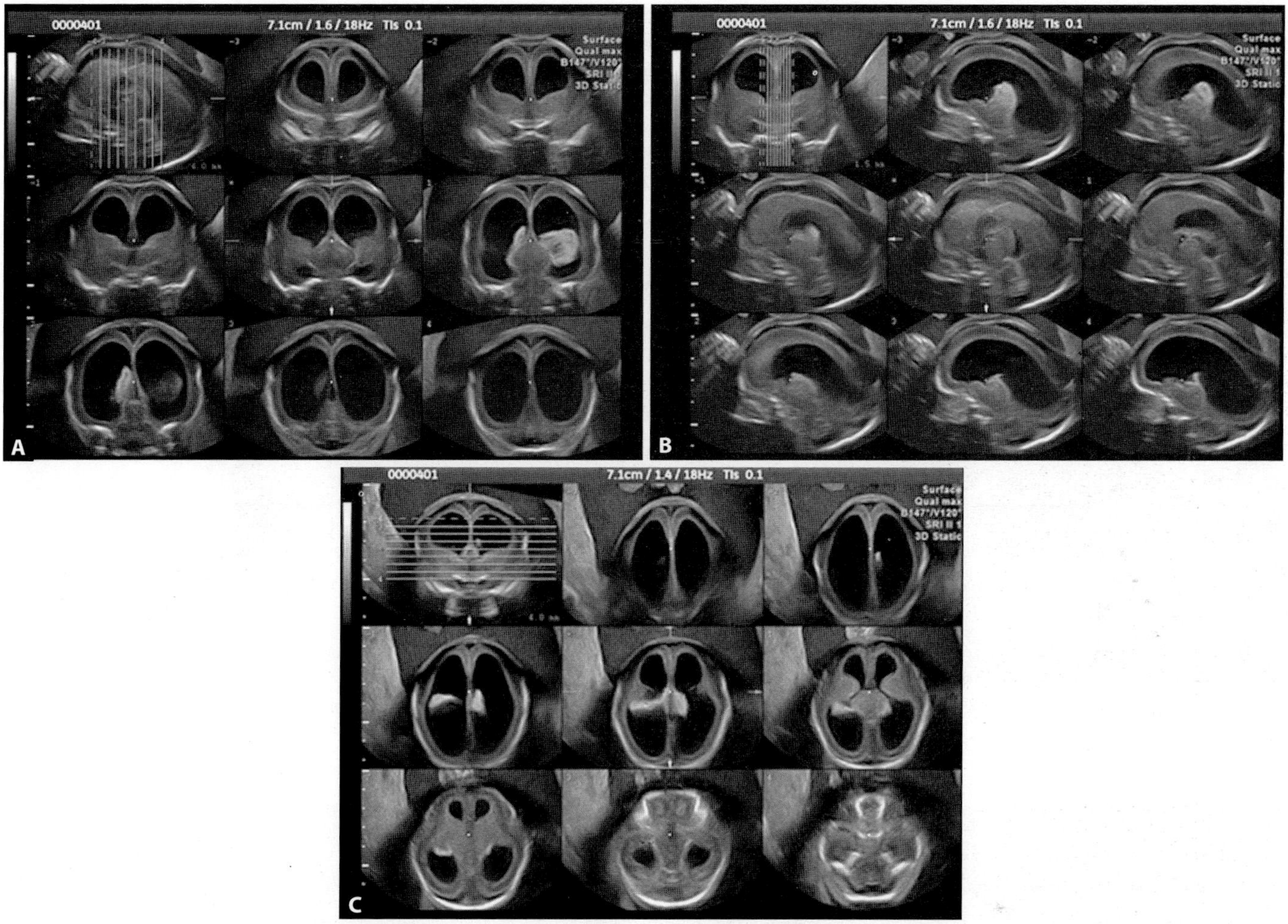

Figs. 17A to C: Hydrocephalus at 20 weeks: Tomographic ultrasound images of coronal (A); sagittal (B); and axial (C) views. Clear visualization of intracranial structure is acquired.

Vertebra and Spinal Cord Abnormalities

Spina bifida is the most common anomaly of the central nervous system. It is often detected during the second and third trimesters. However, the fundamental basis for this anomaly is a failure of the neural tube to close during early embryonic age. Most reports of the diagnosis of spina bifida in utero have occurred after 12 weeks of gestation. Blaas et al.[32] reported an early diagnosis using 2D and 3D ultrasound before 10 weeks of gestation. **Figures 22A and B** demonstrate myelomeningocele at 20 weeks. The vertebral bony structure can be depicted by 3D ultrasound for better understanding the level of spina bifida. Vertebral scoliosis is often seen in cases of limb body wall complex **(Fig. 23)** or cases of hemivertebra as shown in **Figures 24 and 25**. In hemivertebral cases, asymmetrical rib number can be also demonstrated. **Figures 26A to C** show the segmental spinal dysgenesis, characterized by focal agenesis or dysgenesis of the lumbar or thoracolumbar spine, with focal abnormality of the underlying spinal cord and nerve roots.[33]

Abdominal Abnormalities

Ventral body wall defects comprise a group of congenital malformations that includes omphalocele **(Figs. 27 and 28)** and gastroschisis **(Figs. 29A to D)**, which are relatively common. Fetal ascites **(Figs. 30 and 31)** is an uncommon abnormality usually in relation to chromosomal abnormality, intrauterine infections, gastrointestinal processes, genitourinary tract abnormalities, or idiopathic causes.

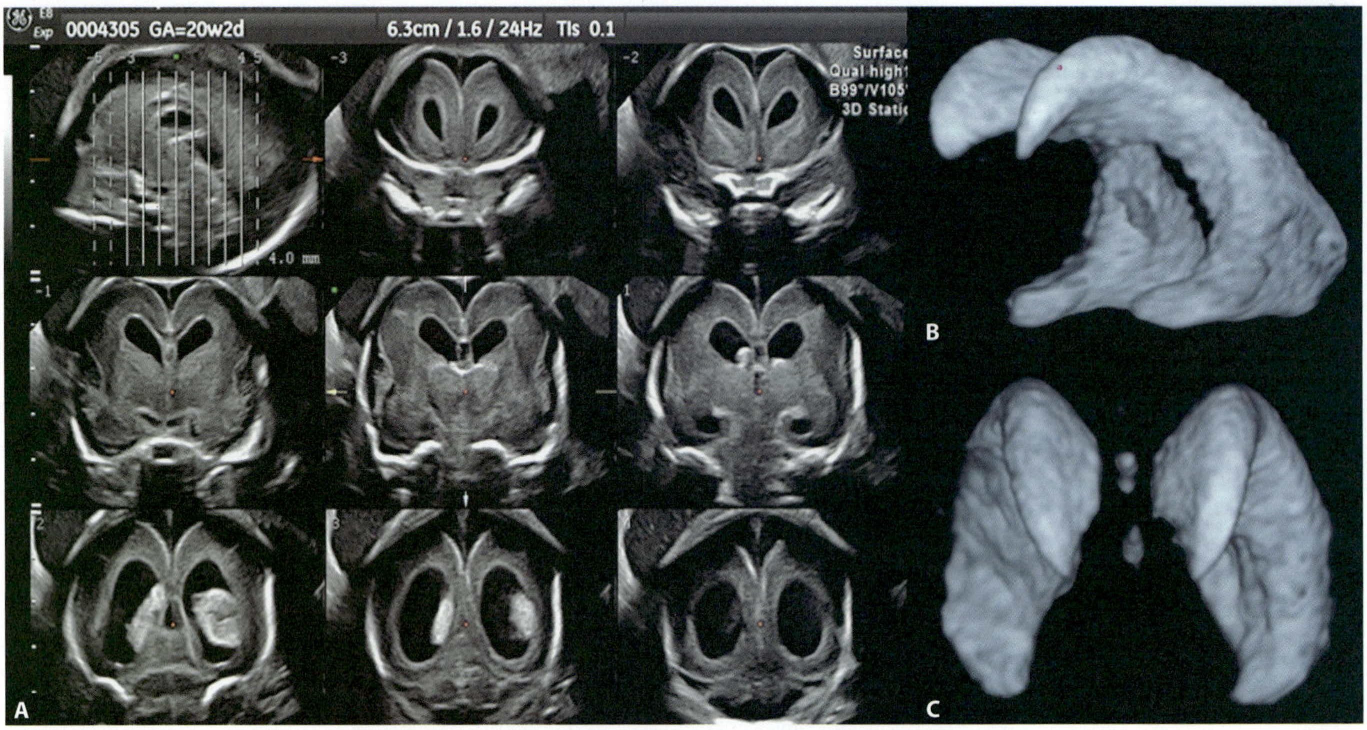

Figs. 18A to C: Ventriculomegaly at 20 weeks: (A) Tomographic ultrasound image of coronal section; (B and C) Demonstrate lateral ventricular appearance by using 3D inversion mode.

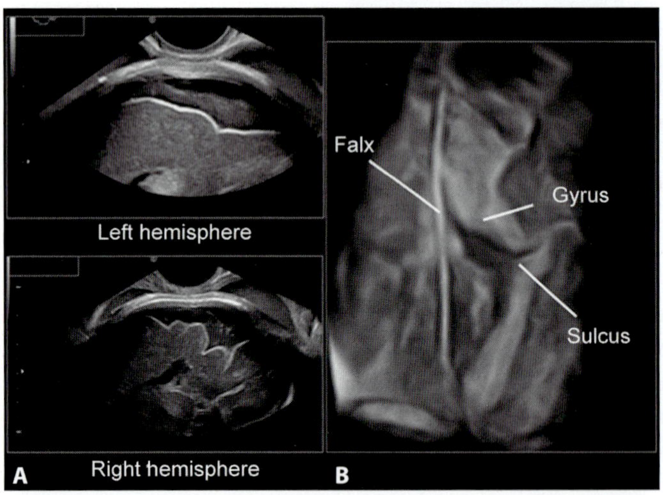

Figs. 19A and B: Asymmetrical cortical formation at 29 weeks: Note the marked difference between left and right cortical appearance (A); (B) Demonstrated asymmetrical superficial image of the brain. Clear visualization of the brain surface with asymmetrical gyral/sulcal formation is acquired.

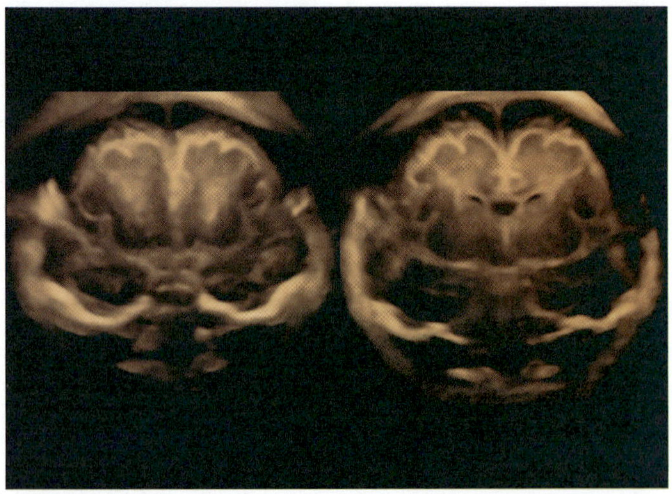

Fig. 20: Hydrocephalus ex-vacuo at 30 weeks: 3D volume contrast images demonstrate the cortical development. Note the abnormal large subarachnoid space around the hemispheres.

Chest-abdominal Abnormalities

Differentiation of congenital diaphragmatic hernia (CDH), congenital cystic adenomatoid malformation (CCAM) and diaphragmatic eventration are important. **Figures 32A to C** is schematic pictures of those chest abnormalities.

Congenital diaphragmatic hernia (CDH) occurs in 1 of every 2,000–4,000 live births and accounts for 8% of all major congenital anomalies.[34] There are three types of CDH; posterolateral or Bochdalek hernia (occurring at approximately 6 weeks' gestation), the anterior Morgagni hernia, and a hiatus hernia. The left-sided Bochdalek hernia occurs in approximately 90% of cases. Left-sided hernias allow herniation of both small and large bowel as well as intra-abdominal solid organs into the thoracic cavity. Early diagnosis of CDH in the first trimester has been reported.[35] **Figure 33** demonstrates 3D image of CDH liver-up type at 15 weeks and **Figure 34** shows the tomographic ultrasound imaging of Bochdalek hernia at 16 weeks. Early diagnosis of this defect is important for the option of fetal treatment. Congenital cystic adenomatoid malformation (CCAM), **(Figs. 35A and B)** is a benign mass of abnormal lung tissue, located usually on one section of the lung. This condition is caused by overgrowth of abnormal lung tissue that may form fluid-filled cysts and has no function of normal lung tissue. Early diagnosis of CCAM by 3D ultrasound was reported.[36] Pleural effusion and ascites **(Fig. 36)** can be easy diagnosed by both 2D/3D ultrasound technologies. In cases of pleural effusion, the lung is floated inside the fluid, whereas in cases of pericardiac effusion, the lungs are oppessed to porsterior portion of the chest **(Figs. 37A to C)**.

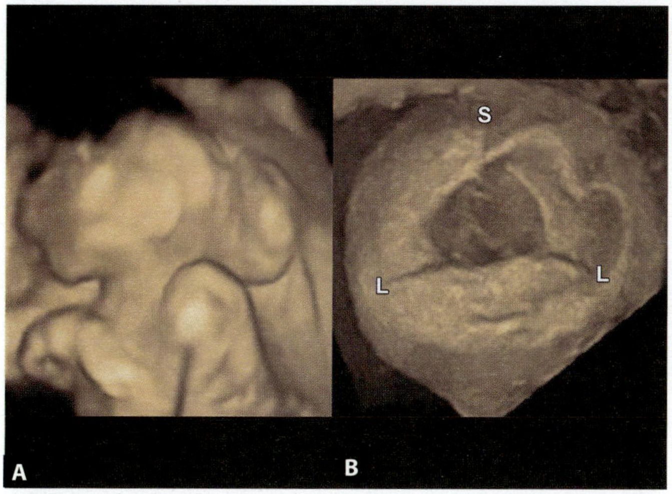

Figs. 21A and B: Encephalocele at 19 weeks: (A) 3D reconstructed lateral image of the fetus. Microcephaly with encephalocele is clearly demonstrated; (B) The posteroanterior view of the cranial bones. The round shaped bony defect is demonstrated. (S: sagittal suture; L: lambdoid suture).

Renal and Urinary Abnormalities

Hydronephrosis **(Fig. 38)** occasionally occurs during pregnancy. The causes are vary, obstruction or stenosis of ureters, posterior urethral valves **(Figs. 39 and 40)** or others. The horseshoe kidney is the most common type of renal fusion anomaly. It consists of two distinct functioning kidneys on each side of the midline, connected at the lower poles by an isthmus of functioning renal parenchyma or fibrous tissue that crosses the midline of the body. **Figures 41 and 42** demonstrate horseshoe kidney by 2D and 3D ultrasound. Multicystic dysplastic kidney (MCDK, **Figs. 43 and 44**) is a form of renal dysplasia characterized by the presence of multiple cysts of varying size in the

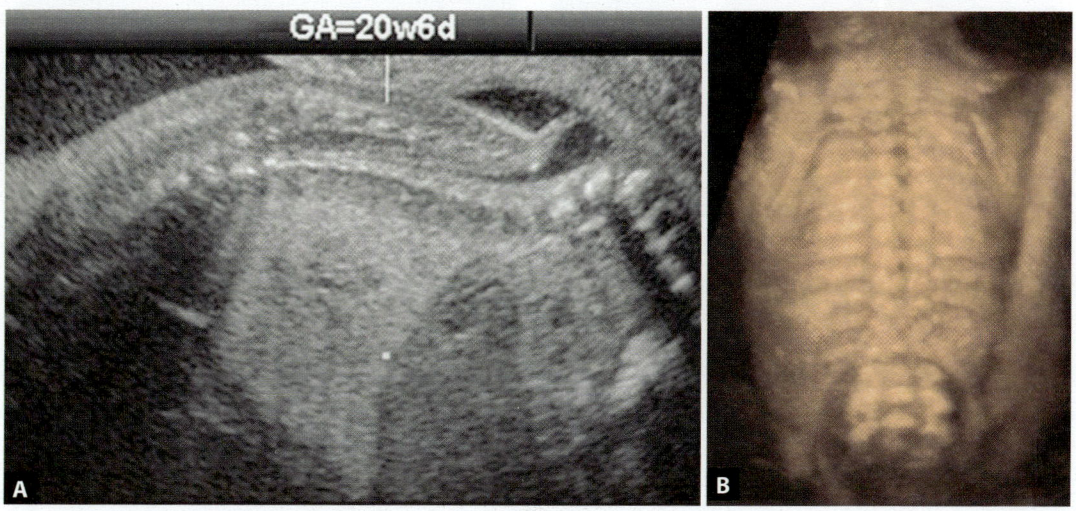

Figs. 22A and B: Myelomeningocele with kyphosis at 20 weeks: (A) Sagittal image of the fetal trunks from 3D orthogonal view. Severe kyphosis and myelomeningocele is seen; (B) 3D reconstructed image of the fetal back. The huge mass is seen from L1 to S region. The ribs are clearly seen and the level of spina bifida is easily understandable.

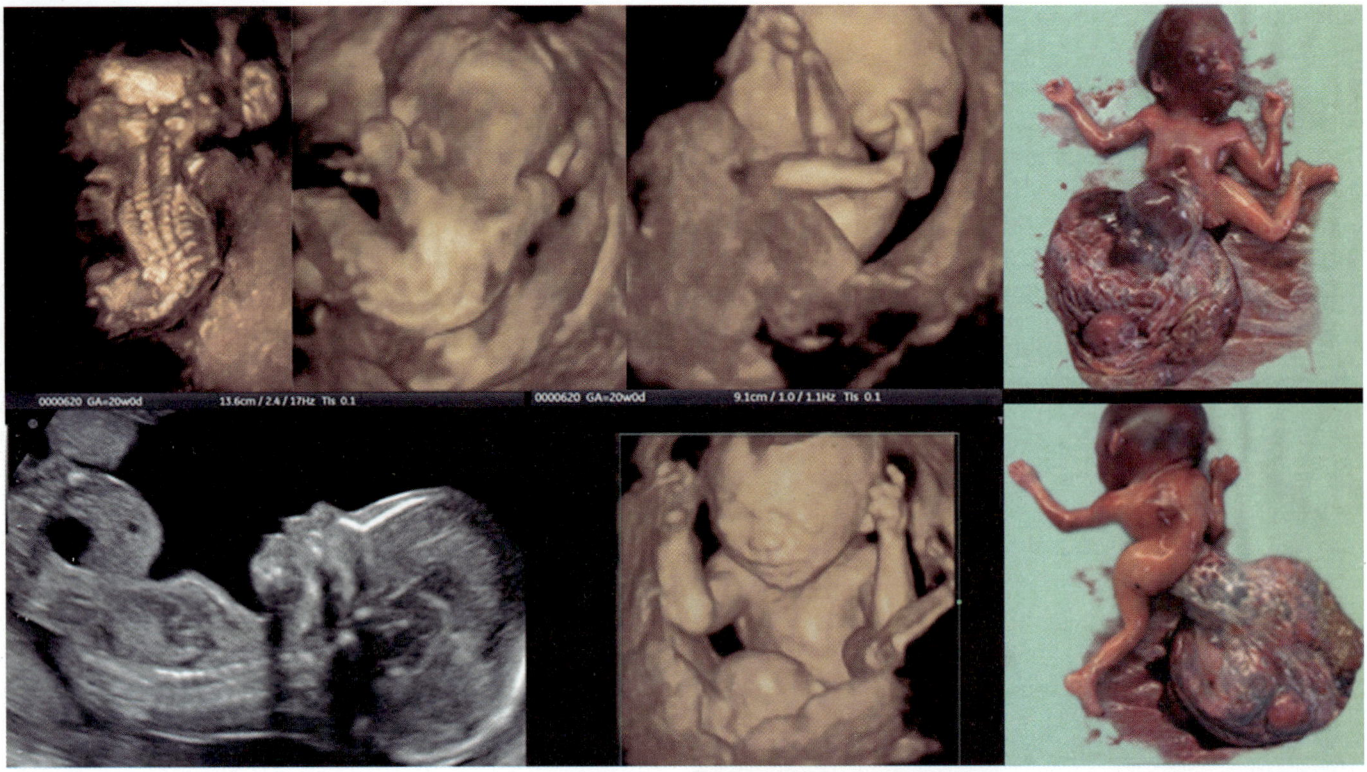

Fig. 23: Vertebral scoliosis associated with limb body wall complex at 20 weeks: Severe vertebral scoliosis, abnormal leg position with one leg missing, Umbilical hernia with short umbilical cord are clearly demonstrated by 2D/3D ultrasound. Right two Figures show the appearance of the aborted fetus.

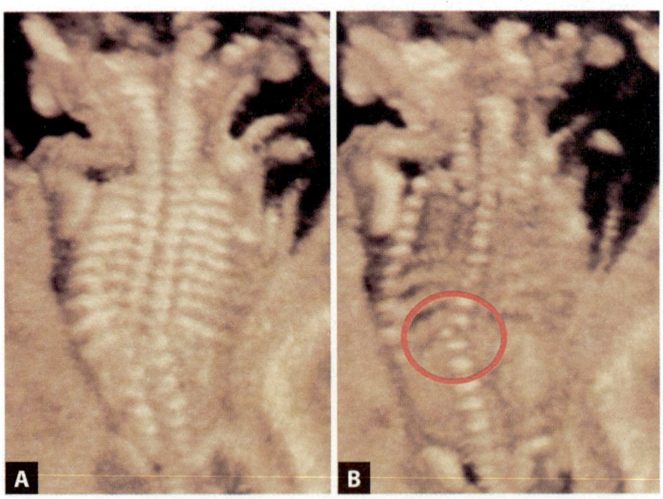

Figs. 24A and B: Hemivertebra at 19 weeks: (A) 3D maximum mode image of the fetal back. Scoliosis with asymmetrical number of ribs (left; 11 ribs, right; 10 ribs) is clearly demonstrated; (B) 3D image of the vertebral body layer reveals Th12 hemivertebra (red circle) and this hemivertebra should be the cause of scoliosis.

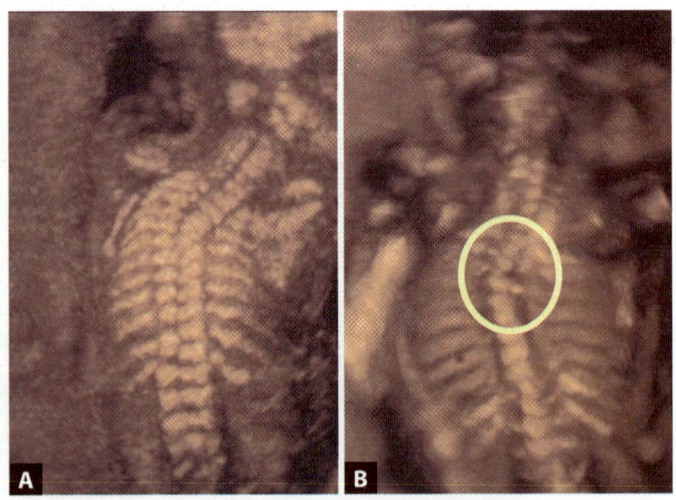

Figs. 25A and B: Three levels hemivertebra at 20 weeks: (A) 3D maximum mode image of the fetal back. Severe scoliosis with asymmetrical number of ribs (left; 12 ribs, right; 9 ribs) is clearly demonstrated; (B) 3D image of the vertebral body layer reveals three levels hemivertebrae (Th1-Th3, yellow circle).

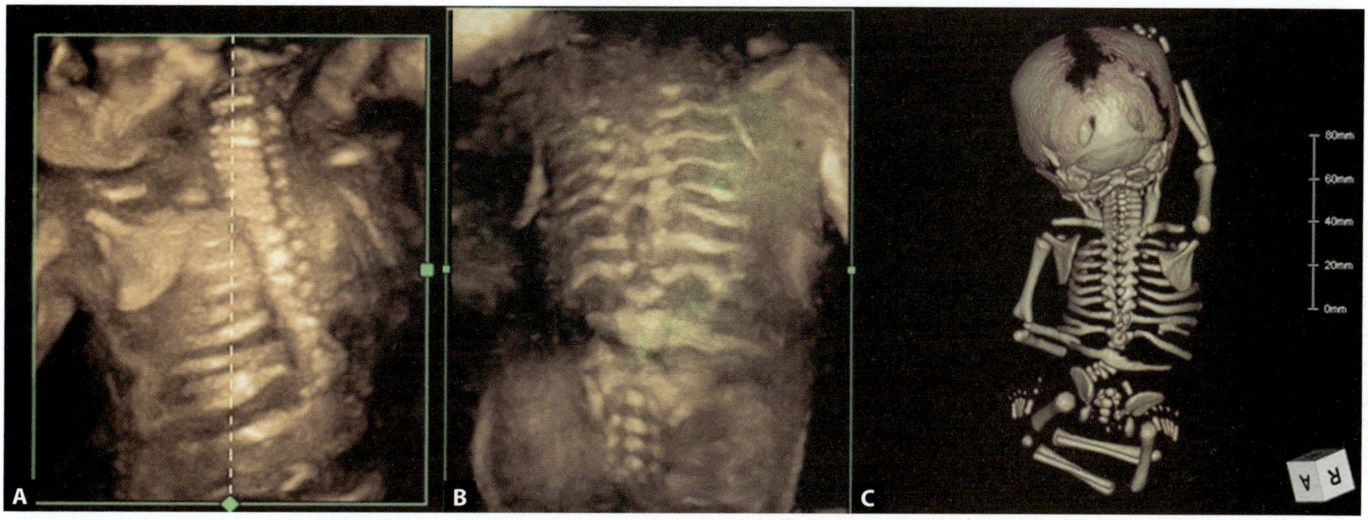

Figs. 26A to C: Segmental spinal dysgenesis at 27 weeks (3D ultrasound and 3D-CT images): (A and B) 3D US reconstructed images. Note the focal dysgenesis of the thoracolumbar vertebra, with rib abnormality which indicates features of segmental spinal dysgenesis; (C) 3D-CT scan image of the same fetus. Clear visualization of the bony structure is acquired.

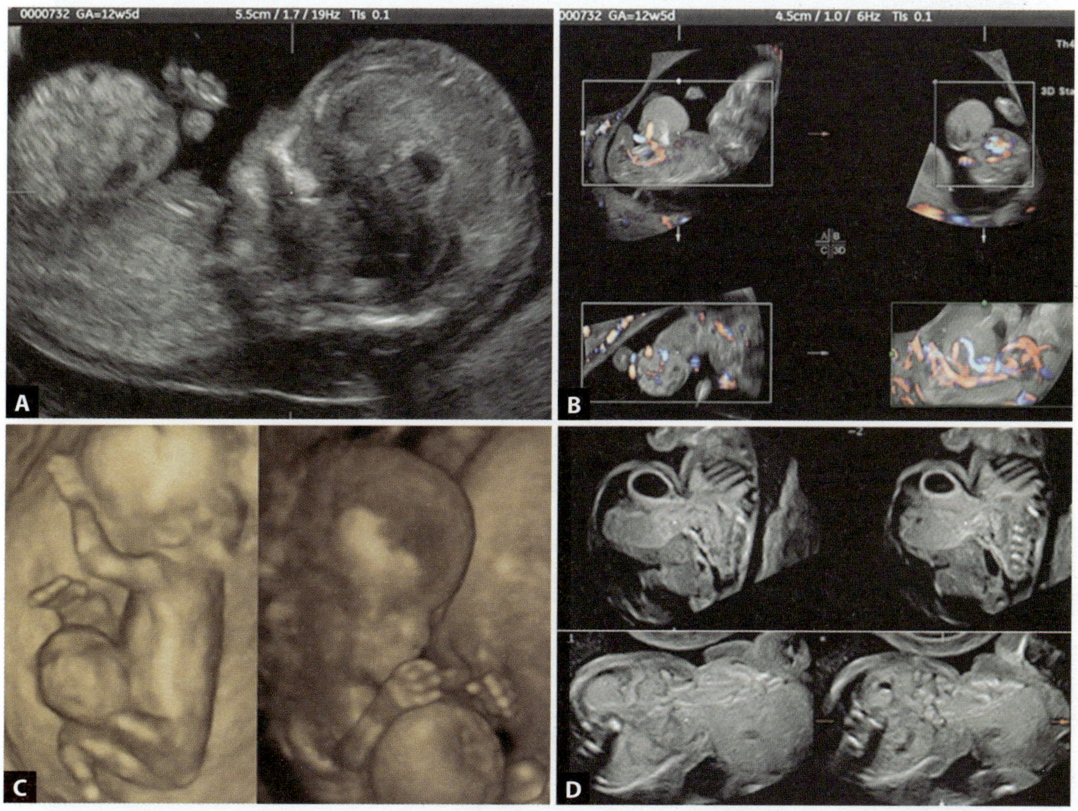

Figs. 27A to D: Huge omphalocele at 12 weeks: (A) Sagittal image from 3D orthogonal view. Increased nuchal translucency is seen; (B) Three orthogonal view and reconstructed image of the fetal circulation. Because of the ectopic liver, the umbilical vein and ductus venosus run outside the body toward the heart inside the body. The ductus venosus reversed flow was seen in this case; (C) 3D reconstructed images; (D) Four selected images from tomographic ultrasound images, demonstrating the relation of ectopic organs and inside organ. After confirming normal chromosome and no other associated anomalies were confirmed, parents decide to continue pregnancy. Postnatal surgery was successful and postoperative course has been favorable.

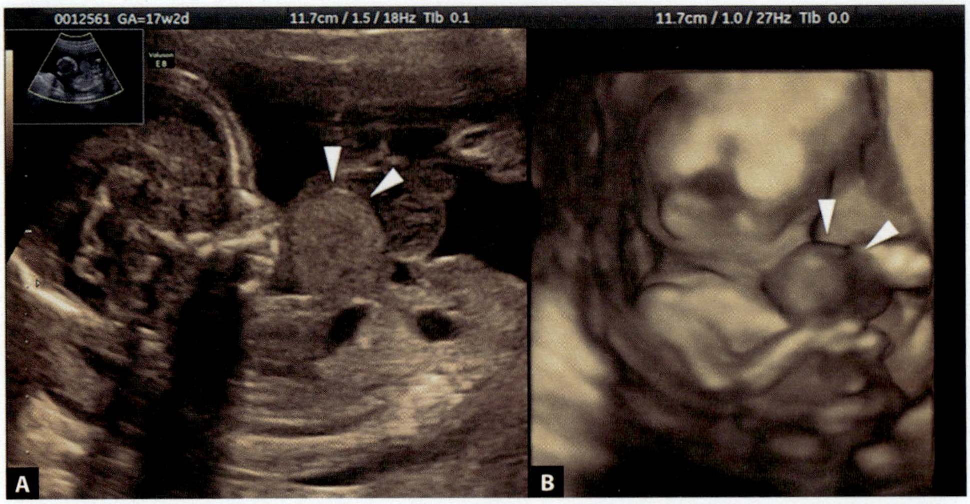

Figs. 28A and B: Omphalocele at 17 weeks: (A) 2D sagittal image. Liver is ectopic (arrowheads); (B) 3D image.

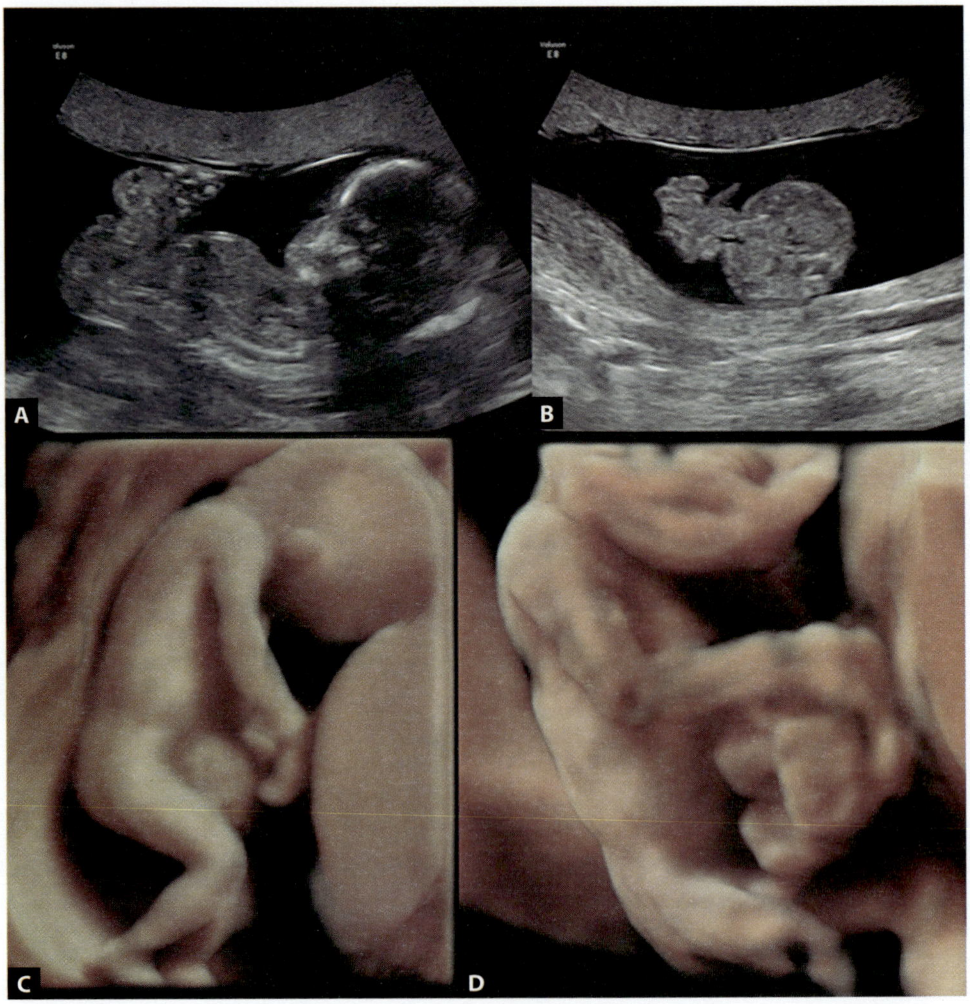

Figs. 29A to D: Gastroschisis at 17 weeks of gestation: (A and B) 2D sagittal and axial images; (C and D) 3D images. Information from A and C, it is difficult to differentiate from umbilical hernia. However, it is easy to diagnose gastroschisis from B and D.

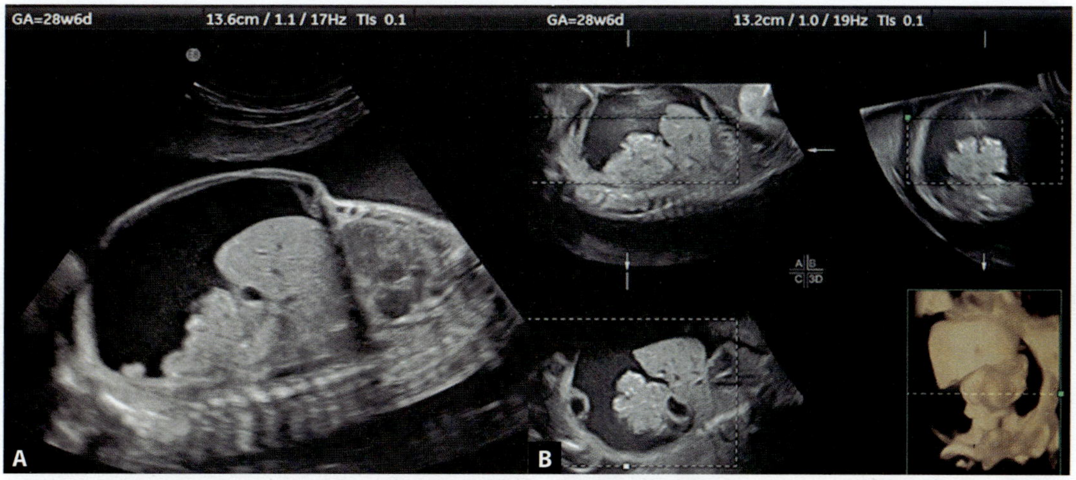

Figs. 30A and B: Severe ascites at 28 weeks: (A) 2D sagittal image demonstrates large amount of ascites; (B) Three orthogonal view with 3D reconstructed image.

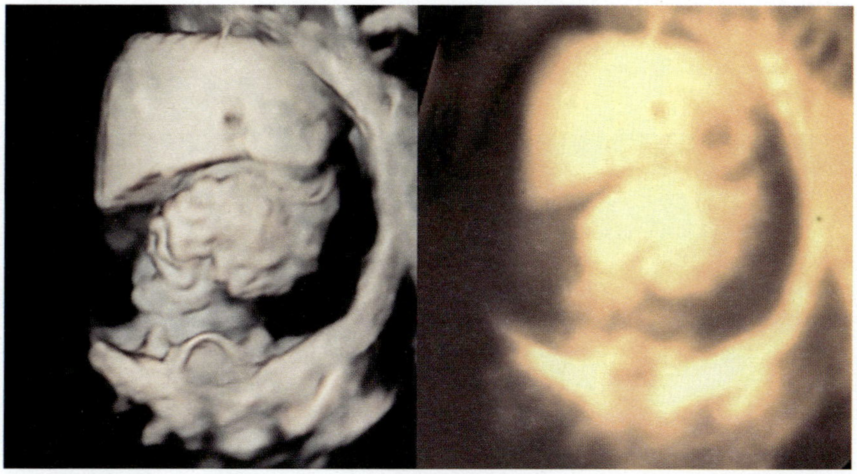

Fig. 31: 3D images of Intra-abdominal organs in a case with severe ascites. Liver, bowels and bladder are demonstrated.

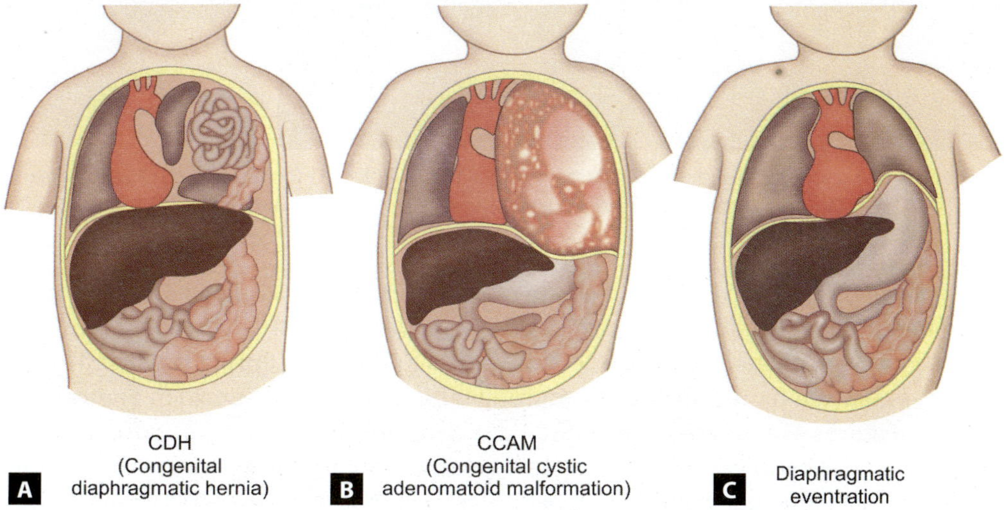

Figs. 32A to C: Schematic pictures of difference among: (A) Congenital diaphragmatic hernia (CDH); (B) Congenital cystic adenomatoid malformation (CCAM); (C) Diaphragmatic eventration.

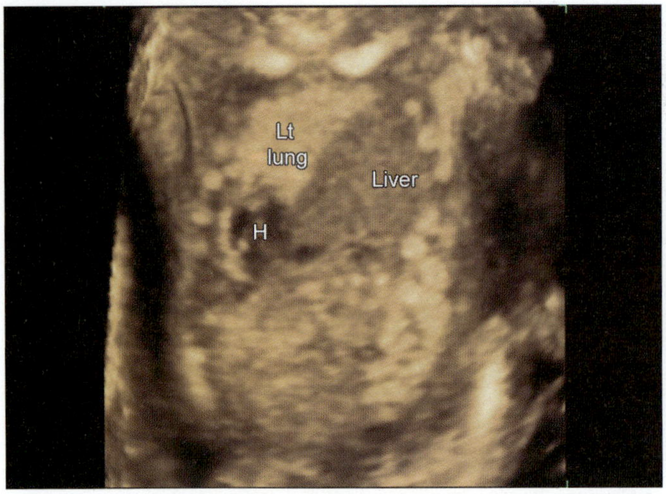

Fig. 33: Congenital diaphragmatic hernia at 15 weeks of gestation. 3D coronal image. Because of huge defect of left side of diaphragm, liver goes up into the chest and the heart (H) and left lung are oppressed to the right side.

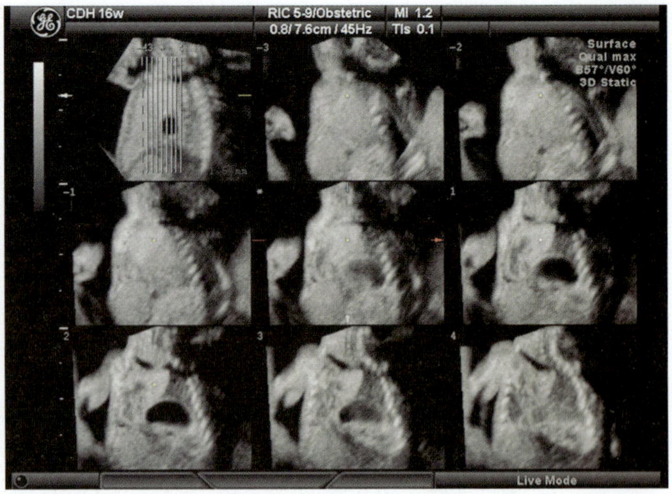

Fig. 34: Congenital diaphragmatic hernia at 16 weeks. Tomographic ultrasound image. Typical Bochdalec hernia is seen. Tomographic image clearly shows oppressed and hypoplastic left lung, heart replacement to the right, and the stomach inside thoracic space.

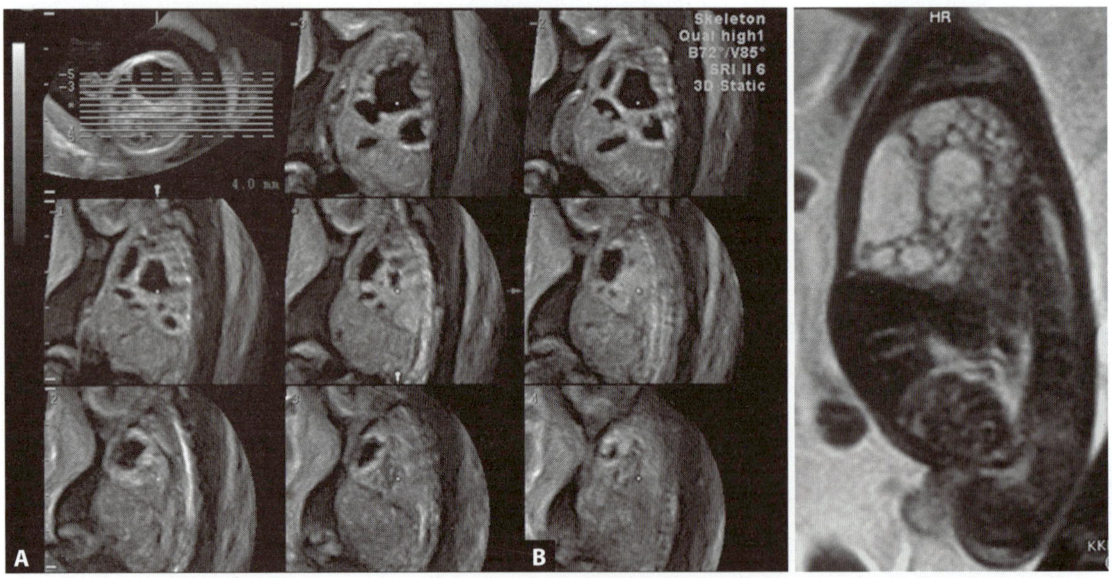

Figs. 35A and B: Congenital cystic adenomatoid malformation (CCAM) at 24 weeks. (A) Tomographic ultrasound sagittal image of fetal chest. Multiple cysts with different size are seen; (B) MR image of the same fetus.

kidney and the absence of a normal pelvocaliceal system. Unilateral MCDK is benign and usually no decreased amniotic fluid is seen. However, bilateral MCDK is lethal anomaly, which causes significant reduction of urine and severe oligohydramnios. **Figures 45A and B** demonstrates development of renal multicysts between 15 and 18 weeks of gestation. Thus, in the early pregnancy, cysts are not conspicuous but during the early second trimester, cysts are increasing in size. Fetal MCDK occasionally decreased its size during pregnancy and it is reported that MCDK size tends to decrease during the first 30 postnatal months.[37] Bladder extrophy as shown in **Figures 46A and B** is rarely seen by ultrasound. A vesico-allantoic cyst is a single communicating cavity consisting of an umbilical cord cyst and the fetal urinary bladder.[38,39] The communication between the allantois and urachus usually closed during

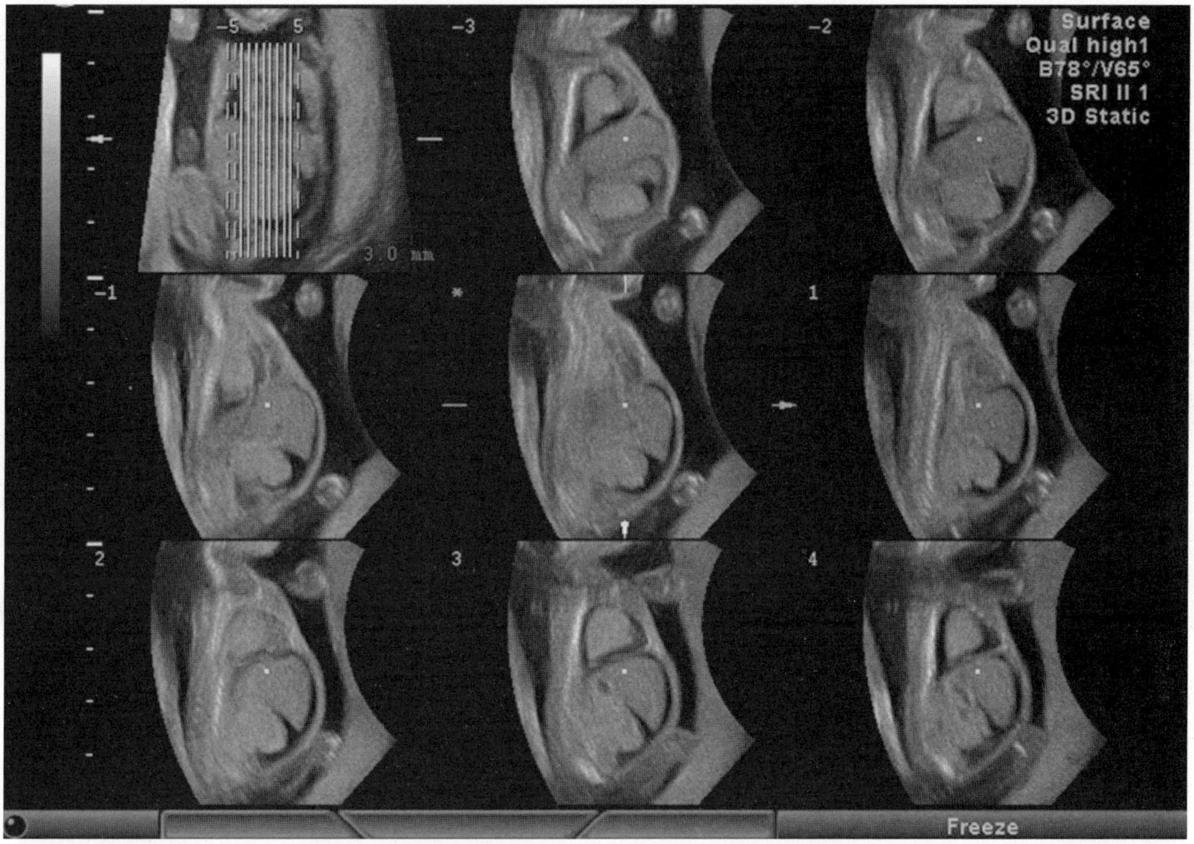

Fig. 36: Pleural effusion and ascites at 19 weeks. Tomographic ultrasound sagittal image of the fetal trunk. Fluid collection in both chest and abdomen are clearly demonstrated.

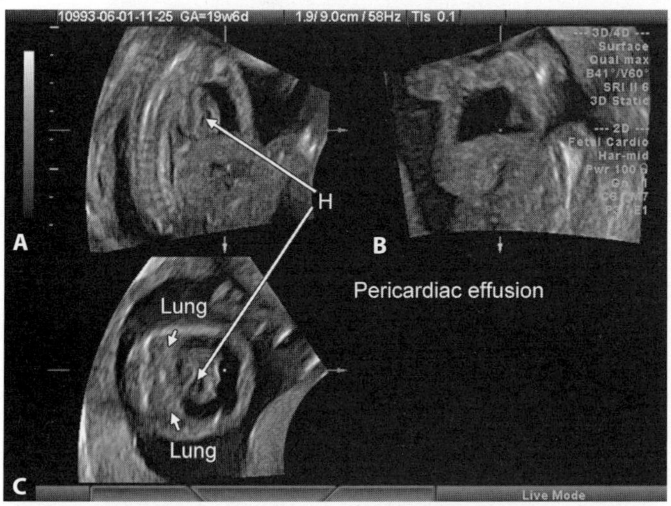

Figs. 37A to C: Pericardiac effusion at 19 weeks. Three orthogonal view of the fetal chest. Due to fluid collection inside epicardium, the lungs are oppressed to posterior potion of the chest. Three orthogonal view (A and C) and 3D reconstructed inverted image of the renal pelvis (B).

the early stage of gestation and when this communication fails to disappear, the fetal urinary bladder, urachus and allantois form a single communicating cavity filled with fetal urine. **Figures 47 and 48** show the vesico-allantoic cyst at 16 and 17 weeks of gestation. Bilateral umbilical arteries along with bladder wall and allantoic cyst proves a single communicating cavity **(Figs. 47A and B)**. Occasionally, the dynamic change of the urachus and the bladder and cyst size change are seen **(Fig. 48)** because of outflow of urine from bladder to the cyst. Maldeveloped external genitalia as shown in **Figures 49A and B** is rarely seen in cases with various anomalies or as a single finding.

Limb Abnormalities and Skeletal Dysplasia

Limb abnormalities can occur as isolated findings or as one component of a syndrome or sequence. However, only 5% of congenital hand anomalies occur as part of a recognized syndrome. **Figures 50A to D** show typical appearance of triploidy with thin limbs and no other abnormalities.

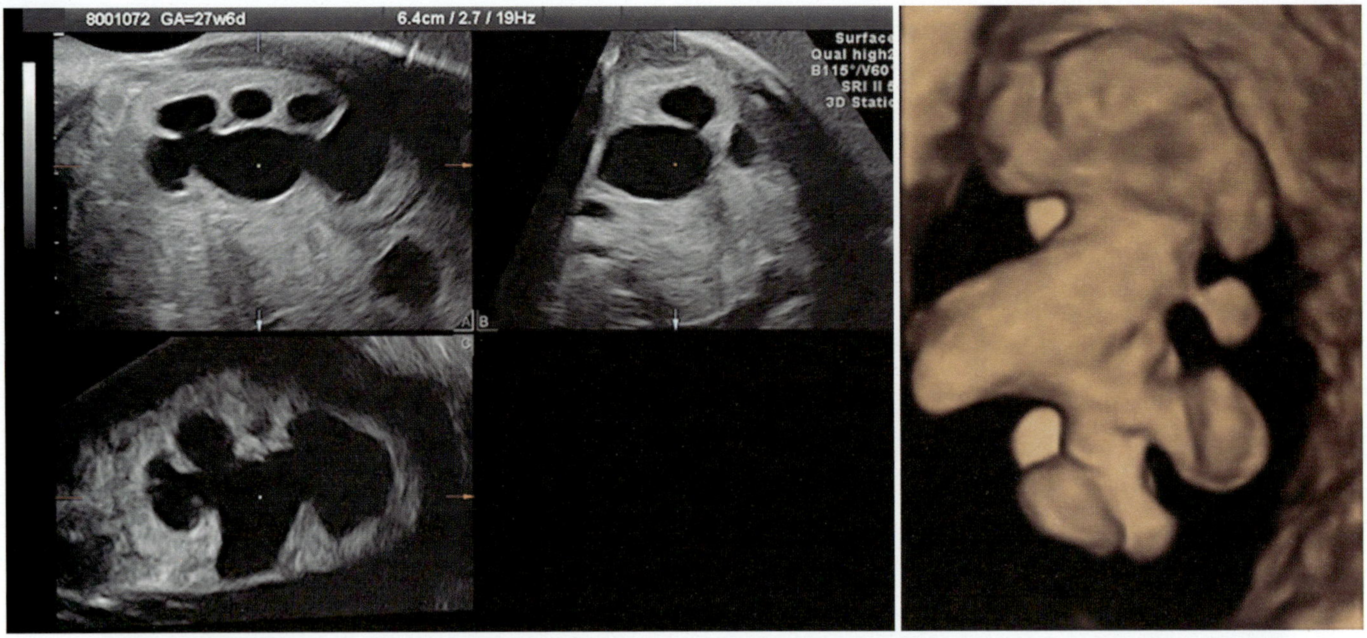

Fig. 38: Mild hydronephrosis at 27 weeks.

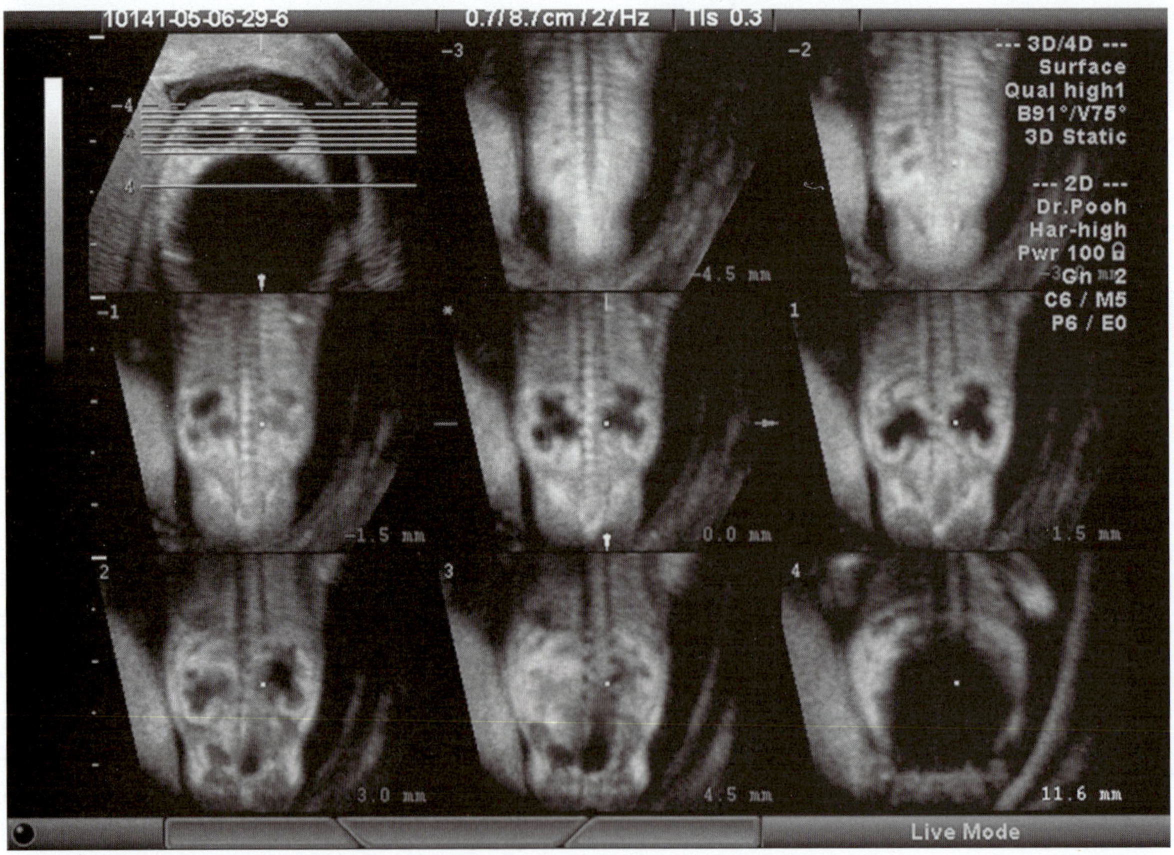

Fig. 39: Bilateral hydronephrosis due to posterior urethral valve stenosis at 15 weeks. Tomographic ultrasound coronal image of the bilateral kidneys. Bilateral hydronephrosis with huge bladder occurred due to poterior urethral valve stenosis. Vesicoamniotic shunt at 17 weeks was successfully performed in this case and postnatal course was favorable.

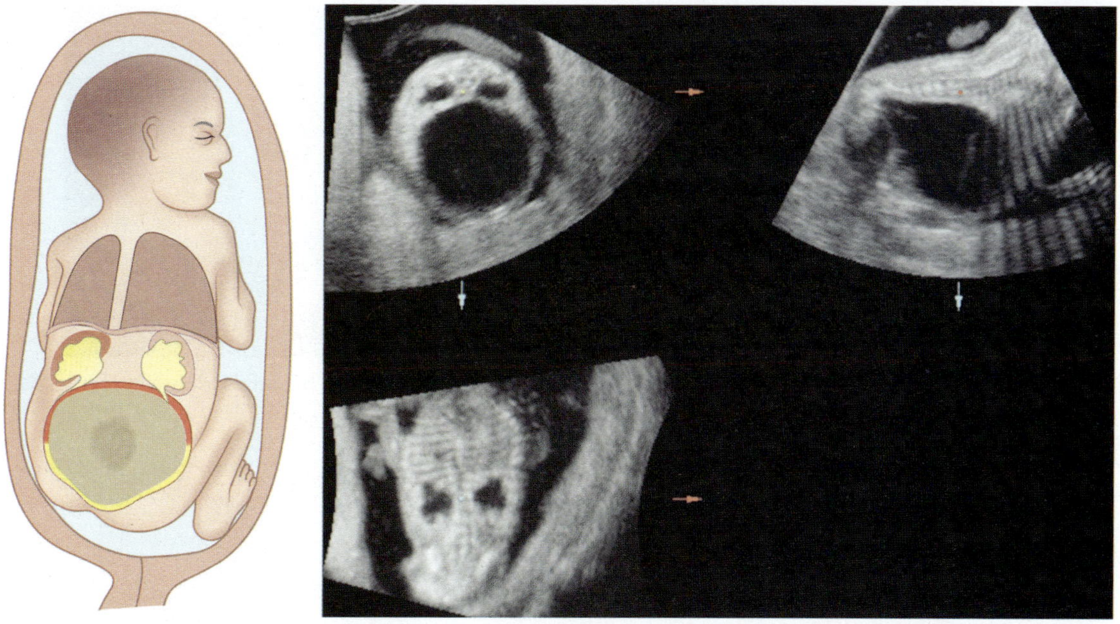

Fig. 40: Megacystis and hydronephrosis due to urethral obstruction at 14 weeks. Multiplanar image. Bilateral hydronephrosis and enlarged bladder is demonstrated.

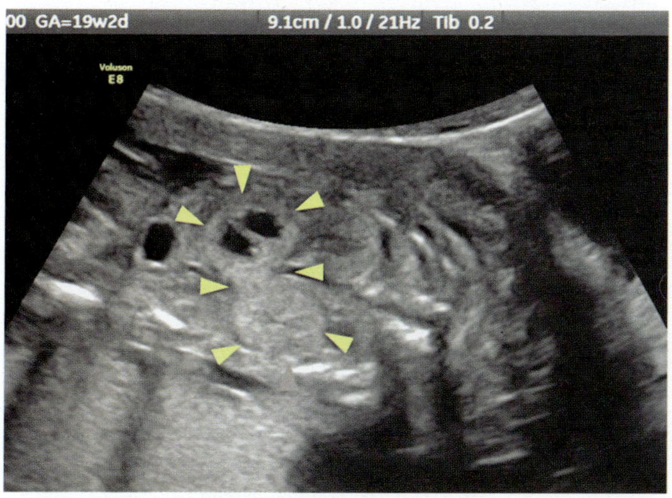

Fig. 41: Horseshoe kidney at 19 weeks. 2D coronal image showing fused bilateral kidneys (arrowheads).

Figure 51 demonstrates 3D ultrasound images and postmortum pictures in a case of lethal pterygium syndrome. Pterygiem is used to describe webbing of the skin across the joint. The term means "wing-like". Limb pterygia at birth indicates an abnormal developmental process probably occurring in the first trimester and involving reduced mobility of the webbed limb. Prenatal diagnosis in the first trimester was reported.[40]

Figures 52A to C show unilateral forearm and thumb abnormality with no other abnormalities in a case of partial chromosomal abnormality.

Genetic disorders involving the skeletal system arise through disturbances in the complex processes of skeletal development, growth and homeostasis and remain a diagnostic challenge because of their variety. The Nosology and Classification of Genetic Skeletal Disorders provides an overview of recognized diagnostic entities and groups them by clinical and radiographic features and molecular pathogenesis. Four hundred fifty-six different conditions were included and placed in 40 groups defined by molecular, biochemical and/or radiographic criteria.[41] **Figure 53** demonstrates two cases of thanatophoric dysplasia (FGFR3 chondrodysplasia) at 19–20 weeks. **Figure 54** shows prenatal diagnosis of severe type of collagenopathy at 20 weeks and **Figures 55 and 56** demonstrate fatal dysplasia of osteogenesis imperfecta at 16 and 20 weeks by ultrasound and 3D-CT.

Clubfoot **(Figs. 57 and 58)** is seen bilaterally or unilaterally, as a single finding or as an association with spina bifida or other congenital abnormalities. **Figure 59** shows rare finding of edematous foot. 3D ultrasound can demonstrate finger/toe abnormality in detail. Overlapping fingers **(Fig. 60)**, polydactyly **(Figs. 61 to 63)**, syndactyly **(Figs. 64 and 36.65)**, clinodactyly **(Fig. 66)**,

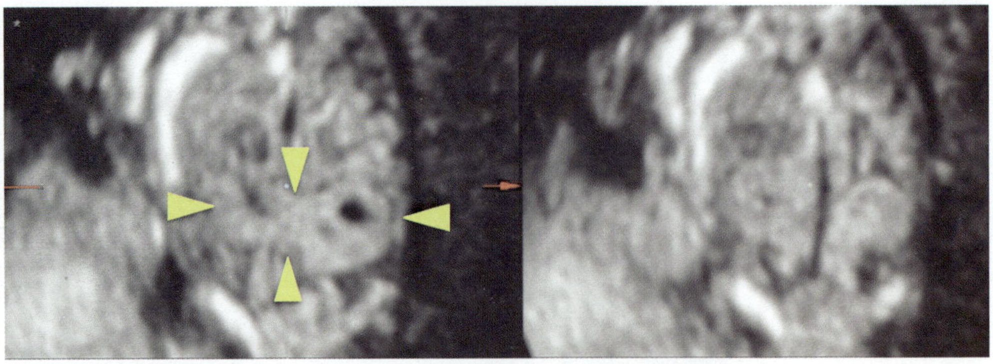

Fig. 42: Horseshoe kidney at 19 weeks. 3D VCI-TUI coronal image shows fused bilateral kidneys (arrowheads).

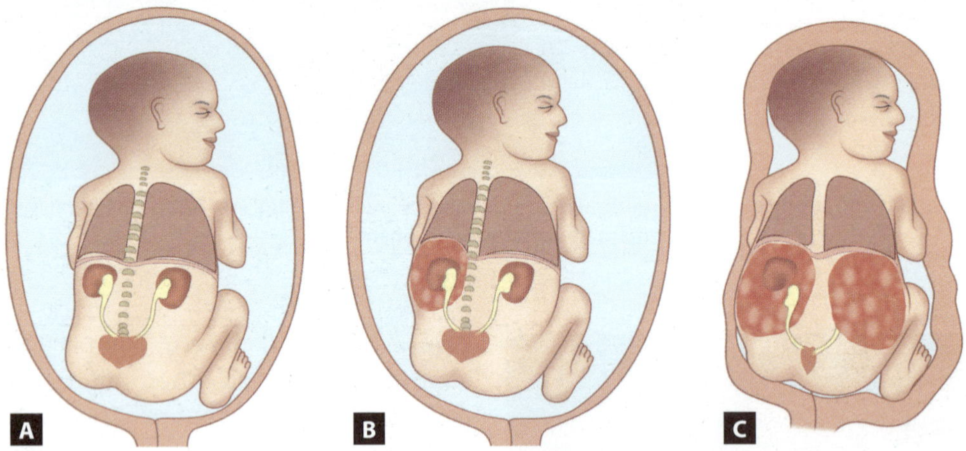

Figs. 43A to C: Schematic picture of normal urinary tract and multicystic kidney. (A) Normal kidneys, ureters and bladder; (B) Unilateral multicystic kidney. The amniotic fluid quantity is normal; (C) Bilateral multicystic kidneys with severe oligohydramnios.

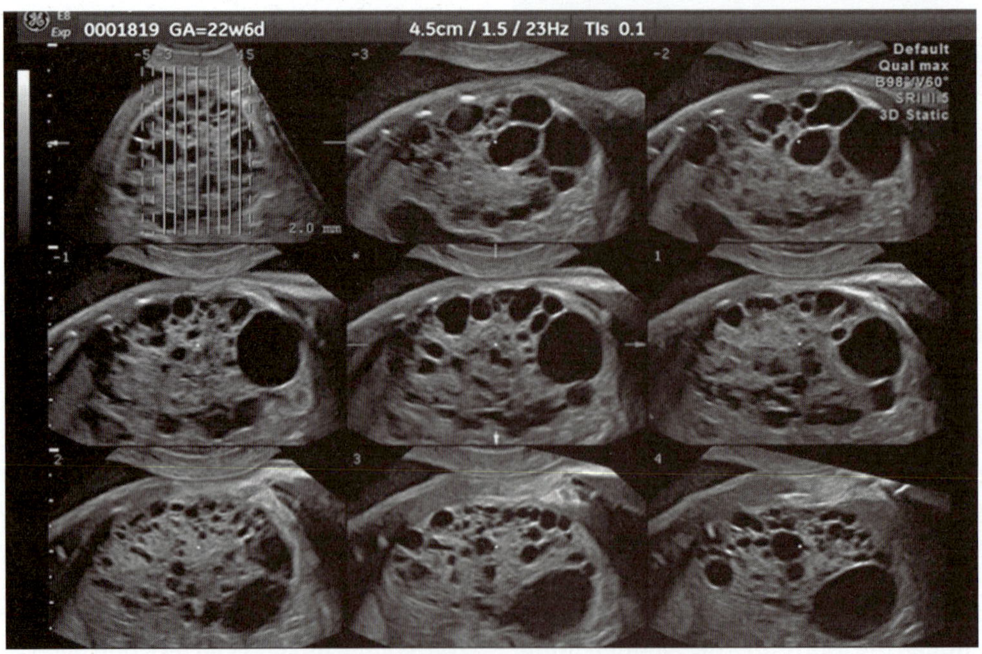

Fig. 44: Multicystic dysplastic kidney (MCDK) at 22 weeks. Tomographic ultrasound image of unilateral MCDK. Note the numerous intrarenal cysts in different size are demonstrated.

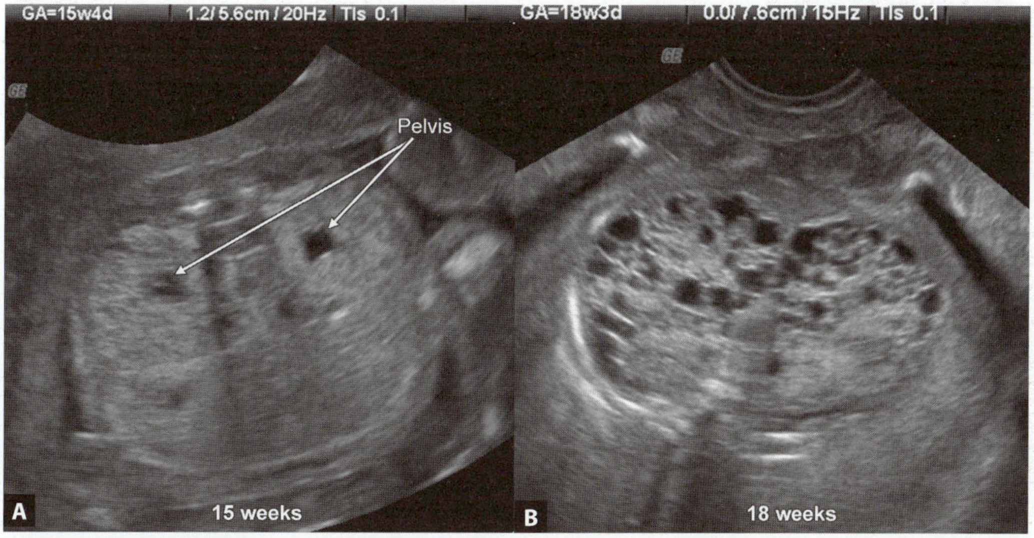

Figs. 45A and B: Bilateral MCDK (multicystic dysplastic kidney) at 18 weeks. (A) 2D axial image at 15 weeks of gestation. At this stage, renal pelvis was visible. Both kidneys are larger than normal and very tiny numerous cystic formation is visible in the kidney; (B) At 18 weeks, multiple cysts are clearly visible in both kidneys.

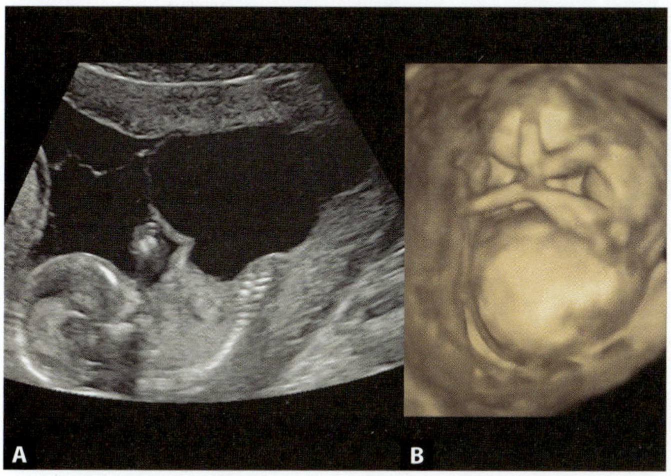

Figs. 46A and B: Bladder extrophy at 15 weeks of gestation. (A) 2D sagittal image. Huge bladder is demonstrated; (B) 3D reconstructed image. Fetus is on the ballooning bladder.

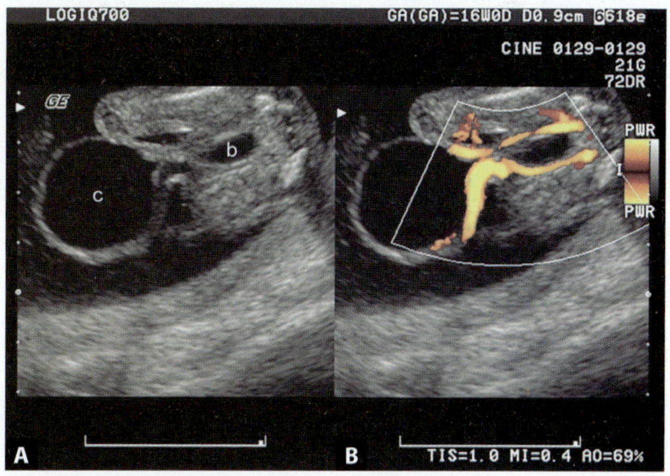

Figs. 47A and B: Vesico-allantoic cyst at 16 weeks of gestation. (A) The extracorporeal cyst (c) is connected with bladder (b); (B) Power Doppler image. Two umbilical arteries are visible along with bladder and allantoic cyst.

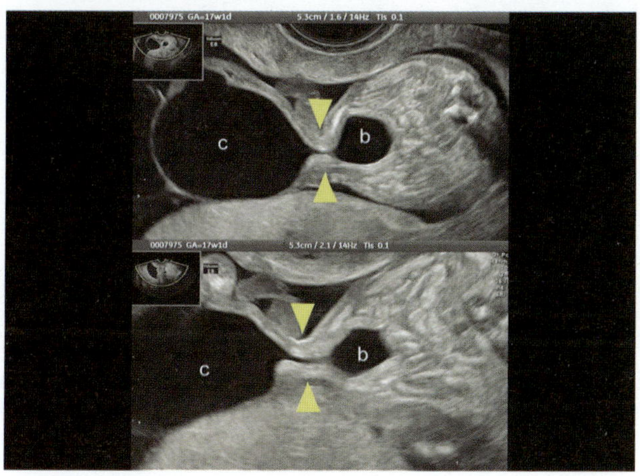

Figs. 48A and B: Vesico-allantoic cyst at 17 weeks of gestation. (A) The extracorporeal cyst (c) is connected with bladder (b); (B) The bladder and cyst size change because of outflow of urine from bladder to the cyst. Note the dynamic change of the urachus (arrowheads).

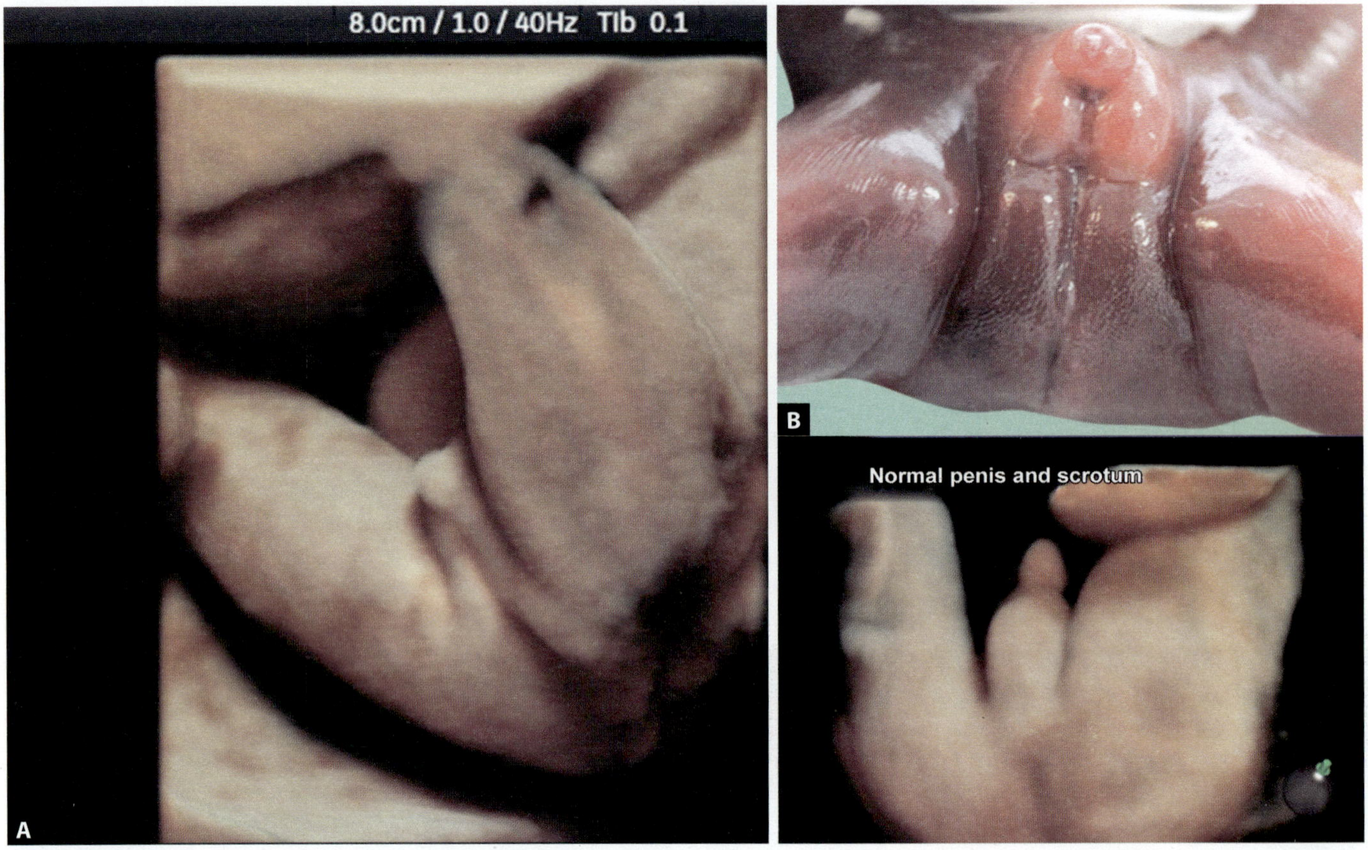

Figs. 49A and B: Hypoplastic external genitalia at 19 weeks. (A) Hypoplastic penis and scrotum is demonstrated in a case of multiple anomalies; (B) Genitalia of the aborted fetus at 21 weeks.
Courtesy: Dr Hideshi Inoshita, Kagawa Inoshita Hospital, Kagawa, Japan.

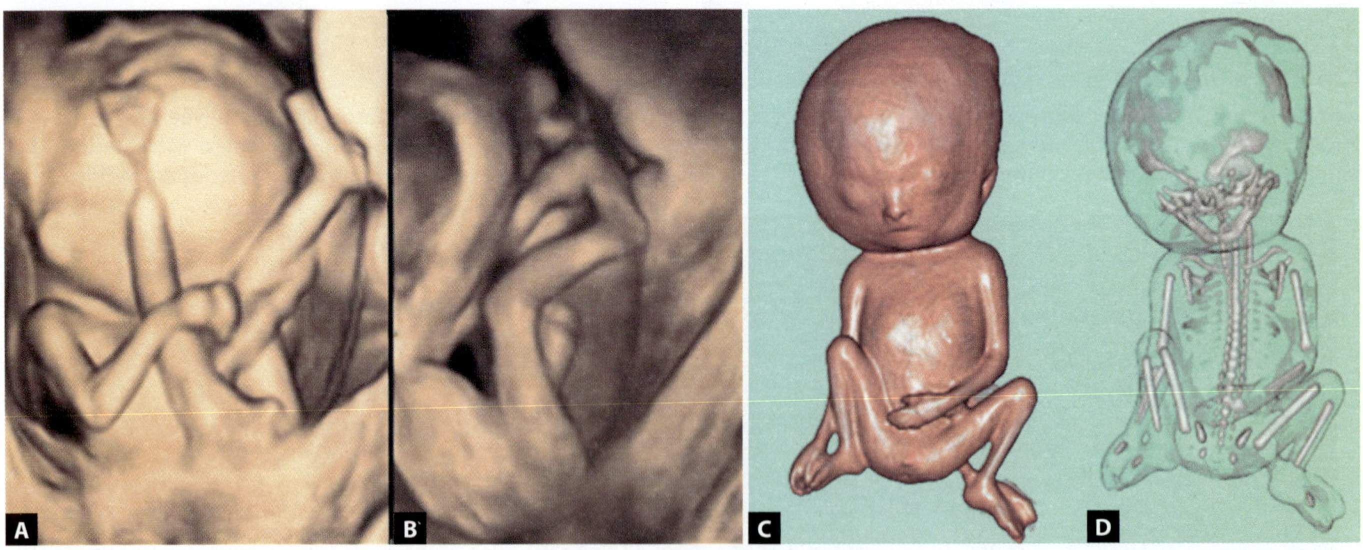

Figs. 50A to D: Thin limbs in a case of triploidy at 17 weeks. (A and B) 3D US reconstructed images. Small for date baby with abnormal proportion, large head and thin limbs and trunk, is demonstrated. Postmortem 3D-CT scan image of surface anatomy (C) and bony structure (D) of the same baby.

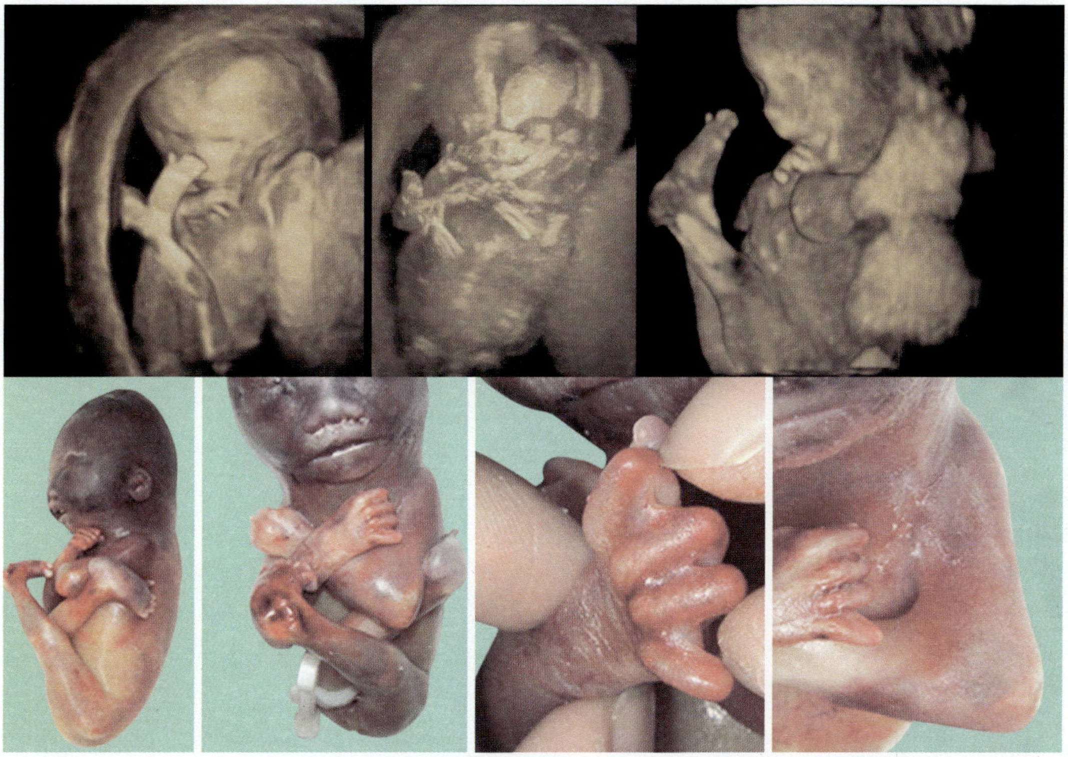

Fig. 51: Lethal pterygium syndrome detected at 14 weeks. Upper Fig.s are 3D reconstructed images. Middle image demonstrated the bony structure by maximum mode. The fetus did not move with the same appearance for weeks. The lower pictures are aborted fetus at 20 weeks. The same appearance as prenatal images is seen. The wing-like shoulders and elbows, finger webs are characteristics of this syndrome.

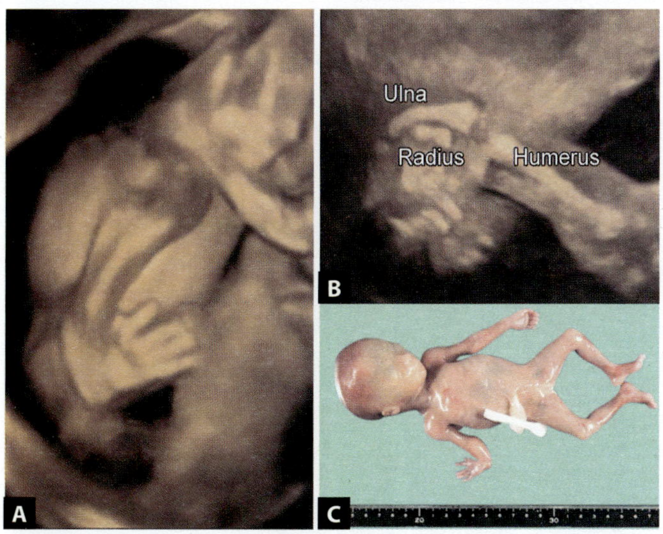

Figs. 52A to C: Right arm abnormality at 18 weeks. (A) Abnormal appearance of right arm by 3D reconstructed image. Short forearm and thumb abnormality are demonstrated; (B) Maximum mode image of the right arm. Short ulna and extremely short radius are clearly demonstrated; (C) Postmortem appearance of the aborted fetus.

Courtesy: Dr H Takemura, Kosaka Women's Hospital, Higashiosaka, Japan. Partial chromosomal abnormality was confirmed.

amputation of fingers **(Figs. 67A and B)**, sandal gap **(Fig. 68)**, and cleft hand/toe **(Figs. 69 to 71)** are clearly seen by 3D ultrasound during pregnancy. Thumb abnormality, especially adducted thumb is one of the important signs for assessment of fetal brain development.[42,43] Genetic hydrocephalus or brain abnormalities which is strongly related to L1CAM gene, are associated with adducted thumbs[44,45] as shown in **Figures 72A to C**. Limb contracture occasionally seen as one of neurological findings is demonstrated in **Figures 73 and 74**.

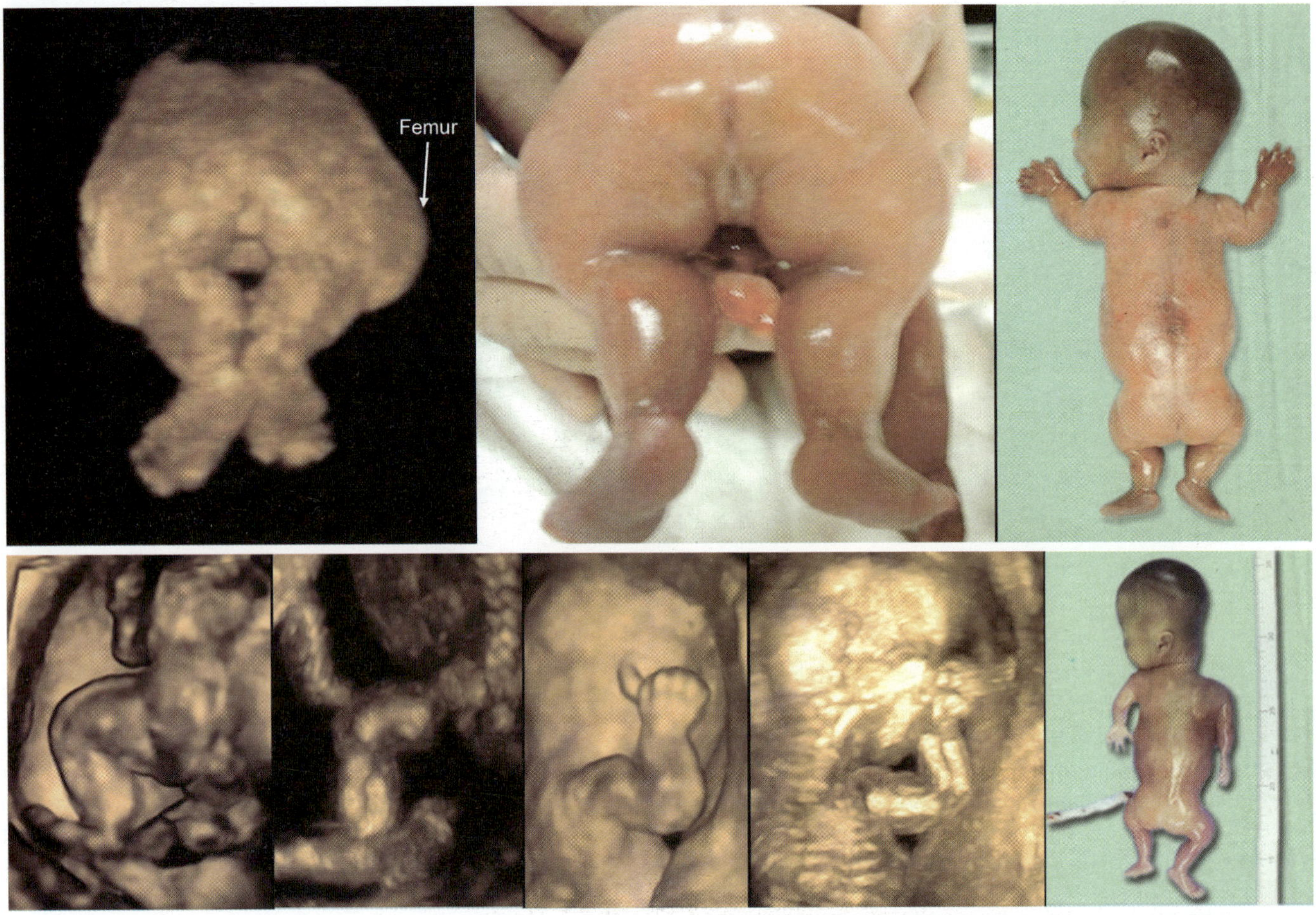

Fig. 53: Thanatophoric dysplasia at 19 weeks. 3D reconstructed images and postmortem appearance of two cases (upper and lower cases) with short limbs and abnormally curved femurs, are shown.

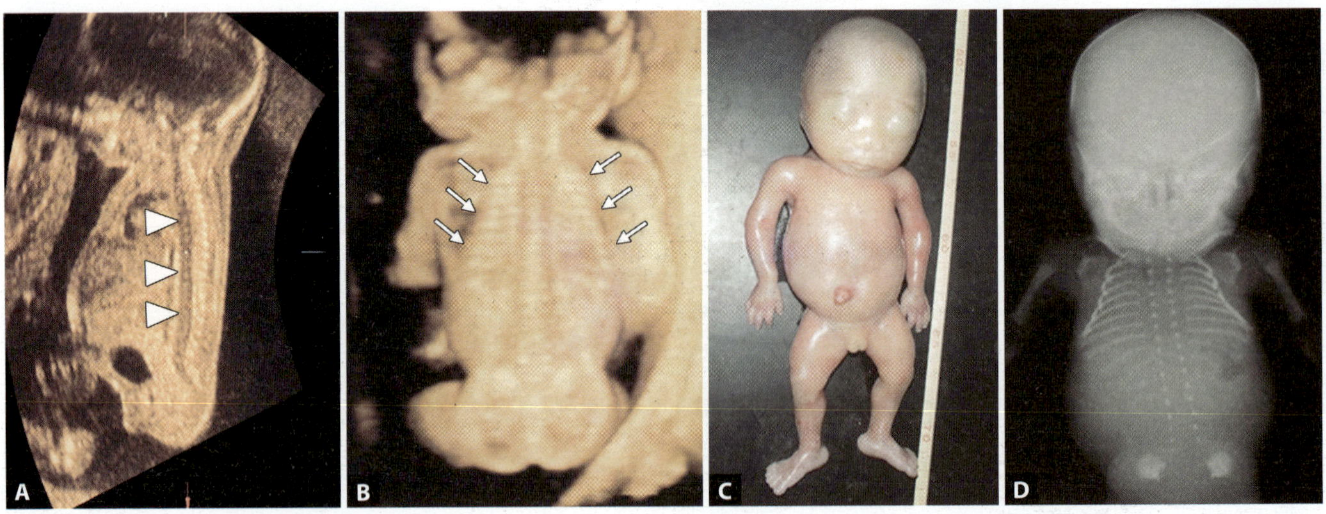

Figs. 54A to D: Short limb, hypoplastic vertebral body with micrognathia seen at 20 weeks. (A) Sonographic image of the fetal body in the sagittal section. Vertebral bodies are not visible (arrowheads); (B) 3D maximum mode in the coronal section. Small thorax is estimated from the shape of ribs (arrows); (C) Macrographic picture of the aborted fetus at 21 weeks. Micrognathia, short trunk, prominent heals are visible; (D) Postmortem X-ray image. Vertebral bodies are not demonstrated. The same appearance of ribs as prenatal 3D ultrasound is seen. This case was confirmed as severe type of collagenopathy by postmortem genetic examination.

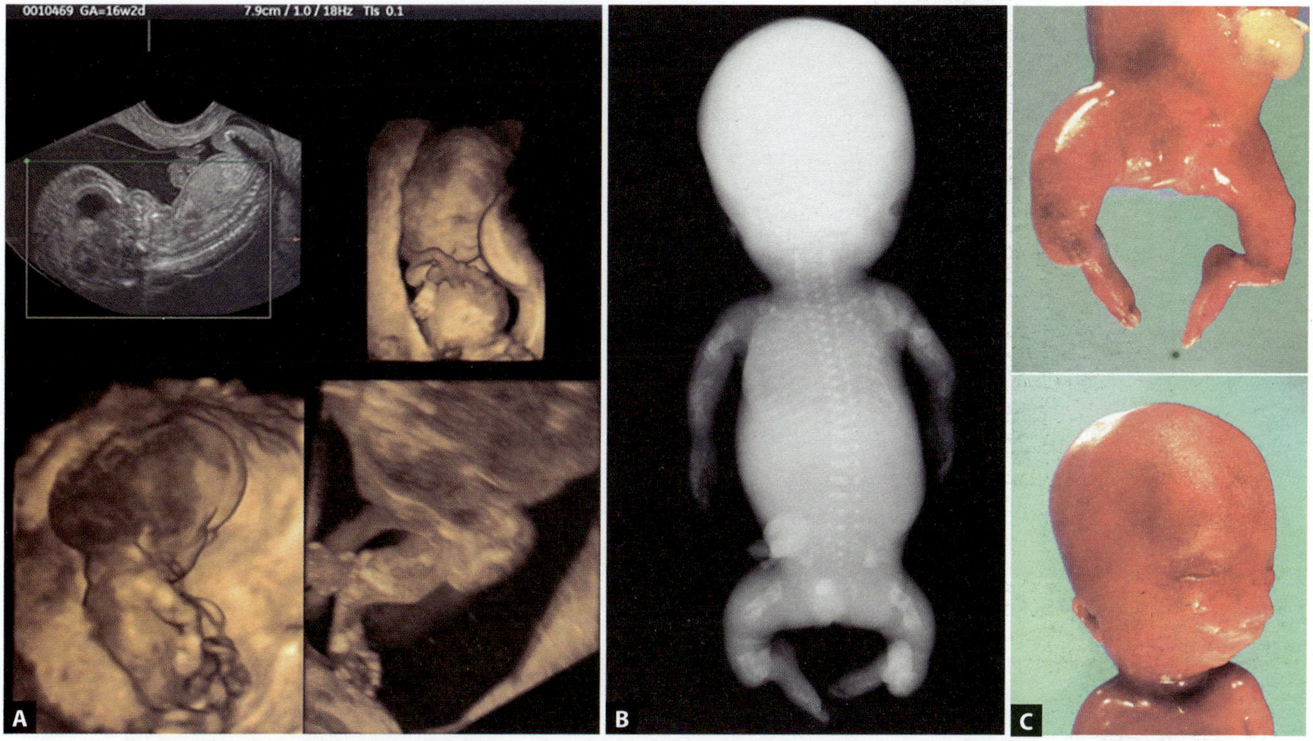

Figs. 55A to C: Severe osteogenesis imperfecta (OI) at 16 weeks of gestation. (A) 3D images at 16 weeks. Abnormally deformed arm is detected (arrows). The long bone development was extremely poor (arrowheads); (B) X ray image of aborted fetus; (C) Aborted fetus.

Courtesy: Dr Takemura, Kosaka Women's Hospital, Osaka, Japan. Molecular genetic exam showed new mutation of COL1A1 was confirmed by Prof Hasegawa, Department of Pediatrics, Keio University, Tokyo, Japan.

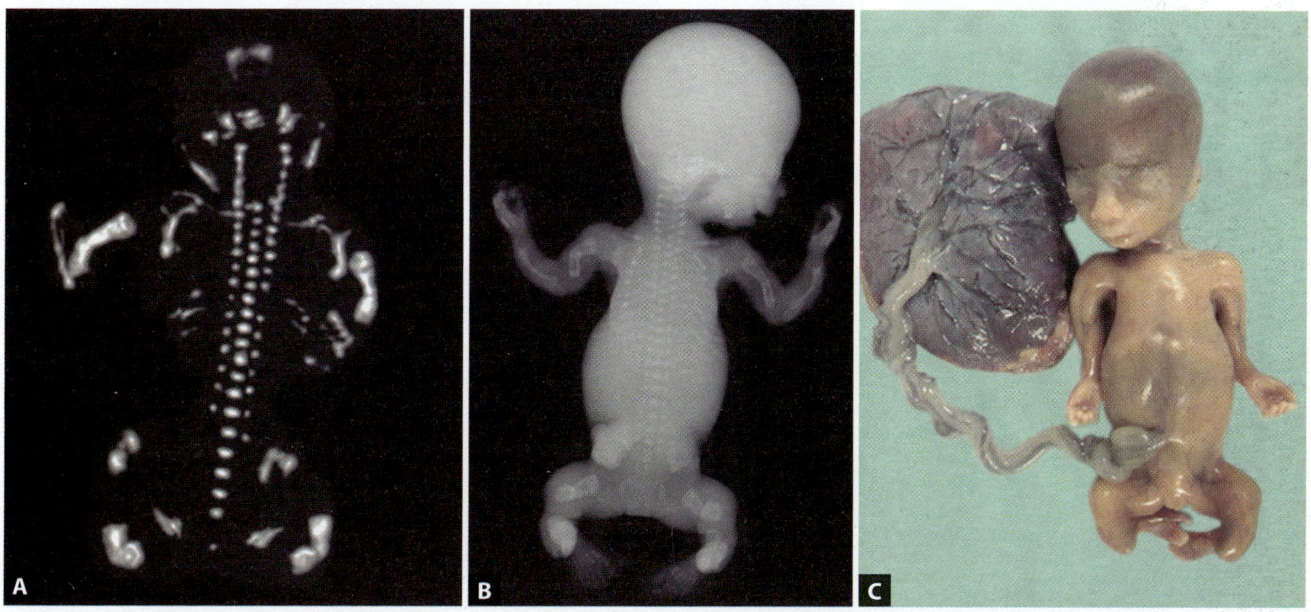

Figs. 56A to C: Osteogenesis imprfecta (OI), fetal 3D-CT and postmortem findings. (A) Fetal 3D-CT image at 20 weeks. Cranial bones were not visualized and short/curved limb bones with hypoplastic vertebral bones indicated OI; (B) Postmortum X-ray. Prenatal findings were confirmed; (C) Macroscopic image.

Courtesy: Dr Hideo Takemura, Kosaka Women's Hospital, Osaka, Japan. In this case, COL1A1gene mutation was confirmed by Prof Hasegawa, Department of Pediatrics, Keio University, Tokyo, Japan.

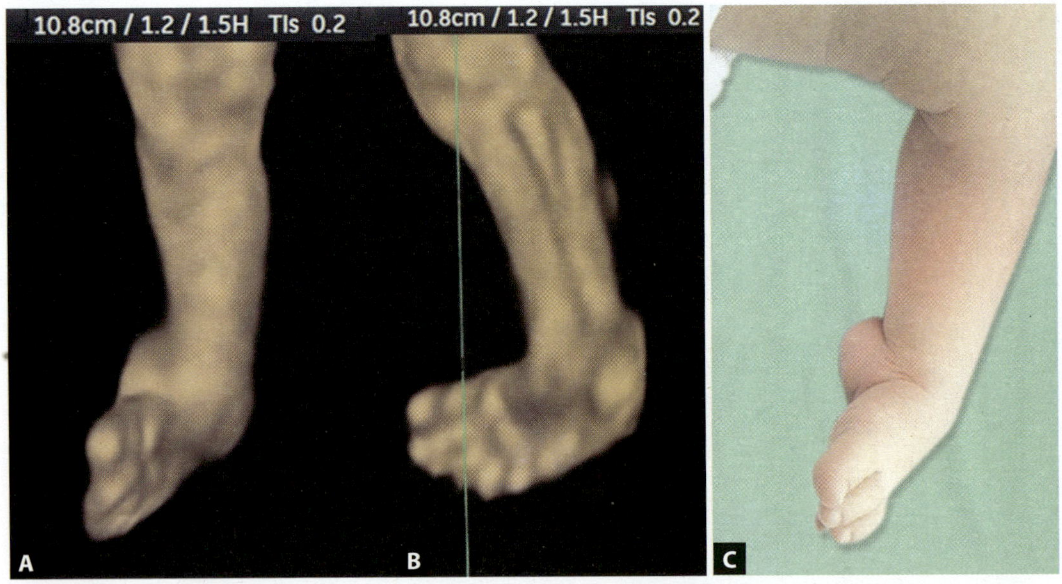

Figs. 57A to C: Clubfoot at 22 weeks of gestation. (A and B) 3D reconstructed images; (C) Postnatal picture.

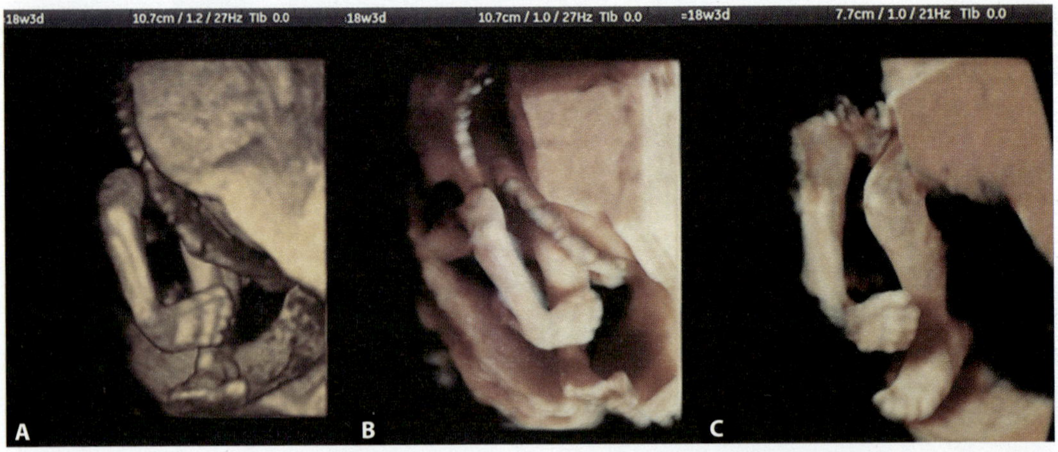

Figs. 58A to C: Unilateral (right side) clubfoot at 18 weeks of gestation. (A) Conventional 3D images; (B and C); HDlive images.

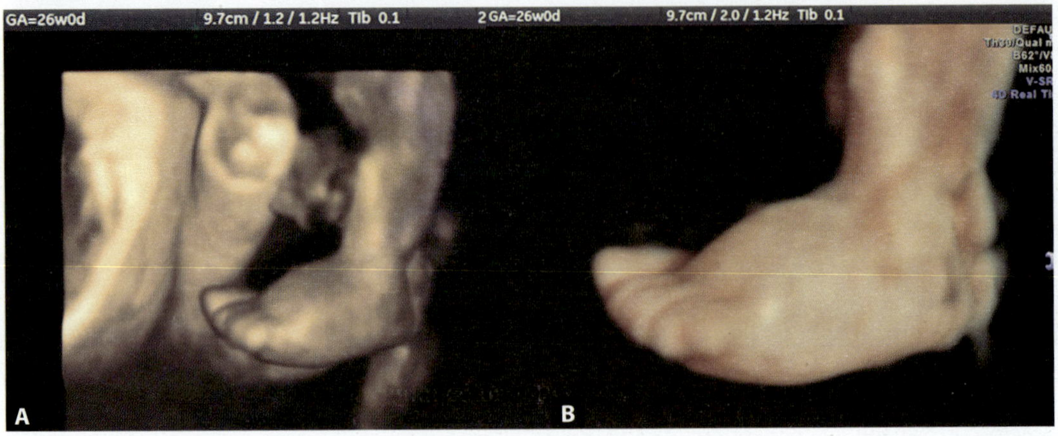

Figs. 59A and B: Edematous left foot at 26 weeks. (A) 3D image; (B) HDlive image. In the first trimester, no increased NT and no abnormalities are seen. The only abnormal finding was left side foot edema at 26 weeks. Although the fetus moved actively and no abnormal sign was found at 26 weeks, sudden intrauterine fetal demise occurred at 33 weeks of gestation.

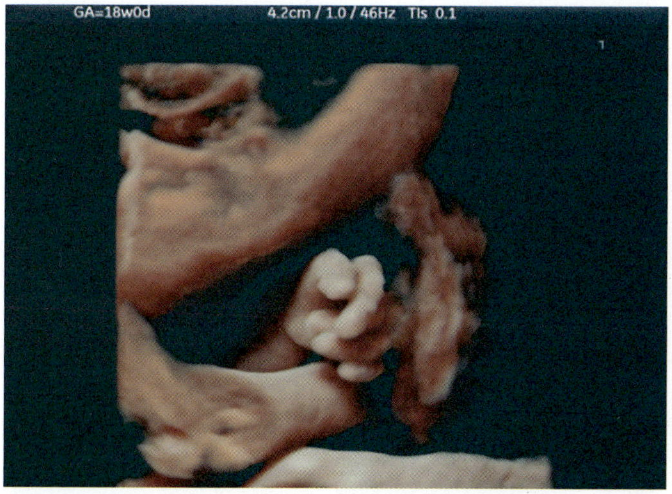

Fig. 60: Overlapping fingers in a case of trisomy 18 at 18 weeks. Typical appearance of overlapping fingers often seen in trisomy 18.

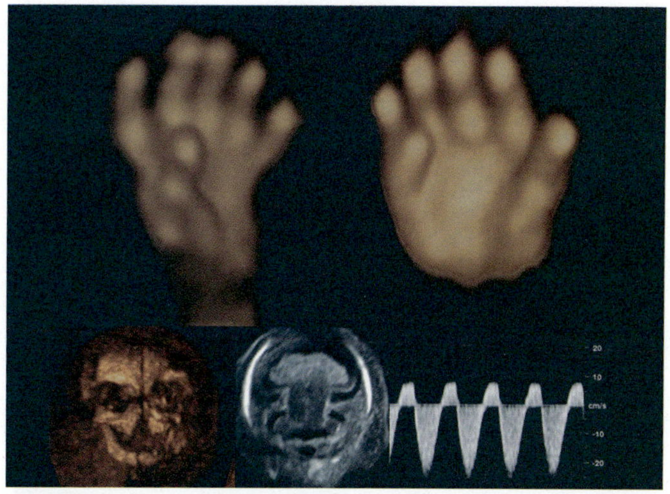

Fig. 61: Polydactyly at 14 weeks. Bilateral polydactyly is clearly demonstrated in upper figures. This case has cleft palate (lower left), holoprosencephaly (lower middle) and umbilical artery reversed flow.

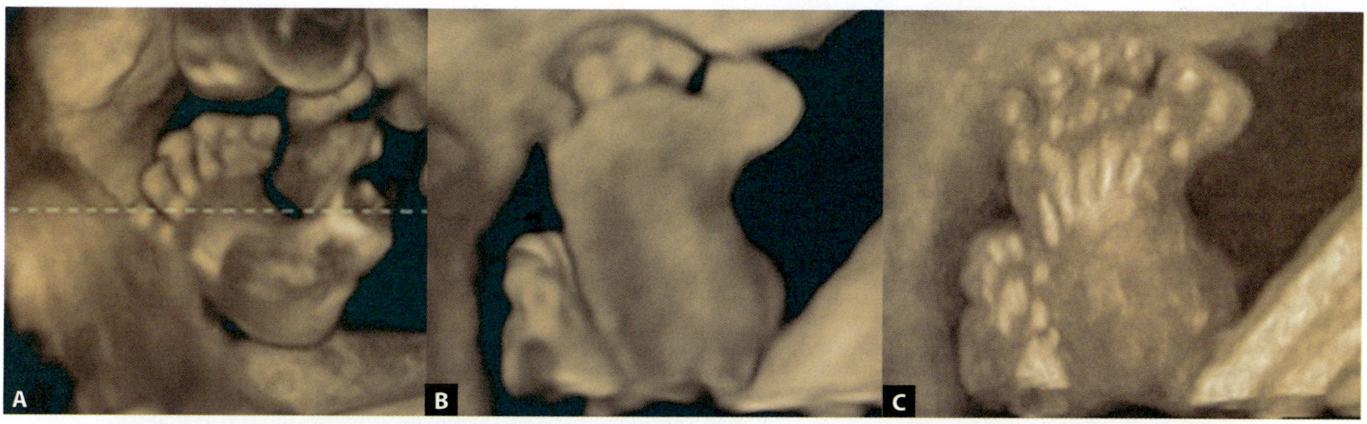

Figs. 62A to C: Polydactyly/syndactyly at 19 weeks. 3D reconstructed images of the right toe. The first big toe is demonstrated in A and B. C clearly shows 6 toe bones.

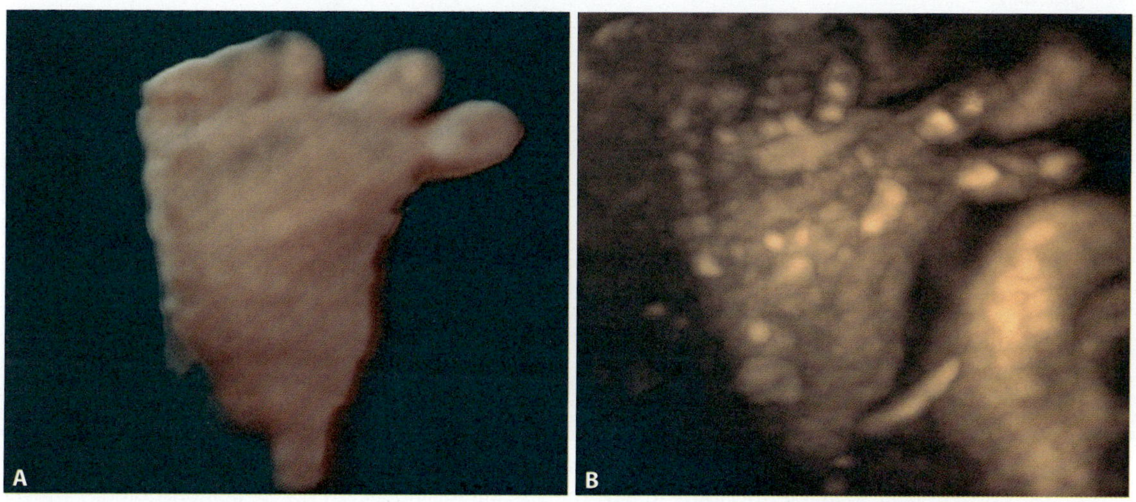

Figs. 63A and B: Polydactyly of the toe at 33 weeks of gestation. (A) HDlive image; (B) Maximum mode image.

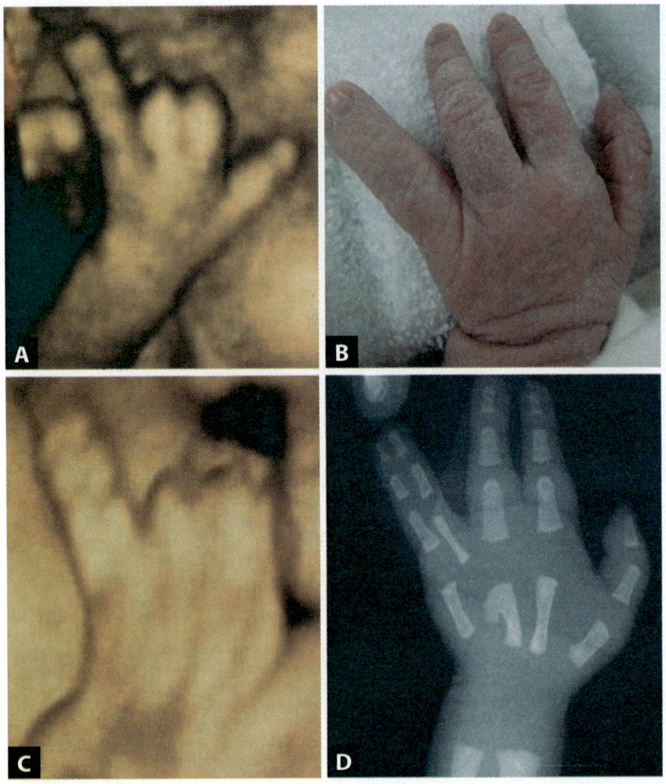

Figs. 64A to D: Syndactyly (single finding) at 28 weeks. (A and C) 3D reconstructed images of the left hand. The forth and fifth fingers are almost the same size and abnormally stretched together. (B) Postnatal hand appearance; (D) Postnatal X-ray image.

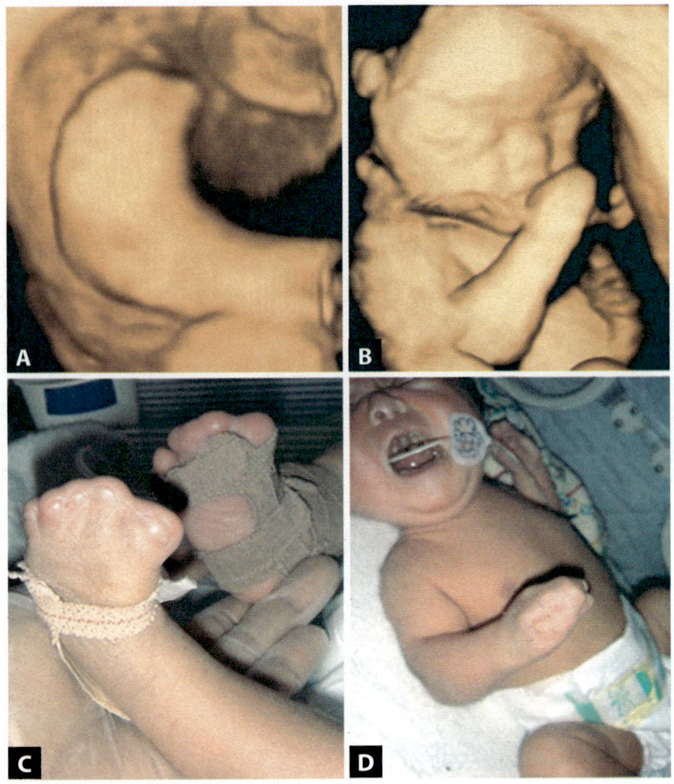

Figs. 65A to D: Syndactyly in a case of Apert syndrome at 31 weeks. (A and B) 3D reconstructed images of the foot and hand. All of toes and fingers are sticked together; (C and D) Postnatal appearance of foot and hand. The same appearance as prenatal imaging is seen.

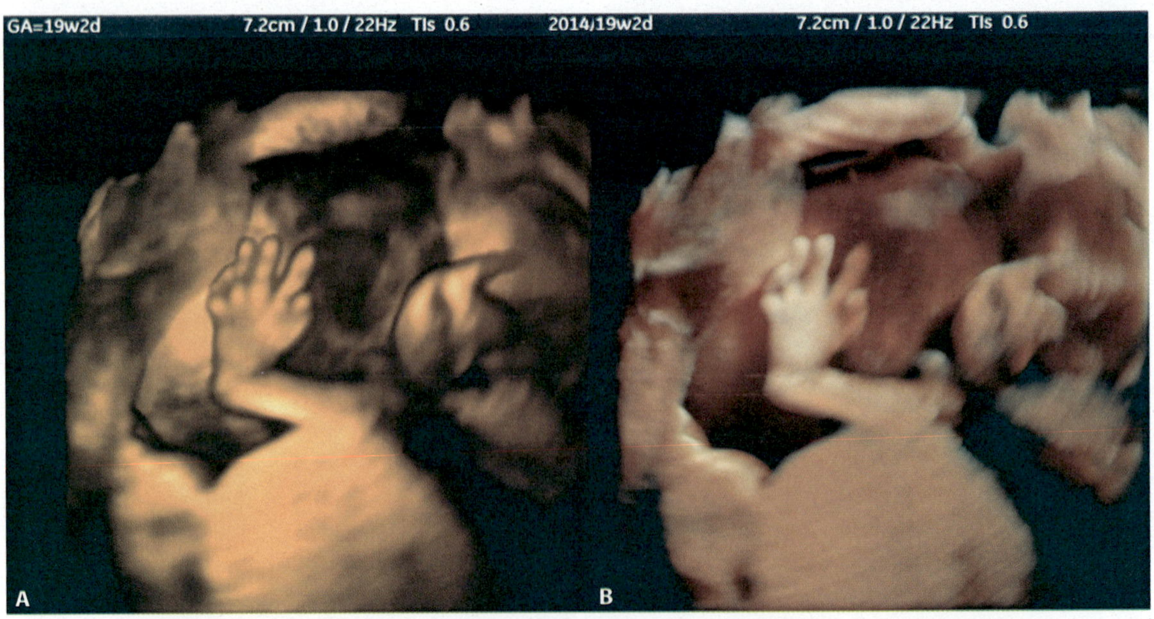

Figs. 66A and B: Clinodactyly seen in a case of Down's syndrome at 19 weeks of gestation. (A); Conventional 3D image; (B) HDlive image. The 5th finger clinodactyly is well-demonstrated.

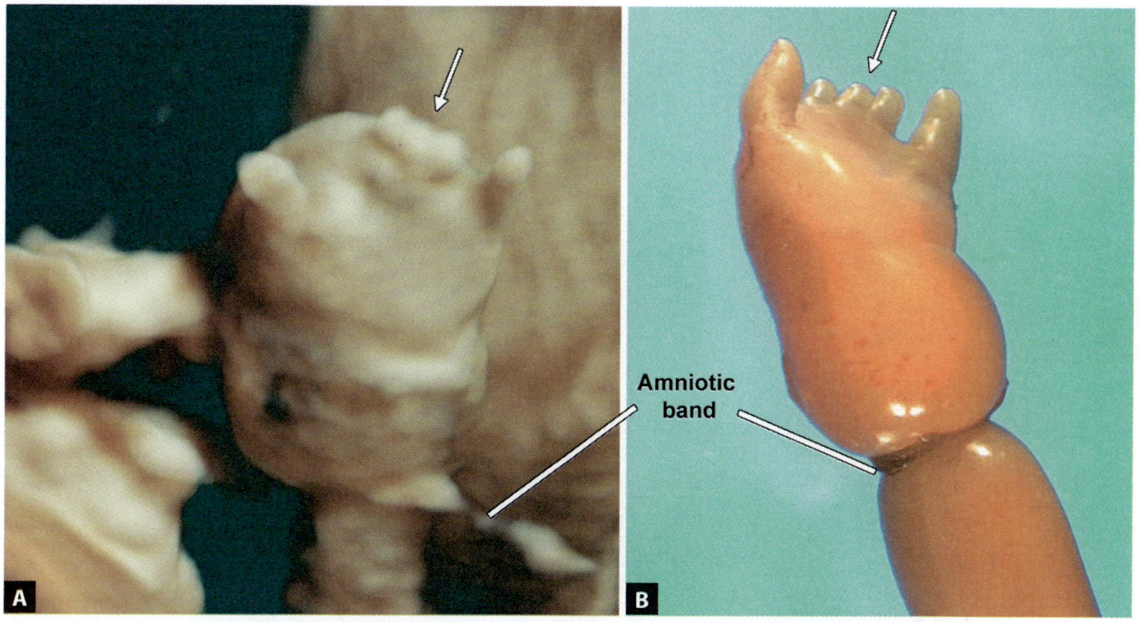

Figs. 67A and B: Amputation of fingers in a case of amniotic band syndrome at 16 weeks of gestation. (A) 3D HDlive image. Edematous left forearm/hand due to amniotic band. Amputation of 2,3,4 digits is depicted (arrow); (B) The left arm of the aborted fetus.

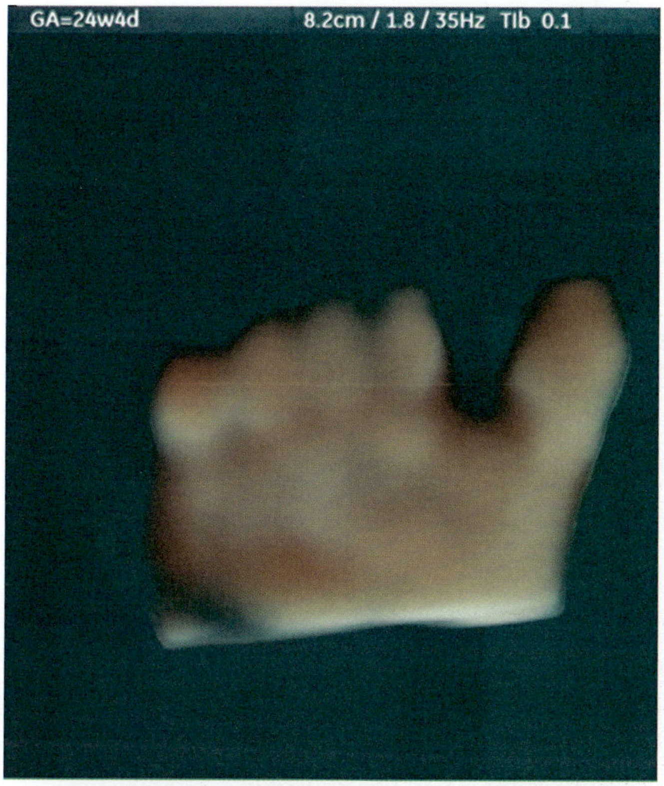

Fig. 68: Sandal gap at 24 weeks. Sandal gap is often seen in Down's fetuses.

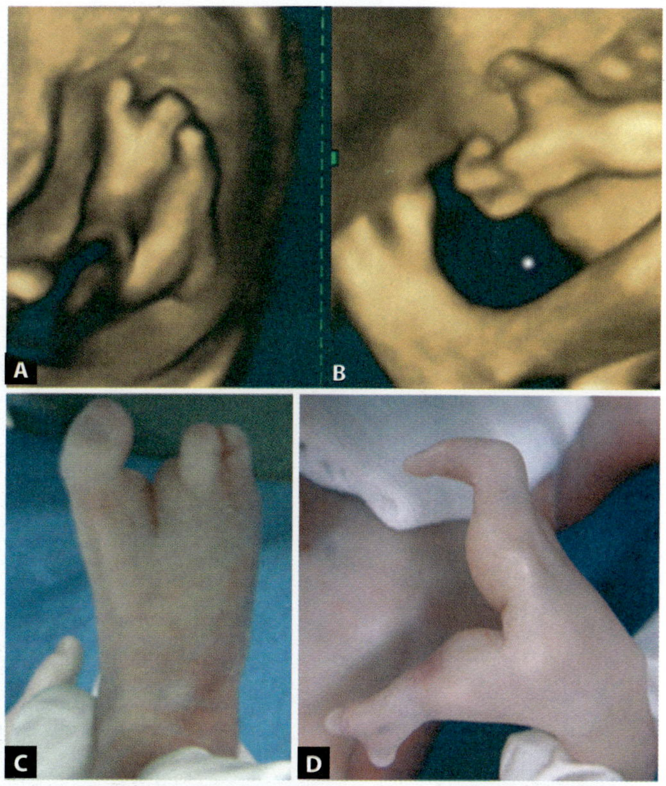

Figs. 69A to D: Cleft foot and cleft hand, oligodactyly/syndactyly at 28 weeks. (A and B) 3D reconstructed images of the foot and hand; (C and D) Postnatal appearance.

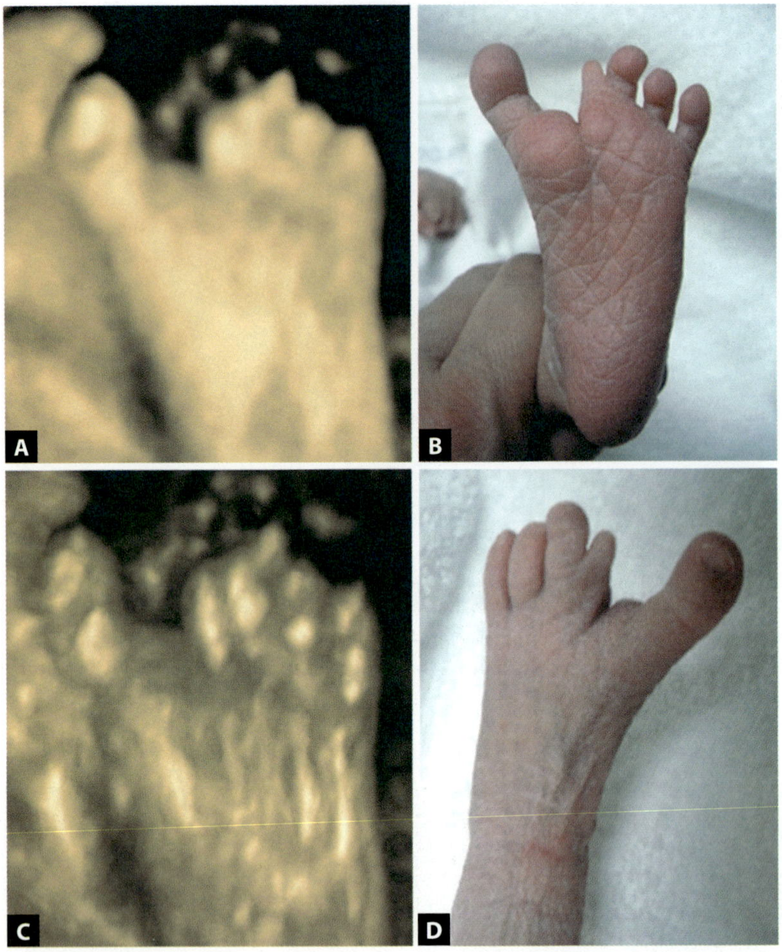

Figs. 70A to D: Cleft foot with toe dysplasia at 35 weeks. (A) 3D reconstructed image; (C) Maximum mode; (B and D) Postnatal appearance.

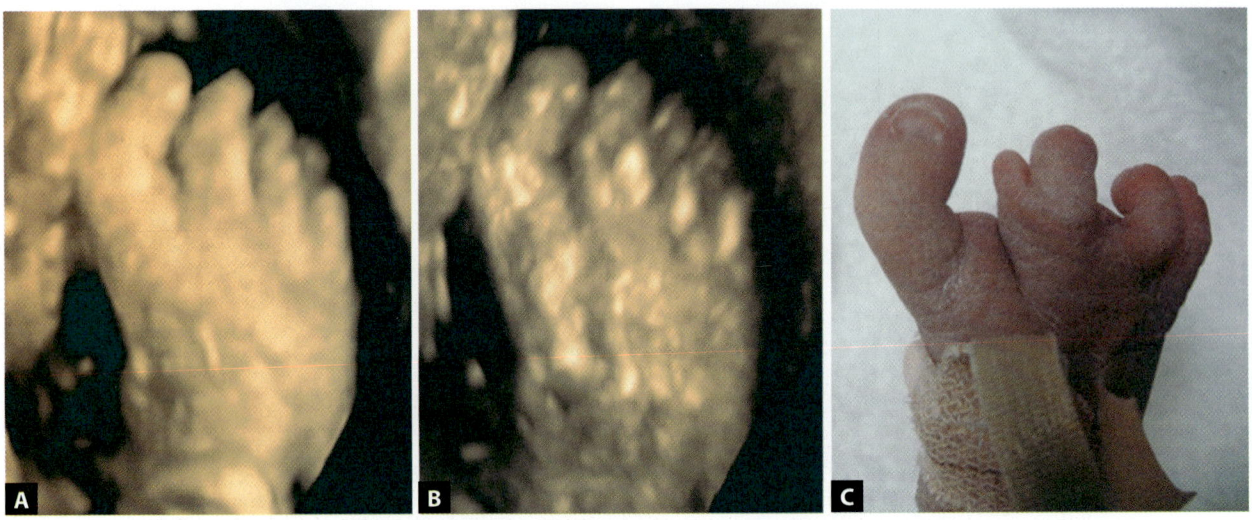

Figs. 71A to C: Cleft foot with toe dysplasia and 1st toe contracture at 35 weeks (same case as Figure 70. (A) 3D reconstructed image; (B) Maximum mode; (C) Postnatal appearance.

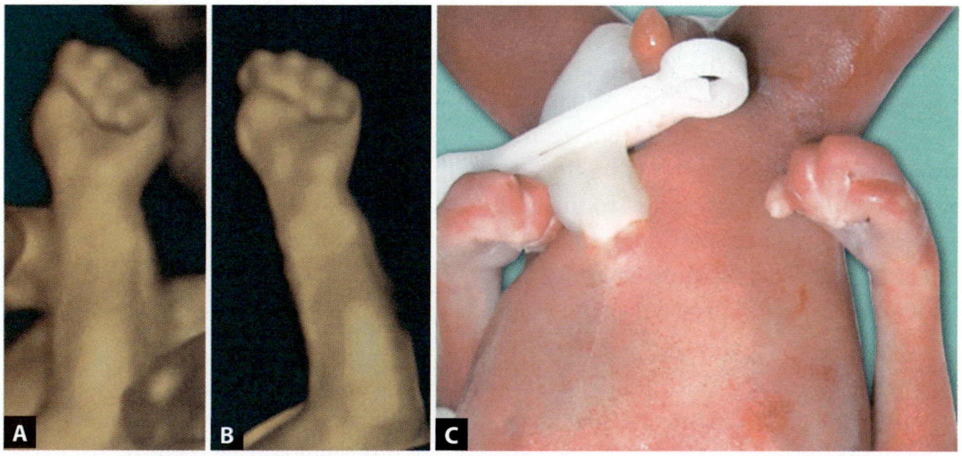

Figs. 72A to C: Adducted thumbs in a case of genetic hydrocephalus. (A and B) 3D reconstructed images of adducted thumb; (C) Postmortem appearance of clenched hands with adducted thumbs. This case is complicated with hydrocephalus, partial agenesis of the corpus callosum. Postmortem genetic test revealed L1CAM disorder.

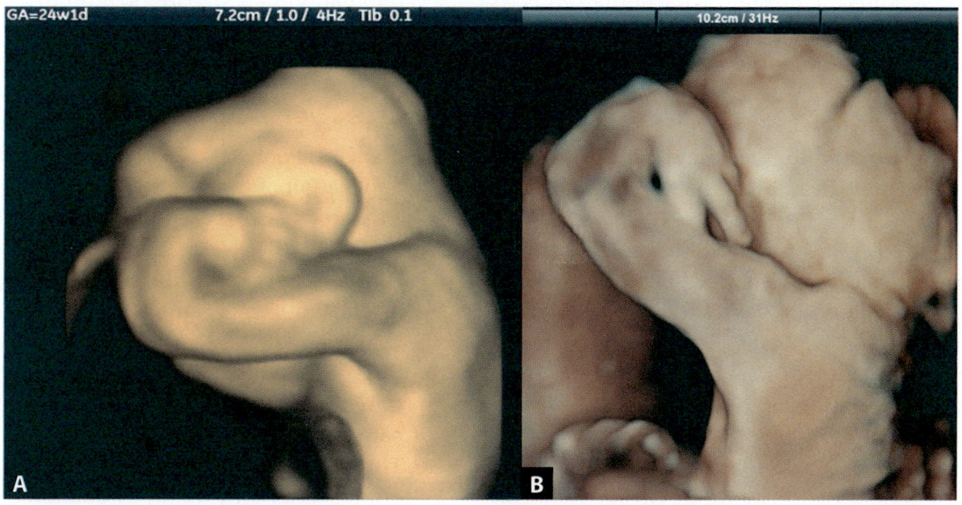

Figs. 73A and B: Short forearm with wrist contracture at 24 weeks of gestation. (A) 3D image; (B) HDlive image. Shoulder joint was movable but elbow and wrist was contracted. Chromosome was normal.

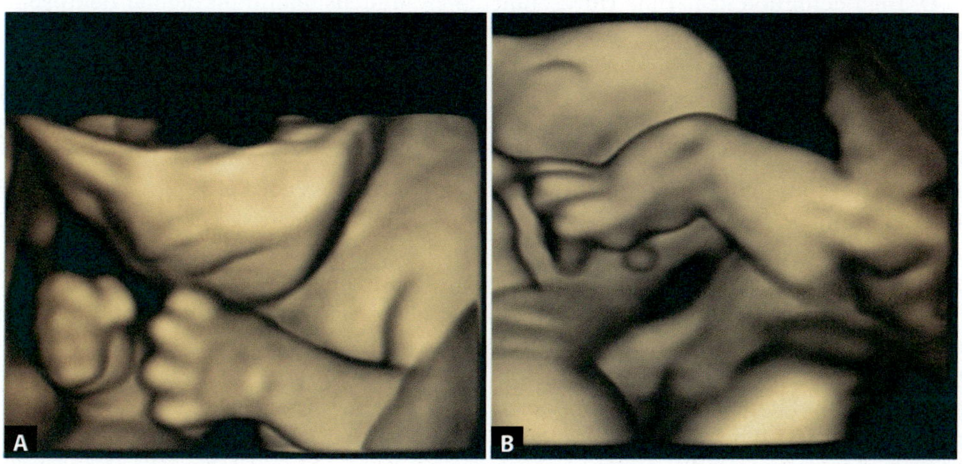

Fig. 74: Hypertonic limb contracture at 26 weeks of gestation. 3D images show hypertonic fingers and wrist. The fetus never unclenched hands throughout pregnancy. Postnatal rehabilitation has improved gradually the limb movements.

CONCLUSION

This article reviews and illustrates the power of high-resolution 3D ultrasound in the definition of normal fetal anatomy as well as in the identification of congenital anomalies. The advances of 3D ultrasound in the last decade have been remarkable and contributed to the field of embryology, fetal physiology and pathology. Further researches by 3D ultrasound will bring more accurate and detailed prenatal diagnosis for better prenatal care.

REFERENCES

1. Kurjak A, Pooh RK, Merce LT, Carrera JM, Salihagic-Kadic A, Andonotopo W. Structural and functional early human development assessed by three-dimensional and four-dimensional sonography. Fertil Steril. 2005;84(5):1285-99.
2. Pooh RK, Shiota K, Kurjak A. Imaging of the human embryo with magnetic resonance imaging microscopy and high-resolution transvaginal 3-dimensional sonography: human embryology in the 21st century. Am J Obstet Gynecol. 2011;204(1):77.e1-16.
3. Pooh RK. 3D Sonoembryology. Donald School Journal of Ultrasound in Obstetrics and Gynecology. 2011;5(1):7-15.
4. Pooh RK. Early detection of fetal abnormality. Donald School J Ultrasound in Obstet Gynecol, 2013;7(1):46-50.
5. Pooh RK, Kurjak A. Editorial. 3D/4D sonography moved prenatal diagnosis of fetal anomalies from the second to the first trimester of pregnancy. The Journal of Maternal-Fetal and Neonatal Medicine 2012;25(5):433-55.
6. Grigore M, Cojocaru C, Lazar T. The role of HD Live Technology in Obstetrics and Gynecology, Present and Future. Donald School J Ultrasound in Obstet Gynecol. 2014;8(3):234-8.
7. Bonilla-Musoles F, Raga F, Castillo JC, Bonilla F Jr, Climent MT, Caballero O. High definition Real-Time Ultrasound (HDlive) of embryonic and fetal malformations before week 16. Donald School Journal of Ultrasound in Obstetrics and Gynecology. 2013;7(1):1-8.
8. Nebeker J, Nelson R. Imaging of sound speed reflection ultrasound tomography. JUM. 2012;31(9):1389-404.
9. Kagan KO, Pintoffl K, Hoopmann M. First-trimester ultrasound images using HDlive. Ultrasound Obstet Gynecol. 2011;38(5):607.
10. Hata T, Hanaoka U, Tenkumo C, Sato M, Tanaka H, Ishimura M. Three- and four-dimensional HDlive rendering images of normal and abnormal fetuses: pictorial essay. Arch Gynecol Obstet. 2012;286(6):1431-5.
11. Pooh RK, Kurjak A. Novel application of three-dimensional HDlive imaging in prenatal diagnosis from the first trimester. Journal of Perinatal Medicine. 2015:43(2);147-58.
12. Pooh RK. First trimester scan by 3D, 3D HDlive and HDlive Silhouette/Flow Ultrasound imaging. Donald School Journal of Ultrasound in Obstetrics and Gynecology. October-December. 2015;9(4):361-71.
13. Pooh RK. 'See-through Fashion' in Prenatal Diagnostic Imaging. Donald School J Ultrasound Obstet Gynecol. 2015;9(2):111.
14. Pooh RK. Brand new technology of HDlive silhouette and HDlive flow images. In: Pooh RK, Kurjak A (Eds). Donald School Atlas of Advanced Ultrasound in Obstetrics and Gynecology. Jaypee Brothers Medical Publishers Private Limited, New Delhi; 2015. pp. 1-39.
15. Teoh M, Meagher S. First-trimester diagnosis of micrognathia as a presentation of Pierre Robin syndrome. Ultrasound Obstet Gynecol. 2003;21:616-8.
16. Tsai MY, Lan KC Ou CY, Chen JH, Chang SY, Hsu TY. Assessment of the facial features and chin development of fetuses with use of serial three-dimensional sonography and the mandibular size monogram in a Chinese population. Am J Obstet Gynecol. 2004;190:541-6.
17. Pooh RK. Three-dimensional ultrasound of the fetal brain. In: Kurjak A (Ed). Clinical application of 3D ultrasonography. Carnforth: Parthenon Publishing, 2000;176-80.
18. Pooh RK, Pooh KH, Nakagawa Y, Nishida S, Ohno Y. Clinical application of three-dimensional ultrasound in fetal brain assessment. Croat Med J. 2000;41:245-51.
19. Blaas HG, Eik-Nes SH, Kiserud T, Berg S, Angelsen B, Olstad B. Three-dimensional imaging of the brain cavities in human embryos. Ultrasound Obstet Gynecol. 1995;5:228-32.
20. Blaas HG, Eik-Nes SH, Berg S, Torp H. In-vivo three-dimensional ultrasound reconstructions of embryos and early fetuses. Lancet. 1998;352:1182-6.
21. Timor-Tritsch IE, Monteagudo A, Mayberry P. Three-dimensional ultrasound evaluation of the fetal brain: the three horn view. Ultrasound Obstet Gynecol. 2000;16:302-6.
22. Monteagudo A, Timor-Tritsch IE, Mayberry P. Three-dimensional transvaginal neurosonography of the fetal brain: 'navigating' in the volume scan. Ultrasound Obstet Gynecol. 2000;16:307-13.
23. Pooh RK, Nagao Y, Pooh KH. Fetal neuroimaging by transvaginal 3D ultrasound and MRI. Ultrasound Rev Obstet Gynecol. 2006;6:123-134.
24. Pooh RK, Pooh KH. Fetal neuroimaging with new technology. Ultrasound Review Obstet Gynecol. 2002;2:178-81.
25. Pooh RK. Fetal brain assessment by three-dimensional ultrasound. In: Kurjak A, Kupesic S (Eds). Clinical Application of 3D Sonography. Carnforth, UK: Parthenon Publishing; 2000.pp.171-9.
26. Pooh RK, Pooh KH. Transvaginal 3D and Doppler ultrasonography of the fetal brain. Semin Perinatol. 2001;25:38-43.
27. Pooh RK, Pooh KH. The assessment of fetal brain morphology and circulation by transvaginal 3D sonography and power Doppler. J Perinat Med. 2002;30:48-56.

28. Pooh RK, Pooh KH. Fetal ventriculomegaly. Donald School J Ultrasound Obstet Gynecol. 2007;2(2):40-6.
29. Pooh RK, Maeda K, Pooh KH. An Atlas of Fetal Central Nervous System Disease. Diagnosis and Management. Parthenon CRC Press, London, New York; 2003.
30. Pooh RK. Neuroscan of congenital brain abnormality. In: Pooh RK, Kurjak A (Eds). Fetal Neurology. New Delhi: Jaypee Brothers Medical Publishers. 2009.pp.59-139.
31. Pooh RK. Fetal Neuroimaging of Neural Migration Disorder. Ultrasound Clinics, Elsevier; 2008;3(4):541-55.
32. Blaas HG, Eik-Nes SH, Isaksen CV. The detection of spina bifida before 10 gestational weeks using two- and three-dimensional ultrasound. Ultrasound Obstet Gynecol. 2000;16(1):25-9.
33. Scott RM, Wolpert SM, Bartoshesky LE, Zimbler S, Karlin L. Segmental spinal dysgenesis. Neurosurgery. 1988;22(4):739-44.
34. Doyle NM, Lally KP. The CDH Study Group and advances in the clinical care of the patient with congenital diaphragmatic hernia. Semin Perinatol. 2004;28(3):174-84.
35. Daskalakis G, Anastasakis E, Souka A, Manoli A, Koumpis C, Antsaklis A. First trimester ultrasound diagnosis of congenital diaphragmatic hernia. J Obstet Gynaecol Res. 2007;33:870-2.
36. Sanz-Cortés M, Raga F, Bonilla-Musoles F. Prenatal diagnosis of congenital cystic adenomatoid malformation using three-dimensional inversion rendering: a case report. J Obstet Gynaecol Res. 2008;34(4 Pt 2):631-4.
37. Siqueira Rabelo EA, Oliveira EA, Silva JM, Oliveira DS, Colosimo EA. Ultrasound progression of prenatally detected multicystic dysplastic kidney. Urology. 2006;68(5):1098-102.
38. Yoo SJ, Lee YH, Ryu HM, Joo MS, Cheon CK, Park KW. Unusual fate of vesicoallantoic cyst with non-visualization of fetal urinary bladder in a case of patant urachus. Ultrasound Obstet Gynecol. 1997;9:422-4.
39. Shukunami K, Tsuji T, Kotsuji F. Prenatal sonographic features of esicoallantoic cyst. Ultrasound Obstet Gynecol. 2000;15:545-6.
40. Gundogan M, Fong K, Keating S, Pierre-Louis J, Chitayat D. First trimester ultrasound diagnosis of lethal multiple pterygium syndrome. Fetal Diagn Ther. 2006;21(5):466-70.
41. Warman ML1, Cormier-Daire V, Hall C, Krakow D, Lachman R, LeMerrer M, et al. Nosology and classification of genetic skeletal disorders: 2010 revision. Am J Med Genet A. 2011;155A(5):943-68.
42. Kurjak A, Miskovic B, Stanojevic M, Amiel-Tison C, Ahmed B, Azumendi G, et al. New scoring system for fetal neurobehavior assessed by three- and four-dimensional sonography. J Perinat Med. 2008;36(1):73-81.
43. Kurjak A, Tikvica A, Stanojevic M, Miskovic B, Ahmed B, Azumendi G, et al. The assessment of fetal neurobehavior by three-dimensional and four-dimensional ultrasound. J Matern Fetal Neonatal Med. 2008;21(10):675-84.
44. Yamasaki M, Thompson P, Lemmon V. CRASH syndrome: mutations in L1CAM correlate with severity of the disease. Neuropediatrics. 1997;28(3):175-8.
45. Kanemura Y, Takuma Y, Kamiguchi H, Yamasaki M. First case of L1CAM gene mutation identified in MASA syndrome in Asia. Congenit Anom (Kyoto). 2005;45(2):67-9.

36

CHAPTER

Fetal Behavior Assessed by Four-dimensional Sonography

Asim Kurjak, Panagiotis Antsaklis, Milan Stanojevic

INTRODUCTION

Recent Advances of 3D Ultrasonography

In utero behavior of the fetus is assessed with the assistance of ultrasound technology, through direct observation in utero of real-time movements and activities of the fetus.[1-3] Ultrasound technology that is now used in everyday clinical practice allows us to study not only the anatomy but also the movements and behavior of the fetus in real time. It has been shown fetal behavior has a specific pattern that corresponds to brain maturation of the fetus at each week or trimester.[4] Both anatomic and functional development of the human brain is a complex and long-lasting procedure that goes through strictly structured developmental stages, which start from the second month of gestational age and continue after birth up to adult life.[4] The cornerstones of human brain development are demonstrated in **Table 1**. This process cannot be always predetermined as it is affected by a variety of genetic and epigenetic factors and can be influenced by incidents that may occur any time during pregnancy. In cases of prematurity, no matter how much intensive neonatal units have progressed, we still have not reached a point where the conditions of ex life are similar to in utero ones, making extremely premature neonates more susceptible to neurological problems.[5,6] The degree at which the brain development will be affected by external factors (genetic factors, external stimuli, pathological conditions, or even environmental changes) is uncertain and cannot be predicted. So, neurological impairment is a great challenge, as its diagnosis in utero is very difficult, and even when we suspect it, again we are often unable to detect the degree at which the fetus will be affected. What is more we cannot be certain of the exact time that the damage occurs: Antepartum, intrapartum, or postpartum, as the diagnosis is most often done after birth.[4] The diagnosis of neurological impairment is one of the greatest challenges in obstetrics and the cause and effect relationship of neurological disabilities most of the times is uncertain. A method that could assess fetal behavior and as a result assess the neurological integrity of the fetus would be a method that would provide many useful information.[6,7] Kurjak's antenatal neurodevelopmental test (KANET) with the use of 4D ultrasound assesses fetal behavior in a similar way that a neonate is assessed postnatally and we now have robust evidence from multicentric studies that it can be used in everyday clinical practice.

TABLE 1: Major events in neural development.[4]

Developmental event	*Peak time of occurrence*
Primary neurulation (dorsal–induction)	3–4 weeks antenatally
Prosencephalic cleavage (ventral induction)	5–6 weeks antenatally
Neuronal proliferation: • Cerebral • Cerebellar	 2–4 months antenatally 2–10 months postnatally
Neuronal migration: • Cerebral • Cerebellar	 3–5 months antenatally 4–10 months antenatally
Neuronal differentiation: • Axon outgrowth • Dendritic growth and synapse formation Synaptic rearrangement	 • 3 months to birth • 6 months to 1 year postnatally Birth to years postnatally
Myelination	Birth to years postnatally

THE EVOLUTION OF FETAL MOVEMENTS AND FETAL BEHAVIOR ASSESSMENT WITH ULTRASOUND

The cerebral growth and maturation of a fetus appear to be represented by its behavior in utero,[8,9] while studies have shown that their movements are very good indicators of neurobehavioral organization and of the future neurological integrity of the fetus.[10-17] Two-dimensional (2D) ultrasound allowed up to a point the complete evaluation of the fetal anatomy and gave the opportunity to view fetal movements. One of the pioneering studies about the importance of fetal movements was published more than three decades ago offering the first knowledge in this new field of fetal medicine and at the same time the inspiration to study the fetal behavior as a whole in utero.[18] de Vries et al. followed and analyzed the qualitative and quantitative aspects of giving more details on the movements and a more methodological way of studying them.[19-21]

Based on the first analysis of fetal movements by 2D ultrasonography, de Vries classified movements into different patterns as follows:

- *Sideways bending:* Started between seventh and eighth gestational weeks, slow and small displacements at one or two poles of the fetus occur, lasting from half a second to two seconds, which usually occur as a single event and disappear through gestation.
- *Startle:* A startle consists of a rapid phase contraction of all limb muscles. It often spreads to the trunk and neck. It occurs frequently in the first trimester from 8 weeks on.
- *General movements (GMs):* These movements are complex movements including neck, trunk, and limbs that are applicable if the whole body is moved but no distinctive patterning or sequencing of the body parts can be recognized. They wax and wane in intensity, force, and speed, and they have gradual beginning and end. These movements are performed from 8 weeks and on.
- *Hiccups:* These consist of a jerky contraction of the diaphragm. Hiccups appear from 9 weeks and on, often in series, for up to several minutes, and isolated arm and leg movements can be observed.
- *Breathing-like:* Fetal breathing-like movements are usually paradoxical in a way that every contraction of the diaphragm (which after birth leads to an inspiration) causes an inward movement of the thorax. The onset of fetal breathing-like is around the 10th week of gestation. Early in pregnancy, they are present continually and are associated with activity in the postural muscles of the neck and limbs.
- *Isolated arm or leg movement:* These movements appear around the 10th week of gestation and they vary in speed and amplitude. They involve extension, flexion, external and internal rotation, or abduction and adduction of an extremity, without movements in other body parts.
- *Twitches:* Twitches are quick extensions or flexions of a limb, or the neck. They are not generalized or repetitive.
- *Clonic movements:* These are repetitive movements of one or more limbs at a rate of about three per second.
- *Isolated retroflexion of the head*: Retroflexions of the head are usually carried out slowly, but they can also be fast and jerky. These movements can be seen around the 10th week of gestation and on.
- *Isolated rotation of the head:* Rotation of the head is carried out at a slow velocity and only exceptionally at a higher speed. The head may turn from a midline position to one side and back.
- *Isolated anteflexion of the head*: Anteflexion of the head is carried out only at a slow velocity. The displacement of the head is small. The duration is about 1 second.
- *Jaw movements*: The onset of irregular jaw opening is at 11th week. The opening may be either slow or quick. The duration of opening varies from <1 to 5 seconds.
- *Sucking and swallowing*: At 13 weeks, rhythmical sucking movements, often followed by swallowing, occur in bursts indicating that the fetus is drinking amniotic fluid.
- *Hand–head contact*: In this pattern of movement, the hand slowly touches the face, and the fingers frequently extend and flex. These movements appear from 10th week onward and at first they usually represent an accidental contact of a hand with the face or mouth. Subgroups of these movements are:
  - *Hand-to-head:* When hand movement ends at contact of fingers with the parieto-occipitotemporal region of the head
  - *Hand-to-mouth:* When hand movement ends at contact of thumb or finger with the mouth, lips, or the immediate oral region
  - *Hand-near-mouth:* When movement ends with fingers in fluid between nose and shoulders/nipples or between both shoulders. Hands must be below eyes and within the area defined by the ears, less than a hand away from the mouth
  - *Hand-to-face:* When movement ends with hand in contact with the face (cheeks, chin, and forehead)
  - *Hand-near-face:* When movement ends with finger in fluid in front of the face but not in mouth region

- *Hand-to-eye:* When movement ends with hand or palm or fingers in the eye region
- *Hand-to-ear:* When movement ends at hand contact with the ear

- *Stretching:* This movement is a complex motor pattern, which is always carried out at a slow speed and consists of the following components: Forceful extension of the back, retroflexion of head, and external rotation and elevation of the arms. It retains an identical movement form into adult life.
- *Yawning:* This motor activity is similar to the yawning observed after birth: Prolonged wide opening of the jaws followed by quick closure, often with retroflexion of the head and sometimes elevation of the arms. This movement pattern is nonrepetitive and it appears around 11th week. The anatomical criterion for fetal yawning is retraction of the tongue, whereas yawning in adults is characterized by an extended tongue.
- *Rotation of the fetus:* Rotation of the fetus occurs around the sagittal or transverse axis. A complete change in position around the transverse axis, usually with a backwards somersault, is achieved by a complex GM, including alternating leg movements, which resemble neonatal stepping.

It has been suggested that distinguishing between types of fetal movements and behavior according to each trimester could help to dissever routine-normal fetal behavioral patterns, from possible pathological patterns.[21-24] The method that brought a revolution to fetal real-time imaging was 4D ultrasonography which offered a more objective and accurate way than 2D ultrasound.[24-27] 3D/4D ultrasound has now become routine in clinical practice and fetal assessment offering better pictures than 2D ultrasound and allowing observation of fetal movements, even detailed ones such as fingers and facial movements.[28,29] Especially for the face, it represents the most visible part of the human being. All major senses are facilitated in this region and expressed through facial expressions. The long-term study of fetuses with 4D ultrasound allowed the production of measurable units that could be finally applied systematically for the assessment of fetal behavior.[30] One of the greatest advantages of 4D ultrasound compared to 2D is the detailed pictures of the fetal face (e.g., smiling, crying, mouthing, and blinking), something that cannot be achieved with 2D ultrasound. When comparing assessment of fetal behavior by 2D and 4D ultrasound, the advantage of 4D is better depiction of fetal facial expressions in three dimensions (3D) with the possibility to assess them in almost real time with the new sophisticated ultrasound machines having fast frame rates.

There are now studies that prove that with the use of 4D differences in fetal behavior can indeed be identified and with these findings eventually abnormal characteristics can be identified.[31-33] The commencement of fetal movements has been shown by ultrasound studies that occurs very early in fetal life and much earlier than pregnant women can start feeling them.[26] Until a mother can start feeling them and until delivery these movements go through a process that they become more organized and with details such as facial expressions.[34] Studies regarding neonatal neurology have shown that the neonatal behavioral examination can give more information about a possible impairment than a typical neurological examination. That initiated a series of studies that aimed to find the exact structure of the development of fetal behavior for each month or each trimester, in order to first of all to define what is a possible normal behavior and then to identify and diagnose abnormal patterns.[1-4,18-23,35] About 5 years ago, the Zagreb group developed a methodical system for assessing the integrity of the nervous system of fetuses, by applying 4D ultrasound.[36] This test was named KANET, standing for Kurjak's antenatal neurodevelopmental test. Its innovation is that it assesses the fetus in the same way that neonates are assessed neurologically after birth, using similar parameters, with the use of 4D ultrasound.[37-39] While 2D ultrasound is used only for the assessment of fetal startles and GMs, introduction of KANET test enabled assessment of not only movements but also some signs used in postnatal neurological assessment like cranial sutures, head circumference, and finger movements of the hand for the detection of neurological thumb (adducted thumb in the clenched feast).

KURJAK ANTENATAL NEURODEVELOPMENTAL TEST: THE ASSESSMENT OF FETAL NEUROBEHAVIOR IN THE 21ST CENTURY

Timely diagnosis of brain impairment is the main reason why so many studies have been conducted regarding the anatomical and functional integrity of the fetal nervous system as well as the understanding of their reactions. The results that these studies showed gave the motivation for the development of a structured way of assessing fetal behavior in a similar way that neonatal assessment is done.[1] KANET is a new pioneering method of fetal evaluation mainly by 4D ultrasound that shows a relationship between fetal behavior and neurodevelopmental processes in different periods of pregnancy, making it possible to distinguish between normal and abnormal brain development.[36,37] It consists of general parameters such as GMs of the fetus and some parameters that are used postnatally for neonatal assessment incorporated by the Amiel-Tison Neurological Assessment at Term (ATNAT) signs.[37,40] The following parameters are included in the KANET test: Isolated head anteflexion, overlapping cranial sutures, head circumference, isolated eye blinking, facial alterations, mouth opening (yawning or mouthing), isolated hand and leg movements and thumb position, and gestalt perception of GMs (overall perception of the body and limb movements with their qualitative assessment).

Studies show a continuity of the behavioral pattern that follows a fetus from its in utero life to its postpartum attitude and it has been observed that all movements which are present in neonates are also present in fetal life, with the exception of Moro's reflex, which cannot be demonstrated in fetuses.[41] The absence of Moro's reflex can be attributed to the differences of the environment in which a fetus develops compared to the postnatal environment, and these differences concern mainly the differences of gravity in the two environments.[6] The parameters finally decided to be used for the KANET test were the result of long-term multicentric studies regarding neurological assessment and the GMs emergence of the fetuses.[40,42]

Kurjak's antenatal neurodevelopmental test is an integrated test consisting of parameters that concern in utero behavior and movements, but also signs which are used postnatally for detection of neurodevelopmental impairment (neurological thumb, overlapping sutures, and small head circumference).[43] KANET is a test that has been standardized, and studies show that it is a method with good reproducibility and the learning curve is very reasonable for physicians and medical staff with good ultrasound background.[43] Regarding the gestational age at which KANET should be performed it has been decided that the best period is the third trimester of pregnancy, and particularly after 28 weeks. The test is proposed to last about 15–20 minutes, and it has been decided that it is best to be performed at periods that the fetus is awake. If this is not achievable because the fetus goes through its sleeping period, the test should be repeated in 30 minutes or the following day, at a minimum period of 14–16 hours.

When the test is abnormal or the score is borderline, it is proposed that test is repeated every 2 weeks until delivery. Very important features are facial movements and eye blinking—"the face is the mirror of the brain". The overall number of movements must be documented in all cases and compared with normal values as presented in previous studied and reviews[40,42] **(Figs. 1 to 6)**.

Examiners who apply KANET should have proper training and adequate experience in low- and high-risk pregnancies. Interobserver and intraobserver variability has to be documented. The suggestion regarding the ultrasonographic machines used is to have a frame rate of at least 24 volumes/sec. KANET consists of eight parameters **(Table 2)**. The results of KANET are divided in three groups: (1) Abnormal, when the score is 0–5, (2) borderline for a score from 6 to13, and finally (3) normal for a score 14–20 **(Table 3)**. A 2-year follow-up should be available and documented for all fetuses that KANET has been applied, in order to draw safe conclusions.

The aim of the KANET test is to evaluate fetal motoric activity and through that the development of the nervous activity. KANET depends on realistic images compared to the traditional 2D ultrasound and maternal perception of fetal movements, as it can demonstrate fetal movements in real time. As mentioned above, parameters used by KANET are a mixture of GMs, some parameters from ATNAT which means that there is a continuity from fetal to neonatal life after delivery, plus the fact that the integrity of fetal nervous system is up to a point represented by the quality and quantity of the movements that a fetus has in utero and its overall behavior.[22,44-49]

Studies show[50-55] that KANET can identify severe motoric impairment in fetuses with already diagnosed anatomical central nervous system (CNS) abnormalities or chromosomal abnormalities. Also it has been proven that the results of KANET in both low- and high-risk populations correspond to a very high extent with the final outcome and particularly in high-risk populations, KANET can be a very useful tool providing information regarding the prognosis and the grade of impairment of these cases.[56] KANET constitutes the first test applying 4D ultrasound, which has been standardized attempting to simplify things and offers a scoring system, with an aim to be introduced in clinical practice.[57-59] Regarding the applicability of KANET, studies show that it is relatively easy to learn and well accepted by pregnant women; it has a reasonable learning curve of about 80 cases and the duration of the KANET appears reasonable, as it should last about 15–20 minutes.[54]

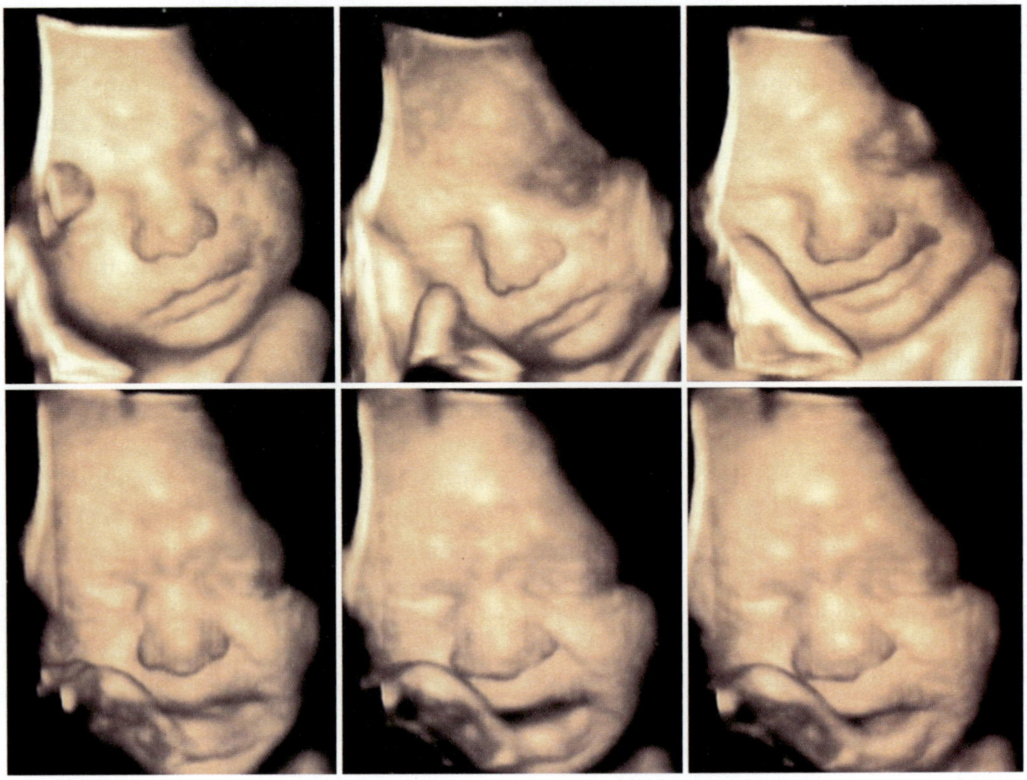

Fig. 1: Typical fetal facial expressions as seen during the performance of Kurjak's antenatal neurodevelopmental test (KANET) and recorded.

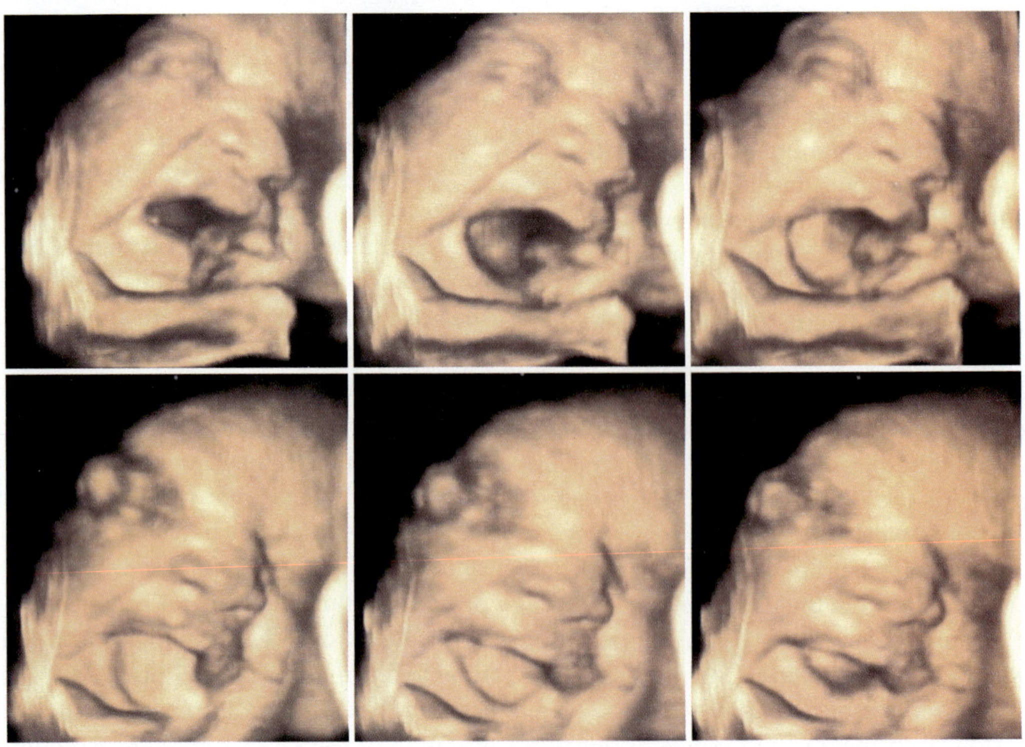

Fig. 2: Mouthing and yawning is an important parameter of Kurjak's antenatal neurodevelopmental test (KANET) and a good sign of neurological development.

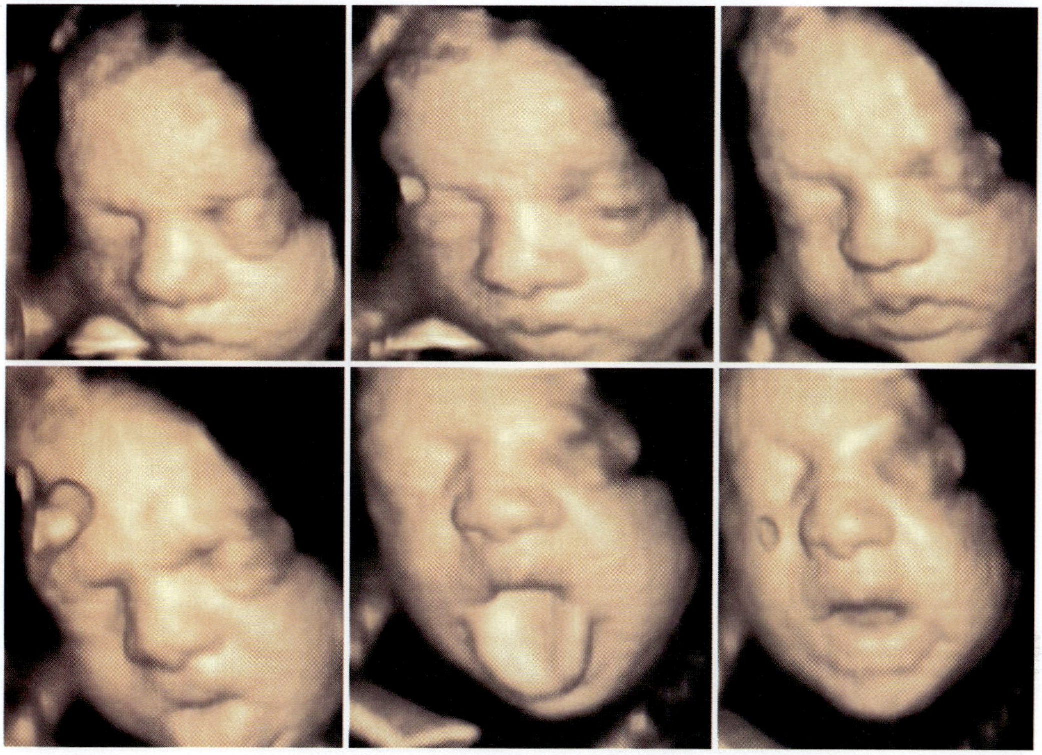

Fig. 3: Typical tongue expulsion while fetus is at an awake state.

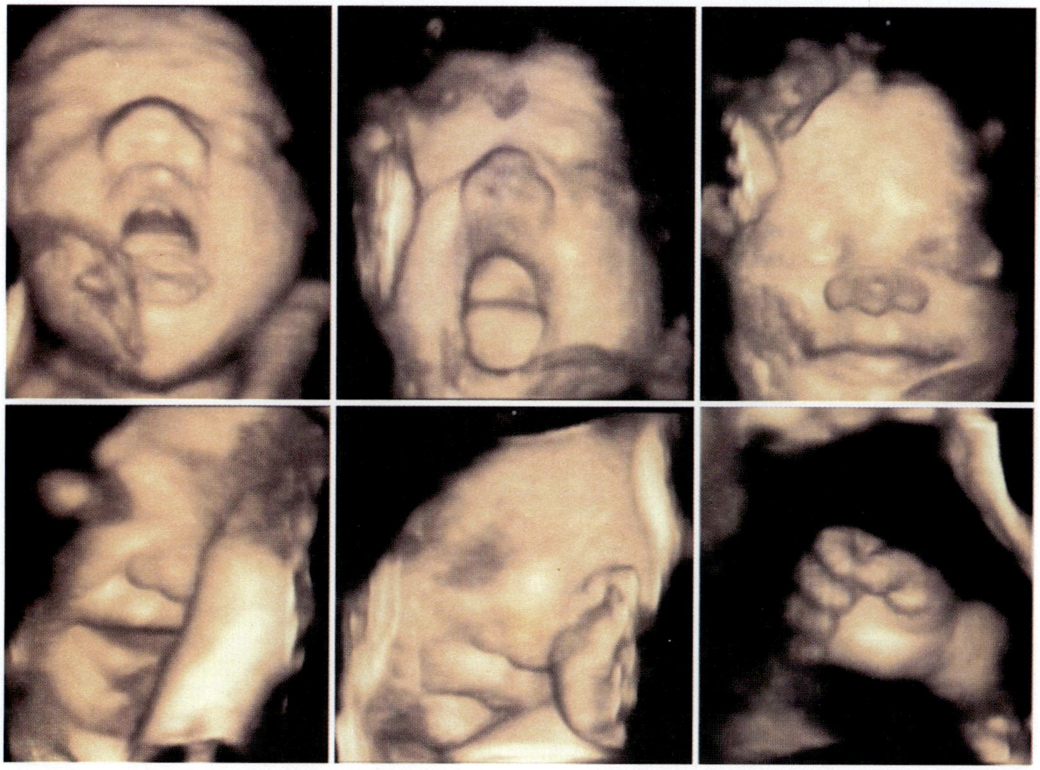

Fig. 4: Mouth opening, yawning, smiling, and finger movements during the performance of Kurjak's antenatal neurodevelopmental test (KANET).

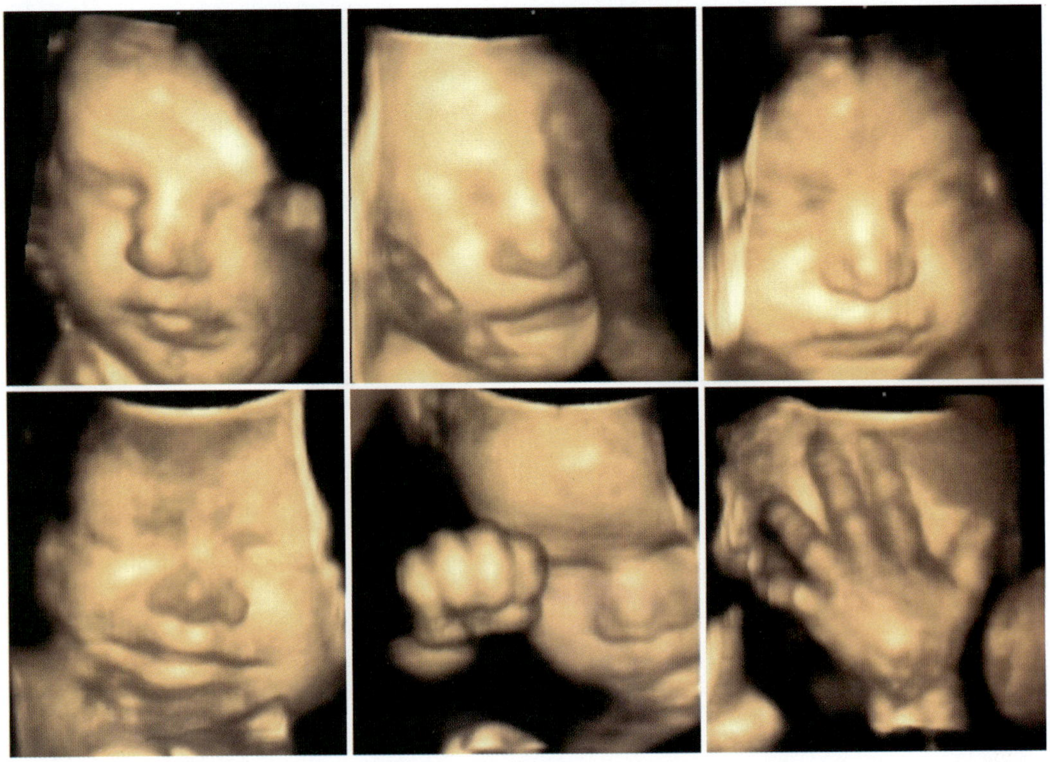

Fig. 5: Facial expressions, eye blinking, and finger movements as part of neurological assessment of the fetus with 4D ultrasound [Kurjak's antenatal neurodevelopmental test (KANET)].

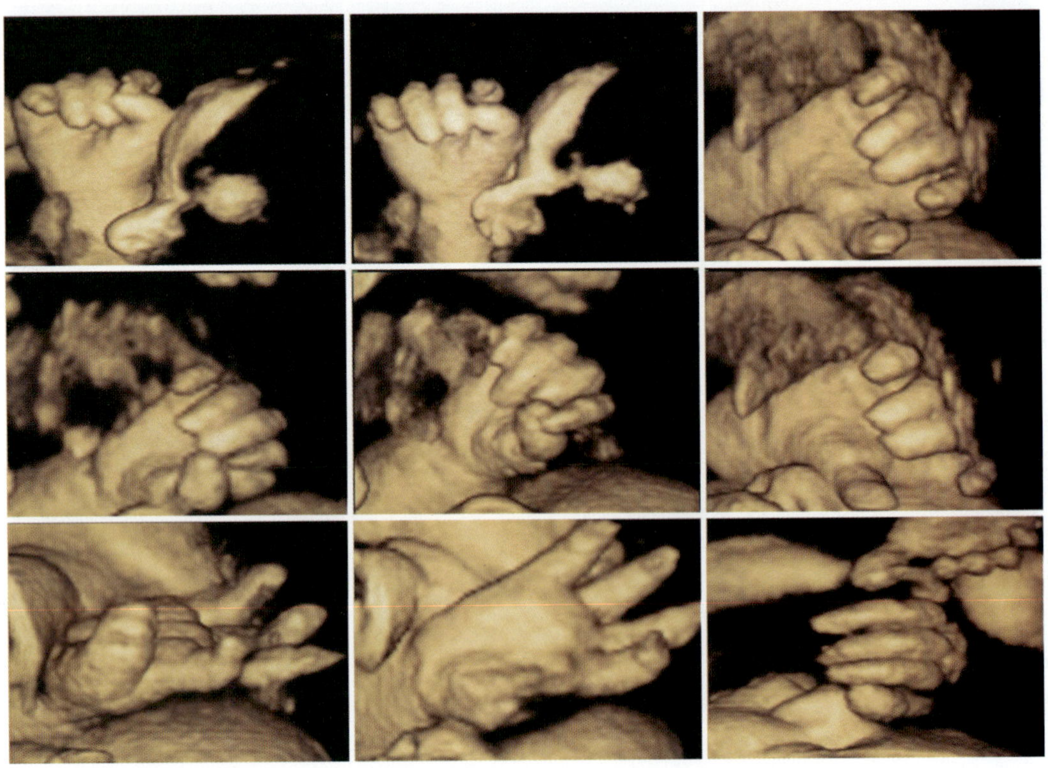

Fig. 6: Fetal hand and finger movements. Detailed movements are very indicative of the neurological maturation and very important parameter of Kurjak's antenatal neurodevelopmental test (KANET).

TABLE 2: The parameters of standardized KANET.[43]

Sign	***Score***			***Sign score***
	0	***1***	***2***	
Isolated head anteflexion 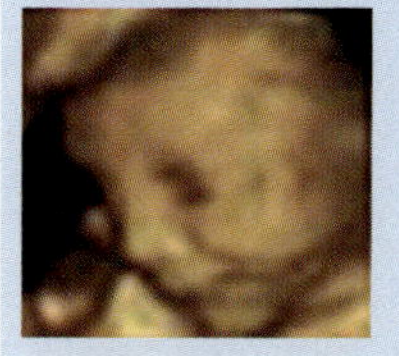	Abrupt	Small range (0–3 times of movements)	Variable in full range, many alternation (>3 times of movements)	
Cranial sutures and HC 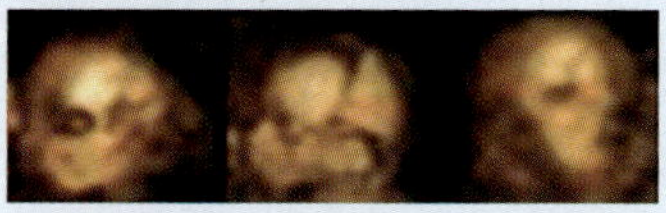	Overlapping of cranial sutures	Normal cranial sutures with measurement of HC below or above the normal limit (–2 SD) according to GA	Normal cranial sutures with normal measurement of HC according to GA	
Isolated eye blinking 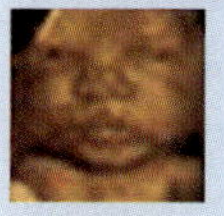	Not present	Not fluent (1–5 times of blinking)	Fluency (>5 times of blinking)	
Facial alteration (grimace or tongue expulsion) 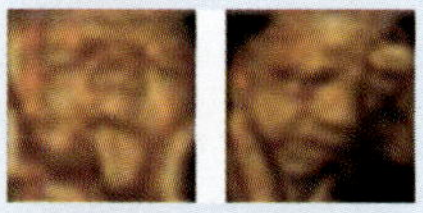	Not present	Not fluent (1–5 times of alteration	Fluency (>5 times of blinking)	
or Mouth opening (yawning or mouthing) 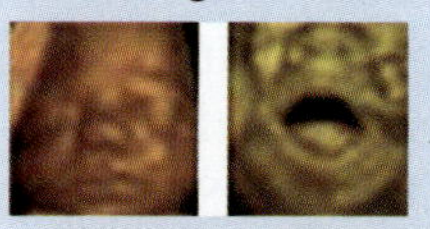				
Isolated leg movement 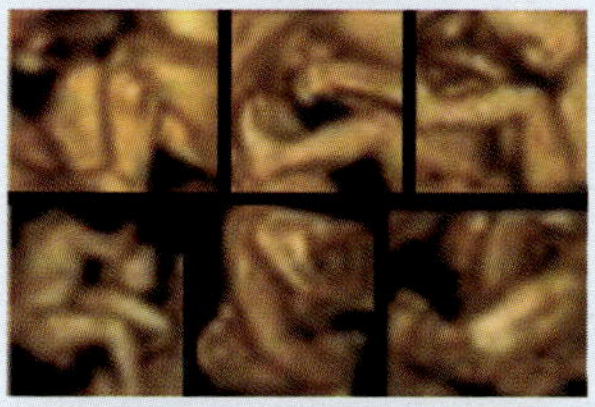	Cramped	Poor repertoire or small in range (0–5 times of movement)	Variable in full range many alternation (>5 times of movements)	
Isolated hand movement 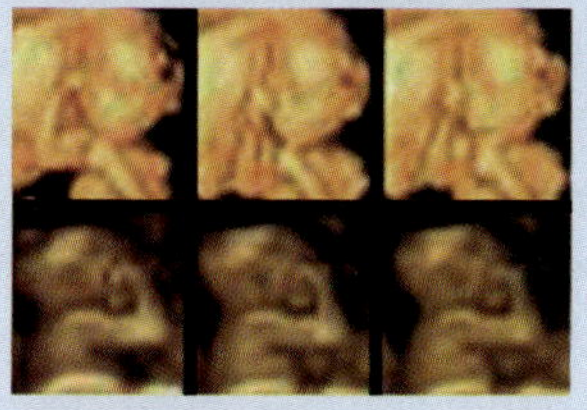	Cramped or abrupt	Poor repertoire or small in range (0–5 times of movement)	Variable in full range many alternation (>5 times of movements)	
or Hand to face movements 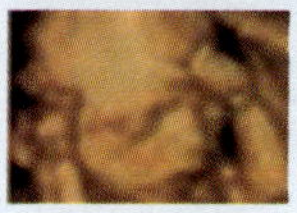				

Contd…

Contd...

Sign	*Score*			*Sign score*
	0	*1*	*2*	
Fingers movements 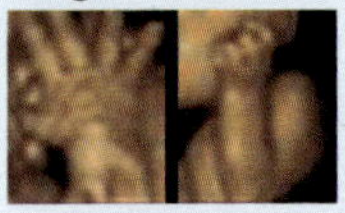	Unilateral or bilateral clenched first (neurological thumb)	Cramped invariable finger movements	Smooth and complex, variable finger movements	
Gestalt perception of GMs	Definitely abnormal	Borderline	Normal	
			Total score	

(GA: gestational age; GMs: general movements; HC: head circumference; KANET: Kurjak's antenatal neurodevelopmental test; SD: standard deviation)

TABLE 3: Kurjak's antenatal neurodevelopmental test scoring system.[43]

Total score	*Interpretation*
0–5	Abnormal
6–9	Borderline
10–16	Normal

Kurjak's antenatal neurodevelopmental test is a new test that takes advantage of the potential offered by the evolution of ultrasound technology, and especially 4D ultrasound for the better assessment of fetal structural and behavioral integrity and especially in order to study details of facial and finger movements. It has been proven that KANET is the method that is well accepted by both examiners and pregnant women, and it has been appropriately standardized. KANET appears to offer useful information about fetal neurobehavior and has the potential to detect and discriminate normal, borderline and abnormal fetal behavior mainly in high-risk pregnancies, so that it can be a valuable diagnostic tool for fetal neurological assessment.[43,60] So far KANET has proven its usefulness in standardization of neurobehavioral assessment, with the potential of prenatal detection of fetuses with severe neuronal dysfunction **(Figs. 7 to 9)**.[60]

According to the Bucharest consensus statement on KANET, it is needed to perform 80 KANET tests by experienced ultrasound specialist in order to be familiar to assess a fetus with 4D ultrasound in 20 minutes. It was calculated that one needs 10–15 cases in 7 days in order to learn the basics of the technique which can be reproducible. The number of tests was comparable with other ultrasound tests like nuchal translucency screening (40 tests by experienced ultrasound specialist) and anomaly scan (100–200 tests by experienced specialist). In a study that 1,712 KANET tests were performed on 655 patients, the success rate of the test ranged between 91 and 95%. Success rate for the assessment of particular signs of the KANET was between 88% for isolated eye blinking and 100% for mouth opening and isolated leg movement. KANET had almost 100% negative predictive value. Interobserver agreement between two examiners for different components of the KANET test were assessed by calculation of Kappa values, which were lowest for the facial expression (K = 0.68) and highest for the finger movements (K = 0.84), proving that KANET test is a reliable method to be used with confidence in everyday clinical practice after appropriate education of experienced examiner. What are the more appropriate educational courses with certificate of completion on the performance of KANET are organized by the Ian Donald School of Ultrasound **(Figs. 10 to 12)**.

Evidence of Prenatal Detection by the Application of KANET According to Multicentric Studies

First form of KANET scoring system was applied by Andonotopo et al.[55] Their aim was to assess whether facial expression and body movements could be of any diagnostic value regarding cerebral palsy (CP) in growth restricted fetuses. They studied 50 pregnancies with intrauterine growth restriction (IUGR) after 28 weeks of pregnancy. They noted decreased behavioral activity in the IUGR fetuses compared to the non-IUGR. This preliminary study motivated further studies about the usefulness of 4D ultrasound for the assessment of fetal behavior. Introduction of KANET as a method could identify characteristics in fetal behavior or movement that manifested some degree of brain impairment. For the development of this test several neonates with variable

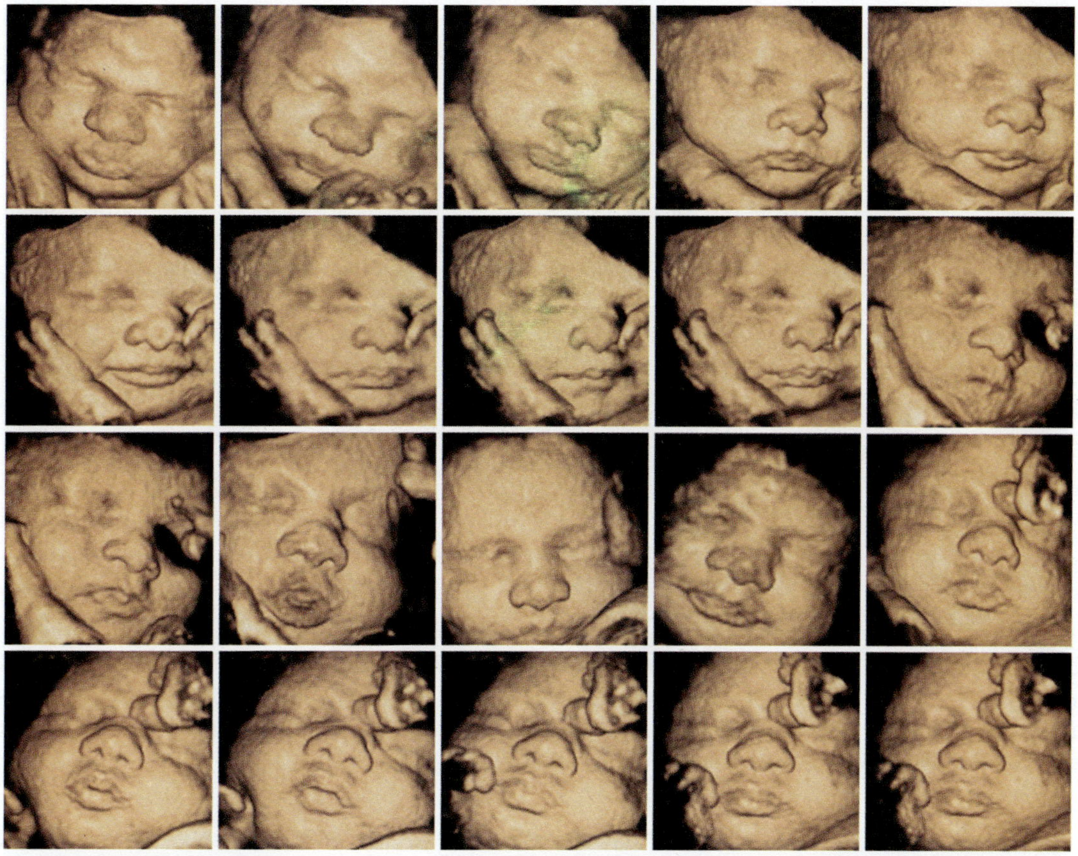

Fig. 7: Normal Kurjak's antenatal neurodevelopmental test (KANET) at 34 weeks of gestation.

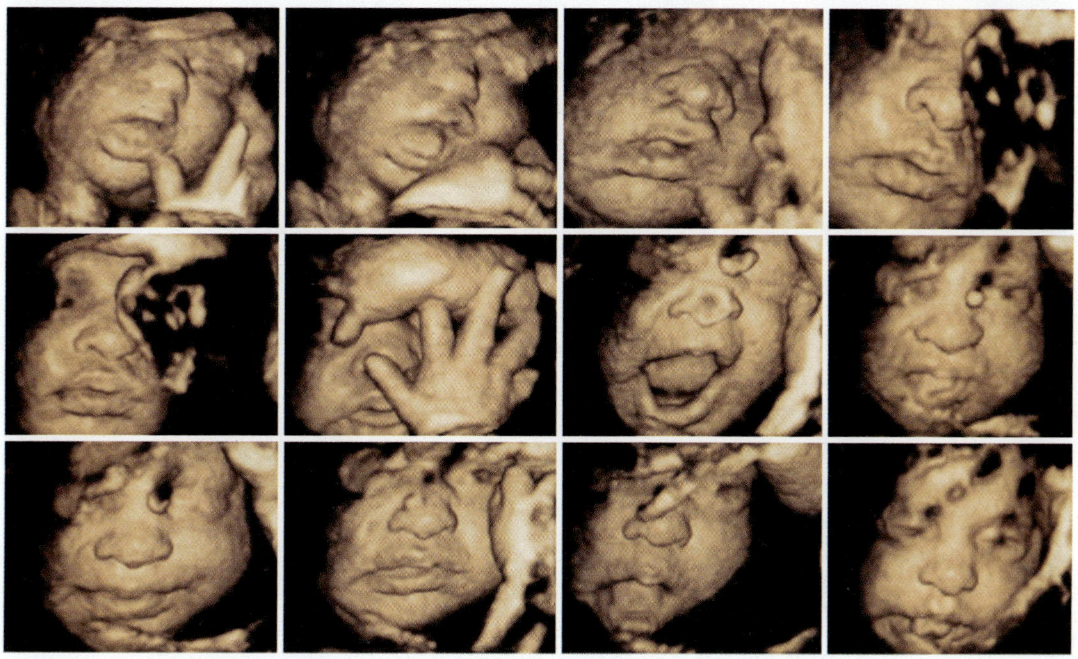

Fig. 8: A complete Kurjak's antenatal neurodevelopmental test (KANET)—facial alterations mouthing, eye blinking, and hand movement.

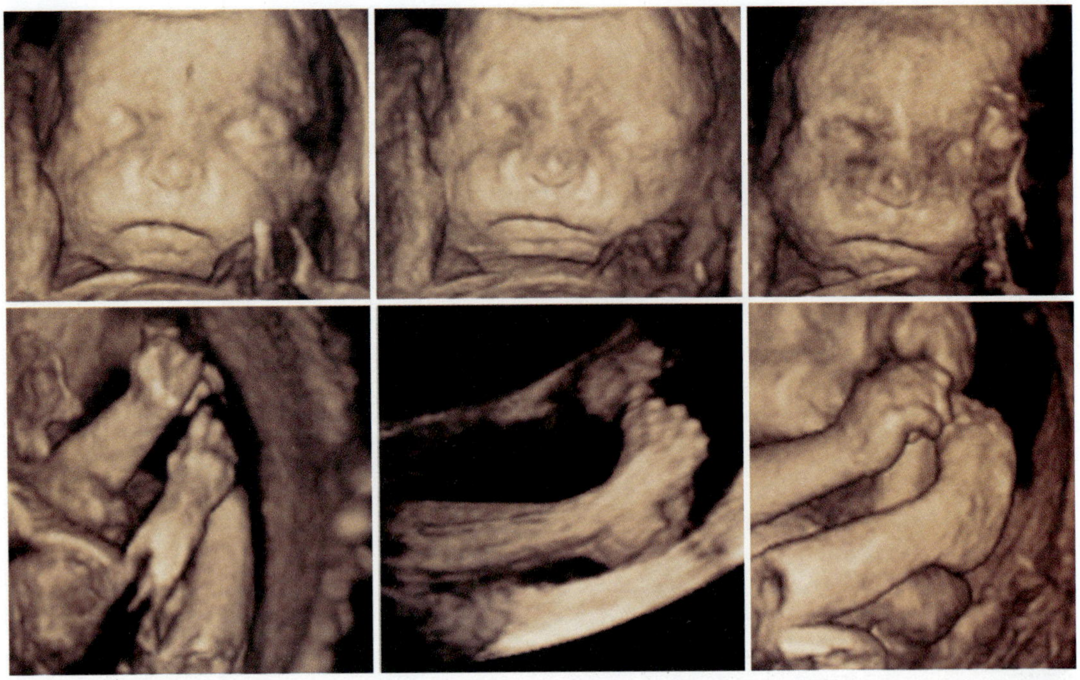

Fig. 9: Abnormal Kurjak's antenatal neurodevelopmental test (KANET) score at 28 weeks of a fetus with severe hydranencephaly after cytomegalovirus (CMV) infection. No facial alterations or mouth movements were identified ("frozen face or face like mask"), fists remained clenched and no leg movements were seen (right foot deviated inward—club foot).

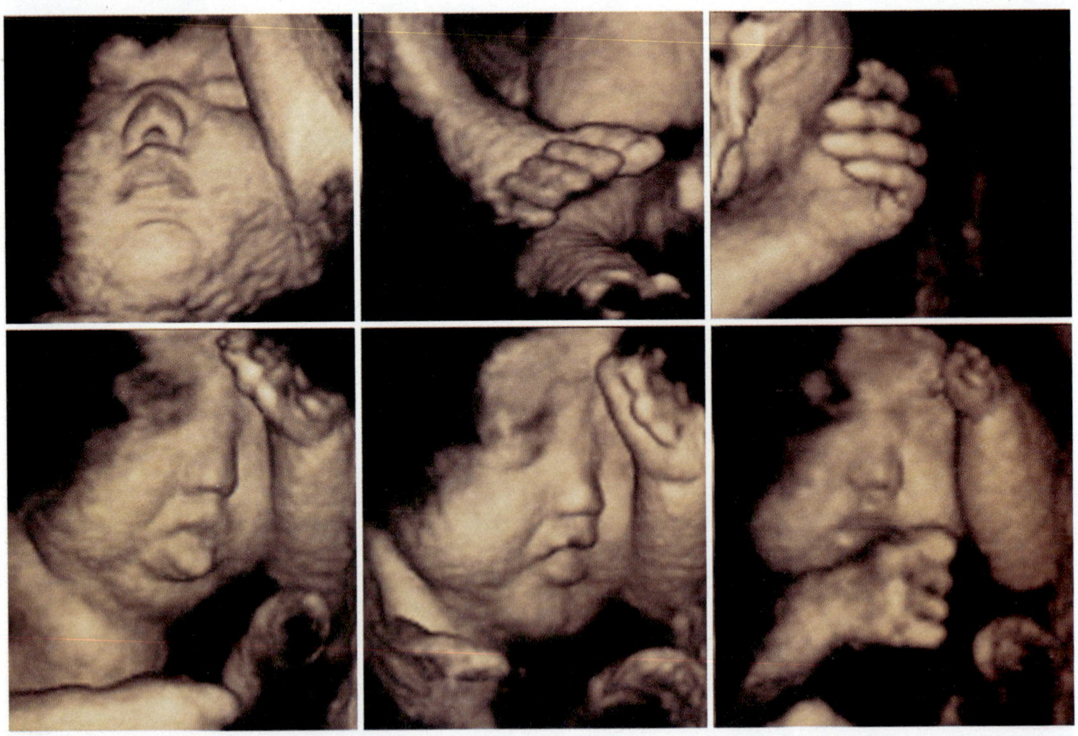

Fig. 10: Abnormal Kurjak's antenatal neurodevelopmental test (KANET) score at 31 weeks of gestation, of a fetus with semilobar holoprosencephaly. Mouth movements were identified (tongue expulsion), but otherwise facial alterations were minimal and the KANET score was abnormal (KANET score = 4). No leg movements were seen and neurological thumb was identified. Neonate died 3 days after delivery.

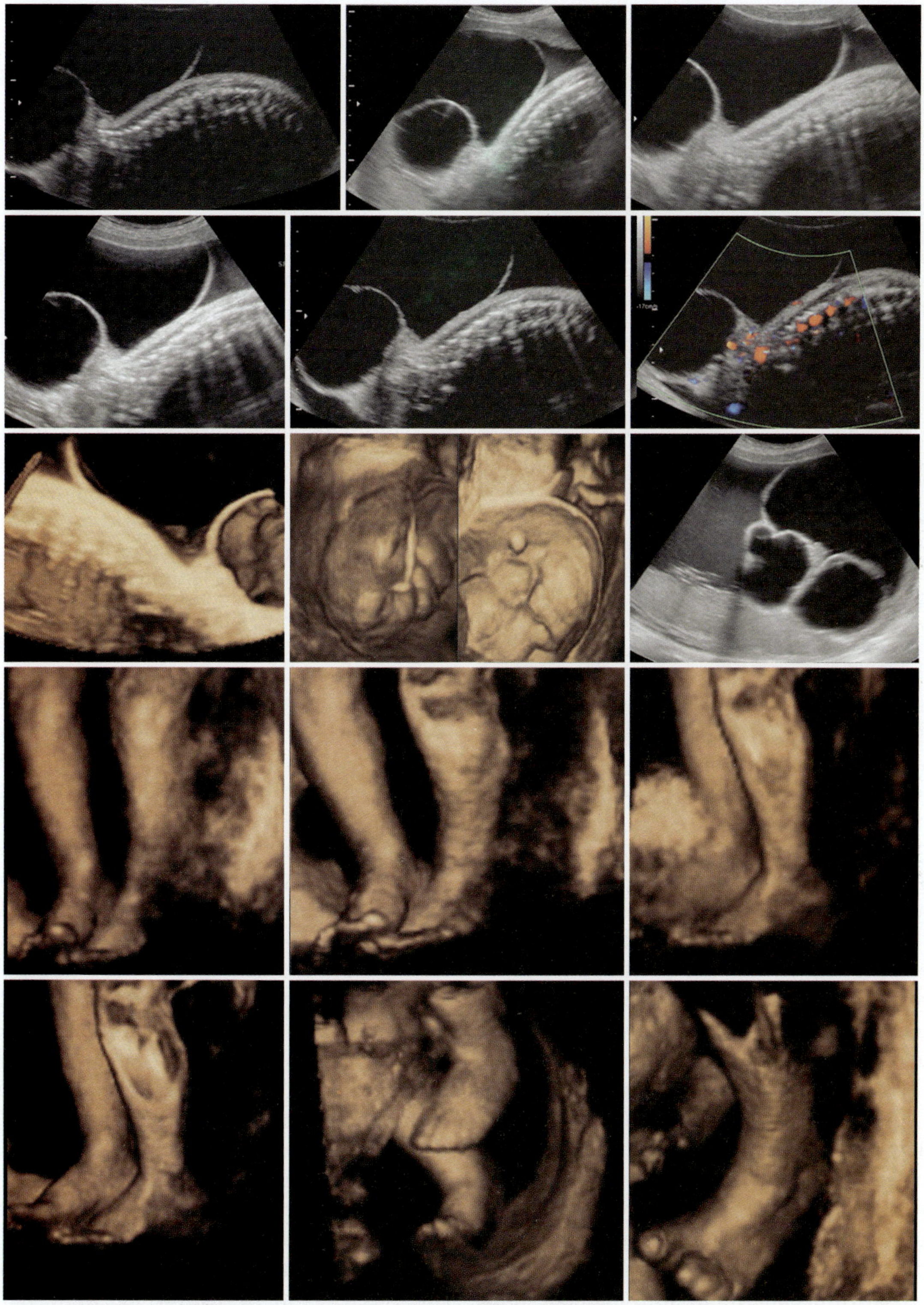

Fig. 11: Special application of Kurjak's antenatal neurodevelopmental test (KANET). This is a patient with sacrococcygeal teratoma. An ultrasound specialist experienced in KANET was asked to assess the integrity of the mobility of the lower extremities of the fetus. The experience acquired as KANET is applied in more and more cases which can offer a wide knowledge of the in utero behavior and motoric activity of the fetus and give answers to special problems.

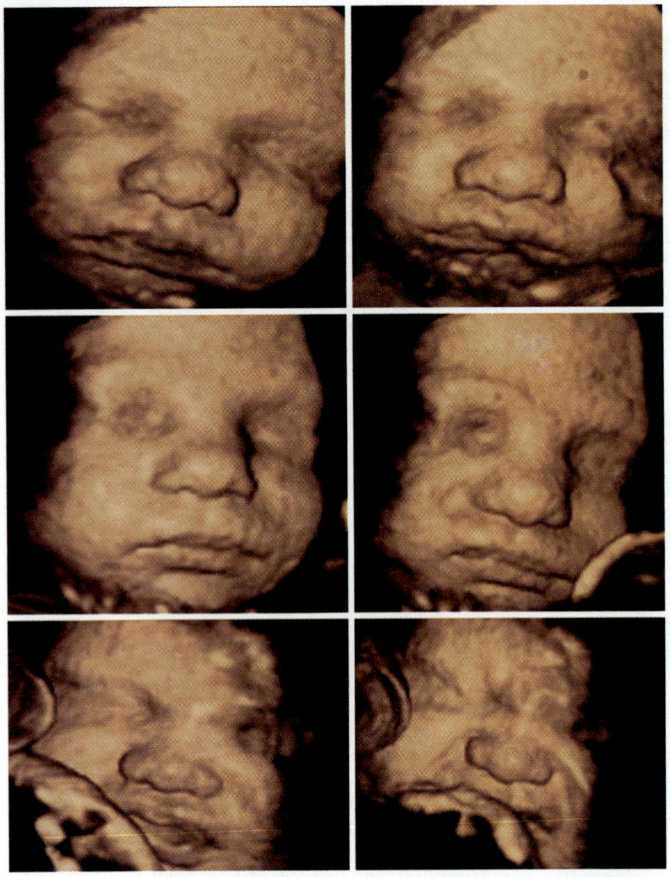

Fig. 12: Kurjak's antenatal neurodevelopmental test (KANET) test—facial alterations and grimacing.

forms of neurological impairment were examined and compared with "normal" neonates. The idea was to try and identify similar differences during in utero life in order to diagnose brain impairment prenatally. KANET was applied retrospectively in 100 low-risk pregnancies and all fetuses were assessed and after delivery, with the score 14–20 characterized as normal. Then the test was applied to 120 high-risk pregnancies according to the postnatal assessment, and neonates were divided into three groups: Normal, mildly or moderately abnormal, and abnormal. According to the results, the scoring system was divided to prenatal score 14–20 (normal), 5–13 (mildly or moderately abnormal), and 0–5 (abnormal). From the abnormal cases, four were diagnosed with alobar holoprosencephaly, one with severe hydrocephaly, one with thanatotrophic dysplasia, and four cases with multiple severe structural abnormalities. Following this preliminary study **(Table 4)**, many studies applied KANET and assessed its usefulness for the detection of neurological impairment during in utero life.[25,32]

In one of the studies out of 288 high-risk pregnancies, seven abnormal cases were included and also 25 cases with borderline KANET score, yielding 32 fetuses at neurological risk. There were also 11 cases with abnormal KANET, of which six fetuses died in utero and five were terminated. The seven remaining neonates with abnormal KANET were followed up postnatally at 10 weeks and from these neonates, three had confirmed pathological ATNAT score postpartum. These three cases included a neonate with arthrogryposis, a neonate with cerebellar vermian complete aplasia and one case with a history of CP in a previous pregnancy.

The main characteristic of these three cases was the facial expressions, which appeared significantly diminished—these faces are characterized as masks due to lack of expressions noted at the time of ultrasound examination. The remaining four cases with pathological KANET did not show abnormal ATNAT postnatally and the examiners characterized the neurological assessment as normal. These four cases included a case of ventriculomegaly, a case complicated by preeclampsia, one case with maternal thrombophilia and one case complicated by oligohydramnios. From the 25 cases diagnosed with borderline KANET result, 22 neonates showed a borderline ATNAT score and were followed up, while the three remaining cases showed normal ATNAT result. These three cases were complicated by ventriculomegaly, chorioamnionitis, and maternal thrombocytopenia, respectively. The cases with pathological prenatal score and normal postnatal ATNAT were characterized by the following risk factors: Ventriculomegaly, Dandy-Walker malformation, skeletal dysplasia, increased amniotic fluid, gestational diabetes, hydrocephaly, thrombophilia, preeclampsia, achondroplasia, oligohydramnios, nonimmune hydrops, chorioamnionitis, growth restriction, Down's syndrome, and thrombocytopenia.

From the three cases with pathological KANET, at neonatal assessment with ATNAT-2 showed confirmed abnormal Prechtl's GMs (these were the cases with arthrogryposis and with cerebellar vermis aplasia) while there were six more cases which were characterized as pathological (history of previous neonate with CP, Dandy-Walker syndrome, hydrocephaly, Down's syndrome, ventriculomegaly, and nonimmune hydrops). From the

TABLE 4: Application of KANET for the detection of neurological impairment.

Author	Year	Study	Study design	Study population	Indication	No.	GA (weeks)	Time (minutes)	Result	Summary
Kurjak et al.[15]	2008	Cohort	Retrospective	High risk	Multiple	220	20–36	30	Positive	Introduction of scoring system was proposed for antenatal assessment of fetal neurobehavior
Kurjak et al.[28]	2010	Multi-center	Prospective	High risk	Multiple	288	20–38	30	Positive	KANET appeared to be prognostic of identification of neurological impairment in utero. KANET also identified fetuses with severe anatomical anomalies, especially related to neurological damage
Miskovic et al.[32]	2010	Cohort	Prospective	High risk	Multiple	226	20–36	30	Positive	Correlation between ante-natal (KANET) and postnatal (ATNAT) results identified. KANET showed variations in the neurobehavior of fetuses from high to low risk cases
Talic et al.[31]	2011	Multi-center Cohort	Prospective	High risk	Multiple	620	26–38	15–20	Positive	KANET test had prognostic value in discriminating normal from borderline to pathological neurobehavior. Abnormal KANET scores were predictable of both intrauterine and postnatal death
Talic et al.[29]	2011	Multi-center Cohort	Prospective	High risk	Ventriculomegaly	240	32–36	10–15	Positive	Statistically significant difference in KANET scores between normal pregnancies and pregnancies with ventriculomegaly. Cases with pathological result and majority of cases with borderline results were noted in cases with severe ventriculomegaly, especially when combined with other anomalies
Honemeyer et al.[61]	2011	Cohort	Prospective	Unselected	Unselected	100	28–38	N/A	Positive	KANET result had a significant predictive value of a good postpartum neurological evaluation
Lebit et al.[27]	2011	Cohort	Prospective	Low risk	Normal 2D examination	144	7–38	15–20	Positive	A specific mode of in utero neurobehavior corresponding to each stage of pregnancy was noted
Abo-Yaqoub et al.[52]	2012	Cohort	Prospective	High risk	Multiple	80	20–38	15–20	Positive	Significant difference in KANET scores was noted. All antenatally abnormal KANET scores had also an abnormal postnatal neurological assessment
Vladareanu et al.[62]	2012	Cohort	Prospective	High risk	Multiple	196	24–38	N/A	Positive	• Most fetuses with normal KANET → low-risk, those with borderline → IUGR fetuses with increased MCA RI and most fetuses with abnormal KANET→ Threatened PTD with PPROM. Difference in fetal movements was identified between the two groups • For normal pregnancies → 93,4% of fetuses had normal score, for high-risk pregnancies → 78,5% of fetuses had a normal score

Contd...

Contd...

Author	Year	Study	Study design	Study population	Indication	No.	GA (weeks)	Time (minutes)	Result	Summary
Honemeyer et al.[63]	2012	Cohort	Prospective	High and low risk	Multiple	56	28–38	30 Maximum	Positive	Introduction of the average KANET score → combination of the mean value of KANET scores throughout pregnancy. Revealed a relationship of fetal diurnal rhythm with the pregnancy risk
Kurjak et al.[64]	2013	Cohort	Prospective	High and low risk	Multiple	869	28–38	20	Positive	Statistical differences regarding the distribution of normal, abnormal, and borderline results of KANET between low-risk and high-risk groups found. Fetal behavior was significantly different between the normal group and the high-risk subgroups
Predojevic et al.[65]	2014	Case study	Prospective	High risk	IUGR	5	31–39	30	Positive	KANET could recognize pathologic and borderline behavior in IUGR fetuses with or without blood flow redistribution. Combined assessment of hemodynamic and motoric parameters could enable in better diagnosis and consultation
Athanasiadis et al.[66]	2013	Cohort	Prospective	Unselected (high and low risk)	Multiple (IUGR, PET, and GDM)	152	Second and third trimester	N/A	Positive	The neurodevelopmental trimester score was statistically significant higher in the low risk in comparison to that of high risk group ($P < 0.0004$). The KANET results in the diabetes subgroup was higher when compared to that of the IUGR and the preeclampsia subgroup ($P = 0.0001$)
Neto et al.[60]	2014	Cohort	Prospective	High and low risk	Multiple	51	Third trimester	20	Positive	Statistical significance between high- and low-risk cases. All abnormal results come from high-risk cases
Hanaoka et al.[67]	2015	Cohort	Prospective	Mixed (Asian and Caucasian)	Multiple	167	Third trimester	N/A	Positive	Differences in pattern movements in different racial groups, so that ethnicity should be considered when performing KANET

(ATNAT: Amiel-Tison Neurological Assessment at Term; GDM: gestational diabetes mellitus; IUGR: intrauterine growth restriction; MCA: middle cerebral artery; No.: number of patients; PET: preeclamptic toxemia; PPROM: preterm premature rupture of membranes; PTD: preterm delivery; KANET: Kurjak's antenatal neurological test) remaining 21 neonates, all of them had normal optimal or suboptimal GMs.

An interesting case was that of a fetus with acrania and by studying this pregnancy they managed to document how fetal behavior altered from 20 weeks of gestation. The remarkable thing was that as pregnancy progressed and the control center of motoric activity shifted from the lower to the upper part the KANET score was becoming lower and lower, suggesting that neurological damage in later pregnancy is possible.[50]

A study with[54] 226 cases, including different study populations, identified three cases with pathological KANET. All three cases had chromosomal abnormalities and all three postnatally had also an abnormal ATNAT. Scores from antenatal KANET and postnatal ATNAT were compared between low and high-risk groups, and showed differences between them, for 8 out of the 10 parameters—these included: Head anteflexion, eye blinking, facial expressions—grimacing, tongue expulsion, mouth movement such as yawning, jawing, swallowing—isolated hand movements, hand-to-face movements, fist and finger movements, and GMs.

The comparison of the two tests revealed correlation between them, proving that the neonatal examination (ATNAT) was a satisfactory confirmation of the prenatal ultrasound examination (KANET), stating that possibly with further studies, this antenatal test could offer useful information about the neurological status of the fetus and be applied in clinical practice.

The largest study of KANET,[53] includes 620 cases, of both low- and high-risk populations (100 low-risk and 520 high-risk cases). This study did not include fetuses with anatomical anomalies that were studied between 26 and 38 weeks of gestation. The high-risk group included the following cases: Threatened preterm delivery with or without preterm premature rupture of membranes (PPROM), previous history of CP, pregnancy hypertension, preeclampsia, gestational diabetes, IUGR, polyhydramnios, Rhesus alloimmunization, placental abruption, and maternal fever >39°C.

Analysis revealed differences in the average KANET scores between high- and low-risk groups. The most cases of pathological KANET were identified in the cases that were characterized by a previous history of CP (23.8%) while the most cases of borderline KANET were noted in cases with maternal fever, which were possibly related to chorioamnionitis (56.4%). The parameters of KANET that were more notably different between the two groups were: Overlapping cranial sutures, head circumference, isolated eye blinking, facial expressions, mouth movements, isolated hand movements, isolated leg movements, hand-to-face movements, finger movements, and GMs. This study concluded that an abnormal KANET score is related with an increased risk of both intrauterine and neonatal mortality, but also with an increased risk of neurological impairment. What they also mentioned is that KANET is indicative of normal but also abnormal fetal neurobehavior, which can be demonstrated in postpartum life.

A study by Honemeyer and Kurjak[61] with 100 cases and a very good postnatal follow up of the neonates not only exactly at the time of delivery, before discharge from the hospital, but also at routine follow up at 3 months of life, showed that a good KANET score confirms up to a great extent and also normal neurological examination of the neonate at the time of delivery and at 3 months of age. A study by Lebit et al.[27] included 144 low-risk pregnancies, which they followed up antenatally from as early as 7 weeks up to 38 weeks, in order to define a specific pattern of fetal behavior that would be characterized as normal and correspond to each trimester. It appears that during the first weeks of pregnancy the number of fetal movements increases as does their complexity. In the second trimester the fetal motoric activity increases in number and different types of movements develop. More detailed movements such as facial grimacing and eye blinking tend to make their appearance during the middle of second trimester. Many women sustain that their perception of fetal movements decrease near term, that is because at that time fetal movements indeed decline in frequency as the duration of fetal rest periods increases as a result of fetal cerebral maturation rather than the fact as many people believe that the amniotic fluid decreases at the end of pregnancy.[25,26] Fetal behavior may reflect the level of CNS maturation and integrity and as a result KANET which assesses fetal behavior may offer useful information.[27] A study which applied KANET in 140 fetuses with ventriculomegaly[56] and compared them with 100 fetuses with normal CNS appearance during 32–36 weeks of gestation showed a big difference of abnormal KANET scores between the 2 groups (6% abnormal KANET in the low risk–control group compared to 34.9% in the group with ventriculomegaly). The greatest the degree of ventriculomegaly, the lowest the KANET score, especially when other anomalies were present.

What is interesting is that no cases of pathological KANET score were identified when the degree of ventriculomegaly was mild or moderate and no other anomalies were present. The study showed agreement of prenatal KANET test with the postpartum neonatal evaluation and also application of KANET in cases of ventriculomegaly offered the opportunity to identify fetuses who would not only have a structural anomaly but also their motoric activity would be affected, so that a complete assessment of the nervous system could be achieved, not only anatomically but also functionally. That is extremely important especially in cases of ventriculomegaly the importance of which and how will it affect a neonate is not always well understood.

A study of[52] 40 cases with increased risk for neurological anomalies applied KANET between 20 and 38 weeks of gestation and compared the results with a control group of 40 low-risk cases. They aimed to define the usefulness and feasibility of 4D ultrasonography in the assessment of fetal neurobehavior and also in the prediction of neurological impairment.

The two groups had significant differences in their KANET scores and the study showed that in all cases where the KANET score was abnormal also postnatally there was some degree of neurological impairment, while when the KANET score was normal or even borderline the neurological outcome postnatally was also normal. The parameters that were significantly different between the two groups were: Isolated head anteflexion, isolated eye blinking, facial expressions, mouth movements, isolated hand movements, hand-to-face movements, finger movements, and GMs. Regarding isolated leg movements and cranial sutures, the difference was not significant.

Vladareanu et al.[62] applied KANET in 196 singleton pregnancies (61 low risk and 135 at risk patients) from 24 to 38 weeks. The study lasted for 3 years. Most fetuses in the study who obtained normal KANET score belonged to the low-risk group. The majority of cases with borderline scores belonged to the IUGR group that also had high resistance index (RI) in the middle cerebral artery (MCA) while the majority of cases with pathological KANET score belonged to cases of threatened preterm labor with PPROM.

There was statistical significant difference in fetal movements in the two groups. In normal pregnancies, most fetuses (93.4%) achieved a normal KANET score compared to 78.5% of the fetuses from high-risk pregnancies. Borderline and abnormal scores were dominant in high-risk pregnancies. In the high-risk pregnancy group, most abnormal KANET scores were noted. In cases of threatened preterm delivery with PPROM (25%), most fetuses with pregnancies complicated by IUGR with MCA resistive index (RI) changes and with hypertension above 160/100 mm Hg achieved borderline score (50%). The highest percentage of normal fetal movements was found in pregnancies complicated by Rhesus alloimmunization without hydrops fetalis (96%). The characteristics of reduced speed and amplitude were found in the threatened preterm delivery group. There was a reduction of both number and duration of GMs in the IUGR group. The IUGR fetuses moved less and their GMs were poorly organized. Alterations in the quality of fetal movements were accompanied by considerable decrease in the quantity of fetal movements. The authors concluded that KANET can be useful in the detection of neurological impairment that could become obvious during the antenatal or postnatal period. Honemeyer et al.[63] studied 56 singleton pregnancies (24 low-risk and 32 high-risk cases) between 28 and 38 weeks of gestation and applied serial KANETs on them, performing a total of 117 tests in total. They did not identify any abnormal KANET scores, but two-thirds of the borderline scores occurred in the high-risk pregnancies. Because they performed more than one KANET in each pregnancy they introduced the average KANET score, which derived from the scores of each fetus during pregnancy. Only one fetus had a borderline average KANET score, and this fetus who belonged to the high-risk group was the only one out of 56 pregnancies who had an abnormal early neurological outcome. When the authors compared all the 18 borderline KANET scores with fetal diurnal rhythm based on maternal observation, they noticed that 89% of the borderline scores of the at-risk group were recorded at times that the mothers characterized them as active periods, compared with 33.3% in the low-risk pregnancies. The authors concluded that KANET is suggestive of expressing the risk for neurodevelopmental fetal disorders, but the connection of fetal diurnal rhythm and pregnancy risk status should be investigated further. Kurjak et al.[64] studied 869 high- and low-risk singleton pregnancies taking under consideration the results of the Doppler studies of umbilical artery and MCA, and noticed that fetal behavior was significantly different between the normal group and the following subgroups of fetuses: IUGR, gestational diabetes mellitus, threatened preterm birth, antepartum hemorrhage, maternal fever, sibling with CP, and polyhydramnios. The authors concluded that their study showed a new clinical application of the KANET test in early identification of fetuses prone to neurological impairment.

Athanasiades et al. studied with KANET 152 pregnancies of both low and high risk. According to the maternal background risk, there were 78 and 74 high-risk pregnancies (12 with IUGR fetuses, 24 with diabetes mellitus, and 38 with preeclampsia). The study showed that the neurodevelopmental score was statistically significant higher in the low-risk group compared to the high-risk group (P <0.0004). The diabetes subgroup score was statistically significantly higher compared to the IUGR and the preeclampsia subgroup (P = 0.0001). The authors concluded that the neurodevelopment fetal assessment by 4D ultrasound appears to be a feasible technique in the evaluation of high-risk pregnancies and the detection of differences in these populations.[66]

Neto Raul performed a pilot study in Brazil by applying KANET to 17 high-risk pregnancies and 34 low-risk pregnancies and compared the results. He noticed that for KANET score 0, 5, out of 8 parameters where significant different: Isolated head anteflexion, cranial sutures and head circumference, isolated hand movement or hand-to-face movements, isolated leg movement, and fingers movements. All abnormal KANET results derived from high-risk pregnancies (17.6%). No low-risk pregnancies presented with KANET score 0, concluding that there were important differences in fetal behavior between low- and high-risk pregnancies.[68]

Hanaoka et al. assessed with KANET 89 Japanese (representative of Asians) and 78 Croatian (representative of Caucasians) pregnant women and studied the total value of KANET score and values of each parameter (eight parameters) in the different populations. Total KANET score was normal in both populations, but there was a significant difference in total KANET scores between Japanese and Croatian fetuses. When individual KANET parameters were compared, significant differences were observed in four fetal movements (isolated head anteflexion, isolated eye blinking, facial alteration or mouth opening, and isolated leg movement). No significant differences were noted in the four other parameters (cranial suture and head circumference, isolated hand movement or hand to face movements, fingers movements, and gestalt of GMs) showing that ethnicity should be considered when evaluating fetal behavior, especially during assessment of fetal facial expressions. The authors concluded that although there was a difference in the total KANET score between Japanese and Croatian populations, all the scores in both groups were within normal range proving that ethnical differences in fetal behavior do not affect the total KANET score, but close follow-up should be continued in some borderline cases.[67]

Advantages of Early Detection of Neurodevelopmental Disorders In Utero

Once the diagnosis of neurological impairment is made in neonates the interventions available in everyday clinical practice are very limited and usually they prove to be ineffective. KANET offers the possibility of very early, prenatal detection of fetus at risk for neurological problems. This very early detection of these high-risk fetuses may be the key for the management of these cases, as the earlier you have a diagnosis, the earlier you may possibly intervene and as a result increase the possibility if not for treatment, for an improved outcome.[69-71] It has been suggested, e.g., for many years that early application of physiotherapy can be of some significance and that it can improve neurodevelopmental outcome. In Cochrane meta-analysis, it has been stated that early intervention programs for preterm infants have a positive influence on cognitive and motor outcomes during infancy, with the cognitive benefits persisting into preschool age. Of course, further research is needed to determine which early developmental interventions really make a difference in improving the cognitive or motoric function of neonates.[64,69-75] In one of the programs the primary caregivers have been educated about evidence-based interventions for improving infant self-regulation, postural stability, coordination and strength, parent mental health, and the parent–infant relationship. A therapy team consisting of a physiotherapist and psychologist delivered the nine sessions of the program (each session was 1.5–2 hours long) in the family home over the infant's first year of life. Infants and their caregivers have selective long-term benefits, with caregivers experiencing fewer anxiety symptoms and lower odds of an anxiety disorder and preschoolers showing fewer internalizing behavior problems.[76,77] It is obvious that we do not have many effective treatment options for cases of neurological impairment, but it appears that the earlier you apply these treatments, the better the results, and the earlier you have a diagnosis then indeed you can apply earlier these treatments to the correct group of people, and this is an area where definitely KANET can be a pioneer.[78,79]

A Decade with KANET: In-depth Analysis and Future Prospects

Over the past decade, KANET has emerged as a groundbreaking diagnostic tool, signaling a paradigm shift in how we approach prenatal diagnostics.[80] Its standout feature is its ability to detect complications that were once considered elusive by contemporary methodologies—most notably, fetal brain impairments and intricate neurodevelopmental variations.[81] As is customary with innovative methodologies, KANET's journey has been one of continuous learning and refinement.[82] Although the initial findings have been promising, the scientific community recognizes the need for larger, more diverse studies.[83] These investigations are crucial not only to corroborate the initial findings but also to identify any nuances or potential limitations of the technique.[84]

One of the most striking findings from preliminary studies is KANET's capability to provide detailed assessments of fetal neurobehavioral patterns.[85] Such insights are pivotal, as they allow medical professionals to identify and possibly intervene in cases where fetuses show signs of severe neurological complications, even before birth.[86] The feasibility of KANET is further accentuated by its potential integration into routine clinical practice.[87] Especially for high-risk pregnancies, the tool offers a ray of hope, ensuring that potential complications are identified early and managed efficiently.[88] Current research efforts are dedicated to optimizing KANET for broader applications. For instance, work is underway to establish comprehensive guidelines for fetal neurosonography and neurobehavior assessments—a step that will standardize procedures and outcomes.[89] A noteworthy aspect of KANET's evolution has been its synergistic relationship with 4D ultrasonography technology.[90] As 4D ultrasonography continues to advance, the granularity of insights that KANET can provide also amplifies.[91] This confluence of methodical fetal neurobehavior study and state-of-the-art technology signifies a promising trajectory.[85] In summary, the decade-long journey with KANET has been transformative. As the tool continues to mature and adapt, driven by rigorous research and technological advancements, the perinatal medicine community is poised to achieve unprecedented understanding and management of the fetal nervous system's functional development and maturation.[92]

NEONATAL ASPECTS OF FETAL BEHAVIOR

As we can learn from the previously presented data, neurobehavior is expression of development of CNS (in particular the brain), which is complex ongoing process throughout gestation and after birth.[92-95] It is important to understand how CNS produces different kind of movements and which of them are important for the assessment of disturbed CNS development. Fetuses and newborns exhibit a large number of endogenously generated motor patterns, which are presumably produced by central pattern generators located in different parts of the brain.[96] Moreover, substantial indications suggest that spontaneous activity is a more sensitive indicator of brain dysfunction than reactivity to sensory stimuli in reflex testing.[96] It has been demonstrated that in newborn infants affected by different brain lesions, spontaneous motility does not change in quantity, but it loses its elegance, fluency, and complexity. As the development of the brain is unique and continuing process throughout the gestation and after birth, it is expected that there is also continuity of fetal to neonatal movements which are the best functional indicator of developmental processes of the brain.[93-97]

Weight, length, and head circumference at birth were not significantly associated with neurodevelopmental outcome at the age of two for small for gestational age (SGA) or appropriate for gestational age (AGA) very low birth weight (VLBW) children.[98] However, weight and length at age two correlated with psychomotor developmental index (PDI) in SGA and AGA children.[98] These findings indicated an association between postnatal growth and neurodevelopmental outcome.[6] Thus, AGA children with catch down growth had the highest risk for mental retardation, motor delay, and CP among all VLBW children.[85] These findings were mostly independent of the diagnosis of CP.[6] The origin of CP in children born at term was considered to be prenatal in 38%, peri-/neonatal in 35% and unclassifiable in 27%, while in children born preterm it was 17%, 49% and 33%, respectively.[99-101]

Heinz Prechtl's work enabled that spontaneous motility during human development has been brought into focus of interest of many perinatologists prenatally and developmental neurologists postnatally.[102,103] According to the research preceding Prechtl's ingenious idea, during the development of the individual, the functional repertoire of the developing neural structure must meet the requirements of the organism and its environment.[102,103] This concept of ontogenetic adaptation fits excellently to the development of human organism, which is during each developmental stage adapted to the internal and external requirements.[102,103] The most important among those movements are so called general movements involving the whole body in a variable sequence of arm, leg, neck, and trunk movements, with gradual beginning and the end.[102,103] GMs are called fetal or preterm from 28 to 36 to 38 weeks of postmenstrual age, while after that we have at least two types of movements: Writhing present to 46–52 weeks of postmenstrual age and fidgety movements present till 54–58 weeks of postmenstrual age.[102,103] According to Hadders-Algra, GMs according to their fluency and complexity could be classified as normal-optimal, normal-suboptimal, mildly abnormal, and definitely abnormal.[103] Abnormality of GM has, however, limited value in the prediction of neurodevelopmental outcome in preschool children.[104]

Are we approaching the era when there will be applicable neurological test for fetus and assessment of neonate will be just the continuation?[64,105] This is still not easy question to answer, because even postnatally there are several neurological methods of evaluation, while in utero we are dealing with more complicated situation and less mature brain.[64,105] Could neonatal assessment of neurologically impaired fetuses bring some new insights into their prenatal neurological status is still unclear and to be investigated?[6,106] New scoring system for prenatal neurological assessment of the fetus proposed by Kurjak et al. will give some new possibilities to detect fetuses at high neurological risk, although it is obvious that dynamic and complicated process of functional CNS development is not easy to investigate.[78,79] Besides that there is an issue of different environments of fetal and neonatal development in term of the influence of the gravity. Data concerning the influence of the gravity on fetal motor development are contradictory. The concept that the fetus floats in a state of weightlessness cannot be applied to the whole pregnancy, and after the fetus is confined by the uterus, it is exposed to the force of gravity.[107-109] The fetus is not in significant contact with the walls of the amniotic sac until the very end of pregnancy, and sensory input arising from antigravity activity is absent, which is similar to the conditions of microgravity.[110] Certain level of mechanical stress is necessary for the physiological development of the fetus. Along with muscle activity, gravitational loading also causes this mechanical stress.[110] Buoyant forces apparently decrease fetal weight and in this way they reduce the effect of gravitation on the musculoskeletal system.[110] The development of antigravity muscular control is critical to normal motor development during the first year of life. After birth the newborn is exposed to the 1G environment. Movement against gravity begins during the first month of life, and by 4 months of age increased flexion control balances the strong extensor muscle patterns.[110] Adequate development of trunk flexion and extension is a prerequisite to the development of anterior and posterior pelvic tilting, lateral trunk flexion, and trunk elongation.[110] These components enable the child to develop weight shifting, which in turn stimulates righting and equilibrium responses.[110]

Concerning the continuity from fetus to neonate in terms of neurobehavior, it could be concluded that fetus and neonate are the same persons in different environment. While in the womb, fetus is protected from the gravity which is not so important for its neurodevelopment, postnatally the neonate is exposed to the gravity during the labor and from the first moments of autonomous life. Development of motor control is highly dependent on antigravity forces enabling erect posture of infant or young child. These environmental differences should be kept in mind during prenatal as well as postnatal assessment. This could be one of the reasons why assessment of GM is not considered as the reliable test for the long-term prediction of neurodevelopmental outcome.

CONCLUSION

One of the greatest challenges of obstetrical ultrasonography is the better understanding of fetal neurological function, a field with still many unanswered questions. The pathogenesis of major neurological conditions, such as CP, is not adequately understood and falsely attributed to accidents during labor, although it has been proven that the majority of CP cases originate sometime during in utero life and are not related to intrapartum events. The distinction between normal and abnormal fetal neurological behavior and the development of an accurate method for the assessment of the function of fetal nervous system is a great challenge in obstetrics, and that was made possible with the introduction of 4D ultrasound, which offered the opportunity to study the fetus in real time and with explicit detail.

Assessment of fetal behavior in utero has been proven by multicentric studies that it is possible with the application of KANET test, so that in many cases we can have an accurate diagnosis regarding some functional neurological abnormalities of fetuses. KANET is the first method that applied 4D ultrasound for the assessment of the fetus in the same way that a neonate is assessed neurologically after birth by neonatologists. KANET offers an objective scoring system that divides the fetuses according to the severity of the ultrasound findings and studies show that it can identify fetal signs that could predict its neurological development. What is more in cases of anatomical findings of uncertain significance and consequences on the neurological integrity of the fetus, like for example, in cases of ventriculomegaly, it offers the possibility of a more complete assessment of the fetus and therefore a more comprehensive counseling of the couples with an affected fetus.

Kurjak's antenatal neurodevelopmental test is currently used by many centers in everyday clinical practice as the investigational tool for normal and high-risk fetuses. It has acceptable sensitivity and specificity, and adequate positive and negative predictive value and also inter- and intraobserver reliability and can be easily learned by ultrasound specialists with access to 4D ultrasound machines. Aim of KANET test is to be widely applied in clinical practice for the selective screening of fetuses with moderate and high neurological risk, and hopefully early detection of these fetuses would firstly allow at last diagnosis of severe cases in utero and secondly an early intervention that could improve the outcome for these neonates.

REFERENCES

1. Yigiter AB, Kavak ZN. Normal standards of fetal behavior assessed by four-dimensional sonography. J Matern Fetal Neonatal Med. 2006;19:707-21.
2. Rees S, Harding R. Brain development during fetal life: Influences of the intrauterine environment. Neurosci Lett. 2004;361:111-4.
3. Joseph R. Fetal brain and cognitive development. Dev Rev. 1999;20:81-98.
4. Kurjak A, Carrera JM, Stanojevic M, et al. The role of 4D sonography in the neurological assessment of early human development. Ultrasound Rev Obstet Gynecol. 2004;4:148-59.
5. Eidelman AI. The living fetus—dilemmas in treatment at the edge of viability. In: Blazer S, Zimmer EZ (Eds). The Embryo: Scientific Discovery and Medical Ethics. Basel: Karger; 2005. pp. 351-70.
6. Stanojevic M, Zaputovic S, Bosnjak AP. Continuity between fetal and neonatal neurobehavior. Semin Fetal Neonatal Med. 2012;17:324-9.
7. Haak P, Lenski M, Hidecker MJ, et al. Cerebral palsy and aging. Dev Med Child Neurol. 2009;51:16-23.
8. Einspieler C, Prechtl HF. Prechtl's assessment of general movements: a diagnostic tool for the functional assessment of the young nervous system. Ment Retard Dev Disabil Res Rev. 2005;11:61-7.
9. Salihagic-Kadic A, Kurjak A, Medić M, et al. New data about embryonic and fetal neurodevelopment and behavior obtained by 3D and 4D sonography. J Perinat Med. 2005;33:478-90.
10. Moster D, Wilcox AJ, Vollset SE, et al. Cerebral palsy among term and postterm births. JAMA. 2010;304:976-82.
11. Almli CR, Ball RH, Wheeler ME. Human fetal and neonatal movement patterns: Gender difference and fetal-to-neonatal continuity. Dev Psychobiol. 2001;38:252-73.
12. DiPietro JA, Bronstein MH, Costigan KA, et al. What does fetal movement predict about behavior during the first two years of life? Dev Phych. 2002;40:358-71.
13. DiPetro JA, Hodson DM, Costigan KA, et al. Fetal antecedents of infant temperament. Child Dev. 1996;67:2568-83.
14. DiPietro JA, Costigan KA, Pressman EK. Fetal state concordance predicts infant state regulation. Early Hum Dev. 2002;68:1-13.
15. Thoman EB, Denenberg VH, Sievel J, et al. State organization in neonate: Developmental inconsistency indicates risk for developmental dysfunction. Neuropediatrics. 1981;12:45-54.
16. St James-Roberts I, Menon-Johansson P. Predicting infant crying from fetal movement data: an exploratory study. Early Hum Dev. 1999;54:55-62.
17. Einspieler C, Prechtl HF, Ferrari F. The qualitative assessment of general movements in preterm, term and young infants—review of the methodology. Early Hum Dev. 1997;50:47-60.
18. Precht HF. Qualitative changes of spontaneous movements in fetus and preterm infant are a marker of neurological dysfunction. Early Hum Dev. 1990;23:151-8.
19. de Vries JI, Visser GH, Prechtl HF. The emergence of fetal behaviour. II. Quantitative aspects. Early Hum Dev. 1985;12:99-120.
20. de Vries JI, Visser GH, Prechtl HF. The emergence of fetal behaviour. III. Individual differences and consistencies. Early Hum Dev. 1988;16:85-103.
21. de Vries JI, Visser GH, Prechtl HF. The emergence of fetal behaviour. I. Qualitative aspects. Early Hum Dev. 1982;7:301-22.
22. Nijhuis JG. Fetal Behaviour: Developmental and perinatal aspects. Oxford: Oxford University Press; 1992.
23. Prechtl HF. State of the art of a new functional assessment of the young nervous system. An early predictor of cerebral palsy. Early Hum Dev. 1997;50:1-11.
24. Kurjak A, Luetic AT. Fetal neurobehavior assessed by three-dimensional/four dimensional sonography. Zdrav Vestn. 2010;79:790-9.
25. Salihagic-Kadic A, Medic M, Kurjak A, et al. 4D sonography in the assessment of fetal functional neurodevelopment

and behavioural patterns. Ultrasound Rev Obstet Gynecol. 2005;5:1-15.

26. Kurjak A, Pooh R, Tikvica A, et al. Assessment of fetal neurobehavior by 3D/4D ultrasound. Fetal Neurology. 2009:222-50.
27. Lebit DF, Vladareanu PD. The role of 4D ultrasound in the assessment of fetal behaviour. Maedica (Buchar). 2011;6:120-7.
28. Merz E, Abramowicz JS. 3D/4D ultrasound in prenatal diagnosis: Is it time for routine use? Clin Obstet Gynecol. 2012;55:336-51.
29. Kurjak A, Vecek N, Hafner T, et al. Prenatal diagnosis: What does four-dimensional ultrasound add? J Perinat Med. 2002;30:57-62.
30. Kurjak A, Vecek N, Kupesic S, et al. Four-dimensional ultrasound: How much does it improve perinatal practice? In: Carrera JM, Chervenak FA, Kurjak A (Eds). Controversies in Perinatal Medicine: The Fetus as a Patient. New York: Parthenon Publishing; 2003. p. 222.
31. Andonotopo W, Stanojevic M, Kurjak A, et al. Assessment of fetal behavior and general movements by four-dimensional sonography. Ultras Rev Obstet Gynecol. 2004;4:103-8.
32. Kurjak A, Carrera J, Medic M, et al. The antenatal development of fetal behavioral patterns assessed by four-dimensional sonography. J Matern Fetal Neonatal Med. 2005;17:401-16.
33. Kurjak A, Miskovic B, Andonotopo W, et al. How useful is 3D and 4D ultrasound in perinatal medicine? J Perinat Med. 2007;35:10-27.
34. Kurjak A, Tikvica A, Stanojevic M, et al. The assessment of fetal neurobehavior by three-dimensional and four dimensional ultrasound. J Matern Fetal Neonatal Med. 2008;21:675-84.
35. Morokuma S, Fukushima K, Yumoto Y, et al. Simplified ultrasound screening for fetal brain function based on behavioral pattern. Early Hum Dev. 2007;83:177-81.
36. Kurjak A, Miskovic B, Stanojevic M, et al. New scoring system for fetal neurobehavior assessed by three- and four-dimensional sonography. J Perinat Med. 2008;36:73-81.
37. Gosselin J, Gahagan S, Amiel-Tison C. The Amiel-Tison Neurological Assessment at Term: Conceptual and methodological continuity in the course of follow-up. Ment Retard Dev Disabil Res Rev. 2005;11:34-51.
38. Amiel-Tison C, Gosselin J, Kurjak A. Neurosonography in the second half of fetal life: A neonatologist's point of view. J Perinat Med. 2006;34:437-46.
39. Tomasovic S, Predojevic M. 4D Ultrasound—Medical Devices for Recent Advances on the Etiology of Cerebral Palsy. Acta Inform Med. 2011;19:228-34.
40. Kurjak A, Stanojevic M, Andonotopo W, et al. Fetal behaviour assessed in all three trimesters of normal pregnancy by four-dimensional ultrasonography. Croat Med J. 2005;46:772-80.
41. Stanojevic M, Kurjak A, Salihagic-Kadic A, et al. Neurobehavioral continuity from fetus to neonate. J Perinat Med. 2011;39:171-7.
42. Kurjak A, Andonotopo W, Hafner T, et al. Normal standards for fetal neurobehavioral developments—longitudinal quantification by four-dimensional sonography. J Perinat Med. 2006;34:56-65.
43. Stanojevic M, Talic A, Miskovic B, et al. An attempt to standardize Kurjak's antenatal neurodevelopmental test: Osaka Consensus Statement. Donald School J Ultrasound Obstet Gynecol. 2011;5:317-29.
44. Pooh RK, Pooh K. Fetal VM. Donald School J Ultrasound Obstet Gynecol. 2007;1:40-6.
45. Kurjak A, Ahmed B, Abo-Yaquab S, et al. An attempt to introduce neurological test for fetus based on 3D and 4D sonography. Donald School J Ultrasound Obstet Gynecol. 2008;2:29-34.
46. Kuno A, Akiyama M, Yamashiro C, et al. Three-dimensional sonographic assessment of fetal behavior in the early second trimester of pregnancy. J Ultrasound Med. 2001;20:1271-5.
47. Koyanagi T, Horimoto N, Maeda H, et al. Abnormal behavioral patterns in the human fetus at term: Correlation with lesion sites in the central nervous system after birth. J Child Neurol. 1993;8:19-26.
48. Kurjak A, Stanojevic M, Andonotopo W, et al. Behavioral pattern continuity from prenatal to postnatal life—a study by four-dimensional (4D) ultrasonography. J Perinat Med. 2004;32:346-53.
49. Stanojevic M, Kurjak A. Continuity between Fetal and neonatal neurobehavior. Donald School J Ultrasound Obstet Gynecol. 2008;2:64-75.
50. Kurjak A, Abo-Yaqoub S, Stanojevic M, et al. The potential of 4D sonography in the assessment of fetal neurobehavior—multicentric study in high-risk pregnancies. J Perinat Med. 2010;38:77-82.
51. Andonotopo W, Kurjak A, Kosuta MI. Behavior of an anencephalic fetus studied by 4D sonography. J Matern Fetal Neonatal Med. 2005;17:165-8.
52. Abo-Yaqoub S, Kurjak A, Mohammed AB, et al. The role of 4-D ultrasonography in prenatal assessment of fetal neurobehaviour and prediction of neurological outcome. J Matern Fetal Neonatal Med. 2012;25:231-6.
53. Talic A, Kurjak A, Ahmed B, et al. The potential of 4D sonography in the assessment of fetal behavior in high-risk pregnancies. J Matern Fetal Neonatal Med. 2011;24:948-54.
54. Miskovic B, Vasilj O, Stanojevic M, et al. The comparison of fetal behavior in high risk and normal pregnancies assessed by four-dimensional ultrasound. J Matern Fetal Neonatal Med. 2010;23:1461-7.
55. Andonotopo W, Kurjak A. The assessment of fetal behavior of growth restricted fetuses by 4D sonography. J Perinat Med. 2006;34:471-8.
56. Talic A, Kurjak A, Stanojevic M, et al. The assessment of fetal brain function in fetuses with ventriculomegaly:

The role of the KANET test. J Matern Fetal Neonatal Med. 2012;25:1267-72.
57. Horimoto N, Koyanagi T, Maeda H, et al. Can brain impairment be detected by in utero behavioural patterns? Arch Dis Child. 1993;69:3-8.
58. Prechtl HF, Einspieler C. Is neurological assessment of the fetus possible? Eur J Obstet Gynecol Reprod Biol. 1997;75:81-4.
59. Nijhuis JG, Prechtl HF, Martin CB, et al. Are there behavioral states in the human fetus? Early Hum Dev. 1982;6:177-95.
60. Neto RM, Kurjak A. Recent results of the clinical application of KANET test. DSJUOG. 2015;9(20):420-5.
61. Honemeyer U, Kurjak A. The use of KANET test to assess fetal CNS function. First 100 cases. Uruguay: Poster presentation. 10th World Congress of Perinatal Medicine 8-11 November, 2011. p. 209.
62. Vladareanu R, Lebit D, Constantinescu S. Ultrasound assessment of fetal neurobehaviour in high-risk pregnancies. Donald School J Ultrasound Obstet Gynecol. 2012;6:132-47.
63. Honemeyer U, Talic A, Therwat A, et al. The clinical value of KANET in studying fetal neurobehavior in normal and at-risk pregnancies. J Perinat Med. 2013;41:187-97.
64. Kurjak A, Talic A, Honemeyer U, et al. Comparison between antenatal neurodevelopmental test and fetal Doppler in the assessment of fetal well-being. J Perinat Med. 2013;41:107-14.
65. Predojević M, Talić A, Stanojević M, et al. Assessment of motoric and hemodynamic parameters in growth restricted foetuses—case study. J Matern Fetal Neonatal Med. 2014;27:247-51.
66. Athanasiadis AP, Mikos T, Tambakoudis GP, et al. Neurodevelopmental fetal assessment using KANET scoring system in low and high risk pregnancies. J Matern Fetal Neonatal Med. 2013;26:363-8.
67. Hanaoka U, Hata T, Kananishi K, et al. Does ethnicity have an effect on fetal behavior? A comparison of Asian and Caucasian populations. J Perinat Med. 2016;44(2):217-21.
68. Neto RM. KANET in Brazil: First Experience. Donald School J Ultra sound Obstet Gynecol. 2015;9(1):1-5.
69. Greenwood C, Newman S, Impey L, et al. Cerebral palsy and clinical negligence litigation: A cohort study. BJOG. 2003;110:6-11.
70. Strijbis EM, Oudman I, van Essen P, et al. Cerebral palsy and the application of the international criteria for acute intrapartum hypoxia. Obstet Gynecol. 2006;107:1357-65.
71. de Vries JI, Fong BF. Changes in fetal motility as a result of congenital disorders: An overview. Ultrasound Obstet Gynecol. 2007;29:590-9.
72. Kurjak A, Predojevic M, Salihagic-Kadic A. Fetal brain function: Lessons learned and future challenges of 4D sonography. Donald School J Ultrasound Obstet Gynecol. 2010;2:85-92.
73. de Vries JI, Fong BF. Normal fetal motility: An overview. Ultrasound Obstet Gynecol. 2006;27:701-11.
74. Rosier-van Dunné FM, van Wezel-Meijler G, Bakker MP, et al. General movements in the perinatal period and its relation to echogenicity changes in the brain. Early Hum Dev. 2010;86:83-6.
75. Hata T, Kanenishi K, Akiyama M, et al. Real-time 3-D sonographic observation of fetal facial expression. J Obstet Gynaecol Res. 2005;31:337-40.
76. Kozuma S, Baba K, Okai T, et al. Dynamic observation of the fetal face by three-dimensional ultrasound. Ultrasound Obstet Gynecol. 1999;13:283-4.
77. Kurjak A, Azumendi G, Andonotopo W, et al. Three- and four-dimensional ultrasonography for the structural and functional evaluation of the fetal face. Am J Obstet Gynecol. 2007;196:16-28.
78. Stanojevic M, Antsaklis P, Salihadic-Kadic A, et al. Is Kurjak Antenatal Neurodevelopmental Test Ready for Routine Clinical Application? Bucharest Consensus Statement. DSJUOG. 2015;9(3):260-5.
79. Spencer-Smith MM, Spittle AJ, Doyle LW, et al. Long-term benefits of homebased preventive care for preterm infants: A randomized trial. Pediatr. 2012;130(6):1094-101.
80. Kurjak A, Antsaklis P. Recent Advances in the Study of Fetal Brain Structure and Function. Sci Arts Relig. 2022;1(1):81-93.
81. Leibovitz Z, Lerman-Sagie T, Haddad L. Fetal Brain Development: Regulating Processes and Related Malformations. Life (Basel). 2022;12(6):809.
82. Dorst MT, Anders SH, Chennupati S, et al. Health Information Technologies in the Support Systems of Pregnant Women and Their Caregivers: Mixed-Methods Study. J Med Internet Res. 2019;21(5):e10865.
83. Johnson-Williams B, Jean D, Liu Q, et al. The Importance of Diversity in Clinical Trials. Clin Pharmacol Ther. 2023;113(3):486-8.
84. American College of Obstetricians and Gynecologists' Committee on Practice Bulletins—Obstetrics; Committee on Genetics; Society for Maternal-Fetal Medicine. Screening for Fetal Chromosomal Abnormalities: ACOG Practice Bulletin, Number 226. Obstet Gynecol. 2020;136(4):e48-e69.
85. Moreira Neto R, Porovic S. Clinical study of fetal neurobehavior by the KANET test. J Perinat Med. 2018;46(6):631-9.
86. Barnes R. Early Intervention in Fetal Neurological Health. Pediatr Med Rev. 2022.
87. Kurjak A, Stanojevć M, Barišić LS, et al. Kurjak Antenatal Neurodevelopmental Test (KANET): A useful tool for fetal neurodevelopmental assessment. In: Schenker JG, Genazzani AR, Sciarra JJ (Eds). Clinical Management of Infertility. Reproductive Medicine for Clinicians, volume 2. Cham: Springer; 2021.
88. Antunes M, Viana CR, Charepe Z. Hope Aspects of the Women's Experience after Confirmation of a High-Risk Pregnancy Condition: A Systematic Scoping Review. Healthcare (Basel). 2022;10(12):2477.

89. Malinger G, Paladini D, Haratz KK, et al. ISUOG Practice Guidelines (updated): sonographic examination of the fetal central nervous system. Part 1: performance of screening examination and indications for targeted neurosonography. Ultrasound Obstet Gynecol. 2020;56(3):476-84. Erratum in: Ultrasound Obstet Gynecol. 2022;60(4):591.
90. Mathews L. Synergy of KANET and 4D Ultrasonography. TechMed Journal. 2022.
91. Leung KY. Applications of Advanced Ultrasound Technology in Obstetrics. Diagnostics (Basel). 2021;11(7):1217.
92. Sandman CA, Davis EP, Buss C, et al. Prenatal programming of human neurological function. Int J Pept. 2011;2011:837596.
93. Schacher S. Determination and differentiation in the development of the nervous system. In: Kandel ER, Schwartz JH (Eds). Principles of Neural Science, 2nd edition. New York-Amsterdam, Oxford: Elsevier Science Publishing; 1985. pp. 730-2.
94. Kostovic I. Prenatal development of nucleus basalis complex and related fibre system in man: A histochemical study. Neuroscience. 1986;17:1047-77.
95. Kostovic I. Zentralnervensystem. In: Hinrichsen KV (Ed). Humanembryologie. Berlin: Springer-Verlag; 1990. pp. 381-448.
96. Kuo AD. The relative roles of feedforward and feedback in the control of rhythmic movements. Motor Control. 2002;6:129-45.
97. Ferrari F, Cioni G, Einspieler C, et al. Cramped synchronized general movements in preterm infants as an early marker for cerebral palsy. Arch Pediatr Adolesc Med. 2002;156:460-7.
98. Latal-Hajnal B, Siebenthal K, Kovari H, et al. Postnatal growth in VLBW infants: Significant association with neurodevelopmental outcome. J Pediatr. 2003;143:163-70.
99. Himmelmann K, Hagberg G, Wiklund LM, et al. Dyskinetic cerebral palsy: A population-based study of children born between 1991 and 1998. Dev Med Child Neurol. 2007;49:246-51.
100. Palmer FB. Strategies for the early diagnosis of cerebral palsy. J Pediatr. 2004;145:S8-S11.
101. Hadders-Algra M. Early diagnosis and early intervention in cerebral palsy. Front Neurol. 2014;5:185.
102. Einspieler C, Marschik PB, Pansy J, et al. The general movement optimality score: A detailed assessment of general movements during preterm and term age. Dev Med Child Neurol. 2016;58(4):361-8.
103. Hadders-Algra M. General movements: A window for early identification of children at high risk for developmental disorders. J Pediatr. 2004;145:S12-8.
104. Bennema AN, Schendelaar P, Seggers J, et al. Predictive value of general movements' quality in low-risk infants for minor neurological dysfunction and behavioural problems at preschool age. Early Hum Dev. 2016;94:19-24.
105. Kurjak A, Talic A, Stanojevic M, et al. The study of fetal neurobehavior in twins in all three trimesters of pregnancy. J Matern Fetal Neonatal Med. 2013;26(12):1186-95.
106. Stanojevic M. Antenatal and postanatal assessment of neurobehavior: Which one should be used? Donald School J Obstet Gynecol. 2015;9(1):67-74.
107. Sekulic SR, Lukac DD, Naumovic NM. The fetus cannot exercise like an astronaut: Gravity loading is necessary for the physiological development during second half of pregnancy. Med Hypotheses. 2005;64:221-8.
108. Assaiante C, Mallau S, Viel S, et al. Development of postural control in healthy children: A functional approach. Neural Plast. 2005;12:109-18.
109. Sellers JS. Relationship between antigravity control and postural control in young children. Phys Ther. 1988;68:486-90.
110. Meigal AY. Synergistic action of gravity and temperature on the motor system within the lifespan: A "Baby Astronaut" hypothesis. Med Hypotheses. 2013;80(3):275-83.

37

CHAPTER

Fetal Brain Function and Artificial Intelligence

Yasunari Miyagi, Toshiyuki Hata, Takahito Miyake

INTRODUCTION

Little is currently known about fetal brain activity. To understand this activity, it is necessary to obtain information from the fetus and for us to understand it correctly and objectively. The perceptions we can recognize are sight, hearing, touch, smell, taste, and depth, but our visual observation of fetal movements is probably the most effective way to recognize fetal brain activity. Noninvasive methods to obtain information on fetal movements are limited, and ultrasound is best suited for this purpose. Observation of fetal facial expressions is particularly suitable for examining fetal brain activity, because facial expressions are considered to reflect brain activity.[1-11]

Fetal expressions can be observed in four-dimensional (4D) ultrasound images[2,12] and are considered to relate to such activity.[1,3] Since understanding of fetal facial expressions depends on the subjectivity of the observer, it is desirable for the judgment criteria to be uniform. For this purpose, the application of artificial intelligence (AI) that can recognize facial expressions is useful. Such AI could be used to investigate the nature of fetal brain activity objectively and quantitatively.

FETAL FACIAL EXPRESSIONS RECOGNIZED BY ARTIFICIAL INTELLIGENCE

There are eight main fetal expressions: Blinking, mouthing, neutral, scowling, smiling, sucking, tongue expulsion, and yawning, excluding rare expressions. Eye blinking (blinking) is a reflex response possibly related to brain function maturation and development that occurs with advancing gestation.[12-16] Mouthing is the most frequent expression and is recognized as a sign of fetal brain maturation if it occurs together with nonrapid eye movement after 35 weeks of gestation.[17] The frequency of scowling, which may indicate fetal suffering in utero such as pain or stress,[18] increases with advancing gestation.[12] Smiling might indicate a state of brain development whereby the fetus can perform complex facial movements.[13,14] The correlation of an expressionless face and tongue expulsion with the brain function is unclear.[12] Yawning may be utilized as an index of fetal development.[19,20] Miyagi et al. (2021) created original AI to classify fetal expressions using pregnant women with a singleton fetus from 19 to 38 weeks of gestation.[21,22] The AI classifier is able to recognize seven facial expressions: Blinking, mouthing, neutral, scowling, smiling, tongue expulsion, and yawning, excluding sucking, for which few cases were observed. The AI classifier can also generate seven different confidence scores as probability values for each of the seven types of facial expressions in a single still image. Sample images classified by AI are shown in **Figure 1**. The AI classifier is composed of a convolutional neural network (CNN).[23-28] CNN comprises layers with a combination of convolutional layers such as pooling layers,[29-31] linear layers,[32,33] flattened layers,[34] batch normalization layers,[35] rectified linear unit layers,[36,37] and softmax layers,[38,39] which present the probabilities of each category, named confidence scores. The accuracy/sensitivity/specificity values were 0.996/0.964/1.000, 1.000/1.000/1.000, 0.996/1.000/0.994, 1.000/1.000/1.000, 1.000/1.000/1.000, 1.000/1.000/1.000, and 1.000/1.000/1.000 for blinking, mouthing, neutral face, scowling, smiling, tongue expulsion, and yawning, respectively **(Table 1 and Fig. 2)**. Other statistical values, such as the negative predictive value, positive predictive value, and area under the receiver operating characteristic (ROC) curve, were over 0.96 in all categories.

The AI classifier was applied for analyzing the seven types of fetal facial expressions in videos from 4D ultrasound equipment for singleton pregnancies at

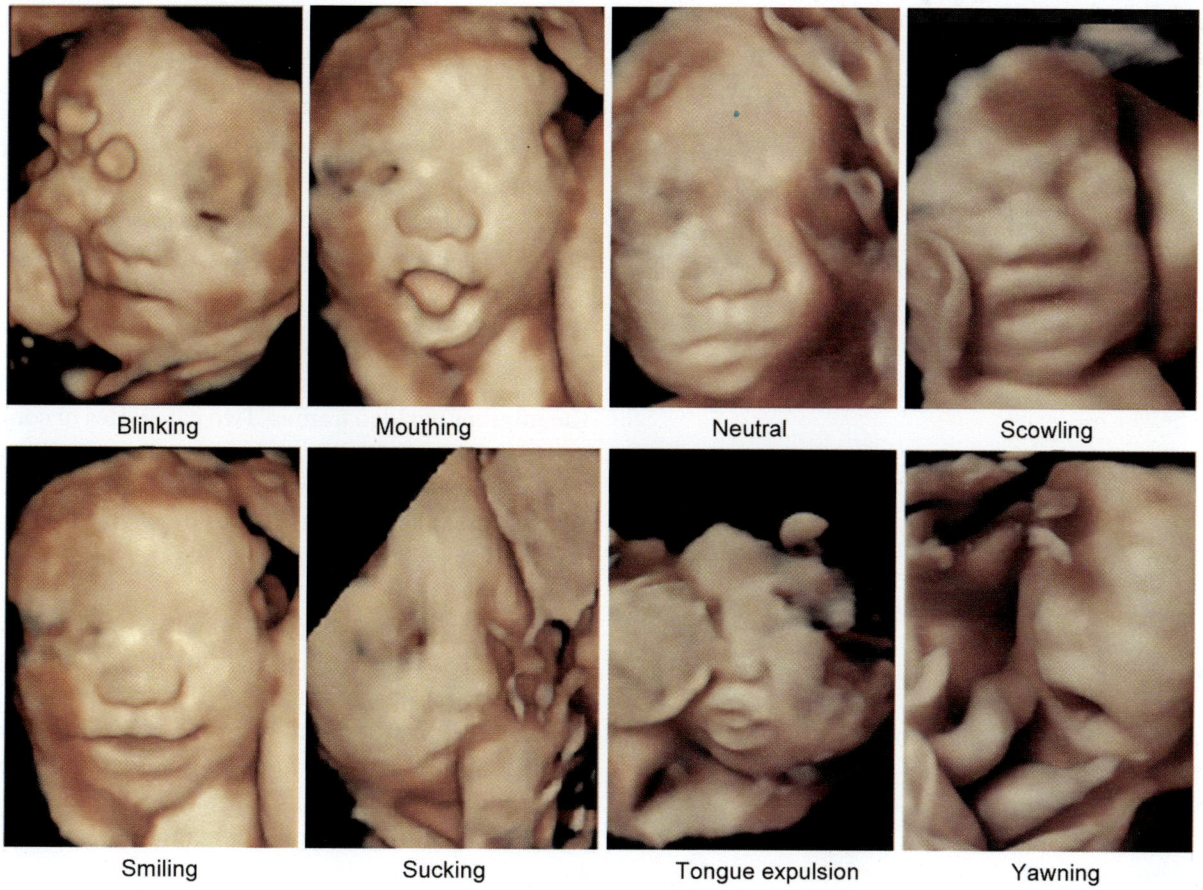

Fig. 1: Sample images of eight fetal facial expressions.

TABLE 1: Statistical results of artificial intelligence (AI) for classifying fetal facial expressions.

Statistic	*Blinking*	*Mouthing*	*Neutral*	*Scowling*	*Smiling*	*Tongue expulsion*	*Yawning*
True positive number	27	90	88	9	4	7	25
True negative number	223	161	162	242	247	244	226
False positive number	0	0	1	0	0	0	0
False negative number	1	0	0	0	0	0	0
Accuracy	0.996	1.000	0.996	1.000	1.000	1.000	1.000
Area under ROC curve	1.000	1.000	1.000	1.000	1.000	1.000	1.000
Negative predictive value	0.996	1.000	1.000	1.000	1.000	1.000	1.000
Positive predictive value	1.000	1.000	0.989	1.000	1.000	1.000	1.000
Sensitivity	0.964	1.000	1.000	1.000	1.000	1.000	1.000
Specificity	1.000	1.000	0.994	1.000	1.000	1.000	1.000

(ROC: receiver operating characteristic)
Source: Miyagi Y, et al.[22]

27–37 weeks of gestation.[21,22] Then, the seven-dimensional time-series confidence score lists were obtained. The seven-dimensional time-series confidence score lists per fetus were as follows:

$$\boldsymbol{x}_j = {}^t\{x_{j_1}, x_{j2}, \ldots, x_{j7}\}$$

There was a significant difference in confidence scores among the categories of facial expressions [$P < 1.00 \times 10^{-11}$ by one-way analysis of variance (ANOVA)]. Mouthing was the most prevalent (47–49%), followed by neutral (37–40%). The frequencies of other facial expressions were <5%; notably, scowling, smiling, and tongue expulsion were all <2%.

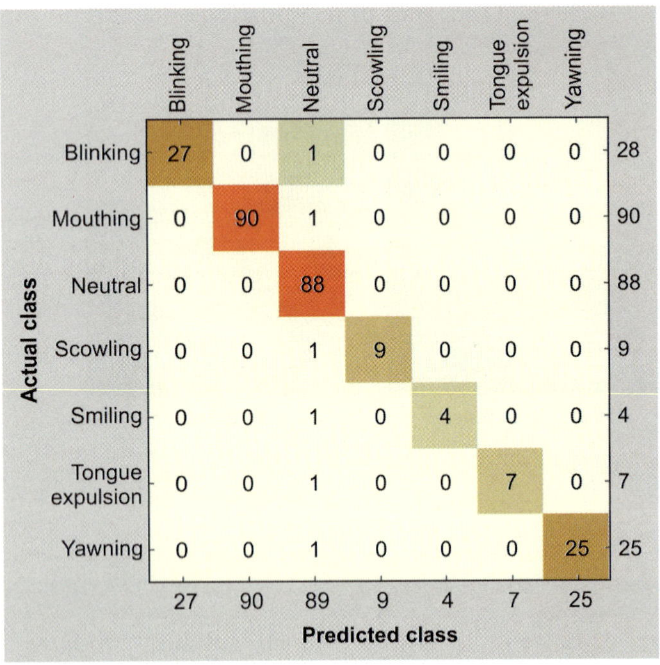

Fig. 2: The confusion matrix plot for the test dataset. The correct predictions were located in a diagonal matrix position.
Source: Miyagi Y, et al.[22]

DISCRETE FOURIER TRANSFORM AND CHAOTIC DIMENSION ANALYSIS

Discrete Fourier Transform

The seven-dimensional vector lists were investigated using discrete Fourier transform (DFT) and chaotic analysis.

The first five power spectra and corresponding periods for each facial category of all the sets were obtained by:

$$\frac{1}{\sqrt{N_j}} \sum_{j=1}^{N_j} {}^t\boldsymbol{x}_j \, e^{2\pi i(j-1)(x-1)/N_j}$$

where $i^2 = -1$, j is the facial category number, and N is the number of video frames. Two categories of confidence score profiles, dense and sparse, were discovered. The dense status showed marked fluctuation of the numerical value, and sparse status showed little fluctuation. **Figure 3** presents a sample profile of confidence scores showing the states.

The period was approximately 70 seconds for all expressions, with no significant differences between them. The power spectrum by DFT showed that mouthing and neutral components were the most dominant. 200 seconds, equal to the frame length, was the maximum period in all categories. Neutral had the largest power spectrum, followed by mouthing. There was a difference between categories for the power spectrum ($P = 0.004$ by one-way ANOVA). There were no differences in periods between the categories.

Chaotic Dimension Analysis

The seven-dimensional vector list was applied to a practical algorithm to determine the character of strange attractors.[40-44] The vector xi by shifting time τ was reconstructed:

$$\boldsymbol{Y}_j = \{{}^t\boldsymbol{x}_{jk}, {}^t\boldsymbol{x}_{j,\,k+\tau}, \ldots, {}^t\boldsymbol{x}_{j,\,k+(m-1)\tau}\}, \ (k = 1, 2, \ldots, N_i)$$

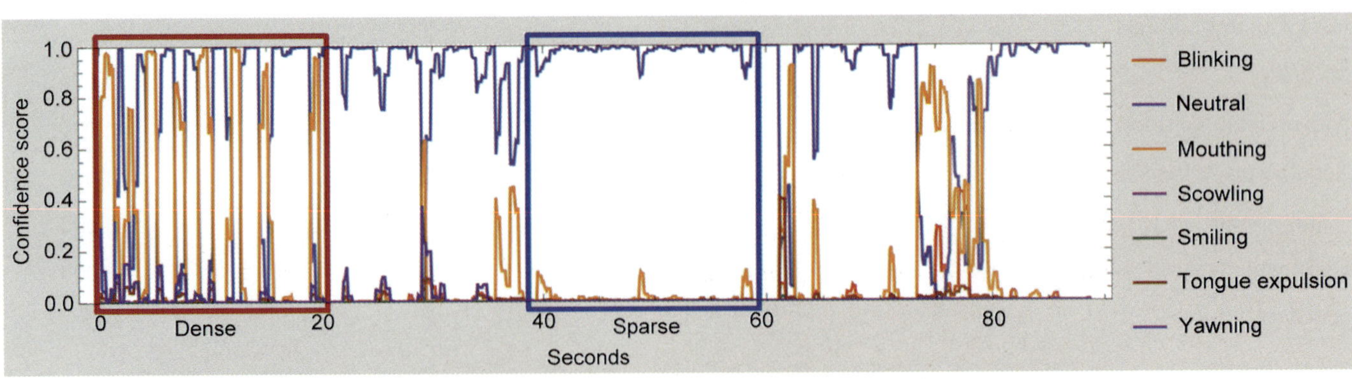

Fig. 3: A sample profile of confidence scores showing the dense and sparse states.

where τ is the time, j is the facial category number, m is the embedding dimension, and N is the number of video frames.

Then, the correlation dimension, D_2, was calculated as follows:

$$C_j(r) = \frac{1}{N_j^2} \sum_{f=1}^{N_i} \sum_{g=1}^{N_i} Q(r - |\boldsymbol{Y}_{jf} - \boldsymbol{Y}_{jg}|)$$

$$p_j = \frac{1}{N_{ij}} \sum_{g=1}^{N_j} Q(r - |\boldsymbol{Y}_{jf} - \boldsymbol{Y}_{jg}|)$$

$$D_{2j} = \lim_{r \to 0} \frac{\log C_j(r)}{\log r} = \lim_{r \to 0} \frac{\sum_{j=1}^{N_j} p_j^2}{\log r}$$

where r is $\{r \in \mathbb{R} \mid r > 0\}$ and Q is a Heaviside step function. The generalized dimension,[45] D_q, was obtained as follows:

$$D_{qj} = \frac{1}{q-1} \lim_{r \to 0} \frac{\log \sum_{j=1}^{n(r)} p_j^q}{\log r}$$

where $n(r)$ is the number of spheres required to cover the object (orbit) with a sphere of radius r, and q is $\{q \in \mathbb{R}\}$.

The capacity dimension, D_0, was obtained as follows:

$$D_{0j} = -\lim_{r \to 0} \frac{\log n_j(r)}{\log r}$$

The information dimension, D_1, was obtained as follows:

$$D_{1j} = \lim_{r \to 0} \frac{\log \sum_{j=1}^{n_j(r)} p_j \log p_j}{\log r}$$

The α-f (α) profile graph was obtained using D_{qj}:[40]

$$D_q = \frac{1}{q-1}\{q\,\alpha(q) - f(\alpha(q))\}$$

These chaos analyses were applied not only for a seven-dimensional vector, ${}^t\{{}^t\boldsymbol{Y}_1, {}^t\boldsymbol{Y}_2, \ldots, {}^t\boldsymbol{Y}_7\}$, but also each element of the vector of category $\boldsymbol{Y}_j$; $\{j = 1, 2, \ldots, 7\}$.

For D_2, there were no significant differences by fetal sex, maternal age, or gestational week (data not shown). There was no significant difference in D_2 between categories ($P = 0.068$), although there was a trend toward a smaller median value for neutral. This tendency suggests that the low D_2 in neutral was the basic state, and the energy needed for fetal development might be lower for neutral in terms of facial muscle movement and brain activity in utero.

D_2 was significantly smaller in the dense state than in the sparse state ($P = 0.047$) **(Fig. 4)**.[46] There was no difference by variance between the two states. **Figure 5** shows the case of a male fetus at 36 weeks of gestation.[46] Fluctuation in D_2 was noted in conjunction with changes in the dense/sparse state. Chaotic analysis of the data objectively and quantitatively showed the existence of fluctuations in fetal brain activity.

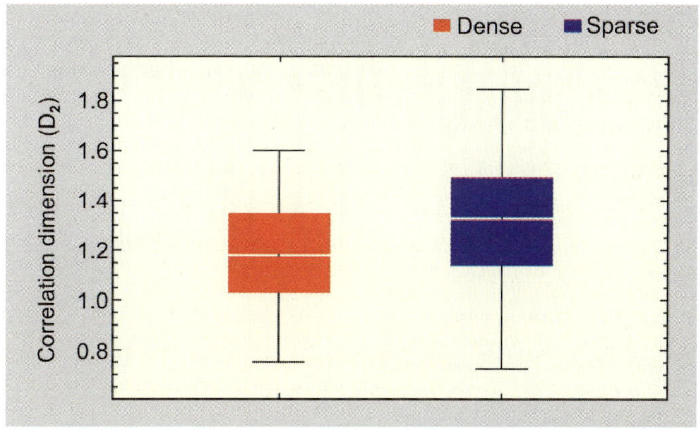

Fig. 4: Comparison of correlation dimension, D_2, in dense and sparse states. D_2 was significantly smaller in the dense state than in the sparse state; $P = 0.035$ and $P = 0.047$ by t-test and Mann–Whitney test, respectively.
Source: Miyagi Y, et al.[46]

THE FREE-ENERGY PRINCIPLE

Miyagi et al. (2023) explained what the fluctuation in D_2 between the dense and sparse status by chaotic dimension analysis meant using a mathematical model based on the free-energy principle.[47] The free-energy principle with active inference is a comprehensive theory that attempts to explain the structure and function of cognition and the brain's behavior.[48-51] The theory is based on a variational Bayesian estimate to provide a comprehensive explanation of action, emotion, perception, sentiment, and decision-making. The agent performs active inference to minimize the system's informational free energy and reduce the prediction error from the current presumption to the generated model for any self-organized system to be in equilibrium within its environment. An agent using a free-energy formulation of perception adjusts its internal states and sampling of the environment to minimize their free energy.[51]

The free energy, F, in generating a fetal expression model using the free-energy principle was applied in order to explain fetal facial behavior, as follows:

$$F(\tilde{o}, \mu) = D_{KL}[Q(\tilde{s}, \tilde{u} \mid \mu) \,\|\, p(\tilde{s}, \tilde{u} \mid \tilde{o})] - \ln P(\tilde{o} \mid mdl)$$

$$\mu_t = \arg\min{}_{\mu} F(\{o0, \ldots, o_{t+1}\}, \mu)$$

$$a_t = \arg\min{}_a \sum_{\Omega} P(o_{t+1} \mid o_t, a) F(\{o_0, \ldots, o_{t+1}\}, \mu_t)$$

$$\boldsymbol{x} \in a$$

$$\tilde{o} = (o_1, o_2 \ldots, o_t)$$

$$\tilde{S} = (s_1, s_2, \ldots s_t)$$

$$\tilde{u} = (u_1, u_{2,} \ldots u_t)$$

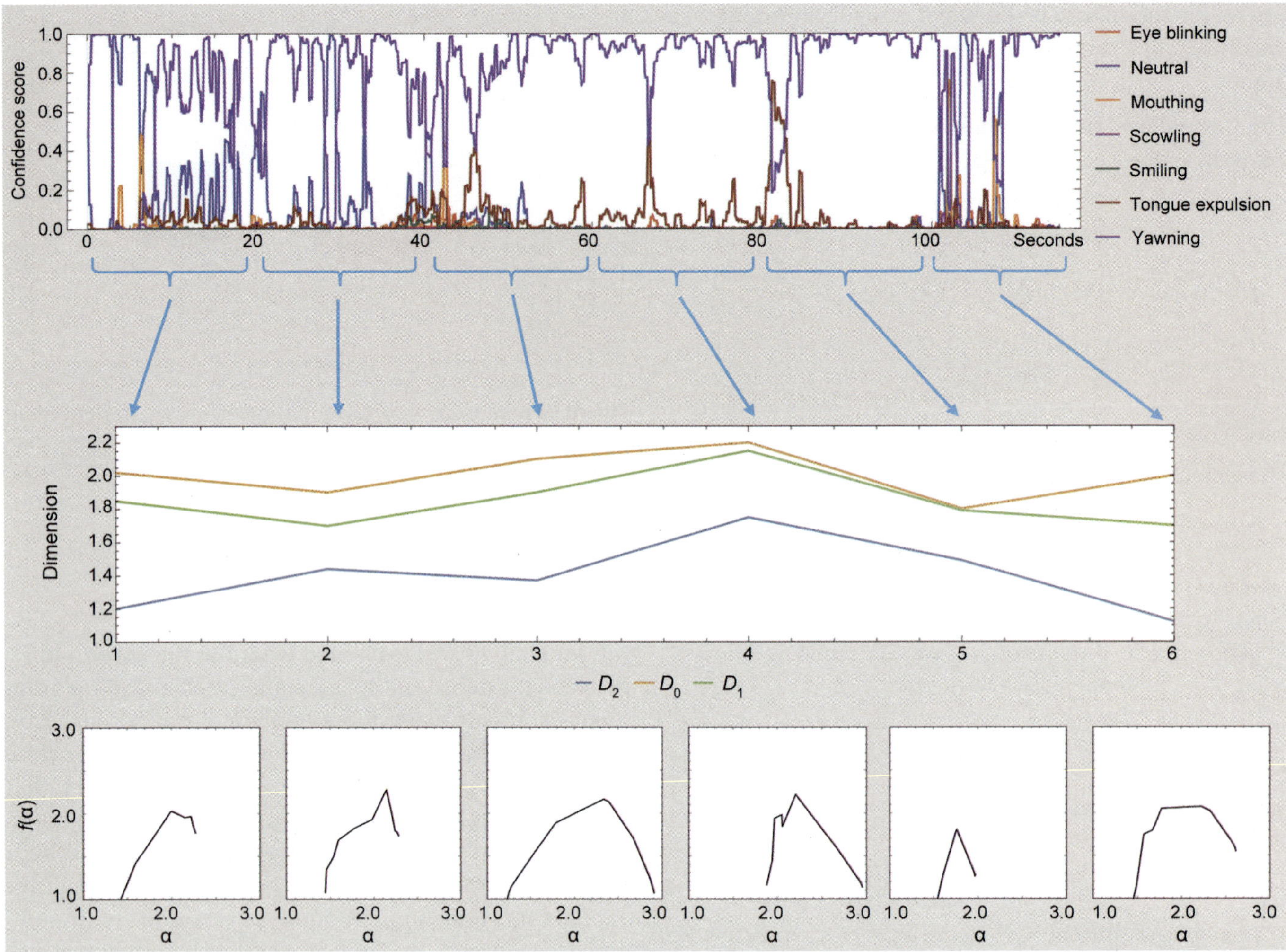

Fig. 5: A male fetus at 36 weeks of gestation. A fetal facial video was divided into 20 seconds intervals. The upper panel shows confidence score profiles of seven facial expression categories in accordance with facial image samples. The dense state was observed during the first 50 seconds, and then the sparse state followed. The dense state appeared again at 100–110 seconds. Fluctuation of the dimensions was observed. The variation profiles of D_0, D_1, and D_2 are shown (middle panel). Variations of the α– $f(\alpha)$ profiles, where $q = \{-5, -4, ..., 5\}$, derived from a seven-dimensional vector with each set, are demonstrated in the bottom panel.
Source: Miyagi Y, et al.[46]

where a is an action, D_{KL} is the Kullback-Leibler divergence,[52] *mdl* is a model, o_t is an observation, P is the generative density, Q is the recognition density, s_t is a hidden state, u is prediction of the result of causing an action,[53] Ω is a set of observations, μ represents sufficient statistics,[49] and μ_t is perception.

When facial expressions of a fetus are focused on:

$$x \approx a$$

Samples of the sparse and dense statuses are shown in **Figures 6 and 7**, respectively. The fetal expression image with the bar chart of the seven confidence scores generated by AI and the line graph of the confidence score time-series profiles are shown in the upper and lower panels, respectively. Each is a still image from a video in the sparse and dense statuses of the confidence score lists. A dense score list shows that the categories of expression categories are dispersed, while sparse shows that the score was concentrated on a specific category of fetal facial expression. The correlation, information, and capacity dimensions of the seven-dimensional time-series lists were 1.85, 2.23, and 2.25, and 0.79, 1.40, and 1.94 in the sparse and dense statuses, respectively. All three dimensions for the sparse status were larger than for the dense status.

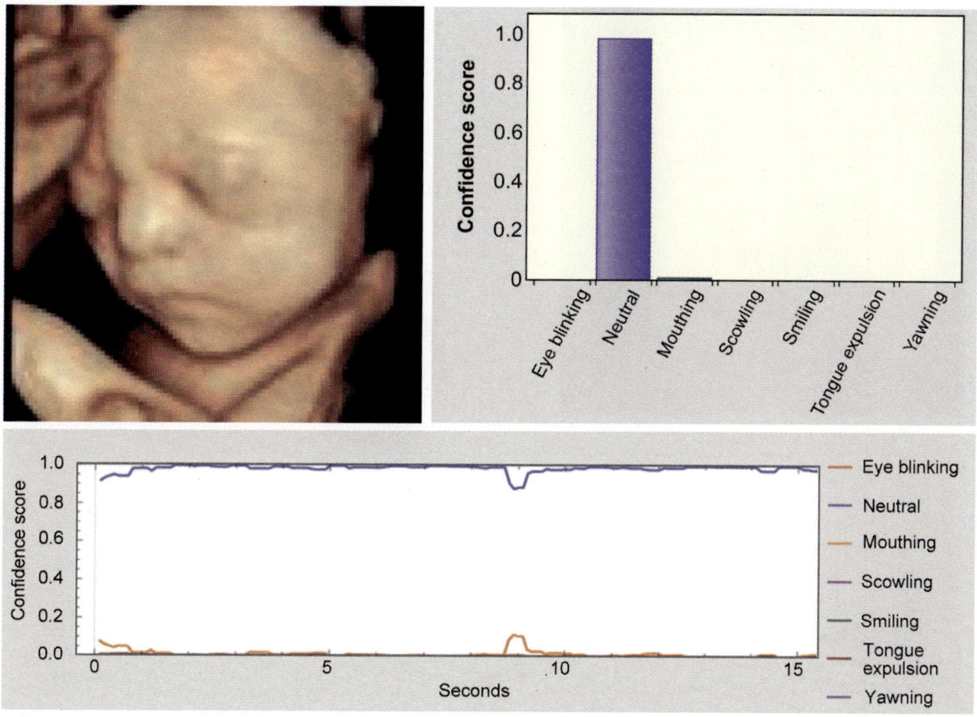

Fig. 6: A sample of the sparse status. A sample of a moment from a video as the sparse status of the confidence score is listed by artificial intelligence. This was a female fetus at 29 weeks and 5 days of gestation. The mother was 26 years old. The confidence score profile is shown on the bar chart in the upper right graph. Time-series changes in the confidence scores are shown in the line graph below. The artificial intelligence determined that neutral dominated the score for this expression. The correlation, information, and capacity dimensions of the seven-dimensional time-series lists were 1.85, 2.23, and 2.25, respectively. The correlation dimensions of eye-blinking, mouthing, neutral, scowling, smiling, tongue expulsion, and yawning were "not available", 1.62, 1.81, 1.80, 1.55, 1.80, and 1.80, respectively.
Source: Miyagi Y, et al.[47]

A simple invented sample case of free energy and fetal facial movement is demonstrated in **Figure 8**. Regarding the interpretation of the model, Miyagi et al.[47] stated that "Assume the fetus is mouthing to swallow amniotic fluid once the stomach is empty. The stomach is emptied as gastric peristalsis expels the stomach contents into the duodenum. The sensory information that the stomach has emptied is sent to the brain, which issues instructions via the motor neurons to the mouthing action to fill the stomach with amniotic fluid. This initiates a decrease in free energy. As the stomach expands, the free energy decreases and reaches a minimum when the stomach is fully distended. At the same time, mouthing activity decreases and facial movements become quiescent. The chronological variations of mouthing activity, volume of fluid in the stomach, and free energy are shown.

Thus, the fetal brain activity using the free-energy principle could be interpreted. There are at least two different states of fetal brain function. The free-energy principle was applied to fetal brain activity, and the chaotic dimension might reflect free energy. The brain function acts in such a way that free energy as a cost function is reduced by active inference, thereby providing a comprehensive explanation of actions. The sparse status can be interpreted as high free energy, because a specific expression accounts for most of the confidence score, suggesting that the consciousness is focused. Therefore, as shown in **Table 2**, when the profile is sparse, the dimension is large, and when the dimension is large, the complexity is large and free energy may be high, while the fetal brain activity may be excited or stressed. When the confidence score list profile is dense, the dimension is small, and when the dimension is small, the complexity is small and free energy may be low; therefore, the fetal brain activity may be relaxed. Although the chaotic dimension does not directly represent the free-energy value, it can be considered to be of an equivalent magnitude. The fact that the chaotic dimension by confidence score profile could be measured indirectly suggests the free energy concept's existence.

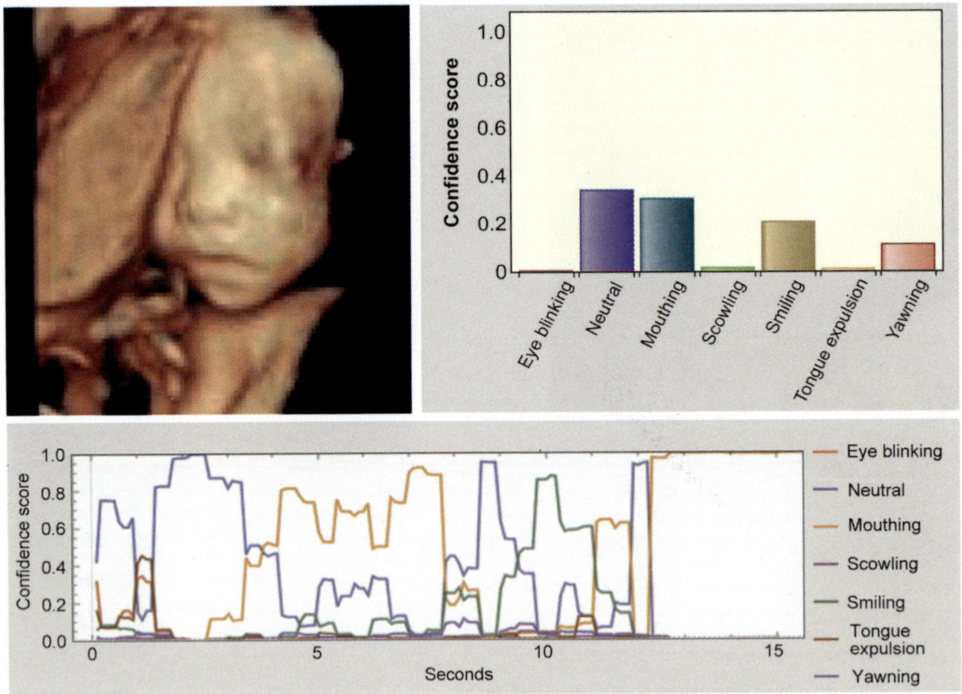

Fig. 7: A sample of the dense status. A sample of a moment from a video as the dense status of the confidence score is listed by artificial intelligence. This was a female fetus at 28 weeks and 4 days of gestation. The mother was 35 years old. The confidence score profile is shown on the bar chart in the upper right graph. Time-series changes in the confidence scores are shown in the line graph below. The artificial intelligence judged that these expressions were distributed among neutral, mouthing, smiling, yawning, etc., and could not be considered specific expressions. The correlation, information, and capacity dimensions of the seven-dimensional time-series lists were 0.79, 1.40, and 1.94, respectively. The correlation dimensions of eye-blinking, mouthing, neutral, scowling, smiling, tongue expulsion, and yawning were 1.50, 0.82, 0.81, 0.91, 1.01, 0.88, and 0.90, respectively.
Source: Miyagi Y, et al.[47]

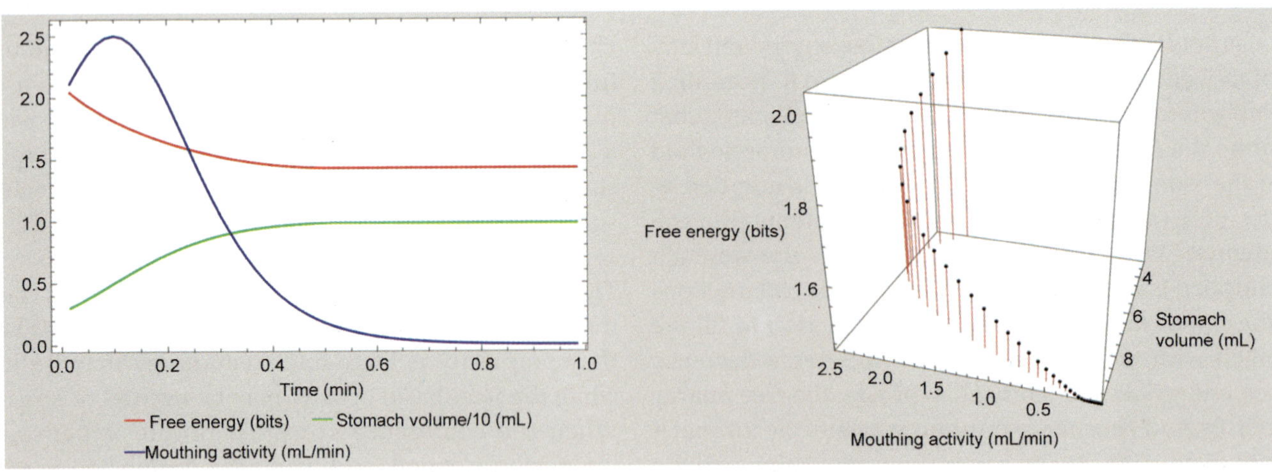

Fig. 8: A simple invented sample case of free energy and fetal facial movement. Assume that the fetus is mouthing to swallow amniotic fluid once the stomach is empty. The stomach is emptied as gastric peristalsis expels the stomach contents into the duodenum. The sensory information that the stomach has emptied is sent to the brain, which issues instructions via the motor neurons to perform the mouthing action to fill the stomach with amniotic fluid. This initiates a decrease in free energy. As the stomach expands, the free energy decreases and reaches a minimum when the stomach is fully distended. At the same time, mouthing activity decreases and facial movements become quiescent. Here, the stomach volume is set to 10 mL. In the left panel, chronological variation of mouthing activity (mL/min), volume of fluid in the stomach (mL), and free energy (bits) are shown in blue, green, and red, respectively. In the right panel, the relationship between mouthing activity, volume of fluid in the stomach, and free energy is shown as dots in a three-dimensional graph. The interval between dots corresponds to 1 second. The red line is the free energy value at each point.

TABLE 2: Estimated relationships of chaotic dimension, free energy, and fetal brain activity regarding confidence score profiles of fetal facial expressions by artificial intelligence (AI).

Confidence score profile	*Chaotic dimension*	*Free energy*	*Brain activity*
Sparse	Larger	Higher	More active
Dense	Smaller	Lower	Less active

Source: Miyagi Y, et al.[47]

Fetal facial expressions can reflect various brain activities, including quale, rather than fetal movements. In living organisms, active inference is important for development and survival, because canonical neural networks that optimize their cost functions implicitly perform active inference.[54] If facial muscle movements and fetal movements are behaviors of self-recognition, active inference may also be a fetal brain function. The change in the chaotic dimension also alters the free energy. Active inference has a purposeful and self-centered aspect with the hallmarks of consciousness.[55] The theory of consciousness from the free-energy principle also states that consciousness is a process of matching recognition density with generative density.[56] If chaotic dimensional change corresponds to free-energy change, this is a discovery of free energy change's process. The discovery of this dynamism can therefore be considered as detecting the existence of consciousness in the fetus after at least 27 weeks of gestation.

CONCLUSION

Fetal brain activity by ultrasonography with AI is an area of future research that is still unknown. There may be a need to cluster cases, examine the association with prognostic factors, and preferably perform follow-up after birth. Although dimensional interpretation of the fetal brain has yet to be established, the method described herein is an objective and quantitative method for understanding the state of the fetal brain based on the free-energy principle.

REFERENCES

1. Hata T, Dai SY, Marumo G. Ultrasound for evaluation of fetal neurobehavioural development: from 2-D to 4-D ultrasound. Inf Child Dev. 2010;19:99-118.
2. Hata T, Kanenishi K, Hanaoka U, et al. HDlive and 4D ultrasound in the assessment of fetal facial expressions. Donald School J Ultrasound Obstet Gynecol. 2015;9:44-50.
3. Hata T. Current status of fetal neurodevelopmental assessment: 4D ultrasound study. J Obstet Gynecol Res. 2016;42:1211-21.
4. Nijhuis JG. Fetal behavior. Neurobiol Aging. 2003;24(Suppl. 1):S41-S46.
5. Prechtl HF. State of the art of a new functional assessment of the young nervous system: An early predictor of cerebral palsy. Early Hum Dev. 1997;50:1-11.
6. de Vries JIP, Visser GHA, Prechtl HFR. The emergence of fetal behaviour. l. Qualitative aspects. Early Hum Dev. 1982;7:301-22.
7. de Vries JIP, Visser GHA, Prechtl HFR. The emergence of fetal behaviour. ll. Quantitative aspects. Early Hum Dev. 1985;12:99-120.
8. Prechtl HF. Qualitative changes of spontaneous movements in fetus and preterm infant are a marker of neurological dysfunction. Early Hum Dev. 1990;23:151-8.
9. Prechtl HF, Einspieler C. Is neurological assessment of the fetus possible? Eur J Obstet Gynecol Reprod Biol. 1997;75:81-4.
10. Kuno A, Akiyama M, Yamashiro C, et al. Three-dimensional sonographic assessment of fetal behavior in the early second trimester of pregnancy. J Ultrasound Med. 2001;20:1271-5.
11. Hata T. Fetal Face as Predictor of Fetal Brain. Donald School J Ultrasound Obstet Gynecol. 2018;12(1):56-9.
12. AboEllail MAM, Hata T. Fetal face as important indicator of fetal brain function. J Perinat Med. 2017;45:729-36.
13. Bodfish J, Powell S, Golden R, et al. Blink rate as an index of dopamine function in adults with mental retardation and repetitive movement disorders. Am J Ment Retard. 1995;99:335-44.
14. Kleven MS, Koek W. Differential effects of direct and indirect dopamine agonists on eye blink rate in cynomolgus monkeys. J Pharmacol Exp Ther. 1996;279:1211-9.
15. Driebach G, Muller J, Goschke T, et al. Dopamine and cognitive control: The influence of spontaneous eyeblink rate and dopamine gene polymorphism on perseveration and distractibility. Behav Neurosci. 2005;119:483-49.
16. Colzato LS, van den Wildenberg WPM, van Wouwe NC, et al. Dopamine and inhibitory action control: Evidence from spontaneous eye blink rates. Exp Brain Res. 2009;196:467-74.
17. Horimoto N, Koyanagi T, Nagata S, et al. Concurrence of mouthing movement and rapid eye movement/non-rapid eye movement phases with advance in gestation of the human fetus. Am J Obstet Gynecol. 1989;161:344-51.
18. Hata T, Kanenishi K, AboEllail MAM, et al. Fetal consciousness 4D ultrasound study. Donald School J Ultrasound Obstet Gynecol. 2015;9:471-4.
19. Walusinski O, Kurjak A, Andonotopo W, et al. Fetal yawning assessed by 3D and 4D sonography. Ultrasound Rev Obstet Gynecol. 2005;5:210-7.
20. Reissland N, Francis B, Manson J. Development of fetal yawn compared with non-yawn mouth openings from 24–36 weeks gestation. PLoS One. 2012;7:e50569.
21. Miyagi Y, Hata T, Bouno S, et al. Recognition of Facial Expression of Fetuses by Artificial intelligence (AI). J Perinat Med. 2021;49(5):596-603.
22. Miyagi Y, Hata T, Bouno S, et al. Recognition of Fetal Facial Expressions using Artificial Intelligence Deep

Learning. Donald School J Ultrasound Obstet Gynecol. 2021;15(3):223-8.
23. Bengio Y, Courville A, Vincent P. Representation learning: A review and new perspectives. IEEE Trans Pattern Anal Mach Intell. 2013;35:1798-828.
24. LeCun YA, Bottou L, Orr GB, et al. Efficient Backprop. In: Montavon G, Orr GB, Müller KR (Eds). Neural Networks: Tricks of the Trade. Heidelberg, Berlin: Springer; 2012. pp. 9-48.
25. LeCun Y, Bottou L, Bengio Y, et al. Gradient-Based Learning Applied to Document Recognition. Proc IEEE. 1998;86:2278-324.
26. LeCun Y, Boser B, Denker JS, et al. Backpropagation Applied to Handwritten Zip Code Recognition. Neural Comput. 1989;1:541-51.
27. Serre T, Wolf L, Bileschi S, et al. Robust object recognition with cortex-like mechanisms. IEEE Trans Pattern Anal Mach Intell. 2007;29:411-26.
28. Wiatowski T, Bölcskei H. A Mathematical Theory of Deep Convolutional Neural Networks for Feature Extraction. IEEE Trans Inf Theory. 2017;64:1845-66.
29. Ciresan DC, Meier U, Masci J, et al. Flexible, High Performance Convolutional Neural Networks for Image Classification. In: Proceedings of the Twenty-Second International Joint Conference on Artificial Intelligence. Barcelona, Spain; 2011. pp. 1237-42.
30. Scherer D, Müller A, Behnke S. Evaluation of pooling operations in convolutional architectures for object recognition. In: Diamantaras K, Duch W, Iliadis LS (Eds). Artificial Neural Networks – ICANN 2010. Lecture Notes in Computer Science. Berlin, Heidelberg: Springer; 2010. pp. 92-101.
31. Huang FJ, LeCun Y. Large-Scale Learning with SVM and Convolutional for Generic Object Categorization. In: 2006 IEEE Computer Society Conference on Computer Vision and Pattern Recognition. New York, USA; IEEE: 2006. pp. 284-91.
32. Mnih V, Kavukcuoglu K, Silver D, et al. Human-level control through deep reinforcement learning. Nature. 2015;518:529-33.
33. Szegedy C, Liu W, Jia Y, et al. Going Deeper with Convolutions. In: Proceedings of the IEEE conference on computer vision and pattern recognition 2015. Boston, USA: Computer Vision Foundation; 2015. pp. 1-9.
34. Zheng Y, Liu Q, Chen E, et al. Time Series Classification Using Multi-Channels Deep Convolutional Neural Networks. In: Li F, Li G, Hwang S, Yao B, Zhang Z (Eds). Web-Age Information Management. WAIM 2014. Lecture Notes in Computer Science. Cham: Springer; 2014. pp. 298-310.
35. Ioff S, Szegedy C. Batch Normalization: Accelerating Deep Network Training by Reducing Internal Covariate Shift. [online] Available from https://arxiv.org/abs/1502.03167v3 [Last accessed April, 2024].
36. Glorot X, Bordes A, Bengio Y. Deep Sparse Rectifier Neural Networks. In Proceedings of the Fourteenth International Conference on Artificial Intelligence and Statistics (AISTATS) 2011. Lauderdale, USA: AISTATS; 2011. pp. 315-23.
37. Nair V, Hinton GE. Rectified Linear Units Improve Restricted Boltzmann Machines. In Proceedings of the 27th international conference on machine learning (ICML-10). Haifa, Israel: Omni press; 2010. pp. 807-14.
38. Krizhevsky A, Sutskever I, Hinton GE. Imagenet Classification with Deep Convolutional Neural Networks. [online] Available from http://papers.nips.cc/paper/4824-imagenet-classification-with-deep-convolutional-neural-networks.pdf [Last accessed April, 2024].
39. Bridle JS. Probabilistic Interpretation of Feedforward Classification Network Outputs, with Relationships to Statistical Pattern Recognition. In Soulié FF, Hérault J (Eds). Neurocomputing. Berlin, Heidelberg: Springer; 1990. 227-36.
40. Miyagi Y, Miyagi Y, Terada S, et al. Variations of multifractal structure in the fetal heartbeats. Acta Med Okayama. 2003;57:49-52.
41. Grassberger P, Procaccia I. Characterization of strange attractors. Phys Rev Lett. 1983;50:346-9.
42. Grassberger P. Dimensions and entropies of strange attractors from a fluctuating dynamics approach. Physica D. 1984;13:34-54.
43. Farmer JD, Ott E, York JA. The dimension of chaotic attractors. Physica D. 1983;7:153-80.
44. Halsey TC, Jensen MH, Kadanoff LP, et al. Fractal measures and their singularities: The characterization of strangesets. Phys Rev A. 1986;33:1141-51.
45. Hentschel HE, Procaccia I. The infinite number of generalized dimensions of fractals and strange attractors. Physica D. 1983;8:435-44.
46. Miyagi Y, Hata T, Bouno S, et al. Artificial intelligence to understand fluctuation of fetal brain activity by recognizing facial expressions. Int J Gynecol Obstet. 2023;161:877-85.
47. Miyagi Y, Hata T, Miyake T. Fetal Brain Activity and the Free Energy Principle. J Perinat Med. 2023;51(7):925-31.
48. Friston K, Kilner J, Harrison L. A free energy principle for the brain. J Physiol Paris. 2006;100:70-87.
49. Friston K. The free-energy principle: A rough guide to the brain? Trends Cogn Sci. 2009;13:293-301.
50. Friston KJ, Daunizeau J, Kilner J, et al. Action and behavior: A free-energy formulation. Biol Cybern. 2010;102:227-60.
51. Friston KJ, Daunizeau J, Kiebel SJ. Reinforcement learning or active inference? PloS One. 2009;4:e6421.
52. Joyce JM. Kullback-Leibler Divergence. In: Lovric M (Ed). International Encyclopedia of Statistical Science. Springer: Berlin, Heidelberg; 2011. pp. 720-2.
53. Inui T. The free-energy principle: A unified theory of brain functions. Brain Neural Networks. 2018;25:123-34.
54. Isomura T, Shimazaki H, Friston KJ. Canonical neural networks perform active inference. Commun Biol. 2022;5:55.
55. Friston K. Am I self-conscious? (or does self-organization entail self-consciousness?). Front Psychol. 2018;9:579.
56. Yoshida M, Taguchi S. Free energy principle and visual consciousness. Brain Neural Networks. 2018;25:53-70.

38

CHAPTER

Ultrasound-guided Fetal Invasive Procedures

George A Partsinevelos, Aris J Antsaklis

INTRODUCTION

The tremendous advances in fetal diagnosis recorded during the last five decades are undoubtedly attributed to the introduction of ultrasonography in fetal imaging. Development of high-resolution ultrasound equipment combined with increasing operator expertise allows early detection and accurate diagnosis of many congenital fetal anomalies. Ultrasound-guided invasive procedures integrate prenatal diagnostic sequels and serve in the in utero management of selected cases of fetal malformations.

In this context, amniocentesis, chorionic villus sampling (CVS), and fetal blood sampling (FBS) have been adequately evaluated in both singleton and multiple pregnancies and have long been applied in the clinical practice. The inception of celocentesis initially in animal models and later in humans might represent an alternative technique for prenatal diagnosis and potentially a mean for in utero gene therapy in immunoincompetent embryos. Ultrasound-guided fetal diagnosis through fetal biopsy and fetal therapy for anemia, thrombocytopenia, obstructive uropathy, pleural effusion, congenital diaphragmatic hernia, and congenital heart defects has also been applied with either acceptable or promising results in selected cases. Finally, interventions in twin-to-twin transfusion syndrome (TTTS), multifetal pregnancy reduction, and selective feticide have been successfully accomplished through sonographic guidance.

Amniocentesis, CVS, and FBS are separately presented in dedicated chapters in this textbook.

CELOCENTESIS

Introduction

Currently, first-trimester screening for fetal aneuploidies and congenital genetic diseases can be performed as early as 10 completed weeks using CVS. The application of this procedure earlier in pregnancy has been linked with fetal anomalies, such as limb reduction syndrome and oromandibular hypoplasia.

Undoubtedly, the earlier in pregnancy fetal diagnosis is achieved, the better for the couple in terms of earlier reassurance of a healthy pregnancy and decision-making in case of fetal aneuploidy or congenital genetic defect. Termination of the pregnancy can be accomplished in the first rather than second trimester of pregnancy in this case, when the complication rates are lower. Moreover, in terms of privacy, the earlier an abnormal pregnancy is terminated the lesser the chance of being widely socially recognized. However, a potential drawback is the termination of a pregnancy, which is otherwise destined to end up with a miscarriage.

In this context, celocentesis was introduced to offer diagnosis of fetal abnormalities earlier than 10 weeks of gestation. Although this approach was initially performed between 6 and 10 weeks, later it was restricted to 7–8 weeks of gestation.

Indications

Fetal sex, β-thalassemia, sickle cell anemia, Marfan syndrome detection, and paternity testing are some of the initial applications of the procedure. The implementation of the technique for fetal karyotyping has not been validated yet and further evaluation of its role is required.[1] Difficulties in culturing celomic cells for conventional cytogenetic analysis obscure its efficacy and hinder the application of celocentesis in the clinical setting.[2]

Technique

The pregnant woman is placed in the lithotomy position, and meticulous cleansing of the vagina and external genitalia with an antiseptic solution is applied. A transvaginal obstetric ultrasound examination is

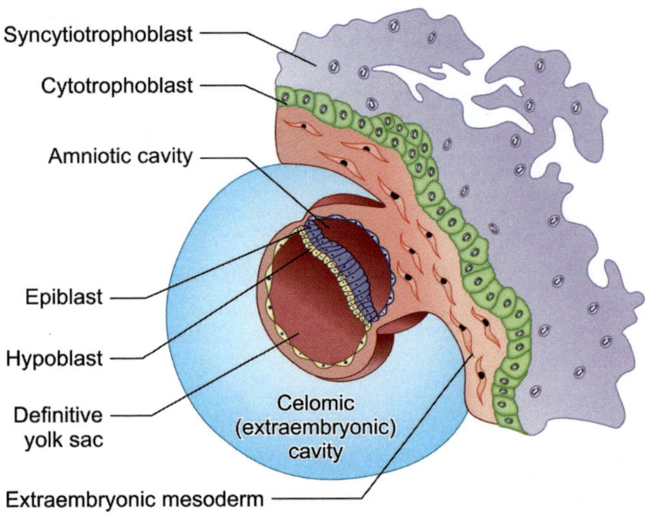

Fig. 1: Celomic (extraembryonic) cavity. The needle is inserted into the celomic (extraembryonic) cavity and 1–2 mL of celomic fluid is aspirated.

preformed and a 20-G needle is advanced transvaginally into the celomic (extraembryonic) cavity, which occupies the vast majority of gestational sac until the 9th week of gestation **(Fig. 1)**. Celomic fluid is aspirated using syringe. The first 0.2 mL of fluid is discarded to avoid contamination with maternal genetic component and a sample of 1–2 mL is subsequently aspirated and sent for biochemical analysis or cytogenetic studies.

Assessment of maternal contamination is considered crucial. According to protocols published, if maternal contamination is absent or very low (<5%), direct DNA extraction, amplification, and sequencing for genetic diseases can be performed. Furthermore, quantitative fluorescence polymerase chain reaction (PCR) of short-tandem repeat sequences in chromosome 13, 18, 21, X, and Y can be applied.[3] If maternal contamination of 5–60% or >60% is found, specific microbeds or micromanipulation can be mobilized to select fetal cells for cytogenetic analysis, respectively.[4]

Complications

A study evaluating short-term safety of celocentesis showed a 2% procedure-related fetal loss rate in women who were subjected to celocentesis 1–3 weeks before termination of pregnancy for social reasons. However, celocentesis was performed at 6–10 weeks of gestation in this study.[5]

A more recent study found 3.2% fetal loss rate, which was decreased to 2.3% after exclusion of the lethal chromosomal abnormalities.[6] Given that no randomized studies assessing procedure-related risk of fetal loss exist, it is reasonable to assume that the risk may be only 1–2%.[6]

In theory, intracelomic hemorrhage may result in fetal hypovolemia and consequently hypoperfusion of the developing fetus. Moreover, postprocedure uterine contractions may lead to hypoxia and vasoactive agents released following intrauterine trauma may have direct action on the heart and the blood vessels.[5] Concerns of potential developmental abnormalities due to these theoretic effects have not been validated so far as no significant hemorrhage or impact in fetal heart has been shown in previous studies.[6,7] However, large scale prospective randomized controlled studies are needed to address the issue of safety of the procedure before it is widely adopted in the clinical practice.

EMBRYOSCOPY AND FETOSCOPY

Introduction

Diagnosis of various fetal congenital anomalies and genetic disorders has substantially improved with the technical advancement in resolution of ultrasonography and the introduction of ultrasound-guided diagnostic procedures. Sonographic and fetoscopic techniques have been used for detailed imaging studies and direct visualization of the fetus, respectively. Ultrasonography serves in fetal diagnosis in all trimesters of pregnancy, whereas fetoscopy is applied beyond 12 weeks of gestation. Earlier than 12 weeks embryoscopy can be used instead.

Over and above diagnosis, both ultrasonography and fetoscopy serve in minimal invasive fetal surgery, with ultrasound-guided percutaneous and fetoscopic procedures progressively replacing most open fetal surgeries.

Both procedures involve the implementation of ultrasonography to various degrees, from amniocentesis, celocentesis, CVS, and FBS, which are fully ultrasound-guided procedures, to fetoscopic endoluminal tracheal occlusion (FETO) in congenital diaphragmatic hernia (CDH) and laser photocoagulation in TTTS, which are ultrasound-assisted interventions.

Historically, in the late 1970s and early 1980s, transabdominal fetoscopy was used during the second trimester of pregnancy for direct visualization of the external anatomy of the fetus and for fetal blood and tissue sampling. Subsequently, high resolution ultrasound imaging rendered second-trimester fetoscopy obsolete. Thus, novel techniques for prenatal diagnosis emerged changing the practice in perinatal medicine.

Recent developments in the field of fiberoptics allowed the introduction of progressively smaller visualization equipment. To this end, the introduction of embryoscopy, which allows direct inspection of the embryo earlier in the first trimester of pregnancy before 12 weeks of gestation, has drawn much interest.

During the past two decades, prenatal diagnosis has increasingly moved to the first trimester of pregnancy with the application of transvaginal sonography, CVS, and transcervical and transabdominal embryoscopy.

Transabdominal Fetoscopy

The terms embryoscopy and fetoscopy correspond to the gestational age at which pregnancy is endoscopically visualized. Although there has been a tendency to refer to embryoscopy as a synonym for the use of transcervical route and fetoscopy for transabdominal approach, we prefer to use gestational age for this terminology.

Transabdominal route for the endoscopic visualization of the fetus was first used by Mandelbaum in 1967. The endoscope carried only optical fibers and the illumination was provided by a device delivered through a second port.

In this technique, endoscopes of 1.7–3.5 mm in diameter have been used. The model we used for several years had an outer diameter of 1.7 mm (Needlescope Dyonics Inc., Woiburn, USA) with an oval outer sheath of 2.2 × 2.7 mm to accommodate a working channel.

In 1980s, advances in ultrasonography allowed ultrasound-guided invasive techniques, which displaced fetoscopy for the majority of clinical purposes, including anatomic visualizations, cordocentesis, and fetal tissue biopsy. Efficacy of ultrasound-guided percutaneous umbilical blood sampling (PUBS) was emphasized, particularly after the Daffos' report (1985) in which "cordocentesis" (a new technique) was performed successfully solely under ultrasound guidance for FBS in >600 pregnancies.[8] However, transabdominal fetoscopy is still a valid invaluable tool with certain indications, such as fetal skin sampling for the diagnosis of certain genodermatoses, liver, kidney or muscle biopsies, and laser photocoagulation of anomalous placental vessel anastomosis in severe cases of TTTS.

Transcervical Embryoscopy

Transcervical endoscopic observation of human fetus was first achieved by Westin in Sweden in 1954.[9] He used a 10-mm rigid hysteroscope to perform transcervical fetoscopy in three patients before termination of pregnancy at 16–20 weeks.

Transcervical endoscopy was first applied for the detection of congenital anomalies in the second trimester of pregnancy by Dubuisson (1979) and Roume (1985), whereas Gallinot (1978) suggested that the fetus could be best visualized beyond 7th week of gestation. Girardini (1991) pointed out that in order to adequately visualize the embryo, the chorionic membrane needed to be perforated. In his early work presented in Athens in 1988, Dumez (1988) successfully performed transcervical endoscopy in >50 continuing pregnancies. Initially, two pregnancies were lost, however no fetal losses were reported in his subsequent work.[10]

Cullen (1990) used a modification of the Dumez's technique to confirm congenital anomalies suspected by ultrasound during the first trimester of pregnancy.[11] The technique for first trimester transcervical embryoscopy is described as follows: the patient lies in the lithotomy position and a rigid fiberoptic endoscope 30 cm in length with a diameter of 2.0–3.5 mm and a 0–30° angle connected to a light source is passed under ultrasound guidance through the cervical canal and apposed by the fetal membranes. The chorionic membrane is penetrated bluntly by a rapid thrust, and the tip of the endoscope enters the coelomic cavity leaving the amniotic sac intact. The yolk sac and the placenta are directly visualized. The embryo can be observed through the transparent amniotic membrane and structural defects of the head, neck, and limbs are expected to be diagnosable with embryoscopy in early pregnancy. Because of the wide in diameter endoscope used, images are very clear and is rarely impossible to obtain a complete anatomic survey of the fetus. In contrast to midtrimester transabdominal fetoscopy, the wide-angle lens and the small size of the embryo during embryoscopy often permit visualization of the embryo in total.

Limitations include trauma to fetal membranes as a result of the relatively large bore of the endoscope, bleeding especially in cases of placenta previa and potential infection. Another drawback is the potential rupture of the amniotic membrane. Finally, severely anteverted or retroverted uterus may be inaccessible to the endoscope. Due to procedure-related limitations, there is no eagerness to offer this procedure to patients at risk for congenital anomalies in ongoing pregnancies.

Thus transcervical embryoscopy was replaced by the less traumatic and more practical transabdominal approach.

Transabdominal Embryoscopy

Considering the limitations of transcervical embryoscopy, in 1993, Quintero developed a transabdominal endoscopic technique to visualize the embryo in the first trimester of pregnancy with the use of the new submillimetric fiberoptic endoscopes.[12] These endoscopes are of such a small diameter that they can be passed through the lumen of a thin needle.

The endoscope is percutaneously introduced into the amniotic cavity through the uterine wall mimicking amniocentesis' technique. The eyepiece of the endoscope is attached to a video camera and the procedure is watched on a video monitor and recorded for subsequent review. During the procedure, successful visualization of both eyes, nostrils, mouth, ears, anterior chest wall, umbilicus, hands, and feet can be achieved.

Thus, abdominal embryoscopy can be performed as early as 3 conceptional weeks' gestation and this technique is useful not only for detecting abnormalities but also for visualizing normal milestones of embryonic development of the trunk and limbs including complete closure of the neural tube and fully development of the hand by the age of 7 conceptional weeks.

Transabdominal embryoscopy is considered invaluable in identifying fetal anomalies nonrecognizable by ultrasound early in pregnancy and confirming others already detected ultrasonographically. An additional application of transabdominal embryoscopy is fetal tissue sampling. This application serves as a basis for further studies into the diagnosis and treatment of congenital diseases early in pregnancy. If the concept of human gene therapy and stem cell transplantation becomes a reality, embryoscopy will permit accessibility to the human embryos, which are immunologically "naive" and may therefore be receptive to grafts.

Potential Applications

Current applications of the technique include accurate endoscopic description of the embryonic development **(Figs. 2A to E)**, first trimester diagnosis of congenital anomalies and intraluminal endoscopic description of blood flow within fetal vessels in the second trimester.

Fetal Therapy

The next step in the evolution of transabdominal embryo fetoscopy is fetal surgery. Fetoscopic ligation of the umbilical cord in case of TTTS, in other words, selective fetal termination, has less complications and does not have the recanalization problems associated with percutaneous

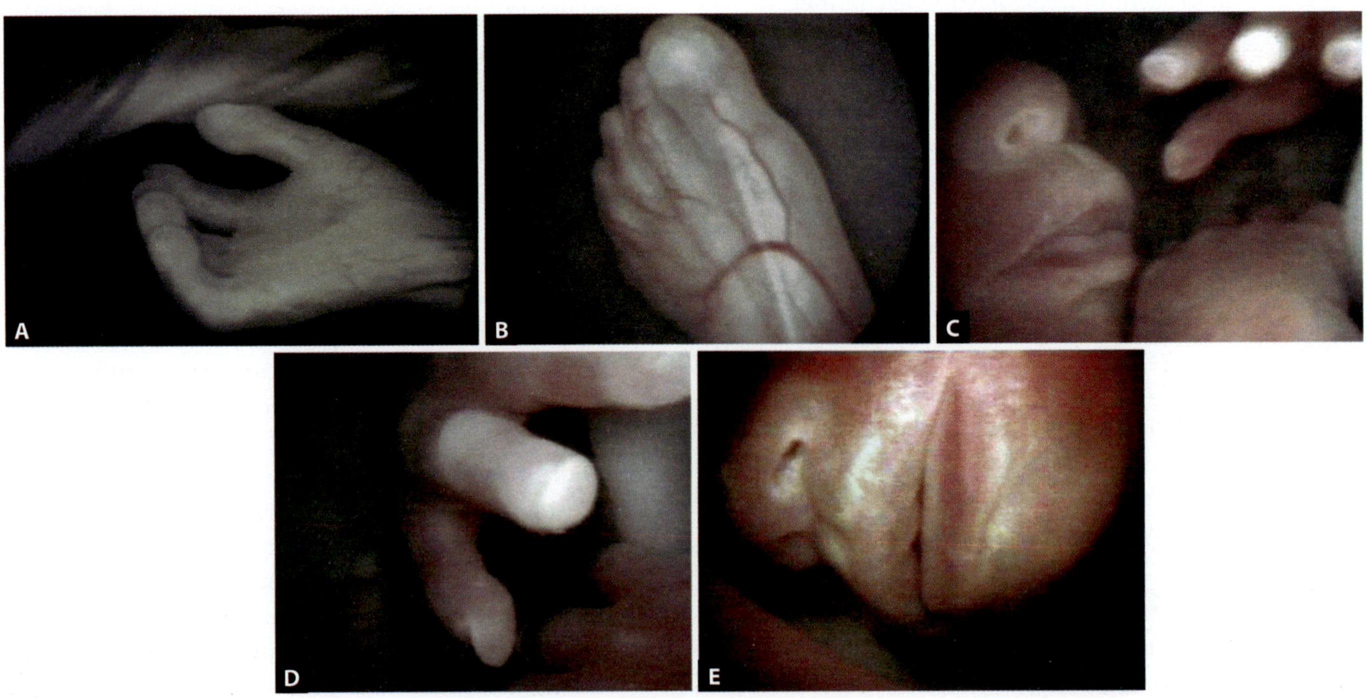

Figs. 2A to E: Fetal imaging through fetoscopy.

ultrasound-guided intra-arterial injection of either thrombogenic coils or fibrin in the umbilical cord.[13]

It has been suggested that fetal cystoscopy using thin transabdominal embryoscopy is useful in the evaluation and treatment of obstructive defects of the urinary system in uteri.[14,15]

The introduction of transabdominal visualization of the embryo in the first trimester using a thin gauge embryoscopy allows earlier diagnosis of congenital anomalies currently beyond the resolution of ultrasound.[16] In addition, it has the true potential of providing access to the fetal circulation at an early age, an accomplishment that would have important diagnostic and therapeutic applications. In the first and second trimesters, operative fetoscopy techniques promise to open new frontiers in the diagnosis and management of fetal surgical and medical conditions.

MULTIFETAL PREGNANCY REDUCTION AND SELECTIVE TERMINATION

The significant increase in the incidence of multiple pregnancies recorded during the last four decades is mainly attributed to the dramatic evolutions in reproductive medicine. Presently, the widespread use of ovulation induction and in vitro fertilization (IVF) techniques account for approximately two-thirds of the increase in multiple gestations in Sweden, whereas the other one-third results from delayed childbearing in increasingly advanced reproductive age.[17] During the last two decades, a substantial effort toward reducing the number of transferred embryos in IVF/intracytoplasmic sperm injection (ICSI) cycles has been made and single embryo transfer at least for women with the best chance of success has been established in many countries nowadays. In addition, close monitoring and cancellation of ovulation induction cycles in case of multifollicular development serve in reducing twin or higher order multiple pregnancy rate.

There is no doubt that multifetal pregnancies are associated with prematurity and low birth weight, which result in increased perinatal morbidity and mortality. In fact, it would appear that despite modern prenatal management, prematurity rate in multiple pregnancies has not changed during the last 50 years, although perinatal mortality rates have declined due to improved neonatal care.[18]

Cerebral palsy, a major component of perinatal morbidity, is related to preterm birth, intrauterine growth restriction (IUGR), and intrapartum complications, factors that are more common in multifetal pregnancies. In particular, the risk of cerebral palsy in twins has been estimated to be five times that in singletons and in triplets increases up to 17- to 20-fold. Nevertheless, antenatal death of the comultiple in utero has been associated with cerebral palsy in the survived co-multiple.[19-22]

In addition to potential fetal complications, multiple pregnancies increase maternal risks. A woman carrying multiples has a higher risk of developing hypertensive disorders in pregnancy and cardiovascular and respiratory system complications. Placenta previa, placental abruption, and postpartum hemorrhage are also increased in these women.[23,24]

Multifetal pregnancy reduction (MPFR) describes the reduction in the number of theoretically normal fetuses mainly in order to lower the likelihood of low birth weight and premature birth. On the contrary, selective termination refers to the "reduction" of the affected fetus and is also called selective feticide, selective embryocide, and selective abortion.

Multifetal Pregnancy Reduction

Introduction

Taking into account increased fetal and maternal risks, pregnant women carrying high order multiples should be offered three options: termination of the entire pregnancy, continuation of the high-risk gestation, and MFPR. The first option is not usually adopted by the couple, especially in case that the conception has been achieved through reproductive medicine technologies following a long period of infertility. The second option requires informed consent due to the potential pregnancy risks and the third aims to lower these risks and optimize the chance of a successful outcome.[25]

Technique

A meticulous ultrasound examination is considered mandatory before proceeding with MFPR. Fetal viability should be assessed, and structural anomalies should be ruled out. Location of the gestational sacs and chorionicity will dictate which fetus/fetuses should be reduced as well as the appropriate method for reduction.

Both transabdominal and transvaginal approach have been employed for this purpose. Historically, cervical dilatation and transvaginal ultrasound-guided aspiration of the gestational sacs was first used in 1986.

Later, transabdominal "free hand" technique for the insertion of a 22-G 9-cm long spinal needle under direct sonographic visualization was applied. The needle targets fetal thorax and 2–3 mL of strong potassium chloride (2 mEq/mL) are injected. If cardiac activity persists for >2 minutes, more potassium chloride is added. A new needle insertion is required for each fetus. As a general rule, termination of >3 fetuses should be performed in two sessions one week apart. Finally, one should avoid reducing the fetus lying over the internal cervical os. The patient is followed-up for 1 hour for signs of uterine contractions, vaginal bleeding, and leakage of amniotic fluid and a repeat ultrasound examination of the nonreduced fetuses integrates the procedure.

Multifetal pregnancy reduction is usually performed between 11 and 14 weeks of gestation. The cut-off of 10 weeks was set to make transabdominal accessibility of the gestational sacs and fetal thorax more feasible, to avoid reducing fetuses that are destined to spontaneous fetal loss later in pregnancy and to have the time for nuchal translucency measurement and a limited ultrasound assessment for signs of fetal anomalies before deciding which fetus is going to be reduced.[26,27] On the contrary, the upper limit of 14 weeks has been applied to reduce the risk of pregnancy loss and premature delivery.

Some physicians recommend first-trimester nuchal translucency measurement accompanied by early anomaly scan to evaluate the risk of chromosomal abnormalities in each fetus prior to MFPR. CVS has been suggested if the calculated risk justifies this invasive diagnostic procedure. An alternative but less popular approach is to perform amniocentesis to the nonreduced fetuses 4 weeks post- MFPR, if indicated.

Complications

Perinatal outcome of reduced twins approaches but never reaches that of spontaneous twins.[28,29] The major risk of MFPR is procedure-related pregnancy loss. It is stated that contemporaneous high-resolution ultrasound combined with increasing operator experience tends to keep the overall miscarriage to an acceptable low rate.[30,31] To this end, transabdominal MFPR has almost entirely replaced the transvaginal alternative due to the lower pregnancy loss rate associated with the former (5.4% vs. 12%).[30,32]

Total pregnancy loss is correlated with the initial and final number of fetuses. In a recent single center study, when >4 fetuses were reduced to twins, there was a 12.1% loss rate. The corresponding features for 4 and 3 fetuses were 5.8% and 4.5%, respectively.[31]

On the contrary, maternal complications and risk of congenital anomalies in nonreduced fetuses are not increased.

It is common sense that MFPR using intrathoracic injection of potassium chloride cannot be applied in monochorionic fetuses, as the risk of an adverse event in the nonreduced fetus is possible due to the presence of placental vascular anastomosis. Actually, 30–50% risk of death or neurological damage has been reported.[33,34] Only newly developed vaso-occlusive techniques available in specific centers could be appropriate in these cases.

Reduction of Triplets to Twins

Although MFPR has been deemed as an effective technique in reducing preterm delivery and perinatal loss in quadruplets and higher order pregnancies, considerable debate exists regarding its efficacy in triplets.[35-37] Increasing knowledge and experience in dealing with multifetal pregnancies along with advances in neonatal care has improved perinatal outcome in triplets.[38,39] Although, there are no randomized control trials questioning the benefit of MFPR in triplet gestations, available evidence indicates that reduction of triplets to twins significantly reduces preterm delivery and low birth weight rate but increases miscarriage rate. In fact, embryo reduction from trichorionic triplets to dichorionic twins decreases preterm birth in 24+0 to 32+6 weeks' gestation from 35% to 13%, but almost duplicates miscarriage rate in 12+0 to 23+6 weeks' gestation (from 3% to 7%). Interestingly, in dichorionic triplets, embryo reduction to monochorionic twins decreases preterm birth from 38% to 23%, but increases miscarriage rate from 9% to 13%, whereas the respective rates for embryo reduction to singleton are from 38% to 9% and from 9% to 18%.[40] Thus, it is a recommendable invasive procedure not only from a medical point of view but also from an ethical perspective based on individual's autonomy and moral and religious beliefs.[41] However, it should be stressed that expectant management of trichorionic triplet pregnancies has a fairly good perinatal outcome.

Reduction to Singleton

In the vast majority of cases, the goal of MFPR is twin pregnancy. However, there are cases where singleton pregnancy is desired. No data have linked this approach with better perinatal outcome in the absence of underlying maternal cardiac disease, history of cervical incompetence, uterine abnormalities, or previous preterm labor. In a recent review, the authors concluded that reduction to a singleton increases the risk of miscarriage, but overall appears to have lowest risk of preterm labor.[42]

In case of nontrichorionic triplets, reduction to singleton using a single intracardiac potassium chloride technique is a feasible option, whereas reducing one of the monochorionic fetuses using modern vaso-occlusive methods, such as bipolar cord occlusion or radiofrequency ablation, will lead to a dichorionic twin pregnancy.

Selective Termination for Fetal Anomaly

Introduction

A dilemma arises in case one of the fetuses in a twin or higher order pregnancy is affected by aneuploidy or severe structural anomaly. Prospective parents need to decide the future of the pregnancy among continuing with both normal and abnormal fetus, terminating the entire pregnancy or selectively terminating the abnormal fetus. The terms selective reduction selective feticide, selective embryocide, and selective abortion of the abnormal multiple have alternatively been used. In selective reduction, a defective fetus is terminated, whereas a healthy one is protected at the same time.[43,44] The main difference from MFPR is that selective termination is usually performed later in pregnancy following diagnosis of abnormal fetus.

Technique

The technique of selective termination is similar to that for first trimester MFPR. Transabdominal insertion of the needle into the fetal thorax is performed under ultrasound guidance, but the potassium chloride must be injected directly into the fetal heart. The dose of potassium chloride increases with gestational age, but rarely exceeds 3 mL.[45]

Determination of chorionicity is mandatory before the procedure, as monochorionicity in case of monochorionic twins or nontrichorionic triplets, is a contraindication for intracardiac potassium injection. Possible mechanism of postprocedure death or neurological damage of the nonreduced twin is agonal twin-to-twin blood transfusion through placental vascular anastomosis from the alive twin to the dying one. This results in hypotension and subsequent brain damage in the surviving fetus.[34,46] Vaso-occlusion techniques can be only applied in these cases. Ultrasound-guided needles 14–18 G are advanced into the fetal abdomen adjacent to the umbilical cord insertion and monopolar diathermy, laser, radiofrequency ablation, and microwave energy can be applied. Ultrasound-guided bipolar forceps for cord occlusion and fetoscopic procedures have also been practiced. Radiofrequency ablation has better results in early- to mid-pregnancy (12–23 weeks) and bipolar cord occlusion in mid pregnancy (18–25 weeks). Laser coagulation is not frequently used nowadays and fetoscopic cord ligation has been rather replaced by ultrasound-guided cord ligation in advanced pregnancies (>26 weeks).

It would appear that a rational approach based on chorionicity would be summarized as follows: in dichorionic twins, delayed termination of the affected fetus at 32 weeks of gestation would protect the healthy multiple of pregnancy loss. On the contrary, in monochorionic twins, the earlier selective feticide takes place the better the prognosis for the unaffected twin.[42]

Complications

Although the aim of selective termination is to reduce the abnormal fetus and protect the healthy one, pregnancy loss is a recognized complication of this procedure. In a review of the literature, radiofrequency was associated with the lower pregnancy loss rate (14%). Corresponding features for bipolar cord occlusion, laser cord coagulation, and cord ligation were 18%, 28%, and 30%. Operator's experience as well as parent's preferences following informed consent should be taken into consideration in decision-making.[47]

TWIN-TO-TWIN TRANSFUSION SYNDROME

Introduction

Multiple pregnancies have long been associated with increased perinatal morbidity and mortality.[48] For example, multiple births represent 3% of all deliveries, but account for 15% of preterm birth and 20% of low birth weight (2,500 g) neonates born in the United States.[49] Pregnancy risks are 3- to 10-fold higher in monochorionic compared to dichorionic twins[50,51] and some of them are unique for monochorionic gestations. TTTS is one of them complicating 5.5–17.5% of monochorionic pregnancies.[52]

Pathophysiology

Three distinct types of anastomoses between placental vessels have been described in monochorionic placentas:

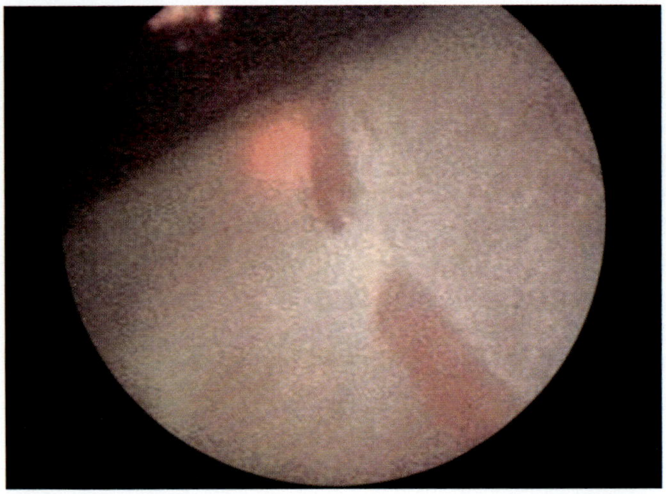

Fig. 3: Fetoscopic aspect of arteriovenous placental anastomoses in twin-to-twin transfusion syndrome.

Source: Adapted from James D (Ed). High-risk pregnancy, management options, 3rd edition. Philadelphia: Elsevier Saunders; 2006.

arteriovenous (AV), arterioarterial (AA) and venovenous (VV) anastomoses. AV anastomoses are deep and unidirectional **(Fig. 3)**. On the contrary, AA and VV are superficial and bidirectional, the direction of blood flow determined by the intervessel changes in hydrostatic pressure. The presence of AV has been considered the cause of unbalanced blood transfusion from the "donor" to the "recipient" fetus, which in the absence of adequate AA and VV anastomoses can result in TTTS. Thus, AV anastomoses appear to be the causative factor, whereas AA anastomoses and to a lesser extend VV anastomoses play a significant protective role in TTTS development and progression.

AV anastomoses are found in almost all monochorionic pregnancies and ex vivo placental studies have shown that they are present in all TTTS placentas, but in 84% of non-TTTS monochorionic diamniotic placentas.[53]

Intertwin unbalanced blood flow through AV leads to hypovolemia and hypoperfusion of the donor twin, which is accompanied by elevation in renin, angiotensin II, and aldosterone.[54,55] At the same time, hypervolemia and hyperperfusion of the recipient twin results in an increase in atrial natriuretic peptide (ANP) release as well as decrease in antidiuretic hormone (ADH) secretion. This sequel is responsible for oligohydramnios (stuck twin), IUGR, and multiorgan malfunction in the donor, whereas polyhydramnios, visceromegaly, cardiac, renal failure, and hydrops are observed in the recipient.[56]

Complications

Monochorionic pregnancies are considered high-risk pregnancies, mainly due to the risk of developing TTTS, which is currently considered one of the most serious perinatal complications. Actually, it has an 80–100% mortality rate and a 15–50% risk of disability, including brain damage, in survivors if left untreated.[48]

Diagnosis

Taking into account that TTTS complicates only monochorionic pregnancies along with gestational age-related limitations of ultrasound diagnostic efficacy in determining chorionicity in multiples, early ultrasound scan at 10–14 weeks' gestation is recommended in these cases. "Twin peak" or "lambda" sign as opposed to "T" sign for dichorionic and monochorionic diamniotic pregnancy, respectively, is diagnostic. Alternatively, intertwin membrane thickness with a cut-off of 2 mm, above which a dichorionic pregnancy is suggested, can be used. Finally, discordance in twins' gender can confirm dichorionicity.

Twin-to-twin transfusion syndrome can develop at different gestational ages. However, it typically develops between 15 and 26 weeks.[57,58]

Sonographic features of TTTS include significant growth discordance (>20%) accompanied by oligohydramnios in donor (maximum vertical pocket of amniotic fluid <2 cm) and polyhydramnios (maximum vertical pocket of amniotic fluid >8 cm before 20 weeks of gestation and >10 cm after 20 weeks) in the recipient. The donor has usually signs of IUGR, small or invisible urinary bladder, and abnormal Doppler studies in the umbilical artery. Circulatory redistribution with abnormal middle cerebral artery and ductus venosus Doppler flow can be evident.

The recipient is often characterized by visceromegaly, abnormal ductus venosus Doppler studies, pulsatile flow in the umbilical vein, and tricuspid regurgitation. An advanced sign of the syndrome is hydrops fetalis in the recipient.

Quintero's staging system for TTTS severity is widely used nowadays as it allows comparison of the outcome of different treatments, which help in decision-making.[59]

Treatment

Amnioreduction

As twin oligohydramnios-polyhydramnios sequence (TOPS) is a common feature of multiple gestations affected by TTTS, serial amnioreduction was traditionally practiced aiming to correct uteroplacental hypoperfusion and relieve maternal discomfort.[60]

An 18-G echotip needle is usually inserted into the polyhydramnios sac under ultrasound guidance and excess amniotic fluid is drained. Local anesthesia and/or sedation can be applied on center's preferences. A maximum vertical amniotic fluid pocket of 5–6 cm indicates the end of the procedure. Repeat of amnioreduction can be performed in case of recurrence. Preterm premature rupture of membranes (PPROM), preterm labor, intrauterine infection, and placental abruption complicate 15–20% of the cases.[61] Retrospective trials have shown that serial amnioreduction results in 66% survival rate of at least one twin at the expense of 15% cerebral palsy rate.[52]

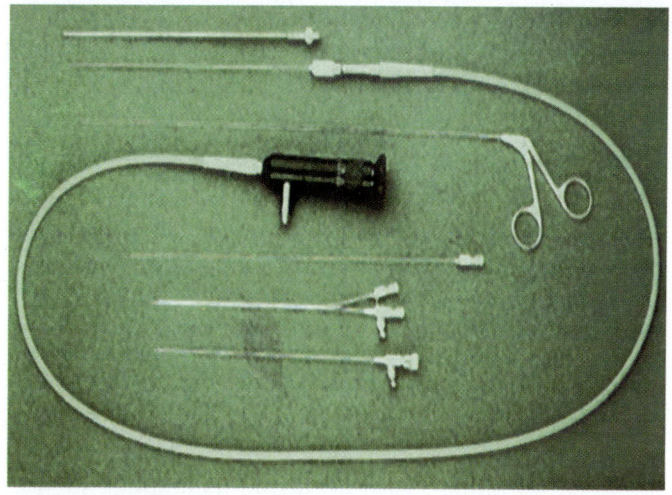

Fig. 4: Fetoscope.
Source: Adapted from James D (Ed). High-risk pregnancy, management options, 3rd edition. Philadelphia: Elsevier Saunders; 2006.

Amniotic Septostomy

This technique, also known as interventional amniotomy, employs a 20–22 G needle to create an opening between the gestational sacs under ultrasound guidance in order to equilibrate intra-amniotic pressures. The benefits of this approach are not quite clear nowadays. One of the drawbacks is the possibility of converting diamniotic to pseudo-monoamniotic twin pregnancy with the accompanied risks for cord entanglement and the formation of the amniotic band syndrome.[62] Another problem is the difficulty in assessing the syndrome's effect in the donor's renal function and also the postseptostomy inability to add laser treatment or serial amnioreduction if needed.[63] Compared to amnioreduction, septostomy seems to have similar results in terms of survival rate, although more than one procedure is usually needed with the amnioreduction approach. However, its use is not supported on an etiological basis and many physicians would probably prefer an alternative treatment option today.

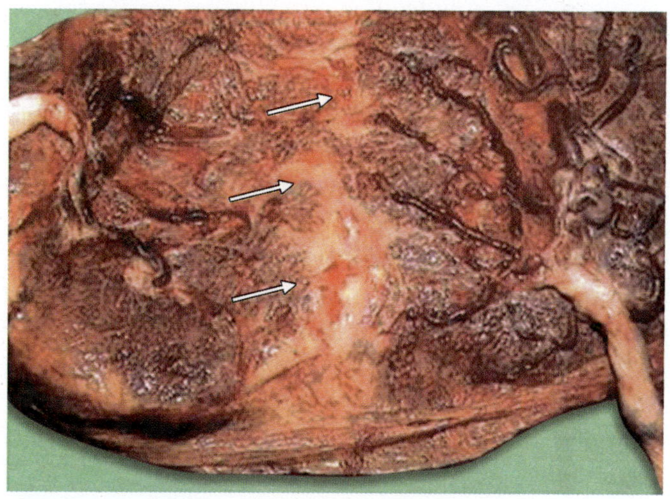

Fig. 5: Placenta following previous laser ablation. Scars are evident.
Source: Adapted from James D (Ed). High-risk pregnancy, management options, 3rd edition. Philadelphia: Elsevier Saunders; 2006.

Laser Therapy

Pathophysiology of the syndrome justifies laser application to divide communicating vessels on the placental surface. This approach was initially performed through laparotomy and later through ultrasound-guided fetoscopy.[64] Nd:YAG or preferably diode laser can be used to perform selective or nonselective coagulation **(Fig. 4)**. In the selective technique, only the anastomotic vessels considered responsible for the syndrome are targeted, whereas in the nonselective all superficial placental vessels approaching or crossing the intertwin membrane (membranous equator) are ablated **(Fig. 5)**. However, in the majority of cases, accurate mapping and characterization of placental anastomosis are not feasible and a combination of selective and nonselective coagulation is usually performed. Solomonization refers to the technique of selectively sealing the blood vessels between the twins, followed by nonselective application of laser, drawing a line across the vascular equator of the placenta, right to the edges, in order to coagulate smaller vessels. This approach seems to reduce the risk for anemia-polycythemia sequence and recurrent TTTS.[65-67] Subsequent amnioreduction integrates laser treatment. The selective technique has been related to higher survival rates compared to the nonselective approach.

Laser coagulation has been linked with at least one surviving fetus in 71–83% of cases[68-70] and also reduced neurological complications ranging from 5% to 11% compared to amnioreduction and amniotic septostomy.[71]

Selective Feticide

Selective termination of the severely affected twin can be an option to salvage the co-twin in strictly selected cases, as an overall intact survival rate of 70–80% is expected in the co-multiple.[57] Vaso-occlusion techniques such as fetoscopic laser cord coagulation before 18–20 weeks or ultrasound-guided bipolar cord coagulation at advanced gestational ages may serve to this end.

Conclusion

Initial evidence implied that amnioreduction might suffice for Quintero stage I and II and about 20% of stage II would recede to stage I after treatment, whereas for stage III laser treatment and subsequent amnioreduction could represent the best option.

Nowadays, accumulated evidence supports fetoscopic laser coagulation for TTTS stages II-IV between 17 and 26 weeks. Furthermore, Quintero stage I complicated by increasing polyhydramnios, progressive shortening of the cervix, and maternal discomfort require prompt laser treatment too. Cardiovascular differences between twins can identify cases that may benefit from laser surgery at an early stage and gestational age.

FETAL BIOPSY PROCEDURES IN PRENATAL DIAGNOSIS

Introduction

Prenatal diagnostic techniques implemented in maternal-fetal medicine during the last 40 years have accomplished the detection of an increasing number of fetal anomalies. In addition to noninvasive diagnostic modalities, interventional approaches have been validated as an invaluable component of modern obstetrics. Amniocentesis, CVS, and FBS are routine prenatal tests nowadays, whereas other invasive diagnostic techniques are applied less frequent. Fetal biopsy procedures are included among them.

Fetoscopy was initially used to access the intrauterine cavity and the fetus. Nevertheless, the introduction of ultrasonography allowed safer approach of the developing embryo for diagnostic purposes. Presently, ultrasound-guided insertion of fetal biopsy needles or forceps is the preferable method for fetal tissue sampling.

Technique

Technical difficulties in accessing fetal organs for biopsy explain the long-learning curve related to this procedure. However, an experienced operator can ensure adequate fetal tissue sampling at an acceptable complication rate.

Fetal skin sampling is deemed as one of the most difficult fetal biopsy procedures in prenatal diagnosis. Kidney and muscle biopsy follows in terms of technical demands and liver sampling seems to be a relatively feasible procedure. With regard to instrumentation, both biopsy forceps and conventional needles with isometric aspiration techniques can be used depending on the tissue targeted. Care to avoid placenta should be taken, if possible. Insertion and thorough advancement of the biopsy instrument should be ultrasound-guided preferably via the free-hand technique. To avoid fetal movements, which may render the procedure difficult and risky, a rational approach is to enter the fetal tissue abruptly as soon as the puncture point has been determined. Anesthesia may be required only in cases of lengthy procedures such as paracentesis of fetal pleural or pericardial effusion.[72]

Skin Biopsy

The procedure should be better performed around 20 weeks of gestation. A skin sample of at least 1 mm in thickness and 1 mm in length is recommended in order to eliminate inadequate sampling rate.[73] Both biopsy forceps and conventional needles can be used. The puncture site should be chosen based on the suspected diagnosis and if possible, more than one biopsy from different skin areas should be obtained.

Liver Biopsy

Again, this procedure is better performed around 20 weeks of gestation. Liver biopsy is considered one of the most feasible in utero biopsy procedures due to the location, the large size, and the texture of the organ. It is succeeded using 18-G biopsy needle and isometric vacuum aspiration. The needle puncture is usually performed at the external third of the right lobe for anatomical reasons.

Kidney Biopsy

A tissue sample of fetal kidney is mainly indicated in cases of obstructive uropathy, which is diagnosed during the second trimester ultrasound screening for fetal anomalies. The aim is to assess a potential detrimental effect in renal function and estimate its reversibility following prompt in utero intervention.

Renal function can also be assessed through analysis of urine obtained by puncture of the distended urinary tracts. Furthermore, renal biopsy can be performed at the same time.

Muscle Biopsy

Muscle biopsy is mainly indicated for the diagnosis of Duchenne muscular dystrophy, in case DNA analysis is not adequately informative. Immunofluorescence is employed to determine the presence of dystrophin, which is absent in the disease.[74-77] External face of the thigh can be punctured using conventional 18-G needle or the sure cut method.[78-82]

Complications

Current practice implies the utilization of conventional needles for fetal biopsy procedures as they are associated with minimal risks compared to forceps inserted through trocars into the amniotic cavity.[80] Obviously, procedure-related miscarriage rate does not differ substantially than that linked to amniocentesis.

CONGENITAL DIAPHRAGMATIC HERNIA

Introduction

Embryologically, diaphragm initially appears at approximately 4 weeks of gestation and completes its development at around 8 weeks with the closure of the pleuroperitoneal canals. Failure of the septum transversum to fuse to the structures surrounding the esophagus and to connect to the pleuroperitoneal membranes results in congenital diaphragmatic hernia (CDH).

Congenital diaphragmatic hernia has an incidence of 1 in 2,000 to 3,000 live births.[83] In the vast majority of cases it is unilateral (95%). Furthermore, 85% of the cases involve the left side, 13% are right sided, and 2% are bilateral.[84] In approximately one-third of cases, CDH is not an isolated malformation and coexist with other fetal anomalies as part of genetic syndromes or chromosomal abnormalities.[85]

The diaphragmatic defect can be repaired in the newborn by primary closure or using a patch. However, the main problem is the associated developmental deficiency of fetal lungs causing pulmonary hypoplasia and pulmonary hypertension. Therefore, in utero interventional procedures have been applied to prevent the consequences of CDH in fetal respiratory system. However, it should be noted that only isolated cases are candidates for such an approach.

Diagnosis

Although the defect exists since the first trimester, CDH is usually detected during second trimester anomaly scan. The severity of the anomaly is assessed using lung-to-head ratio (LHR), which corresponds to the degree of pulmonary hypoplasia. Observed-to-expected LHR and total lung volume have been more recently introduced in CDH severity assessment.[84,86] Magnetic resonance imaging (MRI) has been also employed to confirm the diagnosis of herniated viscera. Fetal karyotype should be always performed in these cases to exclude aneuploidies or genetic syndromes.

Prenatal Intervention

Fetal tracheal occlusion has been shown to reverse CDH-induced pulmonary hypoplasia either by entrapping lung secretions and thereby mechanically stimulating pulmonary development or by the release of growth factors in response to intra-alveolar pressure.[87] The procedure was initially performed by open fetal surgery and later endoscopy using tracheal clips.[88] However, in 2004, these techniques were replaced by percutaneous fetoscopic endoluminal tracheal occlusion (FETO) **(Figs. 6 and 7)**.[89,90] An endotracheal balloon is introduced to occlude the respiratory tract fetoscopically through a single port under ultrasound guidance. The procedure is applied between 26 and 29 weeks of gestation and the balloon can be removed prenatally 4–6 weeks after placement or at 34 weeks' gestation, either by fetoscopy or ultrasound-guided puncture, intrapartum by ex utero intrapartum therapy (EXIT) or postnatally either by tracheoscopy or percutaneous puncture.[91,92]

Complications and Prognosis

Fetoscopic endoluminal tracheal occlusion is associated with the complications of fetoscopy. Concerns regarding the appropriate gestational age at which the procedure

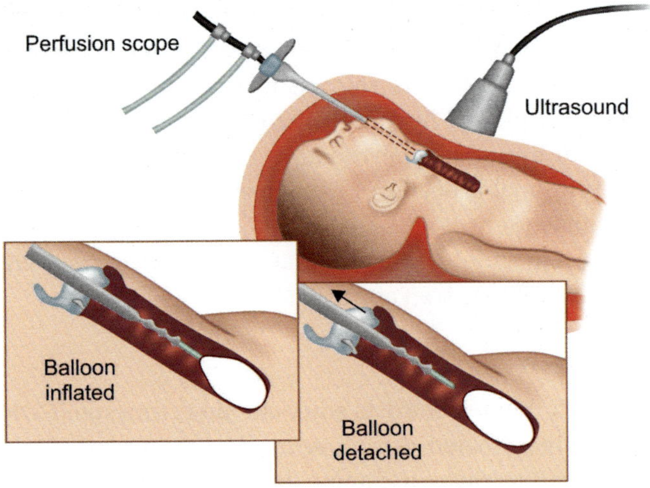

Fig. 6: Schematically percutaneous fetoscopic endoluminal tracheal occlusion (FETO) for congenital diaphragmatic hernia.

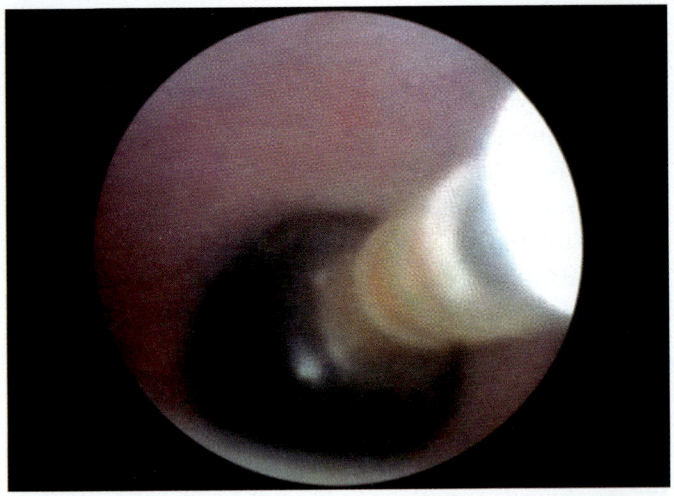

Fig. 7: Fetoscopic image of percutaneous fetoscopic endoluminal tracheal occlusion (FETO) for congenital diaphragmatic hernia.

should be performed have been raised. In theory, the later FETO is performed, the less the risk of preterm birth. However, early FETO starting from 22 weeks' gestation has been tested with a potential additional benefit.[93] Long-term benefit of FETO later in fetal life has not been adequately studied and current evidence dictates that it should be reserved only for milder cases.[94,95]

Although MRI can assess hepatic herniation, which has been related to the severity of the defect, prognosis of CDH is mainly based on sonographically measured LHR. In case of LHR <15%, no chance of survival is expected, whereas in LHR of 15–25%, survival reaches 15%. LHR >25% yields survival rates of at least 60%.[96] However, neonatal survival rates in reference centers may be as high as 80–90%.[97]

FETAL PLEURAL EFFUSION

Introduction

Fetal pleural effusion is a rare condition in fetal medicine with an estimated incidence of 1 in 10,000 to 15,000 pregnancies.[98] It may be either unilateral or bilateral and according to the causative factor is characterized as primary or secondary. Primary results from lymphatic leakage in the pleural cavity and antenatally is called hydrothorax, whereas postnatally chylothorax. Secondary pleural effusion results from generalized fluid retention associated with immune or non-immune hydrops,[98,99] the latter resulting from chromosomal or structural fetal anomalies, such as congenital cystic adenomatoid malformation (CCAM), bronchopulmonary sequestration, and mixed lesions.[100] In the newborn, primary pleural effusion is much more common than secondary. On the contrary, secondary is much more common in the fetus than in the neonate.

Hydrothorax can resolve or progress during pregnancy. Once progression is observed, the mediastinal shift-cardiac compression-vena cava obstruction sequel occurs and subsequent hydramnios and hydrops develop. Furthermore, pulmonary hypoplasia can result from persistent or progressive pleural effusion.

Diagnosis

Ultrasonography can accomplish prenatal diagnosis of pleural effusion as early as 15 weeks of gestation.[101] In the past, the condition was not diagnosed until the third trimester.[98] However, in more recent series, the median gestational age at diagnosis was 20 weeks (range 6–35).[102]

It should be clarified that in order to define a case of pleural effusion as primary, detailed diagnostic approach similar to that for fetal hydrops should be undertaken. Investigations for congenital infections (TORCH), blood type and antibody screen, Kleihauer-Betke test, hemoglobin electrophoresis, middle cerebral artery (MCA) Doppler studies, and fetal karyotype should be performed.[102-107] In 6–10% of cases fetal aneuploidy is expected,[108] whereas structural malformations are detected in 25% fetuses with pleural effusion.[106] Therefore, anomaly scan including echocardiography should focus on potential associated fetal defects.

In Utero Intervention

Expectant management and close follow-up at weekly intervals can be justified in primary small non-hydropic effusions, as spontaneous regression has been reported. However, thoracocentesis or pleuroamniotic shunting can be applied in all other cases to prevent pulmonary hypoplasia and fetal death. Drainage of pleural effusion can result in expansion of fetal lungs and resolve hydramnios and hydrops improving fetal and neonatal survival. In addition, it can allow further investigations in the aspirated fluid.

Thoracocentesis was first applied in 1982 for primary fetal hydrothorax.[109] A 20–22G needle is introduced transabdominally under ultrasound guidance. Although it has been reported that pleural effusion can be treated with one session of thoracocentesis, which is possible to correct the underlying imbalance in fluid development, usually recurrence of the hydrothorax is expected and repeat thoracocentesis is required.[110] Thus, this procedure is reserved for cases where transient decompression is combined with diagnostic evaluation of the aspirated fluid. Furthermore, it can be applied in the immediate prepartum period to facilitate neonatal respiratory function.

Pleuroamniotic shunting was initially described in 1986.[111] It involves the transabdominal introduction of a 3-mm metal trocar with a cannula into the amniotic cavity under direct ultrasound visualization. The mid-axillary line is considered the ideal site for the insertion of the trocar cannula system into the fetal thorax. The trocar is withdrawn and a double pigtail silastic catheter is inserted into the fetal pleural cavity before the removal of the cannula in order to drain pleural fluid to the amniotic cavity. In bilateral pleural effusion, the operator should avoid double uterine puncture and an attempt to access the contralateral thoracic cavity through the same uterine trocar is recommended.

Pleurodesis with the injection of the sclerosant substance OK-432 into the pleural space as an alternative approach has been applied but the initial results were inconclusive, suggesting that more studies are required to clarify its role in hydrothorax management.[112-116]

Complications—Prognosis

Although hylothorax in the newborn is associated with mortality rate, which reaches 15%, a 53% mortality rate has been ascribed to prenatally diagnosed hydrothorax.[98] Nevertheless, secondary pleural effusion associated with hydrops has been linked to a mortality rate as high as 95%.[108]

Catheter migration and shunt obstruction are the most frequent complications of pleuroamniotic shunting.[98,117-119]

Conclusively, in early stages of pleural effusion, conservative management is considered a rational approach, as spontaneous regression of the condition is possible, whereas thoracocentesis may be performed before delivery. On the contrary, in advanced pleural effusion with hydrops, mediastinal shift, and hydramnios diagnosed earlier than 36 weeks of gestation, pleuroamniotic shunting is recommended. In case the diagnosis is made after 35–36 weeks, thoracocentesis and prompt delivery should be the appropriate practice.[98-120]

FETAL LOWER URINARY TRACT OBSTRUCTION

Introduction

Fetal lower urinary tract obstruction (LUTO) is a rare condition in fetal medicine with an estimated incidence of 2.2 in 10,000 live births.[121] It represents the most common type of congenital abnormalities of the kidney and urinary tract (CAKUT). The most common cause is the presence of posterior urethral valves, which occurs almost exclusively in males, whereas the presence of anterior urethral valves, urethral atresia or stenosis, and excessive ureterocele obstructing lower urinary tract are less common underlying causes, which are found in both males and females.[122]

Lower urinary tract obstruction is complicated by oligohydramnios or anhydramnios, given that by 16th weeks' gestation, urine produced by fetal kidneys represents 90% of amniotic fluid volume. As a result, pulmonary hypoplasia and pulmonary insufficiency at birth are expected. Besides, long-lasting obstructive uropathy may result in renal failure. Therefore, fetal intervention has drawn increasing attention to rescue both pulmonary and renal impairment.

Diagnosis

Lower urinary tract obstruction can be identified sonographically as early as the first trimester. A longitudinal bladder diameter of >7 mm, defined as megacystis, may imply this underlying condition, whereas a diameter >15 mm has been associated with 10% incidence of fetal aneuploides.[123] In the second-trimester ultrasound anomaly scan, oligohydramnios or anhydramnios accompanied by dilated urinary bladder, bilateral hydroureters, and hydronephrosis comprise the typical sequence. The "key-hole" sign is characteristic of LUTO and represents dilated posterior urethra.[124] Depending on the duration and the severity of the effect of LUTO to the renal function, kidney hyperechogenicity, renal cortical cysts, and lack of corticomedullary differentiation may be seen.[125]

Magnetic resonance imaging has been also employed to confirm the diagnosis although it cannot always rule out the exact etiology.[126]

As proper selection of candidates for fetal intervention is crucial, detailed ultrasound evaluation of the fetus and invasive genetic testing (amniocentesis or fetal blood sampling) are required to confirm that LUTO is an isolated defect. Besides, fetal renal function assessment through vesicocentesis after 18 weeks' gestation is mandatory to exclude cases with severe renal function failure.[127,128]

In Utero Intervention

Spontaneous regression of the defect and restoration of amniotic fluid volume as well as of the anatomy of urinary bladder, ureters, and kidneys have been reported in the literature, however, occurs in the minority of cases (10%).[128]

Treatment options available for LUTO include repeat vesicocentesis, vesicoamniotic shunting, and fetal cystoscopy.

Vesicocentesis is performed using a 20–22 G needle, which is introduced transabdominally under ultrasound guidance and urine from fetal bladder is drained. Recurrence of the dilated bladder in a few days is expected and repeat vesicocentesis is required, usually several times per week, which increases the procedure-related risks. Thus, this procedure is reserved for cases, where transient decompression is combined with diagnostic assessment of the aspirated urine. It should be noted that at least three vesicocentesis are needed to reliably assess urine biochemistry.[127]

Vesicoamniotic shunting involves the transabdominal introduction of a 3-mm trocar with a cannula into the amniotic cavity under real-time ultrasound visualization. The trocar is withdrawn and a double pigtail silastic catheter is inserted into the fetal bladder before the removal of the cannula in order to drain urine to the amniotic cavity. In cases of severe oligohydramnios or anhydramnios, restoration of amniotic fluid volume through amnioinfusion precedes the procedure.

Fetal cystoscopy is performed under maternal epidural anesthesia and fetal anesthesia. A 2.2-mm trocar in advanced into the fetal bladder under ultrasound guidance, through which a 1.0-1.3 mm fetoscope is introduced. In case membranous urethral obstruction suggesting posterior urethral valves is seen, intervention with hydroablation, laser or mechanical wire-guide application takes place.[129]

Conclusion

Lower urinary tract obstruction is a fetal defect that is responsible for pulmonary hypoplasia and renal failure in the fetus and the newborn. Repeat vesicocentesis was initially applied to treat this condition. Nowadays, vesicoamniotic shunting as well as fetal cystoscopy are preferred in centers with expertise.

Repeat vesicocentesis has been linked with the repeat procedure-related risks of fetal loss, premature rupture of membranes, preterm labor, and chrorioamnionitis. Vesicoamniotic shunting is the most common technique practiced today. It has been associated with increased survival rate. Unfortunately, the PLUTO trial[130] designed to study vesicoamniotic shunting in moderate/severe LUTO faced poor recruitment and the researchers decided early discontinuation the trial.[131] Therefore, inconclusive results came out indicating that, although shunting benefits survival, the chances of renal function restoration may be very low.[125]

Fetal cystoscopy has been associated with fetoscopy risks and risks specific for cystoscopy, such as urinary ascites and fistula formation between urinary and gastrointestinal tract and the skin.[128]

INTERVENTIONAL FETAL CARDIOLOGY

Introduction

Advances in fetal imaging with the use of high-resolution ultrasonography, modern ultrasound techniques, and increasing operator experience allow diagnosis of congenital heart defects as early as 12–14 weeks of gestation. Early identification of cardiac anomalies suggests further detailed imaging of the developing fetus in order to exclude coexistent structural defects. Furthermore, prenatal invasive genetic studies (CVS or amniocentesis) for fetal karyotyping and DNA analysis are required in these cases. The parents are informed about the prognosis of the anomaly and potential available intrauterine interventions aiming to alleviate the consequences of the anomaly to flow-dependent cardiac morphogenesis until birth. Postnatal management options of the affected child are also discussed based on current evidence. Finally, they are offered the option of terminating the pregnancy.

Currently, most of these pregnancies are terminated due to the couple's reluctance to adopt the medical, emotional, and socioeconomic consequences of a child with congenital heart disease.[132] However, modern fetal echocardiography has encouraged the application of intrauterine therapy in some cardiac diseases during the last two decades.[133]

Technique

Till now, intrauterine interventions for fetal cardiac defects have been performed from 20 weeks of gestation onward.[134-140] For intracardiac stenotic lesions, transabdominal or open abdominal transuterine ultrasonography accomplishes the introduction of a needle into the amniotic cavity and subsequently into the fetal heart. The needle facilitates the insertion of a floppy-tipped guidewire and a balloon catheter into the stenotic area and the balloon is inflated to correct the defect.

Fetoscopy assisted by concurrent transesophageal or intra-amniotic fetal echocardiography has been also employed for fetal cardiac surgery. Alternatively, open abdominal surgery with direct fetal exposure has been used, but it has been associated with high complication rates rendering this technique unacceptable for fetal cardiac intervention.[134]

Nowadays, indications for fetal cardiac interventions include critical aortic stenosis, pulmonary stenosis with an intact septum, and restrictive foramen ovale. It is noteworthy that these interventions have been linked with significant morbidity and mortality, which compromise initial enthusiasm since their introduction in the clinical setting.[92]

Complications

Due to the lack of randomized controlled trials, the outcome of prenatal intrauterine interventions for cardiac anomalies has been assessed through case reports and case series. Uncertainties regarding the efficacy of these procedures along with their potential risks for both the fetus and the mother reserve the application of these techniques in an investigational setting. The progress of the cardiac disease later in pregnancy following successful intrauterine intervention is possible.[141] Moreover, additional postnatal procedures may be required to integrate management of the defect.[142] Conclusively, more data concerning the results of intrauterine interventions for fetal cardiac anomalies are needed before this approach is considered as a realistic option in the clinical practice.

CONCLUSION

Since 1961, when Sir William Liley completed the first percutaneous fetal transfusion[143] ultrasound-guided fetal invasive procedures have gained increased interest in modern obstetrics. From celocentesis, embryoscopy/fetoscopy, multifetal pregnancy reduction and selective termination to clinical approach of twin-to-twin transfusion syndrome, fetal biopsy procedures in prenatal diagnosis, treatment of congenital diaphragmatic hernia, fetal pleural effusion, fetal lower urinary tract obstruction and interventional cardiology, ongoing development and implementation of innovative technologies have served in either acceptable or promising results in selected cases. Given that these procedures may be accompanied by maternal morbidity or even mortality, the pregnant woman has a central role in decision making. Therefore, well-designed randomized clinical trials are welcome in the field of closed fetal intervention under ultrasonographic guidance to robust clinical acceptance.

REFERENCES

1. Jurkovic D, Jauniaux E, Campbell S, Pandya P, Cardy DL, Nicolaides KH. Coelocentesis: a new technique for early prenatal diagnosis. Lancet. 1993;341(8861):1623-4.
2. Makrydimas G. Celocentesis: an alternative technique for prenatal diagnosis. In: Antsaklis AJ, Troyano JM (Eds). Donald School Textbook of Interventional Ultrasound. New Delhi: Jaypee Brothers Medical Publishers (P) Ltd. 2008. pp. 57-63.
3. Giambona A, Leto F, Passarello C, Vinciguerra M, Cigna V, Schillaci G, et al. Fetal aneuploidy diagnosed at celocentesis for early prenatal diagnosis of congenital hemoglobinopathies. Acta Obstet Gynecol Scand. 2018; 97(3):312-21.
4. Makrydimas G, Damiani G, Jakil C, Cigna V, Orlandi M, Picciotto F, et al. Celocentesis for early prenatal diagnosis of hemoglobinopathy. Ultrasound Obstet Gynecol. 2020;56(5):672-7.
5. Makrydimas G, Kaponis A, Skentou C, Lolis D. Short-term safety of celocentesis for the mother and the fetus. Ultrasound Obstet Gynecol 2002;19(3):243-5.
6. Lau TK, Fung TY, Wong YF, Fung HY. A study of fetal sex determination in coelomic fluid. Gynecol Obstet Invest. 1998;45(1):16-8.

7. Lestou VS, Desilets V, Lomax BL, Barrett IJ, Wilson RD, Langlois S, et al. Comparative genomic hybridization: a new approach to screening for intrauterine complete or mosaic aneuploidy. Am J Med Genet. 2000;92(4):281-4.
8. Daffos F, Capella-Pavlovsky M, Forestier F. Fetal blood sampling during pregnancy with use of a needle guided by ultrasound: a study of 606 consecutive cases. Am J Obstet Gynecol. 1985;153(6):655-60.
9. Westin B. Hysteroscopy in early pregnancy. Lancet. 1954; 264:872.
10. Dumez Y, Oury J, Duchetel F. Embryoscopy and congenital malformations. Proceedings of the International Conference on Chorionic Villus Sampling and early Prenatal Diagnosis Athens, Greece. 1988.
11. Cullen MT, Reece EA, Whetham J, Hobbins JC. Embryoscopy: description and utility of a new technique. Am J Obstet Gynecol. 1990;162(1):82-6.
12. Jeffcoate TN, Fliegner JR, Russell SH, Davis JC, Wade AP. Diagnosis of the adrenogenital syndrome before birth. Lancet. 1965;2(7412):553-5.
13. De Lia JE, Kuhlmann RS, Harstad TW, Cruikshank DP. Fetoscopic laser ablation of placental vessels in severe previable twin-twin transfusion syndrome. Am J Obstet Gynecol. 1995;172(4 Pt 1):1208-11.
14. Quintero RA, Hume R, Smith C, et al. Percutaneous fetal cystoscopy and endoscopic fulguration of posterior urethral valves. Am J Obstet Gynecol. 1995;172(1 Pt 1):206-9.
15. Quintero RA, Johnson MP, Romero R, et al. In-utero percutaneous cystoscopy in the management of fetal lower obstructive uropathy. Lancet. 1995;346(8974):537-40.
16. Reece EA, Homko CJ, Wiznitzer A, Goldstein I. Needle embryofetoscopy and early prenatal diagnosis. Fetal Diagn Ther. 1995;10(2):81-2.
17. Bergh T, Ericson A, Hillensjö T, Nygren KG, Wennerholm UB. Deliveries and children born after in-vitro fertilisation in Sweden 1982-95: a retrospective cohort study. Lancet. 1999;354(9190):1579-85.
18. Kiely JL, Kleinman JC, Kiely M. Triplets and higher-order multiple births. Time trends and infant mortality. Am J Dis Child. 1992;146(7):862-8.
19. Pharoah PO, Cooke T. Cerebral palsy and multiple births. Arch Dis Child Fetal Neonatal Ed. 1996;75(3):174-7.
20. Yokoyama Y, Shimizu T, Hayakawa K. Prevalence of cerebral palsy in twins, triplets and quadruplets. Int J Epidemiol. 1995;24(5):943-8.
21. Nelson KB, Ellenberg JH. Childhood neurological disorders in twins. Paediatr Perinat Epidemiol. 1995;9(2):135-45.
22. Petterson B, Nelson KB, Watson L, Stanley F. Twins, triplets, and cerebral palsy in births in Western Australia in the 1980s. BMJ. 1993;307(6914):1239-43.
23. Lynch L, Bercowitz R. Multifetal pregnancy reduction. Ultrasound Reprod Med. 1991;2:771-81.
24. Klein VR. Maternal complications associated with triplet pregnancies in triplet pregnancies and their consequences. In: With L, Blickstein I (Eds). The Parthenon Publ Group; 2002.
25. Berkowitz RL, Lynch L, Chitkara U, Wilkins IA, Mehalek KE, Alvarez E. Selective reduction of multifetal pregnancies in the first trimester. N Engl J Med. 1988;318(16):1043-7.
26. Landy HJ, Keith LG. The vanishing twin: a review. Hum Reprod Update. 1998;4(2):177-83.
27. Lipitz S, Shulman A, Achiron R, Zalel Y, Seidman DS. A comparative study of multifetal pregnancy reduction from triplets to twins in the first versus early second trimesters after detailed fetal screening. Ultrasound Obstet Gynecol. 2001;18(1):35-8.
28. Cheang CU, Huang LS, Lee TH, Liu CH, Shih YT, Lee MS. A comparison of the outcomes between twin and reduced twin pregnancies produced through assisted reproduction. Fertil Steril. 2007;88(1):47-52.
29. Lipitz S, Uval J, Achiron R, Schiff E, Lusky A, Reichman B. Outcome of twin pregnancies reduced from triplets compared with nonreduced twin gestations. Obstet Gynecol. 1996;87(4):511-4.
30. Evans MI, Berkowitz RL, RJ W, et al. Improvement in outcomes of multifetal pregnancy reduction with increased experience. Am J Obstet Gynecol. 2001;184(2):97-103.
31. Stone J, Ferrara L, Kamrath J, et al. Contemporary outcomes with the latest 1000 cases of multifetal pregnancy reduction (MPR). Am J Obstet Gynecol. 2008;199:406.e1-4.
32. Melgar CA, Rosenfeld DL, Rawlinson K, Greenberg M. Perinatal outcome after multifetal reduction to twins compared with nonreduced multiple gestations. Obstet Gynecol. 1991;78(5 Pt 1):763-7.
33. Pharoah PO, Adi Y. Consequences of in-utero death in a twin pregnancy. Lancet. 2000;355(9215):1597-602.
34. Ong SS, Zamora J, Khan KS, Kilby MD. Prognosis for the co-twin following single-twin death: a systematic review. BJOG. 2006;113(9):992-8.
35. Evans MI, Krivchenia EL, Gelber SE, Wapner RJ. Selective reduction. Clin Perinatol. 2003;30(1):103-11.
36. Stone J, Eddleman K, Lynch L, Berkowitz RL. A single center experience with 1000 consecutive cases of multifetal pregnancy reduction. Am J Obstet Gynecol. 2002;187(5):1163-7.
37. Boulot P, Vignal J, Vergnes C, Dechaud H, Faure JM, Hedon B. Multifetal reduction of triplets to twins: a prospective comparison of pregnancy outcome. Hum Reprod Update. 2000;15(7):1619-23.
38. Lipitz S, Reichman B, Uval J, et al. A prospective comparison of the outcome of triplet pregnancies managed expectantly or by multifetal reduction to twins. Am J Obstet Gynecol. 1994;170(3):874-9.
39. Albrecht JL, Tomich PG. The maternal and neonatal outcome of triplet gestations. Am J Obstet Gynecol. 1996;174(5):1551-6.
40. The Fetal Medicine Foundation. Fetal abnormalities, Multiple pregnancies, Triplet pregnancies. Management

options at 11–13 weeks. [online] Available from https://fetalmedicine.org/education/fetal-abnormalities/multiple-pregnancies/triplet-pregnancies [Last accessed May, 2024].

41. Yaron Y, Bryant-Greenwood PK, Dave N, Moldenhauer JS, Kramer RL, Johnson MP, et al. Multifetal pregnancy reductions of triplets to twins: Comparison with nonreduced triplets and twins. Am J Obstet Gynecol. 1999;180(5):1268-71.
42. Wimalasundera RC. Selective reduction and termination of multiple pregnancies. Semin Fetal Neonatal Med. 2010;15(6):327-35.
43. Antsaklis A, Politis J, Karagiannopoulos C, Kaskarelis D, Karababa P, Panourgias J, et al. Selective survival of only the healthy fetus following prenatal diagnosis of thalassaemia major in binovular twin gestation. Prenat Diagn. 1984;4(4):289-96.
44. Boulot P, Hedon B, Pelliccia G, Deschamps F, Benos P, Audibert F, et al. Obstetrical results after embryonic reductions performed on 34 multiple pregnancies. Hum Reprod. 1990;5(8):1009-13.
45. Evans MI, Littmann L, King M, Fletcher JC. Multiple gestation: the role of multifetal pregnancy reduction and selective termination. Clin Perinatol. 1992;19(2):345-57.
46. Benirschke K. Intrauterine death of a twin: mechanisms, implications for surviving twin, and placental pathology. Semin Diagn Pathol. 1993;10(3):222-31.
47. Rossi AC, D'Addario V. Umbilical cord occlusion for selective feticide in complicated monochorionic twins: a systematic review of literature. Am J Obstet Gynecol. 2009;200(2):123-9.
48. Martin JA, Hamilton BE, Sutton PD, Ventura SJ, Menacker F, Munson ML. Births: final data for 2003. Natl Vital Stat Rep. 2005;54(2):1-116.
49. Goodnight W, Newman R. Optimal nutrition for improved twin pregnancy outcome. Obstet Gynecol. 2009;114(5):1121-34.
50. Burn J, Corney G. Zygosity determination and the types of twinning. In: MacGillivray I, Campbell D, Thompson B (Eds). Twinning and Twins. Chichester, UK: John Wiley; 1988. pp. 7-25.
51. Pasquini L, Wimalasundera RC, Fisk NM. Management of other complications specific to monochorionic twin pregnancies. Best Pract Res Clin Obstet Gynaecol. 2004;18(4):577-99.
52. Quintero RA. Twin-twin transfusion syndrome. Clin Perinatol. 2003;30(3):591-600.
53. Denbow ML, Cox P, Taylor M, Hammal DM, Fisk NM. Placental angioarchitecture in monochorionic twin pregnancies: relationship to fetal growth, fetofetal transfusion syndrome, and pregnancy outcome. Am J Obstet Gynecol. 2000;182(2):417-26.
54. Van Peborgh P, Morineau G, Bussières L, Escourrou P, Ville Y. Twin-to-twin transfusion syndrome: polyhydramnios-associated changes in maternal plasma volume and maternal plasma aldosterone concentrations: a preliminary study. Fetal Diagn Ther. 1998;13(3):184-6.
55. De Paepe ME, Stopa E, Huang C, Hansen K, Luks FI. Renal tubular apoptosis in twin-to-twin transfusion syndrome. Pediatr Dev Pathol. 2003;6(3):215-25.
56. Bajoria R, Ward S, Sooranna SR. Atrial natriuretic peptide mediated polyuria: pathogenesis of polyhydramnios in the recipient twin of twin-twin transfusion syndrome. Placenta. 2001;22(8-9):716-24.
57. El Kateb A, Ville Y. Update on twin-to-twin transfusion syndrome. Best Pract Res Clin Obstet Gynaecol. 2008;22(1):63-75.
58. Bebbington M. Twin-to-twin transfusion syndrome: current understanding of pathophysiology, in utero therapy and impact for future development. Semin Fetal Neonatal Med. 2010;15(1):15-20.
59. Quintero RA, Morales WJ, Allen MH, Bornick PW, Johnson PK, Kruger M. Staging of twin-twin transfusion syndrome. J Perinatol. 1999;19(8 Pt 1):550-5.
60. Saunders NJ, Snijders RJ, Nicolaides KH. Therapeutic amniocentesis in twin-twin transfusion syndrome appearing in the second trimester of pregnancy. Am J Obstet Gynecol. 1992;166(3):820-4.
61. Mari G, Roberts A, Detti L, et al. Perinatal morbidity and mortality rates in severe twin-twin transfusion syndrome: results of the International Amnioreduction Registry. Am J Obstet Gynecol. 2001;185(3):708-15.
62. Gilbert WM, Davis SE, Kaplan C, Pretorius D, Merritt TA, Benirschke K. Morbidity associated with prenatal disruption of the dividing membrane in twin gestations. Obstet Gynecol. 1991;78(4):623-30.
63. Trevett T, Johnson A. Monochorionic twin pregnancies. Clin Perinatol. 2005;32(2):475-94.
64. De Lia JE, Cruikshank DP, Keye WR Jr. Fetoscopic neodymium:YAG laser occlusion of placental vessels in severe twin-twin transfusion syndrome. Obstet Gynecol. 1990;75(6):1046-53.
65. Chalouhi GE, Essaoui M, Stirnemann J, Quibel T, Deloison B, Salomon L, et al. Laser therapy for twin-to-twin transfusion syndrome (TTTS). Prenat Diagn. 2011;31(7):637-46.
66. Ruano R, Rodo C, Peiro JL, Shamshirsaz AA, Haeri S, Nomura ML, et al. Fetoscopic laser ablation of placental anastomoses in twin-twin transfusion syndrome using 'Solomon technique'. Ultrasound Obstet Gynecol. 2013;42(4):434-9.
67. Slaghekke F, Lopriore E, Lewi L, Middeldorp JM, van Zwet EW, Weingertner AS, et al. Fetoscopic laser coagulation of the vascular equator versus selective coagulation for twin-to-twin transfusion syndrome: an open-label randomised controlled trial. Lancet. 2014;383(9935):2144-51.
68. Ville Y, Hyett J, Hecher K, Nicolaides K. Preliminary experience with endoscopic laser surgery for severe twin-twin transfusion syndrome. N Engl J Med. 1995;332(4):224-7.

69. Ville Y, Hecher K, Gagnon A, Sebire N, Hyett J, Nicolaides K. Endoscopic laser coagulation in the management of severe twin-to-twin transfusion syndrome. Br J Obstet Gynaecol. 1998;105(4):446-53.
70. Quintero RA, Morales WJ, Mendoza G, Allen M, Kalter CS, Giannina G, et al. Selective photocoagulation of placental vessels in twin-twin transfusion syndrome: evolution of a surgical technique. Obstet Gynecol Surv. 1998;53(12 Suppl):S97-103.
71. Papantoniou N. Twin to twin transfusion syndrome. In: Antsaklis AJ, Troyano JM (Eds). Donald School Textbook of Interventional Ultrasound, 1st edition. New Delhi: Jaypee Brothers Medical Publishers; 2008. pp. 100-12.
72. Troyano JM, Alvarez de la Rosa, Martinez-Wallin MI. Fetal biopsy procedures in prenatal diagnosis. In: Antsaklis AJ, Troyano JM (Eds). Donald School Textbook of Interventional Ultrasound. New Delhi: Jaypee Brothers Medical Publishers; 2008. pp. 72-85.
73. Elias S, Emerson DS, Simpson JL, Shulman LP, Holbrook KA. Ultrasound-guided fetal skin sampling for prenatal diagnosis of genodermatoses. Obstet Gynecol. 1994; 83(3):337-41.
74. Evans MI, Farrell SA, Greb A, Ray P, Johnson MP, Hoffman EP. In utero fetal muscle biopsy for the diagnosis of Duchenne muscular dystrophy in a female fetus "suddenly at risk". Am J Med Genet. 1993;46(3):309-12.
75. Kuller JA, Hoffman EP, Fries MH, Golbus MS. Prenatal diagnosis of Duchenne muscular dystrophy by fetal muscle biopsy. Hum Genet. 1992;90(1-2):34-40.
76. Fanin M, Pegoraro E, Angelini C. Absence of dystrophin and spectrin in regenerating muscle fibers from Becker dystrophy patients. J Neurol Sci. 1994;123(1-2):88-94.
77. Lindahl M, Bäckman E, Henriksson KG, Gorospe JR, Hoffman EP. Phospholipase A2 activity in dystrophinopathies. Neuromuscul Disord. 1995;5(3):193-9.
78. Benzie RJ, Ray P, Thompson D, Hunter AG, Ivey B, Salvador L. Prenatal exclusion of Duchenne muscular dystrophy by fetal muscle biopsy. Prenat Diagn. 1994;14(4):235.
79. Evans MI, Hoffman EP, Cadrin C, Johnson MP, Quintero RA, Golbus MS. Fetal muscle biopsy: collaborative experience with varied indications. Obstet Gynecol. 1994;84(6):913-7.
80. Evans MI, Krivchenia EL, Johnson MP, Quintero RA, King M, Pegoraro E, Hoffman EP. In utero fetal muscle biopsy alters diagnosis and carrier risks in Duchenne and Becker muscular dystrophy. Fetal Diagn Ther. 1995;10(2):71-5.
81. Evans MI, Quintero RA, King M, Qureshi F, Hoffman EP, Johnson MP. Endoscopically assisted, ultrasound-guided fetal muscle biopsy. Fetal Diagn Ther. 1995;10(3):167-72.
82. Troyano JM, Padron E, Clavijo M. Fetal biopsy and puncture. Actual status. Balkan Ohrid's School of Ultrasound. Ohrid, Macedonia: Dobri S Filipche; 1996. pp. 51-61.
83. Langham MR Jr, Kays DW, Ledbetter DJ, Frentzen B, Sanford LL, Richards DS. Congenital diaphragmatic hernia: epidemiology and outcome. Clin Perinatol. 1996;23(4):671-88.
84. Deprest J, Jani J, Van Schoubroeck D, Cannie M, Gallot D, Dymarkowski S, et al. Current consequences of prenatal diagnosis of congenital diaphragmatic hernia. J Pediatr Surg. 2006;41(2):423-30.
85. Witters I, Legius E, Moerman P, Deprest J, Van Schoubroeck D, Timmerman D, et al. Associated malformations and chromosomal anomalies in 42 cases of prenatally diagnosed diaphragmatic hernia. Am J Med Genet. 2001;103(4):278-82.
86. Ruano R, Lazar DA, Cass DL, Zamora IJ, Lee TC, Cassady CI, et al. Fetal lung volume and quantification of liver herniation by magnetic resonance imaging in isolated congenital diaphragmatic hernia. Ultrasound Obstet Gynecol. 2014;43(6):662-9.
87. Gratacos E. Congenital diaphragmatic hermia. In: Antsaklis AJ, Troyano JM (Eds). Donald School Textbook of Interventional Ultrasound. New Delhi: Jaypee Brothers Medical Publishers; 2008. pp. 33-41.
88. Sydorak RM, Harrison MR. Congenital diaphragmatic hernia: advances in prenatal therapy. World J Surg. 2003; 27(1):68-76.
89. Deprest J, Gratacos E, Nicolaides KH; FETO Task Group. Fetoscopic tracheal occlusion (FETO) for severe congenital diaphragmatic hernia: evolution of a technique and preliminary results. Ultrasound Obstet Gynecol. 2004;24(2):121-6.
90. Gucciardo L, Deprest J, Done' E, Van Mieghem T, Van de Velde M, Gratacos E, et al. Prediction of outcome in isolated congenital diaphragmatic hernia and its consequences for fetal therapy. Best Pract Res Clin Obstet Gynaecol. 2008;22(1):123-38.
91. Jani JC, Nicolaides KH, Gratacós E, Valencia CM, Doné E, Martinez JM, et al. Severe diaphragmatic hernia treated by fetal endoscopic tracheal occlusion. Ultrasound Obstet Gynecol. 2009;34(3):304-10.
92. Nassr AA, Erfani H, Fisher JE, Ogunleye OK, Espinoza J, Belfort MA, et al. Fetal interventional procedures and surgeries: a practical approach. J Perinat Med. 2018;46(7):701-15.
93. Ruano R, Peiro JL, da Silva MM, Campos JA, Carreras E, Tannuri U, et al. Early fetoscopic tracheal occlusion for extremely severe pulmonary hypoplasia in isolated congenital diaphragmatic hernia: preliminary results. Ultrasound Obstet Gynecol. 2013;42(1):70-6.
94. Cannie MM, Jani JC, De Keyzer F, Allegaert K, Dymarkowski S, Deprest J. Evidence and patterns in lung response after fetal tracheal occlusion: clinical controlled study. Radiology. 2009;252(2):526-33.
95. Deprest J, Jani J, Gratacos E, Nicolaides K. Deliberately delayed and shortened fetoscopic tracheal occlusion: a different strategy after prenatal diagnosis of life-threatening congenital diaphragmatic hernias-Repy. J Pediatr Surg. 2006;41:1345-6.
96. Deprest JA, Flemmer AW, Gratacos E, Nicolaides K. Antenatal prediction of lung volume and in-utero treatment by fetal endoscopic tracheal occlusion in severe isolated

congenital diaphragmatic hernia. Semin Fetal Neonatal Med. 2009;14(1):8-13.
97. Javid PJ, Jaksic T, Skarsgard ED, Lee S; Canadian Neonatal N. Survival rate in congenital diaphragmatic hernia: the experience of the Canadian Neonatal Network. J Pediatr Surg. 2004;39(5):657-60.
98. Longaker MT, Laberge JM, Dansereau J, et al. Primary fetal hydrothorax: natural history and management. J Pediatr Surg. 1989;24(6):573-6.
99. Estoff JA, Parad RB, Frigoletto FJr, Benacerraf BR. The natural history of isolated fetal hydrothorax. Ultrasound Obstet Gynecol. 1992;2(3):162.
100. Khalek N, Johnson MP. Management of prenatally diagnosed lung lesions. Semin Pediatr Surg. 2013;22(1):24-9.
101. Weber AM, Philipson EH. Fetal pleural effusion: a review and meta-analysis for prognostic indicators. Obstet Gynecol. 1992;79(2):281-6.
102. Smith RP, Illanes S, Denbow ML, Soothill PW. Outcome of fetal pleural effusions treated by thoracoamniotic shunting. Ultrasound Obstet Gynecol. 2005;26(1):63-6.
103. Barron SD, Pass RF. Infectious causes of hydrops fetalis. Semin Perinatol. 1995;19(6):493-501.
104. Dupre AR, Morrison JC, Martin JN Jr, Floyd RC, Blake PG. Clinical application of the Kleihauer-Betke test. J Reprod Med. 1993;38(8):621-4.
105. Achiron R, Weissman A, Lipitz S, Mashiach S, Goldman B. Fetal pleural effusion: the risk of fetal trisomy. Gynecol Obstet Invest. 1995;39(3):153-6.
106. Klam S, Bigras JL, Hudon L. Predicting outcome in primary fetal hydrothorax. Fetal Diagn Ther. 2005;20(5):366-70.
107. Waller K, Chaithongwongwatthana S, Yamasmit W, Donnenfeld AE. Chromosomal abnormalities among 246 fetuses with pleural effusions detected on prenatal ultrasound examination: factors associated with an increased risk of aneuploidy. Genet Med. 2005;7(6):17-421.
108. Castagno R, Carreras Moratonas E, Toran N, Higueras MT, Sanchez Duran M A. Fetal pleural effusion. In: Antsaklis AJ, Troyano JM (Eds). Donald School Textbook of Interventional Ultrasound. New Delhi: Jaypee Brothers Medical Publishers; 2008. pp. 113-25.
109. Pétres RE, Redwine FO, Cruikshank DP. Congenital bilateral chylothorax: antepartum diagnosis and successful intrauterine surgical management. JAMA. 1982;248(11):1360-1.
110. Benacerraf BR, Frigoletto FD Jr, Wilson M. Successful midtrimester thoracentesis with analysis of the lymphocyte population in the pleural effusion. Am J Obstet Gynecol. 1986;155(2):398-9.
111. Seeds JW, Bowes WA Jr. Results of treatment of severe fetal hydrothorax with bilateral pleuroamniotic catheters. Obstet Gynecol. 1996;68(4):57-580.
112. Okawa T, Takano Y, Fujimori K, Yanagida K, Sato A. A new fetal therapy for chylothorax: pleurodesis with OK-432. Ultrasound Obstet Gynecol. 2001;18(4):376-7.
113. Tanemura M, Nishikawa N, Kojima K, Suzuki Y, Suzumori K. A case of successful fetal therapy for congenital chylothorax by intrapleural injection of OK-432. Ultrasound Obstet Gynecol. 2001;18(4):371-5.
114. Jorgensen C, Brocks V, Bang J, Jorgensen FS, Rønsbro L. Treatment of severe fetal chylothorax associated with pronounced hydrops with intrapleural injection of OK-432. Ultrasound Obstet Gynecol. 2003;21(1):66-9.
115. Chen M, Shih JC, Wang BT, Chen CP, Yu CL. Fetal OK-432 pleurodesis: complete or incomplete? Ultrasound Obstet Gynecol. 2005;26(7):791-3.
116. Nygaard U, Sundberg K, Nielsen HS, Hertel S, Jorgensen C. New treatment of early fetal chylothorax. Obstet Gynecol. 2007;109(5):1088-92.
117. Nicolaides KH, Azar GB. Thoraco-amniotic shunting. Fetal Diagn Ther. 1990;5(3-4):153-64.
118. Rodeck CH, Fisk NM, Fraser DI, Nicolini U. Long-term in utero drainage of fetal hydrothorax. N Engl J Med. 1988;319(17):1135-8.
119. Weiner C, Varner M, Pringle K, Hein H, Williamson R, Smith WL. Antenatal diagnosis and palliative treatment of nonimmune hydrops fetalis secondary to pulmonary extralobar sequestration. Obstet Gynecol. 1986;68(2):275-80.
120. Cardwell MS. Aspiration of fetal pleural effusions or ascites may improve neonatal resuscitation. South Med J. 1996;89(2):177-8.
121. Anumba DO, Scott JE, Plant ND, Robson SC. Diagnosis and outcome of fetal lower urinary tract obstruction in the northern region of England. Prenat Diagn. 2005;25(1):7-13.
122. Pinette MG, Blackstone J, Wax JR, Cartin A. Enlarged fetal bladder: differential diagnosis and outcomes. J Clin Ultrasound. 2003;31(6):328-34.
123. Liao AW, Sebire NJ, Geerts L, Cicero S, Nicolaides KH. Megacystis at 10–14 weeks of gestation: chromosomal defects and outcome according to bladder length. Ultrasound Obstet Gynecol. 2003;21(4):338-41.
124. Bernardes LS, Aksnes G, Saada J, Masse V, Elie C, Dumez Y, et al. Keyhole sign: how specific is it for the diagnosis of posterior urethral valves? Ultrasound Obstet Gynecol. 2009;34(4):419-23.
125. Morris RK, Malin GL, Quinlan-Jones E, Middleton LJ, Hemming K, Burke D, et al; Percutaneous vesicoamniotic shunting in Lower Urinary Tract Obstruction (PLUTO) Collaborative Group. Percutaneous vesicoamniotic shunting versus conservative management for fetal lower urinary tract obstruction (PLUTO): a randomised trial. Lancet. 2013;382(9903):1496-506.
126. Miller OF, Lashley DB, McAleer IM, Kaplan GW. Diagnosis of urethral obstruction with prenatal magnetic resonance imaging. J Urol. 2002;168(3):1158-9.
127. Nassr AA, Koh CK, Shamshirsaz AA, Espinoza J, Sangi-Haghpeykar H, Sharhan D, et al. Are ultrasound renal aspects associated with urinary biochemistry in fetuses

with lower urinary tract obstruction? Prenat Diagn. 2016;36(13):1206-10.
128. Ruano R, Duarte S, Bunduki V, Giron AM, Srougi M, Zugaib M. Fetal cystoscopy for severe lower urinary tract obstruction: initial experience of a single center. Prenat Diagn. 2010;30(1):30-9.
129. Brunner SE, Durmaz LO, Meinzer A, Arp M, Krebs TF, Bergholz R. Minimally invasive bimanual fetal surgery: a review. Children (Basel). 2022;9(9):1377.
130. Pluto Collaborative Study Group; Kilby M, Khan K, Morris K, Daniels J, Gray R, Magill L, et al. PLUTO trial protocol: percutaneous shunting for lower urinary tract obstruction randomised controlled trial. BJOG. 2007;114(7):904-5.
131. Van Mieghem T, Ryan G. The PLUTO trial: a missed opportunity. Lancet. 2013;382(9903):1471-3.
132. Galindo A, Guttierrez-Larraya F, Velasco J, De la Fuente P. Interventional fetal cardiology. In: Antsaklis AJ, Troyano JM (Eds). Donald School Textbook of Interventional Ultrasound. Jaypee Brothers Medical Publishers; 2008. pp. 15-34.
133. Galindo A, Guttierrez-Larraya F, de la Fuente P. Congenital heart defects in fetal life: an overview. Ultrasound Obstet Gynecol. 2004;4:194-207.
134. Kohl T. Fetal echocardiography: new grounds to explore during fetal cardiac intervention. Pediatr Cardiol. 2002;23(3):334-46.
135. Kohl T, Sharland G, Allan LD, et al. World experience of percutaneous ultrasound-guided balloon valvuloplasty in human fetuses with severe aortic valve obstruction. Am J Cardiol. 2000;85(10):1230-3.
136. Marshall AC, van der Velde ME, Tworetzky W, Gomez CA, Wilkins-Haug L, Benson CB, et al. Creation of an atrial septal defect in utero for fetuses with hypoplastic left heart syndrome and intact or highly restrictive atrial septum. Circulation. 2004;110(3):253-8.
137. Tworetzky W, Wilkins-Haug L, Jennings RW, van der Velde ME, Marshall AC, Marx GR, et al. Balloon dilation of severe aortic stenosis in the fetus: potential for prevention of hypoplastic left heart syndrome: candidate selection, technique, and results of successful intervention. Circulation. 2004;110(15):2125-31.
138. Tulzer G, Arzt W, Franklin RC, Loughna PV, Mair R, Gardiner HM. Fetal pulmonary valvuloplasty for critical pulmonary stenosis or atresia with intact septum. Lancet. 2002;360(9345):1567-8.
139. Galindo A, Gutiérrez-Larraya F, Velasco JM, de la Fuente P. Pulmonary balloon valvuloplasty in a fetus with critical pulmonary stenosis/atresia with intact ventricular septum and heart failure. Fetal Diagn Ther. 2006;21(1):100-4.
140. Quintero RA, Huhta J, Suh E, Chmait R, Romero R, Angel J. In utero cardiac fetal surgery: laser atrial septotomy in the treatment of hypoplastic left heart syndrome with intact atrial septum. Am J Obstet Gynecol. 2005;193(4):1424-8.
141. Jouannic JM, Boudjemline Y, Benifla JL, Bonnet D. Re: in-utero intervention for hypoplastic left heart syndrome: for which fetus and for what? Ultrasound Obstet Gynecol. 2006;27(1):101.
142. Allen HD, Beekman RH 3rd, Garson A Jr, Hijazi ZM, Mullins C, O'Laughlin MP, et al. Pediatric therapeutic cardiac catheterization: a statement for healthcare professionals from the Council on Cardiovascular Disease in the Young, American Heart Association. Circulation. 1998;97(6):609-25.
143. Liley AW. Intrauterine Transfusion of Foetus in Haemolytic Disease. Br Med J 1963;2:1107-9

39 CHAPTER

Chorionic Villus Sampling

Ulla Marton, Asim Kurjak, Milan Stanojević

INTRODUCTION

Development of the relatively new field of fetomaternal medicine with new techniques of prenatal diagnosis, which developed in the last few decades, brought new technical possibilities as well as new dilemmas for parents and physicians. Individual risk assessment for fetuses with triploidy requires a setup capable of offering screening methods to all pregnant women offering them an invasive procedure when the estimated risk is recognized above the certain nonacceptable cut-off within noninvasive biochemical tests for patients and when cell-free DNA tests or ultrasound aberration have been detected. First-trimester ultrasound evaluation of the fetal morphology plus measurement of nuchal translucency (NT) combined with the biochemical testing [pregnancy-associated plasma protein A (PAPP-A) and free beta-human chorionic gonadotropin (β-hCG)] in combination with maternal age has been shown to be very efficient with a detection rate of 90 for a 5% false-positive rate.[1] Individual risk assessment for Down syndrome includes maternal age, previous pregnancy with a chromosomal abnormality, a parent with a chromosomal abnormality or carrier of an autosomal recessive disorder, and a structural fetal abnormality by ultrasound and evaluation of fetal morphology on ultrasound such as nasal bone, ductus venous, tricuspid regurgitation, and facial angle.[1] Development and incorporation of noninvasive prenatal diagnosis (NIPD) in everyday clinical practice has been a breakthrough in the field of fetal-maternal medicine during the last decades with the development of advanced and rapid genome analysis technologies such as chromosomal microarray and next-generation sequencing (NGS). Prenatal diagnostics has expanded from the most common aneuploidies to the detection of many other structural chromosomal abnormalities (DNA copy number variations, deletions, and duplications) as well as monogenic diseases.[1,2] Rapid advancement in the field of prenatal medicine has been achieved due to the technological evolution of ultrasonography that has allowed the recognition of various ultrasonographic findings and their combination with biochemical results and demographic characteristics in order to estimate a final individual risk for a chromosomal anomaly of the fetus plus analysis of short fragments of fetal DNA released into the mother bloodstream through a natural process of cell death. However, invasive testing remains the main clinically available technique for the definite diagnosis of both chromosomal anomalies and many single-gene disorders. This new field of prenatal diagnosis requires medical practitioners with extensive training and expensive, highly sophisticated technology and laboratory techniques.[1] Recognition of congenital structural anomalies includes all procedures that lead to the diagnosis and detection of fetal anomalies. Since the introduction of prenatal diagnosis by amniocentesis to obtain fetal cells for analysis to detect or exclude genetic defects, the most unpleasant aspects of the process have been the time of gestation to have the test and the long wait for results. If the diagnosis of an affected fetus with chromosomal disorder was made, then one of the options for the parents is termination of the pregnancy in the second trimester. Late termination causes significant psychological trauma for couples and involves increased medical risk for the mother compared to the termination of the pregnancy in the first trimester, therefore efforts were made toward developing a technique that could be used in the first trimester to have an accurate diagnosis. The psychological stress is not eliminated, but in some aspects, it is lessened and more acceptable by this option. Chorionic villus sampling (CVS), also called chorionic villous biopsy, has evolved as an essential clinical procedure but is invasive in approach to diagnoses of chromosomal, genetic, and metabolic diseases in the embryonic period.[2,3] CVS is one of the invasive diagnostic methods used to diagnose chromosomal, genetic, and metabolic diseases in the embryonic period. The method itself is an accepted procedure across the world and can be performed through transabdominal (TA) and transcervical (TC) approaches.[1] The American College of Obstetricians and Gynecologists (ACOG) is highly determined in the statement that the women of all ages should be offered assessment for aneuploidy by screening or diagnostic testing regardless of maternal age or other risk factors.[2,3] Therefore, application in the everyday practice of noninvasive prenatal tests with (combined test) for aneuploidy screening by the end of the first trimester and use of cell-free DNA testing from maternal blood has resulted in a significant decline in screen-positive results and therefore fewer invasive prenatal tests are being carried out. However, invasive procedures such as CVS and amniocentesis remain the only definitive diagnostic tests for aneuploidy in pregnancy. CVS, carried out to obtain placental villi for analysis, is usually performed between 11+0 and 13+6 weeks of gestation. Individualized counseling on the benefit of CVS versus amniocentesis should be provided for women considering CVS during this time period.[1-3]

Indications for chorionic villus sampling include:

- Abnormal early genetic screening on a noninvasive prenatal testing (NIPT), first trimester combined screening, or abnormalities detected on ultrasound
- Positive family history of a child with autosomal trisomy or sex chromosome aneuploidy or a structural birth defect
- Advanced maternal or paternal age
- Parental carrier of a chromosomal rearrangement or aneuploidy or aneuploidy mosaicism
- Parental request
- Parental carrier of a genetic disorder (Tay-Sachs, sickle cell disease, or neurofibromatosis, thalassemia, cystic fibrosis, Duchenne/Becker muscular dystrophy, congenital adrenal hyperplasia, hemophilia A/B, other monogenic diseases)[1,3]
- *Diagnosis of inborn errors of metabolism:* Lysosomal storage diseases, for example, mucopolysaccharidoses, disorders of amino acid/peptide/organic acid/ carbohydrate/fatty acid metabolism
- Diagnosis of infectious diseases
- Paternity testing.

CONTRAINDICATIONS FOR THE CHORIONIC VILLUS SAMPLING

A relative contraindication for the CVS procedure is maternal alloimmunization as the procedure may cause more severe fetal hemolytic disease.[4] Awareness should be done in patients who are receiving anticoagulation therapy. Patients with bloodborne infectious diseases such as human immunodeficiency virus (HIV) and hepatitis should be advised of the possible risk of vertical transmission with prenatal diagnostic testing. If invasive diagnosis is necessary, the risk of vertical transitions has to be explained to the women and the procedure should be carried out when the woman is on antiretroviral therapy and the viral load is not detectable in order to reduce the risk of vertical transmission to the fetus as much as possible.[4] Active vaginal bleeding and subchorionic hemorrhage are contraindications for CVS and the TC approach is contraindicated in cases of vaginal infections.

TECHNICAL ASPECTS OF THE PROCEDURE

Chorionic villus sampling procedure is performed under continuous ultrasound guidance in real time using an aseptic technique. The following equipment is required:

- *For the TA approach:*
  - Sterile drape
  - Sterile ultrasound probe cover
  - Chlorhexidine or iodine preparation
  - A local anesthetic of your choice (optional)
  - 10 cc and 20 cc syringe
  - 18-gauge or 20-gauge spinal needle
  - Sample collection container with transport media
- *For the TC approach:*
  - Sterile speculum
  - Single tooth tenaculum
  - Iodine preparation
  - 10 cc and 20 cc syringe
  - TC-CVS catheter
  - Sample collection container with transport media.

Before the procedure, consultation with a fetomaternal specialist should be done to inform parents and discuss all the risks and benefits of the procedure. Counseling should include the nature of the procedure, possible complications, and the success rate of the method. The alternative diagnostic methods should be discussed with parents. The accuracy of the laboratory has to be presented as well as the possibility of ambiguity after the results. Evaluation of the need for

RhoGAM in Rh-negative patients has to be discussed. Careful ultrasound examination has to be done to evaluate the location of the placenta, cord insertion, viability of the embryo, and assessment of gestational age by measurement of the crown–rump length. Insurgent of all necessary materials including transport media should be done. During the procedure, appropriate lighting and a comfortable position of the patient on the examination table are required. With the patient whole procedure should be explained step by step to avoid anxiety and fear of the patient and couple. Preparation of the abdominal wall or vagina with cervix is required before the procedure. CVS is performed on an outpatient basis and the patient is instructed to avoid any strenuous physical activity for a couple of days after the procedure is performed. TA CVS is performed like amniocentesis, as a single or double needle technique. The patient is placed in a supine position on the examination table. The abdomen is cleaned with a chlorhexidine or iodine solution; sterile drapes are placed to create a sterile field. A local anesthetic may be used. Detailed ultrasound evaluation of the embryo, amnion, and location of the chorion should be done before the procedure. The course of the needle to enter the placental tissue should be planned and defined in advance **(Figs. 1 and 2)**. After treating the skin surface with an antiseptic solution, a needle is inserted through the skin into the womb and guided to the trophoblast using the image on the ultrasound scan. Since the introduction of the technique in the early 1970s, several types of instruments (needles, plastic or metal aspiration catheters, and biopsy forceps) have been used, but the choice of the instrument is still made on the basis of the personal preference of the operator rather than scientific evidence data. During the procedure, the direction of the needle should be chosen as much parallel to the long axis of the placental tissue as possible, a sampling path is chosen so that the tip of the needle/instrument should pass within the chorion frondosum parallel to the chorionic membrane.[5] The chorionic villi required for cytogenetic analysis are obtained by aspiration using negative pressure created by a syringe or a vacuum aspirator. Alternatively, some tissue forceps can be used by passing through a trocar guide needle, and a small amount of placental tissue–trophoblast tissue is grasped and removed for analysis. When a single needle technique is used, the needle of 20 gauge is inserted into the chorionic tissue, and a syringe is attached to the needle, which is used to take a small sample of cells from the chorionic villi. After the sample is taken, the needle is removed. At some centers, a double-needle technique is used, an 18-gauge needle is inserted into the chorionic villi, and the stylet is removed.[5] Then a smaller needle (20-gauge) with the aspirating syringe is inserted through this needle to obtain a sample and moderate suction is applied. If the sample is not adequate, the sampling procedure with this smaller needle, through an 18-gauge needle, can be repeated if necessary. Theoretically, the double needle technique is less stressful as the outer trocar remains still during sampling, and therefore procedure can be repeated without reinserting the trocar. The learning period of the operator should be done by double-needle technique as it is the most appropriate approach to make the sampling procedure easy and less traumatic for both the physician and the patient. If the tip of the needle is inserted into the myometrium and leads into the frondosum, then the needle is redirected so that the tip of the needle will course parallel to the membrane through as much trophoblast tissue as possible. Insertion

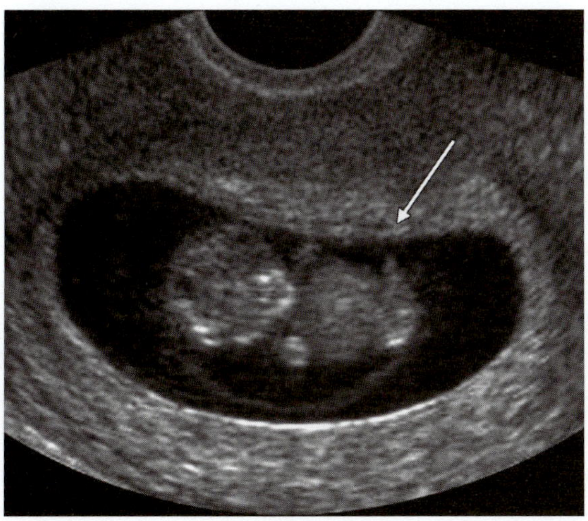

Fig. 1: Route of aspiration of the chorion.

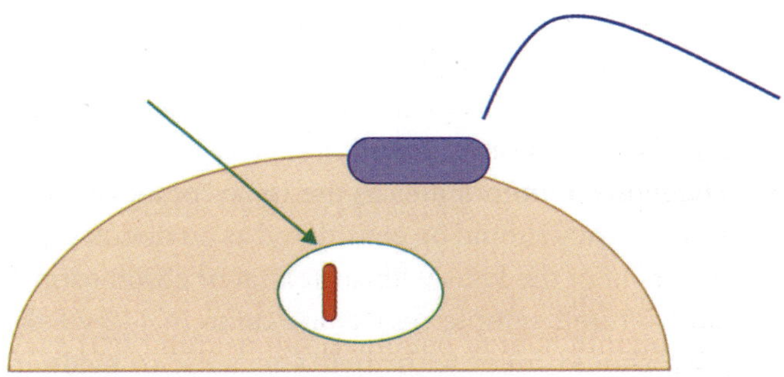

Fig. 2: Scheme of the procedure, freehand technique.

of the needle into the decidua or myometrium, rather than the chorion frondosum, will cause the feeling of "gripping", therefore the adjustment of the tip should be done back into the frondosum. After placement of the tip of the needle in the chorion, the stylet is removed. The syringe of 20 mL containing 2–3 mL of media is attached and negative pressure is applied, the needle is moved up and down several times in the frondosum parallel to the chorionic plate. After the suction, the needle is removed.[5]

If the TC approach is used, the patient is placed in a lithotomy position, and a sterile speculum is inserted into the vagina. The cervix is cleaned with an iodine solution. A single tooth tenaculum may be applied to the anterior lip of the cervix to facilitate the passage of the catheter. Under continuous ultrasound guidance, a TC-CVS catheter is inserted into the chorionic tissue. The catheter contains a malleable guidewire with an echogenic tip, which can be seen on an ultrasound. Once the catheter is in the proper location, the stylet is removed, a 20-cc syringe containing media is attached to the end of the catheter, and negative pressure is created. The sample is evaluated for adequacy before ending the procedure. The TC-CVS can also be performed using small biopsy forceps. After the procedure, the chorionic villi retrieved can be easily confirmed by the operator in the syringe by holding it up to a light or by visualization of the chorionic tissue in a Petri dish. If insufficient chorionic tissue is obtained on the first pass, a second attempt should be made. Chorionic tissue samples are sent to the laboratory for culturing and further testing, including conventional karyotype, fluorescence in situ hybridization, and chromosomal microarray. Rapid assessment results return in 2–4 days providing the ability for the patient's/couple's accurate diagnosis in a short period with the opportunity to seek counseling for obstetric management and recommendations.[1-5] Accurate diagnosis is providing an early referral to fetomaternal and pediatric subspecialistswho can counsel the patient enabling pregnant patient to make informed decision on pregnancy outcome. The moral dilemmas have an essential application in the clinical management of pregnancies complicated by fetal structural or chromosomal abnormalities as the issues of termination of the pregnancy should be considered as an option in the management of the fetus with structural or chromosomal defect. Cultured sample results are done in 1–2 weeks. Couples should meet with their specialist to evaluate results and possible further management and follow-up.

COMPLICATIONS AND FETAL LOSS RISK

The biggest concern for all regarding invasive prenatal diagnosis is the procedure-related risk of fetal loss, especially the loss of a healthy fetus, which is recognized as an agonizing life situation for parents. The risk calculation should have in mind the background risk of miscarriage, which is greater at earlier gestational ages and to exclude all possible additional adverse events. The operator's skill and experience play an important role in achieving the lowest complications and possible loss rates. Published pregnancy loss-rate after the procedure is between 0.5-1.0% eithr for CVS or amniocentesis when performed by experienced experts.[5,6] Performed studies including randomized studies have been conducted and have compared the different methods of CVS sampling with amniocentesis or one CVS method with the other (TC-CVS vs. TA-CVS).[7] Reported postprocedure complications following CVS procedure are rare; vaginal spotting and bleeding are the most common complications, with an incidence of 7–10/100 of TC procedures.[8] In up to 4% of performed procedures, a small hematoma may be identified at the sampling site immediately following the procedure.[9] The nature of the procedure has raised concerns about the possibility of introducing a pathogenic microorganism in the uterine cavity, especially through the TC route. The most common pathogens are those of the vaginal flora when the TC route is performed. Perforation of the bowel could be the main factor of contamination when the TA route is performed. Uterine infection was reported in 0.13% (2/1,501) of TC-CVS and localized peritoneal reaction was reported in 0.3% (3/903) of TA route of CVS.[10] Development of subclinical infection has been related to increased risk of pregnancy loss after the performed procedure. Even in asymptomatic women undergoing CVS procedures, positive vaginal cultures in a group of patients harboring at least one microorganism were found in almost one-third of cases (29.9%). Mycoplasmas alone or in combination with other microorganisms were statistically more frequently isolated after pregnancy losses in the TC-CVS group (37.9%) as well as in the TA-CVS group (20.6%) than in the total group (17.6%).[10] Concerning the TA-CVS performed route group, mycoplasmas could be detected only in cases of late pregnancy losses (abortions >2 weeks after the procedure).[11] Infection may arise from organisms present on the skin, ultrasound probe, and gel, and therefore skin decontamination should be done as well as separate sterile gel sachet has to be used. The ultrasound probe should be in a sterile bag and continuous ultrasound are recommended prior invasive procedures of CVS. If prior the procedure women show any clinical features to suggest acute vaginal infection or intra-amniotic infection, it should be considered to postpone the procedure or consider sending a small quantity of amniotic fluid for microbiological analysis and consider adequate antibiotic treatment. Reduction of amniotic fluid amount, oligohydramnios is registered very rarely. Data published from the Canadian collaborative experience showed no significant increase in fetal loss following CVS when compared to midtrimester amniocentesis.[10] Results showed 7.6% fetal losses (spontaneous abortions, induced abortions, and late losses) in the CVS group compared to 7.0% in the amniocentesis group.[10,11] Results of American collaborative study proved no significant difference in loss between CVS and amniocentesis.[11]

Due to the reported increased risk for limb reduction defects, early CVS <10–11 weeks of gestation is not recommended.[12,13] Early reports identified infants with severe limb malformations among pregnancies after CVS performed prior to 66 days of gestation.[14] Increased risk of limb reduction defects after 10 weeks of gestation was not ducted. Due to the doubtful data below 10 weeks of gestation, it has been suggested to avoid the procedure of CVS before 10 weeks. Only if there is an exceptional medical need to perform the procedure of CVS, patients should be informed about a ≥1% risk of possible limb reduction defects as a probable procedure complication. Four of the reported infants had the oromandibular limb hypogenesis syndrome and one had a terminal transverse limb reduction defect; all of the performed CVS procedures in the affected infants were between 55 and 66 days of gestation and done by TA approach. The report with an overview of the approximate 140,000 CVS procedures reported to the World Health Organization registry demonstrated no increment in the overall incidence of limb reduction defects following CVS between 9 and 12 weeks of gestation.[15] The procedure of choice for the second-trimester invasive diagnostic testing is second-trimester amniocentesis as it turned to be safer than early amniocentesis or TC approach of CVS.[15] The total pregnancy loss after performed invasive prenatal diagnostic procedures (CVS and amniocentesis) should incorporate a procedure-related loss. This data should be added to the background of rates of all fetal loss. The spontaneous fetal loss rate has been difficult to define, as observed populations have not been followed from the early weeks of pregnancy. Previously reported results of certain spontaneous fetal losses may have been prejudiced because of different definitions of fetal demise and provided follow-up. Different approaches in confirming the viability of pregnancy and divergent intervals between the two ultrasound scans showing a live fetus and detection of fetal loss might cause misinterpretation in observed data.[16] The background of fetal demise rate in women in whom invasive procedure may be indicated is related to maternal age, gestational age, and the indication for the testing. The overall calculated risk will, therefore, be different for a unit serving to general population than a referral center serving women who are at high risk. The background fetal demise rate depends on the department where the procedure is performed. In a decisive randomized trial, the estimated incidence of procedure-related pregnancy miscarriage due to amniocentesis performed at a mean gestational age of 16 weeks was 1.0%, when comparing mid-trimester amniocentesis with ultrasonography only in the control group.[17] The miscarriage rate following the CVS procedure was found to be comparable to the fetal loss rate after amniocentesis.[1,3,5] Data from the review showed that the pregnancy loss before 24 weeks was 0.9% following amniocentesis and 1.3% following CVS with a wide variation between studies, depriving invasive procedures to women at a high risk with extended use of NIPT changed the proportion of invasive test from 10.6% to 4.9%.[18] In contrast, due to the introduction of NIPT in everyday practice, the number of Down syndrome diagnosed prenatally has increased. Despite of reported data on the decreasing number of all invasive procedures, the proportion of CVS has been reported as 69% of all invasive tests. The data that can be concluded from systematic reviews and randomized controlled trials as well as a large national registry study show that a procedure-related pregnancy loss rate of 0.5–1.0% for amniocentesis as well as for CVS.[18,19] The data from single-center studies suggests that performance depends on skilled operators. Variation in published results on pregnancy outcomes between studies is due to differences in study organization, including variations in equipment and techniques used. The calculated risk of fetal loss is 0.30% following amniocentesis, and no significant procedure-related risk associated with CVS was found. CVS may appear to be a safer procedure than amniocentesis. Presented results showed that the estimated rates for fetal demise are even lower, with no significant increase in the risk of miscarriage for both invasive procedure amniocentesis and CVS when the analyzed data are limited to studies in which the control study group has a similar risk profile for chromosomal abnormalities as the women underwent an invasive procedure for prenatal testing. Pregnancies with increased fetal NT, a reversed a-wave in the ductus venosus, and decreased maternal serum PAPP-A are at high risk of carrying a fetus with chromosomal abnormalities.[20] CVS in such cases is associated with an increased risk of pregnancy loss.[20] Data from the study demonstrated that the risk of pregnancy loss before 24 weeks gestation in women who underwent invasive diagnostic procedure, amniocentesis or CVS, is not significantly different from women who had any invasive procedure.[20] In conclusion, the proximate loss rate accountable to the invasive procedure is 0.1% for amniocentesis and 0.2% for CVS.[19,20]

These risks may be that are unrelated to the invasive procedure but also may reflect the pregnancy characteristics of the women undergoing invasive testing. It is important that pregnant women should be counseled with accurate estimates of procedure-related risks associated with invasive testing to allow them to make appropriate choices rather than with exaggerated risks based on historical data.

MULTIPLE PREGNANCY

With maternal age, the prevalence of multiple pregnancies is getting higher, the number is increased by assisted reproductive techniques. Screening for chromosomal abnormalities in multiple pregnancies is based on maternal age, evaluation of fetal morphology, and the NT, nasal bone; therefore, it has been possible to calculate the risk of trisomy-21 for each fetus in multiple pregnancies by using this screening method. By evaluation of fetal morphology with ultrasound, some of the major fetal anomalies can be detected by the end of the first trimester and this can put the pregnancy at risk for chromosomal abnormalities. With the CVS invasive procedure, early prenatal diagnosis is possible in multiple pregnancies as early as the end of the first trimester. The fetal demise rate after a CVS procedure in twin pregnancy is high compared to amniocentesis (single entry to sample both sites of the trophoblastic tissue at the same attempt) and rises to 2%.[21,22] When using a two-entry approach and needling technique for both CVS and amniocentesis, the reported fetal loss rate is approximately the same.[21,22] Adequate information and genetic counseling should be given to the family about the risk for chromosomal abnormalities in multiple pregnancies and according to the procedure-related fetal loss rate. With clear and proper information, a couple can make a decision based on sufficient information available. In multiple pregnancies, CVS in the first trimester in a patient at risk for chromosomal abnormality (according to the evaluation of the nuchal fold) gives an ability to make selective feticide if there is a chromosomal abnormality in the fetus. The procedure of CVS has been proven to be both a safe and effective method for sampling in multiple gestations and has the advantage of an earlier diagnosis than amniocentesis.[23] Ultrasound scanning identifies the locations of the individual chorion frondosum sites and confirms the viability and gestational age. The application of ultrasound allows evaluation of the location of the pregnancies, characteristics of the dividing membrane, and chronicity (monochromic or chorionic). The procedure is done by sampling of each gestation by needling each distinct frondosum; to ensure sampling of each chorion frondosum, continuous ultrasound localization of the needle tip is required. Ultrasound evaluation is necessary for both sagittal and transverse views to confirm that individual samples of chorionic tissue are being retrieved. In pregnancies where chorions are fused and the borders of the chorion frondosum are indistinct, sampling near cord insertion sites is suggested. If there is a doubt about the adequate sample, a follow-up procedure should be performed as a repeat CVS sampling performed immediately, or a second-trimester amniocentesis should be suggested.[21,24] Contamination of one sample with villi from the second sac occurs most frequently when sampling is performed close to the dividing membrane. Twin-twin contamination can also occur if a needle is dragged through one frondosum while attempting to sample another villus. In evaluated twin series, fetal karyotype abnormalities occurred in 2.0% and 3.1% of the fetuses.[23,24] Therefore, documentation of the location of the fetuses is most important; if later there is any doubt as to the location of the affected fetus with chromosomal abnormality, a repeat placental biopsy can be performed prior to selective termination of the pregnancy with chromosomal abnormality and a direct villous preparation or fluorescence in situ hybridization (FISH) technique utilized to confirm correct fetal location. There is the possibility of one fetus having an abnormal chromosomal result, it may occur somewhat more frequently with CVS than following amniocentesis as chromosomal abnormalities are more common in earlier gestations.

CONCLUSION

Ultrasound-guided CVS has been demonstrated to be a safe and useful outdoor invasive effective procedure that is capable of providing adequate information for the couple at risk of having a child with a chromosomal aberration. Pregnancy affected with a fetus with chromosomal abnormality is rising a list of possible medical and psychological complications of second-trimester pregnancy termination. Therefore, early diagnosis is more than essential to have a final diagnosis when in utero gene or stem cell therapy is contemplated to correct a genetic defect or to make an end-most decision whether to continue or terminate ongoing pregnancy. For a proper diagnosis or application of the new therapies, advanced and complex technology is required as well dedicated and well-trained experts are needed to provide complete procedure and treatment. First-trimester procedures lowered maternal anxiety levels earlier when they are provided information relevant to decisions about whether to continue a current gestation, which is affected by the congenital disease of malformation, which has a great impact on life quality and spans. Despite the main advantages of the CVS procedure and the ability of early diagnosis, utilization of CVS has failed to become widely available. This lack of complete acceptance of CVS has been primarily due to exaggerated literature data on the risks of pregnancy demise and possible congenital abnormalities as a procedure complication.

The discovery and ability to isolate fetal nucleic acid in maternal plasma have opened in the last decade. Despite the development of noninvasive, risk-free, and accurate screening tests for both mother and fetus, it's important to remember that these tests are only intended for screening purposes and do not provide a definitive diagnosis. However, they offer physicians and future parents a detection rate of 98–99% for chromosomal anomalies. When the outcome of the cell-free DNA test is positive, in most of the positive cases it is usually followed by an invasive diagnostic procedure for a definitive result. Invasive diagnostic procedures such as CVS with a procedure-related fetal loss risk of 0.5–1.0% can be directly attributed to inexperience with the procedure. Performing chorionic villi biopsy is technically demanding, with a relatively long-learning curve. Due to the 0.5–1% risk of fetal loss after invasive prenatal diagnostic testing, tremendous interest in the development of NIPD techniques that may possibly replace invasive procedures such as CVS and amniocentesis in the future is present. Still, at present, we are facing the clinical limitation of the NIPT, therefore CVS is still the method of choice for first-trimester invasive prenatal diagnosis. In experienced hands, it is a safe and reliable method, with a fetal loss risk close to that of amniocentesis. If the procedure is performed after 10 completed weeks of gestation, the risk of limb defects is not greater than the risk in the general population. Complications such as infection, spotting, and light bleeding are rare. CVS remains at present the main method of choice for accurate and definite early prenatal diagnosis. Adequate training, observation of competence, good clinical practice, "centralization" in specialized centers, and continuous control of outcomes are essential to keep its safety.

Prenatal medicine in terms of screening for fetal anomalies, structural and chromosomal, originates from the 60s of the last century. Advancements in technology have enabled first-trimester screenings for chromosomal abnormalities using various factors such as maternal age, nuchal thickness, nasal bone, ductus venosus, tricuspid regurgitation, facial angle, and minor's markers, along with free-β-hCG and PAPP-A. These screenings have brought about a detection rate of 97% for chromosomal abnormalities. With the development of advanced and rapid genome analysis technologies, such as chromosomal microarray and NGS, prenatal diagnostics has expanded from the most common aneuploidies to the detection of many other structural chromosomal abnormalities (DNA copy number variations, deletions, and duplications) as well as monogenic diseases, but still in present CVS is a requested method of early definitive prenatal diagnosis. Women and couples should be reassured that CVS, as an invasive procedure carried out with experienced physicians in specialist centers, is not associated with a significant increase in fetal loss rate, with a risk rate below 0.5%, and that the possible background risk for miscarriage is significantly higher in the presence of fetal anomaly and abnormal karyotype. Ultrasound-guided TA-CVS is a useful outdoor procedure and is considered the method of choice for fetal sampling and accurate early prenatal diagnosis.

REFERENCES

1. Khalil A, Akolekar R, Pandya P, Syngelaki A, Nicolaides K. Chorionic villus sampling at 11 to 13 weeks of gestation and hypertensive disorders in pregnancy. Obstet Gynecol. 2010;116(2 Pt 1):374-80.

2. Navaratnam K, Alfirevic Z; the Royal College of Obstetricians and Gynaecologists. Amniocentesis and chorionic villus sampling: Green-top Guideline no. 8. BJOG. 2022;129(1):e1-e15.
3. ACOG. (2016). Prenatal diagnostic testing for genetic disorders. [online] Available from https://www.acog.org/clinical/clinical-guidance/practice-bulletin/articles/2016/05/prenatal-diagnostic-testing-for-genetic-disorders [Last accessed May, 2024].
4. Floridia M, Masuelli G, Meloni A, Cetin I, Tamburrini E; Italian Group on Surveillance on Antiretroviral Treatment in Pregnancy, et al. Amniocentesis and chorionic villus sampling in HIV-infected pregnant women: a multicentre case series. BJOG. 2017;124(8):1218-23.
5. Nicolaides KH. First-trimester screening for chromosomal abnormalities. Semin Perinatol. 2005;29(4):190-4.
6. Evans MI, Goldberg JD, Horenstein J, Wapner RJ, Ayoub MA, Stone J, et al. Selective termination for structural, chromosomal, and mendelian anomalies: international experience. Am J Obstet Gynecol. 1999;181(4):893-7.
7. Ahmed S. Transabdominal chorionic villus sampling (CVS) for prenatal diagnosis of genetic disorders. J Coll Physicians Surg Pak. 2006;16(3):204-7.
8. Alfirevic Z, Navaratnam K, Mujezinovic F. Amniocentesis and chorionic villus sampling for prenatal diagnosis. Cochrane Database Syst Rev. 2017;9(9).
9. Jackson LG, Wapner RJ. Risks of chorionic villus sampling. Clin Obstet Gynecol. 1987;1(3):513-31.
10. Medical Research Council European Trial of Chorion Villus Sampling. MRC working party on the evaluation pf chorion villus sampling. Lancet. 1991;337(8756):1491-9.
11. Brambati B, Oldrini A, Ferrazzi E, Lanzani A. Chorionic villus sampling: an analysis of the obstetric experience of 1,000 cases. Prenat Diagn. 1987;7(3):157-69.
12. Multicentre randomised clinical trial of chorion villus sampling and amniocentesis. First report. Canadian Collaborative CVS-Amniocentesis Clinical Trial Group. Lancet. 1989;1(8628):1-6.
13. Rhoads GG, Jackson LG, Schlesselman SE, de la Cruz FF, Desnick RJ, Golbus MS, et al. The safety and efficacy of chorionic villus sampling for early prenatal diagnosis of cytogenetic abnormalities. N Engl J Med. 1989;320(10):609-17.
14. Saura R, Gauthier B, Taine L, Wen ZQ, Horovitz J, Roux D, et al. Operator experience and fetal loss rate in transabdominal CVS. Prenat Diagn. 1994;14(1):70-1.
15. Kuliev A, Jackson L, Froster U, Brambati B, Simpson JL, Verlinsky Y, et al. Chorionic villus sampling safety. Report of World Health Organization/EURO meeting in association with the Seventh International Conference on Early Prenatal Diagnosis of Genetic Diseases, Tel-Aviv, Israel, May 21, 1994. Am J Obstet Gynecol. 1996;174(3):807-11.
16. Cederholm M, Axelsson O. A prospective comparative study on transabdominal chorionic villus sampling and amniocentesis performed at 10–13 weeks of gestation. Prenat Diagn. 1997;17(4):311-7.
17. Smidt-Jensen S, Permin M, Philip J. Sampling success and risk by transabdominal chorionic villus sampling, transcervical chorionic villus sampling and amniocentesis: a randomized study. Ultrasound Obstet Gynecol. 1991;1(2):86-90.
18. Mujezinovic F, Alfirevic Z. Procedure-related complications of amniocentesis and chorionic villus sampling. Obstet Gynecol. 2007;110(3):687-94.
19. Akolekar R, Bower S, Flack N, Bilardo CM, Nicolaides KH. Prediction of miscarriage and stillbirth at 11–13 weeks and the contribution of chorionic villus sampling. Prenat Diagn. 2011;31(1):38-45.
20. Spencer K, Cowans NJ, Avgidou K, Nicolaides KH. First trimester ultrasound and biochemical markers of aneuploidy and the prediction of impending fetal death. Ultrasound Obstet Gynecol. 2006;28(5):637-43.
21. Sebire NJ, Snijders RJ, Hughes K, Sepulveda W, Nicolaides KH. Screening for trisomy 21 in twin pregnancies by maternal age and fetal nuchal translucency thickness at 10–14 weeks of gestation. Br J Obstet Gynaecol. 1996;103(10):999-1003.
22. Wapner RJ, Johnson A, Davis G. Prenatal diagnosis in twin gestations: a comparison between second trimester amniocentesis and first trimester chorionic villus sampling. Obstet Gynecol. 1993;82(1):49-56.
23. Gil MM, Rodríguez-Fernández M, Elger T, Akolekar R, Syngelaki A, De Paco Matallana C, et al. Risk of fetal loss after chorionic villus sampling in twin pregnancy derived from propensity score matching analysis. Ultrasound Obstet Gynecol. 2022;59(2):162-8.
24. Elger T, Akolekar R, Syngelaki A, De Paco Matallana C, Molina FS, Gallardo Arozena M, et al. Fetal loss after chorionic villus sampling in twin pregnancy. Ultrasound Obstet Gynecol. 2021;58(1):48-55.

40

CHAPTER

Amniocentesis and Fetal Blood Sampling

Aris J Antsaklis, George A Partsinevelos

INTRODUCTION

The introduction of ultrasonography in fetal medicine has been uniformly recognized as the milestone in prenatal screening for chromosomal abnormalities and congenital fetal malformations. High-resolution ultrasound equipment currently available allows detailed fetal imaging. These facilities combined with increasing operator experience accomplish accurate noninvasive prenatal diagnosis. Nevertheless, invasive diagnostic procedures are required to establish diagnosis in case of suspected aneuploidy or genetic disease. The vast majority of these tests are performed under ultrasound guidance and aim to obtain fetal samples, such as amniotic fluid (amniocentesis), chorionic villi [chorionic villus sampling (CVS)], and fetal blood (fetal blood sampling) for fetal karyotyping and/or DNA analysis. Unavoidably, each of them is linked to certain potential complications and procedure-related risks, while fetal loss represents the worst scenario in these cases. Gestational age, suspected underlying fetal anomaly, and mainly physician's experience should be taken into consideration in decision-making of the method of choice.

AMNIOCENTESIS

Introduction

Amniocentesis is an invasive prenatal diagnostic and therapeutic technique through which amniotic fluid is withdrawn from the amniotic cavity transabdominally via a needle. It is traditionally considered the oldest invasive procedure in pregnancy, which was first applied therapeutically to drain excess amniotic fluid in a woman with polyhydramnios at the end of the 19th century.[1] For diagnostic reasons, it was first used in 1950s to assess the severity of cases of rhesus isoimmunization through spectrophotometric analysis of the amniotic fluid[2] and later in fetal sex diagnosis by the identification of Barr bodies in the noncultured amniocytes.[3] However, amniocentesis for genetic diagnosis through fetal karyotype determination in amniotic fluid cell culture was not applied before mid-1960s.[4] In the late 1960s and early 1970s, this procedure was reserved only for the highest risk patients in the tertiary setting.[5,6] Thenceforth, amniocentesis has been increasingly used as an invaluable diagnostic tool in prenatal invasive genetic studies for fetal abnormalities. To a lesser extent, it is applied in the diagnosis of endometrial infections. Furthermore, its therapeutic role in singleton polyhydramnios and twin-to-twin transfusion syndrome (TTTS) through amnioreduction, that is, the removal of excess amniotic fluid has been validated.

INDICATIONS

Nowadays, the main indication for amniocentesis is fetal karyotyping to exclude numerical and structural fetal chromosomal abnormalities. Although traditionally advanced maternal age (≥35 years) suggested genetic screening with amniocentesis, it is currently stated that maternal age itself should no longer be used as a cutoff to discern pregnant women at those who should be offered noninvasive screening tests (ultrasound and maternal serum biochemistry) versus those who should undergo invasive diagnostic tests (amniocentesis or CVS). Currently, it is recommended that all pregnant women, regardless of age, should be offered noninvasive first-trimester screening for chromosomal abnormalities and those identified with increased risk of carrying an abnormal fetus should be referred for invasive genetic testing. However, all pregnant women irrespectively of age should have the option of invasive testing on maternal request.[7] Furthermore, history of previous fetal aneuploidy, parental balanced translocation, and an ambiguous result from a previous test such as placental mosaicism in CVS represent indications for amniocentesis.

Fetal conventional G band karyotype is performed in cultured amniotic fluid cells and requires up to 14 weeks to obtain results. Fluorescence in situ hybridization (FISH) or quantitative fluorescence polymerase chain reaction (PCR) of short-tandem repeat sequences in chromosome 13, 18, 21, X, and Y does not necessitate cell culture and provides results within 24–48 hours for the most common fetal aneuploidies related with chromosomes 13, 18, 21, and sex chromosomes X and Y. The result of these approaches, however, should always be confirmed with cell culture and conventional cytogenetic analysis. Nowadays, chromosomal microarray detecting microdeletions and microduplications, single gene testing, multigene panel, whole exome sequencing, and whole genome sequencing have progressively replaced conventional G band karyotype and are increasingly applied in prenatal genetic diagnosis. It should be noted that chromosomal microarray can be applied in aspirated amniotic fluid cells without culture, turning out results in up to 5 days. In this respect, chromosomal microarray is advantageous for genetic studies in stillborns.

Amniocentesis also serves in the diagnosis of genetic diseases in the fetus. Beta-thalassemia, cystic fibrosis, and hemophilia can be accurately identified through DNA analysis using FISH. In the past, some metabolic diseases and other pathologic conditions, such as cystic fibrosis and congenital adrenal hyperplasia, were diagnosed using determination of relevant enzymes in the amniotic fluid. In the new era, DNA analysis has replaced this approach ensuring accurate detection of gene mutation in fetal cells collected through amniocentesis.

Quantitative and qualitative characteristics of the amniotic fluid can be used in fetal lung maturity assessment. Lecithin:sphingomyelin ratio, phosphatidylglycerol determination, foam stability index, fluorescent polarization test for surfactant:albumin ratio measurement, lamellar bodies detection in the amniotic fluid, and other tests may indirectly estimate the risk of respiratory distress syndrome in the neonate. However, amniocentesis is rarely used for fetal pulmonary maturity evaluation nowadays, as advances in neonatal care and accuracy in determination of gestational age early in pregnancy with ultrasonography have restricted its necessity.

Congenital fetal infection with *Toxoplasma gondii*, cytomegalovirus (CMV), rubella, etc., can be ruled out in case of maternal infection accompanied by seroconversion via amniocentesis and application of PCR-based technologies in the amniotic fluid. Moreover, Gram stain microscopy and culture of the amniotic fluid may help toward identification of the bacterial agent responsible for premature rupture of membranes (PROMs) and preterm labor in case of underlying chorioamnionitis.

Several indications for amniocentesis used in the past are not valid nowadays. For example, the severity of fetal hemolytic anemia in cases of Rhesus isoimmunization was traditionally assessed using amniotic fluid spectrophotometry. However, this practice has been abandoned, because middle cerebral artery (MCA) Doppler velocimetry offers a noninvasive alternative approach in the evaluation of fetal hemolysis and anemia.

Finally, fetal therapy can be accomplished in several cases using amniocentesis. Polyhydramnios in singleton pregnancies and twin oligohydramnios-polyhydramnios sequence (TOPS) in monochorionic twin pregnancies complicated by TTTS can be treated with serial drainage of excess amniotic fluid (amnioreduction). Furthermore, excess amniotic fluid removal in case of cervical incompetence complicated by prolapsed embryonic membranes before cervical cerclage placement can increase success rate of the procedure. On the contrary, severe oligohydramnios has been managed with amnioinfusion, although further evaluation of the indications and outcome of this technique is needed. Furthermore, infusion of various drugs in the amniotic cavity such as thyroxine to treat fetal goitrous hypothyroidism has been applied.

Technique

Amniocentesis for prenatal screening for chromosomal aberrations and genetic diagnosis of congenital diseases is ideally performed between 15 and 18 weeks of gestation.[8] Early application in 11–14 weeks has been associated with an increased risk of fetal loss, amniotic fluid leakage, and fetal talipes equinovarus, and thus is not recommended.[9]

Genetic counseling based on family history, parents' medical history, maternal age, first and/or second trimester prenatal screening with ultrasonography, and/or maternal serum biochemistry should initially be offered. Counseling is imperative to include efficacy and shortcomings of the technique including procedure-related risks and also expectations from testing. Available options in case of abnormal results should be also discussed.

The procedure is preceded by a detailed ultrasound examination of the pregnancy, which includes determination of the number of gestational sacs and fetuses, mapping of fetuses and placentas in case of multiple pregnancy, assessment of cardiac function, gestational age, amniotic fluid quantity, and identification of possible fetal abnormalities. Moreover, the existence of fibroids and adnexal masses are recorded. The site for the entry of the needle is chosen preferably distally from the fetal face, the umbilical cord, and the placenta. The anterior placenta rarely covers the entire anterior uterine wall, thus a window for lateral approach is almost always available. However, in case a transplacental approach is unavoidable postponing amniocentesis for 1 week has been proposed to allow progression of gestation and potential development of a placenta-free window. Rarely amniochorionic fusion has not been accomplished until 16–17 weeks' gestation. In such a case, delaying amniocentesis by 1 week could allow remission of amniochorionic separation.

Local anesthesia is rarely required. In fact, local anesthetics take of the pain related to the insertion of the needle into the skin, but has no effect on the pain related to the insertion of the needle into the uterus. On the other hand, local anesthetics are themselves painful at the site they are administered. Having discussed these issues, most candidates of amniocentesis opt to proceed without local anesthesia.

Antiseptic solution is applied on the skin and the "free hand technique" (one hand holds the needle and the other the ultrasound transducer) is usually employed using a "parallel" or a "perpendicular" approach. In the "parallel" approach, the needle is inserted at the end of the probe, thus it is fully visualized on the ultrasound monitor. In the "perpendicular" approach, the needle is inserted adjacent to the middle of the probe, thus only the needle tip is followed-up. A disposable 22-G spinal needle is advanced in the selected amniotic fluid pocket. The inner stylet is removed, and a syringe is attached to the needle hub by an assistant. The first 1–2 mL of amniotic fluid is discarded to avoid contamination with maternal cells, which might render results inaccurate (1/600 pregnancies). A new syringe is attached and approximately 20 mL (volume in mL corresponding to the gestational week) of amniotic fluid is drained and sent to the cytogenetic laboratory. In case that amniotic fluid cannot be aspirated, juxtaposes of the needle to the membrane and rotation 180° may remove fetal membranes that have tented over the needle tip and solve the problem. If not, reinserting of the stylet and advancing the needle under ultrasound guidance may help. Selection of a new insertion site should be reserved as the last resort.

A minority of operators, instead of the free-hand technique, use a needle-guiding device, which is attached to the ultrasound probe, and guides the needle to the selected amniotic fluid pocket. This technique is probably preferred by less experienced operators.

When blood or blood-stained amniotic fluid is drawn, the needle tip should be rechecked and slightly moved as it may have not completely transversed the uterine wall. However, the dark or brown color of amniotic fluid indicates the presence of old blood into the amniotic cavity, and this is associated with an earlier vaginal bleeding or a previous unsuccessful amniocentesis. This is more often associated with failure of amniotic fluid cells culture.[10] Furthermore, discolored amniotic fluid has been associated with chromosomal abnormalities[11] and intrauterine infection.[12,13]

Repeat ultrasound assessment confirms fetal heart activity and the absence of intra-amniotic bleeding. Advice to rest and avoid sexual intercourse for several days and information about signs of potential postprocedure complications, such as persistent uterine cramping, fever, leakage of amniotic fluid, or bleeding, are given.

In twins and higher order pregnancies, certain modifications of the technique of amniocentesis have been applied. In particular, three methods of tapping multiple sacs have been described so far. The first one, introduced in 1980, involves two or more needle insertions, one for each sac, also called the technique of double amniocentesis.[14] In a twin or higher-order multiple pregnancy, two or more 22-G spinal needles are separately and sequentially inserted transabdominally under ultrasound visualization into each sac and approximately 20 mL of amniotic fluid is readily aspirated. Another technique described in 1990 is the single needle insertion technique.[15] The needle entry is made into the proximal sac near the insertion of the dividing membrane and 20 mL of amniotic fluid is retrieved. After the stylet is replaced, the needle is advanced through the second sac under direct ultrasound guidance.[16] In order to avoid contamination and subsequent false negative results, the first few milliliters of amniotic fluid are discarded and aspiration of 20 mL from the second sac integrates the procedure. Double simultaneous amniocentesis represents the third approach first applied in 1992.[16]

Two needles are inserted separately into the amniotic sacs under ultrasound visualization and following aspiration of the amniotic fluid from the first sac, the needle is left in place indicating the sampled cavity while the second needle is advanced into the other sac. Each of these techniques has advantages and disadvantages and finally operator's familiarity with the approach might determine his option.

Complications

Amniocentesis has been proven to be a safe technique in fetal diagnosis and therapy. However, as an invasive procedure, it has been linked to a number of complications. Undoubtedly, many of them are directly influenced by the operators' experience.

Fetal loss is considered the major risk of second trimester genetic amniocentesis. It should be noted that in order to assess procedure-related risk of fetal loss, background loss rate associated with maternal age, gestational age, parity, maternal pathologic conditions (uncontrolled diabetes mellitus, severe hypertension related to lupus, etc.), and fetal anomalies (structural aberrations, karyotype abnormalities, etc.) should be taken into account.

Advanced maternal age is associated with increased background fetal loss rate. On the contrary, gestational age at the procedure is inversely related to fetal loss rate. In fact, the earlier the pregnancy, the higher the background risk of miscarriage. In 1988, it was demonstrated that 2% of clinical pregnancies diagnosed sonographically in women younger than 35 years resulted in miscarriage at 9–11 weeks of gestation. The risk of miscarriage was 4.5% among women aged 35–39 years and estimations for a lower background fetal loss rate later in pregnancy were made.[17]

Only one randomized trial has compared the risks of amniocentesis to controls so far. In this study, which was conducted in Denmark approximately 37 years ago, amniocentesis was performed in 4,606 pregnant women at 14–20 weeks of gestation, although most procedures were performed between 16 and 18 weeks.[18] The amniocentesis group had a total fetal loss rate 1% higher than the controls (1.7% and 0.7%, respectively). In the original paper, it was stated that amniocenteses were carried out with an 18-G needle. However, the authors subsequently retracted this statement and indicated that a smaller needle was in fact used. Apparently, this issue cannot be objectively retested in this era, as such a prospective randomized control study is impossible to be repeated due to ethical reasons.

Thenceforth, a lot of studies reported amniocentesis-related fetal loss rate between 0.2% and 0.9%. The difficulties in evaluating the postprocedure miscarriage rate have been clearly shown by the controversial results of several multicenter trials. In 1978, the National Institute of Child Health and Human Development (NICHD) evaluating the safety and accuracy of midtrimester amniocentesis for prenatal diagnosis reported a fetal loss rate of 3.5% in the amniocentesis group and 3.2% in the controls.[19] The same year, the Medical Research Council[20] reported an amniocentesis-related fetal loss rate between 1% and 1.5% and a small but significant association with neonatal respiratory distress syndrome. It was suggested that these complications could be the result of oligohydramnios following leakage of amniotic fluid. This British study also found an increase in postural deformities such as talipes and congenital dislocation of the hip.[16] The possible mechanism of this deformity is compression due to oligohydramnios or tissue injury from the amniocentesis needle. However, the study was later criticized for significant selection biases. In 1996, Brumfield[21] reported a total fetal loss of 0.2% following amniocentesis at 16–19 weeks' gestation. In the Canadian early and midtrimester amniocentesis collaborative study, a total pregnancy loss of 3.2% was reported, but there were no controls.[22] In 1999, Roper et al. reported an 0.9% risk for miscarriage after midtrimester amniocentesis.[23] A systematic review published early this decade showed a procedure-related pregnancy loss of 0.6%.[24] In 2006, patients who participated in the First and Second Trimester Evaluation of Risk for Aneuploidy (FASTER) trial were analyzed and the total spontaneous fetal loss rate earlier than 24 weeks of gestation in the study group was 1.0% and was statistically significant different from the background 0.94% rate seen in the control group.[25] A systematic review of complications related to amniocenetesis and CVS showed a pooled pregnancy loss within 14 days after amniocentesis of 0.6%, and the figure reached 0.9% for pregnancy loss before 24 weeks of gestation.[26]

In a retrospective study conducted in our center involving amniocentesis performed between 1990 and 2006, we found 1.25% pregnancy loss rate in 12,413 women who underwent amniocentesis versus 0.9% in 5,654 women who did not (control group), which corresponds to 0.35% excess rate in the amniocentesis group, though

TABLE 1: Pregnancy outcome after amniocentesis in "Alexandra" Hospital, University of Athens, Medical School (1990–2006).

Pregnancy outcomes	***(n = 12,413)***
Delivery at <24 weeks	0.2%
Delivery at <28 weeks	0.7%
Delivery at <37 weeks	12.8%
Birth weight <1,500 g	1%
Cesarean section rate	43.4%
Mean gestational age at birth	38.2 weeks
Mean birth weight	3,370 g
SCBU admission (>24 hours)	1.9%

(SCBU: special care baby unit)

it did not reach statistical significance (Fisher exact test P <0.214). Moreover, age-specific analysis did not find statistical significance in the fetal loss rate between the two groups [unpublished data]. Delivery rates earlier than 24, 28, and 37 weeks in the amniocentesis group were 0.2%, 0.7%, and 12.8%, respectively **(Table 1)**.

Gestational age at amniocentesis has an impact on fetal loss rate. Estimations of fetal loss rate of <0.5%, 1%, and 3% following amniocentesis at 15, 14, and 13 weeks of gestation, respectively have been made. Blood-stained amniotic fluid and amniotic fluid leakage were strong predictors for fetal loss. Transplacental needle insertion was initially linked with increased fetal loss; however, several studies concluded that transplacental needle insertion does not influence the risk of pregnancy loss.[18,27] With regard to the number of needle insertions, literature yields contradictory results. In particular, no increased risk for pregnancy loss after multiple needle insertions have been reported in some studies, whereas an increased risk has been documented in some others.[19,27] A possible association between history of bleeding and increased risk of pregnancy loss postamniocentesis (+0.6%) has been reported in a previous study conducted by our team.[28] Other factors associated with increased fetal loss following amniocentesis are >3 terminations of pregnancy and/or miscarriages, thyroid disease, elevated maternal serum α-fetoprotein (MSAFP), and usage of needle with diameter larger than 18 G.

In our retrospective study, we found an increased risk of fetal loss with advanced maternal age 34 years [odds ratio (OR) 2.19], history of >3 terminations of pregnancy and/or miscarriages (OR 3.9), mild bleeding in early pregnancy (OR 2.53), severe bleeding in early pregnancy (OR 5.6), blood stained amniotic fluid (OR 3.82), and the presence of uterine fibroids (OR 2.52).

Nowadays, the estimated procedure-related risk of ultrasound-guided amniocentesis performed by an experienced operator, for fetal loss, is probably around 0.1–0.3%.[29] Risk factors for fetal loss include many of the indications for the procedure, such as elevated maternal serum alpha-fetoprotein, sonographically detected fetal anomalies, vaginal bleeding during current pregnancy,[28] and obstetric history of abortion (spontaneous or induced).[28,30]

Other complications related to amniocentesis include preterm delivery,[31] fetal injury ascribed to the amniocentesis needle,[24] vertical transmission of infectious diseases,[32,33] rhesus alloimmunization resulting from fetomaternal hemorrhage,[34-36] neonatal respiratory distress syndrome possibly due to postprocedure chronic oligohydramnios,[37,38] orthopedic abnormalities (talipes equinovarus congenital dislocation and subluxation of the hip) possibly due again to oligohydramnios,[39] and usually self-limited uterine contractions and vaginal spotting (2–3%), and leakage of amniotic fluid (1%).[31]

FETAL BLOOD SAMPLING

Introduction

Fetal blood sampling is an invasive prenatal diagnostic procedure through which fetal blood is drawn for the diagnosis of fetal disorders. Furthermore, this technique can be applied therapeutically, in cases where intravenous administration of medication or blood product transfusion is required.

Although fetal blood was initially obtained in 1972 endoscopically during the second trimester termination of pregnancy by cesarean section, the first successful transabdominal fetoscopic fetal blood sampling was performed 2 years later under ultrasound guidance.[40,41] However, the origin of the technique currently available for fetal blood sampling using a needle, which is introduced transabdominally under ultrasound visualization, goes back in 1983.[42]

Fetal blood sampling is also known as cordocentesis, omphalocentesis, and percutaneous umbilical blood sampling (PUBS) and involves ultrasound-guided puncture of the umbilical vein. However, the intrahepatic portion of the umbilical vein and the left portal vein as well as the right heart ventricle (cardiocentesis) has also been used to obtain fetal blood sample.[43]

In the past, a frequent indication was the need for rapid diagnosis of chromosomal abnormalities (rapid karyotyping), in as much as results were offered in 2–3 days-time, whereas less risky techniques such as amniocentesis and CVS required cell culture usually for at least 2 weeks. Today, novel molecular techniques allow rapid karyotype determination even earlier without culture.

Therefore, currently, amniocentesis and CVS represent first-line invasive diagnostic procedures for prenatal diagnosis, thus limiting fetal blood sampling's application considerably. However, the latter is indicated in case of abnormal findings in amniocentesis or CVS, which require confirmation. Moreover, rhesus isoimmunization, hydrops of unknown origin, and fetal infections are some of the conditions where fetal blood sampling can be indicated. Finally, fetal blood sampling can be practiced in order to inject pharmacologic agents into the fetal circulation or even perform blood product transfusion such as red blood cells or platelets in severe fetal anemia and thrombocytopenia, respectively.

Technique

Three different approaches for fetal blood sampling have been described so far: cordocentesis, intrahepatic fetal blood sampling, and cardiocentesis. Cordocentesis is far more frequently applied, as intrahepatic fetal blood sampling and cardiocentesis have been associated with higher fetal loss rate. Access to the operating theater should have been ensured in case the procedure is performed after fetal viability, so that emergency cesarean section can accomplished in case long-lasting fetal bradycardia emerges. In this respect, antenatal glucocorticoid administration at least 24 hours prior to fetal blood sampling is advised in gestations of 24–34 weeks.

A maternal blood sample is obtained before the procedure and intravenous catheter in placed. Although the benefit has not been proven so far, we have incorporated antibiotic prophylaxis administration in our clinical practice.

A detailed ultrasound examination of the pregnancy is conducted before the procedure to ensure fetal viability and assess normality of the developing fetus. Furthermore, amniotic fluid volume, location of the placenta, and the insertion site of the umbilical cord in the placenta are documented. To this end, color Doppler can be used as it provides useful information regarding blood flow and facilitates identification of the umbilical vein.

Once the insertion site of the needle has been determined, the skin is cleansed with an antiseptic solution. Local anesthesia is not considered mandatory, however, in therapeutic procedures seems to be prudent.[44] Transabdominal ultrasound-guided free-hand technique is usually opted. A 22-G spinal needle 9–15 cm in length is introduced either transplacentally in case of anterior placenta or through the amniotic cavity in case of posterior placenta targeting the umbilical vein proximal to the insertion of the umbilical cord into the placenta (around 1 cm distance; **Figs. 1 and 2**). The needle-within-needle technique, that is, a 20-G needle biopsy guide advanced into the amniotic cavity followed by a 25-G needle inserted through the guide to puncture the umbilical vein is rarely used nowadays. Puncturing free loops of the umbilical cord is much more difficult and often turns out unsuccessful. No more than 4 mL and 6 mL of fetal blood should be withdrawn during the second and third trimester, respectively. A common rule is that no >100 mL of fetal blood per kg of estimated fetal weight should be drawn. The cord puncture site should be sonographically followed-up for 10 minutes for bleeding or hematoma formation and fetal heart rate at least for 30–60 minutes following the procedure.[45]

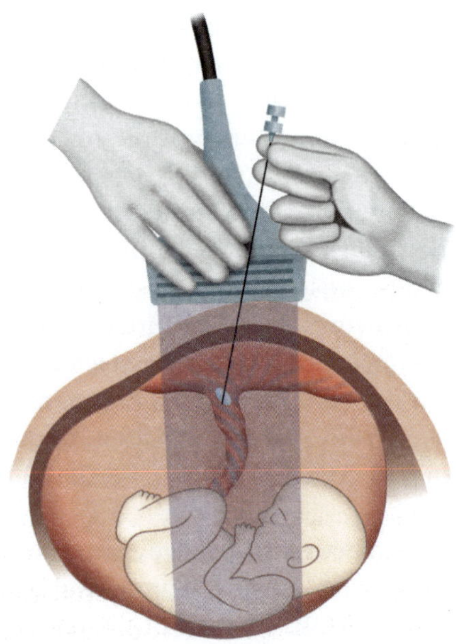

Fig. 1: Transabdominal ultrasound-guided fetal blood sampling in case of anterior placenta.

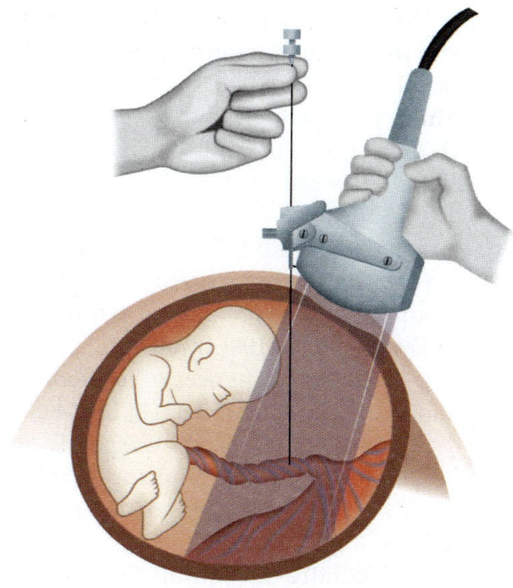

Fig. 2: Transabdominal ultrasound-guided fetal blood sampling in case or posterior placenta.

Complications

The major concern of fetal blood sampling is fetal loss, which has been shown to be higher than other prenatal invasive diagnostic procedures frequently used, such as amniocentesis and CVS.[46] A 0.9–3.2% fetal loss rate has been recorded in previous studies. However, no randomized controlled trials have assessed this risk so far.[42,47] A more recent large cohort study found 1.4–1.9% fetal loss rate, with an excess risk of 0.9% in women with normal results than in controls who were not subjected to fetal blood sampling.[48] Notwithstanding, the relatively increased background pregnancy loss rate associated with pregnancies selected to undergo fetal blood sampling should be always taken into account in assessing adverse pregnancy outcome related with the procedure. In fact, fetal loss rate within 2 weeks postprocedurally was 1% in sonographically normal contrary to 7–13% in sonographically abnormal fetuses,[49] 9–14% in intrauterine growth restricted fetuses[46] and 25–32% in nonimmune hydrops fetalis cases.[50]

Bleeding at the puncture site was initially reported in 41–53% of cases with a mean duration of 35 seconds,[51] although a longer duration of bleeding is expected in cases that umbilical artery has been punctured.[52] It is considered the most common usually benign complication of fetal blood sampling, with more recent data showing that it occurs in 20–30% of cases.[44] Umbilical cord hematoma (17%),[53] transient fetal bradycardia (5–10%),[44] fetomaternal blood transfusion (65.6% in anterior placenta vs. 16.6% in posterior placenta),[54] uterine contractions (7%),[55] and chorioamnionitis due to *Staphylococcus aureus* or bowel bacteria (1%)[45,49,52,56] are all potential complications of fetal blood sampling. Thus, it is prudent to reserve this procedure for cases where the results of other noninvasive and invasive techniques were inconclusive or cordocentesis is the unique option for fetal diagnosis and therapy.

With regard to twin or higher order pregnancies, fetal blood sampling does not differ technically from that in singletons. In a study conducted in 2003, involving 84 twin pregnancies, mainly screened for hemoglobinopathies, the overall procedure-related fetal loss (up to 2 weeks of the procedure) was 8.2%, about fourfold higher than the correspondence risk in singletons. It should be noted that cautious interpretation of these results is needed given the small number of cases and the various indications for fetal blood sampling.[57,58] However, this technique can be used as an alternative to amniocentesis after 20 weeks' gestation to confirm an abnormal karyotype in a dichorionic twin pregnancy, when selective feticide is considered a few weeks after the initial procedure.[59]

CONCLUSION

Since the end of the 19th century when amniocentesis was first applied therapeutically to drain excess amniotic fluid in a woman with polyhydramnios, and 1950s when this technique was used diagnostically to assess the severity of cases of rhesus isoimmunization, the introduction of ultrasonography in prenatal fetal assessment has boosted the implementation of amniocentesis in the clinical setting. Fetal karyotyping and genetic studies for fetal diseases are considered the major indications today. Less frequently, amniocentesis is used for fetal lung maturity assessment and congenital fetal infection. Therapeutic application in polyhydramnios, amnioreduction in TTTS, or prolapsed fetal membranes before placing of a cervical cerclage have also been validated. Either the free-hand technique or the use a needle-guiding device attached to the ultrasound probe have been studied, although the latter is far less popular among clinicians. Complications of amniocentesis are rare, hence this modality is widely accepted in modern obstetrics.

Fetal blood sampling is a more demanding ultrasound-guided fetal invasive procedure, which can be used in case of abnormal findings in amniocentesis or CVS that require confirmation. However, it is mainly used therapeutically for blood product transfusion such as red blood cells or platelets in severe fetal anemia and thrombocytopenia, respectively. Complications associated with fetal blood sampling are considered more frequent compared with amniocentesis, therefore this technique is reserved for cases that cannot be managed alternatively.

REFERENCES

1. Von Schatz F. Gine besondere art von einseitiger polyhydramnie mit anderseitiger oligohydramnie bie eineiigen zwillingen. Arch Gynaecol 1882;19:329.
2. Bevis DC. Composition of liquor amnii in haemolytic disease of newborn. Lancet. 1950;2(6631):443.
3. Fuchs F, Riis P. Antenatal sex determination. Nature. 1956;177(4503):330.
4. Steele MW, Breg WR. Chromosome analysis of human amniotic-fluid cells. Lancet. 1966;1(7434):383-5.
5. Jacobson CB, Barter RH. Intrauterine diagnosis and management of genetic defects. Am J Obstet Gynecol. 1967;99(6):796-807.
6. Nadler HL, Gerbie AB. Role of amniocentesis in the intrauterine detection of genetic disorders. N Engl J Med. 1970;282(11):596-9.
7. American College of Obstetricians and Gynecologists. ACOG practice bulletin—Screening for fetal chromosomal anomalies. Obstet Gynecol. 2007;109:217-26.
8. Emery AE. Antenatal diagnosis of genetic disease. Modern Trends Hum Genet. 1970;1:267.
9. Alfirevic Z, Sundberg K, Brigham S. Amniocentesis and chorionic villus sampling for prenatal diagnosis. Cochrane Database Syst Rev. 2003;(3):CD003252.
10. Golbus MS, Loughman WD, Epstein CJ, Halbasch G, Stephens JD, Hall BD. Prenatal genetic diagnosis in 3000 amniocenteses. N Engl J Med. 1979;300(4):157-63.
11. Isada NB, Koppitch FC 3rd, Johnson MP, Evans MI. Does the color of amniotic fluid still matter? Fetal Diagn Ther. 1990;5(3-4):165-7.
12. Cassell GH, Davis RO, Waites KB, Brown MB, Marriott PA, Stagno S, et al. Isolation of Mycoplasma hominis and Ureaplasma urealyticum from amniotic fluid at 16-20 weeks of gestation: potential effect on outcome of pregnancy. Sex Transm Dis. 1983;10(4 Suppl):294-302.
13. Gray DJ, Robinson HB, Malone J, Thomson RB Jr. Adverse outcome in pregnancy following amniotic fluid isolation of Ureaplasma urealyticum. Prenat Diagn. 1992;12(2):111-7.
14. Elias S, Gerbie AB, Simpson JL, Nadler HL, Sabbagha RE, Shkolnik A. Genetic amniocentesis in twin gestations. Am J Obstet Gynecol. 1980;138(2):169-74.
15. Jeanty P, Shah D, Roussis P. Single-needle insertion in twin amniocentesis. J Ultrasound Med. 1990;9(9):511-7.
16. Bahado-Singh R, Schmitt R, Hobbins JC. New technique for genetic amniocentesis in twins. Obstet Gynecol. 1992;79(2):304-7.
17. Mackenzie WE, Holmes DS, Newton JR. Spontaneous abortion rate in ultrasonographically viable pregnancies. Obstet Gynecol. 1988;71(1):81-3.
18. Tabor A, Philip J, Madsen M, Bang J, Obel E, Norgaard-Pedersen B. Randomised controlled trial of genetic amniocentesis in 4606 low-risk women. Lancet. 1986;1(8493):1287-93.
19. Stone J, Ferrara L, Kamrath J, Getrajdman J, Berkowitz R, Moshier E, et al. Contemporary outcomes with the latest 1000 cases of multifetal pregnancy reduction (MPR). Am J Obstet Gynecol. 2008;199(4):406.e1-4.
20. Pharoah PO, Adi Y. Consequences of in-utero death in a twin pregnancy. Lancet. 2000;355(9215):1597-602.
21. Brumfield CG, Lin S, Conner W, Cosper P, Davis RO, Owen J. Pregnancy outcome following genetic amniocentesis at 11-14 vs. 16-19 weeks' gestation. Obstet Gynecol. 1996;88(1):114-8.
22. Simpson NE, Dallaire L, Miller JR, Siminovich L, Hamerton JL, Miller J, et al. Prenatal diagnosis of genetic disease in Canada: report of a collaborative study. Can Med Assoc J. 1976;115(8):739-48.
23. Wimalasundera RC. Selective reduction and termination of multiple pregnancies. Semin Fetal Neonatal Med. 2010;15(6):327-35.
24. Seeds JW. Diagnostic mid trimester amniocentesis: how safe? Am J Obstet Gynecol. 2004;191(2):607-15.
25. Eddleman KA, Malone FD, Sullivan L, Dukes K, Berkowitz RL, Kharbutli Y, et al. Pregnancy loss rates after midtrimester amniocentesis. Obstet Gynecol. 2006;108(5):1067-72.
26. Mujezinovic F, Alfirevic Z. Procedure-related complications of amniocentesis and chorionic villous sampling: a systematic review. Obstet Gynecol. 2007;110(3):687-94.
27. Marthin T, Liedgren S, Hammar M. Transplacental needle passage and other risk-factors associated with second trimester amniocentesis. Acta Obstet Gynecol Scand. 1997;76(8):728-32.
28. Antsaklis A, Papantoniou N, Xygakis A, Mesogitis S, Tzortzis E, Michalas S. Genetic amniocentesis in women 20-34 years old: associated risks. Prenat Diagn. 2000;20(3):247-50.
29. Practice Bulletin No. 162: Prenatal diagnostic testing for genetic disorders. Obstet Gynecol. 2016;127(5):e108-e122.
30. Odibo AO, Gray DL, Dicke JM, Stamilio DM, Macones GA, Crane JP. Revisiting the fetal loss rate after second-trimester genetic amniocentesis: a single center's 16-year experience. Obstet Gynecol. 2008;111(3):589-95.
31. Medda E, Donati S, Spinelli A, Di Renzo GC; EUROPOP Group Czech Republic; EUROPOP Group Finland; EUROPOP Group France; EUROPOP Group Germany; EUROPOP Group Greece; EUROPOP Group Italy; EUROPOP Group The Netherlands; EUROPOP Group Slovak Republic; EUROPOP Group Spain; EUROPOP Group Sweden. Genetic amniocentesis: a risk factor for preterm delivery? Eur J Obstet Gynecol Reprod Biol. 2003;110(2):153-8.

32. Giorlandino C, Bilancioni E, D'Alessio P, Muzii L. Risk of iatrogenic fetal infection at prenatal diagnosis. Lancet. 1994;343(8902):922-3.
33. Minola E, Maccabruni A, Pacati I, Martinetti M. Amniocentesis as a possible risk factor for mother-to-infant transmission of hepatitis C virus. Hepatology. 2001;33(5):1341-2.
34. Clayton EM Jr, Feldhaus WD, Whitacre FE. Fetal erythrocytes in the maternal circulation of pregnant women. Obstet Gynecol. 1964;23:915-9.
35. Tabor A, Bang J, NOrgaard-Pedersen B. Feto-maternal haemorrhage associated with genetic amniocentesis: results of a randomized trial. Br J Obstet Gynaecol. 1987;94(6):528-34.
36. Murray JC, Karp LE, Williamson RA, Cheng EY, Luthy DA. Rh isoimmunization related to amniocentesis. Am J Med Genet. 1983;16(4):527-34.
37. Midtrimester Amniocentesis for Prenatal Diagnosis: Safety and Accuracy.The NICHD National Registry for Amniocentesis Study Group 1976. JAMA. 1976; 236(13):1471-6.
38. Hunter AG. Neonatal lung function following mid-trimester amniocentesis. Prenat Diagn. 1987;7(6):433-41.
39. An assessment of the hazards of amniocentesis. Report to the Medical Research Council by their Working Party on Amniocentesis. Br J Obstet Gynaecol. 1978;85(2 Suppl): 1-41.
40. Valenti C. Antenatal detection of hemoglobinopathies. A preliminary report. Am J Obstet Gynecol. 1973;115(6): 851-3.
41. Chang H, Hobbins JC, Cividalli G, Frigoletto FD, Mahoney MJ, Kan YW, et al. In utero diagnosis of hemoglobinopathies. Hemoglobin synthesis in fetal red cells. N Engl J Med. 1974;290(19):1067-8.
42. Daffos F, Capella-Pavlovsky M, Forestier F. A new procedure for fetal blood sampling in utero: preliminary results of fifty-three cases. Am J Obstet Gynecol. 1983;146(8):985-7.
43. Antsaklis AI, Papantoniou NE, Mesogitis SA, Koutra PT, Vintzileos AM, Aravantinos DI. Cardiocentesis: an alternative method of fetal blood sampling for the prenatal diagnosis of hemoglobinopathies. Obstet Gynecol. 1992; 79(4):630-3.
44. Society for Maternal-Fetal Medicine (SMFM); Berry SM, Stone J, Norton ME, Johnson D, Berghella V. Fetal blood sampling. Am J Obstet Gynecol. 2013;209(3):170-80.
45. Papantoniou N. Fetal blood sampling. In: Antsaklis AJ, Troyano JM (Eds). Donald School Textbook of Interventional Ultrasound. New Delhi: Jaypee Brothers Medical Publishers (P) Ltd; 2008. pp. 86-99.
46. Antsaklis A, Daskalakis G, Papantoniou N, Michalas S. Fetal blood sampling--indication-related losses. Prenat Diagn. 1998;18(9):934-40.
47. Weiner CP, Okamura K. Diagnostic fetal blood sampling-technique related losses. Fetal Diagn Ther. 1996;11(3): 169-75.
48. Tongsong T, Wanapirak C, Piyamongkol W, Sirirchotiyakul S, Tongprasert F, Srisupundit K, et al. Second-trimester cordocentesis and the risk of small for gestational age and preterm birth. Obstet Gynecol. 2014;124(5):919-25.
49. Maxwell DJ, Johnson P, Hurley P, Neales K, Allan L, Knott P. Fetal blood sampling and pregnancy loss in relation to indication. Br J Obstet Gynaecol. 1991;98(9):892-7.
50. Bigelow CA, Cinelli CM, Little SE, Benson CB, Frates MC, Wilkins-Haug LE. Percutaneous umbilical blood sampling: current trends and outcomes. Eur J Obstet Gynecol Reprod Biol. 2016;200:98-101.
51. Hogge WA, Thiagarajah S, Brenbridge AN, Harbert GM. Fetal evaluation by percutaneous blood sampling. Am J Obstet Gynecol. 1988;158(1):132-6.
52. Weiner CP, Wenstrom KD, Sipes SL, Williamson RA. Risk factors for cordocentesis and fetal intravascular transfusion. Am J Obstet Gynecol. 1991;165(4 Pt 1):1020-5.
53. Jauniaux E, Donner C, Simon P, Vanesse M, Hustin J, Rodesch F. Pathologic aspects of the umbilical cord after percutaneous umbilical blood sampling. Obstet Gynecol. 1989;73(2):215-8.
54. Nicolini U, Kochenour NK, Greco P, Letsky EA, Johnson RD, Contreras M, et al. Consequences of fetomaternal haemorrhage after intrauterine transfusion. BMJ. 1988;297(6660):1379-81.
55. Ghidini A, Sepulveda W, Lockwood CJ, Romero R. Complications of fetal blood sampling. Am J Obstet Gynecol. 1993;168(5):1339-44.
56. Boulot P, Deschamps F, Lefort G, Sarda P, Mares P, Hedon B, Laffargue F, Viala JL. Pure fetal blood samples obtained by cordocentesis: technical aspects of 322 cases. Prenat Diagn. 1990;10(2):93-100.
57. Antsaklis A, Daskalakis G, Souka AP, Kavalakis Y, Michalas S. Fetal blood sampling in twin pregnancies. Ultrasound Obstet Gynecol. 2003;22(4):377-9.
58. Cox WL, Forestier F, Capella-Pavlovsky M, Daffos F. Fetal blood sampling in twin pregnancies. Prenatal diagnosis and management of 19 cases. Fetal Ther. 1987;2(2):101-8.
59. Antsaklis A, Gougoulakis A, Mesogitis S, Papantoniou N, Aravantinos D. Invasive techniques for fetal diagnosis in multiple pregnancy. Int J Gynaecol Obstet. 1991;34(4): 309-14.

CHAPTER 41

Invasive Genetic Studies in Multiple Pregnancy

Aris J Antsaklis, George A Partsinevelos

INTRODUCTION

Multiple pregnancies, including twin and higher order pregnancies *a priori*, are considered high-risk pregnancies. They are mainly associated with prematurity and low birth weight, which undoubtedly increase perinatal morbidity and mortality. In fact, it would appear that despite modern prenatal management, prematurity rate in multiple pregnancies has not changed during the last 50 years. However, perinatal mortality rates have declined due to improved neonatal care.[1]

The risk of complications is not only related to the number of fetuses, but also strongly influenced by chorionicity. Chorionicity refers to placentation, whereas zygosity implies the genetic profile of the pregnancy and therefore determines the degree of risk and whether or not the fetuses may be concordant or discordant for chromosomal abnormalities, and genetic diseases. In terms of physiology, zygosity is associated with the number of fertilized oocytes, which resulted in multiples and chorionicity, reflecting the exact postconception day when the early embryonic splitting took place. Epidemiologic studies have shown that more than 30% of twin pregnancies are monozygotic (MZ) and nearly 70% are dizygotic (DZ).

Monozygotic twins originate from the division of a single fertilized ovum with an incidence rate of about 2.3–4/1,000 pregnancies. The rate of spontaneous MZ twin pregnancies is constant contrary to the increased incidence of MZ twin pregnancies derived from infertility treatment techniques. Monozygotic twins may be dichorionic (DC) or monochorionic (MC), the chorionicity is determined by the period of embryonic development when zygotic division takes place. In about 20–30% of cases, splitting occurs within 3 days of fertilization resulting in separate fetuses with independent placental circulations, therefore, being dichorionic-diamniotic (DC-DA), even if placentas may seem to be in continuity or fused. In the majority of cases (about 70%) splitting within the first week but later than the third day results in a single MC plate and two distinct amniotic sacs, hence monochorionic-diamniotic (MC-DA) twins are generated. Delayed zygotic splitting leads to monochorionic-monoamniotic (MC-MA) twins, accounting for 1% of MZ twins, though later than 13th day is extremely rare, resulting in the formation of the abnormal conjoined (Siamese) twins.

Dizygotic twins result from the fertilization of two distinct ova, thus may be of the same or different sex. The incidence rate varies significantly, influenced by race (higher in blacks, lower in Asians), heredity, maternal age (peak between 35–40 years of age), history of previous DZ twin pregnancy, nutrition habitus and anthropometric features (height and weight) of the woman.

INCIDENCE OF STRUCTURAL FETAL ANOMALIES IN MULTIPLES

The rising rate of multiple pregnancies recorded nowadays is mainly attributed to the widespread use of infertility treatment modalities. *In vitro* fertilization and ovulation induction with or without intrauterine insemination account for approximately two-thirds increase in multiple gestations, whereas the other one-third results from delayed childbearing in increasingly advanced reproductive age.[2]

Advanced maternal age has been associated with higher rate of aneuploidies. Assisted conception has been claimed to result in an increased rate of MZ twins to greater than 10-fold, the latter being at high-risk of functional and structural abnormalities, affecting 10–15% of these twins.[3-5] In particular, neural tube defects, anencephaly, holoprosencephaly, sirenomelia complex, cloacal exstrophy and abnormalities that fit into the expanded VATER/VACTERAL associations are more common in

MZ twins. Abnormalities unique to the MZ multiple conception include conjoined twinning, fetus *in feto*, acardia and fetus papyraceous. A plausible explanation for the increased incidence of abnormalities in MZ twins, involves the role of hemodynamic imbalance between MC twins through placental vascular anastomoses. Hence, the frequency of malformations in MZ twins is two-three times higher than singletons, whereas in DZ twins is thought to be similar to that of singletons (2–3%).

It has been stressed that the risk of fetal abnormalities in twins may be biased because multiple pregnancies are intensively scanned, increasing the chances of detecting underlying anomalies. Moreover, twinning is much more common in women of advanced age, in whom prenatal screening is more likely to yield the diagnosis of fetal defects as far as maternal aging is associated with increased risk for fetal abnormalities.

Conclusively, available data confirm that twin pregnancies *per se* are at increased risk for fetal chromosomal abnormalities than singletons.[6-7] Hence, the increasing incidence of multiple pregnancies highlights a concomitant increase in the need for invasive diagnostic procedures in these pregnancies.

RISK OF ANEUPLOIDY IN MULTIPLES

Contrary to the constant frequency of MZ twinning all over the world, which is independent of the age of the woman, DZ twin rate is strongly related to maternal age possibly attributed to changes in follicle stimulating hormone production to the higher side.

Zygosity represents the genetic make-up of the developing entities, thus determination of this parameter is considered a prerequisite in multiple pregnancy prenatal screening for aneuploidies.

Taking into consideration the incidence of MZ-DC-DA (20–30% of MZ twins, the latter accounting for 30% of all twin pregnancies) and DZ pregnancies, which are always DC-DA (70% of all twin pregnancies), once dichorionicity is diagnosed, the pregnancy is most likely DZ (around 10% chance of monozygosity). Therefore, chorionicity roughly corresponds to zygosity in these cases.[8]

Accurate diagnosis of chorionicity in multiples is limited to the first trimester of pregnancy. To this end, sonographic measurement of the thickness of the intertwin membrane and recognization of "lambda" or "twin peak" sign have been used. A cut-off value of 2 mm for intertwin membrane thickness may discern MC versus DC twinning, though a high inter- and intra-observer variability has been reported. Sonographic detection of the "lambda" or "twin peak" sign is reported as a more reliable indicator of DC placentation with an accuracy of 100% at 10–14 weeks gestation.[9] Delayed in the second-trimester ultrasound assessment is associated with a 10–12% chorionicity misinterpretation rate,[10,11] while after 20 weeks of gestation the determination may be impossible.

In the absence of the "lambda" or "twin peak" sign in a DA twin pregnancy, single placentation and monozygosity is concluded. However, when a single amniotic sac is detected, monochorionicity is indisputable.

Monozygoyic twins are of the same sex and genetically identical. Therefore, the risk for chromosomal abnormalities does not differ from that in singletons. Very infrequently, mutations can cause genetic discordance between MZ siblings, involving mosaicism, skewed-X-inactivation, differential gene imprinting and small scale mutation.[12] Heterokaryotypia, is used to define the rare karyotypic discordance, most commonly expressed by one fetus affected by Turner syndrome, whereas the other presents either a normal male or normal female karyotype.[13-15] Monozygotic discordance for trisomy 21, Klinefelter syndrome, Pateau syndrome, trisomy 1 and 22q11 deletion syndrome have also been described.[15-19] However, these unusual discrepancies are not taken into consideration when calculating aneuploid risk, though it should always be assumed when invasive prenatal diagnosis is performed dictating sampling from both sacs.

In DZ twins, each embryo has an independent risk for aneuploidy and therefore the risk that at least one fetus being affected will be almost twice the maternal age risk for a singleton. The probability of both fetuses being involved is minimal.[20] In cases with uncertain chorionicity and thus zygocity, aneuploidy risk assessment requires an estimation of the most likely zygocity, which may vary according to maternal age and race. In general, given that one-third of all twin pairs are monozygotic, the risk for one twin being aneuploid in case of unknown zygosity is calculated to five-thirds that of the singleton risk.[8,10] Based on these estimations, a 33-year-old woman bearing twins has a risk for at least one aneuploid offspring, comparable to the risk of a 35-year-old woman bearing a singleton. On this assumption, such women should be offered prenatal testing.[21] However, despite these aspects, reported series show a lower risk for fetal chromosomal abnormalities in live-born twins.

INDICATIONS FOR PRENATAL DIAGNOSIS

In fetal medicine, it is common practice to extrapolate the data derived from singletons to multiples. Currently, all pregnancies singletons and multiples should undergo prenatal screening for chromosomal and structural abnormalities. Furthermore, advanced maternal age, a previous conceptus with chromosomal abnormality, a parent with a structural chromosome rearrangement and the presence of gene associated inborn errors of metabolism draw more attention and render prenatal screening imperative. Screening strategies have been extensively studied in singletons. Nuchal translucency (NT) measurement along with maternal serum biochemistry determination have been widely adopted in first trimester risk assessment for fetal aneuploidies, whereas additional sonographic markers, such as absent nasal bone, abnormal Doppler waveform in the ductus venosus and tricuspid regurgitation have been recently validated. In order to apply these screening tests in multiple pregnancies, cautious interpretation of the results is needed to minimize possible erroneous high false-positive rate and subsequent high rate of undue invasive procedures. Fortunately, as non-invasive early pregnancy risk assessment is rapidly gaining popularity, invasive procedures such as chorionic villus sampling (CVS) and amniocentesis are gradually restricted in cases where rationale exists.

In fact, first trimester ultrasound screening for chromosomal abnormalities in DC multiple pregnancies has yielded comparable results to singletons in terms of detection rate as well as false-positive rate.[22] However, in MC twins, a cautious interpretation of increased NT thickness should be adopted in respect to the possibility of an underlying early twin-to-twin transfusion syndrome. A rational approach would be to use the average of NT measurement of both fetuses in risk assessment.[23]

On the other hand, first trimester maternal serum biochemistry, including free β-hCG and PAPPA has been blamed for low sensitivity and specificity in multiple gestations due to the inability to determine the degree to which each fetus contributes to the overall maternal biochemistry level. A reasonable model of "pseudo risk" approach has been proposed based on the utilization of the quotient derived from the division of the biomarkers' level as multiples of the median (MoM) by the corresponding medians for normal twins.[24-26] However, no adequate data has validated this approach so far.

With regards to maternal serum alpha-fetoprotein (MSAFP) level in the second trimester, in twin pregnancy it is measuring twice as high as in a singleton and 40% of twins are associated with MSAFP levels of more than a 2.5 MoM at 16 weeks.[27] Obviously, elevation of this serum marker may be attributed to the existence of more than one fetuses in multiple pregnancies. However, the possibility of an open neural tube defect in one or more fetuses should always be beared in mind. Thereby, amniocentesis performed in twins where MSAFP exceeds 4.5 MoM is probably justified.[28]

Since the implementation of maternal biochemistry in risk assessment for aneuploidies in twin or higher-order multiple gestations remains arguable, ultrasound scan has been proven of greater value for early determination of chorionicity and subsequent standardized NT measurement as well as genetic sonogram, targeting to identify possible sonographic markers of fetal aneuploidy.

INVASIVE PROCEDURES FOR PRENATAL DIAGNOSIS

Amniocentesis

As alluded to earlier, twin or higher order multiple pregnancies are at increased risk of aneuploidies and fetal structural defects compared with singletons. Estimations of a maternal age older than 35 years at which invasive genetic studies would be justified in these pregnancies have been made.

Amniocentesis, performed in the second trimester of pregnancy later than 15 weeks has been proven a safe and efficient procedure for sampling fetuses of a multiple gestation. Ideally, it is performed between 15–18 weeks of gestation.[29] Application of the procedure earlier in pregnancy has been associated with increased risk of fetal loss, amniotic fluid leakage and fetal talipes equinovarus, and therefore is not recommended.[10,30,31]

A detailed ultrasound evaluation of the multiple pregnancy should be performed before amniocentesis to determine chorionicity, amnionicity, and location of the placenta(s), the size, anatomy and position of each fetus. Furthermore, "labeling" of the multiples should be encouraged to ensure correct sampling from each sac. Recently, the role of amniotic fluid alpha-fetoprotein (AFAFP) level was evaluated in confirmation of both the sacs in a DC pregnancy being sampled.[32]

To date, three different approaches for tapping multiple sacs have been described. All of them use a needle to aspirate amniotic fluid transabdominally under ultrasound guidance. The first one, initially described by Elias et al. in 1980, is called the technique of double amniocentesis.[33] It involves two or more separate and sequential needle insertions, one for each sac. In particular, a 22-G 3.5 inch spinal needle is inserted into each sac transabdominally under ultrasound visualization, and about 20 mL of amniotic fluid is readily aspirated and sent for cytogenetic evaluation or fetal karyotyping. The possibility of sampling twice the same amniotic sac is probably the major drawback of this technique. Although, the instillation of a foreign substance into the amniotic cavity is of concern, marking the sampled sac with a dye following aspiration to avoid reinsertion into it and thereby erroneous sampling, has been practiced. In this context, indigo carmine has been successfully used without any adverse event,[34] although a mild vasoconstrictive effect following intravenous injection has been reported. However, indigo carmine tends to concentrate at the bottom of the sac following instillation and takes some time before the stained fluid surrounds the fetus. Methylene blue used as a marker dye in the past has been linked to certain toxic manifestations such as fetal hemolysis, fetal small bowel atresias and fetal death.[35-40] Presently, technologic advances combined with increasing operator experience render the high-resolution ultrasound equipment in expertise hands as an invaluable tool for safer and accurate sampling from each sac,[41,42] reserving the installation of dye for cases of amniotic volume discordance where detection of the septum is uncertain or high-order pregnancies, where preprocedure sonographic mapping and "labeling" of sacs is not feasible.[43]

An alternative approach is the single-needle insertion technique. It was first described by Jeanty et al. in 1990.[44] The needle entry is made into the proximal sac near the insertion of the dividing membrane and 20 mL of amniotic fluid are retrieved. Following replacement of the stylet, the needle is advanced through the second sac under direct ultrasound guidance. In order to avoid contamination, the first few milliliters of amniotic fluid are discarded and aspiration of 20 mL from the second sac integrates the procedure. Many advantages linked to this technique have been reported: requiring only one needle insertion and being swifter and shorter reduces woman's discomfort as well as the risk of postprocedural complications. Moreover, advancing the needle through the septum between the two sacs under ultrasound guidance provides positive proof of tapping both of them, diminishing the need for dye insertion. However, potential disadvantages render this approach less popular. Possible contamination of the second sample with amniotic fluid and fetal cells from the first one may lead to an incorrect diagnosis of mosaicism in the second fetus. This complication can be avoided by strictly adhering to the technique by replacing the stylet prior to intertwin membrane penetration and by discarding the first few milliliters from the second sac. Besides, the possibility of converting DA to pseudo-MA twin preganancy with the corresponding risks for cord entanglement and the formation of the amniotic band syndrome cannot be precluded.[45] In addition, a technical difficulty in penetrating a "tenting" dividing membrane has been reported.

In 1992, a novel approach for amniocentesis was introduced by Bahado-Singh et al. It was described as the double simultaneous amniocentesis technique.[46] Basically, two needles are inserted separately into the amniotic sacs under ultrasound visualization like in the technique of double amniocentesis. The difference is that after aspiration of the amniotic fluid from the first sac, the needle is left in place indicating the sampled cavity and the second insertion is made into the other sac. The main advantage seems to be the documentation of correct sampling from each sac. However, it is not widely used mainly because it is more time-consuming and thereby the experience with this approach is limited.

Procedure-related fetal loss rate in multiple pregnancies has been assessed in various studies. Early reports suggested a higher fetal loss rate in twin pregnancies than in singletons.[47-49] However, these studies did not take into account the possibility that the increased fetal wastage might be attributed to the twin pregnancy itself rather than the invasive procedure. Subsequently, it was reported that the maternal history of twins *per se* carries a pregnancy loss rate up to 24 weeks of about 6.3% and severe prematurity (24–28 weeks) rate of about 8%.[50] Most series of pregnancy outcome following second trimester amniocentesis report loss rates before 20 weeks of gestation of between 1% and 2.5% and a much higher loss rate before 28 weeks. In a multicenter European study, the pregnancy loss rate was estimated to be 2.3% and 3.7% before 20 and 28 weeks of gestation respectively.[51] In a case-control study, a similar fetal loss rate was reported between sampled twins and unsampled matched twin controls (3.5% vs. 3.2%).[52]

In conclusion, amniocentesis in twin pregnancies has been shown to be a safe and accurate diagnostic tool, providing that sampling involves both the sacs regardless of the zygocity and chorionicity.

Chorionic Villus Sampling

Chorionic villus sampling is a standard first trimester invasive approach for genetic studies in case of suspected aneuploidy or congenital genetic disease. It is considered a safe alternative invasive procedure to amniocentesis for prenatal diagnosis in singletons, whenever early diagnosis is needed. Furthermore, CVS has been shown to be safe and effective for sampling twin gestations as well.[53-55]

Chorionic villus sampling is best performed between 11 weeks and 13 weeks of gestation. Genetic results are available either within hours by direct preparations of the cytotrophoblast layer or within 3–7 days by tissue culture of chorionic villus mesenchymal core. Thus, early diagnosis is reached in case that routine first trimester prenatal screening for chromosomal abnormalities yields a high risk for one of the fetuses or in case that an increased risk of a genetic disease such as beta-thalassemia, cystic fibrosis, hemophilia and congenital adrenal hyperplasia are estimated due to the carrier status of one or both the prospective parents. Undoubtedly, early diagnosis provides earlier reassurance of fetal well-being and thereby eliminates both maternal anxiety and uncertainty regarding the present gestation. On the other hand, the diagnosis of one or both abnormal fetuses allows subsequent selective reduction of the affected fetus or termination of the total pregnancy as early as in the first trimester, where complication rates are lower. Moreover, fetal reduction performed earlier in pregnancy is associated with a higher survival rate of the unaffected twin.[56] In terms of privacy and maternal psychology, the earlier an abnormal pregnancy is terminated, the lesser the chance of being widely recognized.

Two different approaches have been used so far for first trimester CVS in multiple gestations, depending on physician's experience and location of the placenta: transabdominal and transcervical. Several pros and cons have been linked to each of them, but it is postulated that irrespective of the route adopted, first trimester CVS is technically more challenging than second trimester amniocentesis. Transcervical CVS is performed either with an aspiration catheter or using biopsy forceps under ultrasound guidance. Technical difficulties and a "learning curve" that involves many patients characterize this approach. Transabdominal technique uses an aspiration needle and is technically more similar to mid-trimester amniocentesis. Subsequently, this technique is more familiar to specialists in fetal medicine and thus more widely adopted by many centers.

Since no marker is available to assure sampling from each chorion, continuous ultrasound localization of the tip of the needle or catheter is required. If in doubt, a follow-up procedure should be performed either by an immediate repeat CVS or by second trimester amniocentesis. A serious drawback of CVS is a potential contamination of one sample by villi belonging to the other chorion leading to a confusing or even misleading diagnosis. Although, early studies suggested a contamination rate as high as 4%, more recent studies report a much lower rate, almost nullified.[57,58] Still, Weisz and Rodeck suggest that it would be prudent to counsel patients that about 2–3% of twin pregnancies having CVS will need resampling because of uncertainty of results.[43] A tip to eliminate this unfortunate possibility is to obtain samples adjacent to the cord insertion site far away from the dividing membrane.

In case that chorions are not readily accessible transcervically, the combined transabdominal-transcervical route can be opted.

Diagnosis of aneuploidy or severe genetic disease in one of the multiples is usually indicative of selective termination of the affected fetus. In such cases, detailed documentation and "labeling" of the fetuses, and the chorions is as equally important with CVS as with amniocentesis in order to diminish the possibility of unintentional erroneous termination of the healthy co-multiple. Although, the position of sacs will remain unchanged during the 2–3 weeks-time following sampling, it is standard practice to reconfirm the original diagnosis in both fetal and chorionic tissues before selective termination of the affected twin. Of note, CVS does not increase pregnancy loss rate before multifetal pregnancy reduction.[59]

The estimated risk of CVS associated fetal loss in singletons varies widely (1.3–4.3%). Two or more samplings during one procedure have been linked to increased risk of post-procedural miscarriage,[60,61] implying that the risk may be higher in twin sampling. Overall, an estimated risk of 2–4% in twin pregnancies has been reported. However, available data demonstrate significant variations. In a study, the risk of CVS associated fetal loss before 28 weeks of gestation did not seem to differ between twin and singleton pregnancies (4.9 vs. 4%).[53] When only chromosomal normal pregnancies are considered, the overall loss rate found in a study of 202 twin pregnancies that underwent CVS became 3.7%, a figure that is considerably less than that of amniocentesis.[53] In another study, the pregnancy loss rate before 20 weeks following CVS was found 3.3% comparable to 2.8% in a control group of twin pregnancies undergone amniocentesis. Hence, it may be claimed that in experienced centers, CVS is as safe as amniocentesis for sampling twins.

The ideal method for prenatal invasive genetic screening in multiple pregnancies is still a matter of debate. Available data confirm that amniocentesis and CVS share the same safety, and efficacy profile in expertise hands. However, amniocentesis is technically easier and widely adopted, whereas CVS results are available about one month earlier, thus therapeutic as well as selective termination is safer. Hence, none of them can be considered superior to the other, if the characteristics of the pregnancy are not taken into account. By all odds, each case should be individualized, and the ultimate choice should be based on several factors, such as gestational age at referral date, placental location, operator's experience and the likelihood of selective feticide. It should be emphasized that if the center is not skilled and experienced in CVS, amniocentesis should be preferred. A rational approach may be as follows: the choice of invasive technique should be based on individual risk calculated from the combination of maternal age and fetal NT thickness measured in the first trimester. When the risk for a chromosomal defect in at least one of the fetuses is greater than one in 50, it may be preferable to perform CVS. For pregnancies with a lower risk, amniocentesis after 15 weeks may be more appropriate.

FETAL BLOOD SAMPLING

The main principles of fetal blood sampling in twins and higher order multiple pregnancies do not differ substantially from those in singletons. However, from a technical point of view, the procedure in multiples is much more challenging.

Traditionally, fetal blood sampling was mainly indicated in cases that amniocentesis or CVS yielded uncertain or equivocal results, necessitating confirmation or clarification respectively. Another indication was the need for a rapid chromosomal diagnosis (rapid karyotyping), in as much as the results are available in 2–3 days time. Nowadays, novel molecular techniques allow rapid karyotype determination using amniocentesis specimen, thereby reserving fetal blood sampling in cases where rationale exists. The main indications today are rhesus isoimmunization, hydrops of unknown origin and fetal infections. From a therepeutic aspect, cordocentesis can serve in injecting pharmacologic agents into the fetal circulation or even blood transfusion in severe fetal anemia.

Similarly to singletons, a meticulous ultrasound examination should precede fetal blood sampling in multiples. In addition to fetal growth, anatomy and position of each fetus, chorionicity, amnionicity, location of the placenta(s), and umbilical cord insertion should be determined. Furthermore, "labeling" of the multiples is needed to assure correct sampling from each fetus.

In a study conducted in 2003, involving 84 twin pregnancies, mainly screened for hemoglobinopathies, the overall procedure-related fetal loss (up to 2 weeks post-procedurally) was 8.2%, about four-fold higher than the correspondence risk in singletons. However, this technique can be used as an alternative to amniocentesis after 20 weeks of gestation to confirm an abnormal karyotype in a DC pregnancy, when selective feticide is considered a few weeks after the initial procedure.[62]

CONCLUSION

Nowadays, there is an increasing demand for invasive genetic studies in multiple pregnancies due to the rising rate of multiple conceptions, the latter mainly attributed to infertility treatment modalities. Diagnosis of fetal aneuploidies and genetic defects can be accomplished either by first trimester CVS or by second trimester amniocentesis, whereas it is claimed that they are equally safe in expertise hands. Hence, the experience of the center performing the procedure should be emphasized in decision making with regards to the procedure opted. The indications of fetal blood sampling are currently limited and progressively replaced by novel molecular techniques implemented in CVS or amniocentesis specimen. High resolution ultrasound equipment available today, together with increasing operator experience gained throughout the years, results in more accurate and effective invasive prenatal diagnosis in twin or higher-order pregnancies, minimizing post-procedural fetal loss risk.

REFERENCES

1. Kiely JL, Kleinman JC, Kiely M. Triplets and higher-order multiple births. Time trends and infant mortality. Am J Dis Child. 1992;146:862-8.

2. Bergh T, Ericson A, Hillensjö T, et al. Deliveries and children born after in-vitro fertilisation in Sweden 1982-95: a retrospective cohort study. Lancet. 1999;354:1579-85.
3. Derom C, Vlietinck R, Derom R, et al. Increased monozygotic twinning rate after ovulation induction. Lancet. 1987;1:1236-8.
4. Wenstrom KD, Syrop CH, Hammitt DG, et al. Increased risk of monochorionic twinning associated with assisted reproduction. Fertil Steril. 1993;60:510-4.
5. Blickstein I. Estimation of iatrogenic monozygotic twinning rate following assisted reproduction: Pitfalls and caveats. Am J Obstet Gynecol. 2005;192:365-8.
6. Kohl SG, Casey G. Twin gestation. Mt Sinai J Med. 1975; 42:523-39.
7. Nicolaides KH, Sebire NJ, Snjiders RJM. The 11–14 Week Scan. The Diagnosis of Fetal Abnormalities. In: Nicolaides K, Sebire NJ, Snjiders RJM (Eds). New York: Parthenon Publishing;1999.
8. Matias A, MontenegroN, Blickstein I. Down syndrome screening in multiple pregnancies. Obstet Gynecol Clin North Am. 2005;32:81-96.
9. Sepulveda W, Sebire NJ, Hughes K, et al. Evolution of the lambda or twin-chorionic peak sign in dichorionic twin pregnancies. Obstet Gynecol. 1997;89:439-41.
10. Jenkins TM, Wapner RJ. The challenge of prenatal diagnosis in twin pregnancies. Curr Opin Obstet Gynecol. 2000;12: 87-92.
11. Wood SL, St Onge R, Connors G, et al. Evaluation of the twin peak or lambda sign in determining chorionicity in multiple pregnancy. Obstet Gynecol. 1996;88:6-9.
12. Machin GA. Some causes of genotypic and phenotypic discordance in monozygotic twin pairs. Am J Med Genet. 1996;61:216-28.
13. Rogers JG, Voullaire L, Gold H. Monozygotic twins discordant for trisomy 21. Am J Med Genet. 1982;11:143-6.
14. Dallapiccola B, Stomeo C, Ferranti G, et al. Discordant sex in one of three monozygotic triplets. J Med Genet. 1985;22:11.
15. Perlman EJ, Stetten G, Tuck-Müller CM, et al. Sexual discordance in monozygotic twins. Am J Med Genet. 1990;37:551-7.
16. Schmid O, Trautmann U, Ashour H, et al. Prenatal diagnosis of heterokaryotypic mosaic twins discordant for fetal sex. Prenat Diagn. 2000;20:999-1003.
17. Wachtel SS, Somkuti SG, Schinfeld JS. Monozygotic twins of opposite sex. Cytogenet Cell Genet. 2000;91:293-5.
18. Lespinasse J, Gicquel C, Robert M, et al. Phenotypic and genotypic variability in monozygotic triplets with Turner syndrome. Clin Genet. 1998;54:56-9.
19. Nieuwint A, Van Zalen-Sprock R, Hummel P, et al. Identical' twins with discordant karyotypes. Prenat Diagn. 1999; 19:72-6.
20. Rodis JF, Egan JF, Craffey A, et al. Calculated risk of chromosomal abnormalities in twin gestations. Obstet Gynecol. 1990;76:1037-41.
21. Weinblatt V, Wapner RJ. Chorionic villus sampling and amniocentesis in multiple pregnancy. In: Creasy RK, Resnik R (Eds). Maternal-Fetal Medicine Principles and Practice, 4th edition. Philadelphia: WB Saunders; 1999. pp. 201-11.
22. Sebire NJ, Snijders RJ, Hughes K, et al. Screening for trisomy 21 in twin pregnancies by maternal age and fetal nuchal translucency thickness at 10–14 weeks of gestation. Br J Obstet Gynaecol. 1996;103:999-1003.
23. Vandecruys H, Faiola S, Auer M, et al. Screening for trisomy 21 in monochorionic twins by measurement of fetal nuchal translucency thickness. Ultrasound Obstet Gynecol. 2005;25:551-3.
24. Spencer K, Salonen R, Muller F. Down's syndrome screening in multiple pregnancies using alpha-fetoprotein and free beta hCG. Prenat Diagn. 1994;14:537-42.
25. Muller F, Dreux S, Dupoizat H, et al. Second-trimester Down syndrome maternal serum screening in twin pregnancies: impact of chorionicity. Prenat Diagn. 2003;23:331-5.
26. Wald NJ, Rish S. Prenatal screening for Down syndrome and neural tube defects in twin pregnancies. Prenat Diagn. 2005;25:740-5.
27. Gardner S, Burton BK, Johnson AM. Maternal serum alpha-fetoprotein screening: a report of the Forsyth County project. Am J Obstet Gynecol. 1981;140:250-3.
28. Wapner RJ. Genetic diagnosis in multiple pregnancies. Semin Perinatol. 1995;19:351-62.
29. Emery AE. Antenatal diagnosis of genetic disease. Modern Trends Hum Genet. 1970;1:267.
30. Jenkins TM, Wapner RJ. First trimester prenatal diagnosis: chorionic villus sampling. Semin Perinatol. 1999;23:403-13.
31. Cleary-Goldman J, D'Alton ME, Berkowitz RL. Prenatal diagnosis and multiple pregnancy. Semin Perinatol. 2005;29:312-20.
32. Delisle MF, Brosseuk L, Wilson RD. Amniocentesis for twin pregnancies: is alpha-fetoprotein useful in confirming that the two sacs were sampled? Fetal Diagn Ther. 2007;22:221-5.
33. Elias S, Gerbie AB, Simpson JL, et al. Genetic amniocentesis in twin gestations. Am J Obstet Gynecol. 1980;138:169-74.
34. Cragan JD, Martin ML, Khoury MJ, et al. Dye use during amniocentesis and birth defects. Lancet. 1993;341(8856): 1352.
35. Nicolini U, Monni G. Intestinal obstruction in babies exposed in utero to methylene blue. Lancet. 1990;336:1258-9.
36. Kidd SA, Lancaster PA, Anderson JC, et al. Fetal death after exposure to methylene blue dye during mid-trimester amniocentesis in twin pregnancy. Prenat Diagn. 1996;16:39-47.
37. McEnerney JK, McEnerney LN. Unfavorable neonatal outcome after intra-amniotic injection of methylene blue. Obstet Gynecol. 1983;61:35S-7S.
38. McFadyen I. The dangers of intra-amniotic methylene blue. Br J Obstet Gynaecol. 1992;99:89-90.
39. van der Pol JG, Wolf H, Boer K, et al. Jejunal atresia related to the use of methylene blue in genetic amniocentesis in twins. Br J Obstet Gynaecol. 1992;99:141-3.

40. Vincer MJ, Allen AC, Evans JR, et al. Methylene-blue-induced hemolytic anemia in a neonate. CMAJ. 1987;136:503-4.
41. Antsaklis A, Souka AP, Daskalakis G, et al. Second-trimester amniocentesis vs chorionic villus sampling for prenatal diagnosis in multiple gestations. Ultrasound Obstet Gynecol. 2002;20:476-81.
42. Taylor MJ, Fisk NM. Prenatal diagnosis in multiple pregnancy. Baillieres Best Pract Res Clin Obstet Gynaecol. 2000;14:663-75.
43. Weisz B, Rodeck CH. Invasive diagnostic procedures in twin pregnancies. Prenat Diagn. 2005;25:751-8.
44. Jeanty P, Shah D, Roussis P. Single-needle insertion in twin amniocentesis. J Ultrasound Med. 1990;9:511-7.
45. Megory E, Weiner E, Shalev E, et al. Pseudomonoamniotic twins with cord entanglement following genetic funipuncture. Obstet Gynecol. 1991;78:915-7.
46. Bahado-Singh R, Schmitt R, Hobbins JC. New technique for genetic amniocentesis in twins. Obstet Gynecol. 1992;79:304-7.
47. Palle C, AndersenJ.W, Tabor A, et al. Increased risk of abortion after genetic amniocentesis in twin pregnancies. Prenat Diagn. 1983;3:83-9.
48. Pijpers L, Jahoda MG, Vosters RP, et al. Genetic amniocentesis in twin pregnancies. Br J Obstet Gynaecol. 1988;323-326:4.
49. Anderson RL, Goldberg JD, Golbus MS. Prenatal diagnosis in multiple gestation: 20 years' experience with amniocentesis. Prenat Diagn. 1991;11:263-70.
50. Yaron Y, Bryant-Greenwood PK, Dave N, et al. Multifetal pregnancy reductions of triplets to twins: comparison with nonreduced triplets and twins. Am J Obstet Gynecol. 1999;180:1268-71.
51. Pruggmayer MR, Jahoda MG, Van der Pol JG, et al. Genetic amniocentesis in twin pregnancies: results of a multicenter study of 529 cases. Ultrasound Obstet Gynecol. 1992;2:6-10.
52. Ghidini A, Lynch L, Hicks C, et al. The risk of second-trimester amniocentesis in twin gestations: a case-control study. Am J Obstet Gynecol. 1993;169:1013-6.
53. Pergament E, Schulman JD, Copeland K, et al. The risk and efficacy of chorionic villus sampling in multiple gestations. Prenat Diagn. 1992;12:377-84.
54. Brambati B, Tului L, Lanzani A, et al. First-trimester genetic diagnosis in multiple pregnancy: principles and potential pitfalls. Prenat Diagn. 1991;11:767-74.
55. Wapner RJ, Barr MA, Heeger S, et al. Chorionic villus sampling: a 10-year over 13,000 consecutive case experience. In: Orlando FL (Ed). American College of Medical Genetics, First Annual Meeting; 1994.
56. Evans MI, Goldberg JD, Horenstein J, et al. Selective termination for structural, chromosomal, and Mendelian anomalies: international experience. Am J Obstet Gynecol. 1999;181:893-7.
57. De Catte L, Liebaers I, Foulon W. Outcome of twin gestations after first trimester chorionic villus sampling. Obstet Gynecol. 2000;96:714-20.
58. Brambati B, Tului L, Guercilena S, et al. Outcome of first-trimester chorionic villus sampling for genetic investigation in multiple pregnancy. Ultrasound Obstet Gynecol. 2001;17:209-16.
59. Ferrara L, Gandhi M, Litton C, et al. Chorionic villus sampling and the risk of adverse outcome in patients undergoing multifetal pregnancy reduction. Am J Obstet Gynecol. 2008;199:408.e1-4.
60. Rhoads GG, Jackson LG, Schlesselman SE, et al. The safety and efficacy of chorionic villus sampling for early prenatal diagnosis of cytogenetic abnormalities. N Engl J Med. 1989;320:609-17.
61. Kuliev A, Jackson L, Froster U, et al. Chorionic villus sampling safety. Report of World Health Organization/EURO meeting in association with the Seventh International Conference on Early Prenatal Diagnosis of Genetic Diseases, Tel-Aviv, Israel, May 21, 1994. Am J Obstet Gynecol. 1996;174:807-11.
62. Antsaklis A, Gougoulakis A, Mesogitis S, et al. Invasive techniques for fetal diagnosis in multiple pregnancy. Int J Gynaecol Obstet. 1991;34:309-14.

CHAPTER 42

Overview of Fetal Therapy

Tuangsit Wataganara

INTRODUCTION

An improving ability to diagnose fetal conditions with higher accuracy prompts an attempt for a salvage treatment in-utero. Fetal conditions amendable for prenatal intervention are limited to only diseases that can either kill the baby in-utero or leave the baby with significant handicap. Therapeutic intervention has to be highly selective. Factors that need to be considered before offering in-utero treatment include the highly investigative nature of certain procedures. For instance, at the time of writing this chapter, fetal endoluminal tracheal occlusion for severe congenital diaphragmatic hernia is still under a randomized controlled investigational trial to validate its potential benefits and risks to the fetus with severe congenital diaphragmatic hernia with suboptimal growth of the residual lung tissue. There are chances of procedure-related miscarriages, preterm premature rupture of the membranes, and maternal morbidity that need to be discussed in an unbiased counseling session. The right balance between potential benefits and harms requires validation with rigid scientific methodology before the practice has become a 'standard of care'. For example, laser photocoagulation of anastomosing chorionic vessels has become a standard of care in many places due to its superior perinatal survival and composite outcomes, particularly for the childhood neurodevelopmental status. With an ongoing technological development, it is foreseeable that there will be more proposals of implementing novel medical technologies to the use of fetal therapy. Currently, there are only a handful of fetal care centers, most of the experienced ones are clustered in developed part of Europe and the United States. Dissemination of this type of service which require years of experiences to develop surgical skill and the support by the most technological advanced instrument and setting is a real challenge that need to be addressed, discussed, and solved as a global agenda.

HISTORY OF FETAL THERAPY

Certain diseases can develop before the baby is born. Serious diseases are not compatible with fetal life. The fetus may survive with significant neurodevelopmental challenges or physical handicaps. Prenatal detection of fetal anomalies or diseases was fostered by an introduction of ultrasound for diagnosis in 1958 by Ian Donald and colleagues.[1] The advent of real-time ultrasound aided in both fetal diagnosis and intervention. The first published report of fetal therapeutic intervention was intraperitoneal blood transfusion for severely anemic fetus from Rhesus disease by Sir Albert William Liley in 1963.[2]

High quality fetal ultrasound has become broadly available since 1980's. Fetal anomaly scan has become a standard in many places, particularly in developed nations. This practice increases the chance to pick up a fetus with conditions amendable for prenatal intervention. Our center (Faculty of Medicine Siriraj Hospital, Bangkok, Thailand) has adopted ultrasound-guided fetal blood sampling and transfusion, and published our first case report and case series in 1987 and 1989, respectively.[3,4] In those years, ultrasound-guided intravascular (umbilical vein) fetal blood transfusion was performed in the main operating theater, as shown in **Figure 1**. Adding Doppler studies in prenatal well-being evaluation protocol allows for better assessment of fetal anemia and oxygenation.[5]

Since then, there has been significant development of various kinds of techniques for prenatal interventions. The interventions can be categorized into: (a) medical treatment, (b) minimally invasive intervention (including ultrasound-guided needle intervention and shunting), (c) fetoscopic surgery, and (d) open fetal surgery. Fetal therapy is driven by progressively sophisticated fetal imaging, i.e., magnetic resonance imaging (MRI) and molecular genetics technology.[6]

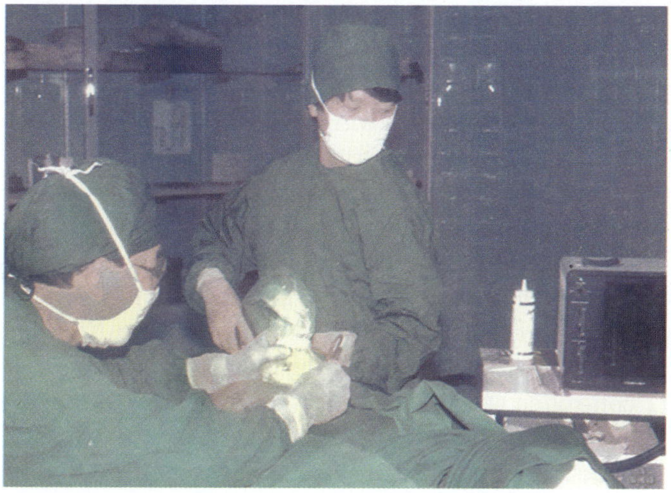

Fig. 1: Historical picture of first in-utero fetal blood transfusion using ultrasound guidance. Note the linear transducer probe being used in the procedure back then.

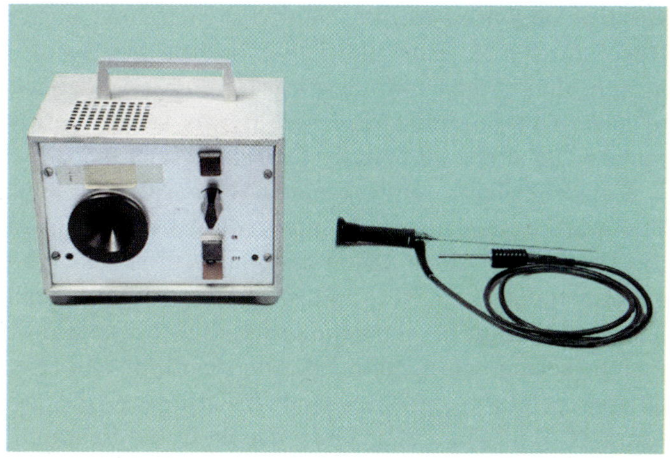

Fig. 2: The first fetoscopy unit used in Department of Obstetrics and Gynecology, Faculty of Medicine Siriraj Hospital. Note the traditional light source, rod lens, and eyepiece. Back then, videoendoscopic unit was not available, and the operator needed to directly look through the eyepiece. This fetoscopy unit was used to sampling blood from chorionic vessel under direct visualization to diagnose severe thalassemia disease of the fetus. It was then replaced by high-resolution ultrasound-guided fetal blood sampling from the umbilical cord vein.

Intrauterine intervention is aiming to improve the outcome of fetal conditions before the baby is born. Prenatal surgery may reduce irreversible damages inflicting on certain developing organs. With this goal in mind, a number of prenatal interventions have been proposed over the past 4 decades. The benefits from most proposed prenatal interventions were not reproducible, and hence they were abandoned. Until recently, only short-term perinatal outcomes have been the benchmarks for the benefits of prenatal interventions. The current evaluation has become more critical. All the new treatments have to undergo a rigorous validation for its true benefits and risks, as well as short-term and long-term health impacts, compared to the conservative or traditional treatments. Most of them are conducted as randomized controlled trial (RCT).

In 1980's, Michael Harrison and his colleagues from University of California at San Francisco (UCSF) have pioneered the use to sheep as an experimental animal model for experimenting fetal intervention. Knowledge from this animal studies has led to the first invasive treatment in human fetus in 1981, which is the placement of a double pigtail shunt in a case of urinary tract obstruction.[7] This intervention is considered the very first minimally invasive intervention performed directly on human fetus. This first fetal patient was born alive, and lived well for at least 25 years later.[8]

Using an ultrasound to guide the shunt placement, this type of procedure was originally called 'image-guided percutaneous fetal access'. 'Open hysterotomy' was subsequently developed for a broader access to the fetus. It is also known as 'open fetal surgery'. Initially, UCSF offered open fetal surgery perform vesicostomy, a surgical procedure to create continuous in-utero bladder drainage for fetuses with lower urinary tract obstruction.[9] In-utero intervention could significantly improve perinatal outcomes and reduce long-term morbidity. However, open hysterotomy was related to higher maternal morbidity and increased risks of premature birth due to its invasiveness.

Videoendoscopic surgery started to gain popularity in the 1990's. Many fetal care centers shifted their practice toward videoendoscopic-assisted access for its minimally invasive nature. Initially, hysteroscope was used to visualize and perform simple intrauterine procedures. Dedicated fetoscope was subsequently commercially developed, and has become the most common access for fetal intervention until today. Fetoscopic approach has overcome the following limitations of open fetal surgery: (a) Because of smaller incision, the chance of preterm premature rupture of the membranes (pPROM) and unstoppable preterm delivery is less; (b) Because of its less invasiveness, maternal morbidity is reduced.

Fetoscopic approach allows for safer operation both mother and fetus. **Figure 2** shows our first fetoscopic surgical unit used in our Faculty of Medicine, Siriraj Hospital over 30 years ago. The fetoscope was used to sample blood from chorionic vessel for prenatal diagnosis of severe thalassemia diseases. It was subsequently replaced by ultrasound-guided fetal blood sampling.

Fetoscopy has recently regained its clinical usefulness. There are quite a few fetal interventions that enjoyed the benefits of direct visualization, small access, and advancement in the technology of laser surgery, such as laser ablation of anastomosing vessels on chorionic plate in severe twin-twin transfusion syndrome and laser ablation of fetal posterior urethral valve. However, the best example of this paradigm shift may lie in the treatment of fetuses with severe congenital diaphragmatic hernia (CDH).

Data on long-term health impact of fetuses with CDH is still lacking. There have been a number of proposed in-utero interventions to improve perinatal outcomes of fetuses with prenatally diagnosed severe CDH. Real benefits of these interventions can only be proven and compared through well-designed RCTs. Interventions for other fetal diseases have also been undergoing rigorous scientific validation, such as laser photocoagulation of chorionic anastomoses in severe mid-trimester twin-twin transfusion syndrome (TTTS), fetal tracheal occlusion (FETO) for severe congenital diaphragmatic hernia (CDH), and open repair of meningomyelocele (MMC).[10-12]

These examples of landmark trials were designed to validate both short-term and long-term benefits of the procedure. Neurocognitive performance is a major indicator of long-term outcome. For instance, FETO can improve neonatal survival in severe left-sided CDH from 24.1% (historical non-interventional controls) to 49.1% (FETO cases) (P <0.001).[13] Many fetal care centers start offering FETO to their patients. The real benefits of FETO should be available after the tracheal occlusion to accelerate lung growth trial (TOTAL trial) led by Eurofetus group is completed.

Some fetal intervention procedures are considered a standard of care, i.e., fetal blood transfusion. Some procedures, on the other hands, were abandoned due to its failure to show genuine benefits to the fetus after rigorous scientific validation. In-utero interventions for fetal lower urinary tract obstruction (LUTO) can be used as a good example here. LUTO is a serious disease. The obstruction results in secondary pulmonary and renal malfunction, which can be reversed only if obstruction is released in utero. Traditionally, vesicoamniotic shunting (VAS) was a standard of care for fetuses with LUTO. The benefits of VAS based on small case series without control groups. A meta-analysis by Clark and colleagues (2003) showed perinatal outcomes of 342 fetuses with severe LUTO diagnosed by ultrasound in the second trimester.[14] Of these, 195 fetuses were from 7 controlled studies and another 147 fetuses were from 9 case series without controls. Fetal bladder drainage procedures, including serial vesicocentesis, VAS, and open fetal vesicostomy, improve overall neonatal survival, particularly in poor prognosis group. The odd ratio (OR) was 26.19 (95% CI: 4.39, 156.2) for poor prognosis (2 controlled studies, 46 fetuses) and 2.25 (95% CI: 0.65, 7.81) for good prognosis (2 controlled studies, 49 fetuses).

The real benefit of VAS was questioned after percutaneous vesicoamniotic shunting in lower urinary tract obstruction (PLUTO) trial was published in 2013.[15] This RCT involving 31 fetuses with LUTO showed a borderline increased survival rate in VAS group, compared to expectant management group [intention-to-treat relative risk (RR) 1.88, 95% CI 0·71-4·96; P = 0·27]. Most babies had impaired renal function irrespective of VAS. Fetoscopic cystoscopy with laser ablation of posterior urethral valve (PUV) has gained an interest recent years. Data showed that laser ablation of PUV can improve the 6-month survival rate and renal function [ARR, 4.10 (95% CI, 1.75-9.62; P<0.01) and 2.66 (95% CI, 1.25-5.70; P=0.01) respectively].[16] RCT to study the real benefit of fetal cystoscopy in management of severe LUTO is underway.

Fetal conditions amendable for in utero treatment are relatively rare. In order to get adequate power, multicenter or international collaboration is frequently needed. There is one significant drawback for this approach. It takes time and experiences for any center to achieve the same outcomes as those previous reported by more established fetal care center. There is a tendency that the complete treatments are concentrated only in a handful of centers, mostly in the United States and Europe.[17]

Newer treatments have been subjected to scientific validation, as to how these new approaches can change the perinatal prognosis. Animal studies and RCTs are generally required prior to clinical implementation of any new technology. Neonatal survival (more than 28 days after birth) used to be the main outcomes to evaluate the benefit of in utero intervention. Improvement of neonatal outcomes can be observed after newer interventions. However, there are some factors that may as well be contributing to the improved outcomes compared to traditional expectant management. These factors include:

- Liberal administration of glucocorticoid to enhance fetal lung maturation
- Advancement of fetal imaging modality, including ultrasound and magnetic resonance imaging (MRI)
- Increased number of experienced pediatric surgeon with formal training
- Upgrade of neonatal intensive care unit (NICU) and availability of more advanced respiratory support, such as high frequency neonatal ventilator.

FETAL THERAPY SEGMENT

In this fifth edition of *Donald School Textbook of Ultrasound in Obstetrics and Gynecology* we systematically explore the principles of fetal therapy in relation to its fetal conditions. Actual benefits and risks of the interventions are discussed based on the evidence obtained from large case series or well-designed studies. Technical aspects of each procedure will be explored. Diagnostic and technical practical points from our own experiences at Faculty of Medicine, Siriraj Hospital in Bangkok are shared for a better understanding of how fetal therapy is being practiced in reality.

PRINCIPLES OF FAMILY COUNSELING FOR FETAL THERAPY

Once fetal disease is suspected from ultrasound examination, it should be confirmed by experienced hands or team approach. Controversial ultrasound findings need to be interpreted for its clinical relevance, as being advised by the recently published recommendation from our Working Group on Ultrasound in Obstetrics of the World Association of Perinatal Medicine (WAPM).[18] Doppler studies and three-dimensional sonography are frequently used for more details. When more advanced sonographic modalities are used, potential thermal effect that may lead to neuronal apoptosis has to be cautioned. This concerned was outlined in another separate publication from our WAPM working group.[19] Occasionally, magnetic resonance imaging, or molecular genetics investigations may be required to reach definitive diagnosis and prognosis.[20]

The patient and her family should be offered a counseling session by multidisciplinary team. Besides emotional stresses that the family needs to deal with, they have to mentally process large and complicated information provided by the medical team. It is important to know that, firstly, people in general can only process a limited piece of information in a single counseling session. Secondly, there are both intuitive and emotional factors involved, when a decision for an unborn child is being made. Lastly, the information on maternal risks is not usually 'weighed' adequately after the first counseling session.

It is important that cultural, religious, legal and technological aspects need to be considered in each counseling session. The ability for people to comprehend and rationalize this piece of information is affected by their intelligence and education level. Even in a country with good educational system like the United Kingdom, only half of the adults can adequately understand medical information after a counseling session.[21]

It has been estimated that over 40 million people in the United States have limited literacy, particularly in ethnic minority group.[21] In addition to this, stress and anxiety created from the distressful information can further add to how people can retain the information when the counseling is over. With all these factors, counseling for fetal disease and its corresponding treatment modality are a real challenge to everyone to reach an informed decision.

PRINCIPLES AND TYPES OF FETAL THERAPY

Only serious diseases are amendable for prenatal treatment. The objectives of initiating the treatment before the fetus is born are to save life and to prevent permanent disabilities. There are many ways to categorize fetal therapeutic interventions. For the purpose of practicality, categorization based on fetal approaches is used in this "fetal therapy segment". The categorization of fetal therapy is as follows.

- Medical treatment
  - Transplacental
  - Transamniotic
  - Intramuscular
  - Intravenous
- In-utero stem cell transplantation and gene therapy
- Minimally invasive fetal intervention
  - Needle-guided intervention
  - Shunting procedure
  - Fetoscopic intervention
- Open fetal surgery.

More details and examples for this categorization are shown in **Table 1**. Fetal therapy is, in fact, a heterogeneous cluster of interventions. It is ranging from simple transplacental medical treatment to invasive surgical

TABLE 1: Types of fetal therapy.

Type	*Examples*	*Remarks*
Medical treatment	Glucocorticoids	Enhance fetal lung maturity
In-utero stem cell transplantation and gene therapy	In utero hematopoietic stem cell transplantation	Severe combined immunodeficiency syndrome (SCID)
Minimally invasive fetal intervention	Laser ablation of chorionic anastomoses	Twin-twin transfusion syndrome
Open fetal surgery	Closure of high-risk meningomyelocele	Improvement of neurological outcomes

TABLE 2: Criteria for invasive fetal intervention.

1. Accurate diagnosis and staging possible, with exclusion of associated anomalies
2. Natural history of the disease is documented, and prognosis is established
3. Currently no effective postnatal therapy
4. In utero surgery proven feasible in animal models, reversing deleterious effects of the condition
5. Interventions performed in specialized multidisciplinary fetal treatment centers within strict protocols and approval of the local ethics Committee with informed consent of the mother or parents

Courtesy: Deprest JA et al. 2010.[24]

intervention. Administration of therapeutic agents to the mother, so that it crosses the placenta to the fetus, carries very small risks to the mother. An example of transplacental medical treatment is maternal administration of antiarrhythmic agent to reverse decompensated fetal arrhythmia. Invasive surgical intervention carries potential maternal morbidity. An example of invasive fetal treatment is open repair of fetal MMC. More invasive procedures are related to a higher chance of membranes rupture and iatrogenic preterm birth.[22]

Fetal therapy used to be offered arbitrarily, based on institutional expert opinion. In 1982, there was the very first congregation of international experts in fetal therapy in Santa Ynez, California.[23] This panel of expert has suggested 5 main rules to guide an optimal clinical application of invasive fetal interventions. This guideline, as shown in **Table 2**, is frequently quoted, and remains the principles of fetal surgical intervention until these days.[24]

ETHICS OF FETAL THERAPY

"The fetus as a patient" is the central ethical concept for fetal medicine.[25] However, this quote should not be taken in an absence of the maternal context. It is imperative during the counseling session that cultural, religious, legal, and technological aspects of fetal disease and the corresponding interventions have to be discussed in an honest way. It is true that in utero intervention can potentially benefit the fetus, but occasionally it comes with an increasing maternal risk.

In terms of research for new fetal therapeutic interventions, investigators should address the initiation and assessment of clinical trials to determine the following issues:

- A standard of care has been established
- An appropriate informed consent process has been used to recruit and enroll subjects
- The selection criteria should include the abortion preferences of the pregnant woman
- The doctors have an obligation to offer referral to such investigation. It means that the doctors have obligations to both the fetal patient and the pregnant woman.

In terms of clinical judgments whether to or not to offer fetal therapy, it is important to know that the definitive goal of fetal interventions is improve the health of children by intervening before birth. Once feasibility and potential benefit of particular procedure are identified, it should be subjected to rigorous scientific validation. "Innovative therapy" is therefore a part of careful care and ongoing research.

Pregnant women receiving fetal treatments entitle for the same legal and health protection as participants in interventional research study. They need to be adequately counseled for the potential risks and benefits of the procedure they are embarking on. These health impacts should be specific from maternal and fetal aspects, or as short- and long-term effects. Written informed consent must be obtained prior to any intervention. The language in this consent must be explicit. The importance of written informed consent for fetal therapy was endorsed in a joint statement from American College of Obstetricians and Gynecologists and American Academy of Pediatrics published in 2011.[26]

Termination of pregnancy, even for medical indications, is not acceptable in many parts of the world. This is important to respect the community's legal and spiritual restrictions. The choice of pregnant women and their family can be limited. In some other communities, termination of pregnancy for fetal indications is possible. Most of fetal indications involve lethal malformations or malformations that result in significant handicap after birth.

In-utero therapy can 'cure' some diseases, such as laser surgery for severe mid-trimester TTTS, but can only palliate in the others, such as FETO in severe CDH. There is a possibility that in-utero therapy may turn deadly disease into lifelong debilitating condition. Experienced doctors know when to offer 'intervention' and 'termination' to avoid that tragic possibility. Upper limit of gestational age legally permissible for termination is varied from one community to the others. Once this legal gestational age is reached, the woman's choice will become limited.

Unbiased counseling is crucial. The counselor has to make sure that the pregnant woman will not undergo fetal treatment without a full awareness of alternative options. Multidisciplinary approach is therefore mandatory in many centers.[27]

CONCLUSION

The world is now globalized. Fetal therapeutic technique created at one place can quickly be communicated and adopted in other places. Effective communication has made the greatest impact in quality health care. Ability to intervene certain fetal diseases prenatally has significantly reduced neonatal and maternal morbidity. Traumatic delivery of an anomalous baby can sometimes be avoided with in-utero intervention.

Quality medical care is a basic service in most developed nations. But in developing nations, even basic second trimester fetal ultrasound is still lacking. Unequal distribution of resources in medicine may obstruct the access of fetal diagnosis and therapy. A good example of how to maximize a limited resource to the benefits of maternal and fetal care can be seen in Africa. This concern has been addressed in our recent publication from Working Group on Ultrasound in Obstetrics of the World Association of Perinatal Medicine (WAPM).[28] Dissemination of technology and funding is crucial to bring down the boundary of fetal care throughout the world.

REFERENCES

1. Donald I, Macvicar J, Brown TG. Investigation of abdominal masses by pulsed ultrasound. Lancet. 1958;1:1188-95.
2. Liley AW. Intrauterine Transfusion of Foetus in Haemolytic Disease. Br Med J. 1963;2:1107-9.
3. Kanokpongsakdi S, Winichagoon P, Fucharoen S, Manassagorn J, Tanphaichitr V. Prenatal diagnosis of the fetus at risk for beta-thalassemia/hemoglobin E disease: a report of the first case in Thailand. J Med Assoc Thai. 1987;70:38-43.
4. Vantanasiri C, Kanokpongsakdi S, Manassakorn J, et al. Percutaneous umbilical cord blood sampling. J Med Assoc Thai. 1989;72:541-4.
5. Wataganara T, Wiwanichayakul B, Ruengwuttilert P, Sunsaneevithayakul P, Viboonchart S, Wantanasiri C. Noninvasive diagnosis of fetal anemia and fetal intravascular transfusion therapy: experiences at Siriraj Hospital. J Med Assoc Thai. 2006;89:1036-43.
6. Wataganara T, Ngerncham S, Kitsommart R, Fuangtharnthip P. Fetal neck myofibroma. J Med Assoc Thai. 2007;90:376-80.
7. Harrison MR, Filly RA, Parer JT, Faer MJ, Jacobson JB, de Lorimier AA. Management of the fetus with a urinary tract malformation. Jama. 1981;246:635-9.
8. Jancelewicz T, Harrison MR. A history of fetal surgery. Clinics in Perinatology. 2009;36:227-36, vii.
9. Harrison MR, Golbus MS, Filly RA, et al. Fetal surgery for congenital hydronephrosis. N Engl J Med. 1982;306:591-3.
10. Senat MV, Deprest J, Boulvain M, Paupe A, Winer N, Ville Y. Endoscopic laser surgery versus serial amnioreduction for severe twin-to-twin transfusion syndrome. N Engl J Med. 2004;351:136-44.
11. Harrison MR, Keller RL, Hawgood SB, et al. A randomized trial of fetal endoscopic tracheal occlusion for severe fetal congenital diaphragmatic hernia. N Engl J Med. 2003;349:1916-24.
12. Adzick NS, Thom EA, Spong CY, et al. A randomized trial of prenatal versus postnatal repair of myelomeningocele. N Engl J Med. 2011;364:993-1004.
13. Jani J, Nicolaides KH, Keller RL, et al. Observed to expected lung area to head circumference ratio in the prediction of survival in fetuses with isolated diaphragmatic hernia. Ultrasound in obstetrics and gynecology: the official journal of the International Society of Ultrasound in Obstetrics and Gynecology. 2007;30:67-71.
14. Clark TJ, Martin WL, Divakaran TG, Whittle MJ, Kilby MD, Khan KS. Prenatal bladder drainage in the management of fetal lower urinary tract obstruction: a systematic review and meta-analysis. Obstetrics and Gynecology. 2003;102:367-82.
15. Morris RK, Malin GL, Quinlan-Jones E, et al. Percutaneous vesicoamniotic shunting versus conservative management for fetal lower urinary tract obstruction (PLUTO): a randomised trial. Lancet. 2013;382:1496-506.
16. Ruano R, Sananes N, Sangi-Haghpeykar H, et al. Fetal intervention for severe lower urinary tract obstruction: a multicenter case-control study comparing fetal cystoscopy with vesicoamniotic shunting. Ultrasound in obstetrics and gynecology: the official journal of the International Society of Ultrasound in Obstetrics and Gynecology. 2015;45:452-8.
17. Ville Y. Fetal therapy: practical ethical considerations. Prenat Diagn. 2011;31:621-7.

18. Ebrashy A, Kurjak A, Adra A, et al. Controversial ultrasound findings in mid trimester pregnancy. Evidence-based approach. Journal of Perinatal Medicine; 2015.
19. Pooh RK, Maeda K, Kurjak A, et al. 3D/4D sonography—any safety problem. Journal of Perinatal Medicine; 2015.
20. Wataganara T, Ebrashy A, Aliyu LD, Moreire dc Sa RA, Pooh R, Kurjak A, et al. Fetal magnetic resonance imaging and ultrasound. J Perinat Med. 2016 Apr 19. pii:/j/jpme.ahead-of-print/jpm-2015-0226/jpm/2015-0226.xml. doi:10.1515/jpm-2015-0226.[Epub ahead of print].
21. Williams MV, Davis T, Parker RM, Weiss BD. The role of health literacy in patient-physician communication. Family Medicine. 2002;34:383-9.
22. Deprest JA, Devlieger R, Srisupundit K, et al. Fetal surgery is a clinical reality. Seminars in Fetal and Neonatal Medicine. 2010;15:58-67.
23. Harrison MR, Filly RA, Golbus MS, et al. Fetal treatment. N Engl J Med. 1982;307:1651-2.
24. Deprest JA, Flake AW, Gratacos E, et al. The making of fetal surgery. Prenat Diagn. 2010;30:653-67.
25. Chervenak FA, McCullough LB. Ethics of fetal surgery. Clinics in Perinatology. 2009;36:237-46, vii-viii.
26. American College of O, Gynecologists CoE, American Academy of Pediatrics CoB. Maternal-fetal intervention and fetal care centers. Pediatrics. 2011;128:e473-8.
27. Noble R, Rodeck CH. Ethical considerations of fetal therapy. Best Pract Res Clin Obstet Gynaecol. 2008;22:219-31.
28. Aliyu LD, Kurjak A, Wataganara T, et al. Ultrasound in Africa: what can really be done? Journal of Perinatal Medicine. 2015.

CHAPTER 43

In-utero Pharmacologic Treatment

Tuangsit Wataganara

INTRODUCTION

In-utero administration of pharmaceutical agents has been broadly practice for either prophylactic or therapeutic purposes. An obvious example is transplacental administration of betamethasone to a fetus at premature gestational age to enhance the function of pneumocyte type II in the lung and to reduce certain complications of preterm delivery, such as respiratory distress syndrome, intraventricular hemorrhage, and necrotizing enterocolitis. Prenatal administration of steroids to reduce the respiratory complications of prematurity might be the most commonly 'fetal therapy' being performed all around the world. Route of administration can be less invasive (i.e., transplacental) or more invasive (i.e., transamniotic and direct intramuscular or intravenous injection to the fetus). There have been a number of reports on fetal conditions that might be benefited from in-utero medical treatment, but most of them are based on a single case report or small case series. This chapter "In-utero Pharmacologic Treatment" chose to discuss three common fetal conditions, including congenital pulmonary airway malformations, arrhythmias, and thyroid disease. These diseases are not uncommon for fetal medicine specialists and their proposed prenatal pharmacologic treatments have undergone scientific validation.

PRINCIPLES AND TYPES OF IN-UTERO PHARMACOLOGIC TREATMENT

Some fetal diseases can be treated prenatally by pharmacologic agents. There are four major routes to administer therapeutic substances to the fetus. The administration can either be indirect (transplacental and transamniotic) or direct (intramuscular and intravenous/intraperitoneal), as shown in **Table 1**.[1]

Medications that can be given through the mother (transplacental) must have a low molecular weight, such as intramuscular injection of betamethasone or dexamethasone to a pregnant woman to facilitate fetal lung maturity. The use of maternal glucocorticoid therapy to reduce respiratory distress of prematurity was first described by Liggins and colleagues in 1972.[2] Prenatal glucocorticoids is also helpful when invasive in-utero interventions are performed, because it may lead to iatrogenic preterm delivery.

Prenatal glucocorticoid therapy significantly reduces prematurity-related morbidity. These include respiratory distress syndrome, intraventricular hemorrhage, and necrotizing enterocolitis. Indications for fetal pharmacologic treatments are expanding based on a variety of medical evidence. Some treatments are regarded as 'standard of care' without critical analysis of the real benefits. Conduct of randomized controlled trial (RCT) to re-visit the real benefits and risks of these treatments may not be possible from ethical point of view.

Examples of these treatments include maternal administration of immunoglobulin to prevent neonatal alloimmune thrombocytopenia, maternal administration of antiretroviral medication to reduce of chance of perinatal infection with human immunodeficiency virus (HIV), maternal administration of antiarrhythmic agents for a conversion to sinus rhythm in a fetus with decompensated

TABLE 1: Routes of pharmacologic administration to the fetus.

Route	*Examples*	*Remarks*
Transplacental	Digoxin	Fetal supraventricular tachycardia
Transamniotic	L-thyroxine	Fetal goitrous hypothyroidism
Intravenous	Amiodarone	Refractory fetal supraventricular tachycardia with hydrops
Intramuscular	Fentanyl	Fetal immobilization

(hydropic) cardiac arrhythmia, or maternal administration of dexamethasone to prevent virilization of female fetus in congenital adrenal hyperplasia (CAH).

Fetal clitoromegaly can appear as ambiguous genitalia, as shown in **Figure 1**. Hypertrophy of fetal clitoris can be prevented by early administration of corticosteroids. Earlier administration of corticosteroids will be more effective. Available reports of other fetal pharmacological treatments are summarized in **Table 2**.[1]

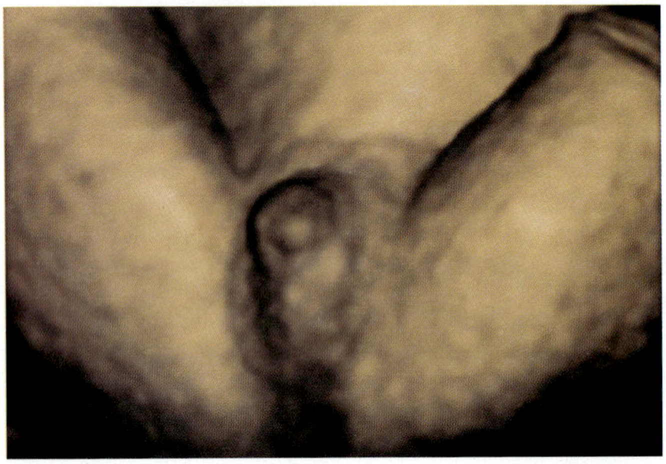

Fig. 1: Three-dimensional, surface-rendered ultrasound picture of ambiguous genitalia in a female fetus affected with congenital adrenal hyperplasia.

Transplacental route can be self-administered, and more convenient, but the final fetal dosage cannot be controlled. Volume of distribution, first pass effect at the liver, and clearance by renal system can affect the final fetal dose. Large-molecule drugs, i.e., levothyroxine, cannot freely distribute through the placental barrier. It has to be injected into the amniotic cavity *(transamniotic route)* for the fetus to swallow.

Ultrasound-guided intramuscular injection *(intramuscular route)* is for giving large-molecule drug at a smaller volume for rapid onset of action. An example is intramuscular injection of 'cocktail' for fetal immobilization to facilitate a complicated prenatal procedure, such as fetal endoluminal tracheal occlusion (FETO). At Faculty of Medicine, Siriraj Hospital, our 'cocktail' is a mixture of pancuronium (0.2 mg/kg), atropine (20 μg/kg), and fentanyl (15 μg/kg). It is delivered through a 20 G spinal needle into the thigh muscle of the fetus under ultrasound guidance.

This chapter will discuss current evidence for prenatal medical treatments in fetuses with congenital pulmonary airway malformation (CPAM), cardiac arrhythmias, and thyroid diseases. Many other in-utero medical interventions did not undergo scientific validation, and the recommendations are based on expert's opinion and personal experiences.

TABLE 2: Available fetal pharmacological treatments.

Fetal condition	*Medication*	*Route*
Congenital pulmonary airway malformation	Betamethasone	Maternal, intramuscular
Congenital adrenal hypersia	Dexamethasone	Maternal, oral
Congenital heart block	Dexamethasone Intravenous immunoglobulin	Maternal, oral Maternal, intravenous
Tachyarrhythmias	Digoxin, solatol, flecainide, amiodarone	Maternal, oral/intravenous Fetal, intramuscular/intravenous
Methylmalonic acidemia	Vitamin B_{12}	Maternal, oral/intramuscular
Multiple carboxylase synthetase deficiency	Biotin	Maternal, oral
3-Phosphoglycerate-dehydrogenase deficiency	L-serine	Maternal, oral
Pyridoxine-dependent seizures	Pyridoxine	Maternal, oral
Smith-Lemli-Opitz syndrome	Fresh frozen plasma (cholesterol)	Fetal, intravascular/intraperitoneal
Fetal goitrous hypothyroidism	Levothyroxine	Fetal, intra-amniotic/intramuscular
Fetal thyrotoxicosis postmaternal thyroid ablation	Propylthiouracil	Fetal intra-amniotic/intramuscular
Polyhydramnios in monoamniotic twins, Bartter syndrome	Nonsteroidal anti-inflammatory drugs, such as sulindac and indomethacin	Maternal, oral

Source: Hui and Bianchi 2011.[1]

FETAL CONGENITAL PULMONARY AIRWAY MALFORMATIONS

Congenital pulmonary airway malformations (CPAMs) is an abnormal proliferation of bronchiolar-like airspace without normal alveoli. It is in fact a harmatomatous tumor of the lung. Tumor size, mediastinum shifting, hydrops, and polyhydramnios are unfavorable prognostic findings.[3] Fetal CPAMs are classified as macrocystic and microcystic types, as shown in **Figures 2 and 3**, respectively. Increased intrathoracic pressure and shifting of the mediastinum from large CPAMs can obstruct cardiac function to the point of decompensation, heart failure, and hydropic change. Sign of fetal decompensation is an indication for in-utero intervention.

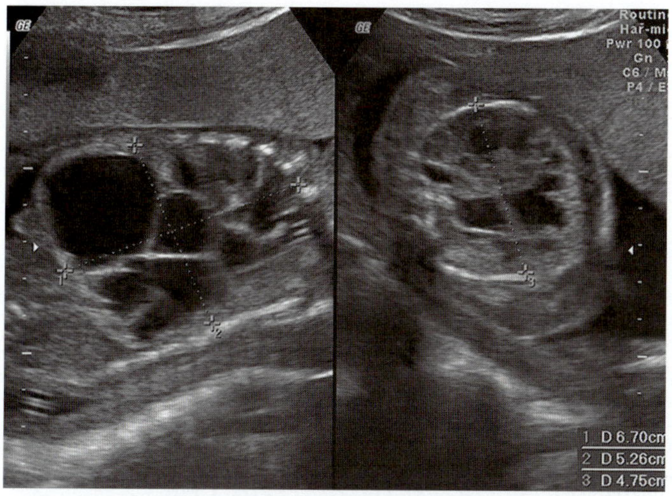

Fig. 2: Congenital pulmonary airway malformation (CPAM): macrocystic type.

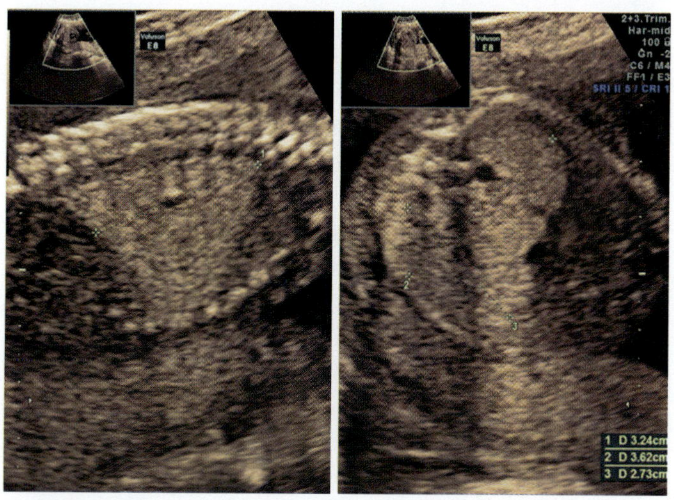

Fig. 3: Congenital pulmonary airway malformation (CPAM): microcystic type.

For macrocystic CPAMs, either needle tapping of the cyst or placement of shunt for decompression can reverse the hydrops. Open fetal resection and ex-utero intrapartum treatment to extracorporeal membrane oxygenation (EXIT to ECMO) can be offered in recurrence and should be performed only in experienced fetal care centers.[4]

For microcystic CPAMs, medical decompression is the first treatment option since mechanical decompression is not technically feasible. Reduction of CPAM size after maternal administration of betamethasone has been reported in small case series.[5-7] Real efficacy of betamethasone in reducing CPAMs size is still conflicting from one case series to another.[8] Meta-analysis of the data from these published reports suggested 80% resolution of hydrops and 87.1% overall survival to discharge in high-risk microcystic CPAM treated with prenatal steroids.[7]

FETAL ARRHYTHMIAS

Fetal Bradyarrhythmia

Fetal bradycardia is defined as a persistent heart rate of less than 100 beats per minute (bpm) with 1:1 atrioventricular (AV) conduction, without structural defect. It indicates fetal hypoxia or acidemia. But if AV conduction is abnormal, then it is called congenital heart block (CHB). The incidence of CHB is 1:15,000 to 1:20,000 of newborns.[9] Most CHBs are caused by maternal transfer of anti-ribonucleoprotein antibodies (anti-SSA and anti-SSB antibodies, or anti-Ro and anti-La, respectively), which can be found in women with Sjogren's syndrome, systemic lupus erythematosus (SLE), and rheumatoid arthritis (RA). Some women never had symptoms of connective tissue disease.

These autoantibodies bind with the AV node, causing focal inflammation and scarring of the myocardium. The estimated chance of fetal CHB in antibody-positive mother is 1 to 2%. The chance is up to 17% if her previous child had CHB.[10] The onset of CHB is in late 2nd trimester. Presence of autoantibody worsen prognosis of CHB (2nd degree AV block).[11] Fetal AV conduction defect can have atypical prenatal findings. Our group at Faculty of Medicine, Siriraj Hospital recently reported a case of 32 weeks' fetus with simultaneous manifestation of 2 different cardiac conduction defects. This complex cardiac arrhythmia was successfully controlled by maternal administration of atenolol (β-antagonist).[12] Examples of 1st, 2nd, and 3rd (complete) degree AV block are shown in **Figures 4 to 6**, respectively.

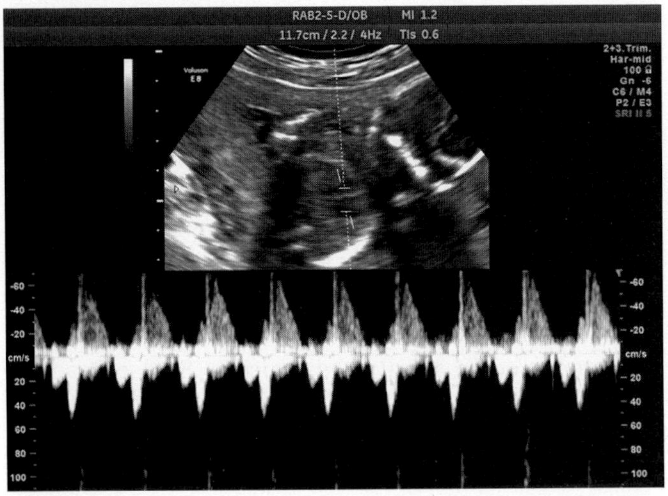

Fig. 4: 1st degree AV block from mitral valve-aorta approach. Note the long delay between mitral A wave and aortic outflow wave. Fetal bradycardia may not be obvious. Fetal hemodynamics are always stable (no hydrops). No intervention is required.

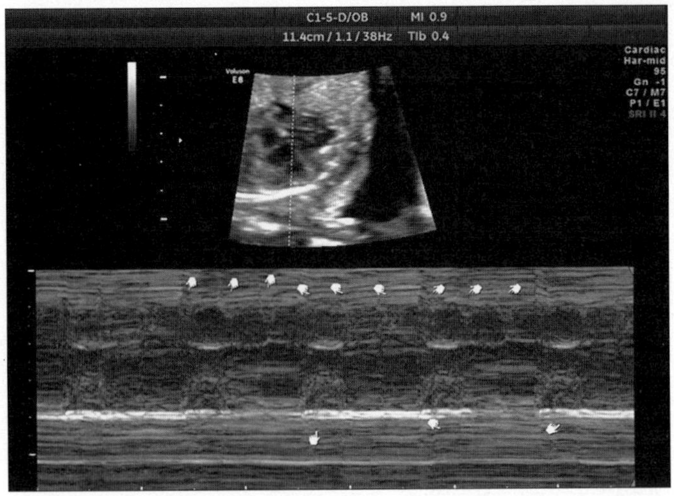

Fig. 6: 3rd degree AV block, so called complete heart block, demonstrated in M-mode. Note the total asynchrony between the atrium and the ventricle. This fetus had an unstable hemodynamics, and subsequently developed hydrops. In-utero intervention or early delivery for pace maker is required.

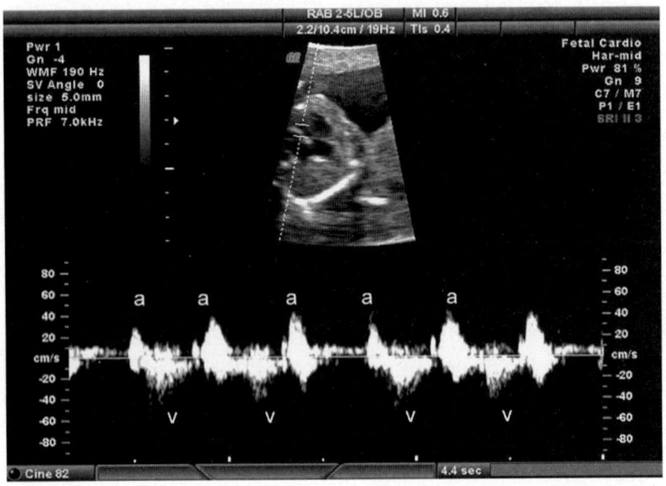

Fig. 5: 2nd degree AV block. Note the missing ventricular beat (v) after one atrial contraction (a). Fetal bradycardia may not be obvious. Fetal hemodynamics are always stable (no hydrops). No intervention is required.

In-utero treatments should be considered in high-risk CHB (for heart failure and fetal death). The following findings suggest for high-risk CHB:

- Fetal hydrops
- Profound bradycardia less than 55 bpm.
- Myocardial dysfunction
  - High myocardial performance index (MPI, or Tei index)
  - Low ejection fraction
- Endocardial fibroelastosis
- Preterm fetus (less than 37 weeks').

In-utero treatments in high-risk CHB are the followings:

- Maternal fluorinated glucocorticoid
  - Dexamethasone
  - Betamethasone
- Maternal β-antagonist, such as atenolol
- Digoxin—direct fetal injection
- Furosemide—direct fetal injection
- In-utero pacing.

Maternal Glucocorticoid and Fetal CHB

Data on the true benefit of maternal glucocorticoid to improve perinatal outcomes in fetuses with CHB are still conflicting. One retrospective review showed 90% neonatal survival from maternal dexamethasone for fetal 3rd degree AV block, compared to 46% survival in untreated group.[13] Breur and colleagues analyzed 93 fetal CHB, and did not find either significant benefit or safety of maternal dexamethasone in the treatment of fetal CHB.[14] There is a safety concern regarding long-term neurodevelopment of after prenatal exposure of dexamethasone.

Because of all the conflicting data, the PR Interval and Dexamethasone Evaluation (PRIDE) study was conducted to validate the efficacy and safety of maternal dexamethasone (4 milligram per day) for fetal CHB.[15] The protocol was changed from RCT to open-label non-randomized trial. There were 40 women enrolled (30 maternal dexamethasone and 10 without treatment). There was no reversal of any 3rd degree AV block.

Marginal benefits of maternal dexamethasone may exist in fetal 1st and 2nd degree AV block.

Maternal Intravenous Immunoglobulin and Fetal CHB

Intravenous immunoglobulin (IVIG) is a standard treatment for fetuses with alloimmune thrombocytopenia, and women with pregnancy-induced thrombocytopenia (ITP). IVIG can convert fetal CHB in a few case reports.[16,17] But 2 multicenter trials the Preventive Intravenous Immune Globulin Therapy for Congenital Heart Block (PITCH) study in United States and another multicenter trial conducted in Europe did not show any benefit of IVIG to fetal CHB, even with early administration at 12 to 24 gestational weeks.'[18,19]

In conclusion, there has been no effective prevention and in-utero treatment of fetal CHB. Close follow up with ultrasound for signs of heart failure and fetal hydrops, timely delivery, and postnatal pacemaker are advisable. Neonatal outcomes may be varied.

Fetal Tachyarrhythmias

Fetal tachycardia is a sustained fetal heart rate of 180 bpm or over, without structural defect. The most common causes are either AV re-entry or atrial flutter, which are more responsive to in-utero medical treatment than the CHB.[20] Conversion of fetal tachyarrhythmias can be achieved by various antiarrhythmic agents. Type of arrhythmia, side effects, and personal experience are considered for choosing the right drug.

Digoxin is generally the first-line for conversion of fetal supraventricular tachycardia (SVT).[20,21] Clinical use of digoxin for conversion of fetal SVTs based on retrospective case reports, and not proper scientific study. Pediatric cardiologists are familiar with clinical use of digoxin; therefore, its adoption was almost spontaneous. Digoxin can be taken orally or intravenously. It passes the placenta, and reaches the fetus at a good concentration, particularly if the fetus is not hydropic. Maternal digoxin therapy can convert SVT to sinus rhythm in over 60% of non-hydropic fetuses. Hydropic fetuses do not respond to maternal digoxin as good, with 20% successful sinus conversion.[22] If fetal SVT cannot be converted after a full dosage of digoxin, 2nd and 3rd line drugs may be considered, which include sotalol,[23-25] flecainide,[22,26,27] and amiodarone.[28,29]

Even in the presence of fetal hydrops, a combination of transplacental drug therapy is still effective.[29-31] Some hydropic fetus may not respond very well to maternal digoxin because of impaired placental drug transfer, then direct fetal injection may be required.[32,33] There are three different injection sites at the fetus: intramuscular, intraperitoneal, and intravenous (umbilical vein). Intramuscular injection is preferred for its convenience. Intravenous administration has risk of fetal exanguination, especially if the agent of choice is amiodarone.[32] Pharmacologic agents that can be used to control fetal heart rate are listed in **Table 3**.

TABLE 3: Pharmacologic agents for fetal bradyarrhythmias and tachyarrhythmias.

Fetal bradyarrhythmias	*Fetal tachyarrhythmias*
• Sympathomimetics • Fluorinated glucocorticoids • Intravenous immunoglobulin	• Digitalis • Furosemide • Flecainide • Verapamil • Amiodarone • Propanolol • Procainamide • Quinidine • Adenosine • Sotalol

FETAL THYROID DISEASES

Fetal Goitrous Hypothyroidism

Fetal goiter results from inadequate maternal transfer of thyroxine, either from defective placental transfer or maternal hypothyroidism.[34-39] Primary fetal hypothyroidism can be due to transplacental passage of maternal antithyroid medication.[37,40]

Goitrous mass can lead to polyhydramnios, hyper-extended neck, and neonatal asphyxia from airway obstruction. Diagnosis can be made by sonography and confirmed by low thyroid hormone level in either fetal blood or amniotic fluid.[41] Intra-amniotic thyroxine therapy, 150 to 600 µg of levothyroxine every week, can reduce the goiter size and its complications. It is a simple procedure, but may require multiple instillations, which can increase the risk of membranes rupture, preterm birth, maternal and neonatal sepsis. Fetal intramuscular injection of thyroxine is also an option to replenish fetal thyroid status in an exceptional case, such as a fetus with severe esophageal obstruction impeding swallowing.[42] Serial assessment of fetal thyroid function from umbilical cord blood sampling is advisable. The benefits of prenatal thyroxine supplementation on long-term neurodevelopmental outcomes, compared to postnatal supplementation, are still elusive.

Fetal Thyrotoxicosis

Fetal thyrotoxicosis can cause growth restriction, high-output cardiac failure, and hydrops. It is most commonly caused by maternal Graves' disease. Maternal-derived thyroid-stimulating immunoglobins (TSIs), traverses the placenta and stimulates fetal thyroid gland. Maternal production of TSIs remains persistent even in her clinical euthyroidism from medicaltion, radioablation, or thyroidectomy.

When a woman with previous history of Grave's disease, particularly those with a documented high level of maternal TSI antibodies, gets pregnant, the fetus should be surveyed for signs of hyperthyroidism, regardless of maternal symptoms. Fetus with hyperthyroidism will have persistent tachycardia, goiter, growth restriction, or hydrops.[43-45] It can be confirmed by thyroid function tests from cord blood sample.

Based on case series, thyrotoxicosis in the fetus can be controlled with transplacental antithyroid drugs, such as 150 mg per day of maternal propylthiouracil (PTU), which is a standard dosage.[43,46-48] PTU may suppress maternal thyroid production, and replacement therapy is given accordingly without the fear of transplacental transfer of thyroid hormone extract. Molecules of thyroid hormone extract are large, and not traversing the placenta.

CONCLUSION

In-utero pharmacologic treatment largely bases on adaptations of postnatal therapy for similar conditions. There is a broad variety of fetal pharmacological treatments being adopted in routine practice, but very few of them have been scientifically proven for its benefits and risks. RCTs have been conducted for selected therapeutic agents, such as glucocorticoids for CHB. The majority of pharmacologic agents for fetal treatment still based on case series and personal experiences.

Certain medications have been used without adequate evidence from quality clinical trial. For example, digoxin has been the first drug of choice for conversion of fetal SVTs. This practice derived from successful reports from small case series and the familiarity of most pediatric cardiologists with this medication. The similar rationale can apply for in-utero treatment of thyroid disease.

Challenges for in-utero medical treatment will be faced in fetuses with extremely rare conditions, such as the inborn errors of metabolism. It is unlikely to conduct a trial to prove the efficacy or safety of medical interventions owing to the rarity of these diseases. Appropriate follow up with ultrasound examination and fetal blood testing are the only way to optimize treatment in this difficult situation.

REFERENCES

1. Hui L, Bianchi DW. Prenatal pharmacotherapy for fetal anomalies: a 2011 update. Prenat Diagn. 2011;31:735-43.
2. Liggins GC, Howie RN. A controlled trial of antepartum glucocorticoid treatment for prevention of the respiratory distress syndrome in premature infants. Pediatrics. 1972;50:515-25.
3. Crombleholme TM, Coleman B, Hedrick H, et al. Cystic adenomatoid malformation volume ratio predicts outcome in prenatally diagnosed cystic adenomatoid malformation of the lung. Journal of Pediatric Surgery. 2002;37:331-8.
4. Grethel EJ, Wagner AJ, Clifton MS, et al. Fetal intervention for mass lesions and hydrops improves outcome: a 15-year experience. Journal of Pediatric Surgery. 2007;42:117-23.
5. Tsao K, Hawgood S, Vu L, et al. Resolution of hydrops fetalis in congenital cystic adenomatoid malformation after prenatal steroid therapy. Journal of Pediatric Surgery. 2003;38:508-10.
6. Peranteau WH, Wilson RD, Liechty KW, et al. Effect of maternal betamethasone administration on prenatal congenital cystic adenomatoid malformation growth and fetal survival. Fetal Diagn Ther. 2007;22:365-71.
7. Curran PF, Jelin EB, Rand L, et al. Prenatal steroids for microcystic congenital cystic adenomatoid malformations. Journal of Pediatric Surgery. 2010;45:145-50.
8. Morris LM, Lim FY, Livingston JC, Polzin WJ, Crombleholme TM. High-risk fetal congenital pulmonary airway malformations have a variable response to steroids. Journal of Pediatric Surgery. 2009;44:60-5.
9. Michaelsson M, Engle MA. Congenital complete heart block: an international study of the natural history. Cardiovascular Clinics. 1972;4:85-101.
10. Llanos C, Chan EK, Li S, et al. Antibody reactivity to alpha-enolase in mothers of children with congenital heart block. The Journal of Rheumatology. 2009;36:565-9.
11. Chang YL, Hsieh PC, Chang SD, Chao AS, Liang CC, Soong YK. Perinatal outcome of fetus with isolated congenital second degree atrioventricular block without maternal anti-SSA/Ro-SSB/La antibodies. European journal of obstetrics, Gynecology, and Reproductive Biology. 2005;122:167-71.
12. Anuwutnavin S, Wanitpongpan P, Chungsomprasong P, Soongswang J, Srisantiroj N, Wataganara T. Fetal long QT syndrome manifested as atrioventricular block and

ventricular tachycardia: a case report and a review of the literature. Pediatric Cardiology. 2013;34:1955-62.

13. Jaeggi ET, Silverman ED, Yoo SJ, Kingdom J. Is immune-mediated complete fetal atrioventricular block reversible by transplacental dexamethasone therapy? Ultrasound in obstetrics & gynecology: the official journal of the International Society of Ultrasound in Obstetrics and Gynecology. 2004;23:602-5.
14. Breur JM, Visser GH, Kruize AA, Stoutenbeek P, Meijboom EJ. Treatment of fetal heart block with maternal steroid therapy: case report and review of the literature. Ultrasound in obstetrics & gynecology: the official journal of the International Society of Ultrasound in Obstetrics and Gynecology. 2004;24:467-72.
15. Friedman DM, Kim MY, Copel JA, Llanos C, Davis C, Buyon JP. Prospective evaluation of fetuses with autoimmune-associated congenital heart block followed in the PR Interval and Dexamethasone Evaluation (PRIDE) Study. The American Journal of Cardiology. 2009;103:1102-6.
16. Kaaja R, Julkunen H. Prevention of recurrence of congenital heart block with intravenous immunoglobulin and corticosteroid therapy: comment on the editorial by Buyon et al. Arthritis and rheumatism 2003;48:280-1; author reply 1-2.
17. David AL, Ataullah I, Yates R, Sullivan I, Charles P, Williams D. Congenital fetal heart block: a potential therapeutic role for intravenous immunoglobulin. Obstetrics and Gynecology. 2010;116 (Suppl) 2:543-7.
18. Friedman DM, Llanos C, Izmirly PM, et al. Evaluation of fetuses in a study of intravenous immunoglobulin as preventive therapy for congenital heart block: Results of a multicenter, prospective, open-label clinical trial. Arthritis and rheumatism. 2010;62:1138-46.
19. Pisoni CN, Brucato A, Ruffatti A, et al. Failure of intravenous immunoglobulin to prevent congenital heart block: Findings of a multicenter, prospective, observational study. Arthritis and Rheumatism. 2010;62:1147-52.
20. Api O, Carvalho JS. Fetal dysrhythmias. Best Pract Res Clin Obstet Gynaecol. 2008;22:31-48.
21. Van den Heuvel DM, Pasterkamp RJ. Getting connected in the dopamine system. Progress in Neurobiology 2008;85: 75-93.
22. Krapp M, Kohl T, Simpson JM, Sharland GK, Katalinic A, Gembruch U. Review of diagnosis, treatment, and outcome of fetal atrial flutter compared with supraventricular tachycardia. Heart. 2003;89:913-7.
23. Oudijk MA, Ruskamp JM, Ververs FF, et al. Treatment of fetal tachycardia with sotalol: transplacental pharmacokinetics and pharmacodynamics. Journal of the American College of Cardiology 2003;42:765-70.
24. Oudijk MA, Michon MM, Kleinman CS, et al. Sotalol in the treatment of fetal dysrhythmias. Circulation. 2000;101:2721-6.
25. Rebelo M, Macedo AJ, Nogueira G, Trigo C, Kaku S. Sotalol in the treatment of fetal tachyarrhythmia. Revista portuguesa de cardiologia: orgao oficial da Sociedade Portuguesa de Cardiologia = Portuguese journal of cardiology: an official journal of the Portuguese Society of Cardiology. 2006;25: 477-81.
26. Frohn-Mulder IM, Stewart PA, Witsenburg M, Den Hollander NS, Wladimiroff JW, Hess J. The efficacy of flecainide versus digoxin in the management of fetal supraventricular tachycardia. Prenat Diagn. 1995;15:1297-302.
27. D'Souza D, MacKenzie WE, Martin WL. Transplacental flecainide therapy in the treatment of fetal supraventricular tachycardia. Journal of Obstetrics and Gynaecology: the Journal of the Institute of Obstetrics and Gynaecology. 2002;22:320-2.
28. Flack NJ, Zosmer N, Bennett PR, Vaughan J, Fisk NM. Amiodarone given by three routes to terminate fetal atrial flutter associated with severe hydrops. Obstetrics and Gynecology. 1993;82:714-6.
29. Strasburger JF, Cuneo BF, Michon MM, et al. Amiodarone therapy for drug-refractory fetal tachycardia. Circulation 2004;109:375-9.
30. Ebenroth ES, Cordes TM, Darragh RK. Second-line treatment of fetal supraventricular tachycardia using flecainide acetate. Pediatric Cardiology. 2001;22:483-7.
31. Merriman JB, Gonzalez JM, Rychik J, Ural SH. Can digoxin and sotalol therapy for fetal supraventricular tachycardia and hydrops be successful? A case report. The Journal of Reproductive Medicine. 2008;53:357-9.
32. Hansmann M, Gembruch U, Bald R, Manz M, Redel DA. Fetal tachyarrhythmias: transplacental and direct treatment of the fetus—a report of 60 cases. Ultrasound in obstetrics & gynecology: the official journal of the International Society of Ultrasound in Obstetrics and Gynecology. 1991;1:162-8.
33. Parilla BV, Strasburger JF, Socol ML. Fetal supraventricular tachycardia complicated by hydrops fetalis: a role for direct fetal intramuscular therapy. American Journal of Perinatology. 1996;13:483-6.
34. Abuhamad AZ, Fisher DA, Warsof SL, et al. Antenatal diagnosis and treatment of fetal goitrous hypothyroidism: case report and review of the literature. Ultrasound in obstetrics & gynecology: the official journal of the International Society of Ultrasound in Obstetrics and Gynecology. 1995;6:368-71.
35. Agrawal P, Ogilvy-Stuart A, Lees C. Intrauterine diagnosis and management of congenital goitrous hypothyroidism. Ultrasound in obstetrics & gynecology: the official journal of the International Society of Ultrasound in Obstetrics and Gynecology. 2002;19:501-5.
36. Hashimoto H, Hashimoto K, Suehara N. Successful in utero treatment of fetal goitrous hypothyroidism: case report and review of the literature. Fetal Diagn Ther. 2006;21:360-5.
37. Miyata I, Abe-Gotyo N, Tajima A, et al. Successful intrauterine therapy for fetal goitrous hypothyroidism during late gestation. Endocrine Journal. 2007;54:813-7.
38. Hanono A, Shah B, David R, et al. Antenatal treatment of fetal goiter: a therapeutic challenge. The journal of

maternal-fetal & neonatal medicine: the official journal of the European Association of Perinatal Medicine, the Federation of Asia and Oceania Perinatal Societies, the International Society of Perinatal Obstet. 2009;22:76-80.
39. Ribault V, Castanet M, Bertrand AM, et al. Experience with intraamniotic thyroxine treatment in nonimmune fetal goitrous hypothyroidism in 12 cases. The Journal of Clinical Endocrinology and Metabolism. 2009;94:3731-9.
40. Borgel K, Pohlenz J, Holzgreve W, Bramswig JH. Intrauterine therapy of goitrous hypothyroidism in a boy with a new compound heterozygous mutation (Y453D and C800R) in the thyroid peroxidase gene. A long-term follow-up. Am J Obstet Gynecol. 2005;193:857-8.
41. Thorpe-Beeston JG, Nicolaides KH, McGregor AM. Fetal thyroid function. Thyroid: official journal of the American Thyroid Association. 1992;2:207-17.
42. Corral E, Reascos M, Preiss Y, Rompel SM, Sepulveda W. Treatment of fetal goitrous hypothyroidism: value of direct intramuscular L-thyroxine therapy. Prenat Diagn. 2010; 30:899-901.
43. Heckel S, Favre R, Schlienger JL, Soskin P. Diagnosis and successful in utero treatment of a fetal goitrous hyperthyroidism caused by maternal Graves' disease. A case report. Fetal Diagn Ther. 1997;12:54-8.
44. Srisupundit K, Sirichotiyakul S, Tongprasert F, Luewan S, Tongsong T. Fetal therapy in fetal thyrotoxicosis: a case report. Fetal Diagn Ther. 2008;23:114-6.
45. Ting MK, Hsu BR, Huang YY, Lin JD, Chen TC. Recurrent fetal thyrotoxicosis in a woman with Graves' disease: case report. Changgeng yi xue za zhi/Changgeng ji nian yi yuan = Chang Gung medical journal/Chang Gung Memorial Hospital. 1999;22:492-7.
46. Wallace C, Couch R, Ginsberg J. Fetal thyrotoxicosis: a case report and recommendations for prediction, diagnosis, and treatment. Thyroid: official journal of the American Thyroid Association. 1995;5:125-8.
47. Bowman ML, Bergmann M, Smith JF. Intrapartum labetalol for the treatment of maternal and fetal thyrotoxicosis. Thyroid: official journal of the American Thyroid Association. 1998;8:795-6.
48. Duncombe GJ, Dickinson JE. Fetal thyrotoxicosis after maternal thyroidectomy. The Australian & New Zealand Journal of Obstetrics & Gynaecology. 2001;41:224-7.

44

CHAPTER

Ultrasound-guided Fetal Intervention

Tuangsit Wataganara

INTRODUCTION

Ultrasound was initially used to provide an accurate appreciation of the fetal anatomy, physiology, as well as its environment (i.e., the womb, placenta, and amniotic fluid). Subsequently, it was used to guide the needle, in real-time fashion, to obtain fetal samples in diagnostic procedure. The ultrasound-guided needle procedures, such as chorionic villus sampling, genetic amniocentesis, and percutaneous umbilical blood sampling, allow for the development of skill that lead to a more complex in-utero intervention. Pleural effusion, an abnormal amount of fluid accumulating in thoracic space, can lead to fetal hydrops and impaired lung development. Ultrasound is an indispensible part for fetal chest paracentesis to obtain the accumulated fluid for both diagnostic and therapeutic purposes. In recurrent massive pleural effusion with hydropic change of the fetus, pleuroamniotic shunting may help maintain the pressure equilibrium between the intrathoracic cavity and the outside amniotic cavity. This can help reverse the hydrops and preserve the physiologic lung development. In-utero shunting may also be applicable in large cystic lung lesion. The patient has to be counseled for chances of complications from in-utero shunting, such as dislodgement and obstruction, and the shunt may have to be re-inserted if fetal condition gets worsen. Solid lung lesion, such as a more solid type of congenital pulmonary airway malformation, can significantly compress the lung, causing obstruction of major venous return, and then hydropic changes of the fetus. A therapeutic combination of transplacental corticosteroids and percutaneous sclerotherapy (under real-time ultrasound guidance) has been successfully to reduce the size of this solid lesion and to reverse the hydrops. Care must be taken for an interpretation of the success from this novel treatment deduced from a small case cohort.

RATIONALE OF ULTRASOUND-GUIDED FETAL INTERVENTION

Ultrasound-guided intervention is a form of minimally invasive fetal therapy. Either needle or shunting instruments are inserted into the affected fetal parts under real time ultrasound guidance. Needle intervention, so called paracentesis or tapping, is generally used to withdraw fluid from a cavity, most commonly pleural. This can be of either diagnostic or therapeutic purpose. Shunting provides a longer drainage, which may be suitable in recurrent case. Most of the published studies in either paracentesis or shunting involve fetal hydrothorax.

Once fetal hydrothorax is diagnosed, associated fetal malformation and chromosomal aneuploidies need to be excluded. In isolated hydrothorax, there are three main treatment options to offer; (1) conservative management, (2) premature delivery, and (3) in-utero treatment. Gestational age of onset, rate of progression (or regression thereof), and signs of fetal decompensation (i.e., hydrops) are three major prognostication factors for fetal hydrothorax.[1] Primary fetal hydrothorax sometimes can spontaneously regress. Slower progression is expected in cases that the effusion is unilateral, small or moderate amount, no mediastinum shifting, and no signs of hydrops. Close monitoring (i.e., weekly ultrasound) is optimal in this type of case, because spontaneous regression is not uncommon. In cases with significant pleural effusion in the third trimester, as shown in **Figure 1**, pleural tapping can be performed immediately before delivery to facilitate neonatal resuscitation.[2]

Rapidly progressive hydrothorax, particularly when develops at earlier gestational, can result in fetal hydrops and demise. Fetal shunting will be warranted in these cases.[3,4] According to our experiences, mediastinum shift occurs not long before fetal decompensation and hydrops, and we offer minimally invasive intervention in these fetuses

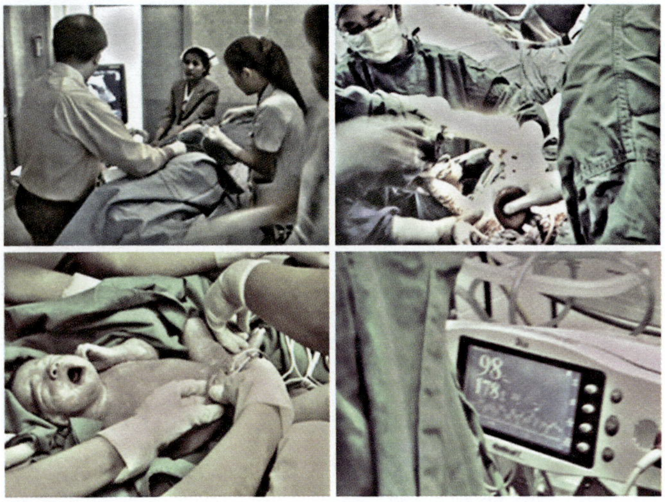

Fig. 1: Pleural tapping immediately before delivery to assist neonatal resuscitation in a case of massive pleural effusion in the third trimester.

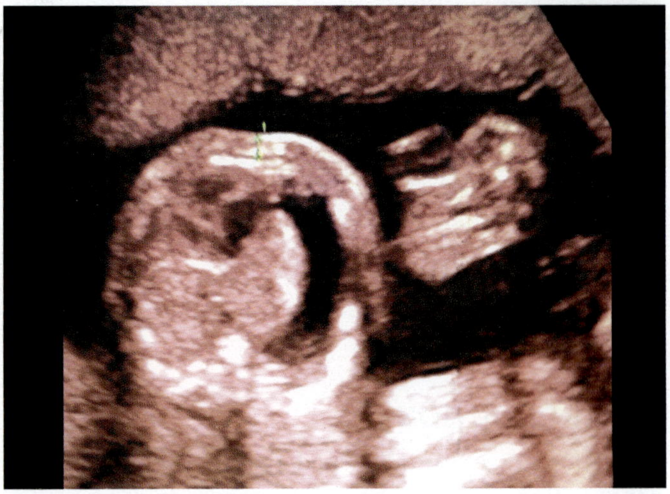

Fig. 2: A 20 weeks' fetus with unilateral hydrothorax. Note that the fetus has shifting of mediastinum and subcutaneous fluid collection as an early sign of hydrops.

even before development of hydrops. If thoracoamniotic shunting is performed, weekly ultrasound follow up is scheduled. Prevention and treatment of fetal hydrops as a result of hydrothorax can reduce incidence of the chance of preeclampsia in the mother.[5] "Mirror syndrome" is a form of preeclampsia that occurs in severe fetal hydrops of any causes.

TABLE 1: Sonographic findings in fetal hydrothorax with bad prognosis.

Sonographic findings in fetal hydrothorax that are related to suboptimal perinatal outcomes
• Rapid progression of effusions • Large amount of effusions • Fetal mediastinal shift • Fetal hydrops • Polyhydramnios

FETAL PARACENTESIS

The most common site for in-utero needle drainage, so called paracentesis, is the pleural cavity. Fetal hydrothorax is not uncommon and the progression is varied. Unilaterality and small amount of effusion are associated with good prognosis, although hydrops can develop very fast, as shown in **Figure 2**. Therefore, it is important to closely monitor a fetus with hydrothorax with weekly ultrasound, at least. Once structural and chromosomal anomalies have been excluded, optimal management depends on gestational age, rate of progression, the development of hydrops and associated maternal symptoms. **Table 1** summarizes sonographic findings in fetal hydrothorax that is associated with bad perinatal outcomes.

The incidence of fetal hydrothorax or pleural effusion is 1 in 10,000 to 1 in 15,000 pregnancies.[1] It may be categorized according to the etiologies as primary and secondary hydrothorax. Primary hydrothorax is a result of immature lymphatic duct, causing leakage into the pleural cavity. It can occur either on one side or both sides of the pleural cavities. Primary hydrothorax is usually called "chylothorax" after birth. Secondary hydrothorax is a result of other systemic fetal diseases, i.e., fetal anemia. Therefore, the prognosis depends on the primary etiology. In-utero intervention to release high-pressure fluid from fetal pleural cavity by either paracentesis or shunting procedure is indicated only in primary fetal hydrothorax. This is to prevent fetal death (as a result of cardiac decompensation from mediastinum shift and hydrops) and neonatal death (as a result of lung hypoplasia and pulmonary hypertension). For secondary hydrothorax, as shown in **Figure 3**, in-utero intervention is aiming the primary etiology, and not simply at releasing the effusion.

The first prenatal detection of fetal hydrothorax by ultrasound was reported in 1977.[6] With broader adoption of high-quality ultrasound in modern obstetrics, increasing cases of hydrothorax are diagnosed prenatally. Prior to the year 1990, fetal hydrothorax cases were diagnosed at an average gestational age of 30 weeks'.[7] Fetal hydrothorax cases were diagnosed at earlier gestational age (median 20 weeks') in a more recent case series from 1997 to 2003.[8] When fetal hydrothorax is detected, possible causes have to be excluded. The suggested list of investigations for

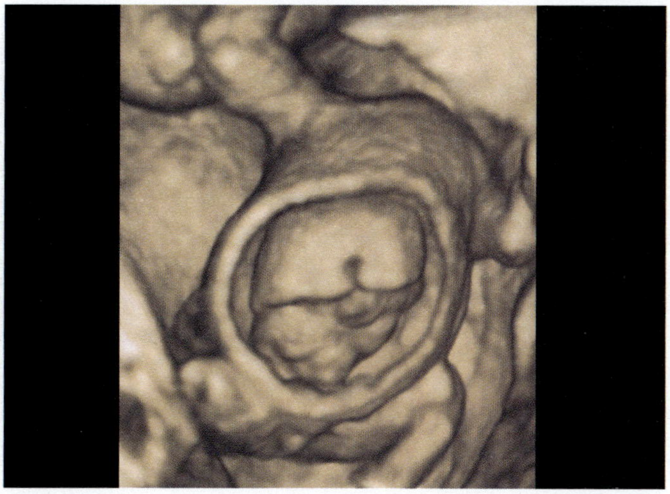

Fig. 3: A 20 weeks' anemic fetus with bilateral hydrothorax, ascites, and subcutaneous edema. This was an anemic fetus as a result from fetomaternal hemorrhage. Fetal anemia will always present with ascites before a pleural effusion appears. Reversal of hydrops was achieved after 2 rounds of intrauterine blood transfusion.

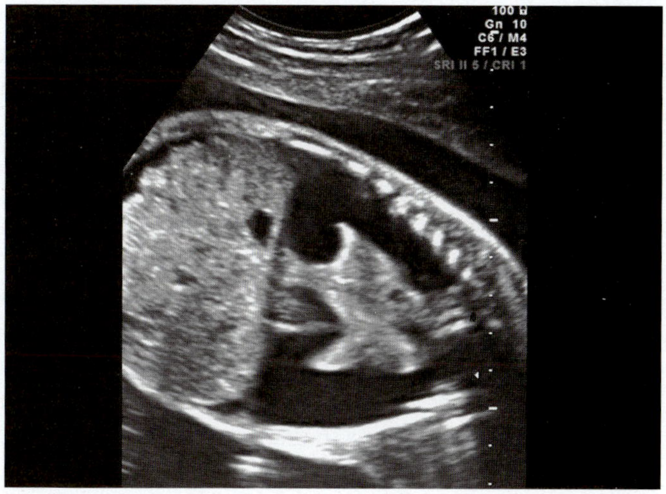

Fig. 4: Large amount of effusion in both pleural cavities in relation to compressed lung volume create a sonographic "bat wing" image.

TABLE 2: Suggested investigations for fetal hydrothorax.

Tests	*Remarks*
Maternal blood serology	To screen for acute infection with toxoplasmosis, rubella, cytomegalovirus, syphilis, and parvovirus B19
Maternal blood type and antibody screening	To differentiate immune and non-immune hydrops
Maternal blood Kleihauer–Betke (acid elution) test	To detect fetomaternal hemorrhage
Detailed fetal ultrasound and echocardiography	To detect associated fetal anomalies
Pulse-wave Doppler studies of fetal middle cerebral artery	To exclude fetal anemia from peak systolic velocity of the middle cerebral artery (MCA-PSV)
Fetal karyotype studies	To exclude fetal aneuploidies

fetal hydrothorax is shown in **Table 2**. Maternal blood works include; serology (for toxoplasmosis, rubella, cytomegalovirus, syphilis, and parvovirus B19), blood type and antibody screening, and acid elution test.[9,10]

Detailed fetal ultrasound and echocardiography are crucial. Approximately 25% of fetuses with hydrothorax have structural or cardiac anomalies.[11] A significant portion of associated malformations is intrathoracic, i.e., congenital pulmonary airway malformation (CPAM), bronchopulmonary dysplasia (BPS), or congenital diaphragmatic hernia (CDH). Peak systolic velocity of the middle cerebral artery (MCA-PSV) is useful to exclude fetal anemia. Fetal karyotype study is recommended. Approximately 6 to 17% of fetuses with hydrothorax have either trisomy 21 or 45, X, particularly those that are hydropic.[8,12] Rapid karyotype studies using either fluorescence in-situ hybridization (FISH) or quantitative fluorescence polymerase chain reaction (QF-PCR) are preferred, particularly when the fetus is already hydropic, and timely intervention is required. In our practice, we sample the amniotic fluid and aspirate the pleural effusion in a single pass with 20-G spinal needle. This is to minimize the miscarriage risk associated with invasive procedure. The effusion is not a preferable specimen for standard karyotype study from cultured cells. The lymphocyte in the effusion specimen is usually not sufficient.[13]

Ultrasound is the primary tool to diagnose, to evaluate associate anomalies, to follow up, and to guide invasive in-utero interventions. Secondary hydrothorax tends to be bilateral, whereas primary hydrothorax tends to be unilateral. At least 22% of primary hydrothorax regresses spontaneously, according to a review of 204 cases published by Aubard and colleagues in 1998.[14] But when hydrops develops, spontaneous regression is unlikely.[15] Usually at this stage of hydrops, bilateral pleural effusion with a disproportionally large, compared to the compressed fetal lung tissue, creating "bat wing" appearance on the ultrasound image, as shown in **Figure 4**.

The sequential deterioration in progressive case of unilateral hydrothorax has been hypothesized as follows:[16]

- Rapid increase of effusion in one pleural cavity, with seeping of fluid on to the contralateral cavity

- Compression of esophagus results in polyhydramnios
- Shifting of mediastinum causes distortion and obstruction of venous return, particularly from superior and inferior vena cava
- Cardiac compression or "temponade like condition" results in low output cardiac failure and hydrops[17]
- External pressure can affect canalicular phase (16 to 24 weeks') of fetal lung development.[18]

There are evidence that prenatal intervention can improve perinatal outcomes in selected cases of primary hydrothorax. Without treatment, approximately 53% (from 32 cases) of fetuses with primary hydrothorax died.[1] Primary hydrothorax that spontaneously regresses, occurs only on one side, and does not hydrops, had a good prognosis, with survival rate of 100% from this series. Preterm delivery of these babies, either iatrogenic or spontaneous as a result of polyhydramnios, worsens the survival rate. Prolongation of pregnancy, as well as reversal of hydrops at the time of delivery can significantly improve the outcome. Thus, in cases of small, non-hydropic primary hydrothorax, conservative management with weekly ultrasound is the most suitable because survival rate in this group is high already.

In-utero intervention to release intrathoracic pressure has a role in cases with rapid elevation of the effusion or when the fetus develops hydrops. Paracentesis was initially proposed in 1982. The benefits from prenatal paracentesis or shunting procedure in fetuses with primary hydrothorax are as follows:

- To decrease intrathoracic pressure, allowing for normalization of lung development. This principle is also applicable to pulmonary lesion, as shown in **Figure 5**.
- Restitution of mediastinum and cardiac axis following the decompression allow for a better visualization of cardiac anatomy
- Failure of lung volume restitution following the decompression may suggest hypoplastic change.[19]
- Reversal of hydrops and decompression of pleural cavity at the time of birth can facilitate neonatal resuscitation
- Prevention of polyhydramnios can prolong the pregnancy and reduce neonatal morbidities related to premature birth
- To obtain the effusion for diagnostic purpose.

Fetal paracentesis, or thoracocentesis in this case, is a simple ultrasound-guided intervention. However, because of the lymphatic system immaturity in primary hydrothorax, the effusion frequently re-accumulates within 48 hours. Repetitive tapping increases the chance of procedure-related miscarriage, compared to a single procedure like shunting.[11]

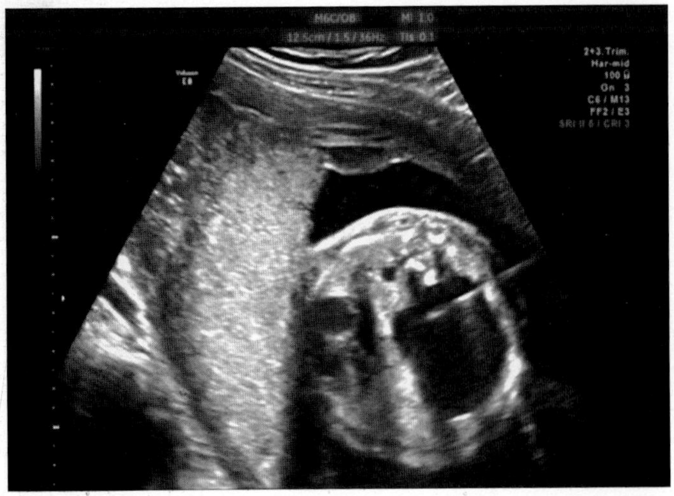

Fig. 5: In-utero thoracocentesis in a fetus at 24 weeks' with large macrocystic congenital pulmonary airway malformation (CPAM) of the left lung. Note the shifting of mediastinum and cardiac axis, and compression of the right lung. Removal of fluid in this case allowed for re-positioning of the mediastinum, allow for normalization of fetal lung growth at this canalicular phase of lung development.

FETAL SHUNTING PROCEDURES

The most common site for fetal shunting procedure is pleural cavity. Survival can be maximized by pleuroamniotic shunting, which can reverse hydrops and hydramnios and prevent pulmonary hypoplasia. Pleuroamniotic shunting can also be used for the treatment of other large cystic lung lesions, such as a macrocystic congenital cystic adenomatoid malformation or bronchopulmonary sequestration, especially when associated with hydrops, as shown in **Figure 6**.

Pleuroamniotic shunting was proposed for the first time in 1986.[20] Fetal shunts that are widely used include Rodeck's rocket shunt, Harrison's bladder shunt, and basket shunt. Our center has been using Harrison's bladder shunt (Cook Medical, Spencer, Indiana, USA) on an off-label basis, most of the time because of its availability.[21] We are performing in-utero shunting procedure in the dedicated part of our maternal-fetal medicine unit. Some centers perform fetal shunting procedures in the operating theater. Maternal and fetal analgesia is mandatory for shunting procedure, unlike laser surgery for twin-twin transfusion syndrome that does not require fetal analgesia.

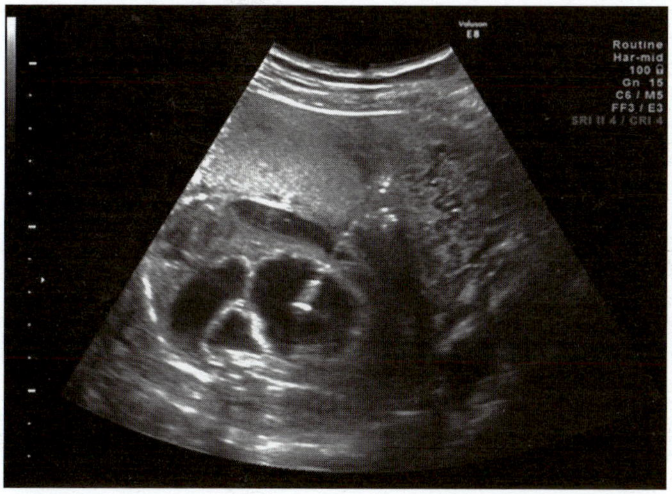

Fig. 6: Insertion of double pigtail shunt into a 24 weeks' fetus with large macrocystic congenital pulmonary airway malformation (CPAM).

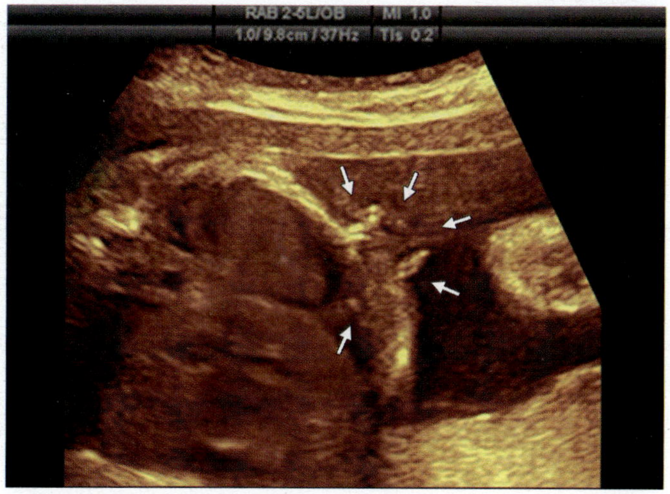

Fig. 7: Pleuroamniotic shunt 1 day after its insertion. Note that the amniotic end, which is double coiled, is seen clutching on the thoracic wall, whereas the fetal end, which is single coiled, is seen on the inside of pleural cavity. The lung is expanded. Some degree of skin edema is still noticeable.

Fetal immobilization with intravenous sedation, such as remifentanil, is recommended by some authors.[22] We always give prophylactic intravenous antibiotics (i.e., cefoxitin 1 gram) and prophylactic tocolysis (i.e., nifedipine 10 milligrams oral) prior to the procedure.

Seldinger technique is applied for this procedure, regardless of the shunt type. This technique was first described in 1953 by Dr Sven Ivar Seldinger, a Swedish radiologist.[23] It allows for a safe access into the blood vessel or hollow organ. Under real-time ultrasound guidance, the amniotic cavity is access with a trocar. Color Doppler is applied onto the chest wall of the fetus for an avascular window between the ribs for the trocar to be inserted. The rationale for choosing the fetal access is as follows:

- Insertion of the trocar from the back of the fetus should be avoided. There are scapula and multiple layers of muscle in the back. There is also a great chance of accentual puncture into great vessels
- Insertion of the trocar from the front of the fetus should be avoided. There is a chance of accidental puncture into the fetal heart. The nipple must be avoided. The shunt may be internally obstructed by the return of mediastinum into proper location after decompression. And the most important issue is, it is convenient for the fetus to grab and pull the shunt
- Insertion of the trocar along the mid-axillary line, at the level of the base of scapula is the most desirable location. Mid-axillary line access does not have the limitations encountered in anterior and posterior chest wall access. The fetus cannot grab the shunt left at this spot easily.

It is important to choose placenta-free area as the uterine access point. Fetal access point should not be too close to the uterine wall. Amnioinfusion with warm lactate Ringer solution is occasionally require for an adequate procedural space and for a better fetal positioning. An adequate amniotic space is required for the deploy of extrafetal end of the shunt. For Harrison's bladder shunt, a guidewire loaded with double pig tail shunt and its obturator is advanced through the trocar's lumen, until the round echoic tip of the guidewire is seen coming out at the end of the trocar sheet. The guidewire is then removed, and the obturator is used to push the fetal end (single coil) of the shunt into the fluid-filled thoracic cavity. The trocar sheet is then gradually withdrawn, while the obturator is fixed to maintain the fetal end position in the cavity. When the sheet is out of the fetal chest wall and into the amniotic cavity, the obturator is pushed again to deploy the amniotic end (double coil) of the shunt until it is all the way out of the sheet and freely floating in the amniotic cavity, as shown in **Figure 7**. Insertion techniques for Rodeck's rocket shunt and basket shunt are similar to that of Harrison's bladder shunt, only with a few modifications. It is important to be accurate and "fast". Once the trocar is in, fluid in fetal pleural cavity starts to leak. This makes deployment of fetal end coil into the pleural cavity more difficult.

For bilateral hydrothorax, fetal access to the contralateral pleural cavity is done by flipping the fetus with the blunt end of the trocar that is still in place and external manipulation. This is to avoid second puncture of

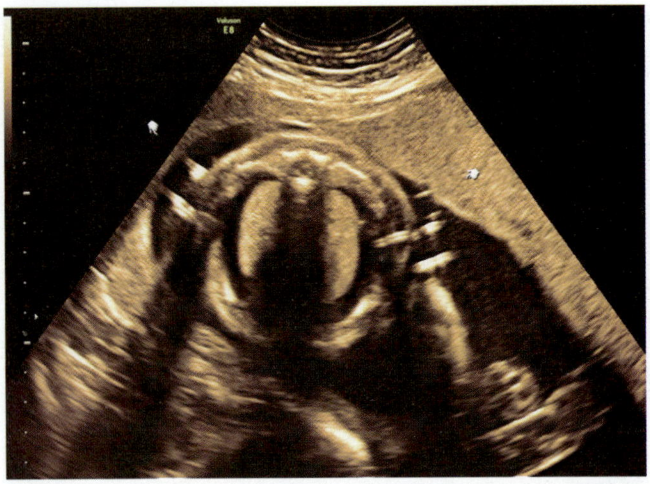

Fig. 8: Insertion of pleuroamniotic shunts in both pleural cavities with 1 puncture of a trocar in a case with anterior placenta. Note the narrow placenta-free uterine access point. There was no second access point, except for puncturing through the placenta. Note the residual skin edema of the fetus.

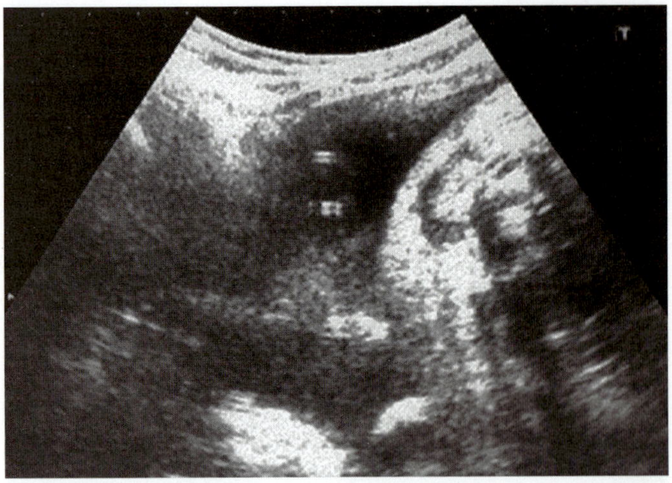

Fig. 9: Displacement of a double pigtail thoracoamniotic shunt. Note the echoic coil of the shunt floating freely near the thigh of the fetus.

the amniotic sac. In certain situation, such as extensively anterior placenta, there is no second amniotic access point without puncturing through the placenta, and fetal manipulation is the only way to put the second shunt in. **Figure 8** demonstrates bilateral insertion of pleuroamniotic shunt with 1 puncture of a trocar in a case with anterior placenta.

At the end of the procedure, shunt location needs to be re-checked before the trocar is removed. The fetal end with single coil must be in the deflated pleural cavity. The amniotic end with double coil must be in the amniotic cavity. We do not use amniopatch to seal the trocar insertion site. Follow-up scan is needed to confirm the pleural decompression and improvement or worsening of hydrops. Shunt can be migrated into the fetal pleural cavity or out to the amniotic cavity, as shown in **Figure 9**. Shunt migration and obstruction can occur up to 20% of a time.[24] The incidence of procedure-related preterm labor and premature rupture of the membranes is approximately 17%.[3] Strictly sterile technique and prophylactic antibiotics are used to prevent chorioamnionitis.

The upper limit of gestational age to perform in-utero shunting and not delivering the baby prematurely to perform postnatal thoracic drainage depends on the experiences of each center. It was suggested in some experts that in-utero shunting should prevail early delivery in up to 36 weeks of gestation.[1,25] If not possible, fetal pleural tapping to decompress the lung within 48 hours before delivery can be helpful. In situ pleuroamniotic shunting is not an indication for cesarean delivery. Newborn resuscitation team needs to be alerted. At the time of birth, the shunt should be clamped immediately to prevent pneumothorax, as shown in **Figure 10**.

PERCUTANEOUS SCLEROTHERAPY (AND PLEURODESIS)

The most common site for in-utero percutaneous sclerotherapy is the lung. There have been some reports of intralesional administration of sclerosing agent to reduce the size of congenital pulmonary airway malformation (CPAM) microcystic type that cause fetal hydrops.[26,27] Fetal decompensation from CPAM is a result of vena caval obstruction and "cardiac tamponade" from mass effect in confined thoracic cage. While most CPAMs are benign, with up to 95% of neonatal survival, CPAM with hydrops is related to almost a 100% neonatal mortality.[28-30] The mother can also suffer from preeclampsia or "mirror syndrome".[31]

With these serious consequences to the mother and the fetus, fetal hydrops associated with large CPAM is amendable for in-utero intervention.[32] For fetal macrocystic CPAM with hydrops, either tapping or shunting is adequate.[32] For fetal microcystic CPAM with hydrops, the management is more challenging. Open surgical removal of CPAM has been attempted in the pioneering fetal care centers. It could improve neonatal survival from nearly 0 to approximately 50%.[30] However, open fetal surgery to remove microcystic CPAM is related

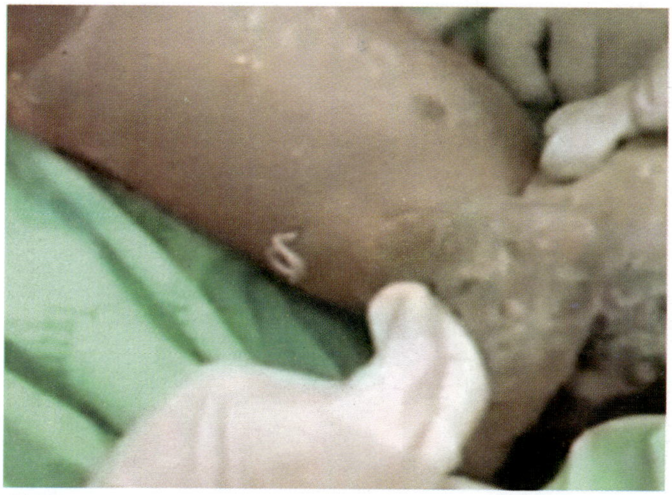

Fig. 10: An intact double pigtail thoracoamniotic shunt from left pleural cavity of the baby. Note an appropriate location of shunt placement, which is along the mid-axillary line. This anatomical landmark is to minimize an accidental injury to intrathoracic organ during the in-utero shunt placement. It can reduce the chance of shunt displacement because the fetus cannot conveniently grab it. The shunt was immediately clamped and removed. Pressure dressing with Vaseline gauze was applied to prevent pneumothorax.

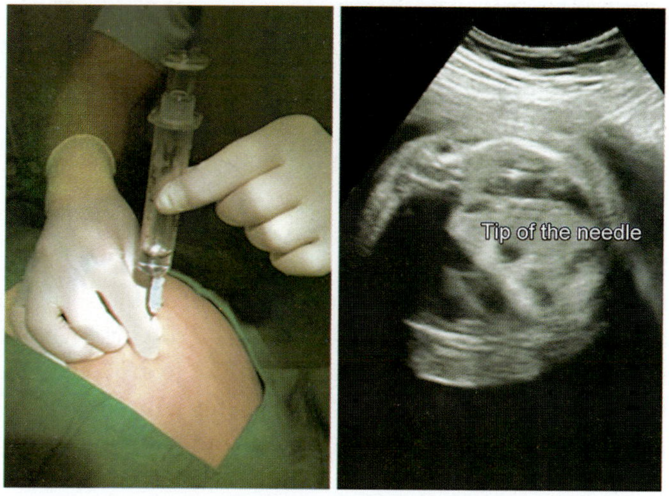

Fig. 11: Successful percutaneous sclerotherapy for a 24 weeks' fetus with large CPAM and hydrops.

to significant maternal morbidities, i.e., bleeding, infection, and uterine rupture. A higher chance of unstoppable preterm labor and preterm premature rupture of the membranes is a trade off for reversal of hydrops after the surgery.[32] Less invasive interventions have been explored. Maternal administration of steroids and intralesional laser ablation has an unpredictable result.[33,34]

There is one case series published in 2008 by Carlos Bermúdez et al. using intralesional injection of sclerosing agents in high-risk fetuses with microcystic CPAM.[26] They have recruited three fetuses with large microcystic (type 2 and 3) CPAM at gestational age below 26 weeks', presented with either hydrops, severe mediastinal shift, or polyhydramnios. Ultrasound-guided intralesional injection of either Ethamolin (ethanolamine oleate) or Polidocanol (aethoxysklerol) reversed hydrops in all three cases, resulting in delivery at term. Our team at Siriraj Hospital used this novel approach to treat a 24 weeks' fetus presented with hydrops from a large microcystic CPAM of the left lung. After a thorough counseling by multidiciplinary team, the patient and her family gave written informed consent for percutaneous sclerotherapy. Under ultrasound guidance, 2 milliliters of aethoxysklerol was given through a 20 G spinal needle, as shown in **Figure 11**. Reversal of hydrops was achieved with residual CPAM still clearly visible, as shown in **Figure 12**. The baby boy was born at term, and

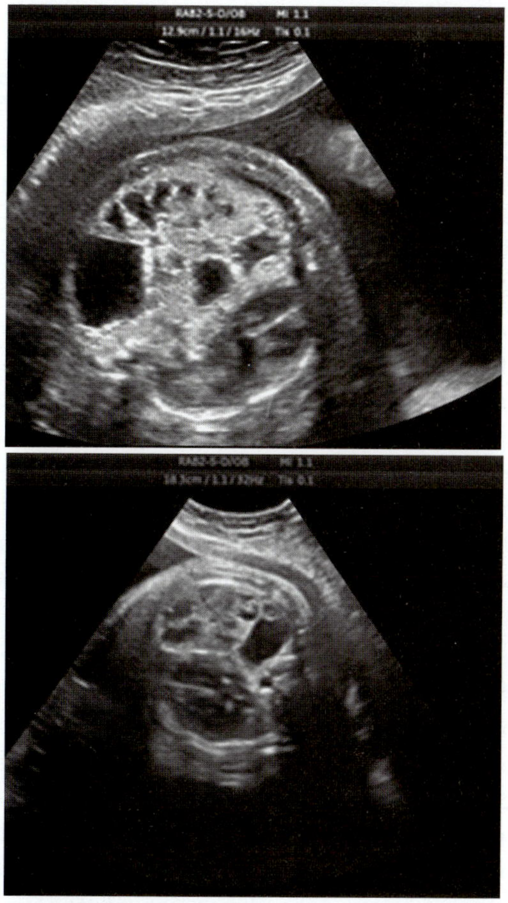

Fig. 12: Reversal of hydrops after percutaneous sclerotherapy in fetal hydrops from large CPAM. The second ultrasound image taken at 36 4/7 weeks' showed reduction in the CPAM size, rerstitution of mediastinum and cardiac axis, and absence of subcutaneous skin edema.

the tumor was soon surgically removed soon after his birth. There was another case series of three fetuses with hydrops from large CPAM receiving percutaneous sclerotherapy with a less favorable outcome.[27]

Regardless of some success in our personal experience and small case series of in-utero sclerotherapy for fetal hydrops from large microcystic CPAM, this result has to be reproducible in a more scientific manner. Criteria for candidacy of this treatment need to be settled. Ethanolamine oleate and aethoxysklerol have been clinically used to collapse varicose vein, hydrocele, and various cystic structures. Their action is by inducing inflammation on the luminal surface, resulting in adhesion. There is some concern that accidental spillage of these substances on to the contralateral fetal lung will do further damage. Adhesion in the CPAM mass caused by these substances may make postnatal surgical removal more difficult. More experiences are needed before this fetal treatment is widely adopted.

Another application of in-utero sclerotherapy is pleurodesis. It has been used in cases of recurrent hydrothorax. OK-432 has been used in a few case series of intrathoracic treatment of recurrent effusion with OK-432.[35,36] This is a biological toxin extracted from group A *Streptococcus pyogenes*. It has been clinically used to collapse lymphangioma.[37] Since there are still limited evidence for OK-432, it is not considered a standard fetal care at a moment. Advantages and disadvantages of intrathoracic OK-432 and shunting in fetuses with recurrent hydrothorax after pleurocentesis need to be explored. Apparently, intrathoracic administration of OK-432 is less technical demanding. Therefore, it can be applied as early as 16 weeks of gestation.[35] Data on long-term effect of OK-432, particularly on the neurodevelopmental milestone of the child, is still lacking.

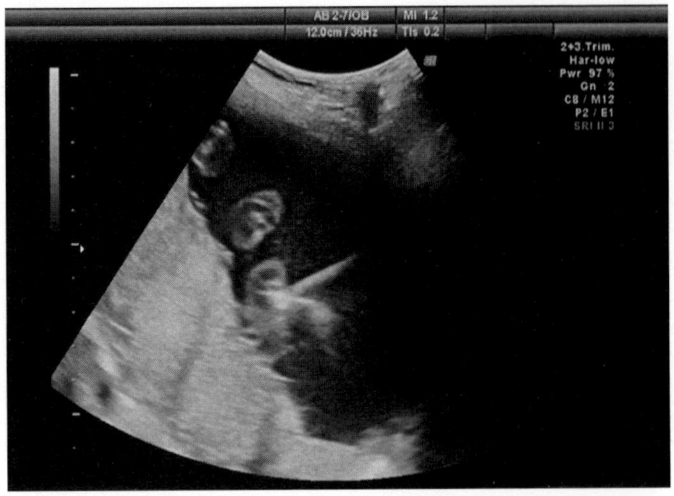

Fig. 13: Fetal blood transfusion. This image shows an access to the umbilical vein using real-time ultrasound guidance.

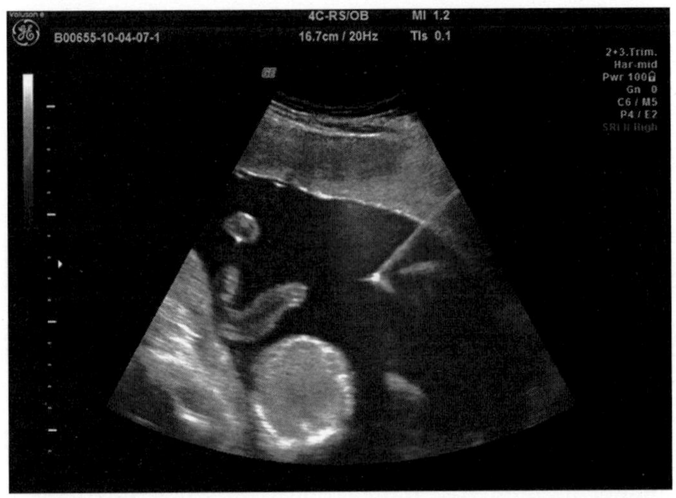

Fig. 14: Amnioreduction has been clinically acceptable method to alleviate the pressure symptoms of pregnant women with polyhydramnios. It is also an acceptable treatment for twin-twin transfusion syndrome stage 1. The procedure is performed with real-time ultrasound guidance.

CONCLUSION

Research in the field of minimally invasive fetal intervention has been very productive. Certain ultrasound-guided in-utero interventions have become accepted without scientific validation. These include intrauterine blood transfusion, amnioinfusion, and amnioreduction. Examples of these procedures are demonstrated in **Figures 13 and 14**. More structured studies are required for any intervention at higher risks, i.e., fetal cardiac intervention. In the next few years after publication of this chapter, more data on percutaneous fetal valvulotomy in fetuses with critical aortic or pulmonic stenosis will be available.[38] Fetal cardiac intervention has been a main research subject in Europe (Association for European Pediatric and Congenital Cardiology: AEPC) and the United States. In-utero management of placental diseases is also a subject of research interest. Our group at Siriraj Hospital has recently published an ex-vivo model to study the effect of radiofrequency ablation to the placental tissue.[39] This is an effort to appropriately utilized this minimally invasive tool to manage chorioangioma. Development of ultrasound technology will certainly foster the adoption of all the minimally invasive intervention and, hopefully, will assist in progressively better post-procedural outcomes.

REFERENCES

1. Longaker MT, Laberge JM, Dansereau J, et al. Primary fetal hydrothorax: natural history and management. Journal of Pediatric Surgery. 1989;24:573-6.
2. Cardwell MS. Aspiration of fetal pleural effusions or ascites may improve neonatal resuscitation. Southern Medical Journal. 1996;89:177-8.
3. Picone O, Benachi A, Mandelbrot L, Ruano R, Dumez Y, Dommergues M. Thoracoamniotic shunting for fetal pleural effusions with hydrops. American Journal of Obstetrics and Gynecology. 2004;191:2047-50.
4. Deurloo KL, Devlieger R, Lopriore E, Klumper FJ, Oepkes D. Isolated fetal hydrothorax with hydrops: a systematic review of prenatal treatment options. Prenat Diagn. 2007;27:893-9.
5. Paternoster DM, Manganelli F, Minucci D, et al. Ballantyne syndrome: a case report. Fetal Diagnosis and Therapy. 2006;21:92-5.
6. Carroll B. Pulmonary hypoplasia and pleural effusions associated with fetal death in utero: ultrasonic findings. AJR American Journal of Roentgenology. 1977;129:749-50.
7. Weber AM, Philipson EH. Fetal pleural effusion: a review and meta-analysis for prognostic indicators. Obstetrics and Gynecology. 1992;79:281-6.
8. Smith RP, Illanes S, Denbow ML, Soothill PW. Outcome of fetal pleural effusions treated by thoracoamniotic shunting. Ultrasound Obstet Gynecol. 2005;26:63-6.
9. Barron SD, Pass RF. Infectious causes of hydrops fetalis. Seminars in Perinatology. 1995;19:493-501.
10. Dupre AR, Morrison JC, Martin JN Jr, Floyd RC, Blake PG. Clinical application of the Kleihauer-Betke test. The Journal of Reproductive Medicine. 1993;38:621-4.
11. Klam S, Bigras JL, Hudon L. Predicting outcome in primary fetal hydrothorax. Fetal Diagnosis and Therapy. 2005;20:366-70.
12. Achiron R, Weissman A, Lipitz S, Mashiach S, Goldman B. Fetal pleural effusion: the risk of fetal trisomy. Gynecologic and Obstetric Investigation. 1995;39:153-6.
13. Teoh TG, Ryan G, Johnson J, Winsor EJ. The role of fetal karyotyping from unconventional sources. American journal of Obstetrics and Gynecology. 1996;175:873-7.
14. Aubard Y, Derouineau I, Aubard V, Chalifour V, Preux PM. Primary fetal hydrothorax: A literature review and proposed antenatal clinical strategy. Fetal diagnosis and Therapy. 1998;13:325-33.
15. Jaffe R, Di Segni E, Altaras M, Loebel R, Ben Aderet N. Ultrasonic real-time diagnosis of transitory fetal pleural and pericardial effusion. Diagnostic Imaging in Clinical Medicine. 1986;55:373-5.
16. Bessone LN, Ferguson TB, Burford TH. Chylothorax. The Annals of Thoracic Surgery. 1971;12:527-50.
17. Bigras JL, Ryan G, Suda K, et al. Echocardiographic evaluation of fetal hydrothorax: the effusion ratio as a diagnostic tool. Ultrasound Obstet Gynecol. 2003;21:37-40.
18. Castillo RA, Devoe LD, Falls G, Holzman GB, Hadi HA, Fadel HE. Pleural effusions and pulmonary hypoplasia. American Journal of Obstetrics and Gynecology. 1987;157:1252-5.
19. Skoll MA, Sharland GK, Allan LD. Is the ultrasound definition of fluid collections in non-immune hydrops fetalis helpful in defining the underlying cause or predicting outcome? Ultrasound Obstet Gynecol. 1991;1:309-12.
20. Seeds JW, Bowes WA Jr. Results of treatment of severe fetal hydrothorax with bilateral pleuroamniotic catheters. Obstetrics and Gynecology. 1986;68:577-80.
21. Harrison MR. The University of California at San Francisco Fetal Treatment Center: a personal perspective. Fetal Diagnosis and Therapy. 2004;19:513-24.
22. Van de Velde M, Van Schoubroeck D, Lewi LE, et al. Remifentanil for fetal immobilization and maternal sedation during fetoscopic surgery: a randomized, double-blind comparison with diazepam. Anesthesia and Analgesia. 2005;101:251-8, table of contents.
23. Seldinger SI. Catheter replacement of the needle in percutaneous arteriography; a new technique. Acta Radiologica. 1953;39:368-76.
24. Sepulveda W, Galindo A, Sosa A, Diaz L, Flores X, de la Fuente P. Intrathoracic dislodgement of pleuroamniotic shunt. Three case reports with long-term follow-up. Fetal Diagnosis and Therapy. 2005;20:102-5.
25. Yinon Y, Kelly E, Ryan G. Fetal pleural effusions. Best practice and research Clinical Obstetrics and Gynaecology. 2008;22:77-96.
26. Bermudez C, Perez-Wulff J, Arcadipane M, et al. Percutaneous fetal sclerotherapy for congenital cystic adenomatoid malformation of the lung. Fetal Diagnosis and Therapy. 2008;24:237-40.
27. Lee FL, Said N, Grikscheit TC, Shin CE, Llanes A, Chmait RH. Treatment of congenital pulmonary airway malformation induced hydrops fetalis via percutaneous sclerotherapy. Fetal Diagnosis and Therapy. 2012;31:264-8.
28. Mann S, Wilson RD, Bebbington MW, Adzick NS, Johnson MP. Antenatal diagnosis and management of congenital cystic adenomatoid malformation. Seminars in Fetal and Neonatal Medicine. 2007;12:477-81.
29. Cavoretto P, Molina F, Poggi S, Davenport M, Nicolaides KH. Prenatal diagnosis and outcome of echogenic fetal lung lesions. Ultrasound Obstet Gynecol. 2008;32:769-83.
30. Grethel EJ, Wagner AJ, Clifton MS, et al. Fetal intervention for mass lesions and hydrops improves outcome: a 15-year experience. Journal of Pediatric Surgery. 2007;42:117-23.
31. Braun T, Brauer M, Fuchs I, et al. Mirror syndrome: a systematic review of fetal associated conditions, maternal

presentation and perinatal outcome. Fetal Diagnosis and Therapy. 2010;27:191-203.
32. Witlox RS, Lopriore E, Oepkes D. Prenatal interventions for fetal lung lesions. Prenat Diagn. 2011;31:628-36.
33. Morris LM, Lim FY, Livingston JC, Polzin WJ, Crombleholme TM. High-risk fetal congenital pulmonary airway malformations have a variable response to steroids. Journal of Pediatric Surgery. 2009;44:60-5.
34. Bruner JP, Jarnagin BK, Reinisch L. Percutaneous laser ablation of fetal congenital cystic adenomatoid malformation: too little, too late? Fetal Diagnosis and Therapy. 2000;15:359-63.
35. Nygaard U, Sundberg K, Nielsen HS, Hertel S, Jorgensen C. New treatment of early fetal chylothorax. Obstetrics and Gynecology. 2007;109:1088-92.
36. Chen M, Shih JC, Wang BT, Chen CP, Yu CL. Fetal OK-432 pleurodesis: complete or incomplete? Ultrasound Obstet Gynecol. 2005;26:791-3.
37. Jorgensen C, Brocks V, Bang J, Jorgensen FS, Ronsbro L. Treatment of severe fetal chylothorax associated with pronounced hydrops with intrapleural injection of OK-432. Ultrasound Obstet Gynecol. 2003;21:66-9.
38. Gardiner H, Kovacevic A, Tulzer G, et al. Natural history of 107 cases of Fetal Aortic Stenosis from a European multicenter retrospective study. Ultrasound Obstet Gynecol. 2016.
39. Satapornteera P, Raveesunthornkiat M, Sukpanichnant S, Tongdee T, Homsud S, Wataganara T. Effects of Power and Time on Ablation Size Produced by Radiofrequency Ablation: In vitro Study in Fresh Human Placenta. Fetal Diagnosis and Therapy. 2015;38:41-7.

CHAPTER 45

In-utero Stem Cell Transplantation and Gene Therapy

Tuangsit Wataganara

INTRODUCTION

Advances in prenatal screening and molecular genetic diagnosis allow for a broader detection of some serious genetic diseases at an earlier gestational age. From theoretical point of view, a fetus up to certain gestational age is considered immune-naïve, and therefore is a perfect recipient for in utero transplantation. It may avoid the need for postnatal treatment and reduce future costs. The concept of prenatal transplantation is relatively new and still in experimental phase. *In-utero transplantation with hematopoietic stem cells* or other kinds of stem cell lines has been attempted with various successes in fetuses with diseases related to the hematology (such as thalassemia and hemoglobinopathies), immunology (such as congenital immunodeficiency disease), and metabolic disorders. It represents a new therapeutic strategy; particularly there is an opportunity to transplant the stem cells across histocompatibility barriers without chemotherapeutic induction. With all the positive prospects of this novel prenatal treatment, so far the clinical success of in-utero allogeneic hematopoietic stem cells transplantation has been limited to only fetuses with severe combined immunodeficiency. Recently, there have been a few successful cases of allogeneic mesenchymal stem cell transplantation that improved phenotype in osteogenesis imperfecta. Faculty of Medicine Siriraj Hospital has recently reported an extraction of human amniotic fluid stem cells as an alternative source for either prenatal or postnatal treatment.

Gene transfer to the cells with long-term transgenic protein expression is now technically feasible. Preliminary reports from animal model have been promising. Ultrasound-guided injection of the transduced cells in sheep model has achieved a lasting production of transgenic protein. It has a potential to be restoring systemic organs that are naturally affected by a number of congenital genetic diseases, such as neurological disorders. Human trials on prenatal gene therapy are not currently available due to an unclear answer in the issue of post-transfer mutagenesis and germ line transfer.

HISTORY OF IN-UTERO STEM CELL TRANSPLANTATION

In-utero hematopoietic stem cell transplantation is an alternative approach for a variety of hematological, metabolic and immunological diseases. It has a dual potential of reconstitution of a defective cell line and clinical amelioration of genetic defects. Transplantation in fetuses in the period of immunologic naïve can avoid myeloablative irradiation or chemotherapeutic immunosuppression, which can lead to serious morbidity commonly found in transplantation in childhood period.[1] Even without complete engraftment, in-utero transplantation can induce prenatal tolerance that facilitates postnatal cellular or organ transplantations.

The first successful human fetal transplantation was reported by Touraine and colleagues in 1989, using human fetal liver cells for transplantation into a fetus with bare lymphocyte syndrome.[2] Their success was not consistently reproducible, except for in patients with severe combined immunodeficiency.[3,4] This is an obvious example of how complex fetal stem cell transplantation is, and it calls for multidisciplinary and international collaboration. The purpose of this chapter in "Fetal Therapy Section" is to set an awareness of certain fetal diseases that may be benefited from in utero stem cell transplantation, and how to detect them with the use of prenatal imaging. Brief review of the theoretical and experimental supports for fetal stem cell transplantation, its proven benefits and limitations, as well as clinical experience to date is provided so that the essential concepts can be materialized. Practical knowledge of these uncommon fetal conditions can facilitate an accurate molecular genetic testing, effective counseling, and timely referral to appropriate facility.

RATIONALE FOR IN-UTERO STEM CELL TRANSPLANTATION

The concept of fetal stem cell transplantation is attractive, but is associated with complicated ethical issues. Women carrying a fetus affected with genetic conditions causing inevitable death or serious neonatal and childhood disability now have an opportunity to explore only two different options; termination of pregnancy or expectant management with postnatal supportive treatment. To date, in-utero transplantation is considered as highly experimental, because the prognosis after transplantation is ambiguous. The possibility of transplantation should be raised only if the parents decide not to terminate the affected fetus.

In theory, the normal biology of the fetus makes it an ideal recipient for stem cell transplantation. Natural embryonic stem cells rapidly expand into anatomical compartments during intrauterine development. From transplantation point of view, the fetus at earlier gestational age is more receptive, and requiring smaller transplant dosage owing to its size.[5] This leads to the concept of "fetal tolerance"; which is an inability to raise an immunological response (or graft rejection) against foreign antigen if the antigen is introduced early enough.[6] According to this principle, any couples at risk of giving birth to a baby with serious genetic condition, should seek prenatal care as early as conception is recognized, or preferably even before conception.

Albeit nicely laid 'fetal intolerance' concept, in-utero hematopoietic stem cell transplantation has been successful only in fetuses with immunodeficiency disorder. In other conditions, fetal immune system is a significant barrier to engraftment. Monocytes and macrophages are the first immunological cell type to appear in fetal circulation.[7] Natural killer (NK) cells also appear in the liver as early as 9 weeks of gestation.[8] At 13 weeks, about 30% of lymphocytes in the fetal circulation are NK cells.[9] These three immunological cell types play an important role in graft failure after in-utero transplantation. From 18 weeks of gestation, the fetal spleen contains equal numbers of T cells, B cells and monocytes/macrophages, and is therefore considered immunocompetent with sufficient accessory cells to initiate T cell activation, and hence 'fetal immunologic barrier' is established.

HUMAN EXPERIENCES OF IN-UTERO STEM CELL TRANSPLANTATION

Clinical experience of intrauterine transplantation is limited, and all of them are highly experimental in nature. The published reports used various sources of the donor cells for a variety of target disease, therefore, general conclusions cannot be drawn. In the present review we have chosen to present these transplantations according to indication. The most successful group of patients transplanted in-utero are those fetuses with immunodeficiencies, i.e., *severe combined immunodeficiency syndrome (SCID)*.[10] In Southeast Asia, the focus has been at preventing new cases of debilitating hemoglobinopathies, which is a major health issue in this region. Successful in-utero transplantation for the treatment of osteogenesis imperfecta has been reported from the region as well.

In-utero Hematopoietic Stem Cell Transplantation

Fetus affected with homozygote alpha-thalassemia 1 has deletion of all 4 alpha-globin genes. The fetus will be progressively anemic starting from early second trimester. Hydropic change can be observed in the second trimester, as shown in **Figures 1 and 2**. Pulse wave Doppler

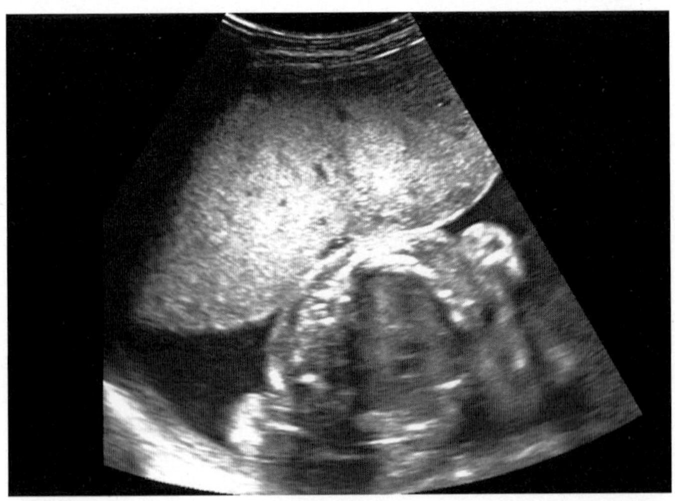

Fig. 1: Ultrasound image, displayed in gray scale mode, of a 24 weeks' hydropic fetus. Note that the fetus had subcutaneous skin edema and pleural effusion. The placenta is thick and appearing 'ground glass'. Analysis of umbilical cord blood showed hemoglobin level of 6 g/dL with hemoglobin Bart's over 90%. The diagnosis was hemoglobin Bart's hydrops. The pregnancy was terminated.

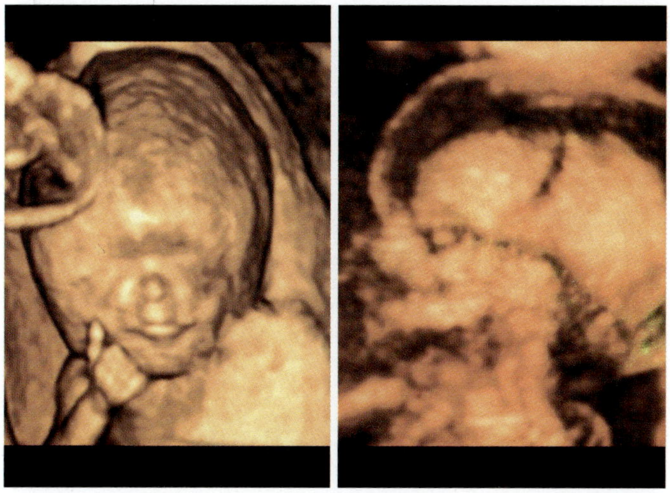

Fig. 2: Ultrasound image, displayed in three-dimensional surface rendered and maximum intensity weighed gradient (X-ray) mode, of a 22 weeks' fetus with anemic hydrops. Subcutaneous fluid collection could be enhanced when its contrast against fetal skull is adjusted.

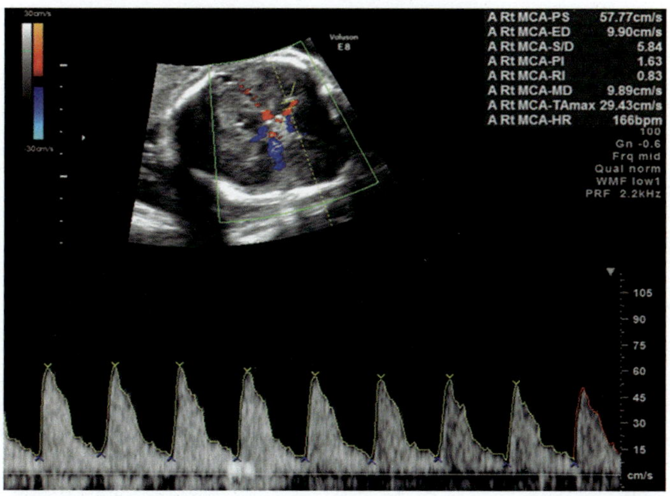

Fig. 3: Pulse wave Doppler interrogation of a 24 weeks' hydropic fetus showed the peak systolic velocity of middle cerebral artery (PSV-MCA) of 57 cm/s (1.5 multiple of the median of PSV-MCA for 24 weeks' is 40 cms/s). Analysis of umbilical cord blood showed hemoglobin level of 6 g/dL with hemoglobin Bart's over 90%. The diagnosis was hemoglobin Bart's hydrops. The pregnancy was terminated.

interrogation of middle cerebral artery shows peak systolic velocity (PSV-MCA) over 1.5 multiple of the median (MoM) has a sensitivity of 100% for prediction of moderate to severe fetal anemia (hemoglobin level in umbilical cord blood less than 7g/dL), as shown in **Figure 3**.[11] This noninvasive screening for fetal anemia has a false-positive rate (the fetus is actually not anemic) of 12%. Women carrying a Bart's hydrops fetus may develop preeclampsia. It is advisable to terminate the pregnancy without offering any fetal intervention. Deletion of three alpha-globin genes results in hemoglobin H disease, which does not cause anemic hydrops. Children with hemoglobin H disease do not require regular blood transfusion, except when there is a hemolytic crisis, usually induced by viral infection. We recently reported a rescue intrauterine blood transfusion in a 32 weeks' fetus with anemic hydrops with PSV-MCA of 100 cm/s.[12] Analysis of umbilical cord blood before transfusion revealed hemoglobin constant spring homozygote. We suspected that intrauterine viral infection may trigger hemolytic crisis in this fetus, but the real causative agent was not identified.

In-utero hematopoietic stem cell transplantations have been attempted predominantly on the fetuses affected with compound heterozygote beta-thalassemia that will be transfusion dependent. Unlike alpha-thalassemia, fetuses with compound heterozygote beta-thalassemia will not be anemic, and will not show any detectable signs from prenatal ultrasound examination. Screening for carrier is a national policy in Thailand. Genetic counseling and prenatal genetic diagnosis is offered in couple at risk of giving birth to a baby with high possibility of transfusion dependent. The onset of anemia is usually in the first year of life with variation in severity according to the point mutation. There is a limited number of published reports on in-utero stem cell transplantation aiming to ameliorate transfusion dependency.[13] There was an evidence of engraftment with microchimerism but all the children are transfusion dependent.

In-utero Mesenchymal Stem Cell Transplantation

Mesenchymal stem cell (MSC) has a broader potential then stem cell of hematopoietic origin. Successful in-utero MSC transplantation cases have been continuously reported in fetus affected with certain congenital skeletal dysplastic disease that either lethal or causing significant childhood morbidity. There are key prenatal ultrasound findings that can help differentiate different types of skeletal dysplasia and predict the prognosis of the fetuses with short bones detected in utero, so that viable candidate for in-utero MSC transplantation can be identified.

Achondroplasia

Is the most common short-limb dwarfism, as shown in **Figure 4**. Affected individuals have normal intelligence

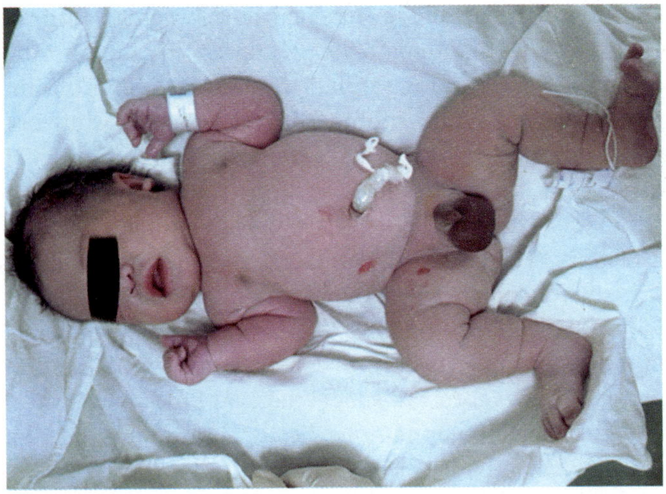

Fig. 4: Postnatal photograph of a term baby with achondroplasia. Note the following features of relatively large cranial vault, prominent forehead, with depressed nasal bridge. There is a slightly thoracolumbar kyphosis. Anterior flaring of ribs is noticeable. Metacarpal and metatarsal bones are short and are of similar length, giving an appearance of 'trident hand'.

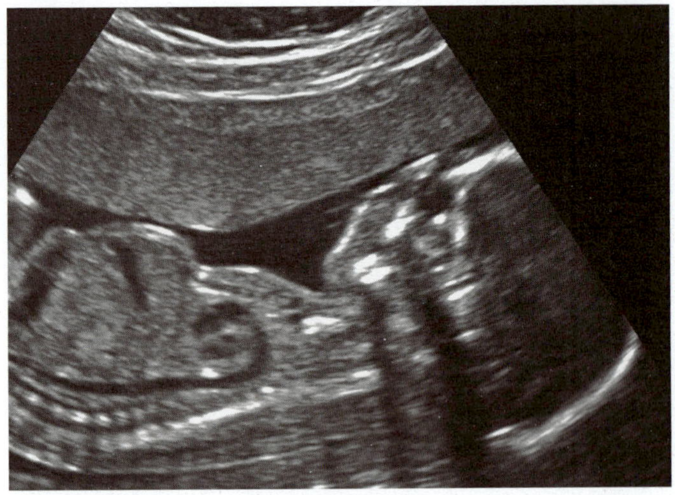

Fig. 5: Ultrasound image, displayed in gray scale mode, of a 24-weeks' fetus with osteogenesis imperfecta type II. Note a small thoracic cage, as a result of multiple fractures causing deformity and shortening of the ribs. Pulmonary hypoplasia is a major cause of death in these babies.

and motor function, except for certain neurologic deficits. Mutation of fibroblast growth factor gene 3 (FGFR3), on chromosome 4p16.3, results in abnormal cartilage formation. Long bones formed by enchondral ossification are affected, whereas skull plates formed by membranous ossification are not affected. Shortening of fetal long bones is not detected until late in the 3rd trimester.[14] Neonatal care in a baby with achondroplasia includes precaution of cervical cord compression due to narrowing of foramen magnum, intracranial shunting, correction of kyphoscoliosis, and respiratory care in homozygous case. Because overall prognosis is good, particularly in heterozygous individuals, in-utero MSC transplantation is generally not required.

Osteogenesis Imperfecta (OI)

It is a cluster of diseases resulting from a mutation in the COL1A1 and COL1A2 genes, which encode the α2 and α2 polypeptide chains that are responsible for over 90% of collagen type 1 synthesis. Most of the inheritance (>95%) is autosomal dominant (>95%), with much smaller numbers from autosomal recessive and sporadic mutations.[15] Affected individuals have osteoporosis and fragile bones at various onsets, which can be divided into 8 major clinical features.[13] Classification system of OI has undergone some major revisions, and the most updated one can be found on an official website of OI.[16] Type II OI is the most severe form, and the most common form of fetal lethal skeletal dysplasia. Prenatal ultrasound examination shows multiple fractures and severe bone deformity, small and deformed thoracic cage, and pulmonary hypoplasia, as shown in **Figure 5**. Intrauterine MSC transplantations have been successful in a few candidate fetuses with osteogenesis imperfecta.[17] MSC seems to have a better fetal engraftment than hematopoietic cell lines. Successful MSC engraftment occurs even late in gestation, well after fetal immune barrier is established. Albeit some initial successes in the prenatal treatment of OI type II by MSC transplantation, there are certain issues before this success can be generalized. Publication bias exists. A number of human in-utero MSC transplantations for the treatment of OI type II failed, and the researchers knew if the transplantation is a success or not only after the baby is born. Most of the failed results are not reported.[18] Standard protocol cannot be materialized yet, due to the limited number of cases. So far, it is advisable to balance the information when it comes to counseling a couple carrying an affected fetus searching for this in-utero MSC transplantation. They have to realize that the benefit from this treatment modality based only on a small number of cases. There are many failed transplantations, and the babies were born with this debilitating disease. Even in cases with successful in utero MSC transplantation, collecting long-term outcome data of these babies is still a work in progress.

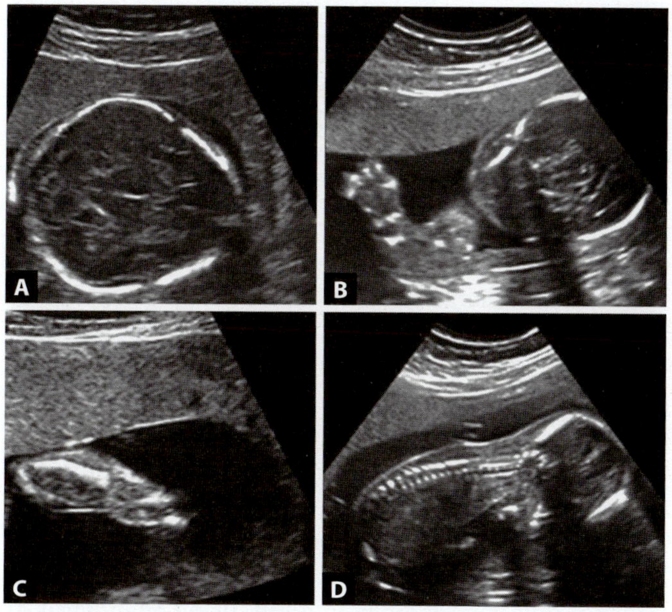

Figs. 6A to D: Ultrasound images, displayed in gray scale mode, of a 23-weeks' fetus with thanatophoric dysplasia. The sonographic features of this disease include: (A) A cloverleaf skull appearance; (B) Thickened soft tissue of the extremities; (C) Short, thick, bowed tubular bones; (D) Redundant skin covering neck and upper back.

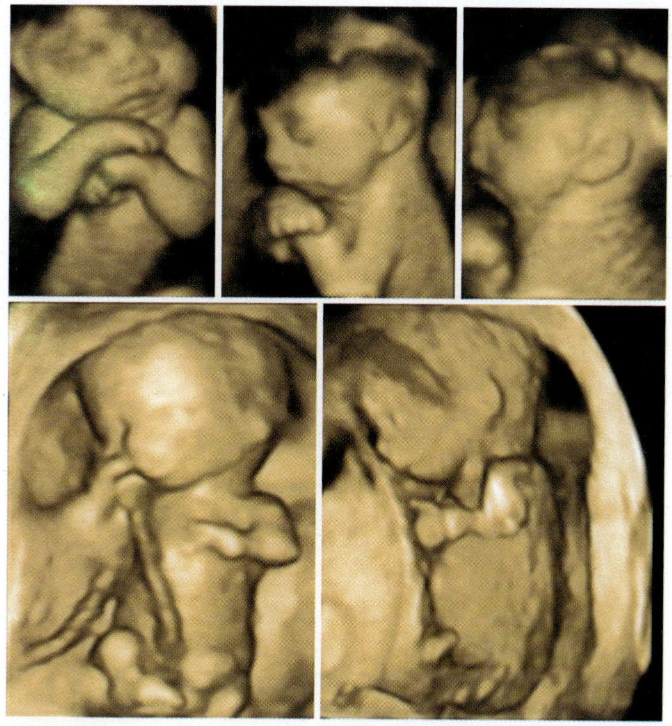

Fig. 7: Ultrasound images, displayed in three-dimensional surface rendered mode, of a 23-weeks' fetus with thanatophoric dysplasia. Shortening of fetal long bones in thanatophoric dysplasia can be noticed late first trimester. Redundant nuchal skin can be observed and suggestive for an early onset nature of this disease. Better communication with the parents is expected when three-dimensional ultrasound images of the sick fetus are used during the counseling.

Thanatophoric Dysplasia

It is the second most common lethal skeletal dysplasia after type II OI. It results from a sporadic mutation of FGFR3, but different from that cause achondroplasia. Short, curved long bones that look like telephone receiver can be visible as early as late first trimester, as shown in **Figures 6 and 7**. The condition is uniformly fatal. The affected baby will die within a few hours of birth from respiratory failure or brainstem compression (narrow foramen magnum). So far, there is no report of successful in utero MSC transplantation to treat a fetus with thanatophoric dysplasia.

Achondrogenesis

It is a very rare type of skeletal dysplasia with extremely poor prognosis. Its responsible genetic mutation and inheritance pattern are not fully understood. Our team at Faculty of Medicine Siriraj Hospital has reported pre- and postnatal imagings of a fetus with achondrogenesis, demonstrated in both gray scale and surface rendered three-dimensional sonographic image, as well as a characteristic postmortem radiograph of this disease.[19] Sonographic findings include nuchal edema in the first trimester. Second trimester ultrasound can reveal extreme micromelia.[20] Generalized absence of ossification except for the calvarium is a diagnostic feature of achondrogenesis, making a floating head appearance on postmortem radiograph, as shown in **Figures 8A to D**. So far, there is no report of successful in utero MSC transplantation to treat a fetus with thanatophoric dysplasia.

HISTORY OF IN-UTERO GENE THERAPY

Gene therapy is the treatment that desirable genetic material, and not the whole cell, is delivered into the targeted cell to correct its function. Appropriate vector is required to deliver the genes into the targeted cells, which technically can be either somatic or germ cells. Currently, germ-line gene therapy is considered unethical due to the concern of potential germ line gene transmission.[21] After 2 decades of human phase trial, most clinical results of in-utero gene therapy have been disappointing. The reasons for this are many and include difficulty targeting the appropriate organ, a robust immune

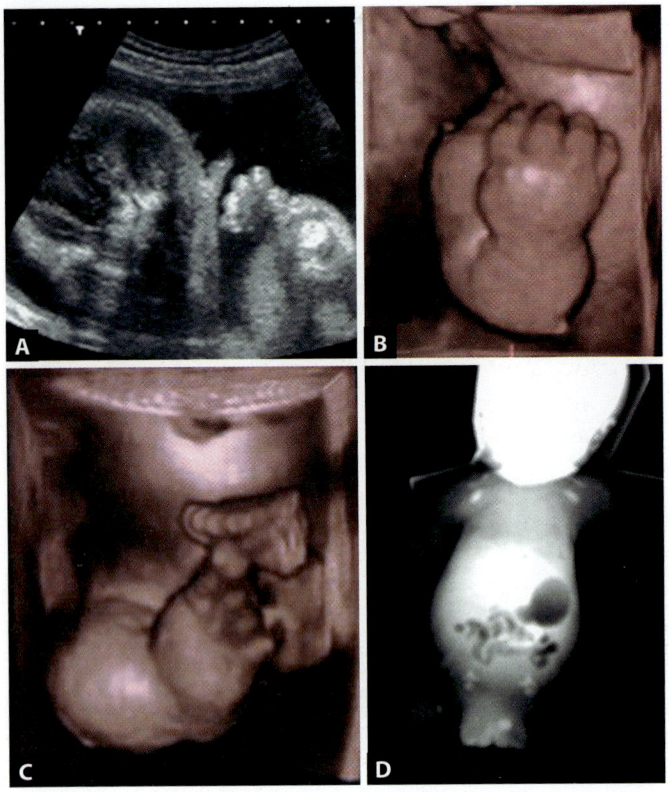

Figs. 8A to D: Pre- and postnatal imagings of a 30-weeks' fetus with achondrogenesis. (A and B) Marked shortening of the arm (rhizomelia), forearms (mesomelia), and fingers (brachydactyly); (C) Shortened and deformed legs with lack of movement; (D) Postmortem radiograph shows nearly total absence of ossification except for skull, clavicles and ilia.

response to the therapy in adults and low level expression of the therapeutic gene product. Some groups have switched their focus to postnatal, rather than prenatal, gene transfer to reduce risks of mutation.

RATIONALE FOR IN-UTERO GENE THERAPY

Certain genetic disorders have an early onset and cause irreversible pathological organ damages. Examples of in-utero damages of specific organs in certain genetic diseases include lung in cystic fibrosis, brain in urea-cycle disorder, and skin in epidemiolysis bullosa. Certain organs are inaccessible after birth. Fetal gene therapy is usually targeting at the rapidly expanding stem cells, so that therapeutic effects can be measurable shortly after administration.

APPLICATION OF IN-UTERO GENE THERAPY

Theoretically, in utero gene therapy is superior to in utero stem cell transplantation or gene therapy, given in postnatal period for certain serious disorders. These candidate diseases are genetic in origin, and destruction of targeted organs started so early from in utero or early postnatal period that postnatal intervention may be too late to preserve the organ function. Obvious examples include hemophilia A and B, cystic fibrosis, and spinal muscular dystrophy.[22,23] The data obtained from animal experiments has not been reassuring enough, most of the trials are unable to reach human subject, except for hemophilia.

Hemophilias A and B are congenital deficiency of coagulation factors IX and VIII, respectively. It has an incidence of 1 in 8,000 adults.[24] Replacement therapy with these factors is expensive and has a number of limitations. The patient may develop anaphylaxis, neutralizing antibodies, or blood borne viruses, i.e., human immunodeficiency virus (HIV) or hepatitis B virus.[25] Adult gene therapy in adult, using adenovirus as a vector to transfect gene of patients with hemophilia B, did not yield a satisfactory result, due to a cell-mediated immune response.[26,27] On the other hand, gene therapy directing into hemophiliac mice fetuses showed permanent phenotypic correction for a longer period of time (14 months).[22]

RISKS OF IN-UTERO GENE THERAPY

Albeit an initial success in proof-of-concept experiments that gene therapy in utero may be associated with high chance and longer duration of phenotypic conversion, most of the experiments have not reached the human phase due to a number of safety concerns. The major concerns include: (1) potential effect of vector to the host, (2) mutagenesis of the transfected gene, and (3) germ line transmission. These issues need to be addressed before such therapy can be embraced clinically.[28]

Potential Effect of Vector to the Host

Vectors being used to transfect the targeted host genes can be categorized into nonviral (i.e., guanidium-cholesterol cationic liposomes) and viral (i.e., adenovirus, retrovirus, or lentivirus). Minimally invasive introduction of these vectors to the fetus, i.e., ultrasound-guided injection or fetoscopic transplantation, can be used. The technique of delivering these vectors without harming the host is of utmost important. From the sheep model, up to 15% of fetal demise was linked to the technique of ultrasound-guided fetal injection.[29] Iatrogenic fetal infection is also not uncommon. Certain targets are more difficult to access.

For example, tracheal injection can result in bleeding complications in the thorax in 6% of the procedures.[29] Intracardiac and intravenous (umbilical) injections in the first trimester of pregnancy also have a high fetal loss rates in sheep model.[30]

Procedure-related complications are higher if the intervention is performed earlier and the target is not readily accessible, i.e., intrapulmonary or intracardiac. Fetal physiology and 'immunologic barrier' have to be taken in context with technical feasibility. Monocytes, macrophages, and NK cells are found in the circulation of human fetus as early as 13 weeks', which soon follows by a progressively increase of T lymphocytes, until 'fetal immunologic barrier' is completed at 18 weeks'.[31] This knowledge suggests that the gene transfection has to be succeeded before particular fetal age. Yet, it has to be balanced with higher procedure-related complications in earlier gestational age.

Mutagenesis of the Transfected Gene

Due to the complexity of gene expression for physiologic organ formation and function, there is a concern that the transfected gene products, or the vector even, can interfere with this developmental cascade. There was evidence from an experiment of in-utero transfection of cystic fibrosis rat with human cystic fibrosis transmembrane receptor gene, using adenovirus as a vector. Significant alterations of fetal lung development, in both anatomical and functional aspects, were observed.[32] While the primary objective of in-utero gene therapy to improve the ciliary function and mucoid secretion in bronchiole of cystic fibrosis rat can be achieved, the collateral effects of a transgenic protein on developmental process of other organs may not be predictable. Transfecting the same target with the same therapeutic gene and the same vector may yield different clinical outcomes if the timing in gestation at the time of introduction is different. This example re-iterates an importance of developing a very stringent protocol, should in-utero gene therapy be practice in human subjects. Long-term monitoring of the clinical outcomes is also mandatory.

Insertional Mutagenesis

Is an established phenomenon. The report of this serious adverse event occur during gene therapy session of a child suffered from X-linked severe combined immunodeficiency (SCID) syndrome. The transgene, with retroviral vector, inserted adjacent to a potential oncogene LMO2 of hematopoietic cell line, and transcribed the products which have been linked to subsequent development of acute leukemia.[33] A number of factors have been analyzed, including type of vector, intrinsic property of the target cells, external factors such as an environment, but no definitive cause was established. Another example of insertional mutagenesis is an observation of high postnatal incidence of liver tumors in the rat born after in-utero treatment with equine infectious anemia virus (EIAV).[34] Apparently, more works are needed in order to clearly understand the relationship between the transgene, the vector, and the target cells in order to reassure the safety of in utero gene therapy.

Germ-line Transmission

By current regulations from professional and ethical organizations, experiments on in utero gene therapy have to exclusively be targeting at somatic cell line. In-utero gene therapy is aiming at that particular fetus, and not at transferring these transgene to the generations to come. However, inadvertent transfer of transgene to fetal or maternal germ-line is possible in theory.[35] In human fetus, gonadal compartmentalization of primordial germ cells is completed by 7 weeks of gestation, and any transfection after this should not transduce the fetal germ-line. Transduction of maternal germ-line should even be less likely, due to the presence of blood-follicle barrier and meiotic metaphase arrest of the eggs until fertilization. A reasonable amount of data from primate animal studies confirmed an absence of fetal or maternal germ-line transduction after fetal gene therapy.[36,37]

CONCLUSION

In recent years, there has been dramatic progress in the technologies available for prenatal diagnosis. With the ability to analyze fetal DNA and fetal cells in maternal peripheral blood, progress with molecular diagnosis of genetic disease, microarray techniques and completion of the human genome project, it is likely that in the near future a majority of human genetic diseases will be diagnosed in early pregnancy. The increased availability of prenatal diagnosis at an early gestational age makes prenatal treatment for several diseases an interesting possibility.[38] When considering diseases that can be lethal or causing irreversible organ damage before birth, this approach seems even more compelling.[39]

In-utero stem cell transplantation and gene therapy provide an alternative option to parents following prenatal diagnosis of inherited disease of serious postnatal clinical consequences. The traditional choices are either termination of pregnancy, which may not be legally or ethically acceptable to either personal or social level, or accepting an affected child that may have a lifelong disability. It is important for the counselor to address the benefits and limitations of these three options in an unbiased fashion. Written informed consent is mandatory in this complex counseling and decision-making process.

Termination of pregnancy is always effective, and is reasonably safe for the mother. Parents who choose to keep the affected baby need to be fully aware of the financial and emotional burdens that will incur on their family, according to the nature of the disease. Social support system should be sought well in advanced. For parents who are interested in fetal therapy, they have to realize that both in-utero stem cell transplantation and gene therapy are still considered highly investigational, unlike termination of pregnancy and expectant management which are considered a standard of care. While the real benefits and long-term outcomes of in-utero genetic treatments are still uncertain, the procedure itself poses some risks of infection, immune reactions, miscarriage, and preterm delivery for the fetus. There is a small, but real, chance of iatrogenic complications to the mother that may impact her future fertility. The 'right of the fetus' has to be exercised in a balanced context with the 'autonomy' of the mother, under legal and religious umbrella of each community. It will take more time, efforts, and funding, before in-utero stem cell transplantation and gene therapy are as effective, reliable, and safe enough to be routinely offered at the same leverage with the previous two options.

In fact, a more appropriate and more effective approach to reduce fetal and neonatal morbidities from serious genetic diseases should be an implementation of comprehensive premarital and prenatal screening policy for common genetic disorders, i.e., thalassemia or cystic fibrosis. Any couples who plan to have a baby should have an access for the carrier screening to know their status. Or they may know their risk from having a previous affected child or from their familial knowledge of certain genetic inheritance. If carrier status is a common knowledge to all the couples, then they will have broader options such as early prenatal diagnosis, followed by early treatment or early fetal intervention, or they can choose to have pre-implantation genetic diagnosis (PGD).

REFERENCES

1. Flake AW, Zanjani ED. In utero hematopoietic stem cell transplantation: ontogenic opportunities and biologic barriers. Blood. 1999;94:2179-91.
2. Touraine JL, Raudrant D, Royo C, et al. In-utero transplantation of stem cells in bare lymphocyte syndrome. Lancet. 1989;1:1382.
3. Flake AW, Roncarolo MG, Puck JM, et al. Treatment of X-linked severe combined immunodeficiency by in utero transplantation of paternal bone marrow. N Engl J Med. 1996;335:1806-10.
4. Westgren M, Ringden O, Bartmann P, et al. Prenatal T-cell reconstitution after in utero transplantation with fetal liver cells in a patient with X-linked severe combined immunodeficiency. Am J Obstet Gynecol. 2002;187: 475-82.
5. Burt RK. Clinical utility in maximizing CD34+ cell count in stem cell grafts. Stem Cells. 1999;17:373-6.
6. Billingham RE, Brent L, Medawar PB. 'Actively acquired tolerance' of foreign cells. 1953. Transplantation. 2003;76:1409-12.
7. Clerici M, DePalma L, Roilides E, Baker R, Shearer GM. Analysis of T helper and antigen-presenting cell functions in cord blood and peripheral blood leukocytes from healthy children of different ages. The Journal of Clinical Investigation. 1993;91:2829-36.
8. Uksila J, Lassila O, Hirvonen T, Toivanen P. Development of natural killer cell function in the human fetus. Journal of Immunology. 1983;130:153-6.
9. Thilaganathan B, Abbas A, Nicolaides KH. Fetal blood natural killer cells in human pregnancy. Fetal Diagn Ther. 1993;8:149-53.
10. Wengler GS, Lanfranchi A, Frusca T, et al. In-utero transplantation of parental CD34 haematopoietic progenitor cells in a patient with X-linked severe combined immunodeficiency (SCIDXI). Lancet. 1996;348:1484-7.
11. Mari G, Deter RL, Carpenter RL, et al. Noninvasive diagnosis by Doppler ultrasonography of fetal anemia due to maternal red-cell alloimmunization. Collaborative Group for Doppler Assessment of the Blood Velocity in Anemic Fetuses. N Engl J Med. 2000;342:9-14.
12. Wataganara T, Wiwanichayakul B, Ruengwuttilert P, Sunsaneevithayakul P, Viboonchart S, Wantanasiri C. Noninvasive diagnosis of fetal anemia and fetal intravascular transfusion therapy: experiences at Siriraj Hospital. J Med Assoc Thai. 2006;89:1036-43.
13. Renaud A, Aucourt J, Weill J, et al. Radiographic features of osteogenesis imperfecta. Insights into imaging 2013;4: 417-29.
14. Schramm T, Gloning KP, Minderer S, et al. Prenatal sonographic diagnosis of skeletal dysplasias. Ultrasound in obstetrics & gynecology: the official journal of the International Society of Ultrasound in Obstetrics and Gynecology 2009;34:160-70.

15. Ablin DS, Greenspan A, Reinhart M, Grix A. Differentiation of child abuse from osteogenesis imperfecta. AJR American Journal of Roentgenology. 1990;154:1035-46.
16. Rauch F, Glorieux FH. Osteogenesis imperfecta. Lancet. 2004;363:1377-85.
17. Le Blanc K, Gotherstrom C, Ringden O, et al. Fetal mesenchymal stem-cell engraftment in bone after in utero transplantation in a patient with severe osteogenesis imperfecta. Transplantation. 2005;79:1607-14.
18. Tiblad E, Westgren M. Fetal stem-cell transplantation. Best Pract Res Clin Obstet Gynaecol. 2008;22:189-201.
19. Wataganara T, Sutanthavibool A, Limwongse C. Real-time three dimensional sonographic features of an early third trimester fetus with achondrogenesis. J Med Assoc Thai. 2006;89:1762-5.
20. Lee HS, Doh JW, Kim CJ, Chi JG. Achondrogenesis type II (Langer-Saldino achondrogenesis): a case report. Journal of Korean Medical Science. 2000;15:604-8.
21. Wilson JM, Wivel NA. Potential risk of inadvertent germ-line gene transmission statement from the American Society of Gene Therapy to the NIH Recombinant DNA Advisory Committee, March 12, 1999. Human gene therapy 1999;10:1593-5.
22. Waddington SN, Nivsarkar MS, Mistry AR, et al. Permanent phenotypic correction of hemophilia B in immunocompetent mice by prenatal gene therapy. Blood. 2004;104:2714-21.
23. Lipshutz GS, Sarkar R, Flebbe-Rehwaldt L, Kazazian H, Gaensler KM. Short-term correction of factor VIII deficiency in a murine model of hemophilia A after delivery of adenovirus murine factor VIII in utero. Proceedings of the National Academy of Sciences of the United States of America. 1999;96:13324-9.
24. Furie B, Limentani SA, Rosenfield CG. A practical guide to the evaluation and treatment of hemophilia. Blood. 1994;84:3-9.
25. Soucie JM, Nuss R, Evatt B, et al. Mortality among males with hemophilia: relations with source of medical care. The Hemophilia Surveillance System Project Investigators. Blood. 2000;96:437-42.
26. Manno CS, Chew AJ, Hutchison S, et al. AAV-mediated factor IX gene transfer to skeletal muscle in patients with severe hemophilia B. Blood. 2003;101:2963-72.
27. Manno CS, Pierce GF, Arruda VR, et al. Successful transduction of liver in hemophilia by AAV-Factor IX and limitations imposed by the host immune response. Nature Medicine. 2006;12:342-7.
28. Fletcher JC, Richter G. Human fetal gene therapy: moral and ethical questions. Human Gene Therapy. 1996;7:1605-14.
29. David AL, Weisz B, Gregory L, et al. Ultrasound-guided injection and occlusion of the trachea in fetal sheep. Ultrasound in obstetrics & gynecology: the official journal of the International Society of Ultrasound in Obstetrics and Gynecology. 2006;28:82-8.
30. David AL, Peebles DM, Gregory L, et al. Percutaneous ultrasound-guided injection of the trachea in fetal sheep: a novel technique to target the fetal airways. Fetal Diagn Ther. 2003;18:385-90.
31. Pahal GS, Jauniaux E, Kinnon C, Thrasher AJ, Rodeck CH. Normal development of human fetal hematopoiesis between eight and seventeen weeks of gestation. Am J Obstet Gynecol. 2000;183:1029-34.
32. Morrow SL, Larson JE, Nelson S, Sekhon HS, Ren T, Cohen JC. Modification of development by the CFTR gene in utero. Mol Genet Metab. 1998;65:203-12.
33. Hacein-Bey-Abina S, von Kalle C, Schmidt M, et al. A serious adverse event after successful gene therapy for X-linked severe combined immunodeficiency. N Engl J Med. 2003;348:255-6.
34. Themis M, Waddington SN, Schmidt M, et al. Oncogenesis following delivery of a nonprimate lentiviral gene therapy vector to fetal and neonatal mice. Molecular therapy: the journal of the American Society of Gene Therapy. 2005;12:763-71.
35. Billings PR. In utero gene therapy: the case against. Nature Medicine. 1999;5:255-6.
36. Tran ND, Porada CD, Zhao Y, Almeida-Porada G, Anderson WF, Zanjani ED. In utero transfer and expression of exogenous genes in sheep. Experimental Hematology 2000;28:17-30.
37. Larson JE, Morrow SL, Delcarpio JB, et al. Gene transfer into the fetal primate: evidence for the secretion of transgene product. Molecular therapy: the Journal of the American Society of Gene Therapy. 2000;2:631-9.
38. Harrison MR, Golbus MS, Filly RA. Management of the fetus with a correctable congenital defect. Jama. 1981;246:774-7.
39. Harrison MR, Filly RA, Golbus MS, et al. Fetal treatment 1982. N Engl J Med. 1982;307:1651-2.

46

CHAPTER

Fetoscopic Interventions

Tuangsit Wataganara

INTRODUCTION

In-utero surgical interventions can be offered in selected cases of twin-to-twin transfusion syndrome (TTTS), congenital diaphragmatic hernia, and other few selected conditions. Randomized controlled trial has shown a clear benefit of laser photocoagulation of chorionic anastomosing vessels in severe TTTS, therefore, the treatment has become a standard of treatment in many places. A significant development in videoendoscopic surgical system has dropped the sizes of lenses, visual systems, and instruments for the purpose of performing in-utero procedures, so called 'fetoscopic intervention'. With this purpose-design surgical equipment, broader indications for fetoscopic surgery have been explored in other conditions, such as amniotic band sequence, posterior urethral valves, and myelomeningocele. However, the evidence for genuine benefits of fetoscopic interventions in the latter conditions is still limited, and conduction of good quality prospective randomized trials for these conditions may not be easy due to rarity of the diseases. This chapter is aiming to describe the latest knowledge in the pathophysiology and treatment approach of three main fetal conditions amendable for fetoscopic interventions: severe TTTS and complicated monochorionic twins, severe congenital diaphragmatic hernia, and lower urinary tract obstruction. Novel techniques for in-utero endoscopic surgery are continuously reported and tested. It is expected that perinatal outcomes will improve with accumulating experiences. Although the maternal morbidity associated with fetoscopy is low, preterm rupture of membranes and preterm delivery remain an important problem. Long-term evaluation of those neonates remains mandatory.

PRINCIPLES OF FETOSCOPY

Traditionally, fetal surgery was performed through a large incision at the uterus (hysterotomy), so called open fetal surgery. Later on, endoscopic surgery has been tremendously developed. It has been replacing many traditional surgical procedures due to its less invasiveness. The advent of better and smaller lenses, development of high-definition camera and visual system, and accumulating experiences of the surgeons, has brought videoendoscopic to the field of fetal intervention. An access to the fetus can now be achieved through a tiny puncture into the amniotic cavity.

Fetoscopic approach has following advantages over traditional open fetal surgery:[1]

- Fetoscopic approach can reduce the chance of preterm labor. Preterm labor is believed to be triggered by the large uterine incision of open fetal surgery.
- Fetoscopic approach can reduce significant maternal morbidity associated with a large laparotomy.

Standardized pre- and postoperative care of pregnant women undergoing fetoscopic intervention has not been established yet. There is a significant variation from one center to another. Generally, preoperative preparation includes premedication with tocolytic agent and broad-spectrum antibiotics. At Faculty of Medicine Siriraj Hospital, we use nifedipine 10 milligrams with 30 milliliters of water taken between 30 minutes to 1 hour prior to the surgery. Intravenous second-generation cephalosporin is used at our center to prevent procedure-related intra-amniotic infection.

The most commonly used anesthetic method is local anesthesia combined with intravenous sedation. Certain intravenous sedative substances are preferred over the others when it comes to fetoscopic intervention, which require simultaneous maternal and fetal effects. For example, remifentanil has been tested against diazepam in a randomized controlled trial for their fetal and maternal effects during laser surgery for twin-twin transfusion syndrome.[2]

Remifentanil is superior to diazepam for fetal immobilization with less suppression of maternal respiration. Suppression of fetal movement can facilitate the procedure, resulting in shorter operating time. In addition, its short duration of action facilitate neonatal resuscitation, if needed. Therefore, remifentanil has become the intravenous sedative drug of choice for in utero intervention by some experienced fetal care centers.[3] General or regional anesthesia may be chosen in more complicated cases, i.e., fetal endoluminal tracheal occlusion (FETO) or ex-utero intrapartum treatment (EXIT).

EQUIPMENTS AND TECHNIQUES

The surgery can be performed in the operating theater, labor and delivery unit, or at the ultrasound suite. Fetal endoscopes have been developed based on experimental animal models. Purpose-designed embryoscopes or fetoscopes typically have remote eyepieces. This design is to reduce weight and facilitate precise movements. Semirigid lens are used liberally in this field. 'Picture-in-picture' system allows for the surgical team to see the ultrasound and fetoscopic images simultaneously.

At the beginning, ultrasound is used to identify an appropriate entry point to avoid the placenta, the fetus, and maternal organs such as bowel and bladder. Fetoscopic intervention is actually a combination between ultrasound guided and endoscopic procedures. Comparison between fetoscopy and laparoscopy is shown in **Table 1**.

Under ultrasound guidance, trocar or cannula can be inserted under direct visualization, or by Seldinger technique. There was a report from one group suggesting the safety, in their hands, of a transplacental approach.[4] Despite their published experience, most operators still attempt to avoid the placenta.

Once amniotic cavity is safely accessed, the trocar is replaced by the fetoscope. Purpose-designed fetoscopes are ranging from 20 to 30 centimeters in length, and 1.3 to 2 millimeters in outside diameter. Rod lens are used in fiberscope with a straightforward view. Angled and semirigid lens are used for better side view visualization. Curved sheaths are use to house the semirigid lens, as shown in **Figure 1**.[5] The sharpness of puncturing tools is very important to minimize amniorrhexis. At our center (Faculty of Medicine Siriraj Hospital, Bangkok, Thailand), fetoscopic interventions are performed in shared obstetrics and gynecology operating theater facility. All of the equipments are highly mobile, as shown in **Figure 2**. The fetoscopic surgical unit can be adapted to a slightly different feature of each operating theater allocated on that day.

Laser is an indispensible part for fetoscopic surgery. Basic principles of laser surgery must be understood. The procedure is performed in water medium. CO_2 medium may be used in exceptional cases, i.e., endoscopic repair of fetal meningomyelocele.[6] There are 2 kinds of laser generators being used in fetoscopic laser surgery: neodymium-yttrium aluminium garnet (Nd-YAG) and diode (semiconductor) laser. The laser generator convert electrical or chemical energy into light energy that is optimal for absorbance in the spectrum of hemoglobin.[5,7] Hemoglobin of red cells in targeted blood vessels absorbs the light, which is turned into heat that coagulates red blood cells. The heat then propagates onto the wall of blood vessels and the adjacent placental tissue. Coagulated tissue is seen as 'whitish' on real time visualization, as shown in **Figure 3**.

TABLE 1: Comparison between fetoscopy and laparoscopy.

Fetoscopy	*Laparoscopy*
• Smaller lens (1.3 to 2 mm) (limited visibility) • Ultrasound guidance ± Seldinger technique • High-protein fluid medium • Developing fetus • Single port (strategic planning for trocar insertion site)	• Larger lens (5 to 10 mm) • Direct puncture ± CO_2 insufflation • CO_2 (laparoscopy) or crystalloid (hysteroscopy) • Multiple ports (fixed anatomical landmark for trocar insertion site)

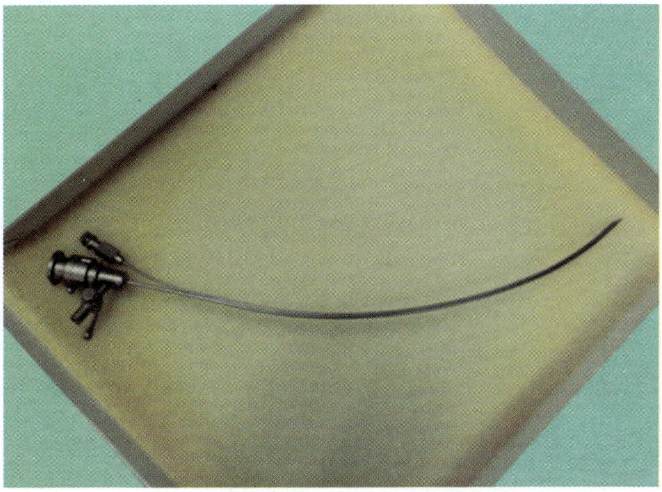

Fig. 1: Curved operating sheath that can house semirigid lens. This instrument allows for a better visualization and approach for in utero target located in difficult angle.

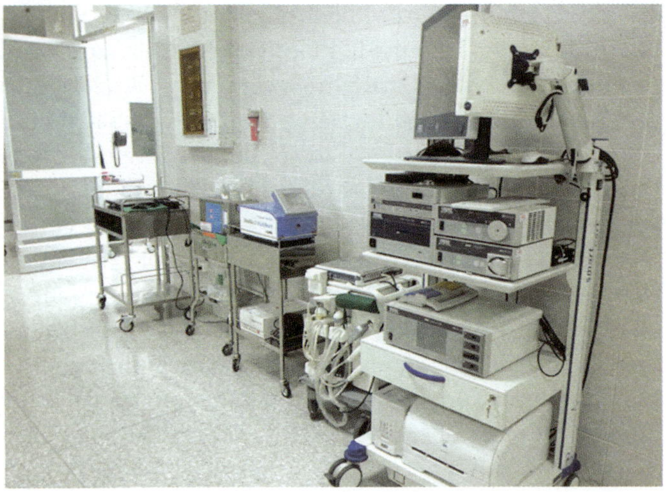

Fig. 2: Equipments of fetoscopic surgery at Faculty of Medicine Siriraj Hospital. The units are highly mobile, and readily adaptable to suit the operating theater allocated on that day. From left to right include laptop computer, warm water bath with lactate Ringer solution, Diode laser generator, compact ultrasound machine, and fetoscopic tower. The tower houses the following units (from top to bottom); touch screen (with picture-in-picture system) with internal hard disc memory system, electrical generator (for bipolar electrical diathermy), light source, pressure controlled fluid infusion pump, and printer.

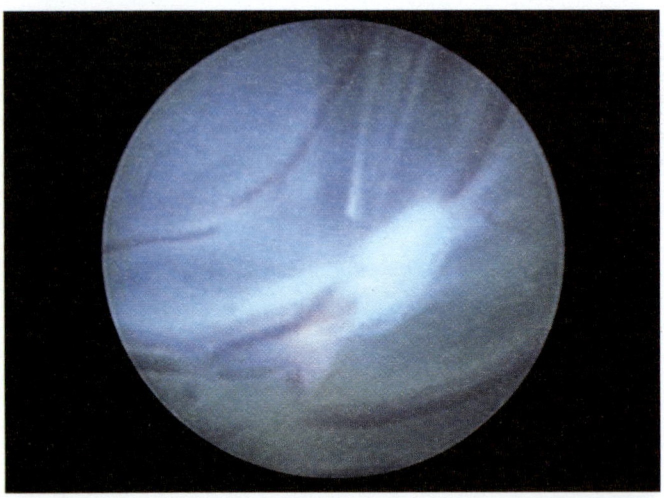

Fig. 3: An endoscopic photo showing 'whitish' coagulation effects of chorionic vessel and surrounding placental tissue from Nd:YAG laser. Size and depth of the lesion depends on the proportion of oxyhemoglobin and the wavelengths used.

Source: Division of Maternal Fetal Medicine, Faculty of Medicine Siriraj Hospital.

Nd:YAG and Diode lasers are equally efficient when tested on an ex-vivo placenta model.[7] Our center has switched from Nd:YAG to Diode laser since 2010 because of the following reasons. Theoretically, Nd:YAG wavelength (λ) is 1,064 nm, which is in infrared range. Nd:YAG is more suitable for thermal intervention, such as interstitial coagulation or ablation of intralesional (or intrafetal) blood vessels.

Diode wavelength is 800 to 980 nm. This wavelength has a high absorption rate for hemoglobin. This quality of Diode laser makes it ideal for soft tissue applications and hemostasis, which is required for coagulation of vascular anastomoses on chorionic plate. In addition, the Diode generator is smaller and cheaper compared to Nd:YAG. The laser energy is transmitted through 400- or 600-mm laser fibers. Lesions of the endothelium together with reduction of vessel lumen were best achieved with a diode laser at 40 Watts.

COMPLICATED MONOCHORIONIC TWINS

Multifetal gestation is considered high-risk. The perinatal risks in monochorionic (MC) twins are 3 to 10 times higher than dichorionic (DC) twins for several reasons.[8] In addition to an increased risk of miscarriages, preterm birth, preeclampsia, intrauterine growth restriction, and other obstetrics complications, its single, shared placenta is also pathogenic by itself. There is an ever present vascular connection between MC twins.[9] Discordance in total blood volume, red blood cell volume, and placental territory can occur, and has been linked to twin-twin transfusion syndrome (TTTS), twin anemia-polycythemia syndrome (TAPS), and selective intrauterine growth restriction (sIUGR), respectively.

Twin-twin Transfusion Syndrome (Table 2)

Twin-twin transfusion syndrome (TTTS) results from imbalance of the net blood flow, mostly from vascular anastomoses on the chorionic plate, between the MC twin pair. It can occur in 5.5 to 17.5% of MC twins.[10] If left untreated, perinatal loss in severe midtrimester TTTS (diagnosed before 26 weeks') can be as high as 80 to 100%, with a 15 to 50% chance of neurodevelopmental delay among the survivors.[4] Knowledge of placental pathology is crucial in order to understand the dynamics of TTTS, as well as to provide causative treatments. Superficial anastomoses (arterio-arterial (AA) and venovenous (VV)) are bidirectional. Deep anastomoses (arteriovenous (AV) and venoarterial (VA)) are unidirectional and lie deep within the placenta at the villous level. Vascular contributions of deep anastomoses, at some point, emerge

TABLE 2: Perinatal outcomes of severe midtrimester twin-twin transfusion syndrome after expectant management, serial amnioreduction, and laser surgery.

	Expectant	*Amnioreduction*	*Laser*
Double survivors	0–10%	26%	35%
Single survivor	0–30%	56–78%	76%
Average gestational age at delivery (weeks')	N/A	27.5–29	33.5
Complications	Cerebral palsy 15%	• PPROM 5–15% • Bleeding • Infection • Cerebral palsy 15%	• PPROM 5–15% • Bleeding • Infection

(N/A: not available; PPROM: preterm premature rupture of the membranes)
Source: Johnson et al. 2001, Senat, et al. 2004, Moise et al. 2005.

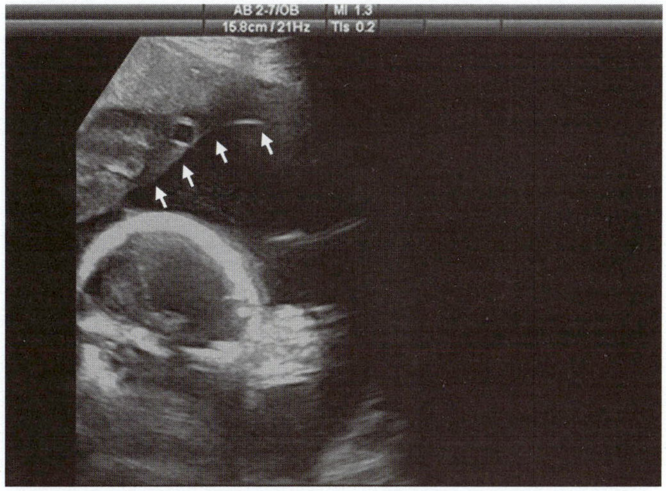

Fig. 5: Ultrasound image of monochorionic twins at 24 weeks' with twin-twin transfusion stage 1, according to Quintero's staging system. Note the oligo-polyhydramniotic sequence, and the 'bulging membranes' toward the donor sac.

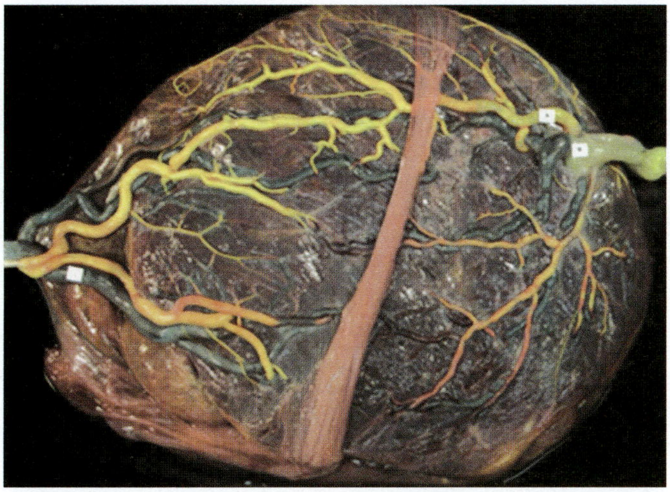

Fig. 4: Photograph of a monochorionic placenta after dye injection study. Note the arterio-arterial (AA) anastomoses (in yellow) at the upper pole of the placenta. AA anastomoses, functioning as bidirectional gradient equilibration, are thought to play protective role for twin-twin transfusion syndrome (TTTS).

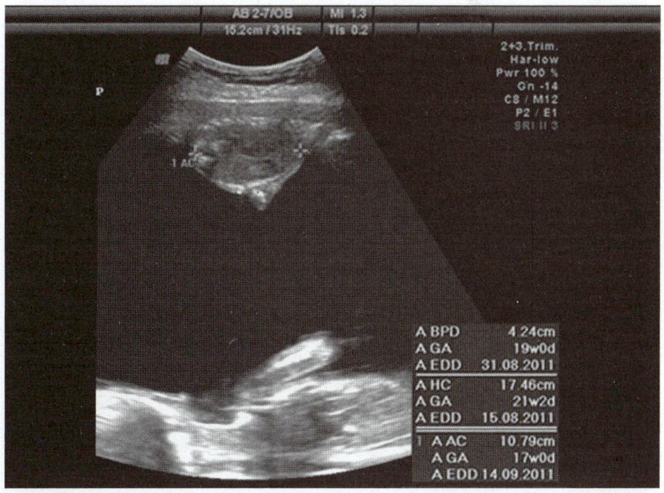

Fig. 6: Ultrasound image of monochorionic twins at 20 weeks' with twin-twin transfusion stage 2, according to Quintero's staging system. The donor sac did not have measurable amount of liquor, compared to polyhydramnios of the recipient, contributes to the 'stuck twin' appearance of the donor.

and run on chorionic surface, and are subjected to be identified and ablated under direct visualization.

TTTS is caused by the relative excess of AV anastomoses.[11] AA anastomoses, as shown in **Figure 4**, maintain the pressure gradient equilibrium between 2 circulations in MC placentas. Reduction of AA anastomoses may increase the chance of developing TTTS.[12] When TTTS develops, the donor twin becomes hypovolemic, oliguric, and oligohydramnios. Dry liquor volume in donor sac makes the fetus appeared 'stuck'. Hypervolemia triggers polyuria and polyhydramnios in the recipient. The recipient eventually will develop high-output cardiac failure and hydrops. TTTS can be categorized according to its ultrasound findings at the time of diagnosis, as proposed by Ruben Quintero and colleagues in 1999, as shown in **Figures 5 to 8.**[13]

At Faculty of Medicine Siriraj Hospital, staging of TTTS based on fetal cardiac performance, as proposed by Fetal Care Center of Cincinnati, is incorporated with the traditional Quintero's staging.[14] This combined staging

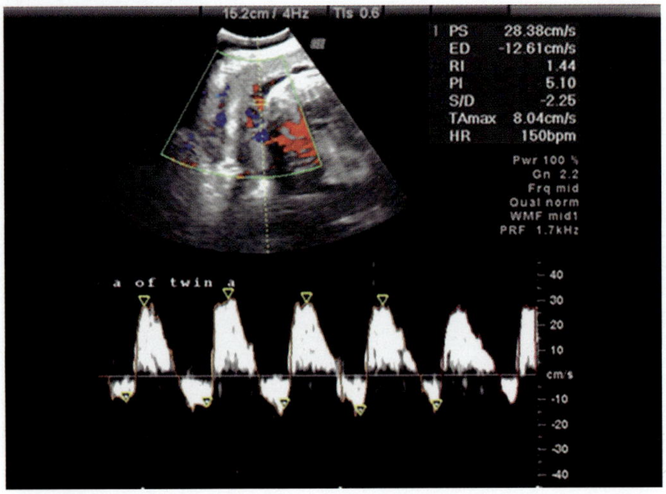

Fig. 7: Ultrasound image of monochorionic twins at 20 weeks' with twin-twin transfusion stage 3, according to Quintero's staging system. Note the reversed end-diastolic flow in umbilical artery of the donor.

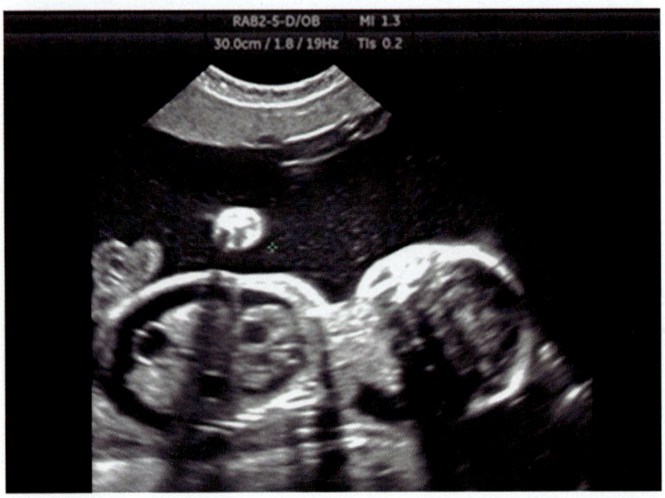

Fig. 8: Ultrasound image of monochorionic twins at 22 weeks' with twin-twin transfusion stage 4, according to Quintero's staging system. Note that the recipient fetus developed hydrops. This is a critical finding, and intervention shall be offered without delay.

TABLE 3: Staging of TTTS: Combination of ultrasound- and fetal cardiac performance-based categorization.

Stage	*Findings*
1	Oligo-polyhydramniotic sequence • Donor DVP <2 cm • Recipient DVP >8 cm at less than 20 weeks' or >10 cm at over 20 weeks'
2	Bladder of the donor is not visible throughout the examination (anhydramnios, 'stuck' twin)
3	Abnormal fetal Doppler studies (at least one) • Absent or reversed end-diastolic flow of umbilical artery • Pulsation in umbilical vein • Reversed a wave in ductus venosus
3A	Abnormal fetal Doppler studies plus at least one of the following cardiac findings of mild cardiomyopathy • Myocardium performance index (MPI or Tei index) of right ventricle >0.5 • Myocardium performance index (MPI or Tei index) of left ventricle >0.42 • Mild ventricular hypertrophy • Mild atrioventricular valve regurgitation
3B	Abnormal fetal Doppler studies plus at least one of the following cardiac findings of moderate cardiomyopathy • Myocardium performance index (MPI or Tei index) of right ventricle >0.56 • Myocardium performance index (MPI or Tei index) of left ventricle >0.53 • Moderate ventricular hypertrophy • Moderate atrioventricular valve regurgitation
3C	Abnormal fetal Doppler studies plus at least one of the following cardiac findings of severe cardiomyopathy • Severe atrioventricular valve regurgitation • Other findings of severe cardiomyopathy
4	Hydrops (either donor or recipient fetus)
5	Demise (either donor or recipient fetus)

system, as shown in **Table 3**, allows for a more detailed categorization of prognosis, especially the survival after laser treatment. Aside from expectant management, treatment options that have undergone rigorous clinical validation and randomized controlled trials are serial amnioreduction, septostomy, and laser photocoagulation of chorionic anastomoses.

Serial amnioreduction used to be the primary treatment of severe midtrimester TTTS. It was suggested that improved placental perfusion following decreased placental resistance with reduction of intra-amniotic pressure is likely to play a key role in the process of mobilizing extravascular fluid towards maternal circulation. It can alleviate maternal symptoms and prolong pregnancy.[15]

Amnioreduction has the advantage of being a simple and inexpensive procedure. It requires minimal skills for ultrasound guidance procedure. At Faculty of Medicine Siriraj Hospital, we use an 18-gauge spinal needle to drain the fluid using vacuum suction until deepest vertical pool is down to 4 to 6 cms, as shown in **Figure 9**. Alternatively, the fluid can be drained slowly by gravitational force.

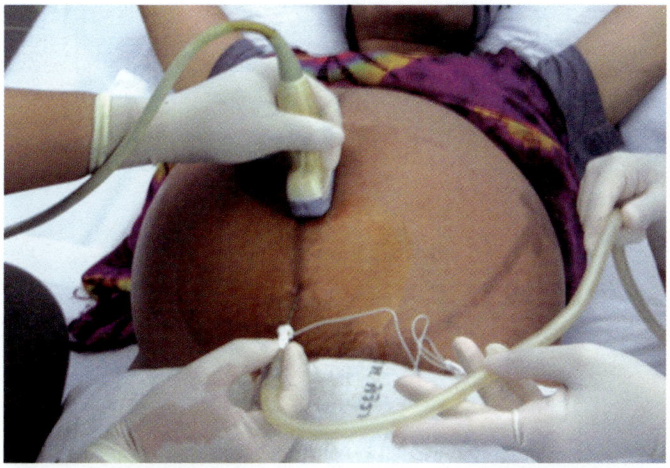

Fig. 9: Photograph of serial amnioreduction in a pregnant woman with Quintero's stage 1 twin-twin transfusion syndrome at 26 weeks'. Note that ultrasound was used to guide the safe entry into amniotic sac of the recipient. Ultrasound monitoring of liquor volume and fetal heart beat activity was carried out until deepest vertical pool of recipient sac reaches 4 to 6 cms, and the needle was removed. Note that the hub of needle is connected to wall suction with surgical suction tube.

Neonatal survival of severe midtrimester TTTS treated with serial amnioreduction is 56 to 78%.[16,17] However, over 80% of the cases required repeated tapping due to rapid reaccumulation of amniotic fluid.[18] This increases risk of preterm premature rupture of the membranes (PPROM) and placental abruption to 15 to 20%.[19] If one of the fetus dies, agonal hypotension can occur in the remaining fetus, which explains a 30% incidence of cerebral palsy in its co-twin.[20]

Septostomy is an ultrasound guided intentional puncture of intervening twin membrane with a small (20 to 22 G) spinal needle, with or without an attempt of amnioreduction. Its goal is to equalize intra-amniotic pressure between the donor and recipient sacs, and to increase perfusion to the donor fetus.[21] Initial experience showed an impressive live birth rate of 83% in MC twins with oligo-polyhydramnios sequence treated with this modality.[21]

The major advantage of septostomy is that it is a single procedure, unlike amnioreduction. Septostomy was then adopted. Small retrospective cohort comparing perinatal outcomes of 14 TTTS cases underwent serial amnioreduction (n = 7) and septostomy (n = 7) showed an equal overall number of survivors (78%) in both groups, eventhough the septostomy group had a significant prolongation of pregnancy (procedure-to-delivery interval of 12 weeks' in septostomy and 6.5 weeks' in amnioreduction group).[22] A randomized controlled trial involving 73 pregnant women showed neonatal survival rates of 80 and 78% in septostomy and amnioreduction groups, respectively ($P = 0.82$).[17] Although overall perinatal survival is not enhanced, patient undergoing septostomy were more likely to require a single procedure for treatment (64% vs. 46%; $P = .04$).[17]

Septostomy has not been well-adopted due to some theoretical criticisms. It is not a causative treatment. The iatrogenic pseudomonoamniotic may result in amniotic band sequence and cord entanglement. The follow up and subsequent laser surgery, if needed, will be more challenging due to an obstructive view from the torn intervening membrane. With all these possible consequences, septostomy has been discouraged from routine clinical practice.

Laser photocoagulation of intertwin anastomoses has become a standard of treatment for severe midtrimester TTTS. The original technique of laser photocoagulation of chorionic anastomoses was described by Julian De Lia and colleagues in 1990.[23] It underwent a significant modification in terms of invasiveness, selectivity, order of coagulation, and completeness of dichorionization.[24-26] Laser coagulation of the anastomoses addresses the underlying pathophysiology of TTTS.

Technical Aspect

Preoperative evaluation consists of a detailed ultrasound examination that includes morphological examination; fetal Doppler evaluation and cardiothoracic index; and location of the placenta, cord insertions, fetal parts and major maternal vessels. Prophylactic antibiotics and tocolysis are administered before laser surgery. Typically, procedures are done under strict aseptic conditions. Local anesthesia is 1% xylocaine without adrenaline injected down to the myometrium. A 2-mm skin incision is made and the trocar is inserted into the amniotic sac of the recipient under continuous ultrasound guidance. The endoscope then replaces the sharp trocar within the introductory sheath. The endoscopes are semi-flexible fiber-endoscopes of either 1.2 mm or 2.0 mm in diameter, with a 0 degree direction of view and an opening angle of 70–80 L. Sheaths can be carefully bent to up to 20 to 35° from the midline axis to provide appropriate curvature also for anterior placentas. This should be done without the endoscope inside.

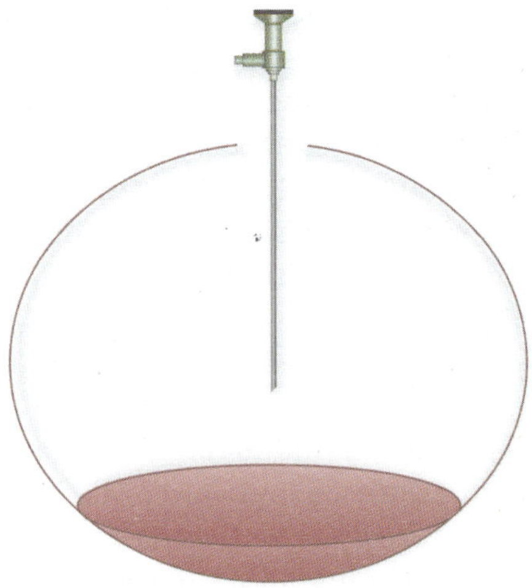

Fig. 10: It is desirable to keep the direction of the scope at entry to be perpendicular to the virtual line joining the 2 cord insertions. This will enhance the chance of visualize the vascular equator in relation to the equator of intervening membranes.

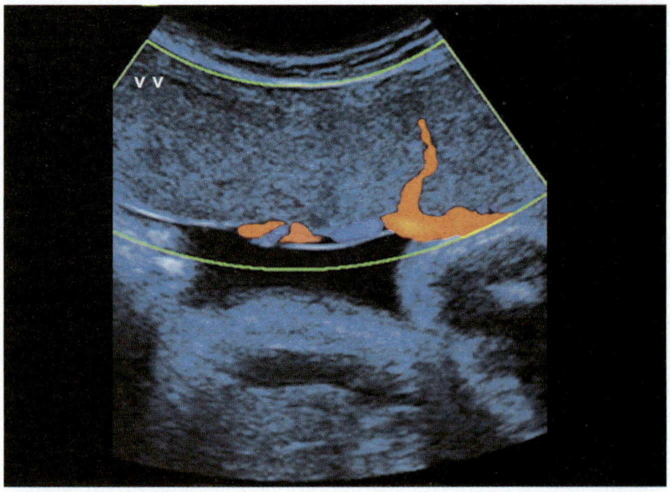

Fig. 11: Identification of arteriovenous anastomosis of in twin-twin transfusion syndrome using an ultrasound examination. Note that this unidirectional anastomosis is deep underneath, but is superficial portions can be identified by direct visualization from fetoscopic examination, and coagulated by laser photocoagulation.

Ideally, the scope should be directed at a 90° to the intertwin membranes, which shall be juxtaposed to the vascular equator. A 3-mm trocar that will house the fetoscope is entered into the recipient's polyhydramniotic sac and directed at right angles to the donor's longitudinal axis. This approach can minimize the movement of scope and trocar during the exploration of chorionic anastomoses. It is desirable to keep the direction of the scope at entry to follow the virtual line joining the 2 cord insertions, as shown in **Figure 10**. This will enhance the chance of visualize the vascular equator in relation to the equator of intervening membranes.

Injection of local anesthesia, such as 1% xylocaine or 1% lidocaine, is used from the skin all the way down to the myometrium. A small skin incision is performed, then the trocar is inserted percutaneously under real-time ultrasound guidance. Some operators may prefer to use silastic cannula and Seldinger technique in addition to this step. Traversing through the placenta should be avoided. After the trocar is in, amniotic fluid is collected. The fluid is sent for chromosome study or additional tests as needed. Being able to freely draw the amniotic fluid also ensure the entrance of amniotic cavity.

The goal of surgical intervention is to ablate all vascular anastomoses between the fetuses, as shown in **Figure 11**. These anastomoses should run on the chorionic surface, and can be categorized as AA, VV, AV, and VA anastomoses, as alluded to in the previous section. The artery is darker and always run over the vein, as shown in **Figure 12**. Identification of these anastomoses, as well as developing the skill to maneuver the instruments appropriately requires training. Our team at Faculty of Medicine Siriraj Hospital has developed a proprietary phantom to enhance the learning experience of the surgeon, as shown in **Figure 13**. The author has described more details about this training strategy in

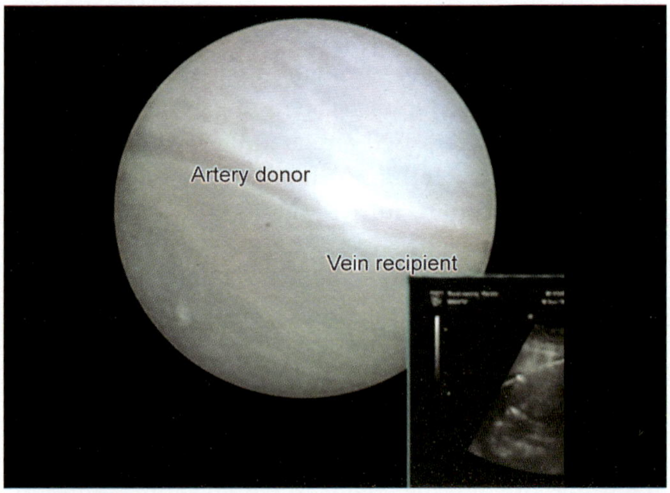

Fig. 12: Endoscopic appearance of arteriovenous anastomosis (superficial portions). Note that the fetal artery (from the donor) is darker, compared to the fetal vein (to the recipient) is brighter. This is pathogenic anastomosis contributing to the occurrence of twin-twin transfusion syndrome. It needs to be ablated with laser photocoagulation.

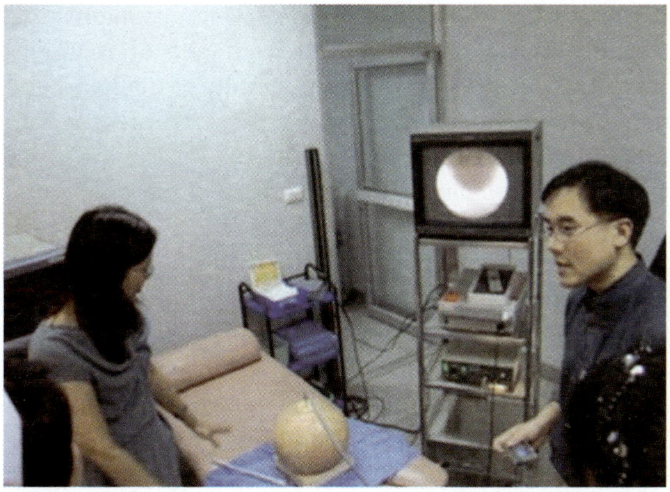

Fig. 13: Learning strategy for fetoscopic interventions using surgical simulator (phantom) at Faculty of Medicine Siriraj Hospital, Bangkok, Thailand.

2013.[27] Visualization of vascular anatomy on the chorionic surface depends of placental location, fetal position, and transparency of the amniotic fluid and the membranes.

In terms of coagulation techniques, the laser beam is fired with non-touch technique to cover 1 to 2 centimeters segment of the targeted vessel until complete cessation of flow is accomplished. It is important to keep the angle of laser beam to be as perpendicular as possible to the target, in order to maximize the laser effect.[5,7,28] Fetal movement, maternal breathing movement, or transmission of maternal aortic pulse can affect the accuracy of laser shot. Fetal immobilization, i.e., with intravenous remifentanil, may help reducing fetal movement, and thus facilitate the procedure.[29]

Rupture of large vessels during laser coagulation is not uncommon. This can be catastrophic. The visibility can suddenly drop. Fetal exanguination can result in demise of both twins. Vessels of higher flow can be coagulated from sideway at the beginning to prevent the rupture. "Double lumen technique" has been described by putting some pressure on the vessel with the trocar to decrease blood flow during the coagulation. Particularly, when the placenta is anterior, access through anterior abdominal wall becomes more difficult. To overcome this obstacle, instrumental designs with curved scopes, deflecting mechanisms, and side-firing fibers have been developed.[30-32] Posterior uterine access through maternal laparotomy has been reported.[33] It was replaced by laparoscopic assistance technique to access the uterus from the back.[34] However, to date, there is no consensus on the best technique for cases with an anterior placenta.

There is also continuing debate on the selection and order in which the chorionic plate vessels should be coagulated. When Julian De Lia and colleagues first photocoagulated vessels, they chose those which appeared suspicious of being anastomoses.[23] This technique was operator-dependent and difficult to reproduce because of the lack of distinct anatomical landmarks for distinguishing anastomoses. Coagulation of all vessels crossing the dividing membranes, so called non-selective technique, has been adopted in many places due to a better reproducibility.[26] Non-selective technique has significant disadvantage of excessive placental infarction. Our team has shown that an elevation of cell-free fetal DNA in maternal circulation, which may be related to degree of ischemic infarction of the placenta, can be predictive of postprocedural fetal demise.[35]

Because the intervening membranes, or membranes equator, is pushed toward the placental territory of the donor, its anatomical location bears very little relationship to the actual distribution of the vascular equator of both twins.[36,37] Identification of the anastomoses led to a more selective approach to coagulate only the vessels involved in blood exchange between the fetuses.[36] Selective approach can help sparing vessels crossing the membrane but that could not be identified as not anastomosing with vessels of the cotwin. This treatment addresses the underlying pathophysiology by disrupting the vascular anastomoses and thus, eliminating intertwin transfusion, resulting in a causal treatment and not just the symptomatic treatment offered by amnioreduction or septostomy.

After successful ablation, the endoscope is withdrawn and the polyhydramnios drained through the cannula under ultrasound guidance. Once the fluid has reached a normal level (deepest vertical pocket of around 5 to 6 cm) the cannula is removed. This amnioreduction reduces the risk of port-site leaking and amniotic fluid irritation of the peritoneal cavity, which may be painful. It may also improve placental perfusion, but regardless, makes the patient more comfortable. In many cases, little or no tocolytic medication is needed, and patients are generally discharged within 24 hours or less of the procedure.

Laser photocoagulation of the anastomosing vessels is the causative treatment for severe TTTS.[38] It can increase neonatal survival to 76%, compared to the neonatal survival rate of 56% after serial amnioreduction.[16] It can also reduce the chance of neonatal handicap as a result of single fetal demise to 11%.[39] This figure is almost equivalent to the incidence of neurological handicap in dichorionic twins of 7%.[40] Iatrogenic rupture of the membranes remains an Achilles heel of fetoscopic surgery, which limits the total success of the diagnostic or therapeutic fetoscopic interventions. Development of adhesive substances to seal small membrane defect have been ongoing.[41] If it is successful, the application of fetoscopic intervention may be broader, and the success rate may be increased.[42]

Twins Reversed Arterial Perfusion Sequence

Twins reversed arterial perfusion sequence (TRAPs) is a rare and severe complication of monochorionic twin placentations. It occurs when the heart of a normal appearing twin serves as the pump for one or more dysmorphic twins. These dysmorphic fetuses have head, thoracic organs, and upper extremities that do not fully develop or do not develop at all. These anomalies are related to secondary atrophy as a result of reversed transfusion of deoxygenated blood from the pump fetus. These fetuses do not have cardiac activity, and hence is commonly called as acardiac fetus. An ultrasound appearance and gross finding of anomalous fetus in TRAPs is shown in **Figures 14 and 15**.

Acardiac twinning affects 1 in 100 monozygotic twin pregnancies and 1 in 35,000 pregnancies overall.[43] There is no familial inheritance. There are 2 major proposed theories for embryopathogenesis of TRAPs. The first theory is that primary cardioembryopathy of the acardiac fetus. The second theory is an abnormal vascular communication between the embryos in the placenta with arterial-to-arterial communication leading to the hemodynamically disadvantaged or recipient twin. This results in secondary atrophy of the heart and dependent organs.[44] An acardiac twin can present with four morphological types:

1. *Acardius anephus:* This is the most commonly found type of TRAPs. There is absence of the head and upper torso and limbs in the acardiac twin with preservation of the lower limbs, genitalia and abdominal viscera.
2. *Acardius anceps:* This is the most developed type of TRAPs. There are rudimentary cranial structures present with otherwise persistent trunk, limbs and organs. However, it still lacks of rudimentary heart.
3. *Acardius amorphous:* This is the least differentiated type of acardiac fetus. It comprises of an amorphous mass of bone, muscle, fat and connective tissue. If rudimentary nerve tissue is present, it is then called acardius myelantencephalus.
4. *Acardius acormus:* This is the rarest type. The only developed structure is the fetal head. All other structures are essentially absent. The umbilical cord insertion is directly into the fetal head pathologically, rudiments of thoracic structures may be present.

Sonographic features of TRAPs can be varied according to each subtype. General features include discordance in fetal shape and size, marked fetal edema (anasarca), and normal or accelerated growth of lower extremities. Umbilical cord to the acardiac twin is often quite short and may be difficult to identify. Single umbilical artery can be found in 66% of the cases.[43] The most important finding is reversed flow in the umbilical artery of the acardiac

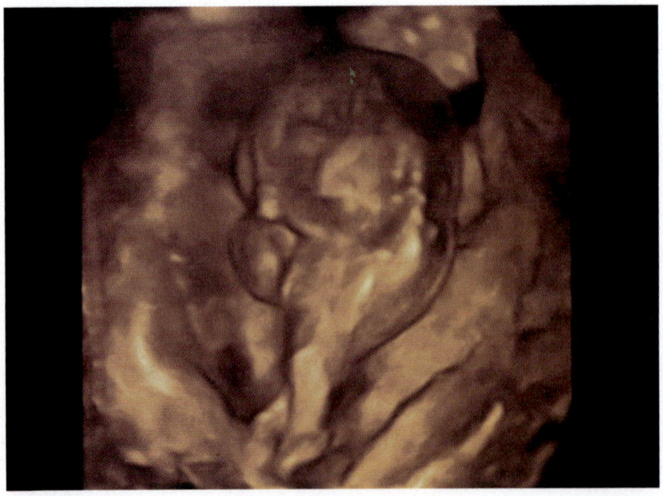

Fig. 14: Three-dimensional ultrasound appearance of acardiac fetus in twin reversed arterial perfusion sequence (TRAPs).

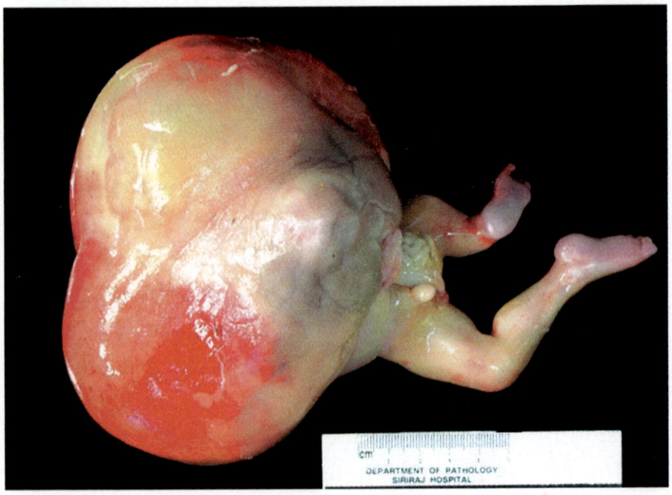

Fig. 15: Gross appearance of acardiac fetus in twins reversed arterial perfusion sequence (TRAPs).

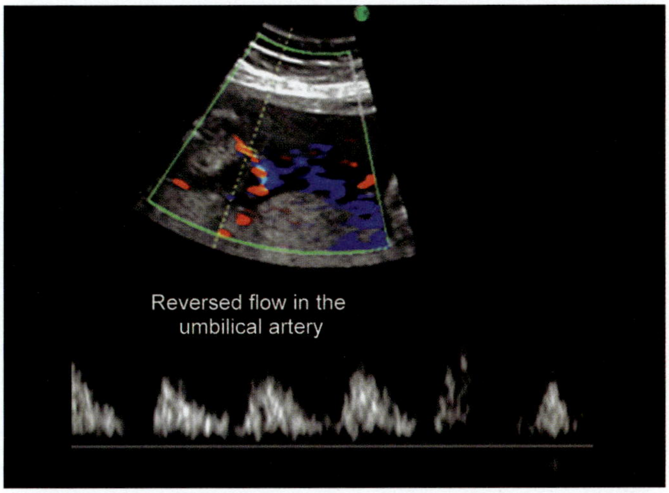

Fig. 16: Pulse-wave Doppler of the umbilical artery of the acardiac fetus in twin reversed arterial perfusion sequence (TRAPs). Note that the direction of arterial pulsatile blood flow toward the acardiac fetus, which is 'reversed' from the nature of fetal artery, which should have had the direction outward from the fetus.

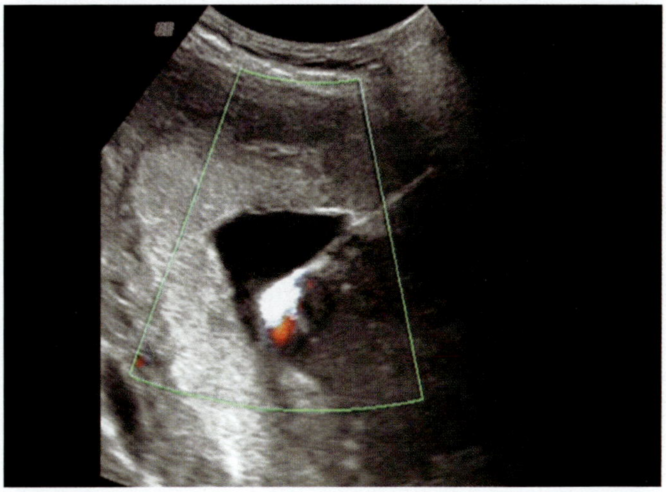

Fig. 17: Ultrasound picture of in-utero bipolar diathermy of the umbilical cord in twin reversed arterial perfusion sequence (TRAPs). Note the echodense signal around the bipolar electrical plate, which is the movement of water molecules when heat is applied. Color Doppler flow is applied to check for complete cessation of blood flow.

fetus, as shown in **Figure 16**. The other donor (pump) twin may develop high-output cardiac failure (hydrops) with a reported mortality of 50–75%.[45]

The acardiac fetus is not viable. Management is aimed at maintaining viability of the other (donor/pump) twin, including close surveillance for development of hydrops. Conservative management with close monitoring appears to be a safe option for TRAP pregnancies in which the acardiac twin is less than 50% the weight of the pump twin.[46] Interrupting blood flow to the acardiac twin may be performed by various methods which include hysterotomy and removal of the acardiac twin (*sectio parva*), umbilical cord occlusion, and ablation of intrafetal vessel.[47]

Umbilical cord occlusion can be accomplished either by ligation or bipolar diathermy.[48,49] Ablation of intrafetal blood vessels can be accomplished with either laser or radiofrequency ablation (RFA). **Figures 17 and 18** show in-utero bipolar cord diathermy of the umbilical cord and radiofrequency ablation of interstitial blood vessels in an acardiac fetus. According to data obtained from 74 cases treated with minimally invasive techniques, intrafetal ablation was associated with later median gestational age at delivery (37 vs. 32 weeks; $P = 0.04$) and higher median treatment-delivery interval (16 vs. 9.5 weeks, $P = 0.02$) compared with cord occlusion techniques. It was also associated with a lower technical failure rate (13% vs. 35%, $P = 0.03$), lower rate of premature delivery or rupture of membranes before 32 weeks (23% vs. 58%, $P = 0.003$) and

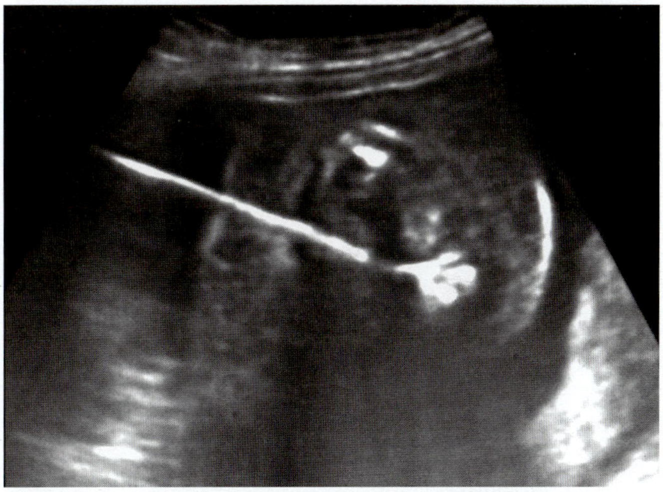

Fig. 18: Ultrasound picture of in-utero radiofrequency ablation (RFA) of intrafetal vessel in twin reversed arterial perfusion sequence (TRAPs). Note the echodense signal around the RFA probe, which is the tissue coagulation effect from the microwave power. Color Doppler flow is applied to check for complete cessation of blood flow at the end of the procedure.

higher rate of clinical success (77% vs. 50%, $P = 0.02$) than cord occlusion techniques.[50]

SEVERE CONGENITAL DIAPHRAGMATIC HERNIA (CDH)

Congenital diaphragmatic herniation (CDH) is one of the most common non-cardiac fetal intrathoracic anomalies.

It is found in 1 of every 2,000 to 4,000 live births. Approximately 84% of prenatally detected cases are left-sided, 13% are right-sided, and 2% are bilateral.[51] However, a significant portion of CDHs are detected soon after birth. Mortality is predominantly due to development of pulmonary hypoplasia, which is thought to be due to mass effect on the developing lung. Such neonates are hypoxic and have persistent fetal circulation due to pulmonary hypoplasia and pulmonary hypertension.

Embryologic development of the diaphragm is usually completed by 9 gestational weeks'. CDH results from failure of fusion of one of the pleuroperitoneal canals at about 8 weeks gestation. They may contain stomach, intestines, liver or spleen. CDH can be classified into two basic types on location:

1. *Bochdalek hernia:* This is a the most common type of fetal CDH. It is more common on the left (75 to 90%). The defect is on posterolateral portion of the diaphragm. It is usually larger, and is associated with poorer outcomes compared to Morgagni hernia. The diagnosis is usually made earlier in gestational age.
2. *Morgagni hernia:* This is less common type of fetal CDH. The defect is on the anterior portion of the diaphragm. The diagnosis is usually made later in gestational age.

While a CDH can occur as an isolated condition, associated anomalies are relatively common. Common associated anomalies with CDH are shown in **Box 1**. Thoracic herniation of abdominal viscera may not be readily visualized during routine ultrasound examination. However, there are certain sonographic findings that are associated with severe midtrimester CDH, and the demonstration of these findings may eventually lead to the diagnosis of CDH. The secondary findings are as follows:

- Polyhydramnios
- Cardiomediastinal shift +/– abnormal cardiac axis
- Inability to demonstrate the normal stomach bubble.

BOX 1: Fetal malformations commonly associated with severe congenital diaphragmatic hernia.

- Pulmonary hypoplasia (as a sequelae)
- Bronchopulmonary sequestration
- Aneuploidy (up to 50%): Trisomy 13, 18, 21, monosomy X
- Syndrome: Pallister-Killian syndrome: tetrasomy 12p, Fryns syndrome, Cornelia de Lange syndrome
- Congenital cardiac anomalies
- Neural tube defects: Anencephaly, meningomyelocele/spina bifida

Sonographic diagnosis of CDH can be made from the following findings shown in **Table 4.**[52,53] Of noted, the study should be performed in the true transverse plane. An example of left- and right-sided CDH is shown in **Figures 19 and 20**, respectively.

Prognostication of prenatally diagnosed CDH relies on the residual lung volume. The observed-to-expected lung-to-head ratio (O/E LHR), as shown in **Figure 21**, may be calculated. O/E LHR ratio correlates with the degree of pulmonary hypoplasia. The degree of lung hypoplasia can be used to predict survival rates and the numbers from the Antenatal-CDH-Registry group that apply to isolated left-sided CDH and liver herniation, as shown in **Table 5.**[51,54]

Fetal magnetic resonance imaging (MRI) may be helpful in further assessing the hernia and any associated pulmonary hypoplasia. Examples of MRI sequences typically performed for assessment of CDH include are shown in **Table 6.**[55,56] A publication from collaboration between our center and Cincinnati Fetal Care Center showed a higher rate of growth in contralateral lung, compared to the ipsilateral lung. Hence, the contralateral lung seems to be the major determination of survival in fetuses with CDH.[57]

TABLE 4: Diagnostic sonographic findings of severe mid-trimester congenital diaphragmatic hernia.

Congenital diaphragmatic hernia (CDH)	
• Absent bowel loops in the abdomen • Intrathoracic herniation of the liver* • Cystic echogenic lung mass**	
Left-sided CDH	***Right-sided CDH***
• Stomach and small bowel (echo-free) at the same transverse level as the heart on four-chamber view*** • Stomach and small bowel superior to the inferior margin of the scapula • Leftward displacement of the gallbladder	• Color Doppler study – Leftward bowing of the umbilical segment of the portal vein – Portal branches to the lateral segment of the left hepatic lobe coursing towards or above the diaphragm • Gallbladder present above diaphragm • Echo-dense space between the left heart border and stomach representing the left hepatic lobe

*Found in 85% of cases, and is associated with a worse prognosis
**The primary diagnosis of a fetal chest mass can change during the course of gestation as the appearance of the chest mass evolves.[100]
***The herniation of echo-free abdominal viscera makes left sided CDH comparatively easier to detect on ultrasound, as opposed to herniation of echo-dense liver on the right side.

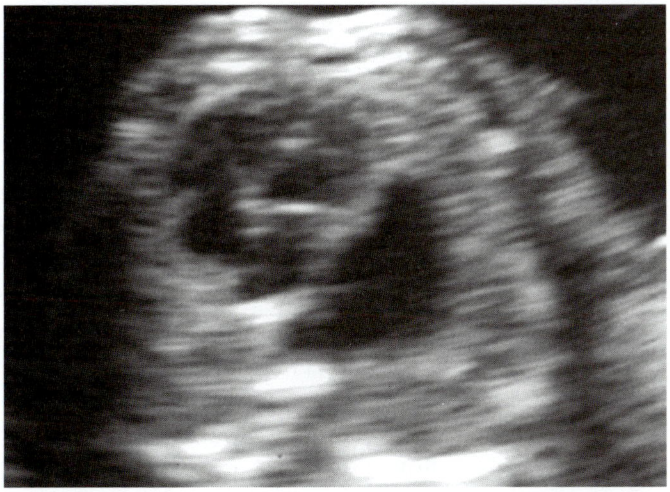

Fig. 19: Ultrasound picture of thorax in axial plane of a fetus at 22 gestational weeks'. Note the herniation of stomach into left hemithorax and shifting of cardiac axis in the presence of left-sided congenital diaphragmatic hernia.

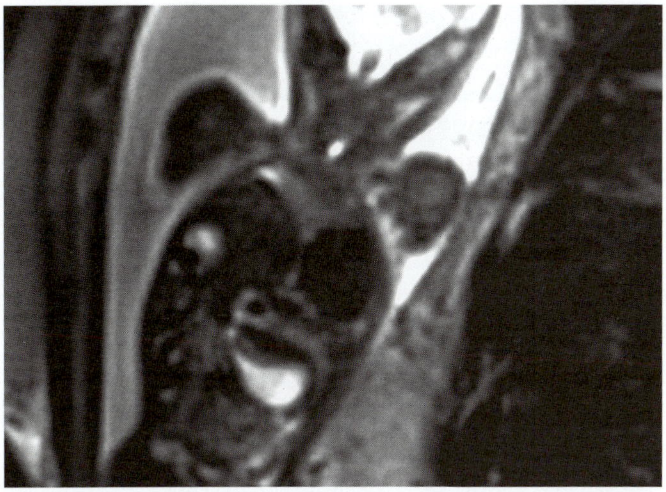

Fig. 20: Magnetic resonance imaging of a fetus with right-sided congenital diaphragmatic hernia at 26 gestational weeks', with T1-weighted fast field echo (FFE). Note the herniation of liver (hypersignal) and gallbladder into right hemithorax. The mediastinum is also shifted.

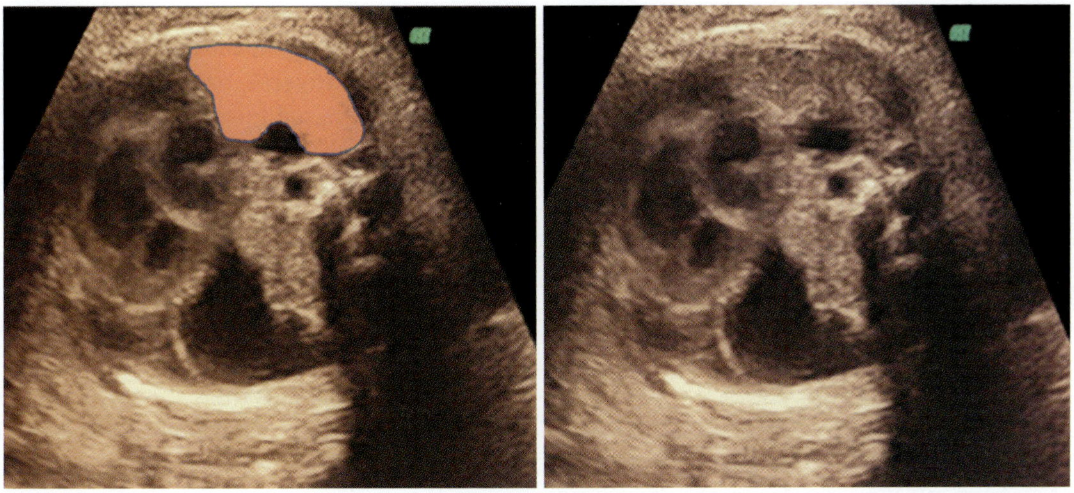

Fig. 21: Sonographic measurement of observed-to-expected lung-to-head ratio (O/E LHR) in a 24-weeks of fetus with left-sided congenital diaphragmatic hernia (CDH). Note that the stomach is herniated into left hemithorax.

Additional Benefits of MRI in Assessment of CDH Fetus

Lung-head ratio can be assessed by either ultrasound of MRI. MRI allows the measurement of total fetal lung volumes (TFLV) which provide an estimate of the severity of pulmonary hypoplasia.[58] The TFLV can be calculated from a contiguous MRI axial cut, then an observed-to-expected TFLV (O/E TFLV) can be derived. It has been found to predict well both mortality and morbidity, including the need for extracorporeal membrane oxygenation (ECMO) and the development of bronchopulmonary dysplasia.[59,60] Using MRI measurement of O/E TFLV early on (22–30 weeks') and later on (>30 weeks') of 47 CDH fetuses, our group in collaboration with Cincinnati Fetal Care Center found that certain fetuses can have deterioration of the contralateral lung growth in the third trimester of pregnancy, and hence this alter the prognosis given from findings in the second trimester.[61]

MRI has been increasing adopted in management scheme of fetus with severe CDH. The roles of fetal MRI

TABLE 5: Prognostication of prenatally diagnosed congenital diaphragmatic hernia based on observed/expected lung-to-head ratio (O/E LHR).

O/E LHR	Degree of lung hypoplasia	Predicted survival
>45%	Mild	>75%
26–45%	Moderate	30–75%
15–25%	Severe	15%
<15%	Extreme	0–15%

TABLE 6: Magnetic resonance (MR) sequences used for imaging of congenital diaphragmatic hernia. Each sequence has its unique features to demonstrate the distortion of fetal thoraco-abdominal structures. These clinical findings are very important in determination of prognosis, as well as to plan for corrective surgery soon after birth.

Magnetic resonance sequence	Features
T1-weighted fast field echo (FFE)	• Liver appears moderately hypersignaled
T2-weighted three-plane single shot fast spin echo (SSFSE)	• Fluid filled stomach and small bowel appear hypersignaled
T2-weighted balanced steady state free precession (bSSFP)	• Flowing blood appears hypersignaled • Portal vessels seen extending toward or above diaphragm
T2-weighted half-fourier acquisition single-shot turbo spin echo (HASTE)	• Lungs, which primarily filled with fluid, appear hypersignaled • Heart, mediastinum and liver appear hyposignaled

in severe CDH were summarized in the recently published recommendation from our Working Group on Ultrasound in Obstetrics of the World Association of Perinatal Medicine (WAPM) (Wataganara et al. JPM 2016 In press). MRI can provide an accurate estimation of lung volume of the fetus. Confirmation of fetal lung hypoplasia should be carried out when there is an oligohydramnios in the second trimester, congenital diaphragmatic hernia (CDH), distortion of thoracic cage in skeletal dysplasia, or tumor mass in the thorax of the fetus.[62] Diagnosis of congenital high airway obstruction syndrome (CHAOS) may not be conclusive on prenatal ultrasound examination. Other conditions, such as congenital pulmonary airway malformation (CPAM), may look almost identical to CHAOS by ultrasound examination. CPAM carries a much better prognosis than CHAOS. MRI can differentiate these 2 conditions, and can locate the level of tracheal or bronchial obstruction in cases of CHAOS.

MRI has been extensively used for further assessment of fetuses with CDH after ultrasound diagnosis. Survival rates of fetuses with isolated left-sided CDH decreases with low observed-to-expected fetal lung to head ratio (O/E LHR) in the second trimester. O/E LHR can be used to guide family counseling for prognosis, prenatal treatment with balloon tracheal occlusion, and immediate postnatal care. Total fetal lung volume (TFLV) measured from MRI is considered as the most accurate prognostic factor for neonatal survival.[63] Observed-to-expected TFLV of less than 35% has been linked with high neonatal mortality.[64] Mayer and colleagues from Eurofetus group concluded that the side of diaphragmatic defect, position of the liver, and O/E TFLV, as determined on MRI were predictive of outcome.[65] The quantitative evaluation of fetal lung using MRI, in association with ultrasound estimates, can help predict the neonatal outcomes of prenatally diagnosed CDH, either with or without prenatal interventions, for the purpose of resource allocation and family counseling.

Additional adverse prognostic findings from MRI include dense signal intensity of contralateral lung field as well as small diameters of pulmonary artery and its branches, which are associated with adverse perinatal outcomes. When fetal tracheal occlusion is indicated, it is advisable to perform MRI prior to the insertion of the balloon. MRI should then be repeated before or soon after the balloon retrieval to evaluate the effect of plugging to fetal lung expansion.[66] MRI picture of fetal airway after balloon tracheal occlusion is shown in **Figure 23**.

CDH cases diagnosed prenatally are more likely to have extradiaphragmatic malformations, particularly in cardiovascular, skeletal, genitourinary, and nervous system.[67] Survival of CDH with associated malformations is poor, compared to the isolated CDH cases. MRI has a benefit of larger field of view that allow for an evaluation of the whole fetus in a single plane. Certain anomalies can cause decreased liquor volume, which hinder the image quality from ultrasound examination. MRI can maintain its soft tissue delineation quality, making the anatomical assessment and plans for neonatal resuscitation in this difficult situation more accurate.

CDH can affect lung development, causing pulmonary hypoplasia and pulmonary hypertension at the time of birth. Fetuses with an antenatal diagnosis of CDH should be delivered in a tertiary referral center with access to neonatal

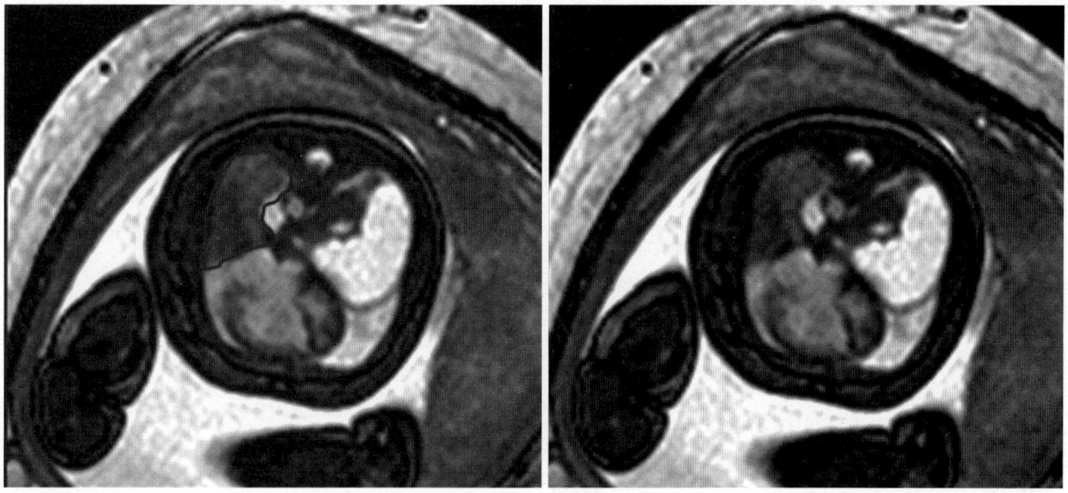

Fig. 22: Magnetic resonance imaging measurement of total fetal lung volume (TFLV) in a 24-weeks of fetus with left-sided congenital diaphragmatic hernia (CDH). This is the same fetus from Figure 21. Note a better soft tissue characterization, and potentially more prognosticative, than measurement with ultrasound.

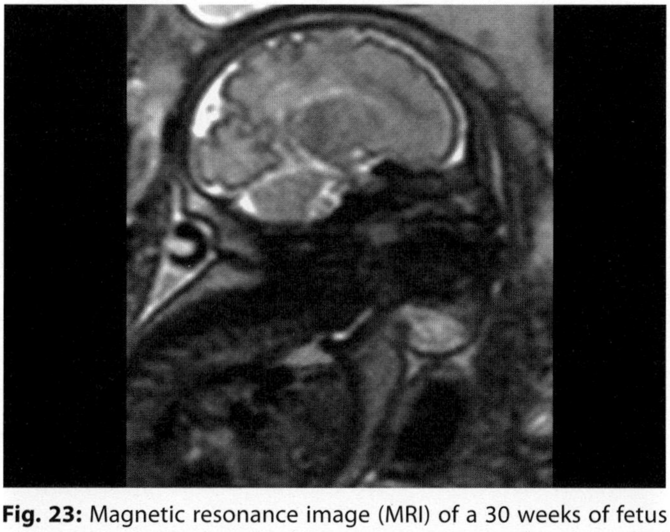

Fig. 23: Magnetic resonance image (MRI) of a 30 weeks of fetus with severe congenital diaphragmatic hernia. Fetal endoluminal tracheal occlusion (FETO) was performed. From the image, note that GoldBalloon was left in the trachea below the glottis and above the carina, which is an appropriate location.

intensive care and pediatric surgical facilities. Prenatal findings of CDH fetuses that suggest for poor prognosis include large defect, bilateral lesions, early gestational age at diagnosis, intrathoracic liver herniation, small contralateral lung, presence of associated abnormalities, and unfavorable lung-to-head ratio. According to our recent joint publication with Eurofoetus group, fetal lung volumes are compromised in the presence of liver and stomach herniation.[68] A composite prognostic index (CDH-CPI) comprising 10 prenatal parameters has been developed and was found to have a stronger correlation with survival and need for ECMO than any one parameter individually.[69] Intrathoracic space has been shown to affect the prognosis of CDH fetus in our recent joint publication with Cincinnati Fetal Care Center.[70]

Right-side CDH (RCDH) is considered a different disease entity from left-sided CDH (LCDH). According to the recent joint publication between our center and Eurofetus group on a retrospective review of 86 fetuses with RCHD.[71] Ten out of 86 cases had associated anomalies. Of the remaining 76 isolated RCDH: 8 opted for termination, 19 opted for expectant management with delivery at 36 +/– 3 weeks'. The expectant management group had survival at discharge of 53% (10/19), with 1 oxygen dependent. The rest (n = 44) opted for fetal endoluminal tracheal occlusion (FETO). This group delivered at 34.5 +/– 3 weeks'. The survival rate was 52%, and 39% were oxygen dependent at discharge. Pooling these data with earlier reported observations by Eurofetus, a 42% survival rate was deduced from 57 fetuses. Lung size on MRI and an interval of over 24 hours between reversal of tracheal occlusion and delivery were predictive of outcome. With these findings, RCDH seems to have a poorer outcome than that reported for fetuses with LCDH with similar lung size before birth. Survival rates after expectant management with observed/expected lung-to-head ratio values less than 45 and less than 30% were 17 and 0%, respectively. There was an increased neonatal survival rate (42%) in RCDH with O/E LHR less than 45% who opted for prenatal intervention.[71]

Prenatal Interventions in Fetus with Severe CDH

Some centers perform in-utero surgery in selected cases with poor prognostication scores. Occlusion of the fetal trachea to allow expansion of the fetal lungs with fluid and consequently, push the herniation back into the abdomen has been attempted, and is currently in a randomized controlled trial phase. Definitive diagnosis is crucial before any invasive procedures can be offered. General imaging differential considerations include:congenital pulmonary airway malformation (CPAM) and pulmonary sequestration. However, either can be found in association with CDH.

FETO has effects on lung proliferation and advanced the morphologic appearance. This effect might be more obvious if the procedure is offered early on in gestational age. Tracheal diameter is a key factor as to how early in gestational age we can plug the trachea. Ruano and colleagues have reported a successful series of early tracheal occlusion as early as 22 to 24 weeks.[72] In a recent joint publication between our center and Eurofetus group, we reported that the lung seems to expand effectively up until 35 to 45 days postocclusion.[73]

At the time this article is written, the "*randomized trial of fetoscopic endoluminal tracheal occlusion (FETO) versus expectant management during pregnancy in fetuses with left sided and isolated congenital diaphragmatic hernia and severe pulmonary hypoplasia'or TOTAL trial* has not finished their enrollment yet. At the conclusion of TOTAL trial, the estimated in-utero lung growth and balloon position will be evaluated. Fetuses with moderate to severe lung hypoplasia resulting from CDH are randomized into expectant management and FETO. These babies will be evaluated for oxygen dependency, need for medication for pulmonary hypertension, need to heart-lung machine, days requiring a ventilator until normal feeding and in the hospital. Day of the surgery and requirement of a patch to close the defect, occurrence of brain problems, infections, prematurity sequelae, and reflux. Long-term evaluation for lung function and neurologic development are made at 1 and 2 years after birth.[66]

Injecting substances that were believed to enhance alveolar and vascular proliferation has been experimented in animal model. For instance, intratracheal infusion of 50 microliters of 20% albumin before plugging the rat trachea resulted in increased cellular proliferation. However, there was an increased fetal loss in albumin-treated group, and this proposed adjunctive therapy cannot reach human trial.[74]

LOWER URINARY TRACT OBSTRUCTION

The incidence of lower urinary tract obstruction (LUTO) is approximately 2 of 10,000 pregnancies. If the obstruction is complete, or near complete, the diagnosis can be readily made by ultrasound examination. The key findings include the presence of a distended bladder, bilateral hydronephrosis, and severe oligohydramnios.[75] Severe LUTO is associated with high perinatal mortality and morbidity due to pulmonary hypoplasia and severe renal pressure damage.[76] The natural history of obstructive uropathy is highly variable and depends on gender, severity, duration, and age of onset of the obstruction. Complete obstruction of the urethra early in gestation can lead to massive distention of the bladder, hydroureter, hydronephrosis, and renal fibrocystic dysplasia. Inability of the urine to enter the amniotic space causes reduction of liquor volume, leading to pulmonary hypoplasia and secondary deformations of the face and extremities (Potter facies). An ultrasound image of a fetus with LUTO is shown in **Figure 24**.

Postnatal survival depends on two factors: pulmonary development and renal function. Of these, pulmonary development may be the more critical for neonatal survival. Pulmonary hypoplasia and prematurity are

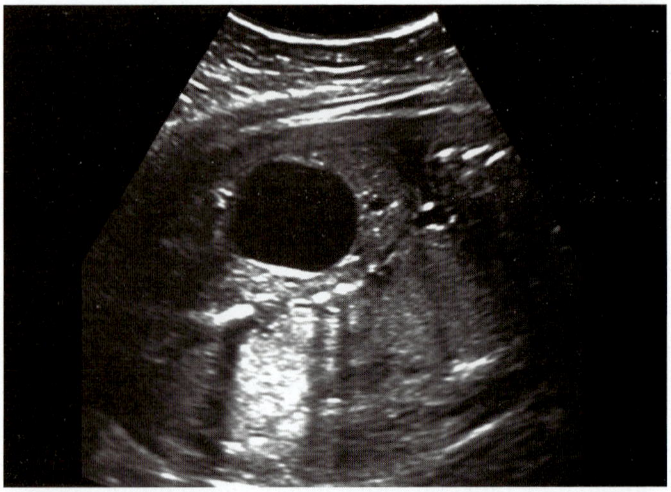

Fig. 24: An ultrasound image in coronal cut of a 26 weeks of fetus with lower urinary tract obstruction. The most obvious ultrasound findings are marked distension of urinary bladder and very low liquor volume. Lung hypoplasia and renal pressure damage are the most important determination factors of morbidity and mortality from this condition.

the leading causes of mortality in obstructive uropathy. In cases of posterior urethral valves (PUVs), about half of the mortality is linked to pulmonary insufficiency.[77] In fact, these statistics do not truly reflect the actual severity of LUTO, since some of the babies cannot make it to the referral center. These 'hidden mortality' also include the LUTO fetuses which died in utero. Earlier finding of oligohydramnios significantly worsens the prognosis. If urethral obstruction is also discovered, the neonatal mortality rate can be as high as 95%.[78]

Macroscopic and Microscopic Sequelae of Severe Second Trimester LUTO

Renal pathologies in fetuses with LUTO were demonstrated in a series of publication using experimental sheep model in 1980s. Ligation of ureter of the sheep fetus at 62 to 84 days of gestation was carried out to mimic obstruction of the urinary tract in human fetus. Of noted, the total pregnancy period of sheep is 144 days, and this sheep ureteral ligation model aimed to mimic the second trimester human fetus.[79] Using a combination of urachal ligation and gradual occlusion of the urethra, the investigators were able to reproduce gross findings of pulmonary hypoplasia, bladder dilatation, hydroureters, and hydronephrosis in a similar fashion of pathophysiologic changes in second trimester human fetus affected with LUTO. Histologically, increased fibrosis was observed throughout the kidney from ureter-ligated group. However, common renal pathologic findings in human fetus, i.e., parenchymal disorganization or cystic changes, are not observed in the sheep's kidney. The common macroscopic and microscopic findings of the kidneys in fetus with severe LUTO are shown in **Figures 25 and 26**, respectively.

Lesson Learned from Experimental Animal Models

This sheep model was then developed to evaluate the beneficial effect of in utero decompression. The urethral obstruction was created at 95 gestational days. After 15 to 27 days of obstruction, half of the animals underwent suprapubic cystostomy allowing for urine to flow freely from the obstructed fetal bladder.[80] In utero cystostomy resulted in survival of all the experimenting animals with minimal need for respiratory support. The study also showed amniotic fluid restoration, that may help with lung growth, and reduce morbidities associated with lung hypoplasia.

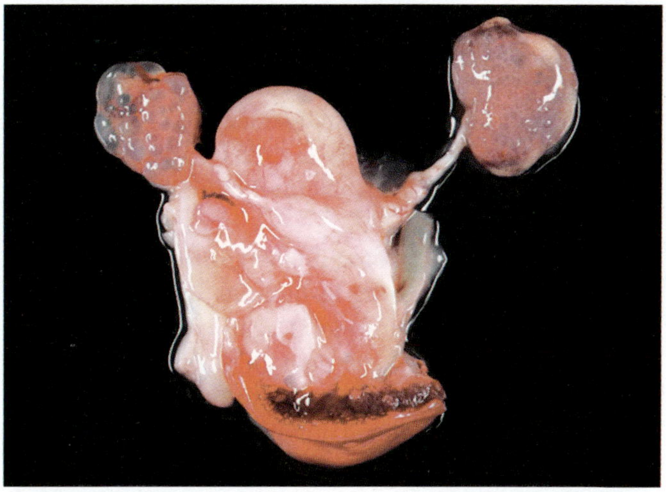

Fig. 25: Macroscopic findings of kidney-ureter-bladder (KUB) from a mid-trimester fetus with severe lower urinary tract obstruction (LUTO). Note the hypertrophic change of the urinary bladder from prolonged obstruction. Thick muscular wall of the urinary bladder can be appreciated from ultrasound examination. Dilatation and tortuosity of the ureters is obvious. Cystic dysplastic change is observed in both kidneys, and it is likely that both of them are non-functioning.

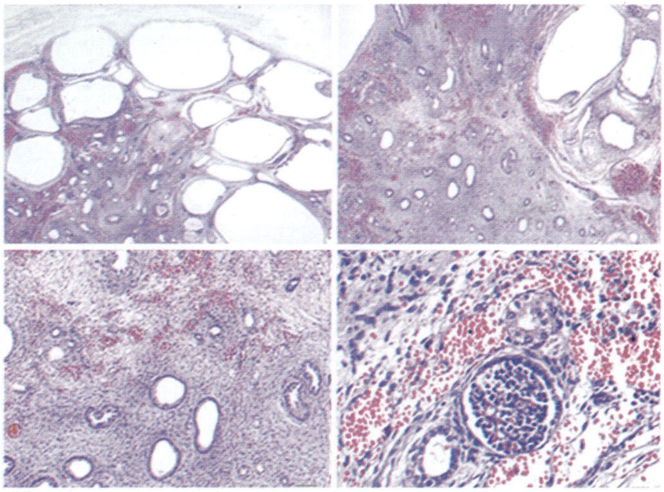

Fig. 26: Microscopic findings of cystic dysplastic kidney from a midtrimester fetus with severe lower urinary tract obstruction (LUTO). This type of renal pathology is characterized by the presence of multiple non-communicating cysts of varying sizes separated by dysplastic renal parenchyma. There was no normal pelvicaliceal system.

Lung hypoplasia and pulmonary vascular hypertension are the major determinants for an early neonatal death. Renal damages are more on the long-term morbidity, i.e., transfusion dependent, recurrent urinary tract infection. Even the perinatal outcomes of in-utero suprapubic cystostomy is good, the urinary bladder and the ureters remained dilated. The survivors will require bladder training to ensure an effective urine flow to prevent secondary infection in the urinary tract. Minimal histologic renal parenchymal damages were still noticeable. Some of the babies require dialysis to help with their faltering renal function.

Renal cystic dysplasia and disorganized architecture similar to those occurring in humans was produced in the sheep model when ureteral ligation was performed earlier in gestation (58–66 days of gestation). Fibrosis and parenchymal disorganization were present, and the medullary region contained abnormal-appearing ducts.[80] To determine whether in utero relief of obstruction would prevent renal dysplasia, unilateral ureteral obstruction at 58 to 66 days of gestation was performed, followed by end-ureterostomy to relieve obstruction at 20, 40, and 60 days after obstruction. Duration of obstruction was directly related to the likelihood of deterioration in renal function and occurrence of histologic change. Decompression, regardless of timing, improved histologic findings and function compared with controls that had not been decompressed, however, and provided evidence that in utero decompression of early obstruction could arrest histologic changes,prevent severe dysplastic damage, and potentially preserve renal function.

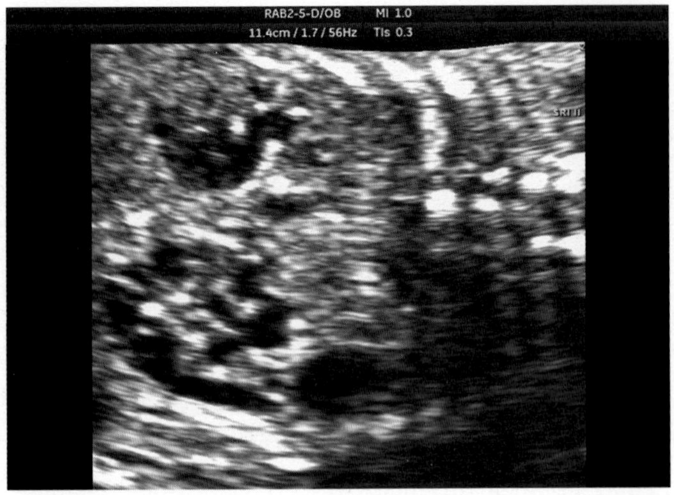

Fig. 27: Ultrasound picture from a 26 weeks' fetus with severe damages of both kidneys. Hyperechogenicity of the renal cortex is a result of extensive fibrosis and scarring. Small cortical cysts are also noted. The pattern of cortex, medully, and pelvicaliceal system is lost. The pregnancy is complicated by anhydramnios, therefore it is very likely that these damaged kidneys are non-functioning already.

Assessment of Residual Renal Function in Second Trimester Fetus with Severe LUTO

Appropriate prenatal management in human fetuses would depend on the ability to determine the presence and extent of functional damage in the kidneys reliably so as to select those that might benefit from intervention to prevent further progressive damage. If severe LUTO is detected too late, then the kidney damages may be irreversible, and rescue intervention shall not be offered. There have been a number of studies exploring different ways to evaluate residual kidney function.[81-83] *Ultrasound appearance of fetal kidneys* has been assessed for its predictive value of renal damage, failure, or non-functioning. Sonographic findings that are suggestive for advanced renal damages include increased echogenicity and presence of discreet parenchymal cysts, as shown in **Figure 27**.[84,85] Differential pattern of renal parenchymal vessels at different stages of obstructive nephropathy is shown and described in **Figures 28A to C**.

Sonographic appearance can be subjective, therefore, this approach did not show a satisfactorily sensitivity, specificity, and accurate correlation with renal function.[84,86,87] Even oligohydramnios is invariably found in fetus with LUTO at late stage, *quantitative assessment of amniotic volume* alone is a poor surrogate of renal function. The reason is it takes both kidneys to be virtually non-functioning, then the fluid will start to drop. In another word, if anhydramnios is found, particularly early on in gestational age, it is very likely that the kidneys are already non-function, which is too late for any intervention or salvage therapy.[88]

Even there is no single marker that can conclusively differentiate viable kidneys from non-functioning one, it is reasonable to accept that a combination of severe oligohydramnios, developed early on in gestational age (early onset), and sonographic appearance of severely damaged kidney (increased echogenicity, discreet intraparenchymal and subcortical cysts) should raise a concerns of bilateral non-functioning kidneys.[85] On the other hand, mild to moderate decreases in amniotic fluid volume and subtle renal parenchymal change on ultrasound are less reliable in predicting renal function and extent of damage, however.

Therefore, a simple and safe method of reliably determining the degree of renal damage was required. The first useful approach was based on the review of *electrolyte patterns from fetal urine* obtained during clinical

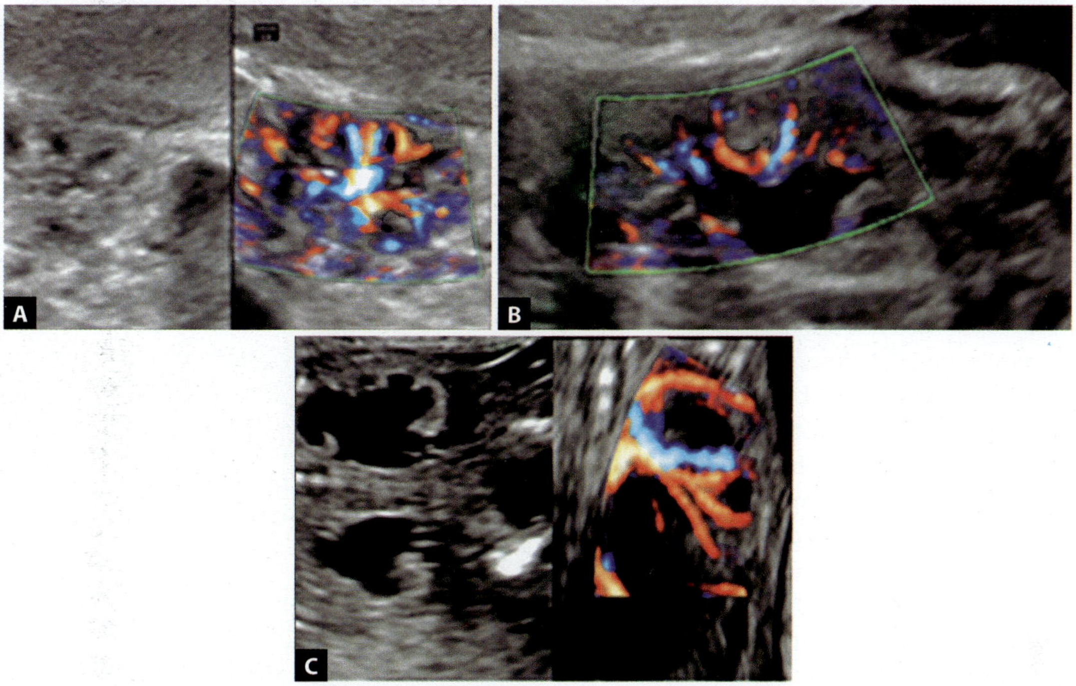

Figs. 28A to C: Renal parenchyma vascular patterns in various degree of nephropathy. Ultrasound image comparing the renal parenchymal vascular patterns in various stages of obstructive uronephropathy (A) Normal kidney of a 26 weeks' fetus. Grey-scale mode shows non-dilated renal pelvis. Renal cortex is normoechoic, and renal medulla is hypoechoic. Color Doppler flow shows multiple intervening vessels with multiple branching evenly in every direction from renal artery at the hilum on to the cortical surface where blood is filtrated through glomeruli. (B) Mild pyelectasis of a 28 weeks' fetus with (tentatively) ureteric immaturity. Grey scale mode shoed mild dilatation of renal pelvis without clubbing of caliceal systems. Renal cortex is getting thin, but normoechoicity of the cortical part and hypoechoicity of the medulla part are still noticeable. Color Doppler flow shows less number of intervening parenchymal vessels with less branching from renal artery at the hilum onto the cortical surface. (C) Severe pyelectasis or hydronephrosis of a 28 weeks' fetus with bilateral ureteropelvic junction (UPJ) obstruction. Grey-scale mode showed ballooning of renal pelvis and clubbing of pelvicaliceal system. Renal cortex is paper thin, and relatively hyperechoic. Medulla cannot be identified. Color Doppler flow shows very few, relatively dilated intervening parenchymal vessels without any branches from renal artery at the hilum straight onto the cortical surface.

evaluation of obstructive uropathies. The University of California, San Francisco (UCSF) group reviewed data from 20 human fetuses and categorized outcomes as "poor function" (N = 510) or "good function" (N = 510) based on renal histologic findings at autopsy or biopsy or on renal and pulmonary function at birth.[89] Groups were compared for (1) amniotic fluid status at initial presentation, (2) ultrasound appearance of the kidney, (3) electrolyte composition of fetal urine obtained by vesicocentesis, and (4) fetal urine output. Fetuses categorized with poor function were found to have moderate to severely decreased liquor volume, echogenic or cystic kidneys on ultrasound, urine outputs less than 2 mL/h, sodium concentrations greater than 100 mEq/L, chloride concentrations greater than 90 mEq/L, and osmolality levels greater than 210 mOsm/L. Measurable parameters in fetal urine that associated with viable kidney are summarized in **Table 7**.

Those fetuses grouped as having good function had normal to moderately decreased amniotic fluid volume, normal to mildly echogenic renal parenchyma, urine output greater than 2 mL/h, sodium concentrations less than 100 mEq/L, chloride concentrations less than 90 mEq/L, and osmolality values less than 210 mOsm/L. Numerous subsequent clinical series have supported and refined these predictive criteria, and evaluation of urinary components has continued to evolve, with the addition of other markers, such as urinary calcium, b2-microglobulin, and total protein.

Recently, there has been investigational interest in fetal cystatin-C in amniotic fluid as another biochemical marker for early identification of obstructive uropathies and postnatal renal function prediction.[90] Cystatin-C is a protein synthesized steadily and continuously by all nucleated cells that does not vary with gestational age and

TABLE 7: Parameters in fetal urinalysis associated with functioning kidney.

Bad prognostication	*Sensitivity (%)*	*Specificity (%)*	*Positive predictive value (%)*	*Negative predictive value (%)*
Sodium <100 mg/DL	56	64	56	88
Calcium <8 mEq/L	100	27	43	100
Osmolality <200 mOsm/L	83	82	71	90
b2-microglobulin <4 mg/L	17	36	100	44
Total protein <20 mg/dL	67	91	80	83

does not cross the placenta.[91] Although promising, its use as a prognostic tool is undetermined. The urine obtained from bladder of a fetus with chronic obstruction is actually a mixture of urine that was produced from back then when the kidneys are not damaged. More recent data shows that use of serial urine aspirations to document change in tonicity after repeated bladder drainage has significantly improved the predictive value.[92] Being able to evaluate the current function of fetal kidney helps to select LUTO fetuses that would benefit from in utero treatment.

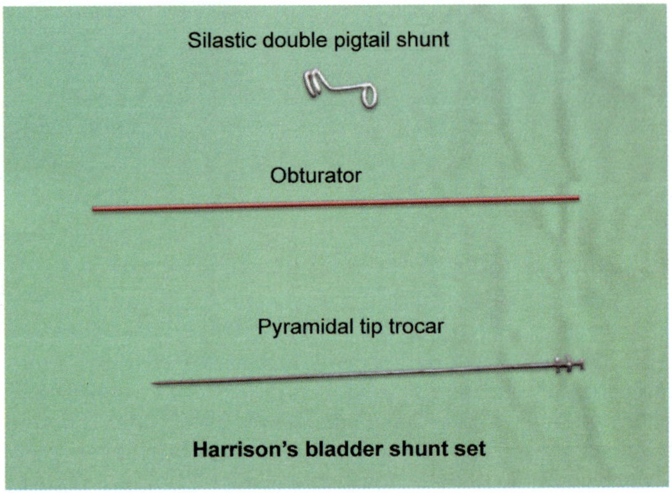

Fig. 29: Harrison's bladder shunt is commonly used for fetal shunting procedures in the Department of Obstetrics and Gynecology, Faculty of Medicine Siriraj Hospital.

Prenatal Interventions in Fetus with Severe LUTO

Managements of fetus prenatally diagnosed with severe LUTO are varied. Some families may choose one extreme measure, which is termination of pregnancy should the prognosis is dismal, i.e., high probability of fetal or neonatal death, or long-term significant renal morbidity. Some may opt for the other extreme, which is expectant management. Some family may choose to have in utero decompression, which can provide dual benefit of preventing further renal damages, as well as to increase liquor volume to enhance fetal lung growth and development.

There are 4 approaches for fetal urine decompression (1) *single or serial vesicocentesis*, (2) *vesicoamniotic shunting (VAS)***,** as shown in **Figure 29**. At Faculty of Medicine Siriraj Hospital, the VAS insertion is performed on an outpatient setting, with strict aseptic techniques and combined maternal and fetal sedation and immobilization, as shown in **Figure 30**. The VAS of choice included Harrison's bladder shunt, Rodeck's Rocket shunt, and Basket shunt. Seldinger's technique is universally applied regardless for the shunt of choice. (3) *Fetoscopic cystoscopy examination and laser ablation of posterior urethral valve*, and (4) *Open fetal vesicotomy*. This last approach has not gained much acceptance due to its invasiveness and risks to the mother.

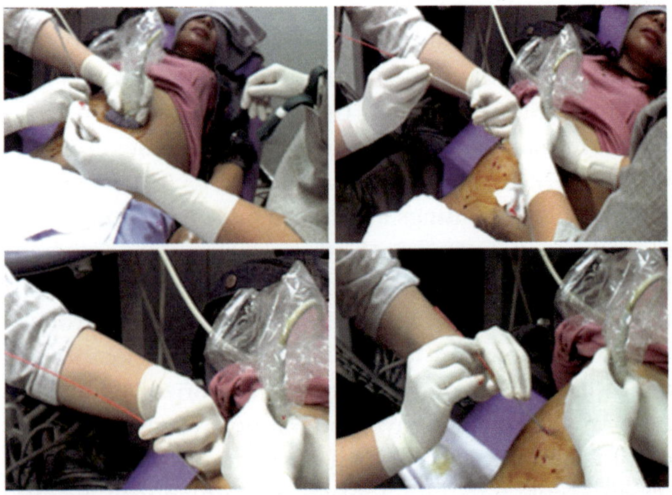

Fig. 30: Vesicoamniotic shunt insertion in the Department of Obstetrics and Gynecology, Faculty of Medicine Siriraj Hospital. It is an outpatient basis, with adequate sedation and pain control for both the mother and the fetus. Seldinger's technique is universally applied.

Percutaneous vesicoamniotic shunting in Lower Urinary Tract Obstruction (PLUTO) trial is a randomized trial aiming to evaluate the real effectiveness of prenatal VAS in LUTO fetus.[91,93] The trial recruited male fetuses with isolated severe LUTO prenatally diagnosed in the UK, Ireland, and the Netherlands. They were randomized into VAS and conservative treatment, with the primary outcome of neonatal survival longer than 28 days. Due to difficult recruitment, only 31 LUTO fetuses were enrolled, and 16 were allocated to VAS, and another 15 were allocated to conservative management. There were 12 livebirths in each group, with a comparable number of fetal demise and medical termination in both groups. Of the 16 LUTO fetuses who received VAS, there were 8/16 that survived longer than 28 days, whereas there were 4/15 neonatal survival longer than 28 days in conservative management group. All 12 deaths were caused by pulmonary hypoplasia in the early neonatal period.

The calculated intention-to-treat relative risk (RR) was 1.88 (95% CI, 0.71–4.96; $P = 0.27$). Analysis based on treatment received showed a larger effect (3.20, 1.06–9.62; $P = 0.03$). Bayesian analysis in which the trial data were combined with elicited priors from experts suggested an 86% probability that vesicoamniotic shunting increased survival at 28 days and a 25% probability that it had a large, clinically important effect (defined as a relative increase of 55% or more in the proportion of neonates who survived). From statistical point of view, the VAS was marginally, and inconclusive, superior to expectant management in terms of neonatal survival of LUTO.

There is a reason to explain the suboptimal neonatal outcomes from VAS. Meta-analysis of neonatal outcomes of 169 LUTO fetuses treated with in utero VAS from 5 case series revealed a total neonatal survival of 79/169 (47%).[94] Shunt dislodgement is not uncommon. Decompression by shunting mechanisms relies heavily on pressure gradient between inside the urinary bladder and the outside amniotic cavity. There is still some residual pressure in the fetal urinary tract system that might further damage the kidney. According to this meta-analysis, the chance that LUTO survivors with VAS will have normal renal function in childhood period is between 50 to 78%.[94] Potential complications of VAS include insertion failure, amniorrhexis, bleeding, infection, shunt migration or obstruction, and rupture of the fetal bladder, as shown in **Figure 31**.

Fetoscopic cystoscopy is a new minimally invasive approach, which allow for visual examination to determine the nature of obstruction, so that specific management may be provided in the same setting. Ultrasound examination can identify level of obstruction by an appearance of 'keyhole', as shown in **Figure 31**. The pathologic lesion at the junction of proximal 1/3 and distal 2/3 of the urethra could be a thin malformed tissue valve, triangular shape, so called posterior urethral valve (PUV). PUV is amendable for decompression procedure with laser ablation under direct visualization.

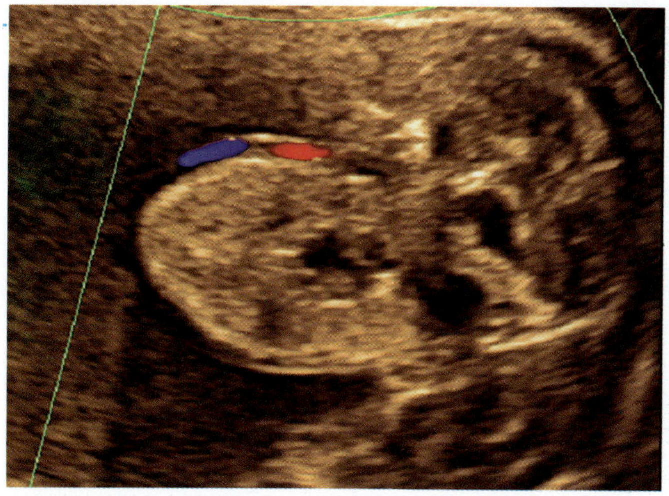

Fig. 31: Ultrasound image of spontaneous ruptured urinary bladder in a 24 weeks' fetus. The fetus was diagnosed with severe lower urinary tract obstruction (LUTO) 2 weeks before. There was urine ascites. Thick muscular wall of the urinary bladder indicates chronic bladder outlet obstruction in this fetus. Rupture of fetal bladder in LUTO can be iatrogenic. It may occur following failed attempts of vesicoamniotic shunting or fetoscopic cystoscopy.

Figure 32 shows the PUV being dissected by Nd:YAG laser fiber (400 µm). The laser output energy should be set to adequately coagulating the bleeding point during dissection. Care must be taken not to set the laser energy up to high, since it might excessively burn the adjacent structure or results in stenotic lesions from fibrosis. But if the pathology of obstruction is either urethral stenosis or atresia, laser surgery will be abandoned. These types of lesion carry a worse prognosis. Shunting can be attempted in the same setting, but with limited success. Preoperative counselling for the parents to realize a different possibilities and the respective outcomes is of utmost importance.

After the PUV is successfully ablated, fetal bleeding points are carefully checked and stopped. Amnioinfusion is done before the instruments are removed. This is to enhance a follow-up ultrasound examination. Follow-up ultrasound examination within 2 days after the procedure.

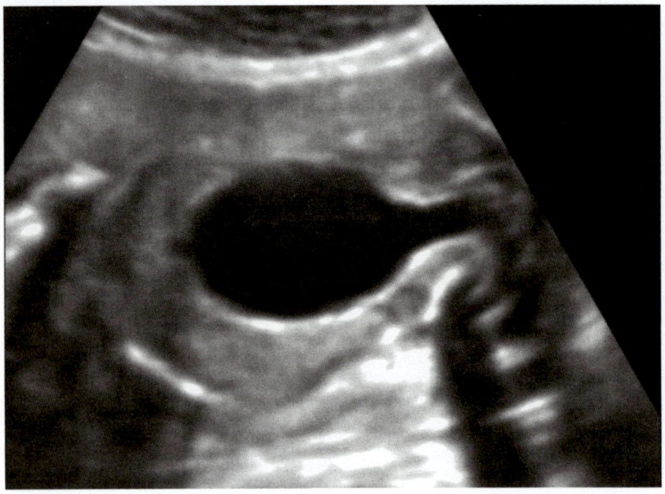

Fig. 32: Ultrasound image of a 24 weeks' fetus with lower urinary tract obstruction (LUTO). The amniotic fluid volume is low. Note the dilatation of urinary bladder and proximal urethra that give an appearance of 'keyhole'. Nature of obstruction cannot be identified exclusively from ultrasound examination.

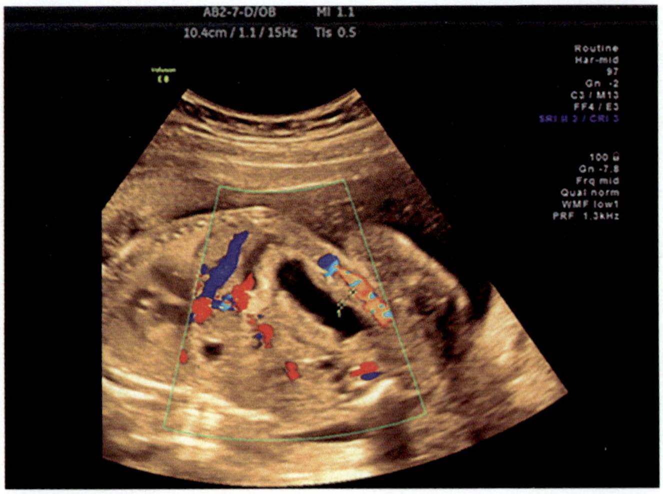

Fig. 33: Ultrasound image of fetal bladder 2 days after fetoscopic laser ablation of posterior urethral valve in a 26 weeks' fetus. The urinary bladder was no longer distended. There was no urine ascites. Amniotic fluid volume was near normal. Thick muscular wall of the urinary bladder (4.9 mm) is still noticeable. These findings suggest for a technical success.

The surgery is technically successful if PUV is adequately examined and precisely ablated. On follow-up scans, urinary bladder, ureters, and renal pelvicaliceal system should be decompressed, although its muscular wall may still retain some thickness, as shown in **Figure 33**. Absence of fetal (urine) ascites and re-accumulation of amniotic fluid are also reassuring.

Recent evidence suggest for superiority in neonatal survival and intact survival rate for in utero treatment of LUTO with laser ablation compared to VAS. Martinez and colleagues reported their 20 PUV fetuses treated with laser at median gestational age 18 weeks' (15–25.6).[95] The proximal urethra were accessible 19/20 times, and they were able to get technical success with responsive postoperative findings in 16/20 (80%). Even with this initial postoperative response, 9 (45%) women subsequently chose to terminate pregnancy, and 11 (55%) of them delivered a liveborn baby at mean gestational age of 37.3 weeks'(29.1–40.2). None of them had pulmonary hypoplasia, but 3 (27.3%) of them had renal failure awaiting for renal transplant. Prediction of postnatal renal function is one of the pre-requisite before this minimally invasive treatment is offered. These tools are not perfect, and it is important to counseled the family for the possibility of long-term renal morbidities in the survivors.

The randomized controlled trial comparing neonatal survival of 111 LUTO fetuses managed (1) expectantly, or (2) VAS, or (3) fetal cystoscopy showed a significantly higher neonatal survival rate with fetal cystoscopy and vesicoamniotic shunting when compared to no intervention (adjusted relative risk (ARR), 1.86 (95% CI, 1.01–3.42; $P = 0.048$) and ARR, 1.73 (95% CI, 1.01–3.08; $P = 0.04$) respectively). A clear trend for normal renal function was present in the fetal cystoscopy group [ARR, 1.73 (95% CI, 0.97–3.08; $P = 0.06$)] but was not observed in the VAS group [ARR, 1.16 (95% CI, 0.86–1.55; $P = 0.33$)]. In cases in which there was a postnatal diagnosis of PUV, fetal cystoscopy was effective in improving both the 6-month survival rate and renal function (ARR, 4.10 (95% CI, 1.75–9.62; $P < 0.01$) and 2.66 (95% CI, 1.25–5.70; $P = 0.01$) respectively) while VAS was associated only with an improvement in the 6-month survival rate (ARR, 3.76 (95% CI, 1.42–9.97; $P < 0.01$)) with no effect on renal function. The authors concluded that fetal cystoscopy and VAS improve the 6-month survival rate in cases of severe LUTO. However, only fetal cystoscopy may prevent impairment of renal function in fetuses with PUV.[96]

Our team at Faculty of Medicine Siriraj Hospital has performed 7 fetoscopic cystoscopy; 1 was diagnostic, and 6 was for PUV ablation. We had 3/6 (50%) deliveries at term: none of them had pulmonary hypoplasia or clinically significant renal impairment. For the 3 failed cases: 2/3 opted for termination of pregnancy, and 1/3 did not get the valve ablation due to technical problem, and the patient opted for termination of pregnancy.

CONCLUSION

Less invasive nature of fetoscopic intervention has broadened the horizon of fetal surgery. Open fetal surgery to repair high-risk meningomyelocele (MMC) has become a commonly offered option to postnatal repair. Significant maternal morbidities, including uterine rupture and potential impairment or loss of future fertility, is not negligible. An alternative approach by fetoscopy is currently ongoing in Germany and Brazil.[97,98] The traditional triple layer closer was replaced by alternative protocol that requires fewer ports and self-locking suture, or covering the defect with biosynthetic cellulose patch.[6,99] Fetoscopy in a CO_2 environment improves visualization, access to tissue, and a wider field of view compared with standard in-amniotic fluid fetoscopy.

Preliminary experience of fetoscopic repair of lumbosacral MMC from Cirurgia Endoscopica para Correcao Antenatal da Meningomielocele (CECAM) trial was recently published.[98] At the conclusion of Phase 1, outcome data was extracted from 10 fetuses enrolled in the trial. The median gestational age at the time of surgery was 27 weeks' (range 25–28 weeks). Endoscopic repair was completed in 8 of 10. The mean gestational age at birth was 32.4 weeks'. There was 1 fetal and 1 neonatal demise, and 1 unsuccessful case underwent postnatal repair. Of the 7 infants available for analysis, complete reversal of hindbrain herniation occurred in 6 of 7 babies. Three babies required ventriculoperitoneal shunting or third ventriculostomy. Functional motor level was the same or better than the anatomical level in 6 of 7 cases. There was no significant maternal morbidity and no evidence of myometrial thinning or dehiscence in all 10 cases.

Phase I trial suggested for a potential of MMC repair through endoscopic approaches. It still requires more data and accumulating surgical experiences before the genuine benefits and risks of this new approach can be materialized. Broader adoption may take even longer time.

REFERENCES

1. Wu D, Ball RH. The maternal side of maternal-fetal surgery. Clin Perinatol. 2009;36:247-53, viii.
2. Van de Velde M, Van Schoubroeck D, Lewi LE, et al. Remifentanil for fetal immobilization and maternal sedation during fetoscopic surgery: a randomized, double-blind comparison with diazepam. Anesthesia and Analgesia. 2005;101:251-8, table of contents.
3. Gratacos E, Deprest J. Current experience with fetoscopy and the Eurofoetus registry for fetoscopic procedures. European Journal of Obstetrics, Gynecology, and Reproductive Biology. 2000;92:151-9.
4. Yamamoto M, El Murr L, Robyr R, Leleu F, Takahashi Y, Ville Y. Incidence and impact of perioperative complications in 175 fetoscopy-guided laser coagulations of chorionic plate anastomoses in fetofetal transfusion syndrome before 26 weeks of gestation. American Journal of Obstetrics and Gynecology. 2005;193:1110-6.
5. Klaritsch P, Albert K, Van Mieghem T, et al. Instrumental requirements for minimal invasive fetal surgery. BJOG. 2009;116:188-97.
6. Belfort MA, Whitehead WE, Shamshirsaz AA, Ruano R, Cass DL, Olutoye OO. Fetoscopic Repair of Meningomyelocele. Obstet Gynecol. 2015;126:881-4.
7. Nizard J, Barbet JP, Ville Y. Does the source of laser energy influence the coagulation of chorionic plate vessels? Comparison of Nd:YAG and diode laser on an ex vivo placental model. Fetal Diagn Ther. 2007;22:33-7.
8. Dube J, Dodds L, Armson BA. Does chorionicity or zygosity predict adverse perinatal outcomes in twins? Am J Obstet Gynecology. 2002;186:579-83.
9. Sebire NJ, Snijders RJ, Hughes K, Sepulveda W, Nicolaides KH. The hidden mortality of monochorionic twin pregnancies. Br J Obstet Gynaecol. 1997;104:1203-7.
10. Quintero RA. Twin-twin transfusion syndrome. Clin Perinatol. 2003;30:591-600.
11. Lewi L, Jani J, Cannie M, et al. Intertwin anastomoses in monochorionic placentas after fetoscopic laser coagulation for twin-to-twin transfusion syndrome: is there more than meets the eye? Am J Obstet Gynecol. 2006;194:790-5.
12. Denbow ML, Cox P, Taylor M, Hammal DM, Fisk NM. Placental angioarchitecture in monochorionic twin pregnancies: relationship to fetal growth, fetofetal transfusion syndrome, and pregnancy outcome. Am J Obstet Gynecol. 2000;182:417-26.
13. Quintero RA, Morales WJ, Allen MH, Bornick PW, Johnson PK, Kruger M. Staging of twin-twin transfusion syndrome. J Perinatol. 1999;19:550-5.
14. Michelfelder E, Gottliebson W, Border W, et al. Early manifestations and spectrum of recipient twin cardiomyopathy in twin-twin transfusion syndrome: relation to Quintero stage. Ultrasound in Obstetrics & Gynecology: the official journal of the International Society of Ultrasound in Obstetrics and Gynecology. 2007;30:965-71.
15. Saunders NJ, Snijders RJ, Nicolaides KH. Therapeutic amniocentesis in twin-twin transfusion syndrome appearing in the second trimester of pregnancy. Am J Obstet Gynecol. 1992;166:820-4.
16. Senat MV, Deprest J, Boulvain M, Paupe A, Winer N, Ville Y. Endoscopic laser surgery versus serial amnio-reduction for severe twin-to-twin transfusion syndrome. The New England Journal of Medicine. 2004;351:136-44.
17. Moise KJ, Jr., Dorman K, Lamvu G, et al. A randomized trial of amnioreduction versus septostomy in the treatment of

twin-twin transfusion syndrome. Am J Obstet Gynecol. 2005;193:701-7.
18. Hecher K, Plath H, Bregenzer T, Hansmann M, Hackeloer BJ. Endoscopic laser surgery versus serial amniocenteses in the treatment of severe twin-twin transfusion syndrome. Am J Obstet Gynecol. 1999;180:717-24.
19. Mari G, Roberts A, Detti L, et al. Perinatal morbidity and mortality rates in severe twin-twin transfusion syndrome: results of the International Amnioreduction Registry. Am J Obstet Gynecol. 2001;185:708-15.
20. Habli M, Lim FY, Crombleholme T. Twin-to-twin transfusion syndrome: a comprehensive update. Clin Perinatol 2009;36:391-416, x.
21. Saade GR, Belfort MA, Berry DL, et al. Amniotic septostomy for the treatment of twin oligohydramnios-polyhydramnios sequence. Fetal Diagn Ther. 1998;13:86-93.
22. Johnson JR, Rossi KQ, O'Shaughnessy RW. Amnioreduction versus septostomy in twin-twin transfusion syndrome. Am J Obstet Gynecol. 2001;185:1044-7.
23. De Lia JE, Cruikshank DP, Keye WR Jr. Fetoscopic neodymium:YAG laser occlusion of placental vessels in severe twin-twin transfusion syndrome. Obstet Gynecol. 1990;75:1046-53.
24. Slaghekke F, Lopriore E, Lewi L, et al. Fetoscopic laser coagulation of the vascular equator versus selective coagulation for twin-to-twin transfusion syndrome: an open-label randomised controlled trial. Lancet. 2014; 383:2144-51.
25. Ville Y, Hecher K, Ogg D, Warren R, Nicolaides K. Successful outcome after Nd:YAG laser separation of chorioangiopagus-twins under sonoendoscopic control. Ultrasound in Obstetrics & Gynecology: the Official Journal of the International Society of Ultrasound in Obstetrics and Gynecology. 1992;2:429-31.
26. Ville Y, Hyett J, Hecher K, Nicolaides K. Preliminary experience with endoscopic laser surgery for severe twin-twin transfusion syndrome. The New England Journal of Medicine. 1995;332:224-7.
27. Wataganara T. Development of fetoscopic and minimally invasive ultrasound-guided surgical simulator: Parts of global education. Donald School J Ultrasound Obstet Gynecol. 2013;7:352-5.
28. Van Peborgh P, Rambaud C, Ville Y. Effect of laser coagulation on placental vessels: histological aspects. Fetal Diagn Ther. 1997;12:32-5.
29. Fink RJ, Allen TK, Habib AS. Remifentanil for fetal immobilization and analgesia during the ex utero intrapartum treatment procedure under combined spinal-epidural anaesthesia. Br J Anaesth. 2011;106:851-5.
30. Deprest JA, Van Schoubroeck D, Van Ballaer PP, Flageole H, Van Assche FA, Vandenberghe K. Alternative technique for Nd:YAG laser coagulation in twin-to-twin transfusion syndrome with anterior placenta. Ultrasound in obstetrics & gynecology: the Official Journal of the International Society of Ultrasound in Obstetrics and Gynecology. 1998;11:347-52.
31. Huber A, Baschat AA, Bregenzer T, et al. Laser coagulation of placental anastomoses with a 30 degrees fetoscope in severe mid-trimester twin-twin transfusion syndrome with anterior placenta. Ultrasound in obstetrics & gynecology: the official journal of the International Society of Ultrasound in Obstetrics and Gynecology. 2008;31:412-6.
32. Quintero RA, Bornick PW, Allen MH, Johson PK. Selective laser photocoagulation of communicating vessels in severe twin-twin transfusion syndrome in women with an anterior placenta. Obstet Gynecol. 2001;97:477-81.
33. De Lia JE, Kuhlmann RS, Harstad TW, Cruikshank DP. Fetoscopic laser ablation of placental vessels in severe previable twin-twin transfusion syndrome. Am J Obstet Gynecol. 1995;172:1202-8; discussion 8-11.
34. Middeldorp JM, Lopriore E, Sueters M, et al. Laparoscopically guided uterine entry for fetoscopy in twin-to-twin transfusion syndrome with completely anterior placenta: a novel technique. Fetal Diagn Ther. 2007;22:409-15.
35. Wataganara T, Gratacos E, Jani J, et al. Persistent elevation of cell-free fetal DNA levels in maternal plasma after selective laser coagulation of chorionic plate anastomoses in severe midgestational twin-twin transfusion syndrome. Am J Obstet Gynecol. 2005;192:604-9.
36. Quintero RA, Morales WJ, Mendoza G, et al. Selective photocoagulation of placental vessels in twin-twin transfusion syndrome: evolution of a surgical technique. Obstetrical and Gynecological Survey. 1998;53:S97-103.
37. Stirnemann JJ, Nasr B, Quarello E, et al. A definition of selectivity in laser coagulation of chorionic plate anastomoses in twin-to-twin transfusion syndrome and its relationship to perinatal outcome. Am J Obstet Gynecol. 2008;198:62 e1-6.
38. Chalouhi GE, Essaoui M, Stirnemann J, et al. Laser therapy for twin-to-twin transfusion syndrome (TTTS). Prenatal Diagn. 2011;31:637-46.
39. Rossi AC, Vanderbilt D, Chmait RH. Neurodevelopmental outcomes after laser therapy for twin-twin transfusion syndrome: a systematic review and meta-analysis. Obstet Gynecol. 2011;118:1145-50.
40. Lenclen R, Ciarlo G, Paupe A, Bussieres L, Ville Y. Neurodevelopmental outcome at 2 years in children born preterm treated by amnioreduction or fetoscopic laser surgery for twin-to-twin transfusion syndrome: comparison with dichorionic twins. Am J Obstet Gynecol. 2009;201:291 e1-5.
41. Haller CM, Buerzle W, Brubaker CE, et al. Mussel-mimetic tissue adhesive for fetal membrane repair: a standardized ex vivo evaluation using elastomeric membranes. Prenatal Diagnosis. 2011;31:654-60.
42. Deprest J, Emonds MP, Richter J, et al. Amniopatch for iatrogenic rupture of the fetal membranes. Prenatal Diagnosis. 2011;31:661-6.
43. Moore TR, Gale S, Benirschke K. Perinatal outcome of forty-nine pregnancies complicated by acardiac twinning. Am J Obstet Gynecol. 1990;163:907-12.
44. Coulam CB, Wright G. First trimester diagnosis of acardiac twins. Early Pregnancy. 2000;4:261-70.

45. Ruiz-Cordero R, Birusingh RJ, Pelaez L, Azouz M, Rodriguez MM. Twin Reversed Arterial Perfusion Sequence (TRAPS): An Illustrative Series of 13 Cases. Fetal Pediatr Pathol. 2016;35:63-80.
46. Jelin E, Hirose S, Rand L, et al. Perinatal outcome of conservative management versus fetal intervention for twin reversed arterial perfusion sequence with a small acardiac twin. Fetal Diagn Thera. 2010;27:138-41.
47. Porreco RP, Barton SM, Haverkamp AD. Occlusion of umbilical artery in acardiac, acephalic twin. Lancet. 1991;337:326-7.
48. Quintero RA, Reich H, Puder KS, et al. Brief report: umbilical-cord ligation of an acardiac twin by fetoscopy at 19 weeks of gestation. The New England Journal of Medicine. 1994;330:469-71.
49. Quintero RA, Romero R, Reich H, et al. In utero percutaneous umbilical cord ligation in the management of complicated monochorionic multiple gestations. Ultrasound in obstetrics & gynecology: the official Journal of the International Society of Ultrasound in Obstetrics and Gynecology. 1996;8:16-22.
50. Tan TY, Sepulveda W. Acardiac twin: a systematic review of minimally invasive treatment modalities. Ultrasound in obstetrics & gynecology: the official journal of the International Society of Ultrasound in Obstetrics and Gynecology. 2003;22:409-19.
51. Gucciardo L, Deprest J, Done E, et al. Prediction of outcome in isolated congenital diaphragmatic hernia and its consequences for fetal therapy. Best practice & Research Clinical Obstet Gynaecol. 2008;22:123-38.
52. Chinn DH, Filly RA, Callen PW, Nakayama DK, Harrison MR. Congenital diaphragmatic hernia diagnosed prenatally by ultrasound. Radiology. 1983;148:119-23.
53. Taylor GA, Atalabi OM, Estroff JA. Imaging of congenital diaphragmatic hernias. Pediatric Radiology. 2009;39:1-16.
54. Done E, Gucciardo L, Van Mieghem T, et al. Prenatal diagnosis, prediction of outcome and in utero therapy of isolated congenital diaphragmatic hernia. Prenatal Diagn. 2008;28:581-91.
55. Mehollin-Ray AR, Cassady CI, Cass DL, Olutoye OO. Fetal MR imaging of congenital diaphragmatic hernia. Radiographics: a review publication of the Radiological Society of North America, Inc. 2012;32:106-84.
56. Victoria T, Danzer E, Adzick NS. Use of ultrasound and MRI for evaluation of lung volumes in fetuses with isolated left congenital diaphragmatic hernia. Seminars in Pediatric Surgery. 2013;22:30-6.
57. Phithakwatchara N, Coleman A, Peiro JL, et al. Differential patterns of prenatal ipsilateral and contralateral lung growth in cases of isolated left-sided congenital diaphragmatic hernia. Prenatal Diagnosis. 2015;35:769-76.
58. Kilian AK, Schaible T, Hofmann V, Brade J, Neff KW, Busing KA. Congenital diaphragmatic hernia: predictive value of MRI relative lung-to-head ratio compared with MRI fetal lung volume and sonographic lung-to-head ratio. AJR Am J Roentgenol. 2009;192:153-8.
59. Walleyo A, Debus A, Kehl S, et al. Periodic MRI lung volume assessment in fetuses with congenital diaphragmatic hernia: prediction of survival, need for ECMO, and development of chronic lung disease. AJR Am J Roentgenol. 2013;201: 419-26.
60. Debus A, Hagelstein C, Kilian AK, et al. Fetal lung volume in congenital diaphragmatic hernia: association of prenatal MR imaging findings with postnatal chronic lung disease. Radiology. 2013;266:887-95.
61. Coleman A, Phithakwatchara N, Shaaban A, et al. Fetal lung growth represented by longitudinal changes in MRI-derived fetal lung volume parameters predicts survival in isolated left-sided congenital diaphragmatic hernia. Prenatal Diagn. 2015;35:160-6.
62. Matsuoka S, Takeuchi K, Yamanaka Y, Kaji Y, Sugimura K, Maruo T. Comparison of magnetic resonance imaging and ultrasonography in the prenatal diagnosis of congenital thoracic abnormalities. Fetal Diagn Ther. 2003;18:447-53.
63. Gerards FA, Twisk JW, Tibboel D, van Vugt JM. Congenital diaphragmatic hernia: 2D lung area and 3D lung volume measurements of the contralateral lung to predict postnatal outcome. Fetal Diagnosis and Therapy. 2008;24:271-6.
64. Cannie M, Jani J, Meersschaert J, et al. Prenatal prediction of survival in isolated diaphragmatic hernia using observed to expected total fetal lung volume determined by magnetic resonance imaging based on either gestational age or fetal body volume. Ultrasound in obstetrics & gynecology: the official Journal of the International Society of Ultrasound in Obstetrics and Gynecology. 2008;32:633-9.
65. Mayer S, Klaritsch P, Petersen S, et al. The correlation between lung volume and liver herniation measurements by fetal MRI in isolated congenital diaphragmatic hernia: a systematic review and meta-analysis of observational studies. Prenatal Diagnosis. 2011;31:1086-96.
66. Deprest J, De Coppi P. Antenatal management of isolated congenital diaphragmatic hernia today and tomorrow: ongoing collaborative research and development. Journal of Pediatric Surgery Lecture. Journal of Pediatric Surgery. 2012;47:282-90.
67. Bollmann R, Kalache K, Mau H, Chaoui R, Tennstedt C. Associated malformations and chromosomal defects in congenital diaphragmatic hernia. Fetal Diagn Ther. 1995;10:52-9.
68. Nawapun K, Eastwood M, Sandaite I, et al. Correlation of observed-to-expected total fetal lung volume with intrathoracic organ herniation on magnetic resonance imaging in fetuses with isolated left-sided congenital diaphragmatic hernia. Ultrasound in obstetrics & gynecology: the official journal of the International Society of Ultrasound in Obstetrics and Gynecology. 2015;46:162-7.
69. Le LD, Keswani SG, Biesiada J, et al. The congenital diaphragmatic hernia composite prognostic index correlates with survival in left-sided congenital diaphragmatic hernia. J Pediat Surg. 2012;47:57-62.
70. Phithakwatchara N, Coleman A, Peiro JL, et al. Expanded intrathoracic space in fetal cases of isolated congenital diaphragmatic hernia contributes to disparity between

percent predicted lung volume and observed to expected total lung volume. Prenatal Diagn. 2015;35:154-9.
71. DeKoninck P, Gomez O, Sandaite I, et al. Right-sided congenital diaphragmatic hernia in a decade of fetal surgery. BJOG. 2015;122:940-6.
72. Ruano R, Peiro JL, da Silva MM, et al. Early fetoscopic tracheal occlusion for extremely severe pulmonary hypoplasia in isolated congenital diaphragmatic hernia: preliminary results. Ultrasound in obstetrics & gynecology: the official journal of the International Society of Ultrasound in Obstetrics and Gynecology. 2013;42:70-6.
73. Nawapun K, Eastwood MP, Diaz-Cobos D, et al. In vivo evidence by magnetic resonance volumetry of a gestational age dependent response to tracheal occlusion for congenital diaphragmatic hernia. Prenatal Diagn. 2015;35:1048-56.
74. Klaritsch P, Mayer S, Sbragia L, et al. Albumin as an adjunct to tracheal occlusion in fetal rats with congenital diaphragmatic hernia: a placebo-controlled study. Am J Obstet Gynecol. 2010;202:198 e1-9.
75. Anumba DO, Scott JE, Plant ND, Robson SC. Diagnosis and outcome of fetal lower urinary tract obstruction in the northern region of England. Prenatal Diagn. 2005;25:7-13.
76. Wu S, Johnson MP. Fetal lower urinary tract obstruction. Clin Perinatol. 2009;36:377-90, x.
77. Nakayama DK, Harrison MR, de Lorimier AA. Prognosis of posterior urethral valves presenting at birth. J Pediatr Surg. 1986;21:43-5.
78. Housley HT, Harrison MR. Fetal urinary tract abnormalities. Natural history, pathophysiology, and treatment. The Urologic clinics of North America. 1998;25:63-73.
79. Harrison MR, Ross N, Noall R, de Lorimier AA. Correction of congenital hydronephrosis in utero. I. The model: fetal urethral obstruction produces hydronephrosis and pulmonary hypoplasia in fetal lambs. Journal of Pediatric Surg. 1983;18:247-56.
80. Glick PL, Harrison MR, Noall RA, Villa RL. Correction of congenital hydronephrosis in utero III. Early mid-trimester ureteral obstruction produces renal dysplasia. Journal of Pediatr Surg. 1983;18:681-7.
81. Kramer SA. Current status of fetal intervention for congenital hydronephrosis. The Journal of Urology. 1983;130:641-6.
82. Bellinger MF, Comstock CH, Grosso D, Zaino R. Fetal posterior urethral valves and renal dysplasia at 15 weeks gestational age. The Journal of Urology. 1983;129:1238-9.
83. Chinn DH, Filly RA. Ultrasound diagnosis of fetal genitourinary tract anomalies. Urologic Radiology. 1982;4:115-23.
84. Glazer GM, Filly RA, Callen PW. The varied sonographic appearance of the urinary tract in the fetus and newborn with urethral obstruction. Radiology. 1982;144:563-8.
85. Adzick NS, Harrison MR, Flake AW, Laberge JM. Development of a fetal renal function test using endogenous creatinine clearance. J Pediatr Surg. 1985;20:602-7.
86. Mahony BS, Filly RA, Callen PW, Hricak H, Golbus MS, Harrison MR. Fetal renal dysplasia: sonographic evaluation. Radiology. 1984;152:143-6.
87. Crombleholme TM, Harrison MR, Longaker MT, Langer JC. Prenatal diagnosis and management of bilateral hydronephrosis. Pediatr Nephrol. 1988;2:334-42.
88. Lumbers ER, Hill KJ, Bennett VJ. Proximal and distal tubular activity in chronically catheterized fetal sheep compared with the adult. Canadian Journal of Physiology and Pharmacology. 1988;66:697-702.
89. Glick PL, Harrison MR, Golbus MS, et al. Management of the fetus with congenital hydronephrosis II: Prognostic criteria and selection for treatment. J Pediatr Surg. 1985;20: 376-87.
90. Mussap M, Fanos V, Pizzini C, Marcolongo A, Chiaffoni G, Plebani M. Predictive value of amniotic fluid cystatin C levels for the early identification of fetuses with obstructive uropathies. BJOG. 2002;109:778-83.
91. Pluto Collaborative Study G, Kilby M, Khan K, et al. PLUTO trial protocol: percutaneous shunting for lower urinary tract obstruction randomised controlled trial. BJOG. 2007;114:904-5, e1-4.
92. Johnson MP, Corsi P, Bradfield W, et al. Sequential urinalysis improves evaluation of fetal renal function in obstructive uropathy. Am J Obstet Gynecol. 1995;173:59-65.
93. Morris RK, Malin GL, Quinlan-Jones E, et al. Percutaneous vesicoamniotic shunting versus conservative management for fetal lower urinary tract obstruction (PLUTO): a randomised trial. Lancet. 2013;382:1496-506.
94. Agarwal SK, Fisk NM. In utero therapy for lower urinary tract obstruction. Prenatal Diagn. 2001;21:970-6.
95. Martinez JM, Masoller N, Devlieger R, et al. Laser ablation of posterior urethral valves by fetal cystoscopy. Fetal Diagn. Ther. 2015;37:267-73.
96. Ruano R, Sananes N, Sangi-Haghpeykar H, et al. Fetal intervention for severe lower urinary tract obstruction: a multicenter case-control study comparing fetal cystoscopy with vesicoamniotic shunting. Ultrasound in obstetrics & gynecology: the official journal of the International Society of Ultrasound in Obstetrics and Gynecology. 2015;45:452-8.
97. Kohl T, Hering R, Heep A, et al. Percutaneous fetoscopic patch coverage of spina bifida aperta in the human—early clinical experience and potential. Fetal Diagn Ther. 2006;21:185-93.
98. Pedreira DA, Zanon N, Nishikuni K, et al. Endoscopic surgery for the antenatal treatment of myelomeningocele: the CECAM trial. Am J Obstet Gynecol. 2016;214:111 e1- e11.
99. Pedreira DA, Zanon N, de Sa RA, et al. Fetoscopic single-layer repair of open spina bifida using a cellulose patch: preliminary clinical experience. The journal of maternal-fetal & neonatal medicine: the official journal of the European Association of Perinatal Medicine, the Federation of Asia and Oceania Perinatal Societies, the International Society of Perinatal Obstet. 2014;27:1613-9.
100. Vettraino IM, Lee W, Comstock CH. The evolving appearance of a congenital diaphragmatic hernia. Journal of ultrasound in medicine: official journal of the American Institute of Ultrasound in Medicine. 2002;21:85-9.

47

CHAPTER

Open Fetal Surgery

Tuangsit Wataganara

INTRODUCTION

Open fetal surgery is a more invasive approach to the fetus via a hysterotomy incision. It has not been commonly practiced due to significant maternal morbidity. Open fetal surgery has gained an attention after a conclusion of a recent randomized controlled trial: Management of Myelomeningocele Study (MoMs trial) that showed a superior benefit of prenatal correction of myelomeningocele (MMC) in terms of (1) decreased the need for ventriculoperitoneal shunting, (2) reversed hind brain herniation (Chiari 2 malformation), (3) improved motor function in lower extremities, and (4) higher rates of independent ambulation at 30 months of age. It has become a new standard of care in many parts of the United States. This chapter is aiming to review the currently available published information on the technical aspects and the evolving indications of open fetal surgery. An alternative approach with fetoscopy is also described and updated. Open fetal surgery used to be an appropriate approach for removal of fetal tumors, and this chapter will describe different kinds of tumors arising in-utero, and how the published data can guide us for an appropriate management.

RATIONALE OF OPEN FETAL SURGERY

Open hysterotomy is aiming to provide a spacious access to the fetus for a more complex surgical management, also known as "open fetal surgery". It was first reported by Michael Harrison et al. from University of California San Francisco in 1982.[1] The first fetal surgery performed through open hysterotomy was fetal vesicostomy. It involved opening of fetal abdominal wall and urinary bladder for semipermanent urinary diversion as a temporizing therapy for a fetus with obstruction below the level of urinary bladder (lower urinary tract obstruction: LUTO).

The indications for open fetal surgery have been evolving in the past 4 decades. Due to its invasive nature to the mother's body, it is mandatory to address all significant potential complications incurring on the mother, the fetus, and the future fertility to the family before going into the fetal part of the surgery.

The key messages during preoperative counseling should include the fact that the mother is about to take the procedure-related risks similar to other major abdominal surgery, but there is no direct physical benefit to the mother herself. The surgical risks to the mother mostly related to large laparotomy, which may put her at a higher chance of excessive bleeding, infection, accidental injury to adjacent organs and respiratory compromise. She is also taking an additional risk associated with aggressive tocolysis therapy and prolonged bed rest. Deep vein thrombosis and pulmonary thromboembolism are not uncommon, particularly if the mother is in hypercoagulable state. The summary of risks to the mother and the fetus related to open fetal surgery are described in **Table 1**. More details on the rationale of various kinds of fetal interventions can be found in our recently published article of Working Group on Perinatal Medicine, under the hospice of World Association of Perinatal Medicine (WAPM) in Journal of Perinatal Medicine in 2015.[2]

TECHNICAL ASPECTS OF OPEN FETAL SURGERY

The patient is usually under a combined general and epidural anesthesia for a complete control of her vital signs. Additionally, the gravid uterus can be more relaxed from the effect of inhalation anesthetics. Detailed protocol for open fetal surgery is available in a landmark publication of Scott Adzick et al., but can be summarized as follows.[3] Broad spectrum antibiotics, i.e., 1 g of intravenous cefazolin, and uterine relaxation agent, such as 50 mg of rectal or

TABLE 1: Risks to the mother and the fetus related to open fetal surgery.

	Remarks
Risks to the mother	• Risks from laparotomy • Bleeding • Infection • Pain • Respiratory compromise • Inadvertent injury to nearby organ • Risks from aggressive tocolysis • Cardiopulmonary failure • Atony bleeding • Risks from large hysterotomy • Rupture of the uterus at hysterotomy scar • Infection • Risks from prolonged bed rest • Thromboembolic events • Respiratory compromise
Risks to the fetus	• Prematurity • Fetal or neonatal sepsis • Permanent disability • Death (from hypothermia or hemorrhage)

oral indomethacin or 10 mg of oral nifedipine are given preoperatively. The indwelling epidural catheter enabled administration of continuous postoperative analgesics.

The gravid uterus was exposed via a low transverse laparotomy incision and exteriorized. A vertical skin incision was used in patients with a BMI over 30 or those with a previous vertical skin scar. Otherwise Kocher transverse skin incision with dissection of rectus muscle will be used. The fetus and placenta are then located by intraoperative ultrasound, The primary surgeon choose the hysterotomy location to avoid them. The fetus was visualized by ultrasound on real-time basis, which help the manually positioning within the uterus to facilitate the intervention. For instance, in case of meningomyelocele (MMC), the sac is positioned in the center of hysterotomy incision. Classical, or vertical, incision of the uterus is required, to make sure that operative space is sufficient. Adequate hemostasis is crucial, and it can be achieved by the use of *uterine stapler*. This device simultaneously cuts and release polyglycolic material to seal the raw surface in the myometrium. The use of uterine stapler is crucial in open fetal surgery due to the following reasons.

- Polyglycolic acid, which is the identical material used for manufacturing suture material such as Catgut and Chromic Catgut, is an absorbable material.
- It helps sealing the end-on arteries and veins within the myometrial wall of the uterus. Hence, it reduces blood loss, as well as helps clearing the visibility of the surgical field. It seals fetal membranes (chorioamniotic sac) with the rim of myometrial incision. Therefore, fetal membranes are not "retracted" following the extension of uterine incision. This certainly helps with the membranes healing after the myometrium incision is restored, preferably in doubly layer fashion, at the conclusion of the procedure.

In the case of a posterior placenta, entry is the amniotic cavity straightforward. Classical or vertical incision is performed on the anterior wall of the uterus. In the case of an anterior placenta, exteriorization of the gravid uterine is needed, so that hysterotomy incision can then be made either at the fundal part or posterior wall of the uterus. Under sonographic guidance, the surgeons place two monofilament traction sutures through the full-thickness uterine wall. Initial uterine entry is accomplished sharply between the uterine traction sutures. Then the uterine stapling device loaded with absorbable polyglycolic acid staples is passed into the uterine cavity. The stapler is palpated manually and ultrasonography was used to exclude the presence of fetal tissue between the instrument's blades and the uterine wall. The stapler is used to create a uterine incision large enough to expose the fetal MMC, which is usually between 6 and 8 centimeters in length. Under direct visualization, the fetus is given an intramuscular injection of a "cocktail" consisting of fentanyl (20 mg/kg) and vecuronium (0.2 mg/kg).

Fetal surgery is then carried out in the hands of either pediatric surgeons or neurosurgeons. Fetal cardiac function is monitored with continuous echocardiography by an individual not involved in the actual prenatal surgery. Postoperatively, the mother is usually given a 24-hour course of tocolysis. Prophylactic antibiotics are continued for 24 hours. The patient also undergoes daily ultrasound by which fetal well-being and fluid volume are assessed. Most patients recover in the hospital for 4–5 days after surgery. The patient is then seen on a weekly basis with ultrasound evaluation. Compared with early experiences with hysterotomy, some of the associated morbidities have now decreased. Significant pulmonary edema or blood loss is now relatively rare.[4]

FETAL MENINGOMYELOCELE

Studies in animal models and clinical case series laid the groundwork for a clinical trial to test the safety and efficacy of fetal meningomyelocele (MMC) repair. The National

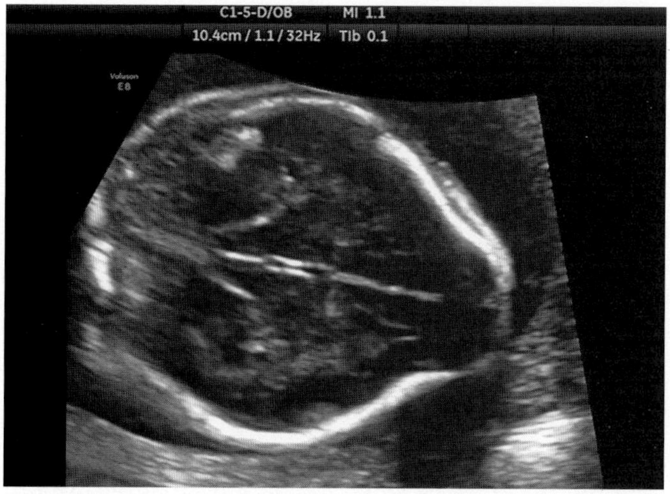

Fig. 1: Ultrasound image of skull and brain of a 24 weeks of fetus with meningomyelocele (MMC). On this axial cut, note an internal curvation of the frontal cranial bones has a similar appearance to lemon, so it is commonly called "Lemon Sign". Borderline cerebral ventriculomegaly, with preferential dilatation of the anterior horn, is another typical intracranial ultrasound finding in a fetus with MMC. This fetus was also microcephalic, with its biparietal diameter and head circumference lower than 5 percentiles of the comparable gestational age.

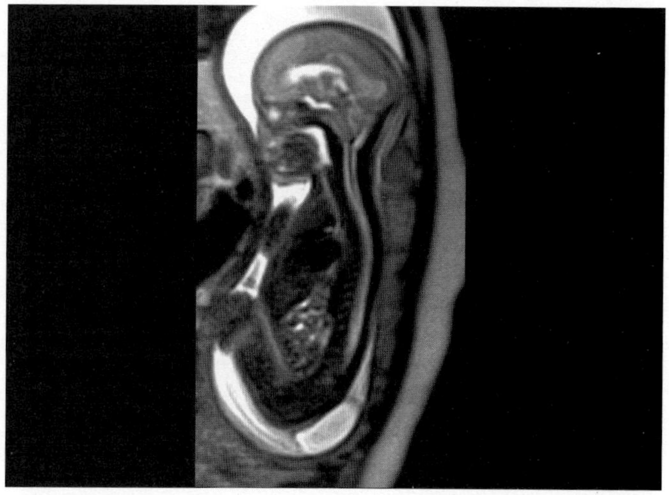

Fig. 2: Magnetic resonance image (sagittal cut, fast T2-weighted single shot technique) of a 24 weeks of fetus with lumbosacral meningomyelocele (MMC). The MMC sac is seen as a thin-walled structure containing hyposignaled fluid content, which is consistent with cerebrospinal fluid. The cavity of this cystic structure is connected to the spinal canal. Downward displacement of cerebellar vermis into spinal canal, so called hindbrain herniation, is noted. Hindbrain herniation contributes to a number of intracranial sonographic findings in fetuses with MMC. It may also necessitate cerebrospinal fluid shunting to relieve intracranial pressure after the baby is born.

Institute of Health-sponsored prospective, randomized Management of Myelomeningocele Study (the MOMS trial) demonstrated that fetal surgery for MMC before 26 weeks' gestation may preserve neurologic function, reverse hindbrain herniation and obviate the need for postnatal placement of a ventriculoperitoneal shunt. There are, however, significant risks related to the uterine scar and premature birth.

Prenatal Diagnosis of MMC

Diagnosis of a fetus with MMC has been fostered by different serum biochemical markers and imaging modalities. Maternal serum a-fetoprotein, as a part of fetal Down syndrome screening program which is widely adopted has allowed for an earlier detection of MMC. Broader availability of high-quality ultrasound, magnetic resonance imaging (MRI), and fetal echocardiogram have helped changing the face of fetal diagnosis, treatment and monitor in the presence of MMC since 1980s.

Fetal cranial scan serves as a practical screening tool for MMC. Certain findings in fetal cranium can be suggestive of MMC, which is not always readily visible. Approximately, 61% and 25% of fetuses with MMC have biparietal diameter and head circumference, respectively, lower than 5 percentile.[5] Ventriculomegaly can be found in 77% of fetuses with MMC. In this case, the anterior cerebral ventricle horns are preferentially dilated, as shown in **Figure 1**.

Frontal cranial bones of a fetus with MMC may have an internal curvation, which makes it look like "lemon" from an axial view, so called "lemon sign". In addition, 4th ventricle and cerebellar might be absent, as a result of protrusion of cerebellar vermix into the spinal canal, as shown in **Figure 2**. Seeing "banana sign", as shown in **Figure 3**, should raise a suspicion for MMC. The incidence and diagnostic accuracy of these intracranial sonographic markers were evaluated in a study of 1,561 patients at high risk for fetal neural tube defects.[6] Of these, 130 fetuses had open spina bifida. There was a relationship between gestational age and the presence of each of these markers. Certain intracranial sonographic markers may disappear with advancing gestational age.

For instance, the lemon sign is present in 98% of MMC fetuses at less than or equal to 24 weeks of gestation, but in only 13% of those at greater than 24 weeks of gestation. Cerebellar abnormalities were present in 95%

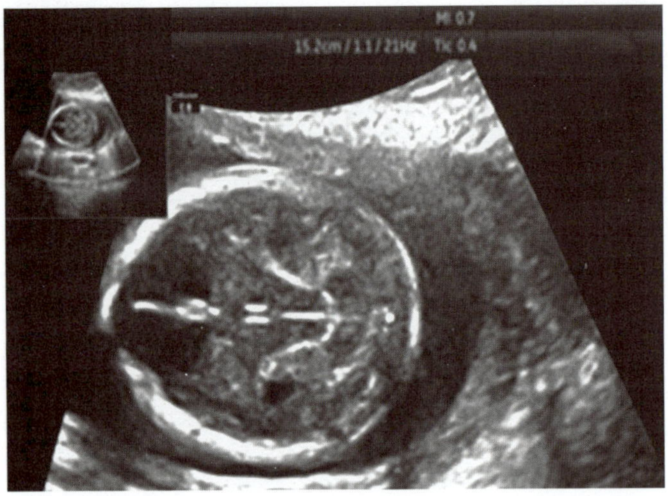

Fig. 3: Ultrasound image of skull and brain of a 24-week of fetus with meningomyelocele (MMC). On this axial cut, with the scanning plan toward caudal to the plane shown in **Figure 1**, it is noticed that the cerebellum is wrapped tightly around the brain stem. The distorted shape of cerebellum has a similar appearance to banana, so it is commonly called "Banana Sign". This is caused by spinal cord tethering and downward migration of posterior fossa content. Cisterna magna is obliterated. These sonographic findings of posterior fossa persists into the second and third trimester.

of fetuses irrespective of gestation; however, the cerebellar abnormality at less than or equal to 24 weeks of gestation was predominantly the banana sign (72%) whereas at gestations greater than 24 weeks was cerebellar "absence" (81%).[5]

Fetal anatomy survey in the second and third trimesters of pregnancy has become a standard of practice in many places. It is essential that every scan includes a complete evaluation of the spine. Images should be recorded in longitudinal, sagittal, coronal and axial planes. The axial view demonstrates three ossification centers, a centrum for the vertebral body and two lateral masses that converge, creating a triangular configuration. The sagittal view demonstrates the spine as two parallel echogenic lines representing the centrum and lamina with a subtle normal lordosis at the cervical and lumbar levels and a subtle kyphosis at the thoracic level, with convergence of these lines distally. Three-dimensional ultrasound image, using gradient weighed and Silhouette mode, to demonstrate a normal fetal vertebral column. In the coronal plane, the posterior elements appear as paired, echogenic lines with subtle flaring at the lumbar level and tapering at the sacral level.

TABLE 2: Eligibility for women carrying a fetus with meningomyelocele (MMC) to be a candidate for open fetal repair

Eligibility	*Contraindication*
• Singleton • Gestational age of 19.0 to 25.9 weeks' • Upper defect boundary between T1 and S1 • Hindbrain herniation • Normal karyotype	• Associated anomalies not related to MMC • Severe kyphosis • Risk of preterm birth (short cervix and previous preterm birth) • Placental abruption • A body-mass index ≥35 • Contraindication to surgery, including previous hysterotomy in the active uterine segment

It has been previously reported that fetal MRI and ultrasound are equally effective in determining the lesion level in the fetus with MMC.[7] However, our experience at Siriraj Hospital in Bangkok does not support this conclusion. Ultrasound is our primary tool to diagnose, confirm, as well as to determine the lesion level. MRI is deemed definitive for the presence or absence of hindbrain herniation, which was crucial in the selection of candidates for in utero surgical repair.[3]

Preoperative Evaluation of Fetal MMC

Eligibility criteria were set to standardize the recruitment of participants to the MoMs trial. The enrollment criteria for participants who carry a fetus with MMC and wish to undergo open fetal surgical repair of this spinal defect are summarized in **Table 2**. This criteria can be applied to other fetal care centers who wish to participate in this type of surgery, even on a service basis. In summary, they have to be a singleton pregnancy, the upper boundary of MMC must be located between T1 and S1 (high-risk lesion), evidence of hindbrain herniation, a gestational age of 19.0 to 25.9 weeks', and normal fetal karyotype.[3] Determination of spinal defect boundary has to be performed from 3 perpendicular axes; sagittal, coronal, and axial, shown in **Figures 4 to 6**. If the boundary of defect is caudal to S1 level, as shown in **Figures 7 and 8**, the risk of open surgical repair is outweighed by the severity of neurological deficit.

Contraindications of open fetal surgical repair of MMC can be categorized into fetal and maternal contraindications. Fetal contraindications include associated anomalies that are not related to MMC and severe kyphoscoliosis **(Fig. 9)**. Maternal contraindications include risk of preterm birth (including short cervix and previous preterm birth), placental abruption, a body-mass index of 35 kg/m^2

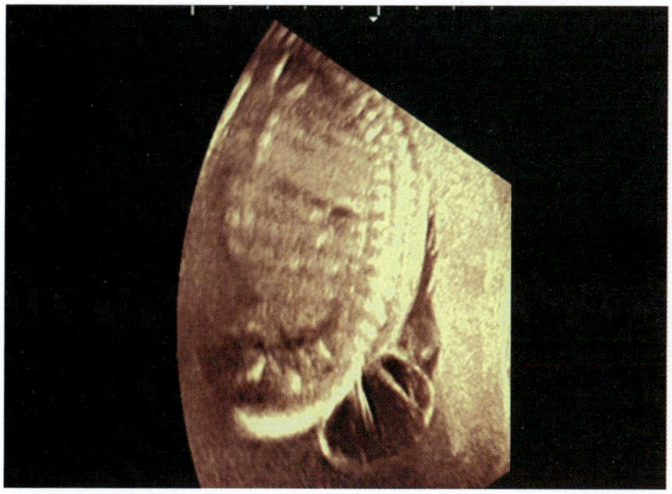

Fig. 4: Ultrasound image of vertebral column of a 26 weeks of fetus with meningomyelocele (MMC). On this sagittal cut, the boundary of defect is from L2 to S1. Note that there is no significant kyphosis or scoliosis, which are the contraindications of open fetal spinal repair. The hyperechoic string-like structures seen in meningeal sac are cauda equina.

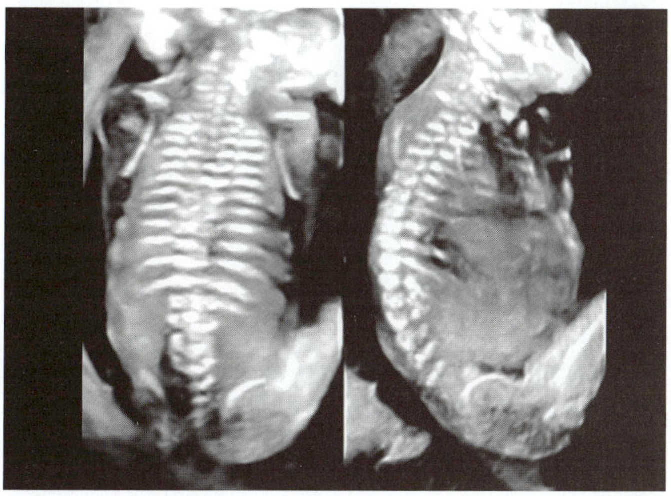

Fig. 5: Three-dimensional ultrasound images, displayed with maximum weighted gradient or X-ray mode, show vertebral column and ribs of a 24-week of fetus in coronal and sagittal planes. Determination of the defect boundary is made simple by the fact that T12 is the last vertebral body with its corresponding ribs, and L1 is the first vertebral body without corresponding ribs.

or more, and other general contraindication to surgery, including previous hysterotomy in the active uterine segment. Woman who is pregnant with a fetus affected with high-risk MMC, but is not eligible for open fetal surgical repair according to the aforementioned criteria, should be offered alternatives, such as termination of pregnancy, pediatric physiotherapy and group support.

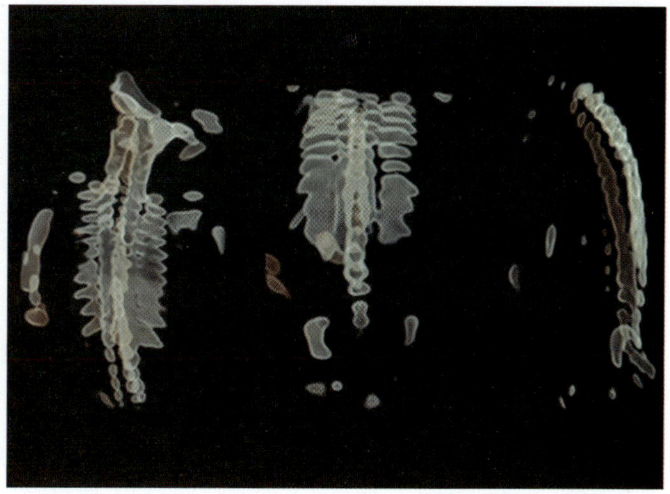

Fig. 6: Three-dimensional ultrasound images, displayed with Silhoutte mode, show vertebral column and ribs of a 25 weeks of fetus in coronal and sagittal planes. There is an alternative approach for sonographic evaluation of fetal vertebral structures.

Open Fetal Surgical Repair of MMC

Technical aspects of prenatal closure of MMC was recently published by the team at Children's Hospital of Philadelphia.[8] Uterine incision is made with uterine stapler. Continuous warm saline irrigation is started. The fetus is positioned accordingly. Fetal heart rate is continuously monitored with ultrasound, with neonatal resuscitation readily available. The surgery starts from closure of the MMC in a standardized manner under magnification. The neural placode is sharply dissected from surrounding tissue and allowed to drop into the spinal canal. The dura is then identified, reflected over the placode and then closed using a fine running suture. In large defect, as shown in **Figure 10**, it is not possible to obtain skin closure, relaxing incisions will be made or artificial skin patch will be used. Tissue-engineered skin patch has been a subject of intensive study.[9] After skin mobilization or artificial patch, the defect is closed using a fine running monofilament suture. The uterine incision is them closed in two layers. The first layer incorporated the absorbable staples and uterine membranes. As the last stitches of this layer were placed, warmed Ringer's lactate, mixed with broad spectrum antibiotics, such as 500 mm silligra of vancomycin, is added to the uterus until the amniotic fluid index is normalized. A second imbricating layer of suture is tied. The abdominal fascial layer and dermis are closed in routine fashion.

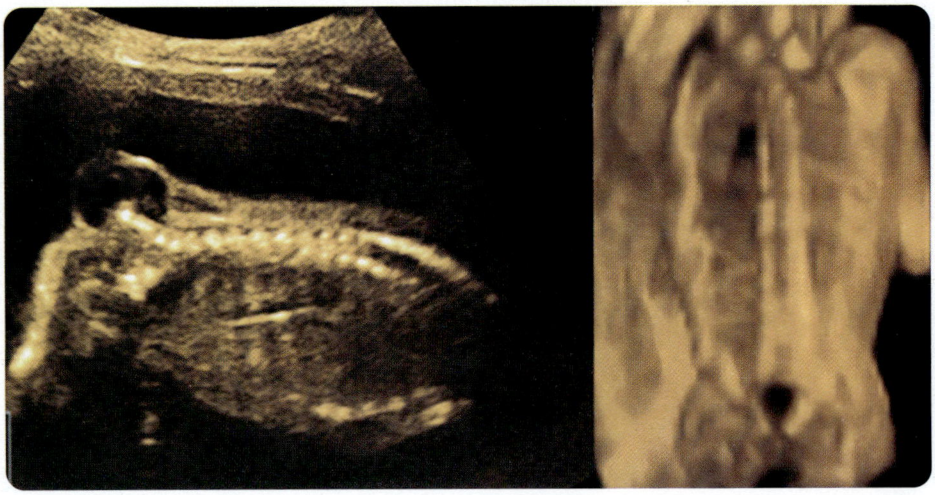

Fig. 7: Ultrasound images, displayed with gray-scale and three-dimensional with surface rendering, show meningomyelocele (MMC) with boundary lower than S2 level. Because of the caudal location of the meningeal sac, may be at the level of or below conus medullaris, often times the sac contain only cerebrospinal fluid, and not spinal cord tissue or nerve root. Meningeal sac without herniated neural tissue is called meningocele, which usually carries a better prognosis. This defect was not covered by skin, hence the dural layer of the meninges is directly exposed.

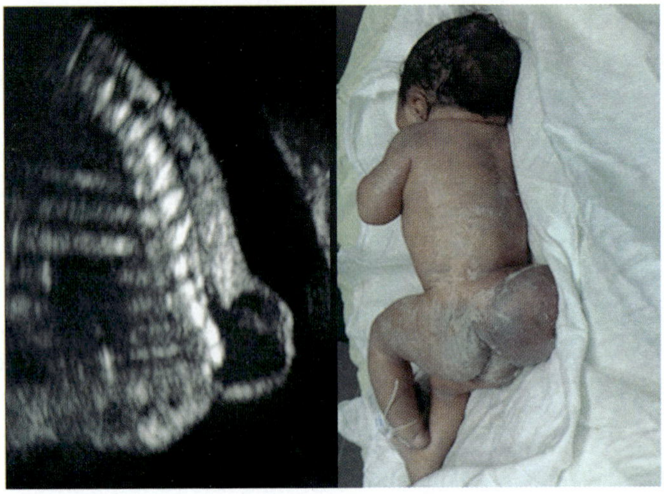

Fig. 8: Ultrasound image, displayed with gray-scale mode, shows meningocele (no herniated neural tissue in the meningeal sac). Full skin coverage of the sac was visible from ultrasound examination, and was confirmed at the time of birth. This newborn baby had a good muscle tone at both lower extremities. Postnatal surgical repair was uneventful.

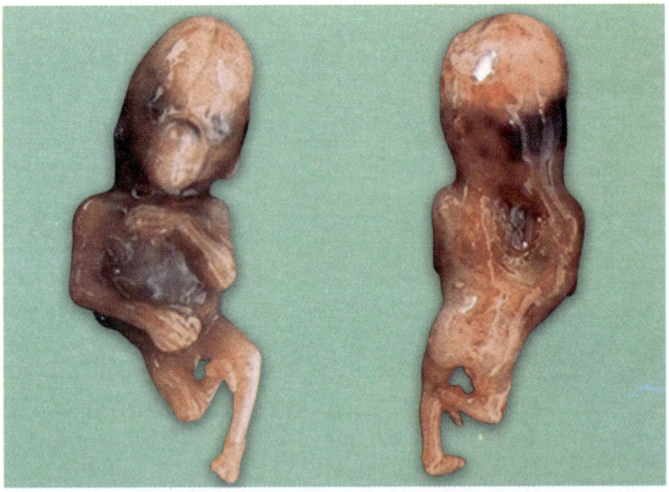

Fig. 9: Photograph of an abortus at 13 weeks' from medical termination of pregnancy due to prenatal detection of major malformation. The abortus has large meningomyelocele (MMC) at thoracic level. The meningeal sac was spontaneously ruptured in the process of miscarriage. Marked scoliosis and contracture of both lower extremities were seen during prenatal ultrasound examination, and was confirmed at the completion of miscarriage. Adverse prognostications in this case included large defect, cephalic location, spinal tissue herniation and scoliosis. Neurological outcomes in childhood period is predictably dismal, and after a thorough counseling, the family opted for termination of pregnancy.

Conclusion

The in-utero repair technique has changed the face of care for fetuses with MMC. There has been accumulating information on the long-term urological functional outcomes. Progressions have been made toward the MMC repair using tissue engineering techniques, as well as shifting the gear from open repair toward the laparoscopic repair of MMC. Data on long-term impact of fetuses that receive the in-utero repair for spina bifida will certainly help guiding and refining the optimal time and techniques of fetal MMC surgery.

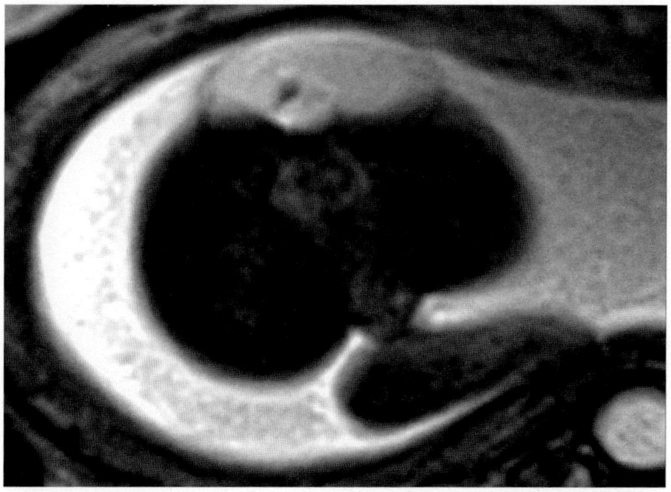

Fig. 10: Magnetic resonance image (axial cut, fast T2-weighted single shot technique) of a 20 weeks of fetus with large meningomyelocele (MMC) at lumbar level. The level is determined from this plane referring to the tip of iliac bones and the level of fetal umbilical insertion. The neural tissue seen inside the meningeal sac is conus medullaris. Note that the defect is wide, and if even after an adequate undermine of musculocutaneous flap, the defect cannot be fully covered, patching the defect with either synthetic or biosynthetic graft should be prepared. This principle is applicable to either prenatal or postnatal repair.

Practicality of the effects from the MOMs trial is worth exploring. After the completion of the MOMs trial, fetal MMC repair has become accepted as a standard of care option in selected circumstances. Recently, a 3-year outcome data from a single experienced center in the United States, following the publication of the MOMs trial was available.[10] It showed that 29% of referral patients met the criteria and underwent in utero repair of MMC. The total number of repair during that period of time was 100 cases. The average gestational age was 21.9 weeks at evaluation and 23.4 weeks at the time of surgical repair. Complications included membrane separation (22.9%), preterm premature rupture of membranes (32.3%) and preterm labor (37.5%). Average gestational age at delivery was 34.3 weeks and 54.2% delivered at ≥35 weeks. The perinatal loss rate was 6.1% (2 intrauterine fetal demises and 4 neonatal demises); 90.8% of women delivered at the Children's Hospital of Philadelphia and 3.4% received transfusions. With regard to the neonates, 2 received ventriculoperitoneal shunts prior to discharge; 71.1% of neonates had no evidence of hindbrain herniation on MRI. Of the 80 neonates evaluated, 55% were assigned a functional level of one or more better than the prenatal anatomic level. Therefore, in an experienced program, maternal and neonatal outcomes for patients undergoing *in utero* MMC repair are comparable to results of the MOMS trial.[10] A recent survey conducted among principal investigators who offer open repair for MMC at their centers showed certain degree of discrepancy in management of MMC post MOMS trial.[11] Quality control and recertification program may help keeping smaller fetal care centers with smaller number of cases and can keep up with the ever demanding standard.

At the time of writing this chapter, a significant progress has been made in developing endoscopic repair of open spina bifida (CECAM trial).[12] Results from the first batch of participants were on the same line with open fetal surgical repair including mean gestational age at delivery, reversal of hindbrain herniation, and neurological outcome in early infancy period. Longer learning curve is expected with endoscopic approach for the pediatric neurosurgical team to get accustomed to the new device and new orientation.

FETAL TUMOR

Most commonly found tumors in prenatal period are teratoma. Teratomas are generic term for tumors that contain tissue from all three germinal layers, namely ectoderm, mesoderm, and endoderm. Teratoma of prenatal onset is most commonly found in the brain, oropharynx (also known as epignathus), sacrococcygeal, mediastinum, peritoneal cavity, and gonad. Teratoma has sonographic appearance of mixed solid-cystic tumor with disorganized internal appearance. Teratoma in fetus is highly vascular, which is not the case of teratoma arising in adult period.

Sacrococcygeal Teratomas

Sacrococcygeal teratomas (SCTs) are the most common neoplasm in the fetus and newborn. The prevalence is 1 in 20,000 to 1 in 40,000, with female predominance in the ratio of 3:1.[13] Teratomas have midline predominance, particularly in the sacrococcygeal area (60%), gonads (20%), and thoracoabdominal cavity (15%). Prenatal ultrasound identifies SCTs as a complex mass at the distal end of the spine containing echoic solid components, as shown in **Figure 11**. Doppler studies can demonstrate its high vascularity, as shown in **Figure 12**, which is a hallmark of SCTs.[14] Malignant transformation of SCTs has been reported in prenatal period.[15] Immature teratoma and endodermal sinus tumor are 2 most common malignant cell types, which yield a high

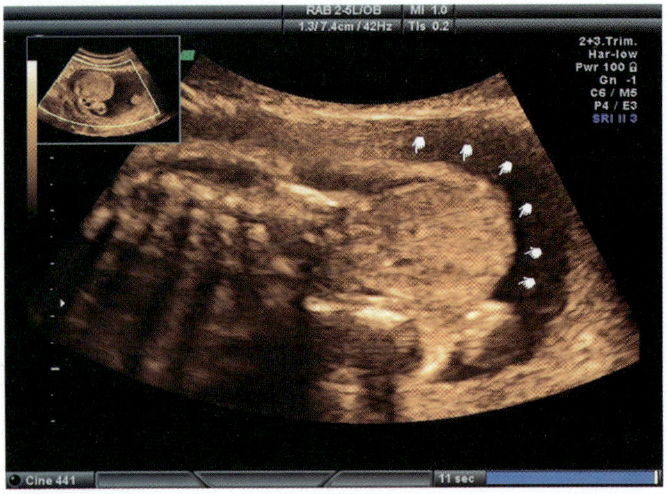

Fig. 11: Ultrasound image, displayed with grey scale, of sacrococcygeal teratomas (SCTs) in a 29 weeks of fetus. Immature teratomas, more common in prenatal life, are mostly solid with high vascularity, whereas mature types, which are more common in adult life, are mostly cystic and not so rich in vascularity, also known as dermoid cyst.

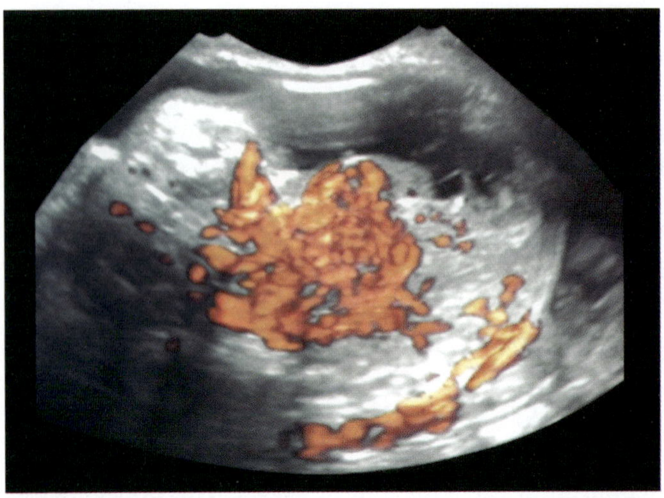

Fig. 12: Color Doppler interrogation image of sacrococcygeal teratomas (SCTs) shows marked hypervascularity with numerous arteriovenous (AV) shunting. Because of its immature nature to begin with, the sonographic appearance of SCTs is readily mimicking malignant tumor (predominantly solid with hypervascularity), and not useful to predict or even diagnose malignant transformation in the fetus. Rapid enlargement of the tumor mass may help raising concern of malignant changes.

remission rate to surgical removal and adjuvant chemotherapy. Prediction or early detection of in utero malignant transformation is difficult, because there is sonographic appearances of the benign immature and the

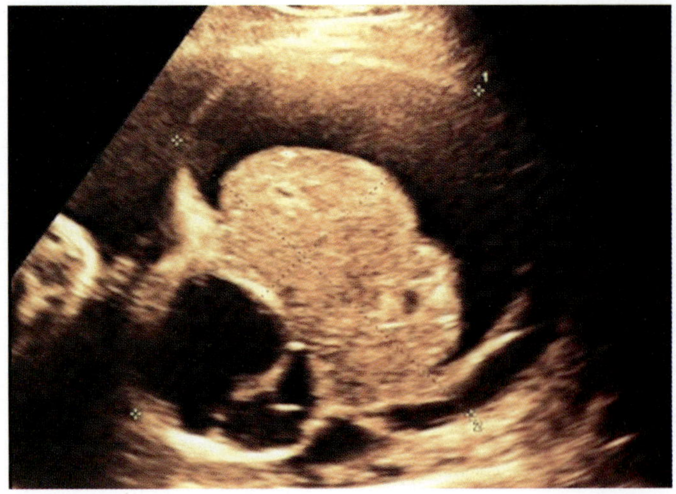

Fig. 13: Ultrasound image, displayed with gray scale, of sacrococcygeal teratomas (SCTs) in a 30 weeks of fetus. The SCTs in this fetus is cystic predominant (over 50% of the tumor mass), which is not usual for SCTs in fetus or neonate. Differential diagnosis from large meningomyelocele (MMC) is possible by demonstration of high vascular flow with multiple arteriovenous (AV) shunting with Color Doppler interrogation.

malignant SCTs are virtually identical.[16] However, rapid growth of the SCTs require closer surveillance **(Fig. 13)**.

Approximately, 10 to 40% of fetuses with SCTs have associated malformation. Possible mechanism is the pressure effect from its natural rapid enlargement, and multiple arteriovenous (AV) shunting. Therefore, it is the internal portion (parts of SCTs in pelvic or peritoneal cavity of the fetus) that is of prognostic importance, and requires vigilant follow-up with ultrasonography. However, most of the prenatal diagnoses are made from visualization of the external portion. The external portion of SCTs can grow so big that it may obstruct vaginal bleeding. Some people advocate cesarean delivery in a fetus with sizable SCTs due to fear of tumor dystocia and catastrophic bleeding.

Some fetal SCTs do not have classic ultrasound appearance of solid tumor with hypervascularity. SCTs are categorized into four different sub-types, based on external and internal (pelvic) components as follows:[17]

- *Type I:* SCTs are completely external. No presacral component
- *Type II:* SCTs are mostly external, with small presacral or internal pelvic component
- *Type III:* SCTs are mostly internal, with an extension into the abdominal cavity
- *Type IV:* SCTs are completely internal pelvic or abdominal (as shown in **Figs. 14 and 15**) No external component

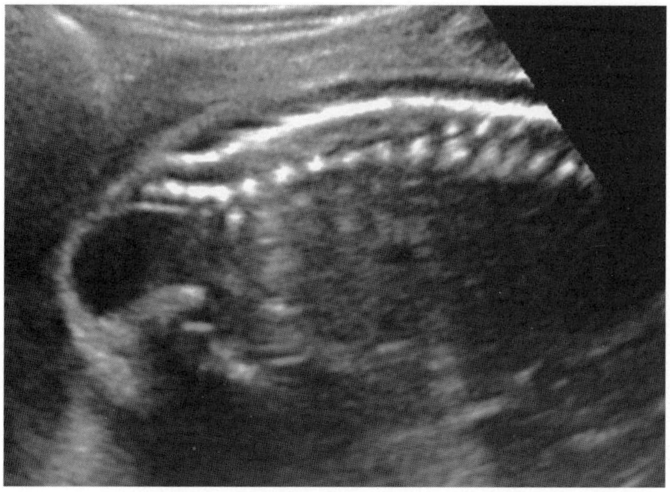

Fig. 14: Ultrasound image, displayed with gray scale, of sacrococcygeal teratomas (SCTs) in a 28 weeks of fetus. This is a type IV SCTs (completely internal pelvic) with atypical single cystic appearance. It has no external component at all. Differential diagnosis from meningomyelocele (MMC) antesacral type may be difficult due to an absence of solid components that contain numerous arteriovenous (AV) shuntings as a diagnostic hallmark. Postnatal examination and imaging is advised if the fetus does not show worsening neurological signs or suffering from pressure effect. In case that the definitive diagnosis is urgently required, then magnetic resonance imaging (MRI) should be informative (*see* **Figure 15**).

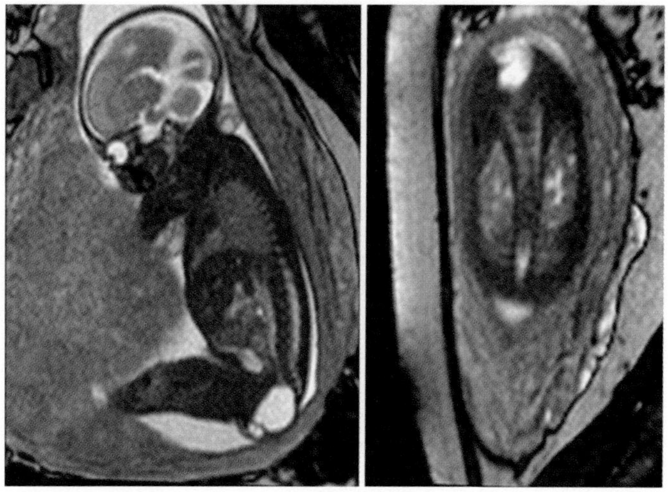

Fig. 15: Magnetic resonance imaging (sagittal and coronal cuts, fast T2-weighted single shot technique) of a 28 weeks of fetus with presacral cystic mass. The cystic content is hyposignaled, and not communicated with cerebrospinal fluid in the spinal canal. It is compatible with sacrococcygeal teratomas (SCTs) type IV with atypical pure cystic presentation. Bilateral pyelectasis without clubbing of pelvicaliceal system is noted, presumably from the mass effect. The size of this SCTs was stable until the delivery date. Vaginal birth was uneventful. Postnatal surgical removal was accomplished, and histopathology was mature teratoma (dermoid cyst).

Ultrasound diagnosis is straightforward in most cases for the unique appearance (solid tumor with hypervascularity) and location (sacrum) of SCTs. However, SCTs with predominant cystic component have to be differentiated from MMC. In selected cases, MRI may provide additional information that potentially can affect the prognosis or change the treatment plan. For instance, with sequence optimization, the superior soft tissue characterization of MRI can provide additional information on the following SCTs tumor mass effects, such as colonic displacement, ureteric obstruction or dilatation, hip dislocation, intraspinal extension, vaginal dilatation, as well as assessment of possible fetal metastasis.[18] Choosing the right MRI sequence, based on the specific type of tissue components of the individual SCTs suspected from ultrasound examination, will help maximizing signal characteristics (Wataganara et al. 2016; In press MRI JPM). SCTs type II, III, and IV are usually dormant and slow growing. Vaginal delivery is possible if the tumor mass is not too large or excessively vascular. On the other hand, SCTs type I has higher chance of causing fetal complications from 2 major mechanisms. First, SCTs type 1 can grow rapidly and compress ureters or intestine. Spontaneous rupture has been reported.[19] Second, sudden proliferation of its AV shuntings, which are numerous in SCTs type I, can cause high output cardiac failure and fetal hydrops.[20] Preeclampsia, so called "Mirror syndrome", can develop and cause maternal morbidity. Alterations in amniotic fluid volume can be variable. Polyhydramnios develops in some cases of fetal SCTs due to increased vascular output of the kidneys and primary production from the SCTs. It can lead to premature birth. Oligohydramnios can be found if the tumor compresses bladder neck causing lower urinary tract obstruction. Dilatation of the urinary bladder will be found in this case. Prognostication characteristics of SCTs are demonstrated in **Table 3**.[21]

In large and hypervascular SCTs (type B) with complications, temporizing treatments may be offered. For instance. percutaneous aspiration of the cystic part (if possible), symptomatic amnioreduction, and amnioinfusion, may help prolonging the pregnancy. Open fetal surgical resections have been attempted on 4 cases, with 3 survivors.[14] These fetuses showed signs of impending

TABLE 3: Prognostic classification of prenatally diagnosed sacrococcygeal teratomas (SCTs)..

Prognostic classification	*Tumor characteristics*	*Natural history*
A	• Diameter less than 10 cm • Absent to mild vascularity • Slow growth	Good maternal and perinatal outcomes
B	• Diameter more than 10 cm • High vascularity • Rapid growth	Worse maternal and perinatal outcomes (high output cardiac failure)
C	• Diameter more than 10 cm • Predominantly cystic • Absent to mild vascularity • Slow growth	Good maternal and perinatal outcomes

high-output cardiac failure at gestational age between 21 and 26 weeks', and the SCTs were in accessible location. The mean gestational age at delivery was 29 weeks, mean birth weight of 1.3 kg and hospital stays ranging from 16 to 34 weeks. The one neonatal death was due to premature closure of the ductus arteriosus with cardiac failure. Another larger series comprising of 41 prenatally diagnosed SCTs cases showed an overall survival of 77%.[20] Fetuses with SCTs require close surveillance, preferably once a week, to evaluate tumor size and characteristics for the chance of bleeding and cardiovascular effect. Sequential fetal echocardiogram is advisable, particularly in the presence of large SCTs with solid components and hypervascularity.

Large, hypervascular SCTs can cause maternal and fetal complications. If the gestational age permits, it is reasonable to deliver the critically ill fetus for ex-utero resuscitation and stabilization, followed by postnatal imaging **(Fig. 16)**, and timely surgical removal **(Fig. 17)**. But if serious fetal complications develop early in pregnancy, minimally invasive interventions have been attempted to improve fetal condition and to prolong the pregnancy. Van Mieghem et al. published systematic review analyzing the success of different types of interventions in salvaging SCTs related fetal hydrops remote from term.[22] There were 20 cases of SCTs related fetal hydrops treated with minimally invasive procedure including fetoscopic laser ablation, interstitial laser ablation, radiofrequency ablation (RFA) and vascular occlusion with coiling. The neonatal survival was 6/20, of which 5/11 survived after RFA or interstitial laser ablation. There were 12 fetal SCTs without hydrops that received minimally invasive treatment, and their survival was 8/12. Mean gestational age at delivery in fetal SCTs receiving minimally invasive intervention was 29.7 weeks'. Open fetal surgical resection

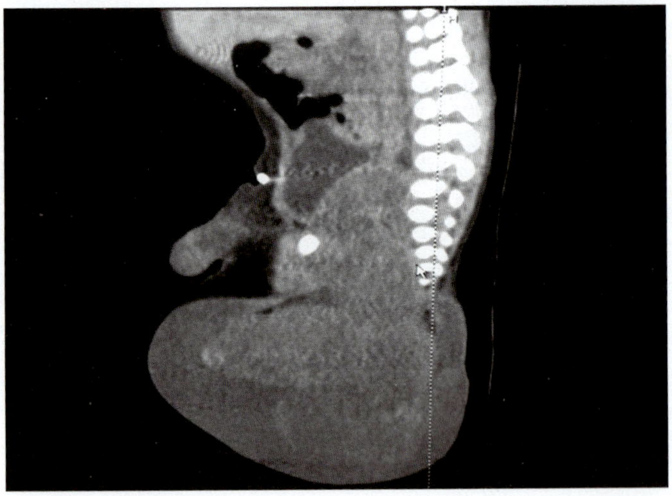

Fig. 16: Magnetic resonance imaging (sagittal cut, T2 weighted single-shot technique) of a neonate born at-term with sacrococcygeal teratomas (SCTs) type II. The purpose of neonatal imaging was to characterize the mass, to delineate its anatomic extent and relationship with other structures. It showed that the mass was predominantly solid with larger extrapelvic and smaller intrapelvic component. There was no involvement of the neural tube.

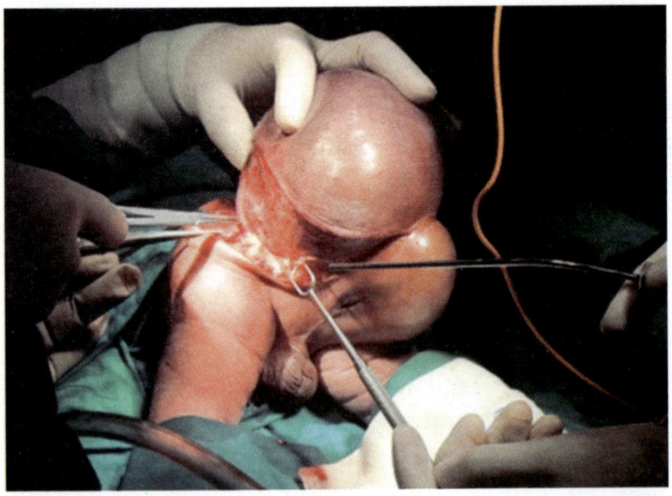

Fig. 17: Photograph of neonatal resection of sacrococcygeal teratomas (SCTs). Special precaution must be exercised to prevent neonatal hypothermia and excessive bleeding. Removal of the coccyx can reduce the recurrence. If malignant transformation is discovered in surgical specimen, adjuvant chemotherapy will be followed. Irradiation may be needed in case of incomplete resection, particularly the internal or intrapelvic portion of the tumor.

was exclusively for fetal SCTs with hydrops (n = 11). The survival was 6/11, with a comparable mean gestational age of delivery at 29.8 weeks.[7]

SCTs is a relatively common tumor arising in the fetus. Large, solid and hypervascular tumor can cause serious maternal and fetal complications. Prenatal intervention can salvage some fetus, but the success rate is still relatively low. Minimally invasive intervention performed solely due to the tumor size seems to be more successful than waiting until the fetus is decompensated. Accidental injury of adjacent organs, i.e., anal sphincter, nerve plexus, from RFA or laser causing long-term morbidity in childhood period cannot be ignored. In large SCTs with fetal decompensation, open fetal surgical excision seems to yield a better perinatal outcome. Interpretation and adoption of this data has to be cautioned, because the analysis is based on a limited number of cases due to the rarity of this tumor.

Teratomas of the Neck

The second most common location of prenatal teratoma is at the fetal neck.[23] It is usually unilateral and well-encapsulated. The tumor can grow quite large, contains solid or solid/cystic and invade the surrounding organs. Teratoma at fetal neck can push fetal head in hyperextended position, which significantly complicate vaginal birth. If the esophagous is compressed by the tumor, polyhydramnios can develop, as seen in **Figure 18**.

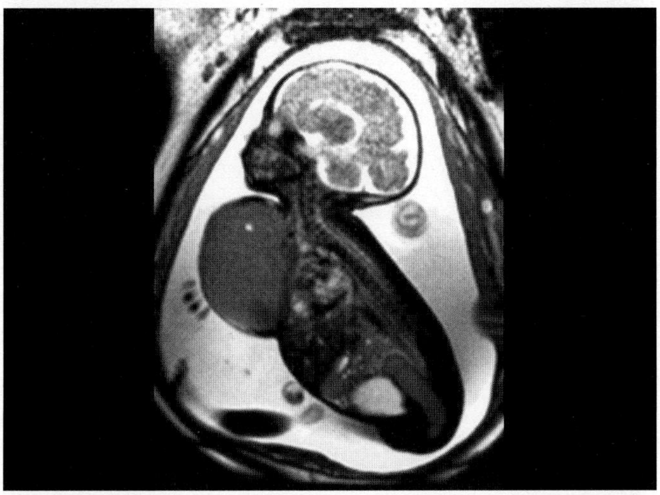

Fig. 18: Magnetic resonance imaging (sagittal and coronal cuts, fast T2-weighted single shot technique) of a 26 weeks of fetus with large solid tumor on the neck and upper chest wall. Note how the tumor mass prevent the fetus from flexing its neck. Increased amniotic fluid volume is also seen.

There are some other kinds of tumor than can arise on the neck of the fetus such as congenital goiter and solid thyroid tumors, neuroblastoma, hamartoma, hemangioma and lymphangioma. These tumors have different aggressiveness, and effective treatment relies heavily on the accurate diagnosis.

Weekly ultrasound surveillance is advocated for a fetus with cervical teratoma. This is a slow growing tumor, but it can always compress the tracheobronchial tree or the esophagous. Fetal echocardiogram can detect hyperdynamic cardiac function well before high output cardiac failure develops. Large, solid, hypervascular tumor can decompensate the fetus, and urgent delivery for ex-utero resuscitation and stabilization is mandated. For safety reason, it is not advisable to offer minimally invasive prenatal ablation with RFA or laser for tumor located in the neck of the fetus.

Multidisciplinary approach is usually required to ensure the safe delivery of a fetus with cervical teratoma, as shown in **Figure 19**. Ex-utero intrapartum treatment (EXIT) delivery shall be considered if there is a possibility that the fetal airway is compromised by the tumor.[24] Advanced airway management can be conducted while the fetus is still on placental bypass. The EXIT protocol at Faculty of Medicine Siriraj Hospital has previously been described.[25]

Intracranial Teratomas

Intracranial teratomas are very rare and have a gender bias to male fetuses at a 10:1 ratio. Fetal intracranial tumors are likely to arise in supratentorial (70%) than infratentorial (30%) part, particularly in the 3rd ventricle. Fetal brain tumors are heterogeneous in cellular origin, but specific to the particular parts of the brain. Most common cell types include craniopharyngioma (base of skull), teratoma (Pineal gland), astrocytoma (cerebral hemosphere), ependymoma (fourth ventricle), and choroid plexus papilloma (choroid plexus).

Similar to other fetal tumor, intracranial tumor can cause complications in both the mother and the fetus. Obstruction of cerebrospinal fluid circulation by the tumor mass can cause obstructive hydrocephalus. **Figures 20 to 22** demonstrate different types of fetal brain tumors. Certain types of fetal brain tumors can be suspected from its origin, echogenicity and internal bleeding, and its growth. Fetus with a brain tumor may develop a number of obstetric complications, including polyhydramnios, fetal hydrops, cephalopelvic disproportion, malpresentation, and

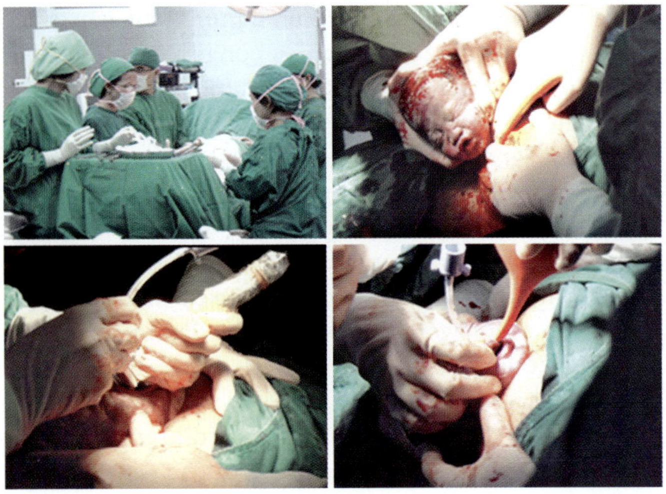

Fig. 19: Photograph of ex-utero intrapartum treatment (EXIT) at Faculty of Medicine Siriraj Hospital. This multidisciplinary team in the operating suite (OS) consisted of obstetrician or maternal fetal medicine (MFM) specialist, neonatologist, pediatric airway specialist, anesthesiologist, and neonatal cardiopulmonary resuscitation (NCPR) team. There is a standard institutional EXIT protocol, but step-by-step delivery plan specific to this fetus had been discussed, and the family had been counseled, before the OS is scheduled. In summary, obstetrician, MFM specialist, and neonatologist scrubbed in. Care must be taken when abdominal cavity and the uterus were accessed, in order to minimize the bleeding. Anesthesiologist turned on inhalation gas after the fetus is partially delivered to the shoulder. This aimed at uterine relaxation to prevent premature separation of the placenta, so that the fetus was still on continuous oxygen support from the placenta. The neonatologist positioned the fetus, direct laryngoscopy to assess the mass effect, then intubate the fetus. After the endotracheal tube was secured, the baby was totally delivered, umbilical cord was clamped and cut. If the fetal airway is significantly distorted, pediatric airway specialist can assist with flexible fiberoptic tracheobronchoscope for a better visualization. On a very rare occasion, on-site neonatal tracheostomy is required.

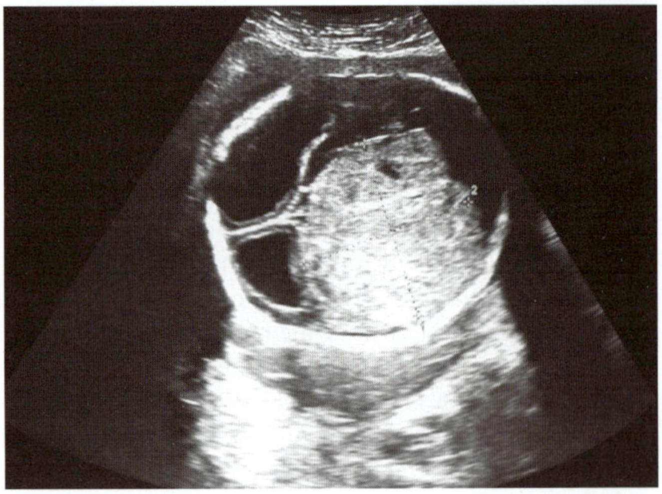

Fig. 20: Ultrasound image, displayed with gray scale, of a 33 weeks of fetus with brain tumor. The tumor originated from the third ventricle, enlarged rapidly with internal hemorrhage and caused obstructive hydrocephalus. Secondary damage from bleeding or pressure (cerebrospinal fluid blockade) can compromise the neurological function, even after the primary tumor was removed. The cell type was ependymoma.

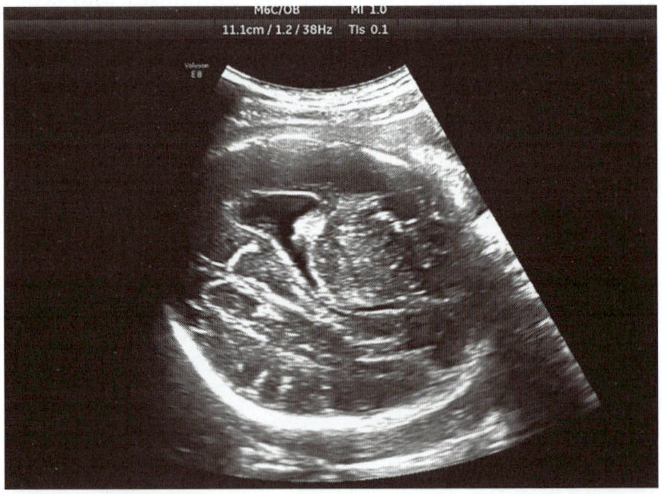

Fig. 21: Ultrasound image, displayed with gray scale, of a 33 weeks of fetus with brain tumor. The tumor originated from cerebral hemisphere, enlarged gradually without internal hemorrhage. It also caused obstructive hydrocephalus. The cell type was astrocytoma.

traumatic delivery to the mother. If fetal head compression is required for maternal safety, cephalocentesis would be appropriate.

There is no effective prenatal intervention for fetal intracranial tumors.

Epignathus

Epignathus is a term given to a very rare form of teratoid tumor that arises from the oropharyngeal region. The estimated incidence is 1 in 35,000 to 200,000 births. The tumor classically presents *in utero* or in the neonatal period. It is often classified under the broader umbrella of cervical teratomas. The tumors are not often consistent in origin, number and differentiation of tissues. They usually have components from all three germ layers and can contain fat, cartilage and bone. The most common origin is palato-pharyngeal region around the basisphenoid (Rathke's pouch) and with progressive growth fills the buccal cavity and finally protrudes out of the mouth.

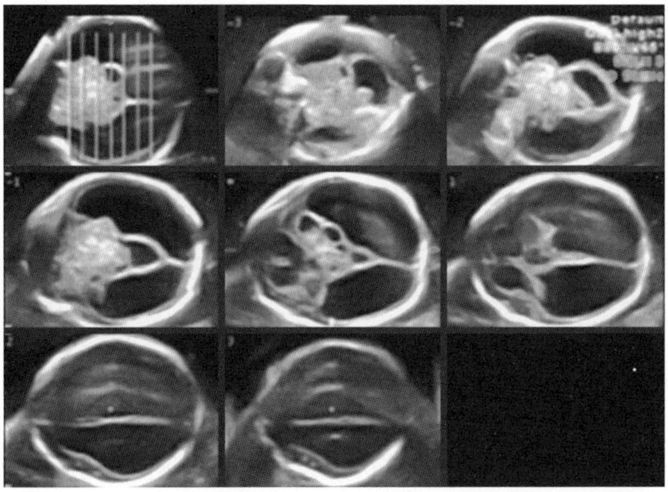

Fig. 22: Three-dimensional ultrasound image, displayed with tomographic ultrasound imaging (TUI), of a 33 weeks of fetus with brain tumor. The tumor originated from base of skull, enlarged gradually without internal hemorrhage. It also caused obstructive hydrocephalus. The cell type was craniopharyngioma.

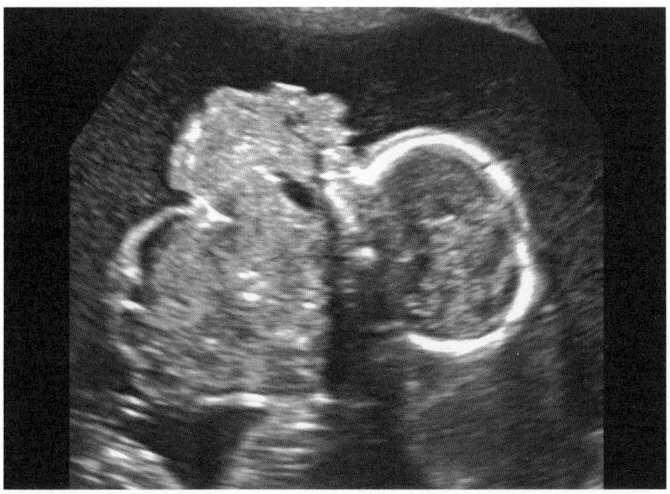

Fig. 23: Ultrasound image, displayed with gray scale mode, of a 22 weeks of fetus with complex expansive mass affecting the fetal face. This mass had coexisting cystic and solid areas that shadowed the fetal face, and had a possibility of invasion to the mandible and base of skull. Color Doppler studies demonstrated hypervascularity with low-impedance flow. This tumor is epignathus, which is a form of teratoma arising in fetus.

Elevation of maternal serum alpha-fetoprotein can be encountered in fetus with epignathus. Prenatal diagnosis of epignathus can be made by ultrasound examination, which finds complex mass protruding from the fetal oral cavity, as shown in **Figure 23**. This mass is usually mixed echoic. Polyhydramnios may be present when there is swallowing impairment. It is common that the fetus may also have associated midline facial defects, cleft lip and/or cleft palate. MRI shall be restricted only when the plan is to keep the baby. Epignathus distorts oropharynx and the airway. MRI can be useful in managing the airway at the time of delivery, and may be used as a guide for EXIT.

Fetuses with epignathus can develop hydrops: due to tumor shunting and using a lot of blood flow. Epignathus can spread upward to destroy the skull base and brain tissue.[26] Fetal hydrocephalous can be a result of secondary brain damage from epignathus. At the time of birth, the affected baby will not be able to breathe because tumor obstructs the airway. Birth asphyxia is the most common cause of death in neonate with epignathus. The prognosis for this tumor is always poor, mostly because of its location that can completely obstruct the airway. Many families choose to terminate the pregnancy due to this condition. Therefore, accurate prenatal diagnosis is crucial. There are a few other childhood tumor that may occur in oropharyngeal area like epignathus, such as rhabdomyosarcoma and myoblastoma. These epignathus mimickers are less vascular, surgical removal is possible and they are responsive to adjuvant therapy with chemotherapy or irradiation.

Cardiac Rhabdomyomas

Cardiac rhabdomyomas are the most common cardiac tumor. It is a hamartomatous change from myocardial cells, and mostly has a benign course. They usually are dormant, more commonly found in left cardiac ventricle.[27] It may obstruct left ventricular outflow or may trigger refractory arrhythmias. This tumor has a clear association with tuberous sclerosis.[28]

Sonographic findings of cardiac rhabdomyxomas are one or more solid hyperechoic masses located in relation to the myocardium, as shown in **Figure 24**. In most cases no treatment is required and these lesions regress spontaneously. Surgical excision is indicated in cases with left ventricular outflow tract obstruction or refractory arrhythmias. The overall prognosis depends on the number, size and location of the lesions as well as the presence or absence of associated anomalies. Fetuses that have cardiac rhabdomyxoma should get a close ultrasound surveillance for an early detection of cardiac arrhythmias, ventricular outflow tract obstruction, valvular compromise, and even disruption of intracardiac blood flow, causing congestive cardiac failure and hydrops, as shown in **Figure 25**.

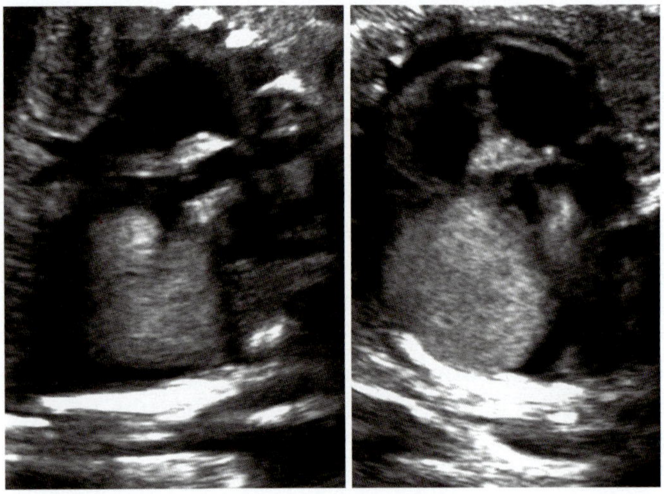

Fig. 24: Ultrasound image, displayed with gray scale, of a 32 weeks of fetus with cardiac rhabdomyxoma. This single, large, hyperechoic tumor originate from myocardial cells on the wall of left cardiac ventricle.

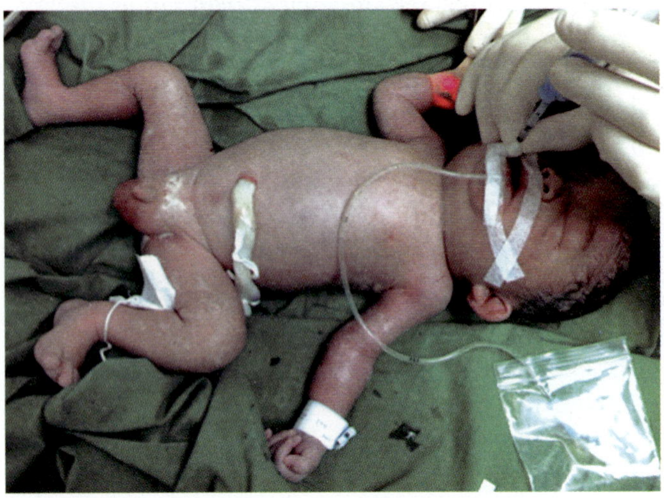

Fig. 25: Photograph of a neonate with superior vena cava (SVC) obstruction syndrome. This neonate has a significant edema limited only to the upper torso. He had a cardiac rhabdomyxoma in his right atrium, which is not a common location for cardiac rhabdomyxoma. Close follow-up with ultrasound examination once a week revealed localized subcutaneous fluid collection, particularly at the scalp. Fetal echocardiography revealed an obstruction of SVC at the right atrial inlet. SVC obstruction syndrome is considered emergency. The baby was delivered by cesarean section, stabilized, and proceeded to surgical removal of the cardiac rhabdomyxoma.

Lymphangioma/Hemangioma

Lymphangioma is a benign malformation composed of dilated cystic lymphatics. They are most commonly seen as a unilateral soft tissue mass of the neck but can also be present in the axilla, thorax and lower extremities. The location of the lymphangioma generally indicates the significance for prenatal surveillance or for perinatal treatment. For neck masses, lymphangioma might result in esophageal obstruction causing polyhydramnios or irreversible facial deformity due to cystic expansion, as shown in **Figure 26**.

Distinguishing between lymphangioma, hemangioma, and cervical teratoma can be extremely difficult. With superb soft tissue characterization of MRI, differential signals in the lumen of lymphangioma are different from that of hemangioma, as shown in **Figures 27A and B**. Fetal/neonatal morbidity and mortality can vary depending on the location of the lymphangioma (larnyx, oral cavity, mediastinum). In utero intervention is not indicated in compensated fetus.

Liver Tumor

Hepatic tumor is rare in fetal and neonatal period.[29] Most common primary hepatic tumors are hemangioma, mesenchymal hamartoma, and hepatoblastoma. Hemangiomas are usually large, well-defined, echogenic intrahepatic masses, often containing echo-free areas. They are generally solid with hypervascularity and AV shunting, which may cause fetal hydrops from hyperdynamic cardiac function. Hemangiomas have also been associated consumptive coagulopathy resulting from disseminated intervascular coagulation with thrombocytopenia and anemia. With the triad of hemangioma, thrombocytopenia, and coagulopathy, then the diagnosis is Kasabach-Merritt syndrome (KMS), as shown in **Figure 28**.

Placenta and Umbilical Cord Tumor

Chorioangiomas are benign vascular tumors of the placenta. They are most commonly encapsulated, round and embedded within the placenta. Chorioangiomas are the most common primary tumor of the placenta. Sonographic appearance of chorioangioma is heterogeneous. Most of time, chorioangioma of the placenta appears as hyperechoic mass within the placenta, as shown in **Figures 29A to D**. Some tumor may be protruding into the amniotic cavity with a location near the placental cord insertion site. This is usually seen after 20 weeks gestation. Tumor vascularity varies but might have the appearance of an arteriovenous malformation. Occasionally, chorioangioma can act as an arteriovenous shunt, with resulting fetal anemia, hydrops, and polyhydramnios. Chorioangioma does not directly

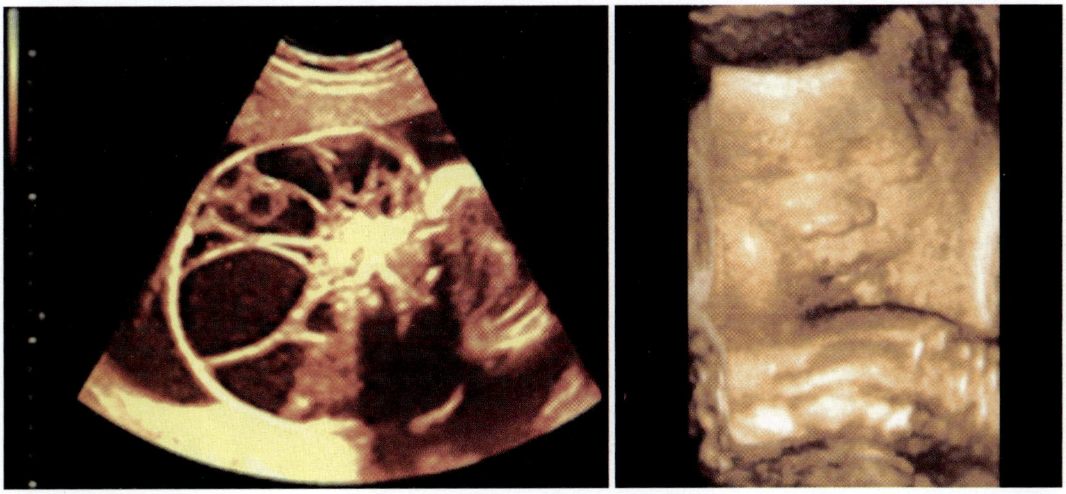

Fig. 26: Ultrasound image, displayed with gray scale, shows large, septated cervical lymphangioma in a 34 weeks of fetus. Three-dimensional, surface rendered displays a dysmorphic appearance of the fetus as a result of excessive expansion.

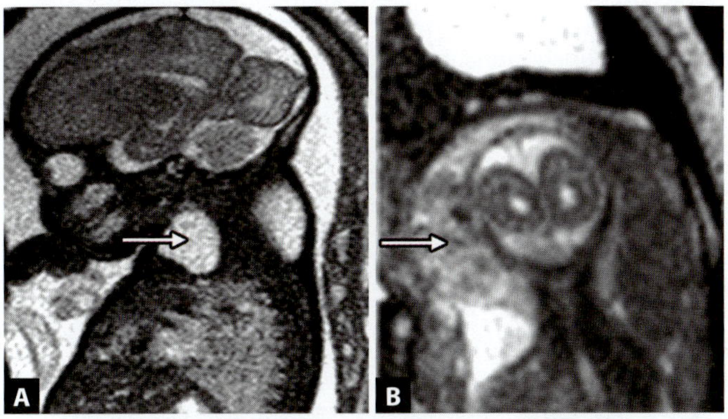

Figs. 27A and B: Magnetic resonance imaging (MRI) (fast T2-weighted single shot technique) (A) A 24 weeks of fetus with cervical lymphangioma. (B) A 20 weeks of fetus with cervical-cephalic hemangioma.

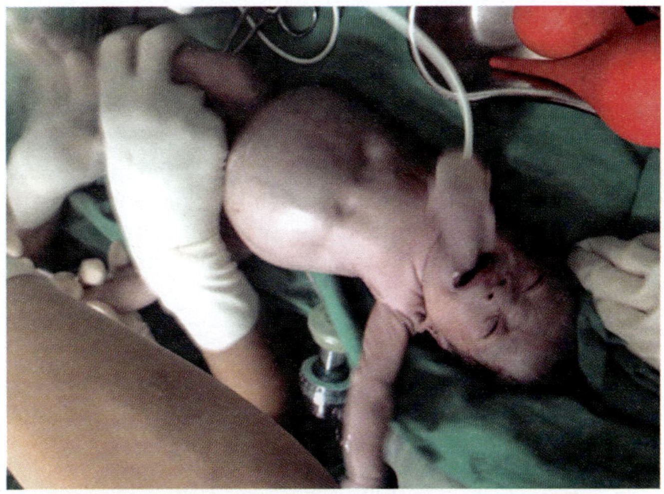

Fig. 28: Photograph of a neonate with congenital hemangioma of liver delivered by cesarean section to avoid the chance of tumor rupture. Blood works showed thrombocytopenia and coagulopathy, which is consistent with Kasabach-Merritt syndrome.

cause obstetric complication, or any complications to the woman. Vaginal delivery is not prohibited. Special precaution needs to apply in delivery complicated with polyhydramnios, fetal anemia and fetal hydrops.

For chorioangioma of the placenta smaller than 6 cm in diameter, the patient should have weekly ultrasound surveillance for the tumor growth and Doppler measurement of peak systolic velocity of fetal middle cerebral artery for an early detection of fetal anemia. If fetal anemia is detected and is linked to the presence of AV shunting within the chorioangioma, fetal blood transfusion is needed. For fetal decompensation remote from term, ablative therapy of the tumor mass has been attempted with various success. Our team at Faculty of Medicine Siriraj Hospital recently published an in vitro experiment of radiofrequency ablation as an energy source to coagulate placental chorioangioma.[30] The designed algorithm, as well as the optimal energy and exposure were experimented. RFA was originally designed to accommodate liver tissue (for minimally invasive ablation of hepatocellular carcinoma). Human liver and placenta have different soft tissue characteristics, therefore, a specific algorithm needs to be developed for a broader use of RFA. Gross findings of chorioangiomas are demonstrated in **Figures 30 and 31** showed mimickers of chorioangiomas.

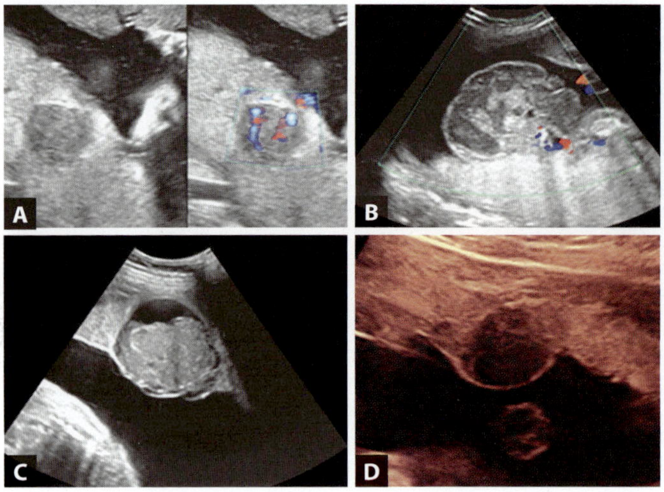

Figs. 29A to D: Ultrasound image, displayed with gray scale, of chorioangioma of the placenta. Chorioangioma is the most common benign tumor of the placenta. The sonographic findings of this tumor are heterogeneous as follows. (A) Well-circumscribed solid mass, located completely beneath the chorionic plate, in the middle of placental tissue, Color Doppler studies demonstrate arteriovenous (AV) shunting in the tumor mass; (B) Sessile mass, located on the chorionic surface, usually very near umbilical cord insertion site and take feeding directly from the umbilical cord; (C) Well-circumscribed mass, predominantly solid, half buried below the chorionic plate; (D) Well-circumscribed, hypoechoic, differentiated from simple cyst of fetal membranes by numerous feeding vessels, some are direct from the umbilical cord insertion.

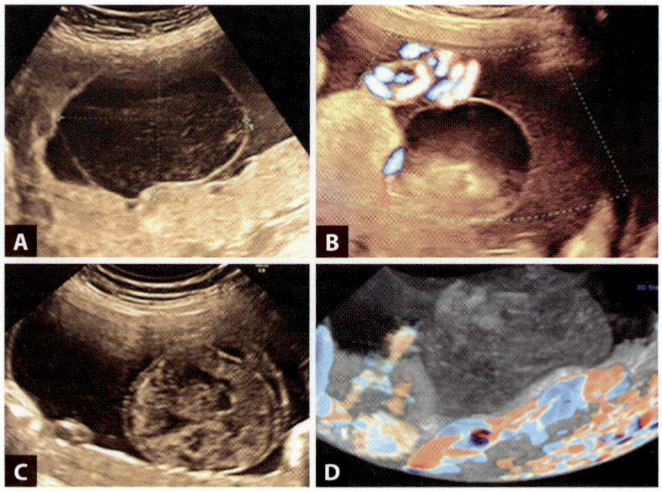

Figs. 31A to D: Photographs of mimickers of chorioangioma of the placenta. (A) Placental cyst is a thin-wall cyst with anechoic content with minimal blood supply; (B) Umbilical cord cyst is within Wharton's jelly and close to umbilical vessel. It may look identical to placental cyst if it is located near cord insertion site at the placenta; (C and D) Subchorionic hematoma has blood clot on the inside that could be mistaken for solid component of the tumor. After the bleeding stops, there will be no flow toward the mass, as demonstrated in (D).

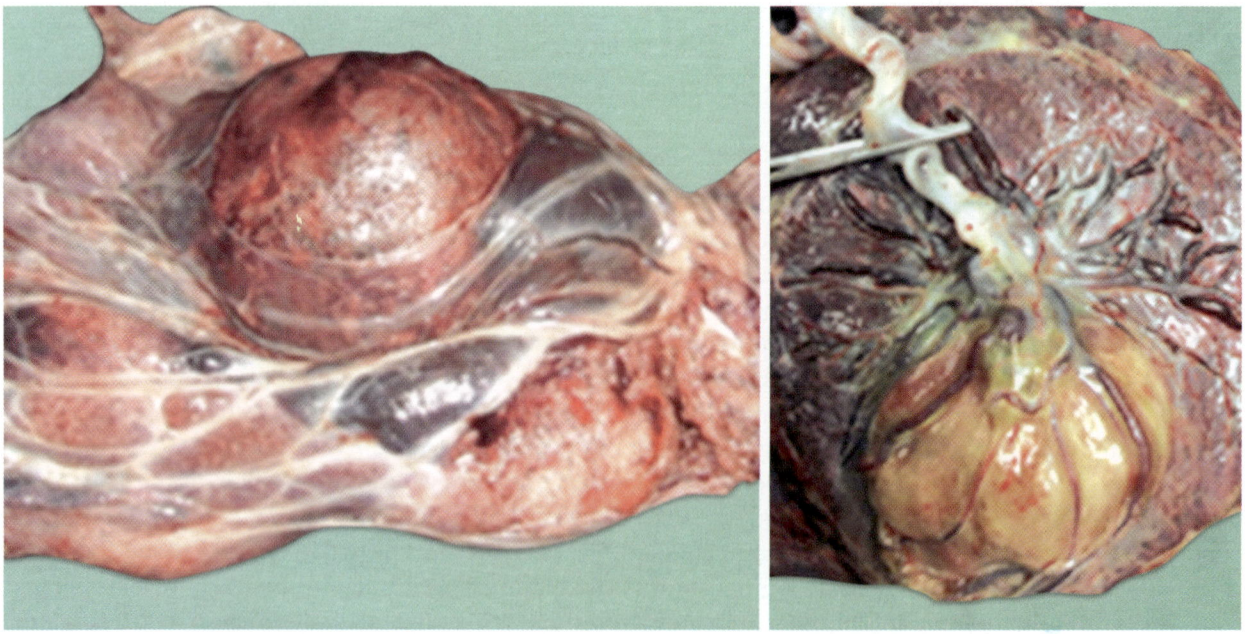

Fig. 30: Photograph of chorioangiomas from different patients. Note the difference in color, size and chorionic covering. With all these difference, these tumors always be found right next to the placental cord insertion.

CONGENITAL PULMONARY AIRWAY MALFORMATION

Congenital pulmonary airway malformation (CPAM) results from failure of normal bronchoalveolar development with hamartomatous proliferation of terminal respiratory units in a gland-like pattern (adenomatoid) without proper alveolar formation. These lesions have intracystic communications and, unlike bronchogenic cysts, can also have a connection to the tracheobronchial tree. There have been a variety of proposal to categorize CPAM, but from sonographic appearance, CPAM can be categorized into macrocystic or microcystic type.[31]

CPAM appears as an isolated cystic or solid intrathoracic mass. Macrocystic CPAM has a benign course of disease. If the fetus is decompensated, minimally invasive interventions, i.e., needle tapping or shunting can be offered with a good outcome. A solid thoracic mass is usually indicative of a microcystic variant and is typically hyperechoic, as shown in **Figure 32**. There can be mass effect where the heart may appear displaced to the opposite side. Alternatively, the lesion may remain stable in size, or even regress. Hydrops fetalis and polyhydramnios may develop, and may be detected on ultrasound as ancillary sonographic features.

Fetus with decompensation from rapid enlargement of microcystic CPAM has a poor prognosis. Microcystic CPAM is similar to solid tumor. Temporizing treatments with corticosteroids and laser ablation have limited success.[32] Open surgical resection of fetal lung lesions has been performed in a small number of fetal treatment centers, mainly in the USA. The largest series to date has been published by the group from Children's Hospital of Philadelphia.[33] They described outcome after fetal lobectomy for massive multicystic or predominantly solid CPAMs in 24 cases between 21 and 31 weeks of gestation. Thirteen (54%) healthy survivors were reported with uneventful follow-up at 1 to 16 years of age. Resolution of hydrops was seen within 1–2 weeks in these cases. Of the 11 nonsurvivors 7 died intraoperatively due to cardiovascular collapse during surgery, 2 became bradycardic and died within the first day after surgery and 3 died of maternal problems (mirror syndrome, postoperative chorioamnionitis and preterm contractions). Recently, an additional 3 successful cases of open fetal surgical lobectomy for microcystic CPAM with fetal decompensation were reported.[34]

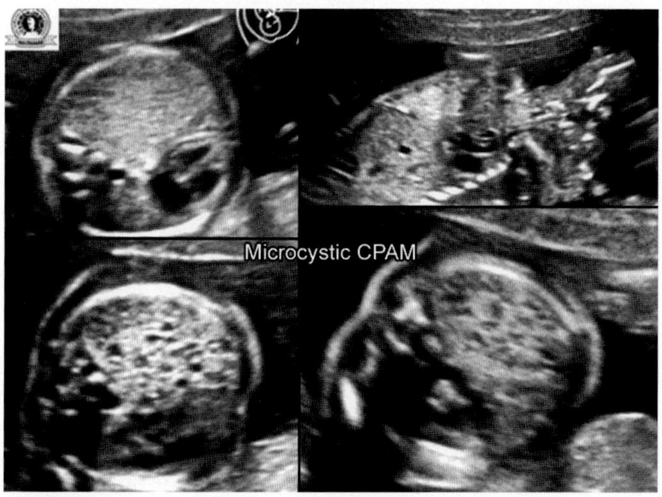

Fig. 32: Ultrasound images, displayed with gray scale, shows a solid thoracic mass is usually indicative of a microcystic variant of congenital pulmonary airway malformation. There can be mass effect where the heart may appear displaced to the opposite side.

CONCLUSION

Approximately, 1 to 3% of babies are born with birth defects. Advancement in fetal imaging technologies, such as high-definition ultrasound machine and dedicated magnetic resonance imaging system, allow for an earlier detection of these defects. Certain defects can be waited and all the necessary treatment, either medical or surgical, can be given after birth. Expanded diagnostic tools have allowed us to identify more precisely when fetal conditions worsen during the developmental process.

Open hysterotomy is an invasive access to the fetus. It is currently reserved for only complex procedure that cannot be performed through endoscopic access. Many groups of expert are working to replace it with endoscopic approach. It means that more skillful surgeons must be trained, more effective instruments must be developed and most important thing is more communications need to be made among the interdisciplinary body of the expert team.

REFERENCES

1. Harrison MR, Golbus MS, Filly RA, et al. Fetal surgery for congenital hydronephrosis. N Engl J Med. 1982;306:591-3.
2. Moreira de Sa RA, Nassar de Carvalho PR, Kurjak A, et al. Is intrauterine surgery justified? Report from the working group on ultrasound in obstetrics of the World Association of Perinatal Medicine (WAPM). Journal of Perinatal Medicine; 2015.
3. Adzick NS, Thom EA, Spong CY, et al. A randomized trial of prenatal versus postnatal repair of myelomeningocele. N Engl J Med. 2011;364:993-1004.

4. Wu D, Ball RH. The maternal side of maternal-fetal surgery. Clinics in Perinatology. 2009;36:247-53, viii.
5. Nicolaides KH, Campbell S, Gabbe SG, Guidetti R. Ultrasound screening for spina bifida: cranial and cerebellar signs. Lancet. 1986;2:72-4.
6. Van den Hof MC, Nicolaides KH, Campbell J, Campbell S. Evaluation of the lemon and banana signs in one hundred thirty fetuses with open spina bifida. American Journal of Obstetrics and Gynecology. 1990;162:322-7.
7. Aaronson OS, Hernanz-Schulman M, Bruner JP, Reed GW, Tulipan NB. Myelomeningocele: prenatal evaluation—comparison between transabdominal US and MR imaging. Radiology. 2003;227:839-43.
8. Heuer GG, Adzick NS, Sutton LN. Fetal myelomeningocele closure: technical considerations. Fetal Diagnosis and Therapy. 2015;37:166-71.
9. Watanabe M, Kim AG, Flake AW. Tissue engineering strategies for fetal myelomeningocele repair in animal models. Fetal Diagnosis and Therapy. 2015;37:197-205.
10. Moldenhauer JS, Soni S, Rintoul NE, et al. Fetal myelomeningocele repair: the post-MOMS experience at the Children's Hospital of Philadelphia. Fetal Diagnosis and Therapy. 2015;37:235-40.
11. Moise KJ Jr, Moldenhauer JS, Bennett KA, et al. Current selection criteria and perioperative therapy used for fetal myelomeningocele surgery. Obstetrics and Gynecology; 2016.
12. Pedreira DA, Zanon N, Nishikuni K, et al. Endoscopic surgery for the antenatal treatment of myelomeningocele: the CECAM trial. American Journal of Obstetrics and Gynecology. 2016;214:111 e1-e11.
13. Adzick NS, Crombleholme TM, Morgan MA, Quinn TM. A rapidly growing fetal teratoma. Lancet. 1997;349:538.
14. Hedrick HL, Flake AW, Crombleholme TM, et al. Sacrococcygeal teratoma: prenatal assessment, fetal intervention, and outcome. Journal of Pediatric Surgery. 2004;39:430-8; discussion-8.
15. Grammatikopoulou I, Kontomanolis EN, Chatzaki E, et al. Immature malignant sacrococcygeal teratoma: case report and review of the literature. Clinical and Experimental Obstetrics & Gynecology. 2013;40:437-9.
16. Sheth S, Nussbaum AR, Sanders RC, Hamper UM, Davidson AJ. Prenatal diagnosis of sacrococcygeal teratoma: sonographic-pathologic correlation. Radiology. 1988;169:131-6.
17. Keslar PJ, Buck JL, Suarez ES. Germ cell tumors of the sacrococcygeal region: radiologic-pathologic correlation. Radiographics: a review publication of the Radiological Society of North America, Inc 1994;14:607-20; quiz 21-2.
18. Danzer E, Hubbard AM, Hedrick HL, et al. Diagnosis and characterization of fetal sacrococcygeal teratoma with prenatal MRI. AJR American Journal of Roentgenology. 2006;187:W350-6.
19. Sy ED, Lee H, Ball R, et al. Spontaneous rupture of fetal sacrococcygeal teratoma. Fetal Diagnosis and Therapy. 2006;21:424-7.
20. Makin EC, Hyett J, Ade-Ajayi N, Patel S, Nicolaides K, Davenport M. Outcome of antenatally diagnosed sacrococcygeal teratomas: single-center experience (1993-2004). Journal of Pediatric Surgery. 2006;41:388-93.
21. Benachi A, Durin L, Vasseur Maurer S, et al. Prenatally diagnosed sacrococcygeal teratoma: a prognostic classification. Journal of Pediatric Surgery. 2006;41: 1517-21.
22. Van Mieghem T, Al-Ibrahim A, Deprest J, et al. Minimally invasive therapy for fetal sacrococcygeal teratoma: case series and systematic review of the literature. Ultrasound in Obstetrics & Gynecology: the Official Journal of the International Society of Ultrasound in Obstetrics and Gynecology. 2014;43:611-9.
23. Tsuda H, Matsumoto M, Yamamoto K, et al. Usefulness of ultrasonography and magnetic resonance imaging for prenatal diagnosis of fetal teratoma of the neck. Journal of Clinical Ultrasound: JCU. 1996;24:217-9.
24. Liechty KW, Hedrick HL, Hubbard AM, et al. Severe pulmonary hypoplasia associated with giant cervical teratomas. Journal of Pediatric Surgery; 2006;41:230-3.
25. Wataganara T, Ngerncham S, Kitsommart R, Fuangtharnthip P. Fetal neck myofibroma. J Med Assoc Thai. 2007;90: 376-80.
26. Clement K, Chamberlain P, Boyd P, Molyneux A. Prenatal diagnosis of an epignathus: a case report and review of the literature. Ultrasound in Obstetrics & Gynecology : the Official journal of the International Society of Ultrasound in Obstetrics and Gynecology. 2001;18:178-81.
27. D'Addario V, Pinto V, Di Naro E, Del Bianco A, Di Cagno L, Volpe P. Prenatal diagnosis and postnatal outcome of cardiac rhabdomyomas. Journal of Perinatal Medicine. 2002;30:170-5.
28. Evans JC, Curtis J. The radiological appearances of tuberous sclerosis. The British Journal of Radiology. 2000;73:91-8.
29. Kamata S, Nose K, Sawai T, et al. Fetal mesenchymal hamartoma of the liver: report of a case. Journal of Pediatric Surgery. 2003;38:639-41.
30. Satapornteera P, Raveesunthornkiat M, Sukpanichnant S, Tongdee T, Homsud S, Wataganara T. Effects of Power and time on ablation size produced by radiofrequency ablation: In vitro study in fresh human placenta. Fetal Diagnosis and Therapy. 2015;38:41-7.
31. Adzick NS, Flake AW, Crombleholme TM. Management of congenital lung lesions. Seminars in Pediatric Surgery. 2003;12:10-6.
32. Ong SS, Chan SY, Ewer AK, Jones M, Young P, Kilby MD. Laser ablation of foetal microcystic lung lesion: successful outcome and rationale for its use. Fetal Diagnosis and Therapy. 2006;21:471-4.
33. Adzick NS. Open fetal surgery for life-threatening fetal anomalies. Semin Fetal Neonatal Med. 2010;15:1-8.
34. Cass DL, Olutoye OO, Cassady CI, et al. Prenatal diagnosis and outcome of fetal lung masses. Journal of Pediatric Surgery. 2011;46:292-8.

CHAPTER 48

Establishment of Fetal Therapy Center

Tuangsit Wataganara

INTRODUCTION

Fetal therapy includes a series of interventions performed to rescue a sick fetus. Currently, fetal conditions amendable for in-utero interventions are limited. The condition has to diagnosable prenatally. There must be features that distinctively differentiate it from other conditions that do not require treatment. And the most important thing is, the natural history of the condition has to be well described to be either deadly or leaving the baby with long-term morbidity. With all these restrictions, only a handful of indications for fetal surgery can be justified. Examples of fetal conditions amendable for prenatal treatment include severe mid-trimester twin-twin transfusion syndrome (TTTS), congenital diaphragmatic hernia (CDH), and lower urinary tract obstruction (LUTO), as previously described in our report from the working group on ultrasound in obstetrics of the World Association of Perinatal Medicine (WAPM).[1]

Fetal treatment, and advanced fetal therapy in particular, is an important crossroads. Before this millennium, intrauterine surgical intervention was semi-experimental. It was limited to a handful of specialized centers because of its complex nature and the significant risks involved with a surgical or medical intervention on a pregnant woman and her fetus. It involves a multidisciplinary team of specialists. Most of these well-established and experienced fetal therapy centers are clustered in North America and Europe. There are a number of restrictions that prevent establishment of new fetal therapy centers, especially in other parts of the world, such as Asia and Africa. It is desirable that a single fetal therapy center can provide both medical and surgical interventions. Some interventions can be handled by one specialist. Examples of these interventions are fetal shunting and fetoscopic laser photocoagulation of anastomosing chorionic vessels for severe TTTS. Other complex interventions may require more than one subspecialist to handle each aspect of the procedure. Examples of these interventions are the ex-utero intrapartum treatment (EXIT) and in-utero repair of myelomeningocele (MMC).

In addition to the fetus, the safety of pregnant woman herself must be taken into consideration when invasive procedure is an option. There is an increasing complexity in counseling of fetal diseases that the natural history is still poorly understood, but there is a real risk of procedure-related maternal morbidity.[2] Maternal morbidity and possible litigation is another factor that prevent establishment of new fetal therapy center. The small number of qualified fetal therapy center limits an access of women to this technological advancement. There is a paucity of information on the published literatures as to how a medical institute can offer invasive fetal therapy in a responsible and ethical manner. This chapter summarizes the essential components in founding a fetal therapy center based on the published information in peer-review medical literatures and direct experience at Faculty of Medicine Siriraj Hospital, Bangkok, Thailand. The objective of this chapter is to promote the knowledge application, to facilitate access to fetal diagnosis and treatment, both for pregnant couples and their physicians.

TRAINING REQUIREMENTS

Medical centers that provides general obstetrics services may not have enough expertise in detecting fetal conditions amendable from intrauterine surgery. Early, and timely, detection of these conditions is as important as the therapeutic part, because some of these conditions can leave a permanent and irreversible damage to the developing organ system of the fetus.[3] In addition to their rarity, the methods used to diagnose these conditions become increasingly sophisticated. We have witnessed development of magnetic resonance imaging sequence protocols for a better soft tissue characterization of the fetus.[4] Molecular genetic tests, such as array comparative hybridization (aCGH), are increasing adopted to improve prognostication.[5]

Even after an extensive research with all these technological advancement, there remain a lot to learn about the natural history of some of these disorders and the safest way to treat them. Teaching of invasive fetal procedures has been a seriously debated issue. Proper training and educational program should be established to avoid unnecessary losses and improve fetal outcome. There have a number of strategies to facilitate the training for fetal therapeutic interventions.

Knowledge sharing remains the critical step for an adoption of any novel procedure. This can be accomplished through lecture, focused roundtable discussion, and medical conference. Networking in the region is not only important for dissemination of novel surgical techniques, because it is also helpful for patient referral for timely intervention. For example, Faculty of Medicine Siriraj Hospital is part of the initiative of fetal therapy network in South East Asia. Teleconference has been scheduled on a regular basis to exchange latest development in the field of fetal therapy in the region, as shown in **Figure 1**.

Although the technical aspects of fetal intervention have improved, there remain substantial gap in the dissemination of the knowledge. Because conditions amendable for in-utero treatment affect only a small minority of fetuses, fetal therapy has a limited impact within a broader public health context. Training of young and aspiring perinatologists to perform an 'exciting' or new invasive procedure that is potentially dangerous has been one of the most important concerns in the past few decades. It is universally agreed that introduction of a new intervention is related to procedure-related complications. 'Learning curve' must be addressed, and it is agreeable that special skills required in performing complex invasive improve with experience.[6]

Currently, there are very few well-established fetal therapy centers eligible for conducting an effective training program. They must have enough volume of fetal procedures per annum. It is also important to realize that only a fraction of referral patients are viable surgical candidates. A recent post-MOMS publication has shown that only 29% of referrals are actually eligible for surgery.[7] High-volume centers are clustered in North American. Europe and Asia have more high-volume centers compared to South America, the Middle East and Australia, of which are mainly low-volume centers.[8]

Therefore, formal fellowship training does not exist in most places, even in fetal therapy centers with high volume of prenatal interventions. Apprenticeship is a traditional way of surgical training. The trainees learn in the workplace by practising on patients under supervision of their mentors.[9] An example of apprenticeship in fetal therapy at Faculty of Medicine Siriraj Hospital is shown in **Figure 2**. However, with a continuously increasing complexity of the procedure, it is not ethically acceptable for inexperienced trainees to practice on the patients in order to develop their expertise.[10] Rigorous patient safety protocols have set significant boundaries to the concept of 'learning by doing'. In addition, apprenticeship training program is limited by restriction of medical licensure, particularly for the foreign trainees. There is an increasing

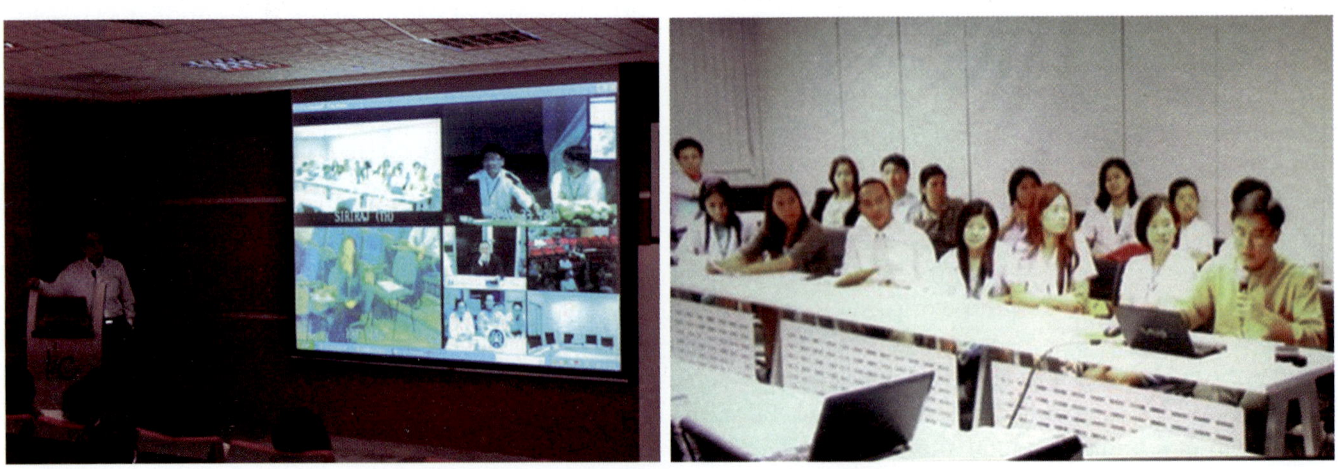

Fig. 1: Teleconference to update latest development of fetal therapy has been regularly scheduled. Participants are fetal therapy centers in South East Asia.

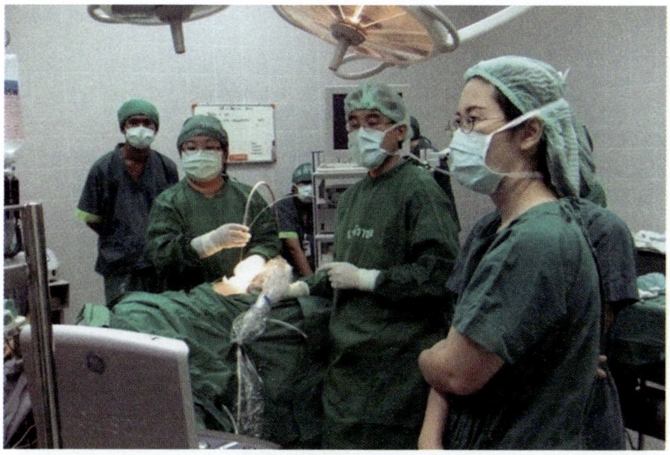

Fig. 2: Training by apprenticeship program at fetal therapy center, Faculty of Medicine Siriraj Hospital.

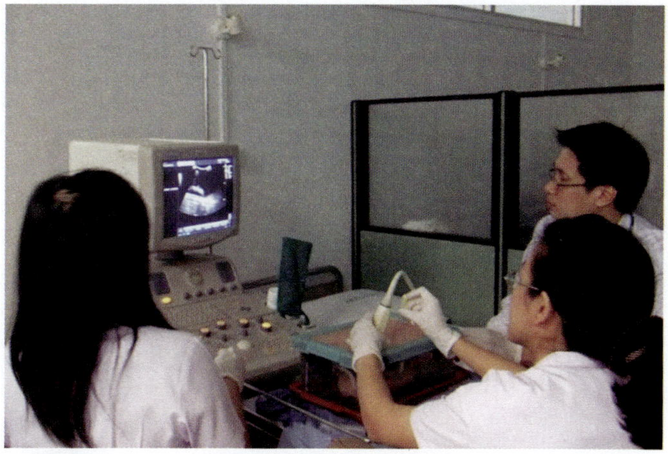

Fig. 3: Basic model used in training of invasive prenatal diagnostic procedures at Faculty of Medicine Siriraj Hospital.

barrier to patient and operating room access, and slower development of surgical and procedural skills is being considered. Alternatives to patient-based training have been proposed in parallel with apprenticeship in order to facilitate the learning of trainees.

In-utero intervention requires complex psychomotor skill of the surgeon. Model training has been developed in other fields of surgery, so that the novice trainees can master their surgical dexterity in a more transparent and more acceptable manner than patient-based training.[11] In order for simulation-based training to be successful, simulators have to be validated appropriately and integrated in a training curriculum. This includes an objective evaluation before and after finishing the simulation training.[12] This approach has been widely used in teaching and training of prenatal diagnostic procedures, i.e. genetic amniocentesis and percutaneous fetal blood sampling.[13] We have adopted the same approach in training the residents in our Department of Obstetrics and Gynecology, Faculty of Medicine Siriraj Hospital. As shown in **Figure 3**, out basic training model is constructed from a fresh human placenta with attached umbilical cord from seronegative woman mounted in plasticine equal to the size of the placenta.[14,15] The plasticine is then filled with tap water to the brim, and covered with our proprietary ultrasound skin. It is important that the placenta has to be collected within 2 days to minimize tissue degradation. The placenta is refrigerated at 4°C, not freezing, until the time of use.

The basic model has limitations for simulation training of fetoscopic laser photocoagulation of chorionic vessels, which is the most frequently performed in-utero endoscopic intervention. The major drawback is the model can simulate the uterus with posterior, but not anterior, placenta. The desired quality of training model for fetoscopic intervention should allow for a flexibility to simulate a broad array of situation expected to be encountered during the surgery. The perfect training curriculum should aiming at improving the novice surgeon's skill on the following; (1) hand-eye coordination, (2) understanding of a three-dimensional intrauterine environment through two-dimensional ultrasound and endoscopic images, and (3) thorough knowledge of fetal and placental anatomy by ultrasound and endoscopic evaluation.[6] Based on these requirements, we have developed another simulator, purpose designed to serve the training of fetoscopy.[16] This 'Siriraj Fetoscopic Surgical Simulator', which is now patented, is shown in **Figure 4**. The whole globe is ultrasound friendly, so that ultrasound-guided skills can be practiced. This training model can simulate the placenta at all locations, and the novice surgeon can master their skills of combining ultrasound and endoscopic views in order to get to the 'vascular equator'. The minimum requirements for in-vitro training under supervision before allowing the training to perform a procedure on an ongoing pregnancy are varied among institutions.

Training of prenatal invasive procedures on an anomalous fetus prior to termination is a poor alternative and not ethically justified. The anomaly often makes the procedure unnecessarily more difficult. Animal models have been used on mostly on experimental, and not for educational, basis when new invasive fetal intervention is conceptualized. The most commonly used animal is pregnant sheep.[17]

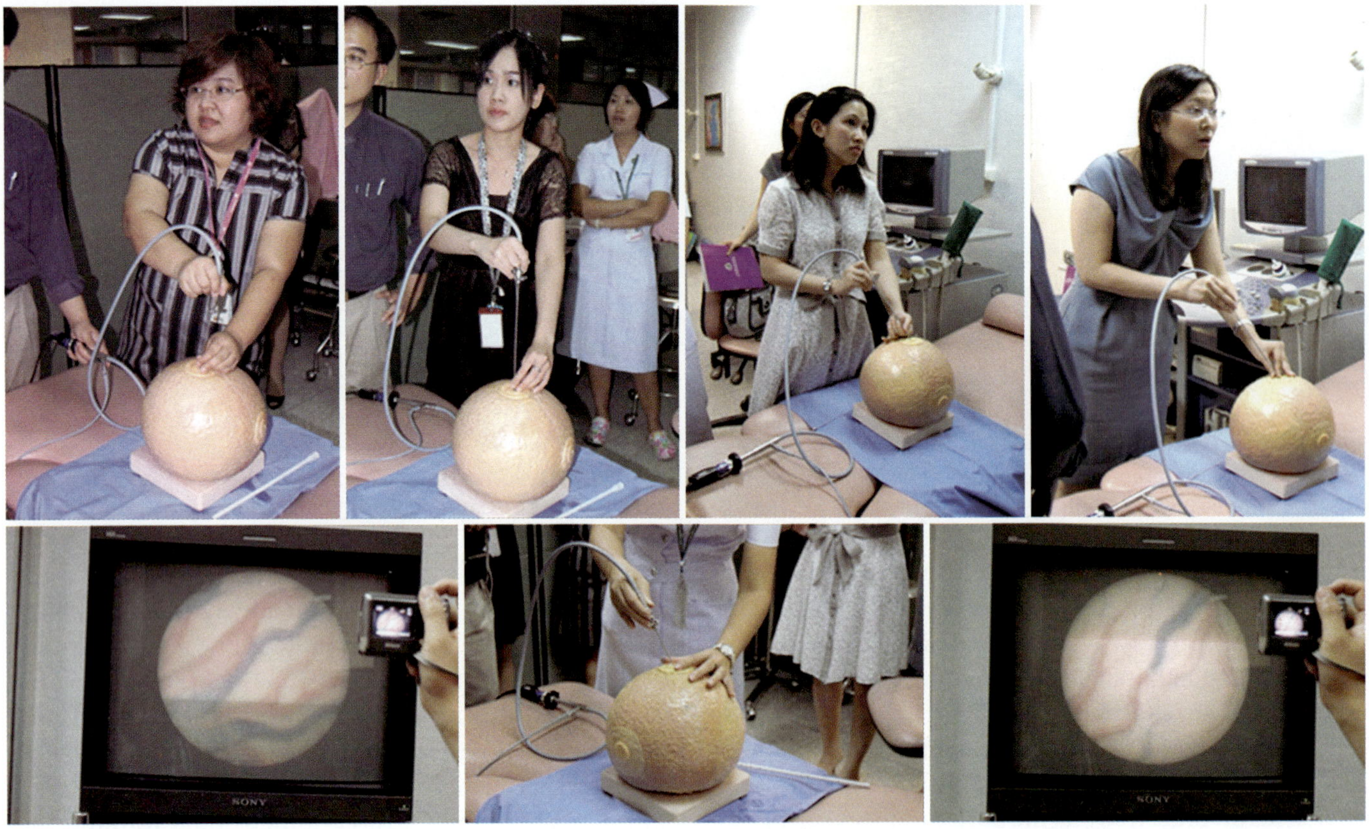

Fig. 4: 'Siriraj Fetoscopic Surgical Simulator' used for training of novice fetal surgeon at Faculty of Medicine Siriraj Hospital.

Training on an ongoing pregnancy should begin with less difficult cases, i.e., stage 2 TTTS with posterior placenta. Naturally, the most difficult and riskiest cases should be performed by the most experienced operator in that fetal therapy center. According to the learning curve statistics of laser surgery for TTTS in established fetal therapy centers in North America, United Kingdom, and Europe, there was a clear and reproducible trend that increasing in experiences of the operator led to improvement of perinatal survival.[18-21] The same trend also observed from a newly established fetal therapy center in Asia.[22] Audit system for the post-surgical outcomes can facilitate the learning.[23] The result for strict audit system can also be used as a quality assurance for the performance of a fetal therapy center.

DEFINITION OF FETAL THERAPY CENTER

So far, the definition and categorization of fetal therapy center have not been universally agreed. According to a publication by Lori Howell and Scott Adzick in 1999 that, based on the mission, fetal therapy center is a specialized center that '*provide comprehensive, multidisciplinary expertise in all facets of prenatal diagnosis, reproductive genetics and prenatal, perinatal, and postnatal treatment for abnormal fetuses*'.[24] It is desirable that the center can integrate cross institutional program for fetal diagnosis and treatment, management of maternal conditions, and high-level of newborn care that can manage major congenital malformations and certain genetic diseases. An effective fetal therapeutic program is the one that can orchestrate subspecialist clinical experts with the clinical and basic science research, with an ultimate goal to improve perinatal outcomes.

Ideally, fetal therapy center should comprise of the major facilities that are closely connected under one roof. These include the clinical services on prenatal diagnosis, counseling, financial arrangement, in-utero surgical intervention, delivery service, maternity facility, and newborn care. Postnatal corrective surgery and childhood rehabilitation program can fulfill the complete picture of fetal-neonatal-pediatric care. These latter two services usually are require in perinatal period or immediately

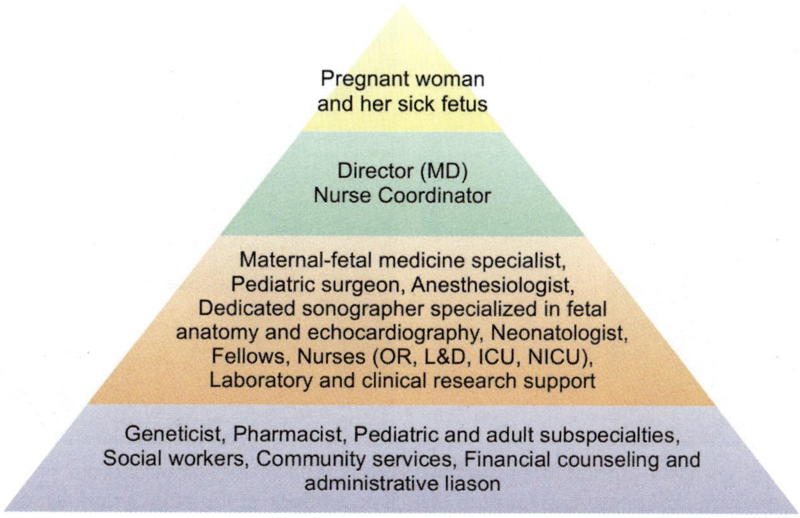

Fig. 5: Specialists and subspecialists required for a high-level fetal therapy center. (Modified from Howell and Adzick, Semin Perinatal. 1999).

after birth. Obviously, it requires people from broad array of medical and social cares to team up and work in harmonious fashion to achieve this goal. Planning for individualized in-utero intervention is a perfect example of complex clinical decisions among specialists with diverse background. It is a challenge for multidisciplinary team at a fetal therapy center to reach a consensus. Components of the multidisciplinary team, as suggested by Lori Howell and Scott Adzick, is summarized in **Figure 5**.[24]

COUNSELING SERVICE AT FETAL THERAPY CENTERS

Counseling the woman and her family is a real challenge. It usually takes place after definitive diagnosis is reached from a targeted ultrasound examination, advanced imaging like MRI, or informative molecular genetics tests. Patients will often minimize the recognized maternal and fetal risks of in-utero intervention to *"try and do whatever possible"* to improve the outcome for their child. This reaction is often due to guilt related to *'if I did not try, how could I live with the life-long consequences that I could have changed for my child'*. Their family and friends can put additional unrealistic pressure on the woman. It requires an approach from various aspects (details in **Figure 5**) for the woman to make an informed decision without under the time constraint.

The counseling sessions provide the family with the results of the evaluation and outline their potential treatment options. Termination of pregnancy is always an option, provided that the local legislation allows. The family can choose to prepare themselves, and their babies, for the best possible care after birth. The third alternative is an operation before birth. If the family chooses to terminate or to continue the pregnancy without in-utero intervention, the team can assist with the arrangements. Most of the time, pregnancy termination or delivery of a baby can be accomplished safely at their local hospital. This will also allow for more support from family and friends. The family will be made aware of a possibility of postnatal referral.

If the family wishes to pursue fetal surgery, an in-depth discussion will be arranged. They have to be given enough time to process the procedure, institutional results, risks to the mother and the baby, and the potential benefits. All available options must be presented, and the counseling has to be conducted in nondirective manner. Institutional conflicts of interest, either financial or research-related, have to be fully disclosed to the family.

After the counseling, if the pregnant woman and her family still elect to proceed, they will be educated for the preparation process by the specialized nurses. Financial arrangement, and assistance in some cases, will be made.

PERSONNEL REQUIREMENTS TO SET UP FETAL THERAPY CENTER

With this type of complex intervention, strong institutional support and commitment are crucial. The components required for critical care can be divided into; *(1) the Surgical Team, (2) the Delivery Team, and (3) Post-operative Team.*

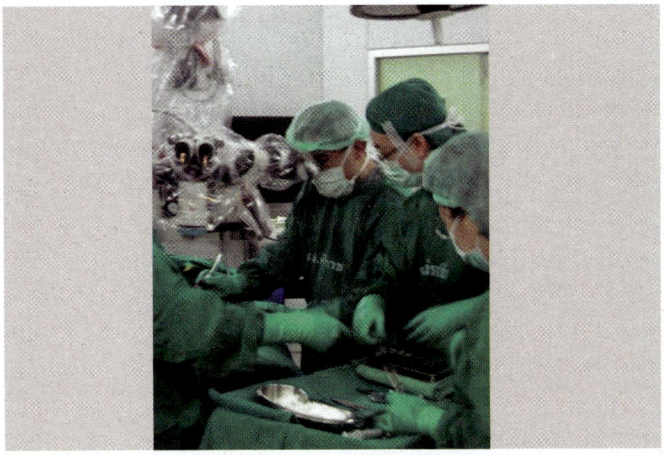

Fig. 6: Maternal-fetal medicine specialist (the author) in the field of postnatal neurosurgical repair of myelomeningocele. This type of practice, or 'fire drill', allows for the team member to maintain their expertise for the procedure that is infrequently performed.

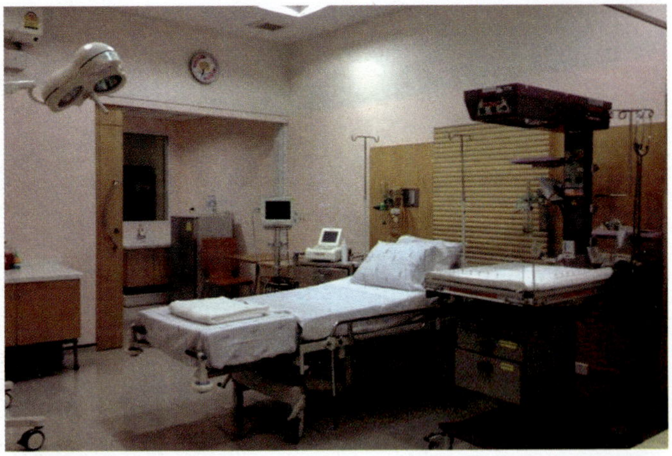

Fig. 7: Specialized labor and delivery unit for high-risk delivery at Department of Obstetrics and Gynecology, Faculty of Medicine Siriraj Hospital. This delivery suite can be transformed into high dependency unit (HDU) to support critical conditions, either of the mother or the newborn.

The *Surgical Team* has to be available at all time. Minimum requirement of specialist team that need to be on-call includes pediatric surgeon, maternal-fetal medicine specialist, fetal or pediatric cardiologist, subspecialty pediatric surgeon, obstetrical or fetal anesthesiologist, dedicated operating room team of scrub nurses (at least 2), circulating nurses (at least 2), and support staff (at least 1). All the 'core members' are committed to maintaining their skills expertise by adequate case volume and regular simulation ("fire drill"). An example of 'fire drill' for open fetal surgery of MMC is shown in **Figure 6**.

The *Delivery Team* and *Post-operative Team*, consists of maternal-fetal medicine specialist and obstetrician who has enough experiences in clinical care of woman during her recovery from fetal surgery. It requires a combination of knowledge, skill, and experience to recognize and manage complications of fetal surgery in a timely fashion. Immediate complications include fetal membrane separation, premature rupture of the membranes, incessant preterm labor that require aggressive tocolysis, rupture or dehiscence of uterine hysterotomy, and massive bleeding from morbidly adherent placenta.

It is desirable to have a *Specialized Labor and Delivery Unit*. The dedicated Labor and Delivery Unit at Department of Obstetrics and Gynecology, Faculty of Medicine Siriraj Hospital is shown in **Figure 7**. There must be a dedicated cohort of nurses who have been trained to recognize immediate complications of fetal surgery. They are able to provide initial resuscitation for either the mother or the high-risk newborn baby. There must be a dedicated cohort of neonatal resuscitation team and in-house. The obstetric anesthesiologist must be familiar with anomaly-specific resuscitation protocols, which have to be regularly standardized and updated.

Eventually, if the fetus cannot be saved, the woman and her family should be guided to bereavement programs, including palliative care and chaplain services. Additional supports from psychosocial workers, maternal advocates, as well as pediatric genetic counseling are always helpful. Fetal pathology should be performed after an informed consent from the family.

MAINTENANCE OF THE EXPERTISE

Quality assurance is mandatory for facilities that offer high-quality medical services, and fetal therapy center is no exception. Once a medical center has decided to make availability of fetal surgery, a dedicated and limited fetal surgical team with established expertise in their specialties must be developed and maintained. The team members are required to be available for emergencies at any time. Newly established fetal therapy center should seek training and guidance from centers with more experiences. Direct involvement through mentorship system is advisable. There has been an ongoing controversy as to what level of experience is necessary to earn designation as a 'qualified' fetal therapy center. Direct experience with 5 to 20 cases of open fetal surgery under supervision or distant monitoring is acceptable by some experts.

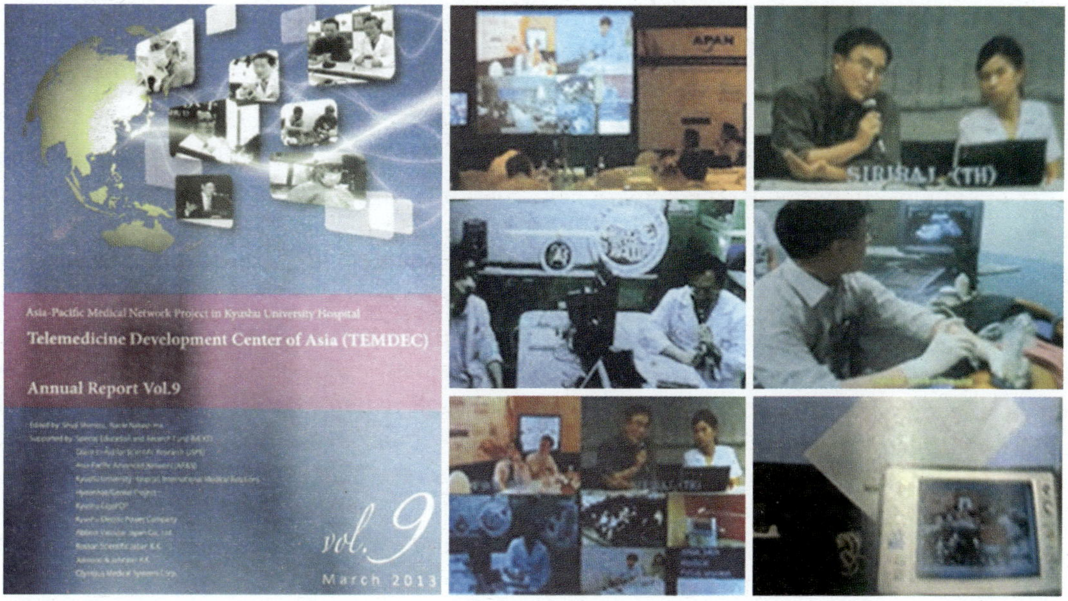

Fig. 8: Documentation of perinatal outcomes subjected for international peer review through telemedicine system.

Once the system is established, maintenance of the necessary case volume and expertise is the next real challenge. There is an increasing competition to get patients among fetal therapy centers. A minimum of 5–10 cases annually is a sufficient referral volume to maintain team skills and experience. However, this goal may not be necessarily achieved, because not all the referred cases are an actual candidate for the surgery. A recent post-MOMS publication has shown that only 29% of referrals are actually eligible.[7] It has not been universally agreed if EXIT deliveries count toward this minimum annual volume requirement.

Some authors suggested that, in order to maintain an adequate referral patients to maintain the skill, the number of fetal therapy center offering invasive procedures should be limited.[25]

QUALITY ASSURANCE OF FETAL THERAPY CENTER

Fetal therapy should have Institutional and Outside Oversight Committees to monitor their outcomes on at least annual basis. This unbiased monitoring is to assure quality of care that meets national standards. If problems are identified, or the practices are not meeting standards, that fetal therapy center would then (1) need to require additional training, or (2) to enforce established protocols, or (3) to consider terminating the program if safety and care benchmarks cannot be met. Finally, either a fetal therapy center can maintain minimum procedures per annum or not, regular practice on simulation ("Fire Drill") is important so that the team members will be reminded and practicing their specific assignment. An example of this fire drill is shown in **Figure 6**.

Alternatively, the 'monitoring' can be achieved by peer review process. For instance, with an advent of high-definition telemedicine system, one fetal therapy center can voluntary share their outcomes to the peers for their constructive input, as well as to reassure that their perinatal outcomes are currently up to an international standard. The results are documented for future reference. Faculty of Medicine Siriraj Hospital has been using this disclosure and peer evaluation since the establishment of fetal therapy program. The documentation is shown in **Figure 8**.

The majority of the published outcome data derive from world's most experienced fetal therapy centers in North America and Europe. These fetal therapy centers often perform international, multicenter trials with equally experienced centers in order to concentrate surgical expertise, to minimize maternal and fetal morbidity, and to optimize infant outcomes. Therefore, it is not unexpected that numerous questions and sceptics arise after the trial completion. There are issues of (1) generalizability of the results from these mega-trials to other fetal therapy centers with less experience, (2) appropriate measures for new fetal therapy centers to develop and maintain similar levels of expertise, (3) establishment of national care standards and benchmarks for fetal surgery, and (4) development of mechanisms to monitor the outcomes.

The number of patients undergoing fetal surgery has risen rapidly. Fetal therapy may still be relatively rare, but it certainly has become a new medical discipline. With this new standard, the multiplication of fetal treatment centers has occurred virtually without any regulations. In August 2004, the National Institutes of Health (NIH), United States, in an urge to take a leading role in developing guidelines for fetal therapy, organized a *'Workshop on Fetal Therapy.'* The workshop delivered a recommendation to establish professional network ('Fetal Therapy Network,' which is now known as 'North American Fetal Therapy Network' or *'NAFNet'*) to promote collaboration in fetal research and to provide national guidelines for the safe and evidence-based use of fetal therapy.

The multidisciplinary *NAFNet* has fostered collaborative research between active fetal diagnosis and treatment centers in the United States and Canada, developed a peer review mechanism for study proposals, explored ways to centralize data collection and study development, and established an educational agenda for medical professionals and the public as well as training of future leaders in the field.

For many reasons, NAFNet has not been able to issue an appropriate protocol for the new fetal therapy centers to properly offering fetal surgery. There are some centers that start to offer novel treatments without unbiased evaluation of inclusion and exclusion criteria as well as operative techniques. A significant variation in practice patterns for offering and performing the open surgery were observed, according to a recent publication by the member of NAFTNet.[26]

NAFTNet has suggested an approach of regionalization of programs to increase access to therapy, and to establish a recognized *'Centers of Excellence.'* Experienced fetal therapy center can help develop the fetal surgery program in the other new center by offering mentoring or training. The minimum resources and necessary clinical expertise criteria should be set to achieve *'Experienced Center'* status. It should be mandatory to have oversight programs for fetal therapy center to monitor outcomes and maintenance of minimal experience to retain 'Center of Excellence' status.

Fetal therapy center with longest experiences may attain *'Develop Center.'* Centers at this level are required to have established programs to gather standardized long-term outcome data. This information (1) will improve an understanding of the composite impact of fetal intervention, (2) can be used for prenatal counseling of candidate patients, and (3) can validate the actual benefits of such interventions. After there are enough number and adequate regional coverage of fetal therapy centers with the same standard and quality, a central national or international registry of cases should be established. Pooling of standardized data from multicenter or multinational collaboration will provide large-scale data to predict perinatal, as well as long-term neurodevelopmental and functional outcomes of fetuses that underwent in-utero surgery. This collaboration will allow for sharing of high-quality data among experienced fetal therapy centers, which may lead to (1) proposal of future research projects to refine prenatal care, or (2) to introduce surgical innovation, or (3) to optimize the management based on scientific validation in controlled clinical trials or studies.

IMPORTANCE OF THE FOLLOW-UP DATA

Systematic collection of follow-up data (or outcome measures) represents quality assurance of that fetal therapy center, as well as a confirmation of successful generalization of mega-trials results. It is likely that fetal therapy centers that begins to offer in-utero interventions will not have sufficient number of patients to for a meaningful outcome data. Selective collection of only key parameters that represent the major outcomes may be enough in the newly found fetal therapy centers. It is important to note that neonatal survival rate alone is no longer adequate to indicate the performance of the treatment or the center.[27]

EXTRINSIC FACTORS THAT CAN AFFECT THE PERFORMANCE OF FETAL THERAPY PROGRAM

There are factors that can be advantageous or setting back the institutional development of fetal surgery. There are advantages and disadvantages of *managed care system* (more prevalent in North America) and *government-subsidized system* (more prevalent in Asia). There is a significant difference in cost-benefit analysis between these two healthcare systems, therefore, it is still uncertain to come up with the number of people needs to be trained for an adequacy of the fetal therapy services in the region. With the government subsidiaries and restrictions in re-imbursement, fetal therapy centers in Asia almost always run a negative financial balance. Hence, there are only a few private medical facilities in Asia that offer in-utero intervention.

Others fetal therapy centers are obliged to affiliate with university hospital so that the program can thrive on research funding. But since very few fetal therapy centers in Asia can make profit out of the service, the competitive feeling to recruit eligible cases is not very intense. Funding problem is universal. Most medical centers in Asia are service-, and not research-oriented. They have to invest in the system of learning and distant coaching from experienced centers from North America or Europe.

Religious belief played a key role in women's decision for pregnancy care when malformation is diagnosed prenatally.[28] Termination of pregnancy is not an option in Catholic and traditional Islamic countries. *Late booking* is not uncommon in countries with low medical resources. First trimester screening for Down syndrome is not universally offered in most parts of the world. Without prenatal screening early on in pregnancy, it is conceivable that a bigger proportion of fetal anomalies are diagnosed when the gestational age is too advanced for legal termination. That leaves either expectant management with planned birthing or in-utero intervention as an option. Unbiased counseling is particularly important in for women from disadvantaged social background, to ensure that the choice they make is well informed.

CONCLUSION

In order to establish a new fetal therapy center, it is important to set a goal. Short and long-term accomplishments should be drafted with realistic timeline. The priority is to determine the true area-specific prevalence of fetal conditions amendable for in-utero treatment. High-quality data from population-based study is still lacking in some regions. Fetal therapy in each region should have a commitment to identify and validate the actual magnitude of prenatally detected conditions with serious consequences. Fetal diseases that either obstructs in-utero development, resulting in significant challenges to maintain optimal quality of life in childhood period deserve this surveillance.

Fetal therapy center is obliged to provide accurate fetal diagnosis at early gestational age by experienced team and adequate imaging technologies. It should make sure that appropriate molecular genetic testings are available. The team has to counsel the pregnant women and her family in an unbiased manner. Diagnostic and therapeutic concepts need to be standardized among regional fetal therapy centers, so that an effective network can be formulated.

It is important to publicize the knowledge to pregnant women and their family, so that they can identify and locate fetal therapy center in their region that is experienced and resourceful for specific fetal disease. This approach is to ensure an adequate number of cases per annum to maintain their skills for the best possible neonatal outcomes. Networking with the areas of high prevalence of fetal conditions amendable for prenatal intervention is also helpful.

In order to obtain high-quality outcome data, it is imperative to standardize the follow-up protocols in childhood period. This includes neonatal survival and morbidity, composite outcomes, and other disease-specific outcomes. This approach can help generating meaningful data that can be used for a counseling, or a benchmark to improve the quality of fetal therapy center.

Adequate training and regular practice for interventionists and their support staffs is crucial. The level of training can be varied, but it is important that everyone in the team is very specific, and very motivated, for their parts. Mentorship system can help new fetal therapy centers that are considerably inexperienced with the procedure to set up the program, in respect to their specific circumstances. The newly adopted complex procedures shall be accompanied by the mentors, until surgical skill satisfactions are met by both parties. Then, remote proctorship may be in place to reassure the proficiency of the new procedure. The number of cases for each step has not been concluded, but it may be varied from one center to another.

New fetal therapy centers are committed to report the neonatal outcomes and procedure-related morbidities in a frank and honest manner. More experienced centers are committed to transfer their knowledge, when requested, to the other less experienced centers. Knowledge sharing can be through lecture, simulation workshop, clinical observership, research fellowship, or even clinical fellowship training.

REFERENCES

1. Moreira de Sa RA, Nassar de Carvalho PR, Kurjak A, et al. Is intrauterine surgery justified? Report from the working

group on ultrasound in obstetrics of the World Association of Perinatal Medicine (WAPM). J Perinat Med. 2015.
2. Golombeck K, Ball RH, Lee H, et al. Maternal morbidity after maternal-fetal surgery. Am J Obstet Gynecol. 2006;194: 834-9.
3. Wataganara T, Grunebaum A, Chervenak F, Wielgos M. Delivery modes in case of fetal malformations. J Perinat Med; 2016.
4. Wataganara T, Ebrashy A, Aliyu LD, et al. Fetal magnetic resonance imaging and ultrasound. J Perinat Med. 2016.
5. Scott DA. Genetics of congenital diaphragmatic hernia. Seminars in Pediatric Surgery. 2007;16:88-93.
6. Ludomirski A. Training in invasive fetal procedures. Ultrasound in obstetrics & gynecology: the official Journal of the International Society of Ultrasound in Obstetrics and Gynecology. 1995;5:150.
7. Moldenhauer JS, Soni S, Rintoul NE, et al. Fetal myelomeningocele repair: the post-MOMS experience at the Children's Hospital of Philadelphia. Fetal Diagnosis and Therapy. 2015;37:235-40.
8. Akkermans J, Peeters SH, Middeldorp JM, et al. A worldwide survey of laser surgery for twin-twin transfusion syndrome. Ultrasound in obstetrics & gynecology: the Official Journal of the International Society of Ultrasound in Obstetrics and Gynecology. 2015;45:168-74.
9. Kneebone RL, Nestel D, Vincent C, Darzi A. Complexity, risk and simulation in learning procedural skills. Medical Education. 2007;41:808-14.
10. Evgeniou E, Loizou P. Simulation-based surgical education. ANZ Journal of Surgery. 2013;83:619-23.
11. Raman M, Donnon T. Procedural skills education—colonoscopy as a model. Canadian journal of Gastroenterology = Journal Canadien de Gastroenterologie. 2008;22:767-70.
12. Boehler ML, Schwind CJ, Rogers DA, et al. A theory-based curriculum for enhancing surgical skillfulness. Journal of the American College of Surgeons. 2007;205:492-7.
13. Nizard J, Duyme M, Ville Y. Teaching ultrasound-guided invasive procedures in fetal medicine: learning curves with and without an electronic guidance system. Ultrasound in obstetrics & gynecology: the Official Journal of the International Society of Ultrasound in Obstetrics and Gynecology, 2002;19:274-7.
14. Tongprasert F, Srisupundit K, Luewan S, Phadungkiatwattana P, Pranpanus S, Tongsong T. Midpregnancy cordocentesis training of maternal-fetal medicine fellows. Ultrasound in obstetrics & gynecology: the Official Journal of the International Society of Ultrasound in Obstetrics and Gynecology. 2010;36:65-8.
15. Tongprasert F, Wanapirak C, Sirichotiyakul S, Piyamongkol W, Tongsong T. Training in cordocentesis: the first 50 case experience with and without a cordocentesis training model. Prenatal Diagnosis. 2010;30:467-70.
16. Wataganara T. Development of fetoscopic and minimally invasvie ultrasound-guided surgical simulator: Part of global education. Donald School J Ultrasound Obstet Gynecol. 2013;7:352-5.
17. Dreyfus M, Becmeur F, Schwaab C, Baldauf JJ, Philippe L, Ritter J. The pregnant ewe: an animal model for fetoscopic surgery. European Journal of Obstetrics, Gynecology, and Reproductive Biology. 1997;71:91-4.
18. Morris RK, Selman TJ, Harbidge A, Martin WI, Kilby MD. Fetoscopic laser coagulation for severe twin-to-twin transfusion syndrome: factors influencing perinatal outcome, learning curve of the procedure and lessons for new centres. BJOG: an International Journal of Obstetrics and Gynaecology. 2010;117:1350-7.
19. Klaritsch P, Albert K, Van Mieghem T, et al. Instrumental requirements for minimal invasive fetal surgery. BJOG: an International Journal of Obstetrics and Gynaecology. 2009;116:188-97.
20. Hecher K, Diehl W, Zikulnig L, Vetter M, Hackeloer BJ. Endoscopic laser coagulation of placental anastomoses in 200 pregnancies with severe mid-trimester twin-to-twin transfusion syndrome. European journal of Obstetrics, Gynecology, and Reproductive Biology. 2000;92:135-9.
21. Rossi AC, D'Addario V. Laser therapy and serial amnioreduction as treatment for twin-twin transfusion syndrome: a metaanalysis and review of literature. Am J Obstet Gynecol. 2008;198:147-52.
22. Chang YL, Chao AS, Chang SD, Hsieh PC, Wang CN. Short-term outcomes of fetoscopic laser surgery for severe twin-twin transfusion syndrome from Taiwan single center experience: demonstration of learning curve effect on the fetal outcomes. Taiwanese J Obstet Gynecol. 2012;51:350-3.
23. Sepulveda W, Wong AE, Dezerega V, Devoto JC, Alcalde JL. Endoscopic laser surgery in severe second-trimester twin-twin transfusion syndrome: a three-year experience from a Latin American center. Prenatal Diagnosis. 2007;27:1033-8.
24. Howell LJ, Adzick NS. The essentials of a fetal therapy center. Seminars in Perinatology. 1999;23:535-40.
25. Bebbington M. Twin-to-twin transfusion syndrome: current understanding of pathophysiology, in-utero therapy and impact for future development. Seminars in Fetal and Neonatal Medicine. 2010;15:15-20.
26. Moise KJ Jr, Moldenhauer JS, Bennett KA, et al. Current Selection Criteria and Perioperative Therapy Used for Fetal Myelomeningocele Surgery. Obstetrics and Gynecology. 2016;127:593-7.
27. Luks FI. New and/or improved aspects of fetal surgery. Prenatal Diagnosis. 2011;31:252-8.
28. McDonnell GV, McCann JP. Issues of medical management in adults with spina bifida. Child's nervous system: ChNS: Official Journal of the International Society for Pediatric Neurosurgery. 2000;16:222-7.

49

CHAPTER

Fetal Face and Four-dimensional Ultrasound

Mohamed Ahmed Mostafa AboEllail, Toshiyuki Hata

INTRODUCTION

The face represents the most visible part of the human being. The five major senses are facilitated in this region. Moreover, tools of communication with the surrounding world are mediated by this vital part of the human body. A universally understood language represented by various facial expressions can be a mirror for most of our feelings. A parent's first impression of their newborn is obtained through looking at their baby's face. Therefore, examination of the face is an essential step during the routine mid-trimester scan using two-dimensional (2D) sonography.[1,2] Moreover a new era of facial examination as an indicator of neurobehavioral development has emerged thanks to new advances in ultrasound machines. In this chapter, we will discuss the role of four-dimensional (4D) ultrasound, which markedly influences fetal facial studies.

FETAL FACE EXAMINATION

Sonographic examination of the fetal face includes two major categories, which are anatomical and functional evaluations. Chronologically, the detection of fetal facial anomalies was the first and main target of sonographers during fetal face visualization. The rapid progress in the field of ultrasound and appearance of new technologies such as three-dimensional (3D)/4D ultrasound as well as new rendering modes such as HDlive and the HDlive silhouette mode helped physicians to use ultrasound to accurately detect fetal facial structural anomalies.[3-12] Moreover, the recognition and diagnosis of fetal chromosomal abnormalities guided by structural fetal facial anomalies as clues for these chromosomal abnormalities were successfully achieved.[13-15]

Concurrently with the appearance of high frame-rate ultrasound machines using the surface-rendering mode of 3D/4D ultrasound, sonographers can now clearly visualize the fetal face **(Fig. 1)**, and observe fine fetal facial movements.[16-21] This was not possible before because the simultaneous detection and evaluation of some fetal facial movements such as swallowing, yawning, and eyelid movements could not be achieved with 2D sonography. 4D ultrasound has the ability to display them all at the same time, and therefore provides an additional advantage.[16]

Neuroscientists found that the maturation and development of the fetal central nervous system can be identified by the evaluation of fetal behavioral patterns.[22-24] Therefore, fetal facial movements can be considered an indicator of the brain function.[11] This opened the field to many studies that aimed at evaluating fetal behavior using the analysis of fetal movements including fetal facial movements as an indicator.[25]

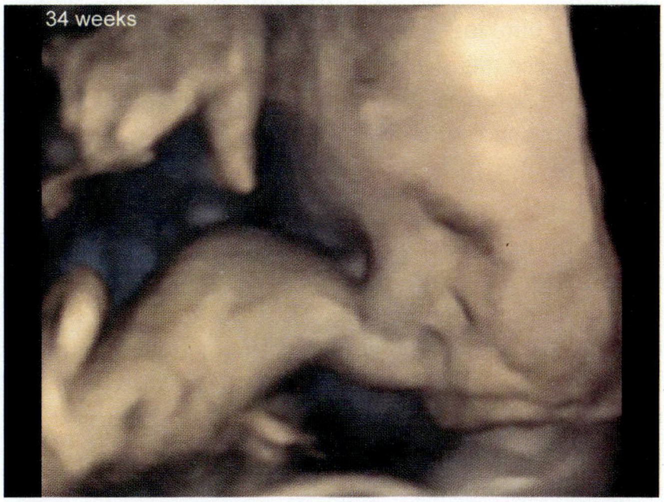

Fig. 1: 4D ultrasound image of a normal fetal face at 34 weeks of gestation. Details of the fetal eyes, nose, mouth, and its angles can be clearly noted.

TIMING OF FOUR-DIMENSIONAL ULTRASOUND VISUALIZATION OF FACIAL MOVEMENTS

Unlike fetal body movements that can be assessed by 4D sonography as early as in the first trimester of pregnancy, the full range of facial movements cannot be assessed at this early time.[26] Mouthing and yawning can be studied at 15–16 weeks of gestation. This does not mean that the onset of fetal facial movements is delayed to this time. The facial and trigeminal cranial nerves appear at 10–11 weeks of gestation,[11] and facial muscles are formed at 16 weeks of gestation.[27] However, at 24 weeks of gestation the deposition of adipose tissue in the fetal face starts, and gradually continues until 36 weeks of gestation.[28] Therefore, it is from around 20 weeks of gestation when the full range of fetal facial movements can be assessed using 4D ultrasound. The onset of fetal facial expressions still remains an unresolved area that needs to be clarified in future research.

DIFFERENT PATTERNS OF FETAL FACIAL MOVEMENTS VISUALIZED BY FOUR-DIMENSIONAL ULTRASOUND

Using 4D ultrasound, various types of fetal facial movement can be observed. High frame-rate machines, as we previously mentioned, can visualize subtle movements. Seven fetal facial movements have comprised the main interest of researchers who study their frequencies throughout gestation as keys to predict fetal brain functions.[20,26-29-33] These movements are: mouthing, yawning, smiling, tongue expulsion, blinking, grimace, and suckling. We will describe each of these facial expressions and the changes in their frequency patterns throughout gestation based on the major published studies.

Mouthing

Mouthing can be defined as a sequence of rhythmic movements involving the jaws, and could be associated with tongue movement **(Fig. 2)**. It can last from 1 to 15 seconds.[30] It has been reported as the most frequent fetal facial movement in all studies examining facial expressions using 4D ultrasound.[29-33] The mouthing movement frequency has been shown to be constant throughout pregnancy,[29-32] while one study showed that its peak is at 24 weeks of gestation, and then it slightly decreases towards the end of pregnancy.[33] Kurjak et al.[20] reported that simultaneous mouthing and eyelid movements dominate

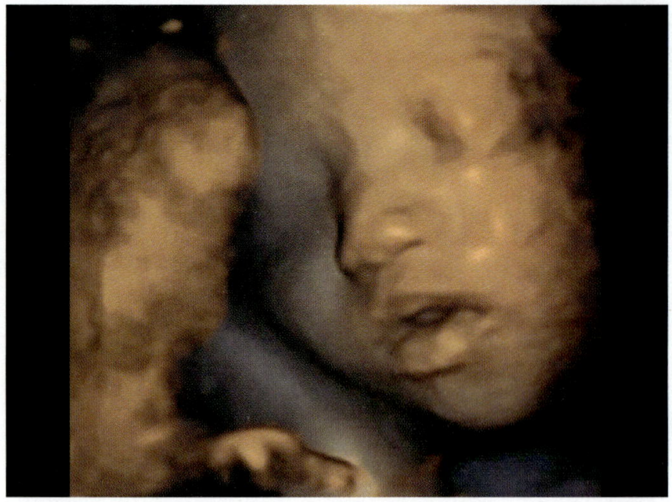

Fig. 2: Fetal mouthing movement at 29 weeks and 5 days of gestation demonstrated by 4D ultrasound.

at 30–33 weeks of gestation. Hanaoka et al.[35] found that this movement frequency showed significant racial differences when compared between Japanese (Asian) and Croatian (Caucasian) fetuses. Reissland et al.[34] conducted an in-depth analysis of this movement. They studied the deviation of fetal mouth movements, and precisely categorized two kinds of movement: mouth stretch and upper lip raise. In mouth stretch movement, 50% of fetuses showed a neutral position, which gradually decreased by 11% for each gestational week, and left lateralization was noted in 68% of the remaining fetuses. Upper lip raising did not change with the gestational age, and showed a predominance on the left side. Therefore, they used mouth movement as an indicator of brain lateralization with advancing gestation, which can be a marker of brain development with the use of 4D ultrasound.

Yawning

It can be defined as prolonged wide and slow jaw opening followed by quick closure with simultaneous head retroflexion **(Fig. 3)**. The function and aim of this movement remains unclear despite different theories on its relation to fetal hypoxia or anemia; however, none have been validated. It is thought to have only a maturational function.[36] It has been reported as the second most frequent fetal facial movement after mouthing.[31,32] Reports on the change in its frequency throughout gestation showed contradictory results. Sato et al.[32] reported its increase with advancing gestation. Yigiter et al.[29] showed that it displays a gradual increase at the second trimester, and then its

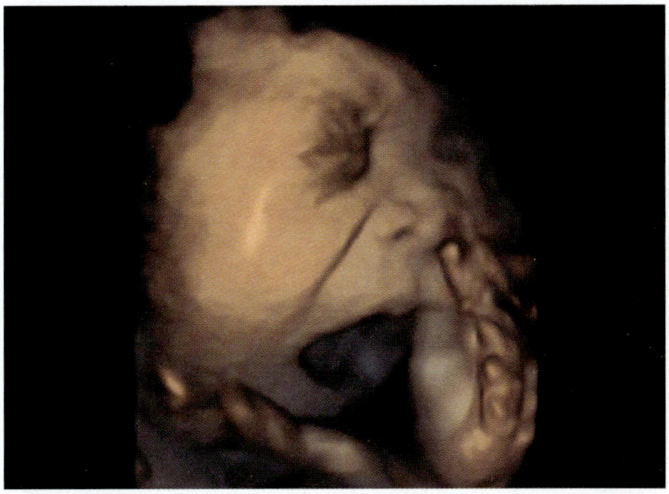

Fig. 3: 4D ultrasound image of fetal yawning at 30 weeks and 3 days of gestation. Wide opening of the jaw with head retroflexion can be recognized.

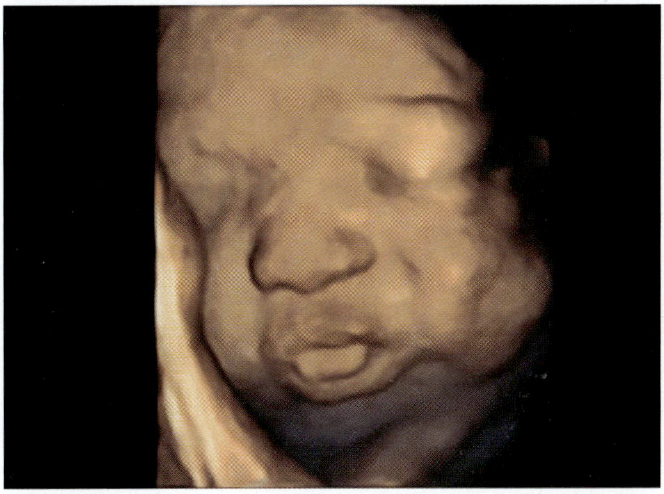

Fig. 4: Fetal tongue expulsion at 36 weeks and 6 days of gestation demonstrated by 4D ultrasound.

frequency does not change with advancing gestation. However, Reissland et al.[36] documented a decrease in the yawning frequency from 28 weeks of gestation and onwards. This discrepancy in the results might be due to difficulty in differentiating yawning from non-yawn mouth opening.

Tongue Expulsion

This is protrusion of the tongue during mouth opening **(Fig. 4)**. It shows a significant increase throughout gestation, as documented in two reports.[29,32] Kurjak et al.[20] stated that it increases at 16–24 weeks and then remains constant, in contrast to Lebit et al.[33] who reported a slight decrease in its frequency at the end of pregnancy.

Blinking

It is a reflex characterized by rapid closing and opening of the eyes **(Fig. 5)**, which occurs involuntarily or as a protective mechanism. Kanenishi et al.[31] reported that it is the least observed facial expression. Kurjak et al.[20] reported its peak at 28 weeks of gestation. Lebit el al.[33] stated that it starts after 23 weeks of gestation, and then its frequency increases until it shows a slight decrease at the end of pregnancy. Yigiter and Kavak[29] stated that it increases throughout the second and third trimesters. Sato et al.[32] were the only group who reported no observable blinking movements in their study at 20–24 weeks of gestation. Generally, blinking shows an increased frequency with advancing gestation. This fetal facial movement needs high frame-rate ultrasound devices to accurately record it.

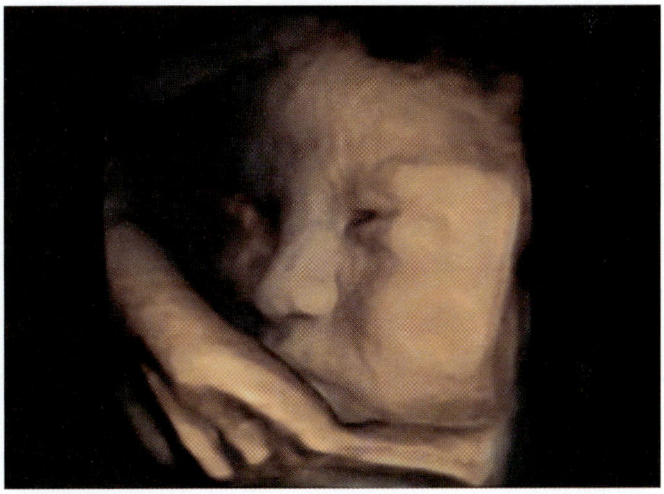

Fig. 5: 4D ultrasound image of fetal eye blinking at 36 weeks and 6 days of gestation.

Sucking

Sucking is a series of opening and closing of the jaws that may be associated with sinking of the cheeks towards the oral cavity. The fetus may suckle one of his fingers, toes, or the umbilical cord. Its frequency remains constant throughout pregnancy.[32] It can be easily observed either by 2D or 4D ultrasound.

Scowling (Grimacing)

It can be described as wrinkling of the bilaterally contracted eyebrows and the muscles between them with a simultaneous drop of the mouth angles bilaterally

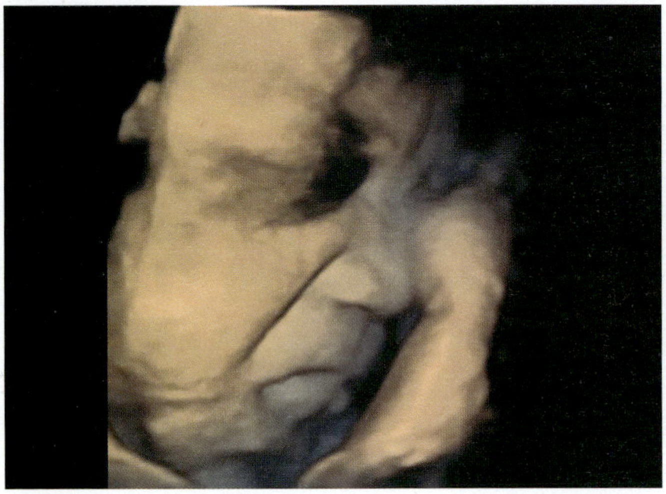

Fig. 6: 4D ultrasound image of fetal grimacing at 36 weeks and 1 day of gestation. Wrinkling of the forehead with a drop of the mouth angles and lip curling is clear.

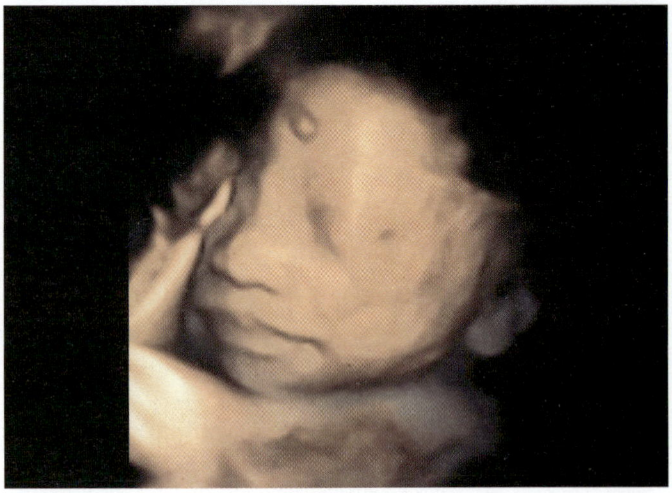

Fig. 7: Fetal smiling at 29 weeks and 1 day of gestation by 4D ultrasound.

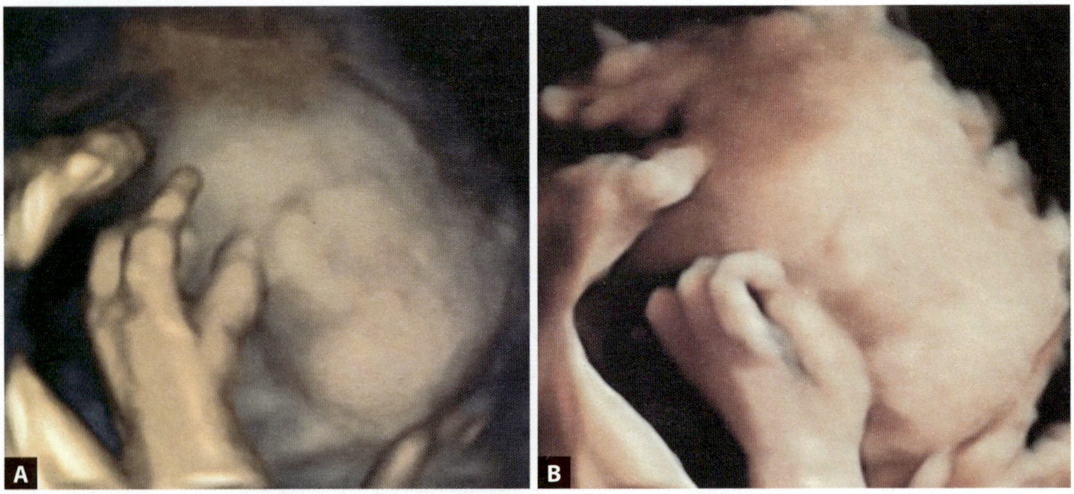

Figs. 8A and B: Sorrow-like movement at 26 weeks and 4 days of gestation demonstrated by 4D ultrasound (A) and HDlive; (B) Does the fetus show emotions?

and curling of one of the lips **(Fig. 6)**. It indicates that the fetus may be suffering from pain or stress. It displays an increased frequency with advancing gestation.[32,37] It starts to be more complex near term as an adaptive process to be used postnataly. Scowling might be associated with other movements which indicate pain, such as as clenching the fists.[37]

Smiling

This movement involves bilateral elevation of the mouth angles **(Fig. 7)**. Its peak frequency was reported to be at 24–32 weeks of gestation,[29] and then it increases throughout gestation.[29,32]

FOUR-DIMENSIONAL ULTRASOUND AND FETAL EMOTION-LIKE MOVEMENTS

Hata et al.[38] extensively studied fetal facial expressions using 4D ultrasound, and elicited some fetal facial movements, which represent emotion-like expressions **(Figs. 8 and 9)**. They raised the question of whether fetuses in utero have emotions or these movements represent reflex behaviors, and whether they should be perceived as emotion-like behavior. 'Most fetal facial expressions may simply constitute a reflexive behavior on the part of the fetus. However, fetal facial expressions and emotion-like behaviors observed by 4D ultrasound may represent some kind of fetal emotions and awareness.'[39]

Further extensive studies in collaboration with neuroscientists and psychologists are advance knowledge on fetal brain and central nervous system functions (including whether or not they have a consciousness) through fetal behavior research using 4D ultrasound.

FOUR-DIMENSIONAL ULTRASOUND OF FETAL FACE AND KURJAK'S ANTENATAL NEURODEVELOPMENT TEST (KANET)

Four-dimensional ultrasound studies of the fetal face have played important roles in the field of fetal neurological assessment. Cerebral palsy is now believed to frequently result from prenatal causes rather than peri- or postnatal ones.[40] Previous studies also showed that investigation of the fetal face can be used to identify normal and abnormal neurological functions in utero; therefore, the antenatal prediction of fetuses at risk of adverse neurological outcomes can be achieved.[41] Kurjak et al. developed the now widely used KANET test to assess neurobehavioral development depending upon 4D ultrasound evaluation of fetal facial expressions and other parameters representing fetal body movements, which were chosen as the most significant indicators of fetal behavioral assessment.[42] Standardization of this test and the postnatal follow-up was achieved in October 2010 during the Osaka consensus meeting.[43] The test should be applied for 15 minutes to awake fetuses with a gestational age of 28–38 weeks. The consensus recommended repeating the test in borderline and abnormal cases with special attention to facial movements, indicating their importance as brain function indicators.

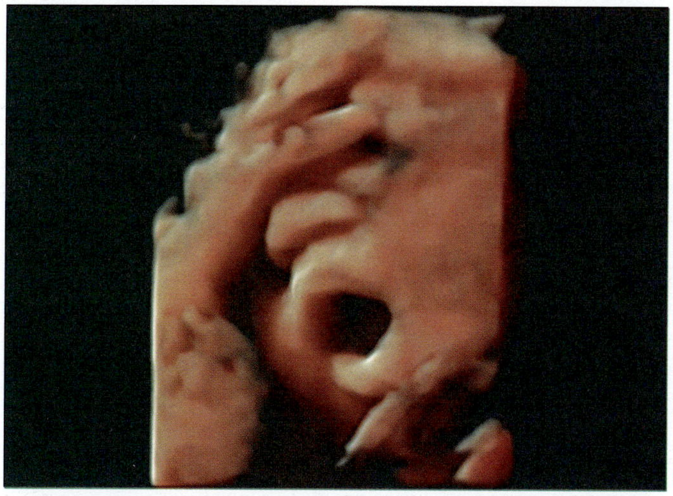

Fig. 9: HDlive image of a fetal face at 35 weeks and 5 days of gestation showing astonished-like expression.

The KANET test has the potential to detect and discriminate normal from borderline and abnormal fetal behavior in normal and high-risk pregnancies, which means that it could become a valuable diagnostic tool for fetal neurological assessment. The components of the KANET test are given in **Table 1**, which shows the criteria used to evaluate the fetus. **Table 2** demonstrates the evaluation of the score as normal, borderline, and abnormal. Caution should be taken when using this test as it showed ethnic differences when applied to Asian and Caucasian fetuses.[35]

TABLE 1: Different parameters of the Kurjak Antenatal Neurological Test (KANET).

	Score			
Sign	***0***	***1***	***2***	***Sign score***
Isolated head anteflexion 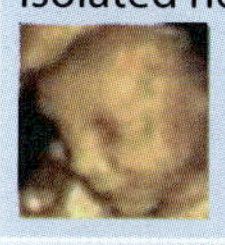	Abrupt	Small range (0–3 times of movements)	Variable in full range, many alternation (>3 times of movements)	
Cranial sutures and head circumference 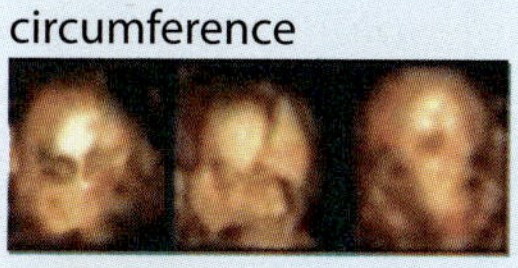	Overlapping of cranial sutures	Normal cranial sutures with measurement of HC below or above the normal limit (-2 SD) according to GA	Normal cranial sutures with normal measurement of HC according to GA	
Isolated eye blinking 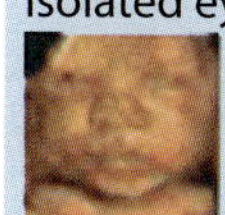	Not present	Not fluent (1–5 times of blinking)	Fluency (>5 times of blinking)	

Contd...

Contd...

Sign	*Score* 0	1	2	*Sign score*
Facial alteration (grimace or tongue expulsion) 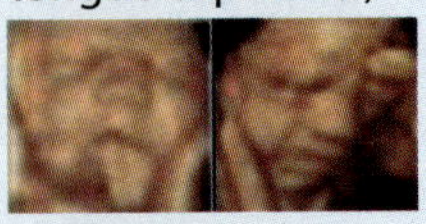	Not present	Not fluent (1–5 times of alteration)	Fluency (>5 times of blinking)	
or Mouth opening (yawning or mouthing) 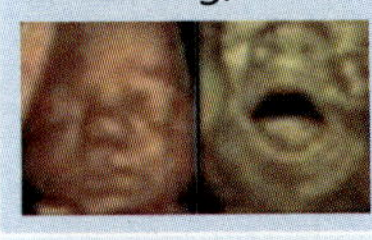				
Isolated leg movement 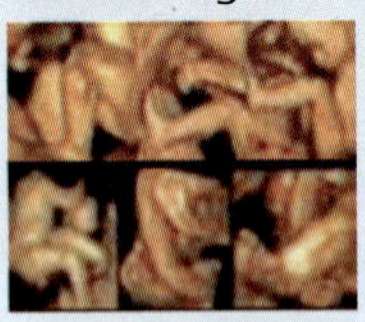	Cramped	Poor repertoire or Small in range (0–5 times of movement)	Variable in full range, many alternation (>5 times of movements)	
Isolated hand movement 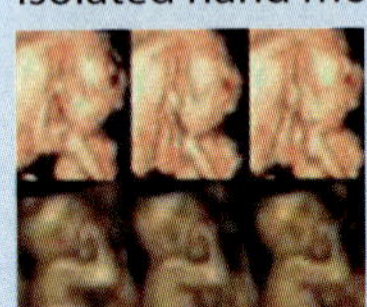 or Hand to face movements 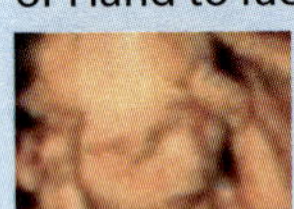	Cramped or abrupt	Poor repertoire or Small in range (0–5 times of movement)	Variable in full range, many alternation (>5 times of movements)	
Fingers movements 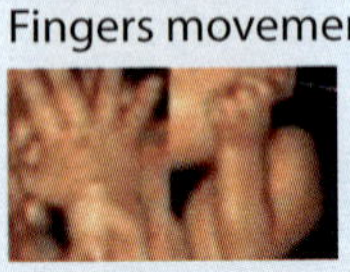	Unilateral or bilateral clenched fist, (neurological thumb)	Cramped invariable finger movements	Smooth and complex, variable finger movements	
Gestalt perception of GMs	Definitely abnormal	Borderline	Normal	
			Total score	

TABLE 2: Interpretation of the total KANET score.

Total score	*Interpretation*
0–5	Abnormal
6–9	Borderline
10–16	Normal

FETAL OBSERVABLE MOVEMENT SYSTEM (FOMS) AND FOUR-DIMENSIONAL ULTRASOUND

Each of the facial expressions used in the evaluation of fetal behavior is a series of movements, which integrate together to form an expression. The problem with fetal neurobehavior is that many scientists consider that the analysis of these expressions is subjective, and they also detect just the quantitative and not qualitative pattern of the movement. Therefore, a need to standardize these facial expressions emerged in order to efficiently pool and compare the results obtained between different centers or even in the same center when the observer of data is not the same. Reissland et al.[44] suggested a coding system resembling those used in children and adults to code facial expressions. It is still not widely used to ascertain if it can solve the problem of the lack of comparison between studies; however, it enables the differentiation of fine movements, such as the ability to differentiate yawning from non-yawn mouth opening.[36] In one of their studies, Reissland et al.[45] used it to indicate that fetuses exposed to stress in the form of nicotine display higher rates of self-touch as an indicator of poor neurodevelopment compared to fetuses of non-smoking mothers. They were also able to differentiate the mouthing movement into mouth stretch and lip raise, and used it in the development of the fetal lateralization theory.[34] This coding system requires a high-scan quality in contrast to KANET, which can use a lower-quality scan. **Table 3** shows scan quality evaluation scoring, which permits coding. This coding system needs to be developed so as to be universally accepted, and facilitate the interpretation of fetal facial expressions.

TABLE 3: Scan quality coding scheme.

Scan quality	*Description*	*What can be coded*
0	Uncodable	Vague outlines of fetal facial configuration discrenible but uncodable using the FOMS system
1	Poor	Allows the coding of only very gross movements
2	Acceptable	Allows the coding of parts of the fetal face
3	Good	A clear view of the fetal face throughout with the few occurrences of uncodable features of the fetal face
4	Very good	A clear view of the fetal face with facioal features and movements being consistently codable

(*Courtesy:* Reprinted with permission from Reissland N et al.)[44]

HDLIVE OF FETAL FACE

The surface-rendering mode of 4D ultrasound is widely used in research, and all investigations documenting fetal behavioral studies were conducted using the surface-rendering mode. Recently, a new technology was developed called HDlive, which is a 3D/4D ultrasound system characterized by an adjustable light source that can be used to create lighting and shadowing effects and, therefore, increase depth perception resulting in skin-like images of the fetal face **(Figs. 10 to 12)**.[45] Although this technique was not used in the neurobehavioral assessment of facial expressions, it showed marked benefit for detecting various congenital anomalies, as reported by Hata and his group who visualized normal and abnormal fetal faces at different stages of pregnancy as well as different structural anomalies.[12-15, 47-51]

LIMITATIONS OF FOUR-DIMENSIONAL ULTRASOUND USE IN FETAL FACE EXAMINATION

Because the 4D ultrasound volume is derived from 2D planes, many of the factors are known to be the same as for 2D sonographic imaging (i.e. maternal obesity, reduced amount of amniotic fluid, fetal position, and shadowing

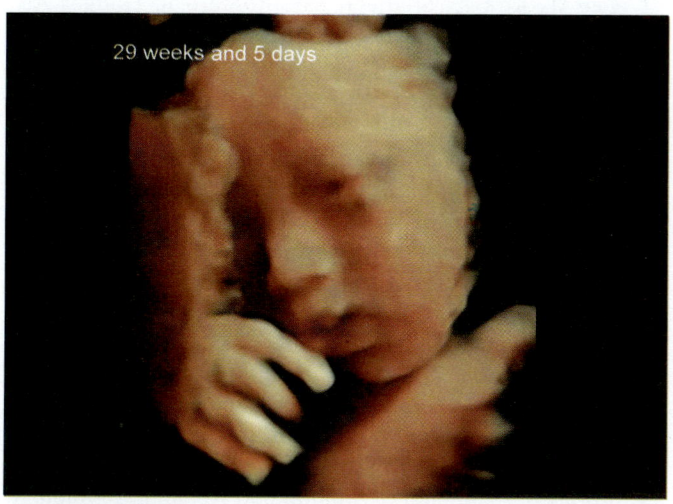

Fig. 10: HDlive image showing eye opening in a fetus at 29 weeks and 5 days of gestation. Demonstration of the eye with identification of the eyelid angles is clearly evident.

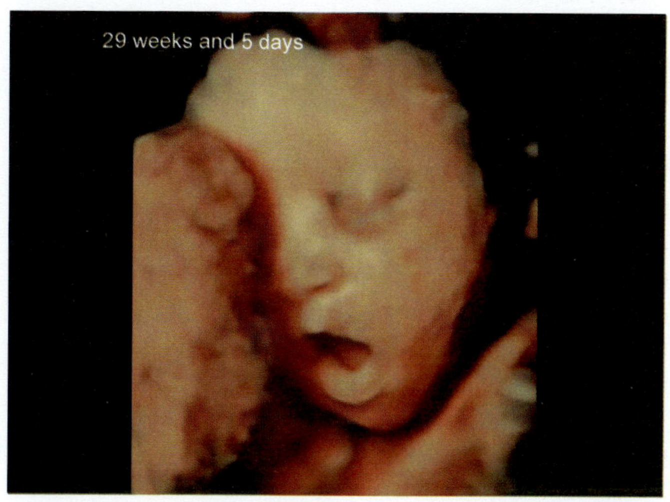

Fig. 11: Fetal yawning movement by HDlive at 29 weeks and 5 days of gestation. An adjustable light source can create life-like images with skin-like colors.

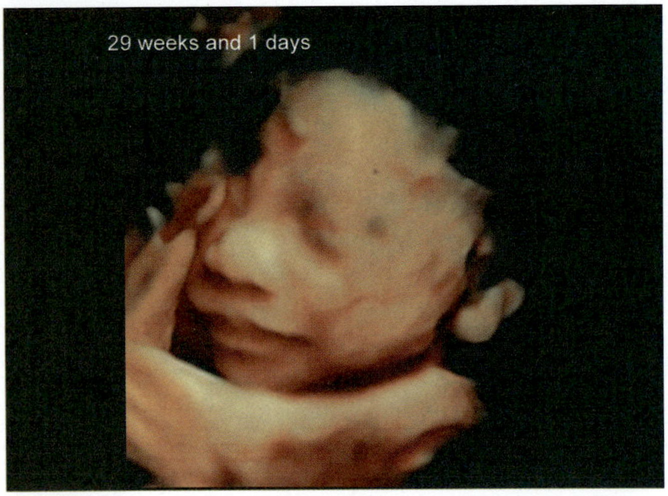

Fig. 12: HDlive image of fetal smiling at 29 weeks and 1 days of gestation.

of overlying structures). Several specific limitations of 4D ultrasound have been noted:

- Time is required for the learning curve of 4D ultrasound scanning
- Motion artifacts can appear during data acquisition
- Limited size of the volume box leads to limitation of the size of the collected volume data
- Volume storage requires a high storage capacity
- After recollection of a stored volume, it can be difficult to achieve orientation. Furthermore, the recognition of an artifact can be hampered when the cause of the artifact has not been stored in the volume.

For good image quality in reconstruction rendering, some contrasts between the boundaries are necessary. Surface reconstruction, for instance, is difficult without some amniotic fluid in front of the structure that is to be displayed.

CONCLUSION

Four-dimensional ultrasound is essential for anatomical evaluation of the fetal face. Moreover, it has opened the door for functional assessment of the fetal brain though the evaluation of different fetal facial expressions. The KANET test is an example of the use of 4D visualization of the face in the field of fetal neurobehavioral assessment. However, it is still limited to research, and larger sample-sized studies with standardization of the ultrasound machine frame rates, examination times, and global standardization of the fetal facial movements by a universally-accepted coding system for these movements can help to pool the data for a better understanding of the relationship between fetal facial movements and the development and functions of different brain areas.

CONFLICT OF INTEREST

The authors have no conflict of interest.

REFERENCES

1. Salomon LJ, Alfirevic Z, Berghella V, Bilardo C, Hernandez-Andrade E, Johnsen SL, et al. ISUOG Clinical Standards Committee. Practice guidelines for performance of the routine mid-trimester fetal ultrasound scan. Ultrasound Obstet Gynecol. 2011;37:116-26.
2. Leung KY, Poon CF, Teotico AR, Hata T, Won H, Chen M, et al. Recommendations on routine mid-trimester anomaly scan. J Obste Gynaecol Res. 2015;41:653-61.
3. Cho FN, Kan YY, Chen SN, Lee TC, Hsu TJ, Hsu PH. Prenatal diagnosis of cyclopia and proboscis in a fetus with normal chromosome at 13 weeks of gestation by three-dimensional transabdominal sonography. Prenat Diagn. 2005;25:1059-72.
4. Merz E, Weber G, Bahlmann F, Miric-Tesanic D. Application of transvaginal and abdominal three-dimensional ultrasound or the detection or exclusion of malformations of the fetal face. Ultrasound Obstet Gynecol. 1997;9:237-43.
5. Dyson RL, Pretorius DH, Budorick NE, Johnson DD, Sklansky MS, Cantrell CJ, et al. Three-dimensional ultrasound in the evaluation of fetal anomalies. Ultrasound Obstet Gynecol. 2000:16:321-8.
6. Tonni G, Centini G, Rosignoli L. Prenatal screening for fetal face and clefting in a prospective study on low-risk population: can three- and four-dimensional ultrasound enhance visualization and detection rate? Oral Surg Oral Med Oral Pathol Oral Radiol Endod. 2005;100:420-6.
7. Lee W, Kirk JS, Shaheen KW, Romero R, Hodges AN, Comstock CH. Fetal cleft lip and palate detection by three-dimensional ultrasonography. Ultrasound Obstet Gynecol. 2000;16:314-20.
8. Wong HS, Parker S, Tait J, Pringle KC. Antenatal diagnosis of anophthalmia by three-dimensional ultrasound: a novel application of the reverse face view. Ultrasound Obstet Gynecol. 2008;32:103-05.
9. Peralta CF, Falcon O, Wegrzyn P, Faro C, Nicolaides KH. Assessment of the gap between the fetal nasal bones at 11 to 13 + 6 weeks of gestation by three-dimensional ultrasound. Ultrasound Obstet Gynecol. 2005;25:464-7.
10. Rembouskos G, Cicero S, Longo D, Vandecruys H, Nicolaides K. Assessment of the fetal nasal bone at 11–14 weeks of gestation by three-dimensional ultrasound. Ultrasound Obstet Gynecol. 2004;23:232-6.
11. Kurjak A, Azumendi G, Andonotopo W, Salihagic-Kadic A. Three- and four-dimensional ultrasonography for the structural and functional evaluation of the fetal face. Am J Obstet Gynecol. 2007;196:16-28.

12. Hata T, Uketa E, Tenkumo C, Hanaoka U, Kanenishi K, Tanaka H. Three- and four-dimensional HDlive rendering image of fetal acrania/exencephaly in early pregnancy. J Med Ultrasonics. 2013;40:271-3.
13. Hata T, Hanaoka U, Tenkumo C, Sato M, Tanaka H, Ishimura M. Three- and four-dimensional HDlive rendering images of normal and abnormal fetuses: pictorial essay. Arch Gynecol Obstet. 2012;286:1431-5.
14. Hata T, Hanaoka U, Uematsu R, Marumo G, Tanaka H. HDlive in the assessment of fetal facial abnormalities. Donald School J Ultrasound Obstet Gynecol. 2014;8:344-52.
15. Hanaoka U, Tanaka H, Koyano K, Uematsu R, Kanenishi K, Hata T. HDlive imaging of fetuses with autosomal trisomies. J Med Ultrasonics. 2014;41:339-42.
16. Kozuma S, Baba K, Okai T, Taketani Y. Dynamic observation of the fetal face by three-dimensional ultrasound. Ultrasound Obstet Gynecol. 1998;13:282-4.
17. Kuno A, Akiyama M, Yamashiro C, Tanaka H, Yanagihara T, Hata T. Three-dimensional sonographic assessment of fetal behavior in the early second trimester of pregnancy. J Ultrasound Med. 2001;20:1271-5.
18. Campbell S. 4D, or not 4D: That is the question. Ultrasound Obstet Gynecol. 2002;19:1-4.
19. Azumendi G, Kurjak A.Three-dimensional and four-dimensional sonography in the study of the fetal face. Ultrasound Rev Obstet Gynecol. 2003;3:160-9.
20. Kurjak A, Azumendi G, Vecek N, Kupešic S, Solak M, Varga D, et al. Fetal hand movements and facial expression in normal pregnancy studied by four-dimensional sonography. J Perinat Med. 2003;31:496-508.
21. Hata T, Kanenishi K. Akiyama M, Tanaka H, Kimura K. Realtime 3-D sonographic observation of fetal facial expression. J Obstet Gynaecol Res. 2005;31:337-40.
22. Prechtl HF. Qualitative changes of spontaneous movements in fetus and preterm infant are a marker of neurological dysfunction. Early Hum Dev. 1990;23:151-8.
23. Prechtl HF. State of the art of a new functional assessment of the young nervous system: an early predictor of cerebral palsy. Early Hum Dev. 1997;50:1-11.
24. Prechtl HF. Is neurological assessment of the fetus possible? Eur J Obstet Gynecol Reprod Biol. 1997;75:81-4.
25. Stanojevic M, Perlman JM, Andonotopo W, Kurjak A. From fetal to neonatal behavioral status. Ultrasound Rev Obstet Gynecol. 2004;4:459-71.
26. Kurjak A, Stanojević M, Andonotopo W, Scazzocchio-Duenas E, Azumendi G, Carrera JM. Fetal behavior assessed in all three trimesters of normal pregnancy by four-dimensional ultrasonography. Croat Med J. 2005;46:772-80.
27. Bosma JF. Anatomic and physiologic development of the speech apparatus. In: Towers DB (Ed). Human Communication and its Disorder. Raven: New York; 1975. pp.469-81.
28. Reissland N, Francis B, Mason J, Lincoln K. Do Facial Expressions Develop before Birth? PLoS One. 2011;6(8): e24081.
29. Yigiter AB, Kavak ZN. Normal standards of fetal behaviour assessed by four-dimensional sonography. J Matern Fetal Neonatal Med. 2006;19:707-21.
30. Yan F, Dai SY, Akther N, Kuno A, Yanagihara T, Hata T. Four-dimensional sonographic assessment of fetal facial expression early in the third trimester. Int J Gynecol Obstet. 2006;94:108-13.
31. Kanenishi K, Hanaoka U, Noguchi J, Marumo G, Hata T. 4D ultrasound evaluation of fetal facial expressions during the latter stages of the second trimester. Int J Gynecol Obstet. 2013;121:257-60.
32. Sato M, Kanenishi K, Hanaoka U, Noguchi J, Marumo G, Hata T. 4D ultrasound study of fetal facial expressions at 20–24 weeks of gestation. Int J Gynaecol Obstet. 2014;126:275-9.
33. Lebit DF, Vladareanu PD. The role of 4D ultrasound in the assessment of fetal behaviour. Maedica (Buchar). 2011;6:120-7.
34. Reissland N, Francis B, Aydin E, Mason J, Exley K. Development of prenatal lateralization: evidence from fetal mouth movements. Physiol Behav. 2014;131:160-3.
35. Hanaoka U, Hata T, Kanenishi K, AboEllail MAM, Uematsu R, Konishi Y, et al. Does ethnicity have an effect on fetal behavior? A comparison of Asian and Caucasian populations. J Perinat Med DOI: 10.1515/jpm-2015-0036.
36. Reissland N, Francis B, Manson J. Development of fetal yawn compared with non-yawn mouth openings from 24–36 weeks gestation. PLoS One. 2012;7:e50569. DOI: 37.10.1371/journal.pone.0050569.
37. Reissland N, Francis B, Mason J. Can healthy fetuses show facial expressions of "pain" or "distress"? PLoS One. 2013;8:e65530. DOI: 10.1371/journal.pone.0065530.
38. Hata T, Kanenishi K, Hanaoka U, Marumo G. HDlive and 4D ultrasound in the assessment of fetal facial expressions. Donald School J Ultrasound Obstet. 2015;9:44-50.
39. Hata T, Kanenishi K, AboEllail MAM, Marumo G, Kurjak A. Fetal consciousness 4D ultrasound study. Donald School J Ultrasound Obstet Gynecol. 2015;9:471-4.
40. Kurjak A, Stanojevic M, Andonotopo W, Salihagic-Kadic A, Carrera JM, Azumendi G. Behavioral pattern continuity from prenatal to postnatal life—a study by four-dimensional (4D) ultrasonography. J Perinat Med. 2004;32:346-53.
41. Einspieler C, Prechtl HFR. Prechtl's assessment of general movements: a diagnostic tool for the functional assessment of the young nervous system. Ment Retard Dev Disabil Res Rev. 2011;5:61-7.
42. Kurjak A, Miskovic B, Stanojevic M, Amiel-Tison C, Ahmed B, Azumendi G, et al. New scoring system for fetal neurobehavior assessed by three- and four-dimensional sonography. J Perinat Med. 2008;36:73-81.
43. Stanojevic M, Talic A, Miskovic B, Vasilj O, Shaddad AN, Ahmed B, et al. An attempt to standardize Kurjak's antenatal neurodevelopmental test: Osaka consensus statement. Donald School J Ultrasound Obstet Gynecol. 2011;5:317-29.
44. Raissland N, Austen JM, Hanaoka U, AboEllail MAM, Uematsu R, Hata T. The potential use of the Fetal Observable

Movement Sysytem (FOMS) in clinical practice. Donald School J Ultrasound Obstet Gynecol. 2015;9:426-33.

45. Reissland N, Francis B, Kumarendran K, Mason J. Ultrasound observations of subtle movements: a pilot study comparing foetuses of smoking and nonsmoking mothers. Acta Paediatr. 2015;104:596-603.
46. Kagan KO, Pintoffl K, Hoopmann M. First-trimester ultrasound images using HDlive. Ultrasound Obstet Gynecol. 2011;38:607.
47. Kanenishi K, Nitta E, Mashima M, Hanaoka U, Koyano K, Tanaka H, et al. HDlive imaging of intra-amniotic umbilical vein varix with thrombosis. Placenta. 2013;34:1110-2.
48. Hata T, Hanaoka U, Tenkumo C, Ito M, Uketa E, Mori N, et al. Three-dimensional HDlive rendering image of cystic hygroma. J Med Ultrasonics. 2013;40:297-9.
49. AboEllail MAM, Tanaka H, Mori N, Tanaka A, Kubo H, Shimono R, et al. HDlive imaging of meconium peritonitis. Ultrasound Obstet Gynecol. 2015;45:494-6.
50. AboEllail MAM, Hanaoka U, Mashima M, Kawanishi K, Hata T. HDlive image of fetal endocardial cushion defect. Donald School J Ultrasound Obstet Gynecol. 2014;8:437-9.
51. AboEllail MAM, Hanaoka U, Numoto A, Hata T. HDlive image of fetal giant hemangioma. J Ultrasound Med. 2015;34:2315-8.

50

CHAPTER

Three-dimensional Ultrasound for the Detection of Fetal Syndromes

Sonila Pashaj, Eberhard Merz

INTRODUCTION

Pediatricians aim to diagnose children with syndromes on the basis of dysmorphic features. These dysmorphic features are classified in four different types.[1-3]

1. Malformation which is a morphologic anomaly of an organ or large area of the body from abnormal embryological development and is due to a genetic etiology.[4] Cleft lip and palate are examples of such a malformation.
2. Deformation refers to abnormal form, shape or position caused by mechanical force antenatal on normal structures, such as clubfoot.
3. Disruption which is a morphological defect of an organ or large area of the body resulting from a breakdown of the previously normal tissue like amniotic bands.
4. Dysplasia which is abnormal growth or organization within the tissue, such as craniosynostosis.

Other terminology that must be known is when dealing with syndromes:[5]

- Association is a nonrandom occurrence of a pattern of multiple anomalies, with unknown pathogenesis, in more than one individual, that are not known as syndrome or sequence. An example is VATER association (vertebral anomalies, anal atresia, tracheoesophageal fistula and renal anomalies).
- Sequence describes multiple anomalies that result from a single initiating event, anomaly or mechanical factor. The best known is Pierre–Robin sequence where the event is micrognathia which will lead to glossoptosis and obstruction of the upper airway. 25% of these sequence will have Stickler's syndrome.[6]
- Syndromes include a pattern of multiple anomalies, resulting from the same etiology.

Knowledge of the pattern of several defects leads to the diagnosis of a syndrome. The London Dysmorphology database and OMIM (Online Mendelian Inheritance in Man) are useful databases that allow the identifications of syndromes. The progress of molecular genetics and the enormous technological progress in three-dimensional ultrasound had enabled the demonstration of subtle findings which lead to the prenatal diagnosis of specific syndromes.

Nevertheless, it is a very difficult task to identify a specific syndrome with ultrasound. A frequently asked question from sonographers performing prenatal ultrasound is regarding to the association observed between a common malformation and a syndrome. To find out the correct diagnosis is a procedure like playing a puzzle. A puzzle requires putting all pieces together in a logical way, in order to find the final picture. When an unusual pattern of different defects is encountered, the question should always be: 'What is the specific syndrome?' instead of just listing the malformations recognized during the ultrasound examination.

Since there are thousands of syndromes, it is important to learn how to find out the correct diagnosis in difficult cases. In this chapter we will discuss the different syndromes associated with face malformations, mainly cleft lip and palate but also micrognathia and maxillary hypoplasia.More than 300 syndromes are associated with facial clefting, e.g., van der Woude, Goldenhar, CHARGE, Treacher–Collins, Nager and Miller syndromes.[7-10]

Embryologically the face is derived from five facial prominences that surround the future mouth, namely the unpaired frontonasal process, the paired maxillary and the mandibular process.[11,12] Any incomplete fusion of the different prominences results in a congenital facial cleft.[11,13]

An internationally accepted anatomical classification system proposed by Tessier[14] is assigning a number to each malformation on the basis of its position relative to the sagittal midline. The different types of Tessier clefts are numbered from 0 to 14. Treacher-Collins syndrome results from a combination of the numbers 6,7 and 8, whereas the Goldenhar syndrome shows number 7.[15]

In the second trimester malformation scan the demonstration of the fetal lips is part of a standard ultrasound examination.[16] The detection rate of orafacial malformations depends on several factors: experience of the operator, ultrasound technology (2D, 3D ultrasound), position of the fetus and amount of amniotic fluid. According to the latest data in literature the prenatal detection rate of CL/CLP ranges from 56%[17] to 85.2 %.[18] However, isolated clefts of the palate remain practically undetected.

Despite the fact that the experienced operator is able to detect CL and CLP with 2D ultrasound,[19] if the fetus is in a good position, the 2D demonstration of a facial defect is difficult to understand for the parents. In contrast to 2D ultrasound 3D ultrasound allows a detailed demonstration of the soft tissue of the fetal face, contributing to a better understanding of the malformation by the physician and the future parents. In particular HDlive technology[20] is now able to provide the operator and the parents with photorealistic pictures of a facial surface defect in the unborn.[21] Using surface rendered images of coronal cut planes we are now able to demonstrate isolated clefts in the hard and soft palate.[21] However, 3D ultrasound is not only advantageous in surface rendering but also in the different demonstration modes allowing a detailed assessment of the fetal face and the oral cavity. These include the triplanar mode that allows the simultaneous display of the 3 perpendicular planes (sagittal, axial and coronal) of the fetal face at the same time on the monitor, the tomographic modus showing parallel planes and the transparency mode with the demonstration of the bony structures of the fetal face only.[22-26] In particular the combination of the different 3D modes provides a detailed examination of the fetal face with a precise evaluation of forehead, orbits, eyes, nose, lips, alveolar ridge, chin, tongue and palate.[21]

In this chapter we will review several syndromes, which are important for physicians involved in prenatal diagnosis, either because they are typical or common or their diagnosis will have an impact on the patient counseling.

APERT SYNDROME

Apert syndrome was first described by Wheaton and later on by the French physician Apert in 1906 (cit. by Azevedo).[27] It is characterized by craniosynostosis (premature fusion of one or more cranial sutures), craniofacial anomalies, such as midfacial hypoplasia and symmetric bony syndactyly of hands and feet.[28] Prevalence is reported 1:64500 births.[29] If the diagnosis is suspected confirmation can be performed by DNA analysis of mutations in the fibroblast growth factor receptor 2 gene (FGFR2).[30] 97% of Apert syndrome cases have 1st or 2nd to 5th finger syndactyly (type 3 and 2). The remaining 3% have 2nd to 4th finger syndactyly (type 1).[31] Apert syndrome is found in 4.5% of all patients with craniosynostotic syndroms.[27] Newborns with Apert syndrome have coronal synostosis and the midline of the calvaria has a gaping defect, extending from the glabelar area of the posterior fontanel, metopic suture, anterior fontanel and sagittal suture area.[32]

Prenatal Diagnosis

The first prenatal diagnosis of Apert syndrome was performed using fetoscopy.[33] In the third trimester, it is suspected in case of craniosynostosis[34-36] **(Figs. 1A and B)**, which may not be present during the second trimester. The typical feature of Apert syndrome is a complete fusion of bones within the second and fourths fingers ("mitten-like syndactyly") which can de deteceted as early as in the first trimester.[37] Midfacial hypoplasia with hypertelorism has been reported.[27] Other facial anomalies are frontal bossing or prominent forehead, acrocephaly (high cranial vault) and depressed nasal bridge **(Figs. 1A and B)**. In the

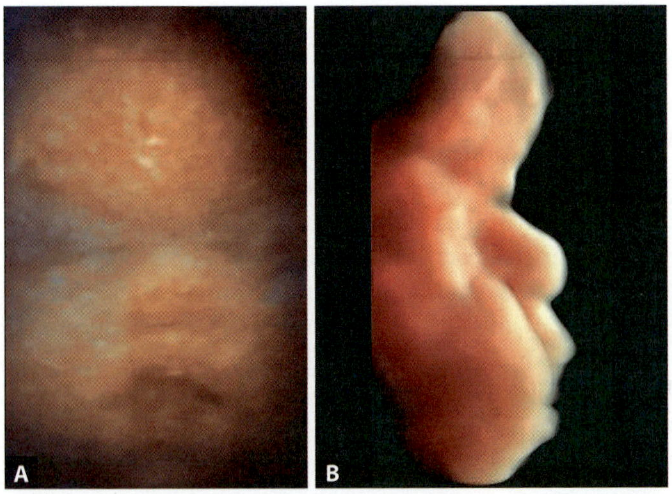

Figs. 1A and B: Apert syndrome at 37 weeks of gestation: (A) Transparency mode, showing complete craniosynostosis of the metopic suture; (B) Surface view of the head from right side, demonstrating frontal bossing and depressed nasal bridge.

three cases reported in the literature, Apert syndrome was associated with increased nuchal translucency.[27,38,39]

Additional sonographic malformations include brain anomalies, such as ventriculomegaly, hydrocephalus, partial or absence of septum pellucidum and pathological corpus callosum.[40,41]

Differential diagnosis include other pathologies with craniosynostosis, but not mitten hands:[42,43]

- Carpenter syndrome (cloverleaf skull deformity),
- Crouzon disease with cranial dysostosis,
- Pfeiffer syndrome,
- Saethre-Chotzen syndrome.

Second to third toe syndactyly, which is an autosomal dominant inherited disease, should also be differentiated from mitten hand of Apert syndrome.

Genetic Counseling

Apert syndrome shows an autosomal dominant heredity. However, most cases are explained by germinal mosaicism.[44] Mutation in fibroblast growth factor receptor gene (FGFR) are associated with skeletal dysplasia.[43] Specific missense mutation involving adjacent amino acids S252W or P253R have been found in 98–99% of cases.[30] An important issue that should be discussed in prenatal counseling is the mental retardation, which is reported in half of the affected individuals.[45,46] A neonate with Apert syndrome will require multiple surgical interventions like craniofacial disjunction or shunting to reduce intracranial pressure or to correct syndactyly.[42]

HOLT–ORAM SYNDROME

Holt–Oram syndrome is an inherited autosomal dominant syndrome, reported for the first time by Mary Clayton Holt and Samuel Oram in 1960.[47] It is characterized by mild to severe congenital cardiac defects, and skeletal abnormalities of the upper limbs.[47,48] There are more than 300 cases reported in the literature, with an estimated prevalence of 1:100,000 of affected live births.[48,49]

Mutations of the T-box genes on the chromosome 12q2 give an embryonic basis for cardiac and skeletal phenotypic appearance.[49,50] Most common heart defects include secundum type atrial septal defect and ventricular septal defect.[48] Skeletal malformations affect the upper limbs in the preaxial radial ray.[49,50] Malformations of the thumb may range from absence to triphalangeal, hypoplastic or completely absent.[49,50]

Prenatal Diagnosis

Prenatal diagnosis of Holt–Oram syndrome is based on congenital heart defects and the upper limb malformations. It was first reported in 1985.[51] In the first trimester, it can be suspected due to the association of heart defects with increased nuchal translucency.[52] Congenital heart defects include atrial septal[53] or ventricular septal defects.[51]

Differential diagnosis includes:[52]

- Fanconi anemia with anomalies of thumbs, forearm and heart with pancytopenia.
- Thrombocytopenia absent radius is characterized by bilateral absent radius, but the thumbs present and thrombocytopenia. Cardiac pathologies are present in up to 33% of the cases.
- Heart-hand syndrome II which includes shortening of the thumb with or without shortening of the fourth and the fifth metacarpals, mild facial dysmorphism and mental retardation.
- Nager syndrome
- Roberts syndrome
- Trisomy 18 (Edward's syndrome).

3D dimensional ultrasound is helpful in the demonstration of the upper limb malformations **(Figs. 2A and B)**.

Genetic Counseling

As an inherited autosomal dominant syndrome, Holt–Oram syndrome has a 50% recurrence rate. Both parents should be evaluated with X-ray examination of the upper

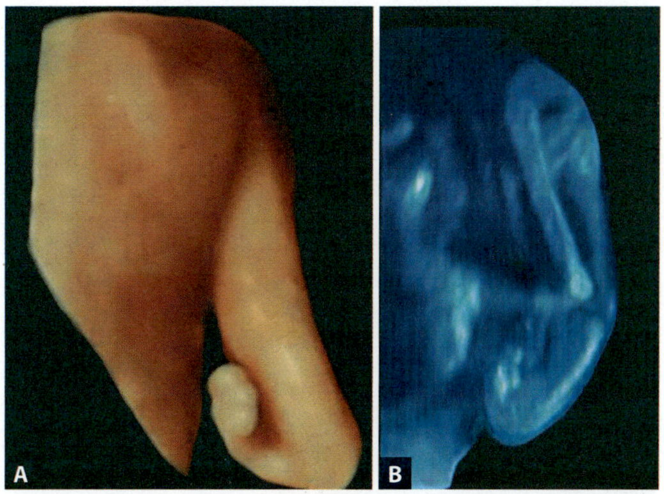

Figs. 2A and B: Holt–Oram syndrome at 23 weeks of gestation: (A) HDlive surface view of the right arm with axis deviation of the hand with only 3 fingers (absent thumb); (B) Translucency mode with demonstration of radius aplasia.

extremities and detailed anatomical evaluation of the heart. Cases of de novo mutations are reported in 30–40% of cases.[54]

WALKER–WARBURG SYNDROME

This lethal autosomal recessive disorder was first reported by Walker in 1942[55] and reviewed by Warburg in 1971.[56] It is characterized by retinal detachment, cataract, microophthalmia, congenital muscular dystrophy and lissencephaly. Brain malformations occur as a result of a failure of neural migration.[57] Hypotonia and muscule weakness are present from birth, which makes feeding difficult. There are also respiratory difficulties. A mutation in gene encoding protein O-mannasyltransferase 1 (POMT1) on chromosome 9q34 is reported.[58]

Prenatal Diagnosis

In prenatal literature it was first reported by Crowe in 1985.[59] A wide variety of brain and facial malformations are reported, including microopthalmia, congenital glaucoma, cataract, optic nerve hypoplasia, persistent hyaloid artery, cleft lip and palate, hydrocephalus, cephalocele **(Figs. 3A and B)**, microcephaly, lissencephaly **(Fig. 4)** and agenesis of the corpus callosum.[60] 3D fetal ophthalmology may be helpful in this diagnosis.

Differential diagnosis includes in utero infections, such as toxoplasmosis, rubella, cytomegalovirus, herpes and other syndromes[61] such as:

- Fryns syndrome.
- Meckel–Gruber syndrome.
- Miller–Diecker syndrome.
- Neu–Laxova syndrome.
- Trisomy 13 and 18.
- Prader–Willi syndrome.

Genetic Counseling

Since it is an autosomal recessive disorder, the risk of recurrence is 25%, if one family had one affected child. Management is supportive and preventive. It is in general a lethal condition, with almost all children dying by the age of three.

VAN DER WOUDE SYNDROME

Van der Woude syndrome is inherited in an autosomal dominant manner and has a high penetrance rate with inter- and intrafamilial variation of the associated phenotype. The prevalence of this syndrome varies from 1:100,000 to 1:40,000 stillborns or live births.[62-66] A significant difference between sexes is not reported.[62,64,67-69]

Van der Woude described for the first time the mode of heredity and introduces the typical clinical entity combining lower lip pits with cleft lip.[70] It is the most frequent form of syndrome clefting, accounting for 2% of all cleft lip and palate cases.[71] Congenital lip pits are developmental defects that occur on the paramedian portion of the vermilion border of the lower lip.[72] According to their location three different types can be recognized: commissural, midline upper lip and lower lip.[73]

A cardinal associated feature is hypodontia.[65,69,74] Other associated malformations include syndactyly of the

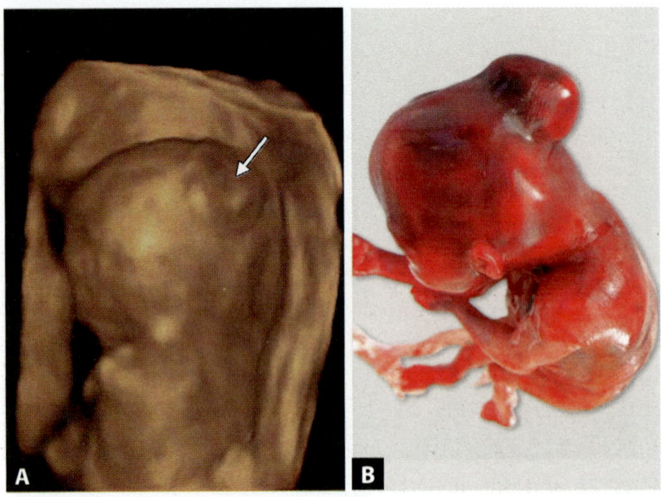

Figs. 3A and B: Walker–Warburg syndrome at 18 weeks of gestation; (A) Surface view of an encephalocele (arrow); (B) Specimen after abortion.

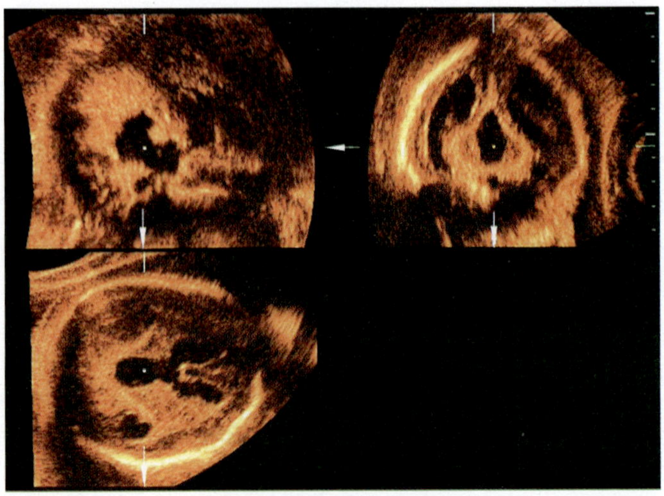

Fig. 4: Walker–Warburg syndrome with lissencephaly at 36 weeks of gestation. The multiplanar mode demonstrates missing gyration of the brain.

hands, polythelia, ankyloglossia and symblepharon,[62,67,75] club foot[76] thumb hypoplasia[77] and congenital heart disease.[78]

Prenatal Diagnosis

Prenatal diagnosis of a cleft lip in the van der Woude syndrome is reported as early as 11 weeks of gestation by embryoscpoy.[79] Cleft lip and palate can be diagnosed by sonography early in the second trimester,[80] but the lower pit lips are difficult to detect during the ultrasound examination.

Differential diagnosis should be performed with:

- Commissural and upper lip pits.[81-84]
- Clefts with no pits, due to variable expressivity of Van der Woude syndrome.
- Popliteal pterygium syndrome which includes the popliteal web, cleft lip and palate, lower lip pits,[85] anomalies of the genitourinary system such as cryptorchidism and bifid scrotum in males and hypoplastic labia majora and uterus in females.[86-89]
- Hirschsprung's disease.[90]
- Orofacial-digital syndrome type 1, an X-linked dominant trait, lethal in males with striking orodental facial, digital, renal and central nervous system abnormalities.

Genetic Counseling

A full family history is recommended before genetic counseling. The disorder results from mutation in gene encoding interferon regulatory factor 6 (IRF6).[91] The affected person is capable of transmitting the malformation to approximately one half of his or her offsprings. There is a significant association between the types of cleft in parent and their children.[62] A severely affected parent appears to have more severely affected offsprings than the mildly affected parents.[67,70]

GOLDENHAR SYNDROME

Goldenhar syndrome also known as hemifacial microsomia is a rare hereditary malformation associated with vertebral, cardiac, renal, central nervous system and gastrointestinal malformations.[92,93] The reported prevalence of Goldenhar ranges from 1:3500 to 1: 5600 births,[92,93] with a male/female ratio of 3:2.[92,94,95] Malformations are unilateral in 85% of cases and bilateral in 10–33% of cases.[95] The etiology of Goldenhar syndrome is not well established.[95,97] Most of cases are sporadic.[92,96-98] In the pathogenesis of the syndrome an autosomal dominant and or sporadic mode of inheritance have been suggested.[92,97] as well as drugs, such as cocaine, thalidomide, retinoic acid, tamoxifene, or maternal diabetes[98,99] and infections, such as rubella and influenza.[100] There may also be fetal hemorrhage in the region of first and second arches at the time of blood supply switches from stapedial artery to external carotid artery.[101]

The disorder was first described by the German-Austrian ophthalmologist Carl Ferdinand von Arlt in 1845 (cit. by Kulkarni).[92] Later on, it became known as Goldenhar–Gorlin syndrome due to the scientist who characterized the syndrome by epibulbar limbal dermoids, periauricular appendage, ear and vertebral malformation.[98]

Facial asymmetry in patients with Goldenhar syndrome results from incomplete development of molar bones, jaws and temporomandibular joint,[102,103] frequently on the right side[94] and in association with hypoplasia of facial muscle.[94]

Vertebral anomalies occur more commonly in cervical spine and include supernumerary vertebrae, hemivertebrae and fused vertebrae.[102,103] Due to absence of genetic analyses and other diagnostic methods, the diagnosis of Goldenhar syndrome is based on clinical and radiologic features.

Prenatal Diagnosis

Sonographic diagnoses have been reported in the second and third trimesters.[40,104-106]

Ear malformation in presence of preauricular tags with unilateral cleft lip or palate should be signs for Goldenhar syndrome **(Figs. 5A and B)**. Other sonographic

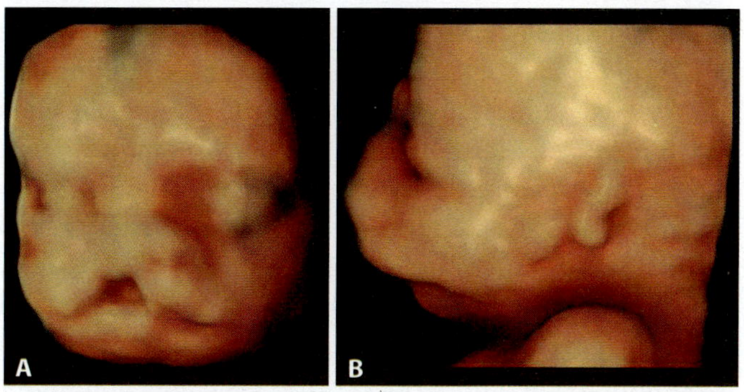

Figs. 5A and B: Goldenhar syndrome at 21 weeks of gestation: (A) Frontal surface view of the fetal face with cleft lip/palate and defect of the right eye lid; (B) Side view of the head with demonstration of a deformed auricle and preauricular tag.

findings include facial asymmetry, unilateral orbital anomalies, retrognathia, lipoma of the corpus callosum, hemivertebrae.[40,104-106]

For differential diagnosis of Goldenhar syndrome should be considered:

- Treacher-Collin syndrome with extreme external ear malformation and an antimongoloid slant of eyes with absence of zygoma in radiograph (autosomal dominant inheritance).
- Hellerman-Streiff syndrome characterized by stunted growth, facial appearance with beaked nose, small mouth, microophthalmia.
- Dellman syndrome includes orbital cyst or microophtalmia, focal skin defects and central nerous system cyst and hydrocephalus.[107]
- Nager syndrome including radial limb defect, hypoplastic thumbs.
- Townes-Brocks syndrome including lop ears, imperforate anus, hypoplastic kidneys, ventricular septal defects, limb anomalies (autosomal dominant inheritance).

Genetic Counseling

The condition occurs sporadically, although a first degree relative's recurrence risk of 2% is estimated.[108] Treatment requires a multidisciplinary approach.

DE GROUCHY SYNDROME

This syndrome was first reported in 1963 by the French geneticist Jean de Grouchy.[109,110] Actually there are more than 150 cases in the literature. The incidence of this syndrome is 1:50,000 live born infants, with a female to male ratio of 3 to 2. Phenotypes of the syndrome vary greatly.[111,112] Deletion of 18p syndrome is due to the absence of all part of the short arm of one chromosome 18. Prenatal karyotypes must be studied to determine if there is a balanced translocation carrier or has the unbalanced 18p-deletion.[113] The main malformation is holoprosencephaly developing an abnormal forebrain and mid face with a large phenotypic spectrum.[114] Facial malformations include severe ones such as cyclopia, cebocephaly, premaxillary agenesis. Bilateral cleft lip and palate are present in 10-15% of cases. Milder forms include hypopituitarism,[115] abnormal corpus callosum, and minor facial features.[40] Cardiac malformations with situs anomaly are also reported.[116] Other malformations are congenital alopecia, mental retardation and dystonia.

Prenatal Diagnosis

De Grouchy syndrome can be detected prenatally by amniocentesis or chorionic villus sampling. This is recommended when one of the parents is heterozygous for a balanced rearrangement involving 18p or carrier of a 18p deletion. Ultrasound findings, such as holoprosencephaly,[114] ventriculomegaly, microophtalmia, brain midline malformation (absent cavum septi pellucidi, corpus callosum hypoplasia) should be followed by fetal karyotyping as a consequence **(Figs. 6A to E)**.[40,117]

Differential diagnosis includes Turner syndrome and trisomy 21.

Genetic Counseling

The recurrence risk is significant if a rearrangement, such as balanced translocation is present in one parent. If one of the parents is carrier of a 18p deletion, the risk of recurrence for siblings may be as high as 50%.[113]

Prognosis

In cases with severe brain malformations the prognosis is poor. In absence of a severe malformation developmental delay is the main concern. Early rehabilitative and educational interventions are recommended, mainly speech therapy and physical therapy for hypotonia.[118,119]

AMNIOTIC BAND SYNDROME

It was first described in 1832 by Montgomery.[120] This congenital pattern of malformation includes annular constriction of multiple extremities, oligodactyly, acrosyndactyly, talipes equinovarus, cleft lip and palate and hemangiomas. The prevalence of amniotic band syndrome ranges from 1:1,200 to 1:15,000 births.[121,122] Various theories (intrinsic, extrinsic, vascular and others) are proposed to explain extremity and central abnormalities, with no firm conclusion.[123]

Amniotic band syndrome is associated with three general types of anomalies: disruptions, deformations and malformations. Disruptions are the breakdowns of the normal tissue which will not have the same exact feature and will not occur consistently.[124] Typical features are constriction bands, amputations and acrosyndactyly. Deformations occur from abnormal forces, for examples, oligohydramnios which is associated with a resultant direct pressure and decreased fetal movement. Typical features are talipes equinovarus, scoliosis and various joint contractures.[124,125] Malformations result from any

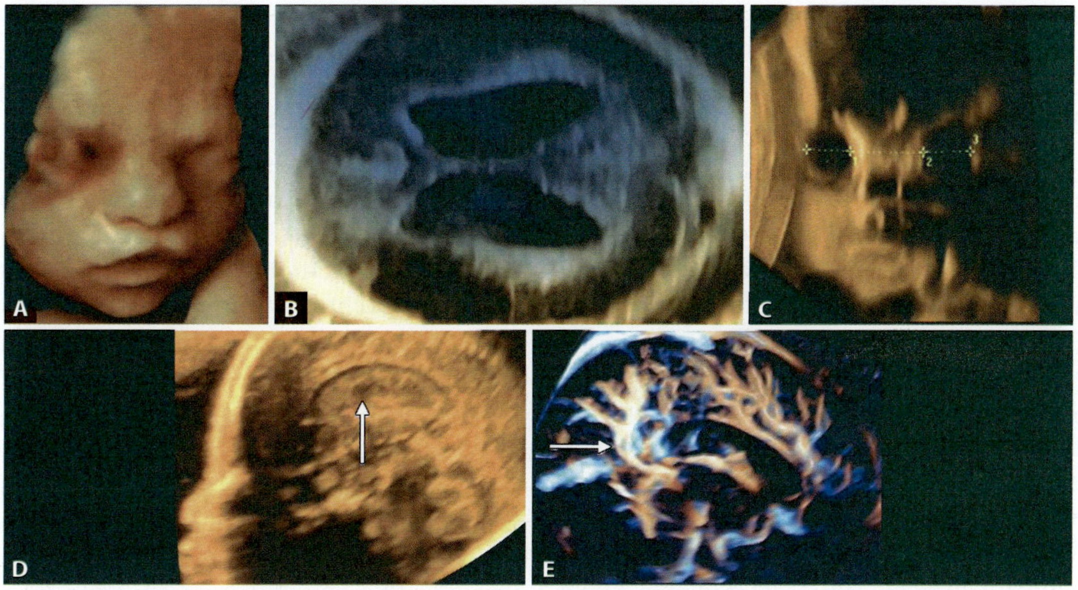

Figs. 6A to E: De Grouchy syndrome with craniofacial and brain malformations at 24 weeks of gestation: (A) Subtle cleft lip; (B) dilatation of the lateral brain ventricles, (C) microophthalmia on the right side, (D) hypoplastic corpus callosum and absence of cavum septi pellucidi (arrow), (E) 3D sonoangiogram of the fetal cerebral arteries. The pericallosal artery (arrow) branches of the anterior cerebral artery, the callosomarginal artery is absent. The posterior part of the corpus callosum is not perfused by the pericallosal artery but by the posterior cerebral artery.

insult early in gestation or an abnormal development of an organ, such as body-wall defects, internal organ abnormalities and craniofacial abnormalities.[126-128]

Prenatal Diagnosis

Sonographers should be familiar with malformations that suggest amniotic band syndrome at prenatal diagnosis. 77% of the cases occur as multiple anomalies.[129] Asymmetric malformations, oligohydramnios and reduction of fetal movements are the typical features of this syndrome. The most important ultrasound diagnostic criteria are visible amniotic bands, constrictions rings on extremities[130] and irregular amputations of fingers and/or toes with terminal syndactyly. Cranial involvement includes encephalocele or anencephaly. Truncal deformities include abdominal wall defects with exteriorization of the heart, liver and bowel. Spinal malformation includes kyphosis, lordosis, scoliosis and marked angulation deformities. Extremities with asymmetrical amputations involve one or more digits or portions of extremities.[131]

Other malformations should be differentiated from the hole spectrum of symmetric fusion defects of middle body line,[132] including amniotic fold, body-stalk anomaly, short umbilical cord syndrome and extra-amniotic pregnancy.[133]

Genetic Counseling

Exclusion of chromosomal pathologies in amniotic band syndrome is important. The recurrence risk is low.[132] Rare sporadic familial cases have been reported in association with epidermolysis bullosum and Ehlers-Danlos syndrome.[130,133-135] Therapy is mostly surgical and multidisciplinary.

NAGER SYNDROME

Nager syndrome is a rare disorder resulting from developmental abnormalities of the first and the second branchial arches.[136,137] It was first described by Nager and de Reyneier.[138] The first arches produce the nerves and muscles for chewing, the lower jaw, two of the three bones in the middle ear and small parts of the ear.[139] Facial defects include downward slanting palpebral fissure, molar hypoplasia, a high nasal bridge, micrognathia and external ear defect with low set ears. The predominant oral findings include cleft palate and an absent soft palate.[140] Typical limb anomalies include preaxial anomalies such as hypoplastic and absent thumbs and radii and proximal radioulnar synostosis.[141] Skeletal anomalies include thoracolumbar scoliosis and cervical vertebra and rib anomalies. A prenatal diagnosis is based in severe micrognathia, abnormal external ear, isolated upper limb reduction defects and polyhydramnios.[142]

Prenatal Diagnosis

For prenatal diagnosis micrognathia and polydydramnios are important signs. Amniocentesis is important to rule out the presence of a chromosomal abnormality. The differential diagnosis is based on the exact sites of limb involvement and presence of facial malformation and includes:[140]

- Treacher–Collins syndrome which have more severe forms of hypoplastic zygoma, downslanting palpebral fissures and hypoplastic maxilla[143]
- Miller syndrome.
- Pierre-Robin syndrome.
- Genée-Wiedemann syndrome is characterized by postaxial limb involvement with defects of ulna, fibula and cup shaped auricles.
- Fontaine syndrome has some features in common with Nager syndrome such as cleft lip and micrognathia, but hand and feet anomalies are different and consist of ectrodactyly and cleft hands and feet.
- Franceschetti-Zwahlen-Klein syndrome.
- Holt-Oram syndrome.
- VATER syndrome.
- TAR syndrome.
- Fanconi syndrome.

Genetic Counseling

In some families the disorder is inherited as a pleiotropic autosomal dominant condition with markedly variable penetrance and expressivity.[144-148] When unaffected parents have more than one affected child, it can have an autosomal recessive inheritance.[143,149,150] Approximately 20% of affected subjects were stillborn or died in the neonatal period due to respiratory distress as a result of mandibular hypoplasia and palate anomalies. Early audiological evaluation and speech therapy are recommended.[151]

TREACHER-COLLINS SYNDROME

Treacher-Collins syndrome is a rare hereditary disorder characterized by symmetrical bilateral malformations that include hypoplasia of the mandibular-zygomatic complex, palpebral fissure, coloboma of the lower eyelid and absence of medial eyelashes at the defect, malformation of the middle and external ears and conductive hearing loss.[152] The syndrome affects approximately 1:50,000 live births, resulting from a disruption of the developing first and second branchial arches.[152]

Genetic Counseling

Its transmission occurs in 40% of cases in a dominant autosomal transmission. The remaining 60% of cases arise as a result of a de novo mutation.[153] The gene which carries the genetic alteration has been mapped in the distal portion of the chromosome 5 long arm (5q31.3–q33.3).[154]

Prenatal Diagnosis

Prenatal diagnosis of Treacher–Collins syndrome using 2D and 3D ultrasound has been reported.[155-161] This syndrome may be suspected from 2D sonography by the presence of polyhydramnion, micrognathia, palpebral clefts and low set ears **(Figs. 7A and B)**. Recently, the quality of ultrasound imaging is improved markedly, allowing not only the demonstration of complex organs, such as ears, but also the auricular biometry.[162,163] An important feature in the diagnoses of this syndrome are the antimongoloid slanted palpebral fissures.[156]

The differential diagnoses include:

- Goldenhar syndrome, which is familial, almost unilateral, involving notching of the upper rather than the lower lid and epibulbar dermoids.[158]
- Nager syndrome in which mandibulofascial dysostosis occurs with preaxial reduction defects of the upper limbs, especially radial defects.
- Pierre–Robin sequence is characterized by early mandibular hypoplasia as a primary anomaly and associated anomalies are limited to this area.[155]
- Oro-mandibular-auricular syndrome.

Genetic Counseling

The gene penetrance of Treacher–Collins syndrome is high, but the severity of the malformations varies very widely within and between families.[164] In a family with a Treacher–Collins syndrome a first trimester invasive procedure for karyotyping is recommended. The parents have to be informed about the respiratory difficulties in the first months complicated with infection. The treatment of this syndrome is multidisciplinary.

TRISOMY 21 (DOWN SYNDROME)

Down syndrome is the most common genetic cause and condition in newborns.[165,166] The incidence of this

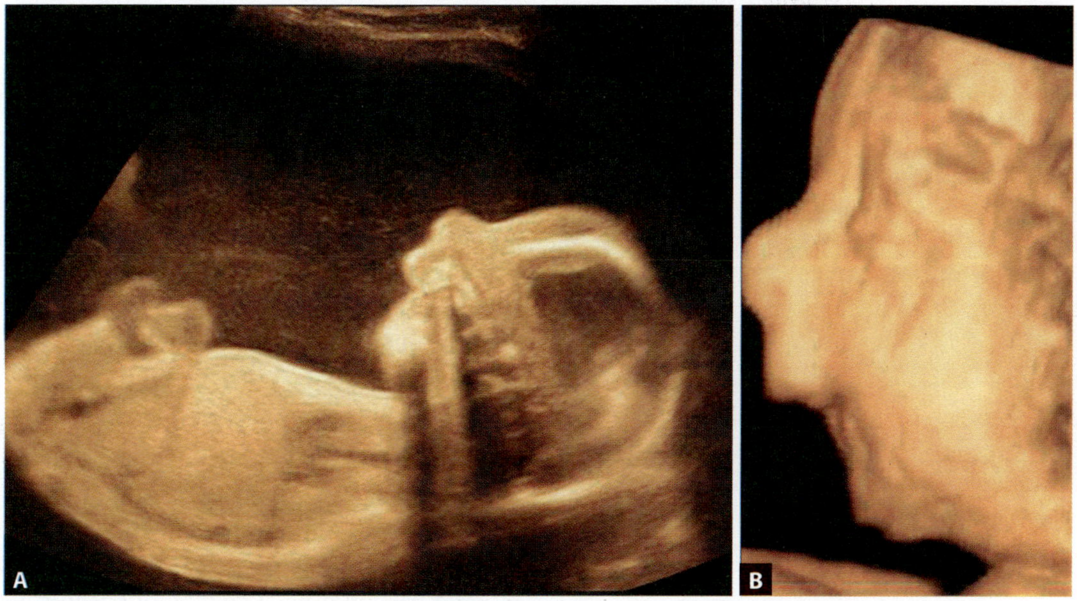

Figs. 7A and B: Treacher–Collins syndrome at 21 weeks of gestation: (A) Polyhydramnios, fetus with absent nasal bone; (B) Side view of the rendered face with marked micrognathia.

syndrome is 1 in 691 live births.[167] It was first described clinically by J Langdon Down in 1866.[168] The genetic basis was published by Lejeune in 1959.[169] Genetically, there are three copies of either the whole or a segment of a long arm of chromosome 21, which can occur as a result of three separate mechanisms: nondysjunction, Robertsonian translocation and mosaicism.[170-172] Clinical signs include intellectual disability, short stature, facial dysmorphism, cardiac, digestive, thyroid malformations and hearing impairment.[173,174] A high rate of miscarriage as high as 30% is reported.[175]

Prenatal Diagnosis

In prenatal diagnosis, there are a number of prenatal screening options available, but the final diagnosis requires an invasive procedure such as chorionic villi sampling, amniocentesis or umbilical blood sampling to evaluate the fetal karyotype.

First-trimester combined screening for trisomy 21 by a combination of maternal age, fetal nuchal translucency (NT) **(Fig. 8)** and maternal serum free β-hCG and PAPP-A[176-178] allows a detection rate for trisomy of about 90% for a false positive rate of 5%.[177] In a recent first trimester screening study the false-positive rate could be decreased until 3.42% with a detection rate for trisomy 21 of 86.8% without additional markers.[178] Using additional sonographic markers, such as nasal bone, ductus venosus and tricuspid regurgitation the detection rate of trisomy is even higher.

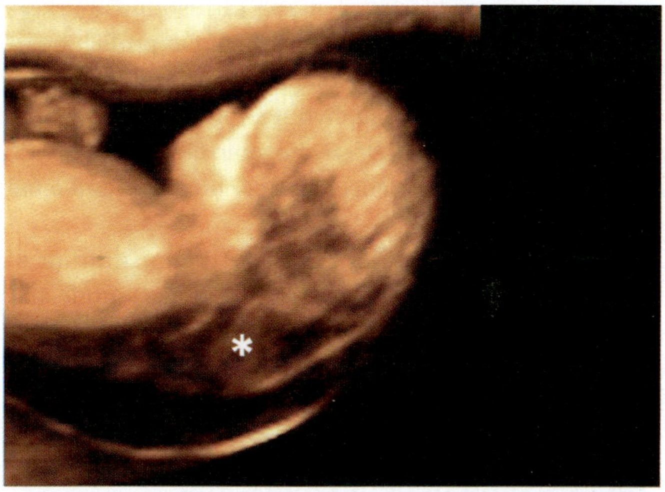

Fig. 8: Surface view of a fetus with trisomy 21 at 11+6 weeks of gestation with increased nuchal translucency (*).

Another screening test for Down syndrome is the integrated test, which combines maternal age, NT and maternal serum of PAAP-A at 11–14 weeks as well as maternal serum alpha-fetoprotein, human chorionic gonadotropin and unconjugated estriol at 15–22 weeks of gestation.[179]

The presence of the cell free fetal DNA in maternal plasma and the development of new counting technologies[180-182] have enabled successfully to detect

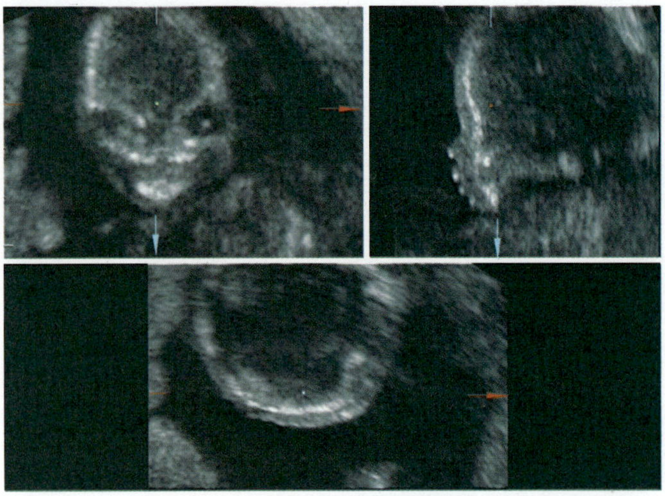

Fig. 9: Multiplanar view of a fetus with trisomy 21 at 17 weeks of gestation. The precise demonstration of the median plane reveals flat profile and absent nasal bone.

noninvasively fetal Down syndrome in the first trimester with a detection rate of 99.5% of the cases.

In the second trimester, many ultrasound markers can be used to detect Down syndrome: flat profile, heart defects (atrioventricular canal and ventricular septal defects), duodenal atresia, hydrops, nuchal thickening, nasal bone hypoplasia, hyperechogenic bowel, echogenic intracardiac focus, shortened femur or humerus and renal pyeloectasis.[183-193]

3D ultrasound enables a precise demonstration of the fetal face in the multiplanar mode, surface mode and transparency mode.[194,195] This enables the demonstration of a flat profile and absent or hypoplastic nasal bone **(Fig. 9)**.

Prognosis and Genetic Counseling

Recent development on ultrasound equipment and sequencing of free fetal DNA from maternal blood are enhancing the prenatal diagnosis. Genetic counseling of the future parents includes information to the various etiologies of Down syndrome and the associated recurrence risk. Down individuals will have a wide range of intellectual disability from mild to moderate and benefit from early intervention including physical, occupational and speech therapy. An 80% of them will have hypotonia. Malformations that will require surgery are heart defects in 40–60% of newborns and gastrointestinal defects in 12% of the babies. Life expectancy extends into the 50s to 60s.[196]

TRISOMY 13 (PATAU SYNDROME)

Trisomy 13, the third most common autosomal trisomy among live births, with an incidence of 1:5,000, was first described by Patau in 1960.[197,198] It is characterized by a number of malformations including brain, face, heart and limbs.[199-201] Whereas autosomic trisomy 13 results from an additional copy of chromosome 13, other forms of mosaicism are also implicated in the etiology.[202]

Prenatal Diagnosis

Prenatal diagnosis can be performed in the first and second trimester. First trimester screening includes the combination of ultrasound markers like increased NT and decreased levels in maternal serum of free ß-human hCG and PAPP-A.[203] Although trisomy 13 is included in all first trimester screenings, the accurate diagnosis is performed by fetal karyotyping. The 90% of trisomy 13 cases result from the free-standing chromosome 13, 10% of them result from unbalanced translocation. This raises the importance of prenatal diagnosis and genetic counseling.[200] Ultrasound markers of trisomy 13 overlap the sonographic appearance of other fetal syndromes.

Sonographic findings include brain malformations, such as holoprosencephaly, ventriculomegaly, abnormal posterior fossa, agenesis of corpus callosum.[200,201,204] Facial anomalies include hypotelorism, cyclopia, midline clefts, microopthalmia and absence of nose[205] **(Fig. 10)**. Congenital heart defects include atrial septal defect, ventricular septal defect, single ventricle, tetralogy of Fallot.[201] Among limb anomalies polydactyly and abnormal limb position can be found.[201,206] Diagnosis of renal malformation, such as large echogenic kidneys raise importance in differential diagnosis from Meckel-Gruber syndrome.[207] Other sonographic markers include polyhydramnios, intrauterine growth restriction, echogenic bowel and echogenic intracardiac focus.[200,201,206,207] Placental malformation like partial mole has also been reported.[208]

For differential diagnosis Smith Lemli-Opitz syndrome and trisomy 18 have to be taken into account.

Genetic Counseling

Fetuses with trisomy 13 have a poor outcome with often intrauterine death and survive only a few months after birth.[209] Individuals with mosaic trisomy 13 may present a range of clinical findings from mental retardation, multiple congenital anomalies to longer survivor.[210] This finding

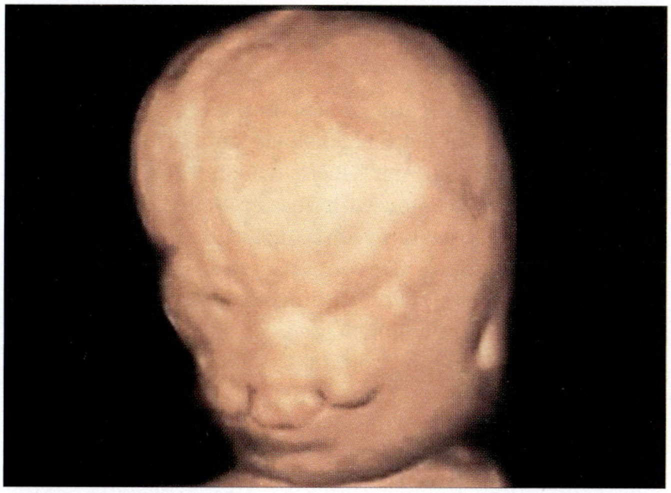

Fig. 10: Surface view of a fetus with trisomy 13 at 13+4 weeks of gestation with bilateral cleft lip and palate.

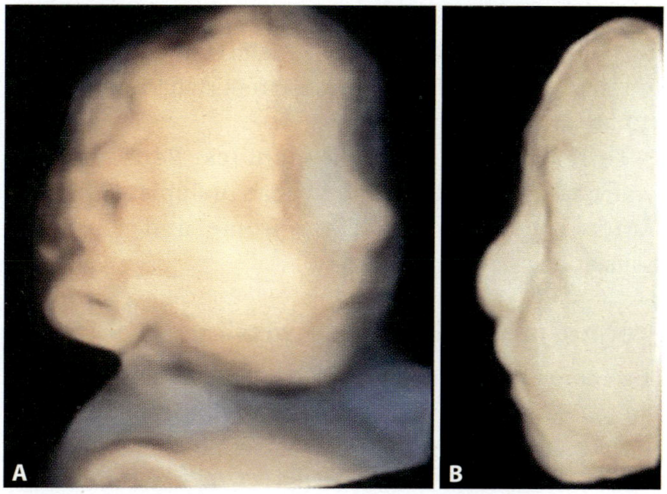

Figs. 11A and B: Surface views of two fetuses with trisomy 18. (A) Side view with demonstration of a low set ear (23 weeks of gestation); (B) Side view of a flat profile at 32 weeks of gestation.

makes the genetic counseling prenatally difficult, due to the isolated finding at the placenta, but not at fetal site. Treatment will be offered according to the severity of the malformations. These babies show muscular hypotonia, develop scoliosis and may have visual problems. Cardiac surgery is withheld due to the high mortality rate in the first months of life.[211]

TRISOMY 18 (EDWARDS SYNDROME)

In 1960 Edwards described genetically and clinically a newborn with congenital malformation, resulting from trisomy 17–18.[212] Smith et al.[213] showed that the additional chromosome was 18. Its prevalence differs among different countries from 1:3600 to 1:8500 live births.[214-217] The clinical diagnosis of trisomy 18 remains challenging, due to the broad spectrum of malformations.[218-221] It includes mental retardation, low birth weight, polyvalvular heart disease, dysmorphic face, kidney malformations, clenched fingers with overlapping of the second over the third and of the fifth over the fourth digit.[218,220]

Prenatal Diagnosis

Prenatal screening for trisomy 18 can be performed throughout the pregnancy. An important role in the first trimester play the screening methods such as nuchal translucency and biochemical analysis which show a reduced level of maternal serum free β-hCG and PAPP-A.[222] Nowadays noninvasive testing (NIPT) from maternal blood results in a high detection rate.

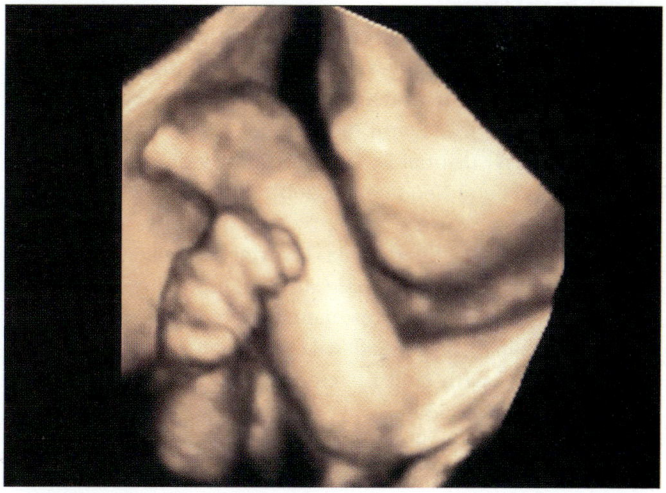

Fig. 12: Surface view of a fetus with trisomy 18 at 33 weeks, showing overlapping fingers.

In the first trimester ultrasound the most common findings are cystic hygromas and lymphangiectasia of the fetal head, neck and scalp.[223]

In the second trimester fetuses with trisomy 18 show intrauterine growth restriction, polyhydramnios, dysmorphic face **(Figs. 11A and B)** and abnormal hand position **(Fig. 12)**. Structural anomalies include abnormal cisterna magna, Dandy-Walker malformation, meningomyelocele and ventriculomegaly.[224-226] Skeletal anomalies include clenched fingers, preaxial limb reduction and pes equinovarus.[227,228] Gastrointestinal tract findings include omphalocele and diaphragmatic hernia.

Different facial anomalies can be diagnosed like cleft lip and palate, low set ears, hypertelorism. Umbilical cord cyst and single umbilical artery are also reported in association with trisomy 18.[229]

Differential diagnosis includes Pena-Shokeir syndrome, trisomy 13, arthrogryposis multiplex congenita (AMC type 1), CHARGE syndrome and VACTERL association.[230]

Prognosis and Genetic Counseling

The majority of fetuses with trisomy 18 die in utero, whereas those born alive usually die within a few days and certainly within the first year of postnatal life.[231,232] The recurrence risk is reported 0.5–1%. In cases of trisomy 18 due to translocations, analysis of the parent's chromosomes is indicated.[233]

REFERENCES

1. Moore KL, Persaud TVN. The developing Human: Clinically Oriented Embryology. WB Saunders: Philadelpia; 1998.
2. Nyhan WL. Structural abnormalities. A systemic approach to diagnosis. Clin Symp.1990;42(2):1-32.
3. Reardon W, Donnai D. Dysmorphology demystified. Arch Dis Child Fetal Neonatal Ed. 2007;92(3):F225-29.
4. Jones KL. Smith's recognizable patterns of human malformation. Philadelphia- Elsevier Inc; 2006.
5. Kummer AW. Cleft Palate and craniofacial anomalies: Effects on speech and resonance. Third edition; 2013
6. Shprintzen RJ, Siegel-Sadewitz VL, Amato J, et al. Anomalies associated with cleft lip, cleft palate or both. Am J Med Genet. 1985;29:585-95.
7. Sulik KK, Smiley SJ, Turvey TA, Speight HS, Johnston MC. Pathogenesis of cleft palate in Treacher Collins, Nager and Miller syndromes. Cleft Palate J. 1989;26:209-16.
8. Stanier P, Moore GE. Genetics of cleft lip and palate: syndromic genes contribute to the incidence of non-syndromic clefts. Hum Mol Genet. 2004;13 (spec no 1): R73-81.
9. Doray B, Badila-Timbolschi D, Schaefer E, et al. Epidemiology of orofacial clefts (1995-2006) in France (Congenital Malformations of Alsace Registry). Arch Pediatr. 2012;19:1021-9.
10. Johnson JM. Moonis G, Green GE, Carmody R, Burbank. Syndromes of the first and second brachial arches. Part 1: Embryology and characteristic defects. Am J Neuroradiol 2011;32:14-9.
11. Moore KL. The developing human clinically oriented embryology. 3rd edition, WB Saunders Co, Philadelphia; 1982.
12. Sperber GH. Craniofacial embryology. 4th edition, London: Wright; 1989.
13. Johnston MC. Embryology of the fetal head and neck. In JG. McCarthy (Ed). Plastic surgery. Philadelphia: WB. Saunders Co; 1990;4:2451-95.
14. Tessier P. Anatomical classification of the facial, craniofacial and latero-facial clefts. J Maxillofac Surg. 1976;4:69-92.
15. Martinez-Wallin L, Ana P, Rayse R, Juan Mario T. Goldenhar syndrome associated with Tessier No. 7: a case report. Ultrasound Obstet Gynecol. 2012;40:261.
16. Merz E, Eichhorn KH, von Kaisenberg C, et al. Updated quality requirements regarding secondary differentiated ultrasound examination in prenatal diagnostics (= DEGUM Level II) in the period from 18+0 to 21+6 weeks of gestation. Ultraschall Med. 2012;33:593-6
17. Doray B, Badila-Timbolschi D, Schaefer E, et al. Epidemiology of orofacial clefts (1995-2006) in France (Congenital Malformations of Alsace Registry). Arch Pediatr. 2012;19:1021-9.
18. Dochez V, Corre P, Riteau AS, Le Vaillant C. Correlation between antenatal ultrasound and postnatal diagnosis in cleft lip or palate: A retrospective study of 44 cases. Gynecol Obstet Fertil. 2015;43:767-72.
19. Wilhelm L, Braumann B. Sonographic evaluation of fetal clefts of the lip, alveolus and palate. Z Geburtsh Neonatol 2012;216:63-72.
20. Merz E. Surface reconstruction of a fetus (28+2 GW) using HDlive technology. Ultraschall in Med. 2012;33:211.
21. Merz E, Pashaj S. Prenatal detection of orofacial clefts. Ultraschall in Med. 2016.
22. Johnson D, Pretorius D, Budorick NE, Jones MC, Lou KV, Nelson TR. Fetal lip and primary palate: three-dimensional versus two-dimensional US. Radiology. 2000:217;236-9.
23. Lee W, Kirk JS, Shaheen KW, Romero R, Hodges AN, Comstock CH. Fetal cleft lip and palate detection by three-dimensional ultrasonography. Ultrasound Obstet Gynecol. 2000;16:314-20.
24. Chaoui R, Levaillant JM, Benoit B, Faro C, Wegrzyn P, Nicolaides KH. Three-dimensional sonographic description of abnormal metopic suture in second- and third-trimester fetuses. Ultrasound Obstet Gynecol. 2005;26:761-4.
25. Andresen C, Matias A, Merz E. Fetal face: the whole picture. Ultraschall in Med. 2012;33:431-440.
26. Merz E, Pashaj S. Current role of 3D/4D sonography in obstetrics and gynecology. Donald School J Ultrasound Obstetrics Gynecology. 2013;7:400-8.
27. Azevedo H, Pereira E, Anderson J, Rosmaninho A, Barbêdo C. Prenatal diagnosis of Apert syndrome without craniosynostosis-case report. Acta Obstet Ginecol. Port. 2012;6(2):79-82.
28. Ferreira JC, Carter MS, Bernstein PS, Jabs EW, Glichstein JS, Marion WR, et al. Second-trimester molecular prenatal diagnosis of sporadic Apert syndrome following suspicious ultrasound findings. Ultrasound Obstet Gynecol. 1999:14:426-30.

29. Cohen MM Jr, Kreiborg S, Lammer EJ, Cordero JF, Mastroiacovo P, Erickson JD, et al. Birth prevalence study of Apert syndrome. Am J Med Genet. 1992;42:655-9.
30. Wilkie AOM,Slaney SF, Oldridge M, Poole MD, Ashworth GJ, Hockley AD, et al. Apert syndrome results from localized mutations of FGFR2 and is allelic with Crouzon syndrome. Nature Genet. 1995;9:165-72.
31. Kim H, Uppal V, Wallach R. Apert syndrome and fetal hydrocephaly. Hum Genet. 1986;73:93-5.
32. Kreiborg S, Marsch JL, Cohen MMJr, Liversage M, Pedersen H, Skovby F, et al. Comparative three-dimensional analysis of CT scans of the calvaria and cranial base in Apert and Crouzon syndromes. J Craniomaxillofac Surg. 1993;21:181-8.
33. Leonard CO, Daikoku NH, Winn K. Prenatal fetoscopic diagnosis of the Apert syndrome. Am J Med Genet. 1982; 11:5-9.
34. Hill LM, Thomas ML, Peterson CS. The ultrasonic detection of Apert syndrome. J ultrasound Med. 1987;6:601-4.
35. Parent P,Le Gren H, Muck MR, Thoma M. Apert syndrome, an antenatal ultrasound detected case. Genet Couns. 1994;5:297-301.
36. Kaufmann K, Baldinger S, Pratt L. Ultrasound detection of Apert syndrome: a case report and review of the literature. Am J Perinatol. 1997;14:427-30.
37. Filkins K, Russo JF, Boehmer S, Camous M, Przylepa KA, Jiang W, et al. Prenatal ultrasonographic and molecular diagnosis of Apert syndrome. Prenat Diagn. 1997;17(11):1081-4.
38. Aleem S, Howarth ES. Apert syndrome associated with increased fetal nuchal translucency. Prenat Diag. 2005;25: 1066-7.
39. David AL, Turnbull C, Scott R, freeman J, Bilardo CM, vanMaarle M, et al. Diagnosis of Apert syndrome in the second trimester using 2D and 3D ultrasound. Prenat Diagn. 2007;27(7):629-32.
40. Pashaj S, Merz E. Detection of fetal corpus callosum abnormalities by mean of 3D ultrasound. Ultraschall in Med. 2015. Doi.org/10.1055/s-0041-108565. (in print).
41. Quintero_Rivera F, Robson SD, Reisse RE, Levine D, Benson C, Mulliken JB, et al. Apert syndrome: what prenatal radiographic findings should prompt its consideration? Prenat Diagn. 2006;26;10:966-72.
42. Kinsman SL, Johnston MV. Congenital Anomalies of the central nercous system. In: Nelson Textbook of Paediatrics. chapt 592. (18th Edition) Kliegman RM, Behrman RE, Jenson HB, Stanton BF. Saunders Elsevier; 2007.
43. Mulvihill JJ. Craniofacial syndromes: no such thing as a single gene disease. Nature Genet. 1995;9:101-3.
44. Allanson JE. Germinal mosaicism in Apert Syndrome. Clin Genet. 1986;29:429-33.
45. Skidmore DL, Pai AP, Poi A, et al. Prenatal diagnosis of Apert syndrome: report of two cases. Prenat Diagn. 2003; 15:23:1009-13.
46. Esser T, Rogalla P, Berg C, Kalache KD. Application of three dimensional maximum mode in prenatal diagnosis of Apert syndrome. Am J Obstet Gynecol. 2005;193:1743-5.
47. Holt M, Oram S. Familial heart disease with skeletal malformations. Br Heart J. 1960;22:236-42.
48. Bossert T, Walther T, Gummert J, Hubald R, Kostelka M, Mohr FW. Cardiac malformations associated with the Holt-Oram syndrome: report on a family and review of the literature. Thorac Cardiovasc Surg. 2002;50:312-4.
49. Basson CT, Cowley GS, Solomon SD, et al. The clinical and genetic spectrum of the Holt-Oram syndrome (heart-hand syndrome). N Engl J Med. 1994;330:885-91.
50. Basson CT, Huang T, Lin RC, et al. Different TBX5 interactions in heart and limb defined by Holt-Oram syndrome mutations. Proc Nat Acad Sci. 1999;96:2919-24.
51. Muller LM, De Jong G, Van Heerden KMM. The antenatal ultrasonographic detection ofthe Holt-Oram syndrome. S Afr Med J. 1985;68:313-5.
52. Sepulveda W, Enriquez G, Martinez JL, Mejia R. Holt-Oram Syndrome. Contribution of prenatal 3-dimensional sonography in an index case. J Ultrasound Med. 2004;23:983-97.
53. Sletten LJ, Pierpont MEM. Variation in severity of cardiac disease in Holt-Oram syndrome. Am J Med Genet. 1996;65: 128-32.
54. Huang T. Current advances in Holt-Oram syndrome. Current Opinion in Pediatrics. 2002;14:691-5.
55. Walker A. Lissencephaly. Arch Neurol Psychiatry. 1942; 48:13-29.
56. Warburg M. The heterogeneity of the microphthalmia in the mentally retarded. Birth defects. 1971;7(3):136-54.
57. Miller G, Ladda RL, Towfighi J. Cerebro-ocular dysplasia-muscular dystrophy (Walker-Warburg) syndrome. Findings in 20 week-old fetus. Acta. Neuropathol (Berl). 1991;82:234-8.
58. Beltran-Valero de Bernabe D, Currier S, Steinbrecher A, Celli J, et al. Mutations in the O. mannosyltransferase gene POMT1 give rise to the severe neuronal migration disorder Walker-Warburg syndrome. Am J Hum Genet. 2002;71:1033-43.
59. Crowe C, Jassani M, Dickerman L. The prenatal diagnosis of the Walker-Warburg syndrome. Prenat Diagn. 1986;6: 177-85.
60. Dobyns WB, Pagon RA, Armstrong D, et al. Diagnositc criteria for Walker-Warburg syndrome. Am J Med Genet. 1989;32:195-210.
61. Monteagudo A, Alayón A, Mayberry P. Walker-Warburg Syndrome. Case report and review of the literature. J Ultrasound Med. 2001;20:419-26.
62. Cervenka J, Gorlin RJ, Anderson VE. The syndrome of pits of the lower lip and cleft lip and/or palate. Genetic considerations. American Journal of Human Genetics. 1967;19:416-32.
63. Gordon H, Davis D, Friedberg S. Congenital pits of the lower lip with cleft lip and palate. South Africa Medical Journal. 1969;43:1275-9.
64. Janku P, Robinow M, Kelly T, Bralley R, Braynes A, Edgerton MT. The van der Woude syndrome in a large kindred:

variability, penetrance, genetic risks. Am J Med Genet. 1980;5:117-23.
65. Rintala AE, Ranta R. Lower lip sinuses. 1. Epidemiology microforms and transverse sulci. British Journal of Plastic Surgery. 1981;34:26-30.
66. Burdick AB. Genetic epidemiology and control of genetic expression in van der Woude syndrome. Journal of Craniofacial Genetics and Developmental Biology Supplement. 1986;2:99-105.
67. Burdick AB, Bixler D, Puckett C L. Genetic analysis in families with van der Woude syndrome. J Craniofacial Genetics and Developmental Biology Supplement. 1985;5:181-208.
68. Burdick AB, lian M, Zhuohua D, Ning G. Van der Woude syndrome in two families in China. J Craniofacial Genetics and Developmental Biology Supplement. 1987;7:413-8.
69. Schinzel A, Kläusler M. The van der Woude syndrome (dominantly inherited lip pits and clefts). J Med Genet. 1986;23:291-4.
70. Van der Woude A. Fistula labii inferioris congenital and its association with cleft lip and palate. Am J Hum Genet. 1954; 6:244-56.
71. Schutte BC, Sander A, Malik M, Murray JC. Refinement of the van der Woude gene location and construction of a 3.5-Mb YAC contig and STS map spanning the critical region in 1q32-q41. Genomics. 1996;36:507-14.
72. Arangannal P, Muthu MS, Nirmal L. Van der Woode syndrome. A case report. J Indian Soc Pedo Prev Dent Sept. 2002;20(3):102-3.
73. Nagore E, Sánchez-Motilla JM, Febrer MI, Serrano G, Bonilla J, Aliaga A. Congenital lower lip pits (Van der Woude Syndrome): presentation of 10 cases. Pediatr Dermatol. 1998;15:443-5.
74. Schneider EL. Lip pits and congenital absence of second premolars: varied expression of the lip pits syndrome. J Medical Genetics. 1973;10:346-9.
75. Neuman Z, Shulman J. Congenital sinuses of the lower lip. Oral Surge. 1961;14:1415-20.
76. Ludy JB, Shirazy E. Concerning congenital fistulae of the lips, their mooted significance; review of the literature; and report of a family with congenital fistulae of the lower lip. New Interna Clin. 1937;3:75-88.
77. Wong FK, et al. Clinical and genetic studies of van der Woude syndrome in Sweden. Acta Odontologica Scandinavica. 1999; 57:72-6.
78. Pauli RM, Hall JG. Lip pits, cleft lip and/or palate and congenital heart disease. American Journal of Diseased Child. 1980;134:293-5.
79. Dommerrques M, Lemerrer M, Couly G, Delezoide AL, Dumez Y. Prenatal diagnosis of a cleft lip at 11 menstrual weeks using embryoscopy in the van der Woude syndrome. Prenat Diagn. 1995;15:378-81.
80. Benacerraf BR, Mulliken JB. Fetal cleft lip/palate: sonographic diagnoses and postnatal outcome. Plast Reconstr Surg. 1993;92:1945-51.
81. Baker BR. Pits of the lip commissures in Caucasoid males. Oral Surgery, Oral Medicine, Oral Pathology. 1966;21:56-60.
82. Gorlin RJ, Cohen MM Jr, Levin IS. Syndromes of the head and neck. 3rd edn. Oxford University press, New York. 1990;629-31, 738-40, 745.
83. Ohishi M, Yamamoto K, Higuchi Y. Congenital dermoid fistula of the lower lip. Oral Surgery. Oral Medicine. Oral Pathology. 1991;71:203-5.
84. Neville BW, Damm DD, Allen CM, Bouquot J E. Development defect of the oral and maxillofacial region. Paramedian lip pits: Oral and maxillofacial pathology. WB Saunders, Philadelpia; 1995. pp. 4-6.
85. Audino G, Tenconi R, Clementi M, Saia OS, Cordioli GP. Popliteal pterygium syndrome presenting orofacial abnormalities. Report of a family. J Maxillofacial Surg. 1984;12:174-7.
86. Klein D, Franceschetti A. Un curieux syndrome héréditaire: chéilo-palatoschizis avec fistules de la lèvre inférieure associé à une syndyctylie, une onychodysplasie particulière, un ptérygion poplité unilateral et des pieds varus équins. Journal de génétique humaine. 1962;11:65-71.
87. Gorlin R J, Sedano H O, Cervenka J. Popliteal pterygium syndrome. A syndrome comprising cleft lip-palate, popliteal and intracranial pterygia, digital and genital anomalies. Pediatrics. 1968;41:503-9.
88. Rintala A, Lahiti A. The facio-genito-poplitea syndrome. Case report. Scandinavian Journal of Plastic and Reconstructive Surgery. 1970;4:67-71.
89. Leck GD, Aird JC. An incomplete form of the popliteal pterygium syndrome? British Dental Journal. 1984;157: 318-9.
90. Schwarz KB, Keating JP, Holtmann B, Ternberg J. Congenital lip pits and Hirschsprung`s disease. J Pediatr Surg. 1979;14:162-4.
91. Little HJ, Rorick NK, Su Li, Baldock C, Malhotra S, Jowitt T, et al. Missense mutations that cause Van der Woude syndrome and popliteal pterygium syndrome affected the DNA-binding and transcriptional activation functions of IRF 6. Human Molecular Genetics. 2009;18:535-45.
92. Kulkarni W, Shah MD, Parikh AA. Goldenhar syndrome (a case report). J Postgrad Med. 1985;31:177-9.
93. Oski FA, de Angelis CA, Feigin RD, Warshaw JB. Sindromes comuns com anomalidades morfológicas Principios e Prática de Pediatria. Rio de Janeiro: Guanabara Koogan. 1990;482.
94. Rios JA. Syndrome de Goldenhar. A propósito de um caso. An Otorrinolaringol Iber Am. 1998;25(5):491-7.
95. Kapur R, Kapur R, Sheikh S, et al. Hemifacial microsomia: a case report. J Indian Soc Pedod Prev Dent. 2008;26:34-40.
96. Reddy MVV, Redy PP, Asha RP, Hema BL. Facio-auricular vertebral syndrome: a case report. Indian J Hum Genet. 2005;11:156-8.
97. Miller TD, Metry D. Multiple accessory tragic as a clue to the diagnoses of the oculo-auriculo-vertebral (Goldenhar syndrome). J Am Acad Dermatol. 2004;50:11-3.

98. Gaukar SP. Goldenhar syndrome. A report of 3 cases. Ind J Dermatol. 2013; 58:244-8.
99. Lessick M, Vasa R, Israel J. Severe manifestations of occuloauriculovertebral spectrum in a cocaine-exposed infant. J Med Genet. 1991;28:803-4.
100. Araneta MR, Moore CA, Onley RS, Edmons LD, Karcher JA, et al. Goldenhar syndrome among infants born in military hospital to Gulf War veterans. Teratology. 1997;56:244-51.
101. Rayan CA, Finer NN, Ives E. Discordance of signs in monozygotic twins concordant for the Goldenhar anomaly. Al J Med Genet. 1986;29:755-61.
102. Martelli-Junior H, Teixeira de Miranda R, Fermandes CM, Bonan PRF, Paranaiba LMR et al. Clinical features with orofacial emphasis. J Appl Oral Sci. 2010;18:646-9.
103. Shawky RM, Zahra SS. Goldenhar syndrome with skin tags on the chest wall. Egyptian J Med Hum Genet. 2011;12: 217-20.
104. De Catte L, Laubach M, Legein J, Goossens A. Early prenatal diagnoses of occuloauriculovertebral dysplasia or Goldenhar syndrome. Ultrasound Obstet Gynecol. 1996;8:422-4.
105. Tamas DE, Mahony BS, Bowie JD, et al. Prenatal sonographic diagnoses of hemifacial microsomia (Goldenhar-Gorlin Syndrome). Am J Obstet Gynecol. 1986;5:461-3.
106. Benacerraf BR, Frigoletto FD. Prenatal ultrasonographic recognition of Goldenhar's syndrome. Am J Obstet Gynecol.1988;159:950-52.
107. Sujit Kumar GS, Haran RP, Rajsheckhar V. Dellman syndrome with Goldenhar' overlap. J Pediatr Neurosci. 2009;4:53-5.
108. Jones KL. Smith's Recognizable Patterns of Human malformation. 1988:584-7.
109. De Grouchy J, Lamy M, Thieffry S, et al. Dysmorphie complexe avec oligophrenie: deletion des bras courts dùn chromosome 17-18. CR Acad Sci. 1963;258:1028.
110. De Grouchy J. The 18p, 18q and 18 Syndromes. Birth defects. Orig Art Ser. 1969;5:74-87.
111. De Grouchy J, Turleau C. Clinical Atlas of Human Chromosomes. 2nd edition. New York. Wiley Medical; 1984.
112. Schinzel A. Catalogue of unbalanced chromosome aberrations in humans 2nd edition. Berlin. Walter de Gruyter; 2001.
113. Turleau C. Monosomy 18p. Orphanet Journal Rare Dis. 2008;3:4.
114. Cohen MM Jr. Holoprosencephaly, clinical, anatomical and molecular dimensions. Birth Defects Res A Clin Mol Teratol. 2006;76:658-73.
115. Schober E, Scheibenreiter S, Frisch H. 18p monosomy with GH-deficiency and empty sella. Good response to Gh-treatment. Cil Genet. 1995;47:254-56.
116. Digilio MC, Marino B, Giannotti A, Di Donato R, Dallapiccola B. Heterotaxy with left atrial isomerism in a patient with deletion 18p. Am J Med Genet. 2000;94:198-200.
117. Taine L, Goizet C, Wen ZQ, Chateil JF, Battin J, Saura R, Lacombe D. 18p monosomy with wide midline defects and a de novo satellite identified by FISH. Ann Genet. 1997;40: 158-63.
118. De Ravel TJ, Thiry P, Fryns JP. Follow up of adults males with chromosome 18p deletion. Eur J Med Genet. 2005;48:189-93.
119. Thompson RW, Peters JE, Smith SD. Intellectual, behavioral and linguistic characteristics of three children with 18p syndrome. J Dev Behav Pediatr. 1986;7:1-7.
120. Montgomery WF. Observations on the spontaneous amputations of the limbs of the foetus in utero, with an attempt to explain the occasional cause of its production. Dublin J Med Chem Science. 1832;1:140-4.
121. Garza A, Cordero JF, Mulinare J. Epidemiology of the early amnion rupture spectrum of defects. Am J Dis Child. 1988:142:541-4.
122. Lindenau KF, Evers G. An unusual case of bilateral and symmetric amniogenic indentations. Padiatr Grenzgeb. 1974;13:61-5. German.
123. Goldfarb CHA, Sathienkijkanchai A, Robin NH. Amniotic Constriction Band: A Multidisciplinary Assessment of Etiology and Clinical Presentation. J Bone Joint Surg Am. 2009;91(4):68-75.
124. Jones K. Smith's recognizable patterns of human malformation. 6th ed. Philadelphia: WB Saunders; 2005.
125. Gorlin RJ, Chohen MM Jr, Hennekam RCM. Syndromes of the fetal head and neck. 4th ed. New York: Oxford University Press; Amnion rupture sequence; 2001. pp.10-3.
126. Graham JM Jr, Higginbottom MC, Smith DW. Preaxial polydactyly of the foot associated with early amnion ruoture: evidence for mechanical teratogenesis? J Pediatr. 1981;98:943-5.
127. Carey JC, Greenbaum B, Hall BD. The OEIS complex (omphlocele, exstrophy, imperforate anus, spinal defects). Birth Defects Orig Artic Ser. 1987:14:253-63.
128. Jabor MA, Cronin ED. Bilateral cleft lip and palate and limb deformities: a presentation of amniotic band sequence? J Craniofac Surg. 2000;11:388-93.
129. Nyberg DA, Mahony BS, Pretorius DH. Diagnostic ultrasound of fetal anomalies. Year Book Medical Publishers, Littleton, Mass; 1990.
130. Buyse ML. Birth defects encyclopedia. Blackwell Scientific Publications. Cambridge. MA; 1990.
131. Mahony BS, Filly RA, Callen PW, et al. The amniotic band syndrome: antenatal sonographic diagnosis and potential pitfalls. Am J Obstet Gynecol. 1985:152;63-8.
132. Bower C, Norwood F, Knowles S. Amniotic band syndrome: a population besed study in two Australian states. Paediatric and Perinatal Epidemiology. 1993;7:395-403.
133. Burk CJ, Aber C, Connelly EA. Ehlers-Danlos syndrome type IV: keloidal plaques of the lower extremities, amniotic band limb deformity and new mutation. J Am Acad Dermatol. 2007:56:S53-4.
134. Marras A, Dessi C, Macciotta A. Epidermolysis bullosa and amniotic bands. Am J Med Genet. 1984:19;815.

135. Young ID, Lindenbaum RH, Thompson EM, et al. Amniotic band syndrome in connective tissue disorders. Arch Dis Child. 1985:60;1061-3.
136. Siluk KK, Smiley SJ, Turvey TA, Speight HS, Johnston MC. Pathogenesis of cleft palate in Treacher Collins; Nager and Miller syndromes. Cleft Palate J. 1989:26:209-16.
137. Vargervik K, Mandibular malformations: Growth characteristics and management in hemifacial microsomia and Nager syndrome. Acta odontol Scand. 1998;56:331-8.
138. Nager FR, de Reynier JP. Das gehororgan bei den angeborenen kopfmissbildungen. Pract Otorhinolaryngol. 1948;10:1-128.
139. Daniel K, Sie D. Cummings otolaryngology, head and neck surgery. Oxford monographs on medical genetics no.19. 3rd ed, New York: Oxford; 1990. pp 652-4.
140. Halal F, Herrmann J, Pallister PD, et al. Differential diagnosis of Nager acrofacial dysostosis syndrome: report of four patients with Nager syndrome and discussion of other related syndrome. Am J Med Genet. 1983;14:209.
141. Kawira El, Weaver DD, Bender HA. Arcofacial dysostosis with severe facial clefting and limb reduction. Am J Med Genete. 1984;17:641.
142. Benson C, Probe B, Hirsh M, Doubilet P. Sonography of Nager acrofacial dystosis syndrome in utero. J Ultrasound Med. 1988;7:163-7.
143. Burton BK, Nadler HL. Nager arcofacial dysostosis. J Pediatr. 1977;91:84-6.
144. Lowry B. The Nager syndrome (acrofacial dysostosis). Evidence for autosomal dominant inheritance. Birth Defects. 1977;13:195-202.
145. Weinbaum M, Russell L, Bixler D. Autosomal dominant transmition of Nager acrofacial dysostosis. Am J Hum Genet. 1981:33:93A.
146. Aylsworth AS, Friedman PA, Powers SK, Kahler SG. New observations with genetic implications in two syndromes: father to son transmission of the Nager acrofacial dysostosis syndrome; and prenatal consanguinity in the Proteus syndrome. Am J Med Genet. 1987;41:43A.
147. Aylsworth AS, Lin AE, Friedman PA. Nager acrofacial dysostosis: Male to male transmission in 2 families. Am J Med Genet 1991;41:83-8.
148. Bonthron DT, Macgregor DF, Barr DGD. Nager acrofacial dysostosis: minor familial manifestations supporting dominant inheritance. Clin Genet. 1993;43:127-31.
149. Pfeiffer RA, Stoess H. Acrofacial dysostosis (Nager syndrome): Synopsis and report of a new case. Am J Med Genet. 1983:15: 255-60.
150. Chemke J, mogilner MB, Ben-Litzhak I, Zurkowski L, Ophir D. Autosomal recessive inheritance of Nager acrofacial dysosotsis . J Med Genet. 1988;25:230-2.
151. McDonald TM, Jerome LG. Nager acrofacial dysostosis. J Med Genet. 1993;30:779-82.
152. Gorlin RJ, Cohen MM, Hennekam RC. Branchial arch and oral-acral disorders, in Syndromes of the fetal head and neck. Oxford University Press. Oxford. UK. 4th edition. 2001;790-849.
153. Edwards SJ, Fowlie A, Cust MP, Liu DTY, Young ID, Dixon MJ. Prenatal diagnosis in Treacher Collins syndrome using combined linkage analysis and ultrasound imaging. J Med Genet. 1996;33:603-6.
154. Arn PH, Mankinen C, Jabs EW. Mild mandibulofacial dysostosis in a child with a deletion of 3p. Am J Med Genet. 1993;46:534-6.
155. Cohen J, Ghezzi F, Gongalves L, Fuentes JD, Paulyson KJ, Sherer DM. Prenatal sonographic diagnosis of Treacher Collins syndrome: a case and a review of the literature. AM J Perinatol. 1995;12:416.9.
156. Ochi H, Matsubara K, Ito M, Kusanagi Y. Prenatal sonographic diagnoses of Treacher Collins syndrome. Obstet Gynecol. 1998;91:862.
157. Crane JP, Beaver HA. Midtrimester sonographic diagnosis of mandibular dysostosis. Am J Med General. 1986;25: 251-5.
158. Meizner I, Carmi B, Katz M. Prenatal ultrasonic diagnosis of mandibulofascial dysostosis (Treacher Collins Syndrome). J Cln Ultrasound. 1991;19:124-7.
159. Milligan DA, Duff P, Harlass FE, Kopelman JN. Recurrence of Treacher Collins syndrome with sonographic findings. Milit Med. 1994:159:250-2.
160. Hsu TY, Hsu JJ, Chang SY, Chang MS. Prenatal three-dimensional sonographic images associated with Treacher Collins Syndrome. Ultrasound Obstet. Gynecol. 2002:19;4: 413-4.
161. Tanaka Y, Miyazaki T, Kanenishi K, Tanaka H, Yanagihara T, Hata T. Antenatal three-dimensional sonographic features of Treacher Collins syndrome. Ultrasound Obstet. Gynecol. 2002;(4):414-5.
162. Merz E, Weber G, Bahlman F, Miric-Tesanic D. Application of transvaginal and abdominal three-dimensional ultrasound for the detection or exclusion of malformations of the fetal face. Ultrasound Obstet Gynecol. 1997;9:237-43.
163. Shih JC, Shyu MK, Lee CN, Wu Ch, Lin GJ, Hsieh FJ. Antenatal depiction of the fetal ear with three-dimensional ultrasonography. Obstet Gynecol. 1998;91:500-5.
164. Dixon MJ, Marres HAM, Eduards SJ, Dixon J, Cremers CWRJ. Treacher Collins Syndrome: correlation between clinical and genetic linkage studies. Clinical Dysmorphology. 1994;3(2):96-103.
165. Murphy CC, Boyle C, Schendel D, et al. Epidemiology of mental retardation in children. Ment Retard Dev Res Rev. 1998;4(1):6-13.
166. Petersen MB, Mikkelsen M. Nondisjunction in trisomy 21: origin and mechanisms. Cytogenetic Cell Genet. 2000;91 (1-4):199-203.
167. Parker SE, Mai CT, Canfield MA, Rickard R, Wang Y, Meyer RE, et al. Updated national birth prevalence estimates for selected birth defects in the United States 2004-2006. Birth

defects Research. Clinical and Molecular Teratology. 2010 (A);88;12:1008-16.
168. Down LJ. Observations on an ethnic classification of idiots. Clin Lectures and reports. London Hospital. 1866;3:259-62.
169. Lejeune J, Gautier M, Turpin R. Etude des chromosomes somatiques de neuf enfants mongoliens. Les Complet Rendus de l`Accadémie des sciences Paris. 1959;248(11):1721-2.
170. De Souza E, Halliday J, Chan A, Bower C, Morris JK. Recurrence risks for trisomy 13, 18 and 21. Am J Med Genet. 2009;149A(12):2716-22.
171. Gardner RJM, Sutherland GR. Chromosome abnormalities and genetic counseling. 2004. New York: Oxford University Press. Inc.
172. Harper PS. Practical genetic councelling. London: Edward Arnold, Ltd; 2004.
173. Cohen WC. Health care guidelines for individuals with Down syndrome: 1999 revision. Down Syndrome Quarterly. 1999;4(3):1-15.
174. Patterson B. Behavioral concerns in persons with Down syndrome. In: Cohen WI, Nadel L, Madnick ME (Eds). Down syndrome. Visions for the 21 st Centery. New York: Wiley-Liss. Inc; 2002.
175. Morris JK, Wald NJ, Watt HC. Fetal loss in Down syndrome pregnancies. Prenat Diagn. 1999;19:142-5.
176. Snijders RJM, Noble P, Sabire N, et al. UK multicentre project on assessment of risk of trisomy 21 by maternal age and fetal nuchal translucency thickness at 10–14 weeks of gestation. Lancet. 1998;351:343-6.
177. Nicolaides KH, Spencer K, Avgidou K, et al. Multicenter study of first-trimester screening for trisomy 21 in 75821 pregnancies: results and estimation of the potential impact of individual risk-orientated two-stage first-trimester screening. Ultrasound Obstet Gynecol. 2005;25(3):225-6.
178. Merz E, Thode C, Eiben B, Wellek S. Prenatal Risk Calculation (PRC) 3.0: An extended DOE- based first-trimester screening algorithm allowing for early blood sampling. Ultrasound International Open. 2016;2:1-8.
179. Wald NJ, Rodeck C, Hackshaw AK, et al. SURUSS. Research Group. First and second trimester antenatal screening for Down's syndrome: the results of the Serum, Urine and Ultrasound screening Study. Health Technol Assess. 2003; 7:1-77.
180. Avent ND, Chitty LS. Non-invasive diagnosis of fetal sex utilization of free fetal DNA in maternal plasma and ultrasound. Prenat Diagn. 2006;26:598-603.
181. Minon JM, Gerard C, Senterre JM, Schaaps JP, Foidart JM. Routine fetal RHD genotyping with maternal plasma: a four year experience in Belgium. Transfusion. 2008;48:373-81.
182. Wright CF, Burton H. The use of cell-free fetal nucleic acids in maternal blood for non-invasive prenatal diagnosis. Hum reprod update. 2009;15:139-51.
183. Benacerraf B, Gelman R, Frigoletto F. Sonographic identification of second trimester fetuses with Down's syndrome. N Engl J Med. 1987;317:1371-6.
184. Gray DL, Crane JP. Optimal nuchal skin-fold thresholds based on gestational age for prenatal detection of Down syndrome. Am J Obstet Gynecol. 1994;171:1282-6.
185. Cicero S, Sonek JD, McKenna DS, et al. Nasal bone hypoplasia in trisomy 21 at 15-22 weeks' gestation. Ultrasound Obstet Gynecol. 2003;21:15-8.
186. Muller F, DOmmergues M, Aubry MC, et al. Hyperecogenic fetal bowel: an ultrasonographic marker for adverse fetal and neonatal outcome. Am J Obstet Gynecol. 1995;173:508-13.
187. Deren O, Mahoney MJ, Copel JA, Bahado-Singh RO. Subtle ultrasonographic anomalies: do they improve the Down syndrome detection rate? Am J Obstet Gynecol. 1998;178: 441-5.
188. Bromely B, Leiberman E, Laboda L, Benacerraf BR. Ecogenic intracardiac focus: a sonographic sign for fetal Down syndrome. Obst Gynecol. 1995;86:998-1001.
189. Sepulveda W, Culen S, Nicolaides P, Hollingsworth J, Fisk NM. Echogenic foci in the fetal heart: a marker of chromosomal abnormality. Br J Obstet Gynaecol. 1995;102:490-92.
190. Vibhakar NI, Budorick NE, Scioscia Al, Harby LD, Mullen ML, Sklansky MS. Prevalence of aneuploidy with cardiac intraventricular echogenic focus in an at risk patient population. J ultrasound Med 1999;18:265-8.
191. Benacerraf BR. The role of the second trimester genetic sonogram in screening for fetal Down syndrome. Semin Perinatol. 2005;29:386-94.
192. Nyberg DA, Resta RG, Luthy DA, Hickok DE, Williams MA. Humerus and femur length shortening in the detection of Down´s syndrome. Am J Obstet Gynecol. 1993:168: 534-9.
193. Corteville JE, Dicke JM, Crane JP. Fetal pyelectasis and Down syndrome: is genetic amniocentesis warranted? Obstet Gynecol. 1992;79:770-2.
194. Merz E, Abramovicz J, Baba K, Blaas HG, Deng J, Gindes L, et al. 3D imaging of the fetal face—recommendations from the International 3D Focus Group. Ultraschall in Med. 2012;33:175-82.
195. Benoit B, Chaoui R. Three-dimensional ultrasound with maximal mode rendering: a novel technique for the diagnosis of bilateral or unilateral absence or hypoplasia of nasal bones in second-trimester screening for Down syndrome. Ultrasound Obstet Gynecol. 2005;25:19-24.
196. Sheets KB, Best RG, Brasington CK, Will MC. Balanced information about Down syndrome: what is essential? Am J Med Genet A. 2011;155A:1246-57.
197. Patau K, Smith DW, Therman E, Inhorn SL. Multiple congenital anomaly caused by an extra autosome. Lancet. 1960;1:790-3.
198. Jones KL. Smith's recognizable patterns of human malformation. Philadelphia: WB Saunders; 1997. p.30.
199. Moerman P, Fryn J, van der Steen K, Kleczkowska A, Lauweryns J. The pathology of trisomy 13 syndrome: a study of 12 cases. Hum Genet. 1988;80:349-56.

200. Papp C, Beke A, Ban Z, Szigeti Z, Toth-Pal E, Papp Z. Prenatal diagnosis of Trisomy 13. J Ultrasound Med. 2006;25:429-35.
201. Watson JW, Miller CR, Wax RJ, Hansen FW, Yamamura Y, Polzin JW. Sonographic detection of Trisomy 13 in the first and second trimester of pregnancy. J Ultrasound Med. 2007;26:1209-14.
202. Chen M, Yeh GP, Shih JC, Wang BT. Trisomy 13 mosaicism: study of serial cytogenetic changes in a case from early pregnancy to infancy. Prenat Diagn. 2004;24:137-43.
203. Brizot ML, Snijders RJM, Bersinger NA, et al. Maternal serum pregnancy-associated plasma protein A and fetal nuchal translucency thickness for the prediction of fetal trisomies in early pregnancy. Obstet Gynecol. 1994;84:918-22.
204. McGahan JP, Nyberg DA, Mack LA. Sonography of fetal features of lobar and semilobar holoprosencephaly. Am J Roentgenol. 1990;154:143-8.
205. Rijhsinghani AG, Hruban RH, Stetten G. Fetal anomalies associated with an inversion duplication 13 chromosome. Obstet Gynecol. 1988;71;991-4.
206. Benacerraf BR, Frigoletto FD Jr, Greene MF. Abnormal facial features and extremities in human trisomy syndromes. Prenatal US appearance. Radialogy. 1986;159;243-6.
207. Nyberg DA, Resta RG, Luthy DA, Hickok DE, Mahony BS, Hirsh JH. Prenatal sonographic findings of Down Syndrome: review of 94 cases. Obstet Gynecol. 1990;76:370-7.
208. Jauniaux E, Halder A, Partingon C. A case of partial mole associated with trisomy 13. Ultrasound Obstet Gynecol. 1988;11:62-4.
209. Lakocschek IC, Streubel B, Ulm B. Natural outcome of trisomy 13, trisomy 18 and triploidy after prenatal diagnosis. Am J Med Genet A. 2011;11:2626-33.
210. Delatycki MB, Pertile MD, Gardner RJ. Trisomy 13 mosaicism as prenatal diagnosis: dilemmas and interpretation. Prenat Diagn. 1998;18:45-50.
211. Batty BJ, Jorde LB, Blackburn BL. Natural history of trisomy 18 and trisomy 13 II: psychomotor development. Am J Med Genet. 1994;15:49:189-94.
212. Edwards JH, Hernden DG, Cameron AH, Crosse VM, Wolf OH. A new trisomic syndrome. Lancet. 1960;1:787-90.
213. Smith DW, Patau K, Theraman E, Inhorn SL. A new autosomal trisomy syndrome: multiple congenital anomalies caused by an extra chromosome. J Pediatr. 1960;57:338-45.
214. Carter PE, Pearn JH, Bell J, et al. Survival in trisomy 18. Life tables for use in genetic counseling and clinical paediatrics. Clin Genet. 1985;27:59-61.
215. Young ID, Cook JP, Mehta L. Changing demography of trisomy 18. Arch Dis Child. 1986;61:1035-6.
216. Goldstein H, Nielsen KG. Rates and survival of individuals with trisomy 13 and 18. Data from 10 year period in Denmark. Clin Genet. 1988;34:366-72.
217. Root S, Carey JC. Survival in trisomy 18. Am J Med Genet. 1994;49:170-4.
218. Hodes ME, Cole J, Palmer CG, et al. Clinical experience with trisomies 18 and 13. J Med Genet. 1978;15:48-60.
219. Marion RW, Chitayat D, Hutcheon RG, Neidich JA, Zackai EH, Singer LP, et al. Trisomy 18 score: a rapid, reliable diagnostic test for trisomy 18. J Pediatr. 1988;113:45-8.
220. Kinoshita M, Nakamura Y, Nakano R, Morimatsu M, Fukuda S, Nishimi, Y et al. Thirty one autopsy cases of trisomy 18: clinical features and pathological findings. Pediatr Pathol. 1989;9:445-57.
221. Zen PR, Rosa RF, Rosa RC, Dale Mulle L, Graziadio C, Pasculin GA. Unusual clinical presentations of patients with Patau and Edwards syndromes: a diagnostic challenge? Rev Paul Pediatr. 2008;26:295-9.
222. Kagan KO, Wright D, Maiz N, Pandeva I, Nicolaides KH. Screening for trisomy 18 by maternal age, fetal nuchal translucency, free beta-human chorionic gonadotropin and pregnancy-associated plasma protein-A. Ultrasound Obstet Gynecol. 2008;32:488-92.
223. Barisic LS, Kurjak A, Pooh RK, Delic T, Stanojevic M, Porovic S. Antenatal detection of fetal syndromes by ultrasound: From a single piece to a complete puzzle. Donald School J Ultrasound Obstet Gynecol. 2016;10(1)1-15.
224. Hill LM, Marchese S, Peterson C, et al. The effect of trisomy 18 on transverse cerebellar diameter. Am J Obstet Gynecol. 1991;165:72-5.
225. Nyberg DA, Mahony BS, Hegge FN, et al. Enlarged cisterna magna and the Dandy-Walker malformation. Factors associated with chromosome abnormalities. Obstet Gynecol. 1991;77:436-42.
226. Chervenak FA, Goldberg JD, Tsung-Hong C, et al. The importance of karyotype determination in fetuses with ventriculomegaly and spina bifida discovered during the third trimester. J Ultrasound Med. 1986;5:405-6.
227. Charlson D, Plat LD, Medearis AL. The ultrasound triad of fetal hydramnios, abnormal hand posturing and any other anomaly predicts autosomal trisomy. Obstet Gynecol. 1992;79:731-4.
228. Sepulveda W, Treadwell MC, Fisk NM. Prenatal detection of preaxial upper limb reduction in trisomy 18. Obstet Gynecol. 1985;85:847-50.
229. Ramirez P, Haberman S, Baxi L. Significance of prenatal diagnosis of umbilical cord cyst in a fetus with trisomy 18. Am J Obstet Gynecol. 1995;173:955-57.
230. Rosa RF, Rosa RC, Zen PR, Graziadio C, Paskulin GA. Rev Paul Pediatr. 2013;31:110-29.
231. Snijders RJM, Sebire NJ, Cuckle H, et al. Maternal age and gestational age-specific risks for chromosomal defects. Fet Diag Ther. 1995;10:356-67.
232. Embleton ND, Wyllie JP, Wright MJ, Burn J, Hunter S. Natural history of trisomy 18. Arch Dis Child. 1996;75:F38-F41.
233. Uehara S, Yaegashi N, Maeda T, Hoshi N, Fujimoto S, Fujimori K, et al. Risk of recurrence of fetal chromosomal aberrations: analysis of trisomy 21, trisomy 18, trisomy 13 and 45X in 1076 Japanese mothers. J Obstet Gynecol Res. 1999;25:373-9.

51

CHAPTER

Ultrasound Role in Perinatal Infection

Alaa Ebrashy

INTRODUCTION

Infections acquired in utero or during the birth process are a significant cause of fetal and neonatal mortality and an important contributor to early and later childhood morbidity. Advances in ultrasound, invasive prenatal procedures and molecular diagnostics have allowed in utero evaluation and given rise to more timely and accurate diagnosis in infected fetuses.

There are two situations where the obstetricians might need to know the role of ultrasound in perinatal infection:

- The first situation is that when the pregnant lady report to her doctor that either she has a rash, or she is exposed to infection by getting near to a diseased person, or she did some investigations raising the suspicion of being attracted infection during pregnancy, etc. In all these conditions the main question is: How could she know that her baby is safe? Can ultrasound give clue to this question?
- The second situation is that during a routine fetal ultrasound examination, Doctor is encountered with some fetal abnormalities that could be related or not to intrauterine infection.

In order to be ready in both situations you should:

- First know a brief knowledge about each organism that cause intrauterine infection and how could it be detected by U/S.
- Second: What are the ultrasound signs that should arouse your suspicion for intrauterine infection.

How to detect, when to detect, modalities of diagnosis, with major emphasis on ultrasound is what will be covered in this chapter:

- First we start with the general ultrasound features of perinatal infection, the role of invasive tests in their diagnosis.
- Second we shall discuss in brief each organism separately together with its ultrasound signs that could be present in case of infection.

ULTRASOUND FEATURES IN CONGENITAL INFECTION

Intrauterine infection can present with a wide spectrum of ultrasound markers and lesions depending on the type of the organism and the age of pregnancy at which the mother contracted the disease and above all the time between acquiring infection and ultrasound examination.

Characteristic ultrasound markers in a mother with a positive TORCH (Toxoplasmosis, other agents, rubella, CMV, herpes simplex) screening test have a high predictive value for congenital infection and may have prognostic significance

Among these markers we can mention early pregnancy loss, nonimmune hydrops fetalis, intrauterine growth restriction, cranial lesions, cardiothoracic lesions, gastrointestinal lesions and other lesions.

Early Pregnancy Loss

Defined as a miscarriage within the first 12 weeks of pregnancy. Infection is considered a rare cause of early pregnancy loss.[1] Among these organisms are toxoplasmosis godii, cytomegalovirus (CMV) and PVB19. ultrasound suggestive of the occurrence of early pregnancy loss include fetal bradycardia, discrepancy between the gestational age and crown lump length. Definite diagnosis depends on the demonstration of an empty sac of more than 15 mm by TVS and embryo with no pulsations documented by Doppler.[2] There is no any recent evidence suggesting that infection could be related to repeated abortion.

Nonimmune Hydrops Fetalis

Hydrops fetalis represents a specific condition characterized by an increase of total body water content. In such a condition, the excess fluid collects by ultrafiltration in body cavities (pleural, pericardial, and peritoneal effusions) and/or in the subcutaneous tissue. Placental edema and polyhydramnios are frequently associated (30–70%). By definition, the term nonimmune hydrops fetalis (NIHF) refers to fluid collections in at least two body cavities or to collection plus diffuse subcutaneous edema.

Etiology and Pathogenesis in Intrauterine Infection

Nonimmune hydrops fetalis (NIHF) is a nonspecific sign of various infections vertically transmitted from mother to fetus, including both viral and nonviral infections.

Severe hemolytic anemia or aplastic anemia that can precipitate heart failure is often the primary cause.[3]

In the case of viral infections, the etiology is probably due to different and synchronous mechanisms: inflammation, myocarditis with pump deficit as in coxsackievirus B or a major cardiac structural defect secondary to a rubella infection during the first trimester. Toxoplasmosis may cause NIHF possibly due to excessive extramedullary hematopoiesis with portal hypertension secondary to liver congestion.

PVB19 is tropic to radidly diving cells in particular the bone marrow red cell precursors causing hemolysis and aplasia of the bone marrow.[4]

The pathophysiology of NIHF in cases of cytomegalovirus CMV or *T. pallidum* is less clear and could be due to combined effect of anemia and hepatic dysfunction resulting in hypoproteinemia and portal hypertension. The viruses most frequently associated with fetal hydrops are: parvovirus B19, coxsackievirus, herpes virus (Varicella), cytomegalovirus (CMV), adenovirus, and influenza virus type B. Among the nonviral infections, the most common are syphilis, listeriosis, and toxoplasmosis.

The final result of the various conditions mentioned above is a breakdown of equilibrium between intra-capillary and extracapillary pressures, with consequent fluid ultra- filtration in the interstitial space.

Nonimmune hydrops fetalis due to fetal infection can occur any time in pregnancy but more common in 2nd and 3rd trimester. The fluid collections in the abdomen, pleura, or pericardium—appear as sonolucent areas with different shapes characteristic of the different locations. Subcutaneous edema appears as a moderately hyperechoic thickening of the soft tissue of the fetal face, trunk, and sometimes limbs. The fluid collection may be limited to one or two sites, and therefore, its diagnosis needs dedicated planes. Axial views of the head, neck and thorax may allow assessment of the extent and severity of the effusions and the subcutaneous edema. With regards to the ascites, it should be noted that, initially, the fluid collects in the pelvis only, and therefore, it should be sought in this region and not at the level of the liver.

Intrauterine Growth Restriction

It is also a nonspecific feature of most congenital infections. It is a more common in rubella, CMV and *T. pallidum*.[5] It also have some relationship with varicella-zoster, human immunodeficiency virus (HIV) and malaria. Intrauterine growth restriction (IUGR) in cases of intrauterine infection may be explained on the ground of capillary endothelial damage during organogenesis, which in turn, induces a decease in the number of cells having a cytoplasmic mass within the normal range together with a cytopathic effect. When the infection is transmitted to the fetus in the 1st trimester, the IUGR will be a manifestation of the 2nd trimester ultrasound (US) usually severe symmetrical pattern and associated with oligohydramnios in most cases hence the fetal anatomy could not be well appreciated. In any case showing symmetrical IUGR early in the 2nd trimester, infection should be always considered and TORCH test is therefore always be performed.[6]

Cranial Lesions

The most common cranial lesions secondary to fetal infection is seen by are—cerebral echogenic foci (calcifications), ventriculomegaly, microcephaly and hydranencephaly. A fetal infection should be suspected when ventriculomegaly is associated with hyperechogenic foci and periventricular cysts.

These lesions are both inflammatory (Gliosis) and destructive lesions. The most common organism that causes cerebral lesions is CMV and less commonly *T. gondii*. The ventriculomegaly that may be seen in such cases is the consequence of aqueductal obstruction. Hydranencephaly observed in cases of congenital infections such as *Toxoplasma* and cytomegalovirus can be explained on the basis of causing necrotizing vasculitis with consequent destruction of the cerebral tissue.[7]

The addition of magnetic resonance imaging (MRI) increases the positive predictive value for diagnosis of fetal brain abnormalities with CMV.[16,22]

Eye Lesions

Eye lesions seen in congenital infection include congenital cataract, micro-ophthalmia and chorioretinitis. They are observed mainly with congenital rubella and congenital toxplasmosis.[8]

Cardiothoracic Lesions

Congenital heart defects mainly as pulmonary valvular stenosis and ventricular septal defect are among the clinical features of congenital rubella syndrome. Similar defects have occasionally been observed following first trimester congenital CMV or toxoplasmosis infection. Cardiomyopathies such as endocardial fibroelastosis (interstitial myocarditis) have been linked to coxsackievirus B and to adenovirus and PVB19.[9] Major heart anomalies are usually complicated by NIHF. Pleural effusion may represent an early stage of NIHF and may be associated with a major fetal infection, usually the heart. Isolated pleural effusion is rarer and has only been observed in one case of adenovirus infection,[10] and one case of PVB19 infection.[11]

Gastrointestinal Lesions

Most congenital infections show abnormal features of the liver, spleen and bowel on ultrasound. The most common sonographically detected markers are peritoneal hyperechogenicities and or hyperechogenic bowel which have been described mainly within the context of congenital cytomegalovirus (CMV), herpes simplex virus (HSV), varicella zoster virus (VZV) and PVB19.[12] True parenchymal liver or splenic hyperechogenicities are far less common and have occasionally been related to congenital infection.[13] The pathophysiology of these echogencities is unclear. Focal lesions are probably secondary to localized ischemia or inflammatory reaction with calcification of the tissue, Diffuse bowel hyperechogenicity could be due to thickened meconium. Congenital infections due to PVB19, CMV, *T. pallidum* or toxoplasmosis may be associated with ascitis and hepatosplenomegaly. These anomalies are secondary to direct infection of the fetal liver parenchyma with secondary enlargement and progressive alteration of liver function.[14] Ascitis can be detected by ultrasound even there is less than 50 mL of intraperitoneal fluid and can be the first presenting sign of congenital infection. Small amounts of ascitis are best visualized at the edge of the liver and may be seen to gradually outline the liver. In severe cases ultrasound picture of the fetal abdomen show free floating or compressed bowel loops. Ascitis is often is early manifestation of serous fluid accumulation in fetuses who later develop full blown hydrops. *Intrauterine fetal infections* are among the most common causes of hepatomegaly. CMV infection, when severe, is commonly associated with hepatosplenomegaly. Fetal infections are also the primary cause of splenomegaly, with or without hepatomegaly. In particular, CMV infection, when severe, is typically associated with splenomegaly, as well as hepatomegaly and ascites. If the enlargement of the spleen and/or liver is severe, the diagnosis of these conditions is straightforward, the two organs occupying most of the abdomen. The recognition of hepatomegaly and splenomegaly is made even simpler if ascites, which acts as an intra-abdominal contrast medium, is associated. If hepatomegaly is very pronounced, the prominence of the liver pushes the anterior abdominal wall, causing a dip at the thoracoabdominal junction, similarly to what happens in cases of severe thoracic hypoplasia, although in this case it is the abdomen that is enlarged rather than the thorax that is hypoplastic. Nomograms of the maximum diameters of the liver and the spleen have been published. 3D ultrasound also have recently been used for estimation of liver and spleen volumes versus gestational age.[15]

Other Lesions

Placental edema and enlargement is commonly found specially in cases of NIHF as in CMV and toxoplasmosis.[15] Urogenital tract lesions have occasionally been reported in cases of CMV and toxoplasmosis. Limb defects have been rarely observed in congenital VZV.

WHAT IS THE ROLE OF INVASIVE PROCEDURES IN THE DIAGNOSIS OF INTRAUTERINE INFECTION?

There are three modalities of invasive procedures for the diagnosis of fetal infection namly amniocentesis, chorionic villus sampling cardiovascular system (CVS) and cordocentesis.

The cardiovascular system can be done after 11 weeks and have been used in particular for first trimester rubella. Its main disadvantage is early diagnosis which may be useful when there is maternal serological evidence of infection early in pregnancy, however, this method poses a theoretical risk to the fetus as it damages the placental barrier, which may result in an increased transfer of viral particles or parasites to the fetus.[17]

Cordocentesis is played a key role in the diagnosis of most common congenital infections in the 1980s and early 1990s. No fetus with a documented infection has a completely normal hematological profile.[5] White blood count total and differential, TORCH specific IgM, fetal liver enzymes measurement all can be assessed in cases of infection. However, with the development of PCR analysis on the amniotic fluid, its role in this context is fading.[5]

The only advantage of cordocentesis is in cases of PVB19 infection in which the fetal hematological profile is crucial in the management of these cases.

We left with the amniocentesis which is now the most common invasive procedure used for diagnosis of fetal infection.[17] PCR is now the preferred method for analysis of the amniotic fluid in cases of fetal infection. The development of quantitative PCR analysis has optimized the specificity of this assay, preventing the false-positive results that were seen with the earlier qualitative PCR analysis. Current studies in case of CMV are know trying to correlate viral load and degree of fetal damage.[18] An essential point to be mentioned here is the timing for amniocentesis to avoid false-negative PCR results. Delays of more than 5–6 weeks between the serological diagnosis of maternal CMV and toxoplasmosis infection and the invasive procedure are recommended to increase the sensitivity of prenatal diagnosis.[19]

PRENATAL MANAGEMENT OF SPECIFIC CONGENITAL INFECTIONS USING ULTRASOUND MARKERS AND INVASIVE PROCEDURES

Cytomegalovirus

Congenital cytomegalovirus (CMV) is the most common intrauterine infection and the leading infectious cause of sensorineural hearing loss and mental retardation. Seroconversion occurs in approximately 1% of pregnant women in UK, more than 2% in other European countries and the USA.[20]

The probability of intrauterine transmission following primary infection is 30–40%, but only 1% after secondary infection.

About 10–15% of congenitally infected infants will have symptoms at birth, and 20–30% of them will die, whereas 5–15% of the asymptomatic infected neonates will develop sequelae later.[21]

Children with congenital CMV infection following first trimester infection are more likely to have central nervous system sequelae, whereas infection acquired in the third trimester has a high rate of intrauterine transmission but a favorable outcome. Overall congenital CMV infection is asymptomatic at birth in 90% of infants infected in utero.[21] The value of quantitative determination of CMV deoxyribonucleic acid (DNA) in the amniotic fluid is not yet confirmed.

The classic triad of blood dyscrasia (petechiae and thrombocytopenia), intrauterine growth restriction (IUGR) and chorioretinitis is uncommon <10% in utero or at birth.[22,23]

Sonographic findings often imply poor prognosis, but their absence does not guarantee a normal outcome. Among the ultrasound markers for CMV infection that could be detected are cranial findings as periventricular echogenicity, ventriculomegaly, intracranial calcifications, intraventricular adhesions, thalamic hyperechogenicity mega cisterna magna, lissencephaly, vermian defect and cerebellar cyst.[22,23]

Other organ signs include, echogenic bowel, enlarged liver and spleen, focal calcification in the liver and mild ascitis, severe IUGR. Placentomegaly is noted in 32% of the time. Those cases showing cerebral manifestations and/or severe IUGR are more prone to develop neurological sequel.[22,23] The addition of MRI to ultrasound increases the positive predictive value for the diagnosis of fetal brain abnormalities in fetuses with CMV. The two techniques appear to be complementary and should not be mutually exclusive in high-risk fetuses. Their high predictive value for the presence or absence of cerebral lesions provides a useful tool for appropriate counseling since current evaluation of the prognosis is based mainly on the presence of fetal brain lesions.[16,24]

Diagnosis of primary maternal CMV infection in pregnancy should be based on de-novo appearance of virus-specific IgG in the serum of a pregnant woman who was previously seronegative, or on detection of specific IgM antibody associated with low IgG avidity. In case of primary maternal infection, parents should be informed about a 30–40% risk for intrauterine transmission and fetal infection, and a risk of 20–25% for development of sequelae postnatally if the fetus is infected. The mere detection of positive IgM and IgG is not indicative of active infection unless we obtain a rising titer within 2 weeks since the IgM could persist in the circulation for more than 18 months from last infection.[25]

The diagnosis of secondary infection should be based on a significant rise of IgG antibody titer with or without the presence of IgM and high IgG avidity. In cases of proven secondary infection, amniocentesis may be considered, but the risk-benefit ratio is different because of the low transmission rate.

Differentiating between primary or secondary infection is somewhat important for assessing the possibility of fetal infection as mentioned earlier. The CMV IgG avidity test is very useful in this domain.[26]

Serial ultrasound examinations should be performed every 2 to 4 weeks to detect sonographic abnormalities, which may aid in determining the prognosis of the fetus, although it is important to be aware that the absence of sonographic findings does not guarantee a normal outcome.[26]

The prenatal diagnosis of fetal CMV infection should be based on amniocentesis performed 7 weeks after the presumed time of infection and after 21 weeks of gestation. Intrauterine infection diagnosis could be achieved through amniocentesis and isolation of the CMV DNA by PCR with a sensitivity of 80–99% of cases.[26] Quantitative determination of CMV DNA in the amniotic fluid may assist in predicting the fetal outcome. Routine screening of pregnant women for CMV by serology testing is currently not recommended. It should be noted that it takes 5–7 weeks after fetal infection for viral replication in the fetal kidneys to be present in sufficient quantity to be secreted into amniotic fluid, also the PCR testing is unreliable prior to the 21st week of pregnancy. This means that amniocentesis for CMV detected by PCR should not be performed before the 21st week and with an elapse of at least 5 weeks from the time of maternal infection.[27]

Serologic testing for CMV may be considered for women who develop influenza-like illness during pregnancy or following detection of sonographic findings suggestive of CMV infection. Seronegative healthcare and childcare workers may be offered serologic monitoring during pregnancy. Monitoring may also be considered for seronegative pregnant women who have a young child in day care.[26]

Treatment of CMV Infection

There is currently no approved treatment for congenital infection. Ganciclovir being effective treatment for CMV, however, not safe in the first trimester.[28] Valaciclovir is showing some promise for use, however, with limited research till now.[28] Valganciclovir (V-GCV), a mono-valyl ester prodrug of GCV, is available as an oral syrup. The existing literature demonstrated that V-GCV is well absorbed from the gastrointestinal tract and is rapidly converted into GCV in the intestinal wall and liver. The mechanism of antiviral action is the same that has been described for GCV.[28] All these characteristics make this formulation particularly suitable for the symptomatic congenitally infected newborns. In neonates, V-GCV oral formulation proved stable and constant GVC plasma concentrations, in the suggested therapeutic range. Hyperimmunoglobulin appears to be an effective drug for fetal, however, also with limited data. CMV infection at birth or in the first 3 weeks of an infant's life is crucial, as this should prompt interventions for prevention of delayed-onset hearing loss and neurodevelopmental delay in affected infants. Newborns suffering from symptomatic congenital cytomegalovirus infection have been typically treated with intravenous ganciclovir (GCV).[31]

Prevention strategies should also target mothers because increased awareness and hygiene measures may reduce maternal infection. Recognition of the importance of CMV in pregnancy and in neonates is increasingly needed, particularly as therapeutic and preventive interventions expand for this serious problem.[29-31]

TOXOPLASMA

Mode of infection: It is caused by the protozoon, *Toxoplasma gondii*. The definitive host is the cat and the intermediate hosts include humans, numerous mammals and birds which acquire the infection from the oocysts contained in cat feces and thus seronegatives are urged to avoid contact with cats, wash fruits and vegetables thoroughly and avoid raw meat.[32]

Transmission: The rate of mother to fetus transmission depends on the gestational age and the time of the initial infection. It is around 15%, 30%, 60–70%, in the 1st, 2nd and 3rd trimesters respectively. However, the reverse is the situation for the severity of infection, being highest in 1st trimester and almost nil in the third trimester.[32]

Ultrasound signs: The main ultrasound signs of prenatal toxoplasmosis infection is ventriculomegaly, intracranial calcification. Chorioretinitis is among the sequelae detected postnatal. other ultrasound markers include hepatosplenomegaly, ascitis.[32]

Testing: If the serologic testing shows that the woman has contracted toxoplasmosis during pregnancy by a positive IgG and IgM with a rising titer, detecting *T. gondii* in the amniotic fluid by PCR through amniocentesis is the preferred methods for assessing fetal infection with a sensitivity >80% and specificity of 96%.[33,34]

Treatment: Spiramycin can decrease the risk of congenital toxoplasmosis by around one half. Taken as 1 g every 8 hours continued until delivery.[32] If acute infection is suspected, repeat testing should be performed within 2 to 3 weeks, and consideration given to starting therapy with spiramycin immediately, without waiting for the repeat test results.

This drug does not cross the placenta, so in the evidence of fetal infection by amniocentesis and PCR, treatment should be in favor of other drugs that are effective and also cross the placenta.[32,34,35]

If maternal infection has been confirmed but the fetus is not yet known to be infected, spiramycin should be offered for fetal prophylaxis (to prevent spread of organisms across the placenta from mother to fetus). A combination of pyrimethamine, sulfadiazine, and folinic acid should be offered as treatment for women in whom fetal infection has been confirmed or is highly suspected (usually by a positive amniotic fluid polymerase chain reaction). This include both pyrimethamine and sulfadiazine. Different regimens are used, however, in all of them folic acid is added as both of them are folic acid antagonist.

Examples are:
Pyrimethamine 50 mg/day + sulfadiazine 1 g tid + folinic acid 10–25 mg/day for 3 weeks alternating with 3 weeks of spiramycin 1 g tid. This regimen is continued until term.[32,34]

A non-pregnant woman who has been diagnosed with an acute *Toxoplasma gondii* infection should be counselled to wait 6 months before attempting to become pregnant.

Routine universal screening for toxoplasmosis is not recommended for pregnant women at low risk. Serologic screening should be offered only to pregnant women considered to be at risk for primary toxoplasmosis.[32]

Parvovirus B19 Infection

It is caused by the human parvovirus B19 which belongs to the parvoviruses group a single DNA strand.[36] The viruses affect the function of the hematopoietic organs through the infection and lysis of erythropoid cells. The disease is very mild for the mother and carries a 33% placental transmission rate following maternal seroconversion at any stage of pregnancy. The virus can cause severe destruction of erythroid progenitor cells in the fetus with the risk of developing fetal anemia, hydrops and intrauterine death.[36]

Transmission: It would lead to fetal anemia in 7–17% of affected cases. It is not associated with a clinically significant risk of malformations.[36]

Ultrasound signs: The hallmark of this infection is fetal hydrops which may be severe in very low hemoglobin levels. It accounts for 10–15% of nonimmune fetal hydrops NIHF.[37,38]

Testing: Nonimmune hydrops should call for a parvovirus B19 IgG and IgM antibody testing in the maternal serum. In 80% of the cases, the virus can be detected in the fetal blood by PCR. In case of NIHF the evaluation of middle cerebral artery reak systolic velocity is an important tool to diagnose and follow-up fetal anemia.[39,40] This should be followed by cordocentesis and intrauterine blood transfusion which is the only way for fetal survival, more than 80% of the fetuses transfused in utero will survive.[40]

Varicella Zoster

DNA virus of the herpes family responsible for chickenpox (varicella), the primary infection, and herpes zoster shingles, a reactivation of the virus occurring at any age but with an increasing incidence in adulthood. Transmission via droplet infection and infection is followed by long-lasting immunity.

Both maternal and fetal infection is important and serious. Pregnancy increases the risk of disease associated complications particulary in late pregnancy. Pneumonia occurs in up to 10% of cases and could be so sever that it necessitates mechanical ventilation.[41]

Fetal varicella syndrome occurs when the fetus is infected during maternal viremia in the 1st 20 weeks of gestation. The risk of fetal varicella syndrome is estimated to be 0.4% in the 1st 12 weeks of pregnancy, 2% between 13–20 weeks of gestation, the syndrome dose not occur if maternal infection occurs after 20 weeks.[42]

Prenatal diagnosis of fetal varicella syndrome depend on serial ultrasound examination 5 weeks or later after primary infection. Among the signs are polyhydramnios, microcephaly, liver calcification, NIHF, limb hypoplasia. Varicella embryopathy is the term used for infants contracted the infection intrauterine.[42] It comprises cutaneous scars, denuded skin, limb hypoplasia, muscle atrophy and rudimentary digits. Other more frequent abnormalities are microcephaly, intracranial calcification, cortical atrophy, cataract, chorioretinitis, microophthalmia and psychomotor retardation.[42]

Management

Exposure before 20 weeks: If the mother is not immune globulin 1000 g IM may be given. If she develops chickenpox, council her for the possibilities of fetal infection, and follow up by serial ultrasound.

Exposure after 20 weeks: There is no fetal infection in these cases, however, the mother may develop some complications mainly pneumonitis, thus if she presented within 24 hours of chickenpox rash: she may be given oral acyclovir 800 mg five times daily for 7 days to reduce the severity and duration of illness. If presented after 24 hours, the acyclovir is of no effect and just follow up the disease progression.[42,43]

In herpes zoster: The fetus is unaffected by maternal herpes zoster unless mother is immunosuppressed.

Rubella

Mode of infection: It is caused by a small RNA togavirus, the rubella virus.

Transmission: Direct contact with infected droplets. If the infection is contracted in the first 6 weeks of gestation, two-thirds of the fetuses will develop a rubella syndrome. Infections in later weeks are associated with lower risks; 25% between 7 and 9 weeks, 20% between 10 and 12 weeks, and 10% between 13 and 17 weeks.[44]

Ultrasound signs: The anomaly typically found in rubella embryopathy is VSD or tetralogy of Fallot. Additional signs include growth retardation and microcephaly. The triad of cataract, cardiac anomalies, and deafness (Gregg syndrome) is a classic embryopathy caused by the infection.[15]

Testing: A normal ultrasound scan cannot exclude fetal rubella infection, thus in cases of primary rubella infection. It is possible to detect the virus in chorionic villi or amniotic fluid. Cordocentesis has reasonable accuracy but should not be performed earlier than 22 weeks since the IgM production may still be too low before 21 weeks. A good strategy in earlier cases is too start with CVS or amniocentesis and if negative, confirm the result by cordocentesis at 22 weeks.[44]

CONCLUSION

- Ultrasound has an important role in the detection and follow-up of intrauterine infection. Transplacental transmission of the virus, even in subclinical maternal infection, may result in a severe congenital syndrome. Prenatal detection of viral infection is based on fetal sonographic findings and PCR to identify the specific infectious agent. Most affected fetuses appear sonographically normal, but serial scanning may reveal evolving findings.
- Common sonographic abnormalities, although non-specific, may be indicative of fetal viral infections. These include growth restriction, ascites, hydrops, ventriculomegaly, intracranial calcifications, hydrocephaly, microcephaly, cardiac anomalies, hepatosplenomegaly, echogenic bowel, placentomegaly and abnormal amniotic fluid volume.
- Some of the pathognomonic sonographic findings enable diagnosis of a specific congenital syndrome (e.g. ventriculomegaly and intracranial and hepatic calcifications in cytomegalovirus or in toxoplasma; eye and cardiac anomalies in congenital rubella syndrome; limb contractures and cerebral anomalies in varicella zoster virus).
- Maternal screen for TORCH and TORCH like infections is recommended in these cases.
- Serial ultrasound should be performed every 2 weeks in pregnancies at risk for congenital infection as in case of exposure to infection or maternal seroconversion.
- Amniocentesis is considered the standard invasive test for the diagnosis of most intrauterine infection where isolation of the virus is done by PCR with a sensitivity now approaching 100%.
- Intrauterine infection are not a cause for recurrent pregnancy loss, so TORCH is not indicated in these cases.

REFERENCES

1. Simposon JL, Mills JL, KimH, Holmes LB, Lee J, Metzger B, et al. Infections processes: an infrequent cause of first trimester spontaneous abortions. Hum Reprod. 1996;3:668-72.
2. Jauniaux E, Gavril P, Nickolaides KH. Ultrasongraphic assessment of early pregnancy. In Jurkovic D, Jauniaux E (Eds). Ultrasound and Early Pregnancy, Carnforth, UK: Parthenon Publishing; 1995. pp.53-64.
3. Iskaros J, Jauniaux E, Rodeck C. Outome of nonimmune hydrops fetalis diagnosed during the first half of pregnancy. Obstet Gynecol. 1997;90:321-5.
4. McCoy MC, Katz VL, Gould N, Kuller JA. Nonimmune hydrops after 20 weeks of gestation, review of 10 years' experience with suggestions for management. Obstet Gynecol. 1995;85:578-82.

5. Weiner CP, Grose CF, Naides SJ. Diagnosis of fetal infection in a patient with an ultrasongraphically detected abnormality but a negative clinical history. Am J Obstet Gynecol. 1993;168:6-11.
6. Kilby M, Hodgett S. Perinatal viral infections cause of intrauterine growth restriction. In: Kingdom J, Baker P (Eds). Intrauterine growth restriction: Aetiology and Management. London: Springer Verlag; 2000. pp.29-49.
7. Holliman RE. Clinical sequelae of chronic maternal toxoplsmosis. Rev Med Microbiol. 1994;5:47-55.
8. Hall SM. Congenital toxoplasmosis. BMJ. 1992;305:291-7.
9. Ranucci-Weiss D, Uerpairojkit B, Bowles N, Towbin JA, Chan L. Intrauterine adenovirus infection associated with nonimmune hydrops. Prenat Diagn. 1998;18:182-5.
10. Lambot MA , Noel JC, Peny MO, Rodessch F, Haot J. Fetal parvovirus B19 infection associated with myocardial necrosis. Prenat Diagn. 1998;18:182-5.
11. Parilla BV, Tamura RK, Ginsberg NA. Association of parvovirus infection with isolated fetal effusions. Am J Perinatol. 1997;14:357-8.
12. Muller F, Dommergues M, Aubry MC, Simon-Bouy, Gautier E, Oury JF, et al. Hyperechogenic fetal bowel: an ultrasonographic marker for adverse fetal and neonatal outcome. Am J Obstet Gynecol. 1995;173:508-13.
13. Mac Gregor SN, Trmura R, Sabbagha R, Brenofer JK, Kambich MP, Pergament E. Isolated Hyperechoic Fetal Bowel: Significance and implications for management. Am J Obstet Gynecol. 1995;173:1254-8.
14. Yaron Y, Hassan S, Geva E, Kupferminc MJ, Yavetz H, Evans MI. Evaluation of fetal echogenic bowel in the second trimester. Fetal Diagn Ther. 1999;14:176-80.
15. Degani S. Sonographic finding in fetal viral infection: a systematic review. Obstet Gynecol Surv. 2006;200661(5): 329-36.
16. Benoist G, Salomon L, Mohlo M, Suarez B, Jacquemard F, Ville Y. Cytomegalovirus-related fetal brain lesions: comparison between targeted ultrasound examination and magnetic resonance imaging. Ultrasound Obstet Gynecol. 2008;32(7):900-05.
17. Jauniaux E. A comparison of chorionic villus sampling and amniocentesis for prenatal diagnosis in early pregnancy. In: Grudzinskas JG, Ward RHT (Eds). Screening for Down syndrome in the first trimester. London RCOG Press; 1997. pp.259-69.
18. Guerra B, Lazzarotto T, Quarta S, Lanari M, Bovicelli L, Nicolosi A, et al. Prenatal diagnosis of symptomatic congenital cytomegalovirus infection.Am J Obstet Gynecol. 2000;183(2):476-82.
19. Nigro G, Mazzocco M, Anceschi M, La Toree R, Antonelli G, Cosmi E. Prenatal diagnosis of fetal cytomegalovirus infection after primary or recurrent maternal infection. Obstet Gynecol. 1999;94(6):909-14.
20. Malm G, Engman ML. Congenital cytomegalovirus infections. Semin Fetal Neonatal Med. 2007;12(3):154-59.
21. Yinon Y, Farine D, Yudin MH. Screening, diagnosis, and management of cytomegalovirus infection in pregnancy. Obstet Gynecol Surv. 2010;65(11):736-43.
22. Malinger G, Lev D, Lerman-Sagie T. Imaging of fetal cytomegalovirus infection. Fetal Diagn Ther. 2011;29(2): 117-26.
23. Nigro G. Maternal-fetal cytomegalovirus infection: From diagnosis to therapy. J Matern Fetal Neonatal Med. 2009;22(2):169-74.
24. Dogan Y1, Yuksel A, Kalelioglu IH, Has R, Tatli B, Yildirim A. Intracranial ultrasound abnormalities and fetal cytomegalovirus infection: report of 8 cases and review of the literature. Fetal Diagn Ther. 2011;30(2):141-9.
25. Omoy A, Diav-Citrin O. Fetal effects of primary and secondary cytomegalovirus infection in pregnancy. Reprod Toxicol. 2006;21(4):399-409.
26. Yinon Y, Farine D, Yudin MH, Gagnon R, Hudon L, Basso M, et al. Fetal Medicine Committee, Society of Obstetricians and Gynaecologists of Canada. Cytomegalovirus infection in pregnancy. J Obstet Gynaecol Can. 2010;32(4):348-54.
27. Karacan M, Batukan M, Cebi Z, Berberoglugil M, Levent S, Kır M, et al. Screening cytomegalovirus, rubella and toxoplasma infections in pregnant women with unknown pre-pregnancy serological status. Arch Gynecol Obstet. 2014;290(6):1115-20.
28. Jacquemard F, Yamamoto M, Costa J, Romand S, Jagz-Algarain E, Dejean A, et al. Maternal administration of Valaciclovir in symptomatic intrauterine cytomegalovirus infection. BJOG. 2007;114(9):1113-21.
29. Stronati M1, Lombardi G, Garofoli F, Villani P, Regazzi M. Pharmacokinetics, pharmacodynamics and clinical use of valganciclovir in newborns with symptomatic congenital cytomegalovirus infection. Curr Drug Metab. 2013;14(2):208-15.
30. Meine Jansen CF1, Toet MC, Rademaker CM, Ververs TF, Gerards LJ, van Loon AM. Treatment of symptomatic congenital cytomegalovirus infection with valganciclovir. J Perinat Med. 2005;33(4):364-6.
31. Naing ZW, Scott GM, Shand A, Hamilton ST, van Zuylen WJ, Basha J, et al. Congenital cytomegalovirus infection in pregnancy: a review of prevalence, clinical features, diagnosis and prevention. Aust N Z J Obstet Gynaecol. 2016;56(1):9-18
32. Paquet C1, Yudin MH. Society of Obstetricians and Gynaecologists of Canada. Toxoplasmosis in pregnancy: prevention, screening, and treatment. J Obstet Gynaecol Can. 2013;35(1):78-81.
33. Gilbert R, Gras L. European multicentre study on congenital toxoplasmosis. Effect of timing and type of treatment on the risk of mother to child transmission of Toxoplasma gondii. BJOG. 2003;110:112-20.
34. Gras L, Gilbert RE, Wallon M, et al. Duration of the IgM response in women acquiring Toxoplasma gondii during pregnancy: implications for clinical practice and

cross-sectional incidence studies. Epidemiol Infect. 2004;132:541-8.

35. Foulon W, Villena I, Stray-Pedrsen B, et al.Treatment of toxoplasmosis during pregnancy: a multicenter study of impact on fetal transmission and childrens sequelae at the age of 1 year. Am J Obstet Gynecol. 1999;180:410-5.
36. Hedrick J. The effects of human parvovirus B19 and cytomegalovirus during pregnancy. J Perinat Neonatal Nurs. 1996;10:30-9.
37. Chisaka H, Morita E, Yaegashi N, et al. Parvovirus B19 and the pathogenesis of anaemia. Rev Med Virol. 2003;13:347-59.
38. AlKhan A, Caliguri A, Apuzio J. Parvovirus B19 infection during pregnancy. Infect Dis Obstet Gynecol. 2003;11,175-9.
39. Cosmi E, Mari G, Chiaie LD, et al. Noninvasive diagnosis by Doppler ultrasonography of fetal anemia resulting from parvovirus infection. Am J Obstet Gynecol. 2002; 187:1290-3.
40. Hernandez-Andrade E, Scheler M, Dezerga V, Carmo A, Nicolaides KH. Fetal middle cerebral artery peak systolic velocity in the investigation of nonimmune hydrops. Ultrasound Obstet Gynecol. 2004;23:442-5.
41. Pretorius DH, Hayward I, Jones KL, Stamm E. Sonographic evaluation of pregnancies with maternal varicella infection. J Ultrasound Med. 1992;11:459-63.
42. AL, Levy M, Schick B, et al. Outcome after maternal varicella infection in the first 20 weeks of pregnancy. N Engl J Med. 1994;330:901.
43. Smego RA, Asperilla MO. Use of acyclovir for varicella pneumonia during pregnancy. Obstet Gynecol. 1991;78: 1112-6.
44. Banatvala J, Brown DWG. Rubella. Lancet. 2004;363:1127-37.

SECTION 3

Gynecology

52

CHAPTER

Normal Female Reproductive Anatomy

Sanja Kupesic Plavsic, Ulrich Honemeyer, Asim Kurjak

INTRODUCTION

Transvaginal ultrasound is superior to transabdominal ultrasound in female gynecologic examination due to: (i) Use of high-frequency transvaginal transducer with better spatial resolution and (ii) no need to fill the urinary bladder. Because of these characteristics, transvaginal ultrasonography became essential in gynecologic ultrasound examination.

Two-dimensional (2D) ultrasound imaging is limited by the movement of the transvaginal transducer in the narrow space of vagina allowing bi-planar display (sagittal and transverse). In stark contrast, three-dimensional (3D) sonography permits multi-planar display (coronal, sagittal and transverse). 3D sonography measures the volume of the studied organ and evaluates it more accurately, stores the data, and allows retrospective analysis and application of tele-consultation in telemedicine. The C-plane, however, as a digital construct of A- and B-plane, shows quite often comparatively to A-and C-plane, degradation of the image quality.

Two-dimensional ultrasound imaging is limited by the movement of the transvaginal transducer in the narrow space of vagina. Therefore, it allows presentation of two planes: sagittal and transverse. Three-dimensional sonography permits multiplanar display of all three sections: Coronal, sagittal and transverse. Using this method, it is possible to measure the volume of the studied organ and evaluate it more accurately. Three-dimensional ultrasound enables storage of the data without degradation of the image quality, retrospective analysis and application of tele-consultation in telemedicine.

Color Doppler capability of the transvaginal probes allows visualization of small intraovarian and endometrial vessels, enabling depiction of normal and pathological changes in reproductive organs.

Three-dimensional color histogram measures the color percentage and flow amplitudes in the volume of interest. Therefore, histogram enables quantification of the vascularization and blood flow within a tissue block, in contrast to 2D color histogram measurements, where only single planes can be investigated. Here, three-dimensional tissue block is swept through with a volume probe to get the 3D information and after that, to border the volume of interest, which contains the color information, resulting in an automatic delineation called "shell imaging".

UTERUS

Position

In the female pelvis, uterus is considered to be a reliable landmark because of its central location, relatively large size and the well-known pear-shape. The cervix is less mobile than the uterine body due to uterosacral ligaments that position the cervix in the midline of the pelvis.

Anteverted uterus projects from the anterior fornix of the vagina and extends anterosuperiorly to the uterine fundus. Retroverted uterus projects from the posterior fornix of the vagina to its posterosuperior extension. Anteflexion of the uterus describes its position when the uterine body is angled forward relatively to the axis of the cervix, while retroversion describes backward angulation.

With transabdominal ultrasound, we encounter difficulties in demonstrating the uterine fundus exists if the uterus is retroverted and retroflexed behind the interposed cervix. Some rare positions of the uterus include its anteverted/retroflexed or retroverted/anteflexed position.

Following a generally accepted convention on image orientation in transvaginal sonography, transducer is pressed on the flexed cervical-corporeal junction, shown at the superior apex of the screen. Fundus of the anteverted uterus is often placed on the left side of the ultrasound screen and anteflexed position is imaged as concave upward. Fundus of the retroverted uterus is placed to the right, with retroflexion concave upward. Transvaginal scanning might be limited due to shadowing and attenuation, when the uterus is in the same axis as the cervix and vagina, and ultrasound beam and uterine position are not perpendicular.

Slight deviations of the uterus to the right or left side are common. Larger deviations, when seen are mostly due to pelvic masses, peritoneal adhesions, or post-inflammatory contraction of the ligament suspension of the uterus. Awareness of the position of the uterus is important during the various invasive procedures (curettage, hysteroscopy, insertion of an intrauterine contraceptive device, embryo transfer) to avoid procedure-related injuries like perforation. Transitory change of uterine position and deviation can be caused by bladder and rectal fullness, patient's posture or external manual pressure.

Size, Shape and Echotexture

The normal size, shape, the length ratio of body and cervix of the uterus and appearance of the endometrium depend on the patient's age and parity.

The dimensions of the uterus can be accurately measured with transabdominal and transvaginal ultrasound. Uterine volume measured using the conventional formula for ellipsoid is less informative because the uterine shape does not approximate an ellipsoid.

Uterus consists of the body and the cervix, having a 2:1 length ratio. Dimensions of the body are approximately 7.5–9 cm length × 4.5–6 cm width × 2.5–4 cm thickness. Multiparity increases dimensions by 1–2 cm in all directions. Dimensions of the cervix are 2.5 cm length and 2.5 cm diameter.

In sagittal section, the endometrial cavity is slit-like, with touching anterior and posterior surface. In coronal section or anteroposteriorly on hysterosalpingography, the endometrial cavity appears triangular (cervical canal opens up to the lateral angels of the cavity containing uterotubal junctions).

The majority of the entire volume of the uterus occupies the myometrium constituting the uterine wall. Normal echotexture of the myometrium is homogeneously echodense. The inner layer of the myometrium can be a little less echogenic, but the junction zone with endometrium is very well demarcated and smooth.

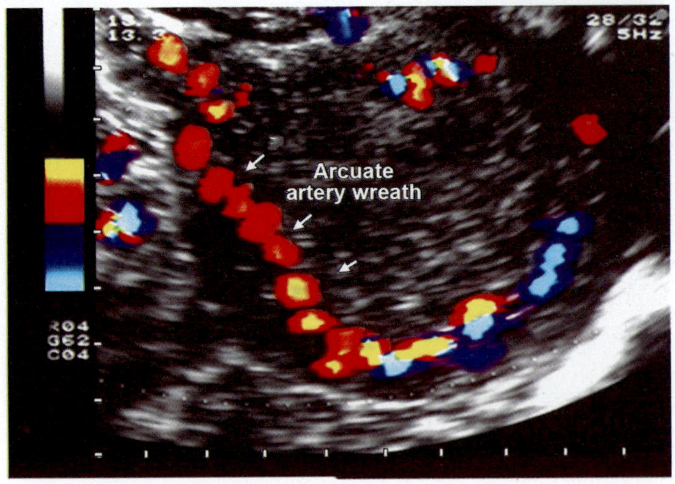

Fig. 1: Transvaginal color Doppler ultrasound of the uterus demonstrating arcuate arteries wreath.

The outer layers of myometrium may contain small circular hypoechoic spaces, calcified with age, which correspond to arcuate arteries in cross-section **(Fig. 1)**. In color Doppler studies, they are represented with slow laminar blood flow signals in color. The development of the endometrium, thickness and echotexture, is highly influenced by circulating ovarian hormones, estrogens and progesterone.

Newborn and Prepuberty

The newborn uterus is tubular in shape with body to cervix length ratio 1:1, and is poorly differentiated. Neonatal uterus can be 0.5–1 cm larger than the uterus in infants due to the influence of pregnancy hormones. Prepubescent dimensions of the uterus are approximately 3 cm length × 2 cm width × 2 cm thickness, tubulary shaped with the same length ratio as in newborns. During puberty, tubular shape of the uterus changes to pear-shape and the corpus enlarges.

Adult

Dimensions of the adult nulliparous uterus are 7.5 × 5 × 2.5 cm, and its position depends on bladder and rectal fullness. Normal uterine size varies with parity, but after postpartal involution it stabilizes at approximately 7.5 cm.[1] During the reproductive period, the pelvic organs (their size and echogenicity) are influenced with cyclic hormonal changes controlled by the ovaries. These changes are especially evident in the uterus. Duration of the normal menstrual cycle is 28 days, with about equal time for the preovulatory (follicular) and postovulatory (luteal) phase. In women with normal fertility, duration of the menstrual cycle can vary with a range between 25 and 36 days. While the follicular phase (proliferative phase of the endometrium) may vary, the luteal phase (secretory phase of the endometrium) remains 14 days.

Approaching the menopause and ovarian insufficiency, the follicular phase becomes shorter, shortening the whole menstrual cycle and bringing the time of ovulation sooner. In contrast, incidence of nonovulatory cycles may prolong menstrual intervals and lead to hypermenorrhea/menorrhagia due to unopposed estrogen influence.

Proliferative Phase

Uterine endometrium consists of two layers: The inner *stratum functionalis*—subjected to the changes during menstrual cycle, peeled off with menstruation, and the outer *stratum basalis*—permanent layer not influenced by cyclic changes, contains glandular buds from which glands develop.

As menstruation ceases, the functional layer of the endometrium responds to small amounts of estrogen secreted by the ovary. Parallel with follicular development and rising estrogen production, the endometrial glands in basal layer proliferate, elongate and become tortuous. The endometrium is best depicted on transvaginal sonography in the sagittal plane. In the sagittal plane, the endocervical canal is seen continuing into the endometrial echo. For most patients who do not have significant amount of intraluminal fluid, the endometrium is measured in a bilayer thickness from the proximal myometrial-endometrial junction to the distal myometrial-endometrial junction. If intraluminal fluid is present, each endometrial thickness should be measured separately, and the combined endometrial thickness should be expressed as a sum of the two layers. In the early proliferative phase endometrium is imaged as a thin echogenic line, measuring 1 to 3 mm. With the progression of proliferative phase the endometrium becomes less echogenic than the surrounding myometrium **(Fig. 2)**. The most characteristic sign of the late proliferative phase is the triple-line endometrium. The central echogenic line represents touching of the anterior and posterior endometrial layers. The two outer hyperechogenic lines represent endometrial-myometrial junction or echo of the basal layer. The endometrial tissue (functional layer) between the two lines becomes hypoechoic and thick during the proliferative phase, continuing to widen in between the basal echogenic line toward uterine cavity and central echogenic zone **(Fig. 2)**.

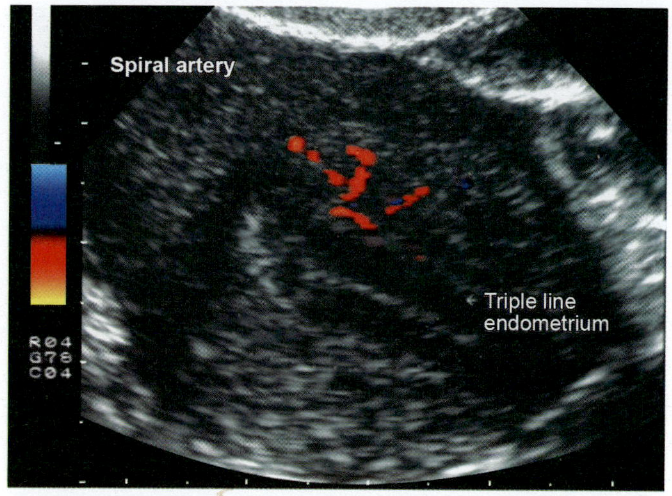

Fig. 2: Transvaginal scan of the uterus in the late proliferative phase of the menstrual cycle. The endometrium is lucent compared with myometrium. Note an echo demarcating the endometrium from the junctional layer, and a third line representing the point of the contact between front and back mucosal surfaces. Color Doppler delineates subendometrial vessels.

The thickness and echogenicity of the endometrium can be used for qualitative assessment of dominant follicle and prediction of the probability of implantation. To achieve a good implantation rate, the endometrium has to be thicker than 7 mm and show a triple-line pattern.[2]

Secretory Phase

Progesterone surge, seen in postovulatory luteal phase ceases epithelial and stromal proliferation of the endometrium and differentiates endometrial glands for secreting glycoproteins, evidenced ultrasonographically as blurring of the three lines in the late proliferative endometrium. The endometrium appears as homogenous and hyperechogenic layer measuring 7 to 14 mm **(Fig. 3)**. Color Doppler reveals subendometrial and intra-endometrial vessels of the secretory transformed endometrium **(Fig. 4)**.

Secretion of endometrial glands is fully developed 7 days after ovulation. Despite the manifestation of stromal edema and predecidual reaction, there is no further change of the ultrasound appearance of the endometrium. If pregnancy occurs, echogenicity and thickness are maintained while decidual reaction to implantation starts to progress. In absence of a pregnancy, endometrium starts to regress in thickness, but not in echogenicity.

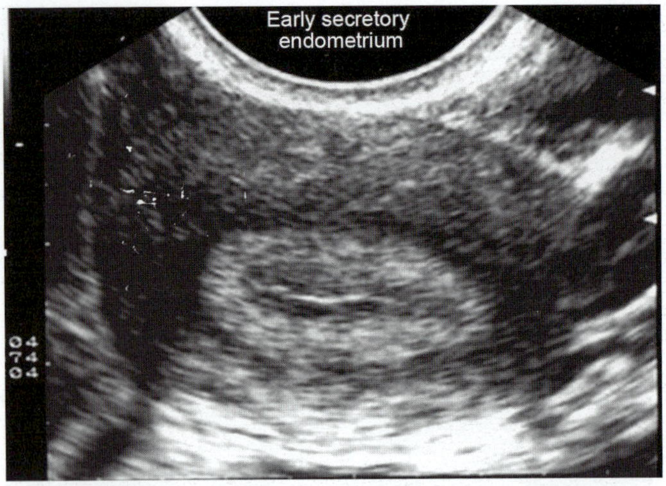

Fig. 3: Transvaginal scan of the uterus with echogenic endometrial lining during the luteal phase of the menstrual cycle.

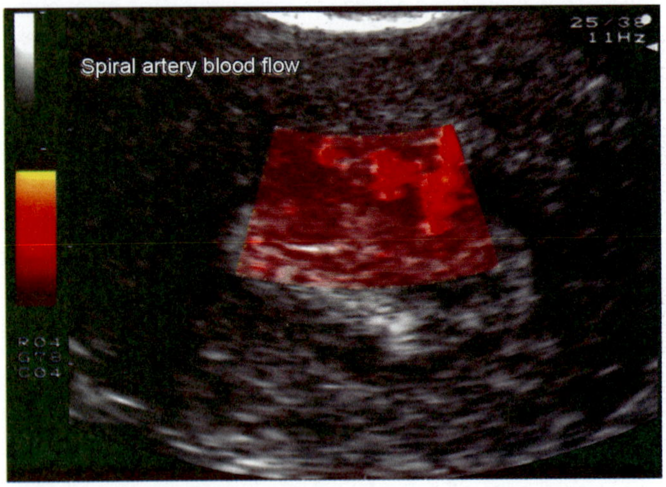

Fig. 4: Color Doppler imaging of the endometrial vessels during the luteal phase of the menstrual cycle.

Menstrual Phase

Menstruation begins when circulating levels of estrogen and progesterone decrease at the end of the ovarian cycle, causing break down of the functional endometrial layer. Ultrasound image varies depending on the amount of blood clots and endometrial fragments which can be seen as echogenic debris. Basal layers are imaged as thin, irregular, and hyperechogenic lines.

Postmenopausal State

The size of the cervix and the body of the uterus decreases gradually after menopause from approximately 6.5 to 3.5 cm.

Due to quiescent ovaries in postmenopausal women, the endometrium is thin and atrophic and not any longer subjected to cyclic changes. The mean endometrial thickness is 2.3 ± 1.8 mm.[3] In postmenopausal state ovaries do not secrete estrogens, but still produce androgen, which together with androgens derived from the adrenal glands are converted to estrogen in peripheral adipose cells (extraglandular conversion). Production of estrogen at that pathway may be responsible for endometrial thickening and proliferation changes shown as glandular hyperplasia or neoplasm. An endometrial thickness cut-off level of >5 mm in a symptomatic patient seems to have a high negative predictive value for the presence of endometrial cancer.[4] Once the endometrial thickness is greater than 8 mm in asymptomatic postmenopausal women not taking hormonal replacement therapy (HRT), an outpatient biopsy is required to exclude endometrial hyperplasia or malignancy. Women taking HRT have an increased endometrial thickness, which changes according to the phase of the cyclical therapy. In continuous combined regimens the endometrium is likely to be relatively thin and echogenic.

Subendometrial Myometrial Waves

Contractions of the hypoechoic junction zone of the myometrium adjacent to the endometrium are very well documented with real-time transvaginal ultrasound and video playback. These contractions have a possible role in propelling sperm to the Fallopian tubes before ovulation as well as in positioning the pre-embryo for proper implantation.[5] The frequency, amplitude and direction of myometrial waves require estrogens, while progesterone decreases its motility. Subendometrial myometrial peristalsis during menstrual bleeding is directed from the fundus toward the cervix.

Cervix

Cervix of the uterus is oval-conic shaped canal measuring approximately 2.5 cm in length, entering the vagina vertically. It consists of the supravaginal and vaginal part or endocervix (cervical canal) and ectocervix (seen clearly in the specula). In midcycle, the endocervix is filled with anechoic mucus due to estrogen produced in pre-ovulatory follicle **(Fig. 5)**. The ectocervix can be visualized on ultrasound better if the fluid surrounds the vaginal fornices. The site where the uterine body turns away from the cervix marks the internal cervical os. This point is

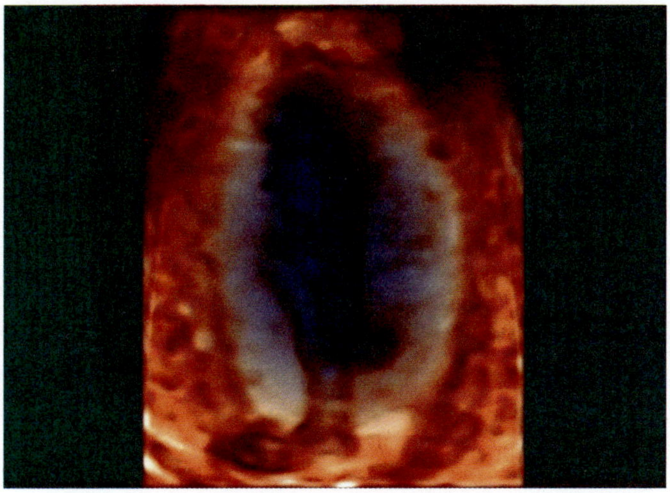

Fig. 5: Three-dimensional ultrasound image of a cervix in mid-cycle.

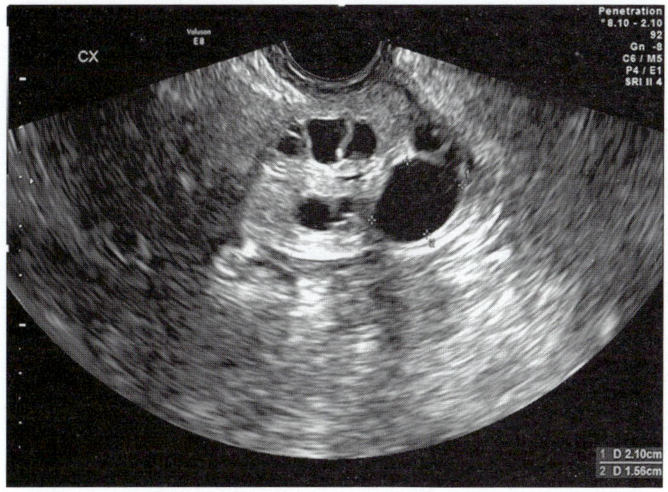

Fig. 6: Cervix with Nabothian cysts.

clearly seen on ultrasound examination of the anteflexed uterus as indentation in the anterior wall. Ovarian hormonal changes do not influence on the epithelium of the endocervical canal, neither histologically nor sonographically. The mucus in the endocervical canal is viscous and echogenic, except at the time of ovulation, when it is diluted and seen as an echolucent area on ultrasound examination **(Fig. 5)**. Nabothian cysts are retention cysts of the cervical glands within the ectocervix undergoing metaplasia from columnar to stratified squamous epithelium. They measure approximately 10 mm in diameter with thin walls and spherical shape containing echolucent fluid. Nabothian cysts have no clinical value even when they are multiple and large in size **(Fig. 6)**.

The Vagina

The vagina is thin walled tubular structure, located antero-inferiorly from the uterine cervix to the perineum, posterior to the bladder and urethra, and anterior to the rectum. It can be visualized by transabdominal ultrasound, with transducer directed caudally, while transvaginal ultrasound is less efficient to demonstrate this structure. Ultrasound determination of the vaginal length is not reliable because of the variable degree of bladder distension. During the menstruation, blood can pool in the vagina and can be visualized as anechoic fluid collection. Similar appearance can be obtained in postmenopausal patient with incontinence that lies in the supine position, due to the collection of the urine in the vagina.

FALLOPIAN TUBE

The fallopian tubes are approximately 10 to 12 cm long and a few millimeters wide. They spread from the lateral uterine angles toward the corresponding ovary. Anatomically, the fallopian tube is divided into: (i) Intramural part—within the uterine wall (1 cm long, less than 1 mm wide); (ii) Isthmic part (2 cm long); (iii) Ampular part (5 cm long, meandering with thin walls, varying in diameter); (iv) Fimbriae and (v) Infundibulum. Fallopian tubes can be only occasionally seen on ultrasound, when distended with fluid (hydrosalpinx), transfused with an echogenic contrast or cannula, or when peritoneal fluid is present surrounding the adnexa. Demonstration of oblique sagittal view during ultrasound scanning enables visualization of the origin of the Fallopian tubes at the lateral uterine angles.

OVARIES

Although both transabdominal and transvaginal ultrasound are able to identify ovaries properly, better resolution, closer focusing, and avoiding the need for a full bladder make trans-vaginal ultrasound much preferable for scanning the ovaries.

Position

Localization of the ovaries is on each side of the cervix, close to the lateral wall of the pelvis in Waldeyer's fossa. Iliac vessels are a reliable landmark for their visualization. Due to mobility of the ovaries and transducer pressure, position of the ovaries is often varying, e.g., in the cul-de-sac, in front of the uterus, above the uterus, or in the abdominal cavity. Sometimes, previous inflammatory disease or surgical interventions might cause origination of pelvic adhesions that fix the position of the ovaries, commonly close to the lateral fornices of the vagina, or posterior to the uterus (endometriosis).

Size, Shape and Echotexture

Normal ovaries are ellipsoid, with dimensions approximately 3 × 2 × 2 cm. Ovarian volume estimated using the ellipse formula (volume = length × width × depth × 0.523) is between 6 and 10 cm^3 (maximum volume 14–16 cm^3).[6]

Ovaries are imaged as homogenous, hypoechogenic ovoid structures with slightly echogenic central part. Ovarian follicles facilitate the identification of the ovaries containing echolucent fluid and varying in size from 2 mm to 25 mm in diameter **(Fig. 7)**. Sites of former ovulations may be identified as echogenic spots. In postmenopausal women detection of ovaries is difficult due to lack of follicles and small size of the ovaries.

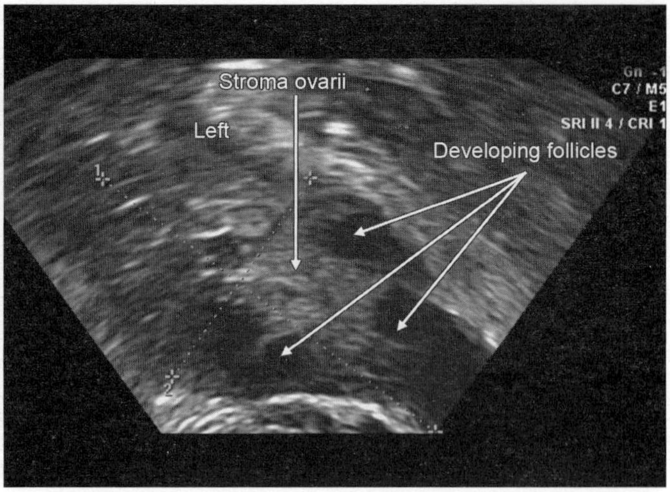

Fig. 7: Normal ovary in a reproductive age patient. Note multiple follicles measuring between 2 and 5 mm.

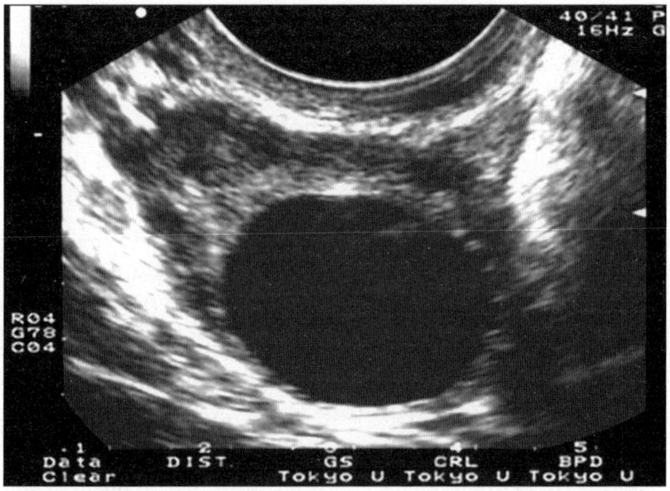

Fig. 8: Transvaginal image of the preovulatory follicle.

Ovarian Cycle

About 7 million of the follicles containing oocytes are present in a female fetus at about 20 weeks of gestation.[7] These follicles, called primordial, are microscopic in size and metabolically quiescent. Later in childhood, reproductive age or during oral contraception therapy, they grow from primordial to primary, secondary and tertiary follicles (microscopic in size) forming a fluid-filled antrum. In adequate hormonal conditions (increased local follicle stimulating hormone-FSH levels) follicles continue to grow until they become sonographically detectable. If endocrine conditions do not support the growth, atresia and permanent loss of the oocytes from the follicular oocyte pool takes place. The majority of follicles will go through the process of atresia, with just a fraction going to ovulation, and until the menopausal period only 100 to 1,000 follicles are left **(Fig. 7)**.

Follicular Phase

The small and transient rise in follicle-stimulating hormone (FSH) serum levels at the end of each ovarian cycle affects the small antral follicles reaching a size of 1 or 2 mm. These follicles have a potential to grow further instead to become atretic. During the early follicular phase of the ovarian cycle, hypophyseal FSH affects follicular cells to secrete estrogen and the peptide hormone inhibin (reduces FSH production as the follicular phase progresses). The smaller follicles go to regression with the drop in FSH levels, while the larger ones grow regardless. One or sometimes two follicles become dominant, producing substantial amounts of estradiol as they grow, while the others become atretic. This turnover happens by the end of the first week of the follicular phase. Atretic follicles can still be visible and can grow, especially in the dominant side, although they are undergoing atresia.

The dominant follicle, also called Graafian follicle, increases in size at a rate of 2.5 mm/day until it reaches about 2 cm in size **(Fig. 8)**, after that it decelerates to 1.3 mm/day.[8] Follicles grow due to increased number

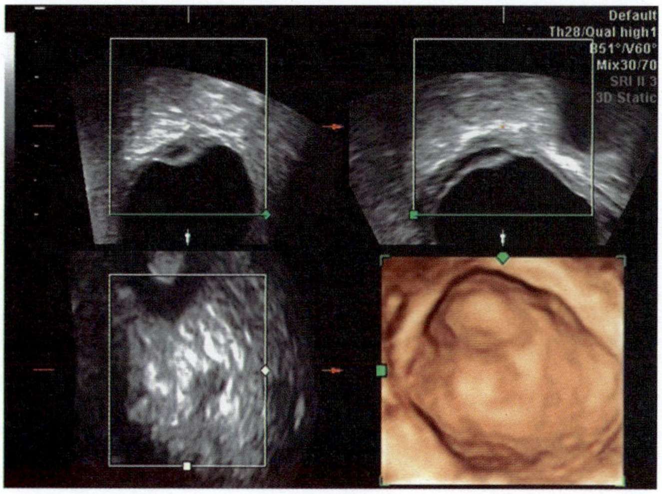

Fig. 9: Three-dimensional ultrasound of preovulatory follicle with cumulus oophorus.

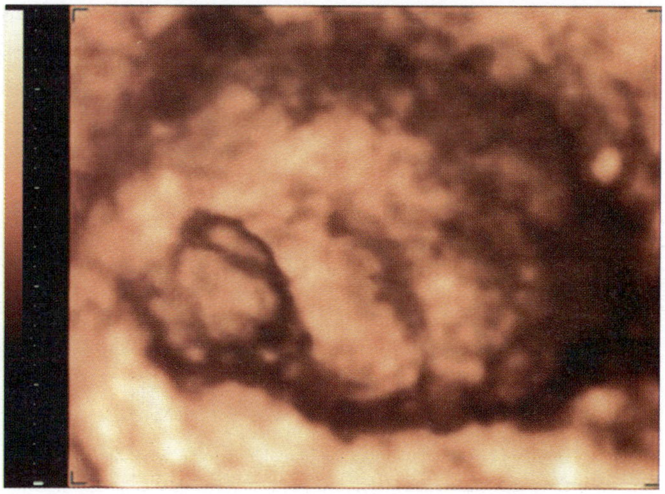

Fig. 10: Surface rendering of preovulatory follicle with cumulus oophorus.

of follicle cells and accumulation of fluid inside the antrum. Cumulus oophorus, consisting of the oocyte and surrounding follicle cells protrudes as a small papillary projection from the follicular wall **(Figs. 9 and 10)**. The side of ovulation in the present and previous ovarian cycle does not have to be the same.

Dominant follicular development is not always sustained by ovulation, especially in early reproductive age when ovulation does not occur. Hence, follicular phase and consequently the entire menstrual cycle may become longer and irregular (oligomenorrhea or amenorrhea).

The multifollicular appearance of the ovaries is explained by persistence of variable sized developing follicles, some of them functioning and some atretic. Difference from polycystic ovaries is the relative lack of hyperechogenic ovarian stroma and central and peripheral location of the follicles. Multifollicular appearance can be normal during adolescence and recovery from weight loss, but in older women it is associated with significant ovulation disorder of primarily ovarian origin and/or beginning of an ovarian failure.

Ovulation

Ovulation occurs with segmental/partial dissolution of the follicular wall, liberation of the oocyte and escape of the follicular fluid into the peritoneal cavity. It takes place about 38 hours after the luteinizing hormone (LH) surge begins, as a consequence of pituitary response to high circulating estrogen levels. At that time, the dominant follicle is 2.1 cm in diameter (range 1.6–3.3 cm), and sometimes contains a triangular structure representing mucus-like cumulus oophorus surrounding the preovulatory oocyte **(Fig. 10)**.[9] The preovulatory follicle luteinizes and begins to secrete progesterone with formation of new blood vessels around the follicle, visible on color Doppler ultrasound examination. High estrogen levels effect on Fallopian tube fluid secretion, and transudation through the follicle, resulting on ultrasonically recognizable accumulation of free peritoneal fluid. Besides the free fluid imaged on ultrasound, ovulation presents as sudden disappearance of the echolucent dominant follicle, and after several days, is followed by formation of the corpus luteum. Corpus luteum maturation into a solid-cystic, steroid-producing "organ" reflects on the rise of the progesterone level in serum.

In cases when ovulation does not take place, the follicle continues to grow and becomes a follicular cyst. On ultrasound scanning it is demonstrated as a thin-walled cystic lesion filled with lucent fluid and very well demarcated from the rest of the ovary. The size of the follicular cyst ranges between 3 and 6 cm in diameter, and it usually regresses spontaneously. Sometimes, it continues to produce estrogens resulting in endometrial hyper-proliferation (glandular cystic hyperplasia).

Luteal Phase

Postovulatory changes include: collapse of (Graafian) follicle wall; secretion of progesterone by follicular/granulosa cells and neovascularization for future corpus luteum. Proliferating capillaries invading theca

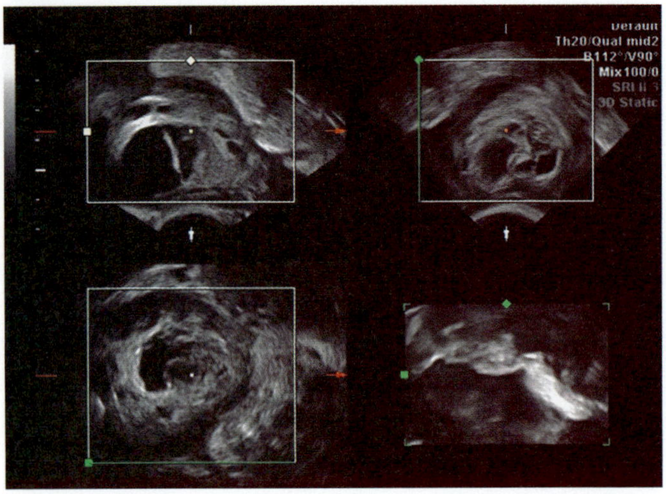

Fig. 11A: Transvaginal three-dimensional ultrasound image of an early corpus luteum. Blood-filled cavity of the former follicle is clearly visualized on three orthogonal planes.

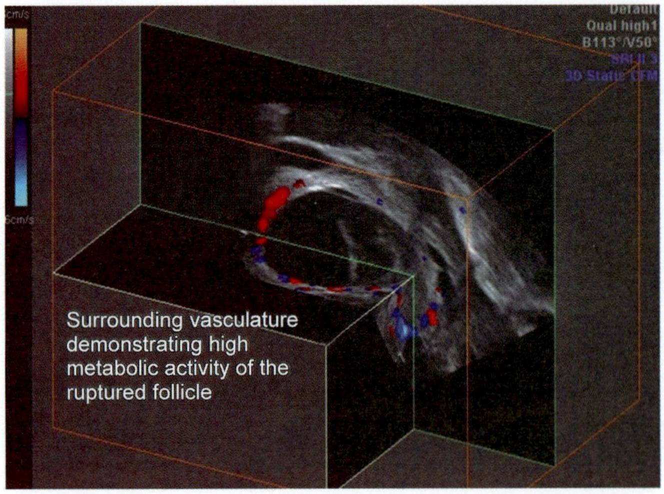

Fig. 11C: Three-dimensional color Doppler ultrasound. Using niche image, capillaries invading the blood filled cavity of the follicle are clearly visualized.

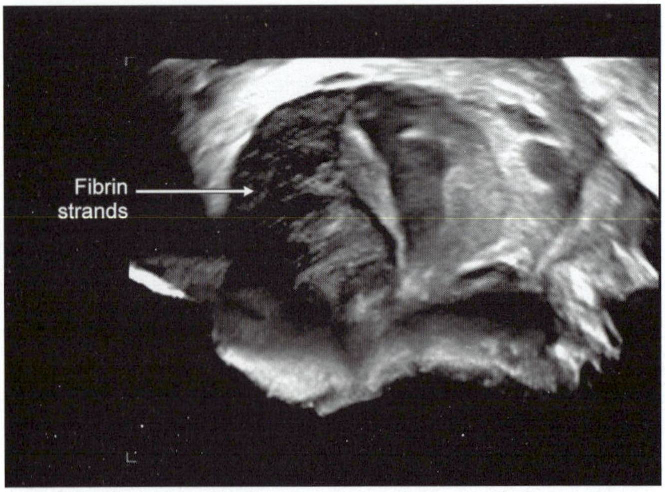

Fig. 11B: Three-dimensional ultrasound of an early corpus luteum.

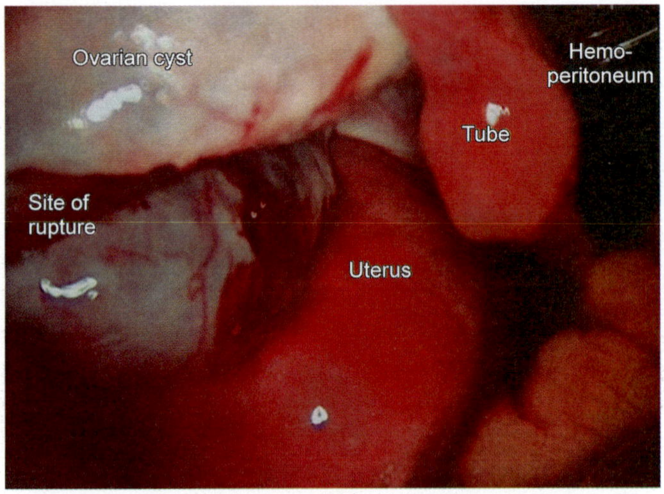

Fig. 11D: Laparoscopy image of the same patient.

interna- and granulosa cell layer are fragile and start to transudate serum or blood. In majority of the ovulatory patients corpus luteum is visualized as a blood filled cavity of the ruptured follicle (**Figs. 11A and B**). Capillaries invade the blood filled cavity of the corpus luteum and give rise to the corpus luteum angiogenesis (**Figs. 11C and D**).

Sometimes, corpus luteum can be hardly seen on transvaginal ultrasound due to variety of echoes in the ovary (**Fig. 12A**). Commonly it is visualized as a structure containing thick hyperechogenic walls enclosing the hypoechoic center. Neovascularization starts about 24 hours after the LH surge and continues to be detectable by the means of transvaginal color Doppler through the entire functional life of the corpus luteum ("ring of fire") (**Figs. 12B and C**).

Sometimes, after follicle ruptures, corpus luteum presents as a hemorrhagic cyst. It can be even 5–6 cm in diameter, and due to its clot component can be mistaken for endometrioma (**Figs. 13A to D**). If the corpus luteum is filled with serous fluid and persists more than 2 weeks, it is called corpus luteum cyst. Cysts which persist more than a month or two in the absence of pregnancy are termed "functional" or "dysfunctional" cysts. While luteal cysts have thicker walls than follicular cysts, it can be very hard to differentiate them. In such cases, record of previous ultrasounds or hormonal studies giving proof of ovulation

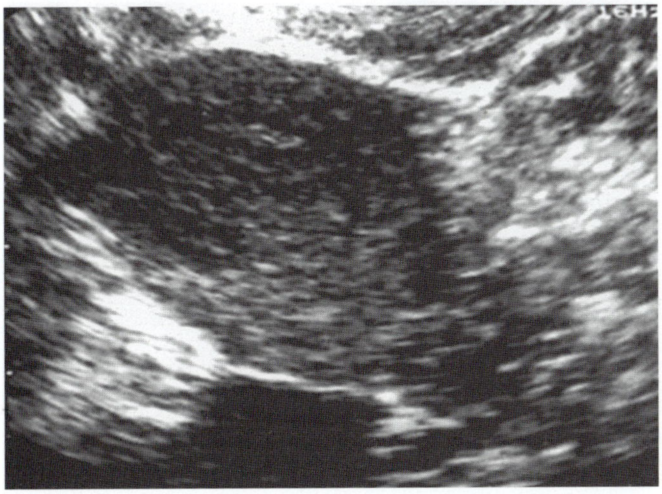

Fig. 12A: Transvaginal scan of the ovary during the luteal phase of the menstrual cycle. Corpus luteum is hardly visible among the stromal ovarian tissue.

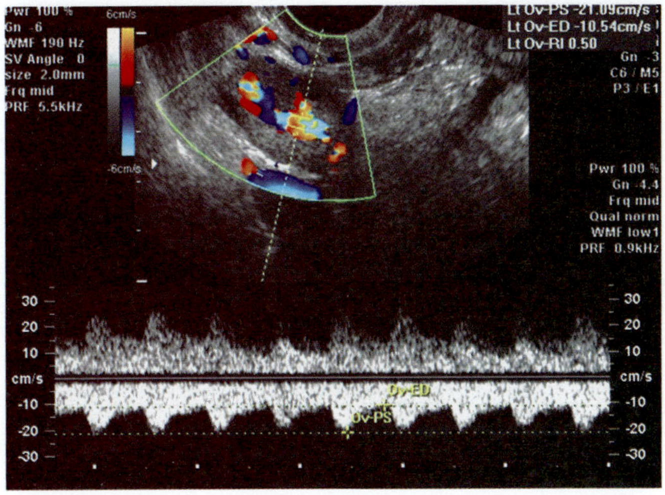

Fig. 12C: The same patient. Angiogenesis signals typical of corpus luteum formation are easily displayed by color Doppler ultrasound.

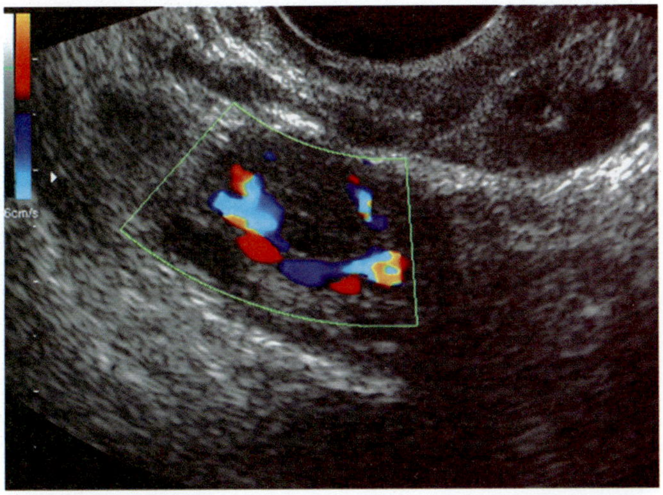

Fig. 12B: Transvaginal color Doppler scan of the corpus luteum, visualized as a ring of angiogenesis within the ovary.

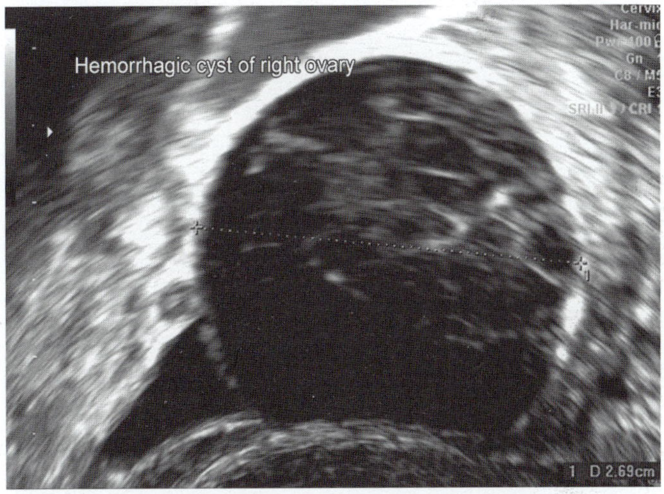

Fig. 13A: Hemorrhagic cyst of the ovary. Note intracystic appearance of a retracting clot and free fluid in the cul-de-sac.

may help. In general, luteal cysts are more painful than follicular cysts. This is especially true if pregnancy occurs due to chorionic gonadotropin stimulation. Luteal and follicular cysts, which do not resolve with time, require hormonal treatment, usually progesterone or OC.

The ultrasound and color Doppler evaluation of ovarian lesions and cysts is best done during the follicular phase of the menstrual cycle due to diagnostic confusion that can be caused by the different appearances of a corpus luteum ("the great imitator") **(Figs. 14 and 15)**.

If the dominant follicle does not release follicular fluid and the oocyte, but luteinization takes place, and growing continues toward a diameter of about 3 cm with echogenic or lucent contents, the structure is called luteinized unruptured follicle (LUF syndrome). Luteinized unruptured follicles occur in about 5% of normal menstrual cycles and in a higher rate of abnormal cycles. Progesterone production in LUF syndrome is less than in a normal luteal phase, and the luteal phase is usually shorter than in a normal cycle.

Newborn

In the newborns, the ovaries can be difficult to demonstrate with ultrasound due to their small size, a need for

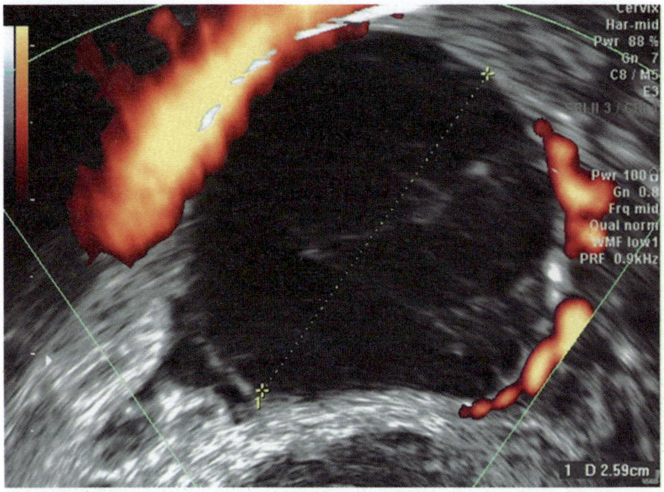

Fig. 13B: Power Doppler ultrasound demonstrates ring of angiogenesis surrounding the hemorrhagic cyst.

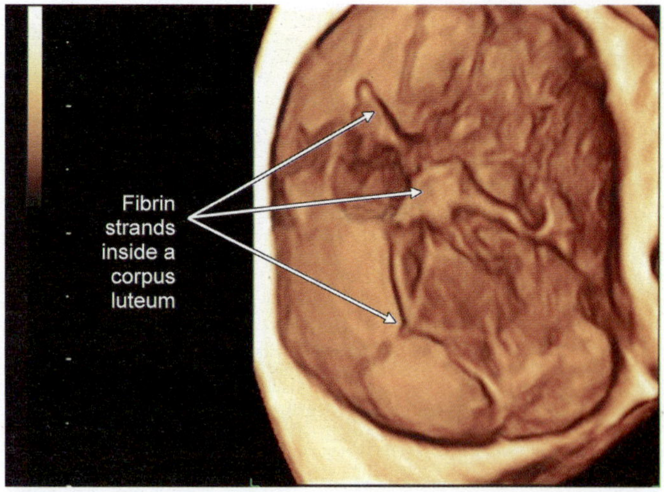

Fig. 13D: Intracystic fibrin strands within the hemorrhagic cyst are better visualized using surface rendering by three-dimensional ultrasound.

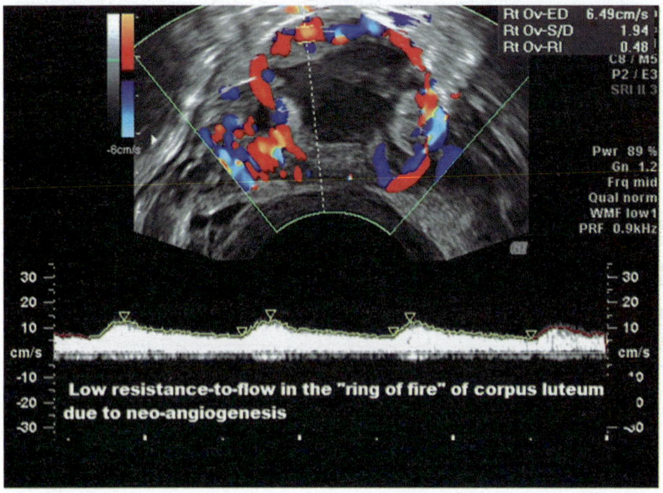

Fig. 13C: Low impedance blood flow signals (RI = 0.48) are isolated from the ring of angiogenesis encircling the hemorrhagic cyst.

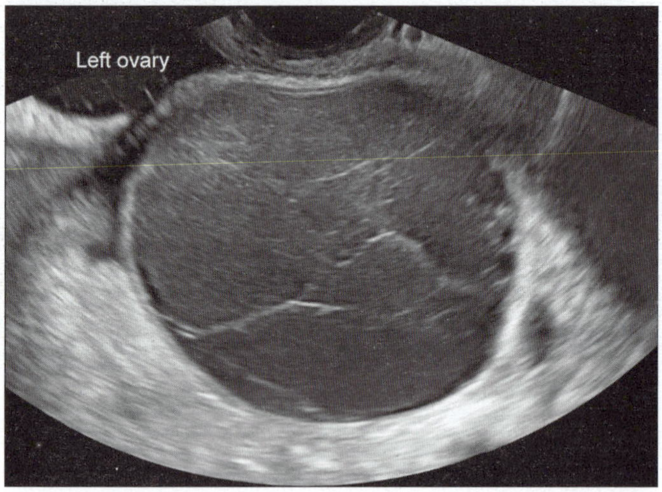

Fig. 14A: B mode transvaginal ultrasound of a hemorrhagic cyst.

trans-abdominal scanning, and difficulty to obtain a full bladder to move the intestines. Developing follicles remain small and invisible to ultrasound resolution. The ovaries continue to decrease in size for the first 2 years of childhood. Cohen et al.,[10] demonstrated that the mean ovarian volume was 1.2 cm^3 among the girls up to 3 months old; 1.1 cm^3 among the girls 4 to 12 months old; and 0.7 cm^3 among the girls 13 to 24 months old. In conclusion, failure to demonstrate the ovaries in newborns does not imply ovarian dysgenesis.

Childhood

The ovaries grow slowly through the childhood, increasing in the mean ovarian volume from 0.5 cm^3 at the age of 3–2.8 cm^3 at the age of 18 years.[11] We can distinguish two periods of the rapid growth: at around 8 years of age during the time of adrenarche and gradually rising levels of FSH; and before and during puberty. It is documented that taller girls have larger ovaries.[11]

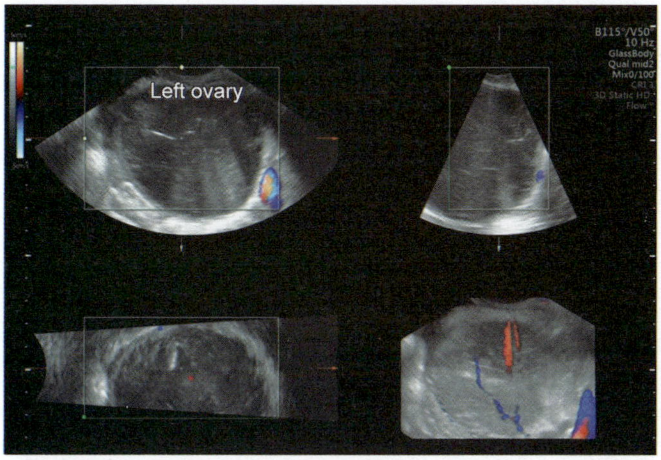

Fig. 14B: Three-dimensional color Doppler image of the same hemorrhagic cyst.

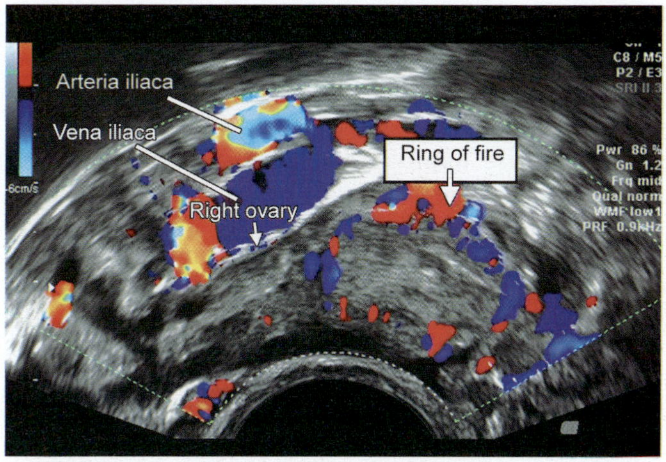

Fig. 15B: Color Doppler image demonstrating "ring of fire" encircling the corpus luteum.

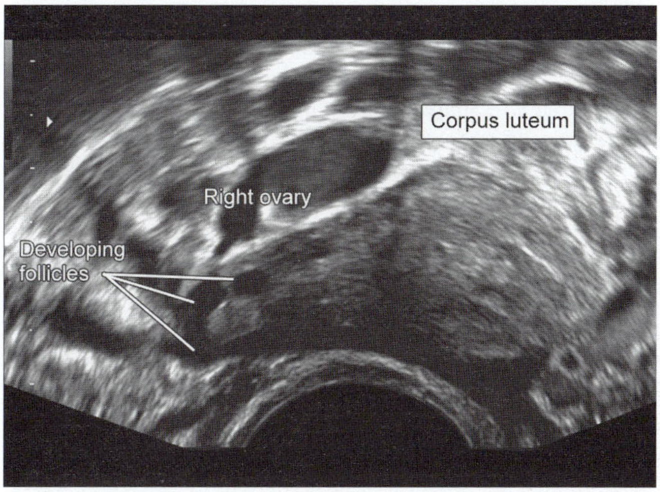

Fig. 15A: Solid appearance of corpus luteum.

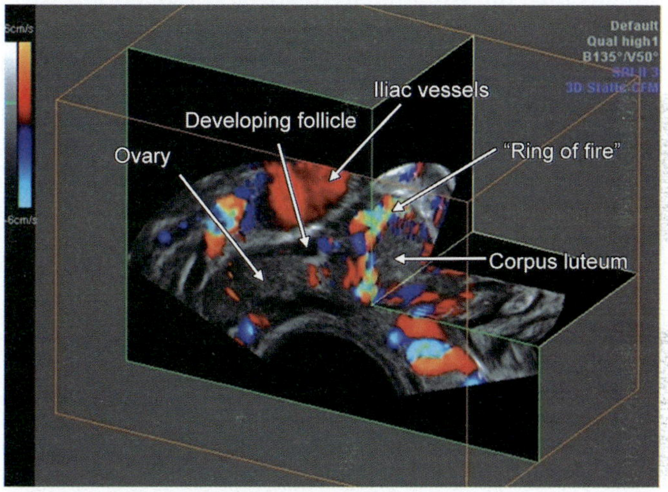

Fig. 15C: 3D color Doppler image demonstrating open cut view to the angiogenesis of the corpus luteum.

Adolescence and Adulthood

This period is characterized by the appearance of the typical ovarian changes through the ovarian cycle. The interruption of normal ovulatory cycle can be caused in both the early and late reproductive age by functional or dysfunctional follicular or luteal cysts, resulting in menstrual irregularities.

The number of follicular "recruits" visible on ultrasound is proportional to the number of primordial follicles present in the ovaries and is inversely proportional to the woman's age.

Perimenopausal and Postmenopausal State

Perimenopausal state is characterized by: (i) Ovarian follicular depletion, (ii) diminishing of antral follicles for

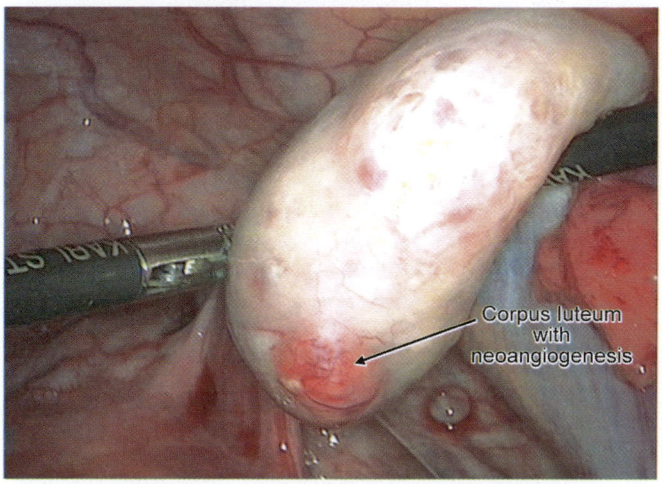

Fig. 15D: Laparoscopy image of the corpus luteum neoangiogenesis.

recruitment, (iii) lower production of follicular inhibin, and (iv) early rise of FSH levels (during the late luteal phase) causing premature start of follicular development of such recruits (before menstruation takes place). As menopause approaches, the follicular phase and menstrual cycle get shorter. During the perimenopausal years, it is common to have multifollicular appearance of the ovaries, as well as functional cysts causing menstrual delay and dysfunctional bleeding.

In postmenopausal state, estrogens and inhibin production falls, but FSH levels increase. The ovaries become small and homogenous with true depletion of follicles.

The addition of color Doppler capabilities to transabdominal and transvaginal probes permits visualization of uterine and ovarian vessels. Recent advances in three-dimensional ultrasound have made accurate noninvasive measurements of the ovarian, follicular and endometrial volumes feasible.[12] Storage capacities, reconstruction of the volume images and simultaneous viewing of all three orthogonal planes are main advantages of this method in gynecology.

REFERENCES

1. Ramsay PA, Jansen RPS. Ultrasonography of the normal female pelvis. In: Anderson JC (Ed). Gynecologic imaging. Churchill Livingstone, London; 1999. pp. 61-80.
2. Abdalla HI, Brooks AA, Johnson MR, et al. Endometrial thickness: a predictor of implantation in ovum recipients. Hum Reprod. 1994;9:363-5.
3. Kurjak A, Kupesic S. Ovarian senescence and its significance on uterine and ovarian perfusion. Fertil Steril. 1995;64:532-8.
4. Wikland M, Granberg S. Endometrial changes as imaged by transvaginal sonography in fertile and infertile women. In: Fleischer A, Kurjak A, Granberg S (Eds). Ultrasound and endometrium. Parthenon Publishing, London, New York; 1996. pp. 17-23.
5. Brosens JJ, de Souza NM, Braker FG. Uterine junctional zone: function and disease. Lancet. 1995;346:558-60.
6. Higgins RV, Van Nagell JR Jr, Woods CH, et al. Interobserver variation in ovarian measurements using transvaginal sonography. Gynecol Oncol. 1990;39:69-71.
7. Faddy MJ, Gosden RG, Gougeon A, et al. Accelerated disappearance of ovarian follicles in mid-life: implications for forecasting menopause. Hum Reprod. 1992;7:1342-6.
8. Nugent D, Smith J, Balen AH. Ultrasound and the ovary. In: Kupesic S, de Ziegler D (Eds). Ultrasound in Infertility. Parthenon Publishing, London; 2000. pp. 23-43.
9. Hamilton CJCM, Evers JHL, Tan FES, Hoogland HJ. The reliability of ovulation prediction by a single ultrasonographic follicle measurement. Hum Reprod. 1987;2:103-7.
10. Cohen HL, Shapiro MA, Mandel FS, Shapiro ML. Normal ovaries in neonates and infants: a sonographic study of 77 patients 1 day to 24 months old. Am J Roentgenol. 1993;160: 583-6.
11. Bridges NA, Cooke A, Healy MJR, et al. Standards for ovarian volume in childhood and puberty. Fertil Steril. 1993;60:456-60.
12. Kupesic S, Kurjak A, Bjelos D. Three- and four-dimensional ultrasound in human reproduction. In: Kurjak A, Jackson D (Eds). An Atlas of three- and four-dimensional sonography in Obstetrics and Gynecology. Taylor & Francis, London, New York; 2004. pp. 19-39.

53

CHAPTER

Uterine Lesions: Advances in Ultrasound Diagnosis

Sanja Kupesic Plavsic, Ulrich Honemeyer, Asim Kurjak

INTRODUCTION

The aim of this chapter is to investigate the role of color Doppler and three-dimensional (3D) ultrasound in the evaluation of the uterine lesions. Morphological and vascular criteria assessed by different forms of ultrasound are listed for each type of the uterine lesions. This chapter is a revision of the previous edition's chapter "Uterine lesions: Advances in ultrasound diagnosis". It includes updated bibliography, and additional high resolution ultrasound images.

The uterus lies in the middle of the pelvis with its long axis perpendicular to the ultrasound probe. Two-dimensional (2D) ultrasound gives an inadequate view of the uterus and uterine pathology as the examination of the uterine lesions is limited to transverse and sagittal planes. Three-dimensional ultrasound provides a simultaneous display of coronal, sagittal, and transverse planes (**Fig. 1A**). Volume data can be viewed using a standard anatomic orientation demonstrating entire volume and continuity of curved structures in a single image. More accurate evaluation of numerous sections through the studied organ becomes possible due to unlimited numbers and the orientations of reformatted planes. When three perpendicular axes are simultaneously displayed on the screen, the sagittal plane is chosen for volume measurements whereas the other two planes are used for pathological determinations. Surface rendering mode allows exploration of the outer or inner contour of the lesion, while "niche aspect" presents detection and analysis of the selected sections of the uterine lesion. Three-dimensional ultrasound offers improved visualization of the lesions, more accurate volume estimation, retrospective review of stored data, and assessment of tumor invasion. Additionally, rendered image can accurately identify location of abnormalities eventually requiring surgical intervention.

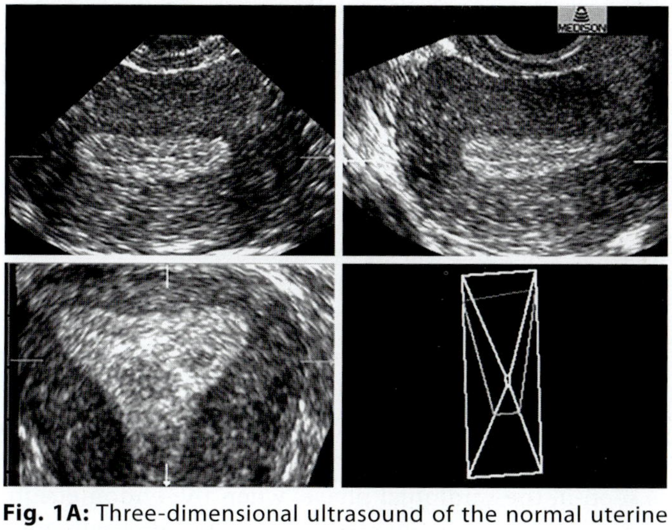

Fig. 1A: Three-dimensional ultrasound of the normal uterine cavity. Note secretory appearance of the endometrium and triangular shape of the uterine cavity in frontal reformatted section (low left image).

Assessment of the uterine cavity can be improved with the use of hysterosonography, a technique that involves distension of the uterine cavity with the injection of sterile saline (saline infusion sonography—SIS). **Figure 1B** shows normal uterine cavity morphology assessed by 3D SIS or hysterosonography. Smooth and echogenic endometrium is visualized along the periphery of the uterine cavity distended with sonolucent fluid. 3D SIS allows simultaneous assessment of the uterine cavity in longitudinal, transverse and coronal planes, and contributes to improved visualization of submucosal fibroids and endometrial polyps.

The three-dimensional power Doppler system improves the information available on normal and abnormal (tumoral) vascularity, enabling visualization of overlapping vessels and assessment of their relationship to other vessels or surrounding tissue. Power Doppler ultrasound, compared to standard color Doppler has

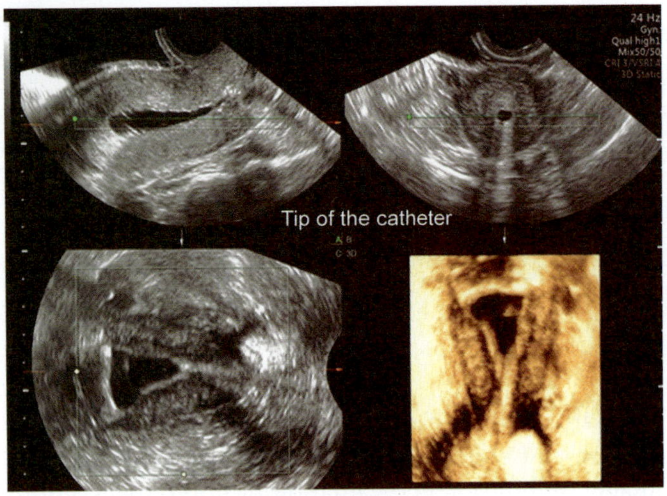

Fig. 1B: Saline infusion sonography or hysterosonography by three-dimensional ultrasound. Tip of the catheter is indicated by arrows.

the advantage of more sensitivity-to-low velocity flow overcoming the angle dependence and aliasing. Using contrast agents it is possible to enhance the three-dimensional power Doppler examination rate of small vessels.

In this chapter findings of uterine lesions with conventional B-mode will be compared with those by transvaginal color Doppler ultrasound and three-dimensional and power Doppler ultrasound.

NORMAL UTERUS

Use of two-dimensional ultrasound imaging of the uterus is limited due to the movement of the transducer allowing sagittal and transverse planes through the uterus. Three-dimensional sonography permits multiplanar display of all three perpendicular sections: coronal, sagittal, and transverse plane **(Figs. 1A and B)**. The coronal plane of the uterus enables simultaneous visualization of endometrial horns and cervix. The normal uterus is usually presented by a convex shape of the endometrium and myometrium in the fundus. Blood vessels of the uterus and endometrium can be detected by color and power Doppler ultrasound where endometrium and myometrium constitute an anatomical and functional unit. Uterine arteries branch off the internal iliac arteries. Ultrasonically, they look like hyperechoic structures running along the cervix and the isthmic part of the uterus. Arcuate arteries are tortuotic anechoic structures that spread through myometrium. Radial arteries penetrate vertically through the myometrial layers of smooth muscle cells. Spiral arteries supply to the *stratum functionale* of the endometrium. Shape and size of this layer of endometrium changes during the menstrual cycle and it sheds during menstruation along with glandular tissue. During pregnancy, these arteries become uteroplacental decidual arteries. Basal arterioles supply to the endometrial *stratum basale*, which remains unchanged during menstruation. Color Doppler research has identified unique waveform from each blood vessel. These waveforms are influenced by several factors including hormones, ischemia, and internal or external vasoactive factors. The vessels in genital tract undergo cyclic changes dictated by the hormonal cycle. During the menstrual phase, due to hormonal deprivation and alterations in the spiral arteriolar system, spiral arteries undergo increased coiling and cause a circulatory stasis that leads to tissue ischemia. Vasoconstriction of the spiral arterioles and necrosis of their walls results in bleeding. Visualization of anechoic areas indicate endometrial breakdown. Subsequently, mixed appearance of anechoic area (indicating blood) and hyperechoic parts (exfoliated endometrium and clots) can be observed. During the late menstrual phase, the endometrium appears sonographically as a thin, single-line, slightly irregular echogenic interface. In this phase, the uterine artery shows high resistance index. In the early follicular phase, the endometrium is imaged as a hyperechoic line with endometrial thickness of less than 5 mm, and visualization of the endometrial-myometrial junction is difficult. As ovulation approaches, glands become numerous and the expected endometrial thickness is about 10 mm. A triple-line endometrium is typical of the peri-ovulatory phase. The hyperechoic echo that represents the endometrial-myometrial junction becomes more prominent and does not produce posterior enhancement. The central echogenic interface probably represents refluxed mucus. Doppler velocimetry of the spiral arteries shows progressive diminution of resistance indices. Secretory phase is characterized by hyperechoic and homogenous endometrium with a loss of the triple-line morphology and surrounding anechoic halo. During this phase of the cycle the ultrasonographic image of the endometrium shows increased echogenicity with respect to the myometrium. The interface of the myometrium with the endometrium is still visible as a hypoechoic zone. Maximum echogenicity is seen in the midluteal phase, when the endometrium appears homogenously hyperechoic. Posterior enhancement is a sonographic characteristic of this phase. Doppler velocimetry demonstrates further decrease of the vascular resistance in uterine and spiral arteries being the lowest in the midluteal phase.

The postmenopausal endometrium typically appears as a thin echogenic line **(Fig. 2A)**. A small amount of endometrial fluid may be seen in postmenopausal patients due to mild cervical stenosis. This fluid should be excluded from the endometrial thickness measurement. A thin endometrium (<4 mm) may be used reliably to exclude endometrial cancer in postmenopausal patients presenting with vaginal bleeding. Postmenopausal endometrium is avascular and occasionally calcifications of the arcuate arteries may be visualized in the outer third of the myometrium **(Figs. 2A and B)**.

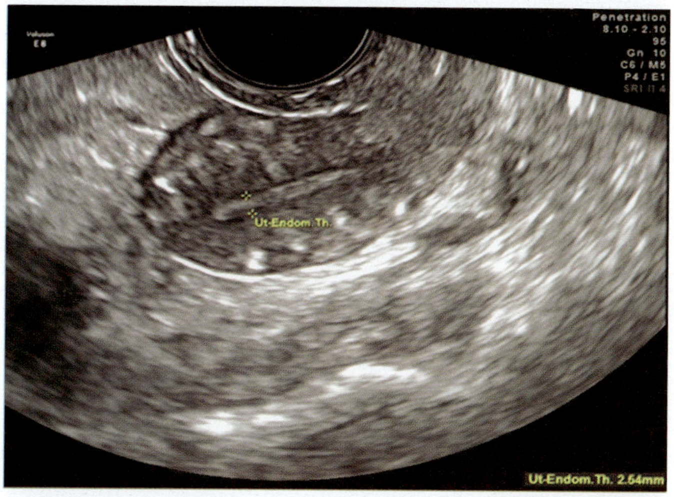

Fig. 2A: Transvaginal ultrasound image of a postmenopausal uterus with thin endometrium (2.5 mm). Calcifications of the arcuate arteries are visualized in the outer third of the myometrium.

Since, changes in the texture and volume of the endometrium can be precisely observed using three-dimensional ultrasound, and retrospectively reviewed by experts, this method may become a method of choice for scanning endometrial pathology in multitude of clinical conditions.

ENDOMETRIAL POLYPS

Endometrial polyps develop as solitary or multiple, sessile or pedunculated soft tumors containing hyperplastic endometrium.[1,2] Patients with endometrial polyps maybe clinically asymptomatic or may present with abnormal genital tract bleeding, infertility, or pain. Ultrasonographic appearance of endometrial polyps is best imaged during the early proliferative phase of the menstrual cycle or during the secretory phase after injection of a negative contrast medium into the uterine cavity **(Fig. 3A)**. The vascularization of polyps is supported by already existing vessels originating from terminal branches of the uterine arteries assessed by transvaginal color Doppler ultrasound **(Fig. 3B)**. It is possible to identify flow in regularly separated vessels and analyze the velocity of blood flow through them. The resistance index is moderate, usually higher than 0.45[1,3] **(Fig. 3C)**. Infection or necrosis of polyps may lower the impedance to blood flow (RI_{MIN} = 0.37). The importance of endometrial polyps lies in the fact that marked reduction in blood flow impedance noted on the periphery and/or within the endometrial polyps may lead an inexperienced ultrasonographer to a false positive diagnosis of endometrial malignancy.

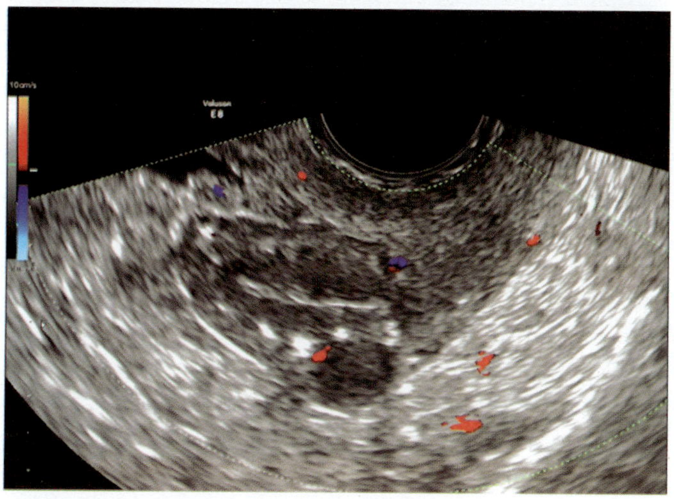

Fig. 2B: Color Doppler ultrasound of postmenopausal uterus. Note thin and hyperechoic avascular endometrium.

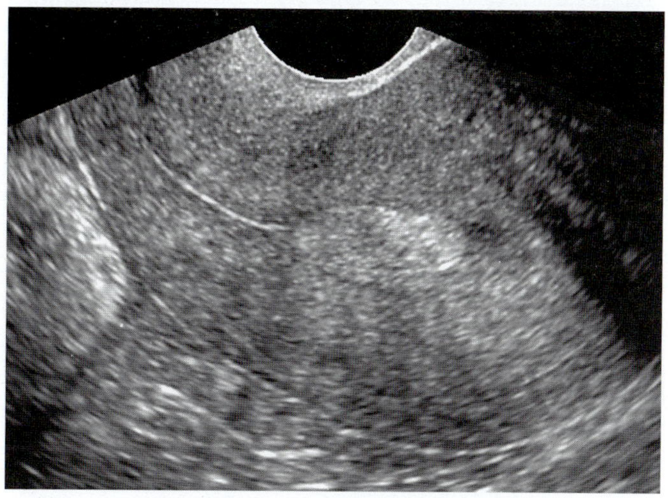

Fig. 3A: Focal endometrial lesion by transvaginal ultrasound.

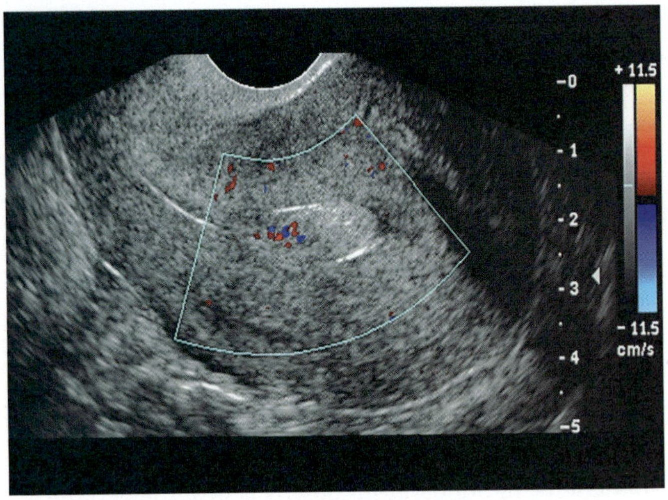

Fig. 3B: Color Doppler scan of an endometrial polyp demonstrating stalk vessels.

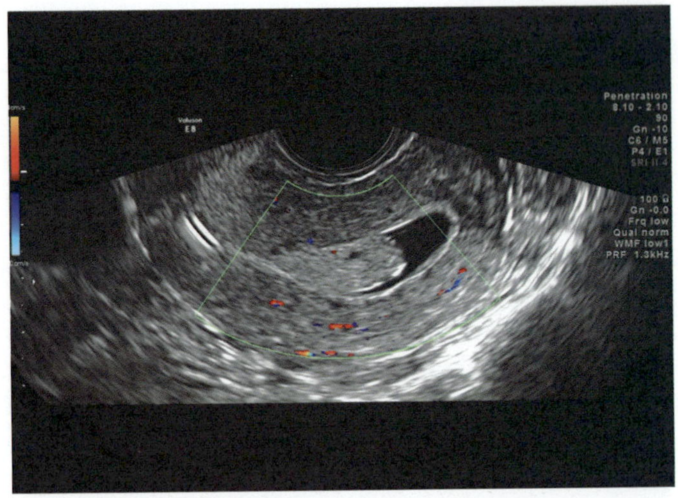

Fig. 3D: Focal endometrial thickening demonstrated by saline infusion sonography with color Doppler ultrasound.

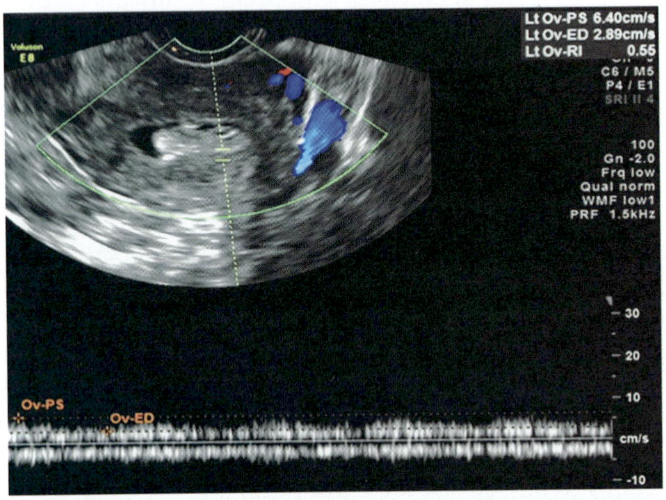

Fig. 3C: Pulsed Doppler waveform signals obtained from regularly separated vessels from the base of an endometrial polyp reveal low velocity and moderate vascular impedance (RI 0.55).

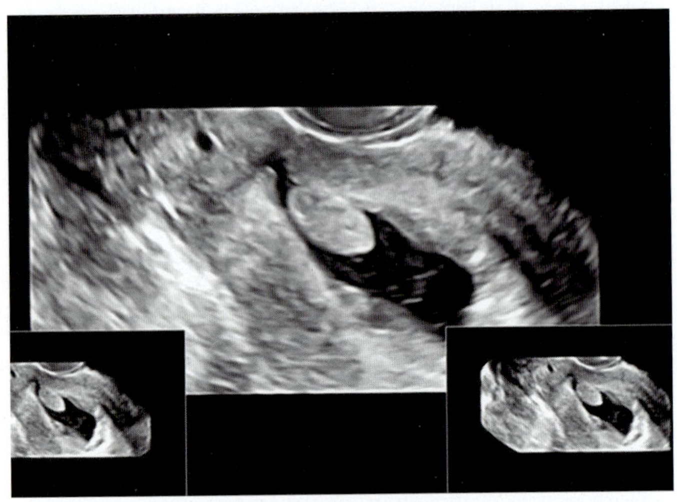

Fig. 3E: 3D saline infusion sonography shows an endometrial polyp protruding into the uterine cavity.

Saline infusion sonography (SIS) and 3D ultrasound are sensitive diagnostic modalities for detection of endometrial polyps, intrauterine adhesions, submucous/intracavitary leiomyomata and congenital uterine anomalies, highly comparable to MRI and hysteroscopy. **Figures 3D and E** illustrate an endometrial polyp protruding into the uterine cavity demonstrated by color Doppler and 3D ultrasound saline infusion sonography.

Tamoxifen is a non-steroidal antiestrogen that is widely used in the hormonal therapy of breast cancer. However, the weak estrogen-like effect that tamoxifen has on the endometrium is a cause of great concern. Patients using tamoxifen should, therefore, be monitored at regular intervals, since several studies have described cases of endometrial cancer associated with this therapy. A wide spectrum of pathological uterine findings has been described in association with long-term tamoxifen therapy at a dose of 20 mg/day.[4] These findings include epithelial metaplasia, simple and atypical hyperplasia, endometrial polyps and endometrial carcinoma.[5] Endometrial changes are characterized sonographically by abnormal endometrial thickening and non-homogenous hyperechogenicity, with multiple, small cystic structures **(Fig. 4A)**.

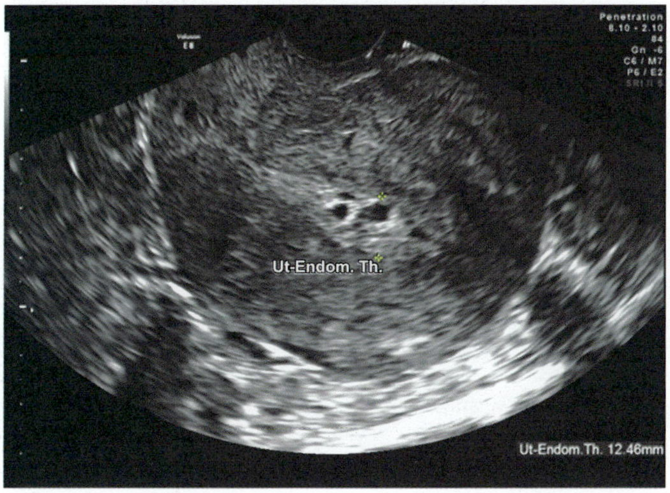

Fig. 4A: Transvaginal ultrasound of a postmenopausal patient using long-term tamoxifen therapy. Note hyperechogenic thickened endometrium with honeycomb appearance.

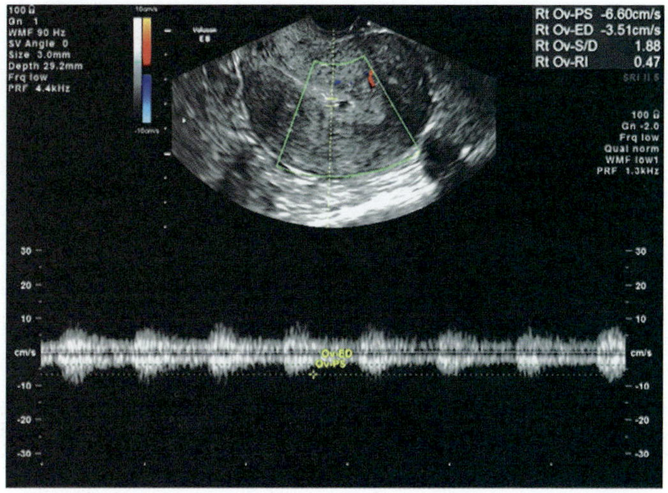

Fig. 4B: The same case as on previous figure. Pulsed Doppler waveform analysis obtained from thickened endometrium reveals low to moderate vascular impedance (RI = 0.47).

At least three studies indicate that tamoxifen treatment in postmenopausal breast cancer patients is associated with a high incidence of endometrial polyps.[6-8] Achiron et al.[7] found that a peculiar endometrial honeycomb appearance, manifested on gray-scale transvaginal sonography, occurred in 44% of this population, and was associated with the same high incidence (40%) of endometrial polyps. The effect of tamoxifen on endometrial blood flow has not been extensively evaluated. Achiron and his group described blood flow changes in the endometrial and subendometrial regions. In asymptomatic postmenopausal patients receiving tamoxifen whose endometrial thickness was less than 5 mm, increased endometrial blood flow with significant reduction of the resistance index compared to untreated, control menopausal women was reported. Another study by the same authors[5] found that women with thick endometrium, and particularly those with endometrial polyps, presented a significantly lower RI, compared to those with thin endometrium (mean RI of 0.39 versus 0.79). The RI values returned to normal following resection of the endometrial polyps, thus supporting a benign transitory effect of long-term tamoxifen therapy on the endometrium **(Fig. 4B)**. The data from Goldstein et al.[9] suggest that the objective assessment of blood flow impedance (resistance index, pulsatility index) in endometrial polyps and the size of these polyps cannot replace surgical removal and pathologic evaluation to predict histologic type. Patients with nonfunctional polyps were older and less likely to have vaginal bleeding.

Perez-Medina et al.[10] evaluated the efficacy of color Doppler exploration for assessing atypia inside endometrial polyps (polyp stalk). Thirty-five polyps (out of 106) with sonographic indications of atypia were pathologically confirmed. Sonographic indications of atypia inside 16 polyps were not confirmed. Three nonquestionable endometrial polyps had atypia inside them. They concluded that low Doppler resistance (RI <0.50) is highly predictive of atypia inside endometrial polyps.

Three-dimensional saline infusion sonography offers a better visualization of the uterine cavity and the endometrial thickness as compared to transvaginal sonography, 2D saline infusion sonography, transvaginal color Doppler, or hysteroscopy according to Bonilla-Musoles et al.[11] Multiplanar views in three-dimensional SIS can be used to visualize polypoid structures allowing optimal plane to present their pedicle. Surface rendering mode can suppress undesirable echoes offering further clarity in visualization of polypoid structure in continuity with the endometrial lining.[12]

Gruboeck et al.[13] performed the measurements of endometrial thickness assessed by conventional two-dimensional ultrasound and endometrial volume assessed with three-dimensional ultrasound in symptomatic postmenopausal patients and compared the results. The volume measurement is performed using longitudinal plane delineating the whole of the uterine cavity in a number of parallel longitudinal sections 1–2 mm apart.

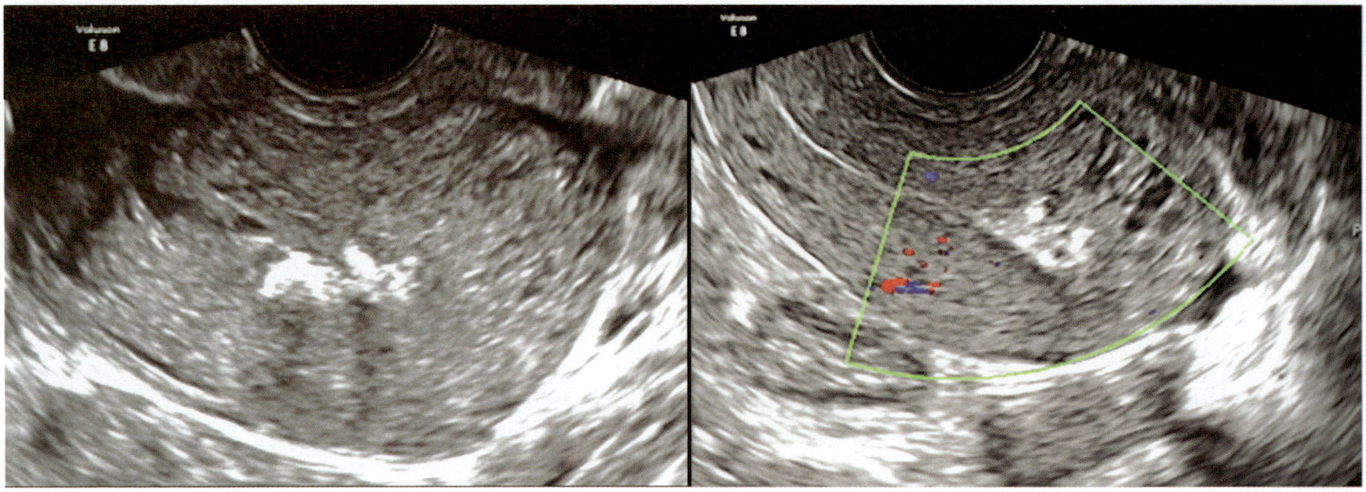

Fig. 5A: Irregular hyperechogenic bridges visualized within the central part of the uterine cavity in a patient with secondary amenorrhea following dilatation and curettage. Intrauterine adhesions do not display increased vascularity on color Doppler examination.

Endometrial volume is then calculated by the software program. The endometrial thickness was similar in patients with endometrial hyperplasia and polyps, but the endometrial volume in hyperplasia was significantly higher than the volume in patients with polyps. Polyps, localized thickenings of the endometrium, do not affect the entire uterine cavity and thus have a smaller volume albeit having similar thickness to that of hyperplasia. In conclusion, differences between endometrial hyperplasia and polyps cannot be detected by sole measurement of endometrial thickness but can be clearly identified based on three-dimensional volume measurement.

INTRAUTERINE SYNECHIAE (ADHESIONS)

Destruction of the basal layer of the endometrium may result in development of bands of scar tissue (synechiae) in the uterine cavity. This damage of endometrium may occur as a result of vigorous curettage of an advanced pregnancy. Infection with tuberculosis may also cause uterine adhesions. Menstrual pattern is characterized by amenorrhea or hypomenorrhea. Ultrasound scan of a patient with Asherman's syndrome shows a mixed picture: in some parts of uterine cavity no endometrium is visualized, whereas in other parts there is appearance of a normal endometrium. Adhesions in the uterine cavity are visualized as hyperechoic bridges. Intrauterine adhesions do not display increased vascularity on color Doppler examination **(Fig. 5A)**. They are better visualized during menstruation when intracavitary fluid outlines them. An alternative is saline infusion sonography or SIS.

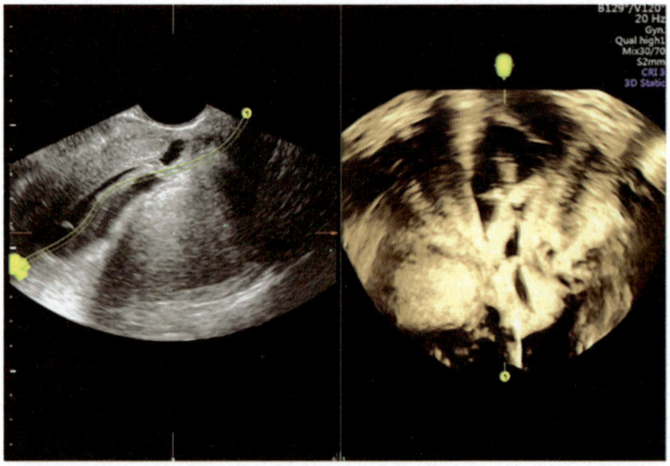

Fig. 5B: Three-dimensional SIS demonstrating a thick adhesion transversing the uterine cavity. 3D SIS determines intrauterine adhesion location and is helpful in surgical planning.

SIS with 3D ultrasound has several advantages over that with conventional 2D ultrasound **(Fig. 5B)**. It gives more accurate information about the location of abnormalities which is very important for preoperative assessment and distinguishing pathologies. Furthermore in SIS, compared to 2D examinations, the uterus is distended for a shorter time translating to better patients' acceptance. However, according to Momtaz et al.[14] in cases of intrauterine adhesions, the use of echogenic contrast media (e.g., Echovist, Schering) is more accurate than 3D SIS. Intrauterine synechiae can be accurately visualized on both multiplanar and rendered imaging traversing the uterine cavity.[12] Weinraub et al.[12] concluded that surface rendering in cases of equivocal signals confirmed their presence, appearance, actual size, volume, and relationship to the surrounding structures.

Three-dimensional SIS is helpful in delineation of intracavitary adhesions and determination of their location which assists in surgical planning. In the cases of bridging adhesions, the degree of cavity obliteration is accurately assessed. Similarly, this technique is beneficial for differentiation between small polyps and adhesions.

ADENOMYOSIS

Adenomyosis of the uterus is a condition in which clusters of endometrial tissue grow into the myometrium. It may be localized close to endometrium, or may extend through the myometrium and serosa. Adenomyosis affects 20% of women, mainly multiparous. The uterus can be normal-sized or enlarged with symptoms such as dysmenorrhea, pelvic pain, and menometrorrhagia.

Two-dimensional ultrasound findings include "Swiss cheese" appearance of the myometrium due to areas of hemorrhage and clots within the muscle **(Figs. 6A and B)**. Disordered echogenicity of the middle layer of the myometrium is usually present in severe cases. Sometimes, the uterus is generally hypoechoic, with the large cysts rarely seen. On SIS or HSG, contrast medium penetrates the myometrium. Color Doppler characteristics present increased vascularity by moderate vascular resistance within the myometrium (RI = 0.56 ± 0.12), while the RI of the uterine arteries show a decreased value compared to controls **(Figs. 6C and D)**.[15] Statistically significant differences exist between adenomyosis and uterine malignancies in both RI and maximum velocity. However, no significant difference was noted between adenomyosis and myoma in RI but slight differences were observed in maximum velocity.[16]

In some cases, transonic areas may not represent adenomyosis, but prominent vessels, or other conditions which give rise to hyperemia. Lee et al.[17] performed the study which confirmed the superiority of 3D power Doppler sonography compared to transvaginal color Doppler ultrasound in the detection of flow in the areas

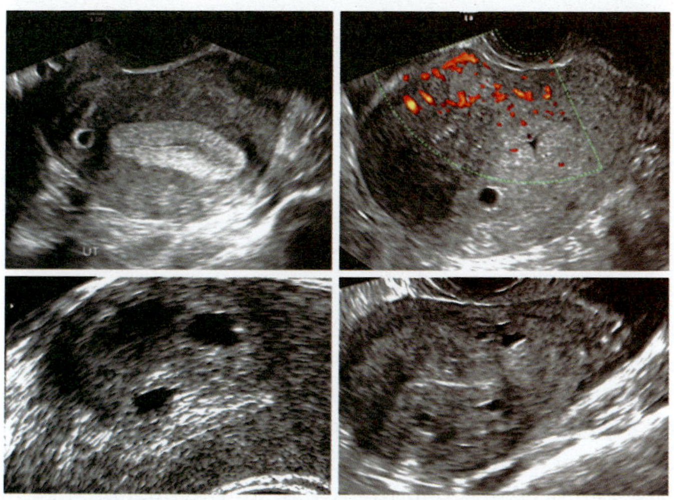

Fig. 6A: Transvaginal sonography of adenomyosis. Solitary focus of adenomyosis localized close to the endometrium is visualized on the upper left image, while multiple cystic structures within all three layers of the myometrium, typical of severe adenomyosis are demonstrated on the lower images.

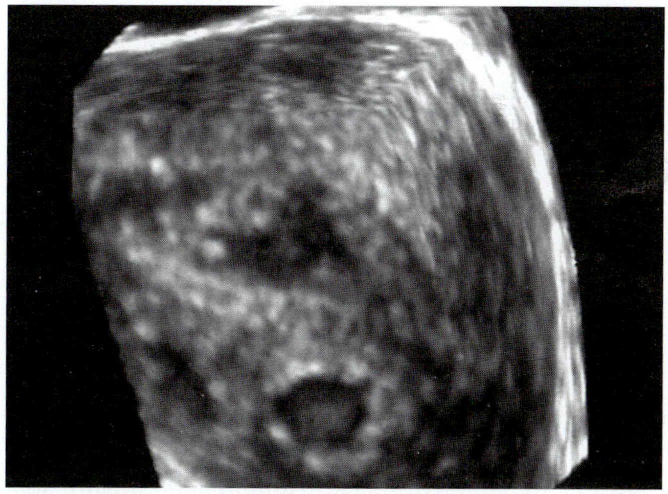

Fig. 6B: "Swiss cheese" appearance of the myometrium on three-dimensional ultrasound is typical of deep adenomyosis. Cystic lesions are visualized within the myometrial layer of the uterus.

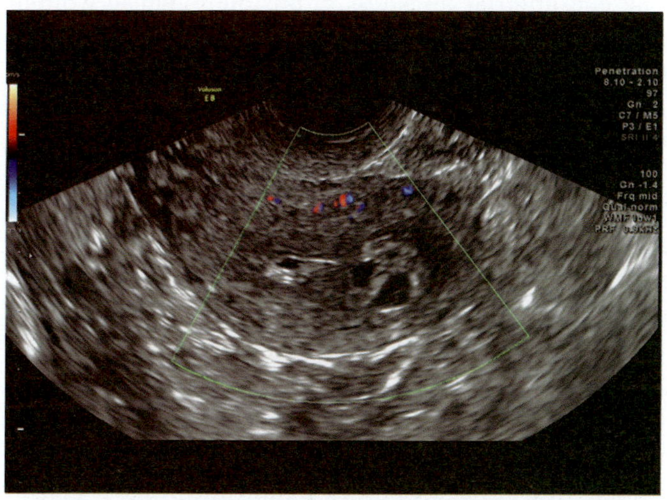

Fig. 6C: Transvaginal color Doppler scan of severe adenomyosis.

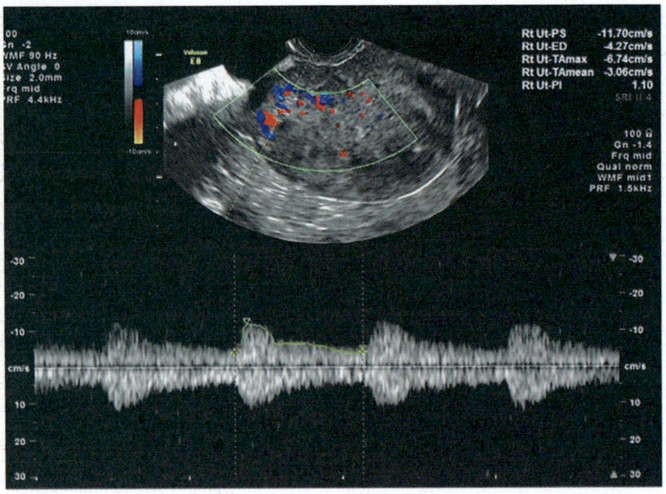

Fig. 6D: Moderate-to-high vascular impedance blood flow signals (RI of 0.56) are detected at the periphery of adenomyotic lesions.

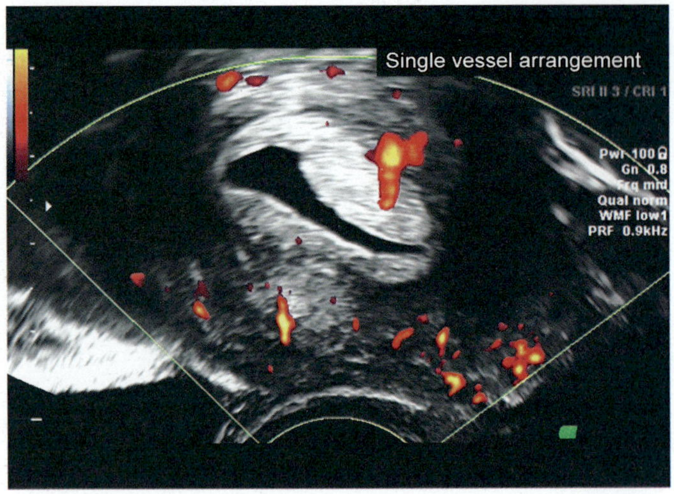

Fig. 7: Single vessel arrangement obtained by power Doppler ultrasound in a patient with endometrial hyperplasia.

of adenomyosis. Women with a provisional diagnosis of adenomyosis listed for hysterectomy were studied. Gray scale ultrasound was first used to screen for the presence of adenomyosis using predetermined ultrasound criteria. Then 3D power Doppler sonography of adenomyotic areas was performed. Ultrasound findings such as distribution of vessels and pattern of flow in adenomyotic foci were compared with histological results. The same method was used for tracing regular vessels' course in this abnormality. Using 3D power Doppler sonography, authors were not only able to demonstrate perfusion in adenomyotic foci but also the vessels' distribution and branching pattern.

ENDOMETRIAL HYPERPLASIA

The endometrial thickness in postmenopausal women is no more than a thin line of 1–3 mm. Abnormal endometrial thickness may be detected in some benign uterine conditions, as well as in the endometrial malignancy. Endometrial thickness greater than 14 mm in premenopausal and greater than 5 mm in postmenopausal women should be further investigated.[1] B-mode transvaginal sonography by itself is insufficient to distinguish between endometrial hyperplasia and carcinoma. More accurate diagnosis of endometrial pathology can be obtained by color and pulsed Doppler sonography[2,3] **(Fig. 7)**. Color Doppler findings characteristically for endometrial hyperplasia include peripheral distribution of the regularly separated vessels with resistance index significantly higher (mean RI = 0.55 ± 0.05) **(Figs. 8A and B)** than in carcinoma

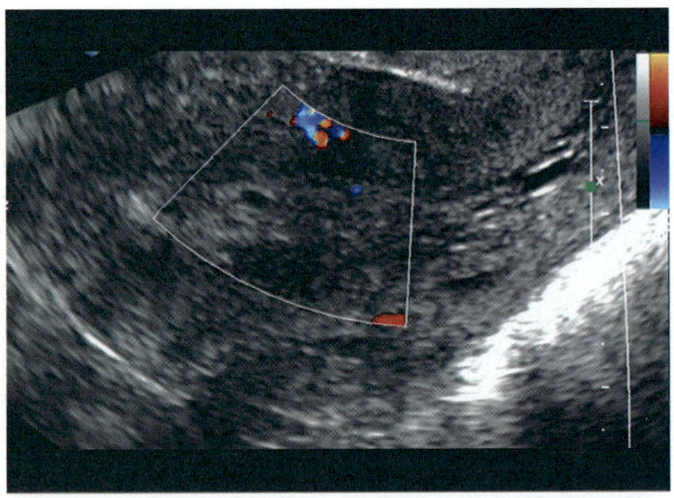

Fig. 8A: Color Doppler ultrasound of endometrial hyperplasia.

(mean RI = 0.42 ± 0.02).[18] However, reliable differentiation between endometrial hyperplasia and carcinoma is not possible due to an overlap in the endometrial thickness measurements, as well as because of the controversial results of blood flow measurements assessed by transvaginal color Doppler ultrasound. Since, there is a positive correlation between arterial blood flow impedance and number of years from menopause,[19] one can presume that the risk of uterine malignancy is increased for postmenopausal patients with decreased uterine artery vascular resistance.

Emoto et al.[20] examined the usefulness of transvaginal color Doppler ultrasound in differentiating between

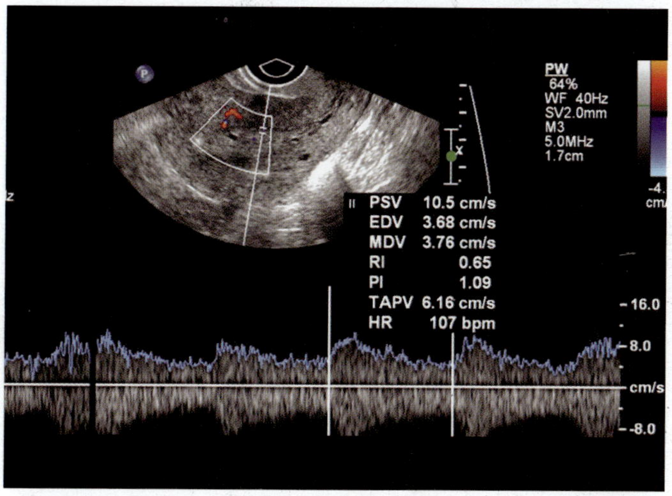

Fig. 8B: Pulsed Doppler waveform analysis of endometrial hyperplasia. Note moderate vascular impedance blood flow signals with RI of 0.65.

endometrial hyperplasia and endometrial carcinoma and in predicting tumor spread in patients with carcinoma. No significant difference was found in the mean value of endometrial thickness between patients with hyperplasia (n = 18 patients; 16.2 mm ± 15.9 mm) and patients with carcinoma (n = 53 patients; 18.7 mm ± 17.1 mm). Intratumoral blood flow was detected in significant numbers of patients who had endometrial carcinoma (71.7% 38 of 53 patients) compared with patients who had endometrial hyperplasia (5.6%; 1 of 18 patients; P <0.0001). This study implies that transvaginal color Doppler may be more useful in differentiating between endometrial hyperplasia and carcinoma than measuring endometrial thickness by transvaginal gray-scale sonography. For patients with carcinoma, the detection of intratumoral blood flow may be helpful in distinguishing between low-grade and high-grade tumors and predicting myometrial invasion. However, intratumoral blood flow analysis using RI, PI, or PSV may not be useful for predicting tumor spread before surgery.

Jarvela et al.[21] evaluated uterine blood flow changes in using transvaginal color Doppler ultrasonography after thermal balloon endometrial ablation therapy. Thermal balloon endometrial ablation induces a rise in uterine blood flow impedance, but not until 6 months after the treatment. The rise in impedance may be due to fibrosis in the uterine cavity which has been attributed to the thermal balloon therapy.

More recently, three-dimensional ultrasound has been successfully used for endometrial volume measurements. According to Gruboeck et al.[13] endometrial volume was measured in 94.2% of patients, while in others the presence of anterior uterine wall myomas caused acoustic shadowing on 3D records. The volume of the endometrium was measured by delineating the uterine cavity on parallel longitudinal sections 1–2 mm apart. The sections were added together using in-built software to calculate the volume. The endometrial volume was significantly lower in patients with benign pathology such as hyperplasia (mean 8.0 mL, SD 7.81 mL) than in patients with endometrial carcinoma (mean 39.0 mL, SD 34.16 mL). Normal endometrial volume in this study was 0.9 mL (SD 1.72 mL).

Kupesic et al.[18] reported on the use of 3D power Doppler sonography in patients with endometrial hyperplasia. They were able to demonstrate regularly separated vessels at the periphery of the examined endometrium.

Bonilla-Musoles et al. suggest that in patients on hormone replacement therapy or tamoxifen, 3D SIS allowed for differentiation of normal proliferative from hyperplastic endometrium.[11]

ENDOMETRIAL CARCINOMA

Endometrial carcinoma is the most common gynecological malignancy in many countries with the reported incidence of about 10% in postmenopausal patients presenting uterine bleeding. Early transabdominal sonographic investigations have demonstrated that increased endometrial thickness is associated with endometrial neoplasms in postmenopausal women, but the quality of transabdominal sonographic images is affected by obesity, retroversion of the uterus, and an unfilled bladder, factors that do not influence transvaginal sonographic visualization of the endometrium. Ultrasound findings assessed by conventional B-mode sonography include increased endometrial thickness >5 mm in postmenopausal women or >8 mm in perimenopausal women, hyperechoic endometrium, free fluid in the cul-de-sac, intrauterine fluid or possible invasion in patients with disrupted endometrial-subendometrial layer. In addition, color and pulsed Doppler improves diagnostic accuracy, because the endometrial carcinoma shows abnormal blood flow due to tumor angiogenesis.[22] Endometrial blood flow is absent in normal, atrophic and most cases of endometrial hyperplasia, while, according to Kupesic's investigation[18] in 91% of the cases of

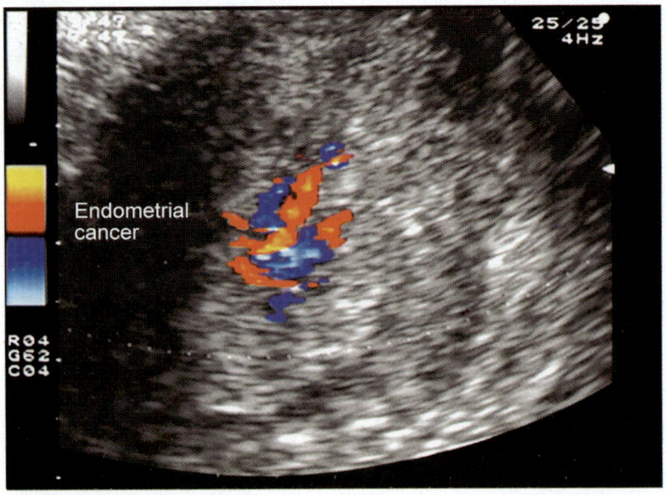

Fig. 9A: Thick heterogeneous endometrium with peripheral and intratumoral neovascularization demonstrated by color Doppler imaging.

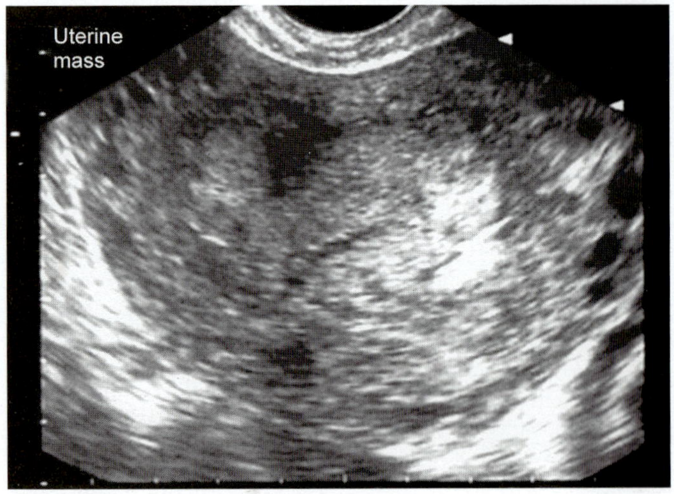

Fig. 10A: Transvaginal scan of a postmenopausal patient with enlarged and heterogeneous uterus. Using transvaginal ultrasound it was impossible to delineate an endometrial lining.

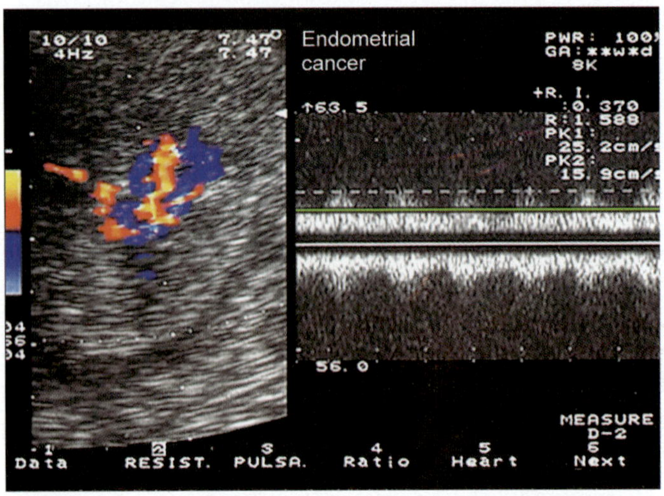

Fig. 9B: Color Doppler analysis shows low vascular resistance (RI 0.37). Endometrial malignancy was confirmed by histology.

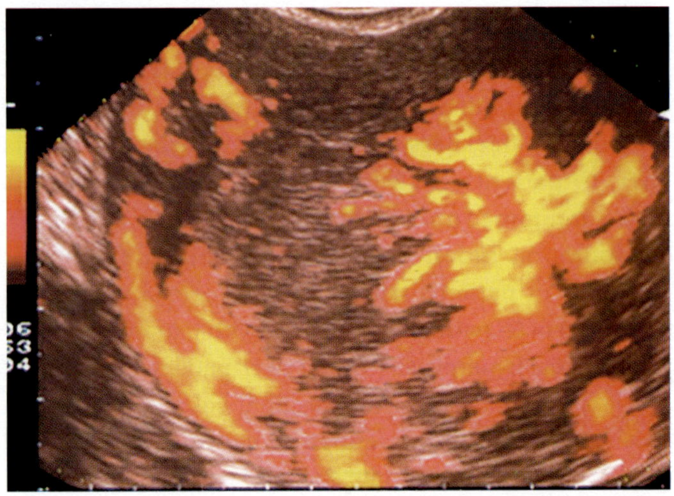

Fig. 10B: Power Doppler imaging demonstrates neovascular areas within the myometrium. Such a finding suggests deep myometrial invasion of an endometrial carcinoma.

endometrial carcinoma areas of neovascularization were demonstrated as intratumoral or peritumoral **(Figs. 9A and B)**. Neovascular signals from the central parts of the lesion demonstrate low vascular resistance (RI = 0.42 ± 0.02), while increased vascularity signals surrounding the lesion indicate tumor invasion. If the myometrial vessels are invaded, low vascular resistance is detected due to incomplete or absent membrane and leaky structure **(Figs. 10A to C)**. Postmenopausal patients with ill-defined endometrium presenting with vaginal bleeding may benefit from color and power Doppler imaging by 2D and 3D ultrasound **(Figs. 11A to C)**.

Conventional 2D ultrasound measurements of endometrial thickness have disadvantages in distinguishing patients with benign and malignant endometrial pathology due to varying thickness, and interference of other pathology like polyps or hypoplasia.

In distinguishing cancer from benign pathology endometrial volume measurements assessed by 3D ultrasound seems to be more helpful. Gruboeck et al.[13] compared endometrial thickness and volume in patients with postmenopausal bleeding and examined the value of each parameter in differentiating between benign and malignant endometrial pathology. Each patient underwent

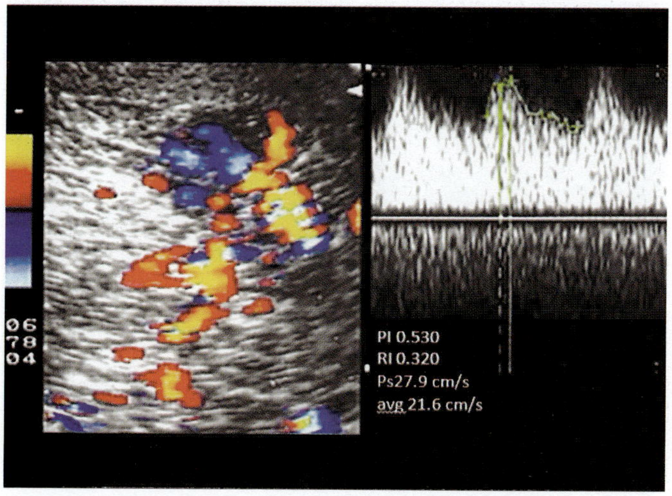

Fig. 10C: Low vascular impedance (RI 0.35) and high velocity of the blood flow (47.7 cm/s) suggest neovascularization within the deep myometrial layer. Histopathology revealed deep myometrial invasion.

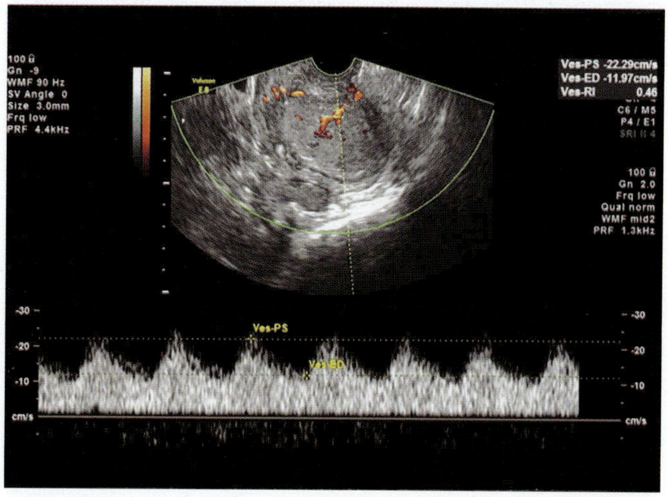

Fig. 11B: The same patient assessed by pulsed Doppler ultrasound. Low to moderate vascular impedance blood flow signals were obtained from the vessels within the proximal myometrial mantle.

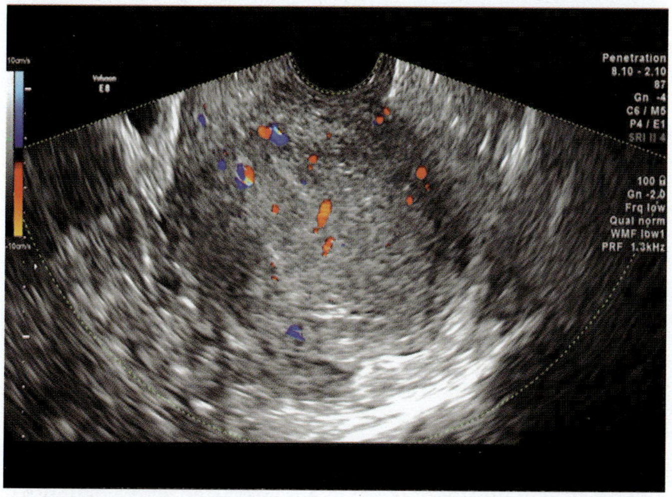

Fig. 11A: Ill-defined heterogeneous endometrium in a postmenopausal patient presenting with bleeding. Multiple randomly dispersed vessels are visualized within the endometrium and myometrium.

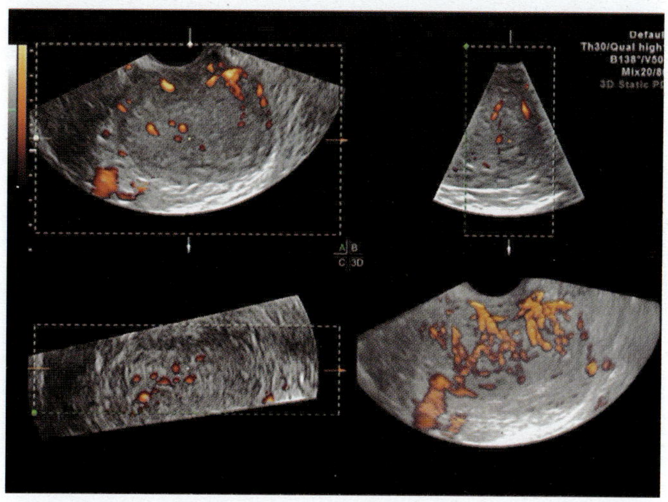

Fig. 11C: The same patient assessed by 3D power Doppler ultrasound shows chaotic vascular distribution and areas of densely packed irregular vessels. Sonographic and Doppler findings are suggestive of invasive endometrial cancer, which was confirmed by histology.

three-dimensional ultrasonography for the measurement of endometrial thickness and volume. The results were compared to the histological diagnosis after endometrial biopsy or dilatation and curettage. The mean endometrial thickness in patients with endometrial cancer was 29.5 mm (SD 12.59) and the mean volume was 39.0 mL (SD 34.16). The optimal cut-off value of endometrial thickness for the diagnosis of cancer was 15 mm, with the test sensitivity of 83.3% and positive predictive value of 54.4%. With a cut-off level of 13 mL, the diagnosis of cancer was made with the sensitivity of 100%. One false-positive result in a patient with hyperplasia gave a specificity of 98.8% and positive predictive value of 91.7%. According to these authors[13] the endometrial volume was significantly higher in patients with carcinoma than those with benign lesions. The measurements of endometrial volume were superior to endometrial thickness as a diagnostic test for the detection of endometrial cancer in symptomatic postmenopausal women. Increased volume size is associated with the severity or higher grade of the endometrial carcinoma,

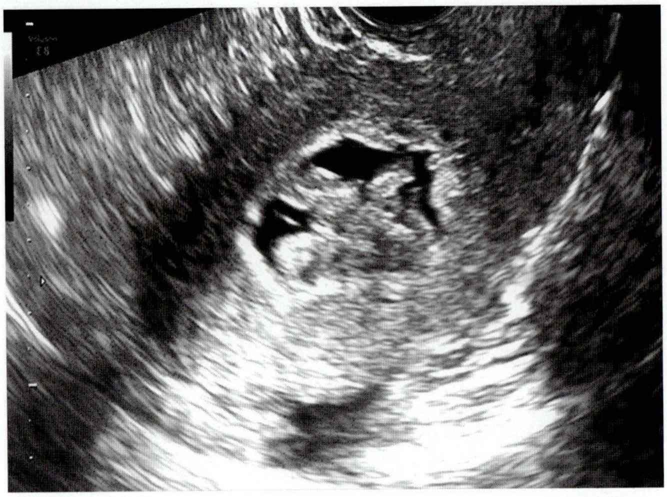

Fig. 12A: Saline infusion sonography reveals irregular polypoid masses originating from the posterios wall of the endometrial cavity.

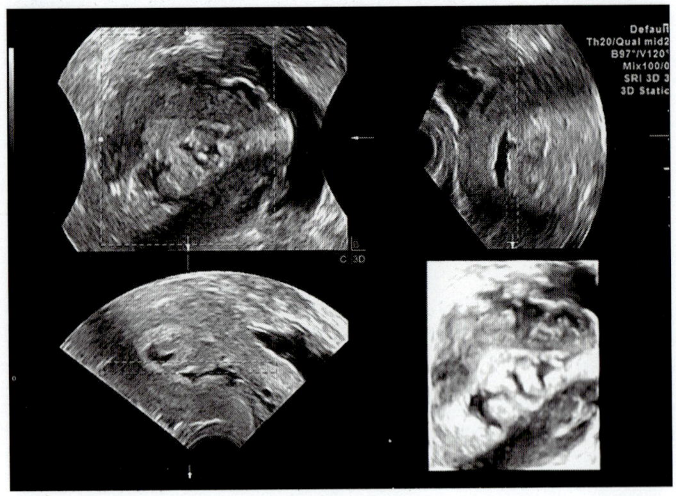

Fig. 12C: 3D saline infusion sonography of the same patient demonstrated irregular polypoid mass that proved to be endometrial carcinoma.

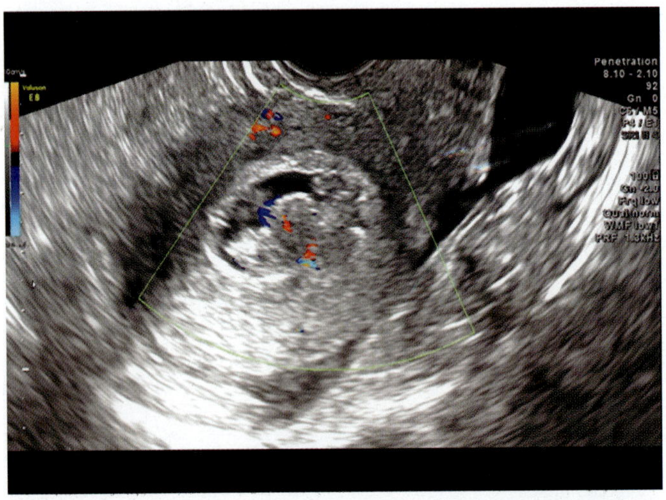

Fig. 12B: The same patient assessed by color Doppler ultrasound. Note multiple vessels with irregular branching pattern.

TABLE 1: Three-dimensional sonographic and power Doppler criteria for the diagnosis of endometrial malignancy.[23]

3D sonographic and power Doppler criteria		*Score*
Endometrial volume	<13 mL ≥13 mL	0 2
Subendometrial hallo	Regular Disturbed	0 2
Intracavitary fluid	Absent Present	0 1
Vessel's architecture	Linear vessel arrangement Chaotic vessel arrangement	0 2
Branching pattern	Simple Complex	0 2
Total score		

Total score = sum of individual scores
Cut-off score = greater or equal to 4 is associated with a high-risk of endometrial malignancy

and progressive myometrial invasion. The depth of myometrial invasion showed a positive correlation with both the endometrial thickness and the endometrial volume. Only patients with tumor volume larger than 25 mL had evidence of pelvic node involvement at operation.

2D and 3D SIS is a sensitive ultrasound technique for differentiating between focal and diffuse endometrial thickening in patients with postmenopausal bleeding **(Figs. 12A to C)**.

Bonilla et al.[11] suggest that 3D hysterosonography allowed for better visualization of myometrial invasion, which may have a significant role in malignant tumors staging. Using simultaneous display of the transverse plane with 3D ultrasound it is possible to detect infiltration of cervical or endometrial carcinoma into the bladder or rectum.

Apart from endometrial volume, Kupesic et al.[23] used 3D power Doppler sonographic criteria for diagnosis of endometrial malignancy together with the assessment of subendometrial halo, endometrial irregularity, presence of intracavitary fluid, chaotic vessel architecture, and branching pattern **(Table 1)**. In patients with endometrial carcinoma, mean endometrial volume was 37.0 ± 31.8 mL

TABLE 2: Volume and vascularity of the endometrial lesions (*N* = 57) obtained by 3D PDS.[23]

Histopathology	*N*	*V (SD) mL*	*Regular endometrial hallo (%)*	*Intracavitary fluid (%)*	*Neovascular signals (%)*
Normal and/or atrophic endometrium	10	0.8 (1.51)	100	20.00	0
Endometrial hyperplasia	27	7.82 (7.60)	100	37.00	0
Endometrial polyp	28	2.63 (2.12)	100	35.71	3.57
Endometrial carcinoma	12	37.0 (31.8)	66.67	41.67	100

TABLE 3: Invasion of endometrial carcinoma assessed with the aid of 3D.[24]

Invasion	*3D power Doppler*	*Pathohistology*
Superficial *	17	18
Deep **	5	4

*Invasion into less than a half of the total myometrial thickness
**Invasion into more than a half of the myometrial thickness

(Table 2). The endometrial volume in hyperplasia had the mean value of 7.82 ± 7.60 mL and was significantly higher than the volume in patients with polyps (mean 2.63 ± 2.12 mL). In patients with normal or atrophic endometrium the mean volume was 0.8 ± 1.51 mL. Subendometrial halo was regular in all patients with benign endometrial pathology, whereas 8 out of 12 patients with endometrial carcinoma had irregular endometrial-myometrial border. Intracavitary fluid was present in 4 patients with benign endometrial lesions and 5 patients with endometrial malignancy. Dichotomous branching and randomly dispersed vessels were detected in 91.67% of the patients with endometrial carcinoma, while single vessel arrangement and regular branching were typical for benign lesions. Three-dimensional power Doppler sonography accurately detected structural abnormalities of malignant tumor vessels such as microaneurysms, arteriovenous shunts, tumoral lakes, elongation and coiling. Combining morphological and power Doppler criteria, the diagnosis of endometrial carcinoma had a sensitivity of 91.67%. One false positive result was obtained in a patient with endometrial hyperplasia and one false negative in a patient with endometrial carcinoma receiving tamoxifen therapy. In this case endometrial lesion demonstrated regularly separated peripheral vessels, and was falsely interpreted as hyperplasia.

Kupesic et al.[24] performed staging of endometrial carcinoma by 3D power Doppler sonography. The objective of their study was to evaluate the accuracy of three-dimensional power Doppler sonography in determining the depth of myometrial invasion in patients in whom the adenocarcinoma of the endometrium has been proven. Sonographic results were compared relative to the amount of myometrial invasion measured by histology **(Table 3)**. Thirty-four patients with histologically proven adenocarcinoma of the endometrium were analyzed. Deep myometrial invasion (>50%) was present at postoperative histology in 5/22 (22.73%) women, while superficial was reported in 17/22 (77.23%). Three-dimensional power Doppler sonography demonstrated a sensitivity of 100% (5/5) and a specificity of 94.44% (17/18) for deep invasion, with a positive predictive value (PPV) of 83.33% (5/6) and a negative predictive value (NPV) of 100% (17/17). In only one patient with adenomyosis, invasion was overestimated by 3D power Doppler. Data showed acceptable accuracy in determining the depth of myometrial invasion in patients with adenocarcinoma. Thus, three-dimensional power Doppler sonography can potentially detect lesions that require aggressive intervention and thus direct to proper treatment.

Lee et al.[25] evaluated the relationship between blood flow in the tumor assessed by color Doppler ultrasound, microvessel density immunohistochemically, and vascular endothelial growth factor levels in endometrial carcinoma. Significantly lower RIs were noted in tumors of stage II or greater (0.37 compared with 0.50, $P < 0.001$), of high histologic grade (grade 3) (0.34 compared with 0.49, $P = 0.004$), with deep myometrial invasion (one-half depth or greater) (0.39 compared with 0.49, $P = 0.002$), with lymphovascular emboli (0.38 compared with 0.49, $P < 0.001$), or with lymph node metatasis (0.30 compared with 0.49, $P < 0.001$) compared with stage I tumors and tumors of histologic grade 1 or 2, with superficial myometrial invasion, without lymphovascular emboli, or with no lymph node metastasis. Increased vascular endothelial growth factor levels and microvessel density also were detected in tumors of stage II or greater, with lymphovascular emboli, or with lymph node metastasis. Resistance index, microvessel density, and vascular endothelial growth factor levels in the tumor showed linear correlations. Blood flow assessed by color Doppler ultrasound has histologic and biologic correlations with angiogenesis and vascular endothelial growth factor levels and may play an important role in predicting tumor progression and metastasis in patients with endometrial carcinoma.

Alcazar et al.[26] correlated intratumoral blood flow as assessed by transvaginal color Doppler ultrasound (resistance index and peak systolic velocity) with tumor histopathologic characteristics, tumoral stage, and risk for recurrence in endometrial carcinoma. Significantly lower RI was found in tumors with the following characteristics: infiltrative growth pattern, grade 3, infiltrating greater than or equal to 50% of the myometrium, cervical involvement, lymph-vascular space invasion, lymph node metastasis, stage greater than or equal to Ic, and high-risk for recurrence. Significantly higher PSV was found in grade 3 tumors, tumors which infiltrated more or equal to 50% of the myometrium, tumor stages greater or equal to Ic, and tumors with a high-risk for recurrence. Their data indicate that a correlation between intratumoral blood flow features and histopathological characteristics, tumor stage, and risk for recurrence exists in endometrial cancer.

Yaman et al.[27] evaluated the reproducibility of transvaginal three-dimensional (3D) endometrial volume measurement in patients with postmenopausal bleeding and compared the reproducibility of this technique to that of two-dimensional (2D) endometrial thickness measurement. Endometrial volume measurement by 3D ultrasound, showed better reproducibility than endometrial thickness measurements by 2D ultrasound.

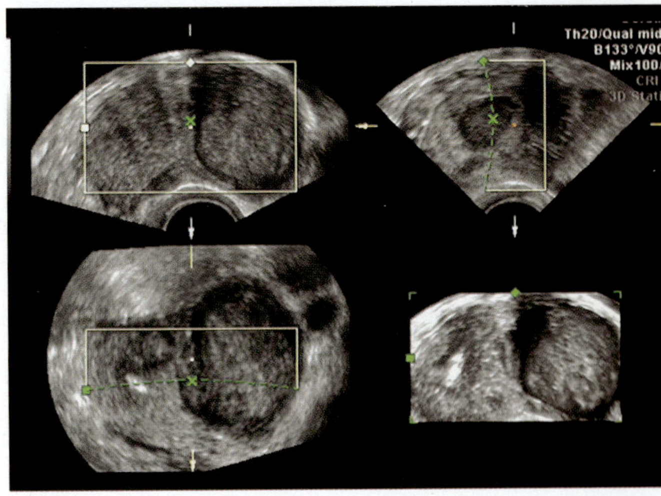

Fig. 13A: Three-dimensional ultrasound image of the uterus with multiple fibroids. A subserosal uterine fibroid is clearly visualized in three orthogonal planes and by surface rendering (right lower image).

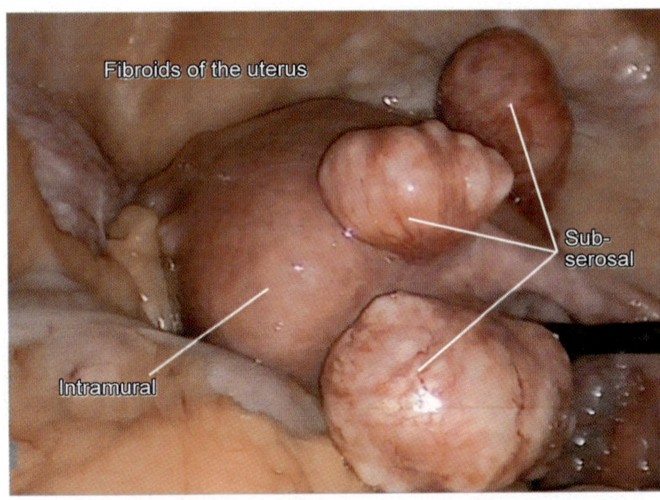

Fig. 13B: Laparoscopic image of the same patient. Note multiple uterine fibroids.

LEIOMYOMA

Leiomyomas are the most common tumors of the female pelvis and occur in 20–25% of women of reproductive age. Leiomyomas mostly arise from the smooth muscle and soft tissue of the uterine fundus and corpus **(Figs. 13A and B)**, while a small fraction originate from the cervix.[28] Myomas are usually multiple and of various sizes. Intramural tumors are the most common **(Figs. 14A and B)**, while the submucosal are the least common. SIS is a supplementary or adjunct imaging modality for characterization of focal uterine lesions diagnosed by transvaginal sonography, assessment of patients presenting with abnormal uterine bleeding, and preoperative mapping of the uterine fibroids **(Figs. 15A to D)**.

If they extend outward, they become either pedunculated or subserosal[29] **(Figs. 16A to C)**. If they extend toward the uterine cavity they become submucosal fibroids. Symptoms of submucosal leiomyomas include metrorrhagia, pelvic pain or infertility, whereas most subserosal leiomyomas are asymptomatic.

On the gray-scale ultrasound the uterine leiomyomas may be represented with uterine enlargement, distortion of the uterine contour, and varying echogenicity depending on the amount of connective or smooth muscle tissue. Transvaginal color Doppler sonography demonstrates vascularization on the periphery of the leiomyoma of uterine origin, with the RI of 0.54 ± 0.08, allowing better

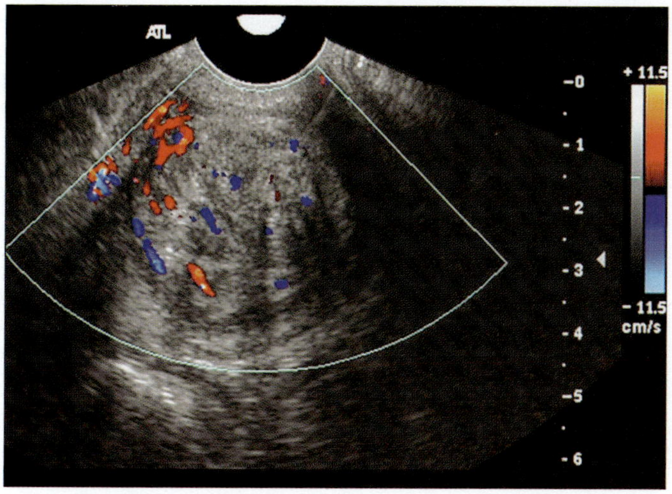

Fig. 14A: Color Doppler scan of an intramural fibroid.

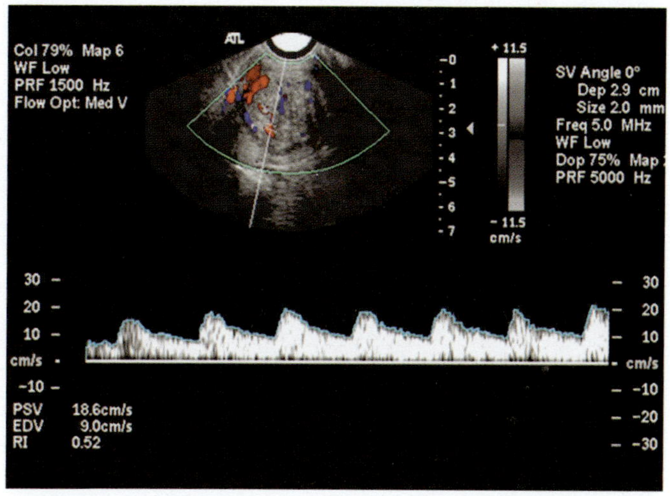

Fig. 14B: Pulsed Doppler waveform analysis demonstrated moderate vascular impedance blood flow signals at the periphery of the uterine fibroid, typical of a benign uterine lesion.

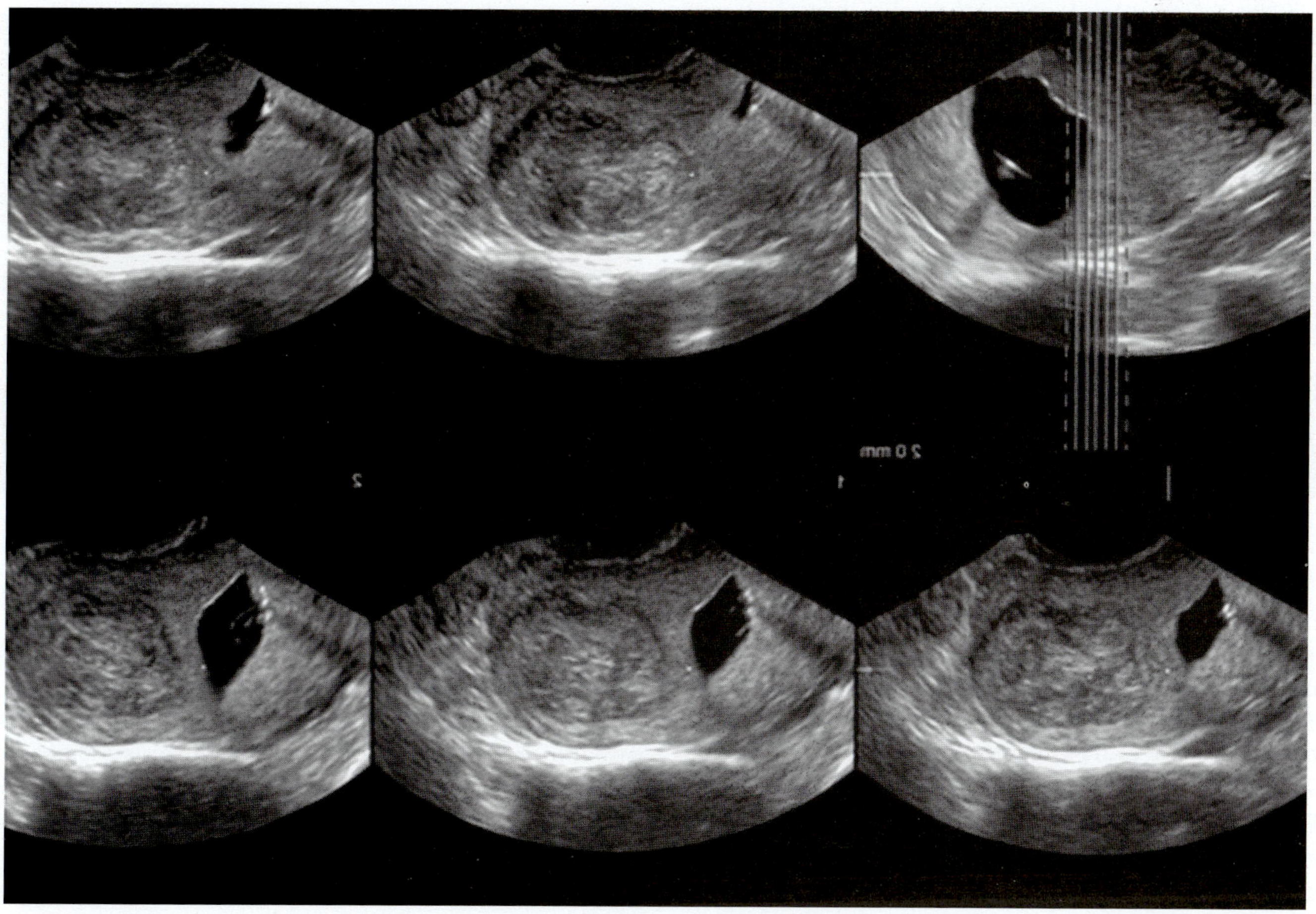

Fig. 15A: Tomographic ultrasound imaging after contrast enhancement with saline. Note distended uterine cavity and intramural/subserosal fibroid.

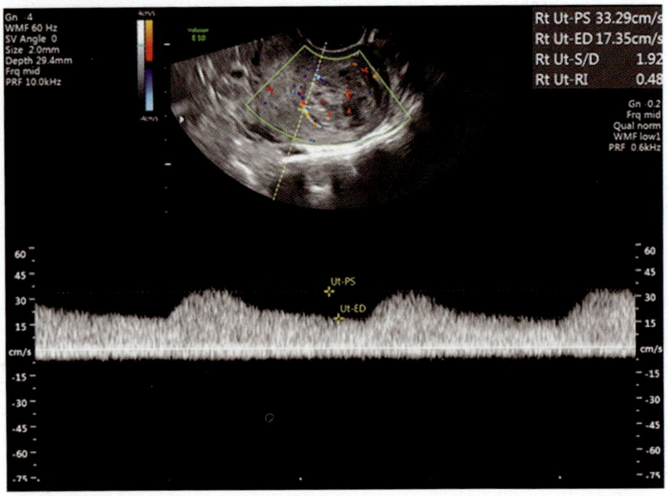

Fig. 15B: The same patient assessed by color and pulsed Doppler ultrasound. Low to moderate vascular impedance is obtained from uterine fibroid peripheral vessels.

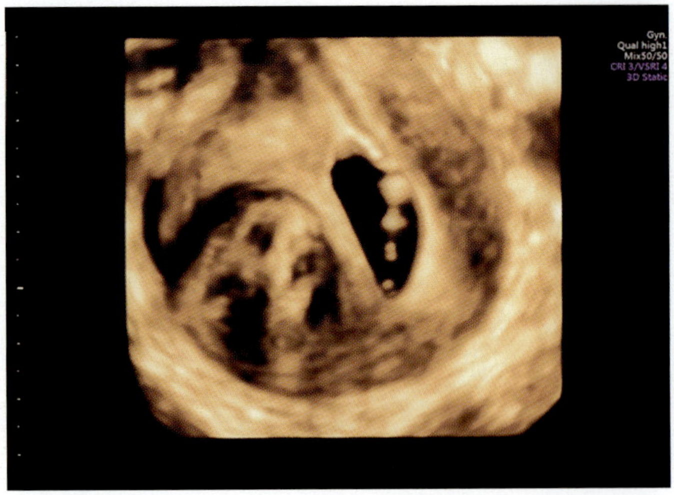

Fig. 15D: Surface rendering of intramural/subserosal fibroid with cystic degeneration following saline infusion sonography. Intrauterine catheter is clearly displayed within the distended uterine cavity.

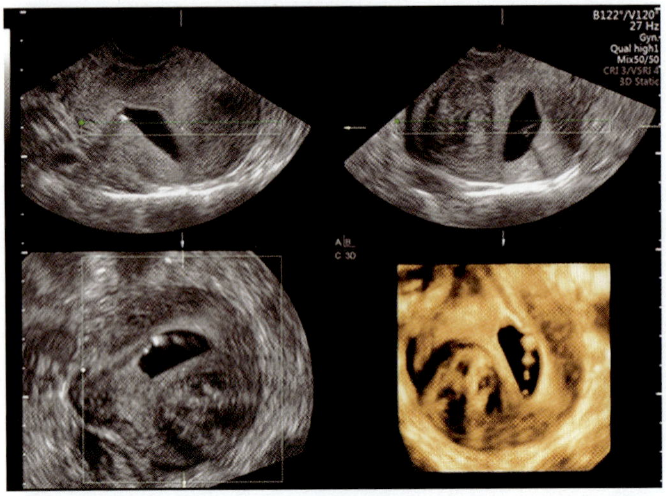

Fig. 15C: 3D saline infusion sonography enables superior mapping of the uterine fibroids.

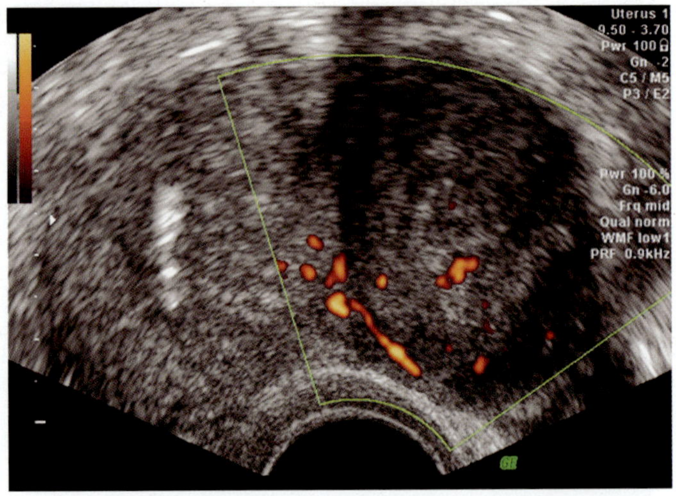

Fig. 16A: 2D color Doppler of the uterine artery branches supplying the subserosal fibroid.

delineation of the tumor **(Fig. 16B)**. Blood vessels in the central part of the myoma in case of necrosis, inflammation or other degenerative changes demonstrate lower RI. Uterine arteries present lower impedance to blood flow in patients with myomas (RI = 0.74 ± 0.09) compared to normal (RI = 0.84 ± 0.09).[30]

Simultaneous display of three perpendicular planes in 3D ultrasound demonstrates accurate location and size of leiomyomas, and their relationship to the endometrium that is very important in therapy planning. Patients receiving medical therapy such as gonadotropin-releasing hormone may be followed with serial 3D ultrasound scans to estimate myoma size and effectiveness of the therapy.

Saline infusion sonography by 3D ultrasound is valuable in obtaining submucosal fibroids **(Figs. 17A to D)**.[11-12,31,32] Balen et al.[31] found that 3D ultrasound and SIS was useful in demonstrating the position of submucosal myomas. They studied both saline and a positive ultrasound contrast agent (Echovist) and found the positive contrast to be superior when visualizing the cavity wall. Weinraub et al.[12] found that the negative contrast was better for accurately evaluating the contents of the uterine cavity

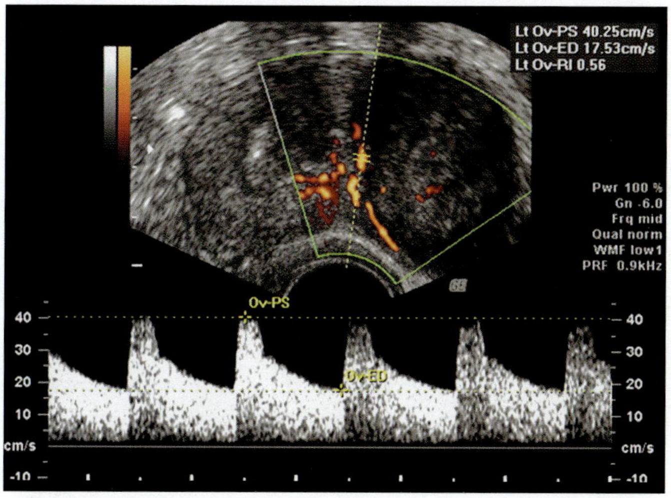

Fig. 16B: Moderate vascular impedance blood flow signals are isolated from the fibroid vessels using pulsed Doppler waveform analysis.

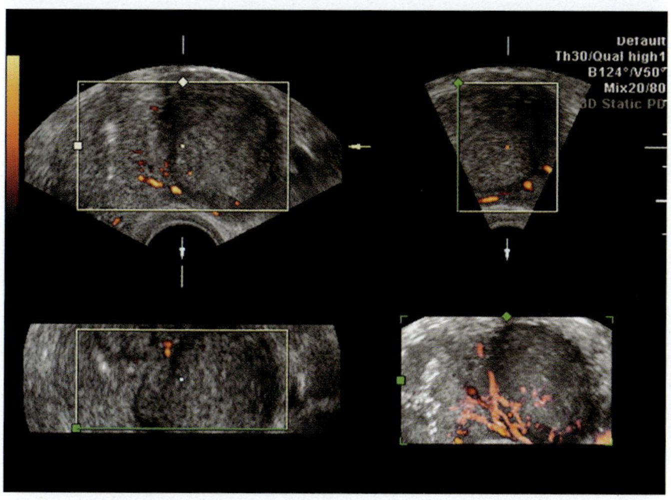

Fig. 16C: 3D power Doppler ultrasound of the subserosal fibroid.

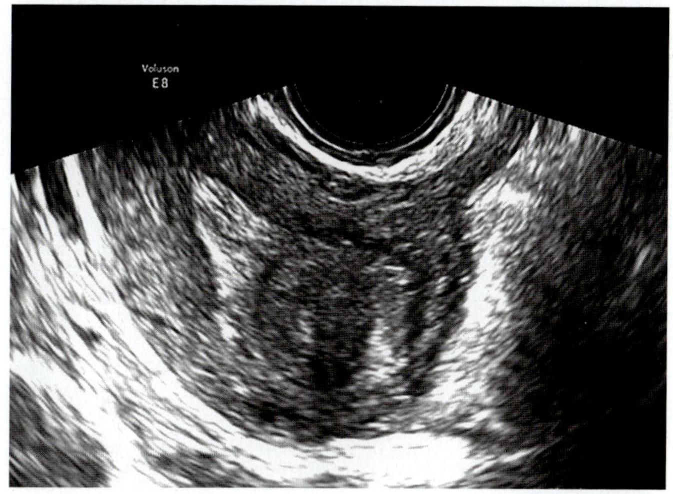

Fig. 17A: Transvaginal ultrasound image of a fibroid with discrete posterior shadowing. Using native scan it is impossible to differentiate between submucosal and intracavitary fibroid.

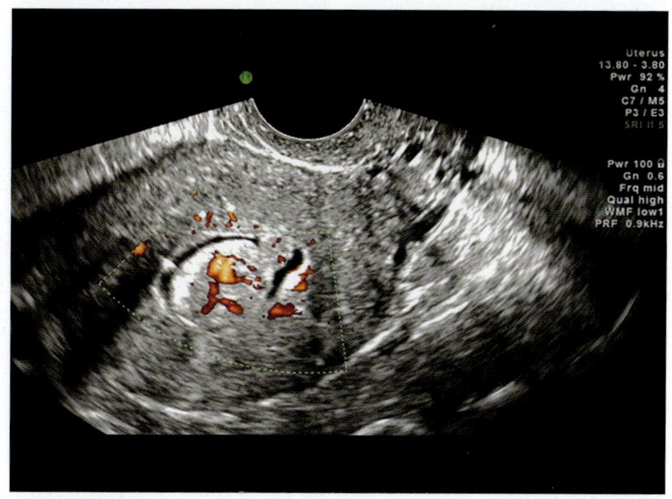

Fig. 17B: Saline infusion sonography with power Doppler imaging of the same patient demonstrates 30 × 25 mm intracavitary uterine fibroid with vascularized pedicle and central vascularization.

delineating of the outer surface of lesions, whereas positive contrast only created a cast of the cavity.

Cervical fibroids are an unusual variation in terms of location for uterine leiomyoma. Clinical symptoms are identical to those of uterine fibroids in other locations and include hypermenorrhea and dysmenorrhea. Sometimes they may protrude into the cervical canal and may be seen as rounded mass centered on the uterine cervix **(Figs. 18A to C)**.

One limitation of scanning the uterus with myomas by three-dimensional or two-dimensional ultrasound is significant shadowing due to calcification. In patients in whom the enlargement of the fibroids has outgrown their blood supply, ultrasound can demonstrate various types of degeneration **(Figs. 19A to G)**, such as cystic degeneration **(Fig. 19D)**, calcification **(Figs. 19E and F)**, hyaline or myxoid **(Fig. 19G)**, and red (hemorrhagic degeneration).

Kurjak and Kupesic[23] evaluated myometrial lesions, morphology, volume, and vascularization with 3D ultrasound and power Doppler sonography. The mean volume of the leiomyomas undergoing surgery was 78.52 ± 50.8 mL. In 84.38%, 3D power Doppler detected regular vascularity at the periphery, while in cases of secondary degenerative lesions the findings were suggestive of

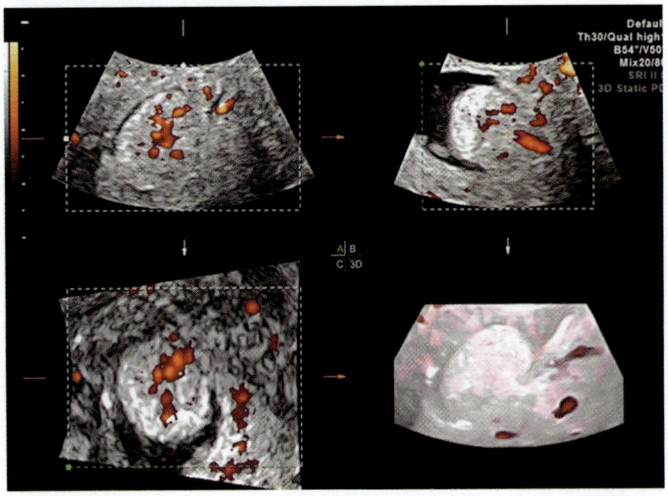

Fig. 17C: 3D saline infusion sonography with power Doppler imaging demonstrates fibroid's arborizing vessels.

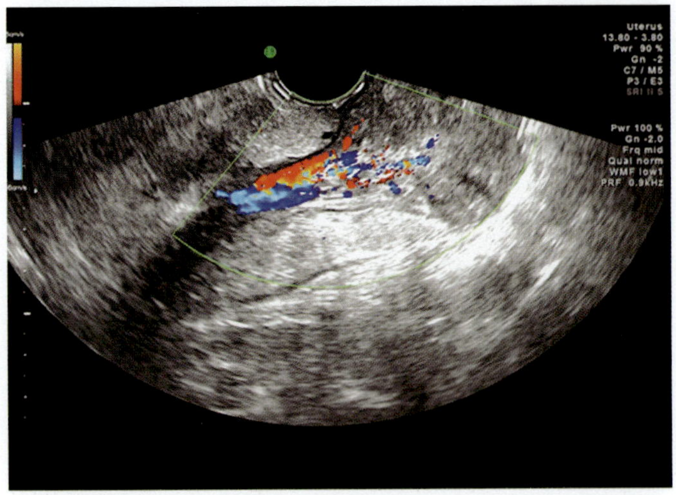

Fig. 18A: Transvaginal color Doppler image of a cervical fibroid demonstrates regularly separated feeding vessels.

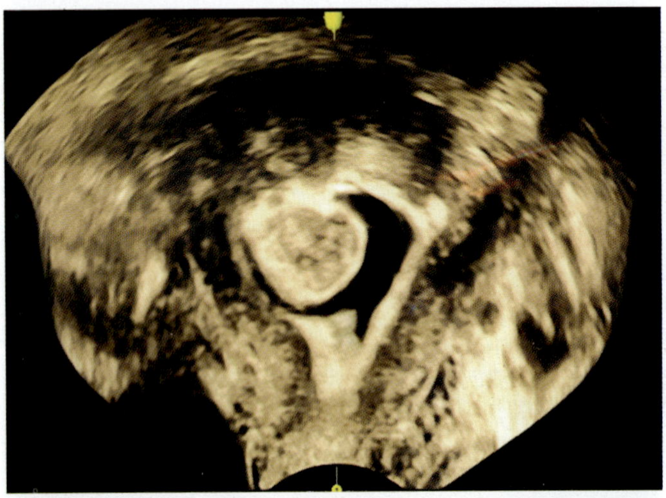

Fig. 17D: Surface rendering of the same patient demonstrates intracavitary fibroid originating from the uterine fundus. A small cervical polyp (not visualized on native ultrasound and 2D SIS) protruding from the internal cervical os is clearly outlined.

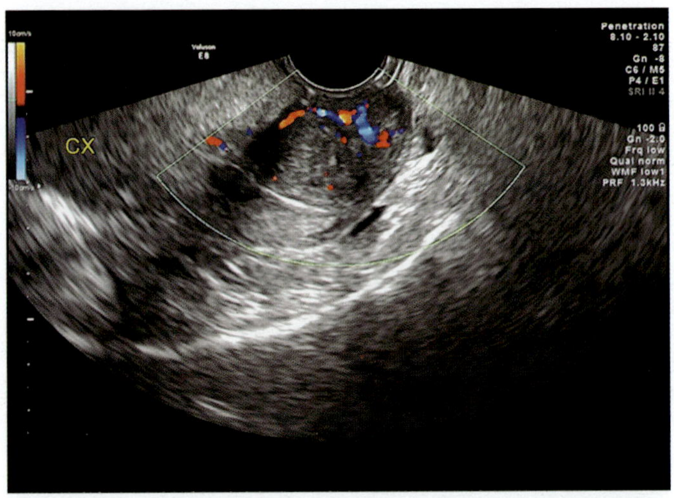

Fig. 18B: Transvaginal color Doppler image of a cervical fibroid demonstrates regularly separated peripheral vessels.

neovascularity, irregular branching and chaotic vascular arrangement, because necrosis, inflammation and degeneration altered the leiomyoma vasculature. The authors concluded that because of the low positive predictive value of 16.7% this method should not be used for the evaluation of myometrial pathology, both benign and malignant.

LEIOMYOSARCOMA

Uterine leiomyosarcoma is a rare tumor, accounting for only 1–3% of all genital tract tumors and 3–7.4% of malignant tumors of the corpus uteri,[33] characterized by early dissemination and poor prognosis for survival. Through the years, several questions regarding these tumors have remained unanswered, and a method for its early and correct diagnosis is still unknown. Furthermore, uterine sarcoma is expected to be more common in the near future, as gynecologists more commonly use the conservative treatment of uterine leiomyomas. Abnormal vaginal bleeding is the most common presenting symptom in patients with uterine sarcoma. Lower abdominal pain or pressure and a palpable abdominal mass are additional

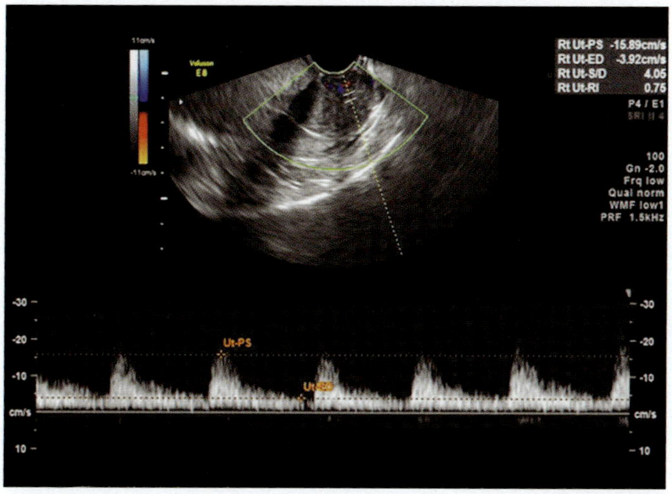

Fig. 18C: Pulsed Doppler waveform analysis demonstrates high vascular impedance depicted from the peripheral vessels of the cervical fibroid (RI = 0.75).

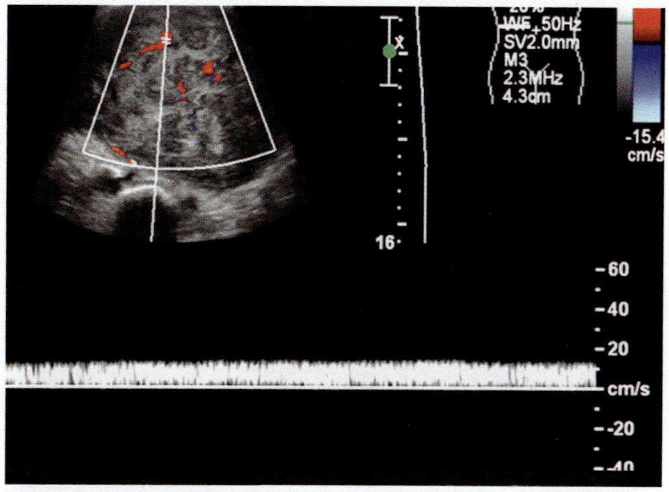

Fig. 19B: Pulsed Doppler ultrasound of a patient with degenerative fibroid. Note venous type of the blood flow signals obtained from the central portion of a degenerative fibroid.

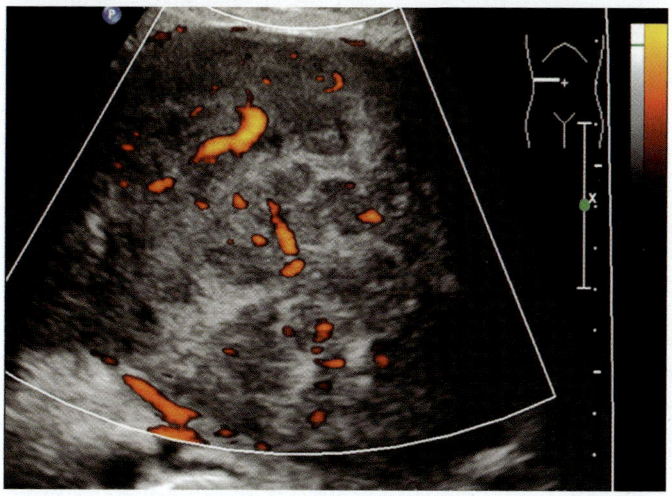

Fig. 19A: Uterine fibroid with secondary degenerative changes. Power Doppler ultrasound displays prominent color/power signals within the central portion of the fibroid.

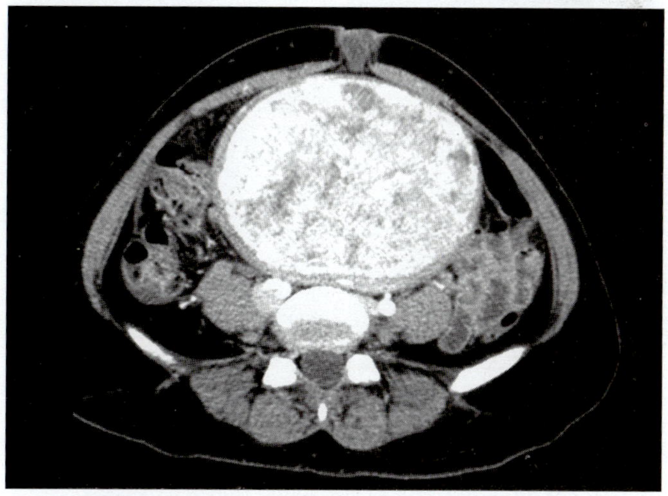

Fig. 19C: CT scan of a large degenerative fibroid.

findings. An enlarged bulky uterus is palpated, and/or the tumor may be seen protruding through the cervix. Dilatation and curettage may be helpful in distinguishing benign from malignant pathology only if the tumor is submucosal. Clinically, a rapid increase in the size of a uterine tumor after the menopause arouses suspicion of sarcoma.

On ultrasound, leiomyosarcoma presents as solid or solid-cystic structure, altering echogenicity of the myometrium. On transvaginal color Doppler, neovascularization of leiomyosarcoma is detected both at the border and in the center of the tumor **(Figs. 20A and B)** with high blood flow velocity and low impedance to blood flow (RI = 0.37 ± 0.03), with irregular, thin, randomly dispersed vessels **(Fig. 20C)**. When cut-off value for RI of <0.40 was used, this method reached the sensitivity of 90.91%, specificity 99.82%, positive predictive value 71.43% and negative predictive value of 99.96%.[34] Because of their rarity, uterine sarcomas are not suitable for screening. Transvaginal ultrasound can detect differences in myometrial tissue density, and therefore can be used for detection of uterine sarcoma, but because of low

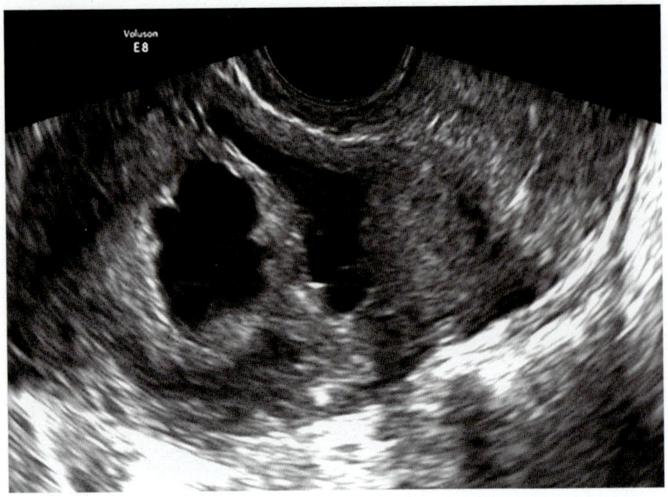

Fig. 19D: Cystic degenerative changes (central dark area) in a patient with intramural uterine fibroid.

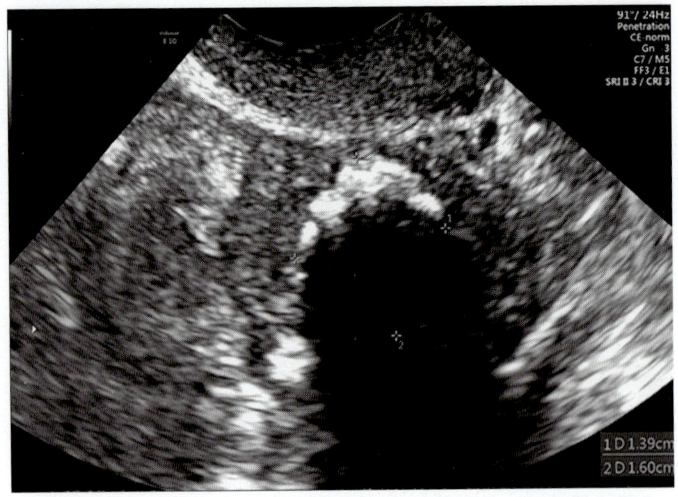

Fig. 19F: Transvaginal ultrasound scan of a calcified uterine fibroid with posterior acoustic shadowing.

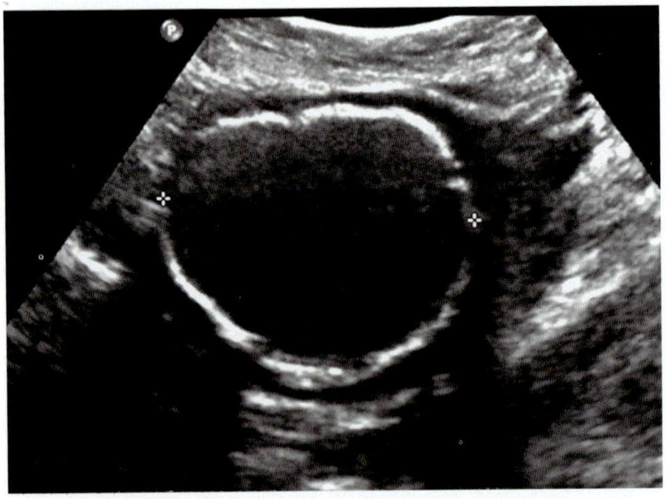

Fig. 19E: Transvaginal ultrasound scan of a calcified uterine fibroid.

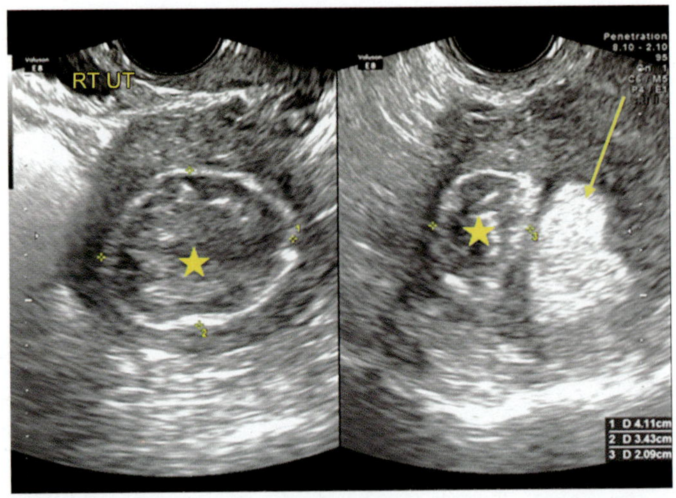

Fig. 19G: Different types of uterine fibroids' degeneration: calcification on the left (marked with an asterix), and hyaline or myxoid degeneration on the right (pointed by an arrow).

specificity this method is not appropriate as a screening procedure.

Szabo et al.[35] investigated uterine vascularity by color and pulsed Doppler in cases of uterine leiomyomas and uterine sarcomas, and determined the efficiency of uterine blood flow analysis in differentiating between them. The mean intratumoral resistance index (RI) and pulsatility index (PI) were significantly lower and the intratumoral peak systolic velocity (PSV) was significantly higher in patients with sarcomas than in patients with uterine leiomyomas. Marked reduction of RI and PI and increased PSV could be found in the leiomyoma cases which showed necrotic, degenerative and inflammatory changes. When a cut-off value of 0.5 for the RI was considered, the detection rate for uterine leiomyosarcoma was 67% and the false-positive rate was 11.8%. These results suggest that the intratumoral RI detected by color and pulsed Doppler ultrasonography cannot be used for preoperative differentiation from uterine leiomyosarcoma.

In our study,[23] one patient with uterine leiomyosarcoma was examined with 3D and power Doppler ultrasound. Enlarged volume of the tumor (97.2 mL) and irregular randomly vessels dispersed both in the central and peripheral parts of the tumor were obtained using this

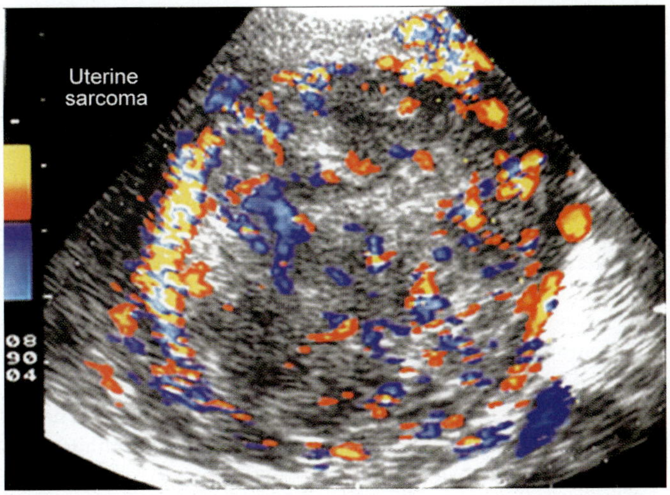

Fig. 20A: Uterine tumor showing highly vascularized area; the tumor proved to be uterine sarcoma.

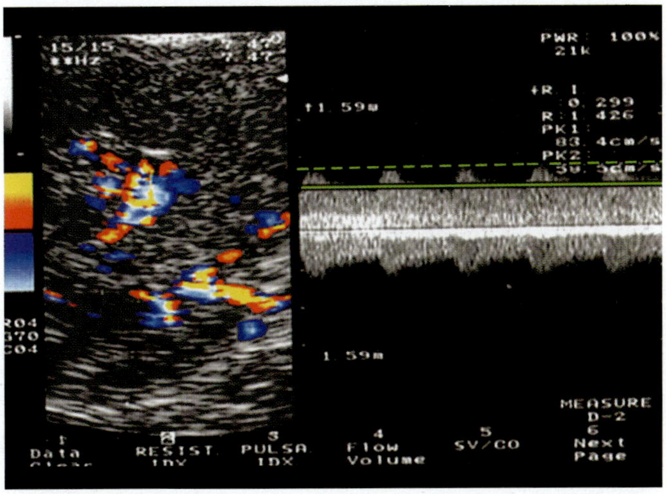

Fig. 20C: Pulsed Doppler waveform analysis demonstrates prominent flow with small systolic-to-diastolic variation and low vascular resistance (RI 0.42), indicative of uterine malignancy. Uterine sarcoma was confirmed by histopathology.

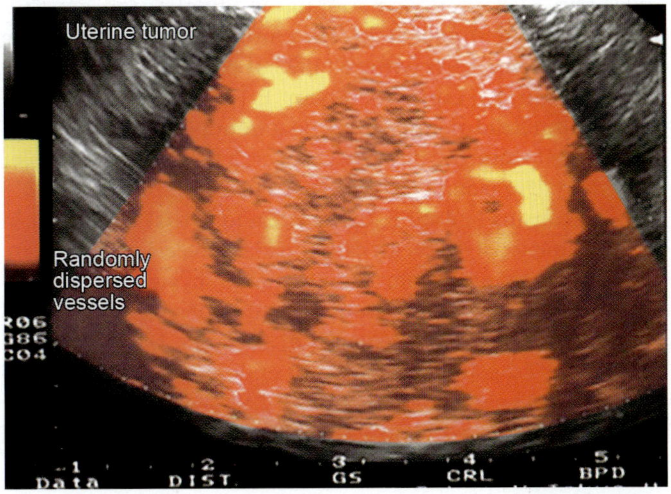

Fig. 20B: Power Doppler facilitates detection of numerous, small, randomly dispersed vessels, typical of uterine malignancy.

method. The diameters of these vessels were "uneven", with numerous microaneurysms and stenosis.

ADVANCES IN ULTRASOUND IMAGING

More recently, an ultrasound algorithm consisting of B mode and Doppler parameters with and without enhancement by gel infusion sonography (GIS) achieved low intra- and inter-observer variability in the prediction of endometrial cancer.[36,37] These studies indicated that the optimal imaging modality for prediction of endometrial cancer is real time 2D GIS. The major advantages of GIS are more detailed visualization of the uterine cavity, minimal leakage and easier application. 3D US parameters, the endometrial volume and 3D vascular indices had no benefit in detection of endometrial carcinoma. Similar results were obtained in a study assessing the diagnostic value of 3D GIS in the planning of hysteroscopy procedures. In daily practice, the addition of 3D GIS to 2D GIS improved the accuracy for the detection of polyps and fibroids, but only marginally improved the planning of hysteroscopic procedures.[38]

CONCLUSION

Transvaginal sonography allows for detailed analysis of the endometrial thickness and texture. Blood flow studies can be efficiently used to monitor endometrial development and distinguish between benign and malignant uterine cavity lesions. An advantage with color Doppler findings is possible reduction in invasive procedures such as dilatation and curettage or hysteroscopy for detection of the uterine cavity lesions. Implementation of these techniques could lower potential risks and economic costs. Saline infusion sonography (SIS) and 3D ultrasound are sensitive diagnostic modalities for detection of endometrial polyps, intrauterine adhesions, submucous/intracavitary leiomyoma and congenital uterine anomalies, highly comparable to MRI and hysteroscopy. In patients with postmenopausal bleeding and thickened endometrium quantification of endometrial vascularity by 2D and 3D color Doppler studies contributes to better discrimination of cancer from other causes of endometrial thickening.

Transvaginal color and pulsed Doppler sonography represents a noninvasive diagnostic tool that can be used repeatedly for assessing vascularity in endometrial lesions. The application of transvaginal color Doppler to the postmenopausal population for the screening of endometrial carcinoma may be a viable option if combined with ovarian screening. In this way, capital costs would be shared and oncological preventive medicine for women could be initiated. Assessment of vascularization of uterine tumors, if used together with analysis of morphology and size, can increase our accuracy in differentiating between uterine leiomyosarcoma and leiomyoma. However, it is unrealistic to expect Doppler studies to clarify confounding histological findings. It seems that the multiparameter sonographic approach, which includes morphology and size depicted by transvaginal ultrasonography and color flow imaging with pulsed Doppler analysis of neovascular signals, can help in the diagnosis of uterine leiomyosarcoma in high-risk groups such as postmenopausal patients with a rapidly enlarging uterus. Therefore, serial measurements are recommended for evaluation of myometrial density, follow-up of the tumoral growth and detection of the impedance to blood flow. Only such complex observations can lead to proper diagnosis of these rare tumors, which have an unpredictable prognosis.

Three-dimensional and power Doppler ultrasound is a new diagnostic technique and its role in the assessment of uterine lesions has yet to be investigated. Three-dimensional ultrasound offers improved visualization of uterine lesions providing simultaneous display of coronal, sagittal, and transverse planes. It displays the entire volume demonstrating continuity of curved structures in a single image, offers more accurate volume estimation using a standard anatomic orientation, retrospective review of data, more complete viewing of pathology using rendered images identifying the location of abnormalities, and assessment of tumor invasion. Three-dimensional saline infusion sonography demonstrates the exact location of intrauterine pathology. Three-dimensional power Doppler sonography provides a better understanding of malignant tumor angiogenesis. Interactive rotation of power Doppler rendered images improves visualization of the tumor vasculature. This method permits the ultrasonographer to view structures in three-dimensions interactively, rather than having to assemble the sectional images in his/her mind. Contrast agents are another possibility for enhancing the three-dimensional power Doppler examination by increasing the detection rate of small vessels.

REFERENCES

1. Kurjak A, Kupesic S, Zalud I, Predanic M. Transvaginal color Doppler. In: Dodson MG (Ed). Transvaginal Ultrasound. New York: Churchill Livingstone. 1995:325-39.
2. Fleischer AC, Kepple DM, Entman SS. Transvaginal sonography of uterine disorders. In: Timor-Tritsch IE, Rottem S (Eds). Transvaginal Sonography, 2nd edn. New York: Elsevier; 1991. pp. 109-30.
3. Kurjak A, Kupesic S. Transvaginal color Doppler and pelvic tumor vascularity: lessons learned and future challenges. Ultrasound Obstet Gynecol. 1995;6:1-15.
4. Ismail SM. Pathology of the endometrium treated with tamoxifen. J Clin Path. 1994;47:827-33.
5. Achiron R, Grisaru D, Golan-Porat N. Tamoxifen and the uterus: an old drug tested by new modalities. Ultrasound Obstet Gynecol. 1996;7:374-8.
6. Lahti E, Blanco G, Kauppila A. Endometrial changes in postmenopausal breast cancer patients receiving tamoxifen. Obstet Gynecol. 1993;81:660-4.
7. Achiron R, Lipitz S, Sivan E. Changes mimicking endometrial neoplasia in postmenopausal, tamoxifen-treated women with breast cancer: a transvaginal Doppler study. Ultrasound Obstet Gynecol. 1995;6:116-20.
8. Exacoustos E, Zupi E, Cangi B. Endometrial evaluation in postmenopausal breast cancer patients receiving tamoxifen: an ultrasound, color flow Doppler hysteroscopic and histological study. Ultrasound Obstet Gynecol. 1995;6:435-42.
9. Goldstein SR, Monteagudo A, Popiolek D, Mayberry P, Timor-Tritsch I. Evaluation of endometrial polyps. Am J Obstet Gynecol. 2002;186(4):669-74.
10. Perez-Medina T, Bajo J, Huertas MA, Rubio A. Predicting atypia inside endometrial polyps. Journal Ultrasound Med. 2002;21(2):125-8.
11. Bonilla-Musoles F, Raga F, Osborne N, Blanes J, Coelho F. Three-dimensional hysterosonography for the study of endometrial tumors: comparison with conventional transvaginal sonography, hysterosalpingography, and hysteroscopy. Gynecol Oncol. 1997;65:245-52.
12. Weinraub Z, Maymon R, Shulman A, et al. Three-dimensional saline contrast hysterosonography and surface rendering of uterine cavity pathology. Ultrasound Obstet Gynecol. 1996;8(4):277-82.
13. Gruboeck K, Jurkovic D, Lawton F, Savvas M, Tailor A, Campbell S. The diagnostic value of endometrial thickness and volume measurements by three-dimensional ultrasound in patients with postmenopausal bleeding. Ultrasound Obstet Gynecol. 1996;8(4):272-6.
14. Momtaz M, El Ebrashi A. 3D sonohysterography in the evaluation of the uterine cavity. Syllabus. Las Vegas, October 1999.

15. Fedele I, Bianchi S, Dorta M, Arcaini L, Zanotti F, Carinelli S. Transvaginal ultrasonography in the diagnosis of diffuse adenomyosis. Fertil Steril. 1992;58:94.
16. Hirai M, Shibata K, Sagai H, Sekiya S, Goldberg BB. Transvaginal pulsed and color Doppler sonography for the evaluation of adenomyosis. J Ultrasound Med. 1995;14:529-32.
17. Lee SL, Busmanis I, Tan A. 3D – Angio of Adenomyotic Uteri. Syllabus. Las Vegas, October 1999.
18. Kupesic-Urek S, Shalan H, Kurjak A. Early detection of endometrial cancer by transvaginal color Doppler. EUROBS. 1993;49:46-9.
19. Kurjak A, Kupesic S. Ovarian senescence and its significance on uterine and ovarian perfusion. Fertil Steril. 1995;3:532-7.
20. Emoto M, Tamura R, Shirota K, Hachisuga T, Kawarabayashi T. Clinical usefulness of color Doppler ultrasound in patients with endometrial hyperplasia and carcinoma. Cancer. 2002;94(3):700-6.
21. Jarvela I, Tekay A, Santala M, Jouppila P. Thermal balloon endometrial ablation therapy induces a rise in uterine blood flow impedance: a randomized prospective color Doppler study. Ultrasound Obstet Gynecol. 2001; 17(1):65-70.
22. Folkman J, Cole D, Becker F. Growth and metastasis of tumor in organ culture. Tumor Res. 1963;16:453-67.
23. Kurjak A, Kupesic S. Three-Dimensional Ultrasound and Power Doppler in Assessment of Uterine and Ovarian Angiogenesis: a Prospective Study. Croatian Medical J. 1999;40(3):51-8.
24. Kupesic S, Kurjak A, Zodan T. Staging of endometrial carcinoma by 3-D power Doppler. Gynecol Perinatol. 1999;8(1):1-5.
25. Lee CN, Cheng WF, Chen CA, Chu JS, Hsieh CY, Hsieh FJ. Angiogenesis of endometrial carcinomas assessed by measurement of intratumoral blood flow, microvessel density, and vascular endothelial growth factor levels. Obstet Gynecol. 2000;96(4):615-21.
26. Alcazar JL, Galan JM, Jurado M, Lopez-Garcia G. Intratumoral blood flow analysis in endometrial carcinoma: Correlation with tumor characteristics and risk for recurrence. Gynecol Oncol. 2002;84(2):258-62.
27. Yaman C, Ebner T, Jesacher K, Obermayr G, Polz W, Tews G. Reproducibility of three-dimensional ultrasound endometrial volume measurements in patients with postmenopausal bleeding. Ultrasound Obstet Gynecol. 2002;19(3):282-6.
28. Kurjak A, Zalud I. Uterine masses. In: Kurjak A (Ed). Transvaginal Color Doppler. Carnforth, UK: Parthenon Publishing; 1991. p. 123.
29. Fleischer AC, Entman SS, Porrath SA, James AE. Sonographic evaluation of uterine malformations and disorders. In: Sanders RC (Ed). The Principles and Practice of Ultrasonography in Obstetrics and Gynecology. Norwalk: Appleton Century Crofts; 1985. p. 531.
30. Kurjak A, Kupesic-Urek S, Miric D. The assessment of benign uterine tumor vascularization by transvaginal color Doppler. Ultrasound Med Biol. 1992;18:645-8.
31. Balen FG, Allen CM, Gardener JE, Siddle NC, Lees WR. 3-Dimensional reconstruction of ultrasound images of the uterine cavity. Br J Radiol. 1993;66(787):588-91.
32. Lev-Toaff AS, Rawool NM, Kurtz AB, Forssberg F, Goldberg BB. Three-dimensional sonography and 3D transvaginal US: a problem solving tool in complex gynecological cases. Radiology. 1996;201(P):384.
33. Olah KS, Gee H, Blunt S, Dunn JA, Chan KK. Retrospective analysis of 318 cases of uterine sarcoma. Eur J Cancer. 1991;27:1095-9.
34. Kurjak A, Kupesic S, Shalan H, Jukic S, Kosuta D, Ilijas M. Uterine sarcoma: a report of 10 cases studied by transvaginal color and pulsed Doppler sonography. Gynecol Oncol. 1995;59:342-6.
35. Szabo I, Szantho A, Csabay L, Csapo Z, Szirmai K, Papp Z. Color Doppler ultrasonography in the differentiation of uterine sarcomas from uterine leiomyomas. E J Gynaecol Oncol. 2002;23(1):29-34.
36. Dueholm M, Moller C, Rydebjerg S, Hansen ES, Ortoft G. An ultrasound algorithm for identification of endometrial cancer. Ultrasound Obstet Gynecol. 2014;43:557-68.
37. Dueholm M, Christensen JW, Rydebjerg S, Hansen ES, Ortoft G. Two- and three-dimensional transvaginal ultrasound and gel infusion sonography for diagnosis of endometrial malignancy. Ultrasound Obstet Gynecol. 2015;45:734-43.
38. Niewenhuis LL, Bij de Vaate M, Hehenkamp WJK, et al. Diagnostic and clinical value of 3D gel installation sonohysterography in addition to 2D gel installation sonohysterography in the assessment of intrauterine abnormalities. Eur J Obstet Gynecol Reprod Biol. 2014; 175:67-74.

54

CHAPTER

Uterine Fibroid

Aleksandar Ljubic, Tatjana Bozanovic

INTRODUCTION

Definition

Uterine fibroids are referred to as fibroid, leiomyoma, leiomyomata and fibromyoma. They are benign (noncancerous) tumors that grow within the muscle tissue of the uterus. Depending on the prevailing type of tissues, i.e. parenchyma or interstitial, they are called differently as myoma, fibroma, fibromyoma, etc. As they are developed mainly from muscle cells, the most correct terminology is considered to be myoma (leiomyoma).

Incidence

The incidence of fibroids in women of reproductive age is reported to be between 20% and 40%.[1] Uterine fibroid is the most common pelvic tumor and they are diagnosed in up to 15–20% of women in pubertal period.[1] Their presence could cause failure to conceive, but no scientific evidence supports improvement after the surgical removal of the fibroid. This was recently highlighted in a review, reporting a pregnancy rate after myomectomy in infertile women varying between 10% and 80%. While many women do not experience any problems, symptoms can be severe enough to require treatment.

Although fibroid (uterine fibroids) is generally considered to be a slowly growing tumor, in 20–40% of women at the age of 35 and more, uterine fibroids of significant sizes with severe clinical symptoms are commonly seen. Moreover, fibroid can be relapsed in 7–28% of patients after surgical treatments and in certain cases it may even turn into malignant tumor.

Etiology and Pathophysiology

Although, the exact etiology of fibroid is not known yet, the growth of uterine fibroid is featured as a benign, hormone sensitive diffuse or nodulus hyperplasia of myometrium, and is characterized by having multiple factors of pathogenesis and systemic changes **(Figs. 1A and B)**.

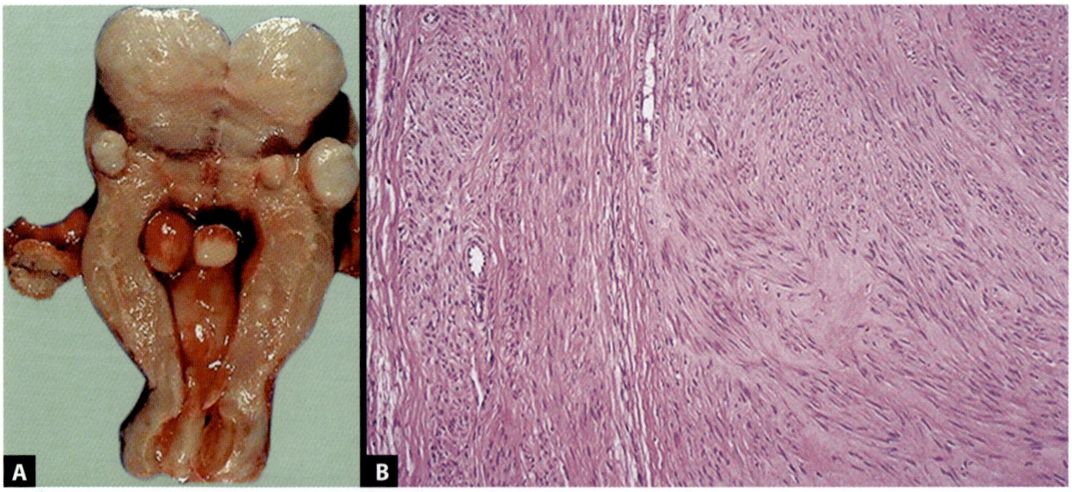

Figs. 1A and B: (A) Various types of fibroid and (B) histopathological picture. Proliferation of muscle tissue surrounded by pseudocapsule can be seen.

Uterine fibroid is developed on the background of hyperestrogens, progesterone deficits and hypergonadotropins. The majority of the researchers consider that the growth of fibroid depends on concentration of cytosolic receptors to the sexual hormones and their interactions with the endogenous or exogenous hormones. In accordance to clinical observations, it can be admitted that both growth and regression of fibroid are estrogen-dependant; the tumor size gets increased during pregnancy and is regressed after menopause.

Genetics

It is not yet clear how an abnormal *HMGA2* gene leads to fibroids. *HMGA2 gene* appears to be involved in body fat metabolism. Likewise, the abnormal gene causing both MCUL1 and HLRCC syndrome was a surprise. The responsible gene was identified by studying large family groups (cohorts) with disease. One research group was following a family affected by MCUL1, and the other was studying HLRCC families. They both found the same gene on chromosome 1, *fumarate hydratase* (*FH*), linked to the clinical findings of the syndrome.[1a,1b] The *FH* gene codes for a protein that is a part of the Krebs cycle, a group of enzymes active in every cell that allows the body to extract energy from molecules. Again, it is not directly clear why this protein would lead to fibroids. However, some recent studies suggest that it may have something to do with fibroid cells being deprived of oxygen (hypoxia) and leading to new blood vessel formation (angiogenesis).[1c]

However, the mutations in the *FH* gene causing HLRCC syndrome lead to nonworking or absent *FH* protein.[1b, 1d] We say that *FH* works as a tumor suppressor gene: normal *FH* suppresses the formation of these tumors, and only when it is inactivated by mutations does a problem arise. Another tumor suppressor gene, phosphatase and tensin homolog (*PTEN*), appears to cause different syndromes. Loss of tumor suppressor genes is a common process in the formation of cancerous tumors as well as benign tumors such as fibroids.

A polymorphism produces a more subtle change. It may change the DNA but keep the protein the same, or it may be outside the gene in the regulatory region so that the gene is more easily turned on or off. There have been some reports of polymorphism of particular steroid-hormone-related genes that appear to increase a woman's risk of developing fibroids.1d, 1e

A number of experiments have also been conducted with gene chips to find whole series of genes that are turned off or on in fibroids compared with normal myometrium. Just as in cancer, there is probably not one master switch involved in fibroid formation. Instead, a series of genetic changes are likely responsible for fibroid formation, fibroid growth, and the production of symptoms.

Possible Causes of Fibroids

Genetics: About 40% of fibroids contain alterations in genes that code for uterine muscle cells. Patients with hereditary leiomyomatosis and renal cell carcinoma (HLRCC cutaneous and uterine leiomyoma) are at risk for papillary renal cell carcinoma (the incidence in women is greater than in men). They also have mutation in fumarate hydratase gene. The chromosomal anomaly (12q13–15) is quite common in myomatous cells. In fact, in 30–40% cases, the predisposition to uterine fibroid is passed down from mothers to daughters on hereditary line. A form of fibroid so called "family type" is present where uterine fibroid are seen in all the family line, i.e. in grandmother, mother, aunts and sisters.

Heredity: If a mother or sister had fibroids, then there is an increased risk of developing them.

Race: Black women are more likely to have fibroids than are women of other racial groups. Also, black women have fibroids at younger age and they are more likely to have more or larger fibroids.

Hormonal imbalance: Estrogen and progesterone appear to promote the growth of fibroids. Fibroids contain more estrogen and estrogen receptors than do normal uterine muscle cells. Other chemicals that help the body maintain tissues, such as insulin-like growth factor, may also affect fibroid growth.

Obesity: Overweight women have a greater risk of developing fibroids.

Fibroids rarely have malignant potential (leiomyosarcoma) **(Figs. 2A and B)**.

Localization

Fibroid may be located in the external, middle or inner layers of uterus (subserous, interstitial and submucous). Nodules can be located in the isthmus (5%) or in the uterine body (95%) **(Fig. 3)**.

Types of Fibroids

Intramural: Fibroids embedded within the myometrium. This is the most common type of fibroid. These develop

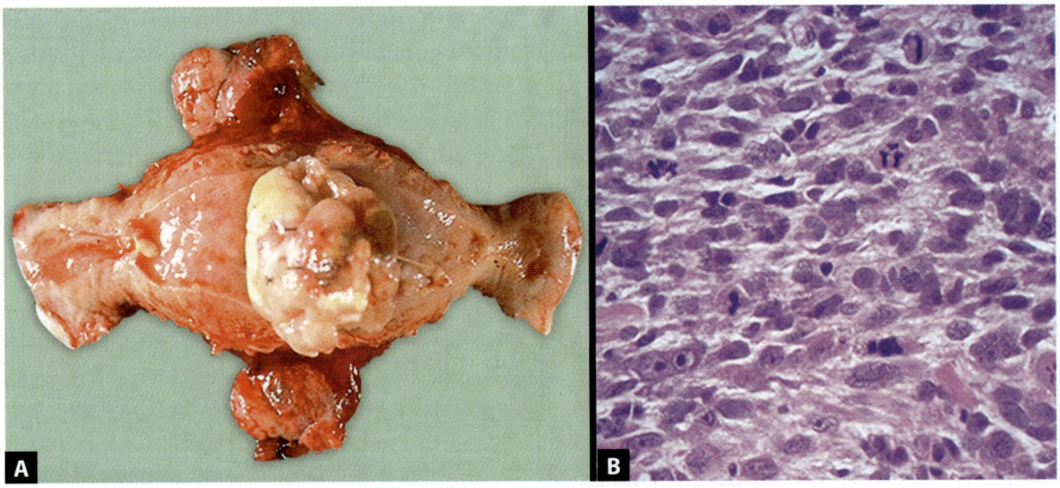

Figs. 2A and B: (A) Leiomyosarcoma with (B) histopathological picture.

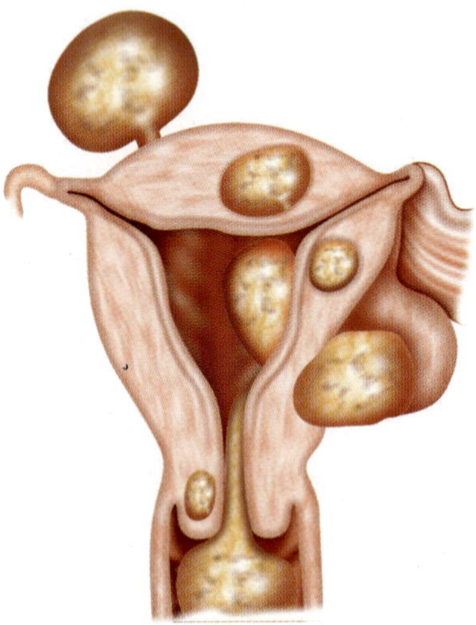

Fig. 3: Different fibroids and their orientation to the uterine wall.

within the uterine wall and expand, making the uterus feel larger than normal (which may cause "bulk symptoms").

Subserosa: Fibroids that bulge on the outside. These fibroids develop in the outer portion of the uterus and continue to grow outward.

Submucosal: Fibroids that grow into the inner cavity. These fibroids develop just under the lining of the uterine cavity. These are the fibroids that have the most effect on heavy menstrual bleeding and the ones that can cause problems with infertility, and miscarriage.

Pedunculated: Fibroids that hang from a stalk inside or outside of the uterus. Fibroids that grow on a small stalk that connects them to the inner or outer wall of the uterus.

Symptoms

Women with fibroids can be asymptomatic (in 50–60% of cases) or may present with menorrhagia (30%), pelvic pain with or without dysmenorrhea or pressure symptoms (34%), infertility (27%), and recurrent pregnancy loss (3%).[1] Much of the data describing the relationship between the presence of fibroids and symptoms are based on uncontrolled studies that have assessed the effect of myomectomy on the presenting symptoms.[2] The prevalence of fibroids in infertile women can be as high as 13%, but no direct causal relationship between fibroids and infertility has been established.[3]

Main fibroid symptoms are bleeding, pressure, pain as well as infertility and pregnancy complications, such as cesarean delivery, breech presentation, malposition, preterm delivery, placenta previa and severe postpartum hemorrhage occur in half of the patients.

Symptoms depend on location, size, growth rate and relation with surrounding organs. Ultrasound is the most important diagnostic tool in determining all previous facts.

Diagnosis

While making an ultrasound diagnosis, it is important to determine size, shape, echogenicity and clear edge with the surrounding tissues. For that purpose, we can use two-dimensional (2D) **(Fig. 4)**, three-dimensional (3D) and four-dimensional (4D) ultrasound. In order to assess the vascularization of the fibroids, color Doppler is used **(Figs. 5A and B)**.

Endometrial and subendometrial blood flow measured by 3D power Doppler ultrasound in patients with small

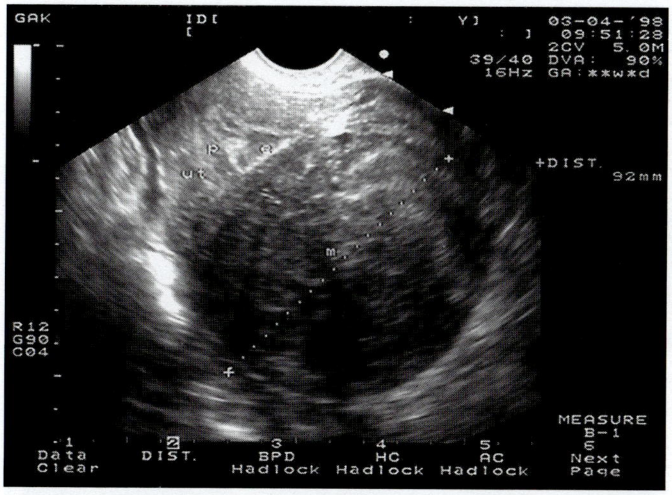

Fig. 4: Two-dimensional ultrasound of intramural fibroid. Possible predictor of the uterine growth is fibroid circulation, which can be assessed by color Doppler examination.[4]

intramural uterine fibroids during in vitro fertilization (IVF) treatment, can be a predictor of a treatment success.[6]

The circulation can be even better assessed using new 3D technologies such as glass body rendering.

Using of 3D and 4D ultrasound enable us in better delineating the fibroid **(Figs. 6 and 7)**.

ELASTOGRAPHY

Elastography is a noninvasive method in which stiffness or strain images of soft tissue are used to detect or classify tumors. A tumor or a suspicious cancerous growth is normally 5–28 times stiffer than the background of normal soft tissue. When a mechanical compression or vibration is applied, the tumor deforms less than the surrounding tissue, i.e. the strain in the tumor is less than the surrounding tissue.

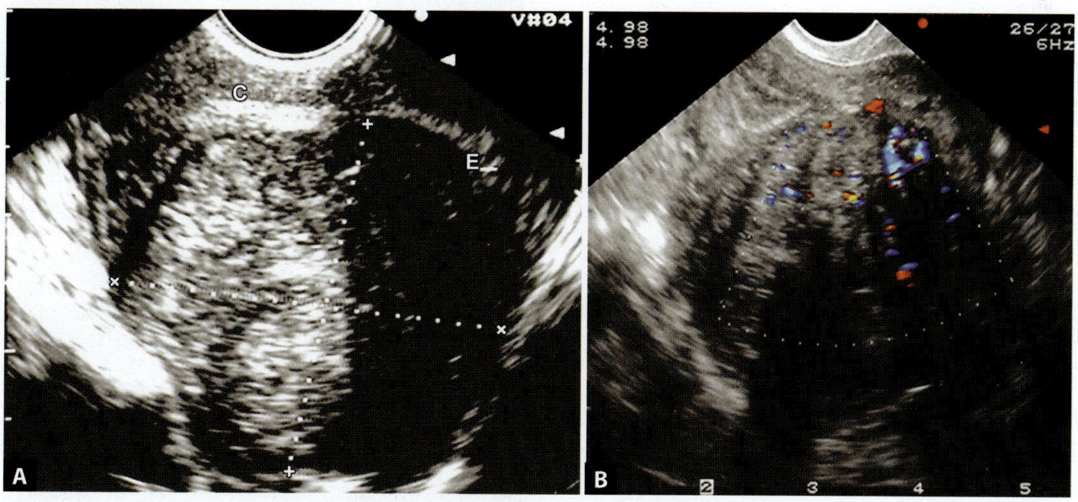

Figs. 5A and B: Examination of the fibroid circulation.

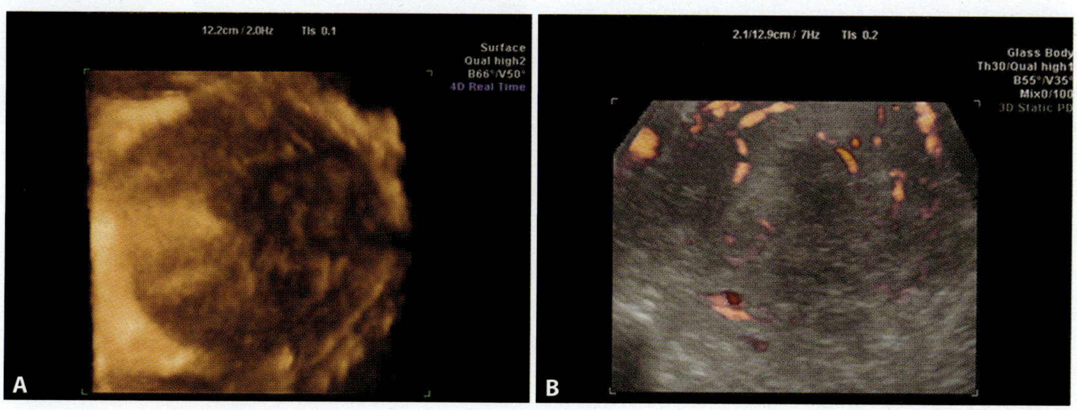

Figs. 6A and B: (A) Three-dimensional and (B) glass body picture of the uterine fibroid.

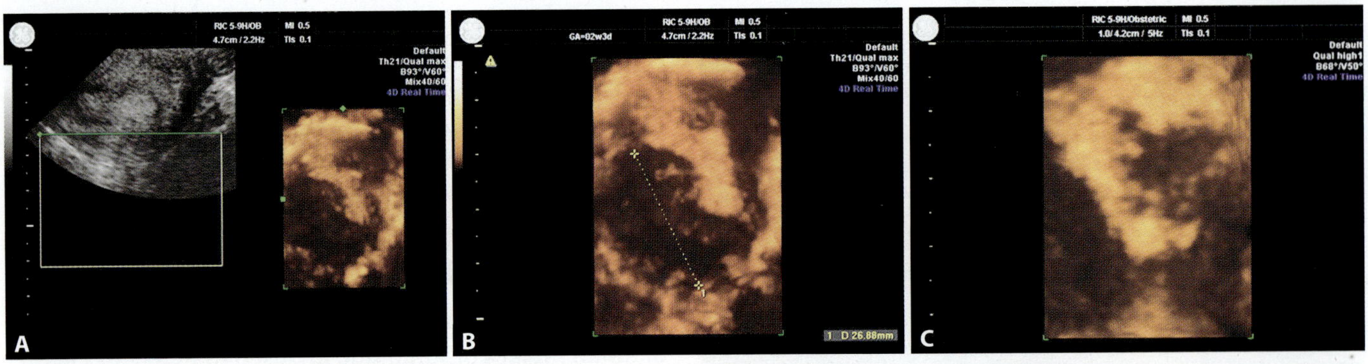

Figs. 7A to C: Three-dimensional ultrasound pictures of the uterine fibroid.

Ultrasonic imaging is the most common medical imaging technique for producing elastograms. Some research has been conducted using magnetic resonance elastography (MRE) and computed tomography. However, using ultrasound has the advantages of being cheaper, faster and more portable than other techniques.

Benefits of Elastoscan

Elastoscan can help gynecologist to find fibroid more easily **(Figs. 8A and B)**.

Uterine fibroids are composed of the same smooth muscle fibers as the uterine wall. They are many times denser than the normal myometrium. This characteristic is frequently responsible for the poor visualization of fibroids on transvaginal ultrasonography, due to strong acoustic shadowing.

As the distribution of fibroids can be difficult to determine on conventional B-mode ultrasonography, their number and size can be underestimated.[6] Three-dimensional ultrasound, computed tomography and magnetic resonance imaging have all been used for better fibroid visualization. However, a new easy-to-use ultrasound tool, real-time transvaginal elastography[7] has been suggested as a new method for evaluating fibroids.[8,9]

With conventional ultrasound, the ultrasound beam is often strongly attenuated by the fibroid. As a result, with low gain, the posterior wall of the uterine fibroid is poorly visualized, but as the gain is increased, noise or artifactual echoes appear inside the mass, obscuring the image of the fibroid.[6] Real-time elastosonography provides an instantaneous color map that precisely delineates the fibroids, thus overcoming the limitations of conventional ultrasound.

The principle of the ultrasonographic technique is based on slight external tissue compression on the

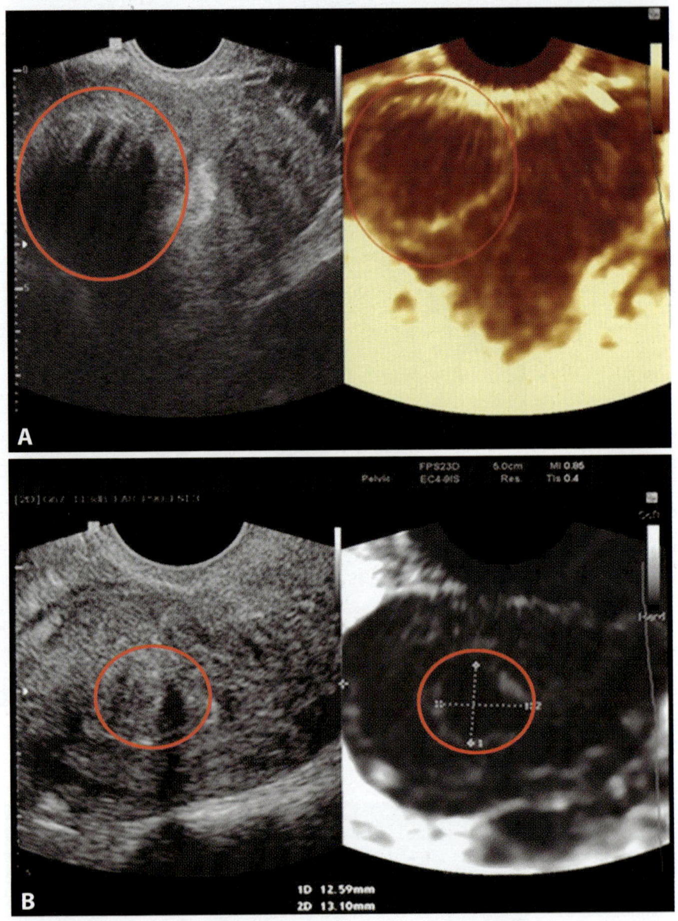

Figs. 8A and B: Fibroid elastoscans.

structures examined, which produces strain (displacement) within the tissue, with subsequent calculation of the strain profile along the axis of compression algorithm to produce the elastographic image. The strain profile is converted into an elastic modules image, i.e. the tissue elasticity distribution, called an elastogram. The calculated elasticity values are then color-coded and superimposed

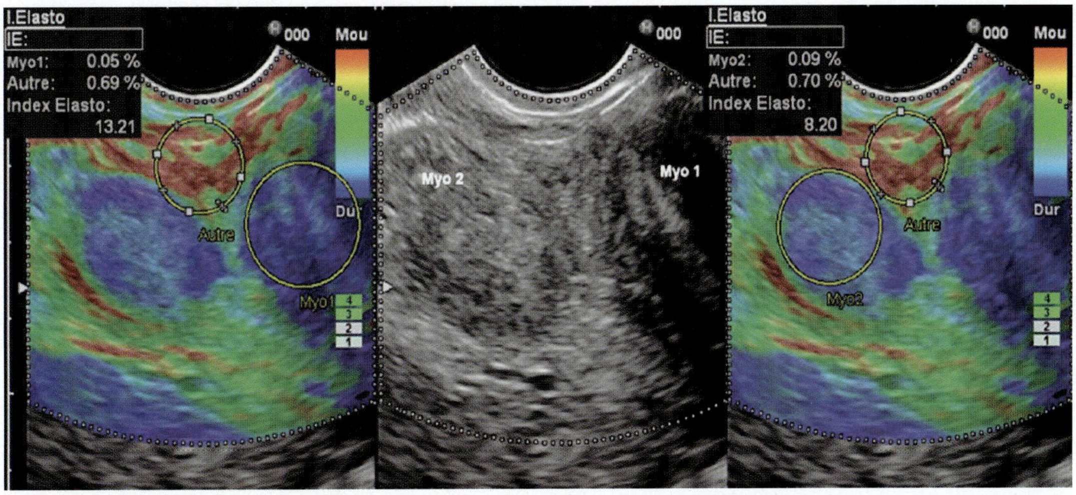

Fig. 9: A real-time elastosonographic images of the two fibroids. The strain ratio is evaluated by comparing the mean strain in a region of interest centered on the fibroid, with the mean strain in a region of interest in the surrounding myometrium close to the probe.[10]

Source: Ami O, Lamazou F, Mabille M, et al. Real-time transvaginal elastosonography of uterine fibroids. Ultrasound Obstet Gynecol. 2009;34:486-8

on the translucent, corresponding B-mode scan image **(Fig. 9)**. The stiffness of the tissue is displayed in a range of color from red (components with the greatest strain, i.e. the softest components) to blue (components with no strain, i.e. the hardest components). The components with average are displayed as green.

All fibroids were seen easily on the color display in elastography mode and their extent was easier to define than it was in conventional B-mode. The distance between the fibroid and the endometrial cavity or uterine serosa could also be measured easily in each case **(Fig. 10)**.[10]

Endovaginal ultrasonography is safe, accessible and inexpensive, and remains the primary imaging method for gynecological evaluation. Real-time elastosonography offers complementary diagnostic and mapping information. It is easy to perform, and the procedure requires only a few seconds of manipulation.

Tables 1 and 2 show the characteristics of different tests in examining uterine changes.[11]

Predictive characteristics of hysteroscopy in the diagnosis of submucosal fibroids comparing to other pathology is given in **Table 3**.[12]

Submucosal fibroids grow into the inner cavity. Ultrasound is of great value in assessing the operability of submucosal fibroids. Contrast ultrasound is of greater efficacy in better diagnosis of submucosal fibroids.[12,13]

Comparison between 3D contrast sonography and diagnostic hysteroscopy in the diagnosis of different types of submucosal fibroids is presented in **Table 4** and **Figures 11A and B**.[8]

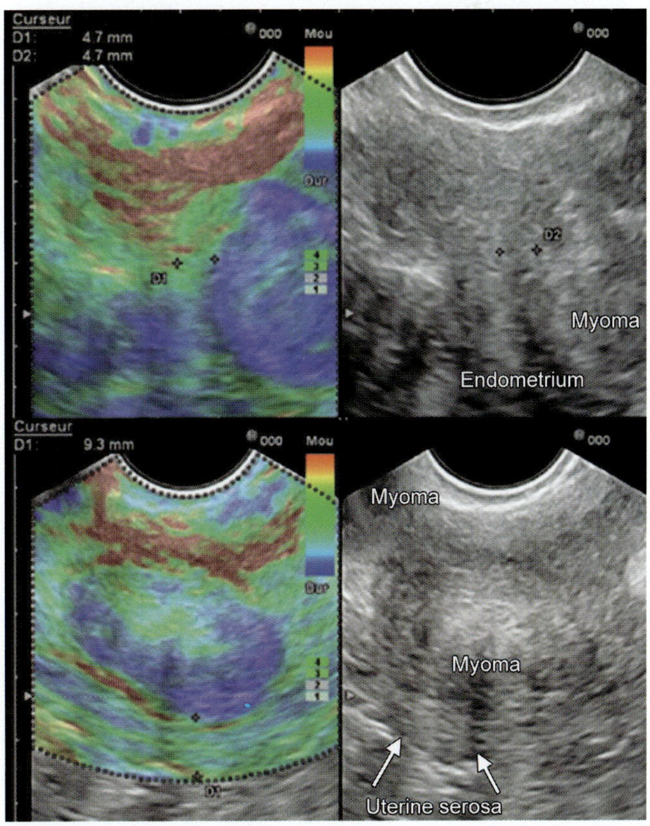

Fig. 10: Color mapping of uterine strain allows precise determination of the so-called "security wall" between the fibroids and the endometrium or uterine serosa before surgical resection with laparoscopy or hysteroscopy respectively.

Source: Ami O, Lamazou F, Mabille M, et al. Real-time transvaginal elastosonography of uterine fibroids. Ultrasound Obstet Gynecol. 2009;34:486-8

TABLE 1: Ultrasound and hysteroscopy: test characteristics.

Features	*Transvaginal ultrasound*	*Saline infusion sonography*	*Outpatient hysteroscopy*	*Evidence and prevailing clinical opinion*
Safety	✓✓✓	✓✓✓	✓✓✓	All safe, with very low rates of adverse effects reported
Acceptability	✓✓✓	✓✓✓	✓✓✓	All acceptable, ultrasound least painful and invasive. Instrumentation and distension of the uterine cavity more painful
Feasibility	✓✓✓	✓✓✓	✓✓✓	Typical failure rates higher in procedures requiring uterine instrumentation—saline infusion sonography (7%) higher than hysteroscopy (4%)
Other	Provides extracavity/ pelvic information	Facilitates diagnosis of intracavity lesions/ provides extra-cavity information	Directed endometrial biopsies and removal of focal pathology possible	Advances in the technology and application of ultrasound (three-dimensional color Doppler) techniques give this modality the greatest future potential in diagnosis. Hysteroscopy has greater therapeutic potential

TABLE 2: Ultrasound and hysteroscopy: test accuracy in abnormal uterine bleeding.

		Accuracy (likelihood ratio[a])		
Endometrial diseases	*Test*	*Positive test [Pooled estimate (95% CI)*	*Negative test if available or range if not]*	*Systematic review*
Cancer	TVS (<5 mm)[b]	2.0 (1.9–2.2)	0.08 (0.04–0.14)	Smith–Bindman (1998)[c]
		2.0 (1.6–2.4)	0.08 (0.03–0.17)	Gupta (2002)[c]
	SIS	–	–	–
	Hysteroscopy	60.9 (51.2–72.5)	0.15 (0.13–0.18)	Clark (2002)
Cancer and/or hyperplasia	TVS (<5 mm)[b]	2.9(2.7–3.2)	0.13 (0.10–0.16)	Smith–Bindman (1998)[c]
		2.2 (1.7–2.7)	0.07 (0.04–0.11)	Gupta (2002)[c]
	TVS (8–14 mm)	2.6–679	0.04–1.0	Farquhar (2003)[d]
	SIS	1.6–70.4	0.14–0.88	Farquhar (2003)[d]
	Hysteroscopy	10.4 (9.7–11.1)	0.24 (0.22–0.25)	Clark (2002)
Polyps	TVS	–	–	–
	SIS	5.2 (4.0–6.9)	0.12 (–0.08–0.17)	de kroon (2003)
	Hysteroscopy	–	–	–
Submucous fibroids	TVS	1.6–62.3	0.03–0.8	Farquhar (2003)[d]
	SIS	29.6 (17.8–49.6)	0.06–0.47	Farquhar (2003)[d]
		11.0 (6.9–17.6)	0.07 (0.03–0.11)	de Kroon (2003)
	Hysteroscopy	29.4 (13.3–65.3)	0.08–0.48	Farquhar (2003)[d]

(TVS: transveginal ultrasound; SIS: saline infusion sonography).

[a]The likelihood ratio (LR) is the ratio of the probability of a positive (or negative) test result in women with disease, to the probability of the same test result in women without disease. The desirable size of a positive likelihood ratio (LR+) is over 10 and of a negative likelihood ratio (LR–) less than 0.1. This is because a test is deemed clinically useful (i.e. substantially increases or lowers the pretest probability, hence ruling in or excluding disease, respectively) at these levels. Likelihood ratios below these levels are at best moderately informative (LR+ 5–10 and LR– 0.1– 0.5) and at worst useless (LR+ <5 and LR– >0.5)

[b]Data from TVS systematic review by Tabor et al. not presented as not stratified by endometrial thickness.

[c]Postmenopausal women only.

[d]Premenopausal women only.

TABLE 3: Predictive characteristics of hysteroscopy in the diagnosis of various conditions in a series of 770 consecutive women with menorrhagia.

Condition	*Sensitivity (%)*	*Specificity (%)*	*Positive predictive value (%)*	*Negative predictive value (%)*
Submucous myomas	95	81	85	93
Endometrial polyps	86	94	91	90
Endometrial hyperplasia	45	99	38	94

TABLE 4: Comparison between three-dimensional saline infusion sonohysterography (3D SIS) and diagnostic hysteroscopy for classification of submucous fibroids.

	3D SIS			
Hysteroscopy	***Type 0***	***Type I***	***Type II***	***Total***
Type 0	11	1	0	12
Type I	0	34	3	37
Type II	0	3	9	12
Total	11	38	12	61

Type 0: fibroid polyp.
Type I: <50% contained within the myometrium.
Type II: >50% contained within the myometrium.

There was agreement between the two methods in 11/12 cases of type 0 fibroids (92%), 34/37 (92%) of type I fibroids and 9/12 (75%) of type II fibroids. The overall level of agreement was good with a kappa value of 0.80.

In differential diagnosis, it is most important not to miss diseases, such as gestational trophoblastic neoplasm or endometrial carcinoma **(Figs. 12A and B)**.

TREATMENT

The uterine fibroid by itself is not an indication for operative method of treatment. Mainly it depends upon the patients' overall health condition, severities of the clinical symptoms and the sizes of the tumor. The major indications for the operative methods of treatment are severe pain, fast

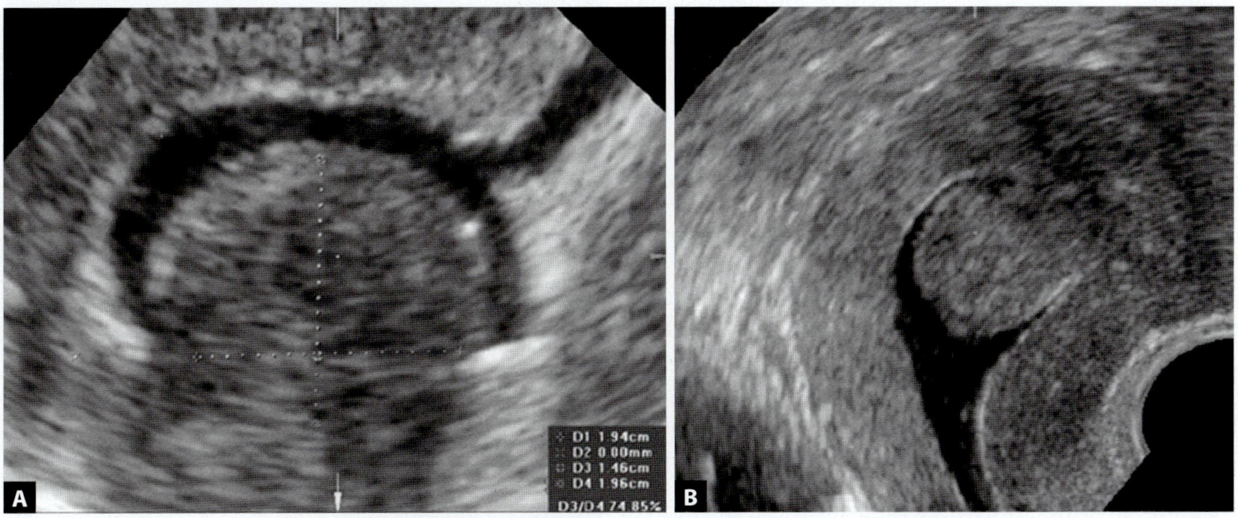

Figs. 11A and B: Contrast sonography in diagnosis of submucosal fibroids.

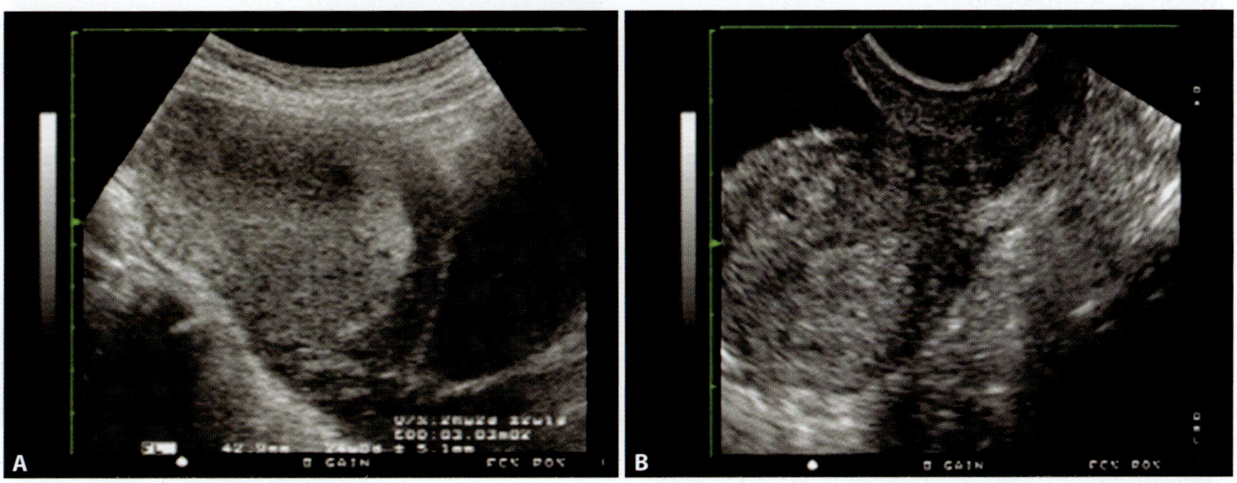

Figs. 12A and B: (A) Gestational trophoblastic neoplasm; (B) Endometrial cancer.

growth rate of the nodules, arising suspicions about the malignancy of fibroid, inflammatory changes in the tumor nodules and dysfunction of closely lying organs (urinary bladder, intestines, etc.) and infertility (when all other reasons are already excluded).

It is necessary to watch the dynamic changes of fibroid (ultrasound examination with vaginal probe), which in most cases gives sufficient information and neither operations nor other therapies are required. First line of therapy is medical therapy which might include the use of nonsteroidal anti-inflammatory drugs, birth control pills or hormone therapy, i.e. GnRH analogs (reduced blood flow with decreasing the size).

Surgical Treatment: Myomectomy

Myomectomy is a surgical procedure that removes visible fibroids from the uterine wall. It leaves the uterus in place and may, therefore, preserve the woman's ability to have children. There are several ways to perform myomectomy, including hysteroscopic myomectomy **(Figs. 13A to C)**, laparoscopic myomectomy and abdominal myomectomy.

Hysteroscopic Myomectomy

Hysteroscopic myomectomy is used only for fibroids that are just under the lining of the uterus and that protrude into the uterine cavity.

Laparoscopic Myomectomy

Laparoscopic myomectomy may be used if the fibroid is on the outside of the uterus **(Figs. 14A and B)**.

Abdominal Myomectomy

Abdominal myomectomy is a surgical procedure, in which an incision is made in the abdomen to access the uterus and another incision is made in the uterus to remove the tumor. Once the fibroids are removed, the uterus is stitched closed. The patient is given general anesthesia and is not conscious for this procedure, which requires a several-day hospital stays. Typical recovery is 4–6 weeks **(Fig. 15)**.

Hysterectomy

In a hysterectomy, the uterus is removed in an open surgical procedure. Hysterectomy is the most common current therapy for women who have fibroids. It is typically performed in women who have completed their child-bearing years.

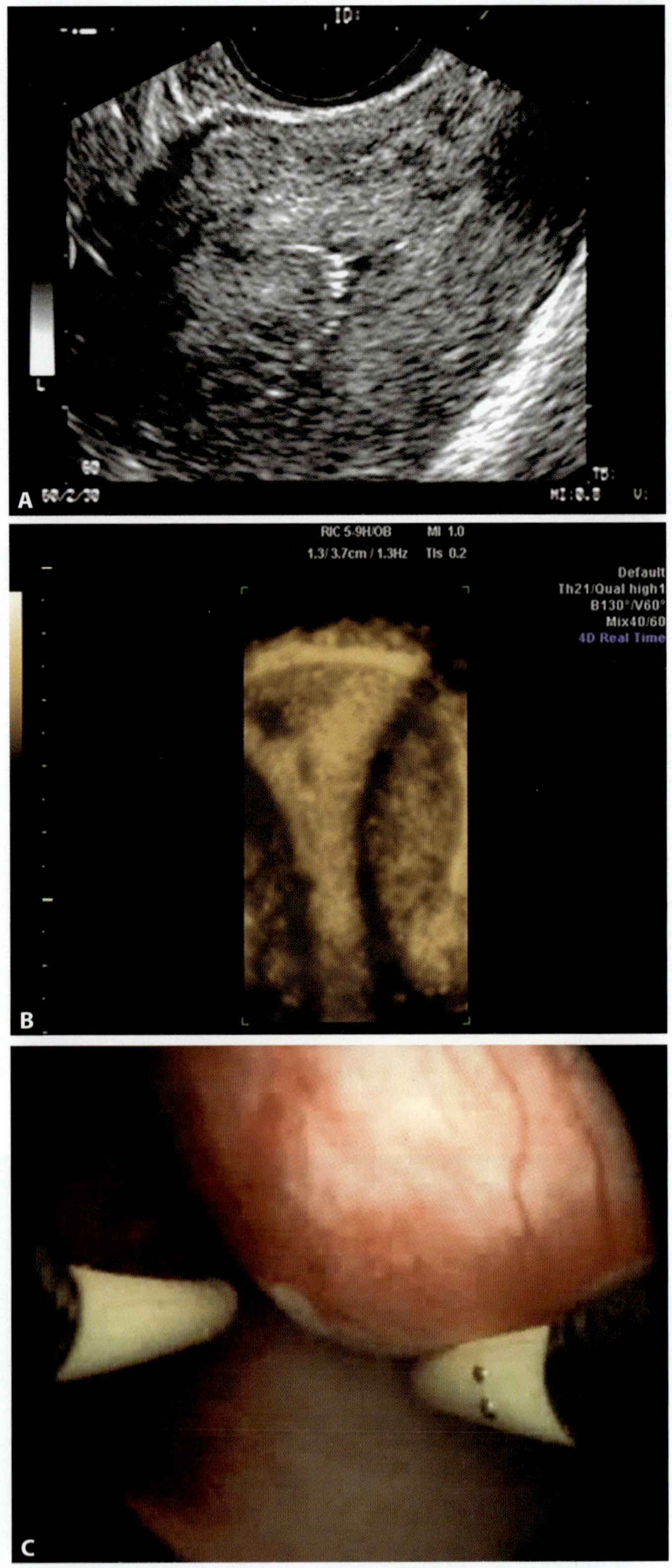

Figs. 13A to C: Contrast 2D, 3D and hysteroscopic view of submucosal fibroid.

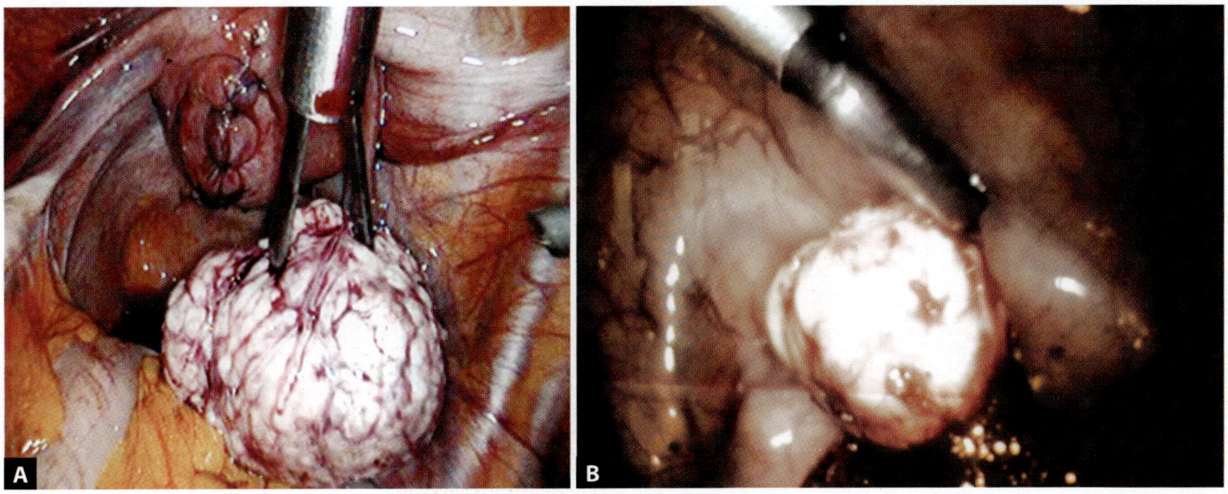

Figs. 14A and B: Laparoscopic myomectomy.

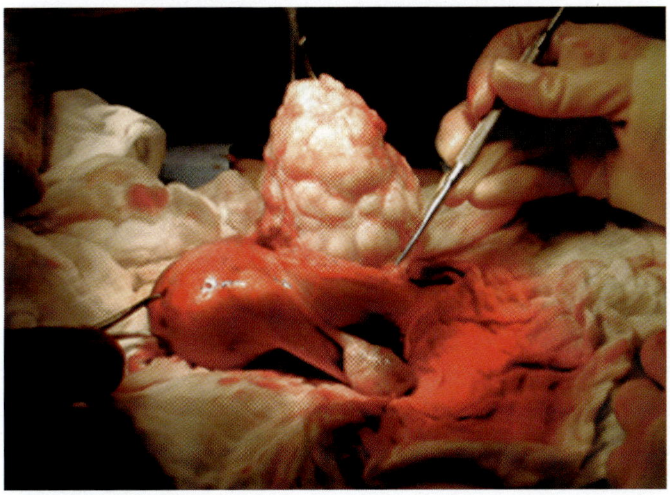

Fig. 15: Abdominal myomectomy.

A generation ago, doctors almost uniformly recommended a hysterectomy—removal of the uterus for the treatment of uterine fibroids. This operation remains the only proven permanent solution for this condition **(Fig. 15)**. Nearly 600,000 women have such surgery each year in the United States and more than one-third of these operations are performed to treat fibroids.

Uterine Fibroid Embolization

Uterine fibroid embolization (UFE) also called uterine artery embolization (UAE) is a minimally invasive surgical procedure used to treat uterine fibroids. This surgery uses a technique called embolization, which blocks the flow of blood through the vessels around the fibroids depriving them of the oxygen they need to grow. The oxygen deprivation results in the fibroids shrinking. Although, a relatively new treatment for fibroids, UFE has been used for years to control heavy bleeding after childbirth. Fibroid embolization is performed by an interventional radiologist who works in consultation with gynecologist. UFE is not recommended for women who are planning future pregnancies because its effects on fertility are not conclusively known. It is the minimally invasive procedure with no need for general anesthesia; treats all fibroids simultaneously; has a short recovery period (1–2 weeks); no abdominal scars and minimal blood loss; infrequent complications and preserved uterus with normal menstrual cycles usually resume after the procedure **(Figs. 16A and B)**.

The disadvantages of UFE are:

- Moderate to severe pain and cramping in the first several hours or days following the procedure
- Postembolization syndrome causing nausea and fever
- Up to 2% technically unsuccessful procedures, 10–15% of procedures do not respond despite technical success and no tissue obtained for pathologic diagnosis
- The risks of UFE are a 1% chance of injury to the uterus, potentially leading to hysterectomy, damage to blood vessels, infection, early-onset menopause (1–5% of women) and allergy to X-ray contrast material (iodine).[14,15]

Magnetic Resonance Guided Focused Ultrasound

Magnetic resonance guided focused ultrasound (MRGFU) is a noninvasive outpatient procedure that uses high intensity focused ultrasound waves to ablate (destroy) the

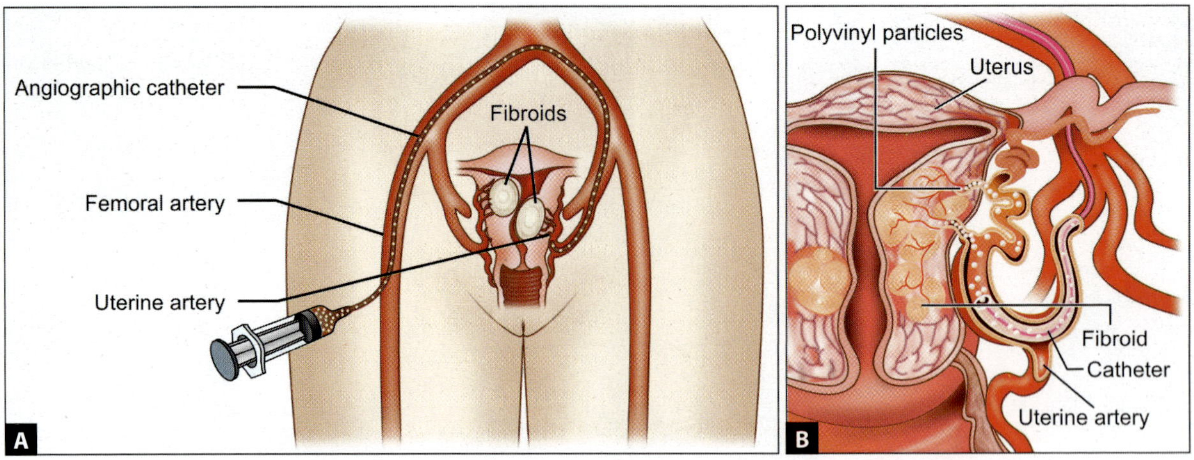

Figs. 16A and B: Schematic representation of uterine fibroid embolization.

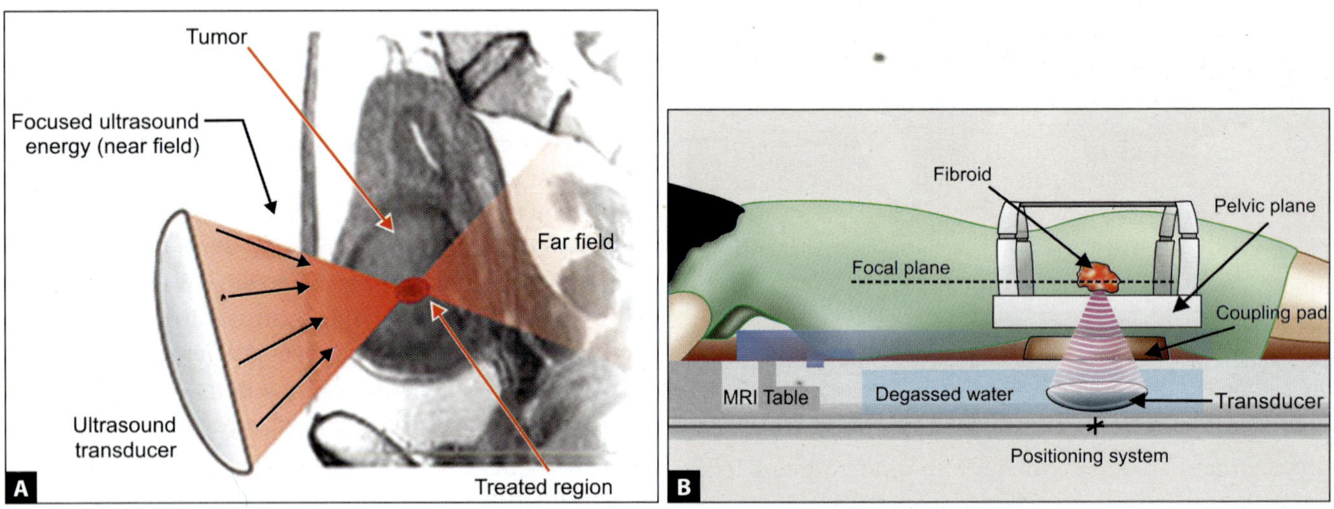

Figs. 17A and B: Schematic representation of a focused ultrasound surgery.

fibroid tissue. During the procedure, an interventional radiologist uses magnetic resonance imaging (MRI) to see inside the body to deliver the treatment directly to the fibroid. The procedure is FDA approved for treating uterine fibroids. Magnetic resonance imaging scans identify the tissue in the body to treat and are used to plan each patient's procedure. It provides a 3D view of the targeted tissue, allowing for precise focusing and delivery of ultrasound energy. It also enables the physician to monitor tissue temperature in real time, to ensure adequate but safe heating of the target. Immediate imaging of the treated area following MRGFU helps the physician determine if the treatment was successful.[16]

The ultrasound energy used in MRGFU can pass through skin, muscle, fat and other soft tissues. High intensity ultrasound energy that is directed to the fibroid heats up the tissue and destroys it. This method of tissue destruction is called thermal ablation **(Figs. 17A and B)**.

Ultrasound-guided Fibroid Sclerosation

Several years ago, authors presented a new method of fibroid therapy: sonographically guided vascular sclerosation. Sclerosation was performed under color Doppler sonographic visualization, generally after circulation mapping. Sclerosation was performed with 96% alcohol and aetoxisclerol (5–15 mL depending on the fibroid volume). There was no difference in age, size, location, vascularization and degeneration of uterine fibroids. Indication for treatment (bleeding, pain and pressure) showed no difference. Sclerosation was intravascular in

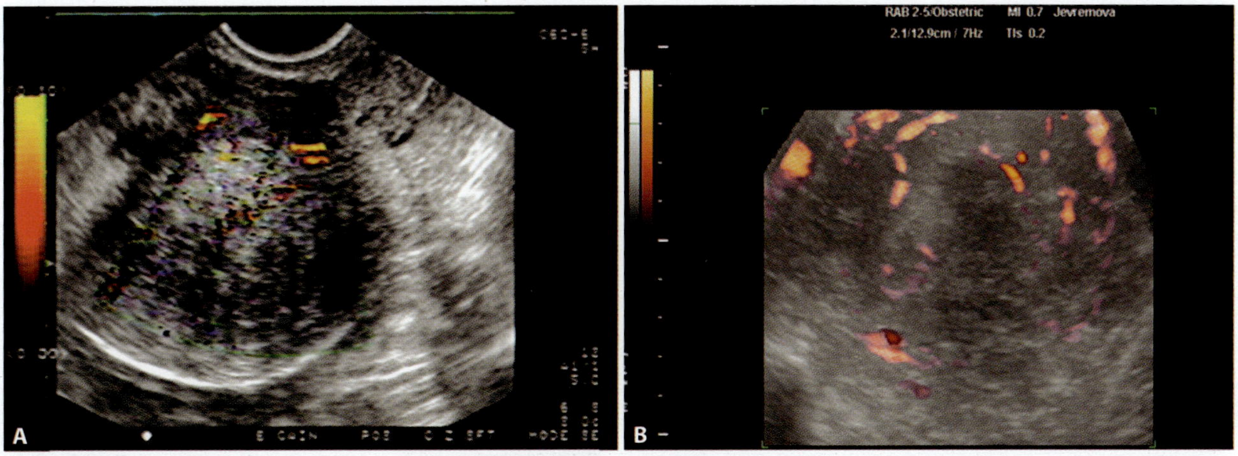

Figs. 18A and B: (A) Vascularization mapping of fibroid; (B) Glass mode with vascular mapping of fibroid.

15% and perivascular in 85% of patients. During procedure, pain was present in 20%, burning in 85% and bleeding in 15% **(Figs. 18A and B)**.

Procedure had to be repeated in 30% and it was done three times in 15% of patients. There was decrease in vascularization (in 85%) and in size (in 95% of patients) after vascular sclerosation. After sclerosation decrease in bleeding occurred in 75% of patients, 65% had less pain and 80% had decreased pelvic pressure. Hospitalization was significantly shorter: 1.5 days and 6.3 days, ICU treatment 0 and 1.5 days, and time to return to work are 3 days and 33 days, in the two groups respectively. Authors have concluded that sonographically-guided vascular sclerosation was safe and effective fibroid treatment. It has less complications and shorter recovery time.[17]

Ultrasound is of great use in making a diagnosis of the uterine fibroids, assessing the circulation, making a treatment choice and monitor the therapy effects.

UTERINE FIBROID AND PREGNANCY

Effects of Pregnancy

Normal rapid uterine expansion that occurs during pregnancy is likely a more complex mechanism mediated in part by estrogen, progesterone, various growth factors especially platelet-derived growth factor and an increase in cells with Ki-67 antigen.[18,19]

These observations support the concept that the same or similar hormonal and growth factors that normally cause uterine growth during pregnancy also stimulate growth of fibroid early in pregnancy. This may serve to explain the paradoxical observations that large fibroids remain unchanged or increase in size late in pregnancy. It is likely that during pregnancy, fibroid estrogen receptors are down regulated due to massive amounts of estrogen. Without effective estrogen receptors and thus estrogen action in the fibroids, epidermal growth factor binding is also decreased.

Effects of Fibroid Size, Location and Number of Pregnancy

Several investigators have attempted to assess the effects of fibroid size, location and number of pregnancy **(Tables 5 and 6)**.

During the first trimester, fibroids of all sizes either remained unchanged or increased in size (early response due to increased estrogen). During the second trimester, smaller fibroids (2–6 cm) usually remained unchanged or increased in size, whereas larger fibroids become smaller (start of downregulation of estrogen receptors). Regardless of initial fibroid size, during the third trimester, fibroids usually remained unchanged or decreased in size (estrogen receptors downregulated) **(Fig. 19)**. The importance of these observations is that an accurate prediction of fibroid growth in pregnancy cannot be made.[20] Pregnancy complications associated with uterine fibroids and relationships of fibroid to placenta are elaborated in **Tables 6 and 7**.

Several conclusions can be delivered:
- Growth of fibroids during pregnancy cannot be predicted
- Placental implantation over or in contact with a fibroid increases the likelihood of placental abruption, abortion, preterm labor and postpartum hemorrhage

TABLE 5: Ultrasonically measured changes in fibroids during pregnancy.

Trimester	Small fibroidsa (n = 111)			Large fibroidsb (n = 51)		
	No change number (%)	Increase number (%)	Decrease number (%)	No change number (%)	Increase number (%)	Decrease number (%)
First	7 (58)	5 (42)	0 (0)	1 (20)	4 (80)	0 (0)
Second	42 (55)	23 (30)	11 (15)	11 (38)	4 (14)	14 (48)
Third	14 (61)	1 (4)	8 (35)	5 (29)	2 (12)	10 (59)

[a]Small fibroids = 2.0–5.9 cm
[b]Large fibroids = 6.0–11.9 cm
Modified from Lev-Toaff and coworkers (1987)

TABLE 6: Pregnancy complications and relationships of fibroid to placenta.

Study	Complication	Fibroid (%)	
		No contact with placenta	Contact with placenta
Winer-Muram et al. (1984)	• Bleeding and pain	5/54 (9)	8/35 (23)
	• Major complications		
	• Abortion	1/54 (2)	9/35 (26)
	• Preterm labor	0	5/35 (14)
	• Postpartum hemorrhage	0	4/35 (11)
Rice et al. (1989)	• Major complications		
	• Preterm labor	19/79 (24)	1/14 (7)
	• Abruption	2/79 (3)	8/14 (57)
Total		48/133 (36)	35/49 (71)

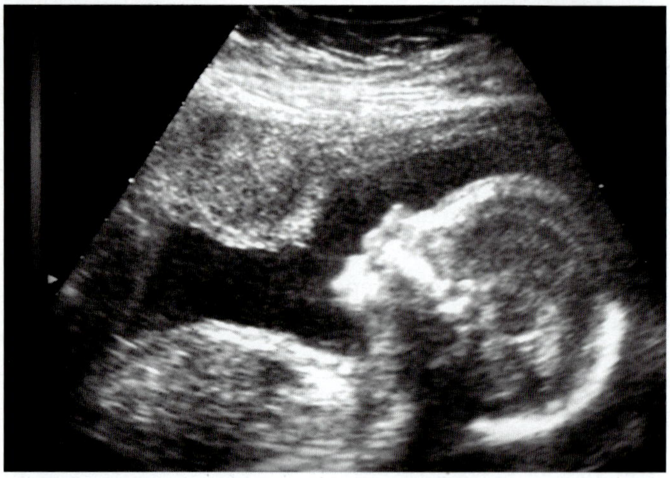

Fig. 19: Anterior wall fibroid and pregnancy.

TABLE 7: Pregnancy complications associated with uterine fibroids.

Study	Complications (%)									
	Antepartum pain and/or bleeding	Placental abruption	Preterm ruptured membranes	Preterm labor	Abortion	Fetal malpresentation	Postpartum hemorrhage	Obstructed labor	Cesarean delivery Indicated	Cesarean delivery Elective
Winer-Muram et al. (1984)	Table 52.6[a]	NS	NS (11)	5/79 (6) 52.6[a]	10/89 (14)	NS	Table	NS	11/79	–
Lev-Toaf et al. (1987)										
Uterine corpus	NS	NS	0/68	NS	6/68 (9)	NS	NS	1/68 (2)	11/68 (16)	10/68 (15)
Lower uterine segment	NS	NS	0/68	NS	0/68	NS	NS	8/45 (18)	15/45 (33)	9/45 (20)
Rice et al. (1989)[a]	Table 52.6[a]	10/93 (11)	NS	20/93 (22)	NS	11/93 (12)	NS	NS	26/39 (38)	–
Katz et al. (1989)	Increased	0/28	6/24 (25)	2/24 (8)	2/24 (8)	4/24 (17)	NS	NS	9/24 (38)	–
Hasan et al. (1990)	NS	NS	NS	16/60	NS (27)	22/60 (37)	10/60 (17)	9/60 (21)	24/60 (40)	20/60 (33)
Davis et al. (1990)	NS	NS	6/85 (7)	15/85 (18)	NS	NS	NS	NS	NS	NS

(NS, not started)
[a]Additional data presented in Table 52.3.

- Multiple fibroids are associated with an increased incidence of fetal malposition and preterm labor
- Degeneration of fibroids may be associated with a characteristic sonographic pattern
- The incidence of cesarean delivery is increased.

FIBROIDS AND STERILITY

Rationale of the association between fibroids and infertility, not completely supported by a clear biological rationale are generally explained with mechanisms by which fibroids may reduce fertility.

Submucous Fibroids

There are several mechanisms by which fibroids can adversely affect implantation, including increased uterine contractility, deranged cytokine profile, abnormal vascularization and chronic endometrial inflammation[21,22]

There is evidence to suggest that submucosal and intramural fibroids that distort the endometrial cavity are associated with decreased pregnancy and implantation rates in women who attempt to conceive spontaneously or who are proceeding with IVF treatment.[23] Several studies suggest that pregnancy rates improve following the resection of fibroids distorting the uterine cavity.[24] Pritts et al. conducted a systematic literature review and meta-analysis of existing controlled studies and concluded that women with submucosal fibroids have decreased clinical pregnancy and implantation rates compared with infertile control subjects.[24] The authors concluded that removal of submucous myomas appeared to improve outcome.[24] Since then, one further randomized controlled trial investigated the effect of hysteroscopic resection of submucous fibroids in women with unexplained primary infertility. This study revealed that hysteroscopic resection of submucous fibroids alone appeared to double cumulative clinical pregnancy rates.[25]

Intramural Fibroids

There is controversy as to whether or not noncavity-distorting intramural fibroids adversely affect IVF outcome. Some studies suggest an adverse effect of noncavity-distorting fibroids on implantation and pregnancy rates in women undergoing IVF, particularly with large fibroids >4 cm, whereas others fail to demonstrate such an association. There are several recent meta-analyses published on this particular subject.[25,26] All these analyses concur that women with intramural fibroids appear to have reduced implantation rates compared with women without intramural fibroids. However, myomectomy did not appear to significantly increase the clinical pregnancy and live birth rates[25] and the most recent meta-analysis cautioned that the available evidence is rather weak because of significant heterogeneity and methodological issues.[26]

TABLE 8: Meta-analysis on the influence of fibrosis on IVF outcome according to the localization of the lesions.

Localization	*Number of studies included*	*Breslow–Day test (P-value)*	*Common OR (95%CI)*
Clinical pregnancy rate:			
• Submucosal			
• Intramucosal	2	0.92	0.3 (0.1–0.7)
• Subserosal	7	0.38	0.8 (0.6–0.9)
• Intramural and/or	3	0.92	1.2 (0.8–1.7)
subserosal	11	0.30	1.0 (0.8–1.2)
• All types	16	0.24	0.8 (0.7–1.0)
Delivery rate:			
• Submucosal	2	0.79	0.3 (0.1–0.8)
• Intramural	7	0.09	0.7 (0.5–0.8)
• Subserosal	3	0.94	1.0 (0.7–1.5)
• Intramural and/or subserosal	11	0.68	0.9 (0.7–1.1)
• All types	16	0.43	0.8 (0.6–0.9)

Results from this meta-analysis are shown in **Table 8**. Overall, the results support the opinion that myomas negatively affect the pregnancy rate. Although based on a small number of studies, submucosal lesions appear to strongly interfere with the chance of pregnancy: the common OR (95% CI) for conception and delivery is 0.3 (0.1–0.7) and 0.3 (0.1–0.8), respectively. The impact of intramural myomas is less dramatic even if also statistically significant: the common OR (95% CI) for conception and delivery is 0.8 (0.6–0.9) and 0.7 (0.5–0.8), respectively. In general, these effects appear to be more relevant when considering the delivery rate rather than the clinical pregnancy rate. Conversely, subserosal lesions do not seem to play a role.[27]

FIBROID-LIKE CONDITIONS

There are several fibroid-like conditions that fall into a clearly different category. Some of the features of these diseases appear to be fibroid-like, and some are more like cancerous tumors.

Intravenous Leiomyomatosis

Intravenous leiomyomatosis (IVL), like fibroids, affects only women. IVL is found in both premenopausal and postmenopausal women. With IVL, the fibroids extend out from the uterus in a "wormlike" (vermiform) fashion through the blood vessels. At its greatest extent IVL can reach all the way from the uterus through the vascular system to the heart. This extension from the uterus to the heart can lead to a number of problems, such as a heart murmur, shortness of breath (dyspnea), heart palpitations, blood clots of the major blood vessels (thrombosis), fainting (syncope), leg swelling, or evidence of right-sided heart failure.

IVL, like ordinary fibroids, appears to be a hormonally responsive disease and has been shown to regress with therapy using a gonadotropin-releasing hormone (GnRH) agonist.[28,29] IVL does not seem to disappear in these instances, merely to shrink so that surgical treatment is more feasible or disease remaining after surgery can be kept at a minimal level. Generally, the vascular disease is removed surgically to prevent some of the more serious complications such as major blood clots.

A particular rearrangement of chromosomes 12 and 14 appears to be associated with IVL.[30] Intravenous leiomyomatosis thus appears to be related to the subgroup of ordinary fibroids that have the chromosome translocations involving chromosomes 12 and 14. Further molecular changes may lead to the more aggressive behavior of IVL. This genetic information also favors the theory that the disease starts with leiomyomas that then become more aggressive through an unknown mechanism.

Leiomyomatosis Peritonealis Disseminata

In leiomyomatosis peritonealis disseminata (LPD), multiple myoma-like nodules are present throughout the abdominal and pelvic cavity. Early reports primarily noted that LPD occurred in women who were pregnant or who were taking oral contraceptive pills. The diameter of lesions can range from 0.1 to 10 cm. At the time of surgery, the number of lesions seen in LPD and the distortion they cause in pelvic structure can make it seem like a cancerous process is occurring. Symptoms appear to wax and wane with LPD, and therefore regression of disease does occur—but recurrence at a later date is common. This makes it very difficult to assess treatments.

The LPD lesions appear to have receptors for estrogen and progesterone as well as luteinizing hormone (LH).[31,32] This may explain why women tend to develop LPD in pregnancy and while taking birth control pills, two states in which the body has high levels of estrogen and progesterone. A case report suggested that treatment with progestins was effective. Biologically, the lesions of LPD appear to be clonal tumors and to have some similarity to leiomyomas.[33]

Lymphangioleiomyomatosis

Lymphangioleiomyomatosis (LAM) is the most serious fibroid-like disease. In LAM fibroid-like lesions are found in the lungs and can lead to significant destruction of lung tissue. This lung disease can be fatal. In LAM, the original tumor is not a fibroid but a similar benign tumor in the kidney, a renal angiomyolipoma. The true inciting event is likely to be a mutation in the *tuberous sclerosis complex 2* (*TSC2*) gene. This gene codes for the protein tubulin, which is a major component of cell structure and also appears to act as a tumor suppressor.

Mutations in the *TSC2* gene as well as a related gene, *TSC1,* cause tuberous sclerosis (TS), a disease that has noticeable overlap with LAM. In TS, many types of benign tumors may appear throughout the body. TS affects both sexes. The lung disease that people with TS develop appears to be the same process that takes place in women with LAM.

Although LAM appears to originate from a benign kidney tumor, it is entirely a disease of women. Most women who develop LAM are premenopausal, but LAM can be diagnosed after menopause, though this is rare. There also appears to be a separate link between fibroids and LAM in that women with LAM were found to be more likely than other women to have a relative with uterine fibroids.

Lung symptoms are the most common initial clues to LAM. Shortness of breath (dyspnea) is often an early symptom; coughing up blood (hemoptysis) is another symptom. The disease leads to the formation of lung cysts and lung collapse, in which the space the lung occupied fills with air (pneumothorax) or fluid (chylothorax). The lung disease appears to be an interstitial pattern more like emphysema, in which the lymphatic spaces (located between the air spaces in the lung) are altered. The lymphatic system takes excess fluid that is located between cells and tissues and collects it into channels similar to blood vessels and eventually deposits the fluid directly into the bloodstream. The lymphatics and the blood vessels travel together in the lung between air spaces just as the pipes for plumbing run between walls and floors in a house; the space where they are located is termed the *interstitial space.*

LAM cells have both the alpha and beta versions of the estrogen receptor and androgen receptors, and estrogenic compounds like estrogen and tamoxifen have been shown to stimulate LAM cells in laboratory studies. These receptors may in part explain why LAM is a hormonally responsive disease. There also appear to be abnormalities in the enzymes that degrade extracellular matrix (ECM) in LAM that leads to cysts forming in the lungs. Just as with fibroids, control of the ECM may provide a future approach to treatment.

Benign Metastasizing Leiomyoma

Benign metastasizing leiomyoma (BML) is characterized by typical leiomyomas in the uterus and what appear to be fibroid-like lesions in a distant location, most often the lung. BML behaves in a relatively benign fashion compared with the deterioration of lung function seen in LAM. In BML the fibroid-like lesions are present in the lung, but the distortion of the interstitial spaces, which leads to so many of the pulmonary problems in women with LAM, is not. There is some evidence that removing the ovaries can cure BML, whereas oophorectomy merely slows the progression of LAM.

Leiomyomas of Uncertain Malignant Potential

Leiomyomas of uncertain malignant potential (UMP) is the easiest fibroid-like disease to understand because there are no associated findings elsewhere in the body. This diagnosis is based purely on the analysis of the fibroid tissue under the microscope. The tissue has some of the markers we associate with sarcomas, but not enough to meet the formal definition.[34]

REFERENCES

1. Buttram VC, Reiter RC. Uterine leiomyomata: etiology, symptomatology and management. Fertil Steril. 1981;6: 433-45.

1a. Tomlinson IP, Alam NA, Rowan AJ, et al. Germline mutations in FH predispose to dominantly inherited uterine fibroids, skin leiomyomata and papillary renal cell cancer. Nature Genetics. 2002;30(4):406-410.

1b. Alam NA, Rowan AJ, Wortham NC, et al. Genetic and functional analyses of FH mutations in multiple cutaneous and uterine leiomyomatosis, hereditary leiomyomatosis and renal cancer, and fumarate hydratase deficiency. Human Molecular Genetics. 2003;12(11):1241-52.

1c. Pollard P, Wortham N, Barclay E, et al. Evidence of increased microvessel density and activation of the hypoxia pathway in tumours from the hereditary leiomyomatosis and renal cell cancer syndrome. Journal of Pathology. 2005;205(1):41-9.

1d. Toro JR, Nickerson ML, Wei MH, et al. Mutations in the fumarate hydratase gene cause hereditary leiomyomatosis and renal cell cancer in families in North America. American Journal of Human Genetics. 2003;73(1):95-106.

1e. Stewart EA, Morton CC. The genetics of uterine leiomyomata: what clinicians need to know. Obstetrics and Gynecology. Apr 2006;107(4):917-21.

2. Lumsden MA, Wallace EM. Clinical presentation of uterine fibroids. Baillieres Clin Obstet Gynaecol. 1998;12:177-95.
3. Valle RF. Hysteroscopy in the evaluation of female infertility. Am J Obstet Gynecol. 1980;137:425-31.
4. Weston GC, Cattrall F, Lederman F, et al. Differences between the pre-menopausal and post-menopausal uterine fibroid vasculature. Maturitas. 2005;51(4):343-8.
5. Ng EH, Chan CC, Tang OS, et al. Endometrial and subendometrial blood flow measured by three-dimensional power Doppler ultrasound in patients with small intramural uterine fibroids during IVF treatment. Hum Reprod. 2005;20(2):501-6.
6. Vitiello D, McCarthy S. Diagnostic imaging of fibroids. Obstet Gynecol Clin North Am. 2006;33:85-95.
7. Janssen J. (E)US elastography: current status and perspectives. Z Gastroenterol. 2008;46:572-9.
8. Hobson MA, Kiss MZ, Varghese T, et al. In vitro uterine strain imaging: preliminary results. J Ultrasound Med. 2007;26: 899-908.
9. Kiss MZ, Hobson MA, Varghese T, et al. Frequency-dependent complex modulus of the uterus: preliminary results. Phys Med Biol. 2006;51:3683-95.
10. Ami O, Lamazou F, Mabille M, et al. Real-time transvaginal elastosonography of uterine fibroids. Ultrasount Obstet Gynecol. 2009;34:486-8.
11. Clark TJ. Outpatient hysteroscopy and ultrasonography in the management of endometrial disease. Current opinion in Obstetrics and Gynecology. 2004;16:305-11.
12. Vercellini P, Cortesi I, Oldani S, et al. The role of transvaginal ultrasonography and outpatient diagnostic hysteroscopy in the evaluation of patients with menorrhagia. Human Reproduction. 2006;12:1768-71.
13. Salim R, Lee C, Davies A, et al. A comparative study of three-dimensional saline infusion sonohysterography and diagnostic hysteroscopy for the classification of submucous fibroids. Human Reproduction. 2005;20(1):253-7.
14. Spies JB, Scialli AR, Jha RC, et al. Initial results from uterine fibroid embolization for symptomatic leiomyomata. Journal of Vascular and Interventional Radiology. 1999;10(9):1149-57.

15. McLucas B, Goodwin S, Adler L, et al. Pregnancy following uterine fibroid embolization. Int J Gynaecol Obstet. 2001;74(1):1-7.
16. Smart OC, Hindley JT, Regan L, et al. Magnetic resonance guided focused ultrasound surgery of uterine fibroids—The tissue effects of GnRH agonist pre-treatment. European Journal of Radiology. 2006;59(2):163-7.
17. Ljubic' A, Šulovic' V. Sonographically guided vascular sclerosation: new method of myoma treatment. Glas SANU. 2002;47:169-79.
18. Mendoza AE, Young R, et al. Increqsed platelet-derived growth factor A—chain expression in human uterine smooth muscle cells during the physiologic hypertrophy of pregnancy. Proc Natl Acad Sci USA. 1990;87(6):2177-81.
19. Kawaguchi K, Fujii S, Konishi I, et al. Immunohistochemical analysis of oestrogen receptors, progesterone receptors and Ki-67 in leiomyomata and myometrium during the menstrual cycle and pregnancy. Virchows Arch A Pathol Anat Histopathol. 1991;419(4):309-15.
20. Lev-Toaff AS, Coleman BG, Arger PH, et al. Leiomyomas in pregnancy: sonographic study. Radiology. 1987;164(2):375-80.
21. Buttram VC Jr, Reiter R. Uterine leiomyomata: etiology, symptomatology, and management. Fertil Steril. 1981;36:433-45.
22. Taylor E, Gomel V. The uterus and fertility. Fertil Steril. 2008;89:1-16.
23. Bernard G, Darai E, Poncelet C, Benifla JL, Madelenat P. Fertility after hysteroscopic myomectomy: effect of intramural myomas associated. Eur J Obstet Gynecol Reprod Biol. 2000;88:85-90.
24. Pritts EA, Parker WH, Olive DL. Fibroids and infertility: an updated systematic review of the evidence. Fertil Steril. 2009;91:1215-23.
25. Shokeir T, El-Shafei M, Yousef H, Allam AF, Sadek E. Submucous myomas and their implications in the pregnancy rates of patients with otherwise unexplained primary infertility undergoing hysteroscopic myomectomy: a randomized matched control study. Fertil Steril. 2010;94:724-9.
26. Metwally M, Farquhar CM, Li TC. Is another meta-analysis on the effects of intramural fibroids on reproductive outcomes needed? Reprod Biomed. Online 2011;23:2-14.
27. Somigliana E, Vercellini P, Daguati R, Pasin P. Fibroids and female reproduction: a critical analysis of the evidence. Human Reproduction Update. 2007;13(5):465-76.
28. Tresukosol D, Kudelka AP, Malpica A, et al. Leuprolide acetate and intravascular leiomyomatosis. Obstetrics and Gynecology. 1995;86(4 Pt 2):688-92.
29. Mitsuhashi A, Nagai Y, Sugita M, et al. GnRH agonist for intravenous leiomyomatosis with cardiac extension. A case report. Journal of Reproductive Medicine. 1999; 44(10):883-6.
30. Dal Cin P, Quade BJ, Neskey DM, et al. Intravenous leiomyomatosis is characterized by a der(14)t(12;14)(q15;q24). Genes, Chromosomes and Cancer. 2003; 36(2):205-6.
31. Akkersdijk GJ, Flu PK, Giard RW, et al. Malignant leiomyomatosis peritonealis disseminata. American Journal of Obstetrics and Gynecology. 1990;163(2):591-3.
32. Butnor KJ, Burchette JL, Robboy SJ. Progesterone receptor activity in leiomyomatosis peritonealis disseminata. International Journal of Gynecological Pathology. 1999; 18(3):259-64.
33. Fujii S, Nakashima N, Okamura H, et al. Progesterone-induced smooth muscle-like cells in the subperitoneal nodules produced by estrogen. Experimental approach to leiomyomatosis peritonealis disseminata. American Journal of Obstetrics and Gynecology. 1981;139(2):164-72.
34. Quade BJ. Pathology, cytogenetics and molecular biology of uterine leiomyomas and other smooth muscle lesions. Current Opinion in Obstetrics and Gynecology. 1995;7(1):35-42.

55

CHAPTER

Three-dimensional Static Ultrasound and Three-dimensional Power Doppler in Gynecologic Pelvic Tumors

Juan Luis Alcázar

INTRODUCTION

Pelvic tumors from gynecologic origin are common disorders in clinical practice.

Ultrasound has been used largely for the differential diagnosis of pelvic tumors such as endometrial, myometrial and adnexal pathologies.

In the case of endometrial cancer, the measurement of endometrial thickness has been proved to be an effective method to exclude malignancy.[1] However, a thickened endometrium is a nonspecific finding. The use of pulsed Doppler remains controversial[2,3] and for this reason some authors have advocated the use of color mapping for differentiating endometrial cancer from other benign conditions.[4] However, this approach is only reproducible in experienced hands.[5]

Uterine myomas are a very common benign disease. The diagnosis use to be easy by ultrasound[6] and there is evidence that uterine blood flow is increased in the presence of fibroids.[7] Some authors have stated that the use of color Doppler may discriminate benign fibroids from uterine sarcomas.[8] However, other authors have challenged this concept.[9,10]

Cervical cancer has been largely obviated from the assessment by ultrasound. However, recently the assessment of tumor vascularization in cancer of the uterine cervix has gained attention from researches, because some studies have shown that may be possible to predict therapeutic response to neoadjuvant chemotherapy or chemoradiation.[11,12]

Adnexal masses are probably one of the most frequent problems in gynecology. Patients with a questionable adnexal tumors should be referred to a gynecologic oncologist specialist[13] whereas benign tumors should be treated with laparoscopic surgery by general gynecologist[14] or even managed expectantly.[15] Morphological ultrasound assessment of adnexal masses can be considered as the primary imaging modality to be used because of its high sensitivity. However, false-positive rate remains high.[16] The role of pulsed Doppler is still controversial.[17]

Some authors have proposed a simpler approach by just looking tumor blood flow mapping with encouraging results.[18]

In the last years, three-dimensional ultrasound has become available in clinical practice, opening a formidable research area.[19]

The objective of the present chapter is to review current evidence of the use of three-dimensional ultrasound and three-dimensional power Doppler ultrasound in the evaluation of pelvic gynecologic tumors.

ENDOMETRIAL CANCER

Few studies have evaluated the role of three-dimensional ultrasound in the diagnosis and assessment of endometrial cancer.

Three-dimensional ultrasound allows the assessment of endometrial volume **(Figs. 1 and 2)**. In our experience this measurement is highly reproducible.[20] The intra-observer

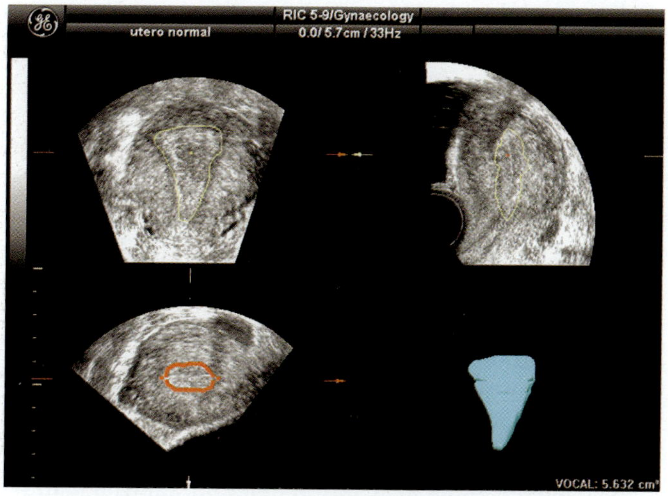

Fig. 1: Endometrial volume calculation by using the VOCAL rotational method.

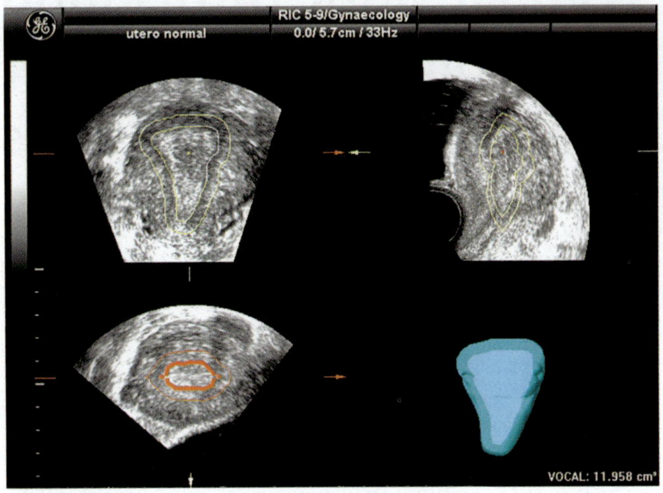

Fig. 2: Subendometrial area volume calculation by using the VOCAL rotational method.

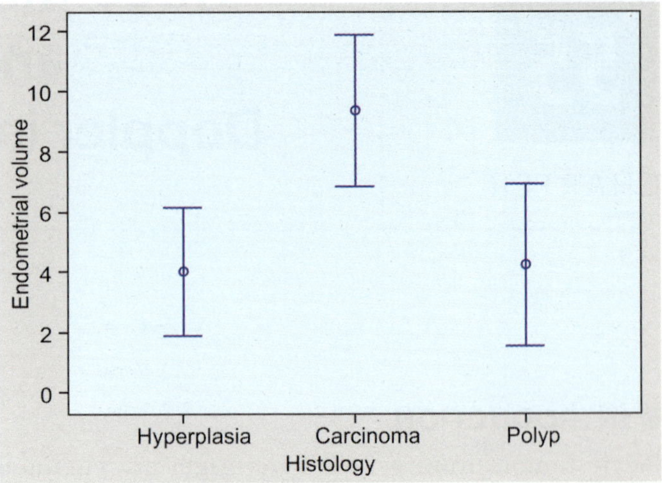

Fig. 3: Mean endometrial volume with 95% CIs in endometrial cancer, hyperplasia and polyps.

intraclass correlation coefficient (ICC) is 0.97 and the interobserver ICC is 0.70.

Gruboeck compared the diagnostic performance of endometrial thickness and endometrial volume in a series of 103 women with postmenopausal bleeding.[21] They found that both mean endometrial thickness (29.5 mm versus 15.6 mm) and mean endometrial volume (39.0 mL versus 5.5. mL)were significantly higher in women with endometrial cancer as compared with whose with benign conditions. Using a cut-off of 15 mm for endometrial thickness and 13 mL for endometrial volume, this parameter was more sensitive (100% versus 83%) and had a higher positive predictive value (91.7% versus 54.5%).

Kurjak et al.[22] evaluating a series of 41 women with suspected endometrial pathology obtained similar results. They reported that endometrial volume as well as endometrial thickness was significantly higher in women with endometrial cancer as compared with those patients with benign conditions, such as polyps, endometrial hyperplasia or cystic atrophy.

More than one decade later, Mansour et al. reached the same conclusions than Gruboeck et al. comparing endometrial volume and thickness in a series of 170 women with postmenopausal bleeding.[23] However, these authors reported that the best cut-off for endometrial volume was 1.35 mL with a sensitivity of 100% and a false-positive rate of 29%, much higher than that reported by Gruboeck. An explanation for that is that Mansour's study included patients with "endometrial atypia" in the group of endometrial cancer.

However, Yaman et al. found that endometrial volume was more specific than endometrial thickness in a series of 213 women, 42 with endometrial cancer.[24] With a cut-off of 2.7 mL, sensitivity was 100% and specificity was 69%. Odeh et al.[25] and Merce et al.[26] have reported similar findings.

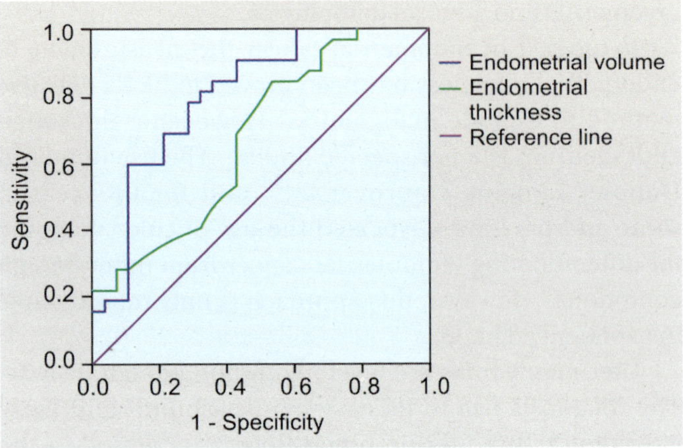

Fig. 4: ROC curves for endometrial thickness and endometrial volume for detecting endometrial cancer in women with postmenopausal bleeding.

Opolskiene et al. did not find differences between endometrial volume and thickness in terms of sensitivity and specificity for diagnosing endometrial cancer.[27]

In our experience,[28] in a series of women with postmenopausal bleeding and thickened endometrium (≥5 mm) we also found that endometrial volume was significantly higher in endometrial cancer as compared with polyps or hyperplasia **(Fig. 3)**. In agreement with previous authors, endometrial volume is more specific than endometrial thickness **(Fig. 4)**. This has been also reported in more recent studies.[29,30]

TABLE 1: Endometrial volume compared with endometrial thickness for diagnosing endometrial cancer in women with postmenopausal bleeding.

				Endometrial thickness		*Endometrial volume*	
Author	***N***	***EC prevalence (%)***	***Cut-off***	***Sensitivity (%)***	***Specificity (%)***	***Sensitivity (%)***	***Specificity (%)***
Gruboeck[21]	97	11	ET 15.0 mm	83	88		
			EV 13 cc			100	99
Mansour[23]	170	16	NA				
			EV 1.35 mL			100	71
Yaman[24]	213	20	ET 7.0 mm	100	43		
			EV 2.70 mL			100	69
Odeh[25]*	56	20	ET 5.5 mm	97	12		
			EV 3.56 mL			93	36
Merce[26†]	84	65	ET 12.1 mm	69	55		
			EV 6.86 mL			63	69
Alcazar[28‡]	99	44	ET 7.6 mm	90	36		
			EV 2.30 mL			93	62
Opolskiene[27‡]	62	20	ET 11.8 mm	85	71		
			EV 5.30 mL			69	88

*Endometrial hyperplasia and cancer included in the same "pathologic" group
†Retrospective study assessing only women with endometrial hyperplasia and cancer
‡Prospective study including only women with thickened endometrium
(EC: endometrial cancer; ET: endometrial thickness; EV: endometrial volum)

These studies are summarized in **Table 1**.

The use of 3D- ultrasound has been also found to be effective to assess myometrial invasion in endometrial cancer by analyzing the myometrial-endometrial interface and to estimate the maximum penetration of the tumor within the myometrium[31,32] **(Figs. 5 and 6)**. Our group described and analyzed the diagnostic performance of a new method for assessing myometrial infiltration preoperatively based on 3D-ultrasound.[33] This new approach was based on a three-dimensional virtual navigation through the uterus for detecting the deepest point of myometrial infiltration in a series of 96 women with endometrial cancer. Sixty-nine women had <50% myometrial infiltration on histologic analysis and 27 had ≥50% myometrial infiltration. The most interesting finding from this study was the negative predictive value reported (100%) using this approach. The false-positive rate reported was 39%. The reproducibility of the method was good.

Similar findings have been reported by other authors.[34] However, another researchers have not found that 3D-ultrasound is better than MRI[35] or 2D ultrasound.[36,37]

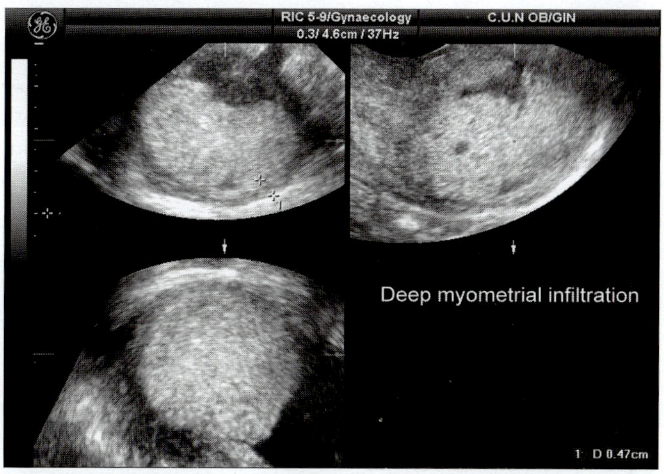

Fig. 5: Estimation of myometrial invasion in endometrial cancer by using 3D multiplanar navigation. In this case, infiltration is considered as deep.

Another possibility for three-dimensional ultrasound is the assessment of tumor vascularity by 3D power Doppler.[38] This technique allows the depiction of vascular network in endometrial lesions as well as the estimation of three vascular indexes (VI, FI and VFI) by the VOCAL rotational method. Vascular network in malignant tumor uses to be irregular with chaotic branching, changes in vessels caliber, pseudoaneurysms **(Figs. 7 and 8)**. On the other hand, these features used to be absent in benign conditions such as polyp **(Fig. 9)** or hyperplasia **(Fig. 10)**.

Kupesic et al. reported that assessing the vascular network by 3D power Doppler they were able to determine correctly the depth of myometrial invasion in 21 out of 22 women with endometrial cancer.[39] They assessed the presence of chaotic vessels in the endometrial-myometrial interface. Depending on whether more than half or less than half of the myometrium was involved by these chaotic vessel, patients were considered as having deep or superficial myometrial invasion **(Fig. 11)**.

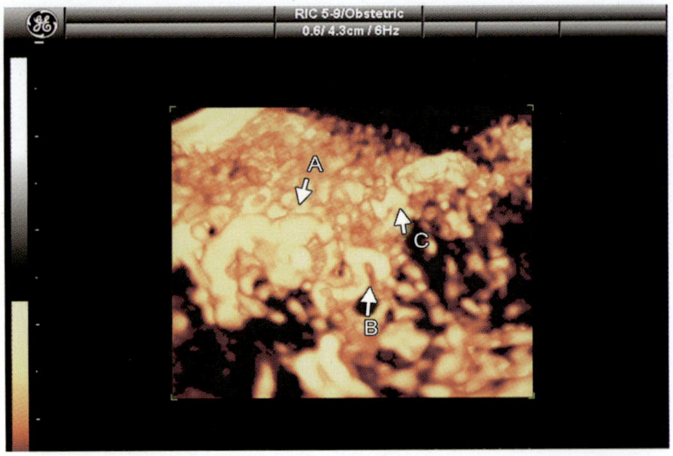

Fig. 8: Same case as **Figure 7**. Different vessel caliber (A), abnormal branching (B) and microaneurysms (C) are seen.

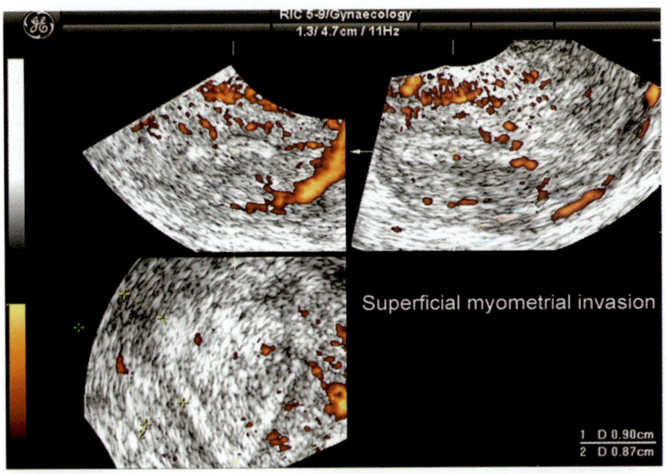

Fig. 6: Estimation of myometrial invasion in endometrial cancer by using 3D multiplanar navigation. In this case, infiltration is considered as superficial.

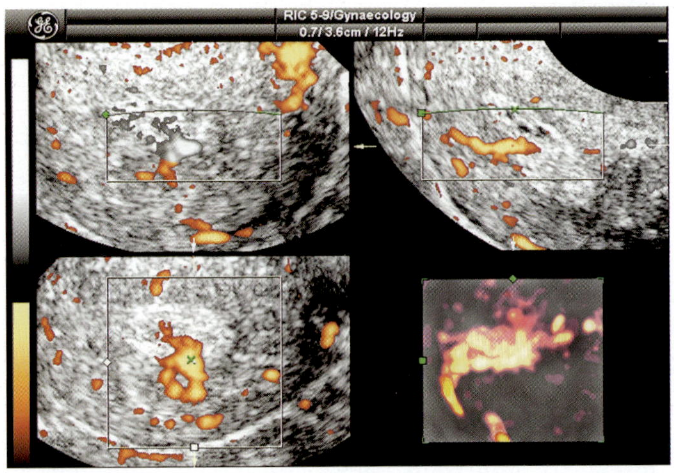

Fig. 9: Vascular pattern for an endometrial polyp. A single predominant vessel is seen within the lesion.

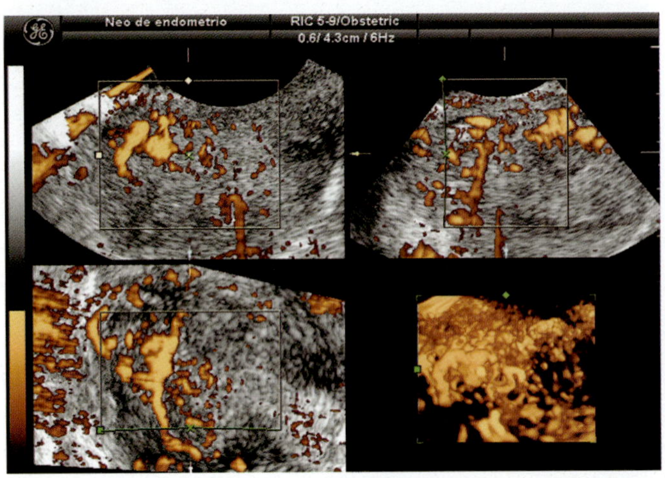

Fig. 7: 3D power Doppler depiction of vascular architecture in a case of endometrial cancer. Chaotic pattern is clearly seen.

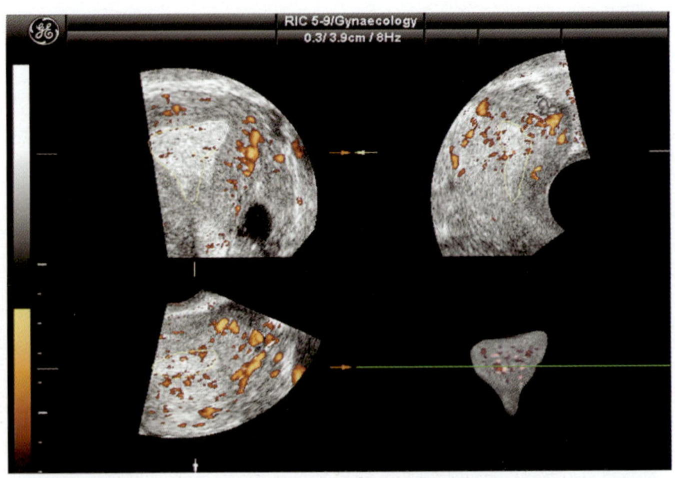

Fig. 10: Vascular pattern for endometrial hyperplasia. Scattered vessels can be seen within the endometrium.

The use of vascular indexes **(Figs. 12A and B)** has not been extensively assessed. Odeh et al. reported that all three 3D-PD indexes were significantly higher in women with endometrial cancer as compared with those with benign pathology.[25] However, they did not compare with conventional 2D-PD and the specificity reported was low. Mercé et al. found that 3D-PD indexes were significantly higher in women with endometrial cancer as compared with those with endometrial hyperplasia.[26] Alcázar et al. also found that 3D-PD indexes were significantly higher in women with endometrial cancer as compared with those with benign pathology,[28] but this study included only women with endometrial thickness above 5 mm and did not compare 3D results with conventional 2D color Doppler. Opolskiene et al reported data in a series of women with postmenopausal bleeding and endometrial thickness ≥4.5 mm.[27] They concluded that, although 3D-PD indexes were significantly higher in women with endometrial cancer as compared with those with benign pathology, this technique adds little information to endometrial thickness or volume. Lieng et al. analyzed a small series of women with endometrial polyps (n = 17) and endometrial cancer (n = 17) comparing 3D-PD indexes within the lesions before and after contrast enhanced examination.[40] They did not find differences between groups in 3D-PD indexes.

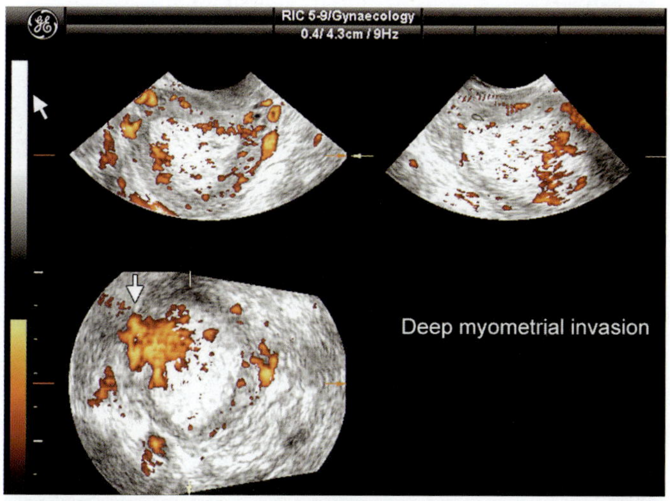

Fig. 11: Assessment of myometrial invasion by 3D power Doppler. In this case, deep myometrial infiltration was considered at the level of the right uterine cornu.

Galvan et al. assessed the correlation between intratumoral 3D-PD indexes and several histological tumor characteristics in a series of 99 women with endometrial cancer.[41] In their analysis, endometrial volume and vascularization index were independently associated with myometrial infiltration and tumor stage, vascularization index was independently associated with tumor grade and endometrial volume correlated with lymph node metastases. Similar findings have been reported by Saarelainen et al.[42]

In conclusion, endometrial volume seems to be a better predictor for endometrial cancer than endometrial thickness in women with postmenopausal bleeding. 3D power Doppler assessment of endometrial vascularity is reproducible, and seems to be useful for differentiating endometrial cancer than benign endometrial conditions. Its performance seems to be better than endometrial volume. This technique also seems to be useful to predict some histological features of endometrial cancers, especially myometrial invasion.

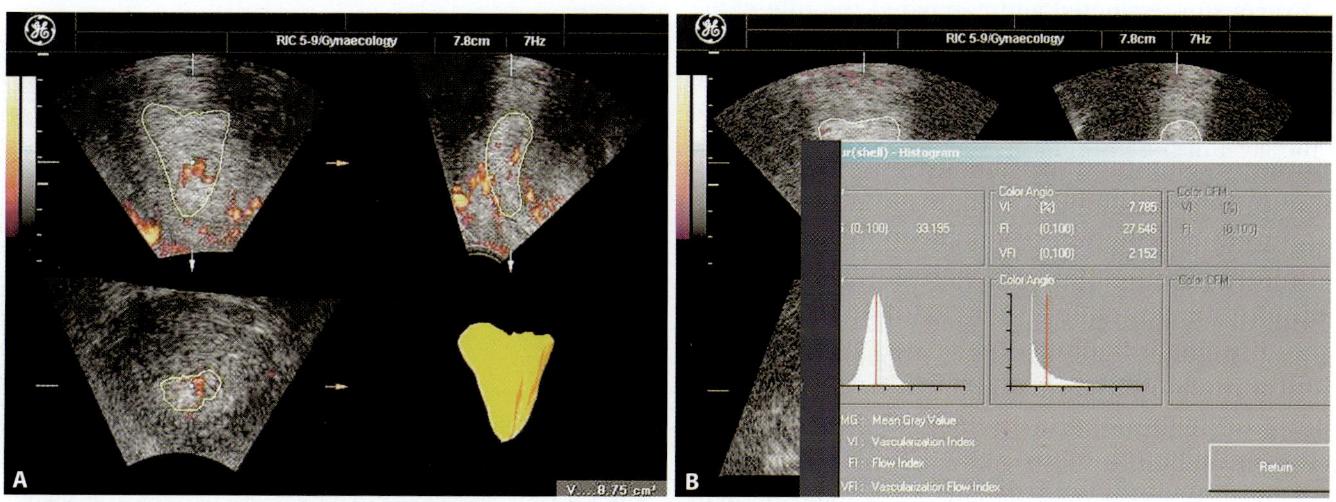

Figs. 12A and B: 3D power Doppler volume (A) and indices (B) calculated in a case of endometrial cancer.

UTERINE LEIOMYOMAS AND SARCOMAS

Uterine fibroids are the most common pelvic tumors of women in reproductive age. The sonographic appearance of uterine leiomyomas use to be a hypoechoic rounded or oval well-defined lesion arising from the myometrium. Sometimes some secondary changes may occur with a wide spectrum of ultrasonic images.

The use of three-dimensional ultrasound in the assessment of uterine fibroids has been evaluated in few studies.

Salim et al. found that 3D sonohysterography is very useful to classify submucous myomas and the agreement with the hysteroscopic classification is high (Kappa index = 0.81)[43] **(Fig. 13)**.

We also have found that 3D multiplanar display of submucous myomas is very useful to determine the myometrial safety margin prior to hysteroscopic resection **(Fig. 14)**.

The assessment of leiomyoma vascularity by 3D power Doppler ultrasound allows the assessment of its vascular network. This assessment clearly shows that typical vascular network of uterine fibroids has a "nest" appearance **(Fig. 15)**. Their findings are is agreement with those studies based on corrosion analysis of vascular network.[44]

One possible clinical application of this technique is its use for predicting response to medical treatment. Muñiz et al. assessed 15 women with uterine fibroids prior to uterine artery embolization by 3D power Doppler ultrasound[45] and concluded that this technique can reveal collateral blood flow not detected by uterine artery arteriography and could predict response to treatment.

Exacoustos evaluated and compared the role of 2D and 3D ultrasound before, during and after laparoscopic cryomyolisis in 10 women with uterine fibroid.[46] The authors used a semiquantitative assessment of blood flow at the level of the fibroid capsule and inside the tumor. This study found that both, 2D and 3D power Doppler ultrasound was useful to assess fibroid vascularization but 3D power Doppler were best to evaluate such a evaluation.

The preoperative diagnosis of uterine sarcoma remains a formidable clinical challenge. Attempts have been made for such diagnosis using 3D power Doppler ultrasound. Kupesic et al. reported that typical vascularization of uterine sarcoma was characterized by irregular vessels that were randomly dispersed both in central parts of the tumor.[47] However, these findings can also be found in growing large benign fibroids **(Fig. 16)**.

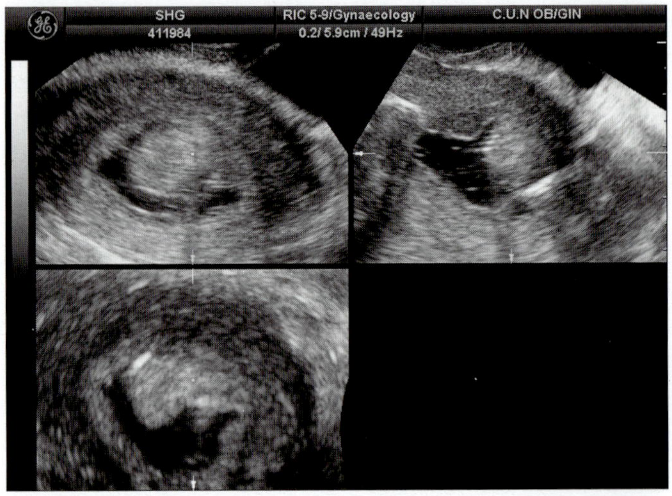

Fig. 13: 3D sonohysterography in a case of submucous myoma.

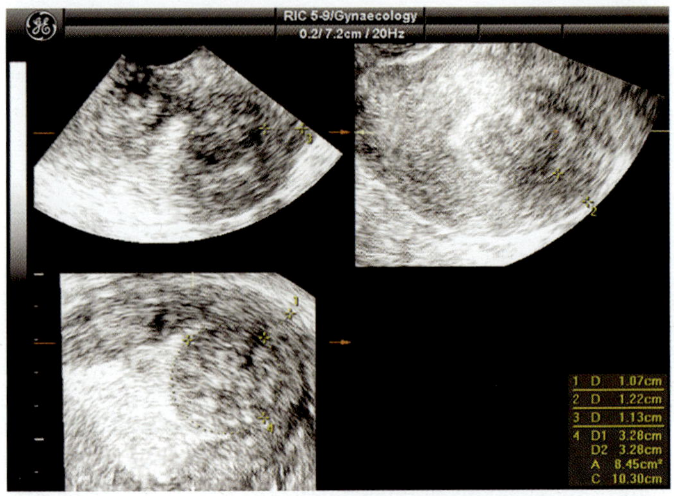

Fig. 14: Estimation of safety margin for hysterosopic resection in a case of submucous myoma using 3D multiplanar navigation.

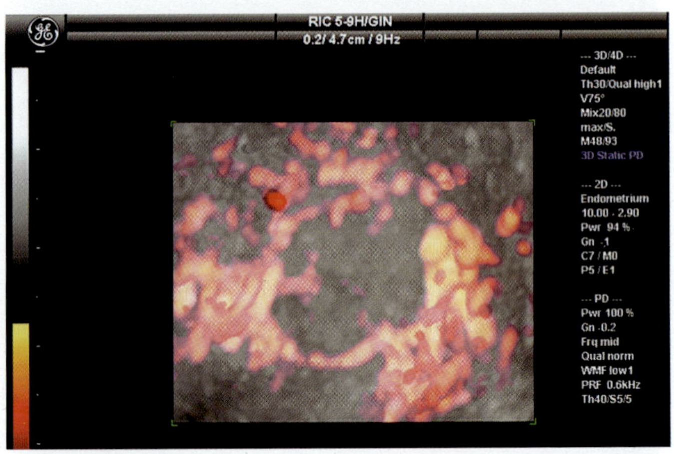

Fig. 15: "Nest" appearance of the vascular network of an uterine fibroid by 3D power Doppler.

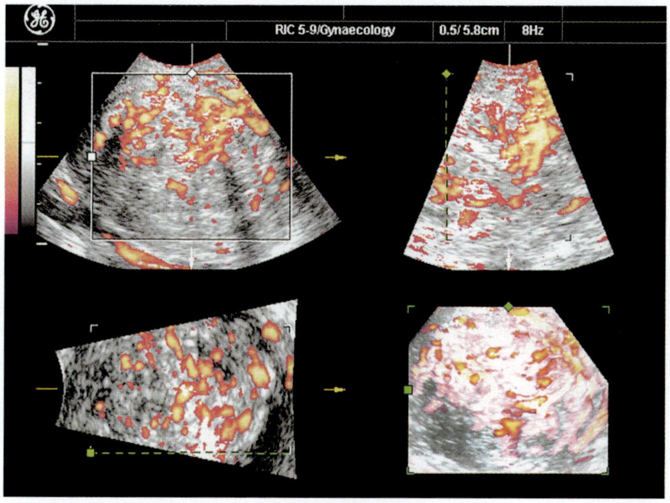

Fig. 16: Chaotic vascular network in a fast growing uterine fibroid.

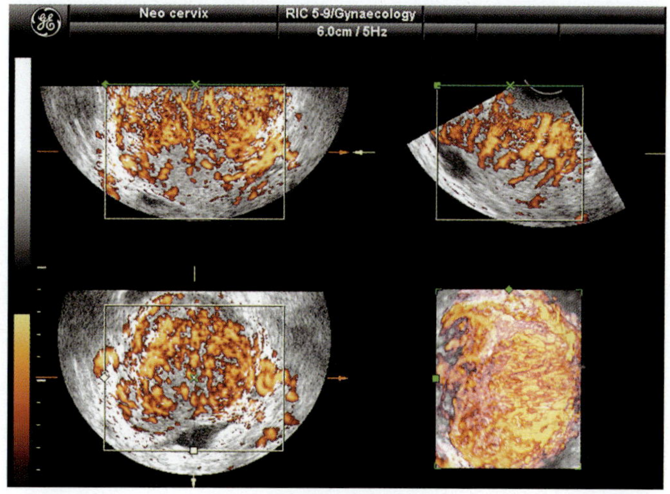

Fig. 18: 3D power Doppler appearance of cervical vascularity in a case of uterine cervical cancer.

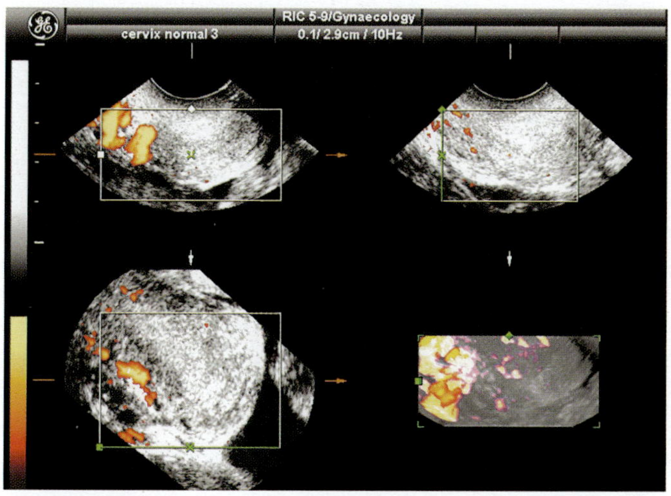

Fig. 17: 3D power Doppler appearance of cervical vascularity in a case of uterine cervix without pathology.

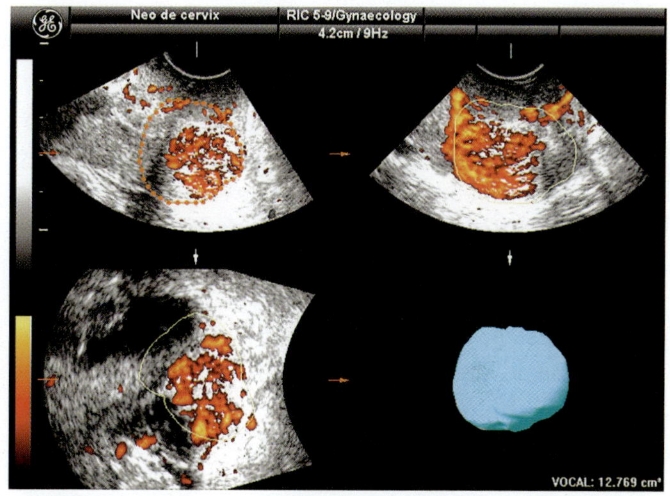

Fig. 19: Tumor volume calculation in cervical cancer by using the VOCAL rotational method.

In conclusion, 3D power Doppler ultrasound seems to be a potential tool for predicting response to medical treatment of uterine fibroids and to assess their growth potential. Its role in the diagnosis of uterine sarcoma remains to be established.

CERVICAL CANCER

Suren et al. were the first to report the assessment of intracervical vascularization by 3D power Doppler ultrasound.[48] They found the typical finding in cases of cervical cancer a chaotic network with tortuous vessels as compared with benign conditions in which the course of vessels has a regular structure **(Figs. 17 and 18)**.

This technique can assess precisely tumor volume and vascularization **(Figs. 19 and 20)**.

Hsu et al.[49] analyzed 141 women with early stage cervical cancer. They described four types of intratumoral vascularity patterns, which were not correlated with VI, FI, and VFI values: localized, peripheral, scattered and single-vessels types. Tumor volume was related to FI ($r = 0.373$, $P < 0.001$), but not with VI or VFI. They concluded that this technique was a useful tool to investigate intratumoral vascularization.

However, Testa et al.[50] did not find differences in 3D power Doppler blood flow parameters in cervical cancer according to tumor diameter, tumor grade and histological

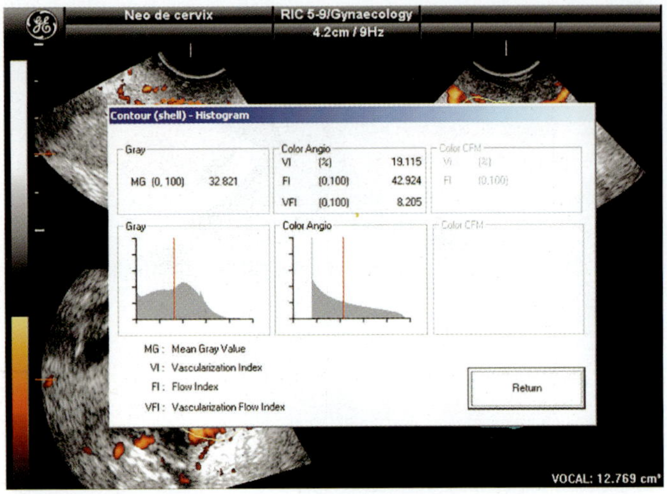

Fig. 20: 3D power Doppler indices calculated in a case of cervical cancer.

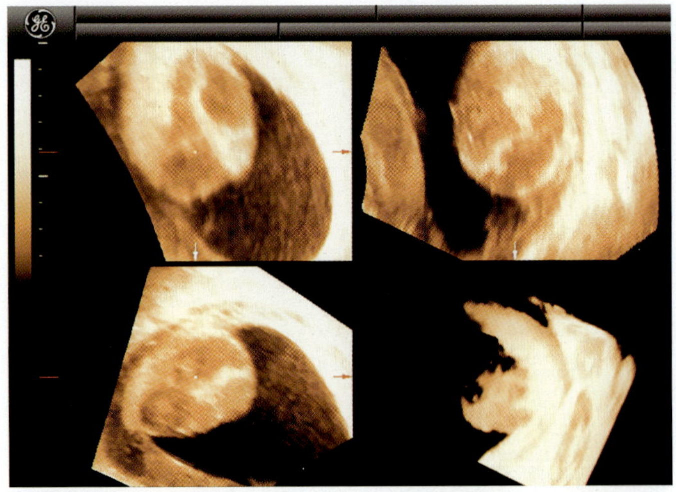

Fig. 21: The use of the "threshold" function allows eliminating some internal echoes in a case of cystic dermoid tumor.

type. They found a marginal statistical significant according to tumor stage, being III/IV stages more vascularized than I/II stages tumors.

In our experience, a progressive increase in VI, VFI and FI exists in patients with no cervical pathology, intraepithelial neoplasia, and invasive cervical cancer.[51] We reported data on 56 women with cervical cancer[52] No correlation was found between tumor volume and 3D-PDA indexes with histologic type, LVSI and lymph node metastases. Moderately and poorly differentiated tumors and advanced stage tumors had larger volume and higher 3D-PDA indexes.

Although the clinical value of 3D-PDA assessment of tumor vascularization in cervical cancer still needs to be established, all these studies pointed out that the non-invasive assessment of tumor vascularity prior to treatment could be useful to identify high-risk patients for recurrence. In fact, some preliminary data show that it may be useful for assessing tumor response to chemoradiation in advanced cancer.[53]

One study described a novel technique using 3D ultrasound for local staging of cervical carcinoma.[54] This method was based on the multiplanar display and was used in 14 women. The concordance of 3D ultrasound and pathology for assessing parametrial, rectum and bladder involvement was 93%, 93% and 100%, respectively.

ADNEXAL TUMORS

Three-dimensional ultrasonography overcomes some limitations of conventional two-dimensional ultrasound

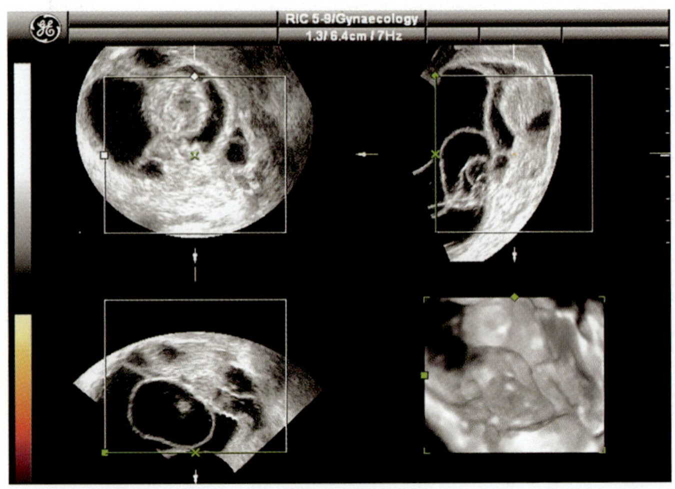

Fig. 22: 3D surface rendering of the internal appearance in an ovarian multilocular cyst with solid components.

allowing a more detailed assessment of morphologic features of the object studied, with no restriction to the number and orientation of the scanning planes.

Among the advantages of three-dimensional ultrasound are the possibilities of obtaining images from all spatial planes and eliminate echoes by using the "threshold" function. The first allows a more detailed assessment of intracystic structures and the second allows eliminating internal echoes mimicking solid tissue, such as clots, debris and fatty and mucinous plugs **(Fig. 21)**. In our experience, surface rendering was the most useful mode for three-dimensional transvaginal ultrasound (3D TVS) evaluation **(Fig. 22)**. The "niche mode" may also be helpful in some instances **(Figs. 23A and B)**. However,

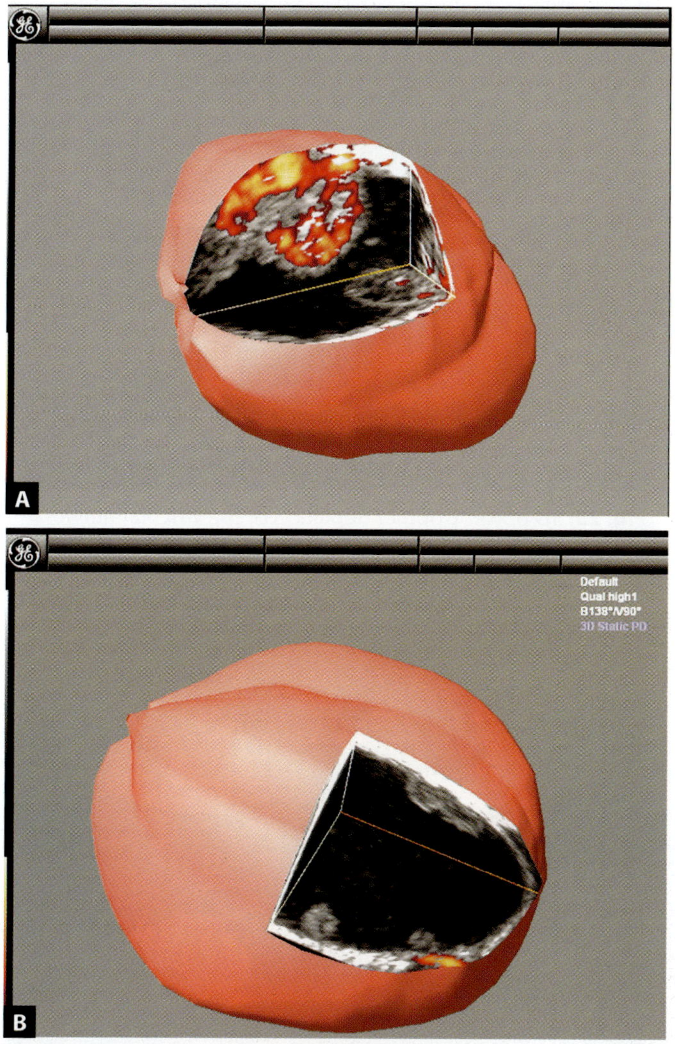

Figs. 23A and B: Two cases of ovarian cyst with a gross papillary projection. (A) In case A "niche" mode allows confirming that vessels coming from the cyst wall enter the papillary projection; (B) In case B, it can be seen how no vessels appear within the papillary projection.

(*Courtesy:* Dr MA Pascual)

some pitfalls when using 3D TVS might be born in mind. By using the surface rendering mode alone some daughter cysts may be interpreted as solid areas. On the other hand, threshold function works similarly to gain in conventional 2D ultrasound. An excessive gain adjusting may eliminate some true solid areas, leading to reclassify as benign an actually malignant lesion.

A new image display modality is the "inversion mode", which can to depict as "solid" cystic components of the tumor. This could be helpful in predominantly cystic complex lesions such as hydrosalpinx **(Fig. 24)**.

Studies evaluating the role of 3D TVS in assessing adnexal masses are scanty and reported controversial results **(Table 2)**.

Bonilla-Musoles et al. evaluated by two-dimensional and three-dimensional ultrasonography 76 women diagnosed as having an adnexal mass. They concluded that 3D TVS was more sensitive than two-dimensional transvaginal ultrasound (2D TVS).[55]

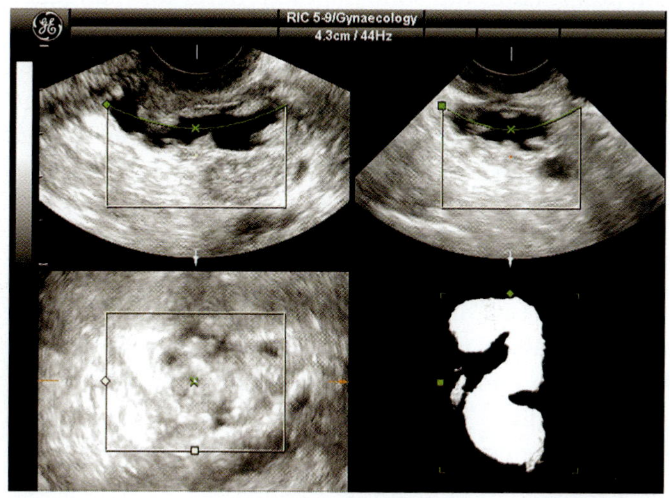

Fig. 24: Three-dimensional reconstruction of a hydrosalpinx by using the "inversion mode". The shape of the tube is clearly shown.

TABLE 2: Three-dimensional versus two-dimensional ultrasound for diagnosing ovarian cancer.

			Sensitivity		*Specificity*		
Author	***N***	***OC prevalence (%)***	***3D (%)***	***2D (%)***	***3D (%)***	***2D (%)***	***P value***
Bonilla[55]	76	7	100	80	100	99	<0.05
Hata[56]	20	25	100	100	92	38	<0.05
Alcazar[57]	49	48	100	90	78	61	NS
Alcazar[58]	82	33	93	89	98	94	NS

(OC: ovarian cancer; 2D: two-dimensional ultrasound; 3D: three-dimensional ultrasound; NS: statistically nonsignificant)

Hata et al. compared 3D TVS with 2D TVS in 20 patients with adnexal masses. They found that 3D TVS was more specific than 2D TVS.[56]

More recently, Kurjak reported the results of a study comparing five different sonographic techniques in a series of 251 adnexal tumors. They found 3D TVS more sensitive than 2D TVS with similar specificity.[22]

We found that 3D ultrasonography had not statistically better diagnostic performance than 2D in a series of 44 selected complex adnexal masses.[57] We found 3D TVS useful to reinforce initial diagnostic impression. In a second series, we found similar results to the previous one.[58] In this second study we showed that 3D-US had a good intra- and inter-observer reproducibility for assessing adnexal masses.[58]

These controversial results might be explained by the fact that in the first two studies the number of malignant tumors was small and, probably, because all of them, except ours, included many not complex tumors. On the other hand, the sonographic criteria for malignant suspicion on 3D US were the same than in 2D US.

With the advent of three-dimensional ultrasound, three-dimensional power Doppler imaging has also become available for clinical practice. This technique allows tumor vascularization assessment, both quantitatively—by means of 3D-PD US derived vascular indexes, and qualitatively—by depicting three-dimensionally the tumor vascular network.

Kurjak et al., in two different studies on 120 and 90 adnexal masses, respectively, concluded that 3D-PD was superior to conventional color Doppler by increasing the sensitivity.[59,60] This same group found that the use on sonographic contrast agents would improve even more the performance of 3D power Doppler.[61] They compared a scoring system that included some morphological features and 3D-PD evaluation of tumor vessels characteristics, such as vessels arrangement and branching pattern, with another scoring system that included the same morphological features with pulsed Doppler velocimetric parameters (RI ≤ 0.42 or > 0.42). They based their diagnostic criteria for malignancy suspicion on vessel architecture as depicted by 3D, such as branching pattern, vessel caliber, and presence of microaneurysms or vascular lakes **(Figs. 25 and 26)**. This was based on the chaos theory,[62] which establish that vascular architecture of a vascular network of newly formed vessels in malignant tumors is built following a chaotic distribution but not in a predetermined fashion. Although, this has been demonstrated in corrosion studies,[63] the reproducibility of this approach is just moderate.[64]

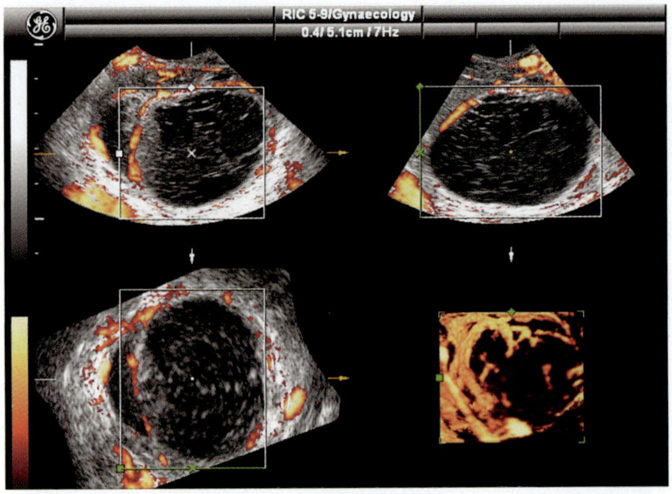

Fig. 25: 3D power Doppler depiction of the vascular network from a benign ovarian cystic tumor.

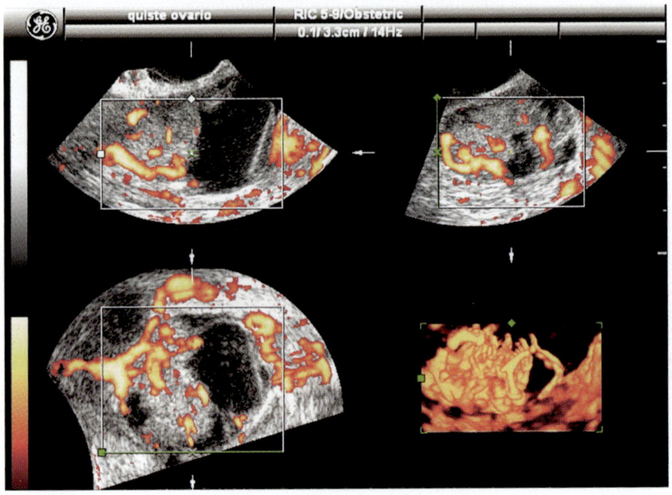

Fig. 26: 3D power Doppler depiction of the vascular network from a malignant ovarian tumor.

Several subsequent studies, using all of them similar criteria for malignancy suspicion, reported similar findings: 3D-PD vascular tree assessment adds little to conventional ultrasound.[65-68] These studies are summarized in **Table 3**. Cohen et al. evaluated the role of 3D-2D in a series of 71 complex adnexal masses on 2D-transvaginal ultrasound.[69] They did not use 2D conventional color Doppler nor 2D power Doppler. In their approach, they combined 2D and 3D morphological features with 3D-PD evaluation of blood flow tumor location, considering a tumor as malignant in the presence of complex morphological pattern and central (in papillary projections and/or septations) blood

TABLE 3: 3D-PD tumor vascular tree assessment for diagnosing ovarian cancer.

Author	N	OC prevalence (%)	Sensitivity		Specificity		P value
			3D-PD (%)	2D (%)	3D-PD (%)	2D (%)	
Kurjak[59†]	120	9	100	91	99	97	NS
Kurjak[60†]	90	10	100	89	99	37	NS
Laban[65†*]	50	62	100	100	74	74	NS
Sladkevicius[66‡]	104	26	96	100	96	90	NS
Alcazar[64§]	39	51	90	95	74	74	NS
Dai[67§*]	36	83	77	97	50	50	<0.05
Mansour[68§]	400	62	88	94	89	73	NS

†Criteria for malignancy suspicion: Scoring system combining morphology and 3D-PD features
‡Criteria for malignancy suspicion: Logistic model combining morphology and 3D-PD features
§Criteria for malignancy suspicion: only 3D-PD features
*Only "complex" masses included in the study
(OC: ovarian cancer; 2D: two-dimensional ultrasound; 3D-PD: three-dimensional power Doppler; NS: statistically nonsignificant)

flow location. They concluded that the addition of 3D-PD improved the specificity of 2D-transvaginal ultrasound (75% versus 54%), without decreasing the sensitivity. Similar results have been recently reported by Geomini et al.[70] These results are not surprising and can also be achieved by using a simpler technique such as color Doppler.[18]

We found that the diagnostic performance of 3D-PD was not statistically better than that of 2D-PD in a series of 69 complex adnexal masses, presenting both techniques similar sensitivity (97.8% for both techniques) and specificity (87% versus 79%).[71] We compared the 2D PD diagnostic criteria proposed by Guerriero et al[18] with the 3D-PD diagnostic criteria proposed by Kurjak et al.[22]

However, when a complex mass with detectable blood flow within solid areas or thick papillary projections is found, it should be categorized mass as "malignant" or "highly suspicious". However, a considerable number of benign tumors may exhibit this appearance. For example, cystadenofibroma, tubo ovarian abscess or solid benign ovarian tumor.

Using conventional 2D color or power-Doppler we have no means to differentiate these benign entities from true malignant tumors. 3D power-Doppler ultrasound provides a new approach to assess tumor vascularization. We have termed this new approach "3D power Doppler vascular sampling".[72] It consists of assessing the vascularization of a given suspicious area in a given tumor by calculating 3D power Doppler derived indexes within these areas **(Figs. 27 and 28)**. In a series of 49 vascularized complex

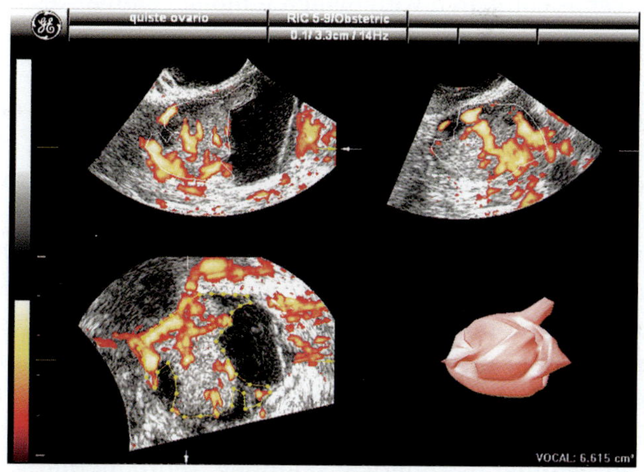

Fig. 27: Volume calculation from the solid portion from a cystic-solid ovarian tumor.

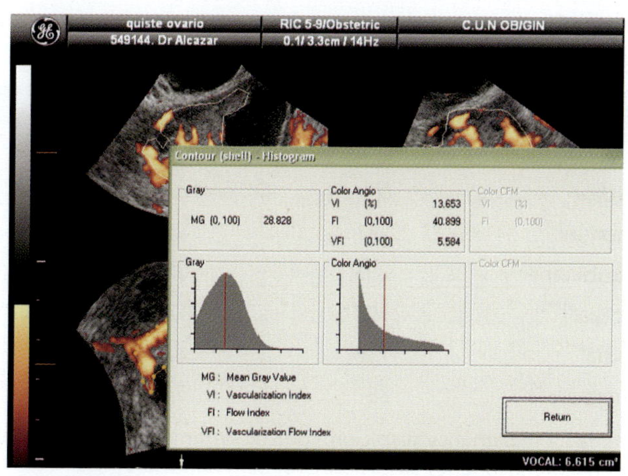

Fig. 28: 3D power Doppler derived vascular indices from the solid component (vascular sampling) from the case of the previous figure.

adnexal masse, we found that 3D power Doppler derived indexes were significantly higher in malignant tumors as compared with benign ones. Pulsed Doppler indexes were not helpful. Almost simultaneously to our study, Testa et al. published a study on 24 solid pelvic masses with basically identical results to ours.[73]

After these pioneering reports, Geomini et al. reported data from a series of 181 women with adnexal masses using the method proposed by Alcazar.[70] This group included any kind of mass diagnosed at transvaginal ultrasound and performed the vascular assessment from the whole tumor. They found that FI, but not VI and VFI, was significantly higher in ovarian cancer.

Jokubkiene et al. proposed a modified approach based on the use of a virtual 5-cc spherical sampling from the most vascularized area from the tumor. They also found that 3D-PD vascular indexes were higher in ovarian cancer as compared with benign tumors.[74] Similar results were reported by Kudla et al., but using a 1-cc spherical sampling.[75]

Only two studies have not shown differences in 3D-PD indexes between benign and malignant ovarian tumors.[76,77] However, the series were too small (only 17 cases) and the methods used were not fully explained.

Alcazar and Prka compared manual and spherical sampling and concluded that both methods are comparable and that spherical sampling is faster to perform but cannot be used in some small tumors.[78] This may be solved using 1-cc sphere.[75]

Several studies have shown that, whatever the approach used, manual or spherical sampling, reproducibility is high between observers.[79,80]

Regarding to the contribution to diagnosis of ovarian cancer, Geomini et al. reported a multicenter prospective study concluding that the use of 3D ultrasound significantly improves the prediction of malignancy as compared to 2D-ultrasonography.[81] Alcazar et al.[82] and Kudla et al.[83] have shown that 3D-PD may decrease false-positive rate of 2D-PD in solid and cystic-solid adnexal masses. However, Joubkiene et al. concluded that 3D-PD does not add more information to gray-scale imaging than that provided by subjective quantification by 2D-PD.[74] Guerriero et al. found that the use of 3D-PD increased the specificity of ultrasound in suspicious masses but also decreased significantly the sensitivity.[84] These studies are summarized in **Table 4**.

Furthermore, we have recently demonstrated that vascularization, as assessed by 3D-PD vascular indexes, is higher in advanced stage and metastatic ovarian cancers than in early stage ovarian cancer.[85] These preliminary results may be valuable for future research. It would be worth exploring if 3D-PD derived vascular indexes in ovarian cancer could be used as prognostic factor in ovarian cancer.

OTHER APPLICATIONS

Three-dimensional ultrasound has been proposed as a means for monitoring the response to treatment in gynecologic malignancies.

Yaman and Fridrik reported on one case of cervical cancer and one case of ovarian cancer evaluated by 3D power Doppler ultrasound before and after treatment with radio- and/or chemotherapy. They observed a reduction of tumor volume, VI, FI and VFI in both cases after treatment.[86]

Su et al. reported on one case of primary papillary serous carcinoma of the peritoneum evaluated by 3D

TABLE 4: 3D-PD vascular sampling for diagnosing ovarian cancer.

Author	N	OC prevalence (%)	Sensitivity		Specificity		P value
			3D-PD (%)	2D (%)	3D-PD (%)	2D (%)	
Geomini[70†]	181	20	57	91	85	63	<0.05
Jokubkiene[74†]	106	25	100	100	92	90	<0.05
Alcazar[82*§]	143	74	95	100	33	0	<0.05
Kudla[83*§]	138	82	91	100	77	0	<0.05
Guerriero[84*§]	35	71	68	100	40	0	<0.05

†Criteria for malignancy suspicion: Logistic system combining morphology and 3D-PD indexes
§Criteria for malignancy suspicion: Only 3D-PD indexes
*Only "complex" masses included in the study
(OC: Ovarian cancer; 2D: two-dimensional ultrasound; 3D-PD: three-dimensional power Doppler)

power Doppler ultrasound before and after treatment with chemotherapy. They also reported that tumor volume and 3D power Doppler indices decreased progressively during treatment.[87]

REFERENCES

1. Smith-Bindman R, Kerlikowske K, Feldstein VA, Subak L, Scheidler J, Segal M, et al. Endovaginal ultrasound to exclude endometrial cancer and other endometrial abnormalities. JAMA. 1998;280:1510-7.
2. Kurjak A, Shalan H, Sosic A, Benic S, Zudenigo D, Kupesic S, et al. Endometrial carcinoma in postmenopausal women: evaluation by transvaginal color Doppler ultrasonography. Am J Obstet Gynecol. 1993;169:1597-603.
3. Sladkevicius P, Valentin L, Marsal K. Endometrial thickness and Doppler velocimetry of the uterine arteries as discriminators of endometrial status in women with postmenopausal bleeding: a comparative study. Am J Obstet Gynecol. 1994;171:722-8.
4. Alcazar JL, Castillo G, Minguez JA, Galan MJ. Endometrial blood flow mapping using transvaginal power Doppler sonography in women with postmenopausal bleeding and thickened endometrium. Ultrasound Obstet Gynecol. 2003;21:583-8.
5. Alcazar JL, Ajossa S, Floris S, Bargellini R, Gerada M, Guerriero S. Reproducibility of endometrial vascular patterns in endometrial disease as assessed by transvaginal power Doppler sonography in women with postmenopausal bleeding. J Ultrasound Med. 2006;25:159-63.
6. Aleen F, Predanic M. Uterine leiomyoma: transvaginal color Doppler studies and new aspects of management. In Ultrasound and the uterus. In: Osmers R, Kurjak A (Eds). Parthenon Publishing Group, London; 1995. pp. 61-70.
7. Alcázar JL, Griffioen M, Jurado M. Uterine artery blood flow in women with uterine myomas. Eur J Ultrasound. 1997;5: 165-9.
8. Kurjak A, Kupesic S, Shalan H, Jukic S, Kosuta D, Ilijas M. Uterine sarcoma: a report of 10 cases studied by transvaginal color and pulsed Doppler sonography. Gynecol Oncol. 1995;59:342-6.
9. Szabo I, Szantho A, Csabay L, Csapo Z, Szirmai K, Papp Z. Color Doppler ultrasonography in the differentiation of uterine sarcomas from uterine leiomyomas. Eur J Gynaecol Oncol. 2002;23:29-34.
10. Aviram R, Ochshorn Y, Markovitch O, Fishman A, Cohen I, Altaras MM, et al. Uterine sarcomas versus leiomyomas: gray-scale and Doppler sonographic findings. J Clin Ultrasound. 2005;33:10-3.
11. Alcázar JL, Castillo G, Jurado M, López-García G. Intratumoral blood flow in cervical cancer as assessed by transvaginal color Doppler ultrasonography: correlation with tumor features. Int J Gynecol Cancer. 2003;13:510-4.
12. Alcázar JL, Jurado M. Transvaginal colour Doppler for predicting pathological response to preoperative chemoradiation in locally advanced cervical carcinoma: a preliminary study. Ultrasound Med Biol. 1999;25:1041-5.
13. Engelen MJ, Kos HE, Willemse PH, Aalders JG, de Vries EG, Schaapveld M, et al. Surgery by consultant gynecologic oncologists improves survival in patients with ovarian carcinoma. Cancer. 2006;106:589-98.
14. Canis M, Rabischong B, Houlle C, Botchorishvili R, Jardon K, Safi A, et al. Laparoscopic management of adnexal masses: a gold standard? Curr Opin Obstet Gynecol. 2002;14:423-8.
15. Alcázar JL, Castillo G, Jurado M, López-García G. Expectant management of sonographically benign ovarian cysts in asymptomatic premenopausal women. Human Reprod. 2005;20:3231-4.
16. Kinkel K, Hricak H, Lu Y, Tsuda K, Filly RA. US characterization of ovarian masses: a meta-analysis. Radiology. 2000;217: 803-11.
17. Tekay A, Jouppila P. Controversies in assessment of ovarian tumors with transvaginal color Doppler ultrasound. Acta Obstet Gynecol Scand. 1996;75:316-29.
18. Guerriero S, Alcázar JL, Coccia ME, Ajossa S, Scarselli G, Boi M, et al. Complex pelvic mass as a target of evaluation of vessel distribution by color Doppler for the diagnosis of adnexal malignancies: results of a multicenter European study. J Ultrasound Med. 2002;21:1105-11.
19. Alcázar JL. Three-dimensional ultrasound in Gynecology: Current status and future perspectives. Curr Women's Health Rev. 2005;1:1-14.
20. Alcázar JL, Mercé LT, García-Manero M, Bau S, López-García G. Endometrial volume and vascularity measurements by transvaginal three-dimensional ultrasonography and power Doppler angiography in stimulated and tumoral endometria: an inter-observer reproducibility study. J Ultrasound Med. 2005;24:1091-8.
21. Gruboeck K, Jurkovic D, Lawton F, Savvas M, Tailor A, Campbell S. The diagnostic value of endometrial thickness and volume measurements by three-dimensional ultrasound in patients with postmenopausal bleeding. Ultrasound Obstet Gynecol. 1996;8:272-6.
22. Kurjak A, Kupesic S, Sparac V, Bekavac I. Preoperative evaluation of pelvic tumors by Doppler and three-dimensional sonography. J Ultrasound Med. 2001;20:829-40.
23. Mansour GM, El-Lamie IK, El-Kady MA, El-Mekkawi SF, Laban M, Abou-Gabal AI. Endometrial volume as predictor of malignancy in women with postmenopausal bleeding. Int J Gynaecol Obstet. 2007;99:206-10.
24. Yaman C, Habelsberger A, Tews G, Pölz W, Ebner T. The role of three-dimensional volume measurement in diagnosing endometrial cancer in patients with postmenopausal bleeding. Gynecol Oncol. 2008;110:390-5.
25. Odeh M, Vainerovsky I, Grinin V, Kais M, Ophir E, Bornstein J. Three-dimensional endometrial volume and 3-dimensional power Doppler analysis in predicting

endometrial carcinoma and hyperplasia. Gynecol Oncol. 2007;106:348-53.
26. Mercé LT, Alcázar JL, López C, et al. Clinical usefulness of 3-dimensional sonography and power Doppler angiography for diagnosis of endometrial carcinoma. J Ultrasound Med. 2007;26:1279-87.
27. Opolskiene G, Sladkevicius P, Jokubkiene L, Valentin L. Three-dimensional ultrasound imaging for discrimination between benign and malignant endometrium in women with postmenopausal bleeding and sonographic endometrial thickness of at least 4.5 mm. Ultrasound Obstet Gynecol. 2010;35:94-102.
28. Alcazar JL, Galvan R. Three-dimensional power Doppler ultrasound scanning for the prediction of endometrial cancer in women with postmenopausal bleeding and thickened endometrium. Am J Obstet Gynecol. 2009;200:44. e1-6.
29. Makled AK, Elmekkawi SF, El-Refaie TA, El-Sherbiny MA. Three-dimensional power Doppler and endometrial volume as predictors of malignancy in patients with postmenopausal bleeding. J Obstet Gynaecol Res. 2013;39:1045-51.
30. Kim A, Lee JY, Chun S, Kim HY. Diagnostic utility of three-dimensional power Doppler ultrasound for postmenopausal bleeding. Taiwan J Obstet Gynecol. 2015;54:221-6.
31. Bonilla-Musoles F, Raga F, Osborne NG, Blanes J, Coelho F. Three-dimensional hysterosonography for the study of endometrial tumors: comparison with conventional transvaginal sonography, hysterosalpingography, and hysteroscopy. Gynecol Oncol. 1997;65:245-52.
32. Su MT, Su RM, Yue CT, Chou CY, Hsu CC, Chang FM. Three-dimensional transvaginal ultrasound provides clearer delineation of myometrial invasion in a patient with endometrial cancer and uterine leiomyoma. Ultrasound Obstet Gynecol. 2003;22:434-6.
33. Alcázar JL, Galván R, Albela S, Martinez S, Pahisa J, Jurado M, et al. Assessing myometrial infiltration by endometrial cancer: uterine virtual navigation with three-dimensional US. Radiology. 2009;250:776-83.
34. Jantarasaengaram S, Praditphol N, Tansathit T, Vipupinyo C, Vairojanavong K. Three-dimensional ultrasound with volume contrast imaging for preoperative assessment of myometrial invasion and cervical involvement in women with endometrial cancer. Ultrasound Obstet Gynecol. 2014;43:569-74.
35. Saarelainen SK, Kööbi L, Järvenpää R, Laurila M, Mäenpää JU. The preoperative assessment of deep myometrial invasion by three-dimensional ultrasound versus MRI in endometrial carcinoma. Acta Obstet Gynecol Scand. 2012;91:983-9.
36. Alcazar JL, Pineda L, Martinez-Astorquiza Corral T, Orozco R, Utrilla-Layna J, Juez L, et al. Transvaginal/Transrectal ultrasound for assessing myometrial invasion in endometrial cancer: a comparison of six different approaches. J Gynecol Oncol. 2015;26:201-7.
37. Christensen JW, Dueholm M, Hansen ES, Marinovskij E, Lundorf E, Ørtoft G. Assessment of myometrial invasion in endometrial cancer using three-dimensional ultrasound and magnetic resonance imaging. Acta Obstet Gynecol Scand. 2016;95:55-64.
38. Pairleitner H, Steiner H, Hasenoehrl G, Staudach A. Three dimensional power Doppler sonography: imaging and quantifying blood flow and vascularization. Ultrasound Obstet Gynecol. 1999;14:139-43.
39. Kupesic S, Kurjak A, Zodan T. Staging of the endometrial carcinoma by three-dimensional power Doppler ultrasound. Gynaecol Perinatol. 1999;8:1-7.
40. Lieng M, Qvigstad E, Dahl GF, Istre O. Flow differences between endometrial polyps and cancer: a prospective study using intravenous contrast-enhanced transvaginal color flow Doppler and three-dimensional power Doppler ultrasound. Ultrasound Obstet Gynecol. 2008;32:935-40.
41. Galván R, Mercé L, Jurado M, Mínguez JA, López-García G, Alcázar JL. Three-dimensional power Doppler angiography in endometrial cancer: correlation with tumor characteristics. Ultrasound Obstet Gynecol. 2010;35:723-9.
42. Saarelainen SK, Vuento MH, Kirkinen P, Mäenpää JU. Preoperative assessment of endometrial carcinoma by three-dimensional power Doppler angiography. Ultrasound Obstet Gynecol. 2012;39:466-72.
43. Salim R, Lee C, Davies A, Jolaoso B, Ofuasia E, Jurkovic D. A comparative study of three-dimensional saline infusion sonohysterography and diagnostic hysteroscopy for the classification of submucous fibroids. Hum Reprod. 2005;20:253-7.
44. Walocha JA, Litwin JA, Miodonski AJ. Vascular system of intramural leiomyomata revealed by corrosion casting and scanning electron microscopy. Hum Reprod. 2003;18:1088-93.
45. Muniz CJ, Fleischer AC, Donnelly EF, Mazer MJ. Three-dimensional color Doppler sonography and uterine artery arteriography of fibroids: assessment of changes in vascularity before and after embolization. J Ultrasound Med. 2002;21:129-33.
46. Exacoustos C, Zupi E, Marconi D, Romanini ME, Szabolcs B, Piredda A, et al. Ultrasound-assisted laparoscopic cryomyolysis: two- and three-dimensional findings before, during and after treatment. Ultrasound Obstet Gynecol. 2005;25:393-400.
47. Kupesic S, Kurjak A. Three-dimensional power Doppler ultrasound examination of uterine lesions. Three-dimensional Power-Doppler in Obstetrics and Gynecology. In: Kurjak A (Ed). Parthenon Publishing Group, London; 2000. pp. 39-52.
48. Suren A, Osmers R, Kuhn W. 3D Color Power Angio imaging: a new method to assess intracervical vascularization in benign and pathological conditions. Ultrasound Obstet Gynecol. 1998;11:133-7.

49. Hsu KF, Su JM, Huang SC, Cheng YM, Kang CY, Shen MR, et al. Three-dimensional power Doppler imaging of early-stage cervical cancer. Ultrasound Obstet Gynecol. 2004;24:664–71.
50. Testa AC, Ferrandina G, Distefano M, Fruscella E, Mansueto D, Basso D, et al. Color Doppler velocimetry and three-dimensional color power angiography of cervical carcinoma. Ultrasound Obstet Gynecol. 2004;24:445-52.
51. Alcázar JL. Transvaginal color Doppler in the assessment of cervical carcinoma. Cancer Ther. 2005;3:139-46.
52. Alcázar JL, Jurado M, López-García G. Tumor vascularization in cervical cancer by 3-dimensional power Doppler angiography: correlation with tumor characteristics. Int J Gynecol Cancer. 2010;20:393-7.
53. Tanaka K, Umesaki N. Impact of three-dimensional (3D) ultrasonography and power Doppler angiography in the management of cervical cancer. Eur J Gynaecol Oncol. 2010;31:10-7.
54. Ghi T, Giunchi S, Kuleva M, Santini D, Savelli L, Formelli G, et al. Three-dimensional transvaginal sonography in local staging of cervical carcinoma: description of a novel technique. Ultrasound Obstet Gynecol. 2007;30:778-82.
55. Bonilla-Musoles F, Raga F, Osborne NG. Three-dimensional ultrasound evaluation of ovarian masses. Gynaecol Oncol. 1995;59:129-35.
56. Hata T, Yanagihara T, Hayashi K, et al. Three-dimensional ultrasonographic evaluation of ovarian tumours: a preliminary study. Hum Reprod. 1999;14:858-61.
57. Alcázar JL, Galán MJ, García-Manero M, Guerriero S. Three-dimensional ultrasound morphologic assessment in complex adnexal masses a preliminary experience. J Ultrasound Med. 2003;22:249-54.
58. Alcázar JL, García-Manero M, Galván R. Three-dimensional sonographic morphologic assessment of adnexal masses: a reproducibility study. J Ultrasound Med. 2007;26:1007-11.
59. Kurjak A, Kupesic S, Sparac V, Kosuta D. Three-dimensional ultrasonographic and power Doppler characterization of ovarian lesions. Ultrasound Obstet Gynecol. 2000;16:365-71.
60. Kurjak A, Kupesic S, Anic T, Kosuta D. Three-dimensional ultrasound and power Doppler improve the diagnosis of ovarian lesions. Gynecol Oncol. 2000;76:28-32.
61. Kupesic S, Kurjak A. Contrast-enhanced three-dimensional power Doppler sonography for differentiation of adnexal masses. Obstet Gynecol. 2000;96:452-8.
62. Breyer B, Kurjak A. Tumor vascularization, Doppler measurements and chaos: what to do? Ultrasound Obstet Gynecol. 1995;5:209-10.
63. Konerding MA, Miodonski AJ, Lametschwandtner A. Microvascular corrosion casting in the study of tumor vascularity: a review. Scanning Microsc. 1995;9:1233-43.
64. Alcázar JL, Cabrera C, Galván R, Guerriero S. Three-dimensional power Doppler vascular network assessment of adnexal masses: intraobserver and interobserver agreement analysis. J Ultrasound Med. 2008;27:997-1001.
65. Laban M, Metawee H, Elyan A, Kamal M, Kamel M, Mansour G. Three-dimensional ultrasound and three-dimensional power Doppler in the assessment of ovarian tumors. Int J Gynaecol Obstet. 2007;99:201-5.
66. Sladkevicius P, Jokubkiene L, Valentin L. Contribution of morphological assessment of the vessel tree by three-dimensional ultrasound to a correct diagnosis of malignancy in ovarian masses. Ultrasound Obstet Gynecol. 2007;30:874-82.
67. Dai SY, Hata K, Inubashiri E, Kanenishi K, Shiota A, Ohno M, et al. Does three-dimensional power Doppler ultrasound improve the diagnostic accuracy for the prediction of adnexal malignancy? J Obstet Gynaecol Res. 2008;34:364-70.
68. Mansour GM, El-Lamie IK, El-Sayed HM, Ibrahim AM, Laban M, Abou-Louz SK, et al. Adnexal mass vascularity assessed by 3-dimensional power Doppler: does it add to the risk of malignancy index in prediction of ovarian malignancy?: four hundred-case study. Int J Gynecol Cancer. 2009;19:867-72.
69. Cohen LS, Escobar PF, Scharm C, Glimco B, Fishman DA. Three-dimensional ultrasound power Doppler improves the diagnostic accuracy for ovarian cancer prediction. Gynecol Oncol. 2001;82:40-8.
70. Geomini PM, Kluivers KB, Moret E, Bremer GL, Kruitwagen RF, Mol BW. Evaluation of adnexal masses with three-dimensional ultrasonography. Obstet Gynecol. 2006;108:1167-75.
71. Alcázar JL, Castillo G. Comparison of 2-dimensional and 3-dimensional power Doppler imaging in complex adnexal masses for the prediction of ovarian cancer. Am J Obstet Gynecol. 2005;192:807-12.
72. Alcazar JL, Merce LT, Garcia Manero M. Three-dimensional power Doppler vascular sampling: a new method for predicting ovarian cancer in vascularized complex adnexal masses. J Ultrasound Med. 2005;24:689-96.
73. Testa AC, Ajossa S, Ferrandina G, et al. Does quantitative analysis of three-dimensional power Doppler angiography have a role in the diagnosis of malignant pelvic solid tumors? A preliminary study. Ultrasound Obstet Gynecol. 2005;26:67-72.
74. Jokubkiene L, Sladkevicius P, Valentin L. Does three-dimensional power Doppler ultrasound help in discrimination between benign and malignant ovarian masses? Ultrasound Obstet Gynecol. 2007;29:215-25.
75. Kudla MJ, Timor-Tritsch IE, Hope JM, Monteagudo A, Popiolek D, Monda S, et al. Spherical tissue sampling in 3-dimensional power Doppler angiography: a new approach for evaluation of ovarian tumors. J Ultrasound Med. 2008;27:425-33.
76. Ohel I, Sheiner E, Aricha-Tamir B, Piura B, Meirovitz M, Silberstein T, et al. Three-dimensional power Doppler ultrasound in ovarian cancer and its correlation with histology. Arch Gynecol Obstet. 2010;281:919-25.

77. Perez-Medina T, Orensanz I, Pereira A, Valero de Bernabé J, Engels V, Troyano J, et al. Three-dimensional angioultrasonography for the prediction of malignancy in ovarian masses. Gynecol Obstet Invest. 2013;75:12-5.
78. Alcázar JL, Prka M. Evaluation of two different methods for vascular sampling by three-dimensional power Doppler angiography in solid and cystic-solid adnexal masses. Ultrasound Obstet Gynecol. 2009;33:349-54.
79. Kudla M, Alcázar JL. Does the size of three-dimensional power Doppler spherical sampling affect the interobserver reproducibility of measurements of vascular indices in adnexal masses? Ultrasound Obstet Gynecol. 2009;34:732-4.
80. Alcázar JL, Rodriguez D, Royo P, Galván R, Ajossa S, Guerriero S. Intraobserver and interobserver reproducibility of 3-dimensional power Doppler vascular indices in assessment of solid and cystic-solid adnexal masses. J Ultrasound Med. 2008;27:1-6.
81. Geomini PM, Coppus SF, Kluivers KB, Bremer GL, Kruitwagen RF, Mol BW. Is three-dimensional ultrasonography of additional value in the assessment of adnexal masses? Gynecol Oncol. 2007;106:153-9.
82. Alcázar JL, Rodriguez D. Three-dimensional power Doppler vascular sonographic sampling for predicting ovarian cancer in cystic-solid and solid vascularized masses. J Ultrasound Med. 2009;28:275-81.
83. Kudla MJ, Alcázar JL. Does sphere volume affect the performance of three-dimensional power Doppler virtual vascular sampling for predicting malignancy in vascularized solid or cystic-solid adnexal masses? Ultrasound Obstet Gynecol. 2010;35:602-8.
84. Guerriero S, Ajossa S, Piras S, Gerada M, Floris S, Garau N, et al. Three-dimensional quantification of tumor vascularity as a tertiary test after B-mode and power Doppler evaluation for detection of ovarian cancer. J Ultrasound Med. 2007;26:1271-8.
85. Alcázar JL. Tumor angiogenesis assessed by three-dimensional power Doppler ultrasound in early, advanced and metastatic ovarian cancer: a preliminary study. Ultrasound Obstet Gynecol. 2006;28:325-9.
86. Yaman C, Fridrik M. Three-dimensional ultrasound to assess the response to treatment in gynecological malignancies. Gynecol Oncol. 2005;97:665-8.
87. Su JM, Huang YF, Chen HHC, Gheng YM, Chou CY. Three-dimensional power Doppler ultrasound is useful to monitor the response to treatment in a patient with primary papillary serous carcinoma of the peritoneum. Ultrasound Med Biol. 2006;32:623-6.

CHAPTER 56

Ultrasound in Human Reproduction

Veljko Vlaisavljevic, Jure Knez

INTRODUCTION

Ultrasound imaging has undergone significant developments through the last decades and today it represents one of the most widely used imaging tools in medicine. Specific to gynecology, the introduction of high-resolution transvaginal ultrasonography has substantially changed the approach to diagnostics of gynecologic conditions. Today, it is an essential tool for assessment of normal and abnormal pelvic anatomy. In patients suffering from reproductive disorders, evaluation of follicular growth pattern, the structure of perifollicular vascular network and endometrium enables close monitoring and prediction of success of medically assisted reproduction.

FOLLICULOGENESIS

Folliculogenesis is a process which starts in the embryonic period and ends with the disappearance of the last functional follicle when woman enters menopause. Before the development of ultrasound (US), the dynamics of follicular growth on primate and human ovarian tissue was first studied by histological methods and morphological classification of follicles was established.[1-5]

During the course of sequential cellular proliferation and differentiation, *primordial follicles* of app. 60 μm in diameter differentiate into *intermediate*, *primary* and eventually into mature *secondary preantral follicles* of 120 μm in diameter, through the phase characterized by the *slow growth*.

The smallest early growing follicles lack an independent blood supply, but secondary follicles 80–100 μm in diameter are supplied by one or two arterioles, terminating in an anastomotic network just outside the basal lamina.[6] After the introduction of colour Doppler ultrasonography it became possible to indirectly assess the process of angiogenesis, vessel maturation and vessel regression, which appeared to play a role in the selection of the dominant follicle, ovulation and corpus luteum formation and function.[7-9] The development of an independent blood supply exposes the follicle directly to the substances circulating in the blood. Secondary preantral follicles with a diameter of app. 120 μm have multiple layers of granulosa cells (GCs) which are coupled by gap junctions, thus forming the functional syncytium and compensating for the otherwise avascular intrafollicular environment.[5]

At this point of development, the follicle begins to change into the antral follicle. After the formation of the antrum (follicle ~0.4 mm in diameter), the rate of follicular growth accelerates and follicle development enters the so-called *accelerated growth phase.*[4,5] The follicles become sensitive to the action of gonadotrophins when they reach 0.2–0.4 mm in diameter.[10] The follicles may develop to early antral stage throughout the fetal and prepubertal life, but they subsequently regress in size. Only with the development of functional hypothalamic-pituitary-ovarian axis at the onset of puberty, follicles can develop to the ovulatory phase. When follicles are recruited from the resting follicle pool, it takes approximately 150 days or roughly 5 menstrual cycles until ovulation occurs.[2,4]

It is still not well-established how the follicles are recruited from the cohort of resting follicles. High-resolution ultrasonography has allowed a deeper insight to this dilemma.[11] Cyclic recruitment of follicles has been demonstrated instead of continuous follicular recruitment, a discovery enabled by serial high-resolution ultrasound and endocrinologic monitoring. Still, there are inconsistencies regarding the number of waves and patterns of wave occurrence during each menstrual cycle in human species. It should be kept in mind, that published studies were performed mostly on follicles larger than 4 mm due to significant measurement errors and technical difficulties measuring smaller follicles.[11,12]

The process of *follicular selection* represents the final selection of the maturing follicular cohort. In humans, follicular selection is presumed to occur during the first five days of the menstrual cycle, at a time when the diameter of a leading follicle is 5–10 mm.[5,11] The follicle destined to ovulate is the *dominant follicle*. After attaining dominance, the follicle grows with an almost uniform rate of 2–3 mm per day, until it reaches a mean diameter ranging from 17 to 27 mm just prior to ovulation.[4,13]

The main pathway of blood supply to the mature follicle is through vascular network around the inner border of the theca interna. From there, the transport of nutrients, oxygen, precursors of steroidogenesis and waste products continues through the avascular granulosa layer to the oocyte by diffusion.

Under the influence of the mid-cycle lutenizing hormone (LH) surge, the dominant follicle undergoes dramatic morphological transformation, the oocyte further matures and finally the follicle ruptures. Mechanically, *ovulation* consists of a rapid enlargement of follicle and it's protrusion from the ovarian surface. The follicular rupture results in the expulsion of an oocyte-cumulus complex into the abdominal cavity.

After ovulation, rapid morphological transformation of the dominant follicle continues. Capillaries and fibroblasts from the surrounding stroma proliferate and penetrate the basal lamina. At the same time mural granulosa cells undergo morphological changes collectively referred to as *luteinization*. Thus, luteinized granulosa cells (GCs), surrounding theca-interstitial cells and invading vasculature intermingle to give rise to the *corpus luteum*. If pregnancy does not occur, the corpus luteum spontaneously regresses after approximately 14 days. At least five cycles later it is replaced by an avascular scar (corpus albicans). If pregnancy does occur, hCG secreted by the trophoblast maintains the life span of corpus luteum and its ability to produce progesterone for at least eight additional weeks.

However, not all cycles are ovulatory. Nonovulatory cycles could be classified into three types: the *cycle without dominant follicle development* (a cohort of selectable follicles starts developing, but the dominant follicle does not emerge); the *cycle with atretic dominant follicle* (the dominant follicle develops, but becomes irregular, continues to grow until mid-cycle and then disorganizes without ovulation); and the *cycle with luteinized unruptured follicle* (the dominant follicle grows till mid-cycle, does not ovulate, oocyte degenerates, luteal transformation of follicular wall occurs).

ULTRASOUND AND FOLLICULAR GROWTH

The ovary is a paired organ with a complex, mosaic-like, constantly changing structure.[14] It is vital to reproduction as the source of oocytes and the main site of sex steroid hormone production in females. Although, follicles were first visualized by ultrasound in the 1970s, the first US studies of follicular growth dynamics were published much later.[15–18] This was possible with significant improvement of ultrasound technique and the introduction of high-resolution transvaginal sonography. From the aspect of assisted reproduction, the ability to perform antral follicle count, monitor follicular growth, predict and confirm the ovulation and to identify clinical parameters of follicle quality is of immense importance.[19–22]

Antral follicles of different sizes are present during all phases of menstrual cycle. The pattern of antral follicle appearance is random, not restricted to a particular location within the ovary. This represents a developmental advantage—if follicles were formed in one particular part of the ovarian cortex only, they would be more easily compromised by pathological processes.[20] Commonly, a diameter of 2 mm is considered as the lower limit at which antral follicles can be visualized, although with improvement of ultrasound machines even smaller follicles can be visualized today.

Visible characteristics of antral follicles which may be used for the prediction of the ultimate fate of a follicle are: *size* (the largest diameter of the follicle), *shape* (round, oval, rectangular, triangular), *echogenicity* (high, medium, low) and *antral edge quality* (smooth, intermediate, rough).[15–18]

In natural cycles, throughout the follicular phase, antral follicle which will gain dominance is usually regularly shaped with regular antral edge and larger than follicles undergoing atresia **(Fig. 1A)**. Dominant follicle has echogenicity in the middle range, whilst follicles destined to become atretic generally display higher echogenicity.[17] Also, early angiographic studies in natural cycles showed that the main characteristics of blood flow in perifollicular tissue of non-dominant growing antral follicles were lower velocity and higher resistance in comparison to perifollicular blood flow of the dominant follicle.[23]

Dominant follicle regulates its own growth and the growth of other follicles from the same cohort by secreting various paracrine regulators. This phenomenon was demonstrated using serial ultrasound and by 3D follicle mapping. Reduction of antral follicles is most

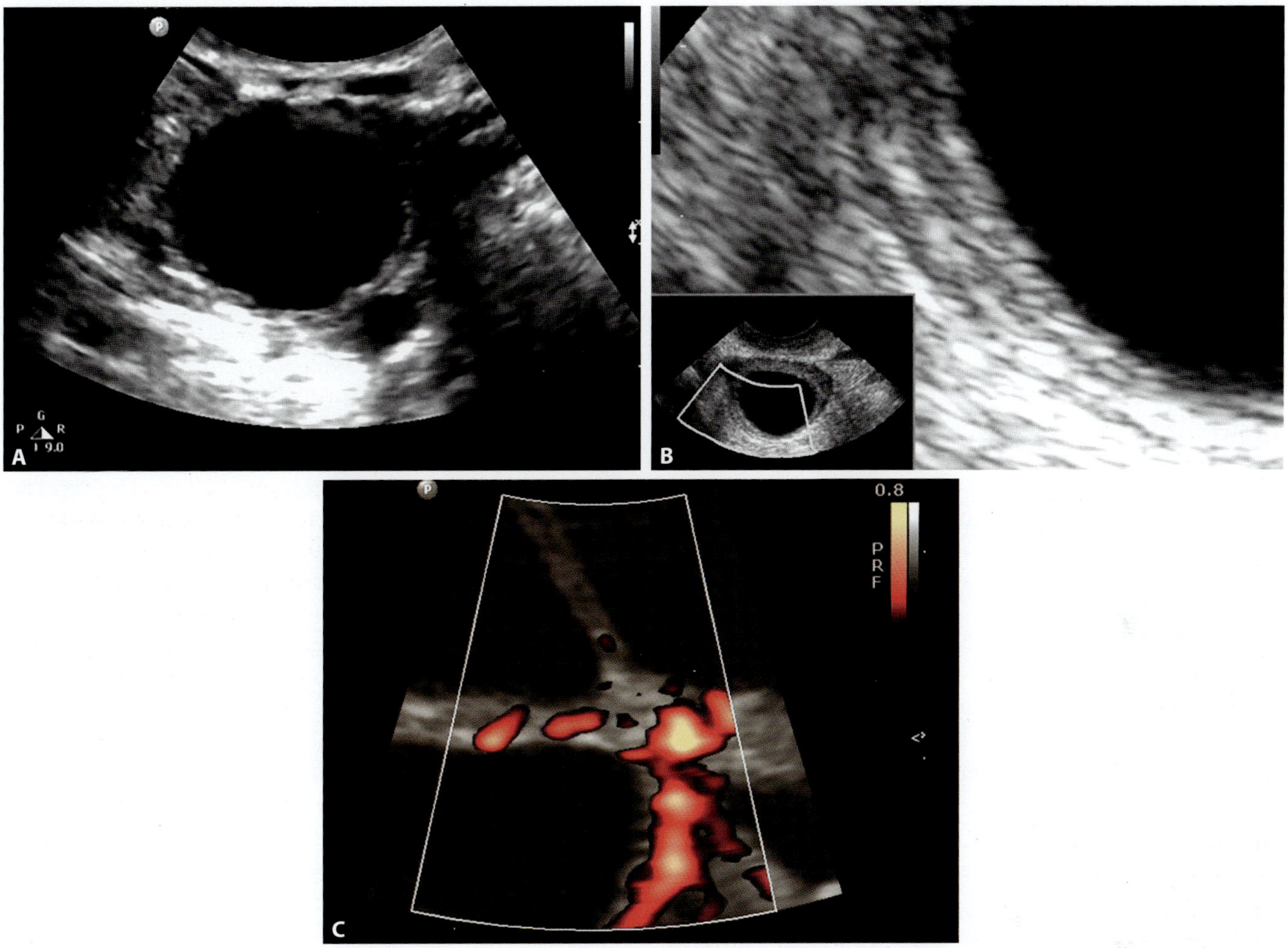

Figs. 1A to C: Dominant follicle. (A) Dominant follicle is regularly shaped with regular antral edge and has echogenicity in the middle range. Reduction in the number of surrounding antral follicles is most pronounced around the midluteal phase; (B) Thickness of the follicular wall is related to the health of the follicle; (C) Increase in perifollicular blood flow of the dominant follicle visualized by power Doppler.

pronounced around the midluteal phase, thereafter their number rapidly increases. Selection of the dominant follicle occurs before the 5th day of the cycle. Its occurrence becomes visually apparent by the 7th day of the cycle due to its *characteristic growth rate.*[20]

Dominant follicle undergoes remarkable changes during the last seven days of its development. There is a marked increase in number and size of granulosa cells and increase in perifollicular blood flow in the vessels of the theca layer **(Figs. 1B and C)**. These changes can be visualized by ultrasound as an increase in diameter and volume of the follicle. Thickness of granulosa layer is directly correlated with the health of the follicle—thin follicular wall is characteristic of an atretic follicle.[24]

ULTRASOUND AND OVULATION

At the time of ovulation, the dominant follicle which has reached its maximal size ruptures, and shortly after, luteogenesis begins. Several sonographic parameters have been investigated as potential markers of ovulation **(Figs. 2 and 3)**:

- *Disappearance of dominant follicle or sudden decrease in it's size* (the most frequent sign of ovulation with sensitivity of 84%).
- *Increase of intrafollicular echogenicity* (non-reliable, because gradual increase of intrafollicular echogenicity may start as far as three days before ovulation, usually with the most pronounced increase during the first day after ovulation).

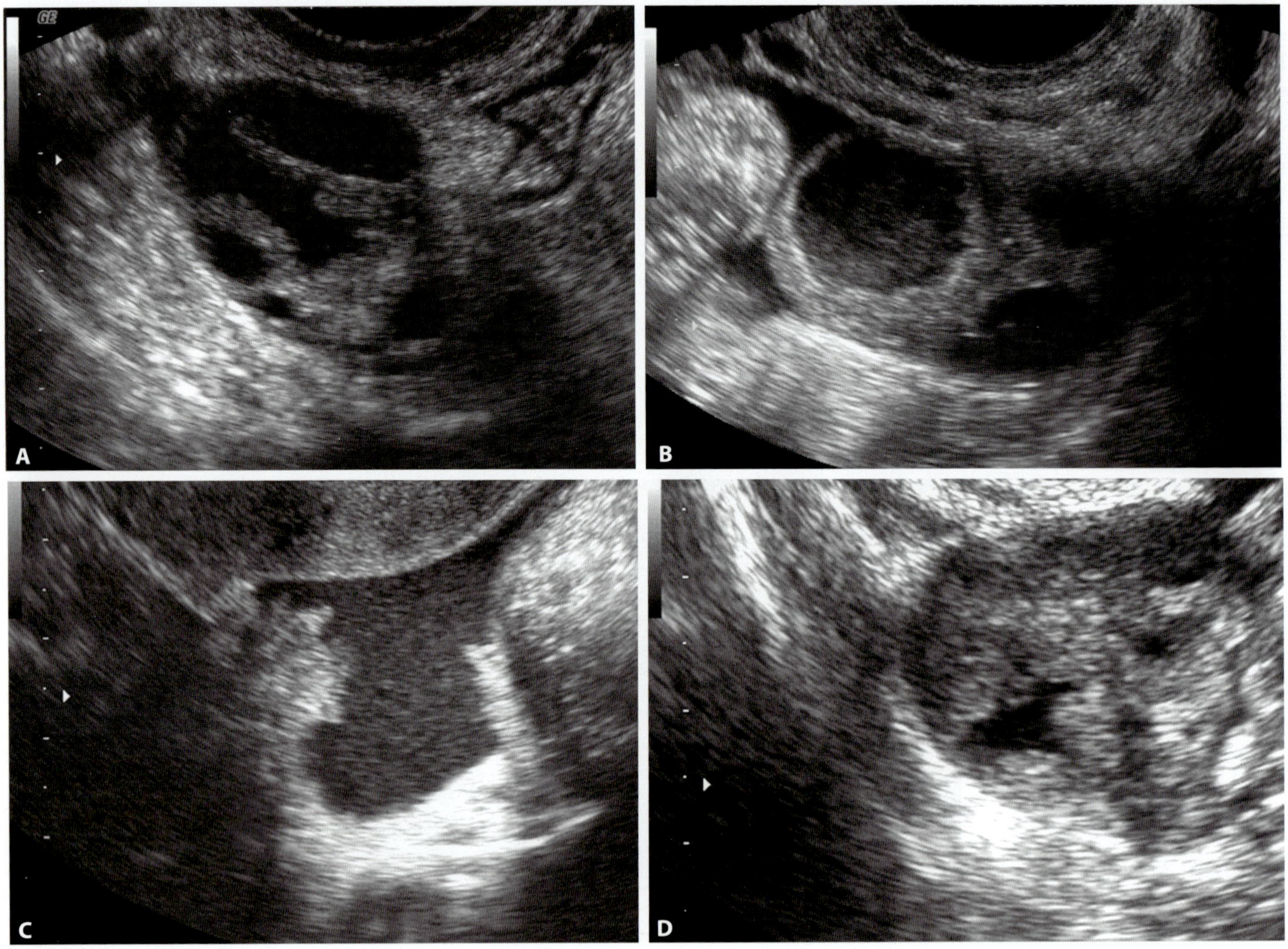

Figs. 2A to D: Ovulation. (A) Collapse of the dominant follicle is a sensitive sign of ovulation; (B) Increased follicular echogenicity can be a sign of forthcoming ovulation; (C) Free fluid in the pouch of Douglas is seen in most women after ovulation; (D) Formation of the corpus luteum at the site of follicular rupture.

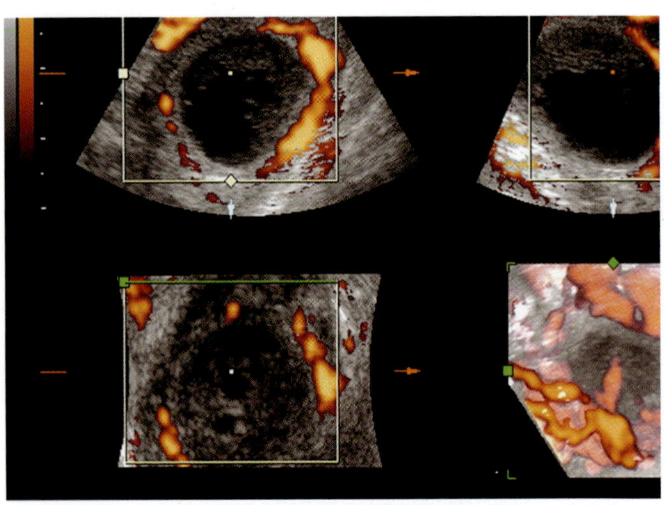

Fig. 3: Characteristic vascularization of the corpus luteum as visualized by power Doppler.

- *Loss of follicular wall regularity* (present in almost 70% of cycles, more reliable than intrafollicular echogenicity).
- *Accumulation of free fluid in the pouch of Douglas* (present in 77% of patients with confirmed ovulation; it could be seen in the pouch of Douglas during all phases of menstrual cycle, but it is a relatively rare finding during the follicular phase (3–11% of the cycles).[25]

During the late follicular phase, the ovary containing the dominant follicle has larger volume and increased perifollicular blood flow compared to the contralateral ovary.[26] With the introduction of advanced ultrasound devices, blood flow assessment at the level of a single follicle and not only at the level of the whole ovary was made possible. Doppler studies of dominant follicles in natural cycles have showed that there is a marked increase of blood flow velocity in perifollicular vessels around the time of ovulation. This increase starts approximately 29 hours before and continues for at least 72 hours after ovulation.[7,27-29] Not all parts of the follicular wall are equally perfused at the time of ovulation—there is a marked decrease in blood flow at the apex of the follicle. The differences in perifollicular blood flow may be of crucial importance for normal release of the mature oocyte.[30]

ULTRASOUND AS THE TOOL FOR PREDICTION OF SUCCESS AND FOR MONITORING IN MEDICALLY ASSISTED REPRODUCTION

Today, ultrasound has a key role in controlled ovarian stimulation monitoring but it is also of significant importance in predicting the success of medically assisted reproduction.

Ultrasound Role in Predicting the Success of Medically Assisted Reproduction

Early follicular FSH is the most widely used marker of ovarian reserve, although it is well-known that it has a relatively limited value in predicting ovarian response. On the other hand, markers such as Anti-Müllerian hormone (AMH) and antral follicle count (AFC) are today well- established as one of the most reliable predictors of ovarian response to exogenous stimulation. Hence, AFC is the most verified sonographic marker, but there are also other sonographic markers that have been investigated, such as ovarian volume and ovarian stromal blood flow.

Antral Follicle Count

The number of antral follicles count (AFC) has been repeatedly established as a reliable marker of ovarian reserve.[31-33] This sonographic criterion is a better predictor of ovarian response to controlled ovarian stimulation compared to ovarian volume or age alone.[34,35] If antral follicle count is less than three, there is a significantly higher chance of cycle cancellation, detection of lower oestradiol (E_2) levels and use of higher doses of gonadotrophins.[36] Some have argued that AFC has higher variability and is less reliable marker of ovarian reserve compared to Anti-Müllerian hormone.[37] However, recently introduced sonography based automated volume count (SonoAVC) algorithm allows for automatic follicle count on ovaries recorded by 3D ultrasound **(Fig. 4A)**. This approach enables lower intra- and interobserver variability, reduces the risk of measurement error, and consequently, could further improve the predictive capability of AFC in women undergoing ovarian stimulation.[38,39]

Ovarian Volume

Ovarian volume (OV) is a parameter easily assessed by ultrasound **(Fig. 4B)**. Using transvaginal sonography, it has been shown that ovarian volume has predictive importance for ovarian response to ovulation induction.[40] Later, an association between ovarian volume and ovarian reserve was recognized, and investigators recommended that this parameter should be measured in all patients prior to MAR.[41] However, later evidence and 3D ultrasound technology has shown that there was no statistically

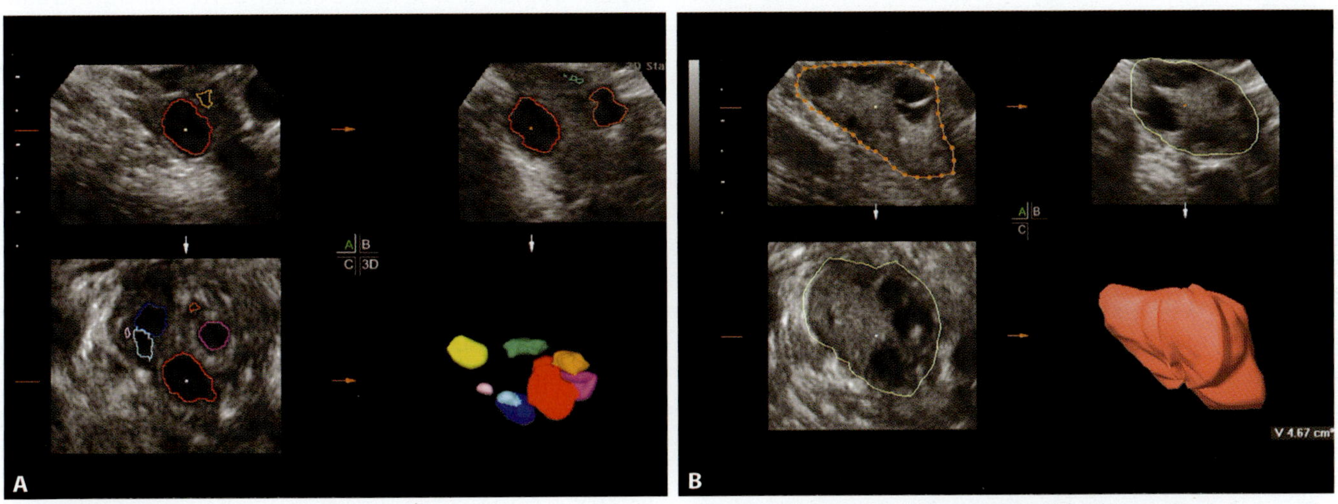

Figs. 4A and B: Markers of ovarian reserve. (A) Antral follicle count (AFC) can be performed automatically with sonography-based automated volume count (SonoAVC); (B) Ovarian volume calculated by virtual organ computer-aided analysis (VOCAL).

significant difference in ovarian volume between low responders and controls on day 3 of the cycle.[42] A meta-analysis assessing ovarian volume as a predictor has shown that AFC is a better predictor for poor response compared to ovarian volume.[35] Hence, despite its early promising predictive importance, it is nowadays accepted that ovarian volume has a relatively limited predictive value for ovarian response to stimulation.

Ovarian Blood Flow Assessment

Stromal blood flow is another aspect of ovarian physiology that was made possible to investigate with the introduction of Doppler technique. Commonly used parameters were stromal peak systolic velocity (PSV), pulsatility index (PI), resistance index (RI) and, lately, vascularization index (VI), flow index (FI) and vascularization flow index (VFI).[43-50] PSV prior to beginning of ovarian stimulation has been associated with the number of retrieved oocytes.[43,44] Early investigations have also suggested the value of ovarian stromal blood flow parameters in predicting the success of MAR,[48] but others have failed to prove their predictive ability.[46,47] Ovarian stromal vessels are thin and torturous and it is impossible to obtain the angle between the ultrasound beam and the intraovarian vessel accurately. This means that the measurement is subjective, depends on the examiner and has low reproducibility.

The introduction of 3D and power Doppler angiography represented significant improvement in terms of ovarian blood flow assessment. It allowed for simultaneous calculation of ovarian volume, AFC and blood flow in a short time and the possibilities of subsequent off-line analysis of stored volumes. This subsequently significantly improved the reproducibility of ovarian blood flow assessment.[51] In the study using 3D ultrasound, it was demonstrated that the mean ovarian stromal flow index (FI) was an important predictor of ovarian response to controlled stimulation.[52] The same authors also concluded that 3D ultrasound enabled more objective assessment of ovarian morphology and ovarian stromal blood flow, shortened the time of examination and increased the patient's comfort during examination.[52] Similar findings of lower VI, FI and VFI in poor responders compared to normal responders were confirmed in another study.[53] In contrary to these findings, it has been shown that all three indices of vascularity (VI, FI, VFI) were significantly increased during gonadotropin stimulation in the group of normal responders compared to the low ovarian reserve group. However, the number of retrieved oocytes correlated only with the antral follicle count and ovarian volume but not with indices of vascularization.[54] Another group has demonstrated that VI, FI and VFI of the ovary were significantly related to ovarian response to stimulation.[55] However, only AFC an OV and none of the blood flow indices were identified as independent predictors of ovarian response and IVF outcome.[55] These findings are coherent with a recent study that compared AFC with OV and ovarian stromal vascularization indices by using 3D and power Doppler as predictors of MAR outcome. Both AFC and OV exhibited strong correlation to the number of retrieved mature oocytes and 3D power Doppler indices displayed only a weak correlation.[56]

Several studies investigated perifollicular blood flow indices in natural menstrual cycles.[27,29,49,57,58] In women undergoing unstimulated IVF cycle, it has been hypothesized that follicles containing oocytes able to produce a pregnancy display more uniform perifollicular vascular network.[29] However, in this setting, none of the studied indices of vascularization (peak systolic velocity (PSV), pulsatility index (PI), resistance index (RI) and the percentage of blood volume showing a volume flow signal (VFS) inside a 5 mm capsule of perifollicular tissue) had clinically useful predictive ability for this outcome.[29]

Ultrasound Monitoring in Controlled Ovarian Stimulation

Ultrasound is the primary tool in monitoring controlled ovarian stimulation for assisted reproduction. Sonographic evaluation of follicle growth and the number of follicles can influence the decision on the dose of administered gonadotropins as well as the timing of hCG administration for triggering final oocyte maturation.

Maturity of the oocyte is closely associated with the follicle *size* and the serum oestradiol levels. Common approaches to controlled ovarian stimulation monitoring involve baseline ultrasound and oestradiol measurements. Afterwards, the approaches vary and usually combine ultrasound and oestradiol monitoring, but the target remains the same—obtaining an adequate number of follicles with oestradiol levels that are consistent with the follicle cohort (serum E2 of at least 200 pg/mL per follicle measuring ≥14 mm).

The growing follicle matures and secretes increasing levels of oestradiol that affects the target organs and promotes proliferation of the endometrium, preparing it for the implantation of the embryo. Direct associations between the diameter of the dominant follicle and the levels of E_2, and between the levels of E_2 and endometrial thickness led to 'ultrasound only' approach to controlled ovarian stimulation monitoring. Abandoning endocrinologic monitoring also makes monitoring less invasive and economical. In 1985 it was suggested that ultrasound alone is sufficient to estimate follicular maturity[59] and reports of simplification of cycle monitoring followed.[60,61] Simplification had to be weighed against possible reduction of the pregnancy rate and increase in the incidence of ovarian hyperstimulation syndrome (OHSS).[62]

OHSS is a potentially life-threatening condition. Risk factors for OHSS are young age, low body weight and polycystic ovary syndrome (PCOS). Further risk factors include the need for high doses of gonadotropins, high absolute (exceeding 2,500 pg/mL) or rapidly rising serum oestradiol levels and previous episodes of OHSS. It is especially important to be aware of the possible risk of OHSS when more than 20 developing follicles are present.[63] OHSS remains the main reason for serial serum E_2 level monitoring. However, considering the low predictability of OHSS, some argue that intensive monitoring (E2 combined with ultrasound) is only justified in cases where risk factors are present.[64] In one retrospective study, the intensive monitoring protocol was compared to ultrasound scanning as the only monitoring tool. There was no difference in the duration of stimulation, the amount of gonadotropins used, the number of oocytes retrieved, fertilization rates and clinical pregnancy rates. Most importantly, the incidence of OHSS in the two approaches did not differ significantly.[65] The assessment of ovarian blood flow is also not effective in predicting the occurrence of OHSS after ovarian stimulation.[66] At present, there is no clear single best approach to monitoring in order to avoid OHSS. Primary prevention by using GnRH antagonist cycles in population at risk is currently the most beneficial strategy.[67] Combined with GnRH agonist triggering for final oocyte maturation, embryo cryopreservation and withholding embryo transfer, this allows for almost complete avoidance of OHSS.[68]

ULTRASOUND MONITORING IN UNSTIMULATED CYCLES

The term "natural cycle" is used to describe spontaneous, unstimulated cycles from which oocytes are recovered for assisted reproduction after human chorionic gonadotropin (hCG) administration.[69] IVF/ICSI in natural cycles is commonly used method for treatment of infertility in selected patients.[70,71] Monitoring of these cycles has greatly extended our knowledge of human reproductive physiology. Assisted reproduction in natural cycles has several advantages compared to ovarian stimulation, but the failure rate is high and delivery rate per recovered oocyte remains unacceptably low. These are the main reasons why unstimulated cycles are not widely used in IVF/ICSI programs.[72]

For evaluation of follicular maturity in unstimulated cycles, serum E2 levels and sonographic monitoring are used. Consensus on the optimal E2 criteria for hCG administration has not been reached and the criteria vary significantly. According to one study, the right time to apply hCG is when the mean follicle diameter reaches 18 mm and serum oestradiol is more than 0.66 nmol/L.[73] Others have proposed E2 levels of 1.1 nmol/L,[74] 0.73–1.1 nmol/L,[75] 0.88 nmol/L,[76] 0.50 nmol/L[77] and 0.40 nmol/L.[78]

The main limitation of using ultrasound only for monitoring of natural cycles is the unpredicted onset of LH surge. Even if follicles are tracked every second day until the diameter of 16 mm and then on a daily basis, spontaneous LH surge or ovulation at the time of oocyte pickup was observed in 40% of patients.[71] Interestingly, further studies have shown that comparable fertilization and implantation rates can be achieved if smaller follicles were aspirated.[79] If hCG was administered when the follicle measured 15 mm and serum E2 was at least 0.49 nmol/L, the aspirated oocytes were suitable for IVF/ICSI and fertilization and implantation rate were satisfactory. Spontaneous LH surge or ovulation before OPU was detected in less than 10% of cases.[79]

THE ROLE OF SONOGRAPHIC EVALUATION OF THE ENDOMETRIUM

For any assisted reproduction procedure, optimally primed endometrium is essential for successful implantation. Endometrial development resulting in endometrial receptivity during the window of implantation requires the subtle collaboration of an extremely large number of different factors. Morphological characteristics of endometrium depend on the circulating levels of oestrogen and progesterone. Transvaginal ultrasonography can provide insight to the state and development of the endometrium and the capability to be receptive for embryos. Anterior and posterior myometrial-endometrial interfaces are easily recognized in all phases of the menstrual cycle. At the end of the menstrual phase, the endometrium appears as a thin, hyperechoic line

(Fig. 5A). During proliferative phase, it becomes thicker (double layer endometrial thickness is normally 5–12 mm) and less echogenic **(Fig. 5B)**. As early as day 6 and as late as one day before the LH peak, the sonographic picture of endometrium changes to the 'triple stripe' pattern. At the time of ovulation endometrium thickness is 10–16 mm.[13,80] After ovulation, in the secretory phase of the menstrual cycle, characteristic 'triple stripe' pattern disappears as the consequence of progesterone influence. Endometrium becomes homogenous and hyperechoic **(Fig. 5C)**. Thickness of endometrium increases only slightly. As a contrast to hyperechogenicity of endometrium, observer could also identify a hypoechoic band at the interface with the myometrium.[81]

Endometrial thickness is defined as the distance between the anterior and posterior stratum basalis layers.[82] Its measurement should be performed in the sagittal plane. During a normal menstrual cycle spontaneous uterine contractions may occur and this may influence the accuracy of measurement.[83,84] Although not commonly used in routine clinical practice, it was proposed that the endometrium should be measured before, during and after these wave-like contractions, and the mean value should be used as the most accurate thickness.[85]

In the luteal phase of the unstimulated cycle endometrium does seem to be thicker in conception compared to non-conception cycles, and in normal pregnancy compared to abnormal pregnancy. However, at

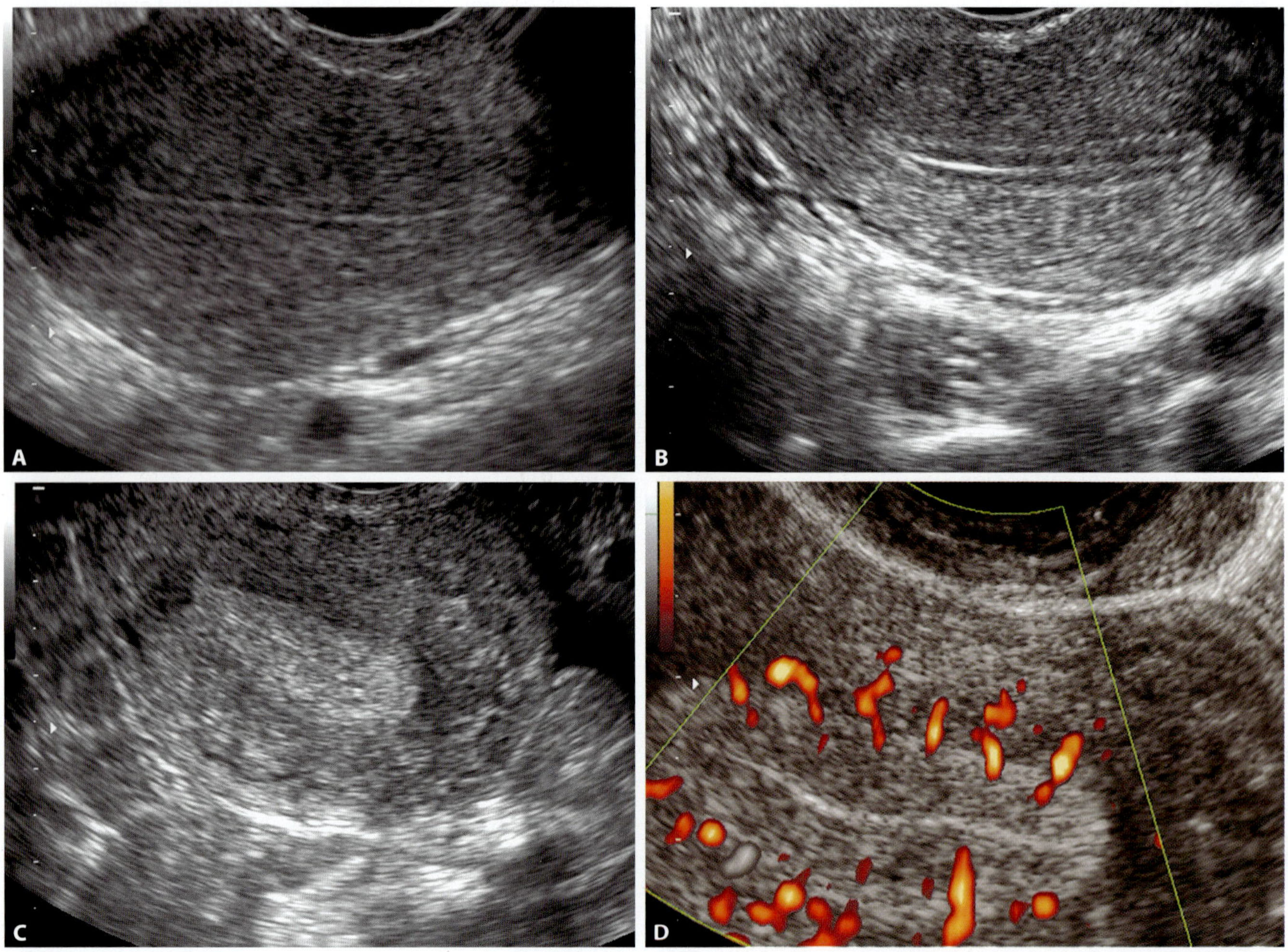

Figs. 5A to D: Sonography of the endometrium. (A) Endometrium in the early proliferative phase appears as a thin, hyperechoic line; (B) Through the proliferative phase the endometrium becomes thicker and less echogenic; (C) Due to progesterone action, the endometrium becomes homogeneous and hyperechoic in the secretory phase of the menstrual cycle; (D) Subendometrial vascularization visualized by power Doppler.

present there is not enough data to confirm that endometrial volume measurement is a useful tool in differential diagnosis of early normal and abnormal pregnancy.[86]

Endometrial thickness measurement is an essential part of evaluation of patients with fertility problems.[87] Although multiple studies investigated the predictive value of endometrial thickness and sonographic appearance in MAR cycles, conclusions remain controversial. A recent systematic review has shown that although frequently used cut-off of 7 mm is related to lower chance of pregnancy, the discriminatory capacity of this value in the prediction of pregnancy is virtually absent.[88] There are also other echographic aspects of endometrium, such as homogenous appearance on the day of hCG administration and uterine artery pulsatility index higher than 3.0 that were associated with poor results of stimulated IVF/ICSI cycle.[89-94] While some investigators suggested that excessive endometrial growth (greater than 14 mm) was also shown to be poor prognostic indicator,[95] others refuted this conclusion.[96,97]

The importance of Doppler angiographic indices as tools for evaluation of endometrium has also been studied **(Fig. 5D)**. Cycle-dependent changes in uterine artery blood flow (velocity and pulsatility index of uterine artery) are evident, but their predictive value is limited due to diurnal variations and difference between the two uterine arteries (ipsilateral or contralateral to the dominant follicle).[89-94]

Although, endometrial measurement represents a routine part of sonographic investigation, the objective importance and prognostic value remain uncertain and the decisions to change stimulation regimen or to cancel the cycle based on these parameters are difficult to justify.[98] Molecular aspects of endometrial receptivity are a subject of extensive current research; however there are currently no clinically validated tools available. Until such determinants are discovered and made clinically applicable and reliable, caution should be used in applying treatment decisions based on ultrasonically assessed parameters of endometrial receptivity.

REFERENCES

1. Gougeon A, Lefèvre B. Evolution of diameters of the largest healthy and atretic follicles during the human menstrual cycle. J Reprod Fertil. 1983;69:497-502.
2. Gougeon A, Chainy GBN. Morphometric studies of small follicles in ovaries of women at different ages. J Reprod Fertil. 1987;81:433-42.
3. Balakier H, Stronell RD. Color Doppler assessment of folliculogenesis in in vitro fertilization patients. Fertil Steril. 62:1211-6.
4. Gougeon A. Regulation of ovarian follicular development in primates: facts and hypotheses. Endocr Rev. 1996; 17(2):121-55.
5. Suh CS, Sonntag B, Erickson GF. The ovarian life cycle: a contemporary view. Rev Endocr Metab Disord. 2002;3(1): 5-12.
6. Bassett DL. The changes in the vascular pattern of the ovary of the albino rat during the estrous cycle. Am J Anat. 1943; 73:252-92.
7. Sladkevicius P, Valentin L, Marsal K. Blood flow velocity in the uterine and ovarian arteries during the normal menstrual cycle. Ultrasound Obstet Gynecol. 1993;3:199-208.
8. Van Blerkom J, Antczak M, Schrader R. The developmental potential of the human oocyte is related to the dissolved oxygen content of follicular fluid: association with vascular endothelial growth factor levels and perifollicular blood flow characteristics. Human Reprod. 1997;12:1047-55.
9. Abulafia O, Sherer DM. Angiogenesis of the ovary. Am J Obstet Gynecol. 2000;182:240-6.
10. Craig J, Orisaka M, Wang H, Orisaka S, Thompson W, Zhu C, et al. Gonadotropin and intra-ovarian signals regulating follicle development and atresia: the delicate balance between life and death. Front Biosci. 2007;12:3628-39.
11. Baerwald AR, Adams GP, Pierson RA. Ovarian antral folliculogenesis during the human menstrual cycle: a review. Hum Reprod Update. 2012;18(1):73-91.
12. Baerwald AR, Adams GP, Pierson RA. Characterization of ovarian follicular wave dynamics in women. Biol Reprod. 2003;69(3):1023-31.
13. Bakos O, Lundkvist O, Wide L, Bergh T. Ultrasonographical and hormonal description of the normal ovulatory menstrual cycle. Acta Obstet Gynecol Scand. 1994;73:790-6.
14. Kratochwil A, Urban G, Fridrich G. Ultrasonic tomography of the ovary. Ann Chir Gynecol Fenn. 1972;61:211-4.
15. Fleisher AC, Darnell J, Rodier J, Lindsay A, James AE. Sonographic monitoring of ovarian follicular development. J Clin Ultrasound. 1981;9:275-80
16. O'Herlihy C, de Crespigny L. Robinson HP. Monitoring ovarian follicular development with real-time ultrasound. Br J Obstet Gynecol. 1980;87:613-8
17. Gore MA, Nayudu PL, Vlaisavljevic V, Thomas N. Prediction of ovarian cycle outcome by follicular characteristics, stage 1. Hum Reprod. 1995;10(9):2313-9.
18. Gore MA, Nayudu PL, Vlaisavljević V. Attending dominance in vivo: distinguishing dominant from challenger follicles in humans. Human Reprod.1997;12(12):2741-7.
19. Bomsel-Helmreich O, Al-Mufti W. Ultrasonography of normal and abnormal follicular development. In: Jaffe R, Pierson RA, Abramowicz JS, (Eds). Imaging in infertility and reproductive endocrinology. 1st edn. Philadelphia: JB Lippincott; 1994. pp. 117-28.

20. Pashe TD, Wladimiroff JD, de Jong FH, Hop WC, Fauser BC. Growth patterns of non-dominant ovarian follicles during normal menstrual cycle. Fertile Steril. 1990;54:638-42.
21. Nayudu P. Relationship of constructed follicle growth patterns in stimulated cycles to outcome after IVF. Human Reprod. 1991;6:465-71.
22. Vlaisavljević V. Analysis of follicular growth in conceivers and nonconceivers after intrauterine insemination. Gynecol Perinatol. 1995;4:49-451.
23. Bourne TH, Jurkovic D, Waterstone J, et al. Intrafollicular blood flow during human ovulation. Ultrasound Obstet Gynecol. 1991;5:53-9.
24. Ecochard R, Marret H, Rabilloud, et al. Sensitivity and specificity of ultrasound indices of ovulation in spontaneous cycles. Eur J Obstet Gynecol Reprod Biol. 2000;91:59-64.
25. Pearlstone AC, Surrey ES. The temporal relation between the urine LH surge and sonographic evidence of ovulation: determinants and clinical significance. Obstet Gynecol. 1994; 83:184-187.
26. Jarvela IY, Sladkevicius P, Kelly S, Ojha K, Nargund G, Campbell S. Three-dimensional sonographic and power Doppler characterization of ovaries in late follicular phase. Ultrasound Obstet Gynecol. 2002;20(3):281-5.
27. Campbell S, Bourne T, Waterstone J, Reynolds K, Crayford T, Jurkovic D, et al. Transvaginal color blood flow imaging of the preovulatory follicle. Fertil Steril. 1993;60:433-8.
28. Kupesic S, Kurjak A. Uterine and ovarian perfusion during the periovulatory period assessed by transvaginal color Doppler. Fertil Steril. 1993;60:439-43.
29. Vlaisavljevic V, Reljic M, Gavric Lovrec V, Zazula D, Sergent N. Measurement of perifollicular blood flow of the dominant preovulatory follicle using three-dimensional power Doppler. Ultrasound Obstet Gynecol. 2003;22(5):520-6.
30. Brannstrorm M, Zackrisson U, Hagstroom HG, et al. Preovulatory changes of blood flow in different regions of the human follicle. Fertil Steril. 1998;69:435-42.
31. Rombauts L, Onwude JL, Chew HW, Vollenhoven BJ. The predictive value of antral follicle count remains unchanged across the menstrual cycle. Fertil Steril. 2011;96(6):1514-8.
32. Broer SL, Dólleman M, Opmeer BC, Fauser BC, Mol BW, Broekmans FJ. AMH and AFC as predictors of excessive response in controlled ovarian hyperstimulation: a meta-analysis. Hum Reprod Update. 2011;17(1):46-54.
33. Broer SL, van Disseldorp J, Broeze KA, Dolleman M, Opmeer BC, Bossuyt P, et al. IMPORT study group. Added value of ovarian reserve testing on patient characteristics in the prediction of ovarian response and ongoing pregnancy: an individual patient data approach. Hum Reprod Update. 2013; 19(1):26-36.
34. Ng EH, Tang OS, Ho PC. The significance of the number of antral follicles prior to stimulation in predicting ovarian response in an IVF programme. Hum Reprod. 2000;15:1937-42.
35. Hendriks DJ, Kwee J, Mol BW, te Velde ER, Broekmans FJ. Ultrasonography as a tool for the prediction of outcome in IVF patients: a comparative meta-analysis of ovarian volume and antral follicle count. Fertil Steril. 2007;87(4):764-75.
36. Chang MY, Chiang CH, Hsieh TT, Soong KY, Hsu KH. Use of antral follicle count to predict the outcome of assisted reproduction technologies. Fertil Steril. 1998;69:505-10.
37. Nelson SM, Klein BM, Arce JC. Comparison of antimüllerian hormone levels and antral follicle count as predictor of ovarian response to controlled ovarian stimulation in good-prognosis patients at individual fertility clinics in two multicenter trials. Fertil Steril. 2015;103(4):923-30.
38. Ata B, Seyhan A, Reinblatt SL, Shalom-Paz E, Krishnamurthy S, Tan SL. Comparison of automated and manual follicle monitoring in an unrestricted population of 100 women undergoing controlled ovarian stimulation for IVF. Hum Reprod. 2011;26(1):127-33.
39. Deb S, Batcha M, Campbell BK, Jayaprakasan K, Clewes JS, Hopkisson JF, et al. The predictive value of the automated quantification of the number and size of small antral follicles in women undergoing ART. Hum Reprod. 2009;24(9): 2124-32.
40. Syrop CH, Willhoite A, Voorhis BJ. Ovarian volume: a novel outcome predictor for assisted reproduction. Fertil Steril. 1995;64:1167-71.
41. Lass A, Skull J, McVeigh E, Margara R, Winston RML. Measurement of ovarian volume by transvaginal sonography before ovulation induction with human menopausal gonadotropin for in vitro fertilization can predict poor response. Hum Reprod. 1997;12:294-97.
42. Pellicer A, Ardiles G, Neuspiller F, Remohi J, Simon C, Bonilla-Musoles F. Evaluation of ovarian reserve in young low responders with normal basal levels of follicle-stimulating hormone using three-dimensional ultrasonography. Fertil Steril. 1998;70(4):671-75.
43. Zaidi J, Campbell S, Pitroff R, Kyei-Mensah A, Shaker A, Jacobs HS, et al. Ovarian stromal blood flow in women with polycystic ovaries—a possible new marker for diagnosis? Hum Reprod. 1995;6:191-8.
44. Engmann L, Sladkevicius P, Agrawal R, Bekir JS, Campbell S, Tan SL. Value of stromal blood flow velocity measurement after pituitary suppression in the prediction of ovarian responsiveness and outcome of in vitro fertilization treatment. Fertil Steril. 1999;71:22-9.
45. Nagrund G, Bourne T, Doyle P, Parsons J, Cheng W, Campbell S, et al. Associations between ultrasound indices of follicular blood flow, oocyte recovery and preimplantation embryo quality. Hum Reprod. 1996;11:109-13.
46. Balakier H, Stronell RD. Color Doppler assessment of folliculogenesis in in vitro fertilization patients. Fertil Steril. 1994;62:1211-6.
47. Tekay A, Martikainen H, Jouppila P. Blood flow changes in uterine and ovarian vasculature and predictive value of transvaginal pulsed colour Doppler ultrasonography in an

in vitro fertilization programme. Hum Reprod. 1995;10(3): 688-93.

48. Coulam CB, Goodman C, Rinehart JS. Colour indices of follicular blood flow as predictors of pregnancy after in vitro fertilization and embryo transfer. Hum Reprod. 1999; 14(8):1979-82.
49. Collins W, Jurkovic D, Bourne T, Kurjak A, Campbell S. Ovarian morphology, endocrine function and intrafollicular blood flow during the periovulatory period. Hum Reprod. 1991;6(3):319-24.
50. Zaidi J, Collins W, Campbell S, Pitroff R, Tan SL. Blood flow changes in the intraovarian arteries during the preovulatory period: relationship to the time of the day. Ultrasound Obstet Gynecol. 1996;7:135-40.
51. Mercé LT, Gómez B, Engels V, Bau S, Bajo JM. Intraobserver and interobserver reproducibility of ovarian volume, antral follicle count, and vascularity indices obtained with transvaginal 3-dimensional ultrasonography, power Doppler angiography, and the virtual organ computer-aided analysis imaging program. J Ultrasound Med. 2005;24(9): 1279-87.
52. Kupesic S, Kurjak A. Predictors of IVF outcome by three-dimensional ultrasound. Hum Reprod. 2002;17(4):950-55.
53. Pan HA, Wu MH, Cheng YC, Wu LH, Chang FM. Quantification of ovarian stromal Doppler signals in poor responders undergoing in vitro fertilization with three-dimensional power Doppler ultrasonography. Am J Obstet Gynecol. 2004;190(2):338-44.
54. JärveläIY, SladkeviciusP, KellyS, OjhaK, CampbellS, Nagrund G. Quantification of ovarian power Dopppler signal with three-dimensional ultrasonography to predict response during in vitro fertilization. Obstet Gynecol. 2003;102(4): 816-22.
55. Mercé LT, Barco MJ, Bau S, Troyano JM. Prediction of ovarian response and IVF/ICSI outcome by three-dimensional ultrasonography and power Doppler angiography. Eur J Obstet Gynecol Reprod Biol. 2007;132(1):93-100.
56. Shaban MM, Abdel Moety GA. Role of ultrasonographic markers of ovarian reserve in prediction of IVF and ICSI outcome. Gynecol Endocrinol. 2014;30(4):290-3.
57. Tan SL, Zaidi J, Campbell S, Doyle P, Collins W. Blood flow changes in the ovarian and uterine arteries during normal menstrual cycle. Am J Obstet Gynecol. 1996;175(3):625-31.
58. Gavrić Lovrec VG, Vlaisavljevic V, Reljic M. Dependence of the in-vitro fertilization capacity of the oocyte on perifollicular flow in the preovulatory period of unstimulated cycles. Wien Klin Wochenschr. 2001;113[Suppl 3]:21-26.
59. Nilsson L, Wikland M, Hamburger L, Hillensjo T, Chari S, Sturm G, et al. Simplification of the method of in vitro fertilization: sonographic measurements of follicular diameter as a sole index of follicular maturity. J In Vitro Fert Emryo Transf. 1985;2:17.
60. Vlaisavljević V, Kovačič B, Gavrić Lovrec V, Reljič M. Simplification of the clinical phase of IVF and ICSI treatment in programmed cycles. Int J Gynecol Obstet. 2000;69:135-42.
61. Vlaisavljević V, Kovačič B, Gavrić V. In vitro fertilization program based on programmed cycles monitored by ultrasound only. Int J Gynecol obstet. 1992;39:227-31.
62. Practice Committee of American Society for Reproductive Medicine, Birmingham, Alabama, USA. Ovarian hyperstimulation syndrome. Fertil Steril. 2008;90(5 Suppl): S188-93.
63. Braude P, Rowell P. Assisted conception. III-problems with assisted conception. BMJ. 2003;327(7420):920-23.
64. Ben-Shlomo I, Geslevich J, Shalev E. Can we abandon routine evaluation of serum estradiol levels during controlled ovarian hyperstimulation for assisted reproduction? Fertil Steril. 2001;76:300-3.
65. Tomaževič T, Meden Vrtovec H. Early timed follicular aspiration prevents severe ovarian hyperstimulation syndrome. J Assist Reprod Genet. 1996;13:282-6.
66. Jayaprakasan K1 Jayaprakasan R, Al-Hasie HA, Clewes JS, Campbell BK, Johnson IR, et al. Can quantitative three-dimensional power Doppler angiography be used to predict ovarian hyperstimulation syndrome? Ultrasound Obstet Gynecol. 2009;33(5):583-91.
67. Griesinger G. Ovarian hyperstimulation syndrome prevention strategies: use of gonadotropin-releasing hormone antagonists. Semin Reprod Med. 2010;28(6): 493-99.
68. Devroey P, Polyzos NP, Blockeel C. An OHSS-Free Clinic by segmentation of IVF treatment. Hum Reprod. 2011; 26(10):2593-97.
69. Paulson RJ. Natural cycle in vitro fertilization. Infertil Reprod Med Clin North Am. 1993;4:653-65.
70. Fahy UM, Cahill DJ, Wardle PG, Hull MGR. In vitro fertilization in completely natural cycles. Hum Reprod. 1995;10(3):572-5.
71. Vlaisavljevic V, Gavric V, Kovacic B. In vitro fertilization in natural cycles: maribor experience. The world congress on in vitro fertilization and assisted reproduction held in Vienna, Austria, 1995 April 3-7.
    Aburumich A, Bernat E, Dohr G, Feichtinger W, Fischl F, Huber J, Mueller E, Szalay S, Urdl W, Zech H, editors. Bologna: Monduzzi Editore: 1995;573-5.
72. Lenton EA, Woodward B. Controversies in assisted reproduction. Natural vs. stimulated cycles in IVF: Is there a role for IVF in natural cycle? J Assist Reprod Genet. 1993;10:406-8.
73. Foulot H, Ranoux C, Dobuisson JB, Rambaud FX, Poirot C. In vitro fertilization without ovarian stimulation: a simplified protocol applied in 80 cycles. Fertil Steril. 1989;52:617-21.
74. Ramsewak S, Cooke I, Li T, Kumar A, Monks N, Lenton E. Are factors that influence oocyte fertilization also predictive? An assessment of 148 cycles of in vitro fertilization without gonadotropin stimulation. Fertil Steril. 1990;54:470-4.

75. Paulson R, Sauer M, Francis M, Macaso T, Lobo R. In vitro fertilization in unstimulated cycles: the University of Southern California experience. Fertil Steril. 1992;57:290-3.
76. Paulson RJ, Sauer MV, Francis M, Macaso M, Lobo R. Factors affecting pregnancy success of human in vitro fertilization in unstimulated cycles. Hum Reprod. 1994;9:1571-5.
77. Reljič M, Vlaisavljević V. The preovulatory serum estradiol pattern in natural IVF/ICSI cycles. J Assist Reprod Genet. 1999;16:535-9.
78. Tomaževič T, Geršak K, Meden-Vrtovec H, Drobnič Š, Veble A, Valenčič B, et al. Clinical parameters to predict the success of in vitro fertilization-embryo transfer in the natural cycle. Assisted Reproduction. 1999;9:149-56.
79. Vlaisavljević V, Kovačič B, Reljič M, Gavrić Lovrec V. Three protocols for monitoring follicle development in 587 unstimulated cycles of in vitro fertilization and intracytoplasmic sperm injection. A comparison. J Reprod Med. 2001:46:892-8.
80. Bakos O, Lundkvist O, Bergh T. Transvaginal sonographic evaluation of endometrial growth and texture in spontaneous ovulatory menstrual cycles: a descriptive study. Human Reproduction. 1993;8:799-806.
81. Quigley MM. In vitro fertilization: a new procedures and new questions. Investigative Radiology 1986;21:503-10.
82. Persadie R. Ultrasonographic assessment of the endometrial thickness: a review. J Obstet Gynecol Can. 2002; 24:131-6.
83. De Vries K, Lyons EA, Ballard G, et al. Contractions of the inner third of the myometrium. Am J Obstet Gynecol 1990;162:679-82.
84. Aguilar HN, Mitchell BF. Physiological pathways and molecular mechanisms regulating uterine contractility. Hum Reprod Update. 2010;16(6):725-44.
85. Dastidar KG, Dastidar SG. Dynamics of endometrial thickness over time: a reappraisal to standardize ultrasonographic measurements in an infertility program. Fertil Steril. 2003;80:213-5.
86. Dmitrovic R, Simunic V. Will Endometrial Volume Measurements Add Something New to the Diagnosis of Early Pregnancy? Current Women's Health Reviews. 2009;5:24-8.
87. Friedler S, Schenker JG, Herman A, Lewin A. The role of ultrasonography in the evaluation of endometrial receptivity following assisted reproductive treatments: a critical review. Human Reproduction Update. 1996;2:323-35.
88. Kasius A, Smit JG, Torrance HL, Eijkemans MJ, Mol BW, Opmeer BC, et al. Endometrial thickness and pregnancy rates after IVF: a systematic review and meta-analysis. Hum Reprod Update. 2014;20(4):530-41.
89. Steer CV, Campbell S, Tan SL, et al. The use of transvaginal color flow imaging after in vitro fertilization to identify optimum uterine conditions before embryo transfer. Fertility and Sterility. 1992;57:371-6.
90. Steer CV, Tan SL, Dillon D, et al. Vaginal color Doppler assessment of uterine artery impedance correlates with immunohistochemical markers of endometrial receptivity for the implantation of an embryo. Fertility and Sterility. 1995;63:101-8.
91. Ueno J, Oehninger S, Bryzski RG, Acosta AA, Philput B, Muasher SJ. Ultrasonographic appearance of the endometrium in natural and stimulated in vitro fertilization cycles and its correlation with outcome. Hum Reprod. 1991;6:901.
92. Check JH, Nowroozi K, Choe J, Lurie D, Dietterich C. The effect of endometrial thickness and echo pattern on in vitro fertilization outcome in donor oocyte-embryo transfer cycle. Fertil Steril. 1993;59:72.
93. Oliveira JB, Baruffi RL, Mauri AL, et al. Endometrial ultrasonography as a predictor of pregnancy in an in vitro fertilization programme after ovarian stimulation and gonadotropin-releasing hormone and gonadotropins. Hum Reprod. 1997;12:2515.
94. Fanchin R, Righini C, Ayoubi JM, et al. New look at endometrial echogenicity objective computer-assisted measurements predict endometrial receptivity in in vitro fertilization-embryo transfer. Fertil Steril. 2000;74:274.
95. Weissman A, Gotlieb L, Casper RF. The detrimental effect of increased endometrial thickness on implantation and pregnancy rates and outcome in an in vitro fertilization program. Fertil Steril. 1999;71:147.
96. Dietterich C, Check JH, Choe JK, et al. Increased endometrial thickness on the day of human chorionic gonadotropin injection does not adversely affect pregnancy or implantation rates following in vitro fertilization-embryotransfer. Fertil Steril. 2002;77:781.
97. Yakin K, Akarsu C, Kahraman S. Cycle lumping or-sampling a witches' brew? Fertil Steril. 2000;73:175.
98. De Geyter C, Schmitter M, De Geyter M, et al. Prospective evaluation of ultrasound appearance of the endometrium in a cohort of 1,186 infertile women. Fertil Steril. 2000;73:106.

57

CHAPTER

New Insights into the Fallopian Tube Ultrasound

Sanja Kupesic Plavsic, Ulrich Honemeyer, Asim Kurjak

INTRODUCTION

The fallopian tubes (oviducts) are embryologically derived from the Müllerian ducts. Anatomically, they arise from the cornual end of the uterus. They act as a conveyer and meeting ground for the oocytes and the sperms. The fallopian tubes are about 9–11 cm long and are covered by peritoneum, which duplicates to form one of its loose attachments (mesosalpinx), to the broad ligament.

The arterial blood supply to the oviducts is derived from the terminal branches of the uterine and the ovarian arteries. The branches of the uterine arteries supply the medial two-thirds of each tube. The ovarian arteries supply the lateral one-third of the tube. The venous drainage parallels the arterial supply.

The ultrasonic scanning and evaluation of the fallopian tube present a true challenge to even the best sonographers. The normal fallopian tube can be imaged only if fluid surrounds it and creates a sonic interface to outline its boundaries.[1] The most proximal part of it can also be imaged in the normal state, since it is held steady by the uterus, which in this case serves as a landmark for finding the proximal part of the tube.

In certain instances some sonolucent fluid is present in the pelvis, which acts as a contrast medium to highlight the normal fallopian tube.

- At times, a certain amount of pelvic fluid is present and this may be enough to highlight portions of the fallopian tube.
- At midcycle, after the release of follicular fluid, at the time of ovulation or immediately after it, parts of the tube may be detectable.
- Blood may be present in the pelvis for various reasons such as rupture of the corpus luteum, or rupture of an ectopic pregnancy. Such larger amounts of fluid in the pelvis may increase the chance to detect one or both fallopian tubes.
- Ascites present in the pelvis arising from ovarian hyperstimulation or other conditions, may serve as an excellent contrast medium around the fallopian tube and the fimbriae in order to highlight them.
- Fluid originating from infectious processes may also enable us to outline the fallopian tubes.

In absence of fluid, placing the patient into an anti-Trendelenburg position may increase the pooling of fluid and therefore, create the acoustic interface for imaging the tube.[2,3]

In this revised chapter the authors include updated references and new high resolution ultrasound images.

PELVIC INFLAMMATORY DISEASE

Pelvic inflammatory disease (PID) is defined as "the acute clinical syndrome associated with ascending spread of microorganisms (unrelated to pregnancy or surgery) from the vagina or cervix to the endometrium, fallopian tubes, and/or contiguous structures".[4] Very rarely, PID can develop as a result of surgical intervention. PID causes more morbidity than necessary for three major reasons: (i) women are not hospitalized when they should be, (ii) many women receive inadequate or inappropriate antibiotic therapy, and (iii) the male sex partner is not treated or is treated inadequately.

PID is mostly considered ascending and polymicrobial. Rarely, the infection is hematogenous, or spreads directly from other abdominal organs (diverticulitis and appendicitis). Among the sexually transmitted pathogens, *Neisseria gonorrhoeae* and *Chlamydia trachomatis* are most commonly identified.

Over half of women suffering from PID develop tubal damage without any symptoms of the disease, Chlamydia being the most frequent cause of this infection. Because of this observation, PID was classified into four major groups:

1. Silent (asymptomatic) PID (tubal scarring occurs without patient's knowledge).

2. Atypical PID (patients have only minimal symptoms).
3. Acute PID (this form is most commonly seen in patients presenting to emergency rooms).
4. PID residual syndrome (patients suffer from chronic pelvic pain, infertility and scar tissue formation).[5]

Chronologically, PID can be divided into: (i) acute PID with formation of pyosalpinx and tubo-ovarian abscess and (ii) PID-residual syndrome with hydrosalpinx and scar tissue formation.

Ultrasound Findings

Fallopian tube pathology is discerned by evaluating the wall of the tube, the luminal content, the tubal motility, as well as its relation with the surrounding pelvic structures.

Early in the course of the acute inflammation, pelvic sonography may be entirely normal. As the process of inflammation progresses, the endometrium becomes hyperechogenic and hyperperfused **(Figs. 1A and B)**, and the tubes become thick-walled, irregular and hypervascular **(Figs. 1A to F)**. The associated pelvic exudate allows better delineation of the gynecologic structures **(Fig. 1G)**. The inflamed tubes are represented by one of the following pictures:[6]

- A dilated fluid filled tubular structure **(Fig. 2)**.
- Echogenic tubal wall which reflects the inflammatory process of the mucosal lining.
- The presence of internal echoes within the dilated tubes and low vascular impedance due to vasodilatation

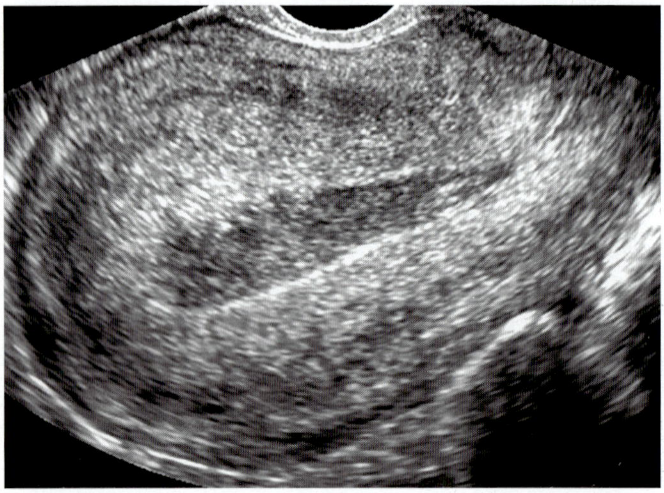

Fig. 1A: Transvaginal ultrasound image of endometritis. Note hyperechogenic endometrium and intracavitary fluid.

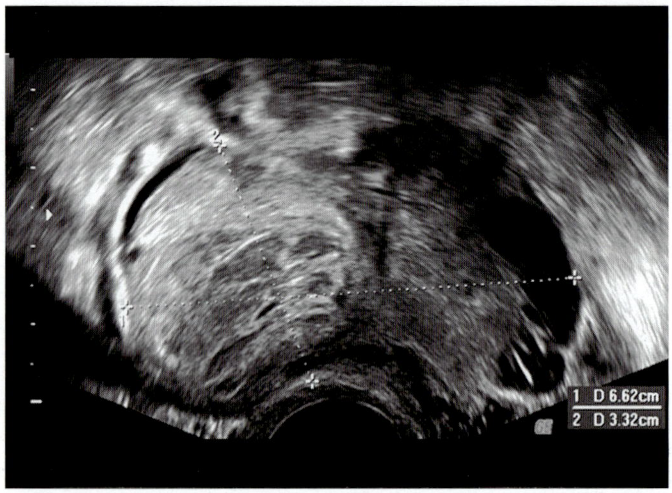

Fig. 1C: Transvaginal ultrasound of a thickened tube filled with echogenic fluid (pus).

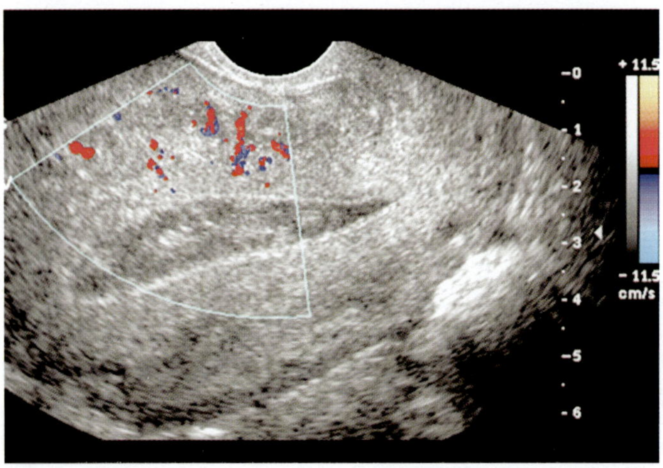

Fig. 1B: The same patient as in previous figure. Color Doppler demonstrates vascularized endometrium.

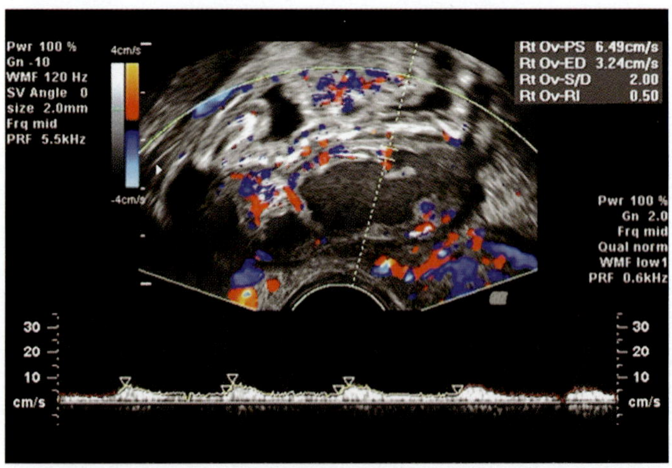

Fig. 1D: Transvaginal color Doppler of the same patient. Note prominent vascularization of thickened tubal walls with low to moderate vascular impedance (RI = 0.50).

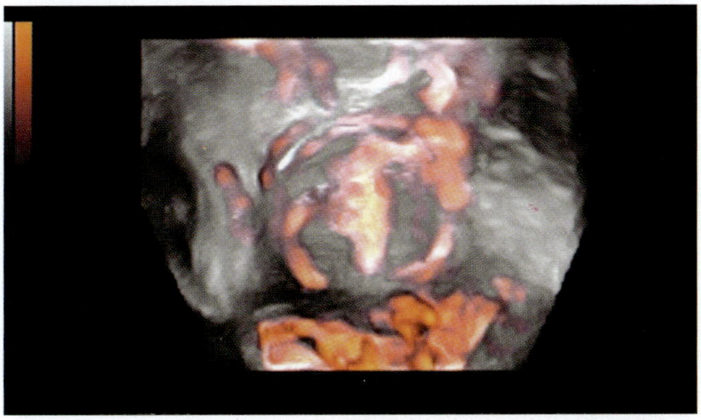

Fig. 1E: Three-dimensional power Doppler image illustrating tubal angiogenesis secondary to inflammation.

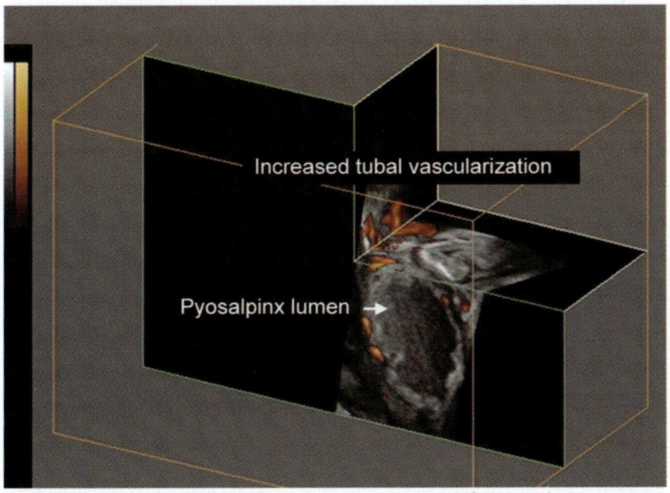

Fig. 1F: Niche mode of an acute PID. Open cut view enables visualization of the tubal lumen and increased vascularization within the tubal wall.

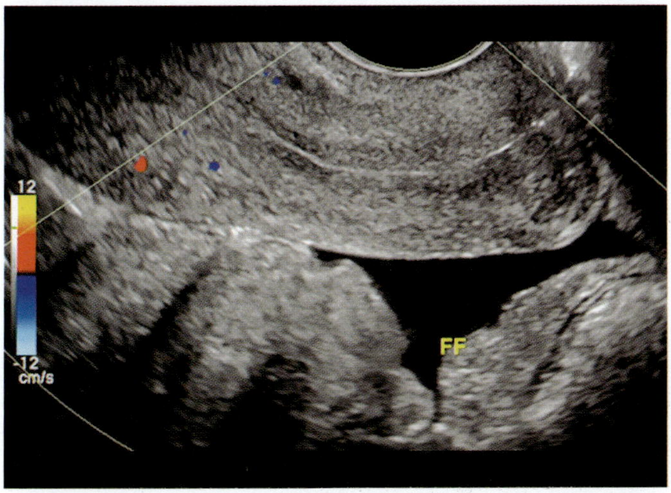

Fig. 1G: Free fluid in the posterior cul-de-sac secondary to peritonitis.

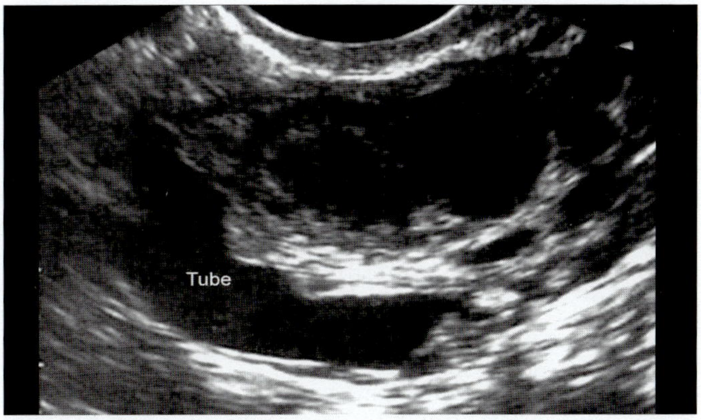

Fig. 2: Complex adnexal mass occupying the pouch of Douglas in a patient with acute pelvic inflammation. Tubal diameter is increased, tubal mucosa is thickened and anechoic fluid fills the tubal lumen. Note enlarged ovary filled with inflamed follicles on the right.

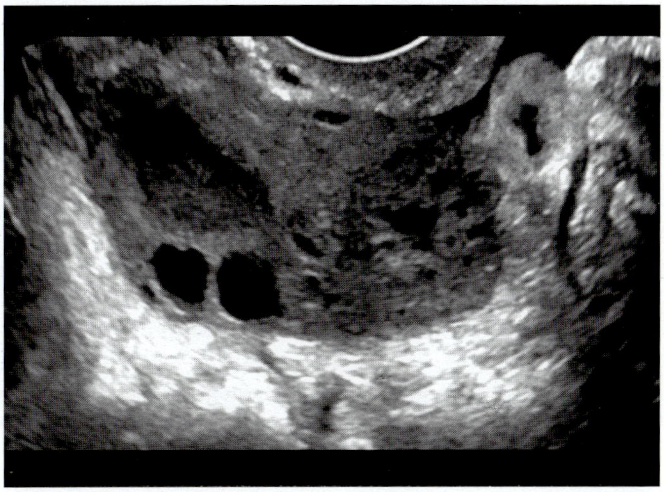

Fig. 3: A complex adnexal mass with thickening of the ovarian capsule and fluid collection are typical features of tubo-ovarian abscess.

indicate pyosalpinx **(Figs. 1C to F)**. Sonographic-guided aspiration of the pus could be helpful for diagnostic purposes and for determining the optimal antibiotic therapy.

- A complex adnexal mass with thickening of the ovarian capsule and loculated fluid collections in the adnexal cul-de-sac represents the tubo-ovarian abscess **(Fig. 3)**.

Sonographic appearance of hydrosalpinx differs depending on the stage of the disease. During the acute phase, the tubal wall is thick and tender to the probe touch **(Figs. 1 to 3)**. In the chronic phase, hydrosalpinx shows a typically thin wall, which is not tender. Chronic

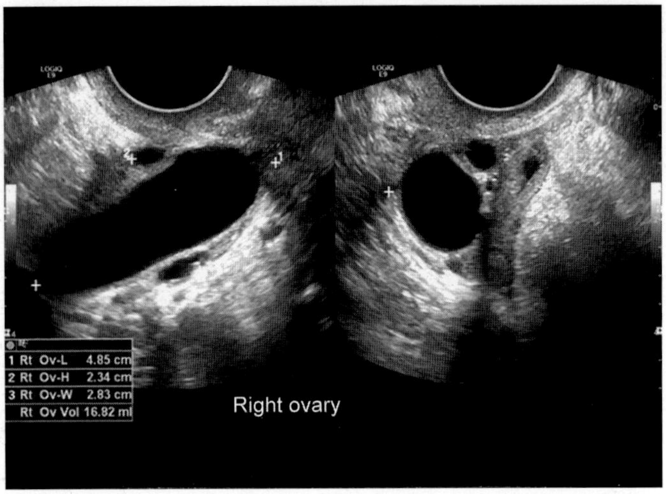

Fig. 4: Transvaginal sonogram of a patient with hydrosalpinx in two different planes. Note the importance of performing different planes, because hydrosalpinx may sometimes be misinterpreted as ovarian or paraovarian cyst.

hydrosalpinx is usually discovered accidentally, on a routine transvaginal scan or during an infertility procedure **(Fig. 4)**. Patients are often unaware of their pelvic pathology, but can recall one or few episodes of pelvic pain and vaginal discharge.

Transvaginal sonography seems to be accurate in identification of fallopian tube pathology by evaluating the structure of the tubal wall and luminal contents. However, it is difficult to differentiate tubal from ovarian pathology when complex masses are found. During the acute stage of pelvic inflammatory disease, the tortuous and dilated fluid-filled tube "embraces" the adjacent ovary. At this time the ovary could not be well delineated, although visualization of the ovarian follicles enables localization of the ovarian component of the mass. During the chronic stage of PID the thin-walled hydrosalpinx is the main sonographic hallmark. Hydrosalpinx produces the typical image of a homogeneous, elongated fluid-filled mass adjacent and medial to the ovary. Incomplete and thin tubal septa are clearly distinguished from the distended tubal wall. However, when hydrosalpinx is presented as a complex lesion with thick walls, septa, suspicious papillary projections and mixed echogenic structures, incorrect diagnosis of an ovarian malignancy could be drawn.

Color Doppler Findings

Introduction of the color Doppler imaging has dramatically changed transvaginal ultrasound imaging. Color Doppler can depict blood flow within the pelvic structure and tell us more about the vessel quality in a particular organ or structure. The same modality can also depict movement of the liquid component such as in case of hydrosalpinx, when tubal content moves and changes the position compressed by vaginal probe or sliding over bowels during peristalsis. Furthermore, color Doppler is very useful in making a differential diagnosis between hydrosalpinx and pelvic congestion syndrome. When color is turned on, pelvic congestion syndrome lights up magnificently on the screen. Contrastingly, hydrosalpinx remains black and white, with specs of color only during peristalsis or deliberate probe movements.

Kupesic et al.[7] evaluated 102 women with laparoscopically proven PID. Seventy-two had acute symptoms, 11 presented with chronic pelvic pain, and 19 were infertility cases suspected of tubal etiology. The mean resistance index in patients with acute symptoms was 0.53 ± 0.09. It significantly differed from those obtained in patients with chronic stage ($RI = 0.71 \pm 0.07$), and infertility cases ($RI = 0.73 \pm 0.09$). Therefore, the bizarre morphology during both the chronic and acute stages of PID if evaluated by color and pulsed Doppler should not cause an overlap with adnexal malignancy, since vascular resistance demonstrates significantly higher values.

Many studies have been undertaken to assess blood flow-related functional changes in the ovaries since our team first introduced the technique.[8] Significant changes have been demonstrated during the menstrual cycle in the active ovary, and most of them were attributed to angiogenesis in the follicle and subsequently, the corpus luteum.[9,10] Transvaginal color Doppler has proved to be an extremely valuable tool in infertility evaluation and management, as well as in the assessment of adnexal masses and early detection of ovarian cancer.[11-14]

Kupesic et al.[7] assumed that an inflammatory process within the pelvis might affect ovarian blood flow. The ovary is in a close proximity to the tube, which is the primary focus of infection, and it shares a significant part of its blood supply with the ipsilateral tube. Therefore, it can be expected that the ovarian blood flow is altered according to the changes in inflammatory process. Indeed, our study[7] demonstrated the correlation of intraovarian blood flow changes with pathophysiological changes. Findings obtained in the acute stage demonstrated rapidly changing patterns. The ongoing vasodilatation mediated by the local products of inflammation causes the decrease in RI **(Figs. 5A to C)**, while the subsequent edema of the ovarian parenchyma causes the increase in the RI

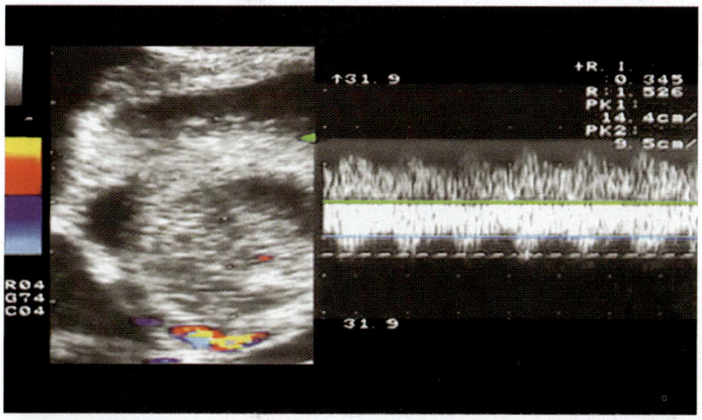

Fig. 5A: Transvaginal color Doppler scan of acute pelvic inflammatory disease. Note hyperechogenic tubal walls and low impedance blood flow signals (RI = 0.35) obtained from tiny tubal arteries.

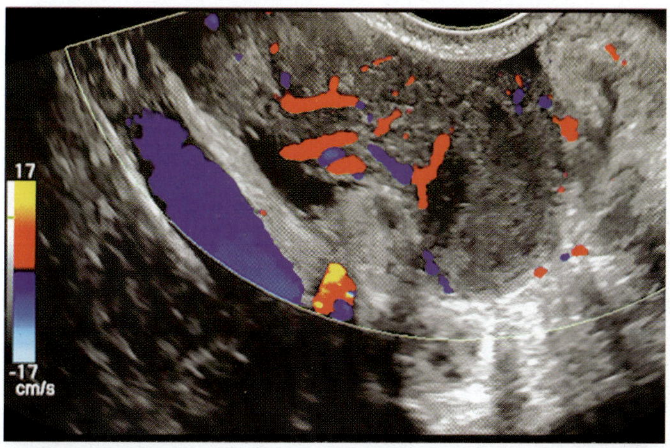

Fig. 5B: Color Doppler ultrasound of a patient with acute PID. Note complex adnexal mass (usually multilocular cystic structure with echogenic fluid and thick septations), and free fluid in the cul-de-sac. Dilated vessels indicate increased angiogenesis.

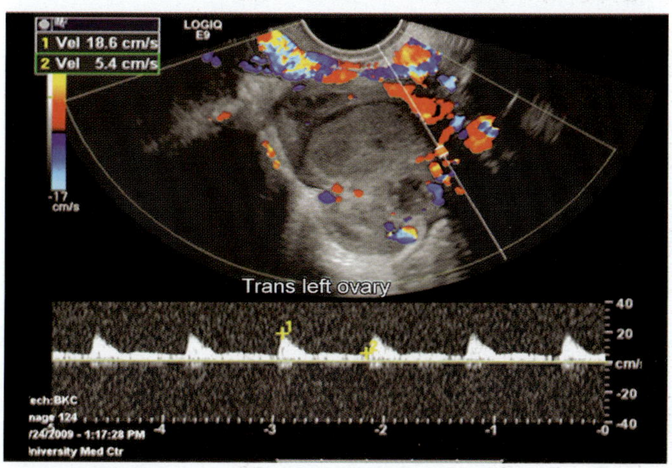

Fig. 5C: The same patient as in previous figure. Pulsed Doppler waveform analysis demonstrates moderate to high vascular impedance blood flow signals.

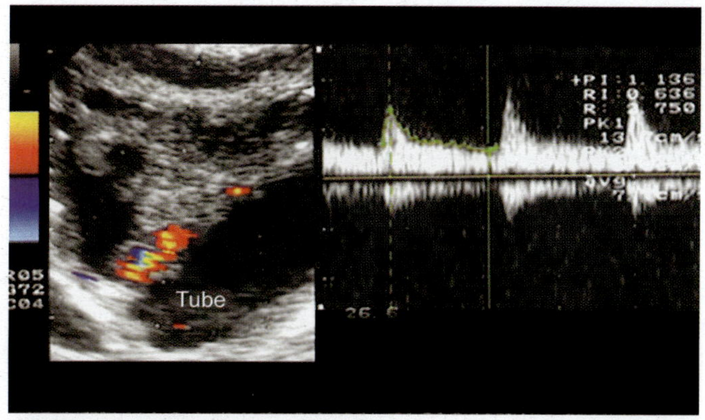

Fig. 6A: Complex adnexal mass containing fluid filled distended tube and pseudopapillomatous vascularized structure protruding into the tubal lumen. Moderate-to-high resistance blood flow signals (RI = 0.64) are obtained from a pseudopapillomatous lesion. This finding suggests subacute PID. Elevation of the vascular impedance is secondary to edema of the ovarian parenchyma.

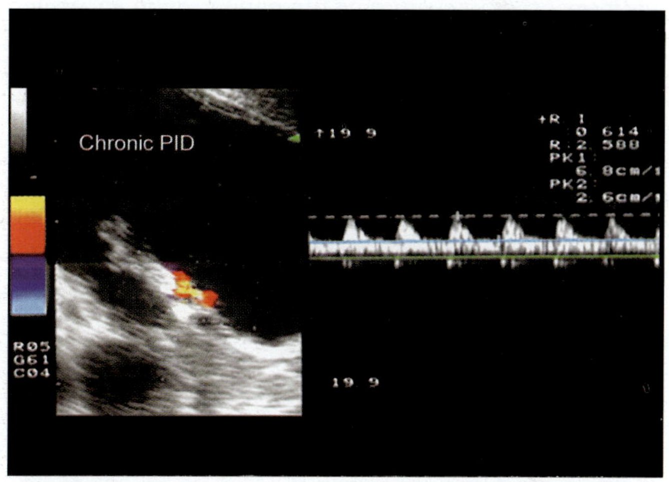

Fig. 6B: Another case of chronic PID. Moderate to high vascular impedance signals (RI 0.61) are clearly displayed from the pseudopapillomatous protrusion.

(Figs. 6A and B). As the ovarian capsule may vary in its rigidity, the intraovarian pressure differs from case to case. It affects the intensity of the intraovarian blood flow, which is reflected by variable values of RI. Furthermore, fluid collection within the tubes may influence the blood flow characteristics by compressing the vessels' wall. As the process advances, the proliferation of the fibroblasts and scarring tissue formation leads toward reduction of the local blood flow, which is demonstrated by the progressive increase in RI **(Fig. 7)**. Very similar results were obtained by other authors, but on small series of patients.[5,15] Clearly,

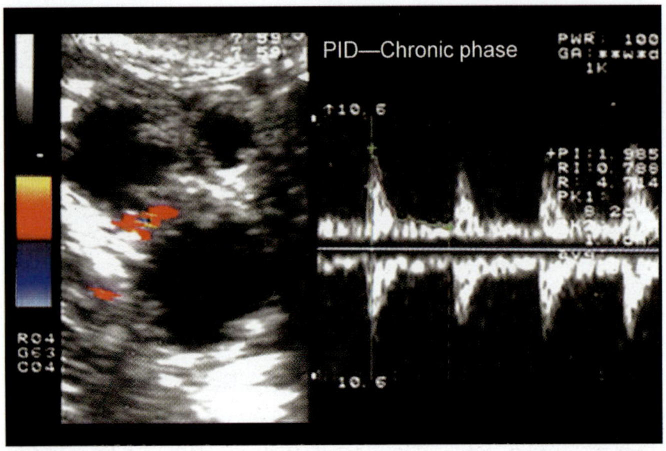

Fig. 7: "Cogwheel" sign produced by hyperechogenic knots and pseudopapillomatous structures is typical of chronic phase of PID. Color Doppler helps to differentiate suspicious morphology.

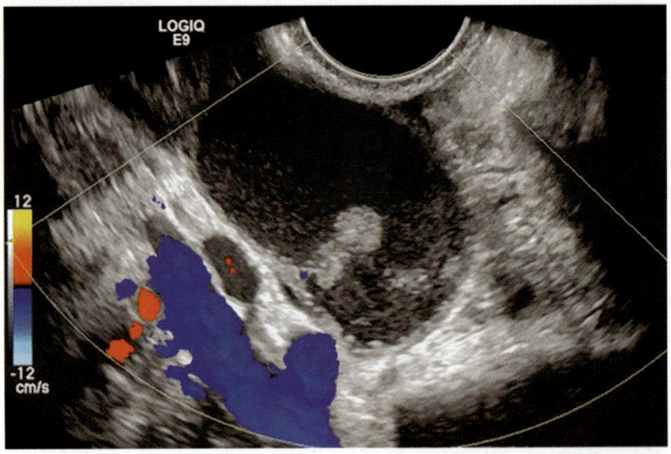

Fig. 8A: Complex adnexal mass in a patient with chronic pelvic inflammatory disease. Hypovascularized papillary protrusion represents tubal mucosal fold.

transvaginal color Doppler imaging can be used as an additional tool in evaluating the patients with suspected PID. Furthermore, we noticed that flow indices returned to normal values after the treatment in 36 (48.65%) patients.

The same method was useful in differentiating pyosalpinx from hematosalpinx in ectopic pregnancy cases. Ectopic pregnancies are characterized with high velocity and low impedance (RI <0.42) blood flow signals which indicate peritrophoblastic flow.[10,16]

As the inflammation may mimic a wide variety of findings, and sometimes even suggest malignancy, serial assessment by color Doppler ultrasound is recommended, always with respect to the patient's age and the phase of the menstrual cycle. Serial examination may demonstrate morphological changes as well as variations in blood flow intensity according to the stage of the disease. Doppler studies are particularly useful in the chronic stage of PID, when pseudopapillomatous structures protruding into the cystic counterpart may morphologically suggest malignancy **(Figs. 8A and B)**. Absence of blood flow, typical for this stage, helps differentiating it from adnexal malignancy. In the acute stage, low resistance to blood flow, suggestive of malignancy may be demonstrated. In those patients, it is useful to do some additional tests (e.g. erythrocyte sedimentation rate, total and differential cells counts, CA-125) that may help in reaching the final diagnosis. Serial ultrasound examination in these cases, reveals the changes that correlate with the pathophysiological stage of the process **(Figs. 9A and B)**. However, there is no single parameter that is sufficiently reliable for the adnexal mass characterization.[17]

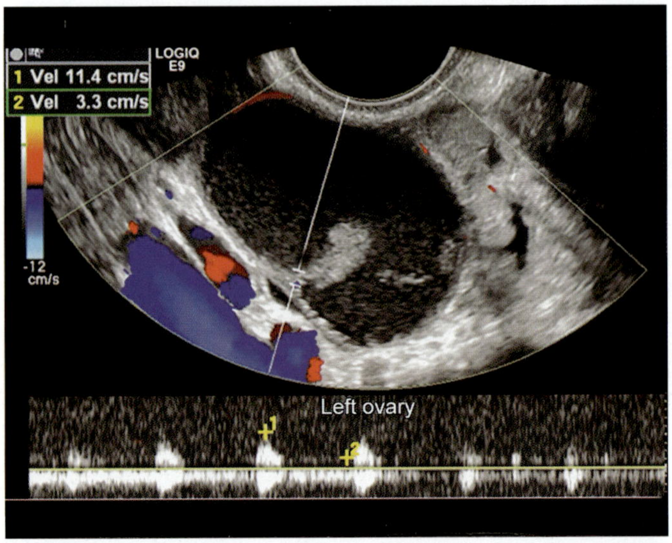

Fig. 8B: The same patient as in previous figure. Moderate to high vascular impedance blood flow signals are obtained from the base of the papillary like structure. Laparoscopy confirmed hydrosalpinx (tubal cause of infertility).

In patients with tubo-ovarian abscess, abscess drainage under transvaginal sonographic guidance can hasten the recovery process and improve the efficacy of the antibiotic therapy.[18] Addition of the color Doppler facilities enables visualization of the large pelvic vessels and thereby may reduce the complication rate of the interventional procedure **(Figs. 10A to C)**. However, a careful clinical examination, transvaginal ultrasound evaluation and blood tests are required before performing the procedure to avoid infection propagation.

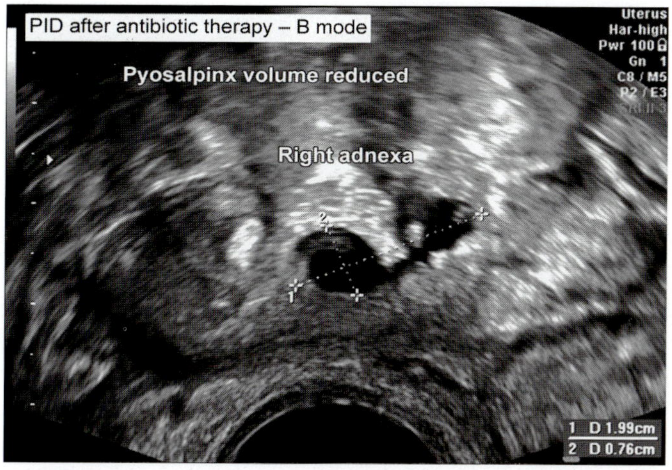

Fig. 9A: Transvaginal ultrasound demonstrates significant reduction of the adnexal mass following the antibiotic therapy.

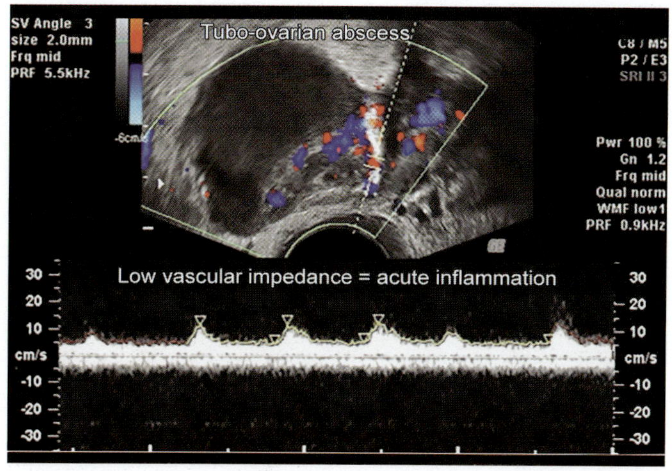

Fig. 10A: Transvaginal color Doppler scan of a tubo-ovarian abscess. Note prominent vascularization and low impedance blood flow signals obtained from the tubal walls and incomplete septations.

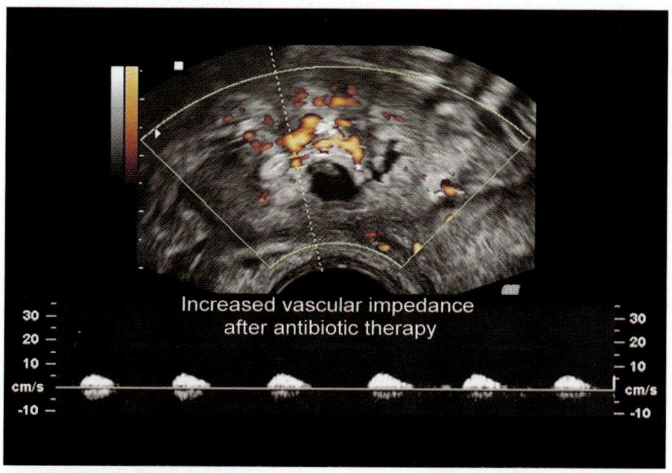

Fig. 9B: Simultaneously with morphologic changes there was an increased RI of the tubal arteries after introduction of the antibiotic therapy.

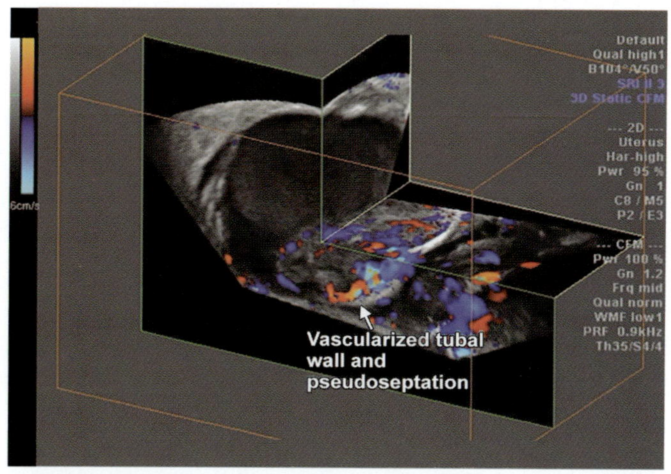

Fig. 10B: The same patient as in previous Figure. Niche mode enables better visualization of the vascularized tubal wall and pseudoseptation.

Three-dimensional Ultrasound

Three-dimensional ultrasound helps in spatial delineation of the inflammatory conglomerates. Any scanned volume can be rotated in all dimensions and thus it is possible to observe borders of tissues and organs **(Figs. 11A and B)**. By conventional B-mode ultrasound hydrosalpinx can be mistaken for a multilocular cyst, but when 3D is applied the true, spatial position and shape of hydrosalpinx is clearly visible **(Figs. 12A and B)**. By using three-dimensional volume sections it is possible to visualize the tortuous structure and contiguous spread of hydrosalpinx. 3D ultrasound enables accurate visualization of three perpendicular planes simultaneously and by moving the cursor, sonographer "sees through" the slices of the hydrosalpinx **(Figs. 13A and B)**. Another useful mode in this clinical situation is the so-called "niche" mode that enables the "cut-into" view of a certain tissue **(Figs. 1F and 10B)**. With the use of this mode, we can show the spatial spreading of hydrosalpinx, and at the same time, visualize its lumen. Furthermore, pseudopapillomatous structures within the tubal lumen can be better assessed. The surface of such papillary protrusions can be thoroughly scanned by surface mode, and its subtype "X-ray mode". When applying this mode, the spaces that appeared anechoic

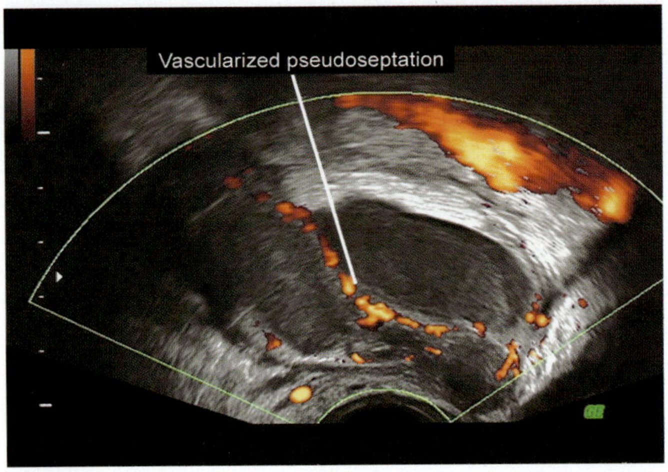

Fig. 10C: Transvaginal power Doppler scan demonstrates tubal and ovarian angiogenesis. Simultaneous visualization of the neighboring pelvic vessels may reduce the complication rate of the ultrasound guided interventional procedure.

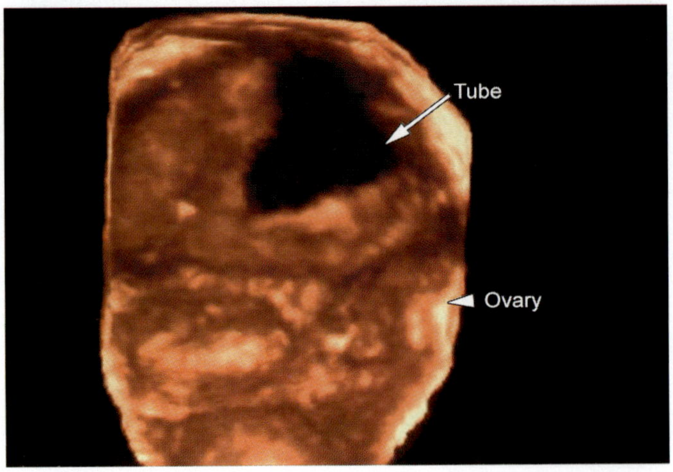

Fig. 12A: Three-dimensional ultrasound of a fluid-filled fallopian tube and ovary in a patient with secondary infertility due to pelvic inflammatory disease.

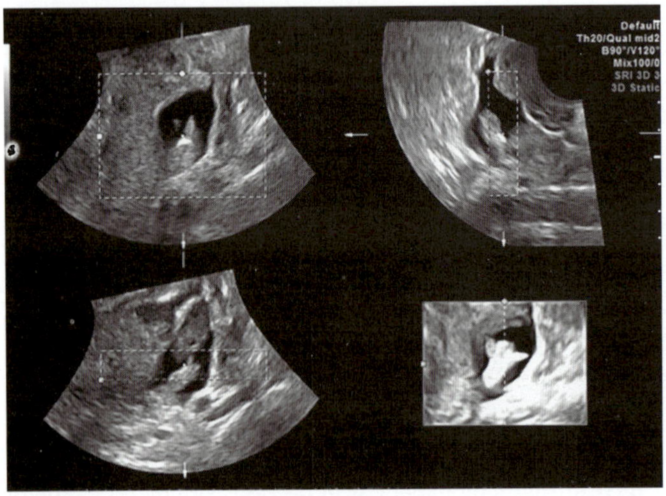

Fig. 11A: Multiplanar imaging of a thick and echogenic fallopian tube in a patient presenting with fever, elevated erythrocyte sedimentation rate and adnexal tenderness. Clinical and sonographic findings are typical for acute salpingitis.

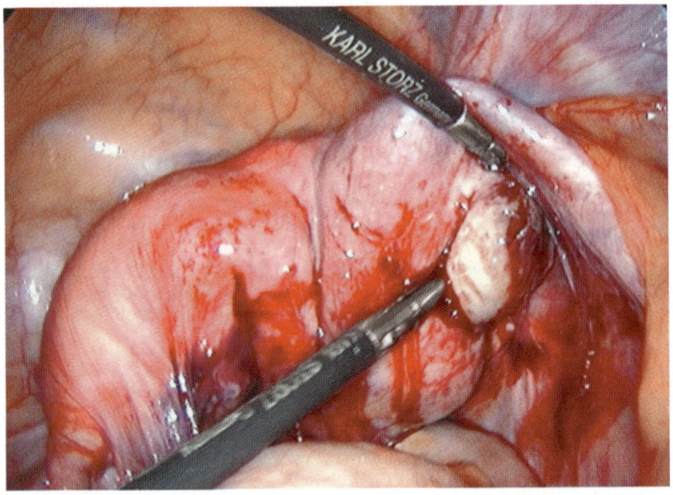

Fig. 12B: Laparoscopic image of the same patient.

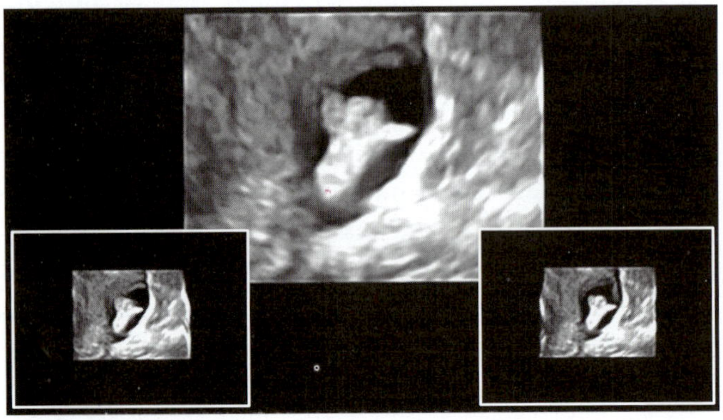

Fig. 11B: 3D surface rendering of the same fallopian tube.

on the conventional ultrasound scan are even darker, while the echoic tissues are shown lighter allowing better sharpness and contrast of the entire image.

Various inflammatory conglomerates sometimes pose a problem to the ultrasonographer. They may form a part of tubo-ovarian abscess or stay encapsulated by two sheets of peritoneum in the retrouterine space. Because of echogenicity and low vascular resistance, such structures may be mistaken for malignant tumors. Various forms of 3D ultrasound can define more clearly the spatial relations of such a structure and its connection or distinction from the surrounding structures **(Figs. 14A to C and 15A)**.

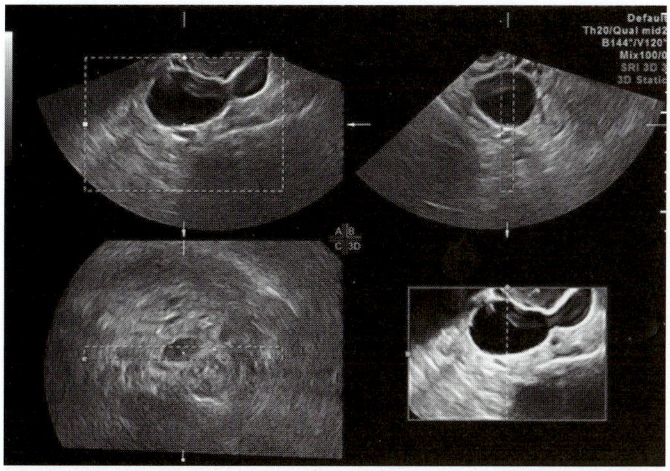

Fig. 13A: Multiplanar imaging of a thick walled elongated tubular fluid-filled structure, distinct from the uterus and ovary.

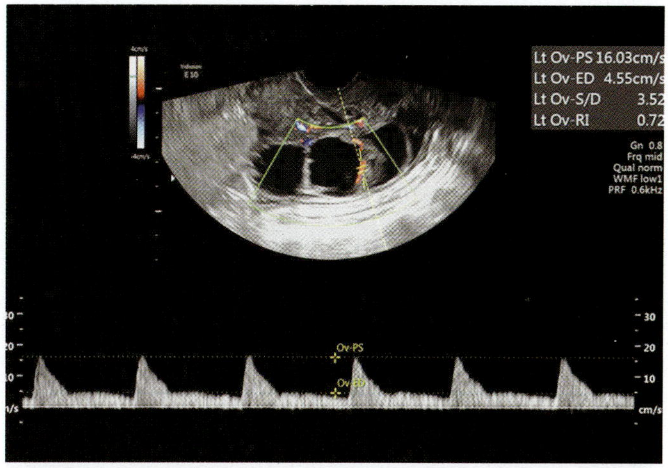

Fig. 14B: Color Doppler ultrasound of the same patient. Pulsed Doppler waveform analysis depicted moderate to high vascular impedance blood flow signals (RI 0.72) within pseudoseptations.

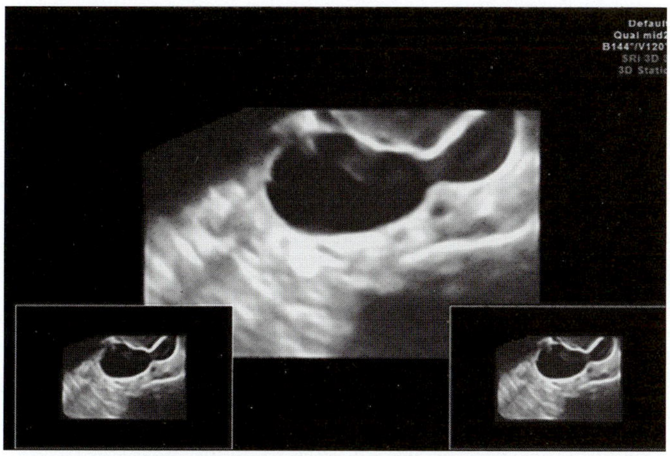

Fig. 13B: 3D surface rendering of hydrosalpinx.

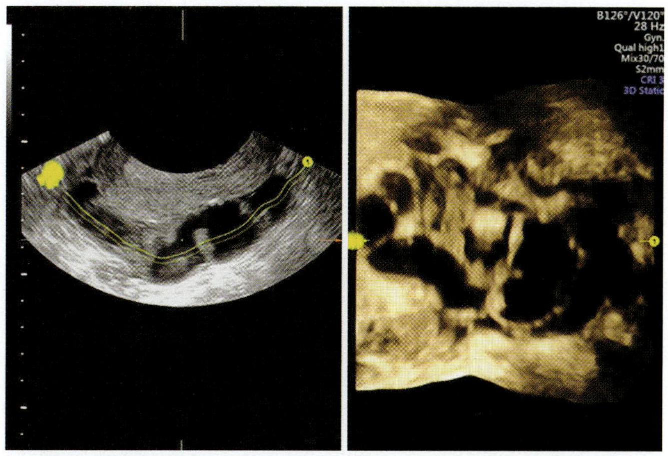

Fig. 14C: 3D ultrasound of the same lesion.

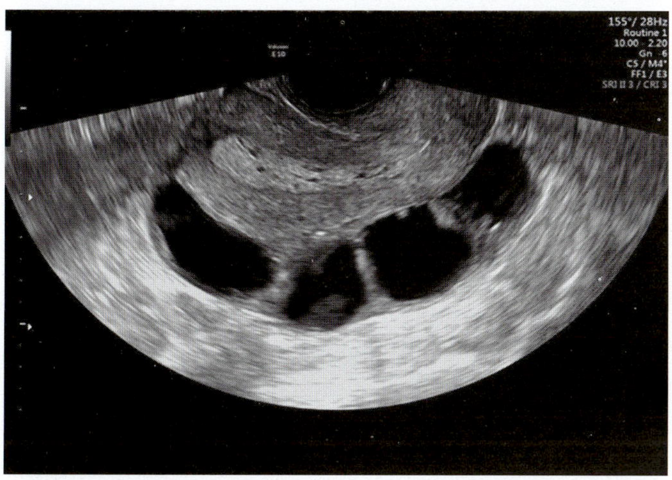

Fig. 14A: B-mode image of hydrosalpinx obtained by 2D ultrasound imitating a multilocular cyst.

The vascularity of the fallopian tube can be assessed using superimposed color and/or power Doppler **(Figs. 15B and C)**. By the use of this modality, it is possible to visualize vascular pattern and to study the branching and shape of the vascular structures. The interesting future possibility for the use of 3D power Doppler in the field of PID stems from work on 3D color Doppler histograms and vascularity index (VI) measurements counting on the number of color voxels in the cube of the tissue, which represent the evolved vessels. Flow index (FI), a mean color value of all blood flow or induced flow intensities, represents the intensity of flow at the time of the three-dimensional sweep. With these indices it would be easier to quantify the flow and conclude on the phase of the inflammatory process. The changes caused by vasodilatation or those caused by scar tissue formation

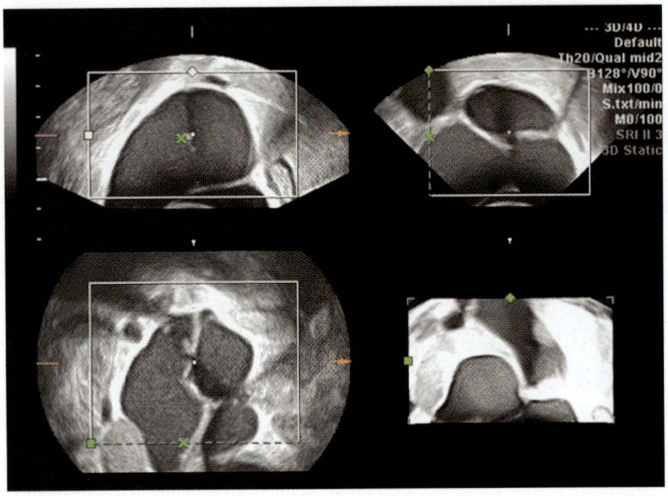

Fig. 15A: Three-dimensional ultrasound of a pelvic inflammatory conglomerate. By conventional B-mode ultrasound hydrosalpinx can be mistaken for a multilocular cyst, but when 3D is applied the true, spatial position and shape of hydrosalpinx is clearly visible.

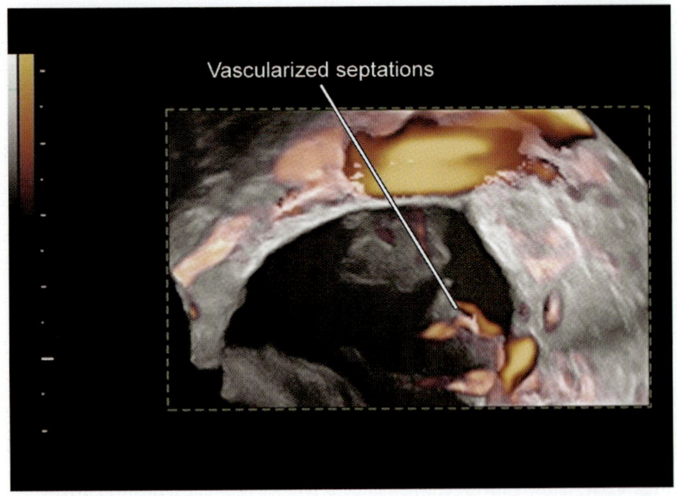

Fig. 15C: The same patient as in Figures 11A and B. Three-dimensional power Doppler ultrasound demonstrates intense vascularization within the tubal pseudoseptation.

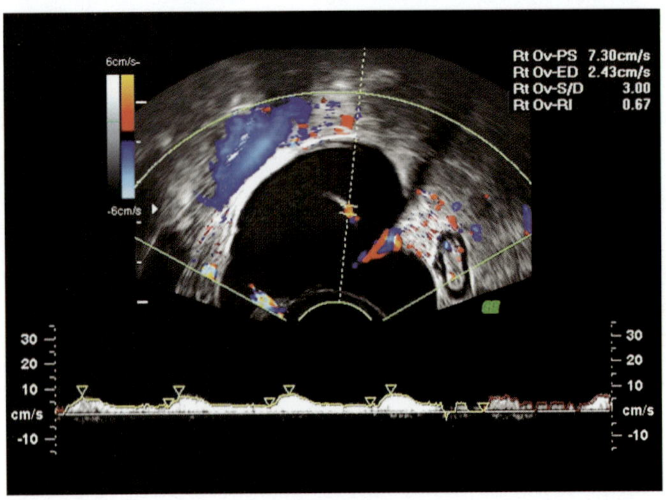

Fig. 15B: Transvaginal color Doppler ultrasound of the same patient as in previous figure. Moderate vascular impedance blood flow signals (RI = 0.67) are isolated from the incomplete tubal septation.

could be better understood following the assessment with 2D and 3D color/power Doppler ultrasound.

Senoh et al.[19] reported on a laparoscopy-assisted intrapelvic sonography with a high-frequency, real-time miniature transducer in the assessment of the fallopian tubes. They developed a special 20 MHz flexible catheter-based high-resolution, real-time miniature (2.4 mm outer diameter) ultrasound transducer and tested it in the population of infertile patients. A total of 21 women (20 infertile, one with unilateral hydrosalpinx, and one tubal pregnancy) were studied with pelvic saline effusion under laparoscopy. The presented technique seems to be useful in the assessment of tubal texture and functional evaluation in tubal disorders, possibly in infertility practice.

BENIGN TUMORS OF THE FALLOPIAN TUBE

Although the muscles of the fallopian tube and the uterus are of the same embryological origin (Müllerian ducts), leiomyoma of the fallopian tube are exceptionally rare. Leiomyomas of the fallopian tube are commonly incidental findings, as they are asymptomatic and small. However, there are reported cases of large tubal myomas associated with acute abdomen consequent to its torsion.[20]

Tubal pregnancy associated with tubal leiomyomas, in which the tubal myoma was the obstructing factor have also been reported.[1,20,21] Kobayashi et al.[22] reported on a case of a 28-year-old woman presented with secondary infertility in which pelvic ultrasound showed a multicystic septated mass extending to the umbilicus. At laparotomy, a 25 × 14 × 4 cm mass originating from the left fallopian tube and the tube was excised. Pathologic examination confirmed an angiomyofibroblastoma of the fallopian tube. Although, angiomyofibroblastoma is a rare tumor that occurs most commonly in the vulva and vagina, this case shows that it can occur in the fallopian tube and should be differentiated form more aggressive angiomyxoma.

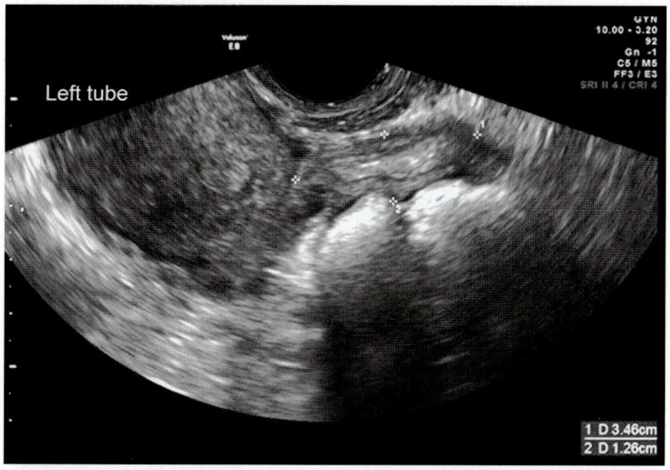

Fig. 16A: B-mode ultrasound of a left fallopian tube in a 48-year-old female. Echogenic lesion is clearly visualized within the tubal lumen.

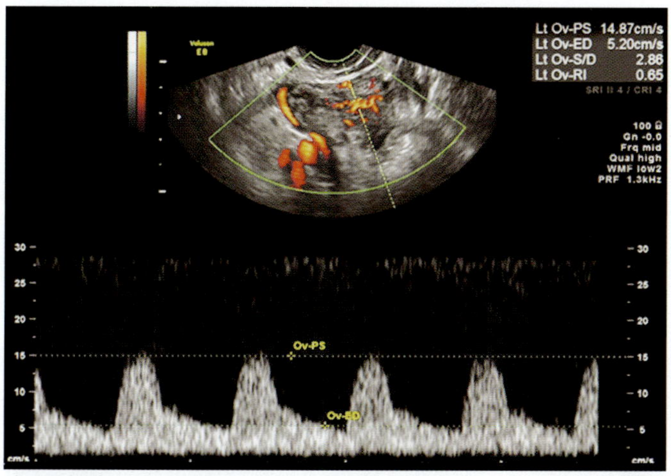

Fig. 16B: Color Doppler revealed moderate to high vascular impedance. Laparoscopy showed dilatation of the left tube with friable white tissue within its lumen. Microscopy revealed fallopian tube papilloma.

Conventional B-mode sonography reveals little of the nature of a benign tubal tumor. A smaller papilla can resemble a chronic PID remnant while a bigger mass in the oviduct can be mistaken for an inflammatory conglomerate **(Fig. 16A)**. Because of its limited imaging possibilities, 2D ultrasound cannot always define the borders of the lesion and delineate it from the surrounding tissue.

Color Doppler can be used for the assessment of vascularity **(Fig. 16B)**. As any other benign tissues, the oviduct papilloma would have a moderate-to-high resistance index. When benign lesions undergo necrosis of inflammation, they can present a true complication in the diagnostic process, caused by a significant reduction of the vascular indices.

3D ultrasound can help in diagnosis of benign ovarian lesions by its possibility to precisely delineate and spatially define a certain tumor. With the use of 3D power Doppler it is possible to visualize regular branching of benign intratubal structures, and distinguish them from uterine and ovarian vascular network.

MALIGNANT TUMORS OF THE FALLOPIAN TUBE

Although rare, tubal malignancy must be considered in the differential diagnosis of an adnexal mass. Of all gynecological cancers, malignancy of the fallopian tube is the most rare. The triad of pain, bleeding and leukorrhea is considered pathognomonic of tubal carcinoma. Sedlis[23] defined parameters for better differentiation between ovarian and tubal malignancies. He postulated that the tumor is of fallopian origin if:

- It derives from the fallopian tube
- Has the same histological structure as fallopian tube mucosa
- There is a clear transition zone between benign and malignant epithelium
- There is no endometrial or ovarian carcinoma.

Ultrasound Findings

The sonographic findings in all reported cases of fallopian tube carcinoma were complex, predominantly cystic adnexal masses and/or sausage-shaped structures apparently separated from the uterus.[24-37]

Table 1 reviews data from the literature on B-mode diagnosis of primary fallopian tube carcinoma.

In a remarkable review of 376 cases of tubal carcinoma, Mc Goldrick et al. found only one diagnosed preoperatively.[38] More recently, Eddy et al. analyzed the data of 74 patients regarding tubal malignancies and only two cases of tubal carcinoma were correctly diagnosed before surgery.[39]

Ayah et al. reported a study of eight cases of primary fallopian tube carcinoma.[24] Dava et al. described six adenocarcinomas of the fallopian tube that resembled the female adnexal tumor of probable Wolffian origin.[25] Microscopically, the tumors were characterized by a predominant pattern of small, closely packed cells punctured by numerous glandular spaces, which were typically small but occasionally were cystically dilated.

TABLE 1: Review of literature on B-mode diagnosis of primary fallopian tube carcinoma.

Reference	*Number of cases*	*Histopathology*
Subramayon et al.[30]	3	Papillary cystadenocarcinoma
Meyer et al.[31]	1	Adenocarcinoma
Kol et al.[47]	1	Adenocarcinoma
Ajjimakorn et al.[32]	4	Papillary cystadenocarcinoma
Granberg and Jansson[33]	1	Adenocarcinoma
Chang et al.[28]	1	Mixed Mullerian tumor
Chiou et al.[27]	1	Mixed Mullerian tumor
Slanetz et al.[34]	9	Adenocarcinoma and mixed Mullerian tumor
Ong[35]	1	Adenocarcinoma

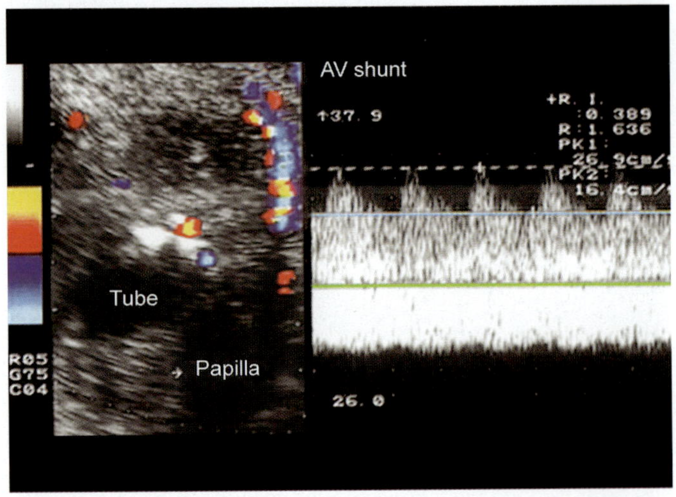

Fig. 17A: Fallopian tube carcinoma as seen by color Doppler ultrasound. Note vascularized papillomatous projection protruding into the distended tube in a postmenopausal patient. Low vascular resistance (RI = 0.38) and arteriovenous shunt indicate tubal malignancy, which was confirmed by histopathology.

Soundara et al. published a review of fallopian tube carcinoma over 20 years.[26] Nine cases of tubal carcinoma were found among approximately 9,000 gynecological malignancies.

Based on the data from the literature[26,38,39] more than 80% of patients have had pelvic mass detected before surgery. However, cervical cytology, X-ray of the pelvis, computed tomography or hysterosalpingography are usually no more specific than the pelvic examination. Conventional transvaginal sonography is one of the most important tools in preoperative diagnosis, but the efficacy of morphologic scoring systems alone is hampered by the degree of overlap between benign and malignant appearing adnexal masses.[35,41,42]

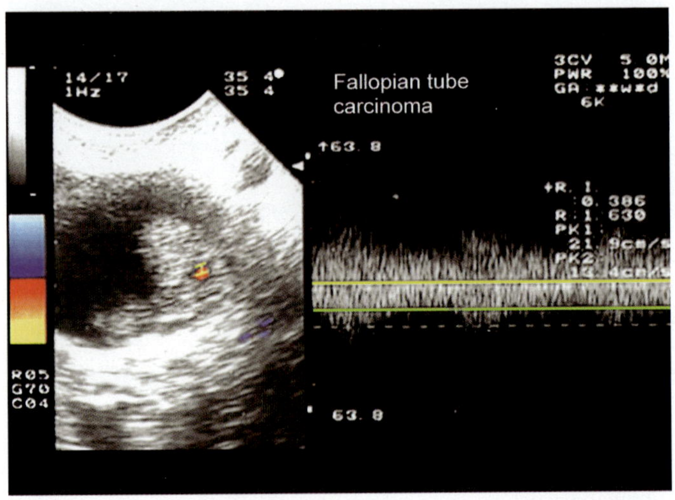

Fig. 17B: The same patient as in previous figure. Cross section through the fallopian tube reveals vascularized carcinoma.

Color Doppler Findings

Kurjak et al. was first to publish a case of primary adenocarcinoma of the fallopian tube (stage I FIGO) preoperatively diagnosed by color and pulsed Doppler ultrasound.[43] Podobnik et al. published the case of a 69-year- old women with a history of right-sided lower abdominal pain accompanied by profuse watery vaginal discharge for the past 3 months.[44] Six years after the initial report Kurjak et al.[45] reported on the series of eight cases of preoperatively diagnosed fallopian tube malignancy. Probably the most illustrative case of successful preoperative diagnosis of the primary fallopian tube carcinoma in his series was a 45-year-old woman treated because of infertility problems. During the routine transvaginal ultrasound examination a pendular myoma and a complex bilateral adnexal mass were discovered. In the left adnexal region a sausage-shaped cystic structure 3.4 × 4.8 × 3.4 cm in size was present. In the upper part of the cyst, a solid papillary protrusion less than 1 cm, richly perfused with the lowest resistance index of 0.37 was detected **(Figs. 17A and B)**. In the right adnexal region, a hydrosalpinx 3.0 × 1.6 cm was delineated from the ovary. Moderate vascular resistance (RI = 0.55) was obtained from the fallopian tube with chronic

TABLE 2: Review of literature on transvaginal color Doppler diagnosis of primary fallopian tube carcinoma.

Reference	*Number of cases*	*RI*	*Histopathology*
Shalan et al.[43]	1	0.35	Adenocarcinoma
Kurjak et al.[45]	8	0.29–0.40	Adenocarcinoma and papillary cystadenocarcinoma
Podobnik et al.[44]	1	0.34	Clear-cell carcinoma

inflammatory changes. According to the visualization of the area of neovascularization and low vascular impedance the authors suspected tubal carcinoma of the left side. Frozen section pathological examination reported papillary fallopian tube carcinoma. **Table 2** reviews data from the literature on color Doppler diagnosis of primary fallopian tube carcinoma.

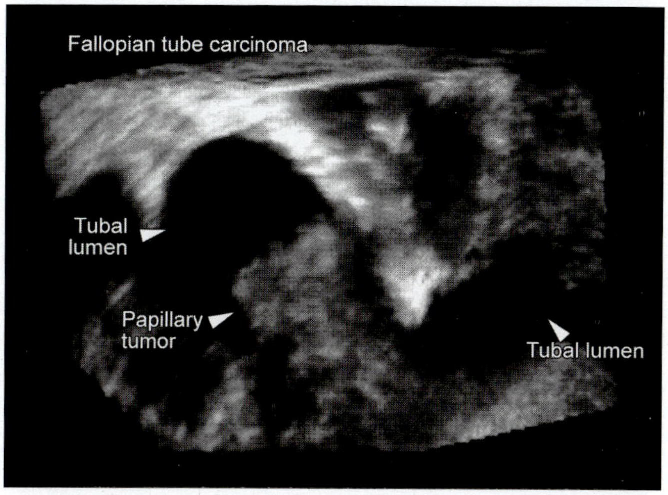

Fig. 18A: Three-dimensional ultrasound image of primary fallopian tube carcinoma. Papillary protrusions suggestive of fallopian tube malignancy are clearly seen within the distended tubal wall.

Three-dimensional Ultrasound

A new progress in diagnostic procedures was made when 3D and power Doppler ultrasound was introduced. Transvaginal 3D ultrasound enables the clinician to perceive the true, spatial relations and thus easily distinguish the origin of an adnexal mass, while 3D power Doppler allows detailed analysis of the neovascularization. Kurjak et al.[46] were the first to report on preoperative diagnosis of the primary fallopian tube carcinoma by 3D power Doppler ultrasound. Three-dimensional ultrasound was used to evaluate 520 adnexal masses prior to elective surgery during a 2-years' period. These lesions were originally detected with conventional transvaginal sonography and/or transvaginal color Doppler. Patients with suspicious morphology and/or Doppler findings underwent a second assessment at the referral center by the investigator performing 3D ultrasound that was unaware of the previous ultrasound examinations. Three-dimensional transvaginal ultrasound was performed using either 5 or 7.5 MHz transvaginal transducers (Voluson 530, Kretztechnik, Austria). Once the region of interest was identified, a volume box was superimposed to scan the image. The patient was asked to lie still on the examination bed, while the ultrasound probe was kept steady in the vagina. Depending on the size of the volume box the scanning procedure lasted between 5 and 13 seconds. The ability to store 3D ultrasound data on a hard disk drive allowed the investigator to keep the examination time short (between 2 and 4 minutes). Detailed analysis of the adnexal tumor was performed after the patient had gone, and lasted between 10 and 20 minutes. Rotation and translation of the stored volumes allowed evaluation of different tumor sections in many planes. The "niche mode" enabled meticulous study through selected sections of the adnexal tumor and was found especially useful in evaluation of the sausage-shaped complex masses. The "surface reconstruction" allowed plastic image of the inner and outer wall of the tumor **(Fig. 18A)**. Demonstration of the complex adnexal mass and/or sausage-shaped cystic lesions with papillary projections was the morphological criteria for detection of the tubal malignancy.

After B-mode analysis, power Doppler imaging was switched on together with the volume mode. In order to reduce the acquisition time, the volume of the color box and sweep angle were reduced. The color frame rate was adjusted as follows: both color density and color quality were as low as necessary to obtain a good color image, while pulse repetition frequency was as high as possible in order to enable the display of targeted flow velocity. The spatial peak temporal average (SPTA) intensity was approximately 80 mW/cm^2. Wall filters (50 Hz) were used to eliminate low-frequency signals. The patient examination time by 3D power Doppler was 3 minutes. Using the fast line density, the average acquisition time was 48 s (range 25–88 s). At the end of each examination combined color and gray rendering mode was used, allowing simultaneous analysis of the morphology, texture and vascularization. The subsequent analysis of the power Doppler reformatted

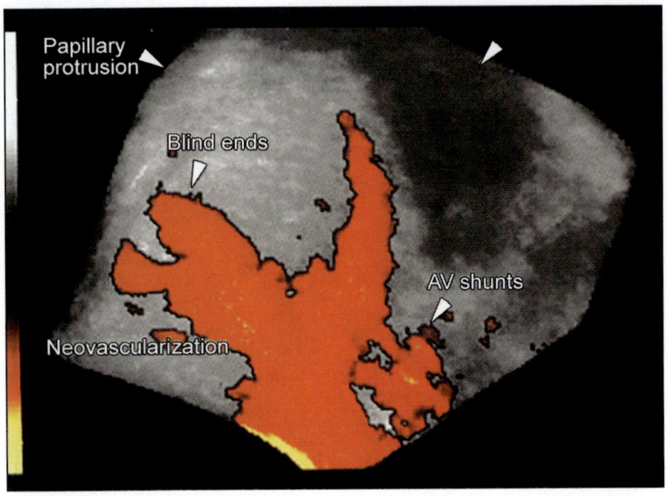

Fig. 18B: Three-dimensional power Doppler imaging enables evaluation of vascular geometry of the newly formed vessels in a case of fallopian tube carcinoma. Note irregular branching of the vessels, blind-ended lakes and disproportional calibration all indicative for tumoral neovascularization.

sections lasted between 5 and 10 minutes. Demonstration of the chaotic, randomly dispersed vessels with irregular branching within the papillary protrusions and/or solid parts was suggestive of tubal malignancy. Other structural abnormalities of the malignant tumor vessels were demonstration of the microaneurysms, arteriovenous shunts, tumoral lakes, disproportional calibration, coiling and dichotomous branching **(Fig. 18B)**. Using the above-mentioned criteria five cases of the fallopian tube carcinoma were successfully identified prior to surgery. They all presented non-pathognomonic appearance by B-mode ultrasound: the image was usually similar to that of pyosalpinx or a fluid-filled tube with a significant solid component adjacent to the tube. Three-dimensional transvaginal ultrasound allowed more precise distinction of the tubal mass from that of the ovary, cervix and uterus. Furthermore, the change in shape and size of the mass and passage of free fluid from tubal mass through the uterine cavity can be documented dynamically. The three perpendicular planes displayed simultaneously on the screen provided the opportunity to obtain multiple sections of the tortuous adnexal lesion by the capacity of rotation and translation in any planes. The ability to reconstruct 3D plastic images improved the recognition of the adnexal lesion anatomy, characterization of the surface features and determination of the extent of tumor infiltration through the capsule.

The "niche" aspect of 3D ultrasound revealed intratumoral structures in selected sections, which was mandatory for evaluation of the tubal pathology. Multiple sections of the tumor, rotation, translation and reconstruction allowed prediction of the tumor spread to the uterus and/or the ovary, or other surrounding structures. Shortened scanning time and detailed analysis of the stored data by trained and experienced ultrasonographer were additional advantages of 3D over 2D sonography.

Tubal malignancy displays angiogenesis that can be detected by color and pulsed Doppler. Reports from the literature demonstrate the potential of transvaginal color Doppler to depict tumor neovascularization and low resistance indices (below 0.42) typical of tubal malignancy.[46-48] Similar color Doppler results were obtained by Gojnic et al.[49] who reported on preoperative diagnosis of two fallopian tube carcinomas in a group of 78 postmenopausal women with adnexal masses. Resistance index ranged between 0.20 and 0.30, and CA 125 was not remarkably elevated.

Consistent sonographic and Doppler findings were reported in a multicenter study involving 13 ultrasound centers and 79 patients with a primary tubal cancer.[50] A well-vascularized ovoid or sausage-shaped structure, either completely solid or complex are the typical ultrasound features of fallopian tube carcinoma. Similarly, a well vascularized solid-cystic tumor, clearly separated from the normal size ovary was visualized in a 67-year-old patient presenting with postmenopausal bleeding with negative hysteroscopy.[51]

Malignant tumor vessels that are usually randomly dispersed within the central and peripheral parts demonstrate irregular course, complicated branching and disproportional calibration, features that can be recognized using 2D color Doppler ultrasound and 3D power Doppler technology. Improved detection and classification of tumor architecture might contribute to better preoperative diagnostics for fallopian tube carcinoma.

FALLOPIAN TUBE TORSION

Isolated fallopian tube torsion is a rare event characterized by the rotation of the fallopian tube on its own axis, without twisting the ipsilateral ovary.[52] Patients typically present with progressive worsening of abdominal and pelvic pain, nausea and vomiting. Recent studies pointed out that this finding was found in 75% of children and adolescent females who practiced sports involving sudden changes in body position.[52,53] Laparoscopy is the intervention of choice for definitive diagnosis and treatment of these cases.[54] Although salpingectomy is the most frequent treatment, detorsion without resection may be considered for selective cases.

CONCLUSION

Transvaginal ultrasound with color Doppler facilities is expedient not only for accurate assessment of the regional blood flow, but also for differentiating benign adnexal conditions from malignant. Based on color Doppler assessment one can distinguish acute pelvic inflammatory disease from the chronic one. The introduction of 3D ultrasound enables spatial delineation of examined structures giving the information whether the pathologic structure is of ovarian or tubal origin. It is expected that wide application of this novel technique will enable early detection of fallopian tube tumors, thus enabling early intervention and increased survival rates.

REFERENCES

1. Timor-Tritsch IE, Rottem S. Transvaginal ultrasonographic study of the Fallopian tube. Obstet Gynecol, 1987;70:424-8.
2. Timor-Tritsch IE, Bar-Yam Y, Elgali S and Rottem S. The technique of transvaginal sonography with use of a 6.5 MHz probe. Am J Obstet Gynecol. 1988;158:1019.
3. Timor-Tritsch IE, Rottem S, Lewit N. The Fallopian tubes. In: Timor-Tritsch IE, Rottem S (Eds). Transvaginal Sonography, 2nd edn, (New York: Elsevier); 1991. pp.131-44.
4. Westroem L, Wolner-Hanssen P. Pathogenesis of pelvic inflammatory disease. Genitourinary Medicine. 1993; 69:9-17.
5. Toth M, Chervenak FA. Color Doppler ultrasound in the diagnosis of pelvic inflammatory disease. In: Kurjak A (Ed). An Atlas of Transvaginal Color Doppler, Parthenon Publishing Group; 1994. pp.215-21.
6. Patten RM, Vincent LM, Wolner-Hanssen P, Thorpe EJr. Pelvic inflammatory disease: endovaginal sonography with laparoscopic correlation. J Ultrasound Med. 1990;9:681-9.
7. Kupesic S, Kurjak A, Pasalic L, Benic S, Ilijas M. The value of transvaginal color Doppler in the assessment of pelvic inflammatory disease. Ultrasound Med Biol. 1995;21(6)733-8.
8. Kurjak A, Zalud I, Jurkovic D, Alfirevic Z, Miljan M. Transvaginal color Doppler for the assessment of the pelvic circulation. Acta Obstet Gynecol Scand. 1989;68:131-4.
9. Collins W, Jurkovic D, Kurjak A, Campbell S. Ovarian morphology, endocrine function and intrafollicular blood flow during the periovulatory period. Hum Reprod. 1991;6: 319-29.
10. Kurjak A, Kupesic S, Schulman H, Zalud I. Transvaginal color Doppler in the assessment of the ovarian and uterine blood flow in infertile women. Fertil Steril. 1991;56:870-3.
11. Bourne T. Transvaginal colour Doppler in gynaecology. Ultrasound Obstet Gynecol. 1992;80:359-73.
12. Kurjak A, Zalud I, Alfirevic Z. Evaluation of adnexal masses with transvaginal color ultrasound. J Ultrasound Med. 1991;10:295-9.
13. Kurjak A, Zalud I, Schulman H. Ectopic pregnancy: Transvaginal color Doppler study of trophoblastic flow in questionable adnexa. J Ultrasound Med. 1991;10:685-9.
14. Kurjak A, Predanic M, Kupesic S, Jukic S. Transvaginal color Doppler for the assessment of adnexal tumor vascularity. Gynecol Oncol. 1993;50:3-9.
15. Tinkannen H, Kujansuu E. Doppler ultrasound findings in tubo-ovarian infectious complex. J Clin Ultrasound. 1993;21:175-8.
16. Jurkovic D, Bourne TH, Jauniaux E, Campbell JS, Collins WP. Transvaginal color Doppler study of blood flow in ectopic pregnancies. Fertil Steril. 1992;57:68-73.
17. Kurjak A, Predanic M. New scoring system for prediction of ovarian malignancy based on transvaginal color Doppler sonography. J Ultrasound Med. 1992;11:631-8.
18. Teisala K, Heinonen PK, Punnonen JR. Transvaginal ultrasound in the diagnosis and treatment of tubo-ovarian abscess. Br J Obstet Gynaecol. 1990;97:178-80.
19. Senoh D, Yanagihara T, Akiyama M, Ohnishi Y, Yamashiro C, Tanaka H, et al. Laparoscopy-assisted intrapelvic sonography with a high-frequency, real-time miniature transducer for assessment of the Fallopian tube: a preliminary report. Hum Reprod. 1999;14(3):704-6.
20. Woodruff JD, Pauerstein CJ. The Fallopian tube. Baltimore: Williams and Wilkins; 1969.
21. Mroueh J, Margono F, Feinkind L. Tubal pregnancy associated with ampullary tubal leiomyoma. Obstet Gynecol. 1993;81:880-2.
22. Kobayashi T, Suzuki K, Arai T, Sugimura H. Angiomyofibroblastoma arising from the Fallopian tube. Obstet Gynecol. 1999;94(5 Part 2 Suppl S):833-4.
23. Sedlis A. Carcinoma of the Fallopian tube. Surg Clinic N Am. 1978;58:121.
24. Ayhan A, Deren D, Yuce K, Tuncer Z and Mecan G. Primary carcinoma of the Fallopian tube: A study of 8 cases. Eur J Gynecol Oncol. 1994;15:147-51.
25. Dava D, Young RH, Scully RE. Endometrioid carcinoma of the Fallopian tube resembling and adnexal tumor of probable Wolffian origin: A report of six cases. Int J Gynecol Pathol. 1992;11:122-30.
26. Soundara RS, Ramdas CP, Reddi RP, Oumachigni A, Rajaram P, Reddy KS. A review of Fallopian tube carcinoma over 20 years (1971–1990) in Pondicherry. Indian J Cancer. 1991;28:188-95.

27. Chiou YK, Su IJ, Chen CA, Hsieh CY. Malignant mixed Muellerian tumor of the Fallopian tube. J Formos Med Associ. 1991;90(8):793-5.
28. Chang HC, Hsueh S, Soong YK. Malignant mixed Muellerian tumor of the Fallopian tube. Case report and review of literature. Chang Keng I Hsueh. 1991;14(4):259-63.
29. Tokunaga T, Miyazaki K, Okamura H. Pathology of the Fallopian tube. Curr Opin Obstet Gynecol. 1991;3(4): 574-9.
30. Subramayon BR, Raghavendra BN, Whalen CA, Ye J. Ultrasonic features of Fallopian tube carcinoma. J Ultrasound Med. 1984;391-3.
31. Meyer JS, Kim CS, Price HM, Cooke JK. Ultrasound presentation of primary carcinoma of the Fallopian tube. J Clin Ultrasound. 1987;15:132-4.
32. Ajjimakorn S, Bhamarapravati Y. Transvaginal ultrasound and the diagnosis of Fallopian tubal carcinoma. J Clin Ultrasound. 1991;19:116-9.
33. Granberg S, Jansson I. Early detection of primary carcinoma of the Fallopian tube by endovaginal ultrasound. Acta Obstet Gynecol Scand. 1990;69:667-8.
34. Slanetz PJ, Whitman GJ, Halpern EF, Hall DA, Mc Carthy KA, Simeone JF. Imaging of the Fallopian tube tumors. Am J Roentgenol. 1997;169:1321-4.
35. Ong CL. Fallopian tube carcinoma with multiple tumor nodules seen on transvaginal sonography. J Ultrasound Med. 1998;17:71-3.
36. Hinton A, Bea C, Winfield AC, Entman SS. Carcinoma of the Fallopian tube. Krol Radiol. 1988;10:113-5.
37. Ekici E, Vicdan K, Danisman N, Soysal ME, Cobanoglu O, Gokmen O. Ultrasonographic Appearance of Fallopian-Tube Carcinoma. International Journal of Gynecology & Obstetrics. 1992;49:325-9.
38. McGoldrick JL, Strauss H, Rao J. Primary carcinoma of the Fallopian tube. Am J Surg. 1943;59:559-63.
39. Eddy GL, Schlaerth JB, Nalick RH, Gadis OJ, Nakamuira RM, Morrow CP. Fallopian tube carcinoma. Obstet Gynecol. 1984;64:556-51.
40. Lerner JP, Timor-Tritsch IE, Federmann A, Abramovich G. Transvaginal ultrasonographic characterization of ovarian masses with an improved weighted scoring system. Am J Obstet Gynecol. 1994;170:81-5.
41. Bourne TH, Campbell S, Steer C, Whitehead MI, Collins WP. Transvaginal color flow imaging a possible new screening technique for ovarian cancer. Br Med J. 1994;299: 1367-71.
42. Kawai M, Kano T, Kikkawa F, Maeda O, Oguchi H, Tomoda Y. Transvaginal Doppler ultrasound with color flow imaging in the diagnosis of ovarian cancer. Obstet Gynecol. 1992;79:463-6.
43. Shalan H, Sosic A, Kurjak A. Fallopian tube carcinoma: recent diagnostic approach by color Doppler imaging. Ultrasound Obstet Gynecol. 1992;2:297-9.
44. Podobnik M, Singer Z, Ciglar S, Bulic M. Preoperative diagnosis of primary Fallopian tube carcinoma by transvaginal ultrasound, cytological finding and CA-125. Ultrasound Med Biol. 1993;19:587-91.
45. Kurjak A, Kupesic S, Ilijas M, Sparac V, Kosuta D. Preoperative diagnosis of primary Fallopian tube carcinoma. Gynecol Oncol. 1998;68:29-34.
46. Kurjak A, Kupesic S, Jacobs I. Preoperative diagnosis of the primary Fallopian tube carcinoma by three-dimensional static and power Doppler sonography. Ultrasound Obstet Gynecol. 1999. (submitted)
47. Kol S, Gal D, Friedman M, Paldi E. Preoperative diagnosis of primary Fallopian tube carcinoma by transvaginal sonography and CA 125. Gynecol Oncol. 1990;37:129-37.
48. Kurjak A, Kupesic S, Breyer B, Sparac V, Jukic S. The assessment of ovarian tumor angiogenesis: what does three-dimensional power Doppler add? Ultrasound Obstet Gynecol. 1998;12:136-46.
49. Gojnic M, Pervulov M, Petkovic S, Barisic G, Stojanovic I, Mostic T, et al. The significance of Doppler flow and anamnesis in the diagnosis of Fallopian tube cancer. Eur J Gynaecol Oncol. 2005;26:309-10.
50. Ludovisi M, De Blasis I, Virgilio B, et al. Imaging of gynecological disease (9): clinical and ultrasound characteristics of tubal cancer. Ultrasound Obstet Gynecol. 2014;43(3):328-35.
51. Arko D, Zegura B, Virag M, et al. Preoperative diagnosis of fallopian tube malignancy with transvaginal color Doppler ultrasonography and magnetic resonance imaging after negative hysteroscopy for postmenopausal bleeding. Coll Antropol. 2014;38(3):1047-50.
52. Romano M, Di Giuseppe J, Serri M, et al. A possible association between sports and isolated fallopian tube torsion in children and adolescent females. Gynecol Endocrinol. 2015;31(9):688-92.
53. Casey RK, Damle LF, Gomez Lobo V. Isolated fallopian tube torsion in pediatric and adolescent females: a retrospective review of 15 cases at single institution. J Pediatr Adolesc Gynecol. 2013;26(3):189-92.
54. Gaied F, Emil S, Lo A, et al. Laparoscopic treatment of isolated salpingeal torsion in children: case series and a 20-year review of the literature. J Laparoendosc Adv Surg Tech A. 2012;22(9):941-7.

58

CHAPTER

Sonographic Imaging in Infertility

Sanja Kupesic Plavsic, Sonal Panchal

INTRODUCTION

Infertility is defined as a failure to conceive a desired pregnancy after 12 months of unprotected intercourse, which affects 10% of married couples. With recent technological advances and the proper use of medically assisted reproduction techniques, one half of these couples will become pregnant.

More than any other new modality, ultrasound has made significant improvements in the modern management of the infertile female patient. Transvaginal sonography provides the reproductive endocrinologist with a tool that cannot only evaluate normal and stimulated cycles but also assists in follicle aspiration and subsequent transfer of the embryo. The addition of color Doppler capabilities to transvaginal probes permits visualization of small intraovarian and endometrial vessels, allowing depiction of normal and abnormal physiologic changes in the ovary and uterus. It may help to predict ovulation and detect certain ovulatory disorders such as the luteal phase defect (LPD). Doppler investigation of ovarian blood flow may improve the early diagnosis of ovarian hyperstimulation syndrome in patients with ovulation induction. Numerous studies conducted during the last two decades have confirmed the initial impressions about the usefulness of blood flow studies in infertile patients.

This chapter is a revision of the previous edition's chapter on "Sonographic Imaging in Infertility". It includes updated bibliography, and additional high resolution ultrasound images. The interested reader should be able to gain an objective point of view on the role of ultrasound in the assessment of ovarian, uterine and tubal causes of infertility, and the current and future role of color Doppler and three-dimensional ultrasound in the field of reproductive endocrinology.

UTERINE CAUSES OF INFERTILITY

The uterine cavity must provide an environment for successful sperm migration from the cervix to the fallopian tube. It is necessary for the uterus to have a normal mucous lining, glandular secretion and vascularity in order to support implantation and placentation. Uterine anomalies, polyps, leiomyomas, neoplasia, infections and intrauterine scar tissue can lead to poor reproductive performance. Attempts have been made to correlate the sonographic parameters (such as thickness and reflectivity) with the endometrial receptivity.

Uterine Perfusion in Infertile Patients

Transvaginal color and pulsed Doppler sonography has been established as an additional tool in the management of infertile patients. In a anovulatory cycles, a continuous increase of the uterine artery resistance index (RI) has been detected **(Fig. 1)**.[1,2] Moreover, in some infertile patients, an end-diastolic flow is absent.[3] The results of some research indicate that absent diastolic flow might be associated with infertility and poor reproductive performance. Therefore, the uterine artery blood flow can potentially be used to predict a hostile uterine environment prior to embryo transfer **(Fig. 2)**. Steer et al.[4] calculated the probability of pregnancy by using pulsatility index (PI) values obtained from the uterine artery on the day of embryo transfer. With the use of these measurements, the highest probability of becoming pregnant was obtained in those patients having medium values of PI for uterine arteries. A mean PI of more than 3.0 before the transfer can predict up to 35% of pregnancy failures. Tsai et al.[5] evaluated the prognostic value of uterine perfusion on the day of human chorionic gonadotropin (hCG) administration in patients who were undergoing intrauterine insemination. They calculated pulsatility index of the ascending branch

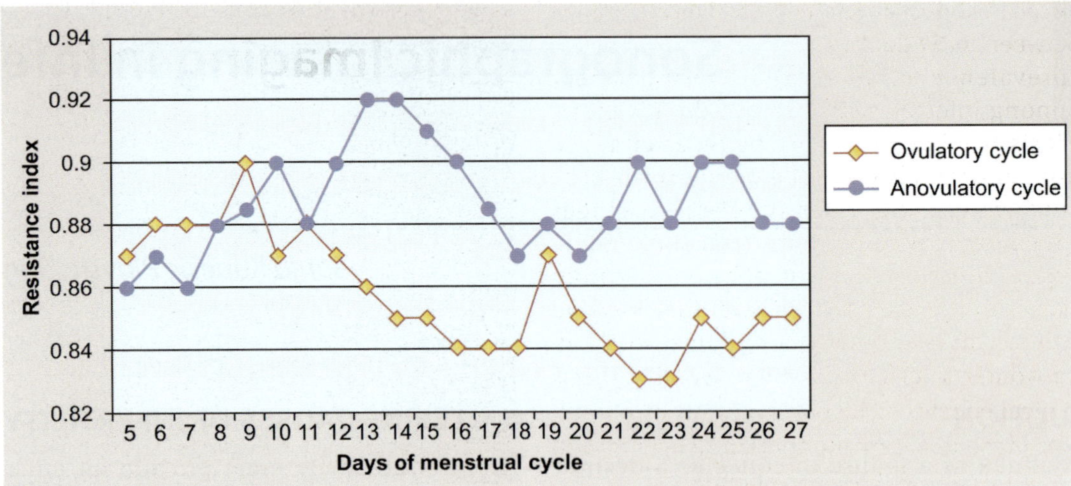

Fig. 1: Changes in the uterine artery blood flow in ovulatory and anovulatory cycles.

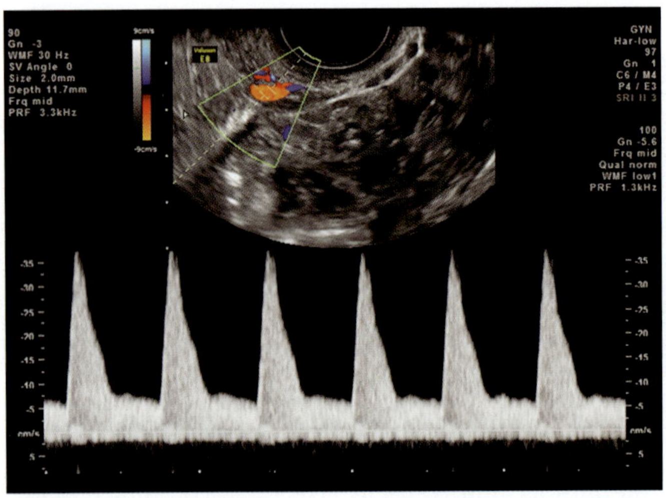

Fig. 2: Uterine artery demonstrated laterally to the cervix at the level of the cervicocorporeal junction. The blood flow velocity form the uterine artery in the secretory phase is characterized by increased end-diastolic velocity and decreased resistance index (RI = 0.76). This is a normal high resistance flow pattern during the non-pregnant state of the uterus.

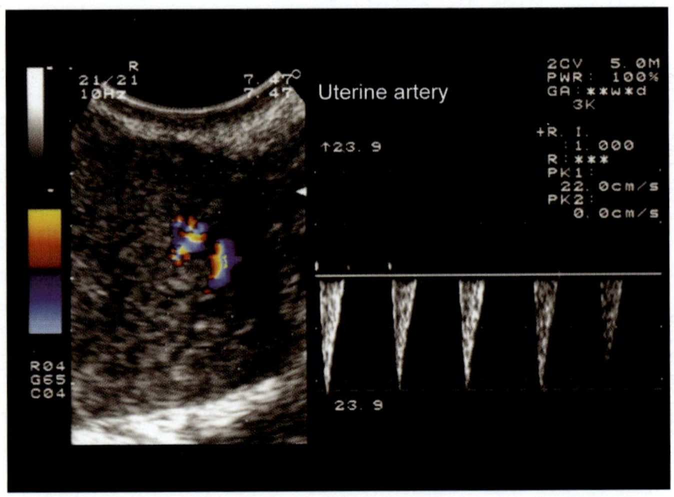

Fig. 3: Absent diastolic flow of the uterine artery may be associated with infertility or poor reproductive performance.

of the uterine arteries on the day of administration of hCG, and compared the uterine artery vascular resistance to the outcome of intrauterine insemination. Pregnancy did not occur when the pulsatility index of the ascending branch of the uterine arteries was more than 3 **(Fig. 3)**. The fecundity rate was 18% when the pulsatility index was less than 2 and 19.8% when the PI was between 2 and 3. Their data suggest that the measurement of uterine perfusion on the day of hCG administration may have a predictive value regarding fertility in patients undergoing intrauterine insemination.

In infertile women, the uterine artery pulsatility indices measured in the midluteal phase of an unstimulated cycles correlates inversely with the endometrial thickness[6] suggesting a direct effect of uterine perfusion on endometrial growth.[7] Furthermore, the pulsatility index correlates directly with the age of patients,[3] suggesting a detrimental effect of age on uterine perfusion. Cacciatore et al.[8] did not find any correlation between uterine artery pulsatility index measured at the time of embryo transfer (ET) and endometrial thickness or the age of the patients. These findings could be explained by the hormonal environment of the superovulated cycles, where the high

E_2 levels achieved in almost all subjects are likely to reduce differences between individuals.

A high prevalence of increased uterine artery impedance among infertile patients with the diagnosis of endometriosis has been reported by Steer et al.[6] In this study, women with a history of endometriosis have significantly higher pulsatility index and resistance index values than the others even after hormonal stimulation. This evidence, although gained in different settings, seem to suggest an adverse effect of endometriosis on uterine perfusion. This is another way endometriosis can compromise a woman's' fertility potential. Whether this is due to mechanical effects on the pelvic vessels as a result of adhesions or is mediated by production of agents with vasoactive properties remains to be explained.

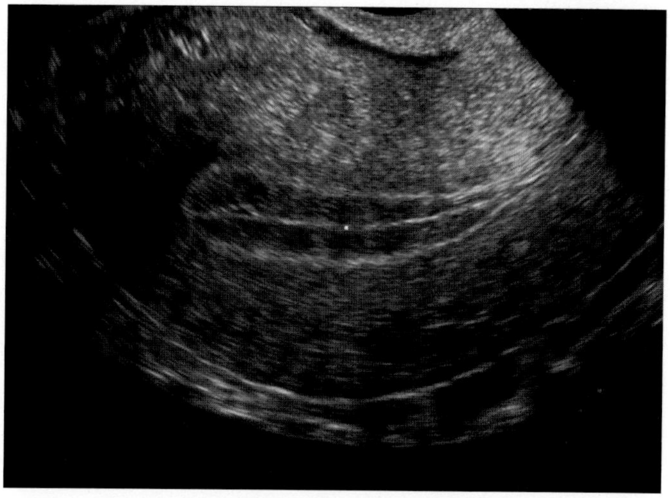

Fig. 4: Multilayered pattern of the endometrium assessed in a longitudinal ultrasound scan.

Endometrial Thickness, Volume and Vascularity

The question of a correlation between endometrial thickness and the likelihood of implantation, in the context of assisted reproduction, remains a contentious issue. However, a very thin endometrium (below 7 mm) seems to be an accepted reliable sign of suboptimal implantation potential.

Recently, Freidler et al.[9] reviewed 2,665 assisted reproduction cycles from 25 reports. Eight reports found that the difference in the mean endometrial thickness of conception and non-conception cycles was statistically significant, while 17 reports found no significant difference. They concluded that the results from the various trials are conflicting and that insufficient data exist describing a linear correlation between endometrial thickness and the probability of implantation. The main advantage of measuring endometrial thickness lies in its high negative predictive value in cases where there is minimal endometrial thickness. Gonen et al.[10] reported an absence of pregnancies in donor insemination cycles when the endometrial thickness did not reach at least 6 mm. Similarly, in a group of oocyte recipients, no pregnancies were reported in women who had an endometrial thickness of less than 5 mm, whereas several pregnancies occurred in patients with an endometrial thickness between >5 mm and 7.5 mm.[11] Finally, in IVF cycles, Khalifa et al. reported a minimal endometrial thickness of 7 mm to be compatible with pregnancy.[12]

Endometrial pattern is defined as the relative echogenicity of the endometrium and the adjacent myometrium as demonstrated on a longitudinal ultrasound scan **(Fig. 4)**.

In a prospective study, Serafini et al.[13] found the multilayered pattern to be more predictive of implantation than any other parameter measured. Sher et al.[14] correlated a non-multilayered echo pattern of the endometrium with advanced maternal age and the presence of uterine abnormalities. In the literature, of the 13 studies that examined the value of the endometrial pattern in predicting pregnancy, only four failed to confirm its predictive value. The endometrial pattern does not appear to be influenced by the type of ovarian stimulation and it is of prognostic value for both fresh IVF, as well as frozen embryo transfer cycles.

Zaidi et al.[15] reported that if subendometrial blood flow is detectable, the endometrial morphology may be less important than previously described and it may be that the absence of blood flow is more significant.

The authors evaluated 96 women undergoing in vitro fertilization (IVF) treatment on the day of human chorionic gonadotropin administration. They assessed endometrial thickness, endometrial morphology, presence or absence of subendometrial or intraendometrial color flow, intraendometrial vascular penetration and subendometrial blood flow velocimetry on the day of hCG administration and related the results to pregnancy rates **(Fig. 5)**. The overall pregnancy rate was 32.3% (31/96) and there was no significant difference between the pregnant and non-pregnant groups with regard to endometrial thickness, subendometrial peak systolic blood flow velocity (V_{max}) or subendometrial pulsatility index. The pregnancy rates based on endometrial morphology

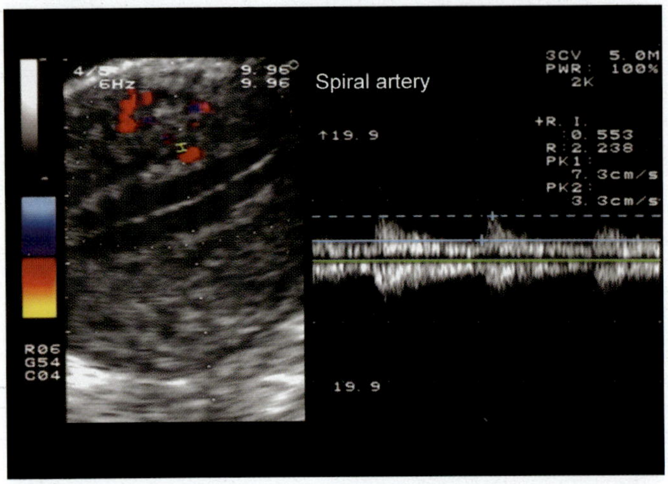

Fig. 5: Blood flow velocity waveforms of the spiral arteries during the periovulatory phase. Note the triple-line endometrium (left) and the moderate resistance index (RI = 0.55) (right) obtained from spiral arteries.

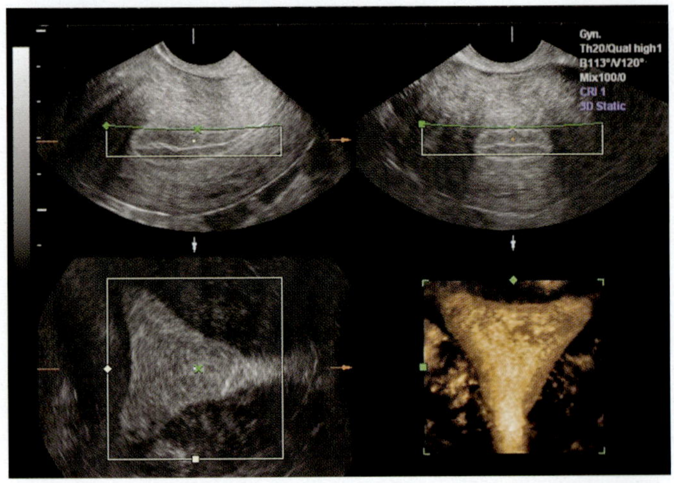

Fig. 6: Three-dimensional ultrasound of normal uterus. Triangular appearance of the endometrium is clearly visualized in coronal and surface rendering images.

were not significantly different, being 17.6% (3/17), 33.3% (2/6) and 35.6% (26/73) for types A (hyperechoic), B (isoechoic) and C (triple-line) endometria, respectively. In eight (8.3%) patients, subendometrial color flow and intraendometrial vascularization were not detected. This absence of blood flow was associated with failure of implantation (p <0.05). The pregnancy rates related to the zones of vascular penetration into the subendometrial and endometrial regions were: 26.7% (4/15) for Zone 1 (subendometrial zone), 36.4% (16/44) for Zone 2 (outer hyperechogenic zone) and 37.9% (11/29) for Zone 3 (inner hypoechogenic zone), and were not significantly different.

Endometrial thickness obtained by two-dimensional sonography is considered the most important parameter of endometrial growth. However, this parameter does not include the total volume of the endometrium. It is useful to have certain diagnostic parameters concerning the endometrium, one of which the endometrial volume measurement can be important **(Fig. 6)**. Furthermore, retarded endometrial development can be associated with primary infertility. In addition to endometrial volume and echogenicity sonographer can evaluate the shape and length of the cervix, as well as determine the presence of the cervical mucus **(Fig. 7)**. The ability to quantify the volume of the endometrium using 3D ultrasound may help to correlate cycle outcome with a quantitative parameter rather than endometrial thickness, which is prone to greater subjective variation in measurement.[16] By stepping through the volume in plane mode, the outer limits of endometrium are traced and in addition, volume calculations can be performed immediately. The accurateness of this method has already been described.[17,18] To obtain the best results, stepping through the volume should be performed in small units. In each new plane, the area tracing has to be corrected to its new extent. Low contrast in ultrasound data can increase the error of volume estimation. In general, the endometrium shows a good contrast to the surrounding myometrial tissue and therefore, in most cases volume estimation can be performed. Measurements can be best reproduced in longitudinal and transverse viewing planes. Other sources of measuring error may derive from the low contrast

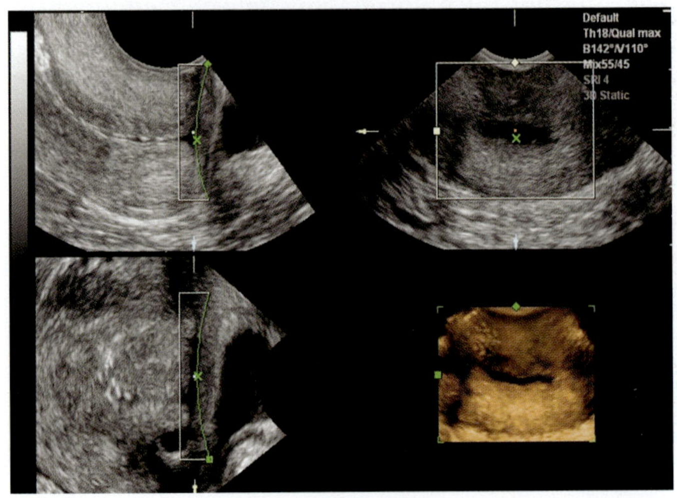

Fig. 7: The same modality can be used for visualization of the cervix and assessment of its mucus.

of the caudal end of the endometrium and the uterus. Endometrial fluid may also increase measuring error because the fluid volume may be too small to be measured accurately by three-dimensional ultrasound.

Lee et al.[19] were first to demonstrate volume estimation of the endometrium by three-dimensional ultrasound. Using the same method Kyei-Mensah et al.[20] assessed the reliability of 3D ultrasound in measuring endometrial volume on twenty patients undergoing ovarian stimulation. Endometrial volumes of these patients were obtained on the day of hCG administration. The intraobserver and inter-observer coefficient of variation was 8 and 11%, respectively. Repeatability within and between investigators was also expressed as the Intra CC and Inter CC. The coefficients describe the proportion of variation in a measurement, which is caused by true biological subject differences. For a single measurement of endometrial volume, the Intra CC was 0.90 and Inter CC was 0.82. These results clearly demonstrate that 3D ultrasound volume measurements are highly reliable, with a small measurement error. However, one could expect higher inter-observer differences in the ability to accurately locate the internal os and endometrial margins. This may explain the greater inter-observer variability for endometrial volume than for ovarian volume. Since, it is applied in the same manner as two-dimensional vaginal ultrasound it does not cause additional discomfort.

It is expected that three-dimensional endometrial volumetry studies will increase diagnostic potential and give additional information to two-dimensional ultrasound. Furthermore, quantification of endometrial volume by 3D ultrasound in combination with blood flow studies may be the best way to predict pregnancy rates.

Kupesic et al.[21] investigated the usefulness of transvaginal color Doppler and three-dimensional power Doppler ultrasonography for the assessment of endometrial receptivity in patients undergoing in vitro fertilization procedures **(Fig. 8)**. The patients were evaluated for endometrial thickness and volume, endometrial morphology and subendometrial perfusion on the day of embryo transfer. Neither the volume nor the thickness of the endometrium on the day of embryo transfer had a predictive value for implantation during in vitro fertilization cycles. Patients who became pregnant were characterized by a significantly lower resistance index (0.53+/-0.04 versus 0.64+/-0.04), obtained from subendometrial vessels by transvaginal color Doppler ultrasonography and a significantly higher flow index

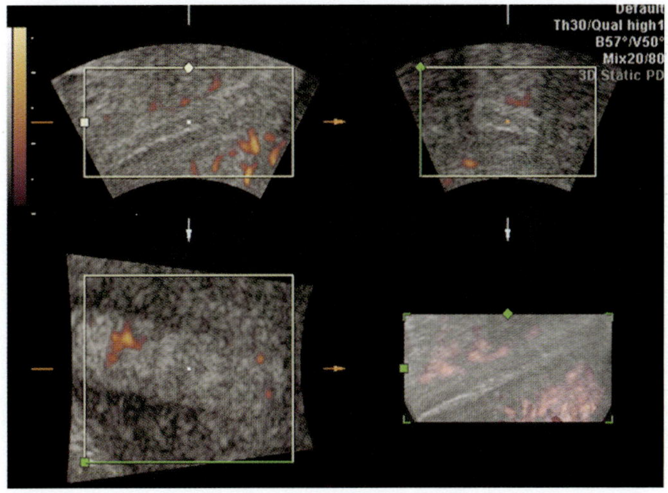

Fig. 8: Three-dimensional power Doppler of the endometrium. Subendometrial flow reflects the degree of endometrial perfusion and may be used as a noninvasive assay of uterine receptivity.

(13.2+/-2.2 versus 11.9+/-2.4), as measured by a 3D power Doppler histogram. No differences were found in the predictive value of scoring systems analyzing endometrial thickness and volume, endometrial morphology and subendometrial perfusion by color Doppler and 3D power Doppler ultrasonography. The high degree of endometrial perfusion shown by both techniques on the day of embryo transfer can indicate a more favorable endometrial milieu for successful in vitro fertilization.

Congenital Anomalies

Congenital uterine malformations are variable in frequency and are usually estimated to represent 3–4% of the general population, although less than half have clinical symptoms.[22-24]

The respective frequency of symptomatic malformations is dominated by the septate uterus.[24,25] During the first trimester of pregnancy, the risk of spontaneous abortion in this group is between 28 and 45%, while during the second trimester the frequency of late spontaneous abortions is approximately 5%.[24] Premature deliveries, abnormal fetal presentations, irregular uterine activity and dystocia at delivery are likely to prevail in cases of septate uterus.[26] Poor vascularization of the septum was proposed as a potential cause of miscarriages.[25] Electron microscopy study conducted by Fedele et al.[27] indicate a decreased sensitivity of the endometrium covering the septa of malformed the uteri to preovulatory changes. This could play a role in the pathogenesis of primary infertility in patients with septate uterus.

It is clear that unfavorable obstetric prognosis can be transformed by surgical correction of the intrauterine septum. Hysteroscopic treatment was currently proposed as the procedure of choice for the management of these disorders. This simple and effective treatment has an obvious advantage that uterus is not weakened by a myometrial scar. Cararach et al.[28] and Goldenberg et al.[29] reported 75% and 88,7% pregnancy rates after operative hysteroscopy, respectively.

The clear simplicity and effectiveness of hysteroscopy makes it necessary for the clinician to arrive at an early and correct diagnosis of uterine anomalies. When used as a screening test for detection of congenital uterine anomalies transvaginal ultrasound had a sensitivity of almost 100%[30,31] However, clear distinction between different types of abnormalities was impossible and operator dependent.[32,33]

X-ray hysterosalpingography (X-ray HSG) is an invasive test, which requires the use of contrast medium and exposure to radiation. Although, HSG provides a good outline of the uterine cavity, the visualization of minor anomalies and clear distinction between different types of lateral fusion disorders is sometimes impossible to visualize. Fifteen years ago hysterosonography has been introduced.[34] This method utilizes the transvaginal ultrasound after distension of the uterine cavity by instillation of a saline solution. This simple and minimally invasive approach allows anatomical images of the endometrium and myometrium, an accurate depiction of the septate uterus and even the measurement of the thickness and height of the septum.[35]

Although some reports have indicated a high diagnostic accuracy of magnetic resonance imaging[36,37] in the diagnosis of congenital uterine anomalies, this technique is rarely routinely used for this pathology. More recently, a three-dimensional ultrasound has been shown to have a high diagnostic accuracy in detection of a septate uterus[38] suggesting that invasive procedures such as CO_2 diagnostic hysteroscopy are not necessary in patients scheduled for corrective surgery.[39]

Kupesic and Kurjak attempted to evaluate the combined use of transvaginal ultrasound, transvaginal color and pulsed Doppler sonography, hysterosonography and three-dimensional ultrasound in the preoperative diagnosis of a septate uterus.[40]

A total of 420 infertile patients undergoing operative hysteroscopy were included in this study. With the use of B mode transvaginal sonography, the morphology of uterus was carefully explored with emphasis on the endometrial lining in both sagittal and transverse sections. The septum was visualized as an echogenic portion separating the uterine cavity into two parts. Once an experienced sonographer completed the B mode examination, another skilled operator who was unaware of the previous finding performed the transvaginal color Doppler examination.

Color and pulsed Doppler was superimposed to visualize intraseptal and myometrial vascularity **(Figs. 9A and B)**. Flow velocity waveforms were obtained from all the interrogated vessels. For each recording, at least five

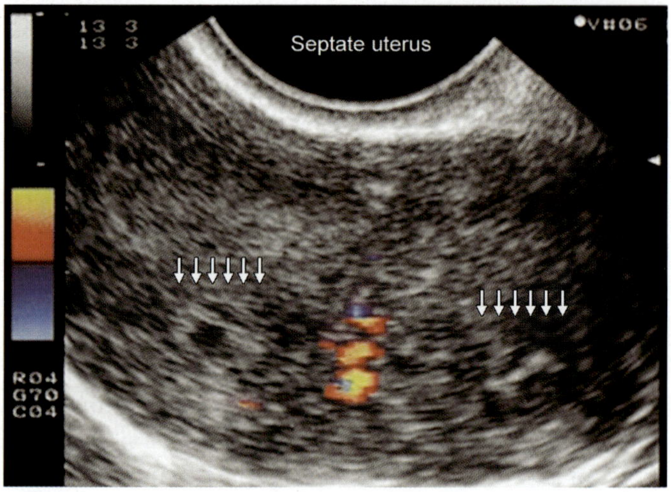

Fig. 9A: Septate uterus demonstrated by color Doppler imaging. Vascularity within the septal area is easily observed by this technique.

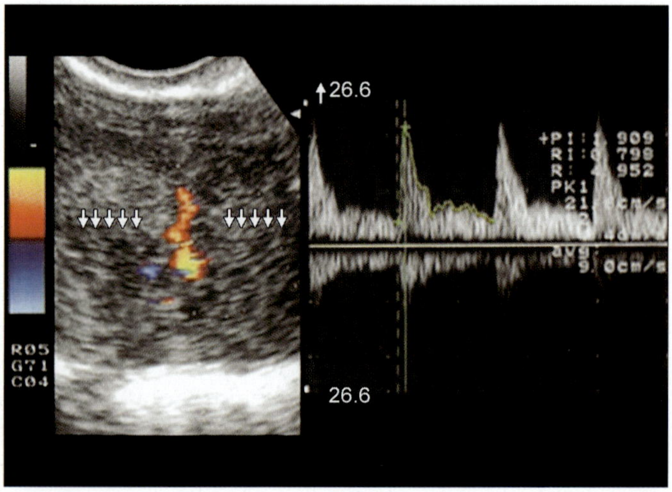

Fig. 9B: Pulsed Doppler waveform analysis (right) reveals moderate to high vascular resistance (RI = 0.79) of the vessels involved in the septum.

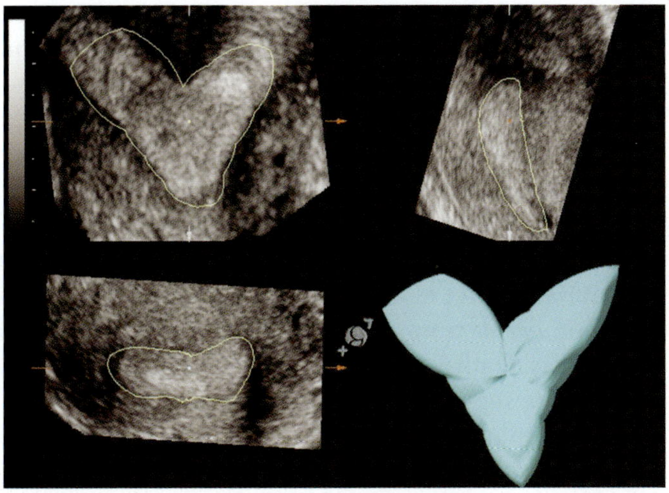

Fig. 10A: Three-dimensional ultrasound of a septate uterus. Note partial division of the uterine cavity and "Y" shape of the uterine cavity. Hysteroscopy confirmed subseptate uterus.

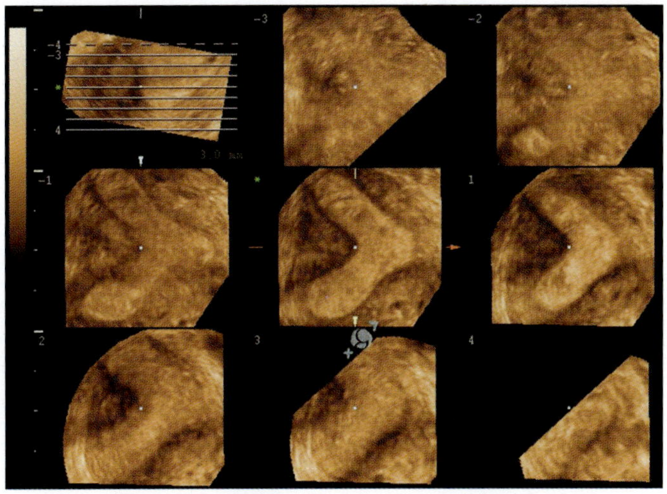

Fig. 10B: Frontal reformatted section and tomographic ultrasound images (TUI) of a septate uterus.

waveform signals of good quality were obtained. During each procedure the resistance index was automatically calculated. The RI was calculated from the maximum frequency envelope and consisted of: peak systolic velocity minus end-diastolic velocity divided by peak systolic velocity. Instillation of isotonic saline (hysterosonography) was carried out on a gynecological examination table. Transverse and sagittal sections were carefully explored, and the septum was visualized as an echogenic portion separating the uterine cavity into two parts.

Eighty-six women undergoing hysteroscopy were examined by a three-dimensional ultrasound. When the patients were evaluated using 3D ultrasound, three perpendicular planes of the uterus were simultaneously displayed on the screen, allowing a detailed analysis of the uterine morphology **(Fig. 10A)**. The frontal reformatted sections and tomographic ultrasound imaging (TUI) were particularly useful for detection of the uterine abnormalities **(Fig. 10B)**. Major advantages of three dimensional ultrasound is simultaneous visualization of the uterine cavity **(Fig. 11A)** and assessment of the fundal shape **(Fig. 11B)**. Diagnosis of a septate uterus is based on visualization of the "V" or "Y" shape of the uterine cavity and convex or planar uterine fundus.

Table 1 summarizes the sensitivity, specificity, positive and negative predictive values of the transvaginal sonography, transvaginal color and pulsed Doppler ultrasound, hysterosalpingography and three-dimensional ultrasound for the diagnosis of a septate uterus. The sensitivity of transvaginal sonography in the diagnosis of

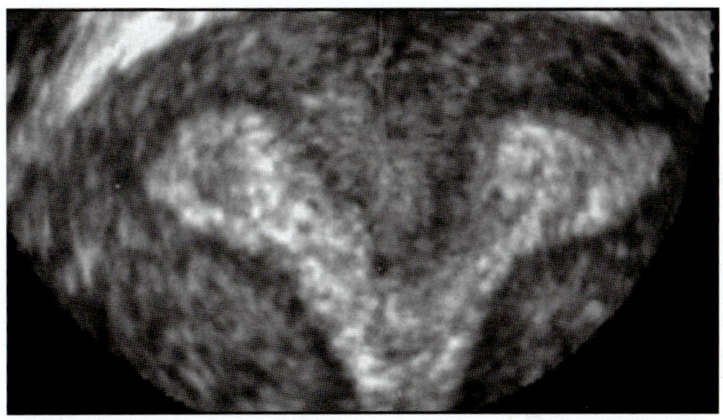

Fig. 11A: Frontal reformatted section of a septate uterus. Note clear division of the uterine cavity in the upper half of the uterine cavity and convex shape of the uterine fundus.

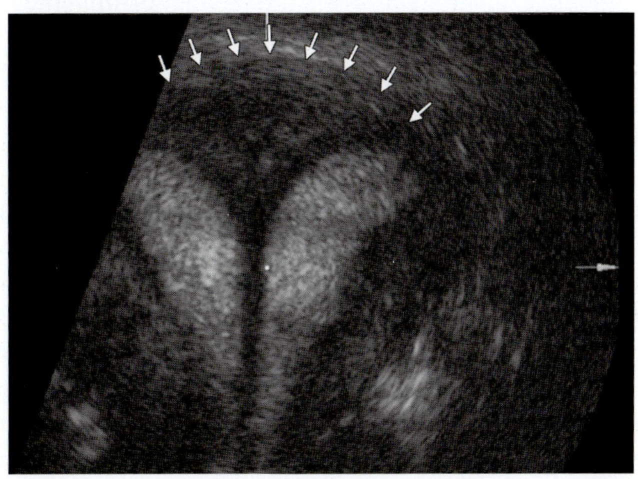

Fig. 11B: Another case of a septate uterus. Note a complete division of the uterine cavity and convex shape of the uterine fundus.

TABLE 1: Sensitivity, specificity, positive (PPV) and negative predictive (NPV) values of various imaging modalities for the diagnosis of septate uterus in 420 patients with history of infertility and recurrent abortions.[40]

Imaging modality	*Sensitivity (%)*	*Specificity (%)*	*PPV (%)*	*NPV (%)*
Transvaginal sonography	95.21	92.21	95.86	91.03
Transvaginal color Doppler	99.29	97.93	98.03	98.61
Hysterosonography	98.18	100.00	100.00	95.45
Three dimensional ultrasound	98.38	100.00	100.00	96.00

septate uteri was 95.21%. Transvaginal color and pulsed Doppler enabled the diagnosis of a septate uterus in 276 cases, reaching a sensitivity of 99.29%. In one patient with an endometrial polyp and one with intrauterine synechiae, a septate uterus was not correctly diagnosed. Therefore, the reliability of color and pulsed Doppler examination was reduced if other intracavitary structures (such as endometrial polyp or submucous leiomyoma) were present.

Color and pulsed Doppler studies of the septal area revealed vascularity in 198 (71.22%) patients. The RI values obtained from the septum ranged from 0.68 to 1.0 (mean RI = 0.84 ± 0.16) **(Figs. 9A and B)**. Hysterosonography reached both a 100% specificity and positive predictive value. In one patient with extensive intrauterine synechiae, hysterosonography did not detect an intrauterine septum.

The sensitivity and specificity of three-dimensional ultrasonography were 98.38% and 100%, respectively. A false-negative result in one patient was caused by a fundal fibroid distorting the uterine cavity. Interestingly, in our study the septate uterus was never mistaken for a bicornuate uterus.

In our study, a transvaginal color Doppler sonography, a hysterosonography, and a three-dimensional ultrasonography were performed. However, in one patient with a bicornuate uterus the transvaginal sonogram was misinterpreted as a septate uterus.

One hundred eighty eight patients underwent X-ray HSG within 12 months prior to our examination. The sensitivity of X-ray HSG for the diagnosis of septate uteri was only 26.06%.

Fedele et al.[27] recently indicated that an intrauterine septum may be a cause of primary infertility. The ultrastructural morphological alterations of the septal area were indicative of irregular differentiation and estrogenic maturation of septal endometrial mucosa. Since, the hormonal levels of the patients enrolled in this study were normal for the cycle phase, the most convincing hypothesis was that the endometrial mucosa covering the septum was poorly responsive to estrogens probably due to scanty vascularization of septal connective tissue.

Dabirashrafi et al.[41] performed a histologic study of the uterine septa from 16 patients undergoing abdominal metroplasty. Statistical analysis confirmed less connective tissue in the septum compared to the amount of muscle tissue, amount of muscle interlacing and vessels with a muscle wall, which was contradictory to the classic view about the histologic features of the uterine septum. Less connective tissue in the septum can be a reason for poor decidualization and placentation in the area of implantation.[35] Increased amounts of muscle tissue and muscle interlacing in the septum can cause an abortion by a higher and uncoordinated contractility of these muscles.

Ultrasound and Doppler studies found no correlation between septal height and thickness and occurrence of obstetrical complications ($p > 0.05$).[40] Pregnancy loss correlated significantly with septal vascularity. Patients with vascularized septa had significantly higher incidence of early pregnancy failure and late pregnancy complications than those with avascularized septa ($P < 0.05$).

A three-dimensional ultrasound enables planar reformatted sections through the uterus, which allows a precise evaluation of the fundal indentation and uterine cavity **(Figs. 12 to 15)**. This approach allows precise assessment of different types of the uterine anomalies such as arcuate, septate and dydelphic uterus **(Figs. 13A and B)**, uterus duplex **(Fig. 14)**, and unicornuate uterus **(Fig. 15)**. Based on our experience, this technique may give a mistaken impression of an arcuate uterus in patients who have a fundal location of a leiomyoma. In these cases the uterine cavity has a concave shape, while the fundal indentation is shallower. Furthermore, shadowing caused by the uterine fibroids, irregular endometrial lining and decreased volume of the uterine cavity (in cases of intrauterine adhesions) are obvious limitations of the 3D ultrasound. More recently three-dimensional power Doppler was used to detect vascularization of the uterine septa in a combined angio and gray rendering mode. This approach allows simultaneous analysis of the morphology, texture and vascularization of the endometrium.

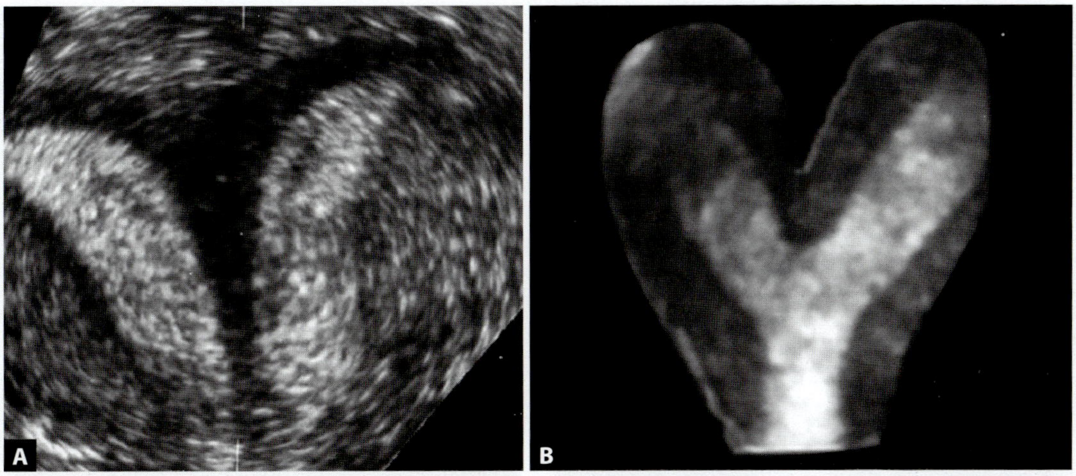

Figs. 12A and B: Frontal reformatted section (A) and surface rendering of a bicornuate uterus (B). Note division of the uterine cavity and fundal cleft exceeding 1 cm. Bicornuate uterus was confirmed by hysterolaparoscopic procedure.

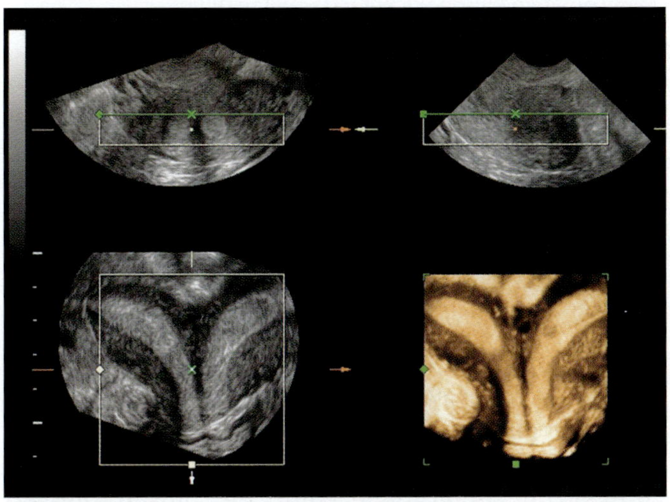

Fig. 13A: Didelphys uterus results from a complete non-fusion of both müllerian ducts. The individual horns are fully developed and almost normal in size. Two cervices are inevitably present.

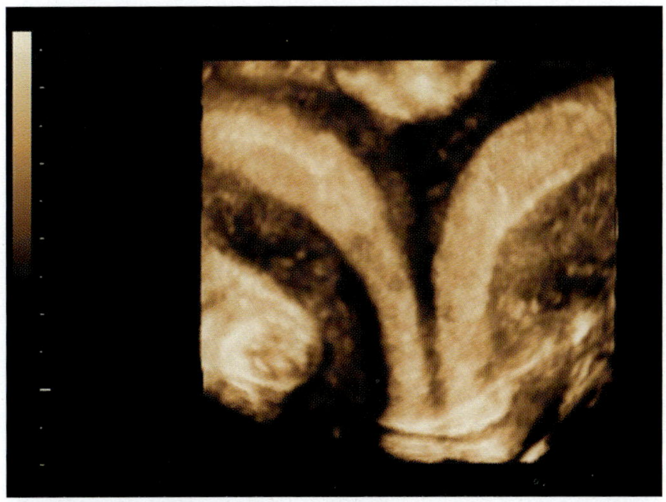

Fig. 13B: Surface rendering image of a dydelphic uterus. Such a frontal view enables better assessment of two cervical canals.

Balen et al.[42] described a technique of three-dimensional reconstruction of the uterine cavity using a positive contrast medium (Echovist). The main problem encountered with Echovist was an acoustic shadowing artifact owing to its highly reflective properties. Despite this, Echovist proved to be superior to saline as an intrauterine contrast agent for 3D reconstruction while testing 10 patients with both methods.

Weinraub et al.[43] used 3D saline contrast hysterosonography on 32 volunteers ranging from 22 to 65 years of age, all in good health and with no evidence of active infections or disease.

Contrast 3D hysterosonography offers a more comprehensive overview of the uterine cavity and surrounding myometrium, and gives access to planes unobtainable by conventional 2D ultrasound examination. Further research is required to document whether contrast instillation contributes to better diagnosis of uterine cavity pathology when compared to unenhanced frontal reformatted section.

Kupesic et al.[44] studied the incidence of surgically correctable uterine abnormalities (congenital uterine anomalies, submucous leiomyoma, endometrial polyps and intrauterine synechiae) in the infertile

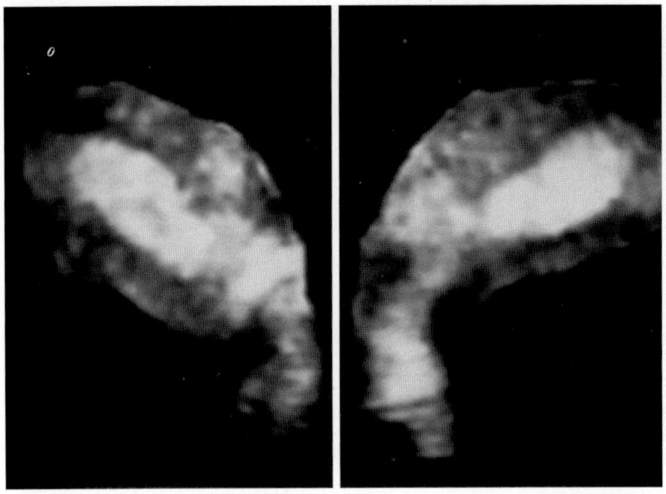

Fig. 14: Three-dimensional ultrasound image of a didelphys uterus. Duplication of the cervix and the vagina is clearly visualized.

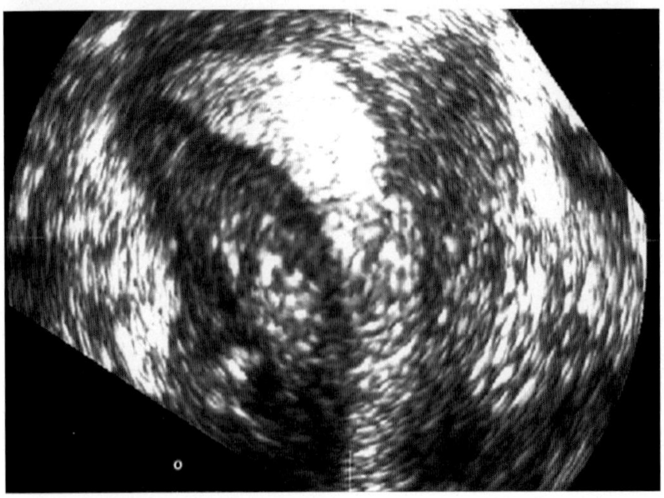

Fig. 15: Three-dimensional ultrasound of an unicornuate uterus.

population attending a tertiary infertility clinic. All of the infertile patients enrolled in the study were evaluated by 3D ultrasound. An additional objective was to assess pregnancy rates before and after operative hysteroscopy in patients affected by uterine causes of infertility. They found the incidence of a uterine septum in their infertile population to be 17.9%. Uterine septum was the most common uterine abnormality accounting for 77.1% of the intrauterine lesions. Out of 310 patients that were followed, 225 (72.6%) patients achieved pregnancy after hysteroscopic metroplasty for an intrauterine septum.

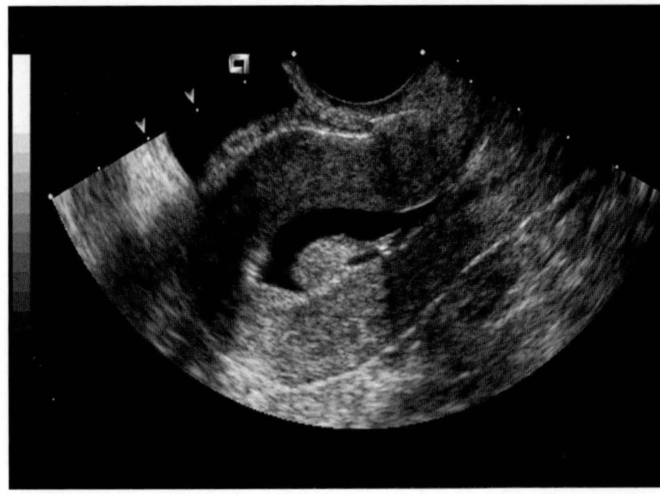

Fig. 16A: Endometrial polyp by saline infusion sonography (SIS). Note focal endometrial thickening typical of an endometrial polyp in a patient with secondary infertility. Hyperechogenic polyp is clearly outlined by sonolucent intracavitary fluid.

Endometrial Polyp

An endometrial polyp is an anatomic defect, which is implicated in the etiology of a recurrent pregnancy loss and infertility. Polyps appear as diffuse or focal thickening of the endometrium **(Fig. 16A)**. Using sonohysterography an intracavitary polyp is seen surrounded by anechoic fluid, at the point of the attachment. If the examination is performed in the follicular phase, the use of a distending medium is not necessary to detect abnormal endometrial thickening. However, during the periovulatory and secretory phase, polyps are better visualized when outlined by fluid.

By using transvaginal color and pulsed Doppler we can study minor arteries supplying the growth of an endometrial polyp **(Fig. 16B)**. Three-dimensional ultrasound allows a detailed analysis of the uterine cavity in frontal reformatted sections, which enables clear demarcation of the polyps **(Figs. 16C and D)**. Small polyps may be found incidentally in subfertile or infertile patients **(Figs. 17A and B)**.

Submucosal Leiomyomas

The diagnosis of a submucosal leiomyoma is based on distortion of the uterine contour, uterine enlargement and textural changes. Since, leiomyomas have a varying amount of smooth muscle and connective tissue, these benign tumors also have a variety of sonographic features. The sonographic texture ranges from hypoechoic to echogenic, depending on the amount of smooth muscle

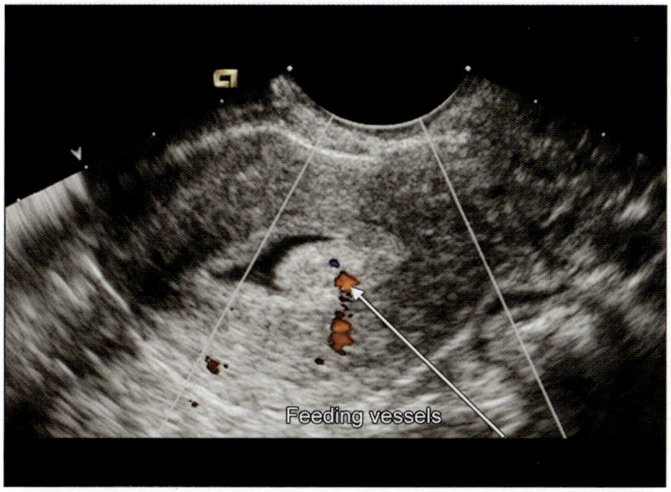

Fig. 16B: Color Doppler image of the same endometrial polyp. Feeding vessels within the stalk are clearly visualized.

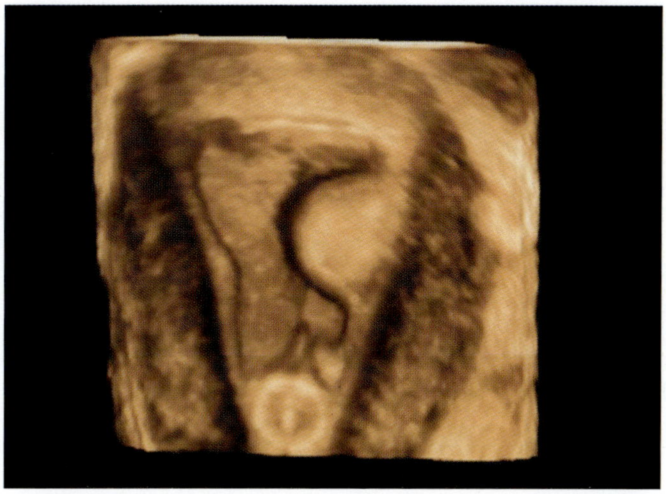

Fig. 16D: Surface rendering of endometrial polyp. This view enables mapping and estimation of the endometrial polyp volume.

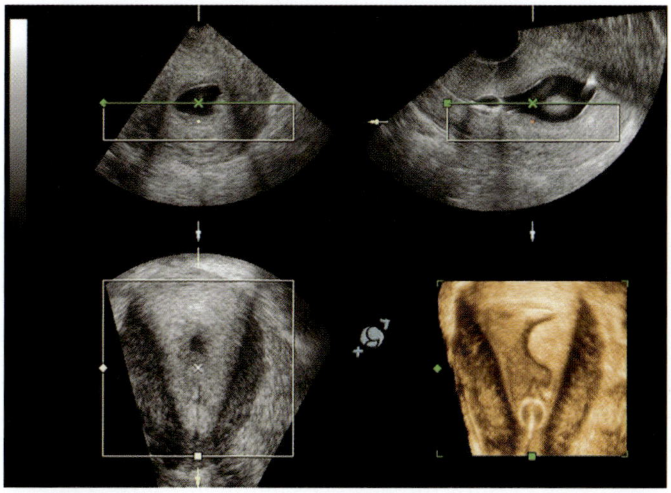

Fig. 16C: Three-dimensional saline infusion sonography (3D SIS). Endometrial polyp protrudes into the uterine cavity.

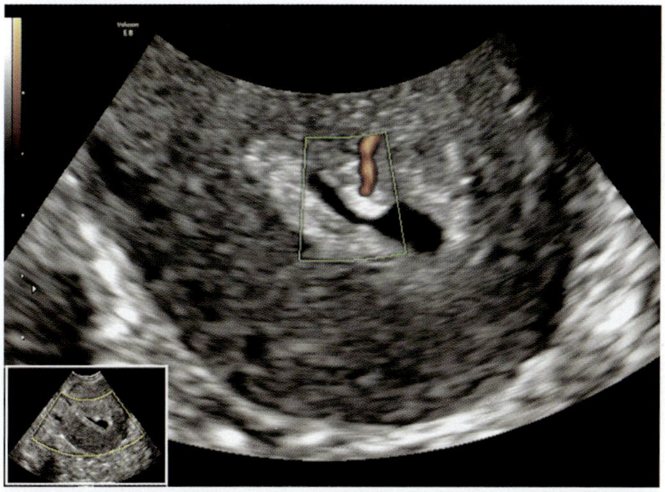

Fig. 17A: B mode ultrasound image of the uterus following saline infusion into the endometrial cavity. Solid echogenic projectile lesion with convex margins is clearly visualized following distension of the uterine cavity with the negative contrast medium (saline). Power Doppler shows a single feeding vessel supplying an endometrial polyp.

and connective tissue. Central ischemia, which is a consequence of tumor enlargement and inadequate blood supply, is usually followed by various stages of degeneration. The most common cause of calcification within the uterus is calcific degeneration within a fibroid. Other types of degeneration include cystic, myxomatous, and hyaline degeneration. Sometimes, because of the variety of appearances, submucosal leiomyomas may be mistaken for endometrial polyps, endometrial carcinoma, blood or mucus. Patients with submucosal fibroids have a uterine environment which is not conducive to nidation of a fertilized ovum. In addition the blood supply might be inadequate. Leiomyomas grow centripetally as proliferation of smooth muscle cells and fibrous connective tissue, creating a pseudocapsule of compressed muscle fibers. Therefore, color Doppler demonstrates most of the myometrial blood vessels at its periphery **(Figs. 18A and B)**. Presence of blood vessels in the central portion of the leiomyomas is usually correlated with necrotic, degenerative and inflammatory changes. These vessels display lower RI values than peripherally located vessels, and sometimes can be misinterpreted for

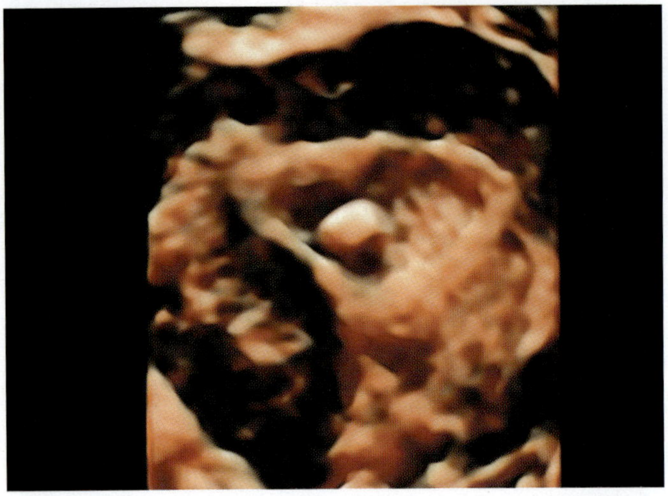

Fig. 17B: The same patient assessed with 3D ultrasound. Depth of the endometrial cavity and the polyp are better perceived by 3D ultrasound surface rendering.

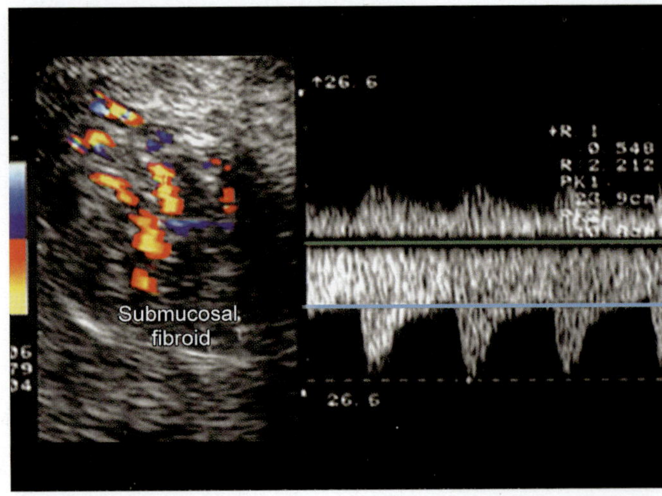

Fig. 18B: Pulsed Doppler waveform analysis of the fibroid feeding vessels. Moderate vascular impedance blood flow signals and resistance index of 0.55 are isolated from the vessels within the capsule of the fibroid.

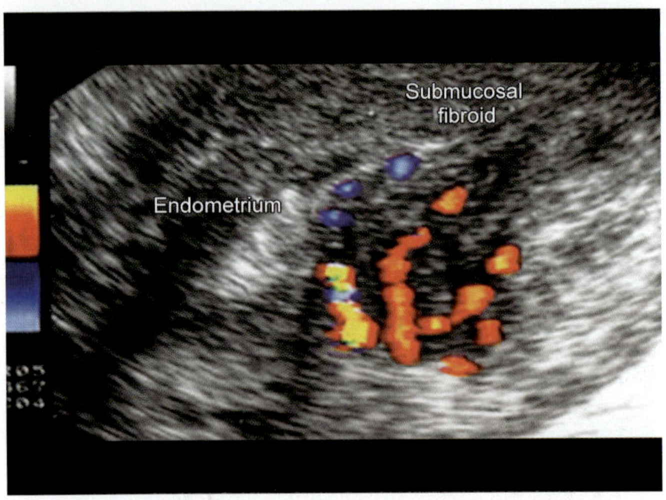

Fig. 18A: Color Doppler ultrasound of submucosal fibroid in a patient with menorrhagia and primary infertility.

malignant neovascular pulsed Doppler signal.[45] Vascular impedance to blood flow in the myometrial supplying vessels depends not only on size but location within the uterus. A significant difference was shown in the blood flow characteristics for the leiomyoma supplying vessels between entirely subserosal versus intramural and submucosal leiomyomas. Lower impedance value for subserosal leiomyomas can be explained by the fact that these leiomyomas are supplied with blood vessels through a very small contact area. These blood vessels are surrounded by loose connective tissue and therefore dilated with a very low vascular impedance to blood flow.

In contrast, submucosal leiomyomas and those located within the myometrium are supplied by blood vessels with higher vascular impedance. A high basal tone of myometrial tissue surrounding intramural or submucosal leiomyomas can cause a difference in hemodynamic parameters. A three-dimensional ultrasound precisely estimates the relationship between the submucosal leiomyoma and the uterine cavity **(Figs. 19A to D)**.

Kurjak et al.[45] performed transvaginal color flow evaluation in 101 patients with palpable uterine fibroids and 60 healthy volunteers. The mean resistance index from the periphery of leiomyoma covered the value of 0.54. Mean PI value was 0.89. The pathohistological finding was benign uterine tumor in all the cases, even when RI was very low. Lowered resistance indices were present in cases with necrosis and secondary degenerative and inflammatory changes within the fibroid. Increased blood flow velocity and decreased RI (mean RI = 0.74) in both uterine arteries occurred in patients with uterine fibroids. Three-dimensional power Doppler ultrasound opens new avenues in evaluation of the patients with uterine fibroids **(Figs. 20A and B)**.

Adenomyosis

Adenomyosis is characterized by the ingrowing of the endometrium into the myometrium. It is usually asymptomatic, but may be present as uterine bleeding, pain and infertility. A diffusely enlarged uterus without discrete fibroids, an intact endometrium and multiple small cysts

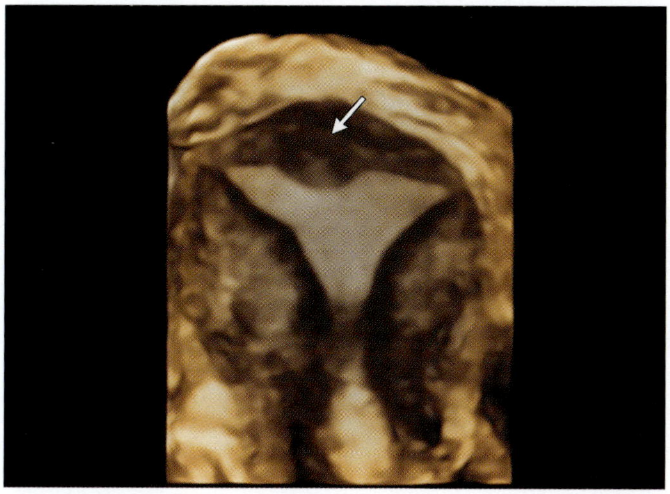

Fig. 19A: 3D ultrasound rendering of the uterus. A concave indentation on the fundal surface of the endometrium, suggestive of a submucosal lesion indenting the endometrium is noted in the coronal plane. In the vicinity of the indentation, within the myometrium an oval hypoechoic area is seen, marginated superiorly by a faint echogenic line (marked by an arrow). Sonographic imaging is suggestive of submucosal fibroid indenting the endometrium.

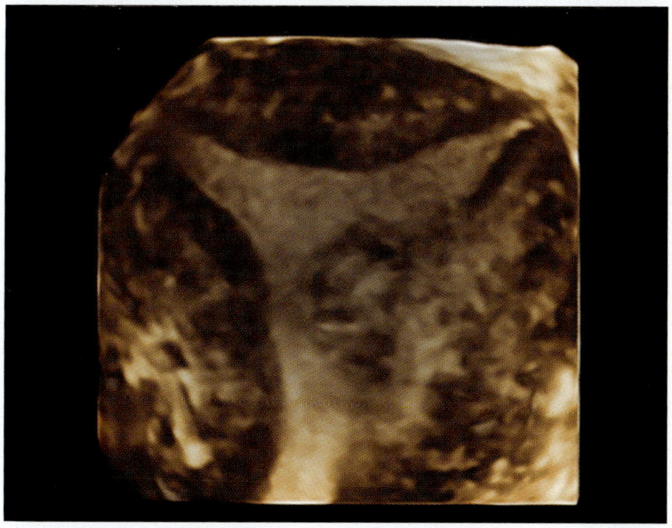

Fig. 19B: 3D ultrasound surface rendered image of the uterus shows concave superior margin suggestive of an arcuate uterus. The body part of the endometrial cavity is grossly indented by an oval heterogeneous lesion. Sonographic finding indicates submucosal fibroid.

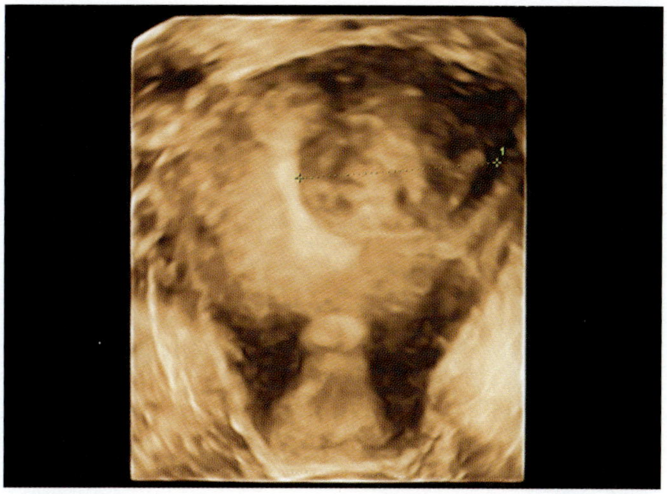

Fig. 19C: 3D ultrasound surface rendered image of the uterus in the coronal plane showing a large round heterogeneous lesion grossly distorting almost the entire the endometrial cavity. Sonographic findings indicate a large fundal submucosal fibroid.

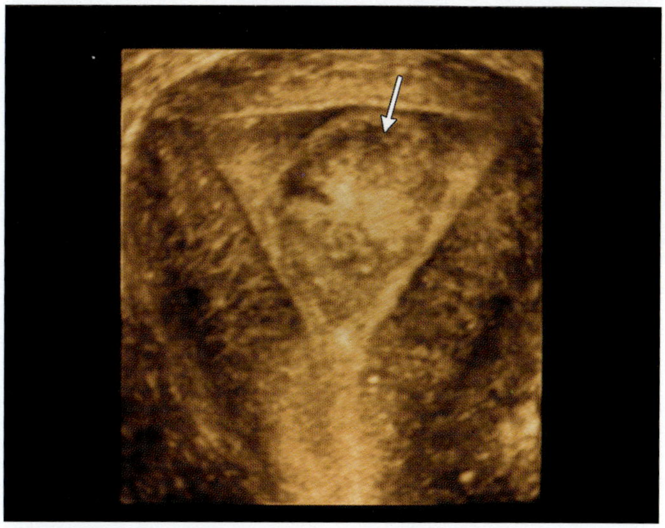

Fig. 19D: 3D ultrasound rendered image of the uterus during the secretory phase demonstrates a round hypoechoic lesion within the endometrial cavity, as marked by an arrow. Round appearance, location, and hypoechoic appearance compared to the endometrium are typical for intracavitary fibroid.

in the myometrium have been reported as a suggestive appearance of adenomyosis **(Fig. 21A)**.[46] Disordered echogenicity of the middle layer of the myometrium is present in some severe cases. Reported sensitivity and specificity of transvaginal ultrasound in detection of this benign entity is 86% and 50%, respectively.[46] Color Doppler may reveal increased vascularity mainly characterized with moderate vascular resistance **(Fig. 21B)**.

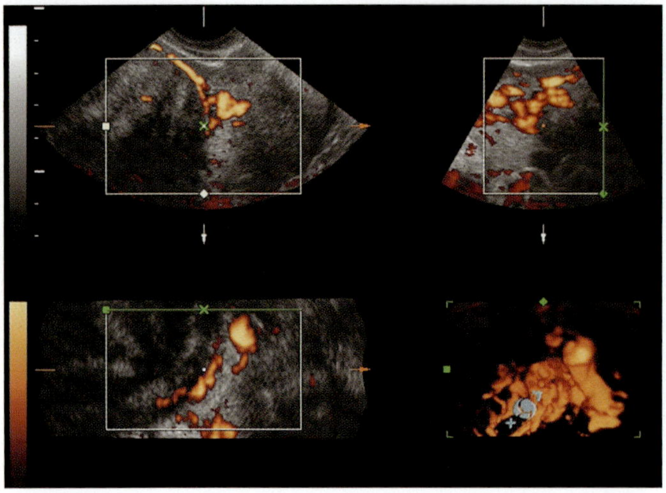

Fig. 20A: Three-dimensional power Doppler ultrasound outlines uterine fibroid feeding vessels within the capsule.

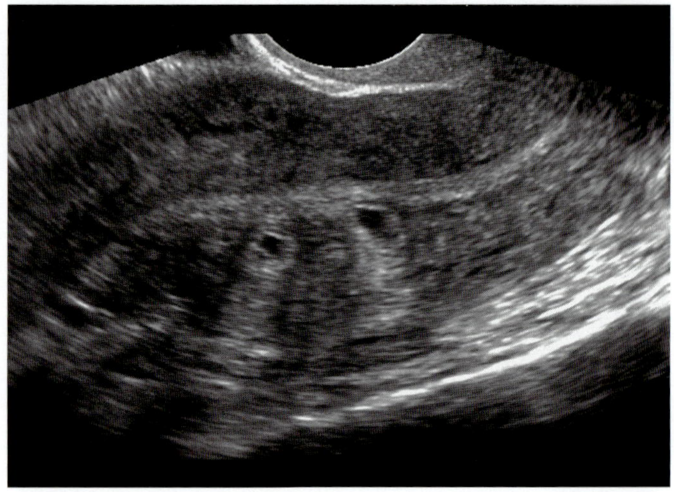

Fig. 21A: Longitudinal plane of the uterus in a patient with superficial adenomyosis. Two adenomyotic implants are visualized within the superficial posterior myometrial layer.

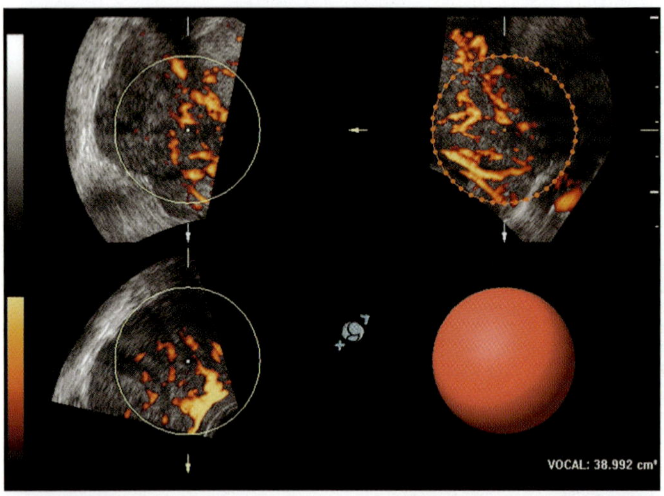

Fig. 20B: Three-dimensional power Doppler ultrasound of the same patient. In addition to vascularity assessment, VOCAL software enables determination of the leiomyoma volume.

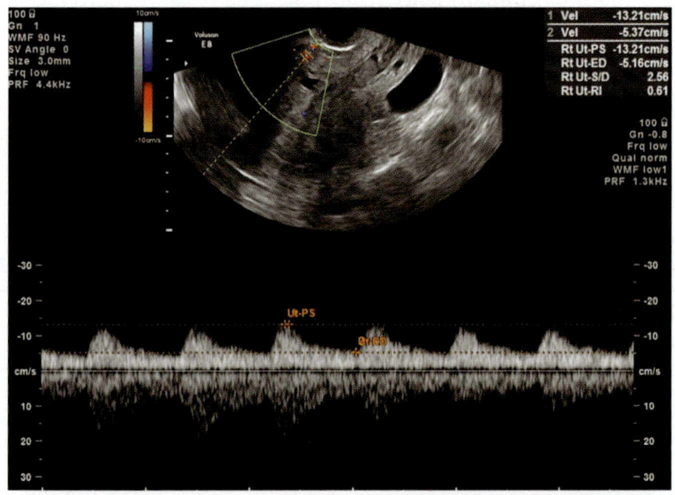

Fig. 21B: Color Doppler reveals increased vascularity characterized with moderate vascular resistance (RI = 0.61).

Endometritis

Acute endometritis is characterized by increased echogenicity, thickness and vascularity of the endometrium **(Fig. 22)**. During the active stage, a pregnancy often terminates as an abortion. In chronic stages, transvaginal sonography reveals deformity of the endometrial cavity suggestive of adhesions. In the absence of a history of prior curettage or abortion the most common cause of a chronic endometrial infection is *Mycobacterium tuberculosis*. Other imaging findings include calcified pelvic lymph nodes or smaller irregular calcifications in the adnexa.

In the acute stage of the endometritis low to moderate impedance blood flow signals are easily obtained on the periphery of the endometrium, as oppose to cases with irreversible tissue damage where blood flow is usually absent. Transvaginal sonography allows elucidation of the abnormal endometrial morphology, after which appropriate cultures should be taken and broad-spectrum antibiotic therapy administered. In order to prevent the development of intrauterine adhesions (especially after D and C) administration of conjugated estrogen for 1 to 2 months is recommended. This therapy allows for the regeneration of a healthy endometrium, which is paralleled

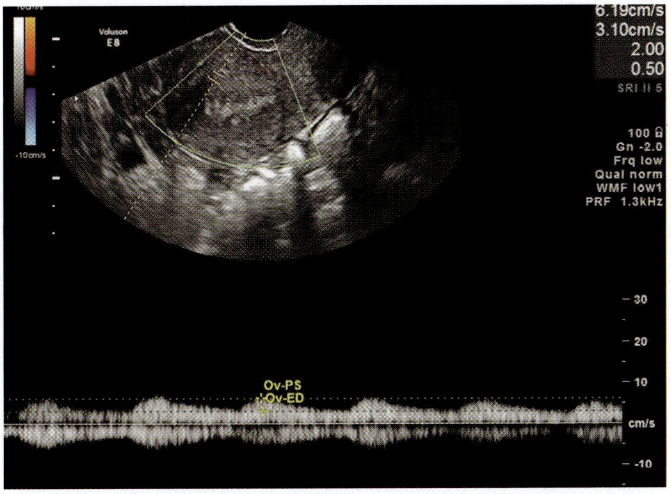

Fig. 22: Color Doppler image of acute endometritis, characterized by increased echogenicity, thickness and vascularity of the endometrium. In the acute stage of the endometritis low to moderate impedance blood flow signals are easily obtained on the periphery of the endometrium (RI = 0.50).

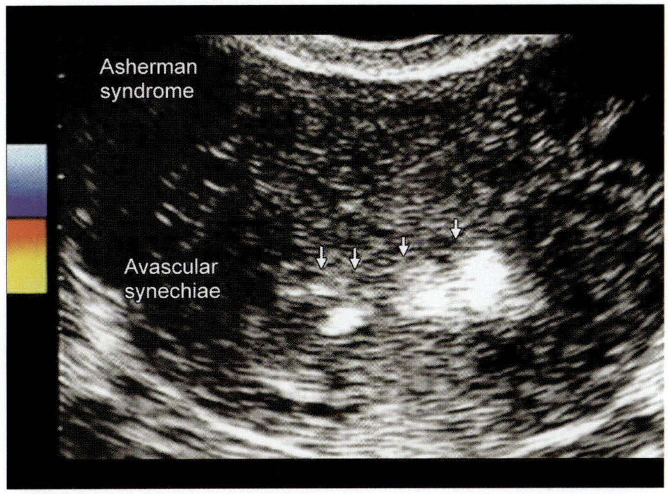

Fig. 23A: Irregular hyperechogenic bridges visualized within the central part of the uterine cavity in a patient with secondary amenorrhea following dilatation and curettage. Color Doppler does not reveal any blood flow signals from the irregular hyperechogenic bridges within the uterine cavity. Hysteroscopy detected intrauterine adhesions (Asherman syndrome).

by a sharp increase in the end-diastolic velocities of the spiral arteries at the time of color flow and pulsed Doppler analysis.

Asherman's Syndrome

Destruction of the endometrium may result in scarring and the development of bands of scar tissue, or synechiae, within the uterine cavity. This destruction may occur as a result of a vigorous curettage of the uterus following an abortion or, more often, after curettage of an advanced pregnancy. Tuberculosis may also cause uterine synechiae, but only in rare cases. This may result in formation of adhesive bands of different sizes, which leads to a subsequent partial or total obliteration of the endometrial cavity. Amenorrhea or hypomenorrhea characterizes the menstrual patterns.

Patients with endometrial adhesions, such as Asherman's syndrome, may have a distorted endometrial pattern consisting of areas where no endometrium can be imaged mixed with areas that appear normal. Adhesions are observed as avascular endometrial irregularities or hyperechoic bridges within the endometrial cavity **(Figs. 23A and B)**.

Schlaff and Hurst[47] analyzed seven amenorrhoic patients with severe Asherman's syndrome. Transvaginal sonography demonstrated a well-developed endometrial stripe in three of the seven women, while three others

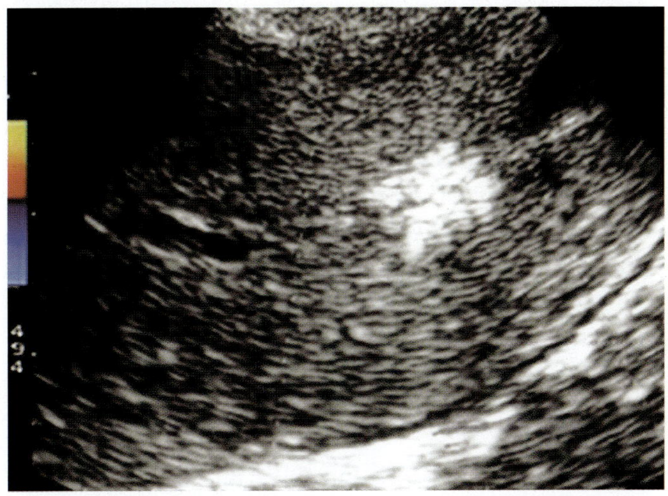

Fig. 23B: Hyperechogenic bridges cranially from the internal cervical os are suggestive of intrauterine adhesions.

had virtually no endometrium seen. All the patients with a well-developed endometrium who were found to have adhesions after undergoing a hysteroscopy for the intrauterine adhesions, who had a normal functioning endometrium, had resumption of normal menses and normalization of the uterine cavity. The women with a minimal endometrium had no cavity identified and thus derived no benefit from surgery. The conclusion of that study was that the endometrial pattern visualized using transvaginal sonography is highly predictive of both

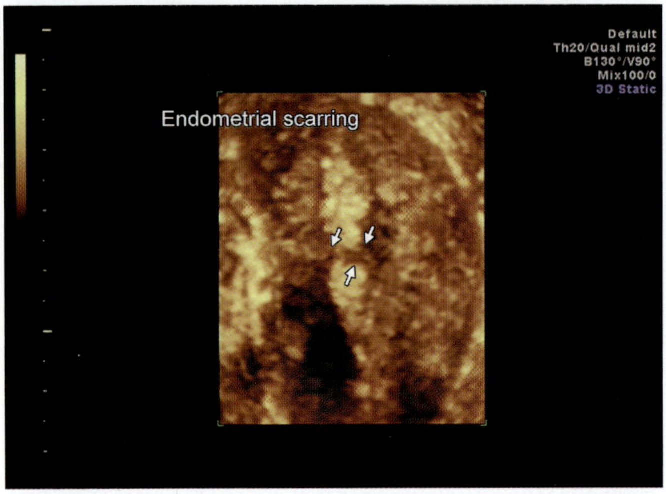

Fig. 23C: 3D ultrasound surface rendered image of the uterus in coronal plane showing nondistended irregular endometrial cavity with a horizontal hypoechoic band in the mid part, typical for intrauterine adhesions (synechia). Sonographic image indicates partial obliteration of the uterine cavity.

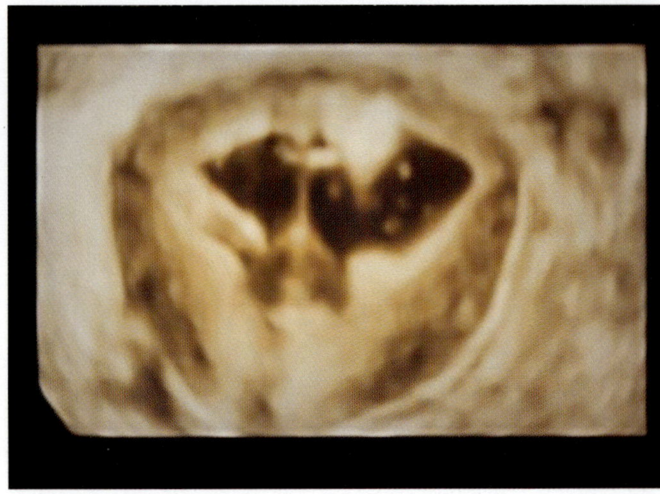

Fig. 23D: 3D ultrasound acquired volume of the uterus with saline infusion hysterography, rendered in coronal plane on surface mode, shows only partial distention of the endometrial cavity. Echogenic strands and irregular echogenicities within the endometrial cavity are typical of multiple endometrial synechia.

surgical and clinical outcomes in patients with severe Asherman's syndrome who are characterized by a complete obstruction of the cavity by a hysterosalpingogram.

Intrauterine synechiae do not present with increased vascularity on color Doppler examination **(Figs. 23A and B)**. They are better visualized during menstruation when the intracavitary fluid outlines them or following a hysterosonography. A three-dimensional ultrasound demonstrates a significant reduction of the endometrial cavity volume in all reformatted sections, and enables superior assessment of the uterine cavity, depiction of intrauterine adhesions and accurate classification the severity of disease **(Figs. 23C to E)**.

OVARIAN CAUSES OF INFERTILITY

The transvaginal sonogram (B mode, color Doppler and more recently three-dimensional and 3D power Doppler ultrasound) is considered the most reliable method for monitoring the follicular growth. It enables an accurate prediction of ovulation and detection of ovulation abnormalities **(Figs. 24 and 25)**.

The success of IVF treatment is dependent on the ability of the ovary to respond to controlled stimulation by gonadotropins and to develop a reasonable number of mature follicles and oocytes simultaneously. Failure to respond is associated with cancellation of the cycle or poor outcome of treatment. Prior prediction of the likelihood of optimal ovarian response is therefore essential in identifying patients who are most likely to benefit from IVF treatment.

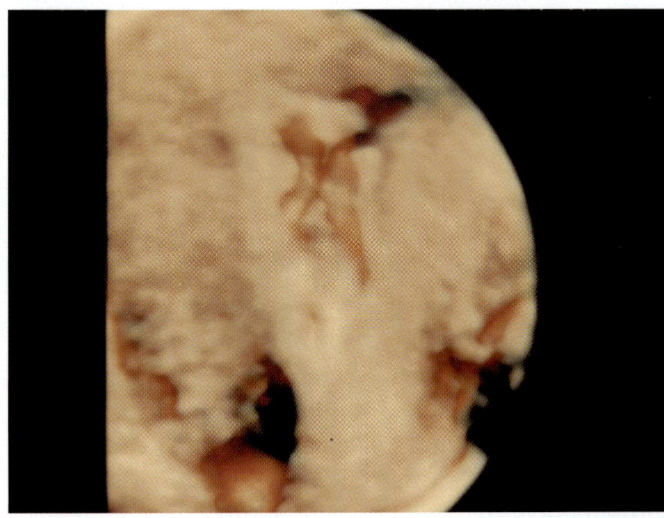

Fig. 23E: 3D ultrasound acquired HDlive rendered coronal plane image of the endometrial cavity shows a thick echogenic fibrotic band (intrauterine synechia) extending from fundus downwards.

Zaidi et al.[48] were the first to show that there was a correlation between ovarian stromal blood flow velocity and ovarian follicular response. They measured the ovarian stromal peak systolic velocity (PSV) in the early follicular phase and showed that poor responders had a low ovarian blood flow PSV. Increased ovarian stromal blood flow

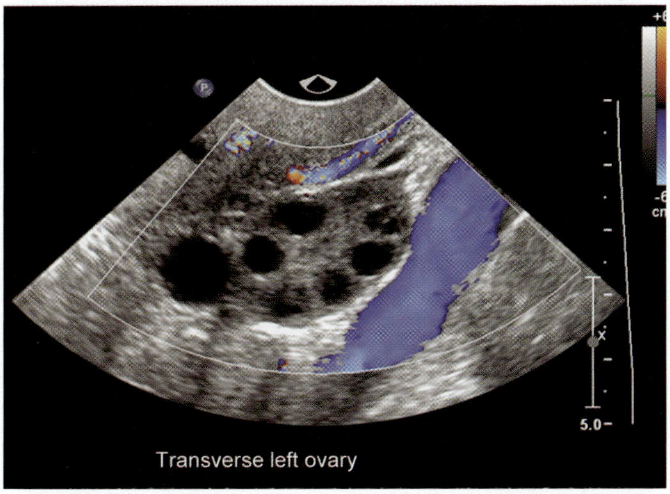

Fig. 24A: Transvaginal color Doppler ultrasound of an ovary containing a dominant follicle on day 10 of the menstrual cycle. Iliac vein is visualized in adjacent to the ovary.

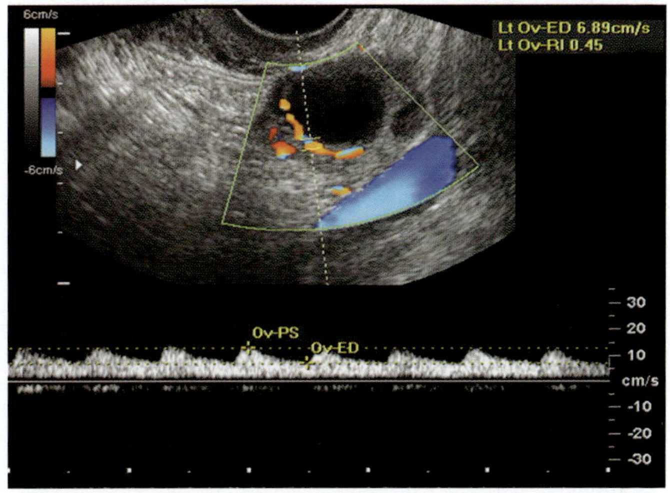

Fig. 24C: Transvaginal color Doppler scan of a dominant follicle. The pulsed Doppler waveform analysis of the follicular vessels shows a resistance index of 0.45. Note that there is a decrease in vascular resistance as ovulation approaches.

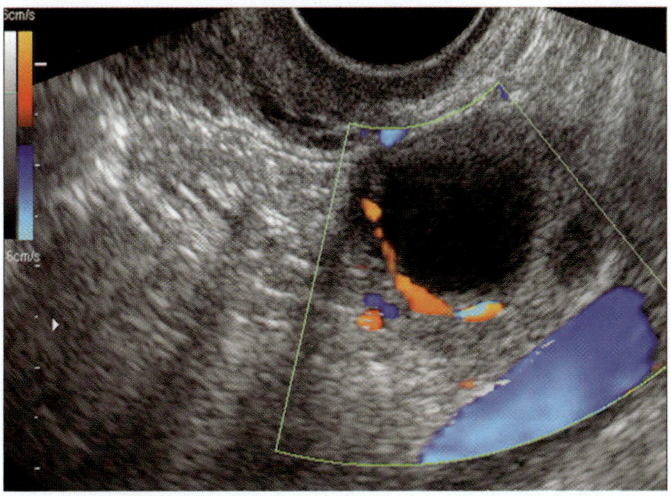

Fig. 24B: Transvaginal color Doppler scan demonstrating a dominant follicle with ring of angiogenesis.

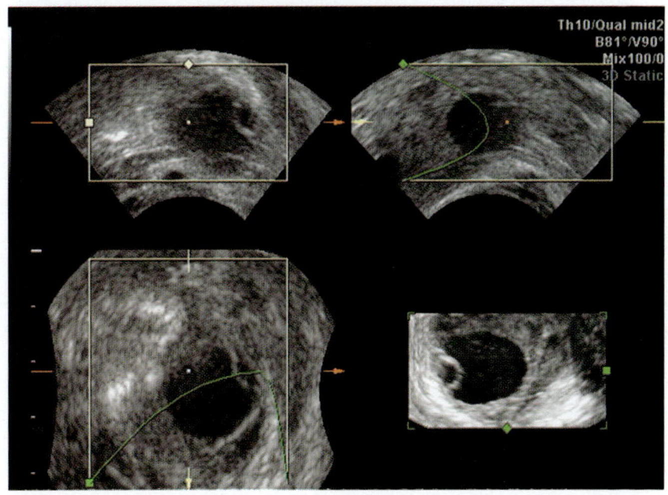

Fig. 24D: Three-dimensional ultrasound of a preovulatory follicle. Careful exploration of its inner wall depicts a cumulus oophorus.

velocity was detected in patients with polycystic ovaries, in combination with a relatively unchanged impedance to blood flow. This may reflect an increased intraovarian perfusion and thus a greater delivery of gonadotropins to the granulosa-theca cell complex with a resultant greater than normal number of follicles being produced. This mechanism may help to explain why patients with polycystic ovaries tend to respond excessively to the administration of gonadotropins,[4856] and may possibly explain their increased risk of ovarian hyperstimulation syndrome.

Documentation of ovarian stromal vascularity at the time of an initial baseline scan may be important and may provide useful information for assisted reproduction techniques. Furthermore, it seems that measurement of ovarian stromal blood flow in the early follicular phase is related to subsequent ovarian responsiveness in IVF treatment.[48] This is particularly useful since the ability to predict ovarian response to stimulation by exogenous gonadotropins is still central to success in any IVF program. Most programs determine the dose of gonadotropins used for the first attempt based on the

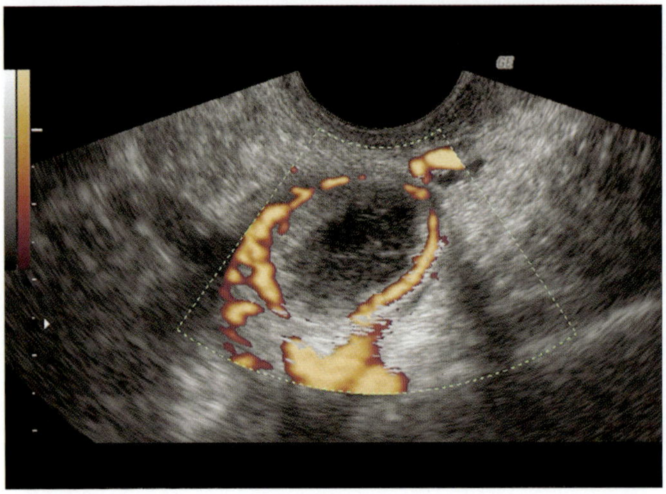

Fig. 25A: Two-dimensional power Doppler ultrasound of corpus luteum.

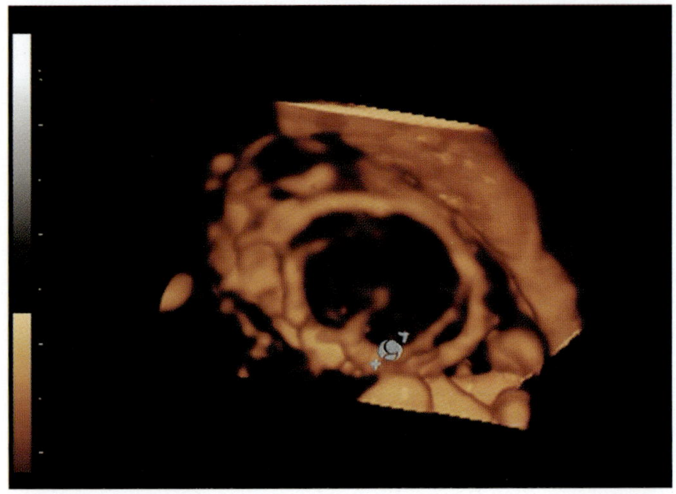

Fig. 25C: Capillary sprouts invading the blood filled cavity of the ruptured follicle are clearly visualized using three-dimensional surface rendering.

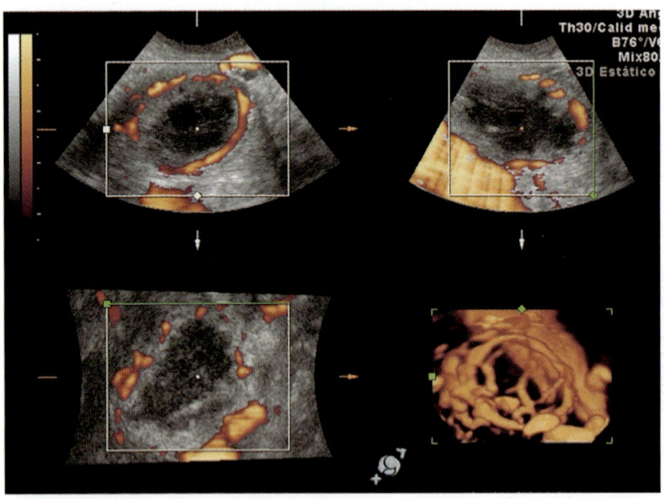

Fig. 25B: Three-dimensional power Doppler ultrasound of corpus luteum.

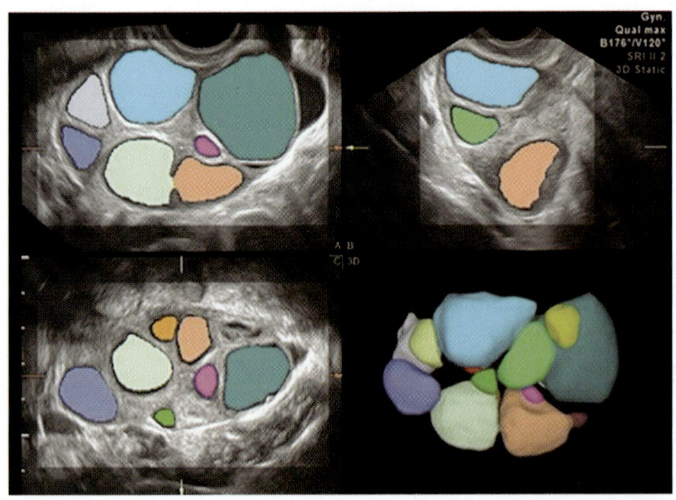

Fig. 26: Three-dimensional ultrasound of the hyperstimulated ovary after ovulation induction. The ovary is enlarged and filled with numerous follicles, that are coded in different colors.

chronological age of the patient, with adjustments being made in subsequent attempts depending on their initial response. Unfortunately the ovarian age (capacity of the ovary to produce fertilizable oocytes) and chronological age are not always synchronous, leading to a degree of unpredictability in the number of developing follicles and collected oocytes. Certainly, if an inadequate dose of gonadotropins is used then there may be a relatively poor response, which reduces the number of oocytes retrieved, whereas if an excessive dose is used, there may be an increased risk of ovarian hyperstimulation syndrome **(Fig. 26)**.

Engman et al.[49] speculated that the ovarian stromal blood flow velocity after 2–3 weeks of pituitary suppression is a true representative of baseline ovarian blood flow because the ovaries are in a quiescent state. The primordial follicles in the ovary have no independent capillary network, lying simply among vessels of the stroma, and therefore depend on their proximity to the stromal vessels for the delivery of nutrients and hormones. The subsequent growth of primary follicles leads to the acquisition of a vascular sheath through the process of angiogenesis. The administration of a GnRH agonist suppresses follicular activity and consequently the ovaries become inactive; ovarian stromal blood flow at this time might be at its lowest and may truly reflect the baseline ovarian blood flow.

Therefore, ovarian stromal blood flow velocity after pituitary suppression is predictive of ovarian responsiveness and the outcome of IVF treatment. One might speculate that by improving the ovarian stromal blood flow velocity, the delivery of gonadotropins to the follicles will be improved and as a result, the number and quality of mature oocytes produced and the implantation rate will improve.

The accuracy of diagnosis and monitoring of infertility treatments such as ovulation induction has increased greatly because of the availability of sophisticated ultrasound technology and equipment.[20] Accurate follicular assessment is essential for a safe and effective infertility treatment. In IVF-ET cycles, follicles with a mean follicular diameter of 12 to 24 mm are associated with optimal rates of oocyte recovery, fertilization, and cleavage.[50] This corresponds to follicular volumes between 3 and 7 mL. In the hands of experienced operators, ultrasound alone suffices for cycle monitoring, without the necessity of additional hormonal estimations.[51-53]

The basic structural information provided by conventional scans in the longitudinal and transverse plan can now be augmented by the new three-dimensional 3D ultrasound systems that provide additional views of the coronal or C-plane, which is parallel to the transducer face.[20] The computer-generated scan is displayed in three perpendicular planes. Translation or rotation can be carried out in one plane, while maintaining the perpendicular orientation of all three so that serial translation will result in an ultrasound tomogram from which volumetric data can be captured.[54] Kyei-Mensah et al.[20] evaluated the accuracy of 3D ultrasound measurement of follicular volume compared with current standard techniques. They compared the volume of individual follicles estimated by both methods with the corresponding follicular aspirates. The volume of follicular fluid aspirated was compared with the corresponding volume of the follicle measured by 3D ultrasound and with the conventional 2D ultrasound volume measurement calculated by using the formula $0.52 \times (D_1 \times D_2 \times D_3)$. Limits of agreement and 95% confidence intervals were calculated and systematic bias between the methods was analyzed. The limits of agreement between the volume of follicular aspirate and follicular volume determined by ultrasound were +0.96 to –0.43 mL for 3D measurements and +3.47 to –2.42 mL for 2D measurements. The high accuracy of 3D measurement of follicular volume is demonstrated clearly in this study by the limits of agreement, which are within 1 mL of the true volume. These limits encompass 95% of the volume measurements. On the other hand, the 2D method produced limits of agreement that was up to 3.5 mL above or 2.5 mL below the true volume of clinical range.

Therefore, the shape and numbers of the follicles influence the reliability of the standard 2D ultrasound technique for follicular volume measurement. There may be technical difficulty in measuring the diameters of a follicle when its shape is distorted because of compression by adjacent follicles. Penzias et al.[55] showed that the mean follicular diameter accurately predicts volume in round and polygonal follicles but not in ellipsoid shaped follicles. Rounded follicles were most prevalent in patients with the fewest follicles. The patients selected for this study had produced fewer follicles than normal and therefore represent the group in which the conventional technique was likely to be most accurate. Kyei-Mensah et al.[20] found that the 3D assessment of follicular volume produced a more accurate reflection of the true volume. This is because the 3D measurement is not affected by follicular shape since the changing contours are outlined serially to obtain the specific volume measurement. The disparity in accuracy between 3D assessment of follicular volume and the conventional approach therefore is likely to increase significantly if there is a florid multifollicular ovarian response because the conventional formula is less precise with ellipsoid follicles, which are likely to predominate in these cases. One limitation of 3D volume assessment is that follicles with a mean diameter of <10 mm cannot be assessed accurately because the limits of agreement are too wide in this range.

Feichtinger et al.[56] found that three-dimensional ultrasound may be useful for the distinction of ovarian cysts from ovarian follicles. Since, both the ovarian cysts and the follicles demonstrate an elevation of the serum estradiol levels, it is difficult to distinguish them by E2 assay alone. For the purpose of the prospective observational study, the authors evaluated 50 IVF patients after ovulation induction. Three-dimensional ultrasound was used to search for the presence of cumuli in follicles greater than 15 mm **(Fig. 19D)**. Only cumuli demonstrable in all three planes by multiplanar imaging predicted mature oocyte recovery. Follicles without visualization of the cumulus in all three planes were not likely to contain mature fertilizable oocytes.

Lass et al.[57] tested the hypothesis that small ovaries measured on transvaginal sonography are associated with a poor response to ovulation induction by human menopausal gonadotropin (HMG) for in vitro fertilization. A total of 140 infertile patients with morphologically normal ovaries undergoing IVF were studied and represented. The mean ovarian volume of each patient was measured on transvaginal sonography before starting HMG. Subsequent routine IVF management was conducted without the knowledge of the transvaginal sonography results. The mean ovarian volume was 6.3 cm^3 (range 0.5–18.9, SD = 3.1). Patients (n = 17; group A) with small ovaries of or = 3 cm^3 represented group B. Both groups were of similar age (mean 35.8 versus 34.4 years). Early basal FSH concentrations were increased in group A (9.5 versus 7.0 mIU/mL, $P = 0.025$). The cycle was abandoned before planned oocyte recovery in nine patients (52.8%) from group A and in 11 patients (8.9%) from group B because of poor response to ovulation induction.

Oyesanya et al.[58] measured the total ovarian volumes before the administration of hCG in 42 women undergoing treatment for infertility by in vitro fertilization and embryo transfer and considered to have an exaggerated response to stimulation (>20 follicles). Seven women who subsequently developed moderate or severe ovarian hyperstimulation syndrome (OHSS) (n = 7; group 1) were compared with 35 matched controls (five matched controls per case; n = 35; group 2) of similar age, number of follicles and duration of infertility who underwent follicular stimulation, oocyte recovery, in vitro fertilization and embryo transfer during the same period but did not develop moderate or severe OHSS. The mean age, duration of infertility and total number of follicles were similar, but the mean total ovarian volume was significantly higher in the group of women who developed moderate or severe OHSS compared with controls (271.00 ± 87.00 versus 157.30 ± 54.20 mL).

Our study was designed to evaluate whether ovarian antral follicle number, ovarian volume, stromal area and ovarian stromal blood flow are predictive of ovarian response and in vitro fertilization outcome.[59] Total ovarian antral follicle number, total ovarian volume, total stromal area and mean flow index (FI) of the ovarian stromal blood flow were determined by three-dimensional (3D) and power Doppler ultrasound after pituitary suppression. Pretreatment 3D ultrasound ovarian measurements were compared with subsequent ovulation induction parameters (peak estradiol on hCG administration day and number of oocytes) and cycle outcome (fertilization and pregnancy rates). The total number of antral follicles achieved the best predictive value for favorable IVF outcome, followed by ovarian stromal FI, total ovarian stromal area and total ovarian volume.

In another study we evaluated whether ovarian antral follicle number, ovarian volume and ovarian stromal blood flow change with a woman's age, and whether these parameters are predictive of ovarian response and in vitro fertilization outcome.[60] Total ovarian antral follicle number, total ovarian volume and mean flow index of the ovarian stromal blood flow were determined by three-dimensional (3D) and power Doppler ultrasound after pituitary suppression. Patients were separated into three groups based upon age and in each group median values of 3D ultrasound parameters (total ovarian antral follicle number, total ovarian volume and mean ovarian stromal vascularity) were measured and presented. Pretreatment 3D ultrasound ovarian measurements were compared with subsequent ovulation induction parameter (number of oocytes) and cycle outcome (fertilization and pregnancy rate). Increasing age is associated with poor ovarian response, smaller ovarian volume, lower antral follicle count and poor stromal vascularity. More studies are needed to determine a place for three-dimensional ultrasound in the assessment of the ovaries prior to and during ovulation induction for medically assisted reproduction.

POLYCYSTIC OVARIAN SYNDROME

Polycystic ovarian syndrome (PCOS) is a major cause of anovulation and oligomenorrhea. In its classic form it is characterized by infertility, oligo- and amenorrhea, hirsutism, acne or seborrhea, and obesity. In 1986 Adams et al., defined the criteria for the ultrasonographic diagnosis of polycystic ovaries: multiple (n >10), small (2–8 mm) peripheral cysts surrounding a dense core of stroma in enlarged (≥8 mL) ovaries **(Fig. 27A)**.[61] However, ovaries which are normal in volume can be polycystic, as demonstrated by histological and biochemical studies. Anatomic structure of the ovaries cannot adequately be assessed with the transabdominal approach in about 42% of cases. Underlying causes are obesity, limited resolution of low-frequency transducers, a full bladder distorting pelvic anatomy, and bowel loops covering the adjacent ovary. More recently, the transvaginal approach for ultrasound scanning of pelvic organs has been used. The high frequency of the transvaginal probe avoids the need for a full bladder and bypasses the problems of attenuation

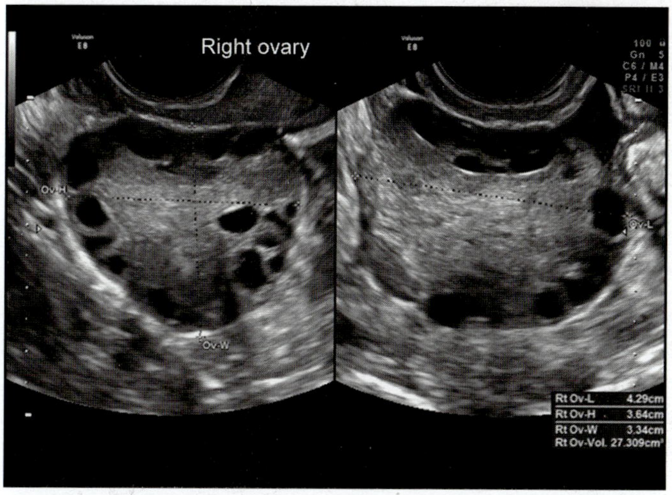

Fig. 27A: B-mode ultrasound image of the ovary in dual frame showing ovary in two orthogonal planes. In both frames the ovary shows multiple small follicles at the periphery of the enlarged and hyperechoic stroma. Both diameters assessed demonstrate more than 10 follicles at the periphery of enlarged ovarian volume 27.3 cc. All these findings are typical for polycystic ovarian appearance.

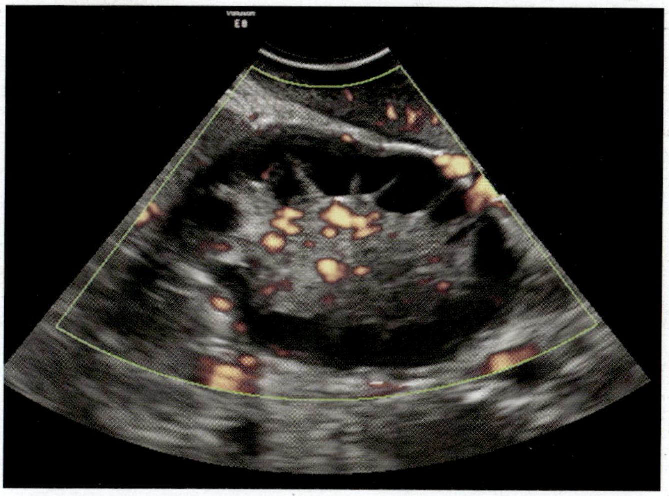

Fig. 27B: Power Doppler scan a polycystic ovary. A large number of small cystic structures are crowded together and stand out from the enlarged ovarian stroma. Stromal vessels are easily visualized by power Doppler imaging.

and artifacts associated with obesity. Furthermore, transvaginal ultrasonography has the advantage of improved resolution, better visualization of pelvic organs, and greater acceptance among patients.

The number of follicles necessary to establish the diagnosis of polycystic ovaries by ultrasonography has been reported to vary between five and fifteen. However, in many reports the highest number of atretic follicles obtained in normal control patients was five per ovary, so it may be established that in polycystic ovaries the number of atretic follicles per ovary would be at least six. Matsunaga et al. identified two types of polycystic ovaries on the basis of ultrasonographic follicular distribution: the peripheral cystic pattern (PCP) and the general cystic pattern (GCP).[62] In the PCP, small cysts are distributed in the subcapsular region of the ovary, whereas in the GCP they are scattered throughout the entire ovarian parenchyma. Recently, Takahashi et al. have shown that these two different ovarian morphologies reflect histopathological differences, and that the PCP and GCP appearances reflect specific endocrine PCOS patterns.[63]

Another parameter considered in the diagnosis of polycystic ovaries is the ovarian volume. However, the wide volume overlap between normal patients and those with PCOS suggests that the discriminative capacity of ovarian volume alone is not sufficient for the ultrasound diagnosis of PCOS.[64] Although, the role of the hyperechogenic ovarian

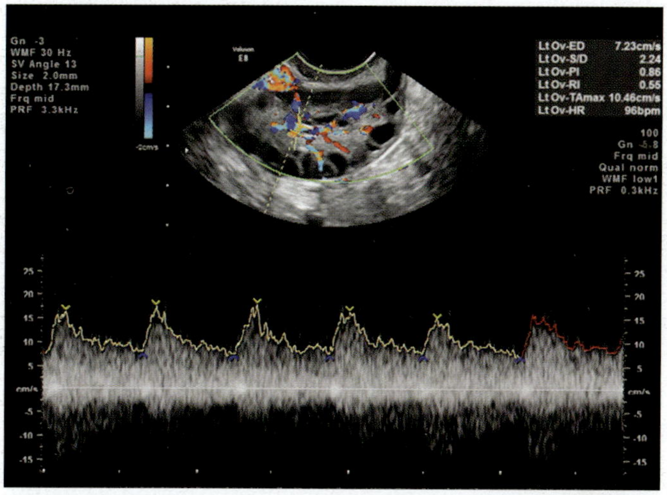

Fig. 27C: Color Doppler and spectral Doppler of the stromal vessels of the same ovary. High velocity and moderate vascular impedance (RI 0.55, PI 0.86) are typical features of flow in polycystic ovaries.

stroma has been emphasized, appraisal of the ovarian stroma echodensity,[65] comparable with computerized quantification,[66] is absolutely subjective and may be interpreted differently by different operators.

Color and power Doppler studies have shown that in patients with polycystic ovarian syndrome important changes in ovarian vascularization occur at the level of the intraovarian arteries **(Figs. 27B and C)**. Although, intraovarian arteries are usually not seen before day 8 to 10 of the 28-day cycle,[67] Battaglia et al. have detected distinct arteries with characteristic low vascular impedance as early as cycle day 3 to 5.[68] In the studied population the results were associated with typical PCOS hormonal parameters and were inversely correlated with the LH/FSH ratio. Tonic hypersecretion of LH during the follicular phase of the menstrual cycle occurs in PCOS and is associated with theca cell and stromal hyperplasia with resultant androgen overproduction.[69] Elevated LH levels may be responsible for increased stromal vascularization by different mechanisms that may act individually or in a cumulative way such as neoangiogenesis, catecholaminergic stimulation, and leukocyte and cytokine activation. In the same study the PCOS patients showed a higher uterine pulsatility index values than nonhirsute normally menstruating women. This finding was correlated with androstenedione levels, confirming a possible direct androgen vasoconstrictive effect due to activation of specific receptors present in the arterial vessel walls and collagen and elastin deposition in smooth muscle cells. The above condition, by reducing the uterine perfusion, has been the theoretical cause that prevents blastocyst implantation, increasing the incidence of miscarriages in PCOS patients. Zaidi et al.[69] and Aleem and Predanic,[70] also having confirmed that the Doppler analysis of stromal arteries in PCOS may be useful in improving the diagnosis and providing further information about the pathophysiology and evolution of the syndrome obtained similar results.

The Doppler evaluation showed that PCP patients, in comparison with GCP patients, present with significantly lower resistance index values at the level of the ovarian stromal arteries. In addition, in 22% of GCP patients, the intraovarian vessels are not recognized[71] and that the GCP appearance of the ovary is more common in the early phase of the disease,[62,63] during the peripubertal period. Thus, the ovarian morphology may evolve from a normal multicystic to polycystic PCP pattern, passing through an ovarian GCP phase. If left untreated PCOS may be regarded as a progressive syndrome. Furthermore, it has recently been shown by comparing oligo- vs. amenorrheic PCOS patients that the amenorrheic patients are older and present with higher PI values in the uterine arteries and lower RI values in intraovarian vessels than oligomenorrheic patients.[72] This finding is associated with a higher plasma LH and androstenedione levels and with a more elevated LH/FSH ratio. Furthermore, significantly higher ovarian volumes and subcapsular small-sized follicles are observed in amenorrheic PCOS patients. This data shows that as the number of ovarian microcysts increases, ovarian volume enlarges and Doppler indices worsen. The clinical and endocrine abnormalities become more remarkable and the menstrual disturbances become more severe.[71]

Recently, it has been demonstrated that obese PCOS women show a higher PI values within the uterine arteries than do lean patients.[73] This is associated with higher hematocrit values, hyperinsulinemia, higher triglyceride levels and lower high-density lipid (HDL) concentrations.

In overweight patients, hyperinsulinemia may be proposed as the uniting factor between increased vascular resistance, obesity, lipid abnormalities and cardiovascular disease.[73,74] Thus, assuming that PCOS patients are at increased risk for cardiovascular disease, it is possible to affirm that obesity may further increase the risk. Unopposed estrogen stimulation is an important contributing factor of endometrial carcinoma and this helps to explain the increased risk in patients with obesity and chronic anovulation.

Recent advances in three-dimensional ultrasound have made accurate noninvasive assessment of the pelvic organs feasible. The ability to visualize the oblique or coronal plane allows accurate volume measurements, especially of irregularly shaped objects.[17,20] Due to the enhanced ability to accurately track an individual's variations in structure during the measurement process, the measurements are considered reliable and highly reproducible.[16]

Wu et al.[75] studied 44 women who presented with a history of irregular menstrual periods; most of the whom women had been diagnosed with polycystic ovary disease (PCOD). The diagnosis of PCOD was based on the clinical symptoms (e.g., menstrual problems, obesity, acne, hirsutism), endocrinologic data (all with reversed serum LH/FSH ratio), and ultrasonographic features (increased ovarian stroma and volume, subcapsular cysts, and thickened capsule). Another 22 women with regular ovulatory cycles were recruited as normal controls. There was no statistically significant difference in age (range, 17–35 years) between these two groups. Three-dimensional ultrasonography was performed to store and document whole volumes of the ovaries for evaluation. Three perpendicular planes of bilateral ovaries were rotated to obtain the largest dimensions. The three-dimensional volume was measured using the trapezoid formula. The ovaries of the patients with PCOD were larger in size, area, and volume than those of normal controls. The mean ovarian volumes (three dimensions;

mean ± SD) were 11.3 ± 3.5 cm^3 in patients with PCOD and 5.5 ± 1.4 cm^3 in the normal controls (P <0.0001). The volumes of the right ovary were 12.2 ± 4.7 cm^3 and 5.3 ± 2.0 cm^3 and the left ones were 10.5 ± 3.6 cm^3 and 5.7 ± 1.6 cm^3 in the PCOD and normal groups, respectively. The right ovary demonstrated a larger volume than the left ovary in women with PCOD (P <0.0001); however, the left ovary was significantly larger than the right one in the normal controls (P <0.0001).

The ovaries in PCOD were significantly increased in size, stroma, and volume (P <0.0001) compared with those of the normal controls. Cut-off values for the ovarian area, stroma, and volume in PCOD were 5.2 cm^2 (sensitivity 93%, specificity 91%), 4.6 cm^2 (sensitivity 91%, specificity 86%), and 6.6 cm^3 (sensitivity 91%, specificity 91%), respectively. The stroma, total ovarian areas, and volume detected by careful rotation and outlining of the longitudinal ovarian cut were increased in 84% (37 of 44), 89% (39 of 44), and 80% (35 of 44) of the patients with PCOD, respectively, in comparison with normal controls. The total ovarian area was highly correlated with the stromal area (r^2 = 0.66).

Undoubtedly, three-dimensional ultrasonography facilitates noninvasive retrospective evaluation and volume calculation. The examination time is short, without increasing the patient discomfort. Three maximal dimensions of the ovaries can be measured easily once the digital volume is documented from either transvaginal or transabdominal three-dimensional ultrasonography, and a superior volume determination can be obtained from the three-dimensional images. The volume measurement in three-dimensional ultrasonography is accurate and highly reproducible **(Fig. 28A)**. The volume of the follicles can be determined precisely, and the volume of the ovary from three-dimensional sonography correlates better with direct measurement of the surgical specimen than that from two-dimensional ultrasonography.[20] The ability of reconstruction increases the diagnostic potential for determining PCOD. The ovaries in PCOD are usually enlarged bilaterally, but they may be about normal size (up to 20% in our study). The stroma areas in PCOD are hypertrophic, and provide yet another subjective ultrasonographic criterion that could differentiate PCOD from the multifollicular ovary. The multifollicular ovary demonstrates a normal or slightly increased size, but an increased number of follicles are noted without an increased amount of stroma. However, the results are usually subjective and not quantitative. Using the

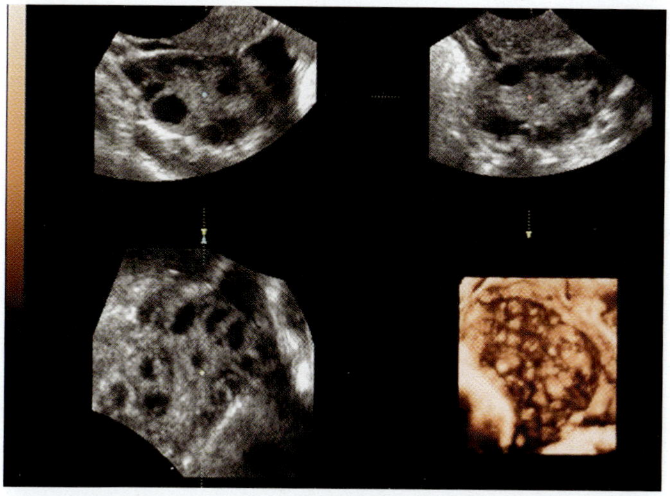

Fig. 28A: Three-dimensional ultrasound image of a polycystic ovary. Surface rendering is demonstrated in the low right image.

computerized quantification measurement, an increased total ovarian area of >5.5 cm^2 highly correlates with increased ovarian stroma at a strict longitudinal ovarian section in the diagnosis of PCOD.

Three-dimensional ultrasonography allows careful and objective evaluation of the ovaries and can repeatedly follow the outline of the ovarian area even after the examination. The value of ovarian stroma can be obtained after subtracting the sum area of ovarian cysts from the total area. The three-dimensional scanning can obtain a more accurate volume data by outlining the contour of the target organ, which is better than traditional two-dimensional ultrasonographic scanning calculated by the ellipsoid formula (height × width × thickness × 0.523). Clearly, three-dimensional ultrasonography can complement two-dimensional ultrasonography for the diagnosis of PCOD since allows excellent spatial evaluation of PCOD with direct quantitative computations from the data.

Apart from morphological and volume measurements assessment of ovarian and uterine vessels can be added to the traditional endocrinologic and ultrasonographic parameters clinically used for the diagnosis of PCOD. Patients with PCOD undergoing ovulation induction for IVF are more likely to develop a greater number of follicles and generate more oocytes compared with women with normal ovaries even though they require less gonadotropin stimulation.[76] Furthermore, since they develop more follicles of all sizes and, in particular small and medium sized follicles, women with PCOD are at greater risk for OHSS.[77] This suggests that the PCOD is more sensitive to gonadotrophin stimulation. The exact mechanism

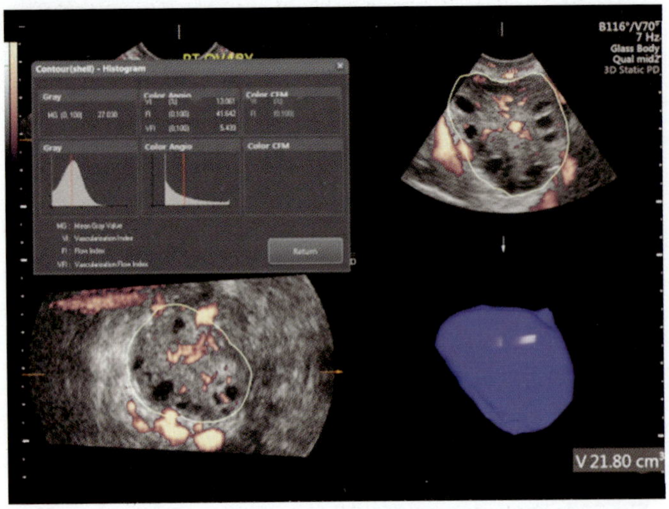

Fig. 28B: 3D ultrasound of the polycystic ovary. VOCAL (Virtual Organ Computer Aided Analysis) calculation of the ovarian volume is demonstrated in the right lower corner. The blue outlines the ovarian contours. The gray box in the upper quadrant of the image is known as volume histogram. The graph on the left shows the average grayness of the calculated volume (density of the tissue ball), and is numerically expressed as a Mean Gray Value (MGV). The right side graph is color angiogram which demonstrates the distribution of color voxels in the calculated volume, describing the abundance of blood vessels in the calculated volume. 3D power Doppler vascular indices (VI, vascularization index; FI, flow index and VFI vascularization flow index) represent 3D power Doppler histogram.

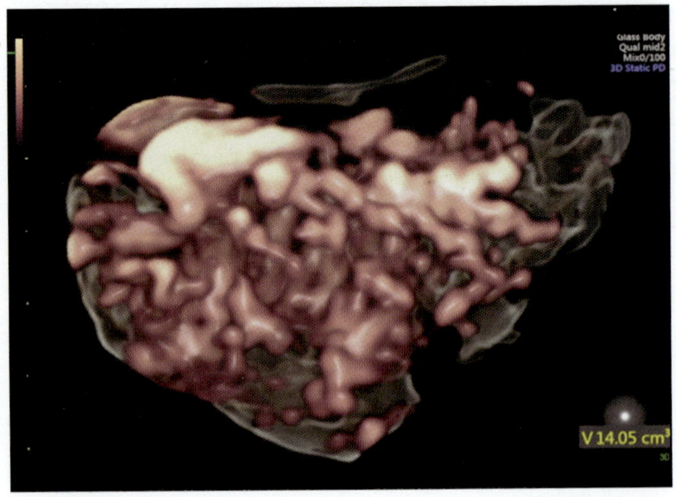

Fig. 28C: Glass body rendering (angio mode) of the 3D ultrasound acquired volume of the polycystic ovary is displayed as power Doppler.

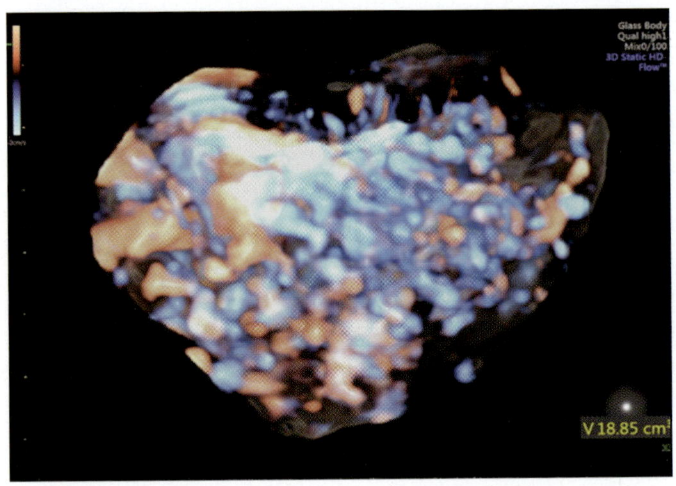

Fig. 28D: Glass body rendering (angio mode) of the 3D ultrasound acquired volume of the polycystic ovary is displayed as high definition Doppler (HD flow).

is unknown although it is possible that the increased ovarian stromal blood flow velocity, in combination with a relatively unchanged impedance to blood flow, may reflect an increased intraovarian perfusion and thus a greater delivery of gonadotropins to the granulosa cells of the developing follicles. This theory may help to explain the greater likelihood of a multifollicular response. Numerous studies showed that women with PCOD have a significantly greater stromal blood flow velocity as detected by transvaginal color Doppler and three-dimensional power Doppler ultrasound **(Fig. 28B)**. The implication of this in ovulation induction treatment is unknown but may help to explain the excessive response often seen in women with PCOD when they are administered gonadotropins. The presence of an increased stromal blood flow velocity in both the PCOD and PCOS groups compared to women with normal ovaries supports the notion that the PCOD is a primary disorder of the ovary. The detection of increased ovarian stromal blood flow velocity by color and pulsed Doppler ultrasound may be a marker in the diagnosis of PCOD. It seems that evaluation of the ovarian stromal vascularity by 3D power Doppler and glass body rendering in angio mode will further increase our knowledge on this enigmatic syndrome **(Figs. 28C and D)**. Using 3D ultrasound technology antral follicles can be counted by using inversion mode rendering, software called SonoAVC (automated volume calculation) or HDlive silhouette mode **(Figs. 29A to D)**.

Luteinized Unruptured Follicle Syndrome

Luteinized unruptured follicle (LUF) syndrome is characterized by regular menses and presumptive ovulation as suggested by a cyclic hormonal profile, similar

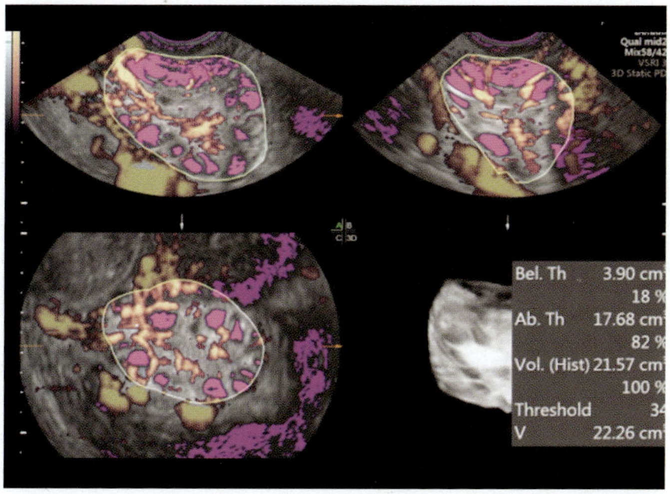

Fig. 29A: 3D ultrasound acquired, VOCAL calculated volume of the ovary. The threshold volume is used to calculate the volume of two structures with different echogenicity in the VOCAL calculated volume. This technique allows calculation of the volume of the follicles and volume of the stroma separately in the total ovarian volume. The pigmented areas (pink color) indicates the threshold which is set at the level of echogenicity of the follicles. The table in the right lower corner illustrates the below threshold volume (Bel. Th.) representing the volume of the pigmented area, which is the follicular volume, and the above threshold volume (Ab. Th.) representing the volume of the ovarian stroma.

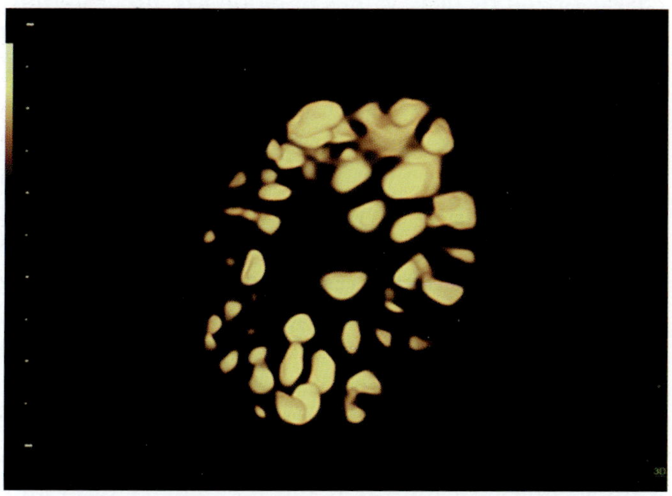

Fig. 29B: 3D ultrasound acquired, VOCAL calculated volume of the polycystic ovary on baseline scan rendered in inversion mode, showing the antral follicles as solid yellow colored balls.

to that seen in normal ovulatory women but without release of the ovum. Although, LUF was first diagnosed at laparoscopy by the absence of an ovulation stigma and the demonstration of lower concentrations of estradiol and progesterone in peritoneal fluid compared with normal

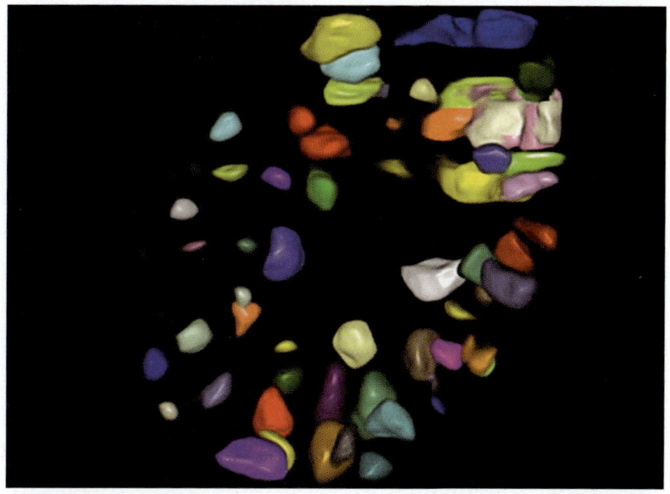

Fig. 29C: The same volume as in previous image. The antral follicle count is here done with SonoAVC (sonographic automated volume calculation). This software color codes the follicles and measures each of them individually.

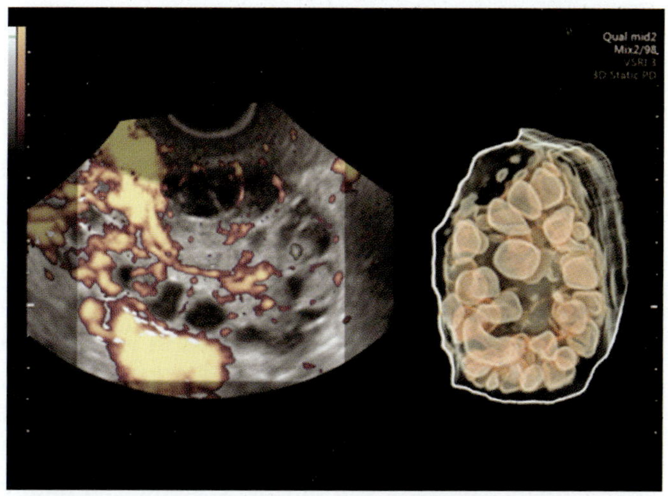

Fig. 29D: 3D ultrasound acquired volume of the polycystic ovary rendered in HDlive silhouette mode, showing numerous follicles scattered throughout the enlarged ovarian stroma.

ovulatory cycles, diagnosis is most commonly made on ultrasound examination, in which there is persistence of the ovarian follicle with progressive loss of its typical echo-free cystic appearance and accumulation of internal echogenicity. The precise etiology of LUF remains uncertain, but impairment of the mid-cycle luteinizing hormone (LH) surge, the absence of the pre-ovulatory progesterone rise, abnormalities of prostaglandin synthesis and a primary abnormality of the oocyte has all been suggested as possible causes. There is a possible association between LUF syndrome and unexplained infertility, chronic pelvic infection and endometriosis. The estimated frequency of this syndrome is between 6 and 47%.

Kupesic et al.[78] tried to evaluate intraovarian resistance index RI in 47 healthy volunteers with ovulatory cycles and compare them to 28 patients with luteal phase defect, and four patients with luteinized unruptured follicle (LUF Sy). Serial sonography allowed daily measurement of the mean follicular diameter and observation of LUF syndrome development which include the follicular collapse, demarcation of the hypoechoic structure with an irregular wall, formation of solid or complex structure representing the corpus luteum, and the extraovarian signs, such as the thickened endometrium and the lack of the free fluid in the cul-de-sac. All these findings were suggestive of ovulation. Doubtful cases (non-visualization of the corpus luteum and/or lack of the serial measurement) were excluded from the current study. LUF syndrome was documented by daily ultrasound observations and endocrinological measurement. During the period of expected ovulation the follicle remained the same size and maintained a tense appearance. Luteinization of the unruptured follicle was seen as a progressive accumulation of the strong echoes located at its periphery.

In the group with regular ovulatory cycles, moderate to high RI (0.56 +/–0.06) was obtained at the rim of the follicle. Significant decline of the RI occurred on the day of LH peak (RI 0.44 +/–0.04). The lowest RI values were obtained during the midluteal phase (RI 0.42 +/–0.06), with a return to higher vascular resistance of 0.50 +/–0.04 during the late luteal phase. In 15 patients, endometrial biopsy was performed, and normal endometrial dating was detected. In the patients with LUF Sy, there was no difference in terms of intraovarian RI which was obtained after the LH peak. Similar RI values were obtained during the follicular and luteal phase (0.55 +/–0.04 vs. 0.54 +/–0.06). Furthermore, there was no difference between the sides in terms of intraovarian vascular resistance. The mean progesterone value in this group was 14.1 ± 6.2 ng/mL, and normal endometrial data was obtained in all patients with LUF Sy.

Similar results were reported by Merce et al.,[79] who did not observe any drop in perifollicular intraovarian resistance after the LH peak. Interestingly, the so called "luteal conversion" did not take place, indicating that the intraovarian and perifollicular neovascularization were either not produced, or were altered in LUF, probably because the follicle failed to rupture.

Indeed, the rise in peri-follicular blood flow during the peri-ovulatory period appears to be primarily regulated by LH. Zaidi et al.[69] reported a decreased blood flow velocity of the peripheral vessels in a patient with LUF Sy after the LH surge to values comparable with those seen in the early follicular phase of the cycle. The reduction in perifollicular blood flow velocity has also been reported in a patient with drug-associated LUF.[80]

Extensive Doppler measurement, biochemical research and three-dimensional ultrasound studies still have to be done to further clarify the causes and consequences of this syndrome.

Luteal Phase Defect

The formation of corpus luteum is an important event in reproductive cycle and one of the crucial factors in early pregnancy support. After ovulation, blood vessels of the theca layer invade the cavity of the ruptured follicle starting the formation of the corpus luteum.

Small luteal cells produce more and more LH receptors and thus amplify the production of progesterone. This chain reaction goes on till the so called midluteal phase which is characterized by peak values of blood LH, progesterone, and the lowest resistance index in corpus luteum blood vessels as proven by transvaginal color and pulsed Doppler by Kupesic et al.[81] Consequently progesterone suppresses the secretion of the gonadotropin, LH and progesterone levels decrease, and RI in the vessels of corpus luteum increases. Whether because of "intrinsic error of mechanism", or because of the interference with external factors (e.g., strenuous exercise, ovulation stimulating drugs), a condition called luteal phase defect occurs. Various names have been assigned to the disorder: short luteal phase, luteal insufficiency, inadequate luteal phase, luteal defect and luteal phase deficiency (LPD). All these names describe the same condition: lack of progesterone, a luteal phase of the cycle shorter than 11 days and, when related to the endometrium, an out-of-phase endometrium by 2 or more days. The new method to detect a corpus luteum abnormality is by ultrasonography. For a better visualization of the corpus luteum a transvaginal approach is used. As an addition to B-mode and real time image, sophisticated ultrasound equipment includes color and pulsed Doppler sonography. The research into the corpus luteum, LPD, early pregnancy and early pregnancy failures has already taken a whole new direction. Until recently, research in this field was carried out mainly using B mode and real time imaging. Glock et al.[82] tried to determine whether the ultrasound appearance size, or change in size of the corpus luteum of early pregnancy correlated with serum progesterone, estradiol E2, or 17-hydroxyprogesterone or were even predictive of pregnancy outcome. Their hypothesis stated: corpus luteum volumes of early human pregnancy would correlate with the serum concentration of steroids produced in the corpus luteum; appearance of the corpus luteum, based on the amount of cystic component, would correlate with serum hormone concentration or pregnancy outcome; and a decrease in corpus luteum volume would be associated with pregnancy loss. Disappointingly, the acquired data showed a lack of correlation between corpus luteum size and steroid products and no correlation between changes in volume and changes in steroid products in early human pregnancy. However, a decreasing corpus luteum volume before 8 weeks' gestation is associated with a higher probability of pregnancy loss. Color flow pulsed Doppler was only used to determine the dominant ovary with corpus luteum and the contralateral one. The dominant ovary showed a low impedance waveform with RI 0.39–0.49, which is characteristic of the blood flow in early pregnancy. The contralateral ovary in each patient demonstrated a high impedance flow RI 0.69–1.0, characteristic of a nondominant ovary. One patient had an RI value of 0.74 in the ovary identified as having a corpus luteum, and RI of 0.79 in the opposite ovary; this high RI in both ovaries was associated with a nonviable outcome.

Kupesic et al.[81] tried to evaluate the intraovarian resistance index RI in 47 healthy fertile volunteers with ovulatory cycles and compare them to 28 patients with luteal phase defect and four patients with luteinized unruptured follicle (LUF Sy). Serial sonography allowed a daily measurement of the mean follicular diameter, visualization of the follicular collapse and demarcation of the hypoechoic structure with an irregular wall, solid or complex structure representing the corpus luteum, as well as observation of the thickened endometrium, and presence of the free fluid in the cul de sac. All these findings were suggestive of ovulation. Doubtful cases (non-visualization of the corpus luteum and/or lack of the serial measurements) were excluded from the current study. LPD was diagnosed by measuring the progesterone levels and performing the endometrial biopsy during the midluteal phase of the menstrual cycle. Sonographic and Doppler findings were correlated to hormonal and histopathological data.

In the group with regular ovulatory cycles (n = 47) different ovarian RI values had been observed. During the stage of the follicular growth and development, moderate to high RI (mean 0.56 ± 0.06) was obtained at the rim of the follicle. Significant decline of the RI occurred for the day of LH peak (RI 0.44 ± 0.04). The lowest RI values were obtained during the midluteal phase (RI 0.42 ± 0.06), with a return to higher vascular resistance of 0.50 ± 0.04 during the late luteal phase. In the LPD group (n = 28) no difference was obtained in terms of intraovarian RI during the follicular phase. However, the mean RI throughout the luteal phase (RI 0.56 ± 0.04) was significantly higher compared to the normals. Furthermore, it did not show any difference between the early, middle and late luteal phase in LPD group.

In the control group, both follicular and luteal RI was significantly lower on the dominant side. However, in the LPD group no difference occurred in terms of intraovarian RI between the sides. The mean progesterone levels were significantly lower in the LPD group (6.9 ± 2.3 ng/mL) than in the controls (24.1 ± 11.4 ng/mL), while histopathology revealed delayed endometrial pattern in all the patients with LPD. The correlation was observed between progesterone and RI during the midluteal phase.

Merce et al.[79] elaborated on all aspects of transvaginal color and pulsed Doppler ultrasonography: its advantages, disadvantages, current possibilities and future directions. In their study of luteal ovarian blood flow they introduced the term "luteal conversion" to describe the Doppler findings during the luteal phase. These Doppler finding include easily obtained Doppler signals, increase in intensity of frequency spectrum, increase in turbulence of the blood flow with extensive dispersion of the maximum frequencies and superposition of multiple waveforms presenting variable maximum systolic velocities and, finally, an increase in the surface and intensity that the color signal occupies in the ovary. The same authors, in their study of LPD, observed that the resistance index of the dominant ovary drops during the luteal phase with respect to the follicular phase, which also occurs in normal cycles and that there were no differences noted regarding this aspect when compared with any phase of the normal cycle. No significant correlation was demonstrated between the index values and serum progesterone levels either.

Glock and Brumsted[83] correlated ovarian blood flow to values of progesterone throughout the cycle. Mean progesterone levels were significantly lower for LPD patients than for normal women throughout the luteal phase. Mean resistance index in LPD patients was significantly higher compared with normal women throughout the follicular and luteal phases. Although, systolic and diastolic velocities were observed to be lower in LPD patients compared with normal women, these differences were not statistically different. High correlations were observed between progesterone and resistance index within each of the luteal time points, achieving its highest value during the midluteal phase luteal. The mean resistance index in the dominant ovary was significantly lower than in the nondominant ovary throughout the cycle in normal women (0.50 versus 0.65), but not in those with LPD (0.60 versus 0.66 $P = 0.37$). In one patient with an anovulatory cycle, the intraovarian resistance index values remained high (mean 0.76, range 0.70 to 0.82).

This study[83] showed a clear correlation between the resistance index of the corpus luteum blood flow and the plasma progesterone in a natural cycle. The strongest correlation was seen in the midluteal phase, the period that corresponds to a peak neovascularization of the corpus luteum. Consistent with this finding, the authors have shown an increase in blood flow impedance in the late luteal phase, the period associated with the onset of the corpus luteum regression. These findings suggest the possibility of using the resistance index of the corpus luteum blood flow as an adjunct to plasma progesterone assay, as an index of luteal function.

Tinkanen,[84] on the other hand found no difference between the blood flow in the corpus luteum in controls with normal luteal phase and infertility patients with an abnormal luteal phase. A short luteal phase, claims the author, is not due to premature vascular regression of the corpus luteum as evaluated by measurement of the vascular resistance.

Strigini et al.[85] observed the change of impedance during the luteal phase of FSH-treated cycles. The uterine pulsatility index during stimulated cycles, both before and after ovulation, was significantly reduced compared with spontaneous cycles. That was explained by an increase of plasma E2. Furthermore, Strigini advocates administration of exogenous progesterone as a supplementation to FSH treated cycles, stating that the uterine pulsatility index after administration of progesterone drops even more than in spontaneous or only with FSH treated cycles.

Kupesic et al.[81] correlated Doppler velocimetry, histological and hormonal markers. They presumed that when combined together, the ultrasound results, the measurement of hormone values and an endometrial biopsy could explain more about LPD. They found out that the mean progesterone levels were significantly lower in the group with luteal phase defect (10.2 ± 4.3 ng/mL) than in controls (21 ± 4.2 ng/mL). The FSH/LH ratio was significantly lower in the group with a delayed endometrial pattern compared to normal subjects during follicular and periovulatory phases (0.70 vs. 1.24; 0.58 vs. 0.75, respectively). There was a close correlation between estradiol levels and the mean diameter of the dominant follicle from days –5 to –1 relative to the days of sonographically observed ovulation. An increase in follicular diameter and endometrial thickness was noted for both normal and luteal phase defect groups.

Intraovarian blood flow resistance showed no difference between the groups during the proliferative phase. A significant decline of the RI occurred in the control group for the day of the LH peak (RI = 0.45 ± 0.04), with a return to the follicular phase level of 0.49 ± 0.02 during the second phase of the menstrual cycle **(Fig. 30A)**. The mean intraovarian RI for the luteal phase defect group (RI = 0.58 ± 0.04) was significantly higher than in the control group throughout the luteal phase **(Fig. 30B)**. Patients in the control group had a significantly lower RI

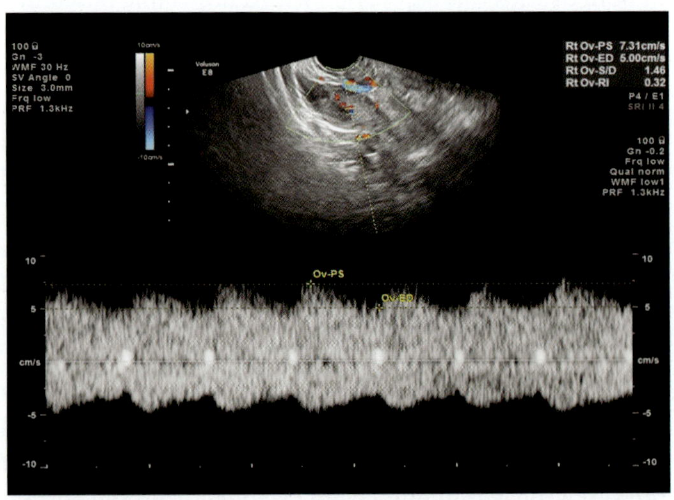

Fig. 30A: Color Doppler ultrasound of a normal corpus luteum. Pulsed Doppler waveform analysis shows high velocity and low resistance index (RI = 0.32), both indicative of a normal corpus luteum function.

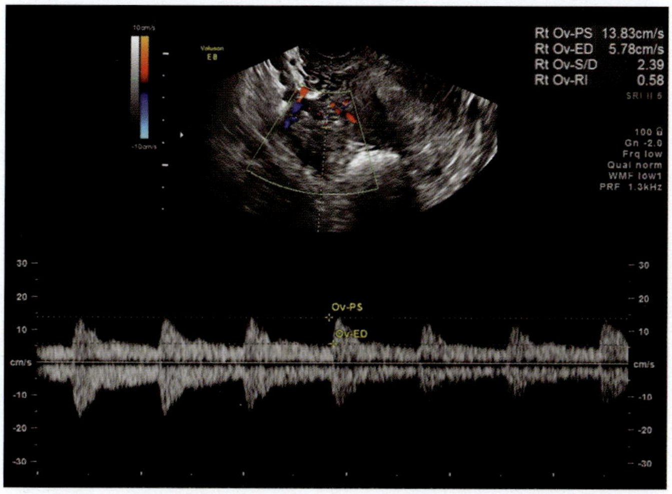

Fig. 30B: Color Doppler ultrasound illustrating luteal phase defect. The increased intraovarian resistance index (RI = 0.58) obtained during the midluteal phase indicates luteal phase defect.

in the dominant than in the nondominant ovary, whereas LPD patients had almost the same RI in both the ovaries. The authors measured blood flow in the spiral arteries as well. The spiral arteries in the control group demonstrated an RI of 0.53 ± 0.04 during the periovulatory phase, and RI values of 0.50 ± 0.02 and 0.51 ± 0.04 were obtained during the midluteal and late luteal phase, respectively. Higher impedance values were obtained from the spiral arteries in the luteal phase defect group during the periovulatory phase (RI = 0.70 ± 0.06, P <0.001), midluteal phase (RI = 0.72 ± 0.06, P < 0.001) and late luteal phase (RI = 0.72 ± 0.04, P <0.001). A close correlation has been found between plasma levels of estradiol and the mean diameter of the follicle. This study clearly demonstrated that patients with normal endometrial development show a similar trend of regression for uterine, radial and spiral artery impedance from the follicular to the luteal phase. In contrast, patients with a delayed endometrial pattern are characterized by an increased uterine vascular resistance during the luteal phase. Since, the most significant difference in terms of RI is obtained for spiral arteries, it might be expected that the endometrial blood flow changes could be used to predict the development of the endometrium and likelihood of pregnancy.

Salim et al.[86] correlated luteal blood in normal pregnancies to the flow in abnormal pregnancies. Their study proved the hypothesis that an absence of luteal flow cannot coexist with a normal pregnancy. The impedance to intraovarian blood flow was significantly higher in patients with an abnormal early pregnancy (missed, incomplete, and threatened abortion) than in women with a normal pregnancy. However, this was not confirmed in patients with a blighted ovum, molar, and an ectopic pregnancy. The impedance to luteal blood flow was almost the same as in normal pregnancy. This difference amongst the subgroups of an abnormal early pregnancy may relate to a different natural history of the disease. Missed and incomplete abortions are manifested as failed early pregnancy with no prospects for further development. A threatened abortion is a potentially similar condition. Whether a decreased corpus luteum blood flow is a potential cause or a consequence of the disease remains unclear. Anembryonic pregnancies, molar or ectopic pregnancies are somewhat different. These pathologic conditions usually are progressive and not self-limited. This can explain why impedance to luteal blood flow in these women is similar to those of women with a normally progressing pregnancy.

Alcazar et al.[87] agree only partially with the results obtained by Salim et al.[86] Alcazar's group found that the mean RI in a missed abortion was higher than in controls. This increased vascular resistance could be explained by the fact that a missed abortion consists of a failure of an early pregnancy to develop, in which the production of human chorionic gonadotropin is impaired, which in turn could have a negative effect on the luteal function. On the other hand, they found no statistically significant difference in RI of patients with a threatened abortion.

Tubal Causes of Infertility

The tubal mucosa responds to the hormonal changes during the menstrual cycle in order to facilitate the transport of sperm and fertilized ova in the process of fertilization. During the luteal phase, decreased tube secretion and more prominent ciliary activity propel the ova into the uterine fundus. If conception does not occur, the secretory and ciliary cells are significantly reduced in number due to withdrawal of endocrine support.

The normal Fallopian tubes are narrow and usually not seen by transabdominal or transvaginal ultrasound unless they contain fluid within their lumina or are surrounded by fluid. The motility and transport function of the oviducts are impaired during all stages of pelvic inflammatory disease. First, during the acute phase, the tube becomes thickened and edematous and contains a large amount of purulent exudate within its lumen **(Fig. 31A)**. Later, the inflammatory process may organize to form a tuboovarian

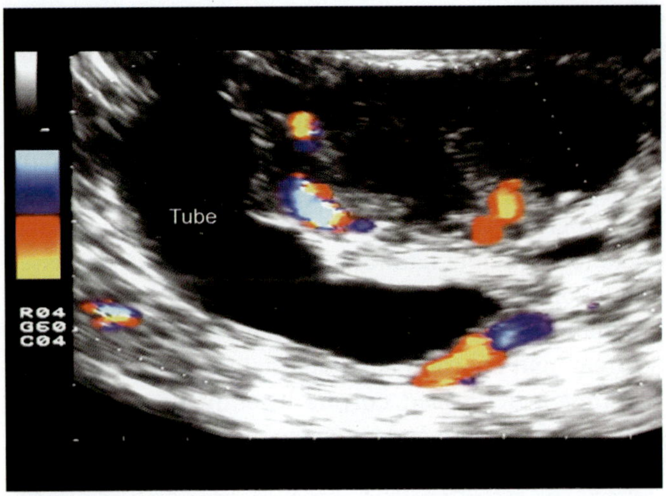

Fig. 31A: Transvaginal color Doppler image of a dilated and fluid filled tube in a patient presenting with acute pelvic pain. Increased vascularization indicates acute pelvic inflammatory disease.

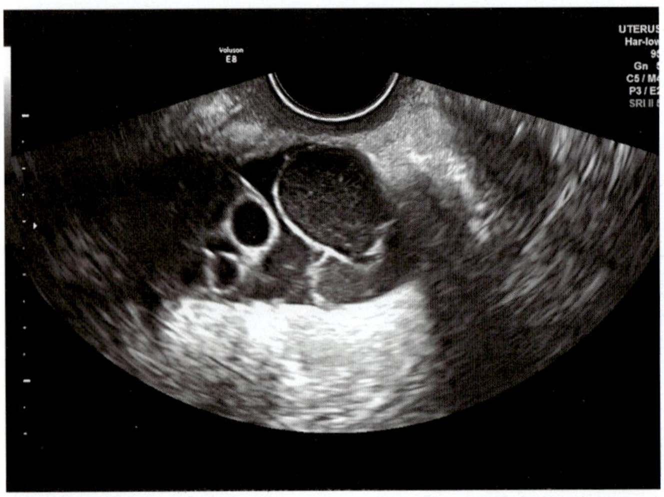

Fig. 31B: B mode ultrasound image of the adnexa showing ipsilateral ovary with follicles (left), and free fluid with low level echogenecities around the ovary. The fluid also shows septations. Low level echogenicities and septated fluid collection are both suggestive of acute pelvic inflammatory condition. If untreated the ovary and the tube may organize to form a tuboovarian abscess.

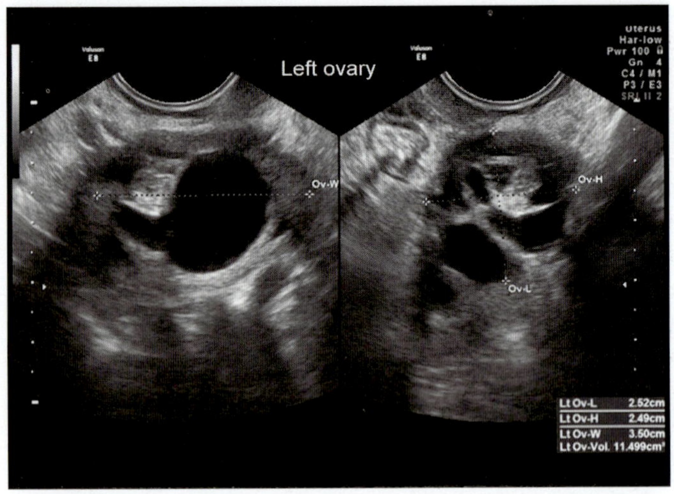

Fig. 31C: Left adnexal mass showing cystic and solid components on B mode ultrasound image. In the left frame the cystic lesion shows a typical shape of a dilated tube-hydrosalpinx and appears adjacent to the ovary. Sonographic findings are typical for chronic stage pelvic inflammatory disease.

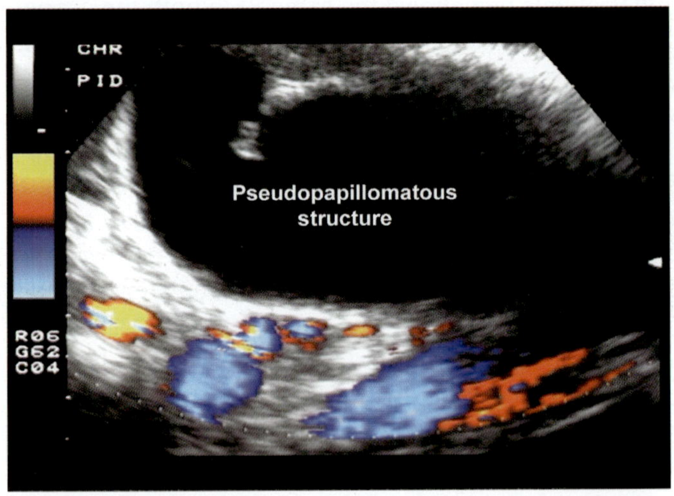

Fig. 31D: Dilated and fluid filled tube with incomplete septation in an infertile patient, caused by a previous pelvic infection.

abscess **(Fig. 31B)**, which will, in most cases lead to scarring and occlusion of the tube **(Fig. 31C)**. Chronic hydrosalpinx is the ultimate remnant of PID: the tube is occluded, thin-walled and filled with fluid **(Fig. 31D)**.

Infertility caused by tubal dysfunction is found in approximately 35% of patients. A history of pelvic inflammatory disease, septic abortion, intrauterine contraceptive device, ruptured appendix, tubal surgery or ectopic pregnancy should alert the physician to the possibility of tubal damage. Amorphous acellular plugs have been identified as the probable cause of obstruction in the proximal tube in nearly 50% of women whose tubes did not opacify on hysterosalpingography. The improved pregnancy rate after uterotubal insufflation and hysterosalpingography suggests that their therapeutic effect may partially result from dislodgment of fallopian tube debris. Reversed spasm at the uterotubal junction is another cause of apparent obstruction on a conventional hysterosalpingogram. In 100 patients with nonfilling on the initial hysterosalpingogram, Lang[88] found that only 39 had persistent occlusion after pharmacologic manipulation and selective tubal salpingography. In the remaining 61 patients the apparent cause of tubal nonfilling was spasm and debris in 49 patients, submucous fibroids in six, synechiae in three, salpingitis isthmica nodosa in two, and a septated uterus in one. Until a few years ago the assessment of the uterine cavity and the Fallopian tube lumen relied on complicated, painful and invasive procedures. The major problem was how to visualize the hollow space within these organs and how to describe the contours of uterine and oviduct walls. The functions of the uterus and the Fallopian tubes depend on their cavities: a uterus filled with endometrial polyp or distorted by a myoma is an obstacle to implantation, while a tortuous and narrow tube with the PID changes does not permit oocytes to descend.

Hysterosalpingography, using radio-opaque dye for X-ray assessment of tubal and uterine anatomy, has been the standard form of investigation for several decades. The disadvantage of this type of investigation is that the ionizing radiation presents a risk to the oocyte: if the conception takes place in the investigation cycle, congenital fetal anomalies may occur. Furthermore, iodine-containing dyes used in X-ray hysterosalpingography can cause an allergic reaction.

In the last two decades, laparoscopy has been the usual procedure for the assessment of tubal status. However, it requires general anesthesia and carries the risk of the anesthetic and of potential surgical complications, such as bowel or vascular injury, false pneumoperitoneum and postoperative discomfort.

Together with the development of ultrasound techniques, a totally new concept of diagnostic procedures has been initiated.[89-91] We have already described in the chapter on hysterosonosalpingography the benefits and limitations of the sonographic evaluation of the tubal patency.

Ovarian Endometrioma

Endometriosis is being increasingly detected amongst infertile patients due to greater use of ultrasound and laparoscopy.[91] On ultrasound ovarian endometrioma has a typical ground glass appearance **(Figs. 32A and B)**. Adhesions can be evaluated by real time transvaginal ultrasound, using the sliding sign technique to determine the likelihood of adhesions. Typical vascular pattern of ovarian endometrioma is considered at the level of ovarian hilus or pericistically **(Fig. 32C)**.[92] Color Doppler ultrasound may detect changes in vascular impedance in the ovaries affected by endometriosis, secondary to interstitial fibrosis and microvascular injury.[93] Surgery is

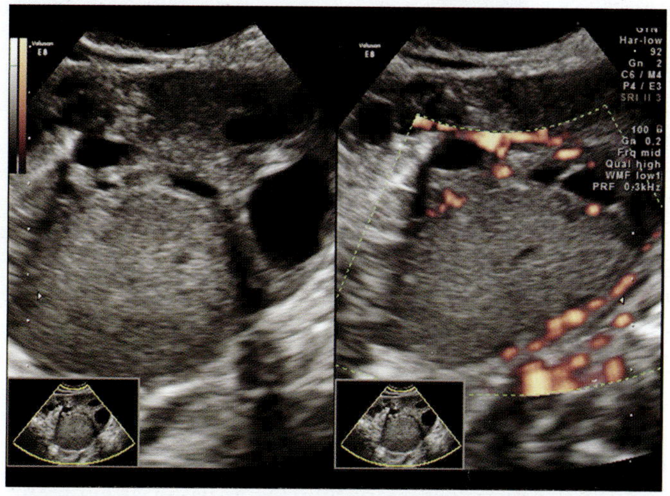

Fig. 32A: Dual frame image – B mode and power Doppler of a well-defined round intraovarian lesion with ground glass echogenicity. Margins show some echogenic flecks. Power Doppler image on the right shows short coursed peripheral vessels. Sonographic and Doppler findings are suggestive of an ovarian endometrioma.

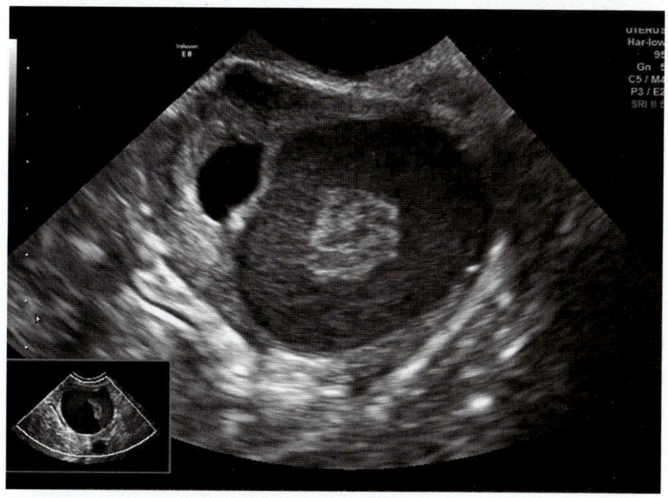

Fig. 32B: B mode ultrasound image of a round, well-defined intraovarian lesion of predominantly ground glass echogenicity. It shows a central, roundish hyperechoic area. The lesion has echogenic flecks in the walls. Posterior acoustic enhancement suggests that the lesion contains fluid. Sonographic findings are suggestive of an ovarian endometrioma. The differential echogenicity can be explained by degenerating blood products in different stages.

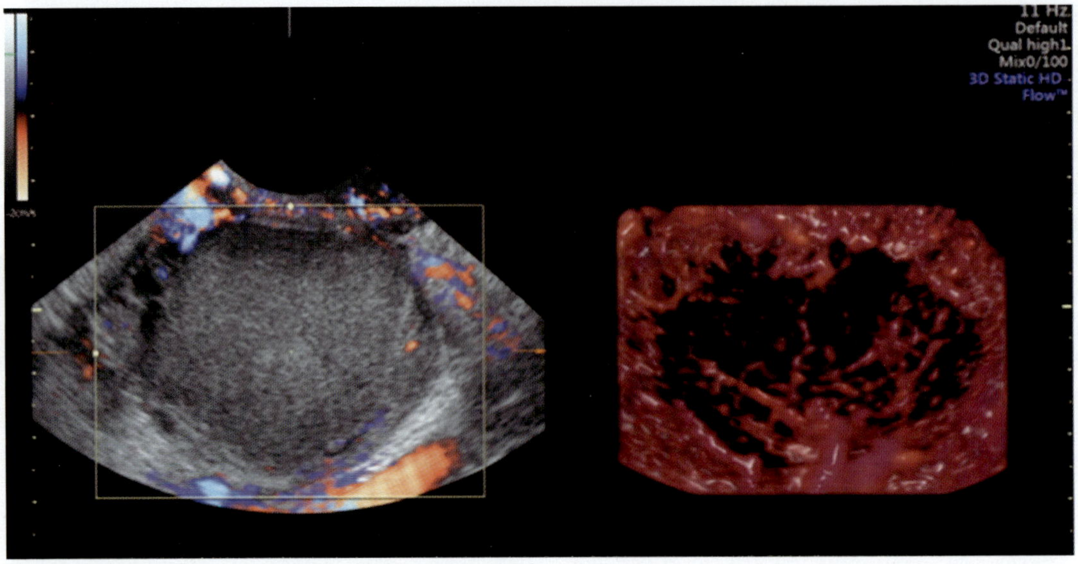

Fig. 32C: 3D ultrasound with power Doppler (HD flow) acquired image of ovarian endometrioma. Angio mode rendering shows short coursed acutely angled vessels, creating an appearance of a "bird's nest", representing typical features of an ovarian endometrioma.

currently being advised only for patients with severe pain or difficult access to growing follicles, and only after careful counselling regarding the potential negative effect on ovarian reserve.[94] Laparoscopic cystectomy demonstrated the highest chance of spontaneous conception, and the lowest risk of postoperative reduction of the ovarian reserve. Medical treatment showed only temporary symptoms relief without improving the fertility outcomes, while the role of ultrasound guided drainage remains to be established.[95]

CONCLUSION

2D and 3D transvaginal sonography with color and power Doppler facilities have made a significant improvement in the assessment of infertility. They may help in the prediction of ovulation and detection of ovulatory disorders.[95] Measurements of uterine perfusion have a predictive value regarding fecundity in patients undergoing different methods of medically assisted reproduction. Absent subendometrial and intraendometrial vascularization on the day of hCG administration appears to be a useful predictor of failure of implantation in IVF cycles, irrespective of the morphological appearance of the endometrium. Studies on uterine and spiral artery perfusion might produce a noninvasive assay of uterine receptivity, giving us more information about the pathophysiology of infertility, especially in the group of patients with unexplained causes.[96-98] Measurement of endometrial and ovarian volumes by three-dimensional ultrasound, assessment of endometrial and ovarian perfusion by 3D power Doppler ultrasound, and screening for congenital uterine anomalies using 3D transvaginal ultrasound play a vital role in infertility management and significantly contribute to better understanding of various disorders that may be encountered in the practice of reproductive endocrinology.[99-101]

REFERENCES

1. Kurjak A, Kupesic-Urek S, Schulman H, Zalud, I. Transvaginal color Doppler in the assessment of ovarian and uterine blood flow in infertile women. Fertil Steril. 1991;56:870.
2. Kurjak A, Kupesic-Urek S. Normal and abnormal uterine perfusion. In: Jaffe R, Warsof LS (Eds). Color Doppler Imaging in Obstetrics and Gynecology, New York: McGraw Hill; 1992. pp. 255-63.
3. Goswamy RK, Silliams G, Steptoe PC. Decreased uterine perfusion a cause of infertility. Hum Reprod. 1988;3: 955-8.
4. Steer CV, Mills CV, Campbell S. Vaginal color Doppler assessment on the day of embryo transfer (ET) accurately predicts patients in an in vitro fertilization programme with suboptimal uterine perfusion who fail to become pregnant. Ultrasound Obstet Gynaecol. 1991;1:79-82.
5. Tsai YC, Chang JC, Tai MJ, Kung FT, Yang LC, Chang SY. Relationship of uterine perfusion to outcome of intrauterine insemination. J Ultrasound Med. 1996;15:633-6.
6. Steer CV, Tan SL, Mason BA, Campbell S. Midluteal phase vaginal color Doppler assessment of uterine

artery impedance in a subfertile population. Fertil Steril. 1994;61:53-8.
7. Kupesic S. The first three weeks assessed by transvaginal color Doppler. J Perinat Med. 1996;24:301-17.
8. Cacciatore B, Simberg N, Fusaro P, Tiitinen A. Transvaginal Doppler study of uterine artery blood flow in in-vitro fertilization—embryo transfer cycles. Fertil Steril. 1996;66(1):130-4.
9. Freidler S, Schenker JG, Herman A, Lewin A. The role of ultrasonography in the evaluation of endometrial receptivity following assisted reproductive treatments: a critical review. Hum Reprod Update. 1996;2:323-35.
10. Gonen Y, Calderon M, Direnfeld M, Abramovici H. The impact of sonographic assessment of the endometrium and meticulous hormonal monitoring during natural cycles in patients with failed donor artificial insemination. Ultrasound Obstet Gynecol. 1991;1:122-6.
11. Abdalla HI, Brooks AA, Johnson MR, Kirkland A, Thomas A, Studd JW. Endometrial thickness: a predictor of implantation in ovum recipients? Hum Reprod. 1994;9:363-5.
12. Khalifa E, Brzyski RG, Oehninger S, Acosta AA, Muasher SJ. Sonographic appearance of the endometrium: the predictive value for the outcome of in vitro fertilization in stimulated cycles. Hum Reprod. 1992;7:677-80.
13. Serafini P, Batzofin J, Nelson J, Olive D. Sonographic uterine predictors of pregnancy in women undergoing ovulation induction for assisted reproductive treatments. Fertil Steril. 1994;62:815-22.
14. Sher G, Herbert C, Maassarani G, Jacobs MH. Assessment of the late proliferative phase endometrium by ultrasonography in patients undergoing in vitro fertilization and embryo transfer (IVF/ET). Hum Reprod. 1991;6:232-7.
15. Zaidi J, Campbell S, Pitroff R, Tan SL. Endometrial thickness, morphology, vascular penetration and velocimetry in predicting implantation in an in vitro fertilization program. Ultrasound Obstet. Gynecol. 1995;6(3):191-8.
16. Kyei-Mensah A, Maconochie N, Zaidi J, Pittrof R, Campbell S, Tan SL. Transvaginal three-dimensional ultrasound: reproducibility of ovarian and endometrial volume measurements. Fertil Steril. 1996;66:718-22.
17. Riccabona M, Nelson TR, Pretorius DH. Three-dimensional ultrasound: accuracy of distance and volume measurements. Ultrasound Obstet Gynecol. 1996;4:29-34.
18. Gilja OH, Smievoll I, Thune N, Matre K, Hausken T, Odegaard S. In vivo comparison of 3D ultrasonography and magnetic resonance imaging in volume estimation of human kidney. Ultrasound Med Biol. 1995;21:25-32.
19. Lee A, Sator M, Kratochwil A, Deutinger J, Vytiska-Binsdorfer E, Bernaschek G. Endometrial volume change during spontaneous menstrual cycles: volumetry by transvaginal three-dimensional ultrasound. Fertil Steril. 1997;68:831-5.
20. Kyei-Mensah A, Zaidi J, Pittrof R, Shaker A, Campbell S, Tan SL. Transvaginal three-dimensional ultrasound: accuracy of follicular volume measurements. Fertil Steril. 1996;65:371-6.
21. Kupesic S, Bekavac I, Bjelos D, Kurjak A. Assessment of endometrial receptivity by transvaginal color Doppler and three-dimensional power Doppler ultrasonography in patients undergoing in vitro fertilization procedures. J Ultrasound Med. 2001;20:125-34.
22. Ashton D, Amin HK, Richart RM, Neuwirth RS. The incidence of asymptomatic uterine anomalies in women undergoing transcervical tubal sterilization. Obstet. Gynecol. 1988;72:28-30.
23. Sorensen S. Estimated prevalence of mullerian anomalies. Acta Obstet Gynecol Scand. 1988;67:441-5.
24. Gaucherand P, Awada A, Rudigoz RC, Dargent D. Obstetrical prognosis of septate uterus: a plea for treatment of the septum. Eur J Obstet Gynecol Reprod Biol. 1994;54:109-12.
25. Fedele L, Arcaini L, Parazzini F, Vercellini P, Nola GD. Metroplastic hysteroscopy and fertility. Fertil Steril. 1993;59:768-70.
26. Heinonen PK, Saarikoski S, Pystynen P. Reproductive performance of women with uterine anomalies. An evaluation of 182 cases. Acta Obstet Gynecol Scand. 1982;61:157-62.
27. Fedele L, Bianchi S, Marchini M, Franchi D, Tozzi L, Dorta M. Ultrastructural aspects of endometrium in infertile women with septate uterus. Fertil Steril. 1996;65:750-2.
28. Cararach M, Penella J, Ubeda J, Iabastida R. Hysteroscopic incision of the septate uterus: scissors versus resectoscope. Hum Reprod. 1994;9:87-9.
29. Goldenberg M, Sivan E, Sharabi Z. Reproductive outcome following hysteroscopic management of intrauterine septum and adhesions. Hum Reprod. 1995;10:2663-5.
30. Valdes C, Malini S, Malinak LR. Ultrasound evaluation of female genital tract anomalies: a review of 64 cases. Am J Obstet Gynecol. 1984;149:285-90.
31. Nicolini U, Bellotti B, Bonazzi D, Zamberleti G, Battista C. Can ultrasound be used to screen uterine malformation? Fertil Steril. 1987;47:89-93.
32. Reuter KL, Daly DC, Cohen SM. Septate versus bicornuate uteri: errors in imaging diagnosis. Radiology. 1989;172:749-52.
33. Randolph J, Ying Y, Maier D, Schmidt C, Riddick D. Comparison of real-time ultrasonography, hysterosalpingography, and laparoscopy/hysteroscopy in the evaluation of uterine abnormalities and tubal patency. Fertil Steril. 1986;5:828-32.
34. Richman TS, Viscomi GN, Cherney AD, Polan A. Fallopian tubal patency assessment by ultrasound following fluid injection. Radiology. 1984;152:507-10.
35. Salle B, Sergeant P, Galcherand P, Guimont I, De Saint Hilaire P, Rudigoz RC. Transvaginal hysterosonographic evaluation of septate uteri: a preliminary report. Hum Reprod. 1996;11:1004-7.
36. Marshall C, Mintz DI, Thickman D, Gussman H, Kressel Y. MR evaluation of uterine anomalies. Radiology. 1987;148:287-9.

37. Carrington BM, Hricak M, Naruddin RN. Mullerian duct anomalies: MR evaluation. Radiology. 1990;170:715-20.
38. Jurkovic D, Giepel A, Gurboeck K, Jauniaux E, Natucci M, Campbell S. Three-dimensional ultrasound for the assessment of uterine anatomy and detection of congenital anomalies: a comparison with hysterosalpingography and two-dimensional sonography. Ultrasound Obstet Gynecol. 1995;5:233-7.
39. Taylor PJ, Cumming DC. Hysteroscopy in 100 patients. Fertil Steril. 1979;31:301-4.
40. Kupesic S, Kurjak A. Septate uterus: detection and prediction of obstetrical complications by different forms of ultrasonography. J Ultrasound Med. 1998;17:631-6.
41. Dabrashrafi H, Bahadori M, Mohammad K, Alavi M, Moghadami-Tabrizi N, Zandinejad R. Septate uterus: New idea on the histologic features of the septum in this abnormal uterus. Am J Obstet Gynecol. 1995;172:105-7.
42. Balen FG, Allen CM, Gardener JE, Siddle NC, Lees WR. Three-dimensional reconstruction of ultrasound images of the uterine cavity. Br J Radiol. 1993;66:588-91.
43. Weinraub Z, Maymon R, Shulman A, Bukovsky J, Kratochwil A, Lee A, et al. Three-dimensional saline contrast rendering of uterine cavity pathology. Ultrasound Obstet Gynecol. 1996;277-82.
44. Kupesic S, Kurjak A, Skenderovic S, Bjelos D. Screening for uterine abnormalities by three-dimensional ultrasound improves perinatal outcome. J Perinat Med. 2002;30:9-17.
45. Kurjak A, Kupesic S, Miric D. The assessment of benign uterine tumor vascularization by transvaginal color Doppler. Ultrasound Med Biol. 1992;18: 645-9.
46. Brosens JJ, de Souza NM, Barker FG, Paraschos T, Winston RM. Endovaginal ultrasonography in the diagnosis of adenomyosis uteri: identifying the predictive characteristics. Br J Obstet Gynaecol. 1995;102(6):471.
47. Schlaff WD, Hurst BS. Preoperative sonographic measurement of endometrial pattern predicts outcome of surgical repair in patients with severe Asherman's syndrome. Fertil Steril. 1995;63:410-3.
48. Zaidi J, Barber J, Kyei-Mensah A, Pittrof R, Campbell S, Tan SL. Relationship of ovarian stromal blood flow at baseline ultrasound to subsequent follicular response in an in-vitro fertilization program. Obstet Gynecol. 1996;88:779-84.
49. Engmann L, Sladkevicius P, Agrawal R, Bekir JS, Campbell S, Tan SL. Value of ovarian stromal blood flow velocity measurement after pituitary suppression in the prediction of ovarian responsiveness and outcome of in-vitro fertilization treatment. Fertil Steril. 1999;71(1):22-9.
50. Wittmack FM, Kreger DO, Blasco L, Tureck RW, Mastroianni L Jr, Lessey BA. Effect of follicular size on oocyte retrieval, fertilization, cleavage, and embryo quality in vitro fertilization cycles: a 6-year data collection. Fertil Steril. 1994;62:1205-10.
51. Golan A, Herman A, Soffer Y, Bukovsky I, Ron-El R. Ultrasonic control without hormone determination for ovulation induction in in-vitro fertilization/embryo-transfer with gonadotropin-releasing hormone analogue and human menopausal gonadotropin. Hum Reprod. 1994;9:1631-3.
52. Shoham Z, DiCarlo C, Pater A, Conway GS, Jacobs HS. Is it possible to run a successful ovulation induction program based solely on ultrasound monitoring? The importance of endometrial measurements. Fertil Steril. 1991;56:836-41.
53. Tan SL. Simplification of IVF therapy. Curr Opin Obstet Gynecol. 1994;6:111-4.
54. Steiner H, Staudach A, Spitzer D, Schaffer H. Three-dimensional US in obstetrics and gynaecology: technique, possibilities and limitations. Hum Reprod. 1994;9:1773-8.
55. Penzias AS, Emmi AM, Dubey AK, Layman LC, DeCherney AH, Reindollar RH. Ultrasound prediction of follicle volume: is the mean diameter reflective? Fertil Steril. 1994;62:1274-6.
56. Feichtinger W. Transvaginal three-dimensional imaging for evaluation and treatment of infertility. In: Merz E (Ed). 3-D Ultrasound in Obstetrics and Gynecology. Philadelphia: Lippincott Williams & Wilkins; 1998. pp. 37-43.
57. Lass A, Skull J, McVeigh E, Margara R, Winston RM. Measurement of ovarian volume by transvaginal sonography before ovulation induction with human menopausal gonadotrophin for in-vitro fertilization can predict poor response. Hum Reprod. 1997;12:294-7.
58. Oyesanya OA, Parsons JH, Collins WP, Campbell S. Total ovarian volume before human chorionic gonadotrophin administration for ovulation induction may predict the hyperstimulation syndrome. Hum Reprod. 1995;10:3211-2.
59. Kupesic S, Kurjak A. Predictors of in vitro fertilization outcome by three-dimensional ultrasound. Hum Reprod. 2002;17(4):950-5.
60. Kupesic S, Kurjak A, Bjelos D, Vujisic S. Three-dimensional ultrasound ovarian measurements and in vitro fertilization outcome are related to age. Fertil Steril. 2003;79(1):190-7.
61. Adams J, Franks S, Polson DW, Mason HD, Abdulwahid N, Tucker M, et al. Multifollicular ovaries: clinical and endocrine features and response to pulsatile gonadotropin-releasing hormone. Lancet. 1985;2:1375-8.
62. Matsunaga I, Hata T, Kitao M. Ultrasonographic identification of polycystic ovary. Asia-Oceania J Obstet Gynecol. 1985;11:227-32.
63. Takahashi K, Ozaki T, Okada M, Uchida A, Kitao M. Relationship between ultrasonography and histopathological changes in polycystic ovarian syndrome. Hum Reprod. 1994;9:2255-8.
64. Battaglia C, Artini PG, D'Ambrogio G, Galli PA, Genazzani AR. Uterine and ovarian blood flow measurement. Does the full bladder modify the flow resistance? Acta Obstet Gynecol Scand. 1994;73:716-8.
65. Ardaens Y, Robert Y, Lemaitre L, Fossati P, Dewailly D. Polycystic ovarian disease: contribution of vaginal endosonography and reassessment of ultrasonic diagnosis. Fertil Steril. 1991;55:1062-8.

66. Robert Y, Dubrulle F, Gaillandre L, Ardaens Y, Thomas-Desrousseaux P, Lemaitre L, et al. Ultrasound assessment of ovarian stroma hypertrophy in hyperandrogenism and ovulation disorders: visual analysis versus computerized quantification. Fertil Steril. 1995;64:307-12.
67. Merce LT, Garces D, Barco MJ, De la Fuente P. Intraovarian Doppler velocimetry in ovulatory, dysovulatory and anovulatory cycles. Ultrasound Obstet Gynecol. 1992;2:197-202.
68. Battaglia C, Artini PG, D'Ambrogio G, Genazzani AD, Genazzani AR. The role of color Doppler imaging in the diagnosis of polycystic ovary syndrome. Am J Obstet Gynecol. 1995;172:108-13.
69. Zaidi J, Campbell S, Pittrof R, Kyei-Mensah A, Shaker A, Jacobs HS, et al. Ovarian stromal blood flow in women with polycystic ovaries - a possible new marker for diagnosis? Hum Reprod. 1995;10:1992-5.
70. Aleem FA, Predanic M. Transvaginal color Doppler determination of the ovarian and uterine blood flow characteristics in polycystic ovary disease. Fertil Steril. 1996;65:510-6.
71. Battaglia C, Artini PG, Salvatori M, Giulini S, Petraglia F, Maxia N, et al. Ultrasonographic patterns of polycystic ovaries; color Doppler and hormonal correlations. Ultrasound Obstet Gynecol. 1998;11:332-6.
72. Battaglia C, Artini PG, Genazzani AD, Florio P, Salvatori M, Sgherzi MR, et al. Color Doppler analysis in oligo- and amenorrheic women with polycystic ovary syndrome. Gynecol Endocrinol. 1997;11:105-10.
73. Battaglia C, Artini PG, Genazzani AD, Sgherzi MR, Salvatori M, Giulini S, et al. Color Doppler analysis in lean and obese women with polycystic ovary syndrome. Ultrasound Obstet Gynecol. 1996;7:342-6.
74. Wild RA, Van Nort JJ, Grubb B, Bachman W, Hartz A, Bartholomew M. Clinical signs of androgen excess as risk factors for coronary artery disease. Fertil Steril. 1990;54:255-9.
75. Wu MH, Tang HH, Hsu CC, Wang ST, Huang KE. The role of three-dimensional ultrasonographic images in ovarian measurement. Fertil Steril. 1998;69:1152-5.
76. MacDougall MJ, Tan SL, Balen A, Jacobs HS. A controlled study comparing patients with and without polycystic ovaries undergoing in-vitro fertilization. Hum Reprod. 1993;8:233-7.
77. MacDougall MJ, Tan SL, Jacobs HS. In-vitro fertilization and the ovarian hyperstimulation syndrome. Hum Reprod. 1992;7:597-600.
78. Kupesic S, Kurjak A. The assessment of normal and abnormal luteal function by transvaginal color Doppler sonography. Eur J Obstet Gynecol Reprod Biol. 1997; 72:83-7.
79. Merce LT, Garces D, De la Fuente F. Conversion lutea de la onda de velocidad de fluio ovarica: nuevo parametro ecografico de ovulacion y funcion lutea. Acta Obstet Gynecol. Scand (ed Esp). 1989;2:113-4.
80. Bourne TH, Reynolds K, Waterstone J, Okokon E, Jurkovic D, Campbell S, et al. Paracetamol-associated luteinized unruptured follicle syndrome: effect on intrafollicular blood flow. Ultrasound Obstet Gynecol. 1991;1:420-5.
81. Kupesic S, Kurjak A, Vujisic S, Petrovic Z. Luteal phase defect: comparison between Doppler velocimetry, histological and hormonal markers. Ultrasound Obstet Gynaecol. 1997;9:1-8.
82. Glock JL, Blackman JA, Badger GJ, Brumsted JR. Prognostic significance of morphologic changes of the corpus luteum by transvaginal ultrasound in early pregnancy monitoring. Obstet Gynecol. 1995;85:37-41.
83. Glock JL, Brumsted JR. Color flow pulsed Doppler ultrasound in diagnosing luteal phase defect. Fertil Steril. 1995;64:500-4.
84. Tinkanen H. The role of vascularization of the corpus luteum in the short luteal phase studied by Doppler ultrasound. Acta Obstet Gynecol Scand. 1994;73:321-3.
85. Strigini FAL, Scida PAM, Parri C, Visconti A, Susini S, Genazzani AR. Modifications in uterine and intraovarian artery impedance in cycles of treatment with exogenous gonadotropins: effects of luteal phase support. Fertil Steril. 1995;64:76-80.
86. Salim A, Žalud I, Farmakides G, Schulmal H, Kurjak A, Latin V. Corpus luteum blood flow in normal and abnormal early pregnancy: Evaluation with transvaginal color and pulsed Doppler sonography. J Ultrasound Med. 1994;13:971-5.
87. Alcazar JL, Laparte C, Lopez-Garcia G. Corpus luteum blood flow in abnormal early pregnancy. J Ultrasound Med. 1996;15:645-9.
88. Lang EK. Organic vs. functional obstruction of the fallopian tubes: differentiation with prostaglandin antagonist- and B2-mediated hysterosalpingography and selective ostial salpingography. AJR. 1991;157:77-80.
89. Kupesic S, Plavsic MB. 2D and 3D hysterosalpingo-contrast-sonography in the assessment of uterine cavity and tubal patency. Eur J Obstet Gynecol Reprod Biol. 2007;133(1):64-9.
90. Tur-Kaspa I, Gal M, Hartman M, Hartman J, Hartman A. A prospective evaluation of uterine abnormalities by saline infusion sonohysterography in 1,009 women with infertility or abnormal uterine bleeding. Fertil Steril. 2006;86(6):1731-5.
91. Mishra VV, Gaddagi RA, Aggarwal R, et al. Prevalence, characteristics and management of endometriosis amongst infertile women: a one year retrospective study. H Clin Diagn Res. 2015;9(6):454-7.
92. Kurjak A, Kupesic S. Scoring system for prediction of ovarian endometriosis based on transvaginal color and pulsed Doppler sonography. Fertil Steril. 1994;62(1)81-8.
93. Qiu JJ, Liu MH, Zhang ZX, et al. Transvaginal color Doppler sonography predicts ovarian interstitial fibrosis and microvascular injury in women with ovarian endometriotic cysts. Acta Obstetr Scand. 2012;91(5):605-12.

94. Psaroudakis D, Hirsch M, Davis C. Review of the management of ovarian endometriosis: paradigm shift towards conservative approaches. Curr Opin Obstet Gynecol. 2014;26(4):266-74.
95. Sun W, Stegmann BJ, Henne M, Catherino WH, Segars JH. A new approach to ovarian reserve testing. Fertil Steril. 2008;90(6):2196-202.
96. Kupesic S. Three-dimensional ultrasound in reproductive medicine. Ultrasound Obstet Gynecol. 2005;5:304-15.
97. Zohav E, Bar Hava I, Meltcer S, Rabison J, Anteby EY, Orvieto R. Early endometrial changes following successful implantation. 2and 3D ultrasound study. Clin Exp Obstet Gynecol. 2008;35:255-6.
98. El Mazny A, About Salem N, Elshenoufy H. Doppler study of uterine hemodynamics in women with unexplained infertility. Eur J Obstet Gyencol Reprod Biol. 2013;171(1):84-7.
99. Bocca SM, Oehninger S, Stadtmauer L, et al. A study of the cost, accuracy and benefits of 3-dimensional sonography compared to hysterosalpingography in women with uterine abnormalities. J Ultrasound Med. 2012;31(1):81-5.
100. Sheikh M, Kupesic Plavsic S. Role of ultrasound in the assessment of female infertility. Donald School J Ultrasound Obstet Gynecol. 2014;8(2):184-200.
101. Tabi S, Kupesic Plavsic S. The role of three-dimensional ultrasound in the assessment of congenital uterine anomalies. Donald School J Ultrasound Obstet Gynecol. 2012;6:415-23.

59

CHAPTER

Two-dimensional and Three-dimensional Saline Infusion Sonography and Hystero-contrast-salpingography

Sanja Kupesic Plavsic, Sonal Panchal

INTRODUCTION

Evaluation of uterine anatomy and tubal status is on one of the initial steps in the diagnostic workup of infertile patients. Saline infusion sonography (SIS) and hystero-contrast-sonography are currently performed as a part of the infertility workup to rule our uterine abnormalities and assess tubal patency, respectively. This chapter is a revision of the previous edition's chapter "2D and 3D Saline Infusion Sonography and Hystero-Contrast-Salpingography". It includes updated bibliography, and additional high resolution ultrasound images. By the end of this chapter the interested reader should be able to gain an objective point-of-view on the role of ultrasound in performing ultrasound assessment of the uterine cavity and the fallopian tubes with contrast enhancement.

The number of cases of tubal sterility is increasing and tubal factors, such as tubal dysfunction or obstruction, account for approximately 35% of the causes of infertility.[1,2] A history of pelvic inflammatory disease (PID), septic abortion, intrauterine contraception device use, ruptured appendix, tubal surgery or ectopic pregnancy should alter the physician to the possibility of tubal damage. One aspect of the infertility investigation which has changed little over the last 20 years is that of the assessment of fallopian tube patency. Until now, the most frequently used procedures to demonstrate tubal patency have been X-ray hysterosalpingography (HSG) and chromopertubation during laparoscopy.[3]

Hysteroscopy is a technique, which complements hysterosalpingography. It can accurately differentiate between endometrial polyps and submucous leiomyomas and can be used for their treatment. The same method is useful in establishing the definitive diagnosis and treatment of intrauterine adhesions and congenital anomalies of the uterus. Risk factors include perforation of the uterus, hemorrhage, infection and eventually anesthetic risk if anesthesia is required.

Hysteroscopy-directed falloposcopy can detect obstruction of the tubal ostium and can be utilized to examine the entire length of the tubal lumen.[4] Treatment of the proximal tubal obstruction can immediately follow the diagnosis. Transcervical tubal cannulation or balloon tuboplasty performed by hysteroscopic approach are the methods of choice.[5]

During the last three decades laparoscopy was used as a gold standard for investigation of the tubal status, but it requires a general anesthesia and carries a risk of surgical complications, such as bowel or vascular injury, hemorrhage, infection, anesthetic risk and postoperative discomfort. With a Jarcho-type of cannula placed in the uterine cavity, one can manipulate the uterus and by instilling indigo-carmine saline, or other tinted saline, can test for tubal competence. Using laparoscopy physician can explore pelvic anatomy and upper abdominal cavity. This approach is useful for evaluation of the ovarian disease, genital anomalies and assessment of tubal patency. Furthermore, it is a valuable tool for staging of endometriosis. Laparoscopy is also used for the assessment of patients with chronic pelvic pain, evaluation and staging of pelvic neoplasia, as well as for a prognostic review of the previous infertility surgical procedure. It has also been helpful in obtaining peritoneal washings and cultures in patients with positive history of PID.

Ultrasound imaging of female pelvis has significantly improved with the use of high-frequency vaginal ultrasound probes. Normal fallopian tubes are usually not seen by vaginal sonography unless some fluid surrounds them. The contrasting fluid may be one of the following: normal serous fluid, follicular fluid during or after ovulation, blood, ascitic fluid, or products of an exudative or infectious process. If the fallopian tube is not filled with fluid its lumen cannot be detected.

Saline infusion sonography of the uterine cavity and hystero-contrast-salpingography (Hy-Co-SY) are

TABLE 1: The accuracy of hystero-contrast-salpingography (Hy-Co-Sy) compared to X-ray HSG.

Authors (year)	Total number	Accuracy N (%)	Sensitivity (%)	Specificity (%)
Richman et al. (1984)[13]	36		100	96
Peters and Coulam (1991)[6]	27	19 (70,37)	–	–
Volpi et al. (1991)[7]	21	19 (92,20)	–	–
Stern et al. (1992)[8]	89	72 (80,90)		
Battaglia et al. (1996)[31]	60	52 (86,66)		

informative variations of X-ray hysterosalpingography, a standard radiographic technique for studying the uterine cavity and fallopian tubes following transcervical infusion of the iodinated contrast under fluoroscopic observation. When sonographic evaluation of the uterine lumen with contrast is combined with evaluation of the tubes, this procedure is called Hy-Co-Sy, sonohysterosalpingography, or sono-HSG. Sonohysterography has also been called hysterosonography and saline infusion sonohysterography. Hy-Co-Sy is based on introduction of a sonographic enhancing positive contrast medium into the uterine cavity and the fallopian tubes. This positive contrast medium is usually used following the instillation of the negative contrast media into the uterine cavity. The advantage of sonolucent fluid is that it better delineates hyperechogenic surface of the endometrium. Positive contrast agents outline the course of the fallopian tubes, producing their hyperechogenic appearance. Microparticles of galactose, micro-air-bubbles and albumin have been extensively studied.[6-9] The most affordable option is to use saline solution with air.

Benefits of Hy-Co-Sy are the following: Avoidance of the ionization and/or idiosyncrasy to contrast media, easy repeatability, and intraprocedural active participation of the patient (increases her knowledge of tubal status). The course of this dynamic analysis of tubal patency and motility can be stored, reviewed, analyzed and interpreted to the infertile couple using CINE mode.

According to Peters et al.[6] and Volpi et al.,[7] the accuracy of Hy-Co-Sy compared to X-ray HSG varies from 70.37 to 92.20% **(Table 1)**. The accuracy of Hy-Co-Sy compared to chromopertubation varies from 81.82 and 91.48% respectively[8, 9] to 100.00[10] **(Table 2)**.

TABLE 2: The accuracy of Hy-Co-Sy compared to laparoscopic chromopertubation.

Authors (year)	Total number	Accuracy (%)
Allahbadia et al. (1993)[33]	27	25 (92,59)
Tüfekci et al. (1992)[20]	38	37 (97,37)
Peters and Coulam (1991)[6]	58	50 (86,20)
Kupesic et al. (1994)[9]	47	43 (91,48)
Stern et al. (1992)[8]	121	99 (81,82)
Deichert et al. (1992)[10]	16	16 (100,00)
Volpi et al. (1996)[7]	29	24 (82.7)
Battaglia (1996)[31]	60	56 (93,33)
Raga (1996)[36*]	42	39 (92)
Sladkevicius (2000)[39*]	67	–
Jeanty (2000)[30]	115	91 (79.4)
Kiyokawa (2000)[42*]	25	–

*three-dimensional Hy-Co-Sy

ULTRASOUND ASSESSMENT OF THE UTERUS AND THE FALLOPIAN TUBES

In 1954, Rubin was the first to assess fallopian tubes by insufflation.[11] Ultrasound visualization of the internal genital tract using exogenous contrast media was first described by Nanini et al., Richman et al. and Randolph et al.,[12-14] who performed abdominal sonography after intracervical injection of the fluid.

Randolph et al.[14] used transabdominal ultrasound for observation of the cul-de-sac after injection of 200 mL isotonic saline through the Rubin catheter. Presence of retro-uterine fluid was accepted as a criterion for patency of one or both tubes. Tubal patency was deduced indirectly from the presence of increasing fluid amount in the pouch of Douglas, without differentiation of the sides.

Lesions projecting into the uterine cavity could not be clearly delineated following the instillation of the echogenic contrast media (e.g., dextran). Therefore, for visualization of the uterine cavity abnormalities, injection of a small amount of sonolucent fluid contributes to better evaluation of the intracavitary lesions. After evaluation of the uterine cavity following saline infusion sonography, sonographer usually continues with instillation of highly echogenic contrast to visualize the lumen of fallopian tubes.[13,15-18] Deichert et al. were the first to analyze tubal patency following transcervical injection of an echogenic and ultrasonic contrast fluid SHU 454 (Echovist; Schering,

Berlin, Germany). The method was named transvaginal hystero-contrast-salpingography.[19]

Tüfekci et al.[20] developed transvaginal sonosalpingography, a technique consisting of intrauterine injection of isotonic saline. This method performed without anesthesia was safe, cost-effective, noninvasive and more convenient when compared with other conventional methods. Due to the use of saline, there is no idiosyncrasy to the contrast agents.

Ultrasound Contrast Agents

Contrast media are divided into two groups: Hypoechogenic and hyperechogenic media.

Isotonic saline, Ringer or dextran solutions belong to the first group. Instillation of these media facilitates the detection of echogenic border surfaces. The main disadvantage is that it is not possible to visualize the phenomena of motion and flow.

Hyperechogenic contrast media enhances echo signals, and allow detection of the flow by both B-mode and Doppler ultrasound. Gramiak and Shah[21] found that small gas bubbles effectively reflect ultrasonic waves. Therefore, all the commercial echo contrast media contain microbubbles. Commercial products Echovist and Levovist (Schering AG, Berlin) represent suspension of microbubbles made of special galactose microparticles. Galactose microparticle granules are suspended either in galactose solution (Echovist) or sterile water (Levovist).[21]

Echovist (SHU 454) is an ultrasound contrast medium consisting of a suspension of monosaccaride microparticles (50% galactose, diameter 2 µm) in a 20% aqueous solution of galactose (w/v). The echogenic suspension is reconstituted immediately before the use from granules and a vehicle solution (200 mg microparticles in 1 mL of suspension).[24] This contrast medium is licensed for gynecological applications and is available on the market since 1995. In addition to galactose, Levovist (SHU 508) microparticle granules contain a very low concentration of physiological palmitic acid.

A few minutes before use, the granules have to be shaken vigorously for 5–10 seconds to be dissolved by an appropriate volume of aqueous galactose solution (Echovist) or sterile water (Levovist). A milky suspension of galactose microparticles in a solution is created after disaggregation of the microparticle "snowball". The suspension of Echovist is stable for about 5 minutes after preparation. Due to its extended stability, Levovist may be administered up to 10 minutes after the suspension procedure. Depending on the indication and the imaging modality (B-mode or Doppler), clinically adequate suspension of Echovist has concentrations of 200 and 300 mg/mL. For Levovist, the maximum concentration is about 400 mg/mL. The predominant limitation at concentrations lower than 200 mg/mL is the decreasing suspension stability. Concentrations exceeding 400 mg/mL are limited by a rapid increase of viscosity.

After intrauterine administration and emergence of Echovist from the fimbriae into the pelvis, the galactose microparticles dissolve. Warming to body temperature and dilution by the peritoneal fluid increases this process. *In vitro,* a rise in temperature of the Echovist suspension to 37°C leads to complete dissolution within 30 minutes. The dissolved galactose is subsequently absorbed and metabolized.

Numerous clinical studies in the field of echocardiography, venous vascular system analysis and HSG showed no evidence of serious side effects. Absolute contraindication for instillation of these contrast media is galactosemia (autosomal recessive disease in which, due to deficiency of galactose-1-phosphate uridyltransferase, galactose cannot be metabolized into glucose).

A second-generation contrast agent, such as SonoVue, provides a substantial harmonic response at a low acoustic pressure. Primarily it is used intravenously to study microcirculation of the liver, breast lesions and various gynecological lesions and it has also been studied extensively in the assessment of myocardial perfusion.[22] Recently, it was introduced for sonographic tubal patency evaluation.[23]

Hy-Co-Sy Requirements

A detailed case history should be obtained from a woman considered for Hy-Co-Sy, to rule out the possibility of the rare condition of galactosemia, which is the only absolute contraindication, apart from acute inflammatory disease of the genital organs. A gynecological and ultrasound examination prior to the procedure is necessary to define the uterine position and anomalies if present. Before any intervention, a pregnancy test should be performed for legal reasons. The possibility of local or systemic infections is excluded by clinical examination (normal body temperature), inspection of the genital tract and assessment of cervical smears. The procedure should never be performed on patients with active pelvic infections, and antibiotic prophylaxis (doxycycline and metronidazole) should be used in patients with a history of PID. Hy-Co-Sy should always be performed during the early follicular phase of the menstrual cycle, after complete cessation of menses. This avoids dispersion of menstrual debris into the peritoneal cavity. Procedures performed during this period allow absorption of the media prior to ovulation, thus avoiding the presence of a foreign substance around the time of an imminent corpus luteum. This decreases any theoretic effect the media may have on tubal transport. Hysterosalpingography performed during the immediate premenstrual phase of the cycle has been advocated to rule out cervical incompetence, as that is the point in the cycle with maximum uterine contractions. Therefore, in order to maximize the information obtained, the indication for the study has influence on timing.

Patients are informed about the benefits and the possible risks of the procedure and the procedure itself is described to them in detail. Anesthesia is generally not required for Hy-Co-Sy and the patient can follow the course of the examination on the monitor. If Hy-Co-Sy is performed without anesthesia, patients occasionally report discomfort, especially if the tubes are occluded. The degree of discomfort depends on the individual response of the patient. Premedication or sedation is routinely used (5–10 mg of diazepam intravenously) especially in anxious patients. Pain signifies the obstruction and potential intravasation or tubal rupture and should not be masked by anesthesia. However, tubal spasm may occur if Hy-Co-Sy is performed without anesthesia and may mimic tubal occlusion. Pretreatment with atropine (0.5 mg) may prevent this complication. Parenteral administration of 1 mg glucagon relieves the spasm and allows the flow of the contrast.

Hy-Co-Sy Procedure

The patient voids and is positioned supine on the gynecological table. With the patient's legs flexed, a speculum is inserted into the vagina and positioned such that the entire cervix is visualized and the os is easily accessible. The cervix and the vagina are then thoroughly scrubbed with Betadine solution. A tenaculum is placed on the anterior lip of the cervix, and the cannula is gently guided into the endocervical canal. Application of the contrast medium is performed via a small and very thin uterine catheter fitted with a balloon for stabilization and occlusion of the internal cervical os. Use of the catheter with stopper or balloon helps anchoring the catheter in the endometrial cavity, so it is not dislocated when removing the speculum or during saline injection. Also, it helps occluding the internal cervical os, preventing reflux of the injected fluid, and allowing better distension of the uterine cavity. After removal of the tenaculum, the transvaginal probe is gently introduced into the posterior fornix of the vagina. The contrast (sterile saline) is then injected slowly, under control of the ultrasound. Usually, no more then 5–10 mL of contrast is instilled into the uterine cavity. The first observation to be made is of the uterine cavity, with verification of the catheter placement **(Fig. 1A)**. In this stage, one can observe the morphology of uterus and endometrial lining. Representative images of the uterus in sagittal and transverse planes allow detection of duplication anomalies **(Fig. 1B)**. Three-dimensional

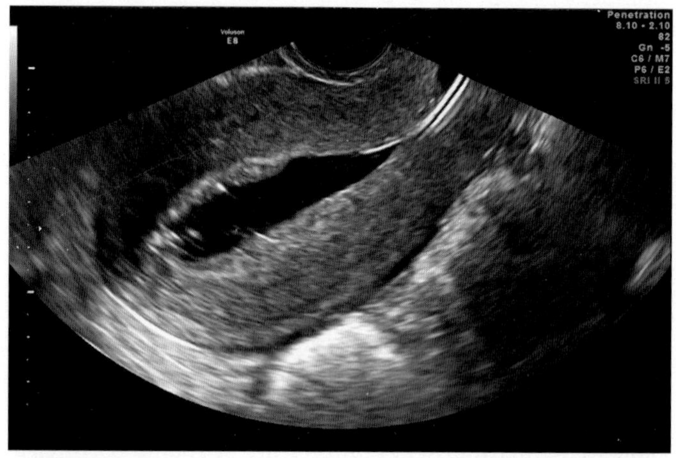

Fig. 1A: Transvaginal ultrasound of the uterus following injection of the isotonic saline solution. The stopper is fixed at the level of the internal cervical os to prevent the reflux of the intrauterine contrast.

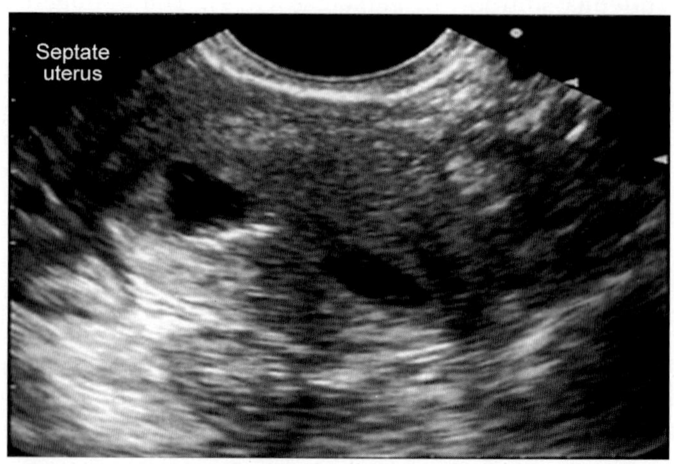

Fig. 1B: Saline infusion sonography demonstrates a division of the uterine cavity. Convex shape of the uterine fundus and hypoechogenic septation indicate septate uterus.

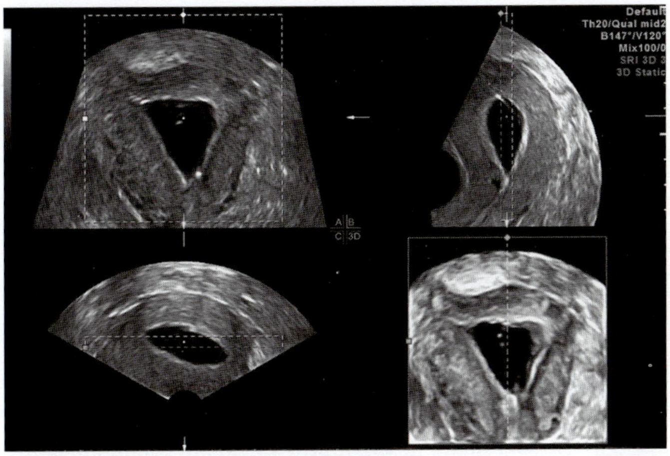

Fig. 1C: Triangular shape of the uterine cavity is visualized in coronal plane (upper left) and surface rendering mode (lower right), and indicates normal anatomy of the uterine cavity.

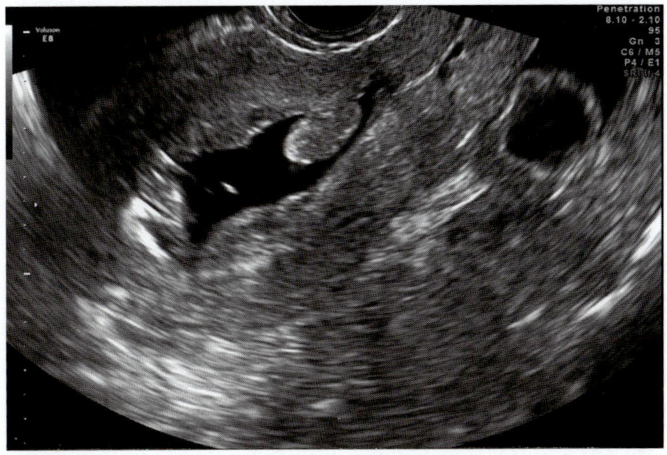

Fig. 2A: Saline infusion sonography enables precise detection and localization of the focal endometrial thickening. Note endometrial polyp protruding into the uterine cavity after injection of isotonic saline.

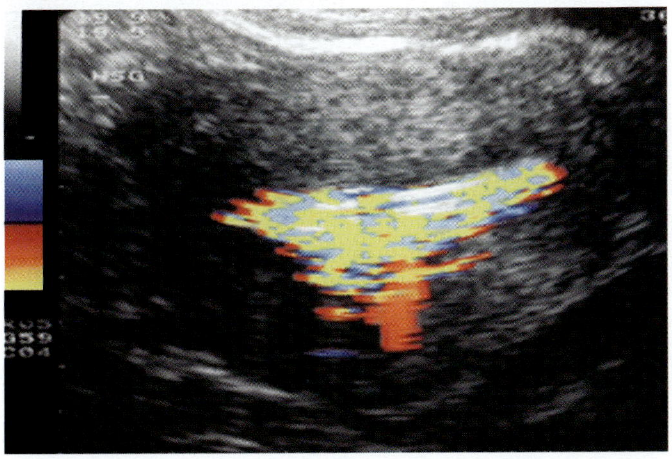

Fig. 1D: Saline infusion sonography by color Doppler ultrasound. Note a triangular shape of the uterine cavity.

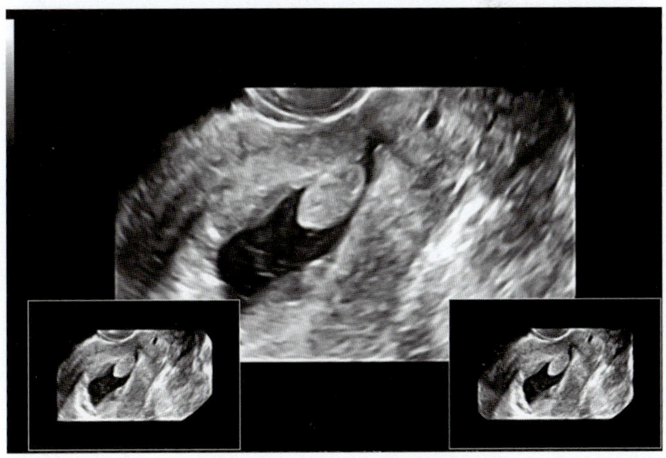

Fig. 2B: Surface rendering of the same endometrial polyp in the lower uterine segment.

ultrasound enables better assessment of the uterine cavity and is superior in detection and classification of the uterine anomalies **(Fig. 1C)**. Similarly, color and/or power Doppler ultrasound can be used for visualization of the shape of the uterine cavity **(Fig. 1D)**. Following distension of the uterine cavity 2D and 3D ultrasound are used to detect focal intracavitary lesions such as endometrial polyp **(Figs. 2A and B)** or submucosal fibroid **(Figs. 3A to C)**. Bands of fibrous tissue bridging the uterine cavity, intrauterine adhesions, are usually not seen on a native ultrasound, but become visible following enhancement with negative contrast medium (saline) **(Fig. 4A and B)**.

If used by a trained physician, Hy-Co-Sy is a well-tolerated and rapid procedure that enables a reliable assessment of tubal patency. In addition, it avoids exposure to X-rays and shows tubal patency to the patient in "real time". Since it is performed without anesthesia, it can be performed as an outpatient procedure. Tubal spasm may sometimes lead to misdiagnosis of tubal occlusion and tubal flow in the proximal part of hydrosalpinx may occasionally give a false impression of tubal patency. To gain familiarity and technical competence, physician has to perform between 10 and 20 investigations. Benefits and limitations of hystero-contrast-salpingography are listed in **Table 3**.

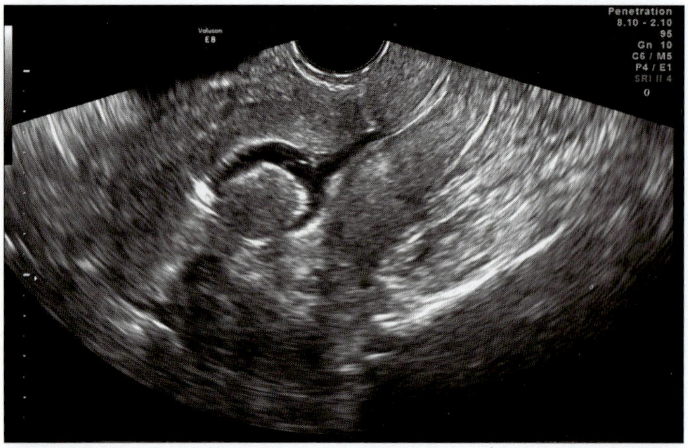

Fig. 3A: Sagittal transvaginal ultrasound image of the uterus obtained as saline infusion sonography demonstrates an echogenic lesion in the uterine fundus, with an appearance suggestive of intracavitary fibroid.

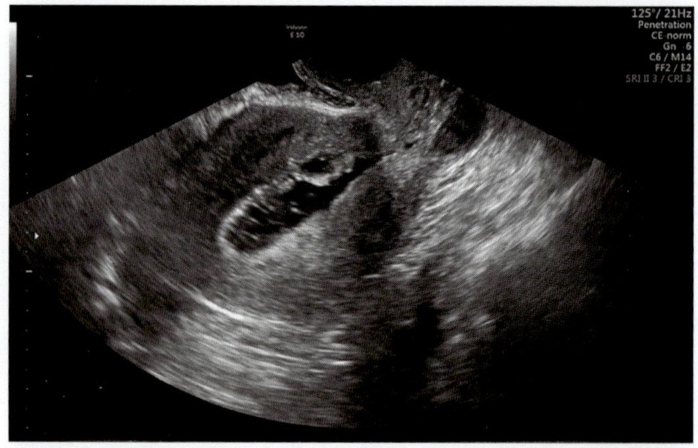

Fig. 4A: Sagittal plane of the uterus following saline injection. Hyperechoic thick band, typical of intrauterine adhesion is visualized in the lower uterine segment.

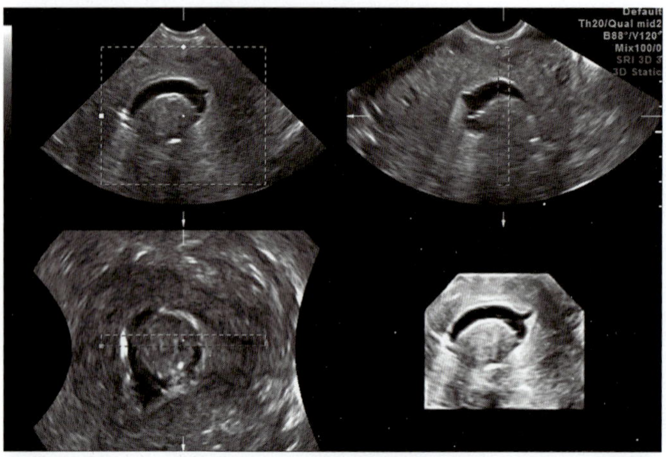

Fig. 3B: 3D ultrasound of the same patient. Point of attachment is better appreciated with multiplanar imaging and surface rendering.

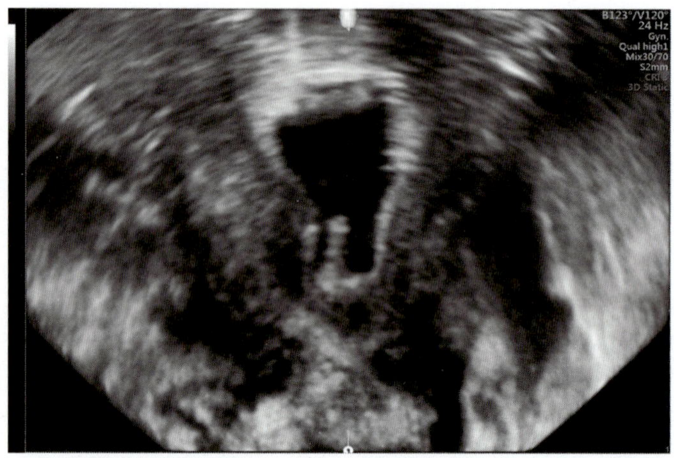

Fig. 4B: 3D surface rendering of the same patient.

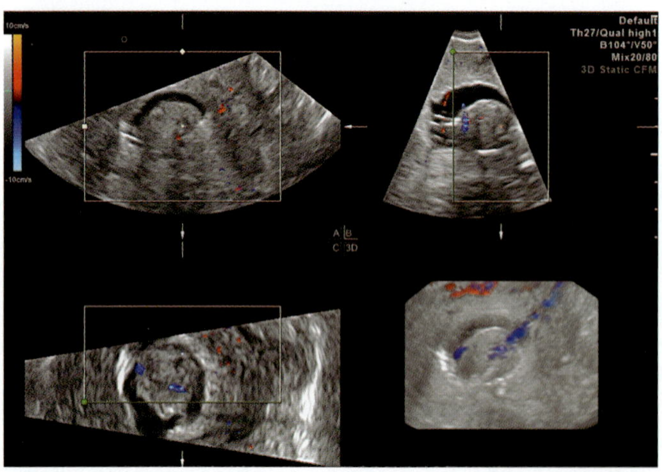

Fig. 3C: 3D power Doppler ultrasound shows regularly separated feeding vessels of the intracavitary fibroid.

TABLE 3: Benefits and limitations of Hy-Co-Sy.

Benefits	***Limitations***
• Reproducible and reliable assessment of tubal patency if used by a trained physician • Avoids exposure to X-rays • Avoids allergic reactions • Avoids general anesthesia • Can be performed as outpatient procedure • Rapid • Well tolerated: little discomfort and few adverse events • Shows tubal patency in "real time"	• Tubal spasm may lead to misdiagnosis of tubal occlusion (spasm also seen with other methods) • In hydrosalpinx, tubal flow may give a false impression of tubal patency • Cannot visualize pelvic and bowel pathology • Requires a degree of technical competence (10–20 investigations are needed to acquire this technique)

Gray-scale (B-Mode) Hy-Co-Sy

Deichert et al.[10,25] described transvaginal Hy-Co-Sy for the assessment of tubal patency with gray-scale imaging (B-mode). The uterine cavity, which in most cases will still be dilated by the Ringer's solution instilled previously, is slowly filled with the echogenic ultrasound contrast medium. If the tube is patent, constant flow in a pattern resembling a point, spot or streak is seen. Further intermittent injections of 1–2 mL of contrast, given slowly and continuously, with further lateral sweeps of the US probe, allow visualization of intraluminal or intratubal flow. For the diagnosis of tubal patency, two or three observation phases per tube are needed, with an observation period of continuous flow of about 10 seconds (during which the contrast medium is slowly injected). Although visualization of a longer segment of the tube beyond the pars intramuralis confirms tubal patency, sonographer should carefully examine the adnexal regions for filling of the distal segments of the tube to exclude sactosalpinx. Examination of the pouch of Douglas for any increase in retrouterine fluid should be compared with the finding at the beginning of the examination.

Pulsed Doppler Analysis of Tubal Patency

Deichert has proposed that B-mode findings should be confirmed by the use of pulsed wave Doppler ultrasound. Every patient with finding suggestive of tubal occlusion should undergo pulsed Doppler analysis of tubal patency.[10,25] After the Doppler gate has been positioned over the area to be examined, the gate width is reduced to measure only the flow noise from the pertubation (not the vascular or any other noise). Tubes are analyzed following brief injections of the contrast medium lasting about 5 seconds. Long sound, drawn-out and initially hissing, and the simultaneous visualization of a broad noise band on the monitor, with band that slowly decreases after injection, indicate that the tube is patent. Thus, unobstructed flow is characterized by a short filling phase with a rapid, steep increase in Doppler shift and a slow, uniform fall in Doppler shift along the time axis, indicates unobstructed free distal outflow. The absence of these acoustic signals or optical tracings indicates obstruction of tubal flow or tubal occlusion. In this case, there is only a short, steep Doppler shift with no subsequent noise signals. This indicates an absence of outflow of the contrast medium distal to the Doppler gate. A sonographic finding of unobstructed tubes on the basis of noise band in pulsed wave Doppler sonography is more impressive than that of a shorter segment of tube in standing B-mode.

Deichert et al. evaluated 17 patients with infertility.[10] Each patient had Hy-Co-Sy by gray-scale ultrasound and pulsed wave Doppler, and follow-up chromolaparoscopy (n = 16) or X-ray HSG (n = 1). The diagnostic efficacies of gray-scale and pulsed wave Doppler were compared with each other and with a conventional control procedure (chromolaparoscopy or X-ray HSG). The gray-scale findings were confirmed by pulsed wave Doppler in five cases on one side; pulsed wave Doppler in seven cases on both sides; corrected by pulsed wave Doppler in one case on one side, and confirmed on the other side by pulsed wave Doppler. In all 17 cases, tubal findings detected by pulsed Doppler waveform analysis were confirmed by chromolaparoscopy or X-ray HSG. The additional use of pulsed wave Doppler in Hy-Co-Sy is recommended as a supplement to gray-scale imaging in cases of suspected tubal occlusion, and in the event of intratubal flow demonstrable only over a short distance.

In more recent study Deichert assessed tubal patency using Hy-Co-Sy, conventional X-ray HSG and laparoscopy with dye in 76 women and 152 fallopian tubes.[25] Hy-Co-Sy showed 87.5% concordance with other techniques, predicted 100% of tubal occlusions and detected 86% of patent tubes.

According to Ayida et al.,[26] when saline infusion sonography is used as a screening test for evaluation of the uterine cavity and results are compared to hysteroscopy findings, SIS has 87.5% sensitivity, 100% specificity, 100% positive predictive value and 91.6% negative predictive value for detection of uterine abnormalities.

Color Doppler Hy-Co-Sy

Transvaginal color Doppler Hy-Co-Sy is a safe and efficacious method for evaluation of fallopian tube patency without exposure to radiation or iodine-based contrast dyes. The cost of this outpatient procedure is significantly lower than for X-ray HSG and does not require collaboration with radiology department. It is advisable that all the scans are recorded on vide-recorder, DVD and/or polaroid films. Similar to X-ray HSG abnormal uterine bleeding, pregnancy and presence of adnexal masses on pelvic or ultrasound examination are contraindications for color Doppler Hy-Co-Sy.

Equipment needed to perform color Doppler Hy-Co-Sy is identical to the equipment needed to perform B mode

Hy-Co-Sy. The only difference is that the monitoring of the procedure is performed using an ultrasound unit with color Doppler capability. The intrauterine cannula is placed into the uterus. One balloon is placed on the level of the internal cervical os, while another one is fixed in the external cervical os. Approximately, 2–5 mL of sterile saline is instilled into the uterine cavity. Sonographer should provide representative images of intracavitary findings. After careful observation of the morphology of the uterus end endometrial lining color Doppler is directed to the cornual region. Color signals passing through the fallopian tubes indicate tubal patency **(Fig. 5)**, while the absence of color signals is interpreted as tubal occlusion.[6,27] Accumulation of the fluid in the cul-de-sac on the side of injection controlled by transvaginal color and pulsed Doppler is an accurate indicator of the ipsilateral tubal patency **(Fig. 6)**. Selective tubal injection using tubal catheter with metal end increases the accuracy of the procedure and appropriateness of the interpretation. In this case, the procedure should be repeated for the contralateral side.

Difficulty in making the diagnosis of tubal occlusion arises in those patients with dilated fallopian tubes (hydrosalpinx), because the flow through the dilated fallopian tube may stimulate spillage in the cul-de-sac **(Fig. 7)**. To avoid this error, careful observation of both adnexa and cul-de-sac should be performed before Hy-Co-Sy procedure. Since, the tubal architecture is not demonstrated with color Doppler or B-mode Hy-Co-Sy, this method is not useful in preoperative salpingoplasty procedures.[28]

Using our modified technique, we compared the findings of color Doppler Hy-Co-Sy from 47 patients with those of chromopertubation at the time of laparoscopy.[9] Forty-three out of 47 (91.48%) color Doppler Hy-Co-Sy findings agreed with observations at laparoscopic chromopertubation. In only one patient, in whom no patency was seen in both tubes under color Doppler evaluation, indirect diagnosis of tubal patency was performed by observation of the accumulation of free fluid in the cul-de-sac. The increased incidence of conception during the 3 months after the procedure (in our study, two patients) may be an effect of a mechanical lavage of the

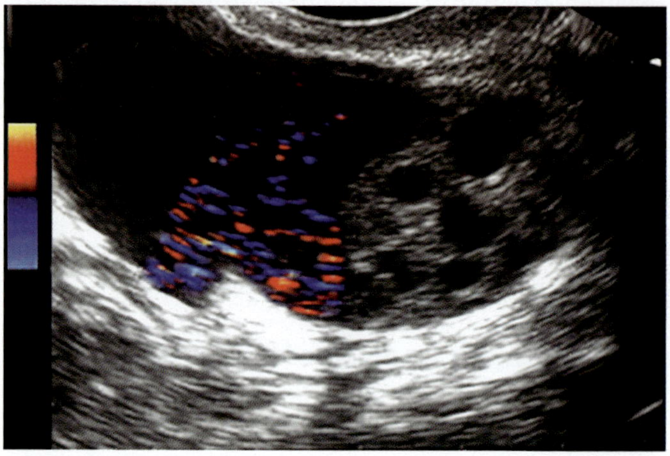

Fig. 6: Color Doppler imaging of the ovary and retrouterine space after injection of the anechoic contrast medium. Color coded signals indicate contrast spillage into the cul-de-sac.

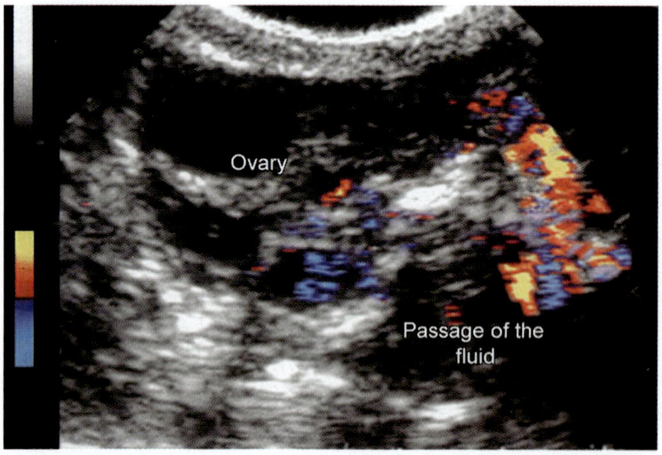

Fig. 5: Transvaginal color Doppler Hy-Co-Sy demonstrates regular tubal patency. Note color flow signals passing through the right tube and simultaneous accumulation of the anechoic fluid in the cul-de-sac.

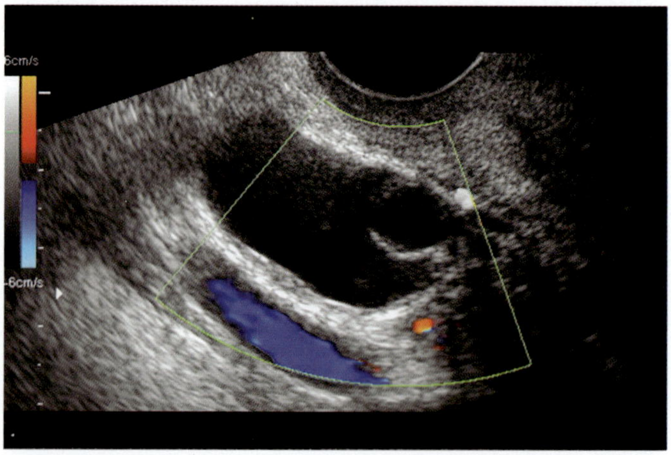

Fig. 7: Transvaginal color Doppler imaging of the distally occluded tube following the injection of the anechoic contrast medium.

uterus by dislodging the mucous plugs, breakdown of the peritoneal adhesions or a stimulatory effect on the tubal cilia. No serious side effects were observed during and after the transvaginal color Doppler Hy-Co-Sy procedure. Eighteen patients complained of a pain that continued for 2–10 minutes after the procedure. No medication was required for these cases. The shortest time taken for the transvaginal color Doppler Hy-Co-Sy was 5 minutes, while the longest time was 14 minutes. After removing the instruments, the cervix should always be inspected for hemostasis and pressure applied to the tenaculum site whenever necessary.

To assess the accuracy of the diagnosis of tubal occlusion with the use of color Doppler flow ultrasonography and HSG, Peters and Coulam (6) studied 129 infertile women. When results of Hy-Co-Sy were compared with those of X-ray HSG and/or chromopertubation, 69 of 85 (81%) studies showed agreement, and 50 out of 58 (86%) Hy-Co-Sy findings agreed with observations at chromopertubation. The frequency of comparable findings between X-ray HSG and chromopertubation was 75%.

Richman et al.[13] evaluated tubal patency in 36 infertile women. They compared Hy-Co-Sy findings with conventional hysterosalpingograms, which had been obtained subsequently. Ultrasound demonstrated bilateral occlusion with a sensitivity of 100% and showed tubal patency with a specificity of 96%.

Tüfekci et al.[20] studied 38 women with infertility complaints. The results obtained by transvaginal Hy-Co-Sy and subsequent laparoscopy were completely consistent for 29 cases (76.32%), and partially consistent for eight cases (21.05%). Only one case showed inconsistent result. Complete consistence means that the passage through both fallopian tubes is identical by both methods. Partial consistence indicated identical results for only either the left or the right tube. Transvaginal Hy-Co-Sy correctly indicated tubal patency or nonpatency in 37 of 38 cases.

Heikkinen et al.[29] evaluated the advantages and accuracy of transvaginal Hy-Co-Sy in the assessment of tubal patency with regards to laparoscopic chromopertubation. Sixty-one fallopian tubes were examined by both techniques, resulting in concordance of 85%. By transvaginal Hy-Co-Sy, 45 tubes were found to be patent and 16 occluded. In chromopertubation, 50 tubes were patent and 11 were occluded. Bilateral tubal patency was detected by transvaginal Hy-Co-Sy in 17 cases and by laparoscopy in 22 cases. Bilateral occlusion was found in three cases using either technique. Based on their results, the authors concluded that transvaginal Hy-Co-Sy with the combination of air and saline is a low-cost, reliable, safe and comfortable examination method that can be used for the primary investigation of infertility on an outpatient basis.

Jeanty et al.[30] assessed the use of air as a sonographic contrast agent in the investigation of tubal patency by Hy-Co-Sy. They examined 115 women assessed for infertility. After saline saline infusion sonography, a small amount of air was insufflated and the tubal passage of bubbles was monitored. Air-sonohysterography and laparoscopy with chromopertubation showed agreement in 79.4%. In 17.2% of patients, the tubes were not visualized by air-sonohysterography when they were patent, which lead to the sensitivity of 85.7% and specificity of 77.2%. In conclusion, air assisted Hy-Co-Sy is a comfortable, simple and inexpensive first line of tubal patency investigation. Similarly, Battaglia et al.[31] confirmed correlation between color Doppler Hy-Co-Sy and X-ray HSG with chromolaparoscopy for 86% versus 93% of patients studied, respectively.

Boudghene et al.[32] compared the efficiency of air-filled albumin microspheres (Infoson) with saline solution in determining fallopian tube patency during Hy-Co-Sy. HyCoSy was performed with a 7-MHz transvaginal probe using both B-mode and color Doppler ultrasound and tubal patency was demonstrated by the appearance of contrast agent in the peritoneal cavity near the ovaries. Infoson enhanced Hy-Co-Sy provided a significantly larger number of correct diagnoses (20/22 fallopian tubes) than did saline Hy-Co-Sy (12/24 fallopian tubes) and the same number of patients as by X-ray HSG. A positive ultrasound contrast agent appears to be more efficient than saline solution at determining fallopian tube patency in infertile women by means of Hy-Co-Sy and as efficient as an iodinated contrast agent in the same population explored by X-ray HSG.

Stern et al.[8] administered saline transcervically during transvaginal color Doppler sonography in 238 women. Traditional X-ray HSG was performed in 89 women, while laparoscopy with chromopertubation was performed in 121 women. Forty-nine women had all three procedures performed. Correlation between color Doppler Hy-Co-Sy and X-ray findings with chromopertubation occurred in 81% versus 60% (P = 0.0008) of all women studied. In forty-nine patients who had all three procedures performed, color Doppler Hy-Co-Sy results correlated with chromopertubation more often than X-ray HSG

(82% versus 57%, $P = 0.0152$). In their previous report,[6] discrepancies between color ultrasound Hy-Co-Sy and chromopertubation findings involved a diagnosis of unilateral patency. Based on their observation, these authors recommend repeating color ultrasound Hy-Co-Sy before making a diagnosis of unilateral occlusion.

Allahbadia[33] reported a 92.6% agreement between color Doppler Hy-Co-Sy compared with X-ray HSG and laparoscopy. The same author described the so-called *Sion* procedure or *hydrogynecography*. This procedure takes about 15 minutes as compared to the 5–6 minutes for Hy-Co-Sy. After accomplishing the first part of the procedure, sterile normal saline is injected until approximately 350 mL have flooded the pelvis. With the adnexa and uterus submerged in a fluid medium, the rescanning of the pelvis is repeated. If there is a bilateral tubal block and reflux of the saline is seen in the stem of the Foley's catheter, filling up the pelvis by alternative means is applied. The saline fills up the pelvis and delineates all sorts of adhesions. All the patients undergoing this procedure are given prophylactic antibiotics.

Contrary to optimistic results of different ultrasound techniques for evaluation of tubal patency, Balen et al.[34] found Hy-Co-Sy using both sterile saline and Echovist contrast media insufficiently accurate and inferior to conventional X-ray HSG. False-positive rates in the range of 9% and false-negative rates in the range of 20% have been reported in the diagnosis of tubal obstruction by color Doppler Hy-Co-Sy.[8] Therefore, all abnormal hysterosalpingograms studies deserve laparoscopic or hysteroscopic follow-up.

Also, normal X-ray or color Doppler Hy-Co-Sy do not rule out the need for diagnostic laparoscopy. While X-ray HSG is the most accurate method of diagnosing intramural or intraluminal abnormalities of the fallopian tube, color Doppler Hy-Co-Sy is the only available noninvasive method for evaluation of the tubal patency and motility.

To obtain maximum information, a well-trained physician who is familiar with the color Doppler investigation and who is capable of manipulating the instruments, the patient's reproductive tract and the rate of injection should perform the procedure.

Sueoka et al.[35] report on the use of the linear everting (LE) catheter to safely guide a falloposcope into the entire length of fallopian tube in order to observe the tubal lumen. This catheter may also be useful therapeutically for the recanalization of occluded tubes. On the basis of tubes attempted, the LE catheter successfully accessed 85.3% (87/102) of the tubes. A follow-up hysterosalpingogram was completed 1–3 months following the falloposcopic tuboplasty (FT) procedure, which revealed an overall patency rate of 79.4% (81/102). In this study, FT was found to be a highly useful, less invasive and novel treatment for tubal infertility.

3D Hy-Co-Sy

Information provided by 2D ultrasound conventional scans in the longitudinal and transverse planes can now be augmented using 3D ultrasound that provides an additional view of the coronal plane, parallel to the transducer face and surface rendering[36,37] **(Fig. 8A)**. The computer generated scan is automatically displayed in three perpendicular planes. Presentation of three orthogonal planes on a screen allows free scrolling of an endless amount of frames through the volume of interest. The coronal or "c" plane view allows more detailed analysis of the uterus and, for the first time, the endometrial cavity between the uterine angles can be visualized. Translation or rotation can be carried out in one plane while maintaining the perpendicular orientation of all three. The images produced by transvaginal ultrasound are superior to those produced by transabdominal ultrasound because vaginal transducers are in closer proximity to the tissues.[37] Because of that, higher frequencies are used and artifactual echoes caused by multiple reflections from intervening tissues are minimized.

Demonstration of the coronal plane is mandatory for the diagnosis of uterine pathology, such as endometrial polyps **(Fig. 8B)** or duplication anomalies of the uterus **(Fig. 8C)**. Also, this plane provides the most exact

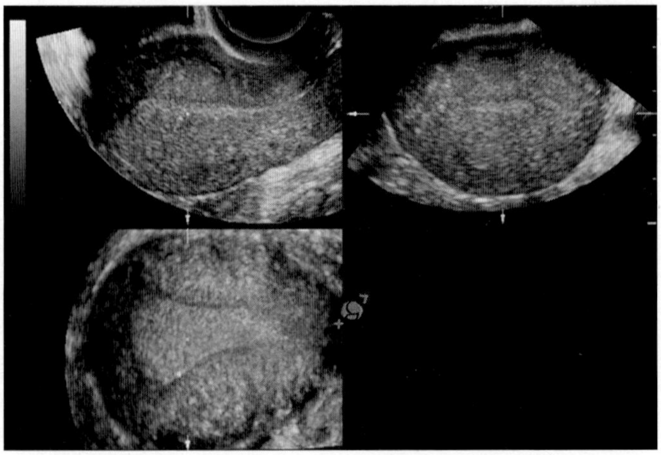

Fig. 8A: Three-dimensional ultrasound image of normal uterine cavity.

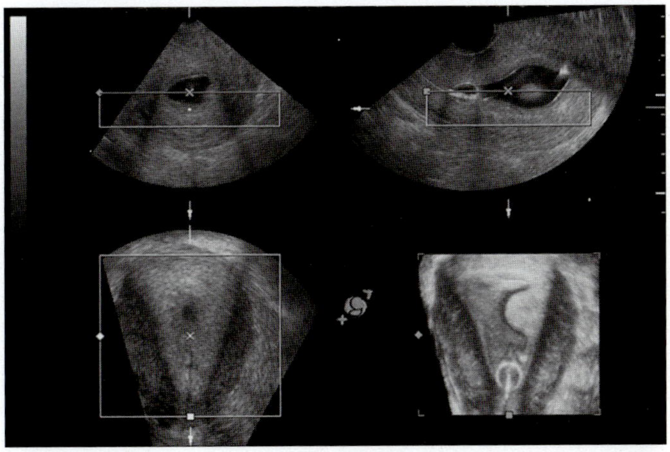

Fig. 8B: Three-dimensional saline infusion sonography of an endometrial polyp protruding into the uterine cavity (lower right image).
Courtesy: Guillermo Azumendi, MD

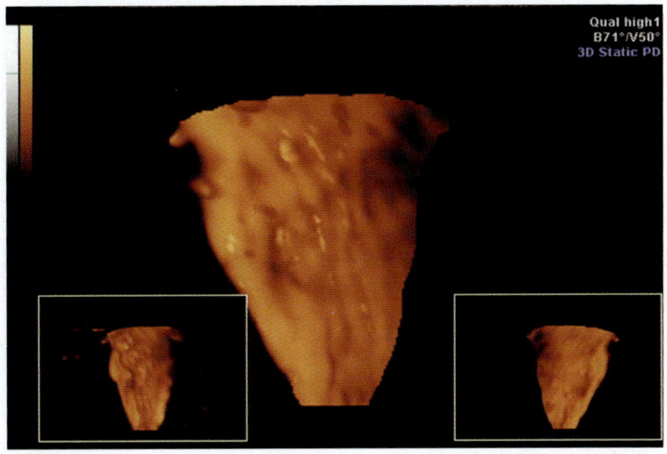

Fig. 9A: Three-dimensional power Doppler image of normal uterine cavity following injection of echogenic contrast medium. This modality facilitates visualization.

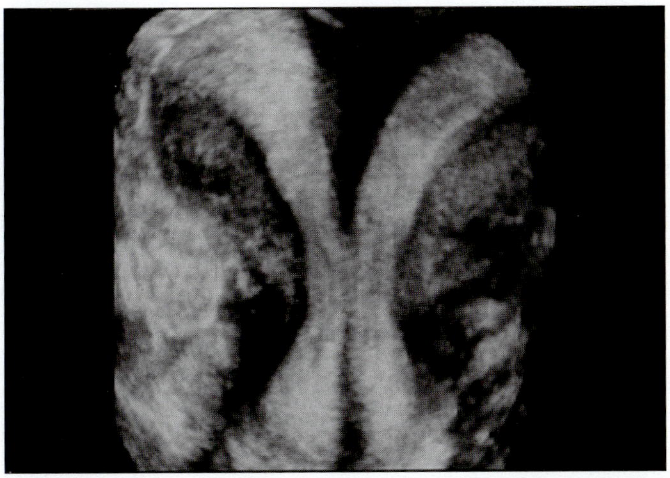

Fig. 8C: Duplication anomaly of the uterus demonstrated in frontal reformatted section.
Courtesy: Guillermo Azumendi, MD

measurement of the endometrial width when transected in a midperpendicular manner. During 3D saline infusion sonography the typical triangulated uterine cavity appears in its full shape[38] **(Fig. 9A)**. Surface rendering and maximal/minimal or X-ray renderings provide even more information on the uterine findings, such as mapping of the endometrial polyp(s) **(Figs. 2A and B, Fig. 8B)** and intracavitary fibroids **(Figs. 3A to C)**. There are two techniques to accomplish this goal: "native" approach, and the use of echogenic contrast medium that is especially useful for demonstration of the uterine cavity shape. Due to its dual consistency the uterus is an excellent ultrasonic medium. Endometrium and myometrium have different acoustic impedance, which permits visualization of the size and shape of the uterus and its cavity. However, contrast medium may be mandatory in cases where a thin endometrium or pathologic content of the uterine cavity precludes its visualization.

Similarly to B-mode and color Doppler Hy-Co-Sy, the negative contrast medium, normal saline, is used for demonstration of the entire uterine cavity, its shape, pathology and the frame of the myometrial mantel, whereas for demonstrating the permeability of the fallopian tubes a positive contrast medium (Echovist) is used.

Weinraub and Herman[38] were the first to report on the uterine cavity assessment by 3D saline infusion sonography. Using three perpendicular planes on one screen, where the left upper plane is coronal and is termed "a", the right upper plane is sagittal and is termed "b" and the left lower plane is transverse and is termed "c" one can detect numerous causes of infertility. Looking at the fundal region in "a" it is very important not to overlook a small indentation, typical of arcuate or subseptate uterus. The maximal endometrial width could be easily measured in sagittal plane. Clear concavity in the middle of the uterine fundus indicates a bicornuate uterus.

The same method is very useful for evaluation of the intracavitary pathology, such as adhesions, submucosal and intracavitary leiomyomas, endometrial polyps, endometrial carcinoma, or location of intrauterine devices (IUDs). Saline infusion sonography with 3D surface rendering is particularly useful in evaluation of the patients with intrauterine adhesions, endometrial polyps and submucosal fibroids.[38]

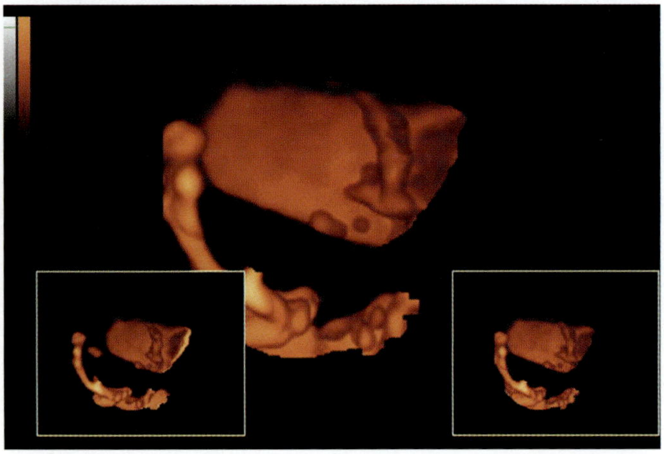

Fig. 9B: Three-dimensional power Doppler Hy-Co-Sy enables simultaneous analysis of the uterine cavity and tubal patency.

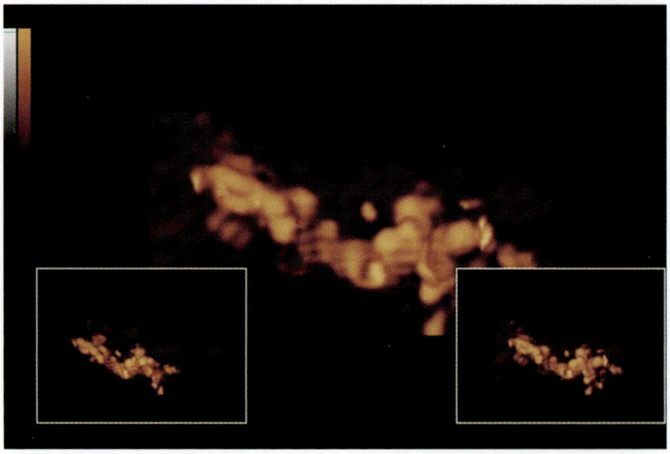

Fig. 9C: Three-dimensional power Doppler image of the entire tubal length and spillage of the contrast medium through the fimbrial end as demonstrated by echo-enhanced 3D power Doppler Hy-Co-Sy.

There are numerous technical difficulties in visualization of the fallopian tubes by 2D Hy-Co-Sy.[37] Due to its tortuosity, tubes are rarely seen completely in a single scanning plane and the echo-contrast medium is, therefore, observed in small sections. The position of the tube is very variable and distended bowel may prevent the visualization of the distal parts of the tubes. In most patients, only the tubal ostia and proximal parts of the tubes are visualized by gray-scale 2D ultrasound imaging. Free spread of the dye is frequently difficult to visualize because of the surrounding bowel, which also produces strong echogenic signals. Instead of visualizing the echo contrast with gray-scale ultrasound, Sladkevicius et al.[39] used 3D power Doppler technology sensitive to slow flow. The aim of the their study was to evaluate the feasibility of three-dimensional power Doppler imaging (3D-PDI) in the assessment of the patency of the fallopian tubes during Hy-Co-Sy procedure. Hy-Co-Sy using contrast medium Echovist was performed on 67 women, and findings on the 2D gray-scale scanning and 3D PDI were compared. The first technique was used to visualize the positive contrast in the fallopian tube, while the second demonstrated flow of medium through the tube. Using 3D-PDI, patent tubes were demonstrated as prominent color coded signals **(Figs. 9A to D)**. Using this technique, free spill from the fimbrial end of the fallopian tubes was demonstrated in 114 (91%) tubes, and in 58 (46%) of the tubes using conventional (2D) Hy-Co-Sy. The mean duration of the imaging procedure was significantly decreased for 3D-PDI, but the operator time, which included post-procedural analysis of the stored information was similar. A significantly lower volume of

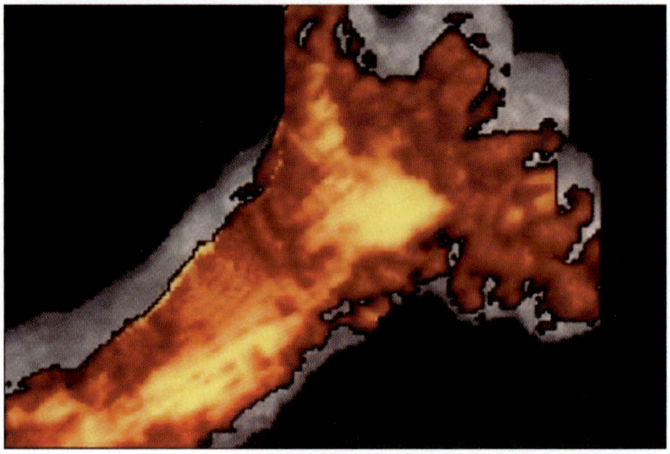

Fig. 9D: Regular spillage of the contrast medium following 3D power Doppler Hy-Co-Sy.

contrast medium (5.9+/–0.6 mL) was used for 3D-PDI Hy-Co-Sy in comparison with conventional 2D Hy-Co-Sy (11.2 +/–1.9 mL). The authors concluded that color-coded 3D-PDI with surface rendering allows visualization of the flow of the contrast medium through the entire tubal length. Using the same technique in majority of cases, the operator can assess the free spill of the contrast was into the cul-de-sac. The 3D-PDI Hy-Co-Sy appeared to have advantages over the conventional technique, especially in terms of visualization of the free spill from the distal end of the tube, which was achieved twice as often with the 3D ultrasound modality **(Figs. 9B to D)**. Although the design of the investigation did not allow the side effects of the two techniques to be compared, the shorter duration of the imaging and lower volume of the contrast medium used suggested that the 3D-PDI Hy-Co-Sy may have a better side-effect profile. Also, the 3D-PDI Hy-Co-Sy allowed better storage of the information for re-analysis and archiving than conventional 2D method.

Ayida et al.[40] compared conventional 2D and 3D ultrasound scanning of the uterine cavity with and without saline contrast medium. Two dimensional ultrasound scanning suggested cavity abnormalities in 4 of 10 women (three fibroids and one hyperechoic thick endometrium). The 3D scanning confirmed these and revealed one additional abnormality suggestive of a uterine septum. The 2D scanning with saline injection diagnosed abnormalities in 5 of 10 patients (one uterine septum, three fibroids and one endometrial polyp). In this study, 3D contrast scanning with saline did not add any further information to 2D contrast scanning with saline. Weinraub et al.[41] have demonstrated the feasibility of combined 3D ultrasound and saline contrast hysterosonography. Since volume sampling has a short pick-up time of a few seconds, the examination is over almost immediately after the uterus is reasonably distended. In such an uncomfortable examination, this type of advantage should not be underestimated. Evaluation of the uterine cavity at a later time allows the operator to manipulate the data at leisure and scrutinize findings in desired planes, which were not available during the initial examination. Simultaneous display of the three perpendicular planes offers a more comprehensive overview of the examined area and gives access to planes unobtainable by conventional 2D examination. Surface rendering may confirm the presence of pathological findings in equivocal cases and characterize their appearance, size, volume and relationship to the surrounding structures. Surface rendering of the polypoid structures shows echogenic masses on a pedicle protruding into the uterine cavity. Submucosal fibroids appear as mixed echogenic sites bulging into the cavity. Intrauterine synechiae appear as bands of varying thickness traversing the uterine cavity. This can be useful when deciding on treatment options, such as conservative management vs. surgery and can be a valuable tool in surgical procedures carried out under ultrasonographic guidance.

Kiyokava et al.[42] evaluated 25 unselected infertile patients for tubal patency and uterine cavity morphology by 3D Hy-Co-Sy with saline as a contrast medium. The efficacy of the procedure was compared with X-ray HSG as a reference. The positive predictive value, negative predictive value, sensitivity and specificity of predicting tubal patency by 3D HyCoSy were 100, 33.3, 84.4 and 100%, respectively. Using 3D Hy-Co-Sy, the full contour of the uterine cavity was depicted in 96% of cases and 64% by X-ray HSG (P <0.005). The uterine cavity area measured by 3D Hy-Co-Sy correlated well with the volume of contrast medium required on HSG. Also, 3D Hy-Co-Sy allowed better assessment of the uterine cavity and tubal patency. In addition, reduced examination time and better tolerance by the patients minimized the need for sedation or anesthesia. Thus, 3D Hy-Co-Sy with saline as a contrast medium is feasible and could comprise a routine outpatient procedure in the initial evaluation of infertile patients.

Unterweger et al.[43] introduced a new method, three-dimensional dynamic magnetic resonance-hysterosonosalpingography (3D dMR-HSG) for imaging of the uterine cavity and fallopian tube patency. The authors used dynamic magnetic resonance (dMR) to assess the visualization of the fallopian tubes following injection of a higher viscosity contrast solution, 20 mL of gandolium-polyvidone. Three-dimensional dynamic magnetic-resonance-HSG may represent a new and promising imaging approach to female infertility patients, primarily because of the avoidance of the ovarian exposure to ionizing radiation. Use of a higher viscosity MR-contrast agent allowed clear visualization of the uterine cavity and fallopian tube patency and morphology.

During the course of last 5 years, 3D ultrasound became more and more utilized for evaluation of tubal patency. Report by Chan et al.[44] quotes the sensitivity, specificity, positive and negative predictive values of 3D Hy-Co-Sy in detecting tubal patency of 100, 67, 89 and 100%, respectively. In their recent study Kupesic and Plavsic[45] analyzed 152 women by 2D B-mode, color and pulsed Doppler Hy-Co-Sy and 116 other women using 3D B-mode and power Doppler Hy-Co-Sy. The diagnostic performance (sensitivity, specificity, PPV and NPV) of 2D and 3D Hy-Co-Sy were assessed and compared to hysteroscopy and laparoscopy and dye test in the assessment of uterine abnormalities and tubal patency. The sensitivity, specificity, PPV and NPV of 2D hysterosonography compared to hysteroscopy were 93.6, 97.3, 98.2 and 97.3%, respectively. The sensitivity, specificity, PPV and NPV of 3D hysterosonography compared to hysteroscopy were 97.9, 100, 97.9 and 100%, respectively. Addition of color and pulsed Doppler to 2D Hy-Co-Sy and power Doppler to 3D Hy-Co-Sy contributed to diagnostic precision in detection of tubal patency. The sensitivity, specificity, PPV and NPV of 3D power Doppler Hy-Co-Sy in detection of tubal patency compared to laparoscopy and dye intubation were 100, 99.1, 99.2 and 100%, respectively.[45] The authors concluded that 3D Hy-Co-Sy was less time consuming than 2D Hy-Co-Sy, since measurements, reconstruction of planes of interest and surface rendering could be performed off-line. Furthermore, half a dose of the contrast medium was needed for 3D B-mode and power Doppler Hy-Co-Sy. By shortening the procedure and using less contrast medium, the discomfort to the patients was significantly reduced. Clearly, smaller contrast volume and slower injection rate have reduced the intraluminal pressure and pain due to the cornual and tubal spasm. 2D and 3D Hy-Co-Sy significantly decreased the cost in comparison with laparoscopy, since it can be done on an outpatient basis. Clearly, Hy-Co-Sy performed by 3D US is a superior screening method for evaluation of infertile patients.[46-47] Screening positives should be directed to operative hysteroscopy and/or laparoscopy.

3D AND 4D HY-CO-SY WITH AUTOMATED CODED CONTRAST IMAGING AND SONOVUE

A new automated 3D coded contrast imaging software (3D CCI by GE) may aid to diagnostic accuracy of 3D Hy-Co-Sy.[47,48] Using this special ultrasound technology that emits an ultrasound beam of a selected frequency and receives a narrow band of harmonic signal avoids the overlap between the tissue and contrast response. CCI software optimizes the use of ultrasound contrast medium by means of low acoustic pressure. Automated 3D volume acquisition permits visualization of the tubes in the coronal view and of the tubal course in 3D space, allowing even less experienced operators to evaluate tubal patency status relatively easily.[48,49] More recently, 4D Hy-Co-Sy with SonoVue (Bracco International BV, Amsterdam, the Netherlands) achieved 81.8% sensitivity, 90.5% specificity and 81.8% PPV compared to laparoscopy,[50] and 84.8% sensitivity, 96.2% specificity, 93.3% positive and 86.2% negative predictive value, respectively.[51] Similar results were obtained by other authors.[52]

Color coded 3D power Doppler imaging (PDI) with surface rendering allows visualization of the flow of the contrast medium through the entire tubal length, and enables detection of the free spill in the majority of cases **(Figs. 10 to 13)**. This method is also superior in

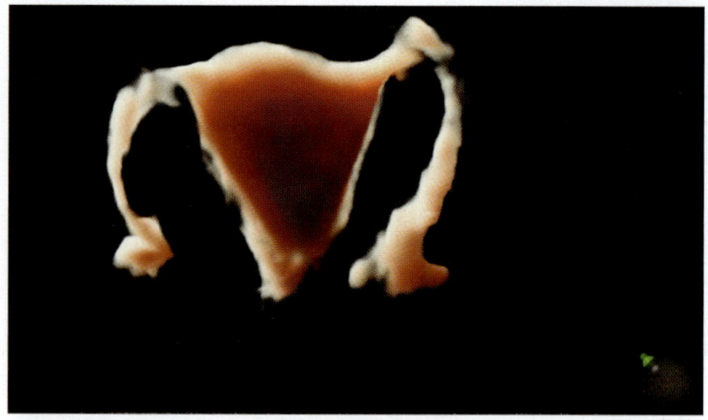

Fig. 10A: 3D Hy-Co-Sy volume rendered with HDlive render mode shows the regular contours of the endometrial cavity and normal patency of both tubes, using SonoVue (Bracco).

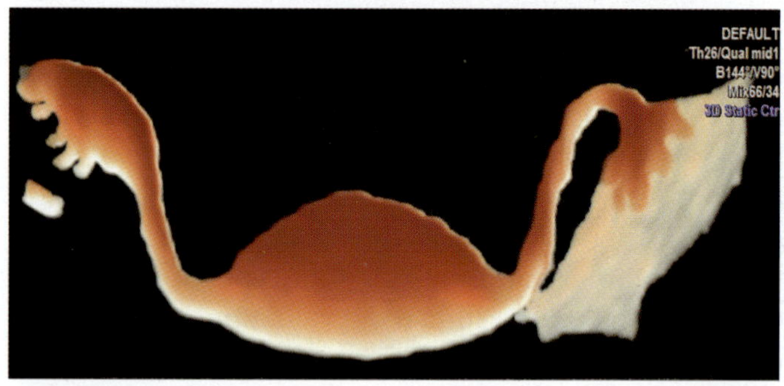

Fig. 10B: 3D Hy-Co-Sy volume rendered with HDlive render mode shows the endometrial cavity in the axial plane. Tubes are filled in their entirety and the fimbrial ends are clearly visualized. Spill is also noticed from the left tube.

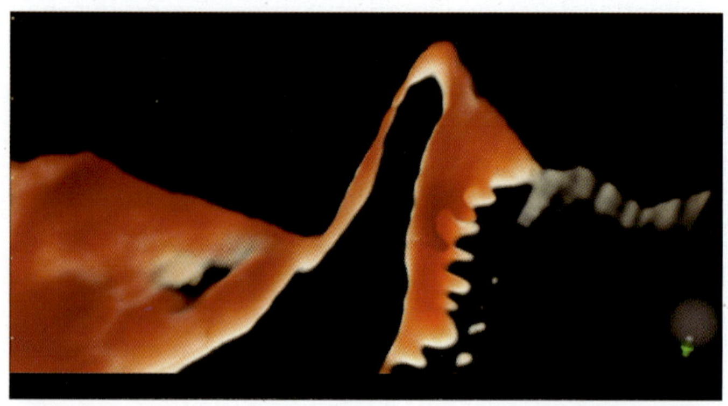

Fig. 11A: 3D ultrasound acquired volume of Hy-Co-Sy with positive contrast in a contrast mode. The B mode image before volume acquisition is zoomed to visualize half of the uterus and ipsilateral ovary on the screen. 3D volume is acquired when the contrast is being slowly injected through the cervix. The image shows half of the endometrial cavity and the entire extent of the ipsilateral tube with the details of the fimbrial end on HDlive render mode.

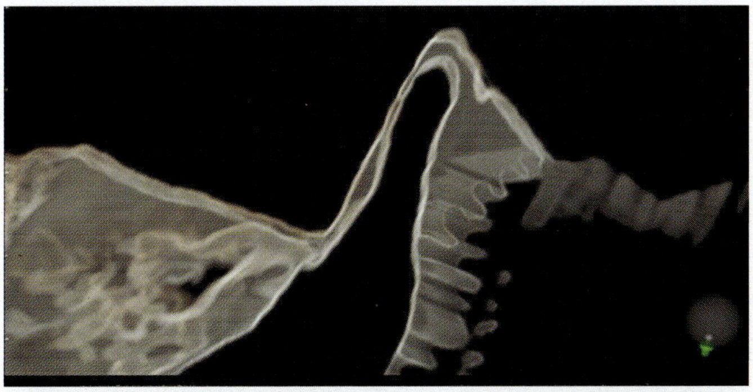

Fig. 11B: The same image is rendered with silhouette mode.

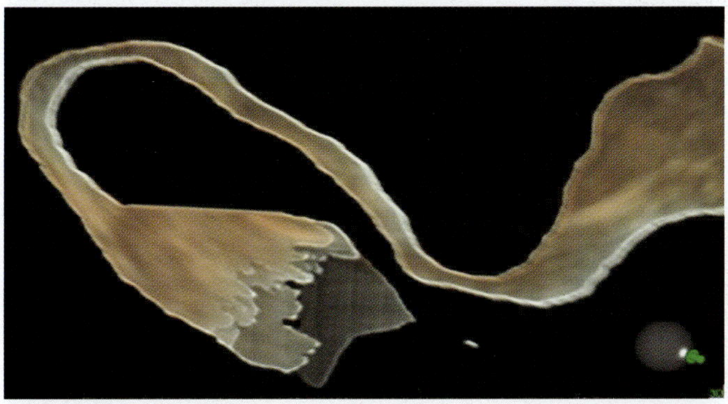

Fig. 12A: 3D ultrasound acquired volume of Hy-Co-Sy with positive contrast in a contrast mode. The B mode image before volume acquisition is zoomed enough to visualize a portion of the uterus and ipsilateral ovary on the screen. 3D volume is acquired when the contrast is being slowly injected through the cervix. The image shows half of the endometrial cavity and the entire extent of the ipsilateral tube with the details of the fimbrial end on HDlive render mode with silhouette.

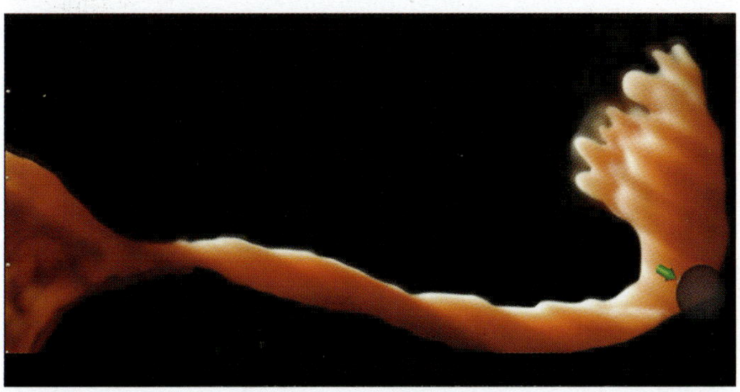

Fig. 12B: 3D ultrasound acquired volume of Hy-Co-Sy with positive contrast in a contrast mode. The B mode image before volume acquisition is zoomed enough to visualize a portion of the uterus and ipsilateral ovary on the screen. 3D volume is acquired when the contrast is being slowly injected through the cervix. The image shows half of the endometrial cavity and the entire extent of the ipsilateral tube with the details of the fimbrial end on HDlive render mode.

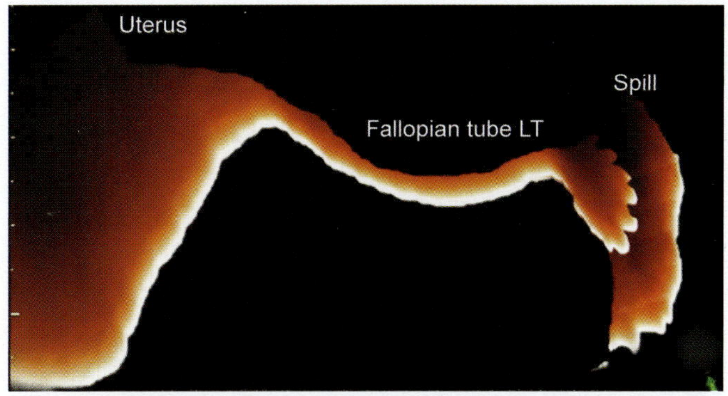

Fig. 13A: 3D ultrasound acquired volume of Hy-Co-Sy with positive contrast in a contrast mode. The B mode image before volume acquisition is zoomed enough to visualize a half the uterus and ipsilateral ovary on the screen. 3D volume is acquired when the contrast is being slowly injected through the cervix. The image shows half of the endometrial cavity and the entire extent of the ipsilateral tube with the details of the fimbrial end in HDlive render mode. Contrast seen outside the fimbrial end of the tube indicates spill.

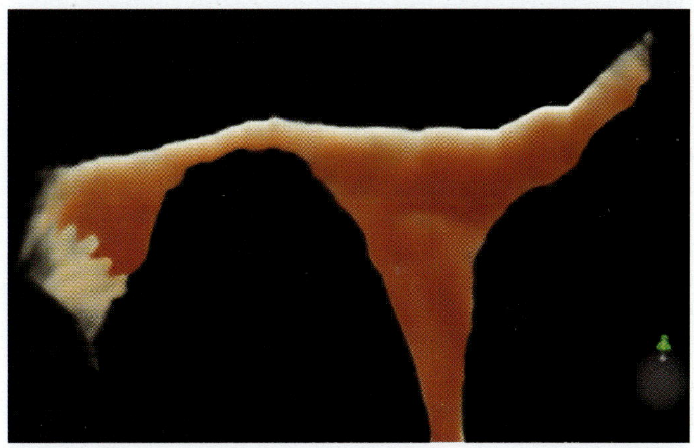

Fig. 13B: 3D ultrasound acquired volume of Hy-Co-Sy with positive contrast in a contrast mode, rendered with HDlive mode. Image shows normal endometrial cavity, normal entire extent and fimbrial end of the right tube with spill. Left tube is seen only in its proximal part, and shows a sudden cut off. Patient had a history of salpingectomy due to left ectopic pregnancy.

demonstration and documentation of tubal blockage **(Figs. 14 to 16)**.

CONCLUSION

Hystero-contrast-salpingography is a safe and efficacious method for evaluation of the fallopian tube patency without exposure to contrast dyes or radiation, which apparently favors the onset of spontaneous pregnancies. Three-dimensional and more recently, four-dimensional technique offers the possibility of simultaneous presentation of the uterine cavity and the fallopian tubes. The acquired volumes of the most appropriate planes of interest can be stored on removable hard disk for additional re-evaluation and documentation. Ultrasonic tomography can be performed using one panel control, producing parallel sections in increments of less than

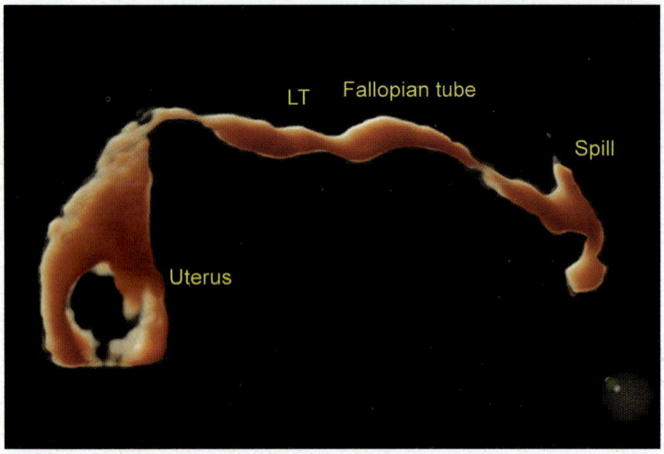

Fig. 14: 3D ultrasound acquired volume of Hy-Co-Sy with positive contrast in a contrast mode, rendered with HDlive mode. The image shows unicornuate (left) uterus with irregular tubal lumen. The fimbrial end also is shrunken and shows abnormal fimbriae. There is a minimal leak from the fimbrial end, but not a normal spill. This is typical of the chronically inflamed tube (the commonest cause in the developing countries like India is tuberculosis). The anechoic area seen in the endometrial cavity is a filling defect caused by an intracavitary fibroid.

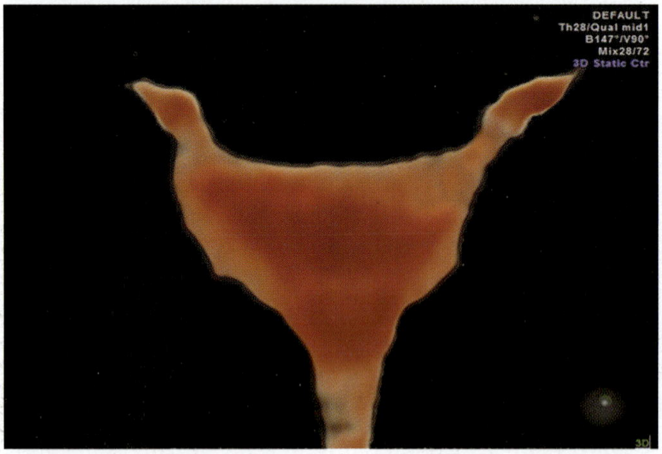

Fig. 15: 3D ultrasound acquired volume of Hy-Co-Sy with positive contrast in a contrast mode, rendered with HDlive mode. Image shows normal endometrial cavity. The proximal part of the tubal lumen is seen bilaterally. The blocked ends of the tube are tapered; Hy-Co-Sy indicates bilateral tubal blockage.

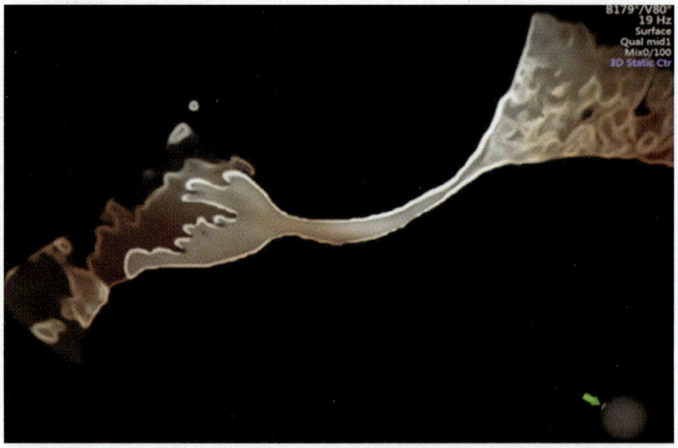

Fig. 16A: 3D ultrasound acquired volume of Hy-Co-Sy with positive contrast in a contrast mode, rendered with HDlive mode with silhouette. This silhouette mode image illustrates right side of the endometrial cavity with normal right tube and fimbriae with free spill.

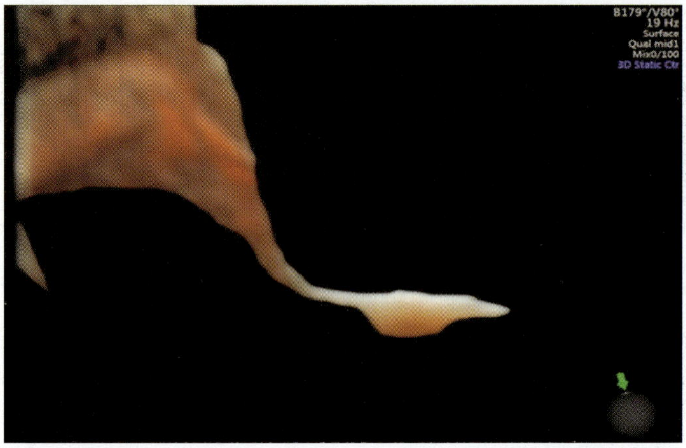

Fig. 16B: The left tube of the same patient in HDlive mode shows a distal tubal block.

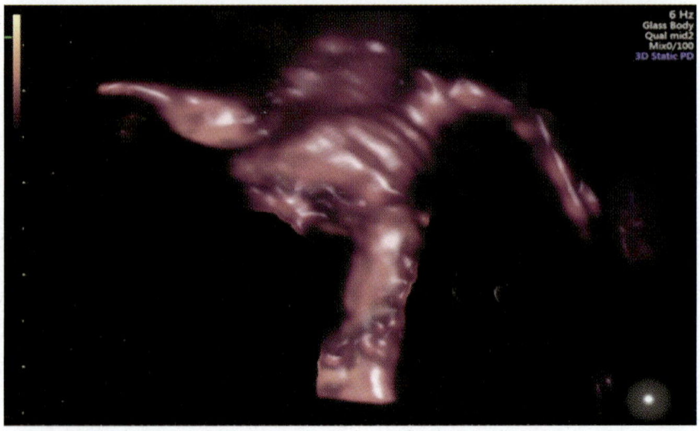

Fig. 16C: 3D power Doppler image of saline infusion salpingography, showing normal uterine cavity. The left tube is filled and lumen appears normal. The right tube shows filling only up to the proximal half. Proximal end of the tube also shows ballooning suggestive of mid tubal block on right side.

1 mm. The ability of 3D ultrasound systems to produce serial scans that can be stored for subsequent analysis, 3D reconstruction, accurate assessment of volume and coronal plane with more detailed analysis of the uterus and endometrial cavity between uterine angles is superior to conventional 2D ultrasound. A new automated 3D coded contrast imaging software and 4D Hy-Co-Sy with SonoVue further increase the accuracy of sonographic tubal assessment.

In conclusion, Hy-Co-Sy performed either by 2-D, 3-D or 4-D US is a practical, minimally invasive, superior screening method for evaluation of the uterine morphology and tubal patency. Screening positives should be directed to operative hysteroscopy and/or laparoscopy.

REFERENCES

1. Hill ML. Infertility and reproductive assistance. In: Neiberg DA, Hill LM, Bohm-Velez M, Mendelson EB (Eds). Transvaginal Ultrasound. St. Louis: Mosby Year Book; 1992. pp. 43-6.
2. Arronet GM, Aduljie SY, O'Brien IR. A 9-year survey of Fallopian tube dysfunction in human infertility: diagnosis and therapy. Fertil Steril. 1969;20:903-18.
3. Page H. Estimation of the prevalence and incidence of infertility in a population: a pilot study. Fertil Steril. 1989;71:571-4.
4. Kerin JF, Williams DB, San Roman GA, Pearistone AC, Grundfest WS, Sucrey ES. Falloposcopic classification and treatment of Fallopian tube disease. Fertil Steril. 1992;57:731-5.
5. Thurmond AS, Rosch J. Non-surgical Fallopian tube recanalization for treatment of infertility. Radiology. 1990;174:371-4.
6. Peters JA, Coulam CB. Hysterosalpingography with color Doppler ultrasonography. Am J Obstet Gynecol. 1991; 164:1530-2.
7. Volpi E, Zuccaro A, Patriarca S, Rustichelli, Sismondi P. Transvaginal sonographic tubal patency testing air and saline solution as contrast media in a routine infertility clinic setting. Ultrasound Obstet Gynecol. 1996;7:43-8.
8. Stern J, Peters AJ, Coulam CB. Color Doppler ultrasonography assessment of tubal patency: a comparison study with traditional technique. Fertil Steril. 1992;58:897-900.
9. Kupesic S, Kurjak A. Gynecological vaginal sonographic interventional procedures—what does color add? Gynecol Perinatol. 1994;3:57-60.
10. Deichert U, Schlief R, van de Sandt M, Daume E. Transvaginal hysterosalpingo-contrast sonography for the assessment of tubal patency with gray scale imaging and the additional use of pulsed wave Doppler. Fertil Steril. 1992;57:62-7.
11. Rubin I. Differences between the uterus and tubes as a cause of oscillations recorded during uterotubal insufflation. Fertil Steril. 1954;5:147-53.
12. Nannini R, Chelo E, Branconi F, Tantini C, Scarselli GF. Dynamic Echohysteroscopy. A New Diagnostic Technique in the Study of Female Infertility. Acta Europ Fertil. 1981;12: 165-71.
13. Richman TS, Viscomi GN, deCherney A, Polan ML, Alcebo LO. Fallopian Tubal Patency Assessed by Ultrasound Fluid Injection. Radiology. 1984;152:507-10.
14. Randolph JR, Ying YK, Maier DB, Schmidt CL, Riddick CH. Comparison of real-time ultrasonography, hysterosalpingography and laparoscopy/hysteroscopy. Fertil Steril. 1986;46:828-32.
15. Davison GB, Leeton J. A case of female infertility investigated by contrast-enhanced echogynecography. J Clin Ultrasound. 1988;16:44-7.
16. Allahbadia GN. Fallopian tubes and ultrasonography. The Sion experience. Fertil Steril. 1992;58:901-7.
17. Broer KH, Turanli R. Überprüfung des Tubenfaktors mitels Vaginalsonographie. Ultraschall Klin Prax. 1992;7:50-3.
18. Bonilla-Musoles F, Simón C, Sampaio M, Pellicer A. An assessment of Hysterosalpingosonography (HSSG) as a Diagnostic Tool for Uterine Cavity Defects and Tubal Patency. J Clin Ultrasound. 1992;20:175-81.
19. Deichert U, Schlief R, van de Sandt M, Junke I. Transvaginal hysterosalpingo-contrast-sonography (Hy-Co-Sy) compared with conventional tubal diagnostics. Hum Reprod. 1989;4:418-22.
20. Tüfekci EC, Girit S, Bayirli MD, Durmusoglu F, Yalti S. Evaluation of tubal patency by transvaginal sonosalpingography. Fertil Steril. 1992;57:336-40.
21. Gramiak R, Shah PM. Echocardiography of the aortic root. Invest Radiol. 1968;3:356-66.
22. Testa AC, Ferrandina G, Fruscella E, Van Holsbeke C, Ferrazzi E, Leone FP, et al. The use of contrasted transvaginal sonography in the diagnosis of gynecologic diseases: a preliminary study. J Ultrasound Med. 2005;24:1267-78.
23. Lanzani C, Savasi V, Leone F PG, Ratti M, Ferrazzi E. Two-dimensional Hy-Co-Sy with contrast tuned imaging technology and a second generation contrast media for the assessment of tubal patency in a infertility program. Fertil Steril. 2009;92:1158-61.
24. Schlief R. Ultrasound contrast agents. Radiology. 1991; 3:198-207.
25. Deichert U, van de Sandt M. Transvaginal hysterosalpingo-contrast sonography (Hy-Co-Sy). The assessment of tubal patency and uterine abnormalities by contrast enhanced sonography. Advances in Echo-Contrast. 1993; 2:55-8.
26. Ayida G, Chamberlain P, Barlow D, Kennedy S. Uterine cavity assessment prior to in vitro fertilization: comparison of transvaginal scanning, saline contrast hysterosonography and hysteroscopy. Ultrasound Obstet Gynecol. 1997;10:59-62.
27. Peters JA, Stern JJ, Coulam CB. Color Doppler hysterosalpingography. In: Jaffe R, Warsof SL (Eds). Color

Doppler in Obstetrics and Gynecology. New York: McGraw Hill; 1992. pp. 283.
28. Groff TR, Edelstein JA, Schenken RS. Hysterosalpingography in the preoperative evaluation of tubal anastomosis candidates. Fertil Steril. 1990;53:417-20.
29. Heikkinen H, Tekay A, Volpi E, Martikainen H, Jouppila P. Transvaginal salpingosonography for the assessment of tubal patency in infertile women: methodological and clinical experiences. Fertil Steril. 1995;64:293-8.
30. Jeanty P, Besnard S, Arnold A, Turner C, Crum P. Air-contrast sonohysterography as a first step assessment of tubal patency. J Ultrasound Med. 2000;19(8):519-27.
31. Battaglia C, Artini PG, D'Ambrogio G, Genazzani AD, Genazzani AR, Volpe A. Color Doppler hysterosalpingography in the diagnosis of tubal patency. Fertil Steril. 1996;65:317-22.
32. Boudghene FP, Bazot M, Robert Y, Perrot N, Rocourt N, Antoine JM, et al. Assessment of Fallopian tube patency by Hy-Co-Sy: comparison of a positive contrast agent with saline solution. Ultrasound Obstet Gynecol. 2001;18(5):525-30.
33. Allahbadia GN. Fallopian tube patency using color Doppler. Int J Gynecol Obstet. 1993;40:241-4.
34. Balen FG, Allen CM, Siddle NC, Lees WR. Ultrasound contrast hysterosalpingography—evaluation as an outpatient procedure. Br J Radiol. 1993;66:592-9.
35. Sueoka H, Asada S, Tsuchiya N, Kobayashi M, Kuroshima Y. Falloposcopic tuboplasty for bilateral tubal occlusion. A novel infertility treatment as an alternative for in-vitro fertilization? Hum Reprod. 1998;13:71-4.
36. Raga F, Bonilla-Musoles F, Blanes J, Osborne NG. Congenital Müllerian anomalies: diagnostic accuracy of three-dimensional ultrasound. Fertil Steril. 1996;65:523-8.
37. Kyei-Mensah A, Zaidi J, Pittrof R, Shaker A, Campbell S, Tan SL. Transvaginal three-dimensional ultrasound: accuracy of follicular volume measurements. Fertil Steril. 1996;65:371-6.
38. Weinraub Z, Herman A. Three-dimensional hysterosalpingography. In: Merz E (Ed). 3-D Ultrasonography in Obstetrics and Gynecology. Lippincott Williams & Wilkins, Philadelphia; 1998. pp. 57-64.
39. Sladkevicius P, Ojha K, Campbell S, Nargund G. Three-dimensional power Doppler imaging in the assessment of Fallopian tube patency. Ultrasound Obstet Gynecol. 2000;16(7):644-7.
40. Ayida G, Kennedy S, Barlow D, Chamberlain P. Conventional sonography for uterine cavity assessment: a comparison of conventional two-dimensional with three-dimensional transvaginal ultrasound; a pilot study. Fertil Steril. 1996;66:848-50.
41. Weinraub Z, Maymon R, Shulman A, Bukovsky J, Kratochwil A, Lee A, et al. Three-dimensional saline contrast hysterosonography and surface rendering of uterine cavity pathology. Ultrasound Obstet Gynecol. 1996;277-82.
42. Kiyokawa K, Masuda H, Fuyuki T, Koseki M, Uchida N, Fukuda T, et al. Three-dimensional hysterosalpingo-contrast sonography (3D-Hy-Co-Sy) as an outpatient procedure to assess infertile women: a pilot study. Ultrasound Obstet Gynecol. 2000;16(7):648-54.
43. Unterweger M, De Geyter C, Fröhlich JM, Bongartz G, Wiesner W. Three-dimensional dynamic MR-hysterosalpingography; a new, low invasive, radiation-free and less painful radiologic approach to female infertility. Hum Reprod. 2002;17(12):3138-41.
44. Comparison of three-dimensional hysterosalpingo-contrast-sonography and diagnostic laparoscopy with chromopertubation in the assessment of tubal patency for the investigation of subfertility. Acta Obstet Scand. 2005;84: 909-13.
45. Kupesic S. 2D and 3D hysterosalpingo-contrast-sonography in the assessment of uterine cavity and tubal patency. Eur J Obstet Gynecol Reprod Biol. 2007;133(1):64-9.
46. Watermann D, Denschlag D, Hanjalic Beck A, Keck C, Karck U, Prompeler H. Hysterosalpingo-contrast-sonography with 3D ultrasound—a pilot study. Ultraschall Med. 2004;25: 367-72.
47. Exacoustos C, Zupi E, Szabolcs B, Amoroso C, Di Giovanni A, Romanini ME, Arduini D. Contrast tuned imaging and second generation contrast agent SonoVue: a new ultrasound approach to evaluate tubal patency. J Minim Invasive Gynecol. 2009;16:437-44.
48. Exacoustos C, Di Giovanni A, Szabolcs B, et al. Automated three-dimensional coded contrast imaging hysterosalpingo-contrast sonography: feasibility in office tubal patency testing. Ultrasound Obstet Gynecol. 2013;41(3):328-35.
49. Luciano DE, Exacoustos C, Luciano AA. Contrast sonography for tubal patency. J Minim Invasive Gynecol. 2014;21(6):994-8.
50. He Y, Geng Q, Liu H, Han X. First experience using four-dimensional hysterosalpingo-contrast-sonography with SonoVue for assessing fallopian tube patency. J Ultrasound Med. 2013;32(7):1233-43.
51. Cheng Q, Wang SS, Zhu XS, Li F. Evaluation of tubal patency with transvaginal three-dimensional hysteron-contrast-sonography. J Chin Med Sci. 2015;30(2):70-5.
52. Zhou L, Zhang X, Chen X, Liao L, Pan R, Zhou N, et al. Value of three-dimensional hysterosalpingo-contrast sonography with SonoVue in the assessment of tubal patency. Ultrasound Obstet Gynecol. 2012;40:93-8.

60

CHAPTER

Guided Procedures Using Transvaginal Sonography

Sanja Kupesic Plavsic, Sonal Panchal

INTRODUCTION

With the recent advances in transvaginal ultrasonographic equipment, settings and technique, guided procedures using transvaginal sonography, in many cases have replaced invasive abdominal procedures. This chapter is a revision of the previous edition's chapter "Guided Procedures Using Transvaginal Sonography". It includes updated references, and additional high resolution ultrasound images. The interested reader should be able to gain an objective point of view on the role of ultrasound in performing transvaginal oocyte retrieval, ovarian cyst aspiration, drainage of pelvic abscess, fetal reduction and ultrasound-guided obstetrical procedures.

In 1974, the first to use ultrasound-guided invasive procedures for both diagnostic and therapeutic goals were Smith and Bartrum.[1] They performed percutaneous aspiration of intrabdominal abscesses. Gerzof et al. used sonography to place an abdominal catheter in order to drain purulent collections.[2,3] The advantages of these procedures over surgery include ease of procedural performance, accurate needle placement, rare injury to adjacent organs, and low cost, shorter time of the procedure, portability and patient comfort. The complications although rare, include: bleeding, infection, unintentional organ puncture and in the case of a fetal reductions, miscarriage. When the tip of a needle is used for a procedure, sonographically, it appears to be within the structure but in reality it is in front of or behind the imaged structure.

When puncture procedures are performed abdominally, one of two techniques is employed: guided needle or free hand. When puncture procedures are performed transvaginally, mobility of the probe is limited, making the free hand approach more difficult. A fixed needle guide attached to the probe shaft facilitates easier visualization of the entire length of the needle within the scanning plane and better control for the exact placement of the needle. Recently developed automated puncture devices attached to the shaft of the vaginal probe, provides extreme accuracy and precision. While its high-velocity release makes the procedure virtually painless thus no anesthesia or analgesia is required. This technique was first used for ovum retrieval during assisted reproductive technology programs, but it was quickly abandoned secondary to the need for reloading and reshooting for each new follicle aspirated. The automated puncture device is crucial when extreme accuracy is needed for any needle placement that is controlled and guided by a transvaginal probe. A manual needle introduction is less accurate and more painful because of the slower forward motion of the needle displacing mobile targets rather than penetrating them.

The punctures are usually performed with the guidance of a 5.0 to 7.5 MHz vaginal transducer probe through a needle guide that is attached to the shaft of the probe. A software-generated fixed "biopsy guided line" is displayed on the ultrasound monitor screen, which marks the path of the entering needle. Needle gauges ranging from 14 to 21 are employed. Depending on the nature of the procedure, the narrowest possible needle able to perform the desired task should be used. For better imaging, the "zoom" feature of the equipment should be used as frequently as possible. After the initial withdrawal of the needle, the pelvic structures and cul-de-sac must be observed sonographically for approximately 10 minutes and rescanned after a 2 to 3 hours period of observation to check for internal bleeding or previously undetected complications.

TRANSVAGINAL PUNCTURE PROCEDURES

This chapter will be describing the more commonly performed transvaginally directed punctures such as:

- Transvaginal oocyte retrieval
- Ovarian cyst aspiration

- Drainage of pelvic abscesses
- Multiembryo reduction
- Culdocentesis
- Obstetrical implications
- Treatment of ectopic pregnancy.

Transvaginal Oocyte Retrieval

For this procedure, experience has shown that the transvaginal technique using a needle-guided transvaginal probe is superior to all other ultrasound-guided techniques.[4]

The proximity of the transducer to the pelvic organs makes possible the use of a high frequency probe, thereby enhancing the resolution and clinical efficiency. The elastic vault of vagina allows for better proximity to the ovaries by the increased pressure on the tip of the probe. Since there is no need for full a urinary bladder, the pelvic anatomy is undistorted and the ovaries are kept beyond the focal zone of the transducer. Obesity or adhesions do not significantly inhibit the visualization of the follicles and are not contraindications for this technique.

Standardized programmed stimulation is monitored by transvaginal sonography.[5] Additional information may be obtained by hormonal estimation and color Doppler studies[6-8] of the ovarian and uterine circulation.

The entire treatment is carried out in an outpatient setting. The patient is placed on a gynecological table in the lithotomy position. Although anesthesia and sedative agents are not being utilized in approximately 50% of IVF programs,[9] sedative medication such as Flunitrazepam, Droperidol and Pentazocine may still be used. Since the mean duration of oocyte retrieval is 10 minutes, most of the patients easily tolerate the procedure. However, the operator should be aware of possible changes in vital signs and discomfort experienced by some patients. Before inserting the probe into the cover, the operator should apply the ultrasonic coupling gel. The cover which is either a sterile condom, surgical rubber glove or specially produced rubber cover is stretched over the gel to expel the air from the tip of the probe. This better prevents artifacts during the procedure. The gel or lubricant should not be used while inserting the probe because of spermicidal action and reported embryotoxicity[10] of the gel. Instead, one can use physiologic saline or a culture medium. Sterile needle guides are used for the transvaginal puncture of the follicles. A sterile cover is applied on to the keyboard of the ultrasound machine, which enables the operator to make any readjustments under sterile conditions. The patient's legs and perigenital area are then covered using the sterile drapes. The vaginal probe is inserted into the vagina after cleaning the vagina with isotonic saline or a cultured medium.

An automatic puncturing device has been developed in order to prevent potential risks of puncture procedures. This device contains a mobile metal tube, a needle carrier into which the aspiration needle is inserted and locked into place by a twisting movement.[4] Before inserting the probe into the vagina with a puncture device, the device should be loaded and secured. After insertion, a detailed ultrasound examination is performed to locate the uterus and the ovaries. The probe is directed to allow the biopsy vector to be placed to the central part of the nearest follicle indicating the direction of the needle **(Fig. 1)**. The operator calculates the distance of the biopsy vector on the screen and "shoots" the follicle either automatically (using a depth limiting screw on "shooting device" or manually. After the needle is rapidly advanced into the follicle, the operator begins to suction the tubing connected with the suction pump. As the follicular fluid is aspirated, one can see the follicle collapsing, while the follicular fluid is pulled into the collecting chamber.[4] A flushing procedure may be employed to improve the retrieval rate of the aspirated oocytes. The flushing medium which contains heparin is injected through the tubing or by using an automated flushing system. All the follicles along the same line are aspirated without withdrawing the needle. Feichtinger et al.[11] reported a low incidence of complications while using the transvaginal technique for oocyte recovery. In 2.4% of patients iliac veins were confused for a follicle and were mistakenly punctured. In all cases, bleeding into the pouch of Douglas was detected on the ultrasound screen and stopped spontaneously. One observation made was that a full bladder may exert pressure on the site and,

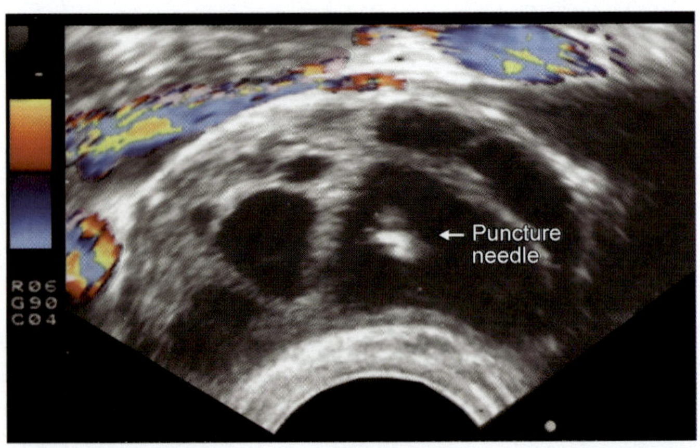

Fig. 1: Transvaginal three-dimensional ultrasound scan of a hyperstimulated ovary at the time of guided aspiration of the oocytes. Note the tip of the needle within the follicle in C plane.

therefore, stop the bleeding. Color Doppler can easily prevent such a complication, since the iliac vessels are easily visualized using this technique **(Fig. 1)**.

The bleeding from the vaginal vault is easily detectable and can be stopped by compression. Pelvic inflammatory disease (PID) is a rare complication of a transvaginal follicle aspiration and is reported in 0.14% of the patients.[9] The disease was mostly caused by infected semen, and occurred in patients with a positive history of PID.

Damario[12] reported a case of 26-year-old patient with Müllerian agenesis who underwent a controlled ovarian hyperstimulation, a transabdominal-transperitoneal ultrasound-guided oocyte retrieval and an embryo transfer of 2 cleavage-stage embryos to the gestational carrier (a 44-year-old woman) resulting in a twin pregnancy. For various reasons, patients with Müllerian agenesis may not be candidates for standard transvaginal ultrasound-guided oocyte retrieval. Although, laparoscopic oocyte retrieval has been frequently used in this setting, the approach of transabdominal-transperitoneal ultrasound-guided oocyte retrieval may offer further advantages in selected cases.

Feichtinger[13] evaluated the possibility of performing follicle puncturing procedures under three-dimensional ultrasound control close to real time using a new commercially available system **(Fig. 2A)**. He has performed a transvaginal needle-guided aspiration of 10 follicles using a newly developed ultrasound machine with a built-in rapid and powerful calculation software program for three-dimensional interactive volume and flow translation during operation. The interactive three-dimensional imaging was carried out during the aspiration of each follicle **(Figs. 2B to D)**. Oocyte recovery was successful for

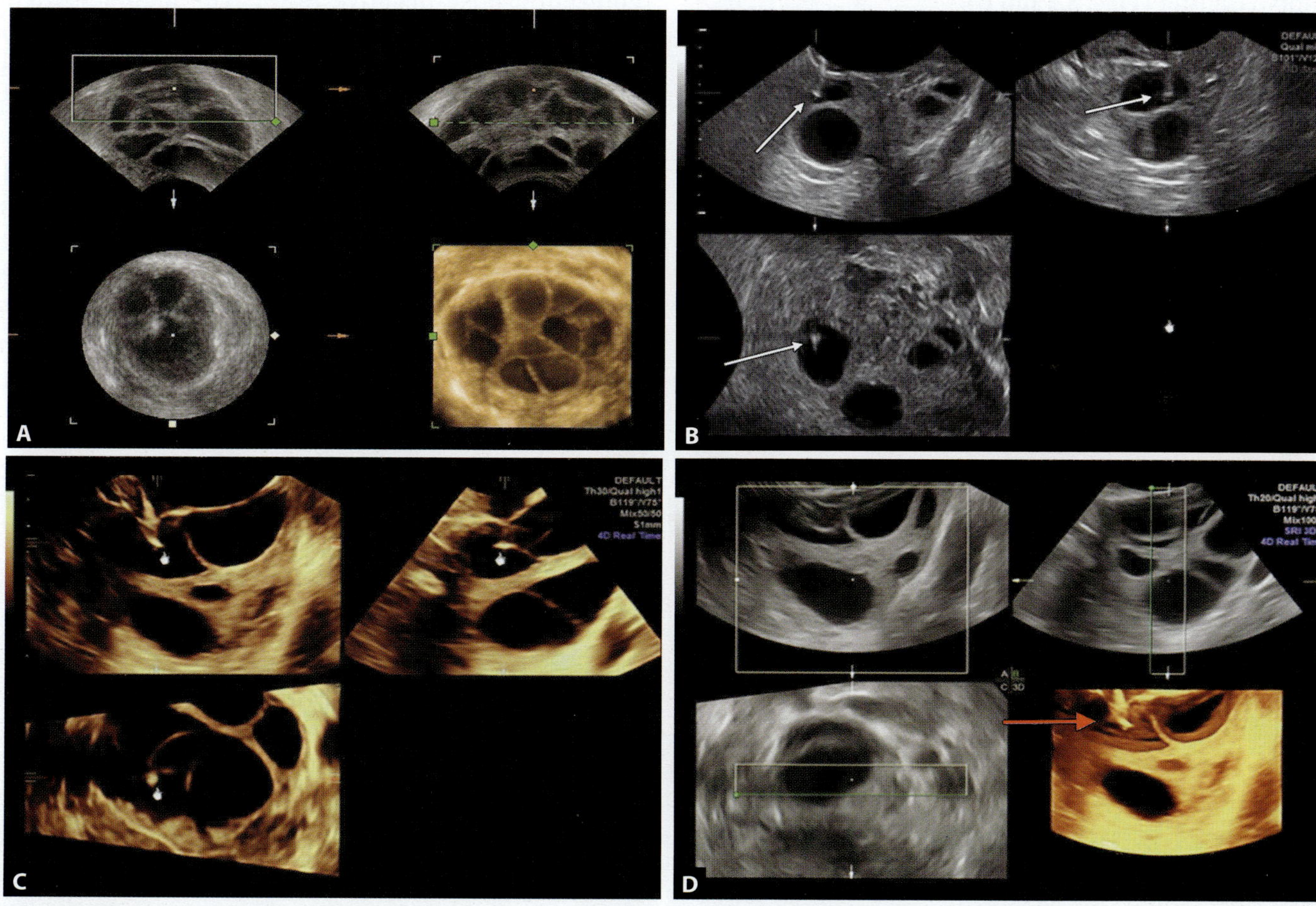

Figs. 2A to D: (A) Transvaginal three-dimensional ultrasound scan of a hyperstimulated ovary at the time of guided aspiration of the oocytes. Note the tip of the needle within the follicle in C plane; (B) 3D volume of the stimulated ovary is acquired at the time of ovum pick up. All the three planes show the needle tip in the follicle as the reference dot is aligned on the needle tip. This confirms the correct needle position in all three planes; (C) The same case as in previous figure. The contrast has been improved by adding volume contrast imaging to the multiplanar image to improve the visibility of the needle point (shown by the pointer); (D) 3D ultrasound acquired volume of the stimulated ovary at the time of pick up. On the rendered image the needle tip is seen in the follicle as marked by the arrow.

all of the follicles. There was a men delay of 5.00+/–1.22 seconds form coasting to resuming real-time ultrasound scanning during the interactive volume calculation and the search for the needle tip in the three-dimensional mode. This did not delay the procedure remarkably but enabled the precise localization of both the needle and its tip after each penetration. The integration of flow signals allowed an impressive color-coded demonstration of the needle within the tissue, but the delay was significantly longer for color-coded volume acquisition (18.40+/–4.56 seconds). This technique seems to be potentially useful in fetal medicine, oncology and surgery.

Intrauterine transfer of fertilized oocytes is not always performed as a sonographically guided procedure but transabdominal, although the available evidence suggests that there is a benefit of using US guidance during embryo transfer **(Figs. 3A and B)**.

A new technique of embryo transfer based on an ultrasound-guided transmyometrial puncture has been performed in 104 cases and described by Kato et al.[14] The use of this technique is proposed to overcome problems of difficult transfers because of cervical abnormalities. Thirty-eight patients conceived for a clinical pregnancy rate of 36.5% per attempt. No serious complications were observed. Tubal catheterization is a diagnostic and therapeutic technique of diagnosing tubal patency via injecting and observing fluid passage into the pelvis. The fallopian tubes can be reached using a transvaginally guided catheter introduced into the cervix. In the same way, fertilized ova may be carried into the ampullary portion of the tube.

Ovarian Cyst Aspiration

Transvaginal guidance permits direct visualization and aspiration of persistent follicular cysts **(Fig. 4A)**.[11] Such cysts may impair folliculogenesis due to release of hormones or as a result of a decreased perfusion by parenchymal compression. In the puncture of an ovarian or paraovarian cyst, the center of the cyst is targeted and the needle is inserted. Such a procedure is highly debated in the literature. The concern of cell spillage from a potentially malignant ovarian cyst into the abdominal cavity prevents many from using it more frequently. Although the aspirated fluid is submitted for a cytologic evaluation, a negative cytologic result may sometimes represent a false-negative result. The high sensitivity and specificity of the transvaginal color Doppler in differentiating between a benign and a malignant adnexal lesion seems to increase the reliability in decision making process as to which cysts should be aspirated **(Fig. 4B)**.

Bret et al.[15,16] published two papers describing their experience using transvaginal sonography in the aspiration of ovarian cysts. They reported a 48% recurrence rate after cyst aspiration in premenopausal patients, and an 80% recurrence rate in postmenopausal women. This group attempted to prevent cyst recurrence by injecting alcohol immediately after cyst aspiration, but this procedure was successful in only 4 out of 7 patients.[16]

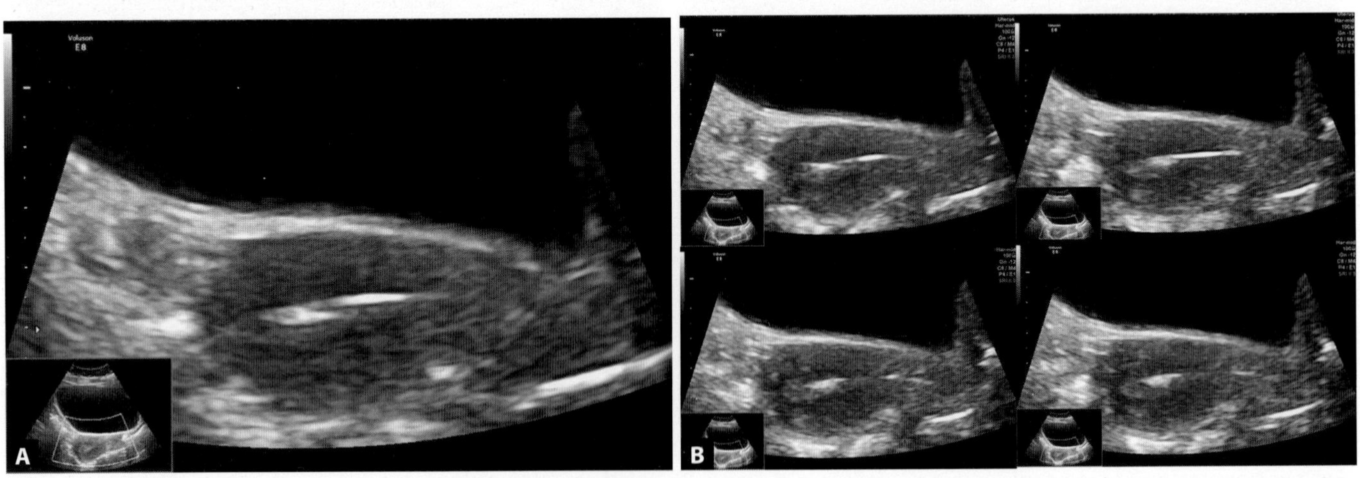

Figs. 3A and B: (A) B mode ultrasound-guided embryo transfer images showing embryo transfer cannula in the uterus with tip close to the fundus. Note echogenic jet with the release of embryos in the medium; (B) Sequence of the images shows gradual withdrawal of the cannula. Finally, right low image shows only retained embryos with air bubble seen as echogenic fleck in the endometrial cavity at fundal end, with no cannula.

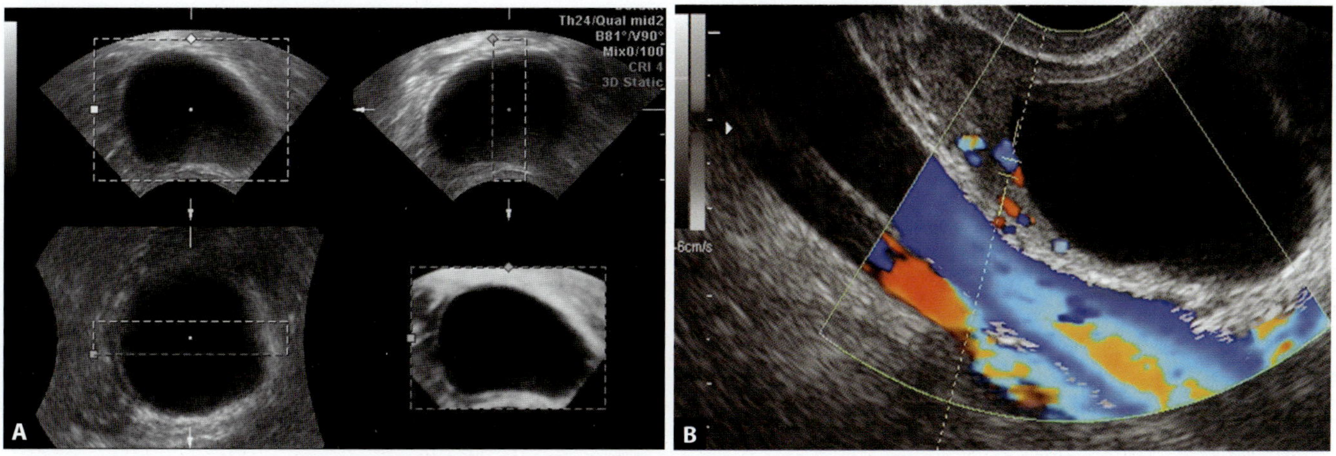

Figs. 4A and B: (A) Three-dimensional ultrasound image of a simple ovarian cyst. Only cysts without papillary protrusions and septa can be treated by transvaginal ultrasound-guided aspiration; (B) Simple ovarian cyst as seen by color Doppler ultrasound. Note the smooth surface of the cyst and extraovarian vessels, while no vascularity is detected within the cystic wall. Color Doppler may help to avoid penetration of the surrounding vessels.

The aspiration of an endometrioma is considered to be relatively contraindicated. Aboulghar et al.[17] studied 21 patients in which transvaginal sonographically-guided aspiration of pelvic and endometriotic cysts was performed. Reaccumulation occurred in only 6 cases during a 12-month follow-up. Certainly, the aspiration of endometriotic cysts is technically simple; however, its overall benefit and safety are still inconclusive due to the lack of experience obtained by evaluating a larger series.[18] In infertility program Vaegemaekers et al.[19] aspirated 32 unilocular anechoic cysts with an average diameter of 45 mm transvaginally. The authors concluded that puncture and aspiration of ovarian cysts in the early follicular phase could diminish the cancellation rate of in vitro fertilization cycles.

Drainage of Pelvic Abscesses

Infertility attributed to tubal obstruction or dysfunction is seen in 30–40% of patients. It is well known that a tubal occlusion is common sequelae of pelvic inflammatory disease. Since recurrent episodes of PID are frequent, one should expect a high incidence of this entity in the infertile population. In patients with a tubo-ovarian abscess, abscess drainage with sonographic guidance can hasten the recovery process and improve the efficacy of antibiotic therapy. Once the needle is placed into the abscess cavity, the fluid can be aspirated and the needle withdrawn **(Figs. 5A and B)**. In addition, an indwelling drainage catheter can be left in place.[11] Teisala et al.[20] used the transvaginal ultrasound-guided aspiration technique to drain 10 tubo-ovarian abscesses on patients receiving antimicrobial treatment. Only light sedation was required, and the procedure was well tolerated by the patients. This technique is accepted as an alternative to open laparoscopy for treating a tubo-ovarian abscess.

Fetal Reduction

During the past 15 years, with the increased use of ovulation inducing drugs, as well as the increased number of medically assisted reproduction procedures, have resulted in a large number of multiple gestations. Multiple pregnancies are associated with high mortality and morbidity rates. In addition, probability of achieving a term pregnancy with healthy neonates is inversely proportional to the number of the fetuses. Therefore, fetal reduction seeks to reduce the number of fetuses to improve survival for the remaining ones.[21] Women with four or more fetuses may be offered selective reduction, with the number of fetuses usually reduced to two.[11] The procedure is normally delayed till 8 weeks, after which the spontaneous loss is relatively low. The transabdominal ultrasound-guided technique was first presented by a French group[22] and adopted by others.[23,24] With the developing use of transvaginal sonography this approach was attempted and successfully applied in fetal reduction, as well. Advantages of this technique are shorter puncture route and a more precise needle placement which reduces the risk of inadvertent injury to the adjacent gestational sacs and or other pelvic structures. Color Doppler may aid in monitoring fetal heart activity during this interventional procedure **(Fig. 6A)**.

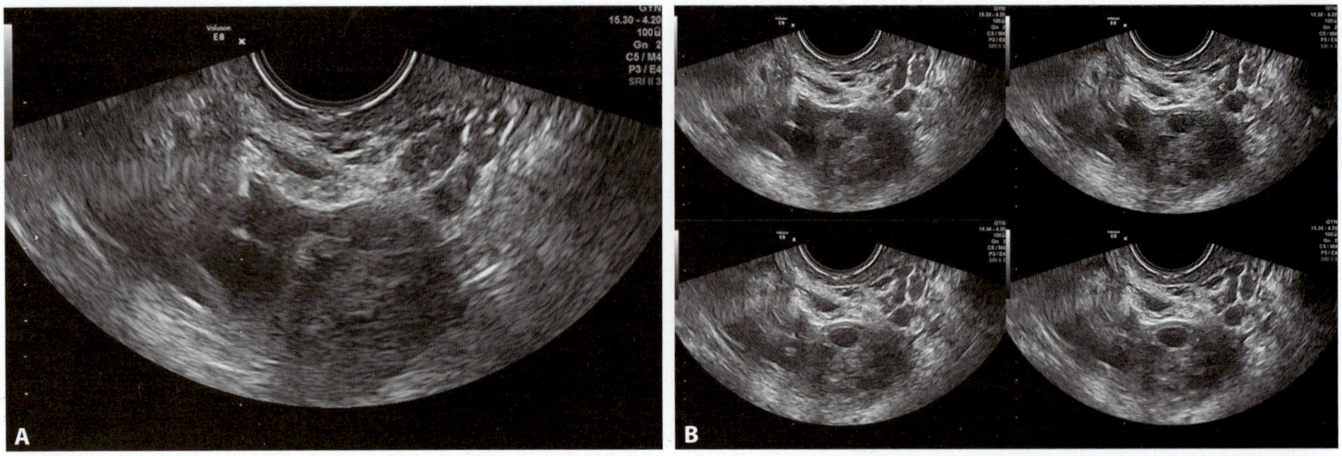

Figs. 5A and B: (A) Low level echogenic fluid is seen in the image around the ovary, with the needle tip seen in the fluid overlapping the biopsy line; (B) Sequence of the images illustrates decreasing amount of fluid following drainage of the pelvic abscess.

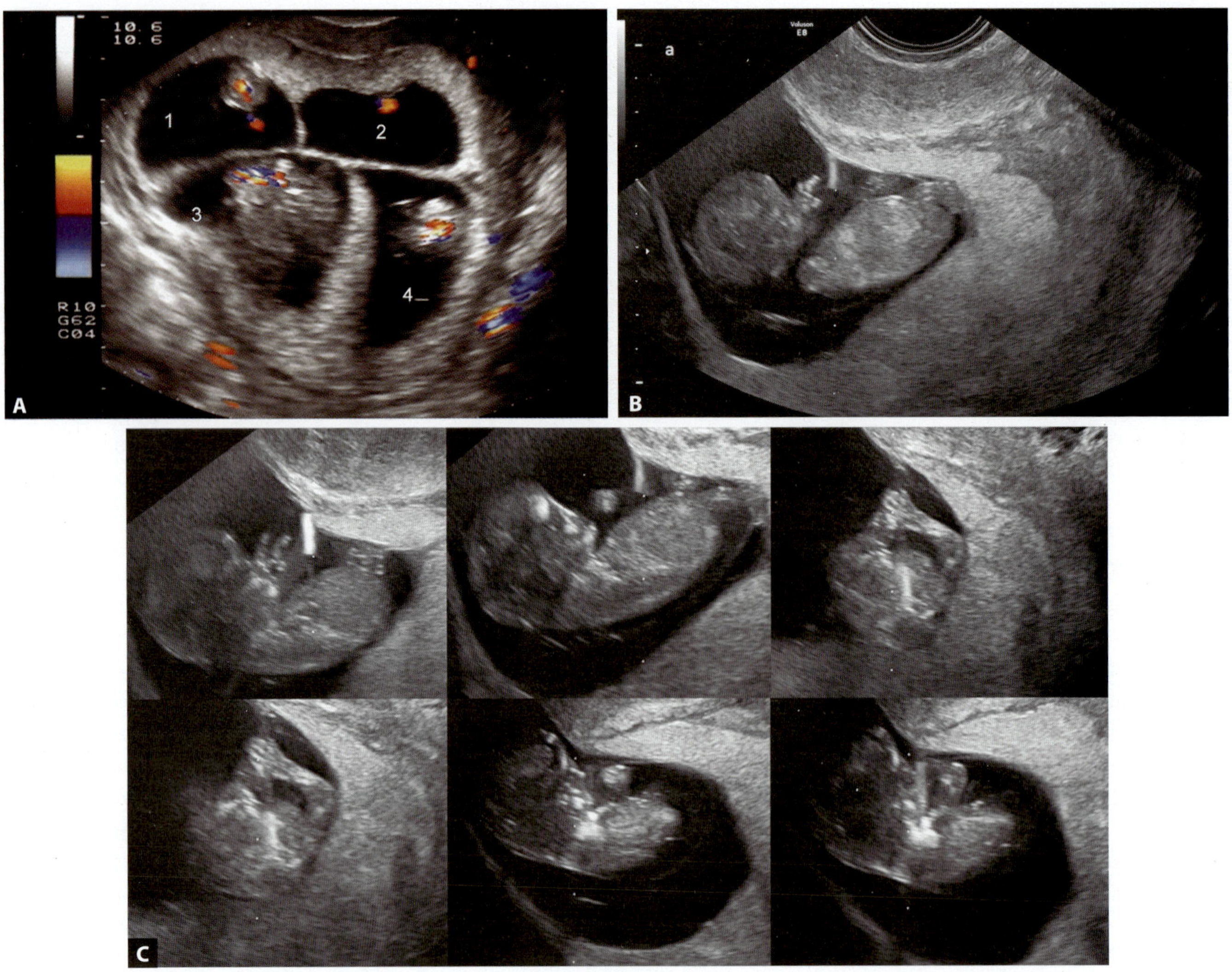

Figs. 6A to C

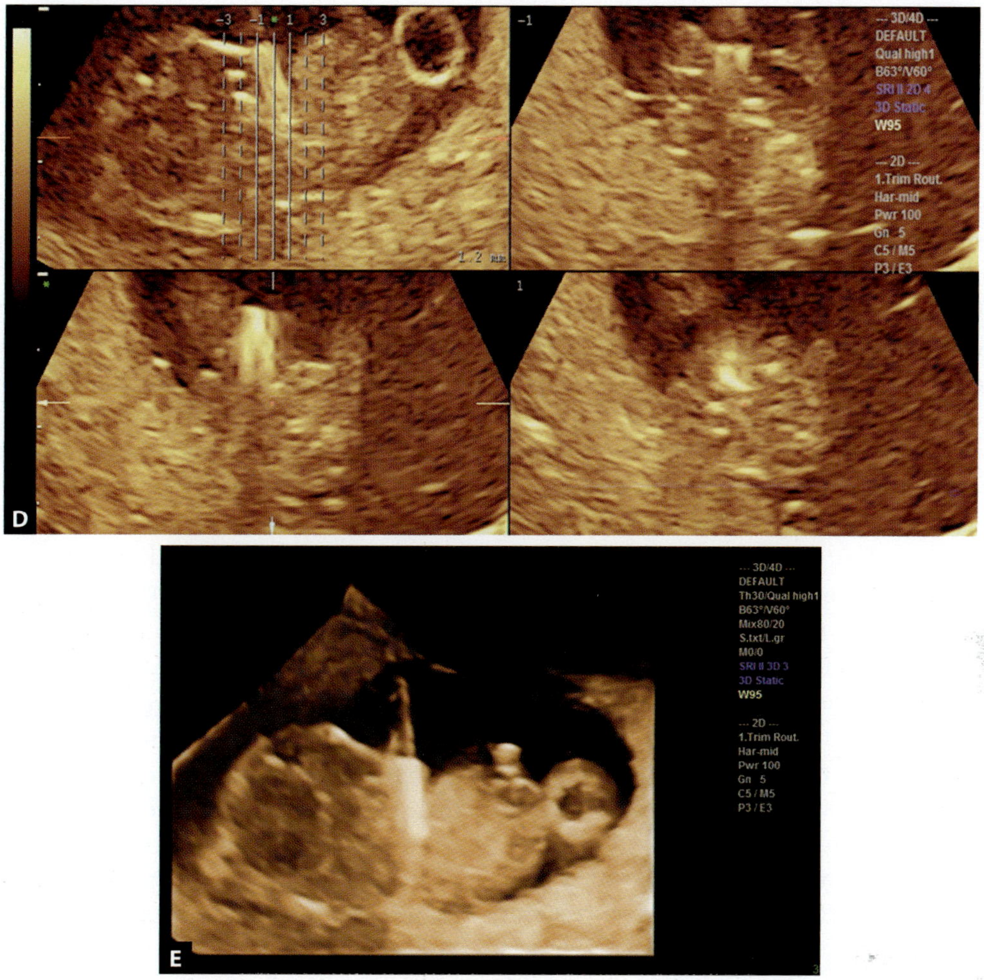

Figs. 6D and E

Figs. 6A to E: (A) Transvaginal color Doppler scan of quadruplet pregnancy. Color Doppler enables visualization and monitoring of heart activity during the procedure of fetal reduction; (B) Fetus in longitudinal axis with a needle tip seen in the amniotic cavity, located close to the fetal thorax; (C) Sequence of images demonstrating fetus in longitudinal and transverse axis with a needle tip approaching fetal thorax. Two right lower images illustrate echogenic jet at the needle tip as KCL is released into the fetal heart; (D and E) Surface rendering is helpful for needle location before injecting the drug for fetal reduction.

A brief explanation of the technique for transvaginal fetal reduction is as follows: baseline mapping procedure of the chorionic sacs, detailed evaluation of the heartbeats of the targeted fetus and placement of the needle with 0.5–1 mL of 2 mEq/mL KCl solution **(Figs. 6B and C)**. The heartbeat of each injected fetus is observed for 5–10 minutes to confirm cessation. The patients should be rescanned 3 hours later and then 1 week after the procedure. The disadvantage of a transvaginal fetal reduction is that at an early gestational age the final number of fetuses is not yet established.[18]

Coffler et al.[25] reported on their experience with 90 women who underwent early (mean 7.5 weeks gestation, range 7.0–8.0 weeks) intracardiac insertion of KCl injected into a selected fetal heart in the vicinity of a non-selected fetal heart for fetal reduction using the transvaginal sonographic approach. The procedure was associated with a total pregnancy loss rate of 11.7%. Early transvaginal fetal aspiration is a simple and relatively safe method for pregnancy reduction. More recently three-dimensional ultrasound is used in fetal reduction, allowing simultaneous and instantaneous assessment of three orthogonal planes and surface rendering **(Figs. 6D and E)**. The overall pregnancy loss rate associated with an early fetal aspiration is similar to that of procedures performed at a later gestational age, but significantly lower when the initial number of fetuses is four or greater. Iberico et al.[26] reported on early transvaginal intracardiac embryo puncture until asystole is verified without the injection of any substances as an effective and safe technique. The baby take-home rate was 89.5% for twins and 80.0% for singletons.

Diagnostic Culdocentesis

The introduction of transvaginal sonography has limited the need for diagnostic culdocentesis. The presence or absence of fluid in the pelvic cavity is easily established by a vaginal approach, but it may be necessary to differentiate between different biological fluids (clear fluid, blood or pus). The wide availability of transvaginal color Doppler sonography to distinguish the dominant pelvic pathology in the presence of pelvic fluid on the basis of different vascularity patterns is very helpful in routine investigations. There are times when the clinician still requires information provided by culdocentesis despite having the knowledge acquired by the history and physical examination, the transvaginal color Doppler and the rapid β-human chorionic gonadotropin (β-hCG) test. Inserting a needle in the cul-de-sac is a simple technique that can be performed safely and accurately with transvaginal ultrasound guidance.[27] High quality B-mode transvaginal sonography with superimposed color Doppler flow allows accurate and simultaneous identification of the main pelvic vessels, physiological angiogenesis (corpus luteum) and ectopic peritrophoblastic blood flow. The color Doppler will help in the accurate placement of the needle, diminishing the risk of injury to adjacent vessels, especially in women who have had previous inflammatory disease of the pelvis with an obliterated cul-de-sac.

Obstetrical Procedures

The high frequency transvaginal probe enables a detailed analysis of embryonic, extraembryonic and early fetal structures. By this method, screening for structural anomalies can be initiated during the first and early second trimester. Recent advances in tissue culture technology have established chorionic villous sampling and early amniocentesis as early invasive diagnostic modalities. Color Doppler imaging has added important information on the functional integrity of the maternal-fetal circulation. The main advantages of the application of color Doppler imaging is in the following invasive transvaginal diagnostic techniques such as:

Chorionic Villous Sampling

The diagnostic accuracy and safety of chorionic villous sampling are nearly the same as those of amniocentesis. Chorionic villous sampling is generally performed with transabdominal ultrasound guidance, with either a catheter placed through the cervix or a needle placed percutaneously through the abdominal wall. The transvaginal route, in which the needle is placed through the vaginal and uterine wall, is usually performed at a gestational age of 8–12 weeks. The ultrasound-guided transmural puncturing procedure promises to be the most accurate, and the least traumatic and painful method. The small depth of penetration under high-resolution ultrasound guidance is the most striking advantage of this method. Color Doppler allows precise sonographic imaging of the placental site by visualization of the umbilical cord and its insertion.

Early Amniocentesis

Using a transvaginal approach and directed needle it is possible to aspirate the amniotic fluid as early as 9 weeks of gestation. The advantages of early amniocentesis are clear images, patient preference for early amniocentesis over chorionic villi sampling, and availability of chromosome analysis and amniotic α-fetoprotein[28] measurement. The main complications during this procedure include fetal demise, rupture of the membranes, bleeding and infection. It seems that color Doppler could decrease the fetal loss rate by a more precise identification of the placental localization and visualization of the umbilical cord.

CONSERVATIVE MANAGEMENT OF AN ECTOPIC PREGNANCY

In the past, the diagnosis of ectopic pregnancy was made at the time of laparotomy, and very often in the presence of a hemodynamically unstable patient. The physician was often left with little choice but to perform a salpingectomy, salpingo-oophorectomy or segmental resection of the fallopian tube. At that time the physician's main concern was to save the patient's life and the potential preservation of the affected fallopian tube was a secondary concern. More recently, by using sensitive pregnancy tests and transvaginal and/or abdominal ultrasonography, it has become possible to diagnose an ectopic pregnancy at such an early stage that currently less radical surgical therapies in addition to medical therapies are being used as the preferred treatment.

The use of a needle, which is inserted into a tubal pregnancy under transvaginal ultrasound guidance, can save a patient from a more invasive procedure. Feichtinger was the first to describe the use of transvaginally guided needle puncture to treat the ectopic tubal gestation.[29] Since then, several centers have used this modality as an additional tool in treatment of patients with an ectopic pregnancy.[28,30-33] One complication that may occur is concurrent or delayed hemorrhaging. Fortunately, this is a very uncommon event, and generally occurs during the first 1 or 2 days postprocedure in approximately 15% of patients.[28] Other complications include a persistence of the trophoblastic tissue within the fallopian tube and a persistent elevation of the hCG levels following the procedure. Many of these cases can be treated in a nonsurgical fashion, using the systemic administration of methotrexate.[34] Systemic use of methotrexate has been documented to be safe, effective and well tolerated.[34,35] Preliminary evidence suggests that the fertility potential after such a treatment is comparable to that following conservative surgery.[34-36]

Since the introduction of transvaginal sonography with color flow imaging within a high frequency probe, a more accurate and faster diagnosis of ectopic pregnancy is feasible. Color Doppler appears to be useful for the positive diagnosis of ectopic pregnancy with ultrasonography when no adnexal gestational sac is observed.[37] Peritrophoblastic flow is prominent, randomly dispersed inside the solid part of an adnexal mass, and clearly separated from the ovarian tissue. A low impedance signal and a resistance index, usually less than 0.45 extracted from the color-coded area indicates an invasive trophoblast. The clinical impression of probable tubal abortion is seen in patients when with no color flow, or an increased vascular resistance of the peritrophoblastic flow and a β-hCG level less than 1,000 IU/mL. Using Doppler it is possible to identify the vitality and invasiveness of the trophoblast. These are the most important characteristics to consider when planning the management of an ectopic pregnancy.

At our department, 11 patients with an unruptured ectopic pregnancy of less than 3 cm in diameter were treated locally with methotrexate. After the patient received slight sedation, the tubal pathology ("tubal ring" containing the ectopic embryo or solid part of the complex adnexal mass) was imaged. Color flow was superimposed on the anatomical structure and a pulsed Doppler waveform analysis showed a low impedance (resistance index cut-off value of 0.45 or less) and a high velocity. Using the equipment's software-generated puncture path line, the needle was introduced in the area of the maximal color signal. We administered methotrexate using the dose of 1 mg/kg of body weight, into the area of active trophoblastic flow. Determination of serum β-hCG levels and transvaginal sonography were performed every second day, until the β-hCG levels reached non-pregnant levels. Color flow imaging, with its excellent potential for tissue characterization, was used for serial determinations of blood flow from the questionable adnexa. In patients with successful salpingocentesis, serially analyzed serum levels of β-hCG returned to non-pregnant levels (n = 9), while pulsed Doppler waveform analysis showed increasing values of impedance to flow. Changes in the vascularity could be correlated with the effect of the medication on the vitality and invasiveness of active ectopic trophoblastic tissue.

Based on our own experience, with regards to an ectopic pregnancy, a transvaginal color Doppler has both a diagnostic and therapeutic potential. By comparing color Doppler findings to declining β-hCG levels, it is possible to follow patients undergoing conservative treatments, safely. Serial β-hCG determinations demonstrated that in patients who underwent successful salpingocentesis, serum levels of β-hCG returned to a non-pregnant levels after 10–22 days. With the use of color flow imaging, it becomes possible to avoid puncturing through a highly vascular area hence bleeding during or immediately following the procedure is significantly reduced. In suspicious cases of tubal pregnancy in which color flow within the tube was absent and β-hCG levels were less than 1,000 mIU/mL, local administration of methotrexate could not be advised.

There is still much to be learned about the diagnosis and management of an ectopic pregnancy. The transvaginal color Doppler represents an important addition in selection of patients for conservative treatment, as well as in defining the individual therapeutic strategy.

In a patient with a history of a previous cervical pregnancy who currently had a cervical pregnancy and a simultaneous intrauterine pregnancy, Monteagudo et al.[38] reported a successful transvaginal ultrasound-guided puncture and injection. They treated the cervical pregnancy by selective reduction using an injection of potassium chloride guided by transvaginal sonography. A cesarean section was performed to deliver the intrauterine gestation at 34 weeks. Timor-Tritsch et al.[39] described a proposed transvaginal ultrasound-guided puncture route to be performed on a cornual ectopic pregnancy by leading the needle into the cornual ectopic pregnancy. To accomplish this procedure the needle would first be traversing the myometrium while simultaneously approaching the gestational sac from the medial aspect. The probe was rotated into a position that enables the software-generated directional puncture lines to "transect" the thick uterine myometrium before reaching the gestational sac. This line approaches the ectopic cornual pregnancy form the medial aspect and avoids the puncture of a stretched out thin myometrium. Only cornual pregnancies with positive heartbeats were considered for puncture. With the use of an automated puncture device, a 21-gauge needle was then introduced into the chorionic sac and the embryo. There was no need for analgesia, as the automated spring-loaded puncture device advances the needle with a high speed, thus making it virtually a painless procedure. The embryo is injected with methotrexate (25 or 50 mg in 1 or 2 mL solvent, respectively) or, in the case of a live heterotopic pregnancy, with potassium chloride. Half of the amount is injected into the embryo to stop the heartbeats and, if possible, the balance into the placental site when the needle is extracted. After completing the procedure the puncture area is observed for approximately 5–10 minutes to detect any moderate post-procedure bleeding. The puncture injection of a cornual pregnancy is a relatively new treatment modality which seems promising because the patient may avoid surgery and the potential outcomes and risks of surgery such as a future cesarean section, uterine scar, and a cornual rupture during a desired future pregnancy. Approaching the cornual pregnancy with its chorionic sac, embryo and placenta form the medial aspect and traversing the thicker myometrium creates a significant and protective safety layer, through which rupture or bleeding are less likely to occur.

OTHER APPLICATIONS

Zanetta et al.[40] reported on the use of transvaginal ultrasound-guided fine needle sampling of deep cancer recurrences in the pelvis. For aspirates and biopsies, the sensitivity was 76 and 91% respectively, while the accuracy was 83 and 91% respectively. This technique is a safe procedure with limited invasiveness and extremely high specificity even when performed on small targets (the median diameter in this study was 30 mm). Whenever possible, biopsies are preferred. A negative fine needle biopsies obtained from a clinically suspicious lesion requires a repeat sampling.

A recent study by Hammoud et al.[41] reported that a ultrasound-guided endometrial biopsy is a viable option for endometrial sampling in patients with a stenotic cervix. Under control of transvaginal sonography, in two postmenopausal patients with vaginal bleeding and a failed endometrial biopsy due to a stenotic cervix, a 20-gauge needle was inserted through the vaginal vault and anterior uterine wall into the endometrium. The endometrium was aspirated and the specimens were submitted for cytology. One patient had an endometrial adenocarcinoma and underwent a staging procedure, while the other patient had a benign cytology and was followed clinically.

Another already reported application of transvaginal ultrasound-guided procedures is aspiration of tubo-ovarian abscesses. Gjelland et al.[42] evaluated 449 transvaginal aspiration performed on 302 women. A total of 282 (93.4%) were successfully treated by transvaginal aspiration of the purulent fluid, together with antibiotic therapy. In the remaining 20 patients, surgery was performed. The main indications for surgery were diagnostic or therapeutic uncertainty, such as suspected residual tubo-ovarian abscess or pain. Sudakoff et al.[43] evaluated the techniques, patient selection, pre- and post-procedural care and monitoring aspects of transrectal and transvaginal ultrasound-guided drainage of the infected pelvic collections. A transrectal ultrasound-guided biopsy of a pelvic mass is also a feasible method of establishing a pathological diagnosis.[44]

CONCLUSION

Although ultrasound-guided procedures are most commonly used in the field of reproductive assistance, it is clear that similar techniques can be applied to other clinical situations as well. The extreme accuracy and high patient tolerance have initiated the widespread use of transvaginally performed puncture procedures. The use of transabdominal and transvaginal sonography has improved the accuracy of embryo placement into the uterine cavity, or via the uterus, into the fallopian tube and guidance of fallopian tube catheterization. Other ultrasound-guided procedures analyzed in this chapter are aspiration of the ovarian cysts, drainage of pelvic collections and abscesses and selective reduction of multiple pregnancies. The advantages of ultrasound-guided procedures are their performance under real-time imaging, relative simplicity, and low procedure-related complication rate. The superior spatial information provided by three-dimensional ultrasound might enhance 2D ultrasound guided procedures in obstetrics and gynecology.

REFERENCES

1. Smith EH, Bartrum RJ Jr. Ultrasonically-guided percutaneous aspiration of abscesses. AJR. 1974;122:308-12.
2. Gerzof SG, Johnson WC, Robbins AH. Expanded criteria for percutaneous abscess drainage. Arch Surg. 1985;120:227-32.
3. Gerzof SG, Johnson WC. Radiologic aspects of diagnosis and treatment of abdominal abscesses. Surg Clin North Am. 1984;64:53-65.
4. Feichtinger W. Transvaginal oocyte retrieval. In: Chervenak FA, Isaacson GC, Campbell S (Eds). Ultrasound in obstetrics and gynecology. (London: Little, Brown and Company); 1993. pp. 1397-406.
5. Kemeter P, Feichtinger W. Experience with a new fixed-stimulation protocol without hormone determinations for programmed oocyte retrieval for in-vitro fertilization. Hum Reprod. 1989;4(suppl.):53-4.
6. Kurjak A, Kupesic S, Schulman H, Zalud I. Transvaginal color Doppler in the assessment of ovarian and uterine blood flow in infertile women. Fertil Steril. 1991;56:870-3.
7. Kupesic S, Kurjak A. Uterine and ovarian perfusion during the periovulatory phase assessed by transvaginal color Doppler. Fertil Steril. 1993;60:439-43.
8. Kurjak A, Kupesic S. Ovarian senescence and its significance on uterine and ovarian perfusion. Fertil Steril. 1995;64:532-7.
9. Feichtinger W, Putz M, Kemeter P. New aspects of vaginal ultrasound in an in vitro fertilization program. Ann NY Acad Sci. 1988;541:125-30.
10. Schwimer SR, Rothman CM, Lebovic J, Oye DM. The effect of ultrasound coupling gels on sperm motility in vitro. Fertil Steril. 1984;42:946-50.
11. Hill ML, Nyberg DA. Transvaginal sonography guided procedures. In: Nyberg DA, Hill LM, Bohm-Velez M, Mendelson EB (Eds). Transvaginal Ultrasound (St. Louis: Mosby Year Book); 1992. pp. 319-29.
12. Damario MA. Transabdominal-transperitoneal ultrasound-guided oocyte retrieval in a patient with Müllerian agenesis. Fertil Steril. 2002;78(1):189-91.
13. Feichtinger W. Follicle aspiration with interactive three-dimensional digital imaging (Voluson): a step toward real-time puncturing under three-dimensional ultrasound control. Fertil Steril. 1998;70(2):374-7.
14. Kato O, Takatsuka R, Asch RH. Transvaginal-transmyometrial embryo transfer: the Towako method; experiences of 104 cases. Fertil Steril. 1993;59(1):51-3.
15. Bret PM, Guibaud L, Atri M. Transvaginal US-guided aspiration of ovarian cysts and solid pelvic masses. Radiology. 1992;185:377.
16. Bret PM, Atri M, Guibaud L. Ovarian cysts in postmenopausal women: preliminary results with transvaginal alcohol sclerosis. Radiology. 1992;184:661.
17. Aboulghar MA, Mansour RT, Serour GI, Rizk B. Ultrasonic transvaginal aspiration of endometriotic cysts: an optional line of treatment in selected cases of endometriosis. Hum Reprod. 1991;6:1408-10.
18. Lerner JP, Monteagudo A. Vaginal sonographic puncture procedures. In: Goldstein SR, Timor-Tritsch IE (Eds). Ultrasound in Gynecology (New York: Churchill Livingstone); 1995. pp. 223-38.
19. Waegemaekers CT, Berg-Helder A, Blankhart A, Naaktgeboren N. Transvaginal ovarian cyst puncture in the early follicular phase of an IVF cycle, indications and results. Hum Reprod. 1988;3(suppl.1):80.
20. Teisala K, Heinonen PK, Punnonen R. Transvaginal ultrasound in the diagnosis and treatment of tuboovarian abscess. Br J Obstet Gynaecol. 1990;97:178-80.
21. Berkowitz RI, Lynch L. Selective reduction: an unfortunate misnomer. Obstet Gynecol. 1990;75:873-4.
22. Dumez Y, Oury JF. Method for first trimester selective abortion in multiple pregnancy. Contrib Gynecol Obstet. 1986;15:50-3.
23. Birnholz JC, Dmowski WP, Binor Z, Radwanska E. Selective continuation in gonadotropin-induced multiple pregnancy. Fertil Steril. 1987;48:873.
24. Brandes JM, Itskovitz J, Timor-Tritsch IE. Reduction of the number of embryos in multiple pregnancy. Fertil Steril. 1987;48:326-7.
25. Coffler MS, Kol S, Drugan A, Itskovitz-Eldor J. Early transvaginal embryo aspiration: a safe method for selective reduction in high order multiple gestations. Hum Reprod. 1999;14(7):1875-8.
26. Iberico G, Navarro J, Blasco L, Simon C, Pellicer A, Remohi J. Embryo reduction of multifetal pregnancies following assisted reproduction treatment: a modification of the transvaginal ultrasound-guided technique. Hum Reprod. 2000;15(10):2228-33.
27. Fleischer AC, Pennel RG, McKee MS, Worell JA, Keefe B, Herbert CM, et al. Ectopic pregnancy: features and transvaginal sonography. Radiology. 1990;174:375-9.
28. Timor-Tritsch IE, Peisner DB, Monteagudo A. Vaginal sonographic puncture procedures. In: Timor-Tritsch IE, Rottem S (Eds). Transvaginal Sonography. New York: Elsevier; 1991. p. 427.
29. Feichtinger W, Kemeter P. Conservative treatment of ectopic pregnancy by transvaginal aspiration under sonographic control and methotrexate injection. Lancet. 1987;1(8529):381-2.
30. Menard A, Crequat J, Mandelbroat L, Hanny JP, Mandelanat P. Treatment of unruptured tubal pregnancy by local injection of methotrexate under transvaginal sonographic control. Fertil Steril. 1990;54:47-8.

31. Egarter C. Methotrexate treatment of ectopic gestation and reproductive outcome. Am J Obstet Gynecol. 1990;62:406-9.
32. Brown DL, Felker RE, Stowall TG, Emerson DS, Ling FV. Serial endovaginal sonography of ectopic pregnancies treated by methotrexate. Obstet Gynecol. 1991;77: 406-8.
33. Mottla GL, Rulin MC, Guzick DS. Lack of resolution of ectopic pregnancy by intratubal injection of methotrexate. Fertil Steril. 1992;57:685.
34. Stowall TG, Ling FW, Gray LA. Single dose methotrexate for treatment of ectopic pregnancy. Obstet Gynecol. 1991;77:754-7.
35. Fernandez H, Baton C, Lelaidier C, Frydman R. Conservative management of ectopic pregnancy: prospective randomized clinical trial of methotrexate versus prostaglandin sulphosterone by combined transvaginal and systemic administration. Fertil Steril. 1991;55:746.
36. Ory SL. Chemotherapy for ectopic pregnancy. Obstet Gynecol Clin N Am. 1991;18:123-4.
37. Kurjak A, Zalud I, Schulman H. Ectopic pregnancy: transvaginal color Doppler of trophoblastic flow in questionable adnexa. J Ultrasound Med. 1991;10:685-7.
38. Monteagudo A, Tarricone NJ, Timor-Tritsch IE, Lerner JP. Successful transvaginal ultrasound-guided puncture and injection of a cervical pregnancy in a patient with simultaneous intrauterine pregnancy and a history of a previous cervical pregnancy. Ultrasound Obstet Gynecol. 1996;8(6):381-6.
39. Timor-Tritsch IE, Monteagudo A, Lerner JP. A "potentially safer" route for puncture and injection of cornual ectopic pregnancies. Ultrasound Obstet Gynecol. 1996;7(5):353-5.
40. Zanetta G, Brenna A, Pittelli M, Lissoni A, Trio D, Riotta S. Transvaginal ultrasound-guided fine needle sampling of deep cancer recurrences in the pelvis: usefulness and limitations. Gynecol Oncol. 1994;54(1):59-63.
41. Hammound AO, Deppe G, Eikhechen SS, Johnson S. Ultrasonography-guided transvaginal endometrial biopsy: a useful technique in patients with cervical stenosis. Obstet Gynecol. 2006;107:518-20.
42. Gjelland K, Ekerhovd E, Granberg S. Transvaginal ultrasound-guided aspiration for treatment of tubo-ovarian abscess: a study of 302 cases. Am J Obstet Gynecol. 2005;193:1323-30.
43. Sudakoff GS, Lundeen SJ, Otterson MF. Transrectal and transvaginal sonographic intervention of infected pelvic fluid collections: a complete approach. Ultrasound Q. 2005;21:175-85.
44. Giede C, Toi A, Chapman W, Rosen B. The use of transrectal ultrasound to biopsy pelvic masses in women. Gynecol Oncol. 2004;95:552-6.

61

CHAPTER

Ultrasound in the Postmenopause

Sonal Panchal, Biserka Funduk Kurjak

INTRODUCTION

The menopause occurs because the ovary has no longer any follicles to respond to hypothalamic/pituitary stimulation. At menarche, there are some 250,000–300,000 oocytes present, which are gradually used up in the succession of menstrual cycle from menarche until around 50 years of age, which is the average age for the menopause in Europe and the United States.[1]

Climacteric defines a more prolonged period of estrogen withdrawal, starting first with the decrease in frequency of ovulation and ending in atrophy of secondary sexual characteristics. A single point in that curve, when insufficient follicle maturity results in inadequate estrogen and no menses is the menopause.[1] The postmenopausal period begins with the last menstrual bleeding (LMB).

Prior to menopause, the remaining follicles begin to perform less well. Release of the hypothalamic and the pituitary gland hormones from inhibition resulted in raised gonadotropins levels, which is a characteristic of the menopause and their level is well above those seen in the menstrual cycle at times other than the luteinizing hormone (LH) surge. Eventually, there is a 10–20-fold increase in follicle-stimulating hormone (FSH) and approximately a threefold increase in LH, reaching a maximal level 1–3 years after menopause, after which there is a gradual but slight decline in both gonadotropins.[1]

Estrogen production by the ovaries does not continue beyond the menopause; however, estrogen levels in postmenopausal women can be significant, principally due to the extraglandular conversion of androstenedione and testosterone, produced by the adrenal gland and the postmenopausal ovary, respectively. The clinical impact of this estrogen will vary from one postmenopausal woman to another, depending upon the degree of extraglandular production, modified by variety of factors, such as body weight, age, and stress.[1]

According to that degree, wide ranges of clinical diversity and symptomatology can be seen in practice.

The genital organs undergo general atrophic changes. The ovaries become shrunken and fibrous. The uterus and tubes shrink, and in the case of uterus the body shrinks to a greater extent than the cervix so that the ratio of the body to cervix becomes 1:1 or even 1:2. The vaginal epithelium shrinks markedly, glycogen disappears from the cells, lactic acid is no longer produced and the environment of the vagina becomes alkaline.[1]

A series of menopausal symptoms arise in many patients. Some concerned directly with hormone deficiency, some possibly concerned with aging, and other are emotion related. Those directly concerned with estrogen lack are vasomotor symptoms and urogenital atrophic changes, which can lead to dyspareunia and incontinence. Demineralization of bone leads to postmenopausal osteoporosis. Cardiovascular changes are evident too. Premenopausal women appear to have some immunity from coronary thrombosis and anginal attacks, which may be causally related to their different lipid background when compared with men. After the menopause, all lipid levels rise, and there is an increase in low-density lipid (LDL) cholesterol with little change in high-density lipid (HDL) cholesterol.

CHALLENGES OF THE POSTMENOPAUSE

For a female, life expectancy in the developed world is approaching 80 years. A woman may, on an average, expect to spend some 30 years or 40% of her active life in the postmenopausal era.[1]

It is probably true that today women have greater expectations of high-quality life than previous generations. Therefore, it seems likely that climacteric and postmenopausal women will continue to place increasing demands on healthcare resources for many years to come.

The gynecological care of the fertile female population has already been well established in most countries. In the not too distant future, postmenopausal women will constitute the major proportion of the gynecological patient population. Preventive medicine and care for elderly will be an essential part of the general gynecological practice. In parallel with the demands, "climacteric and postmenopausal clinics" are being established world-wide with the active participation of gynecologists, cardiologists, rheumatologists, etc.

With better nutrition, health care, and living conditions, more women are living long enough to develop ovarian and endometrial cancers, which are known to be more common after the menopause. Undoubtedly, the care of postmenopausal population must include the early detection of ovarian and endometrial cancers, just as the access to the benefits of hormone replacement therapy (HRT).

Estimating the potential individual benefits and monitoring, the HRT poses further challenges in the medical care of the postmenopausal women.

Vaginosonographic examination has become an examination technique that is very well accepted by postmenopausal women. Recent advantages of transvaginal color Doppler and three-dimensional ultrasound enable the more experienced examiner to visualize even the smallest vessels and investigate blood flow characteristics in the poorly perfused small pelvis in the postmenopause, which helps differentiate between the normal, suspicious, and pathologic variations of the structures or defect, and follow the effects of the HRT on the perfusion of genital tract. In this chapter, we will discuss the role of ultrasound in the management of the postmenopausal women.

INSTRUMENTATION

There are variety of configuration of transvaginal probes, including various number of sizes and shapes. Examining a woman in the postmenopause, the ovaries and the endometrium must be the special field of interest. In general, the curved linear multielement transducers afford the best density and overall field-of-view for imaging.

In elderly women, the stenosis of the upper part of the vagina or adhesions of the vaginal walls can occur in addition to the atrophic changes of the epithelia. One must take special care when introducing the probe into the vagina of a woman in the senescence. Transvaginal sonography (TVS) can induce unnecessary bleeding and pain. Using thinner transducers and lubricant gels could help avoid the unnecessary injuries. The same caution applies to women who have vaginal adhesions secondary to previous surgery for whom the vaginal examination may be painful.

It is advisable to have an additional medical person being present during any kind of vaginal procedure.

SCANNING IN THE POSTMENOPAUSE

The first and perhaps the most important condition for TVS should be a thorough emptying of the urinary bladder. This is the condition which makes the TVS more comfortable for the significant group of incontinent postmenopausal patients, comparing to the transabdominal ultrasonography, which requires full bladder. On the other hand, some elderly patients who are unable to empty their bladder completely may need catheterization for better visualization.

Once the probe is covered with condom, it should be inserted into the introitus with slight downward pressure on the perineum, while gently separating the labia majora with the fingers of the other hand. A small amount of gel applied outside the condom can act as lubricating interface. If the patient desires she can insert the probe herself.

Inserting the probe into the midvagina, the anteflexed uterus can be normally imaged in its sagittal (long-axis) plane. However, in the postmenopause with the loss of the strength of uterine ligaments and the pelvic support, the uterus will frequently alter its position in the female pelvis. With the advanced age, it is usually situated in the midline in a straighten position and can be imaged only after inserting the probe into the fornix **(Fig. 1)**. Additionally, a descended, even a prolapsed uterus let the examiner to be able to orientate only after reestablishing the near normal situation by pushing the uterus upward manually and then holding it there with the help of a probe.

In the long axis, one can appreciate the different interfaces of the endometrium, beginning with the interface of the cervical canal. As the echogenicity of the cervical mucus is very poor and the endometrium may be very thin, and atrophied in the postmenopause, visualization of the endometrium can be difficult **(Fig. 2)**; it usually appears in the form of a thin and echo poor line in the midline of the sagittal plane of the uterus.

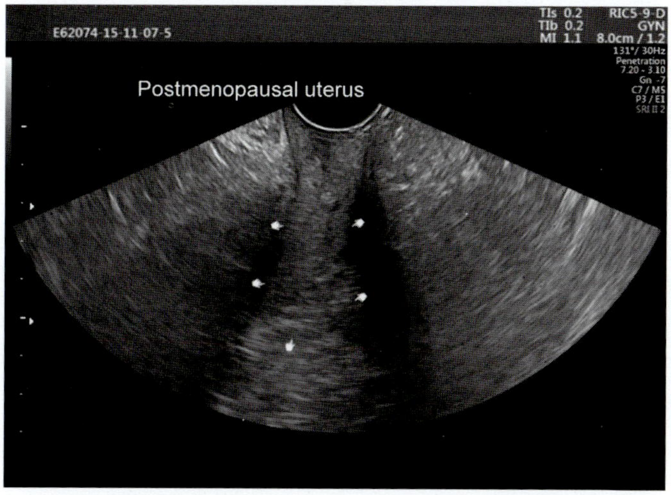

Fig. 1: Small menopausal uterus in the mid position in pelvis and shows very thin barely distinguishable endometrium.

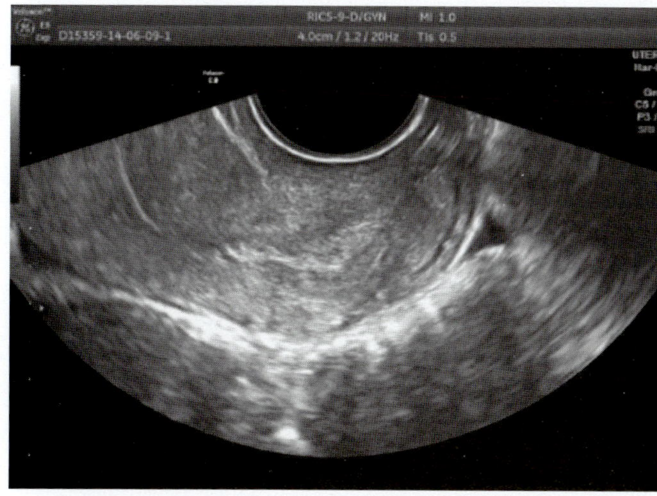

Fig. 3: B-mode ultrasound image of cervix with no mucus (anechoic shadow) in cervical canal.

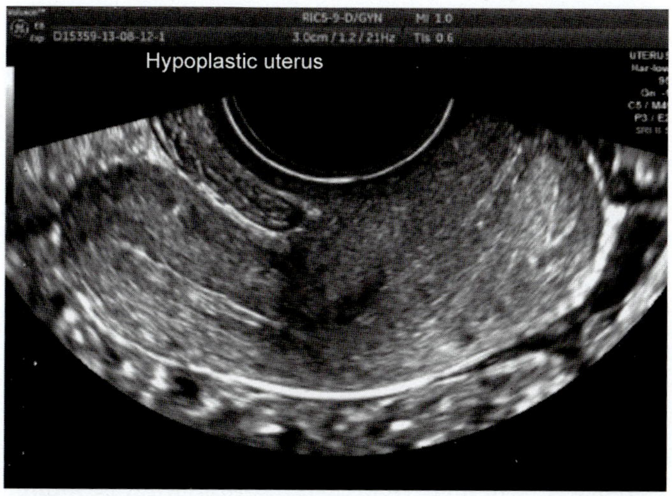

Fig. 2: B-mode ultrasound image of postmenopausal hypoplastic uterus with thin endometrium.

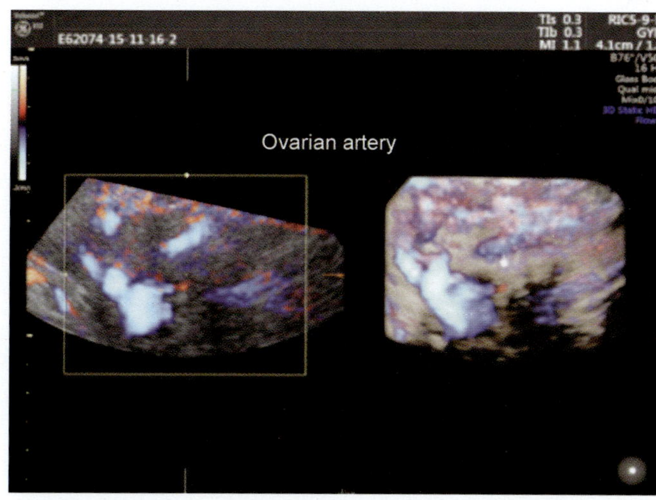

Fig. 4: High-definition (HD) flow and 3D HD flow image of small atrophic ovary showing the ovarian artery entering from the lateral aspect (marked by hand).

After adequate image in the long axis is obtained, the probe can be rotated 90° to image the uterus in a horizontal (semicoronal, semiaxial) plane.

Once the endometrium is adequately depicted in its long and short axes, the probe is withdrawn into the midvagina and images of the cervix can be obtained **(Fig. 3)**.

The ovaries are usually located lateral to the uterus, above and medial to the hypogastric vessels, lying in the area called "Waldeyer's fossa." Their size, morphology, and locations are altered by the age, previous diseases, surgeries, and other factors in the postmenopause. During the reproductive years the follicles serve as "sonographic markers" of the ovaries. After the menopause, it is hard to find them because these "markers" are not present, the ovaries themselves atrophied and there is less pelvic fluid to provide an acoustic interface. Their detection becomes more difficult with advancing age. Beside negative bimanual pelvic examination, nonvisualization of the ovaries can be accepted without serious concern about ovarian pathology. With the introduction of color-coded Doppler flow imaging, by finding the color-coded flow of the ovarian artery or vein, one can better detect the otherwise "sonographically nondetectable" ovaries **(Fig. 4)**. Using the other hand can be very useful for manipulating the ovaries into the "scanning sight"

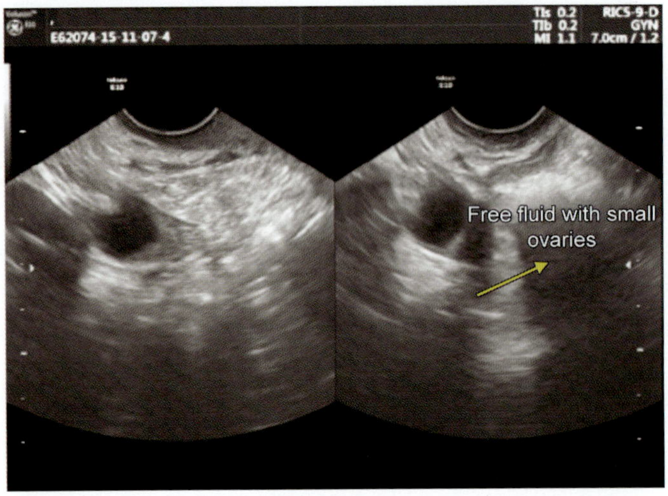

Fig. 5: Small postmenopausal ovary with a single residual follicle seen on B-mode ultrasound. Free fluid is seen close to the ovary.

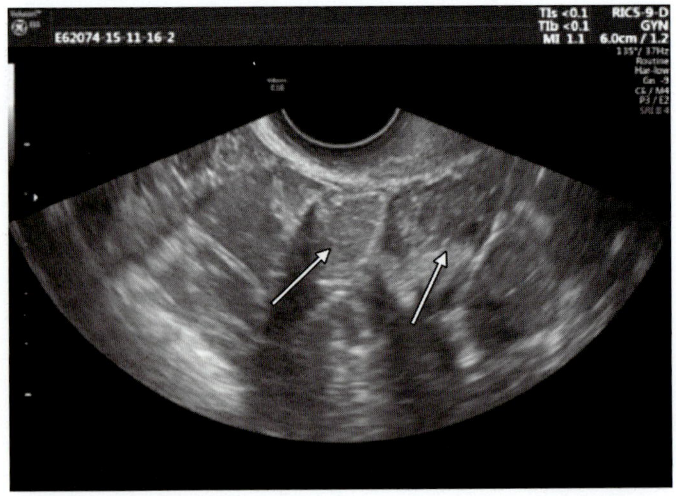

Fig. 6: Bowel shadows appear roundish in cross section and heterogeneous and hypoechoic and can be mistaken for postmenopausal ovary.

of the probe by pushing them slightly downward through the lower abdominal wall into the direction of the tip of the probe.

Detecting some free fluid in the cul-de-sac does not necessarily mean pathological finding, but in its presence ovarian pathology must be searched with special care. The same goes for any palpated or visualized solid structure in the cul-de-sac. The vascularization of these gynecological findings must be examined intentionally by color and pulsed Doppler.

When a large amount of fluid is present, such as in ascites, first questions is whether the **(Fig. 5)** pathological condition arises from an ovarian tumor or is related to a nongynecological disorder. Fluid clearly outlines the boundaries of the structures and ovarian pathology may be revealed. If the ovaries appear normal, one may consider other reasons leading to ascites.

Constipation is not rare in postmenopausal patients. Scybalous should not be confused with pelvic masses. Excluding the vascularization of a structure by the color Doppler helps in differentiating normal to abnormal.

Solid pelvic masses must also be differentiated from the intestines. In real-time mode, the motion of the bowels help distinguish the peristalting intestines from the fixed structures **(Fig. 6)**. In the postmenopause, the peristalsis is frequently inert, which requires proper patience from the examiner. In case of a vascularized mass, color and pulsed Doppler again offers a quick possibility.

From all of the abovementioned techniques, it follows that the sonographer gets to know the finding of bimanual pelvic examination, which should therefore precede the transvaginal ultrasound examination. It strengthens the recommendation that the person, who performs the transvaginal ultrasound examination in a postmenopausal patient, should perform a bimanual pelvic examination before, thus orienteering the anatomical situation and obtaining previous information to decide what are the adequate ways for ultrasonography, or whether there were any suspicious structures palpated. In case of uncertainty of the origin of the palpated or visualized structure, transrectal examination or enema might become necessary.

POSTMENOPAUSAL OVARY

Visualization

In the reproductive years, the normal ovary is relatively easy to detect by TVS. The characteristic small sonolucencies, representing follicles or corpus luteum are missing in the postmenopause. Ovarian volume and diameter decrease with age. The normal atretic ovaries become more difficult to image, but even in the senescence, the small but normal ovaries are sometimes imaged.[2]

The postmenopausal ovaries appear small, uniform and hypoechoic ellipsoidal structures with a smooth outline located above and medial to the hypogastric vessels **(Fig. 7)**.[3] A small amount of pelvic fluid, which

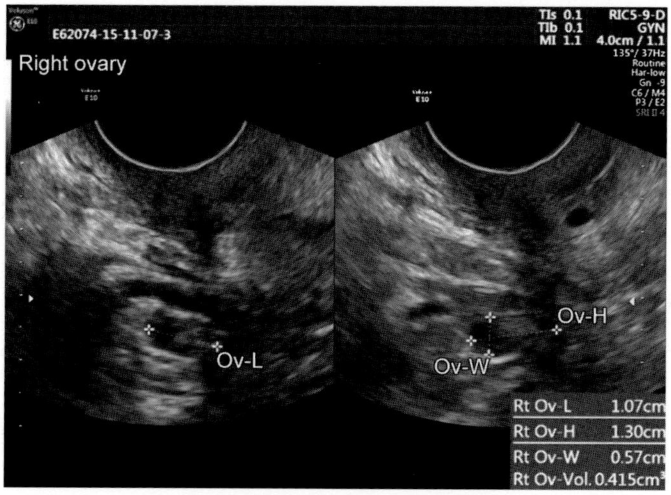

Fig. 7: B-mode ultrasound image of longitudinal and transverse sections of perimenopausal small ovary.

is less frequent in the postmenopause than in the fertile period, may also help to delineate the ovaries. Larger amount of fluid (ascites) makes them easily outlined.

In significant number of patients, the ovaries may not be detected, even after considerable time spent searching for them.

Eventually, the ovary becomes an inert residue that consist of connective tissue, and it clings to the posterior leaf of the broad ligament. Postmenopause, loosing the strength of the ligaments and the support of the pelvic floor the uterus might descent, while the ovaries remain in their position, fixed to the pelvic wall by the atrophic infundibulopelvic ligaments. In this situation, their distance from the fornices increase, thus their transvaginal visualization becomes more difficult and sometimes impossible. This can be the reason that Granberg and Wikland[4] found TVS to be slightly less accurate (23%) than abdominal ultrasound (34%) in visualizing the postmenopausal ovary. The abovementioned use of the abdominal hand might help in directing them into the scanning sight of the transvaginal probe and distinguish them from the bowel.

Previous surgery or the presence of adhesions as the consequences of previous pelvic inflammatory diseases can also fix the ovaries in abnormal locations.

Hall et al.[5] visualized both ovaries in two-third of postmenopausal patients and at least one ovary in three-fourth of patients. Campbell et al.[6] identified both ovaries in 84% of postmenopausal patients by transabdominal sonography. Rodrigez et al.[7] imaged 84% of the postmenopausal ovaries by transvaginal ultrasound. In a study of Fleischer et al.[8] on postmenopausal patients at least one ovary was detected 80% of the time and both ovaries were imaged 60% of the time by transvaginal approach. Healy et al. identified both ovaries by TVS in 71% of women. The right ovary was visualized in 86.3% of women and the left ovary was visualized in 78%.[3]

According to the published data the introduction of the TVS did not result in improvement in the visualization rate of the postmenopausal ovary. However, much clearer images can be obtained using the transvaginal approach when the ovaries are localized. When both the transvaginal and the transabdominal approach were used, the visualization rate came close to 100%.[4] Therefore, in case of any difficulty in detecting the postmenopausal ovary, the techniques of transabdominal and transvaginal ultrasound may be used to supplement each other.[9] In some cases the significantly enlarged ovary can be situated out of the pelvis and out of the range of the transvaginal probe.

There is no consistent view as to whether the inability to visualize the postmenopausal ovary assures a lack of pathology. The general consensus seems to favor the view that lack of visualization of postmenopausal ovaries and a negative bimanual examination suggests ovarian atrophy and lack of disease.[2] In a study Rodrigez et al.[7] were not able to visualize 19 of 104 ovaries preoperatively and during the subsequent histological evaluation all were found to be atrophied without any sign of disease.

Inability to visualize the postmenopausal ovary by experienced examiner can be accepted as normal finding.

Morphology and Biometry

The menopausal ovary tends to atrophy and shrink when the Graafian follicles in the ovary disappear. The tunica albuginea becomes dense, and causes the surface of the ovary to become scarred and shrunken. The cortex is marked with increasing thinning as well as numerous corpora fibrosa and corpora albuginea with areas of dense fibrosis, and hyalinization.[10]

The ovarian weight decreases from an average of 14 g in the fourth decade to approximately 5 g in the postmenopausal state. Whereas the normal ovary measures 3.5 × 2.0 × 1.5 cm after the menopause it shrinks to 2.0 × 1.5 × 0.5 cm and in some instances it may be even smaller. At this point, it can be palpated very rarely.

Several sonographic studies have attempted to define normal ovarian size and the general conclusion is that it should not exceed 2 × 3 × 4 cm.[2,8,11-15] According to the measurements of Fleischer,[8] the mean size of the normal sonographically imaged postmenopausal ovary was 2.2 × 1.2 × 1.1 cm. Others measured postmenopausal ovarian volume rather than size (ovarian volume = d1 × d2 × d3 × 0.523 where d1, d2, d3 are the maximal transverse, anterioposterior, and longitudinal parameters), the mean figure of this parameter was 4.33 cm^3 in the pioneer work of Campbell.[6] In the paper of Goswamy,[12] the mean ovarian volume was reported to measure 3.6 mL after examining 2,246 postmenopausal women by transabdominal ultrasound. Granberg and Wikland[4] found it less smaller (1.4 ± 1.0 cm^3) in a different age group. In the series of Hall et al.,[5] all the ovarian volumes were equal or less than 2.5 cm^3. Pavlik examined 13,963 women and found that mean ovarian volume is 2.2 cm^3.[3,16]

Despite the difference in the size reported for the normal ovary, there is a close correlation between the size of the left and the right ovaries. In the abovementioned work on a large population Goswamy et al.[12] found 0.01 mL difference between the means of the volumes of the left and the right ovaries. Difference in size is particularly important, since each serves to some extent as a normal control for its sister.[9] Campbell et al.[6] recommends that an ovary twice than the size of its pair should be regarded a suspicious finding.

Multiparous women have ovaries that are approximately 12% larger. There seems to be no additional effect of parity if the woman had more than two children. History of breast cancer was associated with an increase in mean ovarian volume of approximately 11%.[12]

Hormone replacement therapy does not seem to influence neither the size nor the perfusion of the postmenopausal ovaries.[17-19]

Ovarian Malignancy in the Postmenopause

Although the ovary becomes too old to function, it is never too old to form a cancer.[10] Visualization and measurement of ovarian volume in the postmenopausal patient are sometimes difficult, but potentially afford early detection of cancer or neoplasm. Ovarian cancer is the fourth leading cause of cancer death in women both in the United States and the UK.[20,21] The incidence increases over the age of 40 years and the peak age for the appearance of common epithelial ovarian cancer is age 56–67 years.[10] The importance of early detection of ovarian cancer is evidenced by the fact that 5-year survival rates for stage I disease are 50–70%, whereas these figures for stage III and IV disease are 13% and 4%, respectively. The 5-year survival rate for women with ovarian cancer has not changed significantly over the past 30 years.[20] The ovarian cancer is asymptomatic until it has reached an advanced stage and mostly it is not diagnosed until the advanced stage. Several attempts were made by different investigators to establish an ultrasound-based safe and cost-effective screening system for ovarian malignancy, including morphological criteria, color and pulsed Doppler, and scoring systems.

Despite of these efforts, currently there are no fully accepted screening methods to detect ovarian cancer at an early stage. On the other hand, ultrasonography offers the capability of detecting even small increase in ovarian size and at least the potential for early diagnosis of ovarian malignancy. It is the responsibility of the examiner to take a chance and search for the ovaries very thoroughly, and measuring them precisely when examining a postmenopausal patient. In case of any suspicious finding, deviation from the normal ovarian morphology or enlargement of the ovarian diameters or volume and change in ovarian volume at repeat scan,[3] the patients must immediately be directed to the higher center and examined in detail according to the established ovarian cancer-detecting protocols.

Postmenopausal Palpable Ovary Syndrome

Enlargement of the ovaries in elderly women was considered pathological by Barber et al. who called this the "postmenopausal palpable ovary" (PMPO) syndrome.[22] For years, surgical exploration and oophorectomy were recommended when PMPO was detected, i.e., the ovary continued to demonstrate the size and consistency of a premenopausal ovary.[23,24]

According to the approach of Barber, in the PMPO, the finding which is interpreted as a normal-sized ovary in the premenopausal patient represents an ovarian tumor in the patient, at least 5 years after the menopause. This statement does not mean that anything that is palpated in the adnexa is abnormal. It only refers to the size and consistency of the ovary.[10,25,26]

Cautious examination of the ovaries by transvaginal color and pulsed Doppler is strongly recommended in PMPO syndrome to resolve the doubts. Mostly ultrasound examination found simple ovarian cyst, which should not necessarily be considered abnormal. For management of simple ovarian cyst, see further.

Unilocular (Simple) Ovarian Cysts in the Postmenopause

The spreading use of the TVS and improved resolution of the equipment led to the detection of more unilocular, simple ovarian cysts in the postmenopausal women than detected by earlier known techniques. The question is "what is the risk of a completely anechoic unilocular tumor being malignant and whether the risk of a simple cystic tumor being malignant increases with age and size?"[27]

Only the cysts without any septation and papillary formations can be regarded unilocular **(Fig. 8)**.[28] Many reports presented on unilocular and anechoic ovarian cysts in the postmenopause diagnosed by ultrasound.[27,29-41] The values in these studies indicate that anechoic unilocular ovarian cysts in postmenopausal women carry a low-risk of malignancy.

Andolf et al. reported 30 simple postmenopausal adnexal cysts (2–8 cm).[31] After the surgical treatment of 15 of them no malignancy was revealed, while the following of another 15 by transvaginal ultrasound, six disappeared after 1 month and altogether 12 disappeared after seven months. After 2 years, only two cases with 2 cm cysts remained. In their next work,[32] they confirmed on a larger number that small anechoic lesions are seldom, if ever, malignant in elderly women. However, among their 33 patients having totally anechoic cysts >5 cm they found three malignancies.

Upon the histological examination of 28 unilocular postmenopausal cysts <5 cm, Goldstein et al.[33] also reported 0% incidence of malignancy. Another 14 patients were followed from 10 to 73 months without any change in size or character of the cyst.

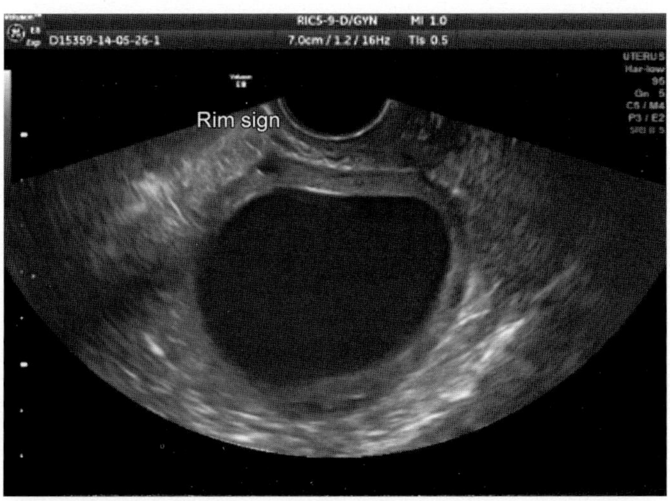

Fig. 8: Large round anechoic intraovarian cystic lesion with no internal echogenicities or solid components—unilocular cyst on B-mode ultrasound.

Parker et al.[34] reported 25 unilocular cyst (3–9 cm, mean 5 cm) diagnosed by transabdominal sonography in postmenopausal women, who later underwent cystectomy by laparoscopy or laparotomy. None of the cysts were malignant.

In their studies Granberg et al.[28,30] examined 140 postmenopausal unilocular cysts, 60 of them were <5 cm in diameter, 51 measured 5–10 cm, and 29 cysts were >10 cm. Only one malignant tumor was found among them, this measured >5 cm in diameter. The sensitivity and specificity for excluding malignancy in an ovarian cyst in postmenopausal women by transvaginal ultrasound was 100%.[27]

Valentin and Akrawi[35] followed 134 postmenopausal women and were found to have an adnexal cyst judged to be benign and not causing any symptoms. Transvaginal ultrasound examinations were performed at 3 months, 6 months, and 12 months' time interval and thereafter every 12 months interval. Median follow-up time was 3 years. In majority of women the cysts disappeared or remained unchanged. With advancing age chance for regression of cyst is declining.

Valentin et al.[36] examined 52 women who died from causes other than gynecological cancer or intraperitoneal cancer of extragenital origin. They found 36 simple cyst. All cysts were benign.

Modesitt et al.[37] examined 15,106 women at least 50 year old; 2,763 women (18%) were diagnosed with 3,259 unilocular ovarian cysts. A total of 2,261 (69.4%) of these cysts resolved spontaneously, 537 (16.5%) developed a septum, 189 (5.8%) developed a solid area, and 220 (6.8%) persisted as a unilocular lesion. During this time, 27 women received a diagnosis of ovarian cancer and 10 had been previously diagnosed with simple ovarian cysts. All 10 of these women, however, developed another morphologic abnormality, experienced resolution of the cyst before developing cancer or developed cancer in the contralateral ovary. No woman with an isolated unilocular cystic ovarian tumor has developed ovarian cancer in this population. The authors concluded that the risk of malignancy in unilocular ovarian cystic tumors of <10 cm in diameter in women 50 year old or older, is extremely low.

Nardo et al.[38] followed-up 226 women with simple cysts for 5 years. The cancer antigen 125 (CA-125) is also measured and found that 54 cysts increase in size. They were removed and two carcinomas were found. Both carcinomas had increased CA-125 levels.

Castillo et al.[39] examined 8,794 asymptomatic postmenopausal women by transvaginal ultrasound. 223 simple adnexal cysts in 215 women were found out (prevalence: 2.5%). Annual incidence did not change significantly. 149 patients with 153 cysts were entered ultimately in the study. 45 (30%) underwent surgery (34 after initial diagnosis and 11 during follow-up). A total of 49 cysts were removed. The most frequent histological diagnosis was serous cystadenoma (84%). There was a case of a stage IA ovarian carcinoma (2% of the cysts removed, 0.6% of all the cysts included in the study). 104 patients with 104 cysts underwent conservative follow-up throughout the study period. 46 (44%) of these cysts were resolved spontaneously (74% of them within 2 years). In 14 (30%) of these women, a new cyst was diagnosed when follow-up went on. In 58 patients, cysts persisted during all study period (median follow-up: 48 months, range: 6–90 months), 69.6% of them remained unchanged, 17.2% increased and 17.2% decreased. Patients in whom cysts resolved spontaneously had a shorter menopausal time ($P = 0.001$) and tend to be younger ($P = 0.06$). No differences were found regarding cyst features.

Dorum et al.[40] examined 234 woman, died from nongynecological causes. They found 36 simple benign cysts.

In a paper from Greenlee et al.,[41] simple cysts were ascertained among a cohort of 15,735 women from the intervention arm of the prostate, lung, colorectal, and ovarian cancer screening trial through 4 years of transvaginal ultrasound screening. Simple cysts were seen in 14% of women, the first time that their ovaries were visualized. The 1 year incidence of new simple cysts was 8%. Among ovaries with one simple cyst at the first screen, 54% retained one simple cyst and 32% had no cyst 1 year later. Simple cysts did not increase risk of subsequent invasive ovarian cancer.

Due to the physics of ultrasound, structures which are farther from probe tip can be easily missed out. The risk of missing papillary formation increases with diameter of the cyst. Most of the authors agree that cyst which is >5 cm cannot be properly examined and therefore should not be considered simple.

The cytological evaluation of the cyst content proved to be very limited value for identifying malignancy even after the irrigation of the cystic tumor and the combination of it with transvaginal ultrasound did not increase the diagnostic accuracy as compared with ultrasound alone.[29,42-44]

Once again, only unilateral cyst smaller than 5 cm, filled with clear anechoic fluid, with entirely smooth and thin walls (up to 3 mm), without any septation and papillary formations can be regarded as unilocular simple cyst.

Royal College of Obstetricians and Gynecologists recommendation for such cyst is ultrasound and CA-125 follow-up in 4 months intervals for a year. If there is no change in cyst morphology and size (or cyst size decrease) and/or CA-125 levels, further follow-up is not necessary.[45] Any change in cyst morphology or increased cyst size or blood flow, or increased CA-125 warranted removing of ovaries.

With its widespread utilization in the near future transvaginal color Doppler will make it possible to increase the reality of ultrasound diagnosis of unilocular cystic ovarian lesions. In their paper of 18 stage I ovarian cancers, Kurjak et al.[46] reported that ovarian cancer stage I was also discovered in two simple unilocular ovarian cysts using transvaginal color Doppler as well as in two morphologically normal ovaries which would have been missed if the morphology alone was considered. This finding would have an important clinical implication as these simple cysts are not always innocent and color Doppler is, therefore, mandatory to rule out the malignant revascularization.

Color Doppler Velocimetry of the Postmenopausal Ovary

The ovarian blood flow is significantly affected by aging and the postmenopausal ovary shows varying degree of avascularity.

The ovarian artery is a tributary of the upper aorta and reaches the lateral aspect of the ovary through the infundibulopelvic ligament. Color Doppler enables visualization of the ovarian artery **(Fig. 9)** at the lateral edge of the ovary. In some patients, especially in the postmenopausal, these vessels are not clearly visualized and the sample volume should be moved across the ligament and then through the ovary until the arterial signal is identified. Signals from the ovarian artery are characterized by low Doppler shifts of a small artery with low velocity.

The first published data from direct and noninvasive measurement of normal ovarian and uterine perfusion in the postmenopause are from Kurjak et al.[47] Unlike in

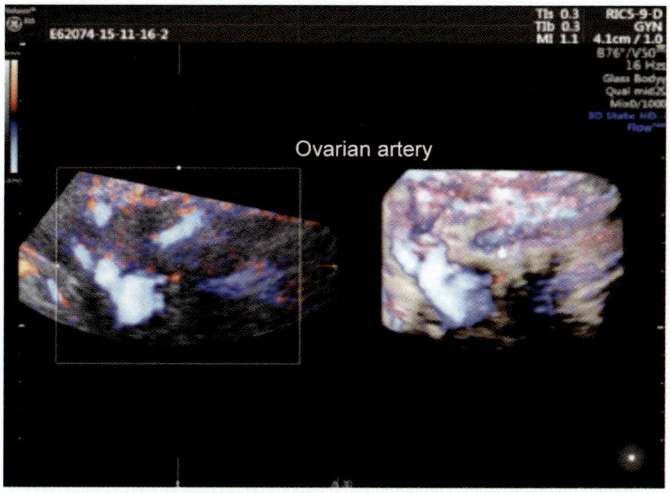

Fig. 9: High-definition (HD) flow and 3D HD flow image of small atrophic ovary showing the ovarian artery entering from the lateral aspect (marked by hand).

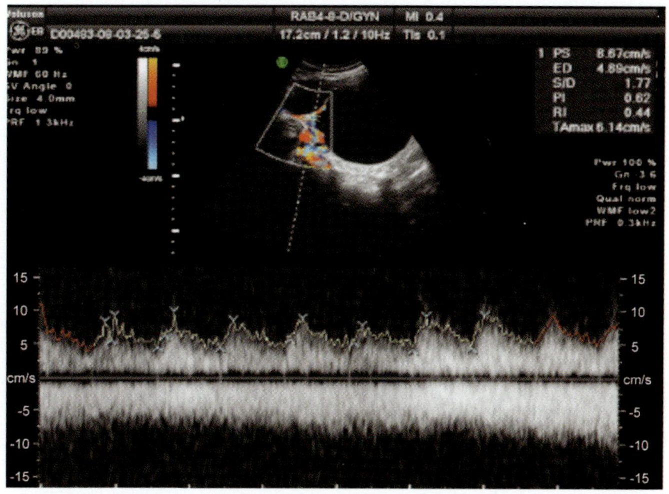

Fig. 10: Color and spectral Doppler image of an intraovarian lesion showing low resistance flow [resistive index (RI) 0.44].

the presence of unilateral folliculogenesis and corpus luteum formation during the normal menstrual periods, there is no difference in the vascular impedance between the left and right ovaries in the postmenopause.[48,49] Significantly, increased ovarian blood flow impedance can be demonstrated already during the climacterium, when compared to that of the "dominant" ovary in a normal menstrual cycle. The mean resistive index (RI) increasing further in the next years of the postmenopause reaching the value of one after 10 years. The absence of the diastolic flow is already common in the early postmenopausal period and constantly found in patients with more than 11 years of postmenopause.

Even with the latest advanced equipment seems to be not possible to detect velocity waveform signals from the ovarian parenchyma in normal postmenopausal patients. This can be the result of the relative increase of the amount of the connective tissue. Therefore, any color flow obtained from a postmenopausal ovary should generate a high index of suspicion for abnormal revascularization and requires detailed pulsed waveform Doppler analysis.[47,50]

In a previous study, Kurjak et al. examined 1,000 postmenopausal women with transvaginal color and pulsed Doppler sonography.[50] A total of 74% were asymptomatic; the others were referred or self referred for symptoms. There were 83 women with findings that resulted in surgery. Separation of the groups into benign and malignant cases did not reveal significant differences in age, duration of the menopause, or symptomatology. A total of 29 tumors were malignant, prevalence rates were 36% in the group underwent surgery and 3% in the total postmenopausal group underwent examination. An ultrasound score was used to analyze the morphology of the tumors. The score was successful in separating benign from malignant tumors with all indices of normality >90%. Color flow was identified in 27 of 29 malignant tumors and 35% of benign masses. A cutoff value in the Doppler RI is 0.40 **(Fig. 10)** in the feeder vessels; it had a sensitivity and specificity of 96% and 95% for separating benign tumors from malignant tumors, respectively. Positive and negative predictive values were 96% and 95%.

In their next retrospective study on this topic already mentioned above, 18 patients with ovarian carcinoma stage I were studied to evaluate the efficiency of transvaginal color Doppler sonography.[46] Four of these patients were asymptomatic and self-referred for their annual check-up. Another four asymptomatic women, two with morphologically normal ovaries and two with simple unilocular cysts, were picked up during the screening program. Ovarian carcinoma stage I was detected in two normal-sized ovaries from only color and pulsed color signals **(Figs. 11A to C)**, which represented tumor angiogenesis and low impedance to blood flow (RI <0.40).

Fleischer et al. published data of nine stage I ovarian carcinomas where three of them had benign appearance but with suspicious blood flow characteristics.[51]

Crade et al. calculated that a postmenopausal woman with a mass >5 cm and an RI <0.50 had a malignancy risk of 66%, while a mass having an RI value higher than 0.60 had only a risk of 2.4%.[52]

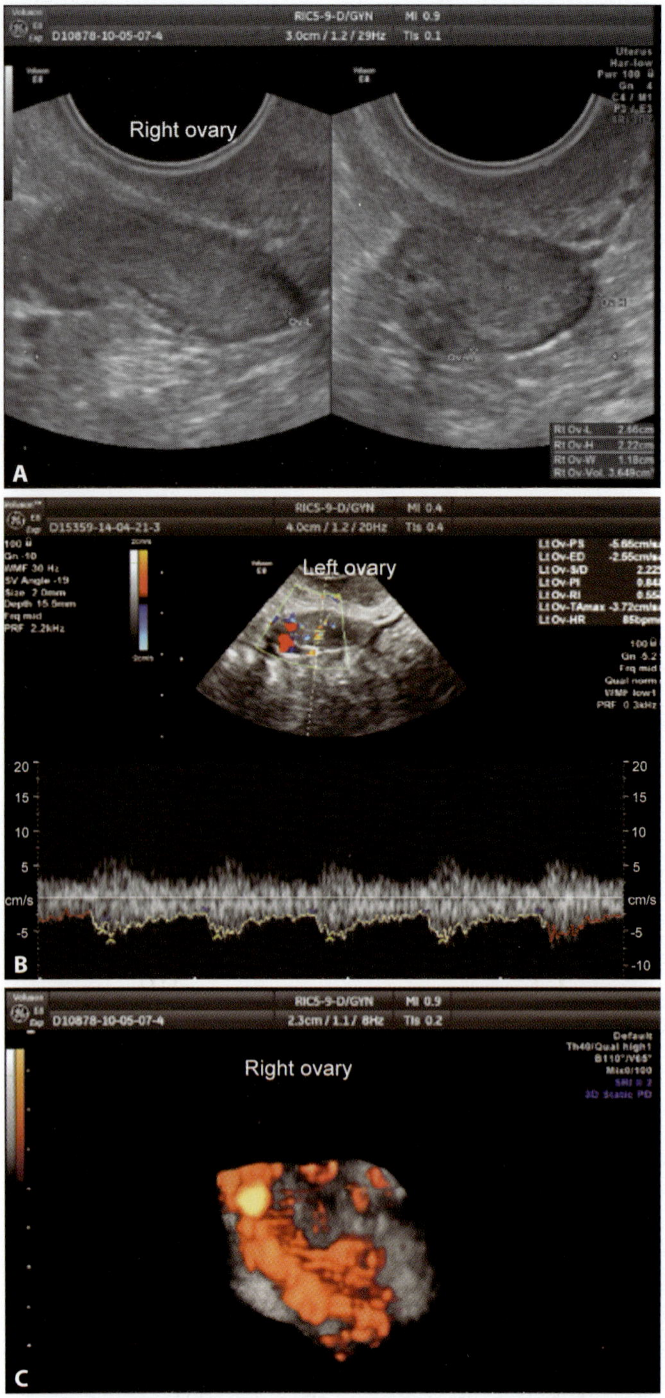

Figs. 11A to C: (A) B-mode ultrasound image of a normal-sized but almost solid looking ovary in longitudinal and transverse sections in a postmenopausal female; (B) Same ovary as in **Figure 11A** on color and spectral Doppler shows moderate resistance flow. As the blood flow is almost absent in postmenopausal ovary normally, this flow may be considered pathological and should raise doubt of malignancy; (C) The same lesion on 3D power Doppler shows rich vascular network with vascular channels of irregular caliber, strongly suggesting the malignant nature of the lesion.

If further investigations by other researchers also confirm these results, transvaginal color Doppler ultrasonography may provide a valuable tool for monitoring the ovarian involution in the postmenopause and objective aid for choosing between the conservative, laparoscopic, or radical management of pelvic masses found in postmenopausal patients.

THE POSTMENOPAUSAL UTERUS

Morphology

The uterus can be imaged in three major scanning planes with TVS. There is generally a homogeneous echo pattern in the postmenopause, and the uterine cavity is not frequently imaged.[53] The uterine wall is smooth and clearly outlined against its surroundings. In the myometrium, toward its periphery and often protruding can be found echoless vessels. In the postmenopause the arteries can calcify in this region. These calcifications appear as small, bright reflections, and regularly spreaded in the uterine wall. They can evoke shadowing, which may impair the assessment of structures lying beyond, e.g., the endometrium.[54] Unlike in all phases of the menstrual cycles, undulatory motions, i.e., uterine contractions,[55] cannot be observed in the postmenopause.

Biometry

As in the case of all genital organs in the female, the development, the maintenance of the fertile size and shape, and the postmenopausal physiologic involution of the uterus are highly dependent on the actual serum level of the estrogen.

Measurement of the uterus in the sagittal plane can be carried out either by determination of the portio-fundus distance, or in postmenopause, the separate measurement of the cervix, and corpus uteri can also be used. It was already mentioned in the introduction that the corpus–cervix ratio of the postmenopausal uterus shows remarkable changes in favor of the cervix. With advanced ages it can even fall below one and can reach a ratio of 1:2 like in childhood.

The sagittal measurement is supplemented by the determination of the largest anteroposterior diameter of the corpus uteri and of the largest transverse diameter of the corpus. The size of the corpus decreases markedly in the postmenopause, shrinking to average size of 4.5 × 1.5 × 2.5, with the cervix predominantly over the corpus in the sense of the elongation of the cervix.[53] The mean length of

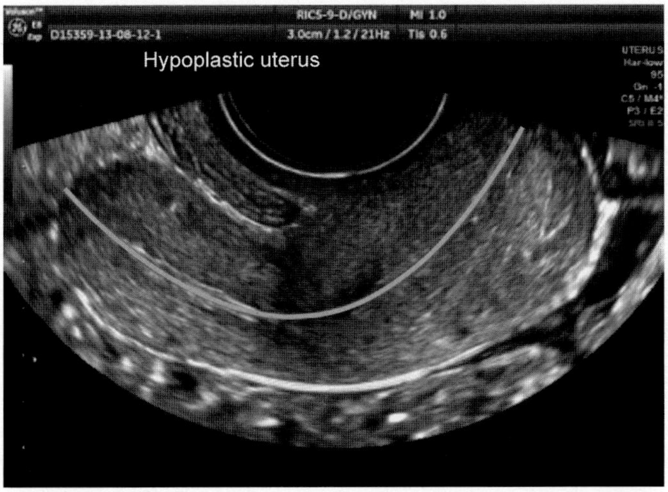

Fig. 12: B-mode ultrasound image of postmenopausal hypoplastic uterus showing measurement of the uterocervical length as a continuous trace.

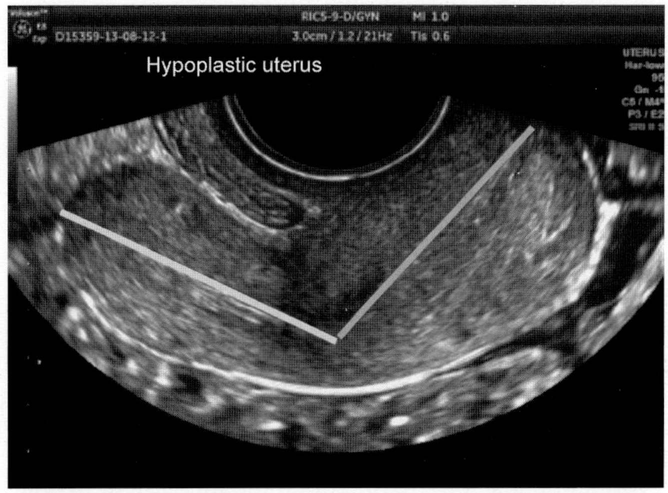

Fig. 13: B-mode ultrasound image of postmenopausal hypoplastic uterus showing separately measured uterine length and cervical length. This is of help for calculating uterocervical ratio.

the postmenopausal uterus was shown to be 59 ± 11 mm by Andolf et al.[56] The upper size limit of the postmenopausal uterus has been suggested to be 3 cm in the anterior-posterior diameter, with a cervical-fundal length of 8 cm. The patient who is only 1–3 years postmenopausal when still has significant endogenous estrogen production by the ovaries or who has significant endogenous estrogen production by fat from adrenal precursors will have larger uterus than the patient who is over 10 years postmenopausal. Clinical judgment is needed in interpreting normality of uterine size in postmenopausal uterine size in the postmenopausal patient **(Figs. 12 and 13)**.[9]

Uterine involution is a slow process. Myometrial thickness is changed as the years of the postmenopause progresses.

Uterus Under Hormone Replacement Therapy

Comparing myometrial thickness between groups of postmenopausal with and without HRT, Zalud et al.[57] did not demonstrate statistical difference, though slight differences were found in favor of women, who received HRT for more than 5 years. These data are not surprising in the mirror of the findings of the same group, namely that the myometrial involution could not be statistically expressed over the years throughout the postmenopause too. The involutional process of the myometrium is very slow and other factors than estrogen can also influence, as the sizes of the uteruses of fertile women can show greater variability too.

Color Doppler Velocimetry in the Postmenopausal Uterus

The vascular supply of the uterus is provided by a complex network of arteries originating from the uterine artery, which is a branch of the hypogastric artery. The color Doppler signal from the main uterine vessels can be seen lateral to the cervix at the level of the cervicocorporal junction of the uterus.[58] Flow velocity waveforms from the radial arteries can be obtained within the myometrial fibers, while spiral arteries are visualized at the level of endometrial-myometrial junction.[48]

Visualization of both uterine artery by transvaginal color Doppler can be achieved even in the advanced years of the postmenopause. In contrary, visualization rate of the myometrial and endometrial vessels are highly dependent on the length of the postmenopausal period.

The aging process affects the uterine perfusion. In general, high impedance and high velocity are the characteristics for the uterine arteries, though the uterine perfusion is largely dependent on age, phase of menstrual cycle, and other conditions (e.g., pregnancy, tumor),[59] and there are complex relationships between the concentration of the ovarian hormones in the serum and uterine artery blood flow parameters.[60-62]

Additionally, there might also be a relationship between the serum gonadotropin levels and uterine perfusion. Examining normal postmenopausal patient and premenopausal patients treated with gonadotropin-releasing hormone (GnRH) analogs, Luzi et al. found that the pulsatility index of the uterine artery in spontaneous menopausal women is significantly higher than that in artificial menopausal women. This phenomenon may be due to a different hormonal pattern which exists in the two groups, i.e., the gonadotropin levels increased in the former and decreased in the latter. The vascular compliance in artificially induced menopause is higher than that observed in spontaneous menopause, as shown by a higher diastolic flow and a less deep notch. The decrease of the vascular compliance in postmenopause can be caused by progressive sclerosis of the vessel walls.[63]

Resistance to blood flow increases in both the main uterine and the radial arteries as the years of postmenopause progress, though the increase of ovarian blood flow impedance is more pronounced. The fact that uterine artery RI does not change significantly in the first year of menopause, strongly support the thesis that ageing process initially affects the uterus less than the ovary.

The diastolic flow decreases in postmenopause and the systolic peak increases.[63] The RI in the main uterine arteries continuously increases with the number of the postmenopausal ages, but unlike in the case of the ovarian artery, it does not reach the maximum in all women even at advanced ages.

Absent diastolic flow in uterine arteries was found in 15% of women with 1–5 years duration of menopause, while clear interruption of diastolic blood flow was observed in the uterine artery of one-third of the women in the next 5 years of the postmenopausal period. More than half of the women have this finding with 11–15 years lasting postmenopause and finally, 80% of women whom LMB occurred more than 16 years ago demonstrated absent diastolic blood flow signal indicative of high vascular impedance.

The changes in flow velocity patterns of the radial arteries in postmenopausal patients parallel the blood flow dynamics of the uterine arteries.

Visualization of clear Doppler signals from the spiral artery is possible only in less than one-third of postmenopausal women, in whom LMB occurred 1–5 years previously. The impedance is significantly increased in these vessels too, when comparing to the premenopausal levels. In normal postmenopausal women already 6 years after the LMB, no blood flow signals can be expected from the inner-third of myometrium and the area of the myometrial–endometrial junction.[62]

Myomas and Malignant Potential After the Menopause

Uterine fibroids of 0.5 cm can be detected by TVS and their relationship to the endometrial cavity can be precisely defined (e.g., submucous, intramural, and subserosus). They appear with TVS as rounded, well-defined space-occupying structures **(Fig. 14)**.[64]

Growth of myomas is known to be estrogen dependent. The management of the myoma around the menopause is highly conservative, since after the menopause they are supposed to regress in the lack of the hormonal support. Myomas with good vascularization can be seen less frequently after the menopause **(Fig. 15)**. They show more hypoechogenic structure, compared to the normal uterine tissue, while homogeneous and hyperechogenic myoma have often undergone regressive changes, and have a large amount of connective tissue. Other regressive changes such as necrosis, caseous, and cystic degeneration can be recognized by the presence of hypoechogenic regions or regions without echogenicity in the myoma. Such a necrotic myoma can be confounded with an ovarian cyst or a colliquated endometrial carcinoma depending on its localization. Hyalinization and calcifications of the myoma responsible for bright reflections can be seen frequently in the postmenopause **(Fig. 16)**.[53]

Transvaginal color Doppler can be used to assess leiomyoma vascularity, as well as the physiological and

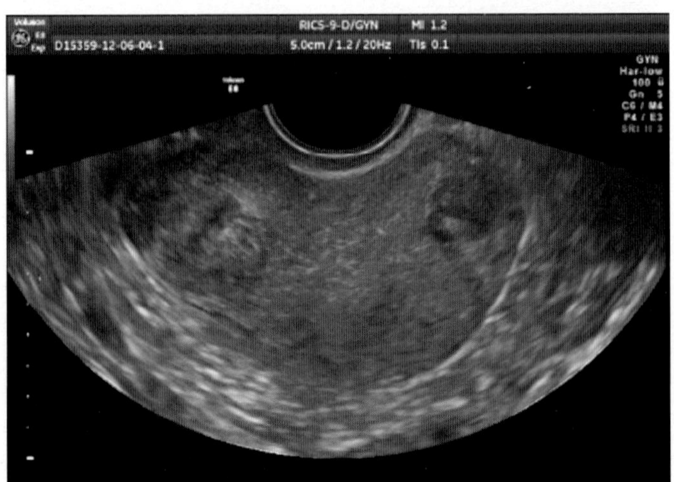

Fig. 14: B-mode ultrasound image of transverse section of uterus showing two intramural myomas one on each side as round well-defined lesions.

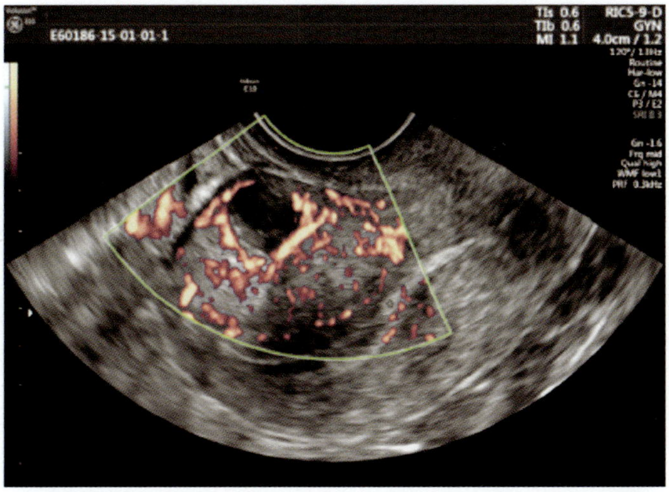

Fig. 15: Power Doppler ultrasound image of the same patient as in **Figure 14**. This image shows uterus in longitudinal section. The myoma is seen in the anterior wall and on power Doppler, typically shows a vascular ring of myoma.

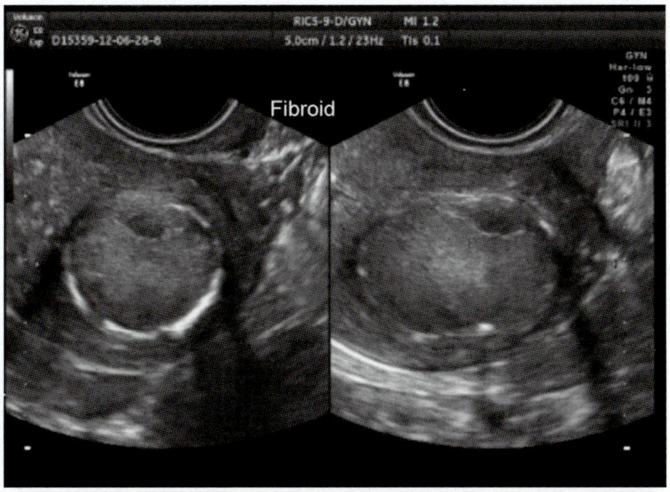

Fig. 16: An echogenic round lesion is seen in the uterus with calcified rim—calcified myoma.

pathophysiological characteristics of uterine arterial blood flow.[65,66] The vascularization of leiomyomas is supported by preexisting myometrial vessels originating from terminal branches of uterine arteries. Since the leiomyoma grows centripetally as proliferation of smooth muscle cells and fibrous connective tissue, the color Doppler demonstrates most of the leiomyometrial blood vessels at its periphery. While their visualization rate is high in the premenopausal period (58–70%),[67-69] it decreases after the menopause with the decreased blood supply of the uterus.[47]

The growing inclination of the myoma is in correlation with the increased blood flow in the uterine network, the latter is thought to be a result of large concentration of estrogen receptors and estrogens.[70-72] Whether the regression of the myoma after the menopause is resulted directly by the fall in estrogen levels, or it is only a secondary consequence of the decreased perfusion, is still not known. Though Doppler studies on the perfusion of the uterine fibroids in the postmenopause are not available yet, it can be anticipated from the Doppler studies on myomas under treatment with GnRH analogs[69,73] that with the decreasing estrogen levels, the previously decreased impedance of the uterine artery and the supplying myometrial vessels are increasing to the level of a normal postmenopausal uterus leading to the involution of the myoma.

It must be emphasized that in case of necrotic and degenerative changes in the myoma, the presence of blood vessels in the central portion is usual and the impedance of them can be so low that it might be misinterpreted as malignant neovascularization.

One can use TVS as a means of monitoring the size and the ability for growth of the leiomyomas around, and after the menopause. If there is evidence of rapid growth of a predescribed myoma in a postmenopausal women and on ultrasound an increase of echoless areas as a sign of necrosis, laparotomy should be performed because of a suspected malignant transformation.

Though the sarcomas accounted for only 1–3% of the malignant tumors of the uterus (including the endometrium), their early diagnosis can greatly depend on an occasional but accurate ultrasound examination, since there are scarcely any symptoms of an early process.[74]

Nevertheless, there are, similar to macroscopic aspects, sonographic indications for the existence of sarcoma. Primary sarcomas in ultrasound examinations appear as poorly outlined masses, partly hyperechogenic, partly irregularly limited, and hypoechogenic or without echogenicity **(Fig. 17)**. Morphological differentiation from myoma can be facilitated by the absence of any systematic structure (onion-skin or whirlpool pattern). Differential diagnosis of inhomogenous, myometrial masses can be myomas undergoing carneous degeneration, with a pool of liquid or bleeding into the myoma.[53]

Application of the color and pulsed Doppler may confirm or preclude the in vivo diagnosis of uterine sarcoma. The presence of irregular, thin, and randomly dispersed vessels in the peripheral and/or central area of tumor, with very low impedance shunts, characterizes

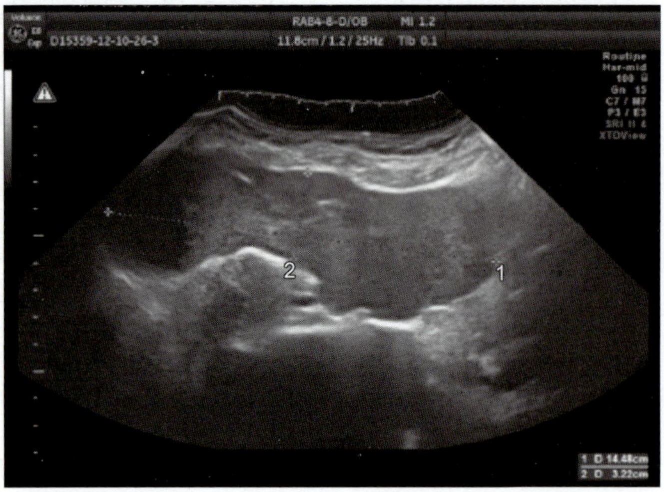

Fig. 17: Large soft tissue mass lesion is seen arising from the uterus. It shows heterogeneous echogenicity and irregular but well-defined margins, suggestive of a large exophytic uterine mass lesion possibly sarcoma.

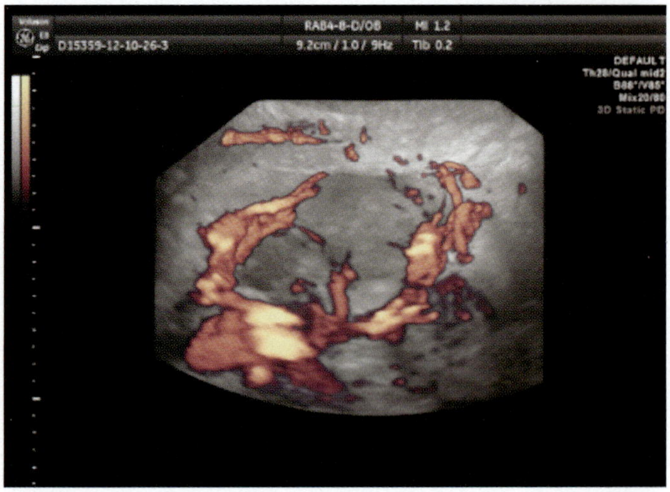

Fig. 18: The same lesion as in Figure 17 is seen on 3D power Doppler, typically shows abundant peripheral and penetrating vascularity with blood vessels showing irregular caliber. This confirms the malignant nature of the lesion.

intratumoral neovascularization (Fig. 18) and is in favor of the malignant transformation. In benign uterine lesions, even if intratumoral vascularization can be detected, the resistance to blood flow was found significantly higher. Furthermore, in the case of the uterine sarcoma, both uterine arteries show a low impedance (Fig. 19) in comparison with that of normal, even the postmenopausal or myomatous uteri.[75,76]

Unfortunately, as a result of the wide range of the biological variations and the vascular characteristics of tumors, an overlap exists between the blood flow patterns of benign and malignant uterine tumors.[76] At the moment, the realistic approach is to consider the abovementioned guidelines only in general, but one has to take the decreased intratumoral impedance and increased vascularity into serious consideration, especially it is accompanied with rapid growth of the tumor during the serial examination.

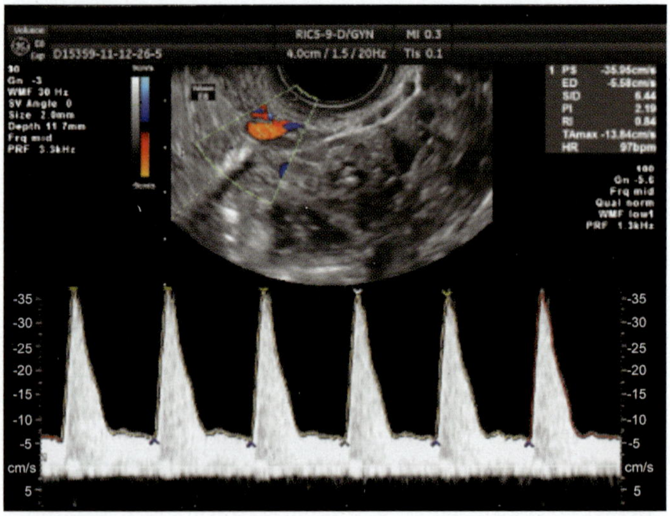

Fig. 19: Color and spectral Doppler assessment of the uterine artery shows significant diastolic flow—low resistance uterine artery flow.

Leiomyomas Under HRT

Leiomyomas are the most common pelvic tumors in women of the reproductive age; 20–25% of women have uterine myomas.[77] Higher concentrations of estrogens[70] and estrogen receptors[71] within leiomyomas than in adjacent myometrium were taken as evidence of the hormone dependence of their growth.

Though they tend to regress after menopause with the decreasing serum level of the promoter estrogen, it is questionable, whether the introduction of the HRT promotes the growing process again. The data are confronting, in some papers myoma growing, in some there is no difference in size, and in some there is even decrease in size.[78-82] However, even if there are increase in myoma size, this does not appear to cause clinical symptoms.

In practice, uterine and fibroid size can be closely monitored by ultrasound, and HRT can be easily discontinued if the fibroid enlarges.

POSTMENOPAUSAL ENDOMETRIUM

Visualization and Morphology

After the menopause, decrease of ovarian estrogen production leads to atrophy of the endometrium. In consequence, the endometrium **(Fig. 20)** of a postmenopausal women is typically thin when examined by TVS, which corresponds to the stratum basale adjacent to the myometrium.[83] Its sonographic feature is very similar to that of the endometrium in the early follicular phase.[84] The endometrial band is sonographically narrowed and the echogenic line of the uterine cavity often cannot be visualized.[54] In the study of Andolf,[56] the endometrium could not be localized in 7% of postmenopausal women without bleeding disorder. Granberg et al. could not visualize 10% of the histologically atrophic postmenopausal endometrium.[85] In addition, shadowing arising from myomas or arteriosclerosis makes visualization more difficult.

Echotexture of the endometrium is usually more echogenic than the surrounding myometrium. In the abovementioned study by Andolf, 85% of the assessable endometrium were less echogenic than the myometrium in asymptomatic postmenopausal women.

The poorly echogenic myometrial zone, the sub-endometrial halo round the endometrium is frequently absent in the postmenopause **(Fig. 21)**.[54] However, the interrupted subendometrial halo was reported as a common sign of the myometrial invasion of the endometrial carcinoma.[86]

Postmenopausal Endometrial Thickness

Contrary to earlier methods of measurement of the thickness of the endometrium, today according to general agreement, measurement should be carried out as follows: The uterus is viewed vaginosonographically in the longitudinal section, and the total thickness of the endometrium is measured in the largest diameter (double layer). In case of any kind of intrauterine fluid collection, the thickness of the fluid pool in the uterine cavity is subtracted from the total thickness.[84]

It is very important to know that transvaginal ultrasound cannot differentiate between focal and symmetrical thickness.[87]

The postmenopausal endometrial thickness is 2–4 mm, with a considerable scatter range of 0–10 mm and consequently; there are different limiting values for the normal state in the literature.

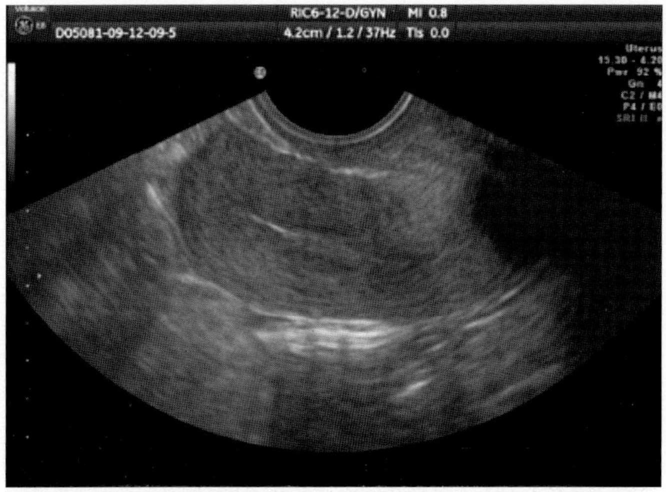

Fig. 20: B-mode ultrasound image of the uterus in sagittal section shows thin endometrium, typical of postmenopausal uterus. This is because of estrogen depletion in menopausal women.

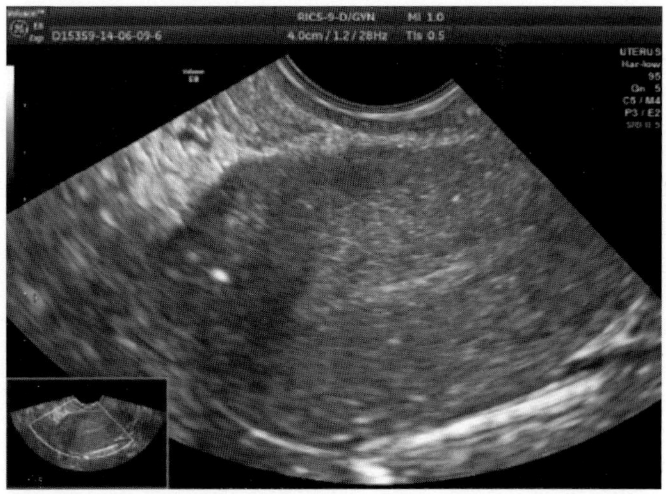

Fig. 21: B-mode ultrasound image of postmenopausal uterus showing thinned endometrium with ill-defined endometrial–myometrial junction. Echogenic spots seen in the myometrium may possibly be due to atherosclerosis of radial and arcuate vessels.

There is a correlation between the endometrial thickness and the body weight. Women with pure estrogen replacement therapy frequently have endometrial thickness exceeding that of postmenopausal women without it.[88]

Suspect Postmenopausal Endometrium

Endometrial carcinoma is the most common invasive gynecological malignancy in the United States and Europe today. The incidence of the disease increases considerably during the fifth decade of life, and the average age at diagnosis is 59 years. In the more cosmopolitan, higher income population, the rate has overcome the 40 cases per 100,000 related to increased longevity, increased cholesterol in diet, and exogenous estrogen supplementation or substances with an estrogen-like effect.[89,90] The 5-year survival rate is related to myometrial invasion, ranging from 93.7% when no invasion is present to 36.2%, if the invasion is deep.[91] When the first clinical sign appears, i.e., vaginal bleeding, the myometrial infiltration depth is already 10 mm on average.[83]

Of endometrial carcinomas, 80–90% present with atypical bleeding demonstrating the ineffectiveness of exfoliative cervical cytology and the need for early recognition of this most frequent genital malignancy.[83,92] Until now curettage and histologic evaluation is the accepted method to assess the background of the atypical bleeding. However, <10% of women with postmenopausal bleeding have endometrial cancer.[85,93] Therefore, a new noninvasive screening method must fulfill at least double requirements: It should be able to recognize the abnormal endometrial process at an earlier stage, when bleeding occurs and it should reduce the number of the "unnecessary" curettage, when postmenopausal bleeding occurs.

Several publications have reported that endosonographically measured endometrial thickness correlates closely with the presence or absence of endometrial cancer in asymptomatic postmenopausal women.[94,95] An endometrium that measures >8 mm from one myometrial–endometrial interface to another in postmenopausal woman without HRT is highly likely to be associated with significant endometrium pathology. Approximately, 10% of asymptomatic postmenopausal women have endometrium exceeding this cutoff level, and 1–3% of them can be expected to have endometrial carcinoma.[96,97] There is, however, a significant false-positive rate. Cutoff level of 8 mm has a very high sensitivity, but a low specificity.[83] The only way to increase the specificity would be to adjust the cutoff value to a higher level, but in this case the sensitivity of the screening would decrease and more positive cases might be overlooked.

Another possible approach to reduce the number of false-positive findings could be the use of color Doppler.

Up to now, there are no sonomorphologic criteria to differentiate between benign and malignant endometrial neoplasm. Therefore, there is no accepted screening method for endometrial cancer.

Postmenopausal Bleeding and Transvaginal Sonography (Transvaginal Sonography versus Dilatation and Curettage)

In atypical bleeding in the postmenopause, besides clinical and cytological examination, careful sonographic assessment should be made of the ovaries and the cervix uteri.[84]

Transvaginal ultrasound has become an important tool for diagnosing endometrial pathology in women with postmenopausal bleeding too. In patients with postmenopausal bleeding, the endometrium is considerably thicker than in asymptomatic women.[98]

Several studies have investigated the effectiveness of the endometrial thickness measurement in detecting malignancy in patients with postmenopausal bleeding, using different cutoff levels.[83,99-105] Summarizing the results of the published works in none of the case was endometrial carcinoma found <4 mm.

Measuring an endometrium <4 mm is safe enough to exclude the possibility of endometrial carcinoma in case of postmenopausal bleeding. Nevertheless, if this method is to be used for identifying those women who will not have a dilatation and curettage (D and C) performed, based on the findings on the endometrium, training is needed to minimize the error. Karlsson et al. found considerable differences, when compared the measurements of experienced and inexperienced examiners.[106]

If endometrial thickness is >4 mm (regardless woman is bleeding or not), it should be differentiated between focal and symmetrical thickness. As is mentioned before ultrasound itself cannot differentiate.

A great help to this is hysterosonography, which can easily differentiate between focal thickness (polyp) and symmetrical thickness.[104] Symmetrical thickness should be further investigated with pipelle biopsy.[107] If there is a polypus structure in the endometrium, hysteroscopy is recommended. Blind curettage is not recommended.[108]

In office setting, alternative method to sonography or hysterosonography is office hysteroscopy.

Postmenopausal Intrauterine Fluid Collection

Occasionally, a small amount of intraluminal fluid **(Fig. 22)** may be detected in the postmenopausal uterus; the detection rate of it can reach 16% in asymptomatic postmenopausal women.[84]

We can only speculate as to the pathophysiology of fluid accumulation in the uterine cavity. Senile cervical stenosis can prevent the drainage of possibly minimal

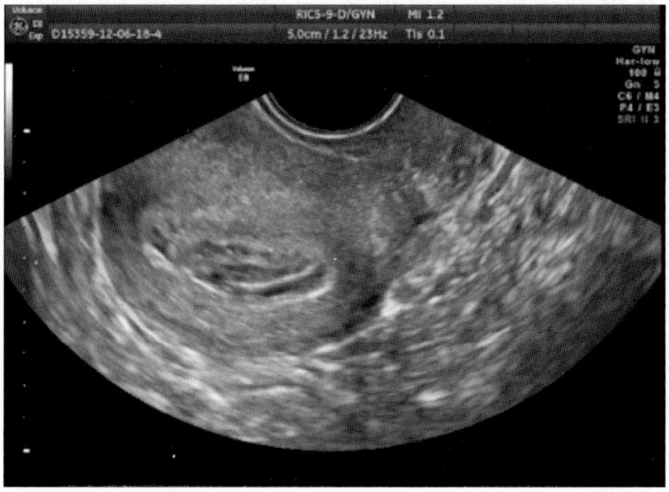

Fig. 22: B-mode ultrasound image of the uterus showing heterogeneous echogenicity in endometrial cavity. This may be due to blood or blood products, which may be a result of cervical malignancy more commonly or may be due to local endometrial cause.

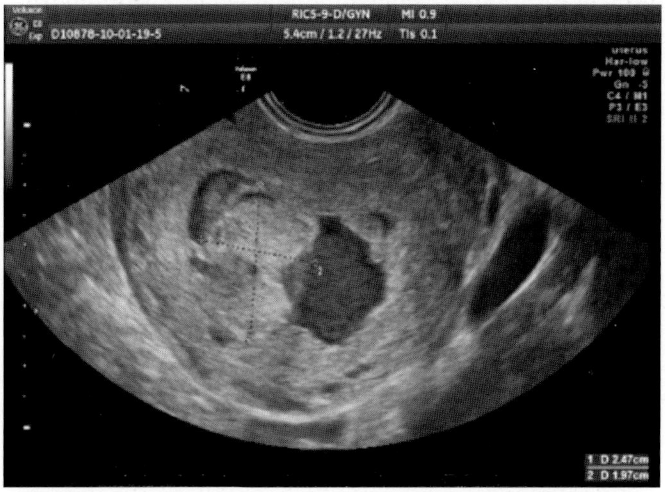

Fig. 23: B-mode ultrasound image of the uterus. Endometrial cavity is filled with fluid with low level echogenicities. A large solid lesion is seen arising from posterior wall of the endometrium. It is a projectile, polypoid growth with well-defined but irregular margins, possibly endometrial malignancy.

endometrial secretion, leading to small intrauterine pools. This, however, speculative as some degree of cervical stenosis is ubiquitous in postmenopausal women, whereas intrauterine fluid is a rare finding. Patients with ascites are more likely to have intrauterine fluid.[109] The possibility of the tubal cancer is rather theoretical than practical, although one case reported by Carlson,[110] cancer of the cervix may obstruct the cervical canal and can cause intrauterine fluid accumulation. However, the main suspected reason must remain the endometrial malignancy.

Although the presence of intrauterine fluid has been considered ominous and related to malignancy by some authors,[111,112] most authors today disagree on this.

In their series of 20 postmenopausal women with intrauterine fluid collection, Pardo et al.[113] revealed three cases of endometrial carcinoma, though it must be emphasized that in all of these positive cases, the endometrial thickness was >4 mm.

Carlson et al. also reported 20 cases of endometrial fluid collection in the postmenopause, of which five proved to be the results of some kind of genital malignancy (two ovarian, one tubal, one endometrial, and one cervical).[110]

However, examining the fluid pools in the uterine cavity, Osmers et al. did not find association with pathological changes in narrow endometrium.[84]

For Schmidt et al.[114] endometrial fluid by itself, without assessment of the endometrium does not indicate the requirement for additional histological clarification. As diagnostics, authors especially suggested the endometrial morphology a better choice.

Bar-Hava et al.[115] examined 1,175 asymptomatic postmenopausal women. They found 166 women with intrauterine fluid accumulation. Of the 166 women with intrauterine fluid accumulation, 91 had an endometrial biopsy, of which 70% were insufficient for evaluation and 30% were normal on histology. They concluded that postmenopausal intrauterine fluid accumulation is a common and mostly benign phenomenon that typically occurs in the late postmenopausal age subgroups.

The extensive use of sonography will lead to an eventual increase in the number of postmenopausal patients diagnosed with intrauterine fluid. In every case, careful scanning is recommended to rule out ovarian and tubal pathology. Certainly, cytological evaluation of the cervix with special regard to the cervical canal is essential. Obviously, the endometrium must be submitted to serious examination by transvaginal ultrasound. Polyploid growths **(Fig. 23)** and irregularity of the endometrial surface are particularly well seen when surrounded by intraluminal fluid. In that case, hysteroscopy is recommended. When thin endometrium surrounds fluid, endometrial sampling is not necessary.[114,115]

Undoubtedly, color Doppler offers an additional help in getting closer to the proper management, as it is able to assess the vascularization around this questionable ultrasound finding of postmenopausal intrauterine fluid collection.

Color Doppler Velocimetry and the Postmenopausal Endometrium

The visualization rate of the postmenopausal endometrial vessels is very low. The visualization rate of the endometrial vessels is in accordance with decreasing endometrial thickness with the postmenopausal years.[62] As it was already mentioned, vascularization of the inner third of the myometrium and the endometrial-myometrial junction is possible only in about or less than one-third out of those normal postmenopausal patient, who had the LMB not more than 5 years previously.[47] No flow can be detected in the normal and atrophic endometrium in the postmenopause.[86]

Although a thick endometrium may be a sign of pathological processes, no morphological features that are unique to malignant disease have been identified.[96] Transvaginal color and pulsed Doppler have shown that the presence of intratumoral vascularization with a low impedance to blood flow can be used as an end point in screening programs for some gynecological malignancies.[93,116,117]

Bourne et al. reported the impedance to blood flow in the uterine arteries and the endometrial thickness in women with postmenopausal bleeding with or without cancer.[90] In the women with postmenopausal bleeding who did not have endometrial cancer and in those without postmenopausal bleeding were similar. Conversely, the highest pulsatility index (PI) in the group with cancer (1.49) was below the lowest value in the group without cancer (1.95). Data from this study suggest that in the presence of malignant tissue, the impedance to blood flow within the uterine artery is reduced significantly when compared to control groups. This observation was later confirmed by others.[118] If color Doppler is used to interrogate the endometrium in such cases, angiogenesis can be demonstrated as areas of color superimposed on the B-mode grayscale image and the sensitivity of the technique is enhanced.[93]

Hata et al. found a feeder artery in patients of endometrial cancer and in 7 out of 9 endometrial cancers even venous blood flow in the endometrium could be detected, while no flow was detected around and within the endometrium in noncancer patients.[119] These findings were confirmed by pelvic angiography.

In the work of Kurjak et al., visualization rate of the abnormal blood flow within the endometrium was 100% in the cases of endometrial carcinoma.[86] Of the cases with detected endometrial carcinoma, 90 had endometrial (tumoral) thickness >10 mm, which is already a suspect sonographic sign alone. However, 10% of these endometrial carcinomas with endometrial thickness 5–10 mm would have been missed without color Doppler.

It was also suggested in the same work that color Doppler should help in distinguishing between cancerous and hyperplastic thickened endometrium. Flow could be detected only in 92% of cases of endometrial hyperplasia. Blood flow patterns were characterized with a low RI near or less than 0.40, which constituted statistically significant difference compared with that of endometrial hyperplasia, if any flow is detected.[86]

By using color Doppler and measurement of the endometrium thickness together whilst maintaining the sensitivity, the false-positive rate of the ultrasound-based test is reduced.[90] If further data confirm, superimposing the color Doppler onto the endometrium at a questionable thickness (5–10 mm) and searching for vascularization in or around the endometrium might help determine the further management of the patient and can lead to a further reduction of the number of D and C in the postmenopause.

Endometrium Under Hormone Replacement Therapy

It is now well established that unopposed exogenous estrogen increases a woman's risk for endometrial hyperplasia and thus has an etiologic role in endometrial carcinoma,[120,121] and that this effect is both dose and duration dependent.[122] Stimulating normal menstrual cycles by the use of progestogens have been found to effectively reduce estrogen-induced breakthrough bleeding, and lower the risk of endometrial hyperplasia and carcinoma.[98,122] Development of a hyperplasia can be prevented and a preexisting glandular cystic or adenomatous hyperplasia can be eliminated by regular administration of gestagens.[84]

Some of the most common adverse effects of postmenopausal estrogen treatment are bleeding disturbances, regardless of whether therapy is sequential or continuous estrogen/progestogen.[123] In those women who receive exogenous hormones continuously, the delicate task of balancing appropriate dosages of estrogen and progestogen may lead to breakthrough bleeding even more often. Since uterovaginal bleeding is the cardinal symptom of endometrial cancer, a disease which has been found to occur more frequently during unopposed estrogen therapy, it is not a surprise that rising estrogen consumption resulted in a need for appropriate invasive examinations to be carried out more frequently. Jensen et al. found that the frequency of D and C and endometrial biopsies in sequentially-treated women as compared with untreated women was 3.1 times higher in the 55–59 age group.[123]

Since TVS has been progressively used as an alternative recourse of monitoring, for the endometrium both in the pre- and postmenopause, it is also suggested that it may be a useful method of monitoring the effects of HRT on the endometrium.[84,124,125] Vaginosonography as a screening method enables us to survey the postmenopausal endometrium, but sonographic assessment of endometrium is a completely different manner. It is therefore desirable to correlate hormone replacement regimens with the sonographic appearance of the endometrium. Establishment of the normal range of endometrial widths for each hormone regimen would help limit unnecessary invasive procedures for suspected endometrial hyperplasia.[88]

Women who are receiving continuous hormone replacement are in favorable position. It is now well established that the kind of therapy is protective for endometrium. There are less cases of endometrial cancer in continuous regime group than in postmenopausal woman without any therapy.[126]

In women receiving sequential hormone replacement, endometrial thickness would be expected to vary throughout the cycle, depending on whether the endometrium was undergoing proliferative or secretory transformation due to estrogenic or progestational stimulation, respectively. For this purpose, the examiner should have the knowledge of the type of HRT and the day of the menstrual cycle, in order to distinguish pathological endometrial findings. It seems to be the best time of examination in the early postmenstrual period.

Contrary, in woman receiving continuous hormone replacement, endometrial thickness should be always the same (thin).

On the basis of the current literature, the following approach can be regarded as guidelines when examining the endometrium of an asymptomatic postmenopausal woman by vaginosonography. The recommendations are only for woman on sequential therapy. Woman on continuous therapy should be regarded and followed as postmenopausal woman without therapy.

- The endometrium of all postmenopausal women should be assessed vaginosonographically before the onset of HRT, whereas the guidelines for assessing the postmenopausal endometrium detailed in the previous chapter should be taken into consideration
- All patients on HRT are advised to have yearly sonographic checks of the endometrium. They should be examined after completion of the progestational phase of the cycle (days 1–2).
- Endometrial thickness up to 8 mm is regarded as normal finding.
- Endometrial thickness of 9 mm and more is regarded suspicious. After administration of an oral gestagen, subsequent to the withdrawal bleeding, a second sonography is performed. If the endometrium still measures >8 mm, hysterosonography is recommended. With endometrial thickness of <8 mm, control sonography in 3 months' time is recommended.

REFERENCES

1. Shifren JL, Shiff I. Menopause. In: Berek JS (Ed). Berek & Novak's Gynecology, 14th edition. Philadelphia: Lippincott, Williams & Wilkins; 2007. pp. 1323-42.
2. Lerner JP, Timor-Tritsch IE. Morphological evaluation of the ovary using transvaginal sonography. In: Kurjak A (Ed): Ultrasound and the Ovary. London, New York: Parthenon Publishing; 1994. pp. 115-28.
3. Healy DL, Bell R, Robertson DM, et al. Ovarian status in healthy postmenopausal women. Menopause. 2008; 15:1109-14.
4. Granberg S, Wikland M. Comparison between endovaginal and transabdominal transducers for measuring ovarian volume. J Ultrasound Med. 1987;6:649-56.
5. Hall DA, McCarthy KA, Kopans DB. Sonographic visualization of the normal postmenopausal ovary. J Ultrasound Med. 1986;5:9-15.
6. Campbell S, Goswamy R, Goessens L, et al. Real-time ultrasonography for determination of ovarian morphology and volume: A possible early screening test for ovarian cancer? Lancet. 1982;1:425-9.
7. Rodrigez H, Platt L, Medearis A, et al. The use of transvaginal sonography of evaluation of postmenopausal ovarian size and morphology. Am J Obstet Gynecol. 1988;159:810-4.
8. Fleischer A, McKee M, Gordon A, et al. Transvaginal sonography of postmenopausal ovaries with pathological correlation. J Ultrasound Med. 1990;9:637-44.
9. Kurjak A, Prka M, Pascual MA, et al. Assessment of normal and abnormal ovaries by transvaginal sonography. In: Kurjak A, Arenas JB (Eds). Donald School Textbook of

Ultrasound in Obstetrics and Gynecology. New Delhi: Jaypee Brothers Medical Publishers; 2005. pp. 446-64.
10. Barber HRK. The postmenopausal ovary. In: Kurjak A (Ed). Ultrasound and the Ovary. London, New York: Parthenon Publishing; 1994. pp. 231-4.
11. Andolf E, Jorgensen C, Svelaneius E, et al. Ultrasound measurement of ovarian volume. Acta Obstet Gynecol Scand. 1987;66:387-9.
12. Goswamy R, Campbell S, Royston J, et al. Ovarian size in postmenopausal women. Br J Obstet Gynaecol. 1988;95:795-801.
13. Wehba S, Fernandes CE, Ferreira JA, et al. Transvaginal ultrasonography assessment of ovarian volumes in postmenopausal women. Rev Paulista de Med. 1996;114:1152-5.
14. Merz E, Miric-Tesanic D, Bahlmann F, et al. Sonographic size of uterus and ovaries in pre- and perimenopausal women. Ultrasound Obstet Gynecol. 1996;7:38-42.
15. Tepper R, Zalel Y, Markov S, et al. Ovarian volume in postmenopausal women—suggestions to an ovarian size normogram for menopausal age. Acta Obstet Gynecol Scand. 1995;74:208-11.
16. Pavlik EJ, DePriest PD, Gallion HH, et al. Ovarian volume related to age. Gynecol Oncol. 2000;77:410-2.
17. Bakos O, Smith P, Heimer G, et al. Transvaginal sonography of the internal genital organs in postmenopausal women on low-dose estrogen treatment. Ultrasound Obstet Gynecol. 1994;4:326-9.
18. Bar-Hava I, Perri T, Zahavi Z, et al. Influence of hormone replacement therapy on postmenopausal pelvic organs. Climacteric. 2001;4:160-5.
19. Manonai J, Chittacharoen A, Theppisai U. Transvaginal color Doppler sonographic assessment of uterus and ovaries in postmenopausal women: the effect of local estrogen treatment. Eur J Obstet Gynecol Reprod Biol. 2006;127:222-6.
20. Davis AP, Oram D. Screening for ovarian cancer. In: Kurjak A (Ed). Ultrasound and the Ovary. London, New York: Parthenon Publishing; 1994. pp. 235-53.
21. Goozner M. Personalizing ovarian cancer screening. J Natl Cancer Inst. 2010;102:1112-3.
22. Barber HRK, Graber EA. The PMPO syndrome. Obstet Gynecol. 1971;38:921-3.
23. Kase NG, Weingold AB. Principles and practice of clinical gynecology. New York: John Wiley and Sons; 1983. p. 579.
24. Barber HRK. Ovarian cancer: Diagnosis and management. Am J Obstet Gynecol. 1984;150:910-5.
25. Barber HRK. The postmenopausal palpable ovary syndrome. Compr Ther. 1979;5:58.
26. Barber HRK. Editorial: A second look at the postmenopausal palpable ovary. Fem Patient. 1988;13:13-4.
27. Granberg S, Wikland M. Endovaginal Ultrasound in the diagnosis of unilocular ovarian cysts in postmenopausal women. Ultrasound Quarterly. 1992;10:1-13.
28. Granberg S, Wikland M, Jansson I. Macroscopic Characterization of ovarian cancer and relation to the histological diagnosis: Criteria to be used for ultrasound evaluation. Gynecol Oncol. 1989;35:139-44.
29. Granberg S, Norström A, Wikland M. Endovaginal ultrasound and cytological evaluation of cystic ovarian tumors: A comparison. J Ultrasound Med. 1991;10:9-14.
30. Granberg S, Norström A, Wikland M. Tumours in lower pelvis imaged by vaginal ultrasound. Gynecol Oncol. 1989;37:224-9.
31. Andolf E, Jörgensen C. Simple adnexal cysts diagnosed by ultrasound in postmenopausal women. J Clin Ultrasound. 1988;16:301-3.
32. Andolf E, Jörgensen C. Cystic lesions in elderly women, diagnosed by ultrasound. Br J Obstet Gynaecol. 1989;96:1076-9.
33. Goldstein SR, Subramanyam B, Snyder JR, et al. The postmenopausal cystic adnexal mass: The potential role of ultrasound in conservative management. Obstet Gynecol. 1989;73:8-10.
34. Parker WH, Berek JS. Management of selected cystic adnexal masses in postmenopausal women by operative laparoscopy: A pilot study. Am J Obstet Gynecol. 1990;163:1574-7.
35. Valentin L, Akrawi D. The natural history of adnexal cysts incidentally detected at transvaginal ultrasound examination in postmenopausal women. Ultrasound Obstet Gynecol. 2002;20:174-80.
36. Valentin L, Skoog L, Epstein E. Frequency and type of adnexal lesions in autopsy material from postmenopausal women: ultrasound study with histological correlation. Ultrasound Obstet Gynecol. 2003;22:284-9.
37. Modesitt SC, Pavlik EJ, Ueland FR, et al. Risk of malignancy in unilocular ovarian cystic tumors less than 10 centimeters in diameter. Obstet Gynecol. 2003;102:594-9.
38. Nardo LG, Kroon ND, Reginald PW. Persistent unilocular ovarian cysts in a general population of postmenopausal women: Is there a place for expectant management? Obstet Gynecol. 2003;102:589-93.
39. Castillo G, Alcazar JL, Jurado M. Natural history of sonographically detected simple unilocular adnexal cysts in asymptomatic postmenopausal women. Gynecol Oncol. 2004;92:965-9.
40. Dorum A, Blom GP, Ekerhovd E, et al. Prevalence and histologic diagnosis of adnexal cysts in postmenopausal women: An autopsy study. Am J Obstet Gynecol. 2005;192:48-54.
41. Greenlee RT, Kessel B, Williams CR, et al. Prevalence, incidence, and natural history of simple ovarian cysts among women >55 years old in a large cancer screening trial. Am J Obstet Gynecol. 2010;202:373.e1-9.
42. Dietrich M, Osmers RG, Grobe G, et al. Limitations of the evaluation of adnexal masses by its macroscopic aspects, cytology and biopsy. Eur J Obstet Gynecol Reprod Biol. 1999;82:57-62.

43. Tahir Z, Yusuf NW, Ashraf M, et al. Fine needle aspiration of unilocular ovarian cysts—a cytohistological correlation. J Pak Med Assoc. 2004;54:266-9.
44. Papathanasiou K, Giannoulis C, Dovas D, et al. Fine needle aspiration cytology of the ovary: Is it reliable? Clin Exp Obstet Gynecol. 2004;31:191-3.
45. RCOG. Ovarian Cysts in Postmenopausal Women: RCOG guideline No. 34. London: RCOG Press; 2003. pp. 1-8.
46. Kurjak A, Shalan H, Matijevic R, et al. Stage I ovarian cancer by transvaginal color Doppler sonography: A report of 18 cases. Ultrasound Obstet Gynecol. 1993;3:195-8.
47. Kurjak A, Kupesic S. Ovarian senescence and its significance on uterine and ovarian perfusion. Fertil Steril. 1995;3:532-7.
48. Kurjak A, Kupesic-Urek S, Schulman H, et al. Transvaginal color Doppler in the assessment of ovarian and uterine blood flow in infertile women. Fertil Steril. 1992;56:870-3.
49. Scholtes MCW, Wladimiroff J, Rijen HJM, et al. Uterine and ovarian flow velocity waveforms in the normal menstrual cycle: a transvaginal color Doppler study. Fertil Steril. 1989;52:981-5.
50. Kurjak A, Schulman H, Sosic A, et al. Transvaginal ultrasound, color flow, and Doppler waveform of the postmenopausal adnexal mass. Obstet Gynecol. 1992;80:917-21.
51. Fleischer AC, Rodgers WH, Kepple DM, et al. Color Doppler sonography of ovarian masses: A multiparameter analysis. J Ultrasound Med. 1993;12:41-8.
52. Crade M, Patel J, Yiu-Chiu V. Evaluation of 103 pelvic masses: Correlation of surgical diagnosis with transvaginal ultrasound size, complexity scores and resistive index values. Ultrasound Obstet Gynecol. 1993;3:23.
53. Kulenkampff D, Puchta J, Osmers R. Sonographic appearance of the myometrium. In: Osmers R, Kurjak A (Eds). Ultrasound and the Uterus. Carnforth, New York: Parthenon Publishing; 1995. pp. 53-9.
54. Rempen A. Normal sonographic features of the uterus. In: Osmers R, Kurjak A (Eds). Ultrasound and the Uterus. Carnforth, New York: Parthenon Publishing; 1995. pp. 1-12.
55. deVries K, Lyons KEA, Ballard G, et al. Contractions of the inner third of the myometrium. Am J Obstet Gynecol. 1990;162:679-82.
56. Andolf E, Dahlander K, Aspenberg P. Ultrasonic thickness of the endometrium correlated to body weight in asymptomatic postmenopausal women. Obstet Gynecol. 1993;82:936-40.
57. Zalud I, Conway C, Schulman H, et al. Endometrial and myometrial thickness and uterine blood flow in postmenopausal women: The influence of hormonal replacement therapy and age. J Ultrasound Med. 1993;12:737-41.
58. Kurjak A, Kupesic-Urek S. Normal and abnormal uterine perfusion. In: Jaffe R, Warsof LS (Eds). Color Doppler imaging on Obstetrics and Gynecology. New York: McGraw Hill; 1992. pp. 255-63.
59. Long MG, Boultbee JE, Hanson ME, et al. Doppler time velocity waveform studies of the uterine artery and the uterus. Br J Obstet Gynaecol. 1989;96:588-93.
60. Goswamy RK, Steptoe PC. Doppler ultrasound studies of the uterine artery in spontaneous ovarian cycles. Hum Reprod. 1988;3:721-3.
61. Goswamy RK, Williams G, Steptoe PC. Decreased uterine perfusion a cause of infertility. Hum Reprod. 1988;3:955-8.
62. Kupesic S, Kurjak A. Uterine perfusion. In: Osmers R, Kurjak A (Eds). Ultrasound and the Uterus. Carnforth, New York: Parthenon Publishing; 1995. pp. 87-90.
63. Luzi G, Coata G, Cucchia GC, et al. Doppler studies of uterine arteries in spontaneous and artificially induced menopausal women. Ultrasound Obstet Gynecol. 1993;3:354-6.
64. Lewit N, Thaler I, Rottem S. The uterus: A new look with transvaginal sonography. J Clin Ultrasound. 1990;18:331-6.
65. Kurjak A, Shalan H, Kupesic S, et al. Transvaginal color Doppler assessment in the pelvic tumor vascularity. Ultrasound Obstet Gynecol. 1993;3:137-54.
66. Hata T, Hata K, Senoh D, et al. Doppler ultrasound assessment of tumor vascularity in gynecologic disorders. J Ultrasound Med. 1989;8:309-14.
67. Kurjak A, Zalud I. The characterization of uterine tumors by transvaginal color Doppler. Ultrasound Obstet Gynecol. 1991;1:50-2.
68. Kurjak A, Kupesic-Urek S, Miric D. The assessment of benign uterine tumor vascularisation by transvaginal color Doppler. Ultrasound Med Biol. 1992;18:645-9.
69. Matta WHM, Stabile I, Shaw RW, et al. Doppler assessment of uterine blood flow changes in patients with fibroids receiving the gonadotropin-releasing hormone agonist Buserelin. Fertil Steril. 1988;49:1083-5.
70. Wilson EA, Yang F, Rees ED. Estradiol and progesterone binding in uterine leiomyomata and in normal uterine tissues. Obstet Gynecol. 1980;55:20-4.
71. Solues MR, McCarthy KS. Leiomyomas: Steroid receptor content. Variations within normal menstrual cycle. Am J Obstet Gynecol. 1982;143:6-11.
72. Filicori M, Hall DA, Loughlin JS, et al. A conservative approach to the management of uterine leiomyoma: pituitary desensitization by a luteinizing hormone-releasing analogue. Am J Obste Gynecol. 1983;147:726-7.
73. Aleem F, Predanic' M. Uterine leiomyomata: Transvaginal color Doppler studies and new aspects of management. In: Osmers R, Kurjak A (Eds). Uterus and Ultrasound. Carnforth: Parthenon Publishing; 1995. pp. 61-70.
74. Meyer WR, Meyer AR, Diamond MP. Unsuspected leiomyosarcoma: treatment with gonadotropin-releasing hormone analogue. Obstet Gynecol. 1990;75:529-34.
75. Kurjak A, Kupesic S, Shalan H, et al. Uterine sarcoma: a report of 10 cases studied by transvaginal color and pulsed Doppler sonography. Gynecol Oncol. 1995;59:342-6.
76. Szabó I, Szánthó A, Csabay L, et al. Color Doppler ultrasonography in the differentiation of uterine sarcomas

from uterine leiomyomas. Eur J Gynaecol Oncol. 2002;23:29-34.
77. Vollenhoven BJ, Lawrence AS, Healy DL. Uterine fibroids: a clinical review. Br J Obstet Gynaecol. 1990;97:285-98.
78. Jirapinyo M, Theppisai U, Leelapatana P, et al. Sonographic findings of uterus and ovaries in normal pre- and post-menopausal women. J Med Assoc Thai. 1998;81:527-31.
79. Fedele L, Bianchi S, Raffaelli R, et al. A randomized study of the effects of tibolone and transdermal estrogen replacement therapy in postmenopausal women with uterine myomas. Eur J Obstet Gynecol Reprod Biol. 2000;88:91-4.
80. Colacurci N, De Francis P, Cobellis L, et al. Effects of hormone replacement therapy on postmenopausal uterine myoma. Maturitas. 2000;35:167-73.
81. Polatti F, Viazzo F, Colleoni R, et al. Uterine myoma in postmenopause: A comparison between two therapeutic schedules of HRT. Maturitas. 2000;37:27-32.
82. Simsek T, Karakus C, Trak B. Impact of different hormone replacement therapy regimens on the size of myoma uteri in postmenopausal period. Tibolone versus transdermal hormonal replacement system. Maturitas. 2002;42:243-6.
83. Osmers R, Kuhn W. Endometrial cancer screening. Curr Opin Obstet Gynecol. 1994;6:75-9.
84. Osmers R, Puchta J, Suren A. Pathological findings of the postmenopausal endometrium. In: Osmers R, Kurjak A (Eds). Ultrasound and the Uterus. Carnforth, New York: Parthenon Publishing; 1995. pp. 31-44.
85. Granberg S, Wikland M, Karlsson B, et al. Endometrial thickness as measured by endovaginal ultrasound for identifying endometrial abnormality. Am J Obstet Gynecol. 1991;164:47-52.
86. Kurjak A, Shalan H, Sosic A, et al. Endometrial carcinoma in postmenopausal women: Evaluation by transvaginal Color Doppler. Am J Obstet Gynecol. 1993;169:1597-603.
87. Kamel HS, Darwish AM, Mohamed SA. Comparison of transvaginal ultrasonography and vaginal sono-hysterography in the detection of endometrial polyps. Acta Obstet Gynecol Scand. 2000;79:60-4.
88. Lin MC, Gosin BB, Wolf SI, et al. Endometrial thickness after the menopause: Effect of the hormone replacement. Radiology. 1991;180:427-32.
89. Lurain JR. Uterine cancer. In: Berek JS (Ed). Berek & Novak's Gynecology, 14th edition. Philadelphia: Lippincott, Williams & Wilkins; 2007. pp. 1343-402.
90. Bourne TH, Campbell S, Whitehead MI, et al. Detection of endometrial cancer in postmenopausal women by transvaginal ultrasonography and colour flow imaging. Br Med J. 1990;301(6748):369.
91. Lehtovirta P, Cacciatore B, Wahlstrom T, et al. Ultrasonic assessment of endometrial cancer invasion. J Clin Ultrasound. 1987;15:519-24.
92. Osmers R. Transvaginal sonography in endometrial cancer. Ultrasound Obstet Gynecol. 1992;2:2-3.
93. Bourne TH. Transvaginal color Doppler in Gynecology. Ultrasound Obstet Gynecol. 1991;1:359-73.
94. Osmers R, Völksen M, Rath W, et al. Vaginosonographic detection of endometrial cancer in postmenopausal women. Int J Gynecol Obstet. 1990;32:35-7.
95. Wikland M, Granberg S, Karlsson B. Assessment of the endometrium in the postmenopausal woman by vaginal sonography. Ultrasound Quarterly. 1992;10:15-27.
96. Osmers R, Volksen M, Schauer A. Vaginosonography for early detection of endometrial carcinoma. Lancet. 1990;1:1569-71.
97. Gambacciani M, Monteleone P, Ciaponi M, et al. Clinical usefulness of endometrial screening by ultrasound in asymptomatic postmenopausal women. Maturitas. 2004;48:421-4.
98. Flowers CE, Wilborn WH, Hyde BM. Mechanisms of uterine bleeding in postmenopausal patients receiving estrogen alone or with a progestin. Obstet Gynecol. 1983;61:135-43.
99. Goldstein SR, Nachtigall M, Snyder JR, et al. Endometrial assessment by vaginal ultrasonography before endometrial sampling in patients with postmenopausal bleeding. Am J Obstet Gynecol. 1990;163:119-23.
100. Varner RE, Sparks JM, Cameron CD, et al. Transvaginal sonography of the endometrium in postmenopausal women. Obstet Gynecol. 1991;78:195-9.
101. Botsis D, Kassanos D, Pyrgiotis E, et al. Vaginal sonography of the endometrium in postmenopausal women. Clin Exp Obstet Gynecol. 1992;19:189-92.
102. Dorum A, Kristensen GB, Langebrekke A, et al. Evaluation of endometrial thickness measured by endovaginal ultrasound in women with postmenopausal bleeding. Acta Obstet Gynecol Scand. 1993;72:116-9.
103. Bakos O, Smith P, Heimer G. Transvaginal ultrasonography for identifying endometrial pathology in postmenopausal women. Maturitas. 1995;20:181-9.
104. Epstein E, Ramirez A, Skoog L, et al. Transvaginal sonography, saline contrast sonohysterography and hysteroscopy for the investigation of women with postmenopausal bleeding and endometrium >5 mm. Ultrasound Obstet Gynecol. 2001;18:157-62.
105. Moodley M, Roberts C. Clinical pathway for the evaluation of postmenopausal bleeding with an emphasis on endometrial cancer detection. J Obstet Gynaecol. 2004;24:736-41.
106. Karlsson B, Granberg S, Ridell B, et al. Endometrial thickness as measured by transvaginal sonography: Interobserver variation. Ultrasound Obstet Gynecol. 1994;4:320-5.
107. Machado F, Moreno J, Carazo M, et al. Accuracy of endometrial biopsy with the Cornier pipelle for diagnosis of endometrial cancer and atypical hyperplasia. Eur J Gynaecol Oncol. 2003;24:279-81.
108. Epstein E, Ramirez A, Skoog L, et al. Dilatation and curettage fail to detect most focal lesions in the uterine cavity in women with postmenopausal bleeding. Acta Obstet Gynecol Scand. 2001;80:1131-6.

109. Fleischer AC, Kepple DM, Entman SS. Transvaginal sonography of uterine disorders. In: Timor-Tritsch IE, Rottem S (Eds). Transvaginal Sonography, 2nd edition. New York: Elsevier Science Publishing; 1993. pp. 109-30.
110. Carlson JA, Arger P, Thompson S, et al. Clinical and pathologic correlation of endometrial cavity fluid detected by ultrasound in the postmenopausal women. Obstet Gynecol. 1991;77:119-23.
111. Brechenridge JW, Kurtz AB, Ritchie WGM, et al. Postmenopausal uterine fluid collection: Indicator of carcinoma. Am J Radiol. 1982;139:529-34.
112. McCarthy KA, Hall DA, Kopans DB, et al. Postmenopausal endometrial fluid collections: Always of indicator of malignancy? J Ultrasound Med. 1986;5:647-9.
113. Pardo J, Kapan B, Nitke S, et al. Postmenopausal intrauterine fluid collection: Correlation between ultrasound and hysteroscopy. Ultrasound Obstet Gynecol. 1994;4:224-6.
114. Schmidt T, Nawroth F, Breidenbach M, et al. Differential indication for histological evaluation of endometrial fluid in postmenopause. Maturitas. 2005;50:177-81.
115. Bar-Hava I, Orvieto R, Ferber A, et al. Asymptomatic post-menopausal intrauterine fluid accumulation: Characterization and significance. Climacteric. 1998;1: 279-83.
116. Kurjak A, Zalud I, Jurkovic D, et al. Transvaginal color flow Doppler for the assessment of pelvic circulation. Acte Obstet Gynecol Scand. 1989;68:131-5.
117. Kurjak A, Shalan H, Kupesic S, et al. An attempt to screen asymptomatic women for ovarian and endometrial cancer with transvaginal color and pulsed Doppler sonography. J Ultrasound Med. 1994;13:295-301.
118. Kupesic-Urek S, Shalan H, Kurjak A. Early detection of endometrial cancer by transvaginal color Doppler. Eur J Obstet Gynecol Reprod Biol. 1993;49:46-9.
119. Hata K, Hata T, Manabe A, et al. New pelvic sonography for detection of endometrial carcinoma: a preliminary report. Gynecol Oncol. 1992;45:179-84.
120. Smith DC, Prentice R, Thompson DJ, et al. Association of exogenous estrogen and endometrial carcinoma. N Engl J Med. 1975;293:1164-7.
121. Ziel HK, Finkle WD. Increased risk of endometrial carcinoma among users of conjugated estrogens. N Engl J Med. 1975;293:1167-70.
122. Whitehead MI, Townsend PT, Pryse-Davies J, et al. Effects of various types and dosages of progestogens on the postmenopausal endometrium. J Reprod Med. 1982;27:539-48.
123. Jensen LC, Obel EB, Linhard E, et al. Frequency of curettage in middle-aged women treated with sequential preparations versus untreated women. Maturitas. 1992;15:61-9.
124. Castelo-Branco C, Puerto B, Durán M, et al. Transvaginal sonography of the endometrium in postmenopausal women: Monitoring the effect of hormone replacement therapy. Maturitas. 1994;19:59-65.
125. Meuwissen JH, van Langen H, Moret E, et al. Monitoring of oestrogen replacement therapy by vaginosonography of the endometrium. Maturitas. 1992;15:33-7.
126. Archer DF, Pickar JH. Hormone replacement therapy: Effect of progestin dose and time since menopause on endometrial bleeding. Obstet Gynecol. 2000;96:899-905.

CHAPTER 62

The Use of Ultrasound as an Adjunct to the Physical Examination for the Evaluation of Gynecologic and Obstetric Causes of Acute Pelvic Pain

Sanja Kupesic Plavsic, Ulrich Honemeyer

INTRODUCTION

Acute pelvic pain may be the manifestation of various gynecologic and nongynecologic disorders ranging from a less alarming rupture of a follicular cyst to life-threatening conditions such as rupture of an ectopic pregnancy or perforation of an inflamed appendix. Pelvic inflammatory disease (PID) presents with many ultrasonographic signs such as thickening of the tubal wall, incomplete septa within the dilated tube, demonstration of hyperechoic mural nodules, free fluid in the "cul-de-sac", etc. Other pathologies such as hemorrhagic ovarian cysts present with a variety of ultrasound findings since intracystic echoes depend upon the quality and quantity of the blood clots. The color Doppler investigation demonstrates a moderate to low vascular resistance typical of luteal flow. Another example that demonstrates another use of ultrasound as an aid in diagnosis is endometriosis. The classic symptom of endometriosis is chronic pelvic pain, in some patients acute pelvic pain does occur. Most of these patients demonstrate an endometrioma or "chocolate" cyst containing diffuse carpet-like echoes. One should be aware that the detection of a pericystic and/or hilar type of an ovarian endometrioma vascularization by color Doppler ultrasound facilitates correct recognition of this entity. Pelvic congestion syndrome is another condition that can cause an attack of acute pelvic pain. It usually occurs as a consequence of dilatation of venous plexuses, arteries or both systems. By switching to color Doppler, gynecologist can differentiate pelvic congestion syndrome from multilocular cysts, pelvic inflammatory disease or adenomyosis. Acute pelvic pain may occur even in normal intrauterine pregnancy. This may be explained by hormonal changes, rapid growth of the uterus and increased blood flow. Ultrasound is mandatory for distinguishing normal intrauterine pregnancy from a threatened or spontaneous abortion, ectopic pregnancy or other complications that may occur in patients with a positive pregnancy test.

Detection of uterine dehiscence and rupture in patients with history of prior surgical intervention on uterine wall relies exclusively on correct ultrasound diagnosis. In patients with placental abruption the sonographer can detect a hypoechoic complex which may represent a retroplacental hematoma, a subchorionic hematoma or a subamniotic hemorrhage.

In this revised chapter, the authors include updated references and new high resolution ultrasound images.

GYNECOLOGIC ETIOLOGIES OF ACUTE PELVIC PAIN

Acute pelvic pain may be the manifestation of various gynecologic and nongynecologic disorders ranging from life-threatening conditions such as rupture of an ectopic pregnancy or the perforation of an inflamed appendix to the less alarming setting of a rupture of a periovulatory follicle. The astute clinician must bear in mind all of the possibilities when evaluating patients presenting with acute pelvic pain.[1,2] Localizing the site of pain in combination with an ultrasound examination of the affected area leads to prompt and accurate clinical diagnosis. Ultrasound has become a valuable tool in evaluating the patient presenting with acute pelvic pain of both gynecological and nongynecological origin such as appendicitis or urinary stones.[3] It would be advisable to offer some type of an algorithm for the differential diagnosis that could guide physicians through the management of such a problem.

A ruptured ectopic pregnancy, salpingitis and hemorrhagic ovarian cysts are the three most commonly diagnosed gynecologic conditions presenting with an acute abdomen. Degenerating leiomyomas and adnexal torsion occur less frequently.[4] In order to have a systematic approach, gynecologic causes of acute pelvic pain can further be divided into two categories those with a negative pregnancy test, and those with a positive pregnancy test.

Acute Pelvic Pain with a Negative Pregnancy Test

Pelvic Inflammatory Disease

Pelvic inflammatory disease is defined as the acute clinical syndrome associated with spread of micro-organisms (unrelated to pregnancy or surgery) from the vagina or cervix to the endometrium,[5] fallopian tubes and or the contiguous structures.[6] This disease can lead to infertility, ectopic pregnancy and chronic pelvic pain.[7,8] Sexually active adolescents are at the greatest risk for PID. Other risk factors include multiple sexual partners, a high number of sexual partners throughout an individual's lifespan, the use of an intrauterine device (IUD), an untreated infected male sex partner (s), a history of previous PID, presence of *Neisseria gonorrhoeae* or *Chlamydia trachomatis* in the reproductive tract and frequent vaginal douching.[7] PID causes more morbidity than necessary for three reasons: women are not hospitalized when they should be, many women receive inadequate antibiotic therapy and the male partner was not treated or is treated inappropriately.[9] PID may manifest itself by various clinical presentations: silent (asymptomatic), atypical, acute and chronic. The patient present with acute PID complains mainly of low abdominal tenderness. Some of them may have an increased body temperature, but it is not unusual to have patients with a normal temperature. Laboratory findings show an increased sedimentation rate and white blood cell count. The next step is to evaluate the pelvis ultrasonographically keeping in mind that the sonographic findings may be normal in the early course of the disease.[10]

Acute PID usually presents with:

- Thickening of the tube wall of[3] more than 5 mm.
- Incomplete septa correlating with the mucosal folds in the dilated tube that is sonolucent or contain low-level echoes (This finding does not discriminate between acute and chronic cases).
- "Beads-on-a-string" sign, which defines hyperechoic mural nodules measuring about 2 to 3 mm, visualized on the cross-section of a fluid-filled distended tube.
- Formation of the tubo-ovarian complex (the ovary cannot be separated from the tube by pushing it with the vaginal probe).
- Fluid in the cul-de-sac.
- Low-to-moderate resistance index (RI = 0.53 ± 0.09) obtained from the adnexal region. **Figures 1A to C** demonstrate complex adnexal mass in a patient with acute PID.

Chronic PID can develop either as the consequence of an acute, symptomatic infection or as a consequence of a silent asymptomatic disease in patients without any clinical evidence of salpingitis. The most common ultrasound appearance is the hydrosalpinx, formed when the fimbrial part of the tube is closed because of pelvic adhesions causing the accumulation of tubal mucus. Chronic hydrosalpinx is usually discovered accidentally on a routine transvaginal ultrasound scan or during the assessment of infertile patients **(Table 1)**.

Hemorrhagic Ovarian Cysts

Cyclic causes of pelvic pain include crampy abdominal pain due to normal menstruation and development of the corpus luteum cyst. Corpus luteum cyst may be painful either due to the large size of the cyst, or due to the hemorrhage within the cyst. Patients with a hemorrhagic ovarian cyst may experience abrupt onset of low abdominal or pelvic pain and in this case the complete blood count may demonstrate a low hematocrit value. Cyst rupture with hemorrhage into the peritoneum is a rare cause of pelvic pain. Functional cysts other than corpus luteum can also be complicated by hemorrhage and rupture. Hemorrhage is excellent evidence that an ovarian mass is benign. Of the hemorrhagic cysts reported in the sonographic literature 98% were non-neoplastic and the remaining 2% were benign tumors.[11-13] The ultrasonographic appearance of the hemorrhagic cysts has different characteristics due to the retracting blood clots. They can look solid or have focal thickening of the walls with a fluid level sometimes resembling an endometrioma. Some hemorrhagic ovarian cysts can mimic sonographic features of solid ovarian masses, such as a teratoma. In most cases, the degree of through transmission is greater than in truly solid masses, and the mass regresses in size over a 2 to 3 week period. On sonography, the most common appearance is a complex mass with internal echoes, and enhancement through transmission **(Figs. 2A to G)**. Although the fibrinolized clot is typically hypoechoic, an acute intraparenchymal hemorrhage frequently appears as an irregular echogenic area **(Fig. 2D)**. The cyst wall may be irregular in contour due to a clot that is adherent to it. Occasionally, a mildly echogenic interface can be seen within a hemorrhagic cyst, most likely representing

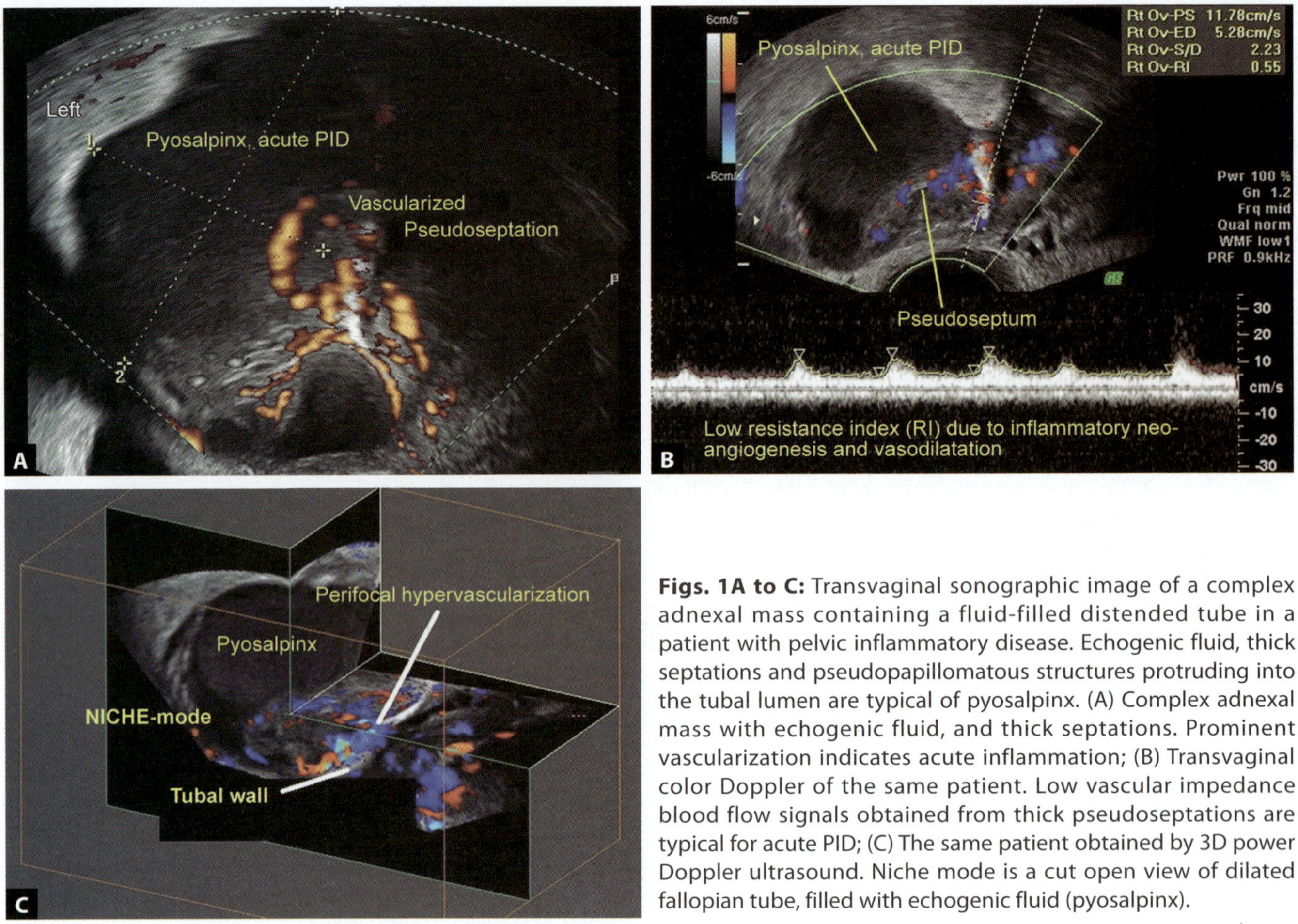

Figs. 1A to C: Transvaginal sonographic image of a complex adnexal mass containing a fluid-filled distended tube in a patient with pelvic inflammatory disease. Echogenic fluid, thick septations and pseudopapillomatous structures protruding into the tubal lumen are typical of pyosalpinx. (A) Complex adnexal mass with echogenic fluid, and thick septations. Prominent vascularization indicates acute inflammation; (B) Transvaginal color Doppler of the same patient. Low vascular impedance blood flow signals obtained from thick pseudoseptations are typical for acute PID; (C) The same patient obtained by 3D power Doppler ultrasound. Niche mode is a cut open view of dilated fallopian tube, filled with echogenic fluid (pyosalpinx).

TABLE 1: A suggested algorithm for the diagnosis of pelvic inflammatory disease.

Diagnosis	*Clinical signs*	*Ultrasound findings*	*Color Doppler findings*
Acute salpingitis	• Low abdominal tenderness • Increased/Normal body temperature • SE, L	• Tubes filled with inflammatory secretions • Retort-shaped tubes	• Low-to-moderate resistance index (RI = 0.53 ± 0.09)
Tubo-ovarian abscess	• Severe pain in the lower abdomen • High fever • SE, L	• Multilocular or unilocular fluid-filled structure • Air bubbles in case of gas-producing bacterial infection	• Low vascular resistance signals obtained from the septa or periphery of the lesion (RI = 0.40 ± 0.08)
Chronic salpingitis	Mild or absent symptoms Infertility	• "Cogwheel sign" • Distended tubes with incomplete septa • Hyperechogenic knots may be visualized every few millimeters in a transverse section	• High vascular resistance (RI = 0.71 ± 0.09) • Absence of diastolic flow, indicating irreversible scarification (RI = 1.0)

(SE: erythrocyte sedimentation rate; L: white blood cell count)

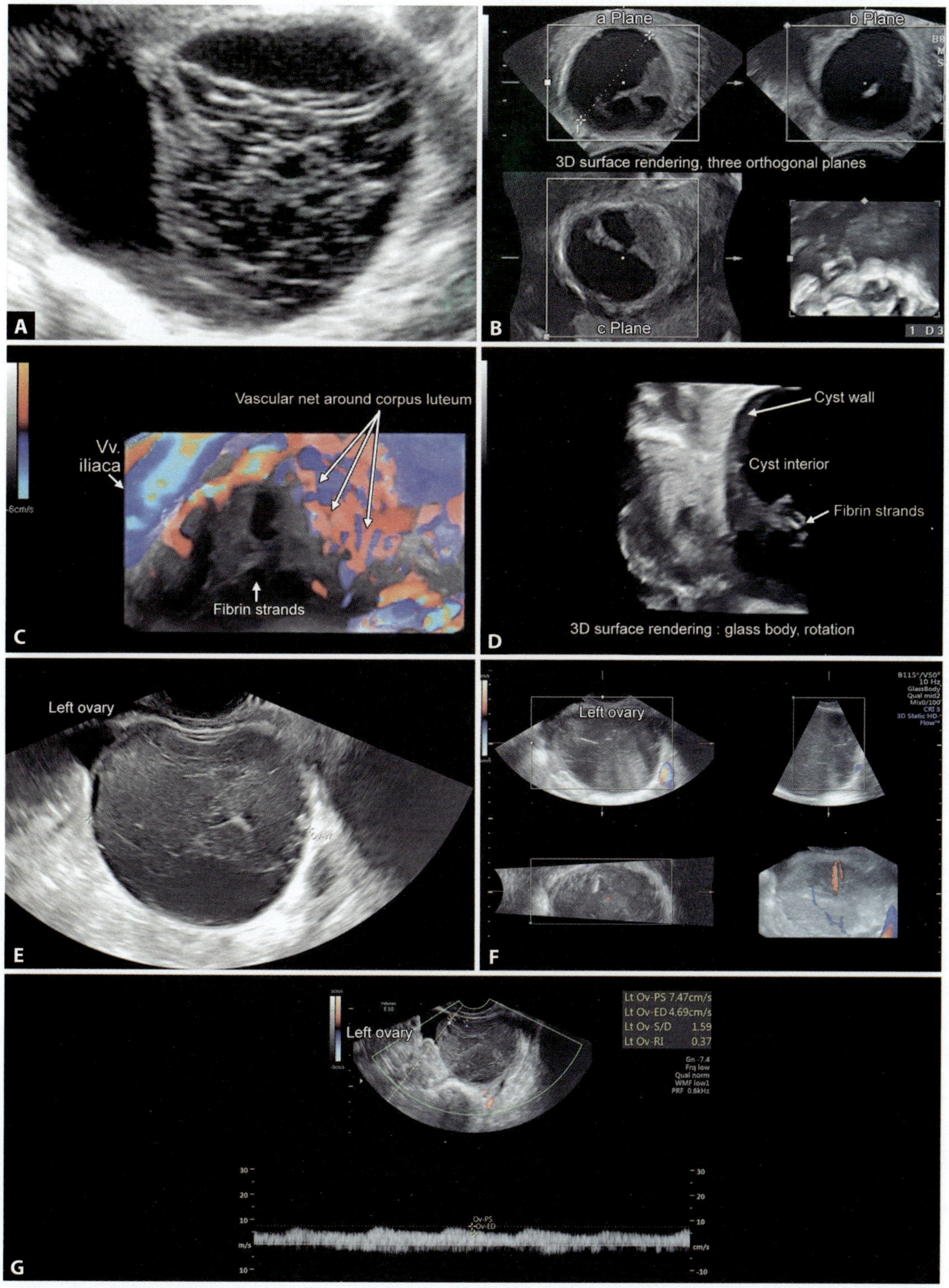

Figs. 2A to G: Transvaginal ultrasound of a hemorrhagic ovarian cyst. Echogenic content represents a retracting clot within the blood-filled cavity of the former follicle. (A) Corpus luteum hemorrhagic cyst obtained by 2D ultrasound. Internal echoes represent retracting clot; (B) Three-dimensional ultrasound of a hemorrhagic cyst. Three orthogonal planes (a, b and c) and surface rendering (right lower image) demonstrate a complex cystic lesion; (C) Color Doppler image of the same patient. Prominent blood flow signals visualized at the periphery of the cystic lesion indicate corpus luteum angiogenesis; (D) Three-dimensional ultrasound of the same patient. Note fibrin strands protruding from the wall of the cystic structure; (E) B mode transvaginal ultrasound of a complex left adnexal with thin avascular pseudoseptations; (F) Three-dimensional power Doppler image of the same patient illustrating regularly separated vessels; (G) Pulsed Doppler waveform analysis reveals low vascular impedance (RI = 0.37) obtained from peripheral vessels.

a partially solid clot.[12,13] Hemorrhagic cysts show low-to-moderate vascular resistance (RI = 0.50 ± 0.08) from the peripheral vessels, while the solid component representing a blood clot remains avascular.

Degenerating Leiomyomas

Leiomyomas are the most common tumors of female pelvis and occur in 20–25% of women of reproductive age. Clinically, symptoms such as metrorrhagia, pelvic pain and infertility are usually present in patients with submucosal leiomyomas, whereas subserosal leiomyomas are mainly asymptomatic. Subserosal leiomyomas may cause lumbar pain and urinary or bowel symptoms due to compression.[14] Acute symptoms are usually seen in leiomyomas undergoing torsion or necrosis.[15] The ultrasound appearance of leiomyomas depends on its size, site and age of the tumor. They are usually spherical in shape and sharply demarked from the myometrium, unlike adenomyosis. Sonographic texture of leiomyomas ranges from hypoechoic to echogenic, depending on the amount of smooth muscle and connective tissue. If present, secondary changes such as necrosis, hemorrhage, degeneration and/or calcification are represented by a wide spectrum of ultrasonic images. A leiomyoma undergoing cystic degeneration (hemorrhagic or proteolytic) presents as a complex or anechoic uterine mass **(Figs. 3A to E)**, which demonstrates far acoustic enhancement. There might be highly echogenic portions and an associated acoustic shadowing from areas of calcification, varying from small focal deposits to extensive calcifications, usually seen in older women.[16] Color flow detects the myoma's feeder vessels that arise from the myometrial vasculature and form a regular ring of angiogenesis and central vessels that develop as a response to the angiogenic activity of the tumor cells, perhaps due to a necrotic or inflammatory process. Resistance index (RI) of the myometrial blood flow in the patients with leiomyoma is 0.54 ± 0.12. Very low resistance indices are usually present in cases with secondary degenerative or inflammatory changes within the leiomyoma. In such cases, it is essential to differentiate this benign condition from a uterine sarcoma that shows rapid increase in size and lower RI of the tumoral blood flow (RI = 0.37 ± 0.03) and RI of the uterine artery (RI = 0.62 ± 0.07, in comparison to the RI of the uterine artery in myomatous uterus that shows a RI of 0.74 ± 0.09),[17] or normal uterus (RI = 0.84 ± 0.09).[18] The difference in vascular signatures noted in this study may have a predictive value in the growth rate evaluation of these benign uterine masses.

Adnexal Torsion

Torsion of the ovary and the fallopian tube is a gynecological emergency that manifests itself with acute pelvic pain.[19] It mostly occurs in patients with adnexal lesions measuring 4–8 cm in diameter. Masses which measure smaller than this do not typically cause torsion, while larger masses are not mobile enough to cause torsion.[20] The recent literature has reported the occurrence of tubal torsion following tubal ligation and laparoscopic tubal cauterization.[21] Adnexal torsion is associated with massive edema and/or hemorrhage within the ovary. The Doppler features relate to the grade and chronicity of the torsion.[22-24] In the initial stage of the torsion, venous blood flow is reduced while arterial signals demonstrate high-impendence blood flow signals indicating that venous and lymphatic occlusion occur first. It is useful to bear in mind that ovarian flow, both venous and arterial may be present in the setting of an ovarian torsion. This is due either to partial torsion of the vascular pedicle or to the dual blood supply of the ovary (from the adnexal branch of the uterine artery and the ovarian artery). In extreme cases, reverse diastolic flow of the intraovarian arteries can be detected.[25] At a late stage when the occlusion is total and involves the arterial circulation, no adnexal blood flow is seen **(Figs. 4A to E)**. Expeditious and early diagnosis of adnexal torsion is highly dependent on the operator's experience. Color Doppler allows prompt and early diagnosis of adnexal torsion before irreversible ischemic changes occur, leading to necrosis and gangrene of the involved organs. This may contribute to conservative treatment by minimally invasive surgery and may prevent surgical removal of the affected structures.[26]

Endometriosis

Endometriosis is defined as a condition resulting from the ectopic location of the endometrial tissue outside the uterine cavity (peritoneal cavity, abdominal and pelvic organs and pelvic ligaments).[27] The precise etiology of this disease is still to be determined. Many theories, some of them more probable than the others have been proposed to explain the pathogenesis of endometriosis. The metastatic theory postulates the importance of the transportation of the viable endometrial cells regurgitated through the fallopian tubes at the time of menstruation. The metaplasia theory explains the origin of endometriosis by metaplastic

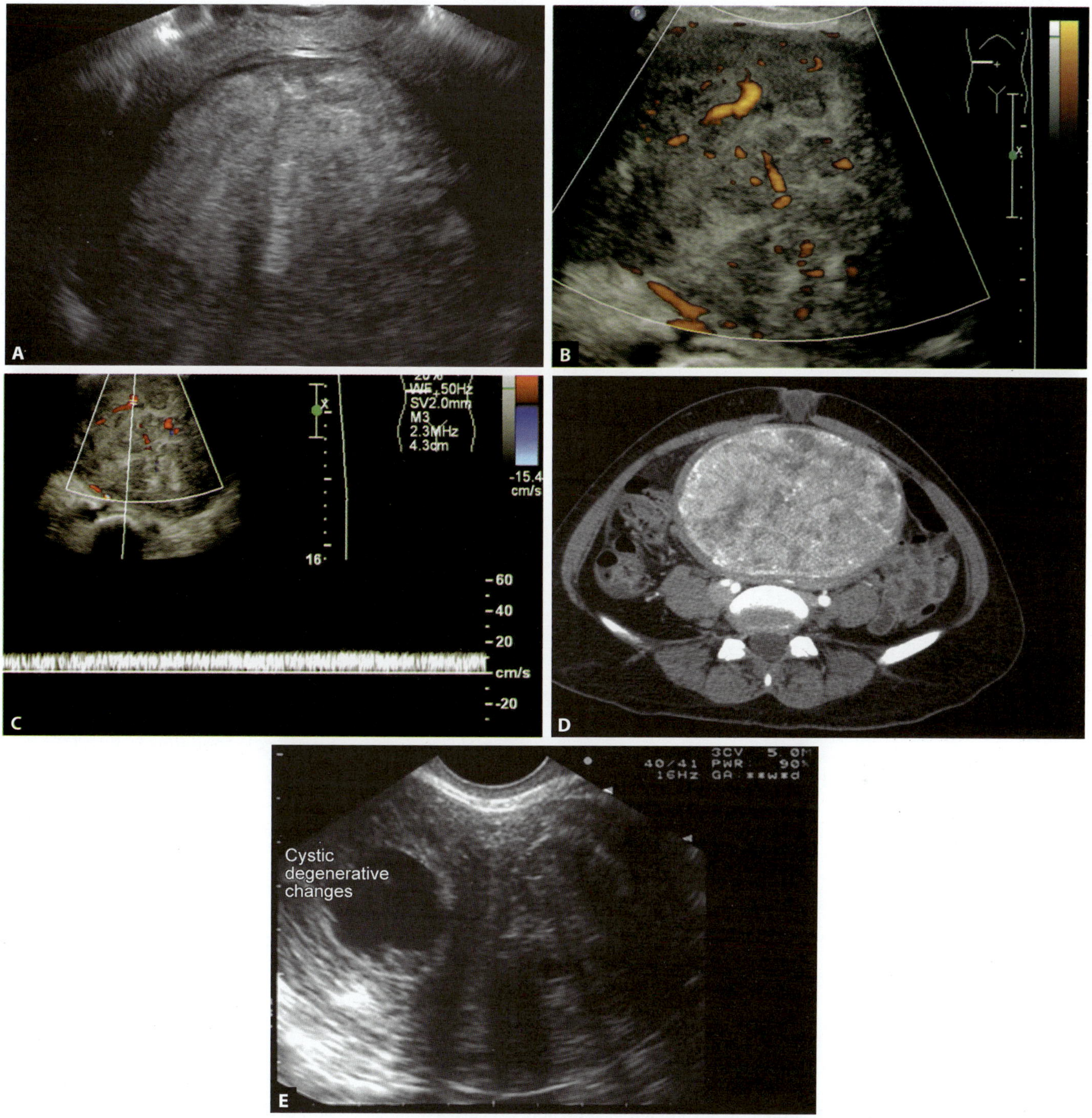

Figs. 3A to E: Transvaginal ultrasound demonstrating degenerating leiomyoma with complex appearance and cystic appearance (central necrosis). (A) Transvaginal sonogram of a degenerative fibroid; (B) Power Doppler ultrasound of the degenerative fibroid vasculature. Prominent color/power signals are visualized within the central portion of the fibroid; (C) Pulsed Doppler ultrasound of a patient with degenerative fibroid. Note venous type of the blood flow signals obtained from the central portion of a degenerative fibroid; (D) CT scan of the same degenerative fibroid; (E) Transvaginal ultrasound scan demonstrating a leiomyoma with central necrosis.

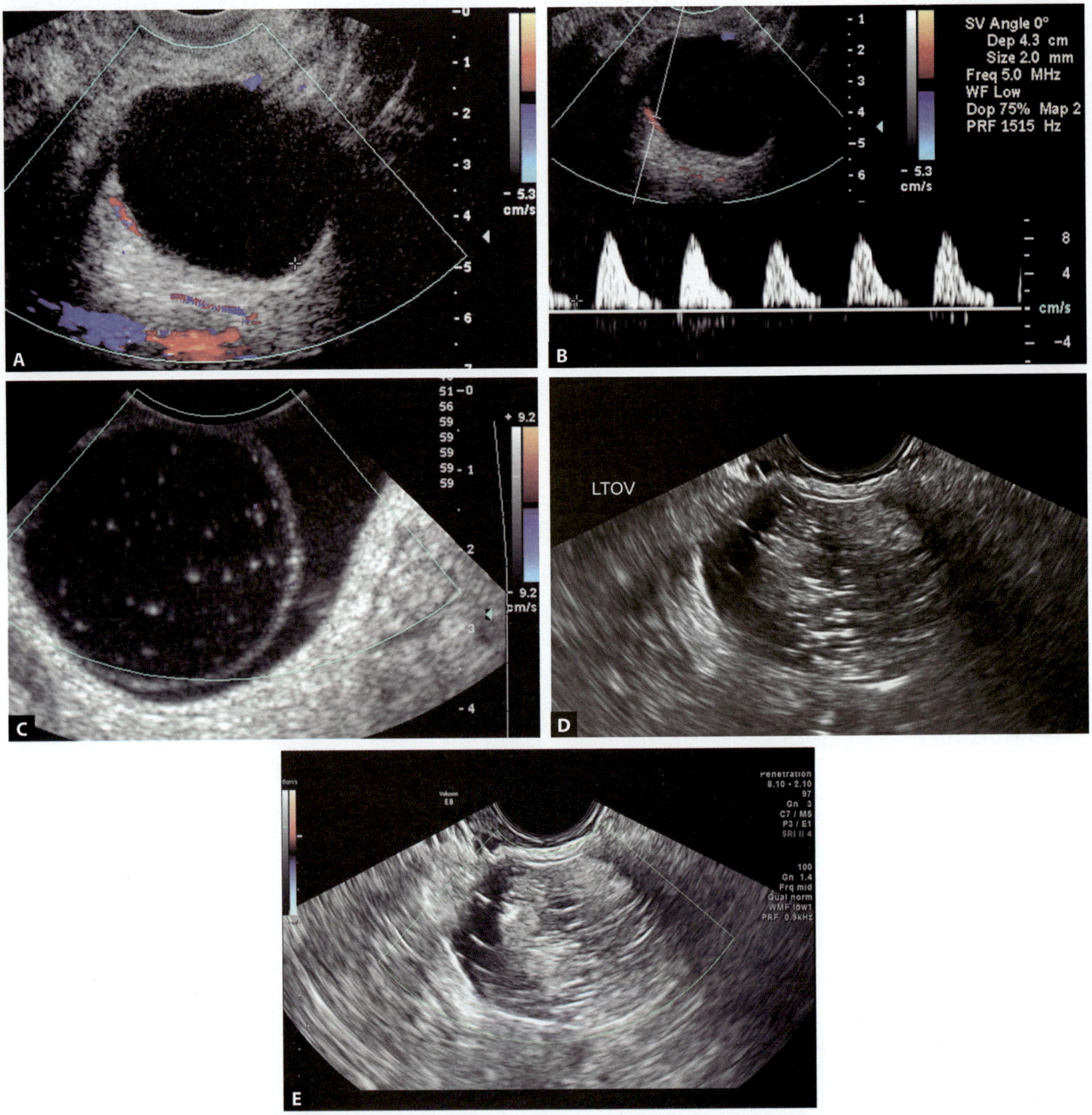

Figs. 4A to E: Transvaginal color Doppler images of adnexal torsion. (A) Partial adnexal torsion of a simple ovarian cyst in a patient presenting with pelvic pain. Discrete blood flow signals are detected at the periphery of the ovarian cyst; (B) The same patient as in previous figure. Pulsed Doppler waveform analysis demonstrates arterial type of blood flow signals with absence of diastolic flow. Sonographic and Doppler findings are suggestive of partial adnexal torsion. Venous type of blood flow signals were also obtained; (C) Color Doppler scan of a complete adnexal torsion. Note the absence of both the venous and arterial blood flow signals; (D) Transvaginal B mode ultrasound image of a complex left adnexal mass with multiple thin echogenic bands caused by hairs in the cyst cavity. This dot-dash pattern is typical for a dermoid cyst; (E) Color Doppler ultrasound of the same patient reveals no adnexal blood flow. This finding is suggestive of a late stage of adnexal torsion, involving both venous and arterial circulation.

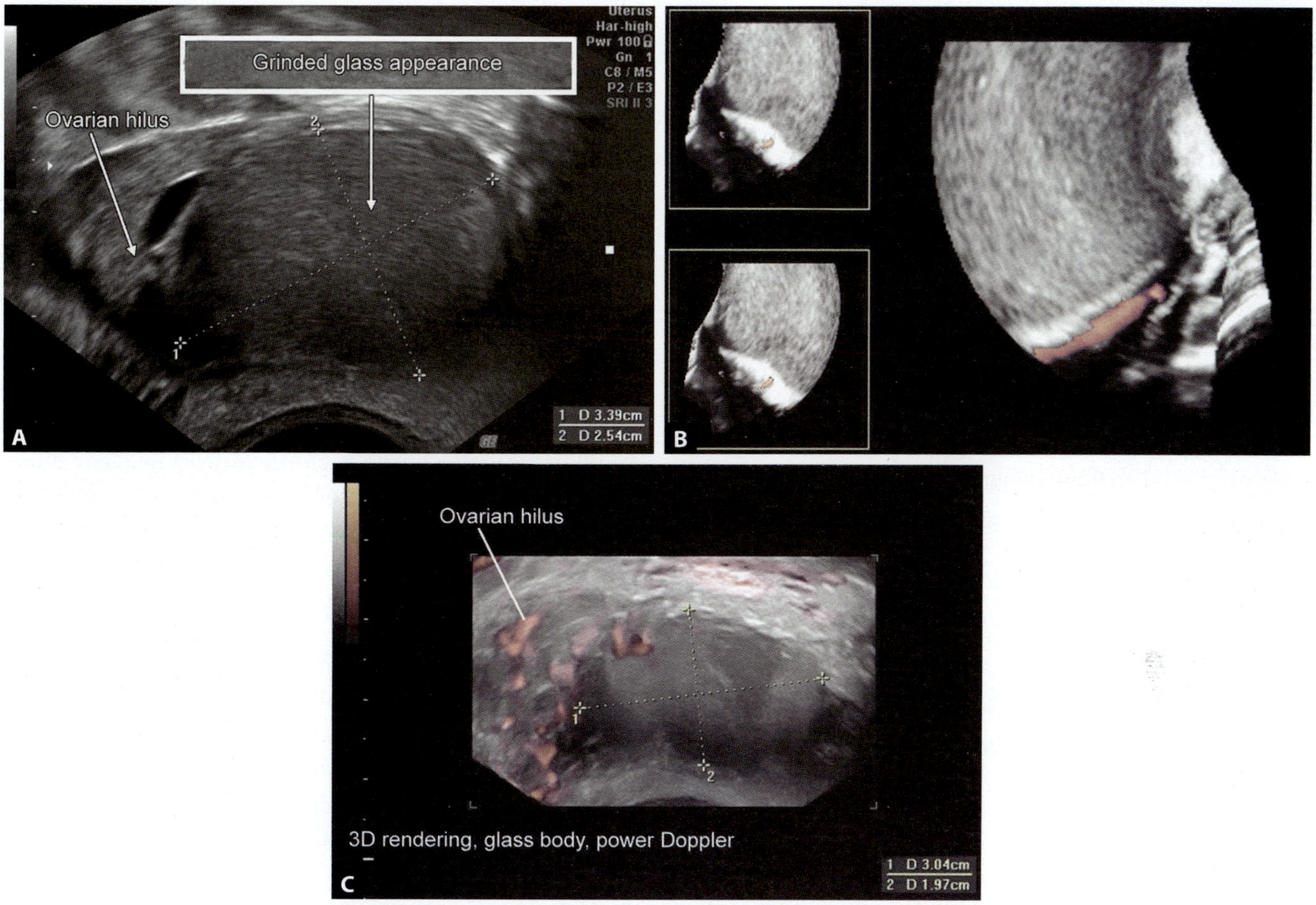

Figs. 5A to C: Two-dimensional, three-dimensional and color Doppler ultrasound images of ovarian endometrioma. Note the parenchymatous texture of the cystic content and single vessel arrangement at the periphery of the ovarian lesion. (A) Transvaginal ultrasound scan of ovarian endometrioma. Grinded glass appearance of cystic content is typical for ovarian endometrioma; (B) Color and/or power Doppler identifies peripheral vessels; (C) Another vascular pattern commonly seen in patients with ovarian endometrioma is vascularization within the ovarian hilus.

differentiation of the original celomic membrane with prolonged irritation and/or estrogen stimulation of the endometrium-like tissue. It is proposed that the adult cells undergo de-differentiation back to their primitive origin and then transform into endometrial cells. The third theory, which is the genetic theory, postulates that there may be a genetic component in the pathogenesis of endometriosis. This is because it has been shown that there is a statistically higher incidence of endometriosis in first-degree relatives of patients with this disorder.[28] The classic symptom of endometriosis is chronic pain associated with menstruation and or the immediate premenstrual phase, or persistent pain without the cyclicity.[29] Even though the classic symptom of endometriosis is chronic pain, in 21% of the cases it manifests itself with acute pelvic pain.[30] Other symptoms associated with this condition frequently noted are dysmenorrhea, dyspareunia, atypical bleeding, premenstrual spotting, menometrorrhagia, while rectal bleeding or hematuria although pathognomonic are rarely encountered. An endometrioma (so called "chocolate cyst") has a variety of ultrasonographic appearances ranging from an anechoic cyst, cyst containing diffuse low-level echoes with or without solid components, to a solid-appearing mass **(Figs. 5A to C)**. "Carpet-like" echoes or "grinded glass appearance" are found in 82% of endometriomas.[31] Sometimes it is difficult to differentiate an endometrioma from a hemorrhagic ovarian cyst, or corpus luteum cyst but the sonographer should always bear in mind the typical morphological features of endometrioma which are thick walls, homogenicity of the echogenic content, bilaterality and multiplicity of the lesions.[32] In order to facilitate recognition

TABLE 2: The combined scoring system for an ovarian endometrioma.[33]

Parameters	*Score*
Reproductive age	2
Chronic pain (premenstrual or menstrual)	1
Infertility	1
B-mode sonography	
• Position	2
• Multiplicity	1
• Serial sonography positive	2
• Thick walls	2
• Homogeneous echogenicity	2
• Clear demarcation from surrounding structures	1
Transvaginal color Doppler sonography	
• Vascularization	2
• Pericystic/hilar location	2
• Regularly separated vessels	2
• Existence of notching	1
Resistance index <0.40 (menstrual phase)	2
Resistance index 0.40–0.60 (late follicular/corpus luteum phase)	2
CA 125 range 35–65 IU/mL	2

of endometriosis, Kurjak and Kupesic[33] developed a new noninvasive scoring system using clinical symptoms, CA 125 level, sonographic findings and transvaginal color and pulsed Doppler parameters **(Table 2)**.

Pelvic Congestion Syndrome

Pelvic congestion syndrome is a condition characterized by formation of pelvic varicosities with concomitant vascular stasis and congestion. There are three possible mechanisms of pelvic congestion. Varicose veins are thought to result from the effects of gravity and defective valves. Worsening of pelvic pain in the erect position in women with pelvic pain syndrome and improvement of the pain upon lying down supports this concept. The second possibility is that an abnormal increase in blood flow through a region with many arteriovenous connections could lead to a state of chronic pelvic venous dilation. The third possibility is that pelvic varicosities may occur as a result of relaxation of the smooth muscle in the walls of the pelvic veins caused by some vasoactive substance as yet unidentified.[34] Pelvic congestion syndrome's clinical presentation is that of abdominal pain in the small pelvis. It is more common in the right iliac fossa, although some patients complain of left-sided pain with movement of the pain from one side to the other. Arterial type of congestion causes predominantly acute symptoms, while venous congestion presents mainly with chronic pain.[35] Changes in position or abdominal pressure alter the symptomatology.[36] This syndrome tends to be accompanied by a polysymptomatic picture in which backache and headache occur together with leukorrhea, dysmenorrhea and functional bleeding like changes in frequency, amount and duration of bleeding or intermenstrual bleeding (result of a minute hemorrhage from the excessively congested endometrium or endocervix which is not hormone conditioned). A leukorrhoic discharge is characterized by clear mucus due to hypersecretion uncomplicated by infection. Many methods have been employed to diagnose this condition such as contrast-enhanced computed tomography, nuclear magnetic resonance,[37] angiography,[38] ultrasound and color Doppler sonography.[39,40] However, laparoscopy remains an essential component when investigating pelvic pain.[41] The sonographic findings of pelvic congestion syndrome include multiple serpentine, anechoic structures within the pelvis.[39] Although real-time sonography depicts this feature, the findings of multiple cystic lesions in the pelvis suggest the occurrence of other entities as well, including hydrosalpinx, multilocular ovarian cysts, or fluid-filled loops of bowel. Transvaginal color Doppler was shown as the safest and most definitive diagnostic technique within the gynecologist's reach **(Figs. 6A to F)**. Its use has allowed a demonstration of the existence of vascular dilatation that affects not only the veins but also the arterial system.[35] The venous plexuses are more thick and in most of cases, observable with vaginal sonography **(Fig. 6E)**. This is not true for the arteries which are thinner and have a tendency to show their dilatation in intraparenchymatous locations usually visible only after switching to color Doppler **(Fig. 6F)**. Sometimes both systems are affected, with the vascular disturbance being more intense and more widespread because of the involvement of myometrial vessels as well. Therefore, cross-sections of the dilated intramyometrial vessels may be misinterpreted as a "Swiss cheese" appearance of the myometrium as in the case of adenomyosis **(Fig. 6D)**.

Ovarian Vein Thrombosis

This uncommon and potentially fatal disorder occurs most often in the postpartum period, but it has been reported after surgical intervention of the pelvis, trauma

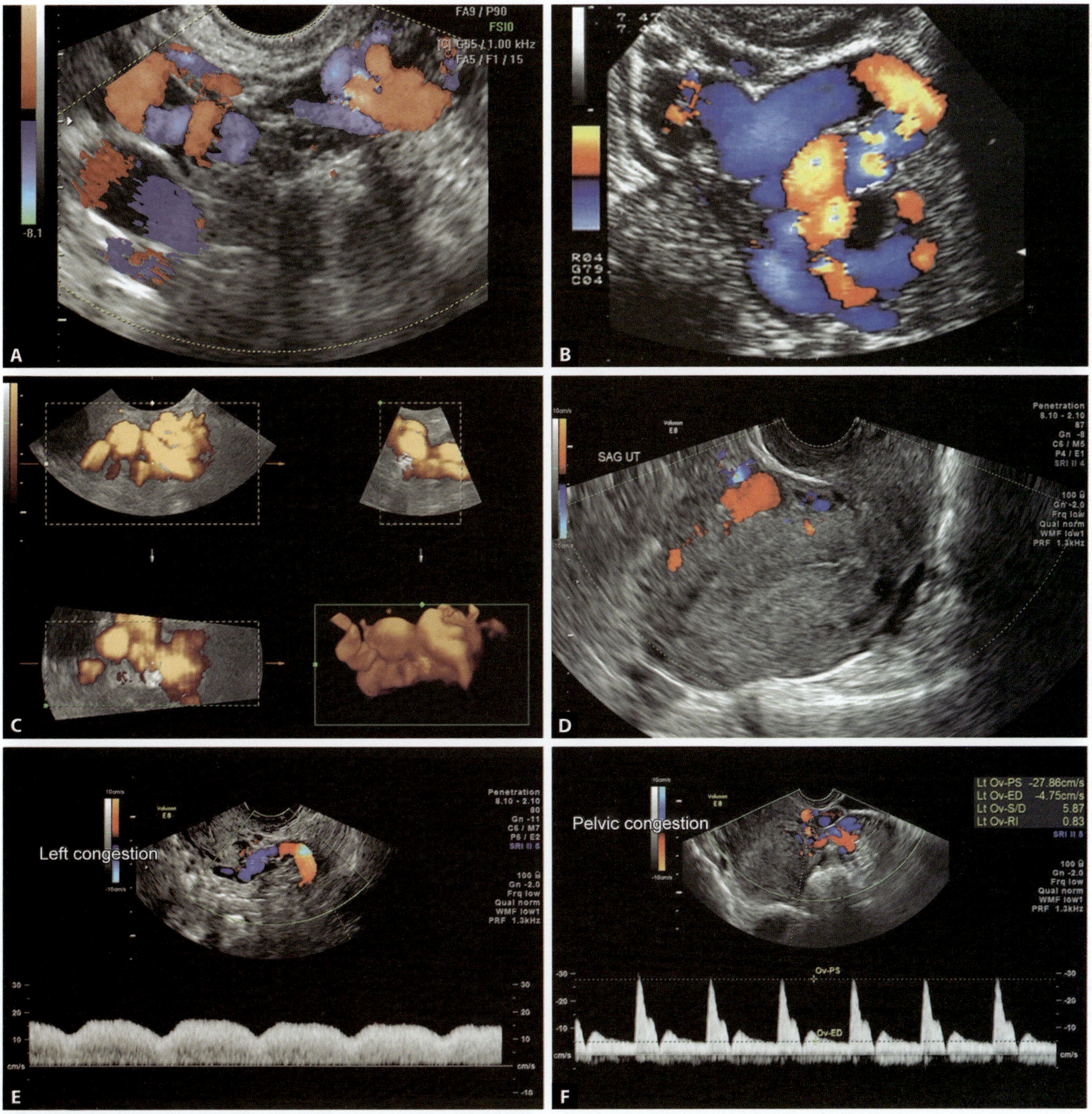

Figs. 6A to F: 2D and 3D color Doppler and power Doppler images of pelvic congestion syndrome. Bright color signals extracted from a bizarre adnexal mass represent pelvic congestion syndrome. (A) Color Doppler ultrasound of dilated periovarian and periuterine veins in a patient with pelvic congestion syndrome; (B) Tortuous and dilated pelvic venous plexuses may mimic complex adnexal mass; (C) Three-dimensional power Doppler ultrasound of pelvic varicosities in a patient with chronic pelvic pain; (D) Transvaginal color Doppler image of intraparenchymatous type of pelvic congestion. Cross-sections of the dilated intramyometrial vessels may be misinterpreted as a "Swiss cheese" appearance of the myometrium as in the case of adenomyosis; (E) Pulsed Doppler signals depicted from the venous plexuses; (F) Pulsed Doppler signals depicted from the arterial plexuses.

of the pelvis or PID.[42] Pelvic vein thrombosis may occur in nonpuerperal patients with hypercoagulable blood and has significant sequelae.[43] Ovarian vein thrombosis affects the right side in 80–90% of cases even though it has been described on the left side and bilaterally.[44-46] Right-sided predominance is explained by dextrotorsion of the gravid uterus compressing the right ovarian vein and causing retrograde flow in the left ovarian vein.[47,48] Most cases occur during the first week after delivery, however, rare antepartum and delayed postpartum cases have also been reported.[45] During a full-term pregnancy ovarian veins reach the three times their normal diameter. Immediate collapse of the dilated veins observed after delivery results in low-pressure state and combined with hypercoagulability increases the risk of ovarian vein thrombosis.[49] Infection and stasis associated with the hypercoagulable state in pregnancy have been cited as additional etiologic factors,[44,49] as well as coexisting endometritis.[50] Whether thrombosis follows or precedes infection is unknown.

Acute Pelvic Pain with a Positive Pregnancy Test

Normal Intrauterine Pregnancy

Normal intrauterine pregnancy is probably the most common cause of pelvic pain in the first trimester. Crampy pelvic pain is due to hormonal changes, rapid growth of the uterus and increased blood flow. Besides clinical and laboratory signs (β-hCG), the transvaginal ultrasound examination may give additional information on the presence, location and development of the pregnancy.

Spontaneous Abortion

Threatened and spontaneous abortion are the most common complications of early pregnancy. Thirty to forty percent of pregnancies fail after implantation, and only 10–15% manifest with clinical symptoms.[51-53] Patients with a spontaneous abortion usually present to a clinic/healthcare facility with symptoms of vaginal bleeding and abdominal pain, with or without the expulsion of the products of conception 8–10 weeks from their last menstrual period.[54] The decreased diameter of the gestational sac and/or its irregular shape, and early intrauterine growth retardation registered on the basis of decreased crown-rump length (CRL) values are indicative for making the diagnosis of early pregnancy failure. Absences of clear visualization of the embryonic parts as well as absent embryonic heart activity are clear signs of a nonviable gestation. There are two specific manifestations of early pregnancy failure, which is important to describe, an anembryonic pregnancy (blighted ovum) and a missed abortion. An anembryonic pregnancy is defined as a gestational sac in which an embryo either failed to develop or died at the stage too early to be visualized. The diagnosis of an anembryonic pregnancy is based on the absence of embryonic echoes within the gestational sac large enough for the embryonic structures to be visible, independent of the clinical data or the menstrual cycle.[55] In these patients, the gestational sac represents only an empty chorionic cavity. The studies conducted regarding the intervillous circulation demonstrated a lower PI value of the artery-like signals in patients with blighted ovum when compared to those with normal pregnancies (0.80 ± 0.04), and missed abortion (0.75 ± 0.04).[56,57] A lower PI value from the intervillous space of the anembryonic pregnancy group may reflect changes in the placental stroma, where the individual villi are prone to edema. The diagnosis of missed abortion is characterized by the identification of the fetus, which does not demonstrate any heart activity[58] **(Fig. 7)**. It is also described as a type of spontaneous abortion when after fetal demise, spontaneous expulsion of the conceptus outside the uterus does not occur.[59] Ultrasound findings can differentiate changes that occur in the gestational sac as time passes from the incident that caused the fetal demise and circulation break. The gestational sac image differs from a normal shape

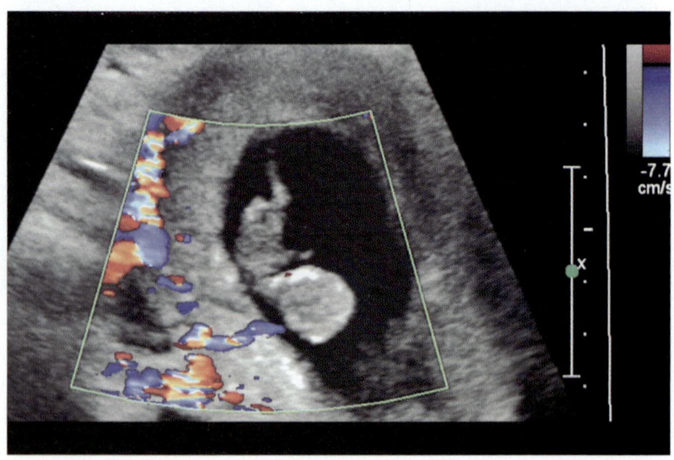

Fig. 7: Transvaginal power Doppler scan of a missed abortion at 8 weeks of gestation. The flow pattern reveals blood flow within the maternal vessels and absence of the flow in fetal vessels. Ultrasound findings should always be correlated with the patient's symptoms, gestational age, and beta (β)-hCG values.

(a recent fetal demise) to a collapsed and altered shape and size (in later stages of fetal demise). The basic ultrasound finding is an embryo without heart activity and dynamics. If the event occurred recently the morphology might be preserved, but with time the embryo morphology is altered (completely amorphous or fragmented) and the size gets smaller. Another characteristic ultrasound finding of this condition is changes of trophoblast tissue. Such changes include an inhomogeneous, degenerative (hydropic or calcified) trophoblast tissue, with the presence of intrauterine hematomas and separation of membranes.

It is relatively easy to make this diagnosis by means of the transvaginal color Doppler facilities. The main parameter is the absence of the heart activity and the lack of color flow signals at expected position of the embryonic/fetal heart after the 6th gestational week.[60] However, one should be aware that the length of the time elapsing between arrest of embryonic development and clinical presentation determines the sonographic image, and therefore, is open for interpretation.

Ectopic Pregnancy

An ectopic pregnancy occurs when the fertilized ovum implants itself in places other than the uterine cavity. Although an ectopic pregnancy is most often localized in the fallopian tube (95%), a zygote implantation may also occur in abdominal, ovarian, intraligamentous, cornual, intramural or cervical sites.[60-64] An ectopic pregnancy is called "the great masquerader" since its clinical presentation can vary from light vaginal spotting to vasomotor shock and hemoperitoneum. The classic triad of delayed menses, irregular vaginal bleeding and abdominal pain is often not encountered. Patients presenting with acute symptoms (frequently in emergency departments) are usually at a more advanced gestational age compared to the asymptomatic infertility patients who are closely followed because of their increased risk for an ectopic pregnancy. Physical examination reveals abdominal tenderness or peritoneal irritation in the presence (or sometimes the absence) of a palpable adnexal mass. The astute clinicians should consider all presenting signs and symptoms as a possible ectopic pregnancy case until an intrauterine pregnancy or an ectopic pregnancy is diagnosed.[62]

The absolute values of the β-hCG levels in circulation are much lower than the levels of the same hormone present in a normal intrauterine pregnancy of the same gestational age. The dynamics of the titer show a slower increase of circulating concentrations which prolongs the doubling time values.

The most important use of the quantitative β-hCG determination in conjunction with ultrasonography is in understanding the value of the β-hCG "discriminatory zone". The discriminatory zone represents that level of β-hCG above which all normal intrauterine chorionic sacs will be detected by ultrasound. Now, there is almost a universal consensus as to the discriminatory zone level to be between 1,000 and 1,500 mIU/mL with the use of transvaginal probe of at least 5 MHz.[65-68] Ultrasonography, more precisely, transvaginal sonography has become the "gold standard" modality for the effective and fast diagnosis of an ectopic pregnancy.

The ultrasonographic criteria for an ectopic pregnancy can be divided into uterine and extrauterine signs (keeping in mind that all of them can be suggestive or diagnostic).[69]

The most common sign of ectopic pregnancy is the empty uterus, with or without increased endometrial thickness. A central hypoechoic area or a sac-like structure inside the uterine cavity is the so-called pseudogestational sac. In some cases, a concurrent intrauterine pregnancy can be found together with an ectopic pregnancy, but this is extremely rare. It usually occurs in patients undergoing some form of an assisted reproduction technique.

Adnexal sonographic findings in women with an ectopic pregnancy are variable. A gestational sac in the adnexal region with a clear embryonic echo and heart activity directly proves an ectopic pregnancy. This is only seen in 15–28% of the cases **(Figs. 8A to C)**. A gestational sac with or without an embryonic echo can be detected in the adnexal region in 46–71% of reported cases, if the tube is unruptured. The tubal ring is generally 1–3 cm in diameter, consisting of a concentric ring of echogenic tissue measuring 2–4 mm surrounding the hypoechoic center. Very often an unspecific adnexal tumor can be visualized. In 40–83% of ectopic pregnancy cases, free fluid is detected in the retrouterine space. The color Doppler is an excellent and rapid guide for identification of the peritrophoblastic tissue in patients with an ectopic pregnancy. The color flow pattern usually presents as randomly dispersed multiple small vessels showing high velocity and low resistance signals. The sensitivity of transvaginal color and pulsed Doppler ranges from 73 to 96% and the specificity ranges from 87 to 100%. Demonstration of a "hot flow pattern" shortens the diagnostic procedure and enables an earlier clinical decision to be reached for the treatment

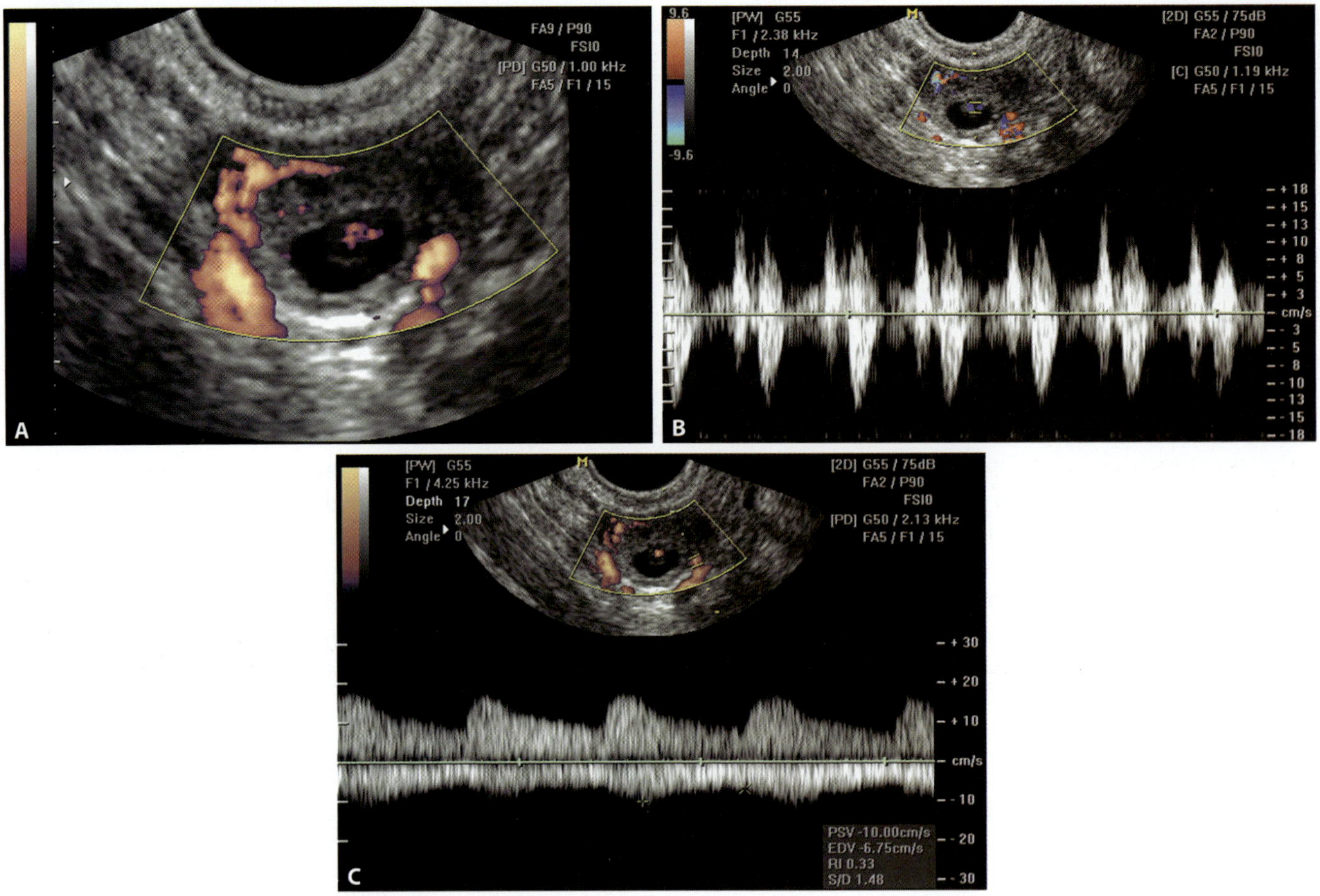

Figs. 8A to C: Transvaginal color, power and pulsed Doppler images of ectopic pregnancy. (A) Prominent blood flow signals derived from ectopic gestational sac indicate invasive trophoblast; (B) The same patient as in Figure A. Pulsed Doppler waveform analysis obtained from the living embryo demonstrates rhythmic heart activity; (C) The same patient as in **Figures A and B**. Pulsed Doppler waveform analysis demonstrates low resistance index (RI = 0.33).

of an ectopic pregnancy. Ultrasound may aid in triage of the patient who may benefit from medical treatment and detection of those who need immediate surgery **(Figs. 9A and B)**.

Corpus Luteum Cysts

Pelvic pain during pregnancy is usually attributed to the adnexal masses and the most common cause considered is a corpus luteum cyst. Pain is typically lateralized and may be either due to the size of the cyst, hemorrhage within the cyst or torsion. The corpus luteum cyst typically presents as a small, rounded, complex cystic structure. It may feature a thick, hyperechoic wall and sponge-like avascular contents, which represent hemorrhage and/or a retracting clot. Doppler imaging frequently reveals a characteristic "ring of fire" pattern with peripheral low-impedance blood flow, reflecting its role in hormone production. Corpus luteum cysts usually resolve by the second trimester.

Leiomyoma

Because leiomyomas are hormonally responsive, they usually grow and change their echotexture during early pregnancy.[70] Their rapid growth with degeneration can lead to pelvic pain localized to the site of the leiomyoma. Leiomyomas have a variable sonographic appearance ranging from hypoechoic to hyperechoic and complex, depending on their composition and the degree of degeneration. The size of leiomyoma increases with the gestational age, mainly due to pregnancy hormones. Leiomyomas also cause some blood flow changes in the uteroplacental circulation during pregnancy. Our study[71] showed an increase of the flow velocity in radial arteries supplying the uterine leiomyoma (P <0.01) from the 10th

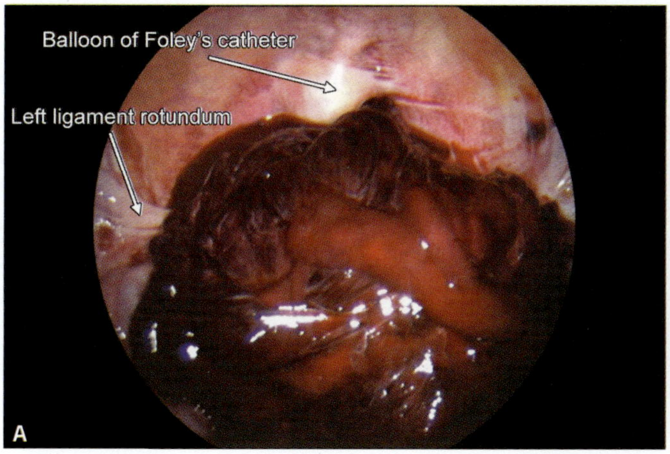

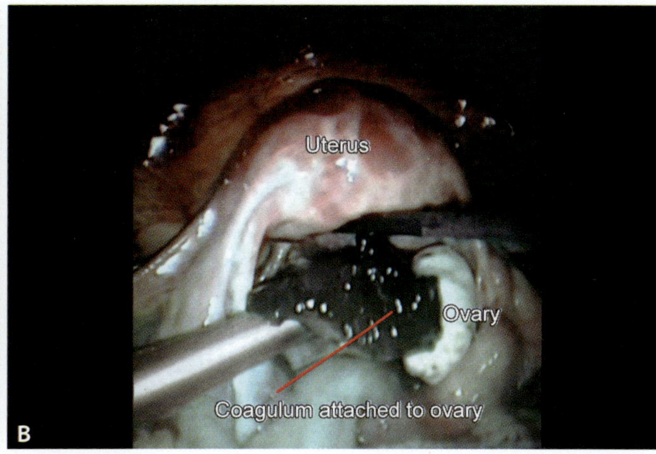

Figs. 9A and B: Laparoscopy images of ectopic pregnancy. (A) Laparoscopy image of a large ectopic pregnancy complicated by bleeding; (B) Coagulum containing ectopic gestational sac in the left adnexal region.

to 13th gestational week. This finding is most likely a consequence of higher levels of the estriol hormone that is metabolized in placenta. All these changes, however, do not influence the blood flow in spiral and uterine arteries.[71]

Uterine Dehiscence and Rupture

Uterine dehiscence and rupture are uncommon obstetric complications with potentially devastating outcome for both the mother and the baby. The term rupture describes a complete separation of the uterine wall (endometrium, myometrium and serosa),[72] while dehiscence represents separation that involves only a portion of the uterine scar.[73] Patients at high risk for uterine dehiscence and rupture have a history of prior surgical intervention on the uterine wall leading to a thinning of the myometrium. In a uterine dehiscence, the scar most likely stretches to the point of translucency, but does not rip. This condition does not necessarily cause a problem. A uterine rupture represents a splitting of the uterus, exposing the fetus to the hostile environment of the intrabdominal cavity and consequently to oxygen deprivation. Oxygen deprivation greater than 7 minutes results in irreversible brain damage, with outcomes ranging from learning disabilities, cerebral palsy, permanent vegetative state, to death. On the maternal side, a uterine rupture can cause internal hemorrhage, which, if not rapidly diagnosed, leads to death in minutes.

Many obstetric and nonobstetric conditions may mimic the symptoms and signs of uterine rupture or dehiscence, especially during the third trimester of pregnancy. Sonography may be useful in the diagnosis of these cases.[74] Diagnosis of this life threatening condition is based upon extrusion of the uterine contents into the abdominopelvic cavity.

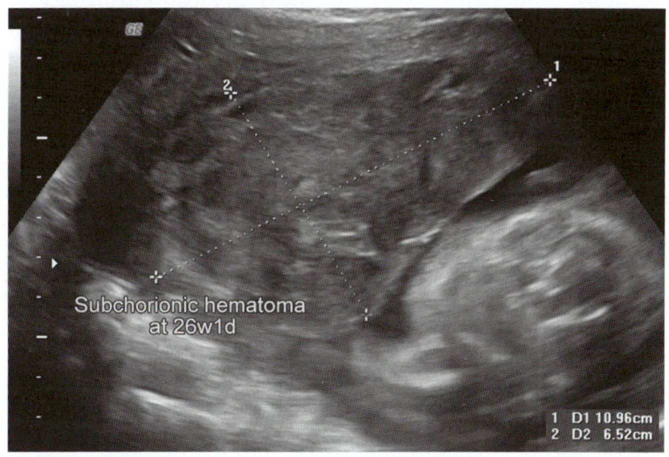

Fig. 10: Ultrasound image of subchorionic hematoma in a patient presenting with vaginal bleeding, abrupt pain and hypovolemic shock. Note subchorionic hematoma measuring 10.9 × 6.5 cm at 26 weeks of gestation. Finding indicates placental abruption.

Placental Abruption

Placental abruption is a condition caused by the acute separation of the placenta accompanied by vaginal bleeding, pain, uterine tenderness and hypovolemic shock. Placental abruption should always be considered if the retroplacental hypoechoic complex mass (composed of uteroplacental vessels-predominantly veins) measurement exceeds 1 to 2 cm in thickness **(Fig. 10)**. Uterine contraction may create focal thickening of this area.

Differentiation from placental abruption may be made on the basis of a transient nature of the contraction and by switching on the color Doppler. Uterine leiomyomas can also be mistaken for the retroplacental hemorrhage, but are generally more rounded in shape and demonstrate greater vascularity on color Doppler.

Patient with conditions such as maternal hypertension, preeclampsia, abdominal trauma, cocaine abuse, cigarette smoking, advanced maternal age, multiparity, twin pregnancy, diabetes, previous history of placental abruption and male fetuses (intriguing but unexplained phenomenon) are at increased risk of this complication.[75,76] The ultrasound presentation of a placental hemorrhage depends on the gestational age, location, and patient's hematocrit. We can differentiate three types of abruption considering the location of the separation: (1) retroplacental hematoma; (2) subchorionic (marginal) hematoma, and (3) subamnionic hemorrhage. A retroplacental hematoma is caused by hemorrhage from the spiral arteries and leads to separation of the basal lamina from uterine/ retroplacental hematoma and is caused by hypertension or overdose of anticoagulants. A subchorionic hematoma is caused by hemorrhage from marginal veins and leads to a separation of the chorionic membrane from the decidua at the edge of the placenta, while a subamnionic hemorrhage is caused by hemorrhage from the fetal blood vessels at the fetal surface of the placenta. It is useful to perform a nonstress test to check the baby's heart rate and look for signs of fetal distress. Placental abruption may have various effects on the baby such as increased risk of stillbirth, premature delivery and low birth weight among infants born to mothers who experience separation of the placenta before delivery.[77] If a large amount of the placenta separates from the uterus, the baby will probably be in distress until delivery. The baby may be premature and need to be placed in the newborn intensive care unit. If the fetus is in distress in the uterus, the newborn baby may have a low blood pressure or a low blood count. If the separation is severe enough, the baby could suffer brain damage or die before or shortly after birth.[78]

CONCLUSION

Acute pelvic pain as a clinical presentation can be a consequence of various pathological conditions. A prudent approach is to select the best imaging modalities which can depict a particular subset of clinical conditions to help narrow the differential diagnosis. The advantages of ultrasound are its low cost, portability, nonionizing radiation, accessibility and widespread use, while the main disadvantage is the subjectivity and limited number of trained radiologist, gynecologist and sonographers.[79,80] The perceptive clinician must consider all possible causes of acute pelvic pain in order to submit the patients to the proper diagnostic and therapeutic procedures.[81] The combined use of the clinical examination and the ultrasound as an adjunct to the physical examination along with laboratory tests increases the sensitivity and specificity in arriving at the correct diagnosis in patients presenting with gynecologic and/or obstetric causes of acute pelvic pain.[80,82] The primary goal of imaging in obstetric and gynecological (OB/GYN) practice is to distinguish between adnexal causes of adnexal pain that may be managed conservatively or medically and those requiring emergency/urgent surgical or percutaneous intervention.[83]

The 3D inversion technique is a simple way to render fluid-filled spaces, such as hydrosalpinges and view them separate from the ovarian cystic structures.[84] Conventional ultrasound supplemented with 3D ultrasound and 3D power Doppler ultrasound facilitates the preoperative classification of complex benign ovarian lesions associated with acute pelvic pain.[85] Three-dimensional ultrasound with Virtual Organ Computer Aided AnaLysis (VOCAL) is a valid technique for measuring trophoblast volume in patients presenting with vaginal bleeding and pain during the early first trimester of pregnancy. Initial study reported that pregnancies ending in miscarriage had smaller trophoblast volumes and reduced trophoblast growth compared with those that resulted in live birth.[86] Another parameter that may be helpful in predicting the outcome of pregnancy is the measurement of the difference between the gestational sac volume and amniotic sac volume.[87] Maximum thickness of the uterine junctional zone assessed by three-dimensional ultrasound was significantly thickened in patients with recurrent miscarriage compared to normal fertile controls.[88]

Ultrasound technology has advanced very quickly and many obstetricians and gynecologists have not achieved comfort with novel methods of ultrasound imaging such as 3D and 3D power Doppler imaging.[89] In order to implement the innovations which 2D and 3D is offering in the assessment of pregnant and nonpregnant patients presenting with pelvic pain, and by eliminating the need for more costly and complex cross-sectional imaging techniques systematic dissemination of knowledge is required.

REFERENCES

1. Baines PA, Allen GM. Pelvic pain and menstrual related illnesses. Emerg Med Clin North Am. 2001;19:763-80.
2. Hewitt GD, Brown RT. Acute and chronic pelvic pain in female adolescents. Med Clin North Am. 2000;84:1009-25.
3. Bau A, Atri M. Acute female pelvic pain: ultrasound evaluation. Semin Ultrasound CT MR. 2000;21:78-93.
4. Bennett GL, Slywotzky CM, Giovanniello G. Gynecologic causes of acute pelvic pain. Radiographics. 2002;22:785-801.
5. Kupesic S, Kurjak A, Zodan T. Color Doppler ultrasound in the diagnosis of pelvic inflammatory disease. In: Kurjak A (Ed). An Atlas of Transvaginal Color Doppler. The London-New York: Parthenon Publishing Group. 2000. pp. 127-35.
6. Westroem L, Wolner Hanssen P. Pathogenesis of pelvic inflammatory disease. Genitourin Med. 1993;69:9-17.
7. Expert Committee on Pelvic Inflammatory Disease. Research directions for the 1990s. Sex Trans Dis. 1991; 18:46-64.
8. Gales W, Wasserheit JN. Genital chlamydial infections: epidemiology and reproduction sequelae. Am J Obstet Gynecol. 1991;164:1771-81.
9. Toth M, Chervenak FA. Infection as the cause of infertility. In: Kupesic S, De Ziegler D (Eds). Ultrasound and Infertility. Carnforth, UK: Parthenon Publishing; 2002. pp. 205-14.
10. Patten RM, Vincent LM, Wolner-Hanssen P. Pelvic inflammatory disease: endovaginal sonography with laparoscopic correlation. J Ultrasound Med. 1990;9:861-5.
11. Reynolds T, Hill MC, Glassman LM. Sonography of hemorrhagic ovarian cyst. J Clin Ultrasound. 1986;14:449-53.
12. Baltrarowich OH, Kurtz AB, Pasto ME. The spectrum of sonographic findings in hemorrhagic ovarian cyst. Am J Roentgenol. 1987;148:901-5.
13. Bass IS, Haller JO, Freidman AP. The sonographic appearance of the hemorrhagic ovarian cyst in adolescents. J Ultrasound Med. 1984;3:509-14.
14. Kupesic S, Kurjak A. Color Dopler assessment of uterine leiomyoma and sarcoma. In: Kurjak A (Ed). An Atlas of Transvaginal Color Doppler. London-New York: The Parthenon Publishing Group; 2000. pp. 179-86.
15. Siskin GP, Bonn J, Worthington-Kirsch RL. III. Uterine fibroid embolization: pain management. Tech Vasc Interv Radiol. 2002;5:35-43.
16. Richengerg J, Cooperberg P. Ultrasound of the Uterus. In: Callen P (Ed). Ultrasound in obstetrics and gynecology. Philadelphia: WB Saunders Company; 2000. pp. 814-46.
17. Kurjak A, Kupesic S, Shalan H, Jukic S, Kosuta D, Ilijas M. Uterine sarcoma: a case report of 10 cases studied by transvaginal color and pulsed Doppler sonography. Gynecol Oncol. 1995;59:342-6.
18. Kurjak A, Kupesic-Urek S, Miric D. The assessment of benign uterine tumor vascularization by transvaginal color Doppler. Ultrasound Med Biol. 1992;18:645-8.
19. Kupesic S. Kurjak A. Color Doppler assessment of patients with pelvic pain. In: Kurjak A (Ed). An Atlas of Transvaginal Color Doppler. London-New York: The Parthenon Publishing Group; 2000. pp. 241-4.
20. Worthington-Kirsch RL, Raftopoulos V, Cohen IT. Sequential bilateral torsion of normal ovaries in a child. J Ultrasound Med. 1986;5:663-4.
21. Sozen I, Kadako R, Fleischman S, Arici A. Diagnosis and laparoscopic management of a fallopian tube torsion following Irving tubal sterilization: a case report. Surg Endosc. 2002;16:217-21.
22. Fleischer A, Stein S, Cullinan J, Warner M. Color Doppler sonography of adnexal torsion. J Ultrasound Med. 1995;14:523-8.
23. Rosado WM, Trambert MA, Gosnik BB, Pretorius DH. Adnexal torsion: diagnosis by using Doppler sonography. Am J Roentgenol. 1992;159:1251-3.
24. Van Voorhis BJ, Schwaiger J, Syrop CH, Chapler FK. Early diagnosis of ovarian torsion by color Doppler ultrasonography. Fertil Steril. 1992;58:215-7.
25. Lineberry TD, Rodriguez H. Isolated torsion of the fallopian tube in an adolescent: a case report. J Pediatr Adolesc Gynecol. 2000;13:135-7.
26. Kupesic S, Plavsic BM. Adnexal torsion: color Doppler and three-dimensional ultrasound. Abdominal Imaging. 2010;35:602-6. DOI 10.1007s00261-009-9573-0.
27. Kurjak A, Kupesic S. Benign ovarian lesions assessed by color and pulsed Doppler. In: Kurjak A (Ed). An Atlas of Transvaginal Color Doppler. London-New York: The Parthenon Publishing Group; 2000. pp. 191-202.
28. Simpton JL, Elias S, Malinak LR, Buttram VC Jr. Heritable aspects of endometriosis I: genetic studies. Am J Obstet Gynecol. 1980;137:327-31.
29. Barlow D, Kennedy H. Endometriosis: clinical presentation and diagnosis. In: Shaw RW (Ed). Endometriosis. Carnforth, UK: Parthenon Publishing; 1989. pp. 1-10.
30. Bai SW, Cho HJ, Kim JY, Jeong KA, Kim SK, Cho DJ, et al. Endometriosis in an adolescent population: the severance hospital in Korean experience. Yonsei Med J. 2002;43:48-52.
31. Kupfer MC, Schwimer RS, Lebovic J. Transvaginal sonographic appearance of endometriomata: spectrum of findings. J Ultrasound Med. 1992;11:129-32.
32. Atri M, Nazarnia S, Bret P. Endovaginal sonographic appearance of benign ovarian masses. Radiographics. 1996;14:747-9.
33. Kurjak A, Kupesic S. Scoring system for prediction of ovarian endometriosis based on transvaginal color and pulsed Doppler sonography. Fertil Steril. 1994;62:81-8.
34. Beard RW, Highman JH, Pearce S, Reginald PW. Diagnosis of pelvic varicosities in women with chronic pelvic pain. Lancet. 1985;2:956-9.
35. Kurjak A, Kupesic S. Congestion syndrome of the uterus. In: Osmers R, Kurjak A (Eds). Ultrasound and the Uterus. Carnforth, UK: Parthenon Publishing; 1995. pp. 115-8.

36. Bonilla-Musoles F, Ballesteros MJ. Transvaginal color Doppler in the diagnosis of pelvic congestion syndrome. In: Kurjak A (Ed). An Atlas of Transvaginal Color Doppler. Carnforth, UK: Parthenon Publishing; 1994. pp. 207-15.
37. Fakhri A, Fisherman EK, Mitchel SE, Siegelman SS, White RI. The role of CT in the management of pelvic arteriovenous malformations. Cardiovasc Intervent Radiol. 1987;10: 96-9.
38. Bottomley JP, Whitehouse GH. Congenital arteriovenous malformations of the uterus demonstrated by angiography. Acta Radiol. 1975;16:43-8.
39. Diwan RV, Brennan JN, Selim MA. Sonographic diagnosis of arteriovenous malformations of the uterus and pelvis. J Clin Ultrasound. 1983;11:295-8.
40. Juhasz B, Kurjak A, Lampe LG. Pelvic varices simulating bilateral adnexal masses: differential diagnosis by vaginal color Doppler. J Clin Ultrasound. 1992;20:81-4.
41. Promecene PA. Laparoscopy in gynecologic emergencies. Semin Laparosc Surg. 2002;9:64-75.
42. Kurman RJ (Ed). Blaustein's Pathology of the Female Genital Tract, 4th edition. New York: Springer-Verlag; 1994. pp. 532-5.
43. Visaria SD, Davis JD. Pelvic vein thrombosis as a cause of acute pelvic pain. Obstet Gynecol. 2002;99:897-9.
44. Munisck RA, Gillanders LA: A review of the syndrome of puerperal ovarian vein thrombophlebitis. Obstet Gynecol Surv. 1981;36:57-61.
45. Simons GR, Piwnica Worms DR, Goldhaber SZ. Ovarian vein thrombosis. Am Heart J. 1993;136:641-3.
46. Khurana BK, Rao J, Friedman SA. Computed tomographic features of puerperal ovarian vein thrombosis. Am J Obstet Gynecol. 1998;159:905-7.
47. Cranston PE, Hamrick-Turner J, Morano JU. Pseudothrombosis of the right ovarian vein: Pitfall of abdominal spiral CT. Clin Imaging. 1995;19:176-9.
48. Dure-Smith P. Ovarian syndrome: Is it a myth? Urology. 1995;13:355-8.
49. Toland KC, Pelamder WM, Mohr SJ. Postpartum ovarian vein thrombosis presenting as urethral obstruction: a case report and review of literature. J Urol. 1993;149:1538-42.
50. Savader SJ, Otero RR, Savader BL. Puerperal ovarian vein thrombosis: Evaluation with CT, US and MR imaging. Radiology. 1988;167:637-9.
51. Hakim RB, Gray RH, Zacur H. Infertility and early pregnancy loss. Am J Obstet Gynecol. 1995;172:1510-7.
52. Wilcox AJ, Weinbert C, O'Connor JF. Incidence of early loss in pregnancy. N Engl J Med. 1988;319:159-64.
53. Alberman E. The epidemiology of repeated abortion. In: Beard RW, Bishop F (Eds). Early pregnancy loss: mechanism and treatment. New York: Springer-Verlag; 1988. pp. 9-17.
54. Cetin A, Cetin M. Diagnostic and therapeutical decision-making with transvaginal sonography for first trimester spontaneous abortion, clinically thought to be complete or incomplete. Contraception. 1998;57:393-7.
55. Kurjak A, Kupesic S. Blood flow studies in normal and abnormal pregnancy. In: Kurjak A, Kupesic S (Eds). An Atlas of Transvaginal Color Doppler. London-New York: Parthenon Publishing Group; 2000. pp. 41-51.
56. Kurjak A, Kupesic S. Doppler assessment of intervillous blood flow in normal and abnormal early pregnancy. Obstet Gynecol. 1997;89:252-6.
57. Kurjak A, Kupesic S. Parallel Doppler assessment of yolk sac and intervillous circulation in normal pregnancy and missed abortion. Placenta. 1998;19:619-23.
58. Jaffe R, Warsof SL. Color Doppler imaging in the assessment of uteroplacental blood flow in abnormal first trimester intrauterine pregnancies: and attempt to define etiologic mechanism. J Ultrasound Med. 1992;11:41-4.
59. Kos M, Kupesic S, Latin V. Diagnostics of spontaneous abortion. In: Kurjak A (Ed). Ultrasound in Gynecology and Obstetrics. Zagreb: Art Studio Azinovic; 2000. pp. 314-21.
60. Szulman AE. The natural history of early human spontaneous abortion. In: Barnea ER, Check JH, Grudzinkas JG, Marvo T (Eds). Implantation and early pregnancy in humans. Carnforth, UK: Parthenon Publishing; 1993. pp. 309-21.
61. Ectopic pregnancy. In: Speroff L, Glass RH, Kase NG (Eds). Clinical Gynecologic Endocrinology and Infertility. London: Williams and Wilkins. 1999:1149-67.
62. Timor-Tristch IE, Monteagudo A. Ectopic pregnancy. In: Kupesic S, de Ziegler D (Eds). Ultrasound and infertility. London-New York: Parthenon Publishing Group; 2000. pp. 215-39.
63. Kurjak A, Kupesic S. Ectopic pregnancy. In: Kurjak A (Ed). Ultrasound in Obstetrics and Gynecology. Boston: CRC Press. 1990:225-35.
64. Kupesic S, Kurjak A. Color Doppler assessment of ectopic pregnancy. In: Kurjak A, Kupesic S (Eds). An Atlas of Transvaginal Color Doppler. London-New York: Parthenon Publishing Group; 2000. pp. 137-47.
65. Timor-Tristch IE, Rottem S, Thale I. Review of transvaginal ultrasonography: description with clinical application. Ultrasound. 1988;6:1-32.
66. Peisner DB, Timor-Tritsch IE. The discriminatory zone of beta-hCG for vaginal probes. J Clin Ultrasound. 1990;18:280-5.
67. Fossum GT, Dvajan V, Kletzky DA. Early detection of pregnancy with transvaginal ultrasound. Fertil Steril. 1988;49:788-91.
68. Bernascheck G, Euaelstorfer R, Csaicsich P. Vaginal sonography versus serum human chorionic gonadotropin in early detection of pregnancy. Am J Obstet. 1988;158:608-12.
69. Kurjak A, Zalud I, Volpe G. Conventional B-mode and transvaginal color Doppler on ultrasound assessment of ectopic pregnancy. Acta Med. 1990;44:91-103.
70. Rosati P, Bellatti U, Exacoustos C. Uterine myoma in pregnancy: ultrasound study. Int J Gynecol Obstet. 1989;28:109-17.

71. Kurjak A, Predanic M, Kupesic S, Zudenigo D, Matijevic R, Salihagic A. Transvaginal color Doppler in the study of early cornual pregnancies and pregnancies associated with fibroids. J Matern Fetal Invest. 1992;2:81-5.
72. Depp R. Cesarian delivery. In: E Gabbe SG, Niebyl JR, Simpson JL (Eds). Obstetrics: Normal and Problem Pregnancies. 3rd edn. New York, Churchill Livingstone Inc; 1986. pp. 606-7.
73. Cunningham FG, MacDonald PC, Gant NF. Obstetrical Hemorrhage. Williams Obstetrics. 20th edn. Stamford Conn, Appleton and Lange; 1997. pp. 772-8.
74. Huang WC, Yang JM. Sonographic Findings of Uterine Dehiscence in the Early Third Trimester: Report of a Case. J Med Ultrasound. 2000;8:116-19.
75. Annath CV, Savitz DA, Luther ER. Maternal cigarette smoking as a risk factor for placental abruption, placenta previa and uterine bleeding in pregnancy. Am J Epidemiol. 1996;144:881-5.
76. Kramer M, Usher R, Pollack R. Etiologic determinants of abruptio placentae. Obstet Gynecol. 1997;89:211-5.
77. Ananth CV, Johnson RW. Placental abruption increases risk of stillbirth and preterm delivery. JAMA. 1999;282: 1646-51.
78. Brown HL. Trauma in pregnancy. Obstet Gynecol. 2009; 114(1):147-60.
79. Kupesic S, Aksamija A, Vucic N, Tripalo A, Kurjak A. Ultrasonic assessment of acute pelvic pain. Acta Medica Croatica. 2002;56:171-80.
80. Kupesic S, Aksamija A. Sonographic evaluation of gynecological and obstetric causes of acute pelvic pain. Ultrasound Rev Obstet Gynecol. 2003;5:192-202.
81. Neis KJ, Neis F. Chronic pelvic pain: cause, diagnosis and therapy from a gynaecologist's and an endoscopist's point of view. Gynecol Endocrinol. 2009;25(11):757-61.
82. Nikola R, Dogra V. Ultrasound: the triage tool in the emergency room: Using ultrasound first. Br J Radiol. 2016;89(1061):20150790. doi.10.1259/bjr.20150790.Epub 2015 Dec 2015.
83. Dupuis CS, Kim YH. Ultrasonography of adnexal causes of pelvic pain in premenopausal non-pregnant women. Ultrasonography. 2015;34(4):258-67.
84. Timor-Tritsch IE, Monteagudo A, Tsymbal T. Three-dimensional ultrasound inversion rendering technique facilitates the diagnosis of hydrosalpinx. J Clin Ultrasound. 2010;38(7):372-6.
85. Vrachnis N, Sifakis S, Samoli E, Kappou D, Pavlakis K, Iliodromiti Z, et al. Three-dimensional ultrasound and three-dimensional power Doppler improve the preoperative evaluation of complex benign ovarian lesions. Clin Exp Obstet Gyneco. 2012;39(4):474-8.
86. Reus AD, El-Harbachi H, Rousian M, Willemsen SP, Steegers-Theunissen RP, Steegers EA, et al. Early first trimester trophoblast volume in pregnancies that result in live birth or miscarriage. Ultrasound Obstet Gynecol. 2013;42(5):577-84.
87. Odeh M, Ophir E, Grinin V, Tendler R, Kais M, Bornstein J. Prediction of abortion using three-dimensional ultrasound volumetry of the gestational sac and the amniotic sac in threatened abortion. J Clin Ultrasound. 2012;40(7):389-93.
88. Lazzarin N, Exacoustos C, Vaquero E, De Felice G, Manfellotto D, Zupi E. Uterine junctional zone at three dimensional transvaginal ultrasonography in patients with recurrent miscarriage: a new diagnostic tool? Eur J Obstet Gynecol Reprod Biol. 2014;174:128-32.
89. Benacerraf BB, Abuhamad AZ, Bromley B, Goldstein SR, et al. Consider ultrasound first for imaging the female pelvis. Am J Obstet Gynecol. 2015;212:450-5.

63

CHAPTER

Ultrasound in Urogynecology

Ashok Khurana

INTRODUCTION

Over the past two decades ultrasound scans have rapidly replaced conventional radiology as the modality of choice for imaging the female patient with a voiding dysfunction. This is consequent to remarkable technological advances combined with innovative techniques of obtaining relevant morphological and dynamic information. Transabdominal ultrasound has now been complemented by a wide variety of ultrasound techniques which include transurethral ultrasound, introital ultrasound, perineal ultrasound, endoanal and transrectal scanning, power Doppler information and 3D and 4D technology. This chapter reviews basic concepts and newer developments in the context of their applications in routine and specialized practice and attempts to put the plethora of presentations in recent literature in clinical perspective.

CLINICAL CONSIDERATIONS

Urogynecological problems that need investigation include recurrent lower urinary tract infections, persistent dysuria, urgency and frequency, urinary incontinence and genitourinary prolapse. Occasionally, urological problems are associated with flatus or fecal incontinence, and this needs to be addressed as well. These problems, particularly in the aging female, need appropriate management because of their social and economic impact. This is consequent not only to direct costs related to matters, such as absorbent pads, diapers, medication, surgery and fractures from falls as a result of nocturnal urgency, but also indirect costs and intangible costs. Examples of indirect costs include loss of productivity at home and at work, time spent on elaborate clinical investigations and clinic visits. Intangible factors include suffering from illness, deterioration of lifestyle, reduced sexual activity, low self esteem, depression, and, social isolation consequent to desperation for rest rooms and a urinary body odor.

Clinical history can often in itself be conclusive as in the diagnosis of stress urinary incontinence. In most cases, of course, it is useful to enumerate symptoms with duration and intensity and patient perception of distress. Other important information includes assessing fluid intake (e.g., caffeine), voiding difficulty, previous treatment, obstetric history, pelvic and abdominal surgery, drug therapy, pelvic organ prolapse and concomitant fecal incontinence.[1] A voiding diary is an excellent method of guiding further investigation and treatment regimens in patients with incontinence.

Physical examination is aimed at evaluating concomitant pathology, such as atrophic changes, vulvovaginitis, organ prolapse and pelvic masses, as also neurologic disease and general debility. Stress urinary incontinence can be observed on a cough stress test. The tone and strength of the pelvic floor muscles should be assessed. This can be done by inspection (drawing up of the anus, lifting of the posterior wall of the vagina and narrowing of the vaginal introitus), digital palpation (e.g., the Oxford score) or more advanced techniques, such as perineometry and electromyography.[1]

INVESTIGATIONS

Urinalysis is usually the first investigation in most patients and offers pointers to the diagnosis by identifying hematuria, glycosuria, pyuria and bacteriuria. Ultrasound scans reveal anatomical details of the kidneys, ureters, urinary bladder, postmicturition residual urine, uterus and adnexae.

Urodynamic studies are not recommended as part of the initial workup of urogynecological problems except if there is a significant postmicturition residue or if incontinence is so severe that surgical methods are considered as a first-line option. Uroflometry can detect obstructed voiding. The technique is a nonimaging, noninvasive method which measures urinary flow rate and volume voided per second. Urethral pressure profilometry is a graphic observation method that can provide information on urethral function and can often be useful, even though it is not always reproducible. Videocystourethrography is the gold standard investigation. In the filling phase, increases in detrusor pressure associated with urgency are indicative of detrusor overactivity. Urinary bladder volumes at which first, strong and urge sensations are noted, help in diagnosis. Incontinence can be recorded during stress maneuvers. During voiding, poor contractility of the detrusor muscle can be assessed. This helps in differentiating poor detrusor function which is a low pressure/low flow state from outlet obstruction which shows high pressure and low flow. It is of note that all these studies are markedly operator dependent.

Specialized ultrasound studies are considered before or after urodynamic evaluation and will be discussed further. Magnetic Resonance Imaging with its capabilities of soft tissue delineation is currently being evaluated against information from three-dimensional (3D) and real-time three-dimensional (4D) ultrasound and will be discussed as well.

TECHNICAL CONCEPTS, PROTOCOLS, NORMS AND ULTRASOUND FINDINGS

The utility of transabdominal ultrasound in assessing the bladder and urethra in women with incontinence was described as far back as 1980.[2] Standardized protocols were published much later[3] and incorporated newer techniques, such as introital and perineal ultrasound scans.

Transvaginal, introital and perineal ultrasound can all be performed with the same transducer. This should be an end-firing intracavitary transducer with an emission angle of at least 90°. The availability of higher frequencies up to 12 MHz permits better resolution of superficial structures and the use of lower frequencies such as 5 MHz allows a better assessment of large pelvic masses and a very large uterus. The transducer is prepared as with standard transvaginal scanning. Warm gel prevents involuntary and voluntary tightening of the perineal musculature by the patient. The examination is best performed in a semireclining position because in a completely supine position, the patient may not be able to press adequately when asked to, and because in a standing position the transducer is difficult to place and maintain in position.[4] There is no significant difference in the dynamic assessment of the bladder neck in the semireclining and standing position.[5] For introital scans, the transducer is placed over the external urethral orifice with the long axis of the transducer along the long axis of the body **(Fig. 1)**. After orientation, the transducer can be angulated and also moved vertically, horizontally and obliquely to assess the urethra, urinary bladder, periurethral tissues, the entire endopelvic fascia, vagina and rectum **(Figs. 2 and 3)**. Studies are done at rest, with contractions,

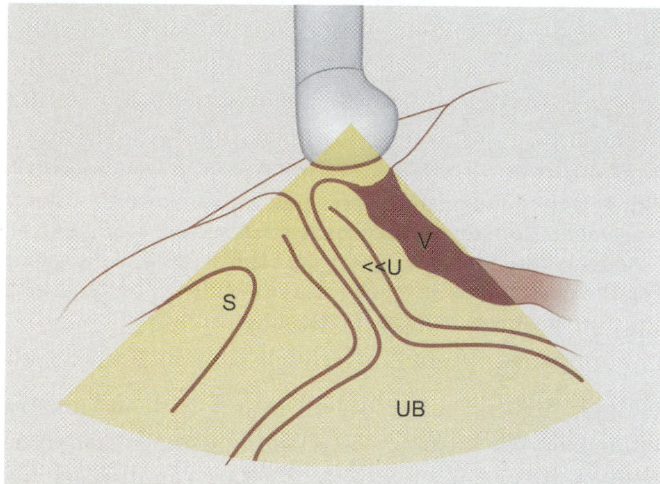

Fig. 1: Graphic representation of introital scanning showing transducer position and the structures to be included in an ideal view. Note that the beam includes the inferior extent of the symphysis pubis (S), the urethra along its long axis (U), the urinary bladder (UB) and its neck and the vagina (V). Posterior angulation would help include the rectum when necessary.

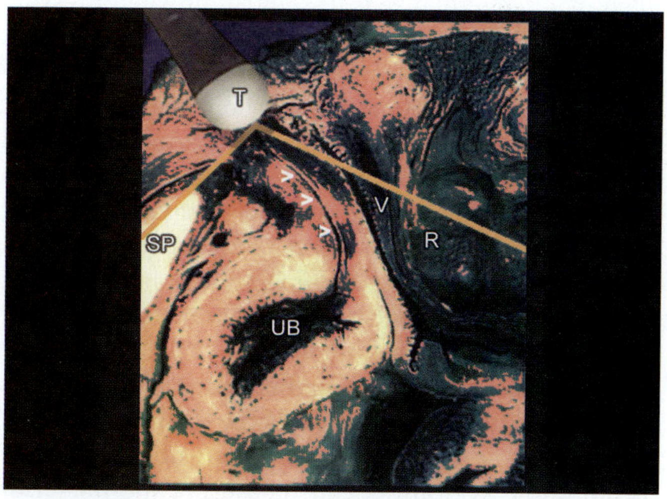

Fig. 2: Long axis through the midline in a cadaver pelvis to show the orientation of the pelvic viscera and transducer position. The transducer (T) is placed as shown and the beam insonates the symphysis pubis (SP), the urethra (>>), urinary bladder (UB), vagina (V) and rectum (R).

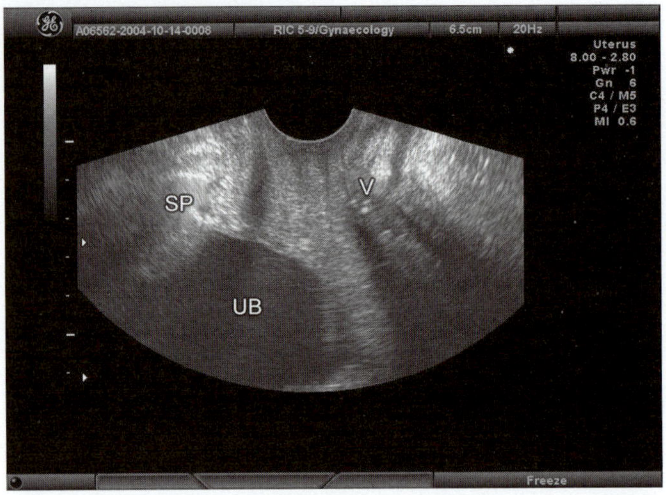

Fig. 3: Ultrasound image as obtained with an ideal transducer placement. Note the hypoechoic symphysis pubis (SP) with an echogenic inferior margin, the urinary bladder (UB) and the vagina (V). The normal urethra is seen as a markedly hypoechoic, long structure and the bladder neck is closed.

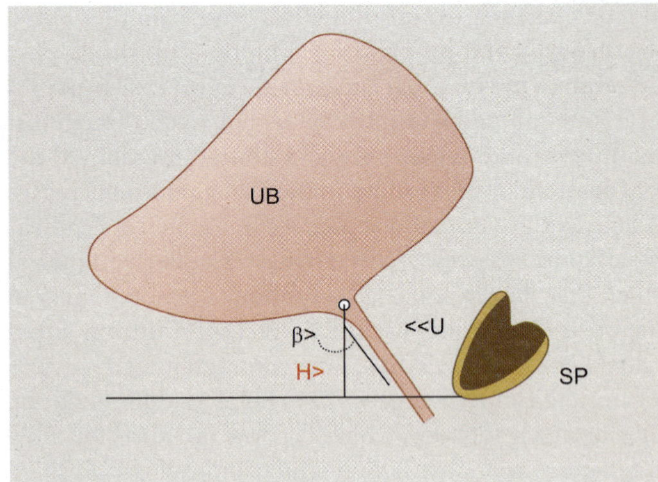

Fig. 4: Graphic representation of quantification of the orientation and length of the urethra. The scan should necessarily include the symphysis pubis (SP), urethra (<<U) and urinary bladder (UB). A horizontal line is drawn at the level of the inferior extent of the symphysis pubis and the vertical height (not the oblique extent) H is calculated as the length of the perpendicular extending upwards from the horizontal line to the bladder neck. The angle beta (β) is the angle between the line H and the bladder neck.

while coughing, with pressure and with a Valsalva maneuver. For introital scans, the transducer has to be held gently because excessive pressure can displace the bladder neck. Recommended bladder filling to ensure reliability and reproducibility of obtained data is about 300 mL.[3,6] In clinical practice, a significant number of patients may become incontinent before achieving this volume and this standard may need to be compromised. Urethral funneling is more pronounced in an appropriately filled bladder.[7] Prolapse is less apparent when pressing with a full bladder than with a partially full bladder.[7] In perineal ultrasound the transducer is placed just over the labia. In this technique, there is a complete visualization of the symphysis pubis from its upper to its lower end whereas in introital ultrasound only the lower edge is seen. Both are equally good in depicting the cystourethral junction. Several studies[8-11] have compared introital and perineal ultrasound with conventional lateral chain cystourethrography and colpocystourethrography and confirmed its reliability.

Quantification of imaging findings **(Fig. 4)** involves measuring the height H which is the distance between the bladder neck and a line through the lower edge of the pubic symphysis and measuring the posterior urethrovesical angle β which is the angle between the urethral long axis and bladder floor. These are determined at rest and during contraction, coughing, and pressing.[3] Changes in these parameters during contraction and pressing, and in particular, visual real-time ultrasound assessment serves to evaluate the reactivity of the pelvic floor muscles and the adequacy of the connective tissue supportive structures of the urogenital organs.[4] In women without stress urinary incontinence and prolapse, the posterior urethrovesical angle is 96.8° at rest and 108.1° during pressing, with a distance H between the bladder neck and lower edge of the pubic symphysis of 20.6 mm and 14.0 mm, respectively.[3,12-14] There are no significant age-related changes in these normal values.[5]

Normal mobility of the bladder neck is influenced by body habitus, pregnancy and delivery. Racial differences in bladder neck mobility between white and black nulliparous continent women have been identified.[15] In volunteers, pelvic floor awareness education alone can significantly reduce bladder neck mobility in nulliparous women.[16,17] Vaginal and instrumental deliveries are associated with a hypermobility of the bladder neck.[18-20]

Bladder wall thickness is best measured after micturition in a lithotomy position with a transvaginal image.[21] These measurements are taken at the thickest part of the trigone, dome and anterior wall of the urinary bladder.

The bladder neck is closed at rest and funneling is not evident in normal individuals **(Fig. 5)**. The anterior

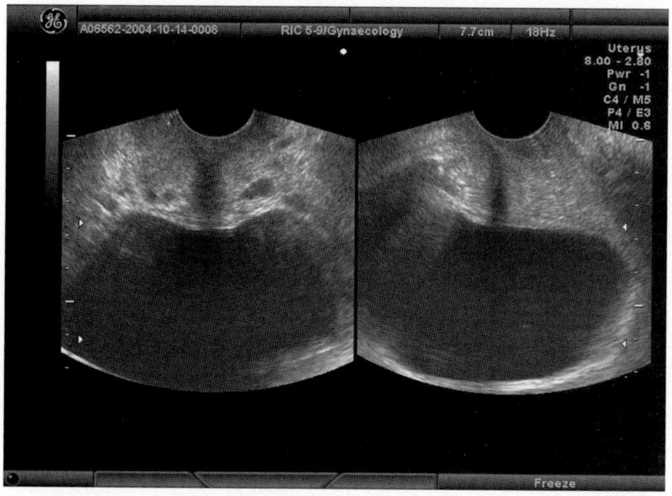

Fig. 5: Anteroposterior (left) and long axis (right) views of a normal urethra with a normal bladder neck. The long hypoechoic area represents the anterior and posterior walls and the urethral lumen. The bladder neck is closed and normal.

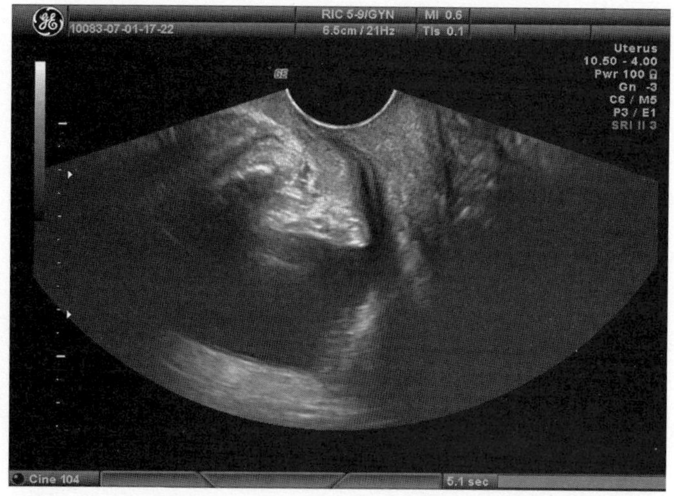

Fig. 6: Longitudinal midline section showing an abnormal bladder neck with funneling. The bladder neck is open in this patient at rest, and there is urine in the urethra. If this opening of the bladder neck and filling of the urethra and incontinence coincide with straining or Valsalva maneuver, a diagnosis of genuine stress incontinence may be made. If the bladder neck opens at rest, further investigation is warranted to differentiate urge and mixed incontinence.

and posterior urethral walls appear as a hypoechoic zone. The morphological layers of the urethra cannot be differentiated in the midsagittal plane due to artifacts. In most cases the mucosa and submucosa are uniformly depicted as a hypoechoic structure and may mimic an open lumen if the gain settings are inappropriate. Failure to demonstrate funneling of the urethra in patients with incontinence is usually a reflection of poor examination technique, such as studies in a recumbent position, insufficient force during Valsalva or an empty bladder.[4]

Bladder neck hypermobility and funneling of the urethra[22-24] **(Figs. 6 and 7)** are typical findings in incontinence but do not always correlate with urodynamic parameters.[25] Mobility of the bladder neck is of two varieties. One of these is a rotational posteroinferior descent[26,27] with the inferior limit of the symphysis pubis as a pivot **(Fig. 8)**. The other is a vertical descent along the urethral axis[28] **(Fig. 9)**. A vector-based assessment of the magnitude and direction of the bladder neck has been assessed.[29] The results of bladder neck and pubic-point movement were as follows (extent in mm +/-SD): strain and bladder neck 16.9 +/-6.1, pubic point 4.8 +/-3.9, cough bladder neck 10.2 +/-5.4, pubic point 2.9 +/-3.4 and Kaegel's exercise bladder neck 7.0 +/-3.6 and pubic point 7.0 +/-1.4.[30]

Urinary continence in the female is consequent to several factors.[30] The endopelvic fascia and the anterior vaginal wall form a supportive layer upon which the urethra courses across.[31,32] When intra-abdominal pressure is

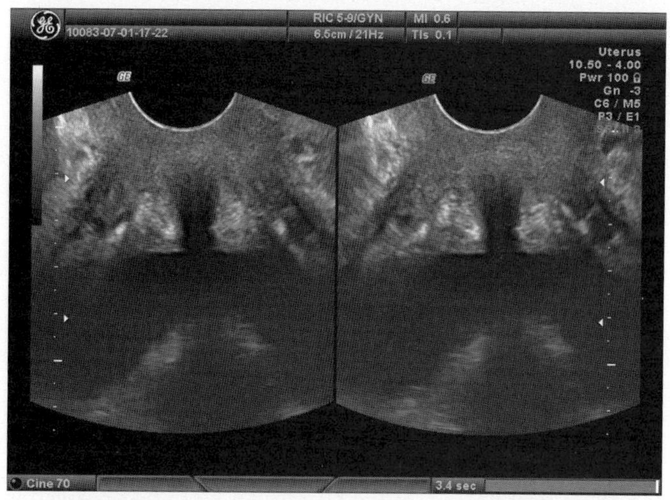

Fig. 7: Anteroposterior view of an open bladder neck.

increased the urethra is compressed against this layer and incontinence is prevented. The endopelvic fascia consists of smooth musle and fibrous connective tissue and inserts into the fascial coverings of the obturator internus and levator ani muscles. The part of the fascia that lies between the vagina and the urinary bladder and supports the bladder is called the pubocervical fascia. Interruption of the support mechanism results in a prolapse, genuine

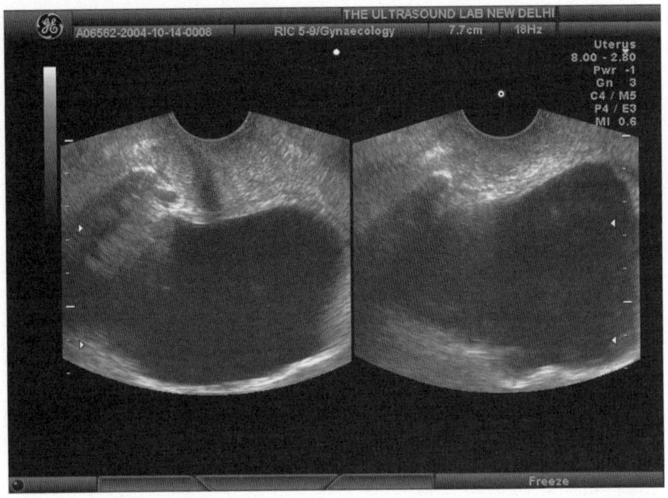

Fig. 8: Rotational hypermobility of the bladder neck is commonly evident in incontinent patients. The scan shows postero-inferior descent of the bladder neck and bladder base to a level below that of the symphysis pubis. The frame on the left is taken at rest and the one on the right is taken during straining, Valsalva or observed incontinence. The inferior limit of the symphysis pubis is seen as an echogenic rim capping the anechoic pubic bone.

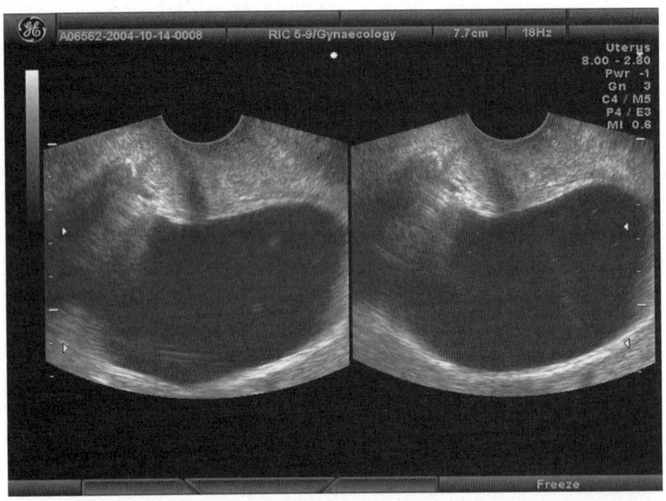

Fig. 9: Vertical descent of the bladder neck can be observed in incontinent patients. The finding is convincingly evident when a scan at rest (left) is compared side-by-side with an image during straining or coughing (right).

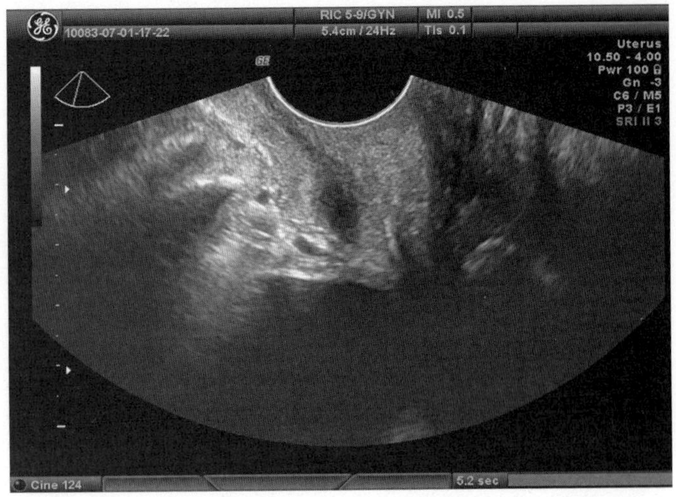

Fig. 10: Assessment of levator ani reactivity. Image at rest for comparison with **Figure 11**.

stress incontinence, incontinence cystocele, urethrocele or both. Knowledge of anatomy, physiology and a detailed ultrasound evaluation can distinguish between these defects.[30] Unilateral or bilateral separation of the pubocervical fascia from the arcus tendineus fascia covering the obturator internus and levator ani muscles is often accompanied by stress urinary incontinence and cystourethrocele.[33-35] Paravaginal defect repair operations and Burch colposuspension restore position and normal mobility of the urethrovesical junction and correct the cystourethrocele and the posterior urethrovesical angle.[30] Differentiation of a lateral defect from a central defect of the anterior compartment is important to decide whether a colposuspension or a tension-free vaginal tape would relieve stress urinary incontinence.[22] Reactivity of the pelvic floor can be assessed by observing the height of the bladder neck relative to a line through the lower edge of the symphysis pubis at rest and during voluntary contractions of the pelvic floor muscles. An increased distance **(Figs. 10 and 11)** reflects good levator ani reactivity.[36] Intraoperative ultrasound can help prevent the development of de novo incontinence by optimizing surgical elevation of the bladder neck during open colposuspension.[37]

Whereas, magnetic resonance imaging (MRI) has been the modality for visualizing the pelvic floor, in recent years 3D ultrasound sectional images are replacing MRI **(Fig. 12)** because of an equivalent resolution **(Figs. 13 and 14)** and the added advantage of ease of utility,[38] dynamic display[39] and vascular display. Anatomical atrophy of the endopelvic fascia, change in the configuration of the vagina **(Fig. 15)** and paucity of vasculature **(Fig. 16)** can be documented with amazing clarity and reproducibility. The deep muscles of the pelvic floor are referred to as the levator ani or the pelvic diaphragm. The muscles that comprise the levator ani include the pubococcygeus,

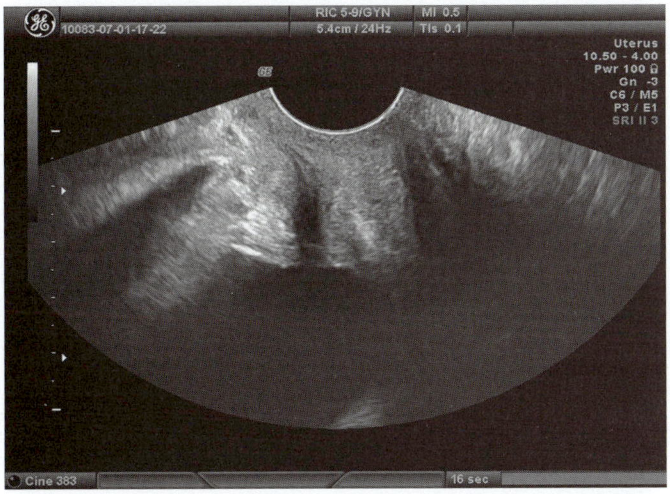

Fig. 11: Increased distance of the bladder neck from the symphysis pubis in a patient with good levator ani reactivity. Image obtained during voluntary contractions of the pelvic floor. For comparison with **Figure 10**.

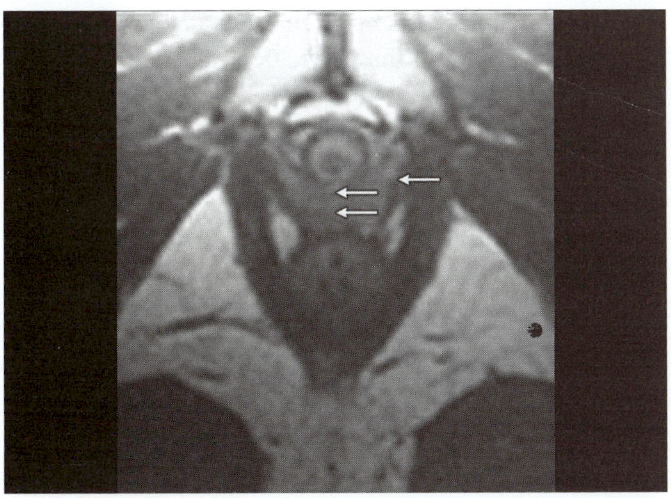

Fig. 12: Magnetic resonance image (MRI) of the pelvis showing in the midline, the urethra anteriorly, the pubocervical ligament (two arrows), the levator ani (single arrow), the vagina and rectum.

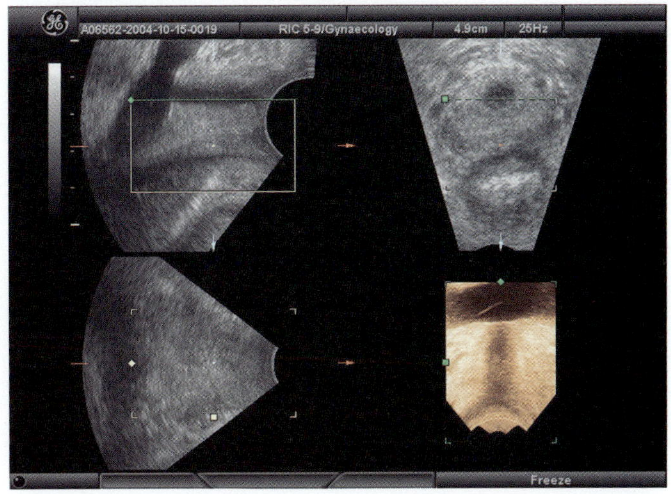

Fig. 13: Three-dimensional (3D) images of the endopelvic fascia showing the region in three-orthogonal planes and one rendered plane. The top left image shows (from top to bottom) the urethra, vagina and rectum in the midline and the fibromuscular tissue laterally. The rendered image (bottom right) shows the urethra flanked by the endopelvic fascia.

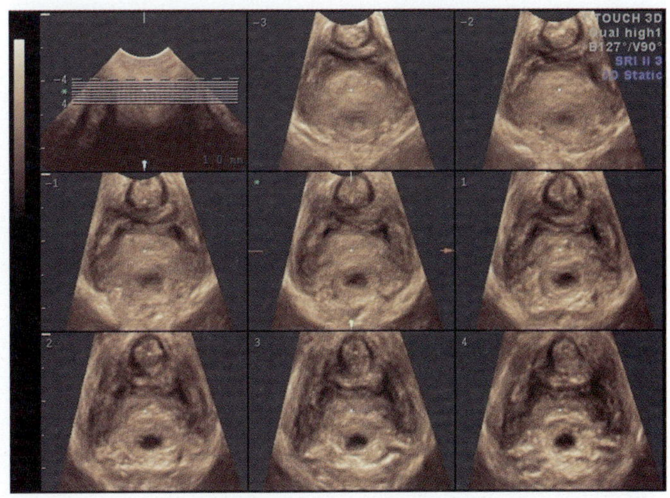

Fig. 14: 3D tomographic ultrasound imaging (TUI). Currently available 3D transducers acquire information in sweeps across the region of interest. Each signal thus acquired can be rendered in an infinite number of planes. TUI allows a choice of plane direction and thickness in much the same format as CT or MRI. Note the exquisite soft tissue detail of the urethra, vagina, rectum and endopelvic fascia. The vagina has an H-shaped configuration as evident in sections 1–4.

puborectalis, and iliococcygeus. These muscles span the space between the obturator internus muscle laterally, the pubis symphysis anteriorly, and the coccyx posteriorly. The superficial muscles of the pelvic floor make up the urogenital diaphragm and include the ischiocavernosus, bulbospongiosus, and the transversus perinea superficialis.[40] The levator hiatus is a space between the various muscle groups that form the levator ani through which the urethra, vagina, and anal canal pass.[41] The puborectalis is the inferior-most muscle of the pelvic floor and is composed of two limbs attached to the two pubic rami anteriorly; they merge posterior to the anal canal.[42] The important role of the pelvic floor musculature is to

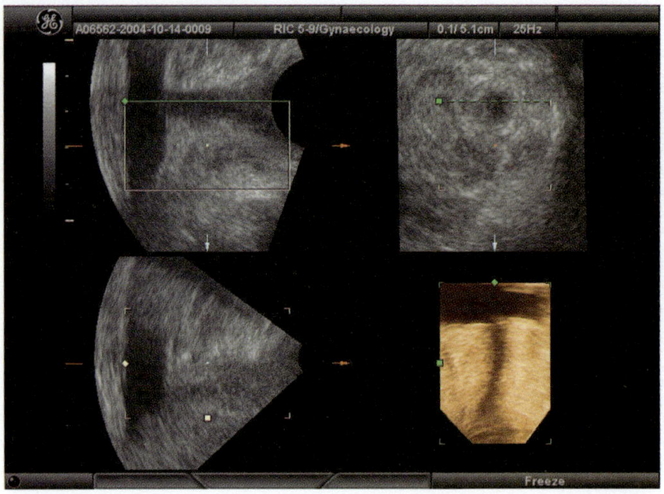

Fig. 15: Complete loss of anatomical delineation of the vagina, rectum and endopelvic fascia in postmenopausal atrophy in a patient with incontinence. The difference is striking when the plane displayed in the top right area is compared with its counterpart in **Figure 13**.

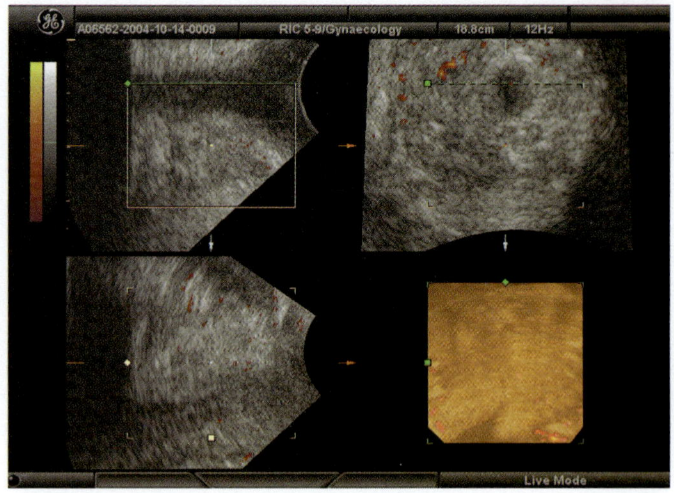

Fig. 17: 3D tomographic ultrasound imaging with 2D and power Doppler information in a patient on perineal exercises and local estrogen cream application. Note the increased vascular signals in the top right frame when compared with **Figure 15**.

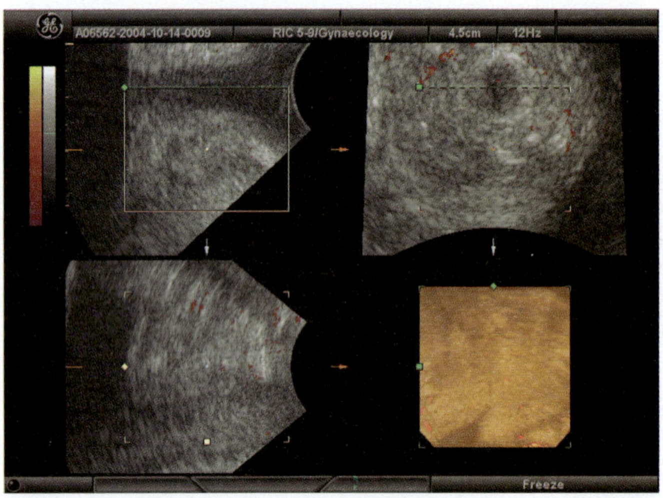

Fig. 16: 3D tomographic ultrasound imaging with grayscale and power Doppler information. Note the scanty vascular signals seen in the top right image and the complete absence of vascular signals in the other orthogonal planes.

perform voluntary contractions as well as involuntary, or reflex, contractions preceding or at the time of increased abdominal pressure. These types of contractions preserve fecal and urinary continence. In response to increased abdominal pressures, the superficial pelvic muscles, such as the anal and urethral sphincters resist these pressures, and the levator ani muscles support the pelvic floor and counteract these pressures by contracting and creating a circular closing of the levator hiatus and an upward movement of the pelvic floor and perineum.[43-46] The puborectalis provides pelvic floor support and ensures continence. When it contracts, the length of its limbs is reduced, and this change lifts the anal canal anteriorly, compressing the structures within the levator hiatus against each other as well as the back of the pubic symphysis.[47] Three-dimensional ultrasound can also visualize anatomic defects of the individual components of the anal sphincter.[48] Patients with anatomical defects of the puborectalis have longer anterior–posterior lengths of the pelvic floor hiatus compared with controls.[39] Other measurements that can be obtained with three-dimensional ultrasound include the muscular component of the levator hiatus (the length of the suprapubic arch subtracted from the hiatal circumference) and the muscle strain on contraction (hiatal circumference subtracted from the hiatal circumference at rest). These images offer an excellent display of avulsion injuries, which appear as abnormal insertion or interruptions of the puborectalis.[48] Vascular response to perineal exercises and local estrogen application **(Fig. 17)** can be demonstrated by serial scans done 6 weeks to 12 weeks apart. Transanal and transrectal side-firing linear transducers now offer detailed delineation of the anal and urethral sphincters and sphincter mechanisms and in the future are likely to find increased application. 3D provides objective

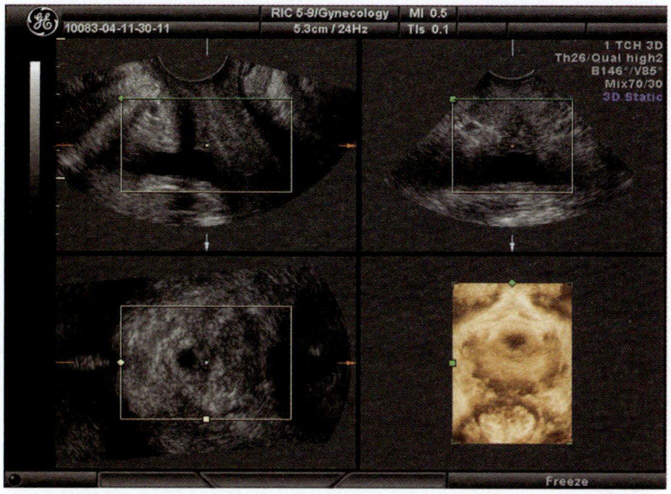

Fig. 18: 3D tomographic imaging with a display of three-orthogonal planes and one rendered (bottom right) image. Note the complete distortion of vaginal echoes best evident in the rendered image in this patient with atrophy.

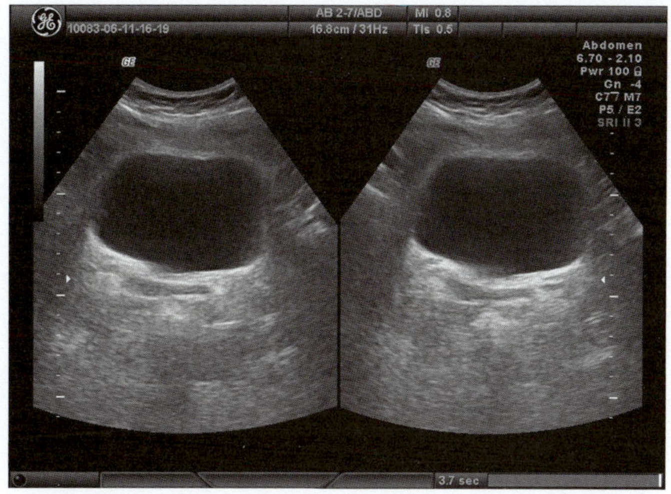

Fig. 19: Significant post-micturition residue in a patient with recurrent urinary tract infection. The upper limit of normal post-micturition residue is 15 mL.

evaluation of outcomes from urethral bulking agent therapy using collagen injections[49] and helps in assessing failure and the need for re-injection. Tension free vaginal tape slings are highly echogenic and can be assessed by 3D ultrasound.[50] Tape movement occurs in an arc around the posterior aspect of the posterior symphysis which serves as the fulcrum. Mechanical compression of the urethra by the tape is evident as a reduction in the gap between the tape and the symphysis pubis.

Most disorders of voiding dysfunction are characterized by a group of ultrasound findings that not only confirm clinical suspicion but also facilitate treatment decision options.

Recurrent lower urinary tract infections are marked by atrophied endopelvic fascia **(Fig. 18)** and increased residual urine **(Fig. 19)** consequent to a distension cystocele or surgical overcorrection of the urethra. Occasionally, bladder diverticuli, urethral diverticuli, intravesical calculi, foreign bodies or an abnormally located intrauterine device may be in evidence.

Patients with urgency and frequency may show periurethral or intravesical masses, bladder and urethral diverticuli, anterior uterine fibroids, and a discordant funneling of the proximal urethra **(Fig. 20)**.

In patients with dysuria and dyspareunia, urethral diverticuli, periurethral masses and migrating old intrauterine contraceptive devices may be in evidence.

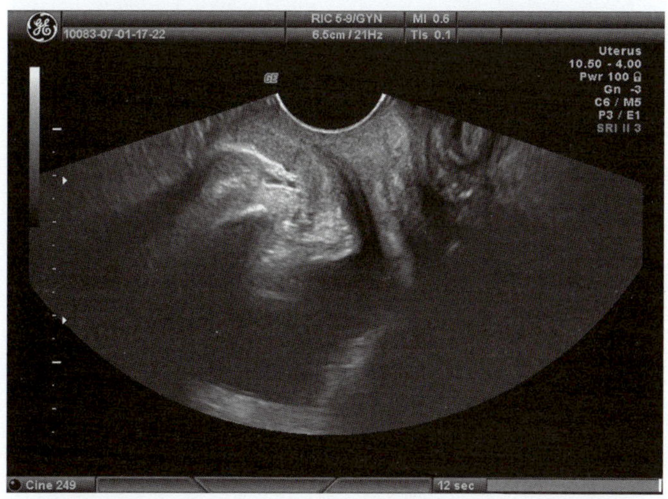

Fig. 20: Funneling of the urethra in a patient with severe genuine stress incontinence.

Urge incontinence is marked by a thickened bladder wall **(Fig. 21)**.

Stress urinary incontinence shows either a fixed or a hypermobile urethra **(Fig. 22)**, reduced or absent pelvic floor reactivity or a cystocele and a funneling of the urethra during stress **(Fig. 23)**.

In the first few years after it was introduced, the utility of pelvic floor ultrasound was confined largely to answering clinical queries related to urinary incontinence and the

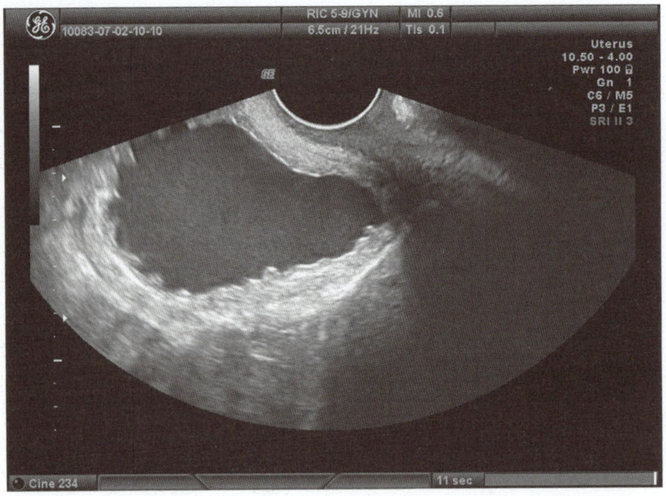

Fig. 21: Markedly thickened wall of the urinary bladder. The normal thickness of the wall is 01–03 mm. Patient of post-viral asthenia.

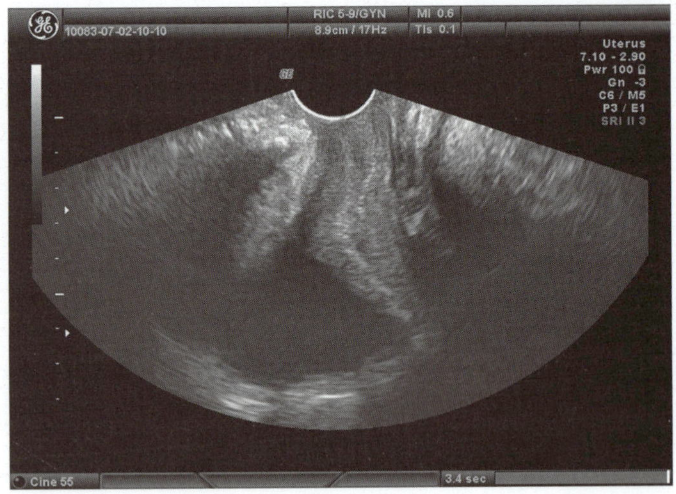

Fig. 23: Same patient as in **Figure 22** showing funneling of the bladder neck, hypermobile urethra and absent pelvic floor reactivity.

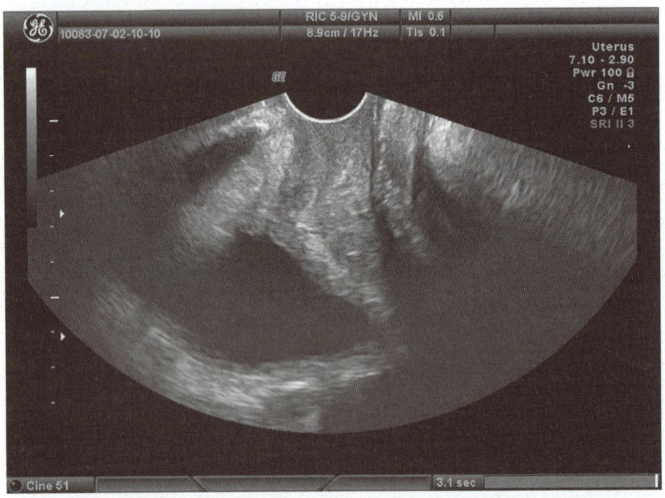

Fig. 22: Incontinent patient showing findings at rest, for comparison with **Figure 23**. The bladder neck is closed.

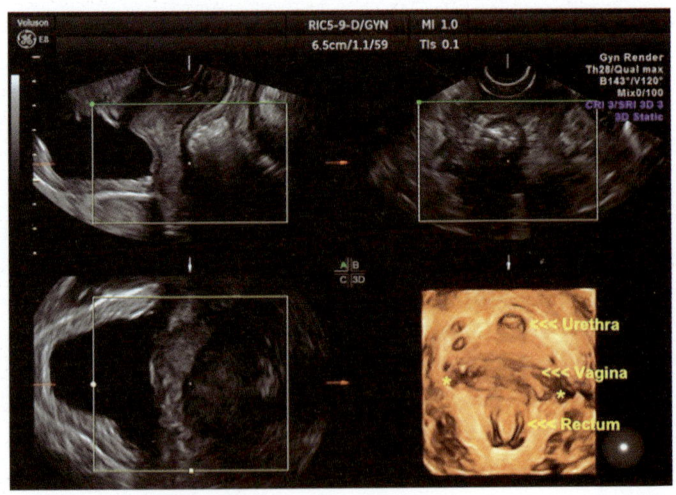

Fig. 24: 3D rendering of the pelvic floor including the symphysis pubis, urethra, vagina and rectum. Note the interruption of the levator ani complex at the 9 o'clock and 3 o'clock position (*).

focus was on the urinary bladder and the bladder neck. Over the past one and a half decade this has evolved because prolapse has emerged as a major clinical problem.[51] The emergence of meshes and slings as therapeutic alternatives has also accelerated the use of pelvic ultrasound as a problem solving modality.[52,53] Meshes and slings can be assessed reliably by ultrasound[54,55] and this is superior to MRI.[56]

The availability of pelvic floor ultrasound has also revolutionized the understanding of morphological anomalies of the levator ani. These abnormalities have now been understood to be consequent to traumatic avulsion of the muscle **(Figs. 24 and 25)** from the sidewall and not as a result of pudendal nerve trauma.[53] Levator trauma during birth is now well recognized.[57] This type of trauma is strongly associated with anterior and central compartment prolapse, but not with stress incontinence.[58] Newer rendering engines in 3D ultrasound demonstrate these defects dramatically. The availability of multislice 3D imaging akin to CT and MRI has enhanced detailed

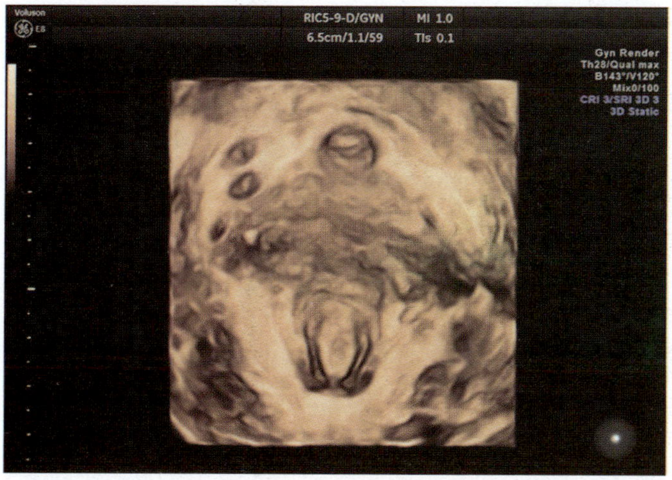

Fig. 25: Same case as in **Figure 24** with a magnified rendered 3D image and the same findings.

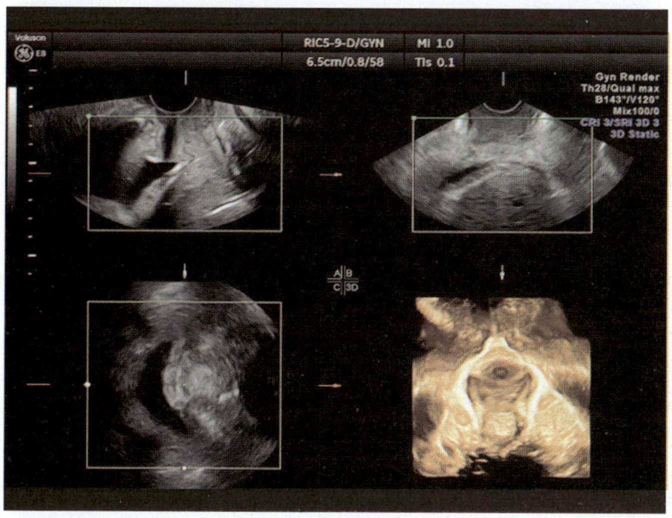

Fig. 26: Normal pelvic floor seen with 3D ultrasound. This format shows three-orthogonal planes and 3D rendering. The rendered plane is indicated by the green line. Such a format displays a single plane. Compare with multislice imaging shown in **Figure 27**.

evaluation of the levator ani complex **(Figs. 26 and 27)**. The choice of multislicing in orthogonal planes with comparable resolution in all reconstructed planes has markedly diminished the need for front firing dedicated transducers **(Figs. 28 to 30)**. Newer software also permits a slice any which way technique that permits visualization in any imaginable plane within the acquired volume **(Figs. 31 to 33)**. Newer options in image enhancement readily and more reliably permit recognition of the levator ani complex **(Figs. 34 and 35)**.

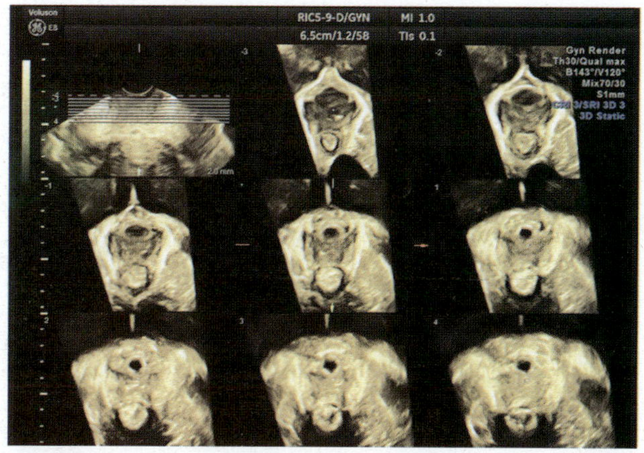

Fig. 27: Same case as in **Figure 26**. The top left frame shows the reference slices displayed in the rest of the image. Software allows a choice of number of slices and distance between slices. This format permits slicing through an entire volume of interest and ensuring visualization of structures throughout that volume.

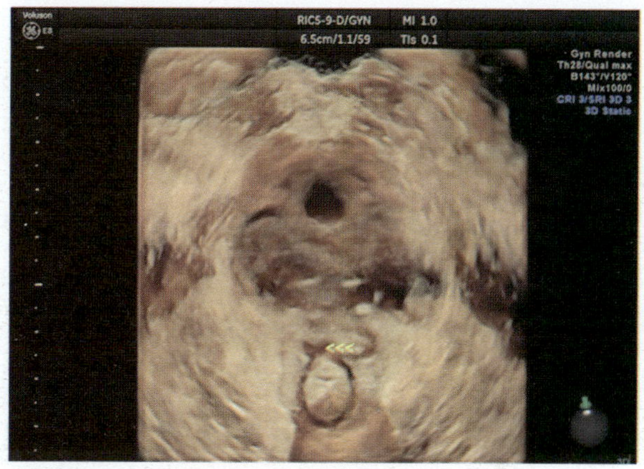

Fig. 28: 3D rendered image of the pelvic floor. Note the tear in the anal sphincter at the 11 o'clock position.

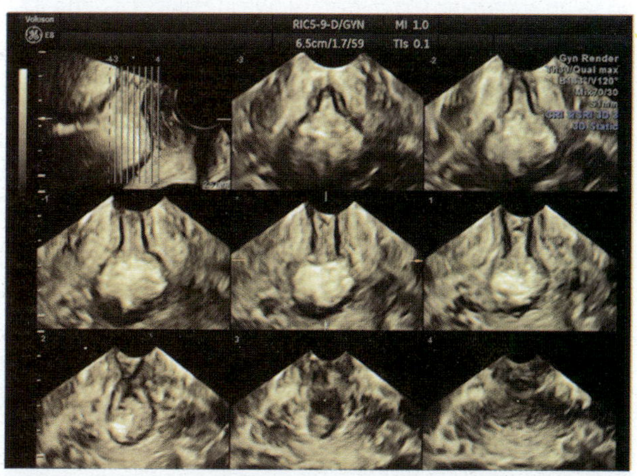

Fig. 29: Multislice display in the longitudinal plane of the same case as in **Figure 28**. Note that the tear will not evident in all slices. There is an excellent visualization of anal morphology in its long axis. This reconstruction diminishes the need for a dedicated front firing transducer.

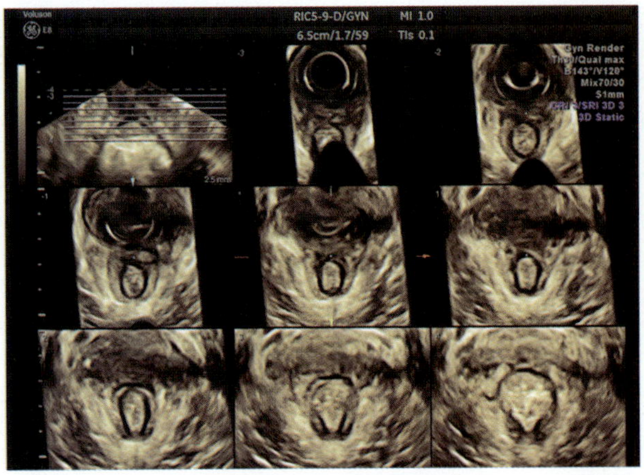

Fig. 30: Same case as in **Figures 28 and 29**. Transverse multislice view. Note that the tear at the 11 o'clock position is now evident in the appropriately located slices. This software is easy to use with the help of one touch controls on the machine desktop.

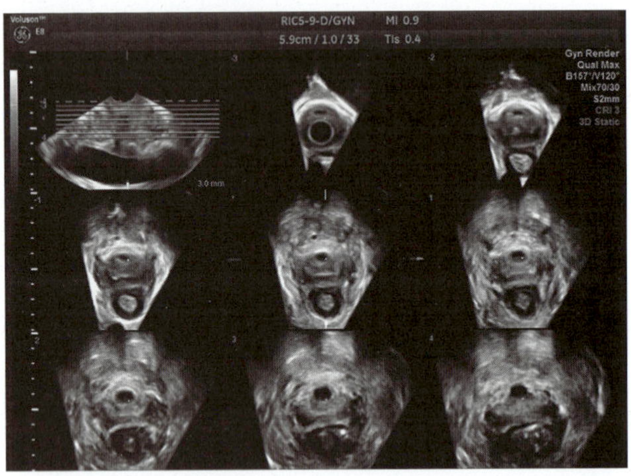

Fig. 31: Advanced 3D software now permits any volume to be sliced in many ways. This is a multislice format. The same volume can be sliced using additional software as shown in **Figures 32 and 33**.

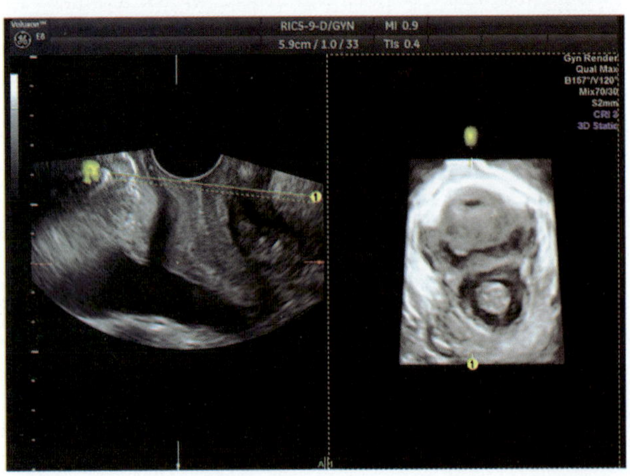

Fig. 32: Same case in **Figure 31**. This viewing format allows a line or curve to be drawn across any part of the volume. This makes it easy to overcome normal variants of the human form. This is particularly useful in postmenopausal patients and in prolapse.

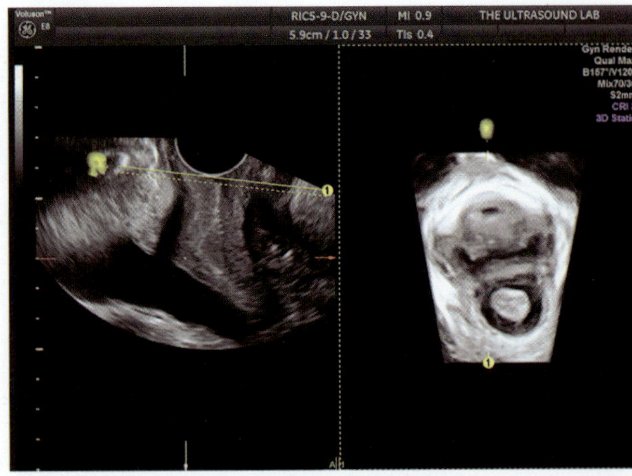

Fig. 33: Same case as in **Figures 31 and 32**. The selected slice is caudal to that shown in **Figure 32**. The urethra, vagina and anal sphincter are far better visualized in this plane.

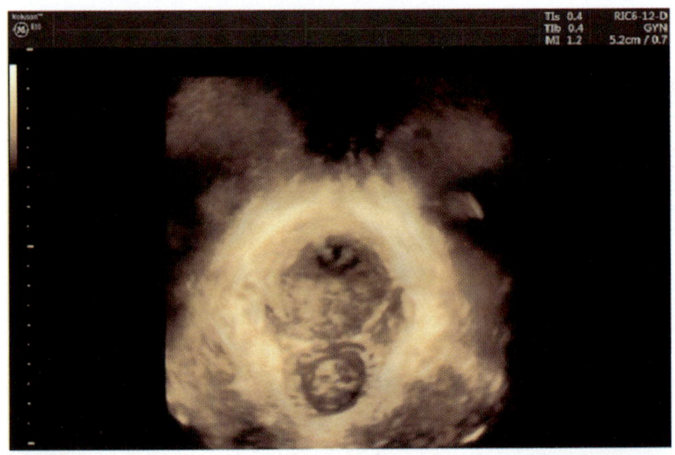

Fig. 34: Conventional rendering engine used for the pelvic floor. Compare with **Figure 35**.

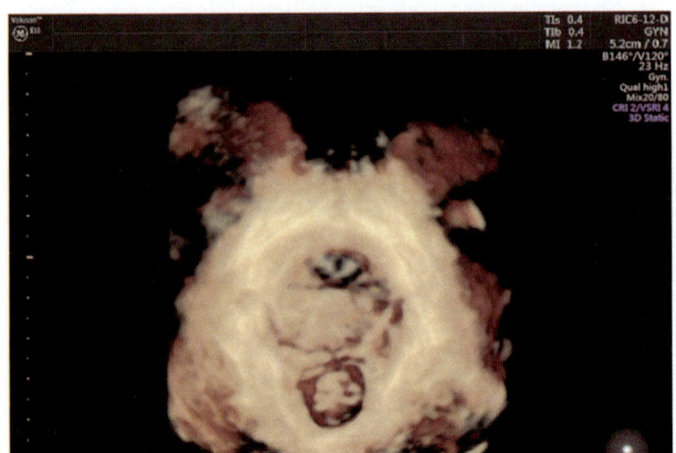

Fig. 35: Newer rendering engine applied on the data shown in **Figure 34**. Note the enhanced detail of the levator ani complex.

CONCLUSION

Several years after its introduction, technical advances and remarkably reproducible objective parameters have put ultrasound and in particular, 3D evaluation, in a unique position for clinical support. Enhanced tissue contrast and proven safety have thrown open numerous imaging protocols which are being perfected rapidly.

REFERENCES

1. Pantazis K, Freeman RM. Investigation and treatment of urinary incontinence. Current Obstetrics and Gynecology. 2006;16(6):344-52.
2. White RD, McQuown D, McCarthy TA, et al. Real-time ultrasonography in the evaluation of urinary stress incontinence. Am J Obstet Gynecol. 1980;138(2):235-7.
3. Schaer G, Koelbl H, Voigt R, Merz E, Anthuber C, Niemeyer R, et al. Recommendations of the German Association of Urogynecology on functional sonography of the lower female urinary tract. Int Urogynecol J Pelvic Floor Dysfunct. 1996;7(2):105-8.
4. Tunn R, Petri E. Introital and transvaginal ultrasound as the main tool in the assessment of urogenital and pelvic floor dysfunction: an imaging panel and practical approach. Ultrasound Obstet Gynecol. 2003;22(2):205-13.
5. Bader W, Degenhardt F, Kauffels W, et al. Morphologic parameters of female stress incontinence. J Ultrasound Ultraschall Med. 1995;16(4):180-5.
6. Schaer GN, Koechli OR, Schuessler B, et al. Perineal ultrasound: determination of reliable examination procedures. Ultrasound Obstet Gynecol. 1996;7(5):347-52.
7. Dietz HP, Wilson PD. The influence of bladder volume on the position and mobility of the urethrovesical junction. Int Urogynecol J Pelvic Floor Dysfunct. 1999;10(1):3-6.
8. Kohorn EI, Scioscia AL, Jeanty P, et al. Ultrasound cystourethrography by perineal scanning for the assessment of female stress urinary incontinence. Obstet Gynecol. 1986;68(2):269-72.
9. Koelbl H, Bernaschek G, Wolf G. A comparative study of perineal ultrasound scanning and urethrocystography in patients with genuine stress incontinence. Arch Obstet Gynecol. 1988;244:39-45.
10. Gordon D, Pearce M, Norton P, et al. Comparison of ultrasound and lateral chain urethrocystography in the determination of bladder neck descent. Am J Obstet Gynecol. 1989;160(1):182-5.
11. Mouritsen L, Strandberg C. Vaginal ultrasonography versus colpo-cysto-urethrography in the evaluation of female urinary incontinence. Acta Obstet Gynecol Scand. 1994;73(4):338-42.
12. Weber AM, Abrams P, Brubaker L, Cundiff G, Davis G, Dmochowski RR, et al. The standardization of terminology for researchers in female pelvic floor disorders. Int Urogynecol J Pelvic Floor Dysfunct. 2001;12(3):178-86.
13. Khullar V, Cardozo LD, Salvatore S, et al. Ultrasound: a noninvasive screening test for detrusor instability. Br J Obstet Gynaecol. 1996;103(9):904-8.
14. Schaer GN, Koechli OR, Schuessler B, Haller U. Perineal ultrasound for evaluating the bladder neck in urinary stress incontinence. Obstet Gynecol. 1995;85(2):220-4.
15. Howard D, Delancey JO, Tunn R, Ashton-Miller JA. Racial differences in the structure and function of the stress urinary continence mechanism. Obstet Gynecol. 2000;95(5):713-7.
16. Peschers UM, Vodusek DB, Fanger G, Schaer GN, DeLancey JO, Schuessler B. Pelvic muscle activity in nulliparous volunteers. Neurourol Urodyn. 2001;20(3):269-75.
17. Miller JM, Perucchini D, Carchidi LT, et al. Pelvic floor muscle contraction during a cough and decreased vesical neck mobility. Obstet Gynecol. 2001;97(2):255-60.
18. Peschers U, Schaer G, Anthuber C, et al. Changes in vesical neck mobility following vaginal delivery. Obstet Gynecol. 1996;88(6):1001-6.
19. Wijma J, Weis Potters AE, de Wolf BT, et al. Anatomical and functional changes in the lower urinary tract during pregnancy. BJOG. 2001;108(7):726-32.
20. King JK, Freeman RM. Is antenatal bladder neck mobility a risk factor for postpartum stress incontinence? Br J Obstet Gynaecol. 1998;105(12):1300-7.
21. Khullar V, Salvatore S, Cardozo L, Bourne TH, Abbott D, Kelleher C. A novel technique for measuring bladder wall thickness in women using transvaginal ultrasound. Ultrasound Obstet Gynecol. 1994;4(3):220-3.
22. Tunn R, Perucchini D. Morphologic assessment for diagnosing urogynaecologic disorders. Zentralbl Gynakol. 2001;123(12):672-9.
23. Schaer GN, Perucchini D, Munz E, Peschers U, Koechli OR, Delancey JO. Sonographic evaluation of the bladder neck in continent and stress-incontinent women. Obstet Gynecol. 1999;93(3):412-6.
24. Schaer GN, Koechli OR, Schuessler B, Haller U. Improvement of perineal sonographic bladder neck imaging with ultrasound contrast medium. Obstet Gynecol. 1995;86(6):950-4.
25. Dietz HP, Clarke B. The urethral pressure profile and ultrasound imaging of the lower urinary tract. Int Urogynecol J Pelvic Floor Dysfunct. 2001;12(1):38-41.
26. Petri E, Koelbl H, Schaer G. What is the place of ultrasound in urogynecology? A written panel. Int Urogynecol J Pelvic Floor Dysfunct. 1999;10(4):262-73.
27. Yang JM, Huang WC. Discrimination of bladder disorders in female lower urinary tract symptoms on ultrasonographic cystourethrography. J Ultrasound Med. 2002;21(11):1249-55.
28. Yang JM, Yang SH, Huang WC. Dynamic morphological changes in the anterior vaginal wall before and after laparoscopic Burch colposuspension in primary urodynamic stress incontinence. Ultrasound Obstet Gynecol. 2005;25(3):289-95.

29. Reddy AP, DeLancey JO, Zwica OM, et al. On-screen vector-based ultrasound assessment of vesical neck movement. Am J Obstet Gynecol. 2001;185(1):65-70.
30. Martan A, Massata J, Halaska M, et al. Ultrasound Imaging of paravaginal defects in women with stress incontinence before and after paravaginal defect repair. Ultrasound Obstet Gynecol. 2002;19:496-500.
31. DeLancy JOL. Structural support of the urethra as it relates to stress urinary incontinence: the hammock hypothesis. Am J Obstet Gynecol. 1994;170:1713-20.
32. DeLancy JOL. Stress urinary incontinence: Where are we now, where should we go? Am J Obstet Gynecol. 1996;175:311-9.
33. Gosling JA. The structure of the bladder neck, urethra and pelvic floor in relation to female urinary continence. Int Urogynecol J. 1996;7(4):177-8.
34. Monga A. Fascia—defects and repair. Curr Opin Obstet Gynecol. 1996;8(5):366-71.
35. Martan A, Masata M, Halaska M, Voigt R. Ultrasound imaging of the urethral sphincter. Ceska Gynekol. 1997;62(6):330-2.
36. Dietz HP, Wilson PD, Clarke B. The use of perineal ultrasound to quantify levator activity and teach pelvic floor muscle exercises. Int Urogynecol J Pelvic Floor Dysfunct. 2001;12(3):166-8.
37. Viereck V, Bader W, Skala C, Gauruder-Burmester A, Emons G, Hilgers R, Krauss T. Determination of bladder neck position by intraoperative introital ultrasound in colposuspension:outcome at 6-month follow-up. Ultrasound Obstet Gynecol. 2004;24(2):186-91.
38. Umek WH, Laml T, Stutterecker D, Obermair A, Leodolter S, Hanzal E. The urethra during pelvic floor contraction: observations on three-dimensional ultrasound. Obstet Gynecol. 2002;100(4):796-800.
39. Dietz HP, Shek C, Clarke B. Biometry of the pubovisceral muscle and levator hiatus by three-dimensional pelvic floor ultrasound. Ultrasound Obstet Gynecol. 2005;25(6):580-5.
40. Unger CA, Weinstein MM, Pretorius DH. Pelvic Floor Imaging. Ultrasound Clinics. 2010;5(2):313-30.
41. Kruger JA, Heap SW, Murphy BA, et al. Pelvic floor function in nulliparous women using three-dimensional ultrasound and magnetic resonance imaging. Obstet Gynecol. 2008;111(3):631-8.
42. Weinstein MM, Jung SA, Pretorius DH, Nager CW, den Boer DJ, Mittal RK. The reliability of puborectalis muscle measurements with 3-dimensional ultrasound imaging. Am J Obstet Gynecol. 2007;197(1):68.e1-e6.
43. Deindl FM, Vodusek DB, Hesse U, Schüssler B. Activity patterns of pubococcygeal muscles in nulliparous continent women. Br J Urol. 1993;72(1):46-51.
44. Peschers UM, Voduek DB, Fanger G, Schaer GN, DeLancey JO, Schuessler B. Pelvic muscle activity in nulliparous volunteers. Neurourol Urodyn. 2001;20(3):269-75.
45. Yang JM, Yang SH, Huang WC. Biometry of the pubovisceral muscle and levator hiatus in nulliparous Chinese women. Ultrasound Obstet Gynecol. 2006;28(5):710-6.
46. Sapsford RR, Hodges PW, Richardson CA, Cooper DH, Markwell SJ, Jull GA. Co-activation of the abdominal and pelvic floor muscles during voluntary exercises. Neurourol Urodyn. 2001;20(1):31-42.
47. Jung SA, Pretorius DH, Padda BS, Weinstein MM, Nager CW, den Boer DJ, et al. Vaginal high-pressure zone assessed by dynamic 3-dimensional ultrasound images of the pelvic floor. Am J Obstet Gynecol. 2007;197(1):52.e1-e7.
48. Abdool Z, Shek KL, Dietz HP. The effect of levator avulsion on hiatal dimension and function. Am J Obstet Gynecol. 2009;201(1):89.e1-e5.
49. Poon CI, Zimmern PE. Role of three-dimensional ultrasound in assessment of women undergoing urethral bulking agent therapy. Curr Opin Obstet Gynecol. 2004;16(5):411-7.
50. Dietz HP, Wilson PD. The 'iris effect': how two-dimensional and three-dimensional ultrasound can help us understand anti-incontinence procedures. Ultrasound Obstet Gynecol. 2004;23(3):267-71.
51. Dietz HP, Haylen BT, Broome J. Ultrasound in the quantification of female pelvic organ prolapse. Ultrasound Obstet Gynecol. 2001;18:511-4.
52. Dietz H. Ultrasound Imaging of the pelvic floor. Part 1: two-dimensional aspects. Ultrasound Obstet Gynecol. 2004;23:80-92.
53. Dietz H. Ultrasound imaging of the pelvic floor. Part 2: three-dimensional or volume imaging. Ultrasound Obstet Gynecol. 2004;23:615-25.
54. Masata J, Martan A, Svabik K, Drahoradova P, Pavlikova M. Ultrasound imaging of the lower urinary tract after successful tension-free vaginal tape (TVT) procedure. Ultrasound Obstet Gynecol. 2006;28:221-8.
55. Tunn R, Picot A, Marschke J, Gauruder-Burmester A. Sonomorphological evaluation of polypropylene mesh implants after vaginal mesh repair in women with cystocele or rectocele. Ultrasound Obstet Gynecol. 2007;29:449-52.
56. Schuettoff S, Beyersdorff D, Gauruder-Burmester A, Tunn R. Visibility of the polypropylene tape after TVT (tension-free vaginal tape) procedure in women with stress urinary incontinence- a comparison of introital ultrasound and MRI in vitro and in patients. Ultrasound Obstet Gynecol. 2006;27:687-92.
57. Dietz H, Lanzarone V. Levator trauma after vaginal delivery. Obstet Gynecol. 2005;106:707-12.
58. Dietz HP, Steensma AB. The prevalence of major abnormalities of the levator ani in urogynaecological patients. BJOG. 2006;113:225-30.

64

CHAPTER

Three/Four-dimensional, Vocal, HDlive and Silhouette Ultrasound in Obstetrics, Reproduction and Gynecology

Juan Carlos Castillo, Francisco Raga, Oscar Caballero, Francisco Bonilla Jr, Fernando Bonilla-Musoles

OBSTETRICS: FIRST AND SECOND TRIMESTER NORMAL FETAL SCAN

INTRODUCTION

In recent years, the three/four-dimensional ultrasound (3D/4D US) has reached a worldwide spread in the obstetric and gynecology fields, and nowadays, it takes part of all diagnostic areas that aim to be comprehended.

The existing world literature on this subject is so vast that, in our view, a new review is meaningless unless, as we intend, it brings something to improve the image quality to make the diagnosis easier.

The image quality only improved dramatically when we began to use higher sound frequencies and, more recently for the fact of having applied the most modern ultrasound, such as the 3D/4D and their modes (STIC, spatial temporal image correlation; AVC, automatic volume calculation; VOCAL, virtual organ computer-aided analysis and the inverse mode), and more recently the HDlive and radiance system architecture (RSA) also called silhouette.

In this chapter, we are going to show normal images and curious cases of malformations that have been observed recently with the use of 3D/4D, HDlive and silhouette. They can demonstrate that these new technologies are really useful.

Referring to the 3D/4D bibliography, we have only showed quotations by some authors, among us; the most published ones in this field.

Concerning the HDlive in Obstetrics, the literature, even being poor, is enough to show that in fact the HDlive improves the quality of the images whose beauty and sharpness are superior to the 3D/4D sonographic ones.

These reviews in early and advanced pregnancies include both normal and pathological features, images on the fetal development and behavior, isolated cases of singleton or normal twin pregnancies, facial expressions, morphological studies of the heart, and sight of the uvula. Moreover, some specific pathology such as hygroma colli, sirenomelia without skulls/exencephaly, meconium peritonitis, twin reversed arterial perfusion (TRAP) sequence, Turner syndrome or placental abnormalities, such as circumvallate placenta or thrombosed placental varicose vein. Concerning the silhouette, there is only a mention, with a small picture, in the case of circumvallate placenta recently described by AboEllail et al.

NORMAL HDLIVE IMAGE

We started presenting isolated images of normal pregnancies, which were examined with HDlive, and compared with conventional 3D, in order to show the high quality of the obtained images. If the use of 3D has already been a noticeable improvement, this new technology, which is easily applicable, is exceptional **(Figs. 1 to 3)**.

PATHOLOGICAL IMAGES USING 3D/4D ULTRASOUND AND HDLIVE

We will introduce some other examples of isolated malformations of the first and second trimester, which were studied with 3D/4D ultrasound and HDlive.

Double Yolk Sac

We show a 6-week gestation image of a double yolk sac in AVC, which can be clearly seen in red and blue. The HDlive allows us to see the embryo anchored to the endometrium, with the amniotic sac and the pathological vesicle **(Fig. 4)**.

Hygroma Colli

Figure 5 shows a typical case at 12 weeks of gestation with 2Dt, surface 3D and, cutting the cephalic pole through a ventricle and the lateral plexuses, the HDlive with

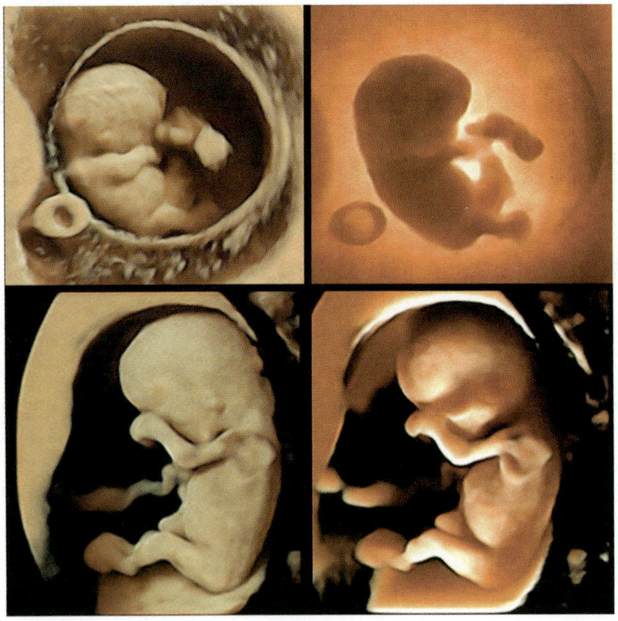

Fig. 1: Above, a 9-week-pregnancy HDlive shows the embryo profile with the virtual light source from the left. We show the whole embryo and the yolk sac from behind, with maximum luminescence. Besides the very pretty image of the embryo, we can see all the amnion and extraembryonic mesenchyme, which as you know, is not a fluid accumulation, but a mesenchyme with fibrillar part which is clearly seen in the picture; Below, a 14-week gestation, where there is a comparison between the fetal silhouette with lower (on the left) and higher brightness (on the right). The virtual light focus direction is from the left side of the fetus.

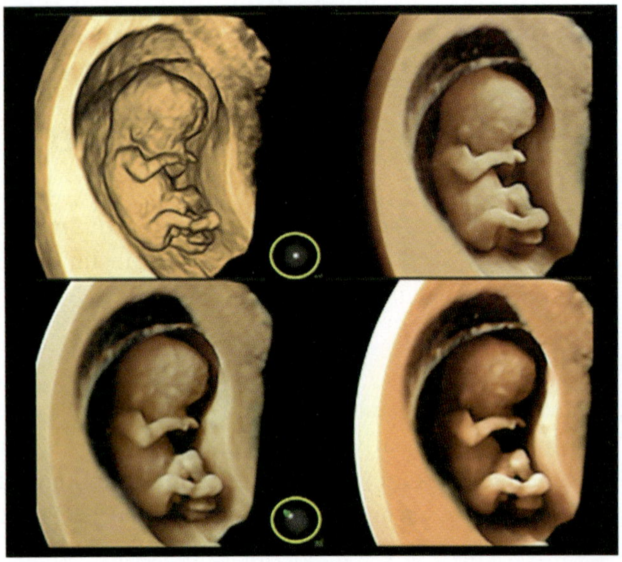

Fig. 2: A complete 13-week-gestation that is shown to compare the 3D (up and on the left) with the HDlive, using different light intensities and locations of the virtual light source (yellow circles). The anatomical details, which have been obtained in both the fetus in the amnion and the extracoelomic mesenchyme, are impressive.

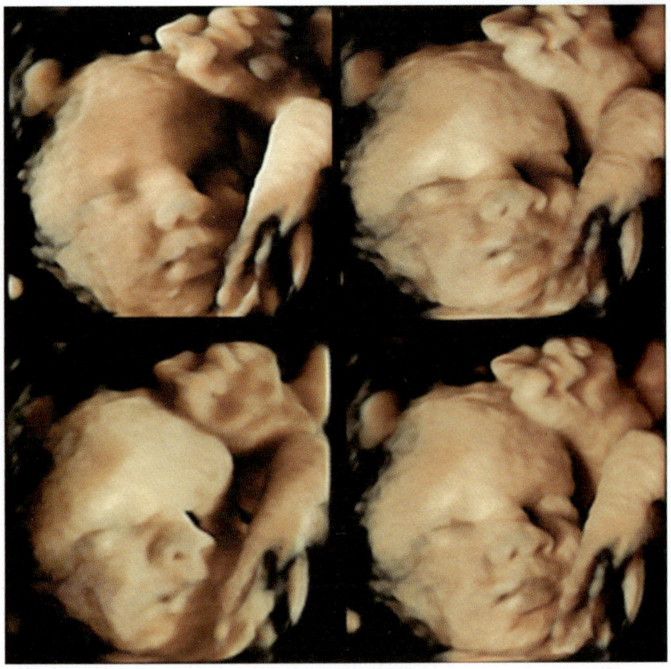

Fig. 3: Variable locations of virtual light source were used to take, with an HDlive, for 36-week facial profiles of the same fetus. The expressions obtained are incredibly beautiful.

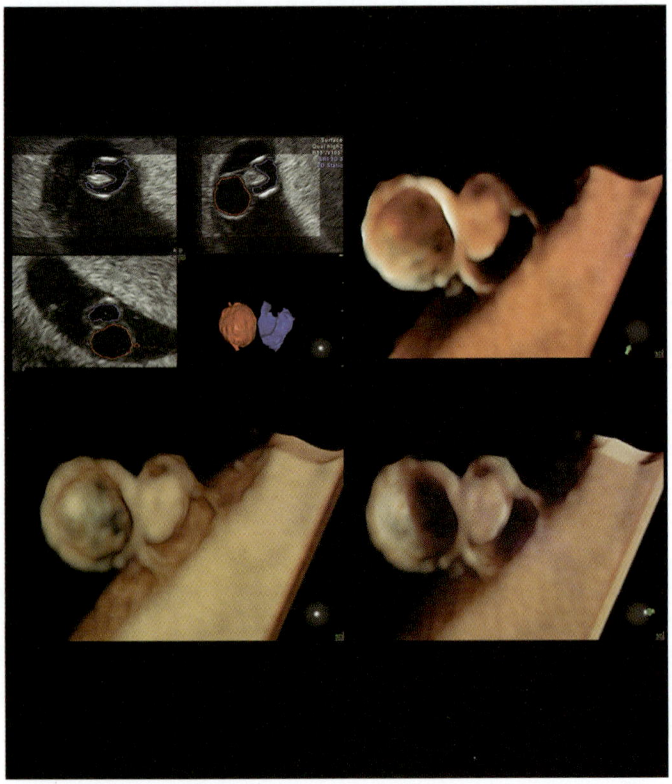

Fig. 4: A 6-week gestational image in orthogonal planes with TUI, AVC, and HDlive, clearly shows two yolk sacs.

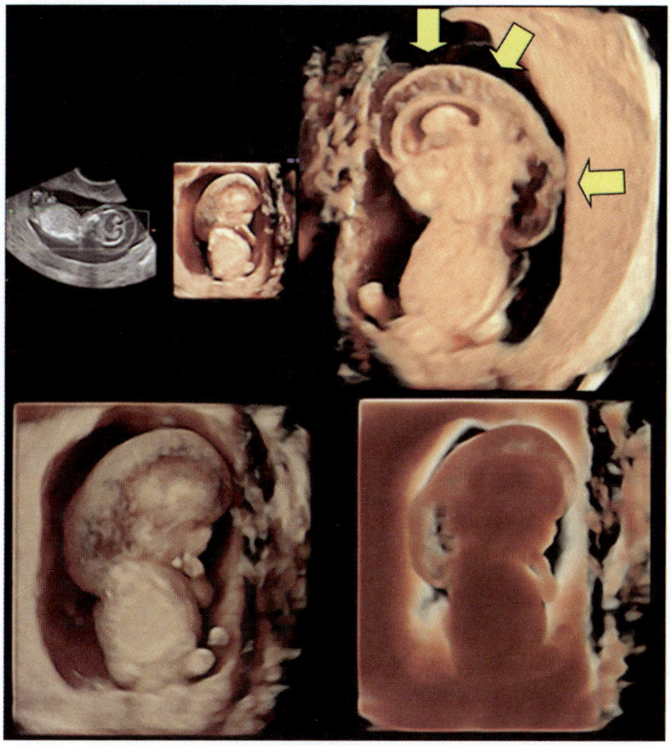

Fig. 5: Hygroma colli. Notice the easy perfect profile in HDlive. In yellow arrows, we have set the thin walls that mold in the magma of hygroma.

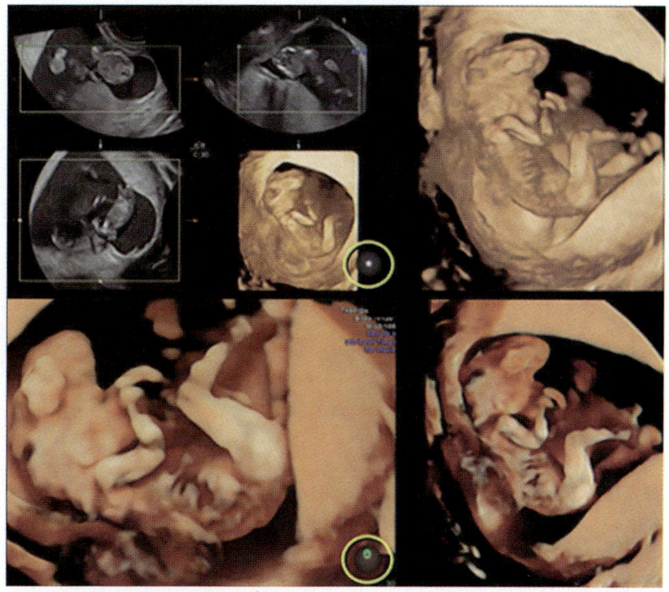

Fig. 6: Comparative study of anencephaly/exencephaly. 2D orthogonal planes (above and on the left), 3D (above and on the right), and HDlive (the two pictures below) of a 14-week fetus diagnosed with exencephaly are shown. The definitive diagnosis is obtained in the pathology of the fetal cranial pole. We can see the HDlive image with the "shadows and the chiaroscuros", which is infinitely superior to 2D/3D ultrasound.

maximum brightness. The HDlive image is extremely beautiful, the whole hygroma colli observed, and the most interesting is how it contains in its interior in addition to an accumulation of fluid, small partitions. These partitions follow the 45XO karyotypes almost in a pathognomonic way.

Anencephaly/Exencephaly/Acrania

This group of malformations has common origin which is the lack or incomplete development of the fetal scalp. Initially, there is a lack of bone development of frontal, temporal and occipital areas, generally the occipital, although it can affect even more skull bones.

In the early stages, the meningeal membranes are preserved, but they usually break in contact with the amniotic fluid.

The encephalic mass come into direct contact with the liquid, and expands and dilates outside the cephalic pole (exencephaly). Then, a nonbacterial encephalitis occurs with atrophy of the brain mass and change into an acrania. Precisely saying about this natural evolution, most of the acrania cases are diagnosed during an advanced pregnancy period. In this way, the diagnosis of exencephaly cases are rare and precocious, and even fewer the anencephaly ones **(Figs. 6 and 7)**.

Encephalocele (Cranium Bifidum)

It is a very rare congenital malformation, in which a diverticulum of the brain tissue and the meninges protrude through defects in the cranial vault.

It is derived from a failure of the closing of neural tube during embryonic development that takes place during the fourth week of gestation. Although its origin is not precisely known, it has been associated with a maternal deficiency in the levels of folic acid during pregnancy, as well as consequence of a trauma.

The brain and its coating stay outside the cranial pole, forming a protrusion, generally in occipital but also in the frontal or sincipital region. If only the ventricle protrudes, we call it as hydroencephalocele. If the meninges also protrude, we call it as meningohydroencephalocele. The tumor, almost permanently, is located in the occipital bone, from where part of the brain mass outputs **(Fig. 8)**.

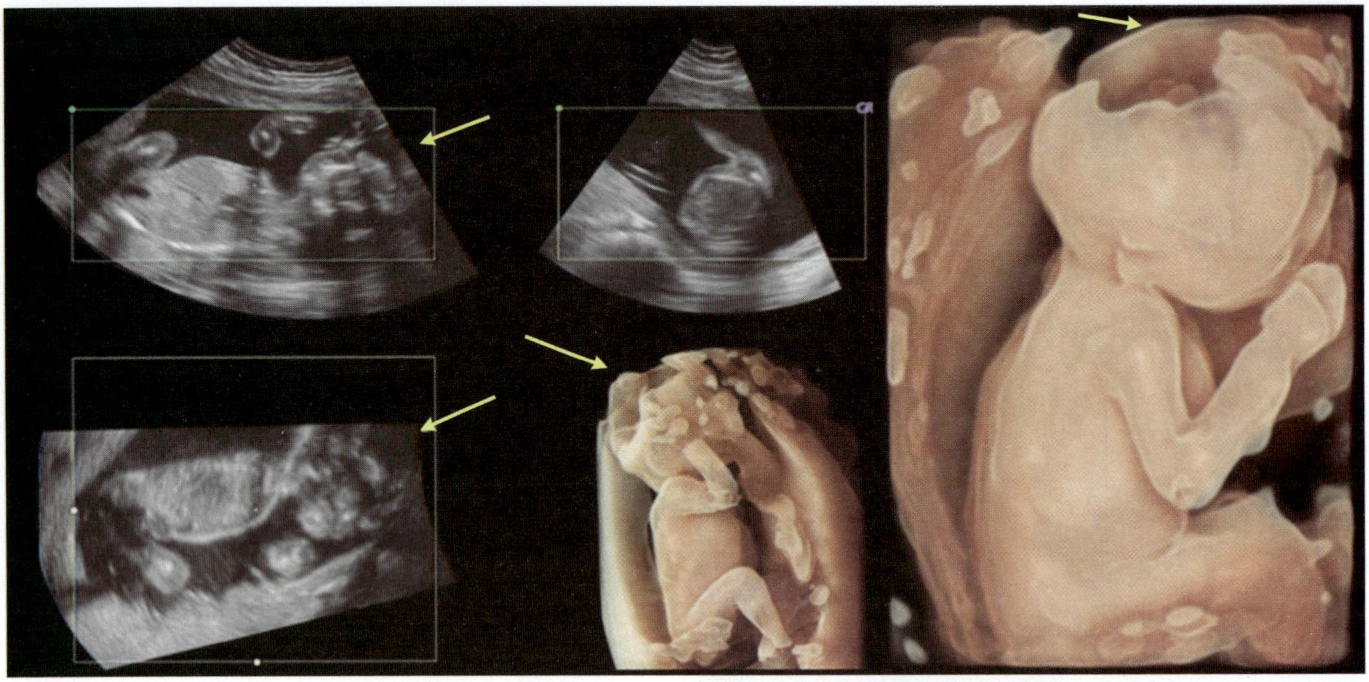

Fig. 7: Silhouette image of an acrania case. The yellow arrows show 2D orthogonal planes (on the left) and 3D radiance view of the cranial bone defect. This new technology that defines the edges very well allows us to see the defect clearly.

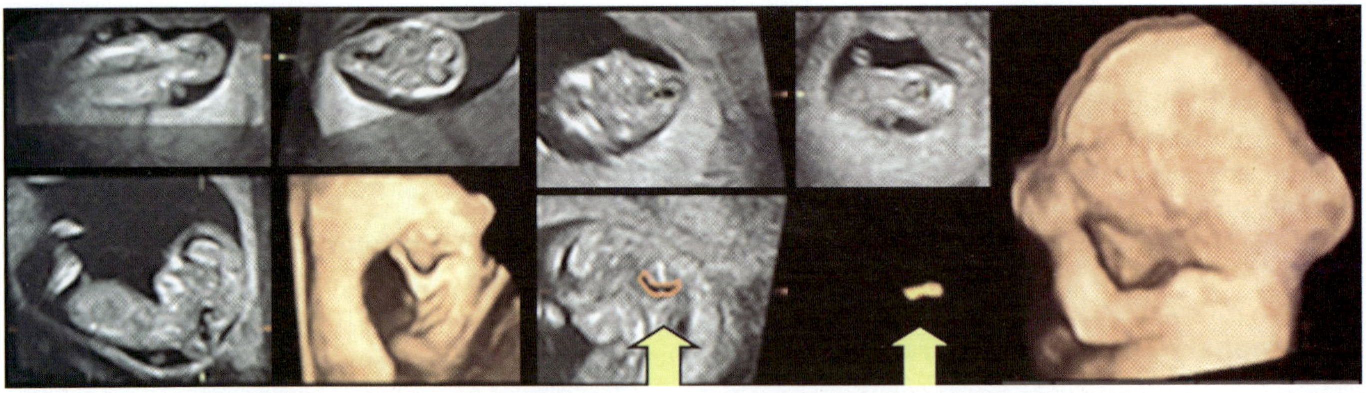

Fig. 8: Encephalocele (arrows). The image using 2D/3D ultrasound shows the occipital tumor.

Abdominal Wall Malformations

It includes:

- Omphaloceles
- Gastroschisis
- Cantrell pentalogy
- Extrophies
  - Vesical
  - Cloacal
- Ectopia cordis
- Limb-body wall complex
- Body-stalk complex

The most common defects are the omphalocele **(Fig. 9)** and gastroschisis **(Fig. 10)**.

Omphalocele

The omphalocele is caused by a closing defect of the two abdominal lateral valves. The defect is covered by an amniotic membrane, similar to the amnion from where the intestinal loops and/or liver go out. This anomaly almost always accompanies trisomy 18 **(Fig. 9)**.

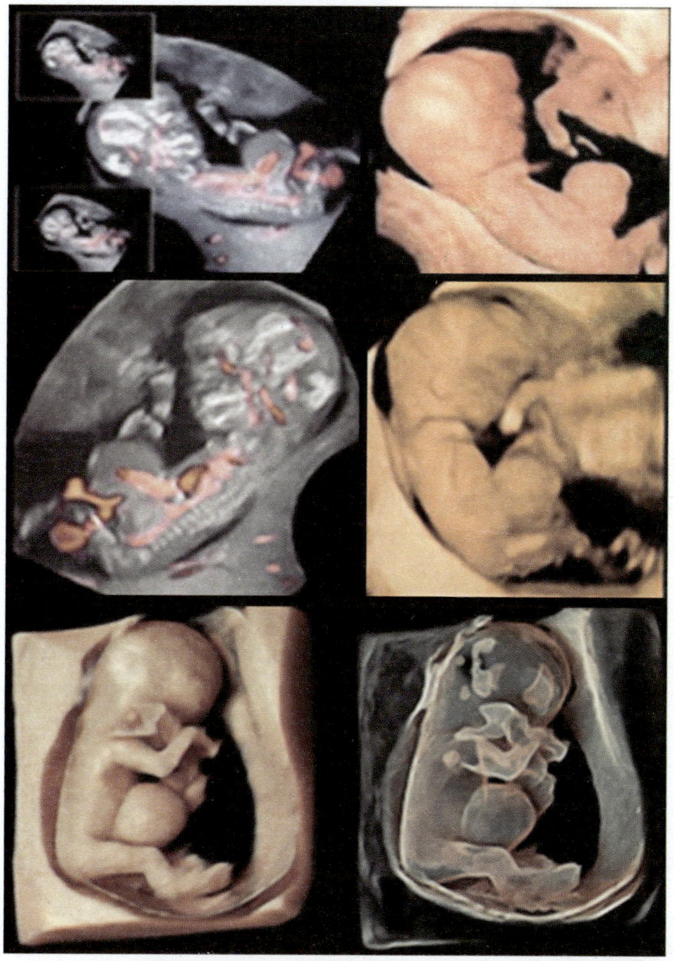

Fig. 9: Omphalocele examined on the 14th week, using a 2D glass-body rendering with Doppler angiography (above left), HDlive (above right) and 3D ultrasound (on the right and meddle). When using silhouette, we can more clearly notice the tumor in the abdominal wall, and how the vessels penetrate its interior because the liver occupies the tumor.

Gastroschisis

Gastroschisis is an authentic abdominal wall defect appearing on the left side of the umbilicus. Generally, it is small, not bigger than 1 cm, and produced by the atresia of one of the umbilical arteries. From the beginning of the intestinal peristalsis, around 14th week, the exit of the intestinal loops to the outside can be produced. They swim freely in the amniotic fluid. Only few exceptionally accompany chromosomopathies **(Fig. 10)**.

Cantrell Pentalogy

Characteristics of Cantrell pentalogy are listed as follows:
- Defect of the supraumbilical abdominal midline
- Defect of the lower sternum
- Defect of the anterior portion of the diaphragm
- Defect of the diaphragmatic pericardium and
- Intracardiac congenital malformations.

The frequency of the disease (2 in 1,700/2,000) is low with a reported prevalence of 0.079 per 10,000 live births.

The etiology is unknown, and it has been associated with the followings:
- Chromosomopathies such as Turner syndrome and trisomy 18
- The teratogen exposure, such as quinidine, warfarin, thalidomide
- Infectious agents, such as influenza infection
- Even vitamin A deficiency.

Although generally is considered as multicausal **(Fig. 11)**.

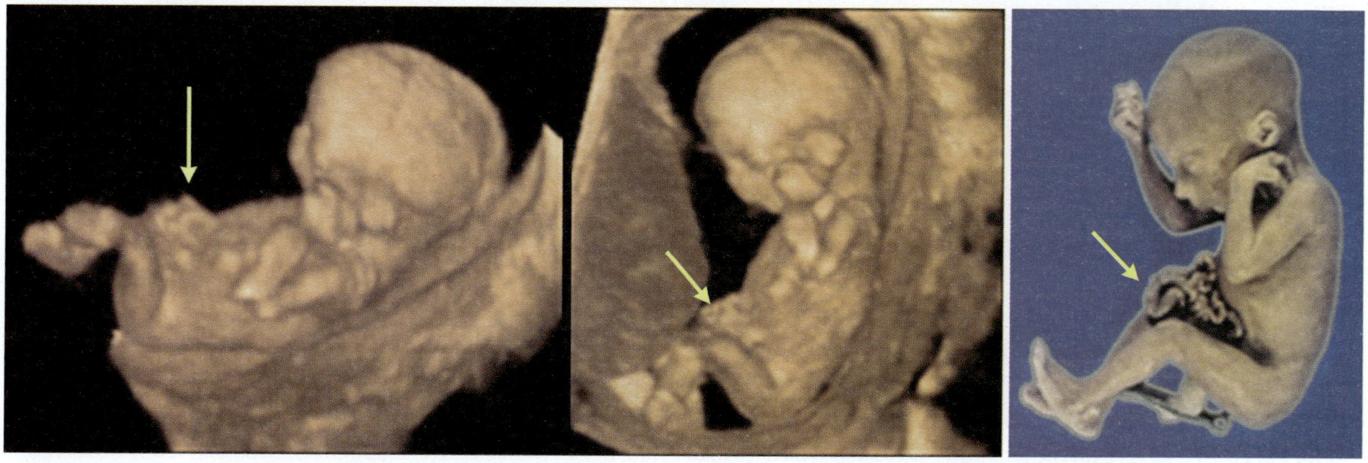

Fig. 10: A 16-week precocious case of gastroschisis (yellow arrows) seen with 3D ultrasound.

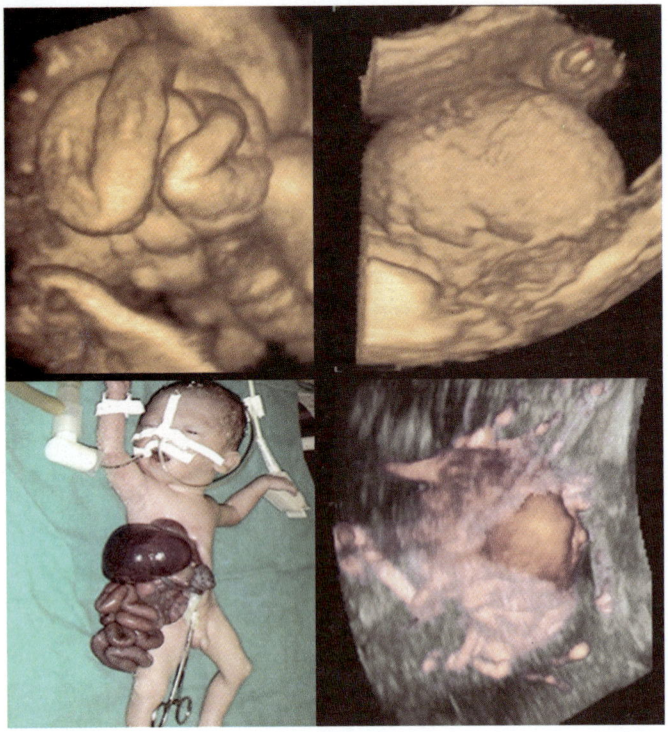

Fig. 11: Cantrell pentalogy depicted with 3D US (above) and 3D Doppler angiography (below right). We can observe the cardias exstrophy, the gastroschisis with liver and intestines protrude due to defect in the diaphragm and abdominal wall. The sternal injury is not shown in this case.

Prune Belly Syndrome

It is a rare congenital urologic obstructive defect with a megacystic bladder and visible deformity of the abdominal wall. The sonographic characteristic triad includes:

- Anterior abdominal wall distention with deficiency or absence of abdominal wall musculature.
- Megacystis, and
- Pulmonary hypoplasia.

Typical prune-belly syndrome has been considered secondary to connective tissue and smooth muscle abnormalities, which cause bladder distention, and result in oligohydramnios.

The major features are dilatation of the fetal urinary bladder and proximal urethra with thickening of the bladder wall.

The bladder wall hypertrophy is the result of the intra-vesical pressure generated secondary to obstruction. The urinary bladder fills the pelvis and the abdomen, and does not empty more often. The ureters are usually dilated, and hydronephrosis of variable degrees may be present.

A keyhole sign, which is a dilated prostatic urethra, frequently with distention of the prostatic utricle (utriculus prostaticus) and thickening of the bladder neck, is present **(Fig. 12)**.

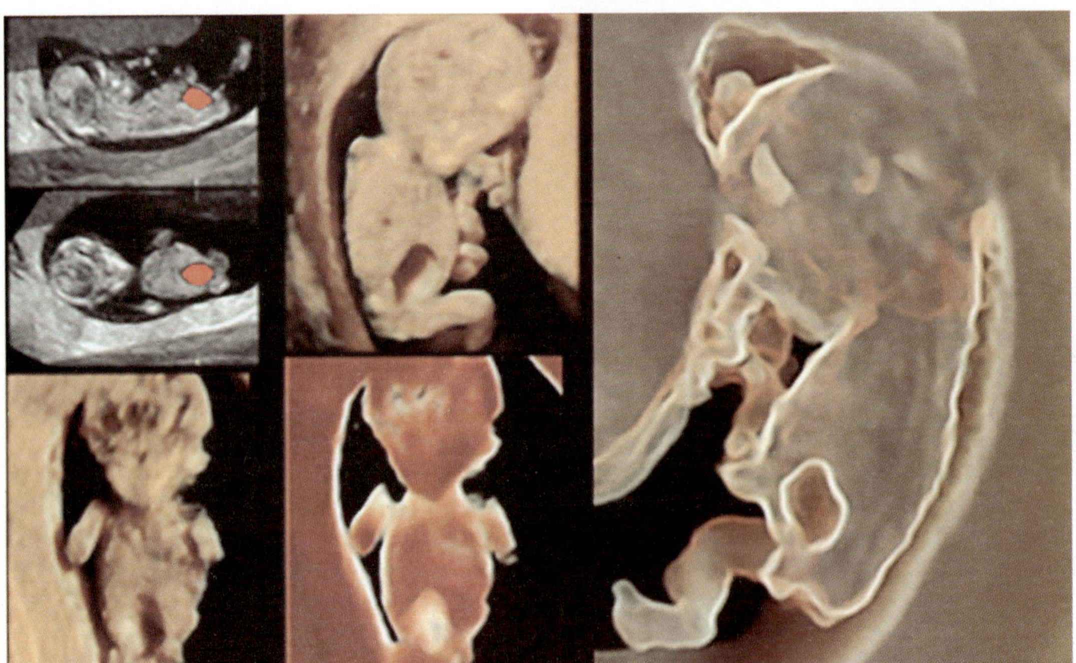

Fig. 12: 2D AVC (above on the left) and HDlive of a typical case of Prune Belly syndrome. The bladder distention is clearly observed, especially when using maximal luminiscence (below right) and silhouette (right).

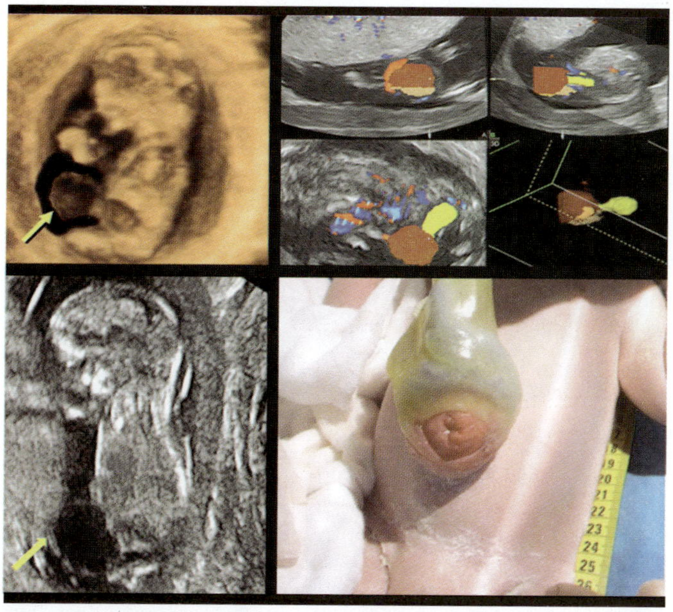

Fig. 13: Comparative images in 2D, 3D, Doppler, and inversion mode. The 3D image (above on the left) shows the tumor. The 2D image (below on the left) shows the tumor and how it communicates with the bladder (AVC). The inverse mode (above on the right) indicates clearly that these are two communicating cysts. The Doppler shows the vessels around the bladder and of the cyst moving towards the umbilical cord. SonoAVC image and correlation with the birth anomaly found the tumor in the base of the umbilical cord. We can see the vesical prolapse, and its mucosa going outside.

Persistent Urachus with Bladder Prolapse: Bladder Exstrophy Variety

It is a rare abnormality that occurs in 1/100,000 newborns. Urachal anomalies occur due to the failure of obliteration, resulting in different pathologies, such as its persistence, cysts, sinus or bladder-urachal diverticula.

The ultrasound most common feature is the presence of a cystic mass located at the base of the umbilical cord, communicating with the bladder and flanked by the umbilical arteries. The use of the Sono AVC, allows us to identify and quantify hypoechoic areas, evaluating their absolute dimensions, average diameter and volume **(Fig. 13)**.

Pyelocalyceal Ectasia

Of all the urinary anomalies, the dilatations are the most common, and can affect the pelvis, calices, ureters and bladder. To carry out an evaluation, it is required to take into account the followings:

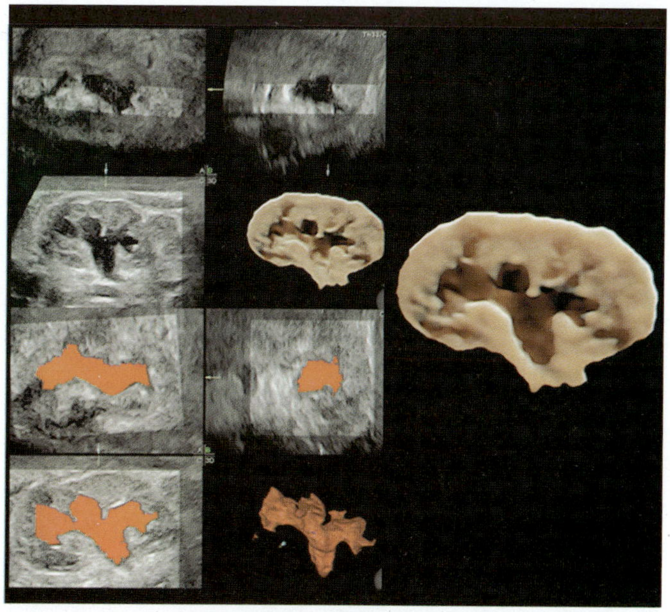

Fig. 14: Pyelocalyceal dilation studied with 2D sonography, sonoAVC (on the left), and with HDlive (on the right).

- *Intensity of dilation level:* The larger, the more likely to be associated with an obstructive process, but the dilation is not synonymous to obstruction
- *Dilation: Unilateral or bilateral*
- *Characteristics of the renal parenchyma:* The presence of a renal dysplasia is associated with poor prognosis
- *Fetal renal function:* It is estimated by analyzing the volume of the amniotic fluid and the analytical study of the fetal urine. The appearance of an oligohydramnios or the presence of fetal hypertonic urine indicates kidney malfunction.

The use of 3D/4D US and their different modes is very useful in the study of internal organic malformations. **Figure 14** shows a 30-week fetal kidney studied in 2D, Vocal and HDlive, presenting a remarkable pelvic dilatation.

RADIANCE SYSTEM ARCHITECTURE (RAS) OR SILHOUETTE HDLIVE

In the literature, there are only a small number of references to this new mode:

- A case of circumvallate placenta
- A right aortic arch with an aberrant left subclavian artery
- A jejunal atresia
- An outstanding review of the normal embryo and fetuses.

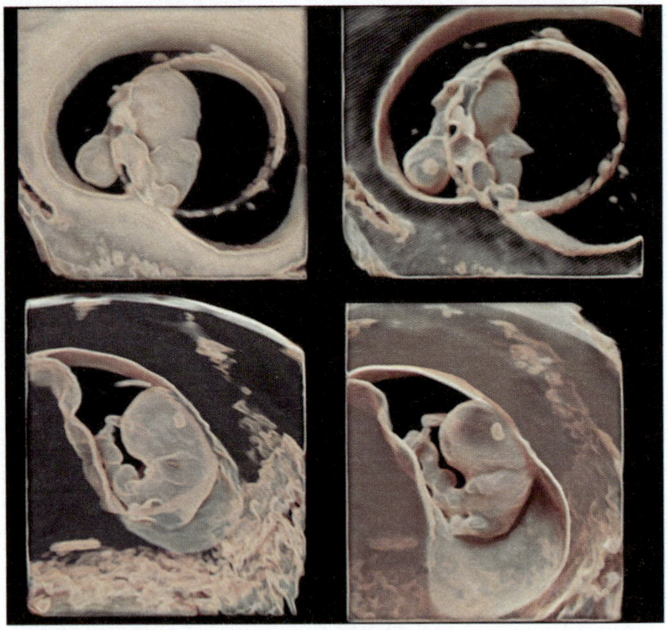

Fig. 15: Nine-week gestation with four images with lower and higher "brightness". Observe the perfect definition of contours of the fetus, the amnion, the yolk sac, and the gestational sac. We are standing in front of a new sonographic view of the gestation.

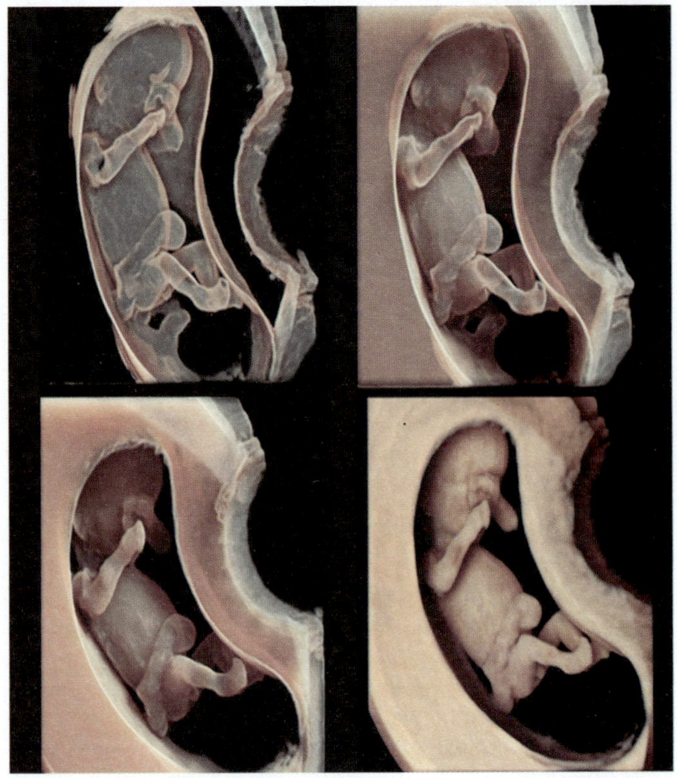

Fig. 16: Silhouette (above), and HDlive (below) pictures of a normal 10-week gestation. It is really amazing the obtained definition of the fetal image. It can be clearly observed the delimitation of the hands, cord, and the physiologic herniation.

Before their description in a series of pregnancy images studied week by week (see below), we provide some pictures of the first- and second-trimester normal pregnancy, in order the readers can have an idea of it diagnostic possibilities, which at first sight, seem to revolutionize the results **(Figs. 15 to 20)**.

COMMENTS TO THESE NEW US MODES

Despite the remarkable improvement in the image quality that involves the introduction of these new technologies shown in this article, they do not invalidate the entire "prenatal diagnosis level I and II" of 13–14 and 18–24 weeks, which will keep on being held by the 2D ultrasound. What these new applications show are the fantastic advance in image quality which supposed, on one hand, the introduction of 3D/4D ultrasound, and on the other hand, more recently, the new HDlive and "silhouette" modes. We think that the latter two technologies should be used in clinical practice, and that they can be arranged in those hospitals with the facilities of specialized "prenatal diagnosis" units.

The 3D/4D ultrasound has already been practically a routine, but not the last two we highlighted and that we think, are going to be essential in the very near future.

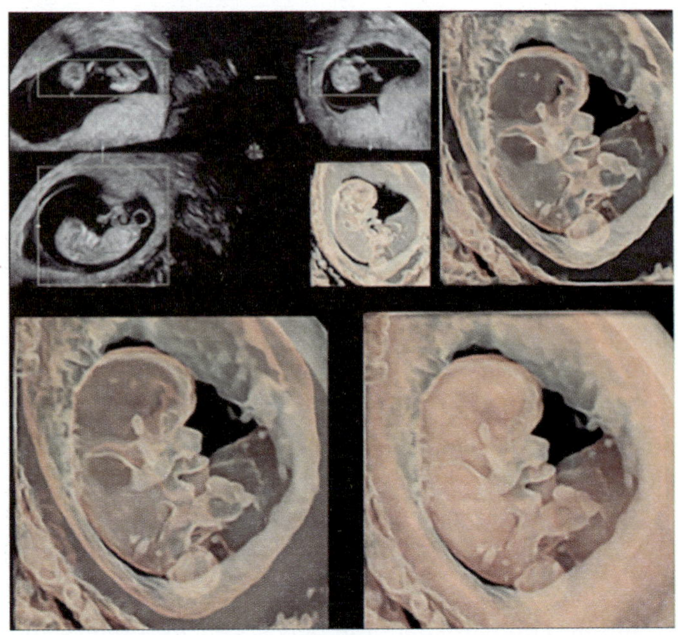

Fig. 17: Normal fetal images in 2D orthogonal planes and "radiance" with less and more "brightness" at 10 weeks of gestation. We can see all its external and internal structures.

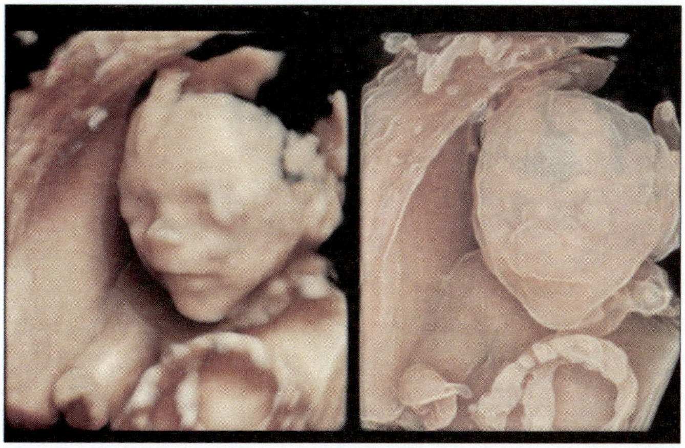

Fig. 18: Compare the HDlive (left) and the silhouette (right) fetal images at 22 weeks of gestation. The most striking aspect is the perfect delimitation of all the structures such as the umbilical cord.

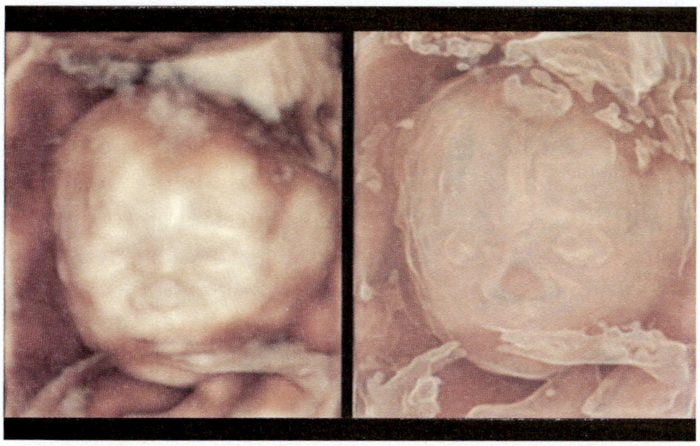

Fig. 19: Two faces of the same 24-week fetus with less (left, HDlive) and more luminous "brightness" (right, RAS). Highlight for the perfect delimitation of its structures is evident.

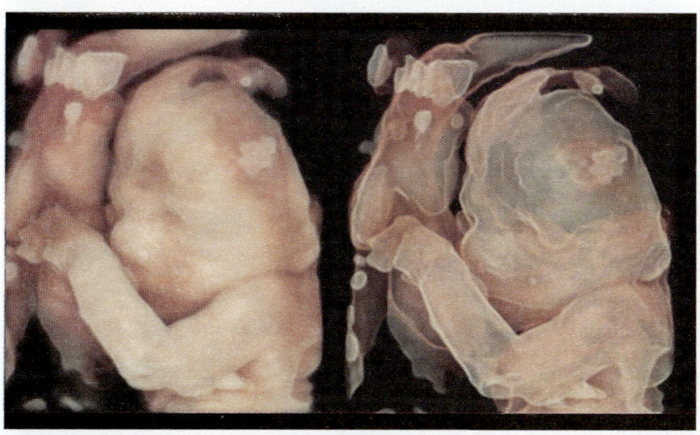

Fig. 20: Complete 25-week gestation fetal profile observed with the "radiance" system which allows us to clearly see all surface delimitation.

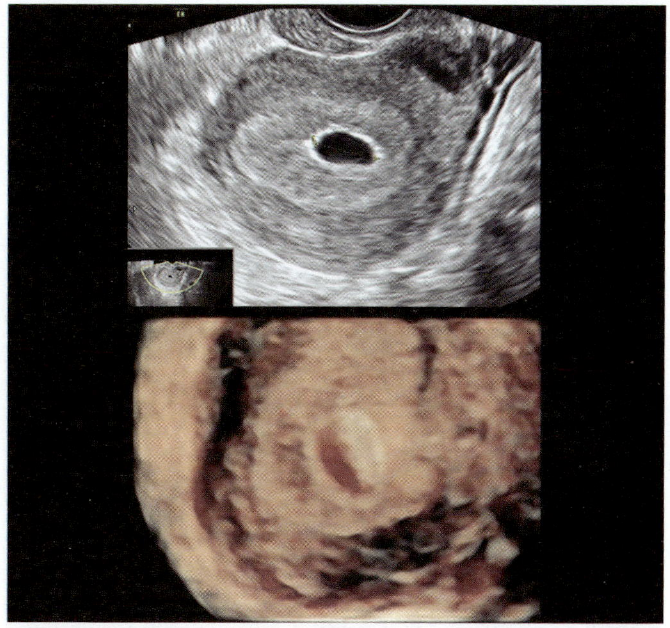

Fig. 21: A pregnancy of 31-day showing a well-delimited single intrauterine gestational sac. Left: 2D US and right: 3D view.

Any high-level hospital (Level III) has obstetrics of such prenatal diagnosis units, therefore, they must adapt.

We focus this work just to show these advances, instead of trying to make a new "descriptive summary" of existing malformations, and they can be seen with 3D/4D ultrasound. The reason is that it is sufficient to observe the reduced bibliography we have brought (a small sample of the existing one), that we have studied only three authors who have worked hard in this area (Hata, Kurjak, and our group) to show the readers that it is not more accurate and descriptive work malformations that this is the right direction to follow.

Herein, we will describe important features during pregnancy by using these new technologies.

DAY-BY-DAY ULTRASONOGRAPHIC CHARACTERISTICS BETWEEN THE 28 DAYS AND 35 DAYS OF PREGNANCY (4TH TO 5TH WEEK)

Day 28: The patient becomes amenorrheic. The endometrium looks decidualized. An active corpus luteum is pathognomonic. Neither of these findings constitutes a definitive diagnosis of pregnancy.

Day 31: The gestational sac appears **(Figs. 21 and 22)**. This finding constitutes the first ultrasonographic evidence of a pregnancy.

Day 32: The yolk sac appears and the omphalomesenteric duct can be seen **(Figs. 23 to 26)**.

Day 33: The embryonic disk appears **(Figs. 26 to 29)**.

Day 35: The embryo heart beat can be observed by using 2D/3D and Doppler US.

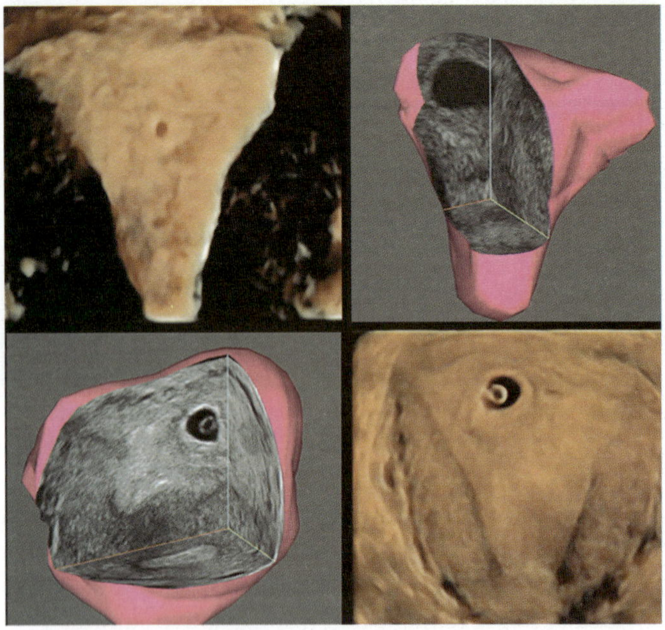

Fig. 22: Upper left: HDlive image showing a 2–3 mm gestational sac (corresponding to a 31–32 days pregnancy). Upper right: Gestational sac on "niche" mode. Bottom: Outstanding images of a gestational sac with the yolk sac.

On day 32 the most characteristic feature is the visualization of the yolk sac which appears as a round structure occupying the major part of the gestational sac. It is always round with clear boundaries. The yolk sac is the first embryonic structure seen on a US scan, not because being the first in appearing but the biggest at this stage **(Fig. 23)**.

On days 33–35 the most important features are:

- The visualization of the embryonic disk **(Figs. 24 to 29)**
- The embryo becomes visible when measuring 2–3 mm **(Figs. 28 to 29)**
- The embryo develops at a rate of 1 mm/daily
- The embryo heart beat appears within the endocardiac tubes on day 34–35.

ULTRASONOGRAPHIC CHARACTERISTICS BETWEEN THE 5TH AND 6TH WEEK

The gestational sac develops at a rate of 1.15 mm daily; whereas the embryo develops at a slower rate: 1 mm/day and the yolk sac at 1 mm per week. Thus, in only few days the embryo appears bigger than the yolk sac. Simultaneously, the omphalomesenteric duct (the future umbilical cord) develops very fast; this feature allows for a better visualization of the embryo and the yolk sac **(Fig. 30)**. Finally the embryo becomes larger due to the development of the notochord.

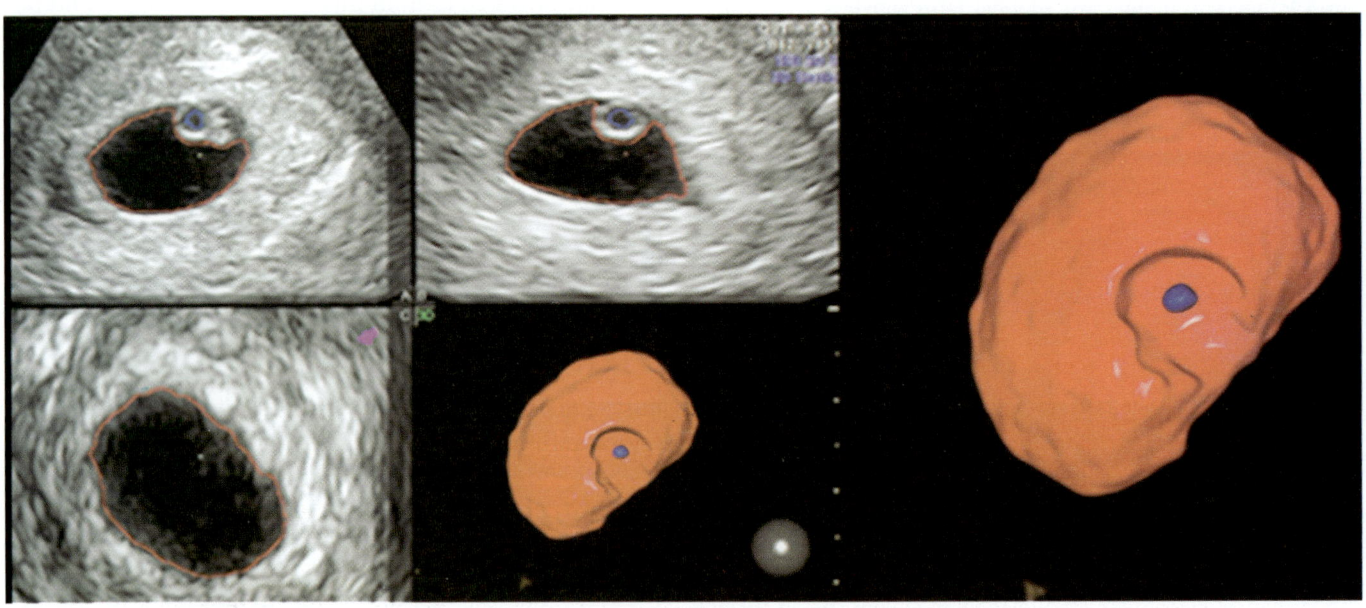

Fig. 23: Orthogonal plane and VOCAL 3D rendering of a gestational sac (red) with a yolk sac (blue).

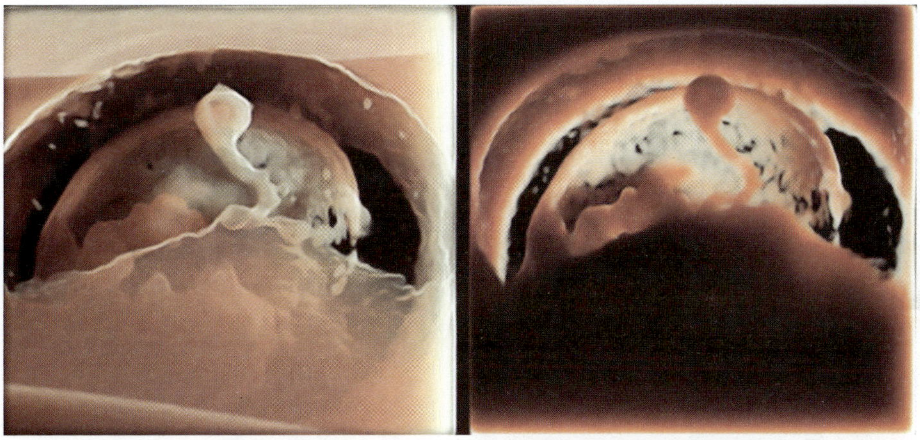

Fig. 24: HDlive silhouette: Yolk sac and amnios.

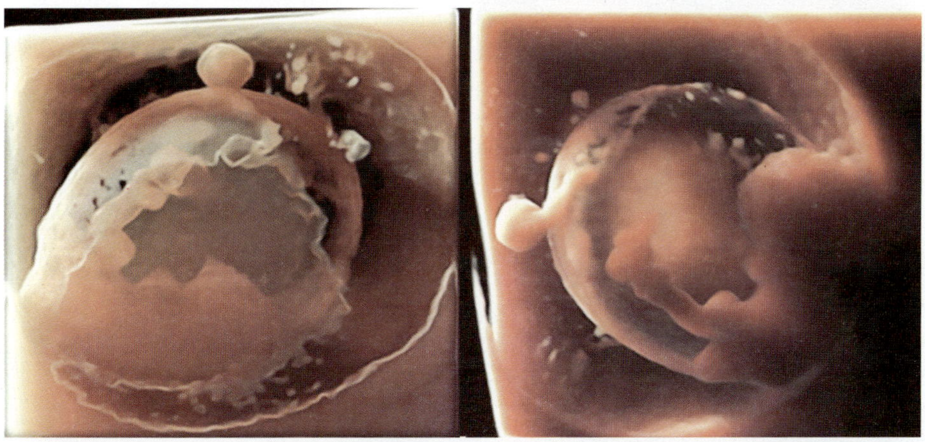

Fig. 25: HDlive silhouette: Outstanding image of an embryo, the omphalomesenteric duct, the yolk sac and the amniotic sac.

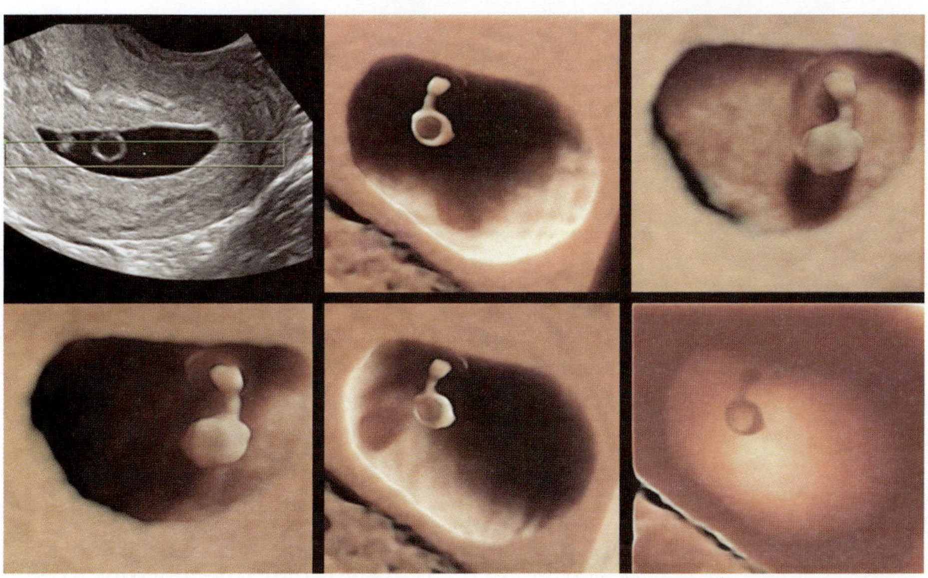

Fig. 26: 3D HDlive: A beautiful image of a gestational sac with an embryonic disk and the yolk sac. Notice the omphalomesenteric duct connecting the embryo to the yolk sac. The amniotic sac is also clearly depicted.

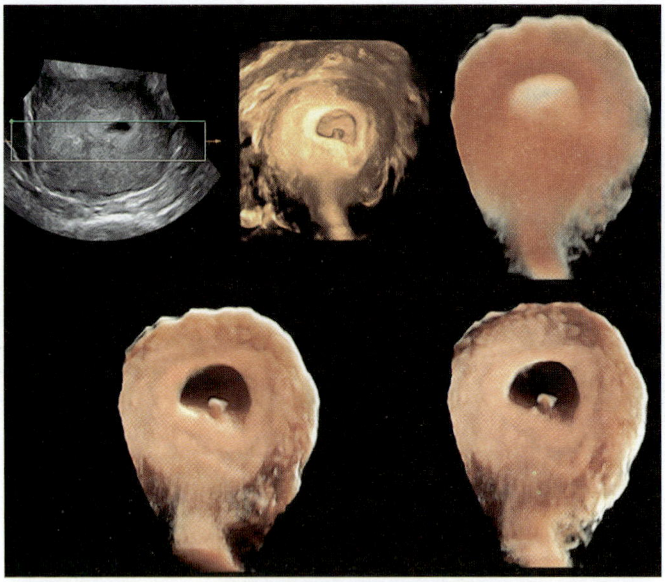

Fig. 27: A pregnancy of 34 days. Multimodalic view of the embryonic disk and the gestational sac. Upper left: 2D. Upper middle: 3D standard. Upper right: HDlive transparency mode Bottom: HDlive.

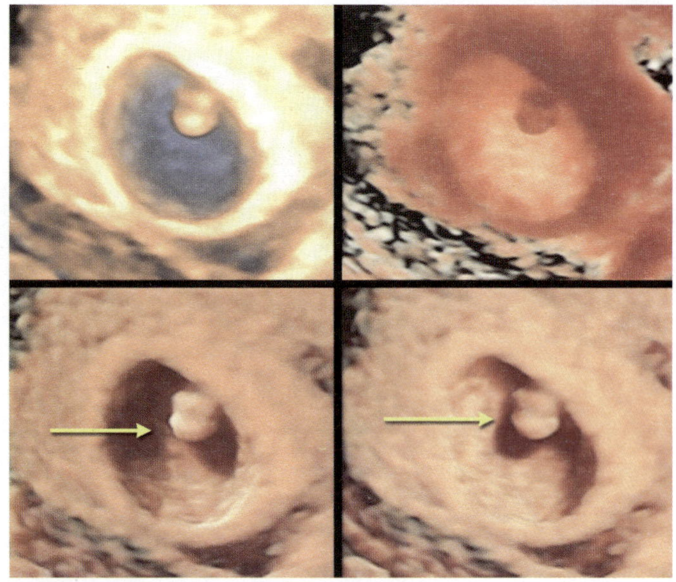

Fig. 28: Multimodalic view of a gestational sac containing the embryo (yellow arrow) and the yolk sac; both structures are about the same size.

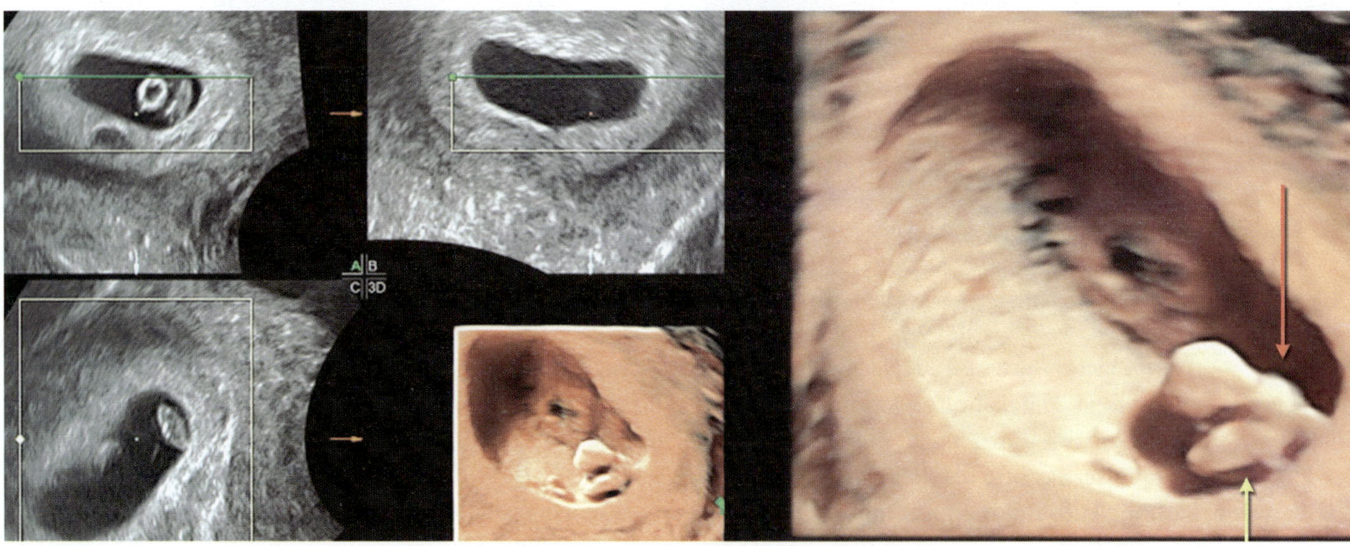

Fig. 29: A 38-day pregnancy. The embryonic disk (yellow arrow) is located beneath the yolk sac. The omphalomesenteric duct is also depicted (pink arrow).

ULTRASONOGRAPHIC CHARACTERISTICS BETWEEN THE 6TH AND 7TH WEEK

The key features are as follows:

- A fast development of the gestational sac and embryo
- The embryonic disk presents a caudal and cranial pole
- The cauda appears in the caudal pole **(Fig. 31)**
- In the opposite zone of omphalomesenteric duct the embryonic disk
- The amnion membrane covers the embryo. It fills with the amniotic fluid which causes the amnion to expand and become the amniotic sac. The yolk sac is displaced towards the extraembryonic coelom
- At the end of this week it is possible to watch the limb buds **(Fig. 32)**.

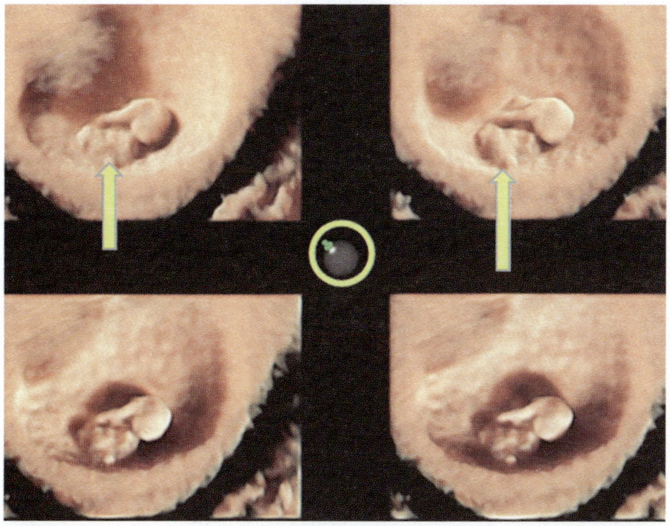

Fig. 30: HDlive view showing a large omphalomesenteric duct located above the embryonic disk (yellow arrow); whilst the yolk sac appears lateral to the right.

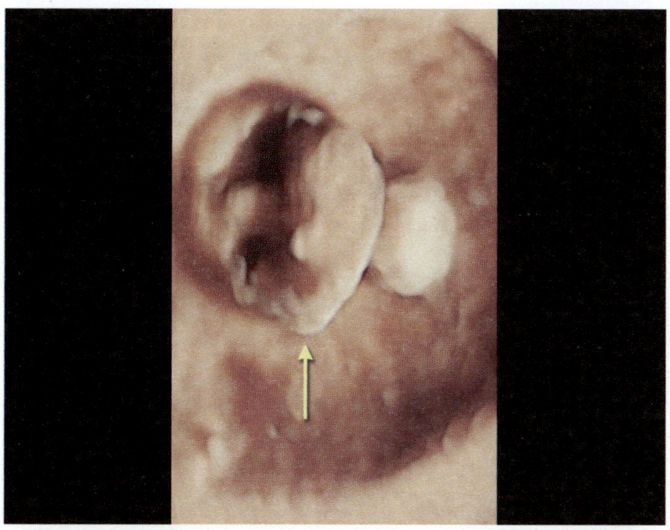

Fig. 31: HDlive view. Notice the embryo with the cranial and caudal pole, the limb buds, the omphalomesenteric duct and the yolk sac. The cauda is evident in the caudal pole (yellow arrow).

ULTRASONOGRAPHIC CHARACTERISTICS IN THE 7TH WEEK

Figures 32 to 34 show the main ultrasonographic differences compared to the previous week.

- The embryonic disk is bigger
- There is a clear definition of the fetal poles. In fact, there is a distinct zone between the cranial pole and the chest (the neck)
- The early spine is seen on the back of the embryo

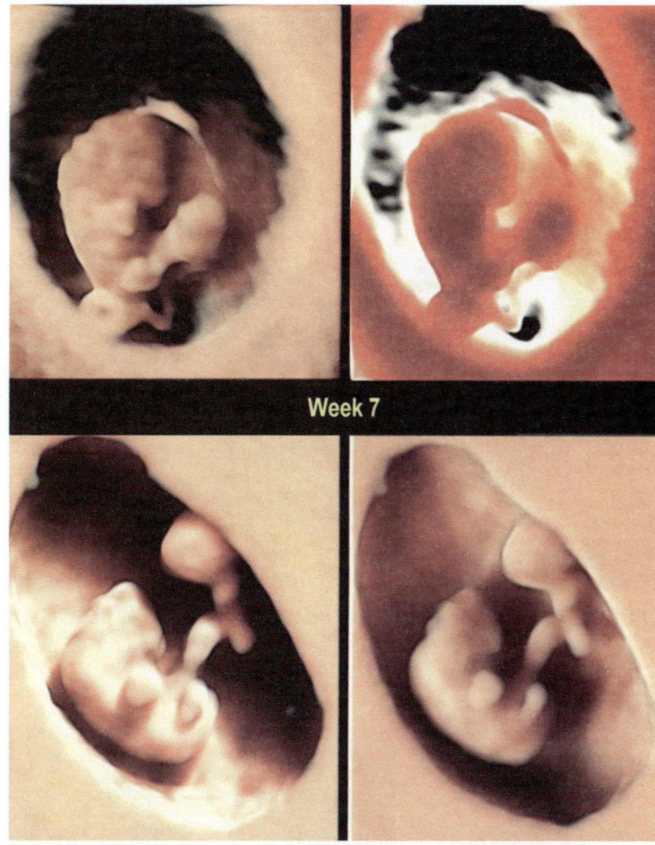

Fig. 32: Notice the bigger embryonic size. The separation of the cranial pole and chest by of the neck becomes evident. The limb buds become bigger and gross. Underneath the lower limb buds the cauda appears. The amnion is clearly seen (upper images). The yolk sac is located adjacent to the right gestational sac wall.

- The most characteristic feature is the visualization of the limbs
- The embryo is able to arch its back and neck and shows sudden and fast movements
- The embryo is closely covered by the amnion.

ULTRASONOGRAPHIC CHARACTERISTICS IN THE 8TH WEEK

The key-features are as follows **(Figs. 35 to 41)**:

- The clear visualization of the cranial pole
- The visualization of the embryonic movements
- A clear visualization of the limb buds, including the hand buds
- The physiologic herniation appears.
- The rhombencephalon or hindbrain also kwon as the "posterior cephalic cyst" continues its development **(Fig. 37)**
- The amnion reaches full development **(Fig. 35)**.

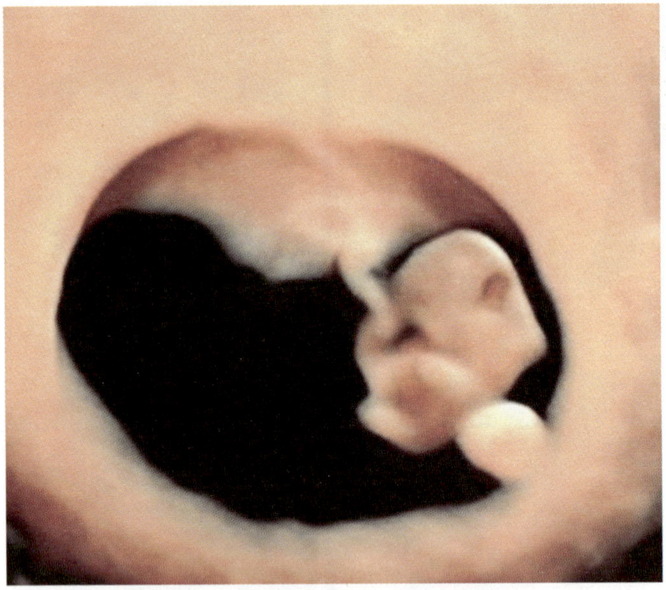

Fig. 33: An embryo of a gestational age of 7 weeks and 5 days. The rhombencephalon appears as a "hole" within the cranial pole.

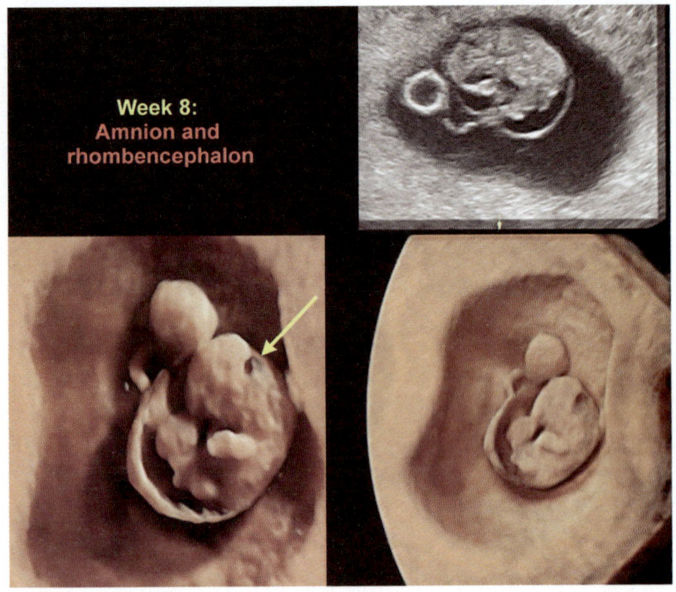

Fig. 35: An embryo of a gestational age of 8 weeks. A side view showing the limb buds, the rhombencephalon (yellow arrow) and the amnion.

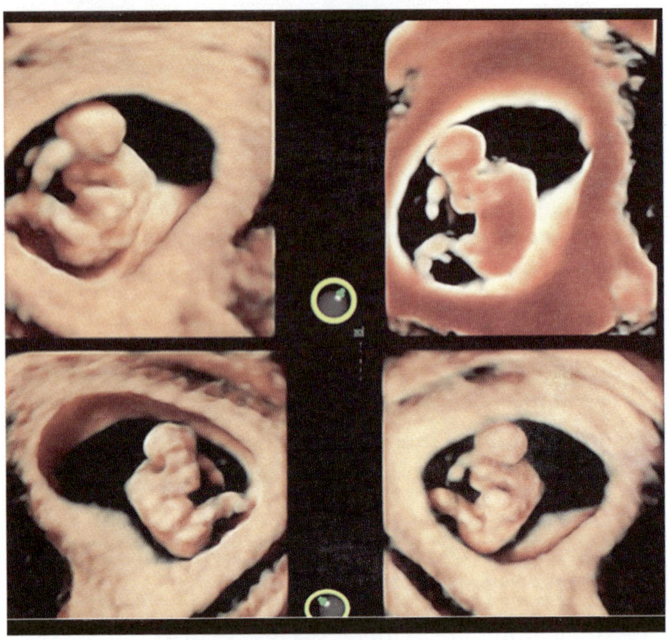

Fig. 34: Outstanding HDlive images using virtual light and translucency modes. Notice the yolk sac and the limb buds.

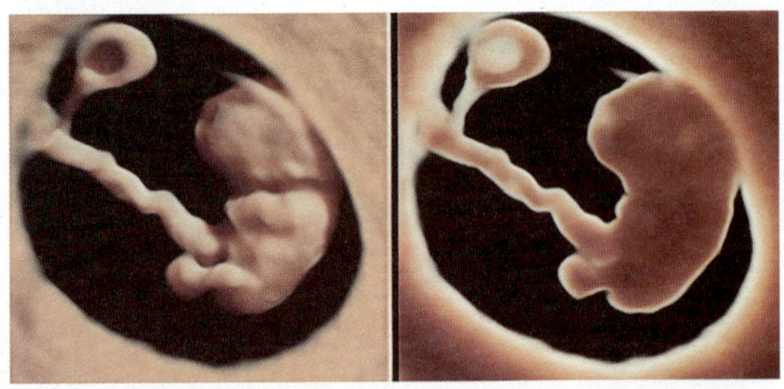

Fig. 36: An embryo of a gestational age of 8 weeks. Complete visualization of the hand and foot buds. Also the ear buds can be depicted. The umbilical cord is already spiralized and the yolk sac is located within the extraembryonic coelom.

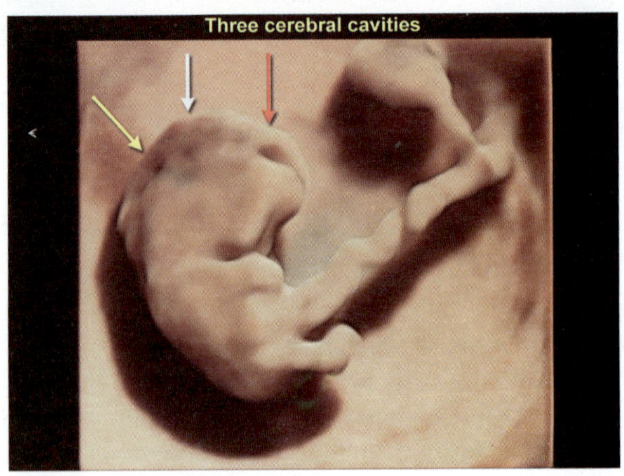

Fig. 37: HDlive view of the rhombencephalon (yellow arrow), the mesencephalon (white arrow) and the diencephalon (red arrow).

ULTRASONOGRAPHIC CHARACTERISTICS IN THE 9TH WEEK

The key-features are the visualization of the fetal face, the stomach and bladder **(Figs 42 to 47)**.

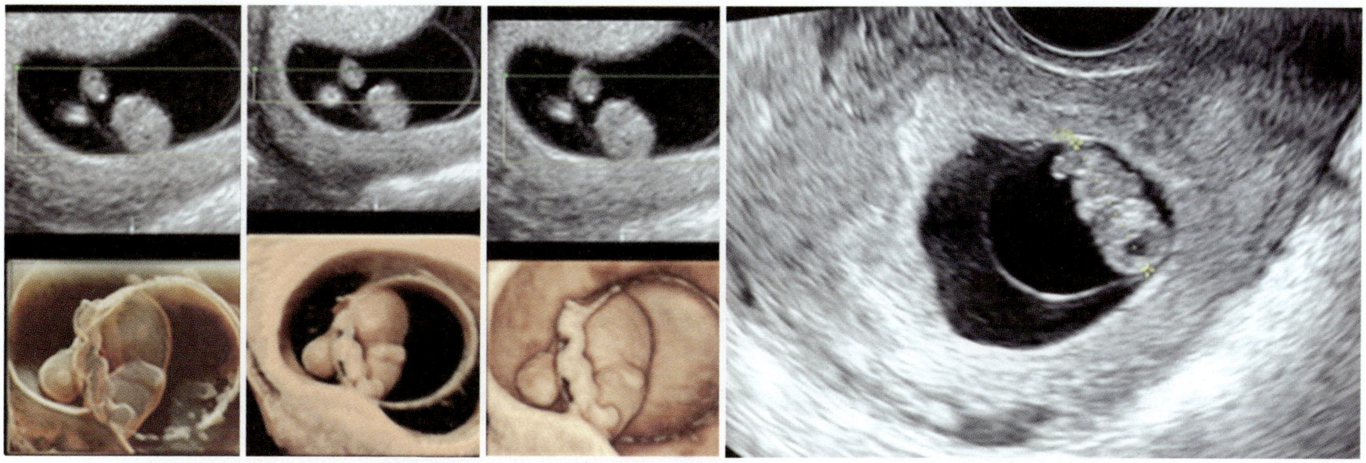

Fig. 38: Comparative multimodal images of an embryo of 8 weeks of gestational age. Right: 2D standard view. Right bottom: HDlive silhouette view.

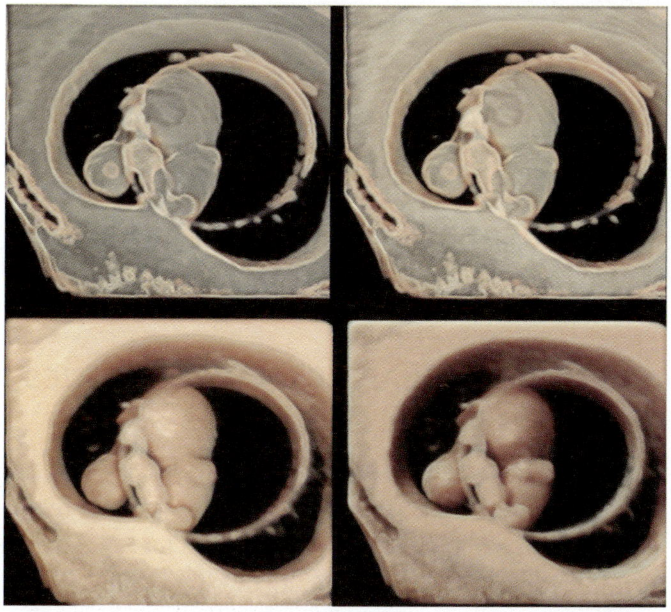

Fig. 39: HDlive silhouette images. Upper: Images in maximum brightness. Bottom: High definition with high (left) and low (right) light intensity. Notice the clear definition of the embryo, the yolk sac, the amnion and the extraembryonic coelom.

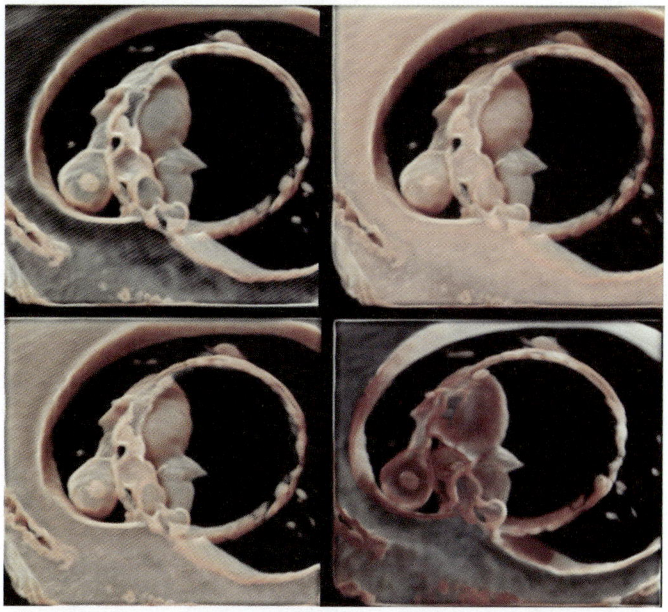

Fig. 40: HDlive silhouette images in maximum brightness. Notice the primordial umbilical cord showing early coiling.

ULTRASONOGRAPHIC CHARACTERISTICS IN THE 10TH WEEK

In this week, the face, orbits, ears, mouth and maxilla are clearly visualized.

The only valuable measurement is the crown-rump length to determinate the gestational age. In 3D US real-time, we will detect the fetal "slow and lazy" movements **(Figs. 48 to 53)**.

ULTRASONOGRAPHIC CHARACTERISTICS IN THE 11TH WEEK

The important features at this week are the disappearance of the physiologic herniation, the visualization of fingers and toes and the coiling development within the umbilical cord (one new spiral coil and one extra-centimeter in length for every gestational week approximately) **(Figs. 54 to 58)**.

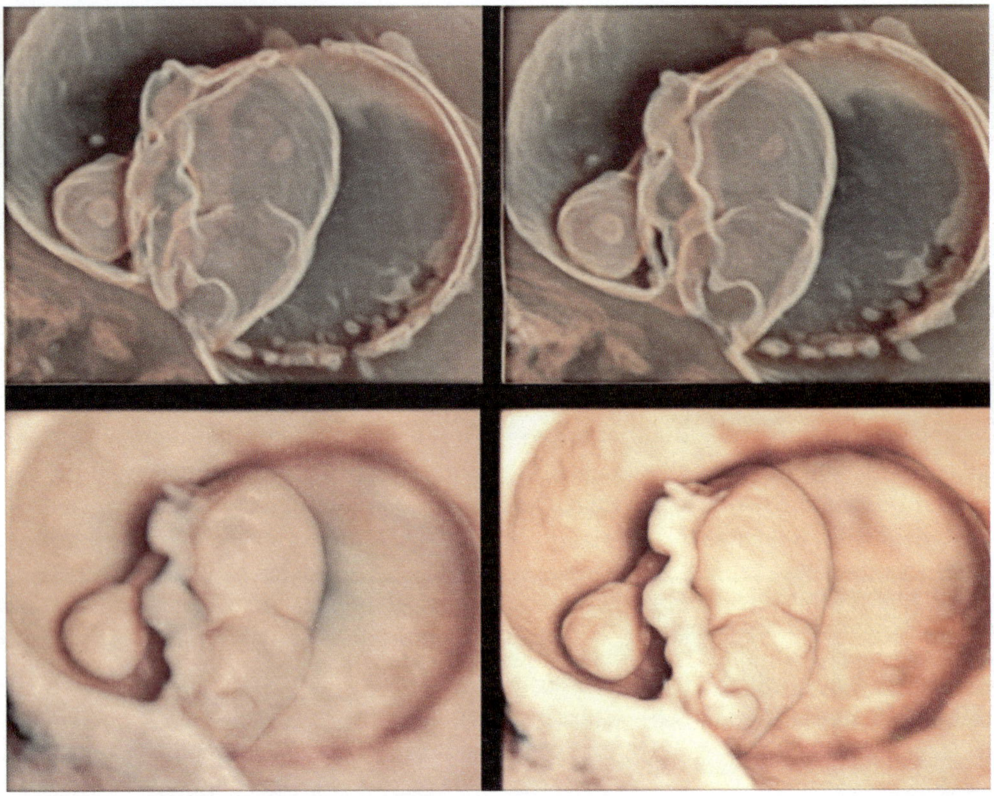

Fig. 41: HDlive silhouette images. Upper: Images in maximum brightness. Bottom: High definition with low (left) and high (right) intensity of virtual light. Notice the embryonic disk, the yolk sac, the omphalomesenteric duct and the amnion.

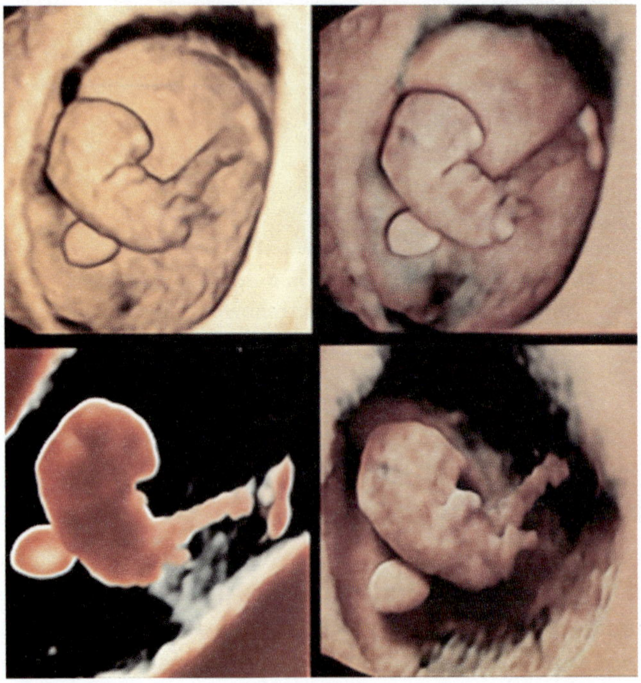

Fig. 42: An embryo of a gestational age of 9 weeks. Notice the fetal limbs, a large omphalomesenteric duct and a distant yolk sac.

ULTRASONOGRAPHIC CHARACTERISTICS IN THE 12TH WEEK

The following images show the typical findings at this gestational age; from this moment onwards the crown-rump length constitutes the key measure for an accurate gestational age. The biparietal diameter, abdominal circumference and femur length measures are also routinely included in the evaluation; it is also possible to detect intra-abdominal structures, such as kidneys and liver **(Figs. 59 to 67)**.

ULTRASONOGRAPHIC APPEARANCE FROM THE 13TH WEEK ONWARDS

From this week onwards, we present outstanding images of fetuses at different gestational ages. The ultrasonographic criteria are exactly the same as with conventional 2D evaluation; however, the images are of remarkable better quality **(Figs. 68 to 74)**.

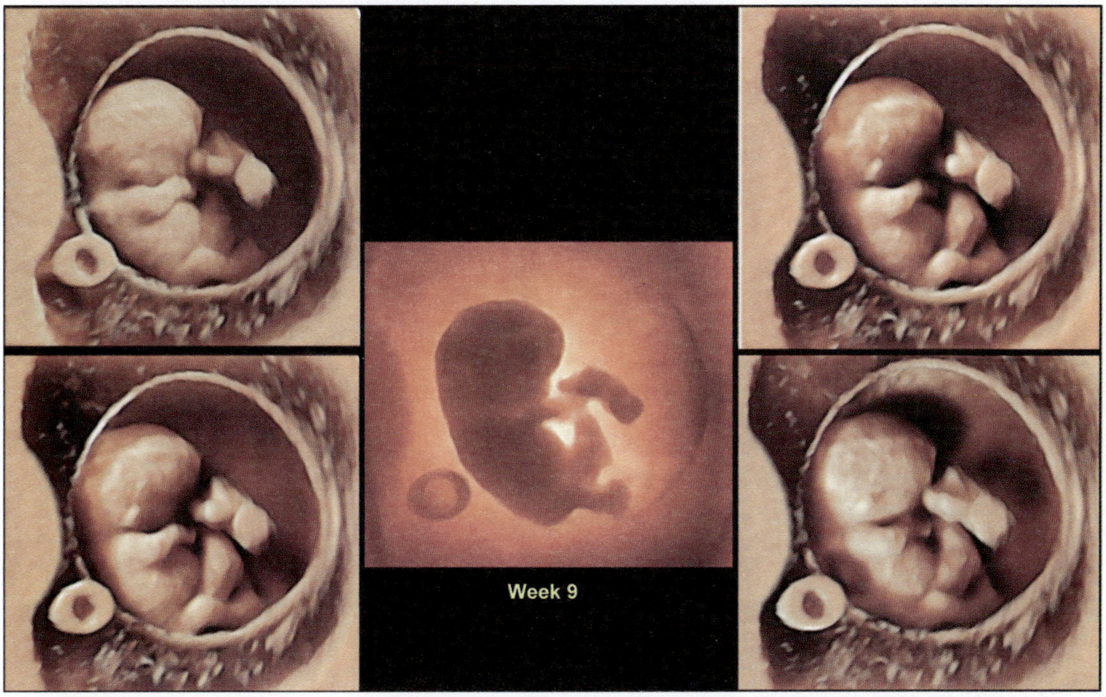

Fig. 43: HDlive view of an embryo of a gestational age of 9 weeks. Notice the cephalic and abdominal poles and the ear buds. The amnion is fully developed and the yolk sac is clearly seen within the extraembryonic coelom. Middle image: maximum transparency.

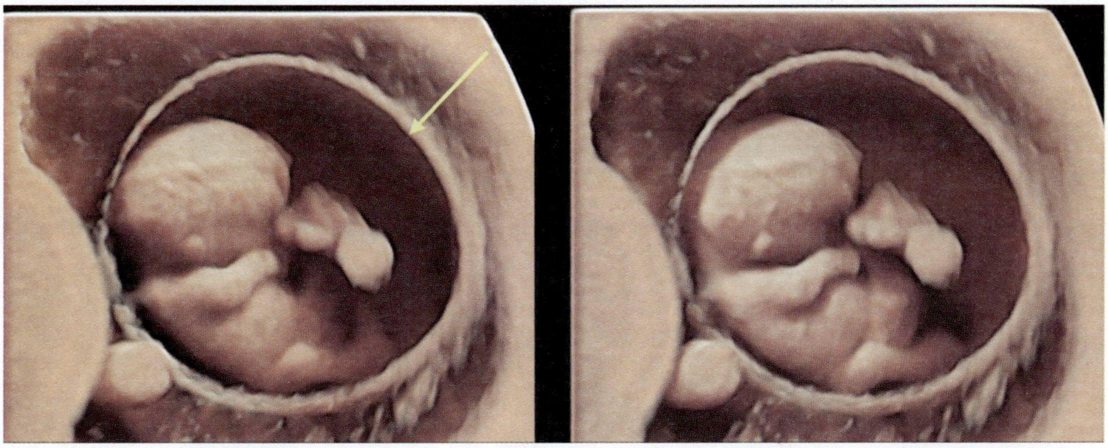

Fig. 44: Week 9. Amnion fully developed. Yolk sac within the extracoelomic space. The fetal arms appears to cover the fetal face.

FINDINGS IN THE 15TH WEEK

We have selected two photographs **(Figs. 69 and 70)** to show very precise details of structures, so that compared the 2D with 3D **(Figs. 75 to 86)**.

Figure 29 shows the front view of a 15-week fetus with HDlive. Note the amount of detail that can be achieved with this system at these gestational ages. Particularly striking is the clarity with which the cord that runs from the navel up is observed, it is grasped and embraced by both hands to go to lead to fetal side of the placenta.

MISCELLANEOUS

The atlas is completed with the following series of images showing beautiful details of specific fetal structures evaluated with this new technology: the umbilical cord, placenta, fetal genitalia, the nuchal translucency and the

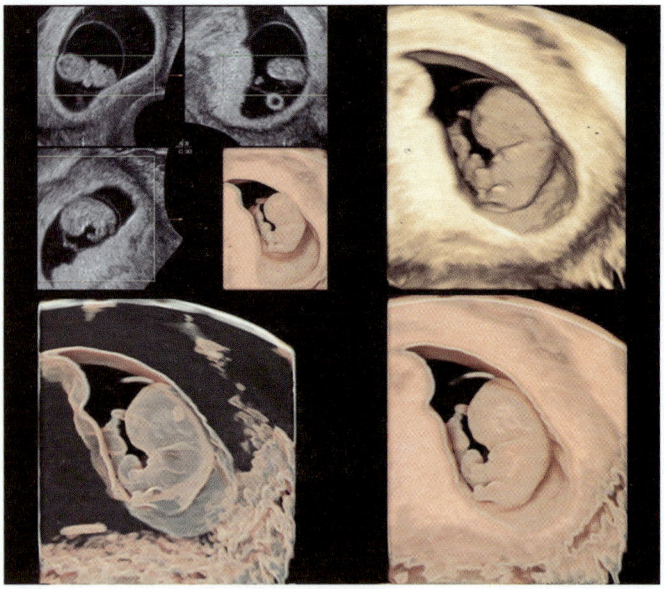

Fig. 45: 9 weeks. Upper left: Orthogonal plane. Upper right: Standard 3D view. Bottom left: HDlive silhouette. Bottom right: HDlive. Notice the embryonic "delimitation", and the limb buds, even the decidua layer can be perfectly visualized.

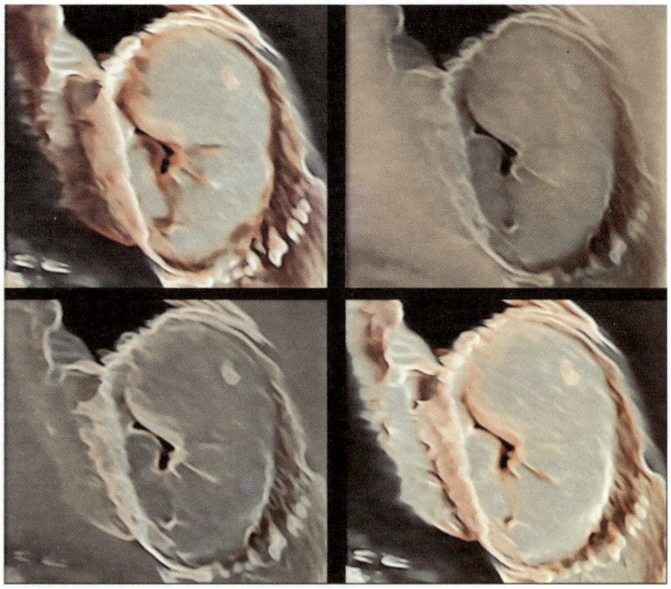

Fig. 47: Images using HDlive silhouette and maximum brightness in a crystal-blue background that shows a beautiful embryonic transparency.

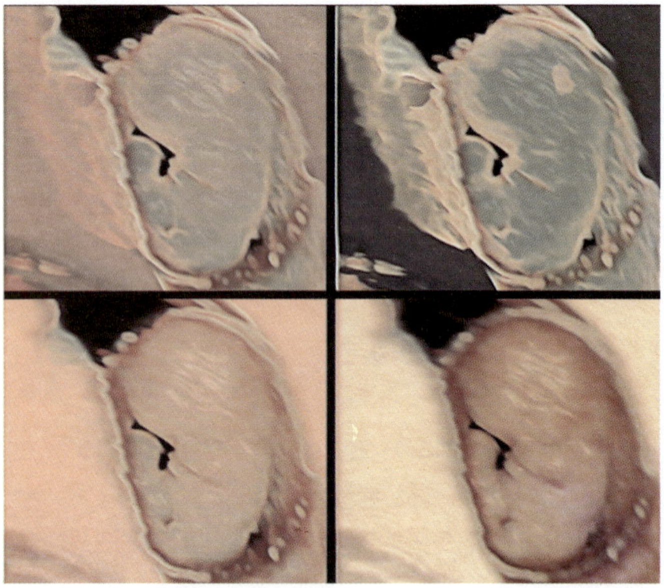

Fig. 46: Images with HDlive silhouette maximum brightness using different grades of virtual light illumination. Notice the complete fetal body and the umbilical cord going upwards to the cranial pole.

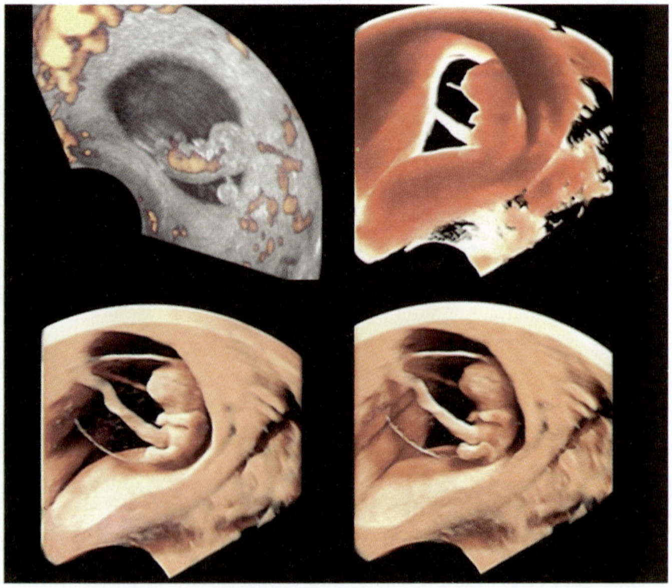

Fig. 48: Power Doppler and HDlive images with/without maximum brightness of a 10-week old gestation.

twin pregnancies; a possible application for the study of fetal anomalies has been also proposed.

COMMENTS

HDlive technology appeared in late 2011; however, the application of the technique was slow. The software was only adaptable to the Voluson™ E8 (General Electrics) machine, thus, it was a quite expensive technology. HDlive silhouette is an step forward within the HDlive technology, in fact, to the best of our knowledge, the technical details of the software are not disclose and again the software is only adaptable to the Voluson™ E10 device (General Electrics).

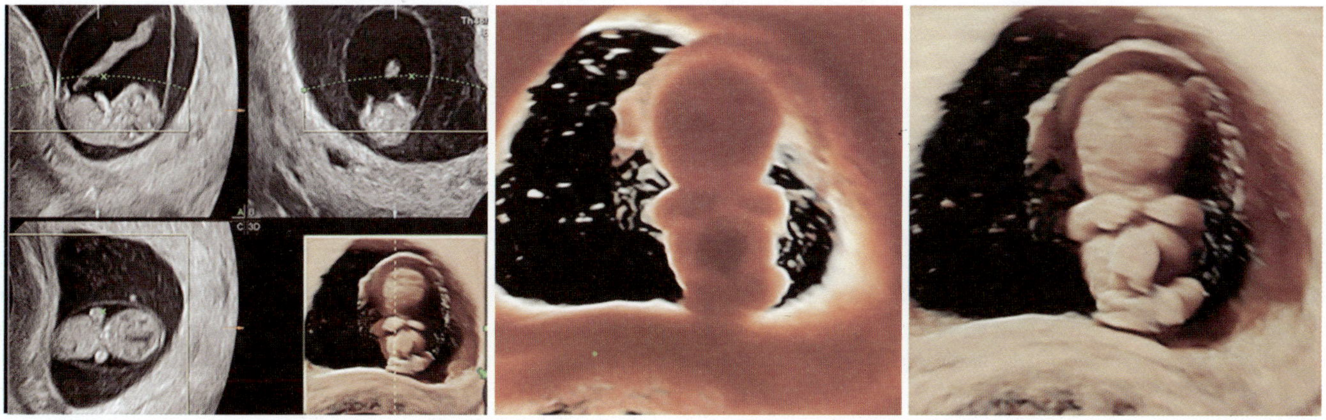

Fig. 49: A 10-week old fetus, sited on a "Buda position", looking at us, head down and with superior and inferior limbs flexed over the abdomen. Notice the amnion surrounding the fetal body and the extraembryonic coelom. The physiologic herniation is seen in the middle part of the abdominal wall as a "round balloon".

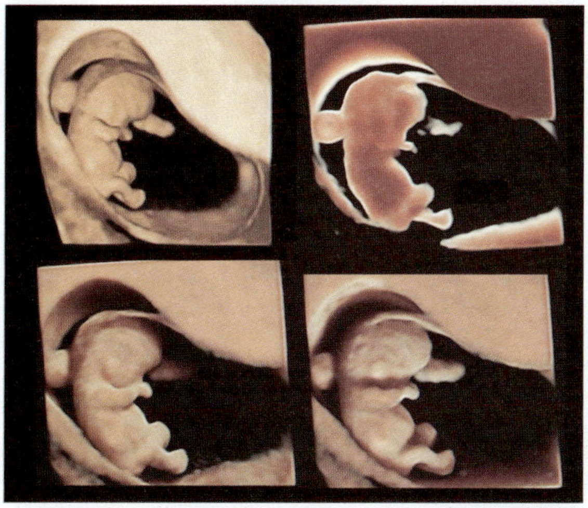

Fig. 50: A 10-week old fetus with perfectly delimited limb buds and a yolk sac. Notice that the fetus is completely surrounded by the amnion.

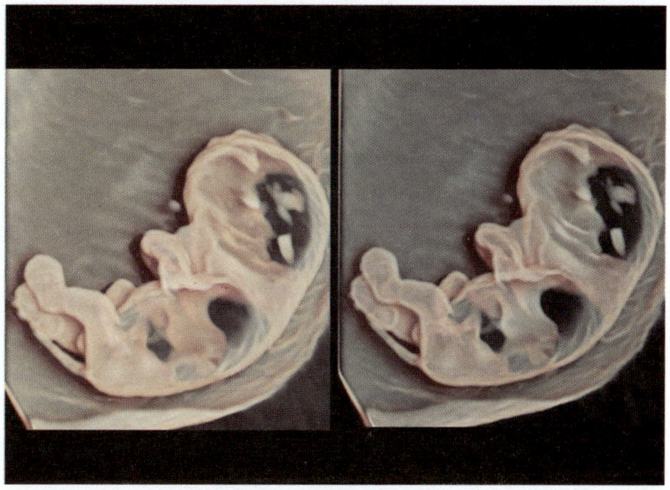

Fig. 52: HDlive silhouette image showing internal and external parts of the fetus. Notice the three brain cavities (compare to **Figure 17**) in outstanding definition. The chest cavity and the stomach are clearly depicted as well.

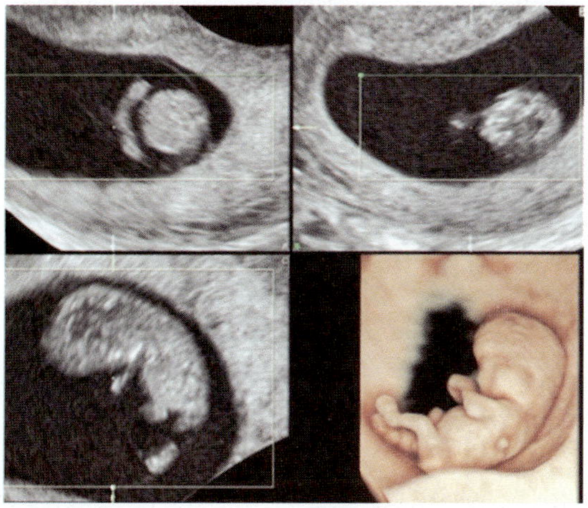

Fig. 51: Orthogonal plane and HDlive image of a large fetus. Notice the clear view of the nose, mouth, limbs, elbows, knees and feet.

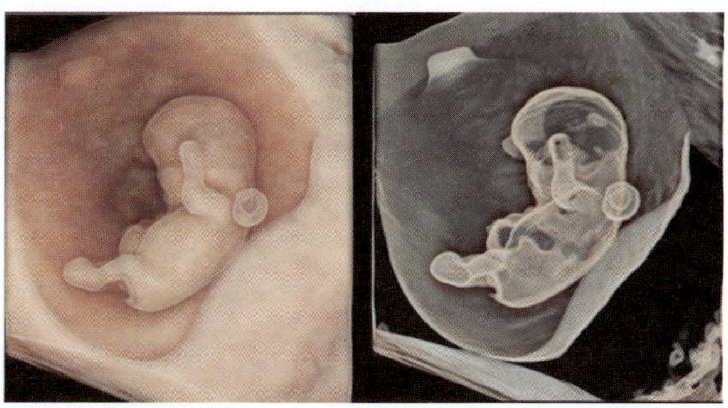

Fig. 53: HDlive silhouette image of a large fetus "lying" on the posterior wall of the gestational sac. The fetal side face, rhombencephalon, lungs and primordial intestines are depicted in outstanding images.

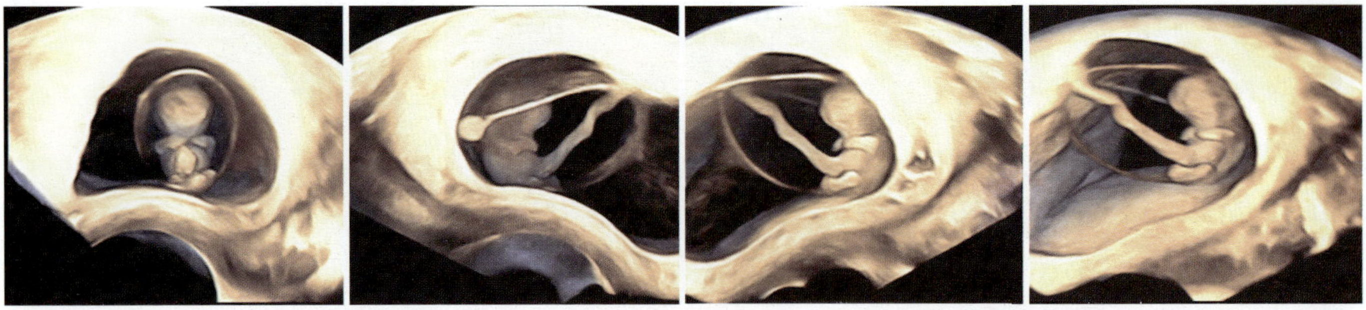

Fig. 54: HDlive silhouette image of an 11-week-old fetus. Notice the clear visualization of the fetal body, the location and characteristics of the physiologic herniation, the hands, legs and feet in remarkable detail. Of outstanding clarity is the visualization of the amnion, the cord and the yolk sac.

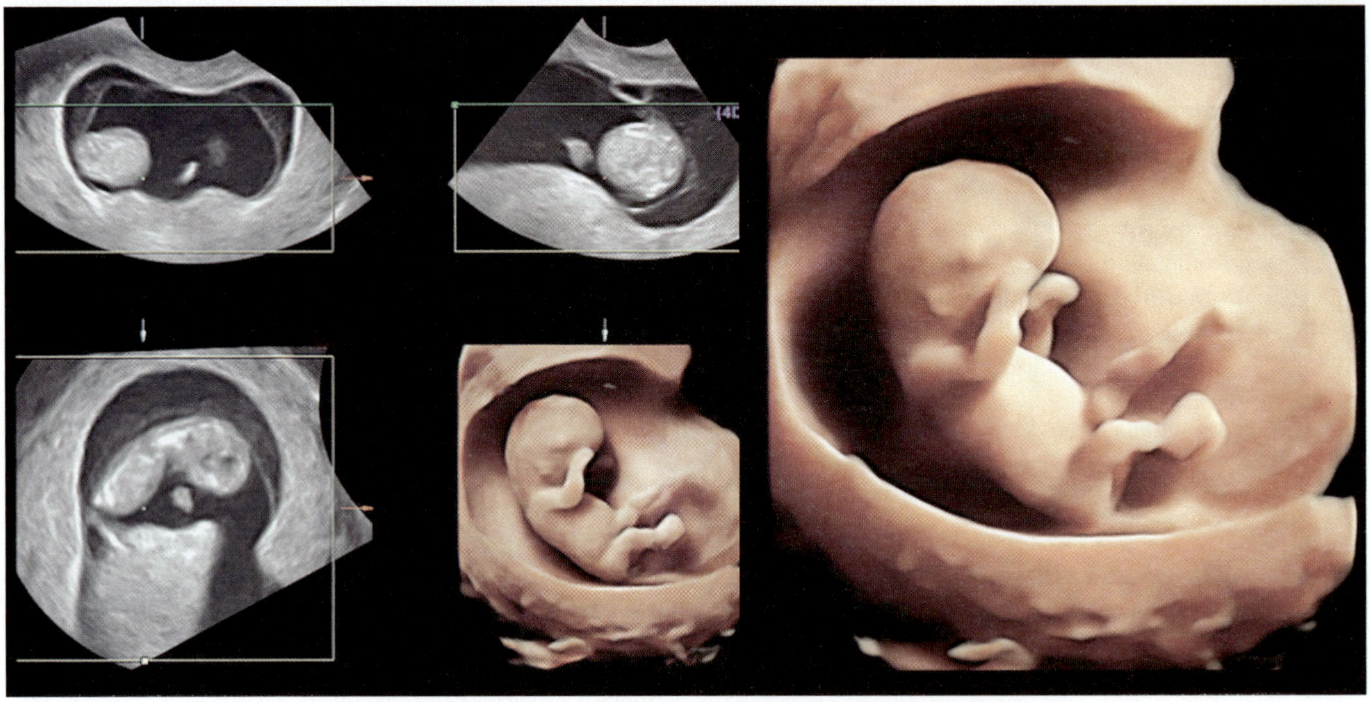

Fig. 55: Orthogonal plane and HDlive image of and 11-week-old fetus. Notice the hand buds and feet with incipient toes.

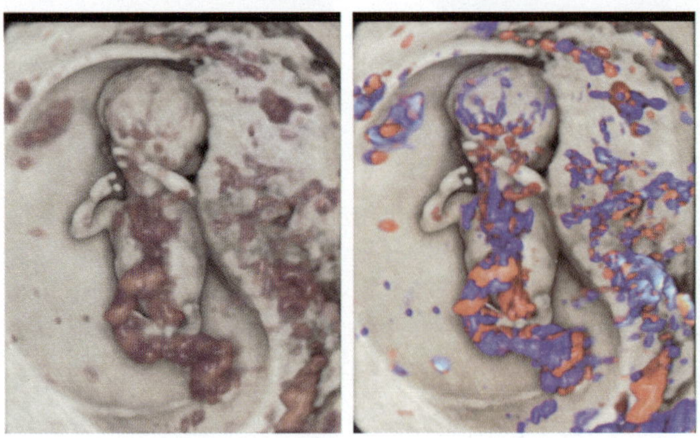

Fig. 56: Orthogonal plane and HDlive with Doppler images showing the fetal vascular tree. Notice the umbilical cord and placenta located to the right.

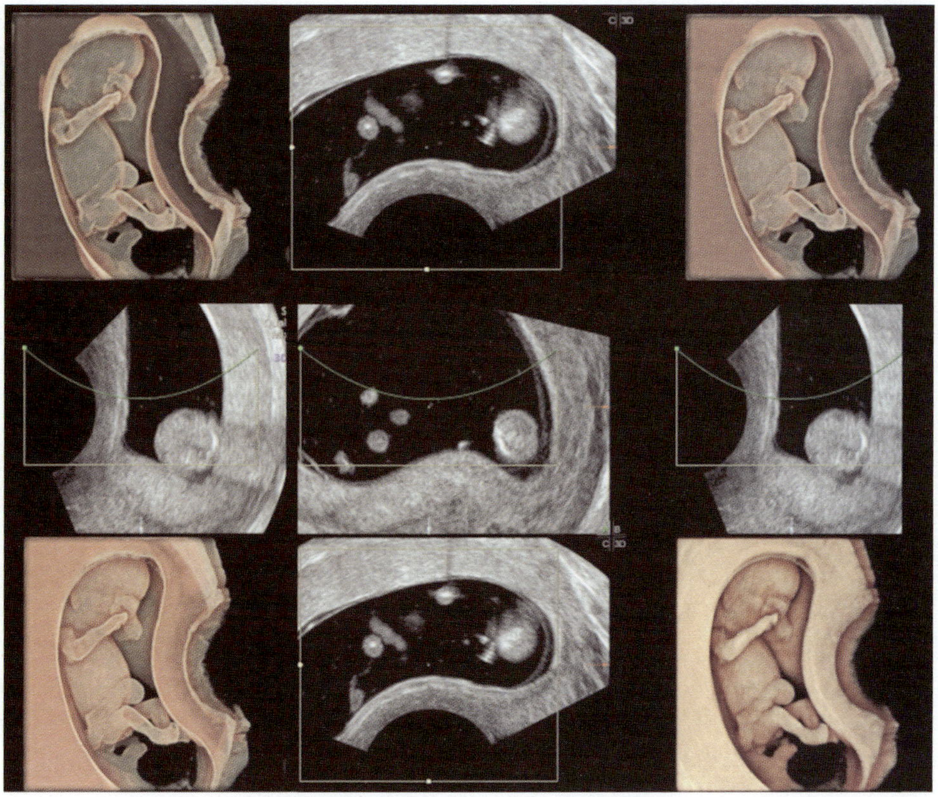

Fig. 57: Fetal images in 2D orthogonal planes and HDlive maximum brightness. The combination of these technologies allows for a better image quality and diagnosis enhancement.

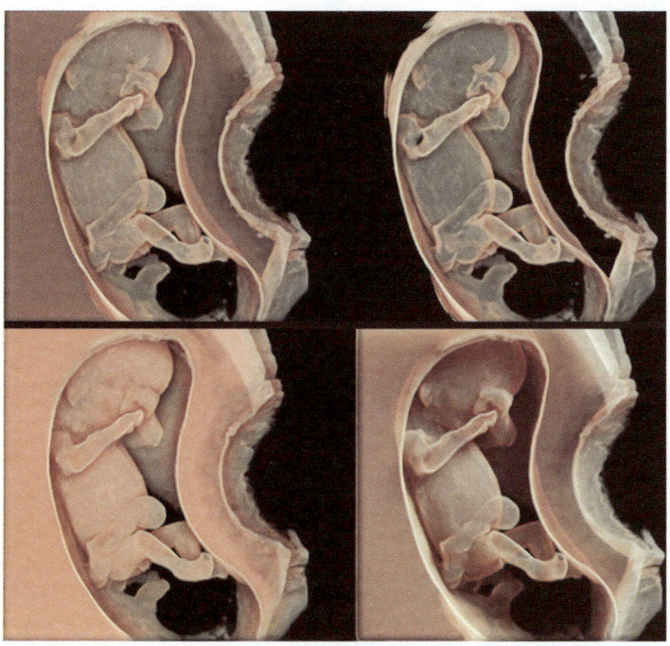

Fig. 58: An 11-week-old fetus evaluated with HDlive. Outstanding images of the fetal body, notice the shape on the hands and the clear delimitation of the umbilical cord, abdominal wall and physiologic herniation.

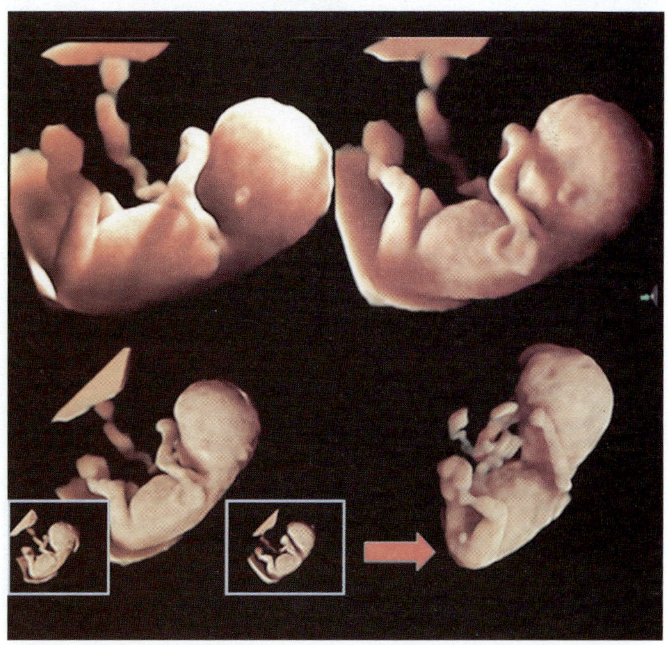

Fig. 59: HDlive evaluation of a 12-week-old fetus. Notice the fetal body including the genital area, the ultrasonographic appearance of the genitals at this age is similar in both genders.

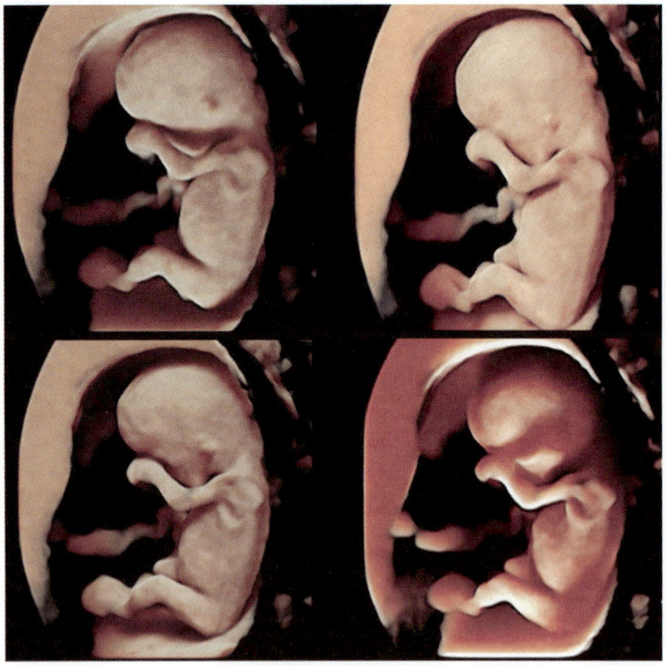

Fig. 60: Side-face view of a 12 week-old fetus. HDlive shows the entire fetal anatomy in impressive detail.

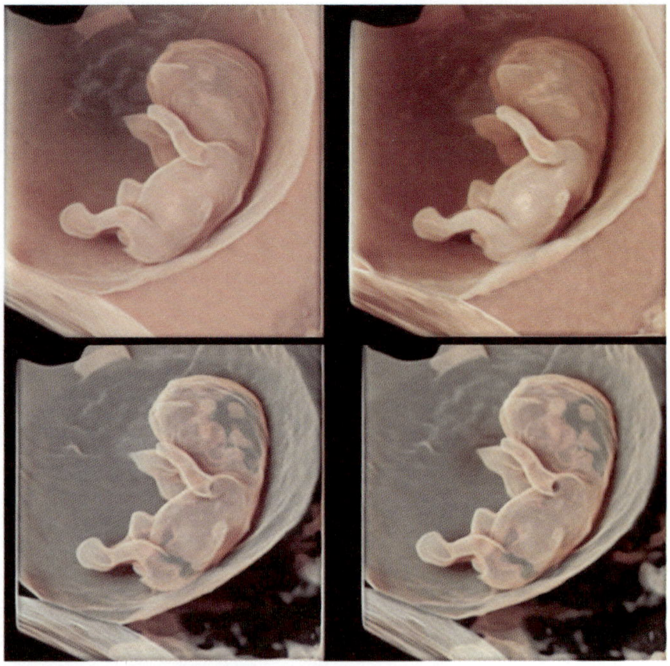

Fig. 62: HDlive silhouette images of a 12-week-old pregnancy. Outstanding pictures of the entire fetal surface, notice the limbs, hands and feet.

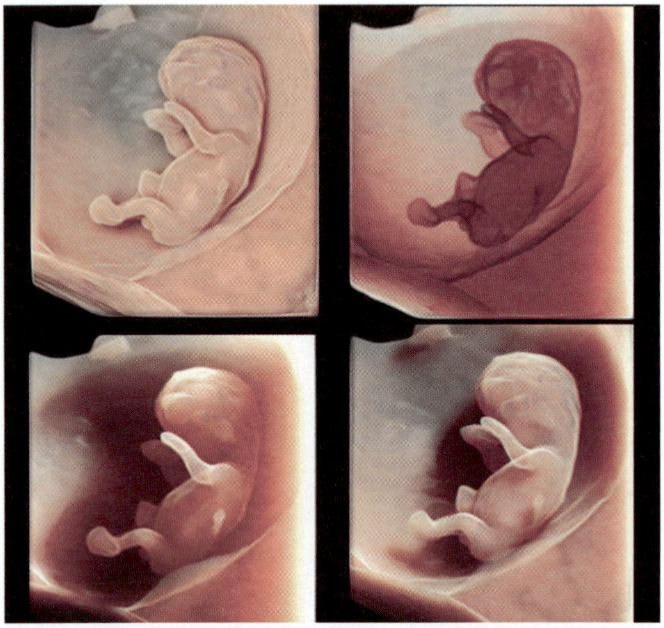

Fig. 61: HDlive silhouette images of a 12 week-old pregnancy. The fetus appears side-face and "laying over" the posterior uterine wall. Notice the fetal anatomy in great detail when evaluated using the maximum brightness tool.

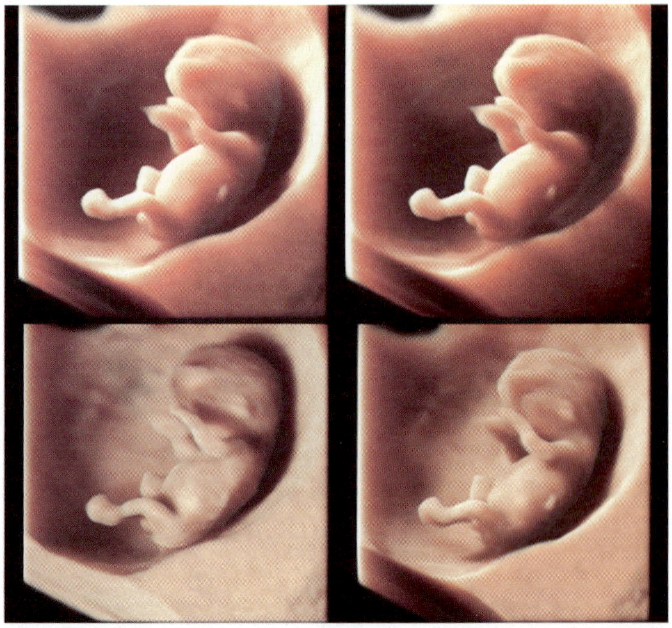

Fig. 63: HDlive images showing the fetal anatomy in different angles of virtual light. This modality allows for a detailed evaluation of the region of interest only by focusing the virtual light in the preferred position.

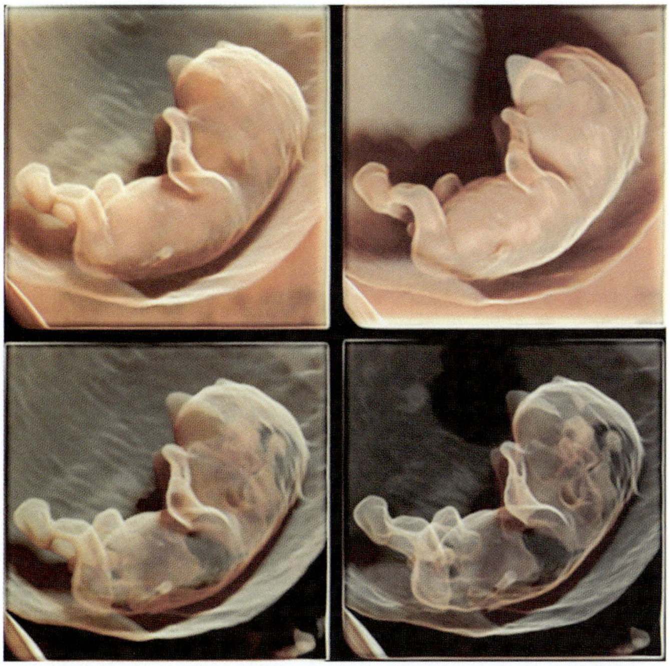

Fig. 64: HDlive silhouette with (bottom images) and without maximum brightness (upper images). The upper images show the surface of the fetal body whereas the lower images give us an approach of the inner fetal structures.

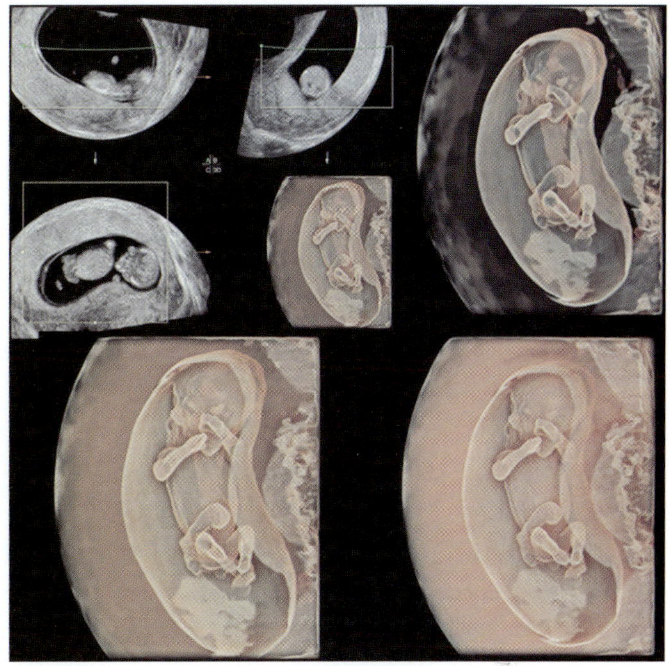

Fig. 66: Outstanding images in orthogonal planes and HDlive silhouette rendering of a 12-week-old fetus.

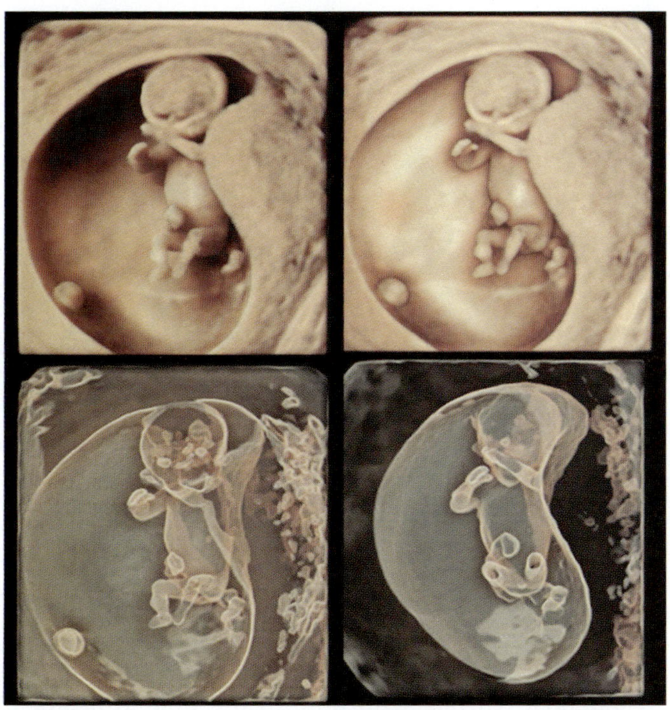

Fig. 65: Comparative images using HDlive and HDlive silhouette. The upper images clearly show the abdominal area and the insertion of the umbilical cord, while the hands are covering the facial area. The bottom images show the fetal body and also notice the silhouette of the placental vascularization.

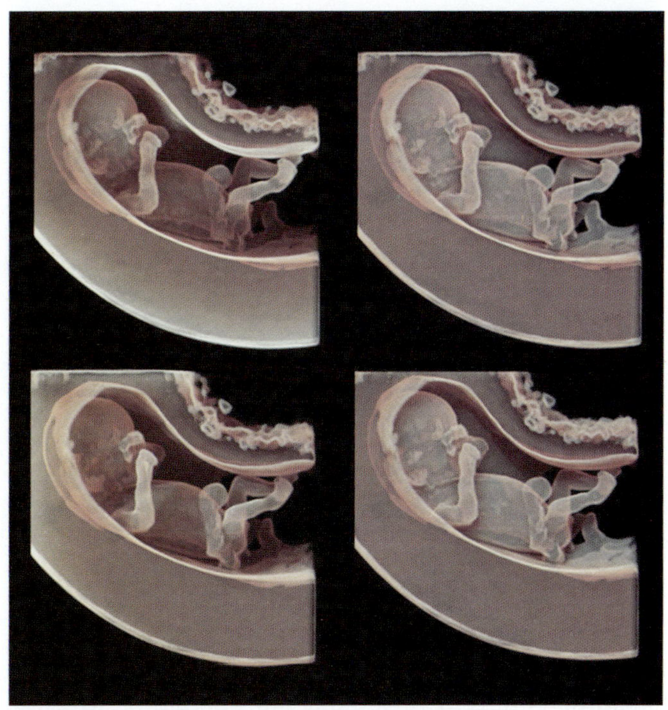

Fig. 67: HDlive silhouette image showing the entire gestational sac, the fetus laying over the posterior aspect of the placenta, the hands are covering the face, notice the early fingers and toes, the abdomen and legs. This picture is really remarkable.

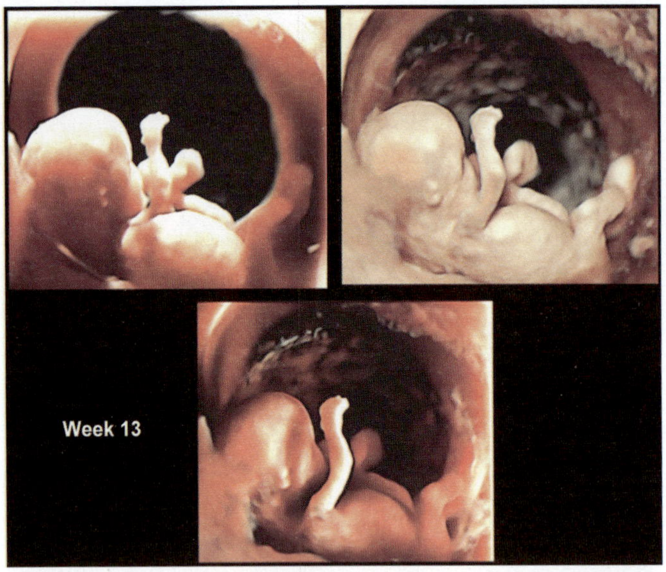

Fig. 68: HDlive images of a 13-week-old fetus. The head is well developed, the fetal body is clearly observed in 3D aspect. Notice the fingers.

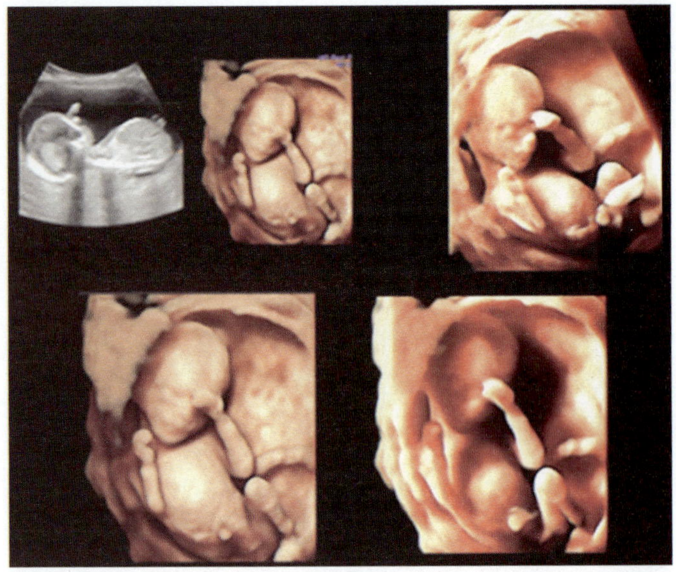

Fig. 70: HDlive image of a 15-week-old fetus. The fetal anatomy is clearly seen; notice the head laterally flexed over the left shoulder and the clear visualization of the face, hands and fingers; the left hand seems to be "scratching" the face.

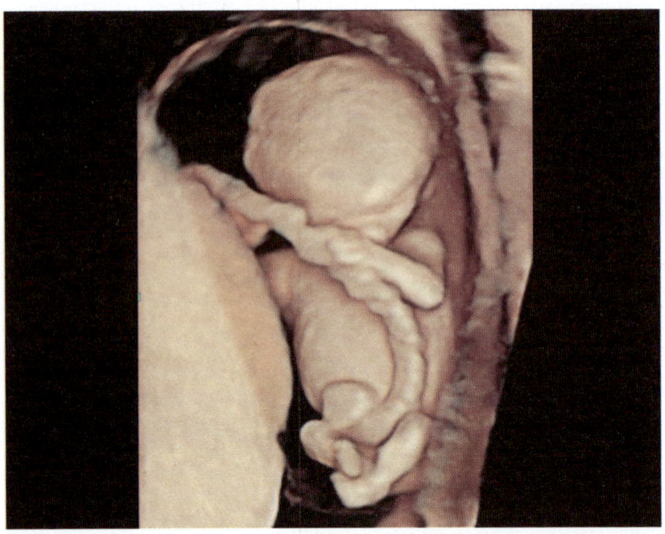

Fig. 69: HDlive image of a 15-week-old fetus. A frontal view in 3D showing the fetal anatomy. The entire umbilical cord is clearly depicted, notice the fetus "holding" the cord with the left hand.

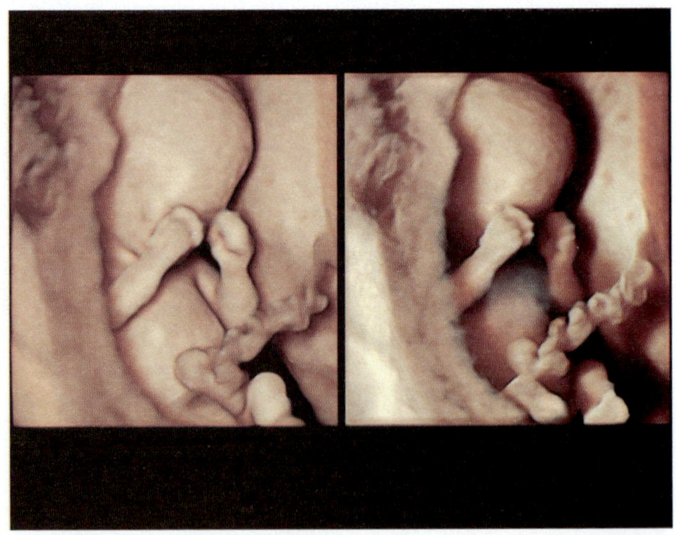

Fig. 71: HDlive image of a 16-week-old fetus. This image shows in great detail both fetal hands covering the face in "boxing fighter" position.

The publications including these novel techniques in Obstetrics are scarce and published as case reports by Japanese groups or reviews by our group. It is worth to mention the review in obstetrics and the clinical reports on circumvallate placenta, intra-amniotic umbilical vein varix with thrombosis, a fetus with meconium peritonitis, the TRAP syndrome, an antenatal diagnosis of jejunal atresia, an antenatal diagnosis of right aortic arch with an aberrant left subclavian artery and the use HDlive technology to diagnose Turner syndrome in the first trimester of pregnancy. In gynecology, HDlive is described for the diagnosis of polycystic ovarian disease, dermoid tumors, ovarian malignancy, leiomyoma degeneration (Raga 2015) and ovarian cancer (Bonilla-Musoles 2015 in press).

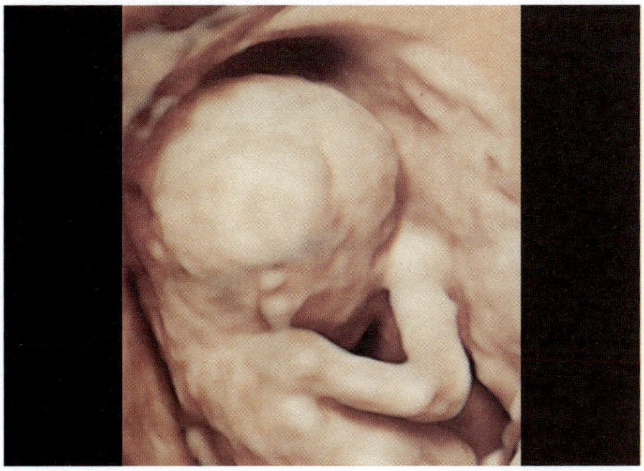

Fig. 72: HDlive image showing the right fetal ear in great detail.

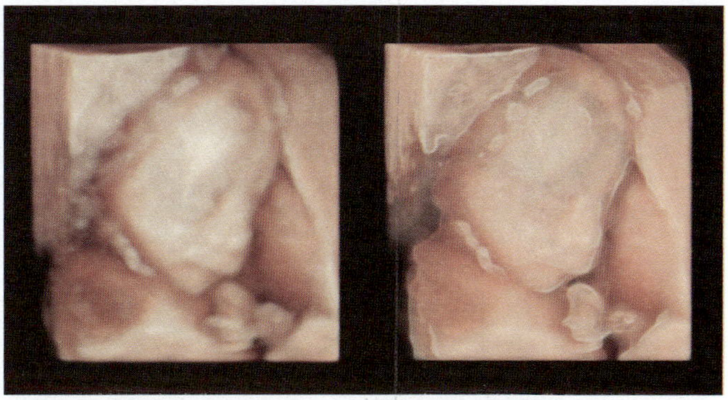

Fig. 74: HDlive silhouette image of a 21-week-old fetus. The fetal face is depicted in great detail; the eyes and mouth are closed. The nose is shown with great definition. Notice the forehead including the anterior fontanel; around the neck a portion of the umbilical cord is also seen.

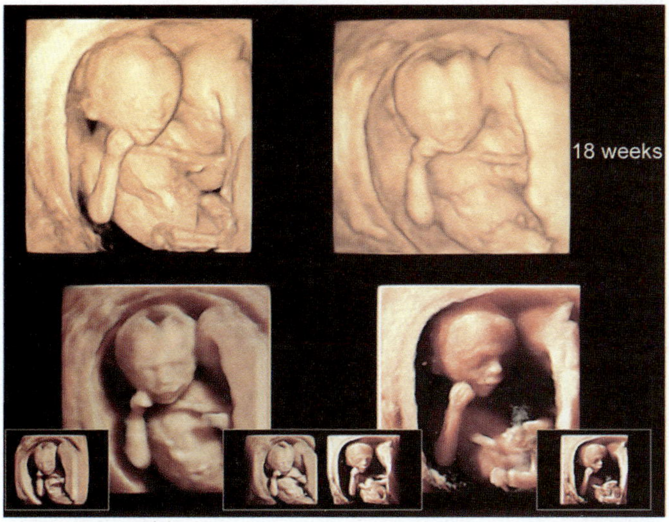

Fig. 73: 3D evaluation of an 18-week-old fetus. Upper: Standard 3D image of the fetal anatomy. Bottom: HDlive images of the same case. HDlive allows for a better visualization of the external fetal anatomy.

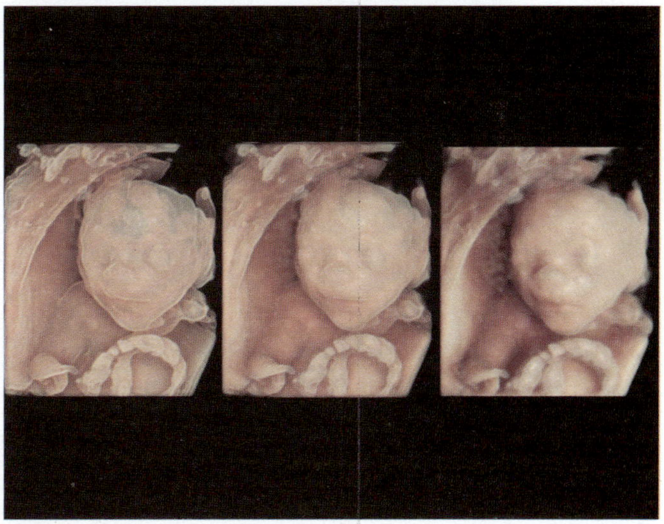

Fig. 75: Fetus at 22 weeks. The fetal face rendering images were obtained with different illumination tones. The fetus (profile) is shown smiling, and the eyes, nose and mouth are depicted in great detail. Notice the umbilical cord coiling.

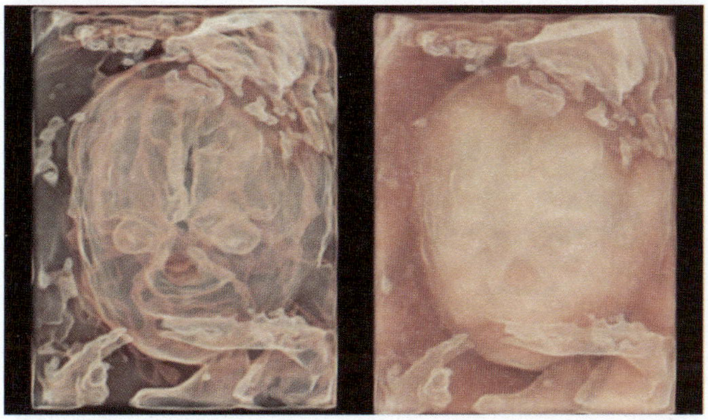

Fig. 76: Fetus at 24 weeks. Comparative evaluation with different intensities of maximum brightness. Notice the following structures: eyes, eyeballs, nose, lips and anterior fontanel.

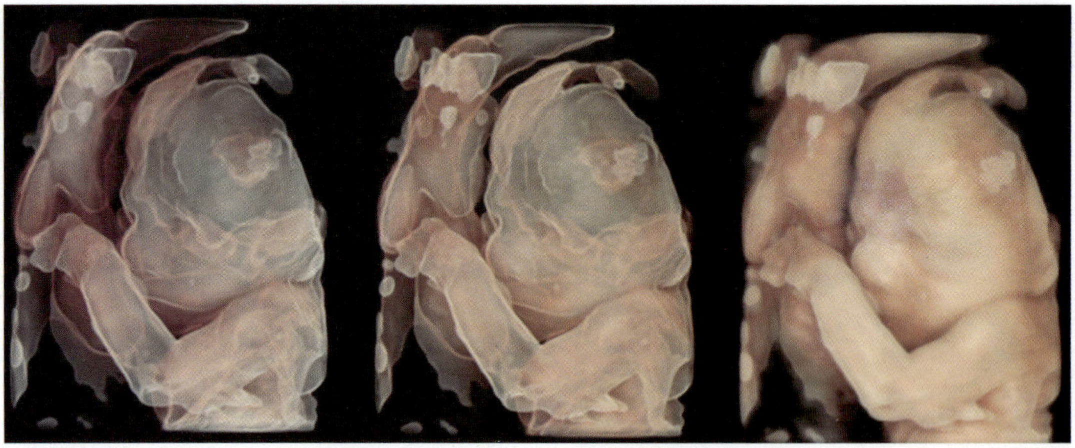

Fig. 77: Fetus at 25 weeks. HDlive silhouette of fetal side-face showing in detail the nose, eyes and forehand; also the left arm, forearm, elbow and hand can be seen.

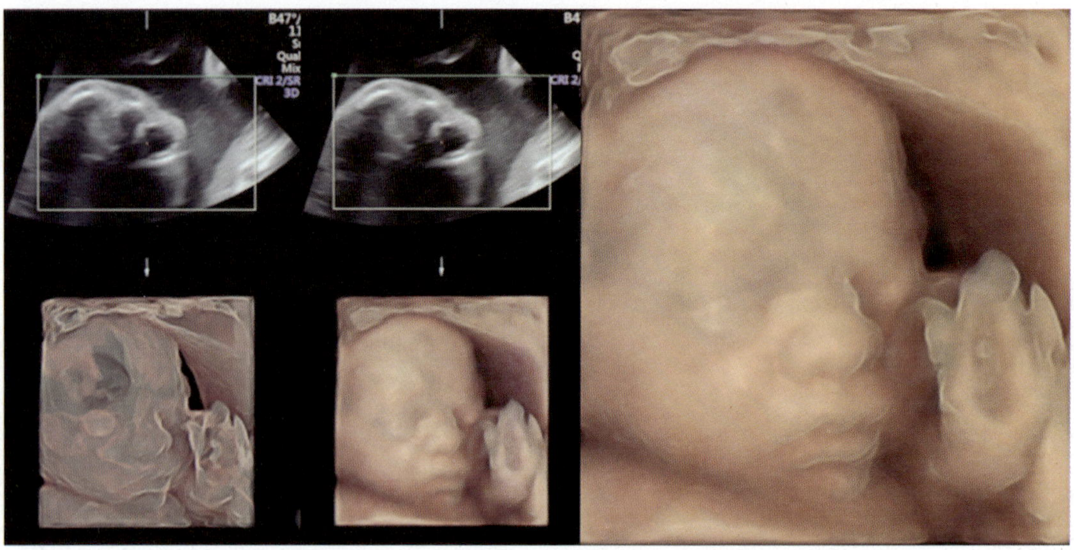

Fig. 78: Fetus at 26 weeks. HDlive silhouette rendering image of the fetal face in outstanding definition, even a portion of the cord cord is depicted.

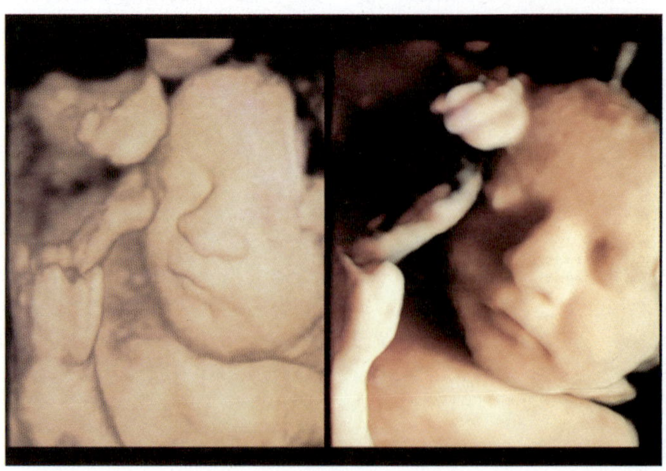

Fig. 79: Fetus at 35 weeks. Comparative images: Conventional 3D (left) and HDlive (right) and rendering image of the fetal face. The pictures are truly "realistic".

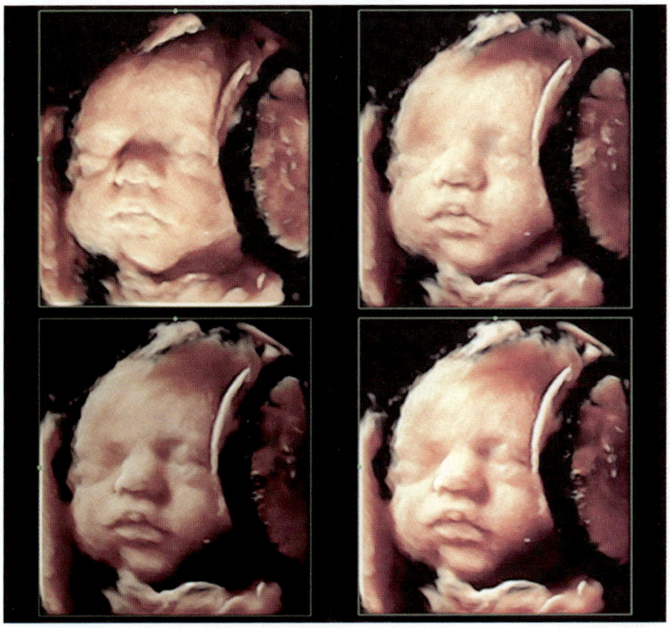

Fig. 80: HDlive images of a 35 week-old fetus in different light projections. The images seem "photo-like" pictures of a newborn.

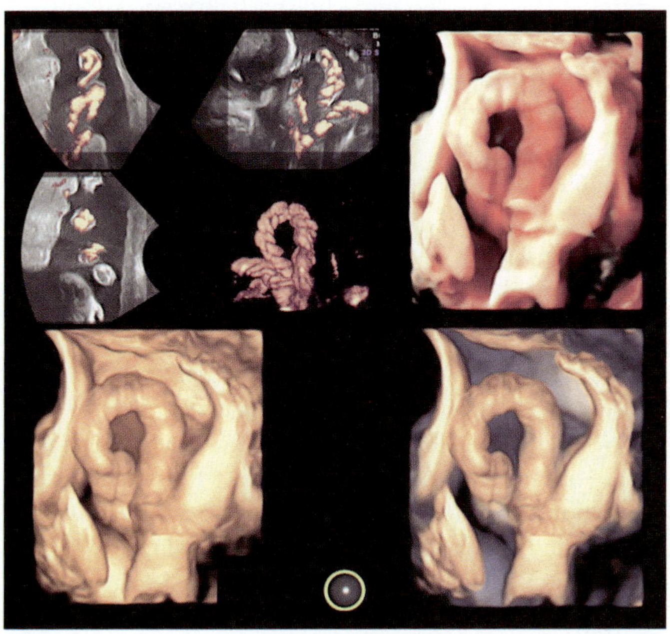

Fig. 81: 3D multimodalic view of the umbilical cord. Upper left: Orthogonal planes plus Doppler and 3D HDlive rendering image of the cord. Upper right: The cord in HDlive imaging. Bottom: Conventional 3D images. Notice the umbilical cord coiling in outstanding detail.

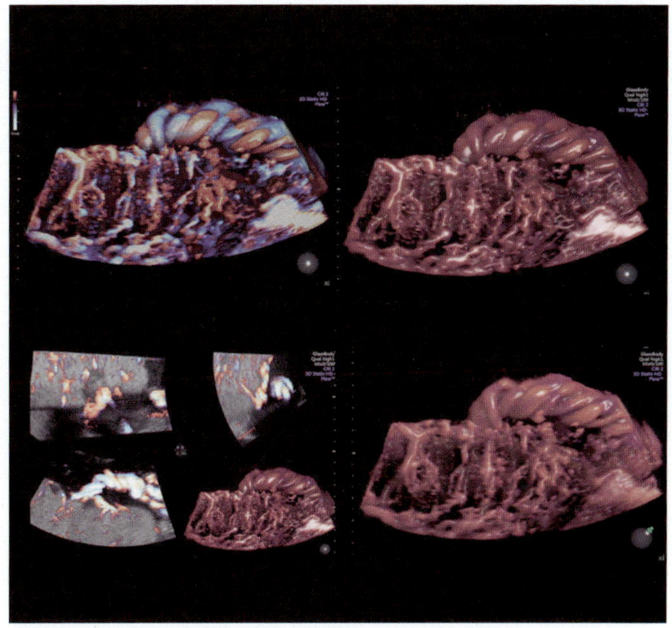

Fig. 82: 3D vascular study of the cord and placental site. Notice in great detail the origin of the umbilical cord on the fetal placental site, the intervillous space and the umbilical cord coiling.

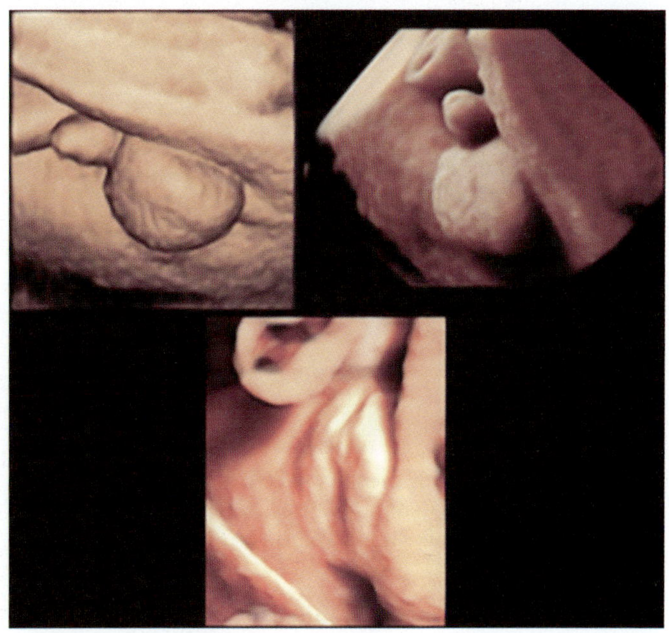

Fig. 83: Fetal genitalia: Upper left: Male fetus genitalia seen in conventional 3D US. Upper right: Male fetus genitalia using HDlive. Notice the clear anatomy of testicles and penis. Bottom: Female genitalia seen with HDlive. Notice the labia majora and clitoris in outstanding detail.

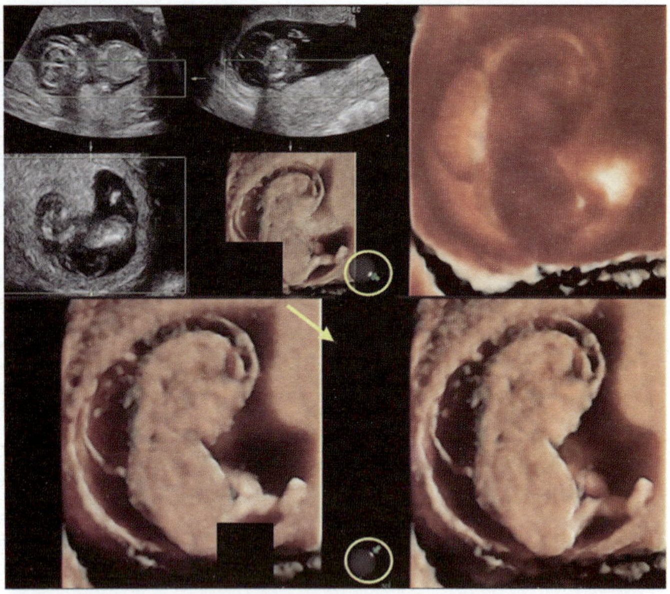

Fig. 84: Orthogonal planes and HDlive imaging showing the nuchal translucency. HDlive allows for a detailed evaluation of the region of interest, of notice the presence of septum within the NT that may worsen the prognosis (yellow arrow).

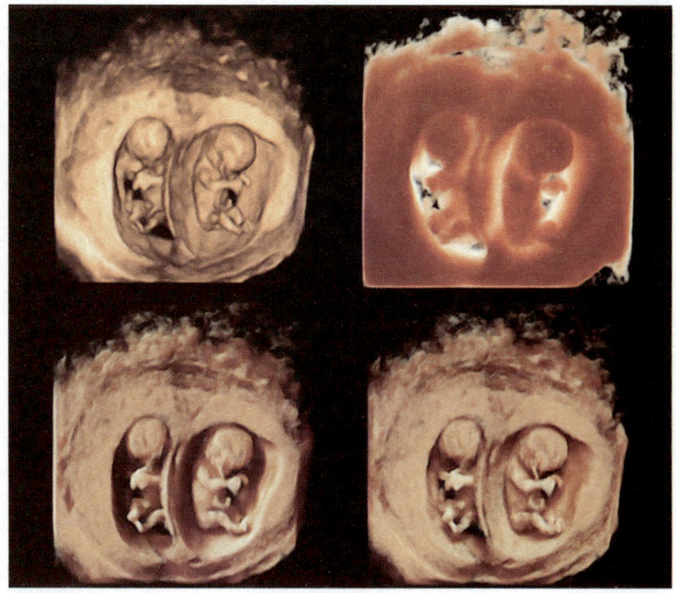

Fig. 86: Multimodalic view of a twin pregnancy. Upper left: Conventional 3D US. Upper right: HDlive maximal translucency. Bottom: HDlive with virtual light positioned in different angles.

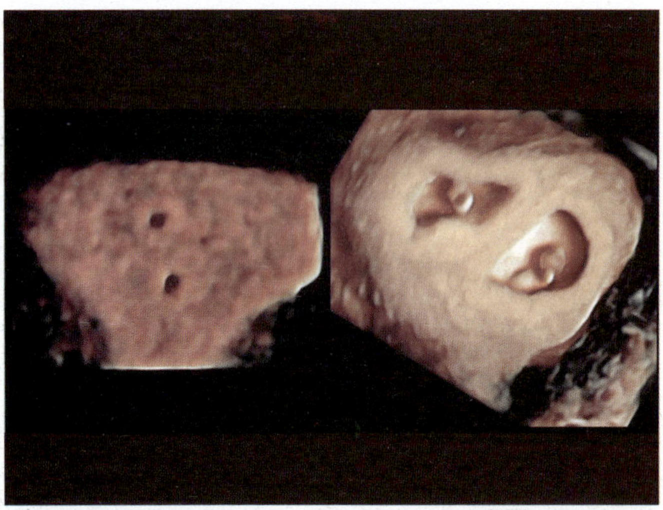

Fig. 85: HDlive of an early pregnancy. Left: A 35-day-old gestation showing the two sacs. Right: A 42-days-old pregnancy showing the gestational sacs, yolk sacs and embryos.

Whilst everyone is convinced (especially after the present publication) that HDlive improves the image quality; yet we recognize that all the routinary prenatal ultrasonographic screening between in the second and third trimester is and will be performed in standard 2D ultrasonography. However, the present publication shows the substantial improvement in quality image achieved by modern 3D US modes, particularly HDlive and silhouette. Finally, based on the available data and the body of evidence from medical publications, this technology should be offered to patients as part of the obstetric care when available, the addition of such technologies may result in an improved obstetric and neonatal care.

SUMMARY

- Modern 3D ultrasound modes, especially HDlive, improve the image quality in obstetrics
- Such technologies, where possible, should be made available for routine obstetric practice
- Whilst outstanding pictures of normal pregnancies are obtained with the application of these techniques, fetal malformations might constitute an ideal area for in-detail evaluation and patient counseling
- Prenatal ultrasonographic screening in the second and third trimester should be basically performed in standard 2D ultrasonography; however, HDlive may offer advantages for first trimester ultrasonographic evaluation
- The cost of the technique is still an important obstacle for a wide clinical use.

REPRODUCTION

NORMAL CYCLE

Ultrasound evaluation is considered an essential tool in the diagnosis of normal ovaries, ovarian, endocrine and tumoral pathologies. Diagnosis of primary and secondary infertility and in ART-related procedures (controlled ovarian stimulation monitoring, oocyte recovery and US-guided embryo transfer).

In ART clinical practice, image quality is extremely important when describing normal structures, but also in order to delineate the origin and extension in case of pathologic findings.

HDlive in Natural Cycles and Corpus Luteum Evaluation

Timed sexual intercourse remains a valid conservative infertility treatment option. Transvaginal ultrasound is used to monitor follicular growth in order to predict ovulation and timed coitus. HDlive allows a clear visualization of the dominant follicle early in the cycle **(Figs. 87 and 88)**.

It allows also a clear and detailed visualization of even small structures such as the cumulus and the beginning of the granulose spring **(Figs. 89 and 90)**.

First-line studies for infertile couples includes the evaluation of a correct ovulation and luteal phase; the measurement of progesterone levels (P4) in the middle of the luteal phase is the most used test to determine ovulation; however, US scans is also a valuable tool due to its capacity is monitoring follicular development, detection of the dominant follicle and visualization of the corpus luteum after ovulation **(Figs. 91 and 92)**.

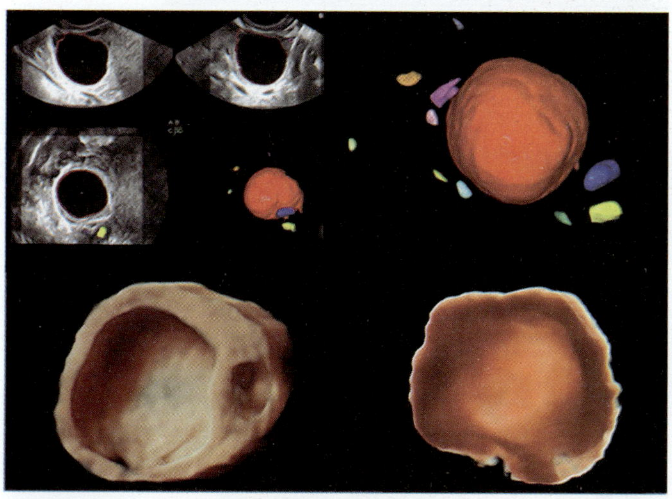

Fig. 87: Ovarian US multimodalic view showing a dominant follicle in a regular menstruating 22-year-old woman (cycle day 13th). From left to right: Conventional 2D ultrasound and AVC (above) imaging showing the dominant and other small follicles. HDlive with maximal luminescence (below).

IVF STIMULATION CYCLES

Ultrasound is an essential monitoring tool for IVF cycles. Basal transvaginal US is useful to predict the ovarian response and total FSH dosage according to the ovarian reserve in terms of number of antral follicle count **(Fig. 93)**. Once under FSH stimulation the ultrasonographic monitorization allows for a timely administration of medication to prevent spontaneous LH surge and also to proceed with the final follicular maturation when at least two follicles reaches 17 mm in diameter **(Fig. 87)**. HDlive shows realistic pictures of the stimulated ovaries, showing cases of low (ovarian failure), normal or high response (hyperstimulation) **(Figs. 93 and 94)**.

EVALUATION OF GYNECOLOGICAL PATHOLOGIES RELATED WITH INFERTILITY

Several gynecological conditions may impair fertility potential. Ultrasonography is the essential component of the initial fertility workup.

Polycystic ovarian syndrome is present in up to 30% of female infertility. In 2003, the Rotterdam consensus established the ultrasonographic criteria to diagnose this pathology; while 2D ultrasound is enough to make a correct diagnosis, the evaluation with HDlive allows a better image quality of this condition, enhancing diagnosis confidence **(Figs. 91 to 96)**.

Silhouette (Voluson E10 GE®), a new software to depict and delineate AF and ovarian cortex, increases much more the image quality and antral follicle delimitation **(Figs. 97 to 99)**.

However, 3D US and all these new modes, cannot be recommended for routine clinical practice until:

- Additional data on reliability are available.
- The high cost of 3D imaging equipments may be reduced.
- Nevertheless, manual follicle counts from stored 3D data currently provide the optimal method of AFC assessment and would minimize many of the practical pitfalls of conventional 2D US evaluation.

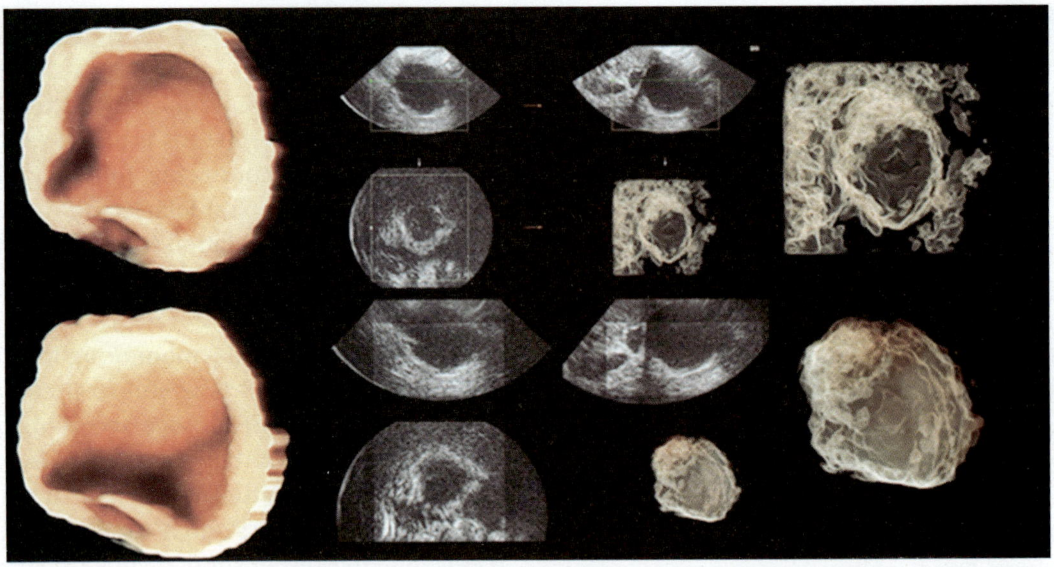

Fig. 88: Antral follicle in HDlive orthogonal 2D planes and silhouette.

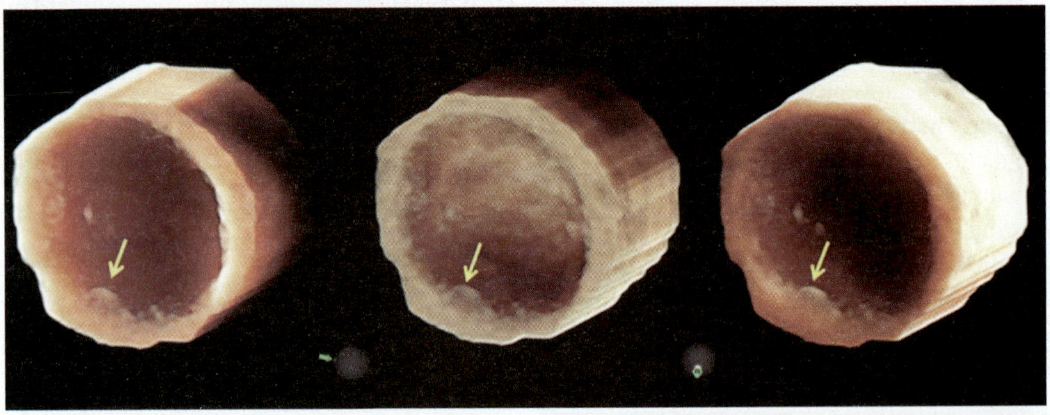

Fig. 89: HDlive imaging of the dominant follicle on the 14th day of spontaneous menstrual cycle. The magic cut software allows a detailed exploration of the region of interest, in this case we clearly observe the growing follicle and also the cumulus complex can be seen within the follicle (yellow arrows). Notice the different HDlive virtual light positioning (green arrows).

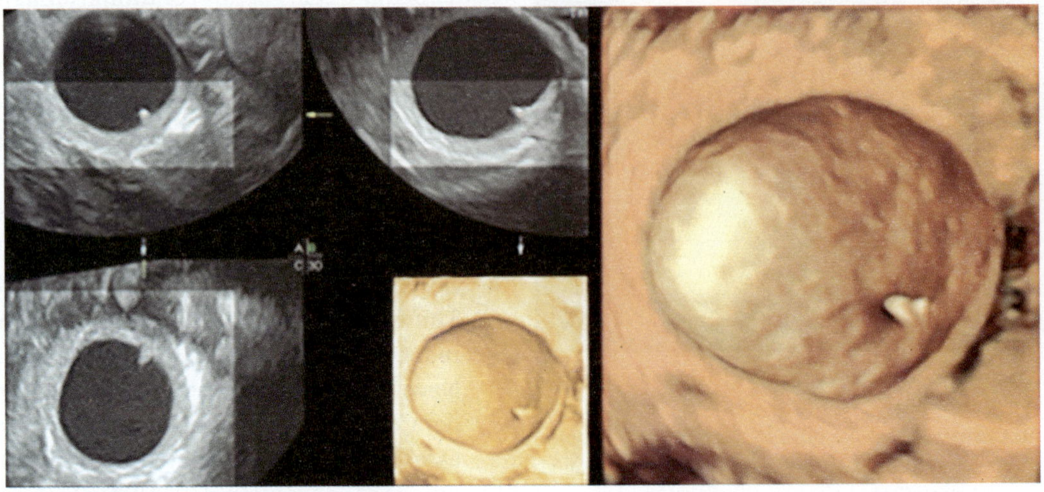

Fig. 90: Cumulus oophorus. This US finding is extremely infrequent using transvaginal 2D.

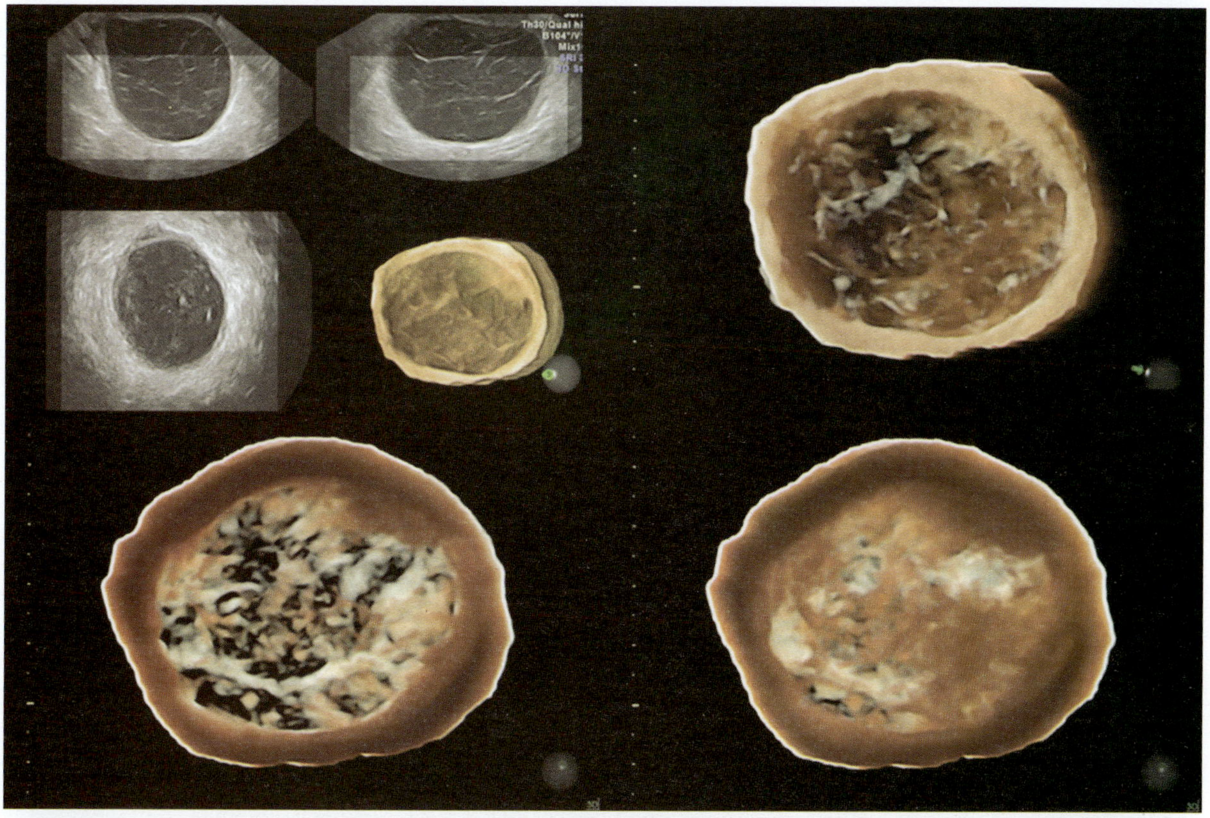

Fig. 91: HDlive view of a "corpus luteum reticularis". Notice the different positions of the virtual light that gives different shadows and images. The translucency mode is show in the upper right image.

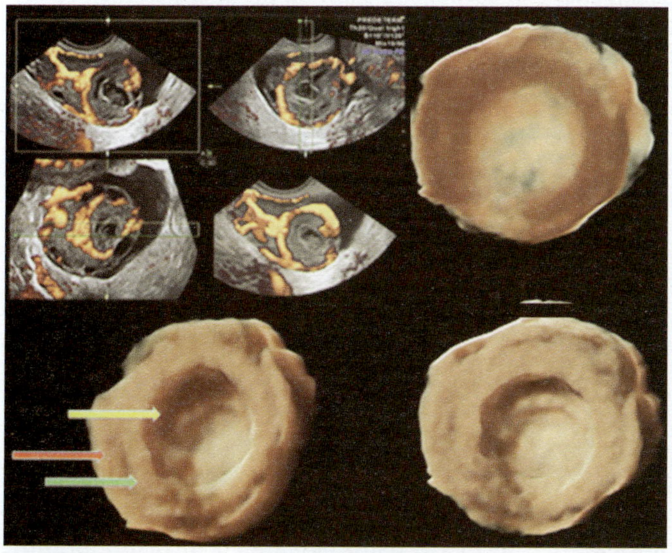

Fig. 92: Corpus luteum depicted with 2D angiography and HDlive showing the follicle cavity (yellow arow), the granulose (green) and the teca (red).

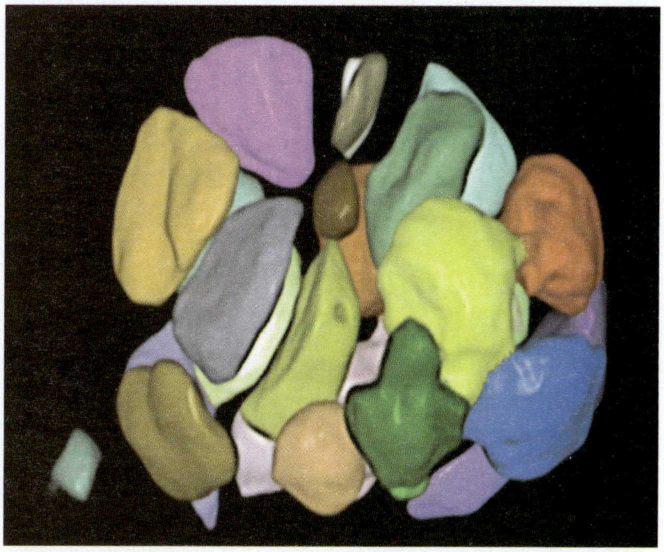

Fig. 93: Antral follicle count (AFC) using AVC mode. Each follicle takes a different color. The computer makes measurements of the different diameters and total volume of each follicle.

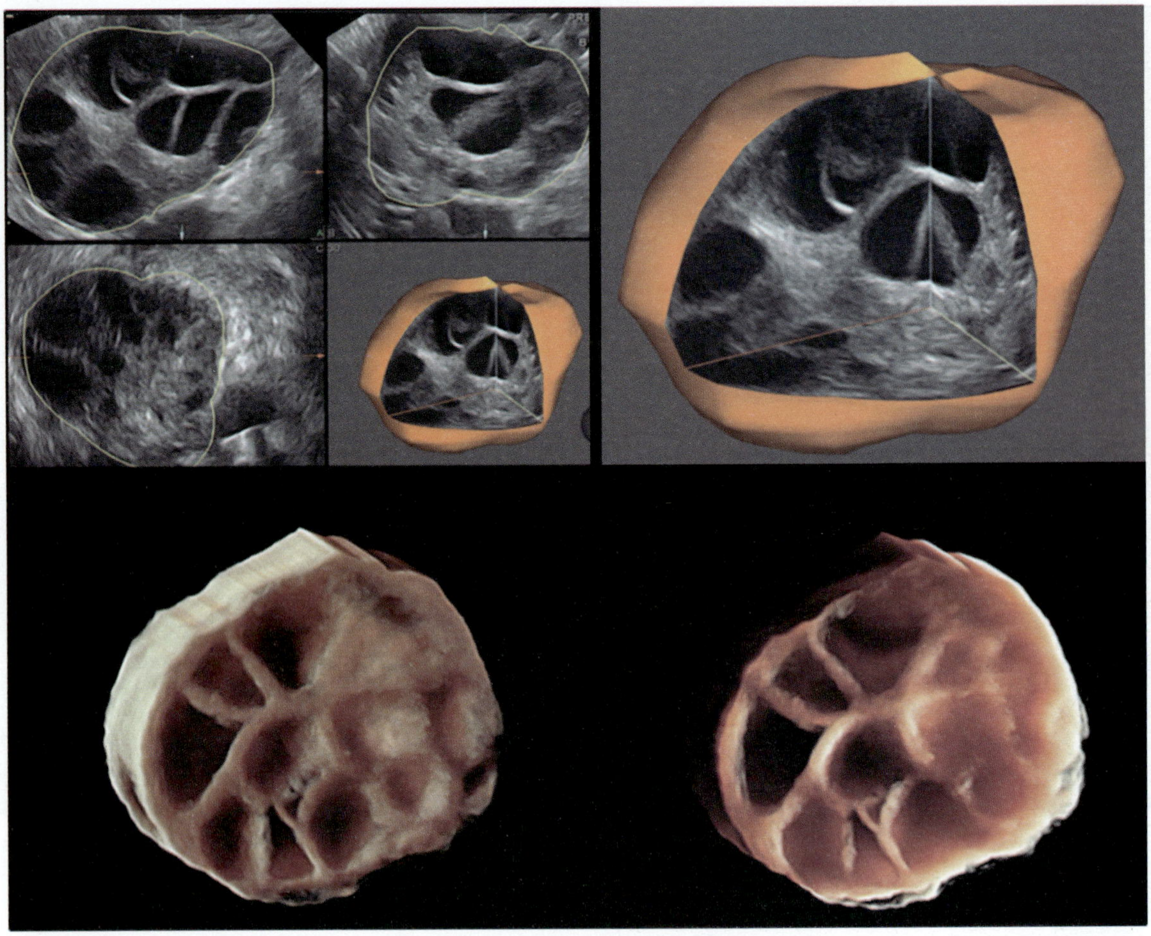

Fig. 94: Antral follicle count: Hyperstimulation. Above 2D orthogonal planes and shell mode showing the whole ovarian surface and the internal structures. Below 4D HDlive. Comparative ovarian view. The figure shows a comparative US (day 9 of menses) of a hyperstimulated patient.

- Nonetheless, it was agreed that the use of real-time 2D US imaging is adequate for measurement and counting of AF in routine clinical practice.

POLYCYSTIC OVARIES AND THE ULTRASONOGRAPHIC EVALUATION

With the advent of ultrasonography, follicle excess has become the main aspect of polycystic ovarian morphology (PCOM) (1) as well as the main aspect of PCOS diagnosis.

Since 2003 Rotterdam criteria (5), the following transvaginal US criteria were recommended (6) and most clinician have been using:

- A threshold of 12 follicles, measuring 2–10 mm in diameter per whole ovary
- And an ovarian volume of ≥10 mL
- But that now seems obsolete.

STATE OF THE ART: NEW CRITERIA AND US MODES

We remark newly 3D US criteria that should be used and the modern 3D US modes introduced that whenever possible- should be employed.

POLYCYSTIC OVARIAN MORPHOLOGY

A PCOM designates the morphologic appearance of the polycystic ovaries under transvaginal sonographic view. Herein, we have described specific morphologic appearance in PCOS using advanced ultrasonographic software. This morphologic descriptions strictly correlates to current diagnostic criteria, and moreover is, in our opinion, more specific than the description given in Rotterdam criteria.

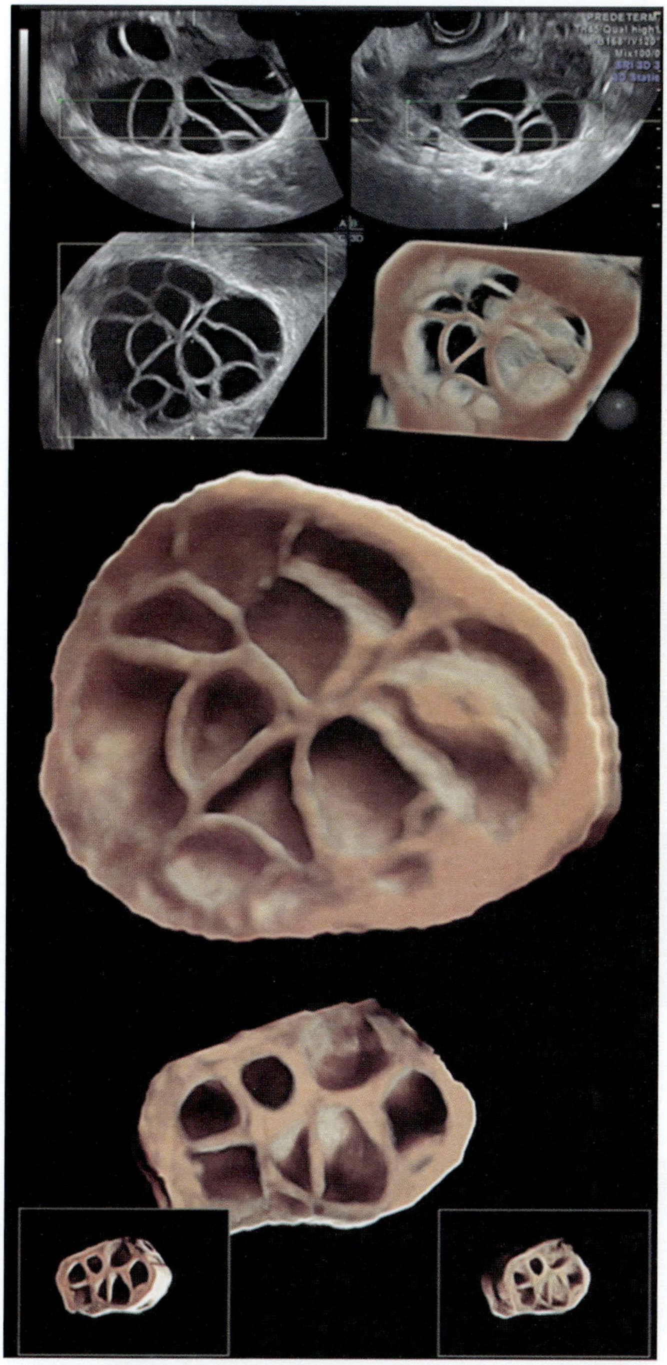

Fig. 95: HDlive in ovarian stimulation. Above 2D and HDlive scan. Center: US control 6 days after stimulation with FSH 150 UI/day. Notice the multifollicular development in a photo-like image. Below: HDlive view of a stimulated ovary in IVF cycle. Notice that the virtual light is positioned in the bottom left corner.

- Polycystic ovaries always show an ovarian surface, the albuginea, which is very thin and highly bright **(Figs. 97 to 99)**, unfortunately little diagnostic value is given to this feature
- The follicular distribution is located, almost in all cases, surrounding the ovarian cortex **(Figs. 87, 88, 90, 92, 93, 96, 99 and 102)**.

Although this peripheral distribution is a typical feature of PCOM (in our opinion of outstanding interest for diagnosis), some previous considerations should remain:

- It is not always present in both ovaries and can be unilateral
- Can be diffuse occupying the whole ovary
- The size of the AF ranges between 2 and 9 mm, and is frequently similar in both ovaries **(Figs. 91 to 97)**
- All these morphologic characteristics are usually present in both ovaries providing that the etiologic factors act over both ovaries. However, it is accepted that the presence of these morphologic features only in one ovary is enough for diagnosis. Unilateral polycystic ovary is an infrequent but still clinically significant finding
- Although chronologic age is the most important predictor of both the qualitative and quantitative ovarian reserve, there is considerable variability in the timing of the female reproductive ageing process.

Taken together, assessment of ovarian follicle number has become the main item of PCOM. Establishing the normal values for follicle number per ovary (FNPO), as well as for ovarian volume, and especially the setting of accurate thresholds for distinguishing normal ovaries from PCOM is still a great controversy.

The total number of AF present is highly variable, but in order to reach a correct diagnosis, it is still enough to find over 12 follicles at least in one ovary.

However, it seems that this cutoff limit is not accurate; in fact, when new ultrasonographic technologies are applied to AFC, this cutoff limit seems to be underestimated.

Several studies in the last two decades, have addressed comparatively 2D vs 3D scan accuracy, and the results clearly showed than 2D underestimate in 12–13% the exact number of AF available. Moreover, recent studies report even higher differences of up to 25–30% of underestimation. Modern 3D ultrasonographic modes like AVC and inverse mode seem to be more accurate when measuring AFC; likewise, VOCAL appear to be very important for volumetry.

Recent publications focused on PCOS patients showed a mean number of AFC of 19–26 follicles. This situation has arisen from the marked improvements in the level of spatial resolution afforded by newer ultrasound scanners.

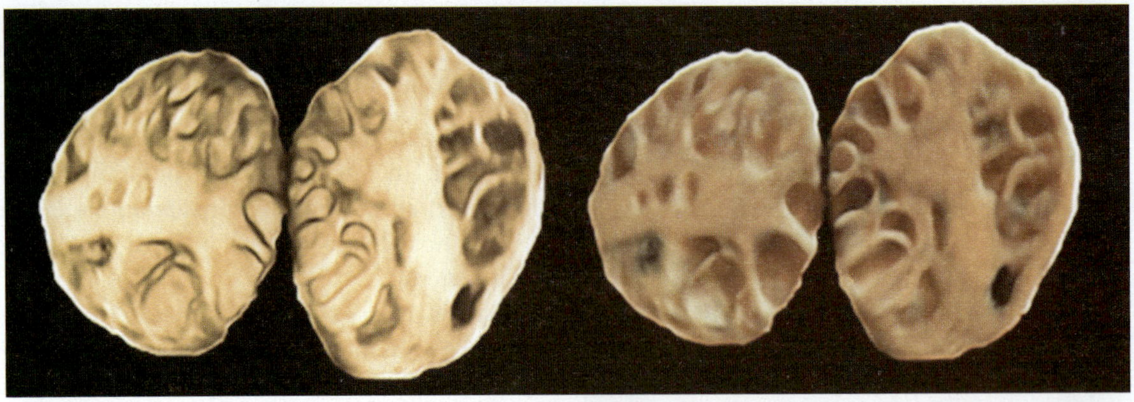

Fig. 96: Comparison of conventional 3D US (above) vs 3D HDlive (below) images of PCOS. HDlive increases the quality imaging view of 3D US.

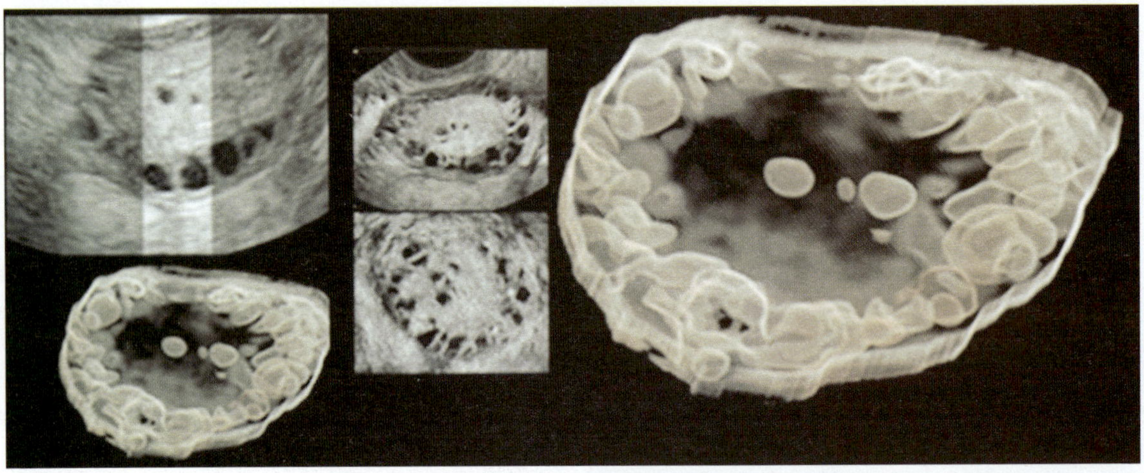

Fig. 97: Radiance System Architecture (Voluson E10 GE®) of an ovary with PCOS (right), compared to 2D US (left). This is the most advanced 3D US mode which allows a wonderful view of the isolated antral follicles and the ovarian tunica albuginea.

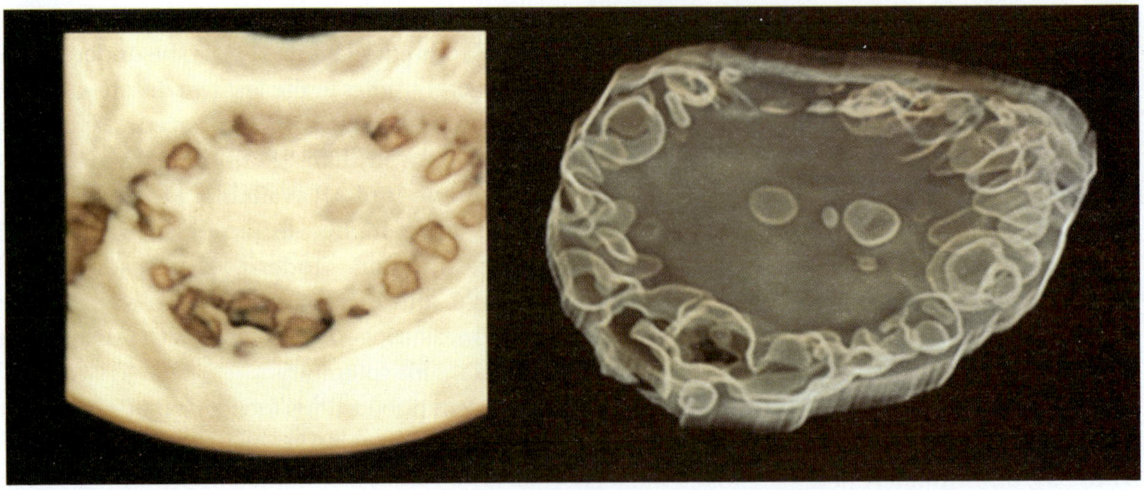

Fig. 98: A PCOM depicted using 3D HDlive (left) versus Radiance System Architecture (right).

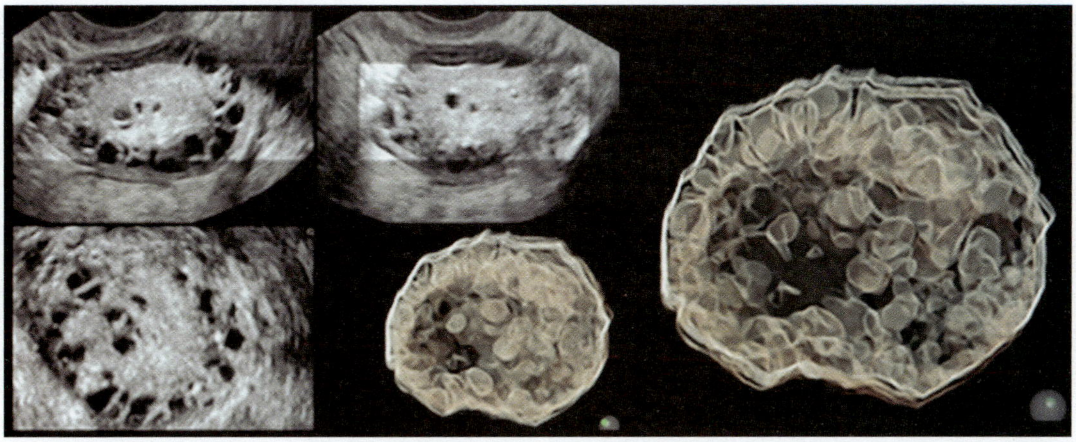

Fig. 99: PCOS-related ovarian morphology image using Radiance System Architecture. Each AF is clearly depicted with much better resolution than with standard 2D US.

Ovarian volume (OV) or area (OA) were also included as mandatory diagnostic criteria by ESHRE.

An OV appears to be a good surrogate marker of PCOM although, when compared with FNPO, it has less sensibility for discriminating between patients with PCOM and controls in all the studies comparing both parameters. As the AFC declines progressively over time, it provides a more useful clinical marker of ovarian responsiveness than ovarian volume.

Large-scale studies over the three last decades have shown that ovarian volume is inversely correlated with age (climacteric and menopause) intake of anovulatory pills, GnRH-agonist and antagonist and diabetes but positively correlated to puberty (beginning of hormonal secretion) and normal ovarian cycles.

2D transvaginal scan measures two planes in order to obtain the ovarian area, and three planes for obtaining the volume of the ovary after the application of the ellipsoid formula ($v = 4/3 \pi$ LD + APD + TD/2); however, there is a high probability of interobserver variations.

Based on all the previous considerations, our critical review shows that OV has less diagnostic potential for PCOM compared to AFC. The usefulness of OV compared to follicle excess remains unclear.

ESHRE and latter studies, suggested maintaining the threshold for increased OV ≥10 mL. By using AVC and VOCAL the measurement of the ovarian volumetry can be more exactly obtained. If such technology is not available, then OV is recommend rather than FNPO for the diagnosis in routine daily practice but not for research studies that require the precise full characterization of PCOM in each patient.

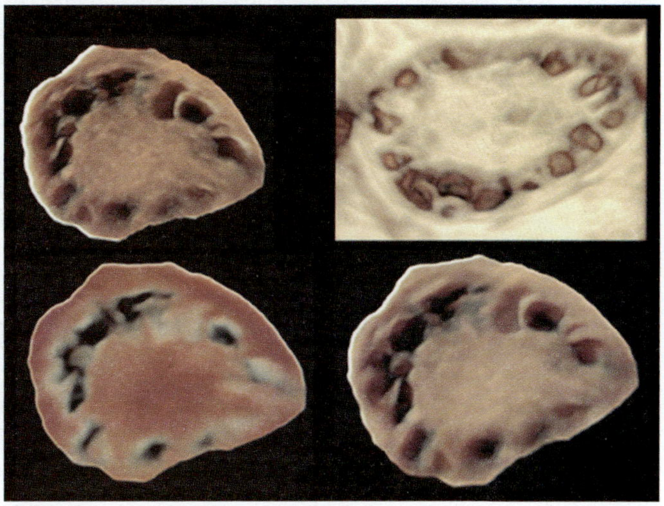

Fig. 100: Left: PCOM using HDlive without (upper left) and with (bottom left) maximum transparency. Note the increased thickness of the medulla and the AF located peripherally in the ovarian cortex.

OVARIAN MEDULLA

Surprisingly, Rotterdam criteria do not consider the characteristics of the ovarian medulla as relevant for diagnosis.

Decades ago specific characteristics of this ovarian zone for PCOS patients were described, including an increased vascularization, thickness and echogenicity. Some authors considered it as an additional feature of PCOS **(Figs. 100 and 101)**.

This review emphasizes that both ultrasonographic features—thickness of the medulla and antral follicles distribution and count—should be included for a correct

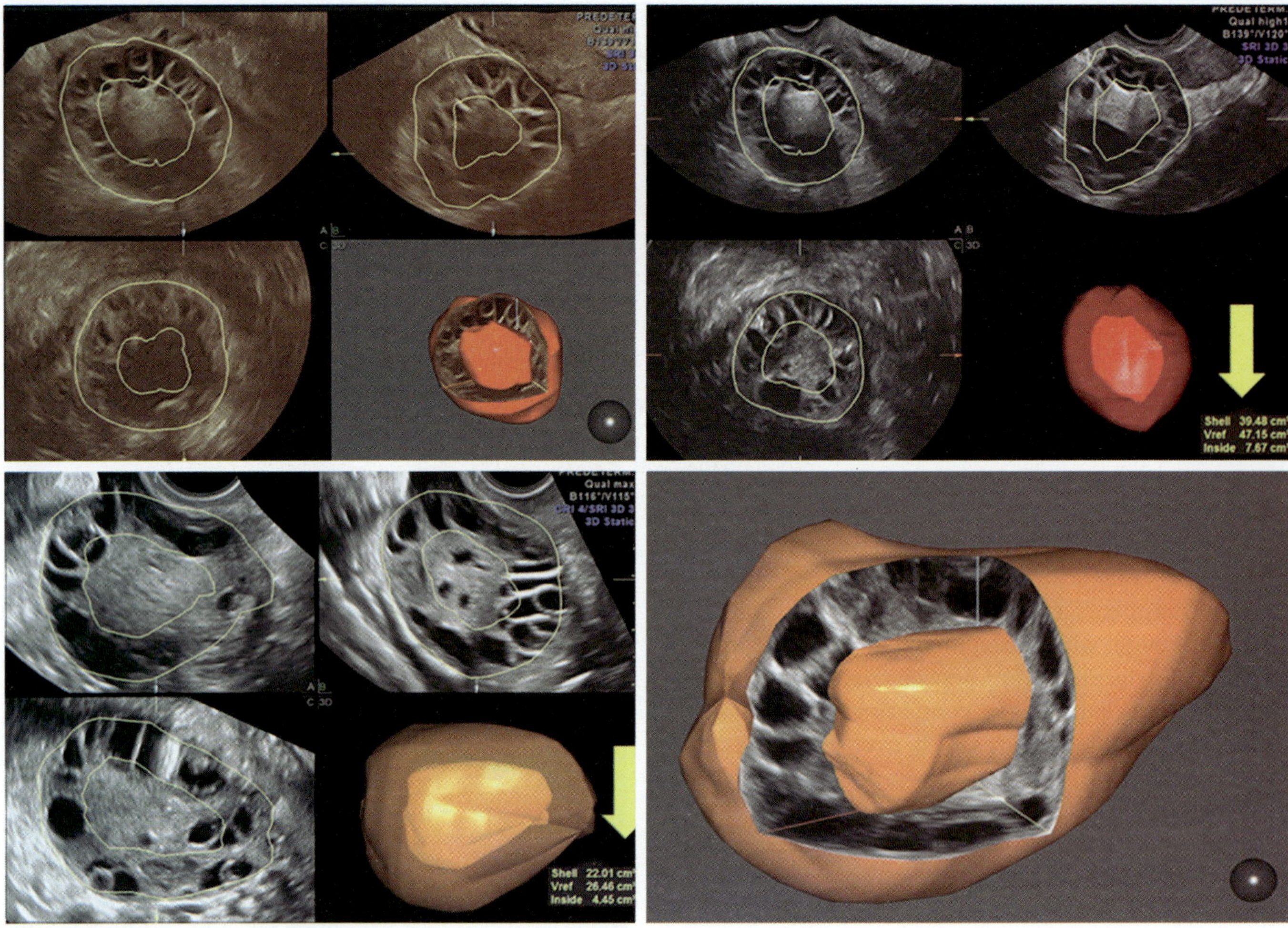

Fig. 101: Double VOCAL and NICHE modes showing the medulla of the ovary in red and orange. Around this structure numerous small AF. The yellow arrows depict total ovary and medullary volumes. The software shows calculates the volumes automatically.

description of PCOM. However, regarding the thickness of the ovarian medulla, there was a lack of consensus on quantitative measure for standardization. The ratio of ovarian stroma to total ovarian size may be a good criterion for the diagnosis of PCOS, with a cut-off value of 0.32 and has been suggested that its size is associated with more hyperandrogenemia.

Nowadays, a new way to quantify the thickness of the medulla is to use the double VOCAL technique or combining it with the niche mode. The software quantifies at the same time the medullar volume as well as the total ovarian volume **(Fig. 101)**.

MEDULLA VASCULARIZATION

PCOS patients shows an enhanced vascularization of the ovarian medulla which remains constant during the menstrual cycle. This feature is not seen in patients having normal hormonal periods which show cyclic changes.

With the pioneering studies focused on Doppler, it was observed that resistance and pulsatility indexes were very low in PCOS patients - related to good vascularization, but without changes throughout the cycle, this feature seems to be characteristic of PCOM, although it is not internationally accepted. This situation might change with the introduction of 3D digital Doppler angiography. This new 3D US mode has allowed observing the following key events in this group of patients:

- A markedly increase in vascularization **(Fig. 102)**.
- 3D parameters (vascular, flow, vascularization/flow indexes) significantly higher
- These features deserve further study to be included as new markers for PCOM.

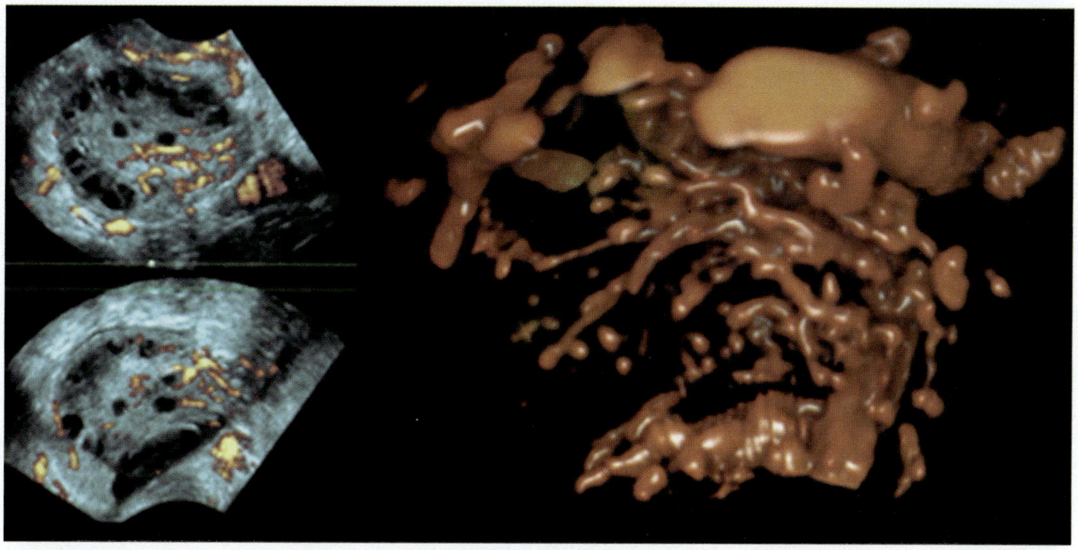

Fig. 102: Vascularization of the medulla in PCOS patients. Note the increased vascular component, gross and long vessels and the absence of changes in flow velocity.

Several studies have compared these vascular indices between normo and hyperandrogenic women having PCOS. The results showed statistically differences as well as a direct relationship between increased flow and hyperandrogenemia.

Besides its enormous interests, we may underline that other several authors remark the lack of uniform data and absence of cutoff values which would still make vascular parameters by Doppler impractical for discriminating between PCOM and normal ovarian morphology.

In our opinion, 3D digital Doppler angiography should be considered as a valuable and potent diagnostic tool.

Comparison between normoandrogenic and PCOS patient

Features	*Normoandrogenic patients*	*PCOS patients*
Vascularity index	2,79%	3.85%
Flow index	(0–100) 31.79	(0–100) 33.54
Vascularity-flow index	(0–100) 0.85	(0–100) 1.27

INTRAUTERINE DEVICES

Correct diagnosis of the intrauterine devices (IUD) placement is crucial to detect gynecological problems of bleeding or pelvic pain. Improvements in 3D, allow us detailed examination of the position of this kind of devices. The introduction of the HDlive technique give us more clear images of IUDs, especially of MIRENAs ones.

The IUDs play an important role in reducing unintended pregnancies and have a higher continuation of use than implants and depots. They are safe, highly effective and a prevalent way of birth control. However, they need to be controlled because:

- Uterine cavity differs considerably in size and shape during the menstrual cycle, also after miscarriages and pregnancies
- After implantation, may occur some complications, e.g., menstrual disorders, pelvic pain, dysmenorrheal, migration, infections, pelvic inflammatory disease, perforation of the uterus **(Fig. 103)** pregnancy **(Fig. 104)**.

IUDs are classified as follow:

- Inert: Ring-shaped (Grafenberg), Lippes Loop, Saft-T-Coil, Chinese Ring
- Cooper-containing IUDs: T or 7-shaped, Cooper-T-380A, Ancora or multiload
- Hormone-containing IUD's: natural progesterone or progestogen-levonorgestrel.

The evaluation of the uterus before and after the IUD includes:

- Vaginal and cervical examination by speculum
- 2D transvaginal US for evaluating the type, placement and complications: displacement, descent, malposition and incarceration **(Fig. 105)**.
- The correct detection of abnormally located IUDs is really important, since many patients with pelvic pain or bleeding have a misplaced IUD. US methods used

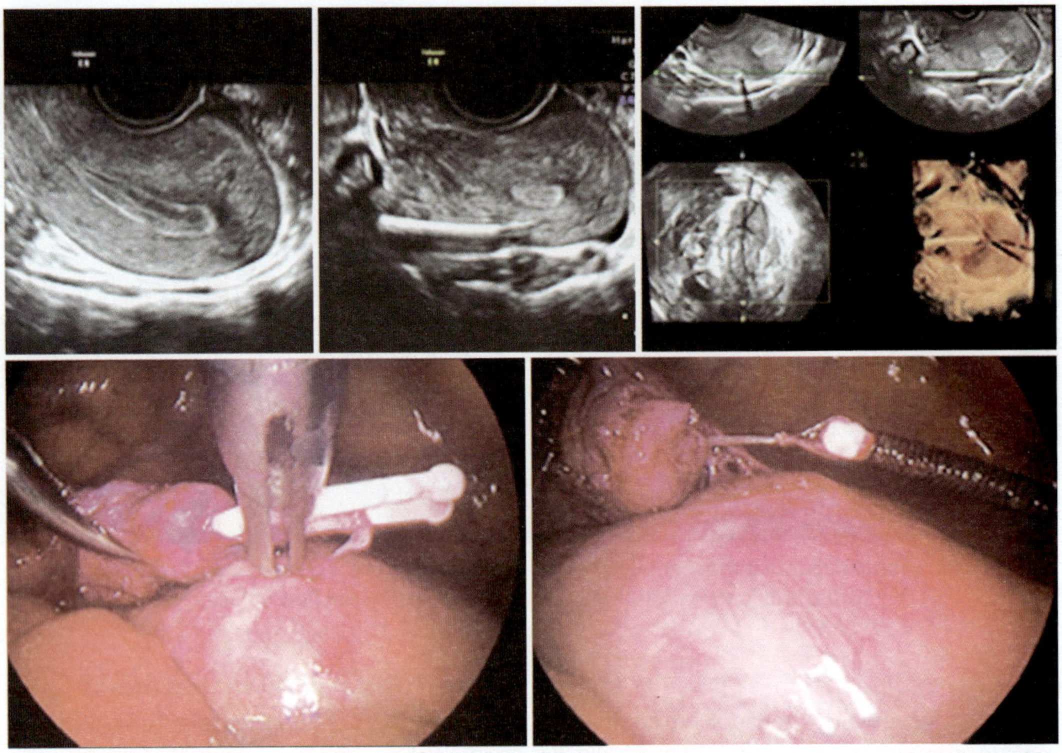

Fig. 103: Above 2D (left) and HDlive (right) of a perforated uterus by a IUD with its laparoscopic image.

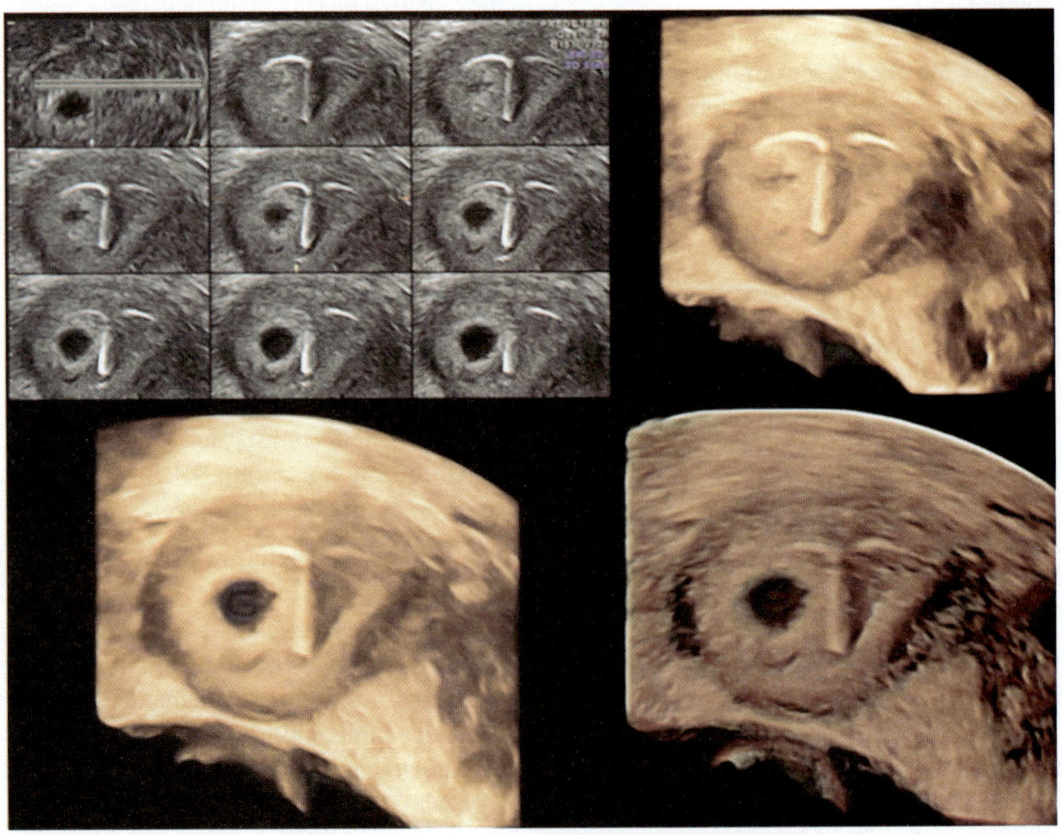

Fig. 104: *Copper T-* IUD and pregnancy. The gestational sac is clearly depicted with a ParaGard T-IUD at its right side.

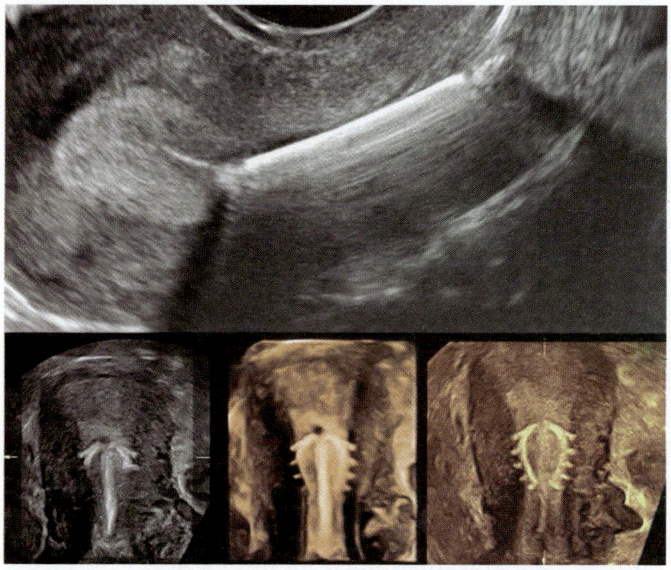

Fig. 105: *Ancora IUD* bad positioned, descended into the cervical canal. Above 2D. The shape is not clearly defined. Below 3D/4D HDlive. The Ancora is clearly defined and observed, as above, in the cervical canal.

for the correct diagnosis of the IUD placement are crucial

- Two-dimensional transvaginal US is the most employed technique.

IDENTIFICATION OF THE IUD TYPE

Copper T

Nonhormonal copper releasing IUD that measures 32 mm horizontally and 36 mm vertically. It has a 3 mm diameter bulb at the tip of the vertical stem and a straight shaft and cross-bars that form the shape of a T. The T frame is made of polyethylene, and a total of 380 mm^2 of copper wire is coiled around the stem and the two horizontal crossbars, which improves sonographic visualization **(Fig. 106)**.

By using HDlive, a clearer and more perfect IUD visualization is seen. The perfect image can be obtained by correctly locating the light source behind the IUD device and/or changing the surface mode for maximum/

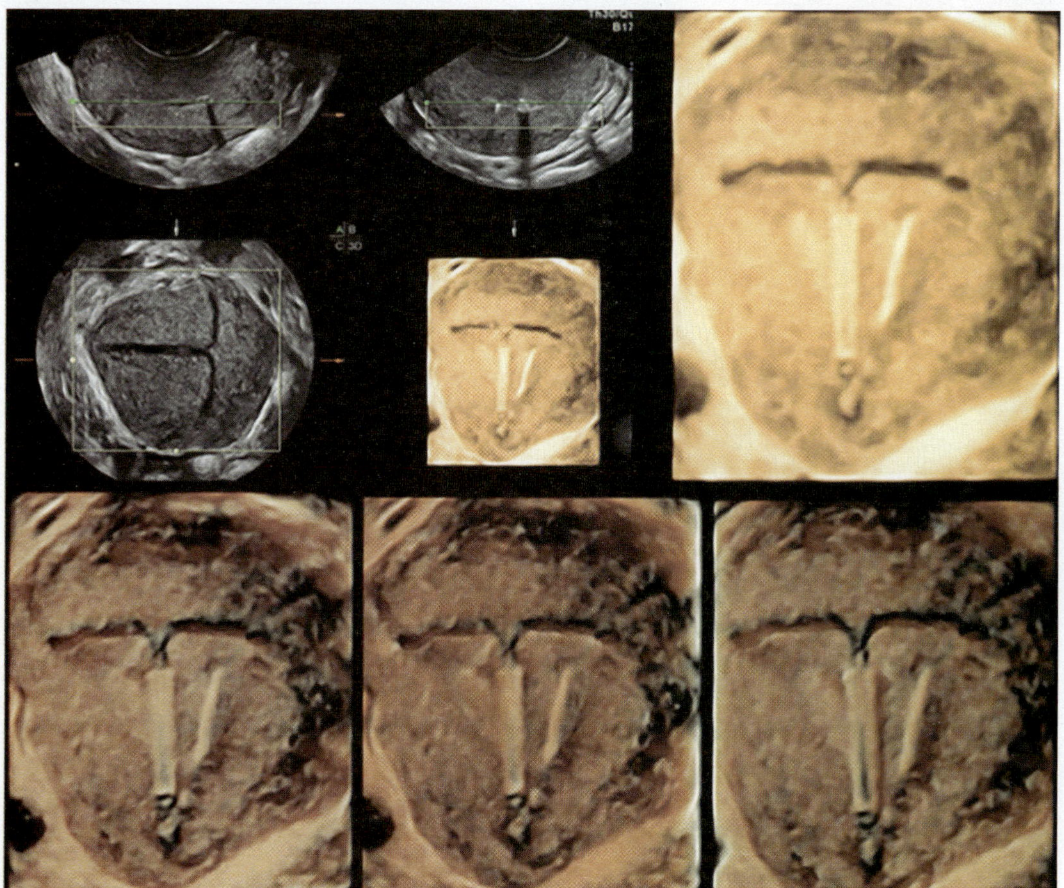

Fig. 106: Orthogonal 2D planes, 3D and HDlive visualization of a copper T-IUD. The ultrasounds show the crossbars that form the shape of the T (below), the copper coiled around the stem and the cord located in the uterine cavity.

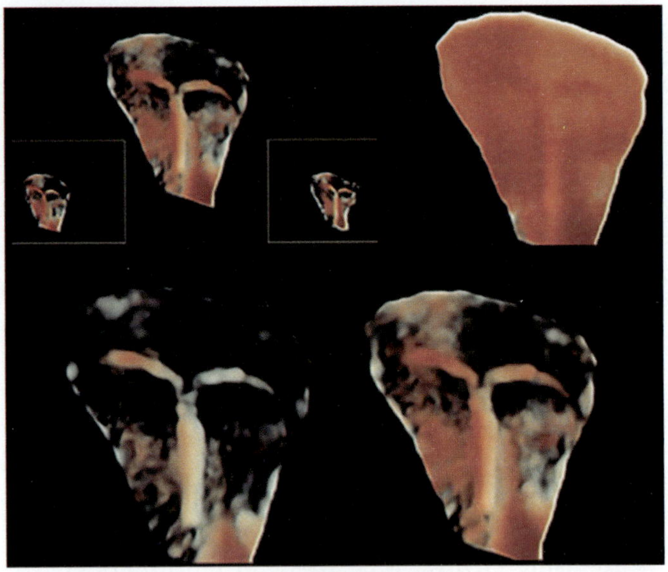

Fig. 107: Maximal translucency and transparence US modes allow the perfect visualization of a copper T- IUD.

minimum transparence modes. Also, other images can be obtained by isolating the endometrium from the myometrium with the cutoff system **(Fig. 107)**.

The HDlive system, permits also the detection of the copper corrosion when it starts.

Multiload/Ancora

Consists on a polyethylene structure with a copper wire spiral rolled along its vertical axis and a polyethylene thread attached to its lower end **(Fig. 108)**.

CONCLUDING REMARKS

Recent papers have been published focusing on the (re)efinition of PCOS; nevertheless, the Rotterdam consensus remains as the most widely accepted across Europe, Asia and Australia and, until a new Consensus, should be still used.

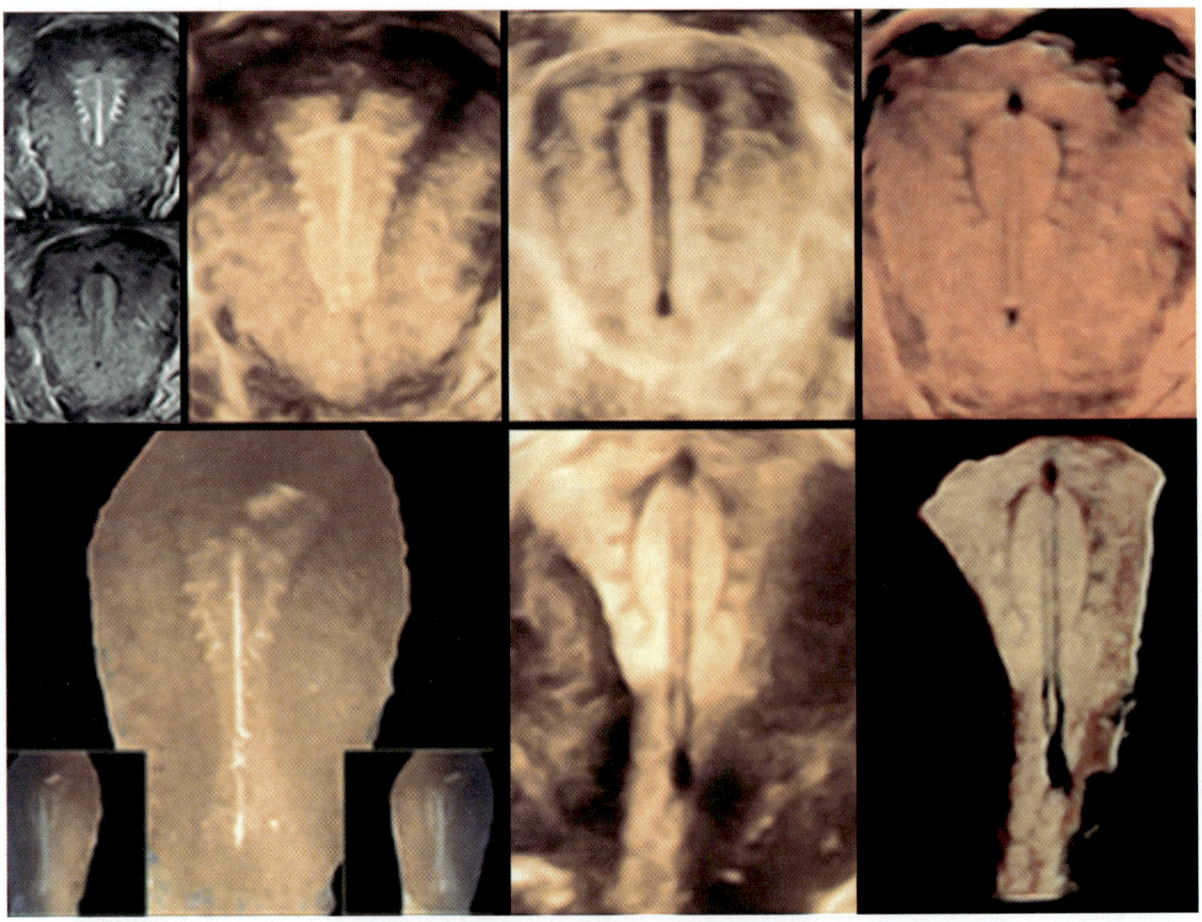

Fig. 108: Ancora multiload IUDs (Euro gine).

Initial investigations must exclude other endocrinological abnormalities: thyroid function, prolactin luteinizing (LH) and follicle stimulating hormone (FSH) levels.

Ovarian US morphology as diagnostic criteria (Rotterdam consensus) plays, in our consideration, a central role, superior to hyperandrogenemia; however, as shown in this review, there is a lack of consensus.

Indeed, PCOS and control populations share a significant overlap in ovarian morphology, and a large proportion (estimates range from 10 to 48%) of adolescents who do not have PCOS may have polycystic-appearing ovaries.

A PCOS should never be considered in young women until 2 years of establishing normal menstruations.

There are cases with typical PCOM and hyperandrogenemia but with ovarian volume less than 10 cc. Ovarian volume and/or area are not as interesting as published by the Rotterdam consensus.

The measurement of the medulla, especially if combined with 3D angio-Doppler is a good adjunctive tool in diagnosing PCOS.

TUI is only of modest interest for PCOM evaluation. It is neither necessary nor recommended.

Inversion mode and AVC are much more specific, reliable and recommended than the simple transvaginal 2D for AF counting.

3D US HDlive and silhouette software improve image quality and should be used if available.

Anovulatory drugs: This medication may interfere with the ultrasonographic appearance of the AF, presumably due to a reduction in testosterone levels, thus, the hormonal and ultrasonography assay are recommended after 3 months of cessation.

The finding of PCOM in ovulatory women not showing clinical or biochemical androgen excess may be inconsequential.

Finally, the new 3D US modalities seems to be superior to the standard 2D transvaginal scan, and should be employed when available.

GYNECOLOGY

NORMAL UTERUS AND BENIGN UTERINE TUMORS

Vaginal two-dimensional (2D) ultrasound is the gold standard technology on which diagnosis, control and management in gynecological tumors is based.

Based on specific case reports of normal uteri and gynecological tumors we are showing the improvement in image quality obtained using the HDlive images

UTERUS

The uterine and endometrial morphology **(Fig. 109)** can be examined as well as with 2D or 3D US, but the quality of the obtained images is clearly superior if 3D US is used. 2D/3D US scans can be employed for the knowledge of the endometrial receptivity during the follicular development and ovarian stimulation in IVF-ET (i.e., failure of receptivity).

Other US modes (AVC, VOCAL, "shell" and double shell techniques), are helpful for uterine measurements, volume calculation and perfect differentiation between myometrium and endometrium **(Fig. 110)**.

ENDOMETRIAL AND MYOMETRIAL PATHOLOGIES

Endometrial pathologies as polyps), mucometra **(Fig. 111)** and myomas **(Figs. 112 and 113)** are discussed shown in **Figures 111 to 113**.

MÜLLERIAN MALFORMATIONS

They are a heterogeneous group of congenital uterine anomalies produced as a failure of one of the three paramesonephric or Müllerian ducts development:

- Organogenic phase: One or both Müllerian ducts are not complete the developed, giving rise to anomalies like agenesis or uterine bilateral or unilateral aplasia (unicornuate uterus)
- Fusion phase: A failure or an abnormal fusion of the distal müllerian segments is produced
- Septal reabsorption phase: After the fusion phase the central septum is reabsorbed appearing unique uterine and cervical cavities.
- Finally and independently from the three mentioned phase defects, there are combinations between them and with kidney anomalies.

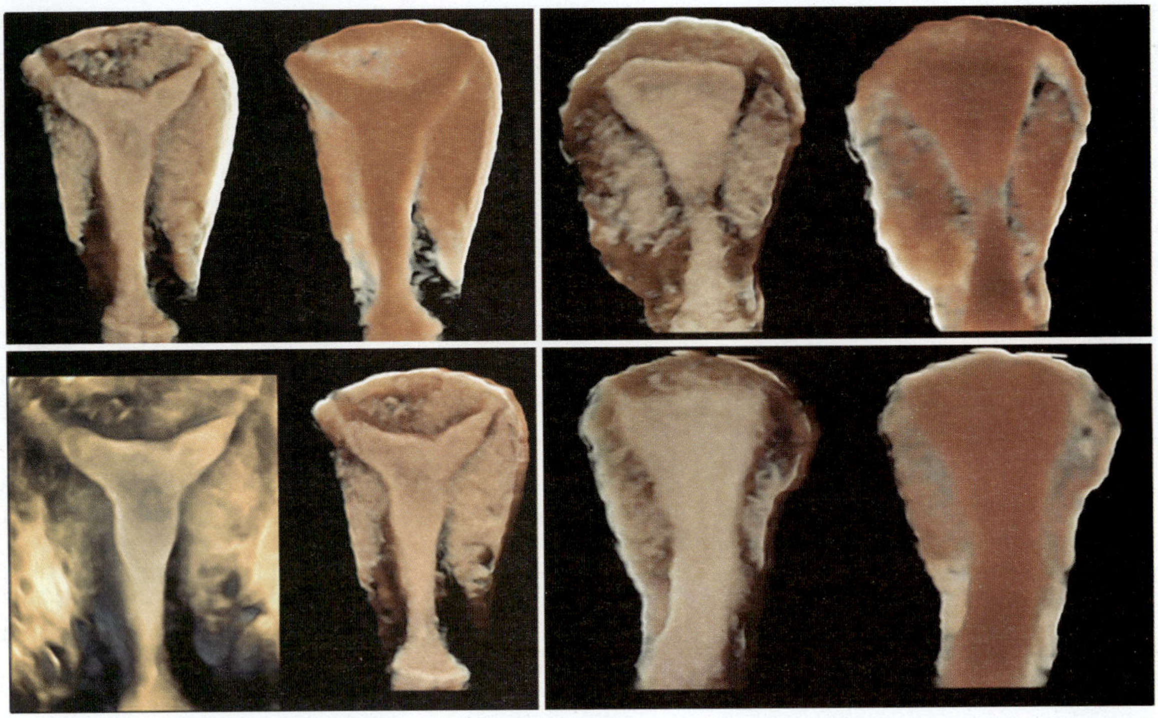

Fig. 109: The uterus (to the left): Normal uterine morphology. Infantile uterus with T endometrial shape. Comparison of 3D (below left) with HDlive. Virtual light entering through different angles and with maximal transparency (above right). It results evident that image quality is much better even when compared with conventional 3D US. The endometrium (to the right). The picture shows the endometrial morphology and homogeneity in the proliferative (above) and secretory hormonal phase (below). The figure shows myometrial and endometrial views in different light angles and maximal luminescence.

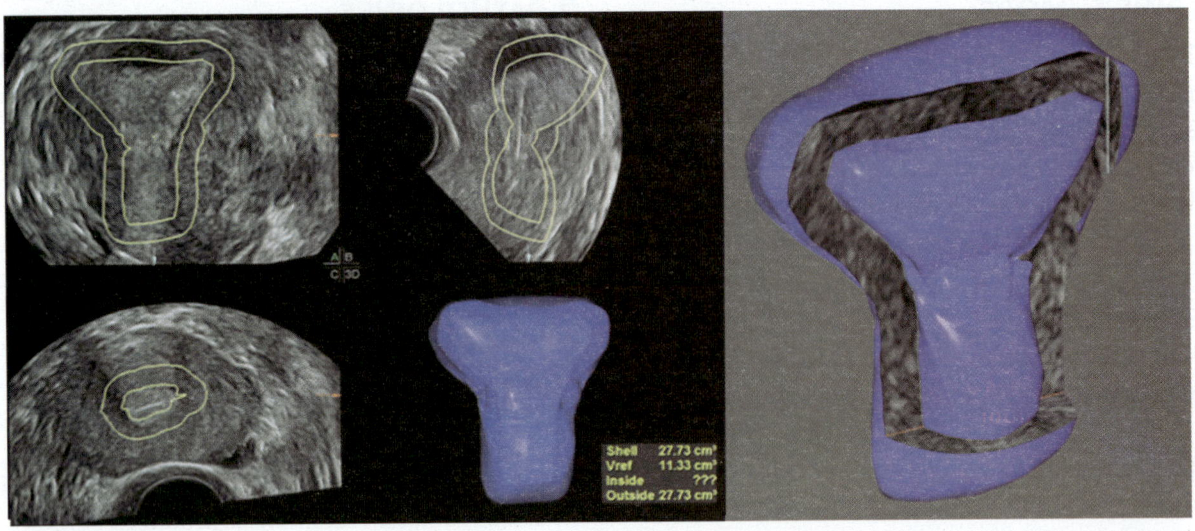

Fig. 110: Limits between myometrium and endometrium. "Shell mode" of a normal uterus with the calculated volume of the endometrium and the myometrium. The image shows endometrium (in blue) and myometrium (in gray).

Classification

These figures are selected according to the most used International Müllerian Malformations Classification, the one of the American Fertility Society dated in 1983 **(Figs. 114 to 122)**.

All these types can be clearly observed with HDlive 4D US.

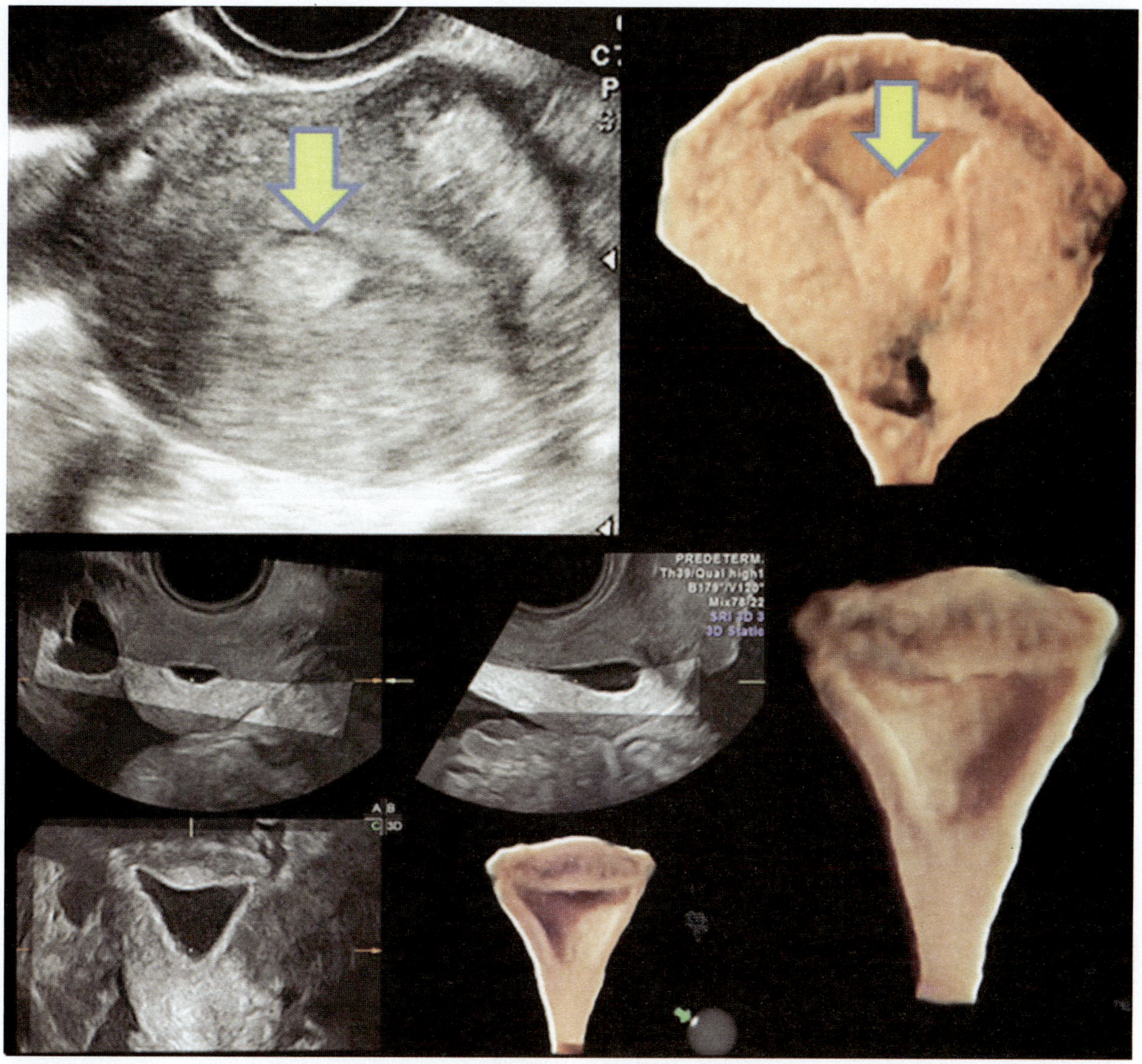

Fig. 111: A polyp observed with 2D and 3D HDlive (above). Mucometra: the uterine cavity is filled with mucus. The whole endometrial cavity can be visualized (below).

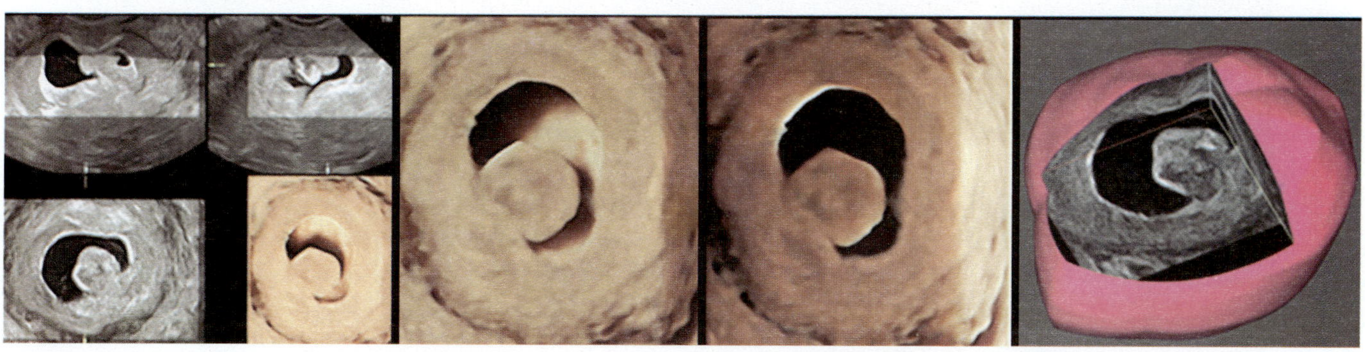

Fig. 112: Submucous myoma examined with 2D/3D, HDlive and shell VOCAL.

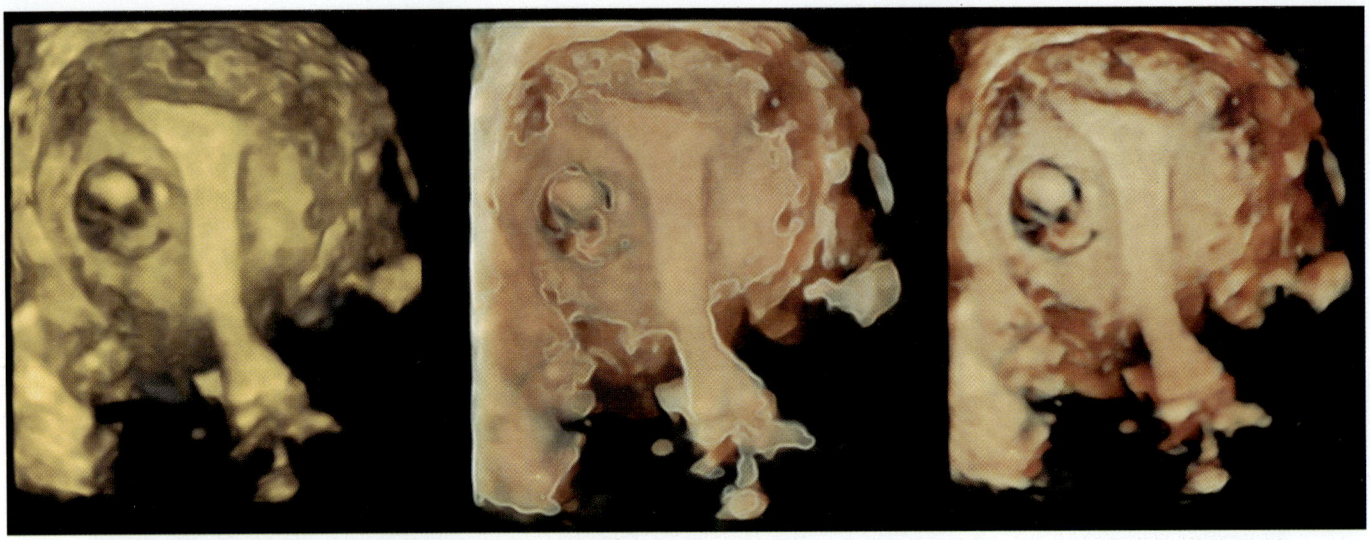

Fig. 113: 3D (left) and silhouette of an intramural myoma.

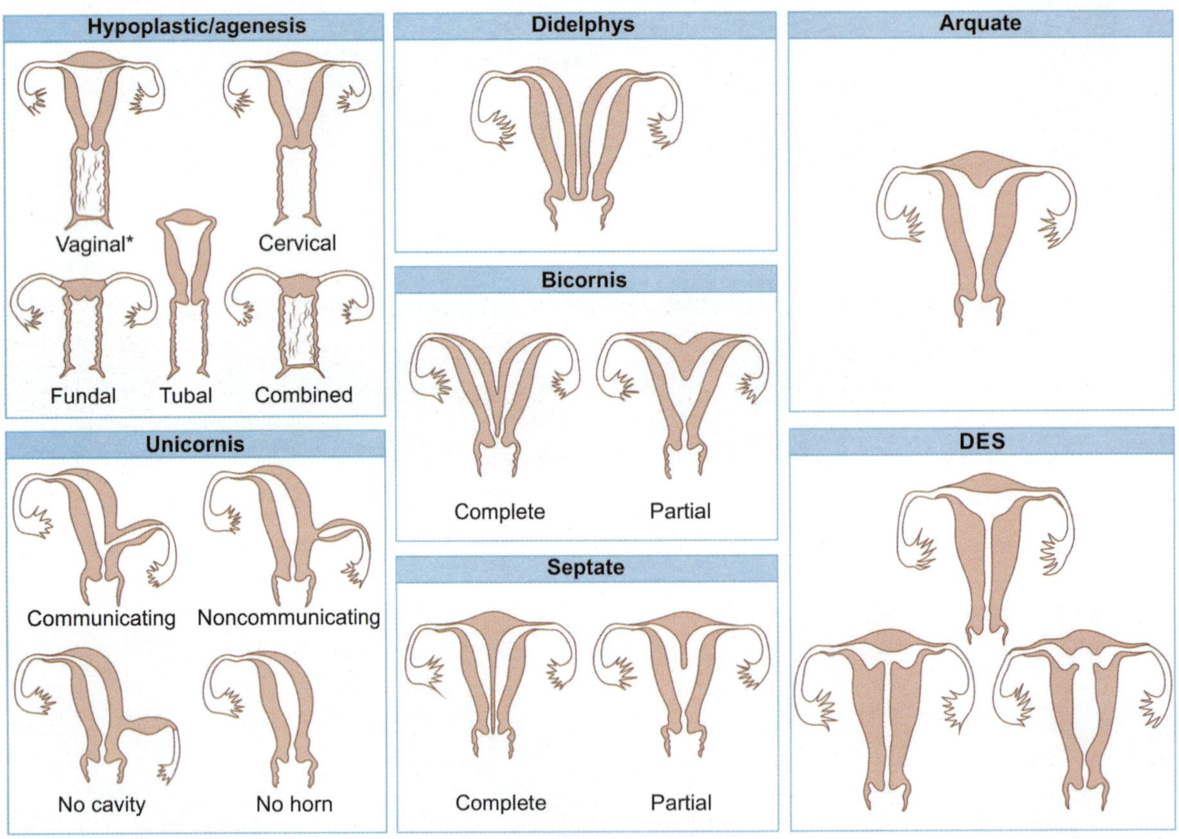

Fig. 114: International classification.

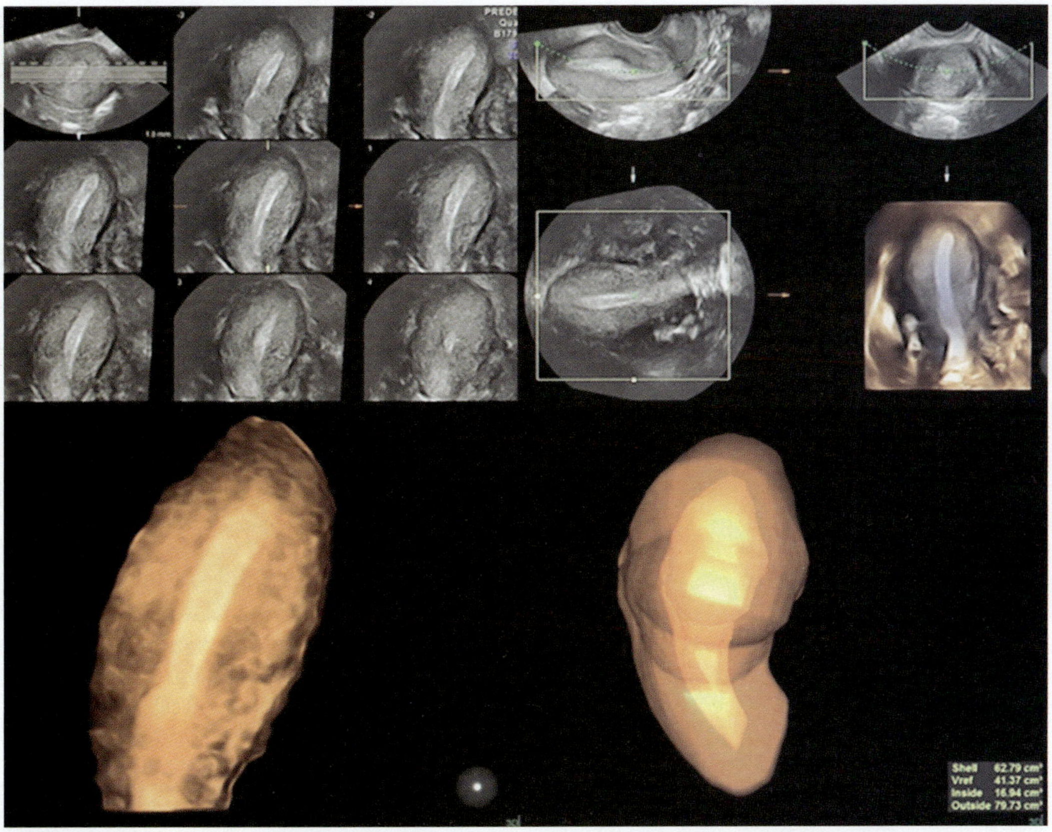

Fig. 115: Pure uterus unicornis. It is the most infrequent variety. Above TUI and 4D HDlive. Below 4D magic cut and VOCAL.

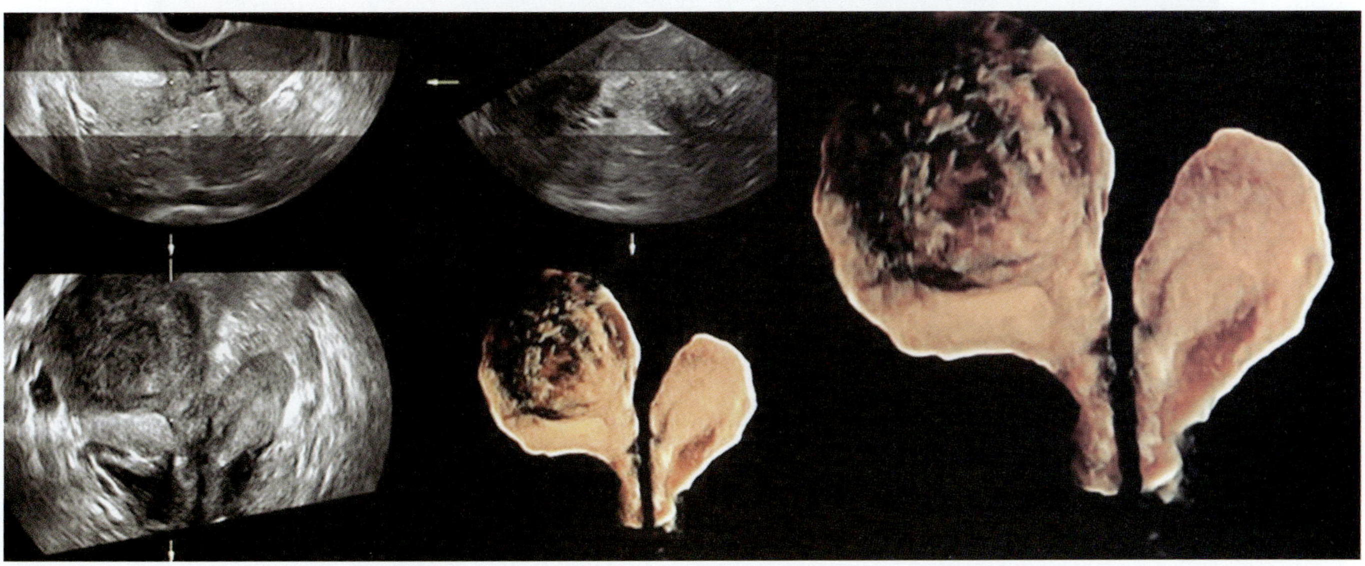

Fig. 116: Uterus didelphys with a myoma at the left corn.

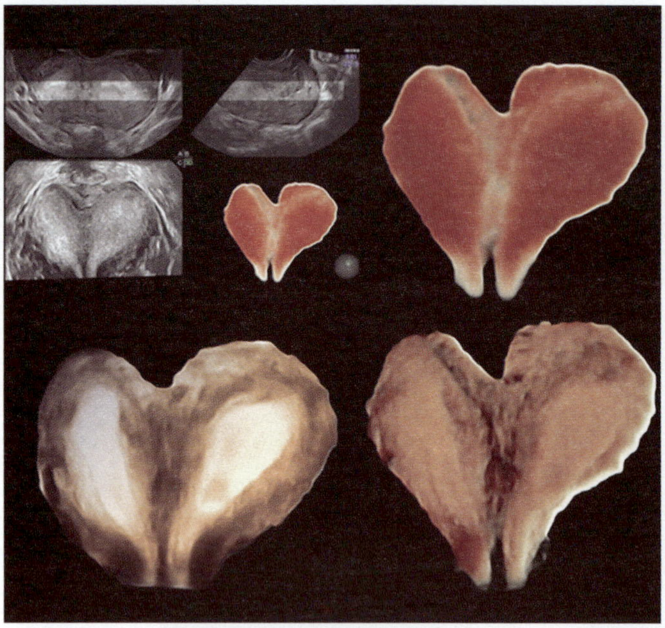

Fig. 117: Uterus bicornis totalis. HDlive and maximum translucency. The uterine separation arrive until cervix (variety IVc).

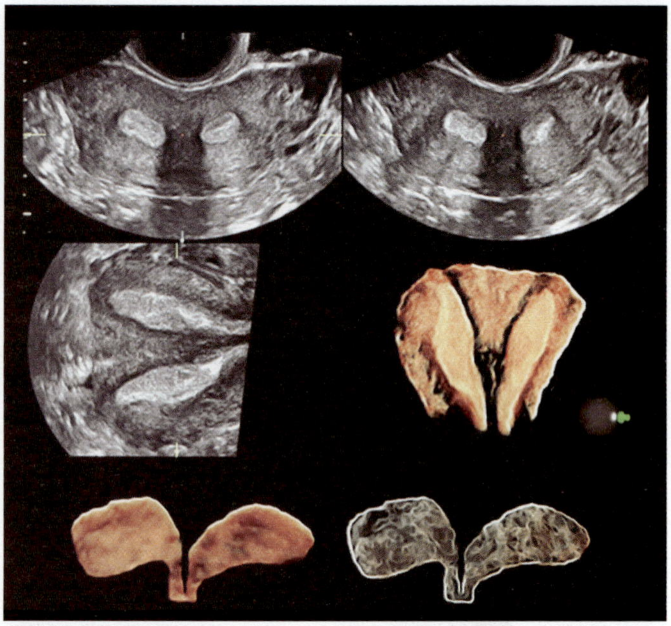

Fig. 118: Above: Complete septate uterus with cervical and vaginal septum. TUI plus HDlive. Below: an incomplete septate uterus depicted with HDlive and silhouette.

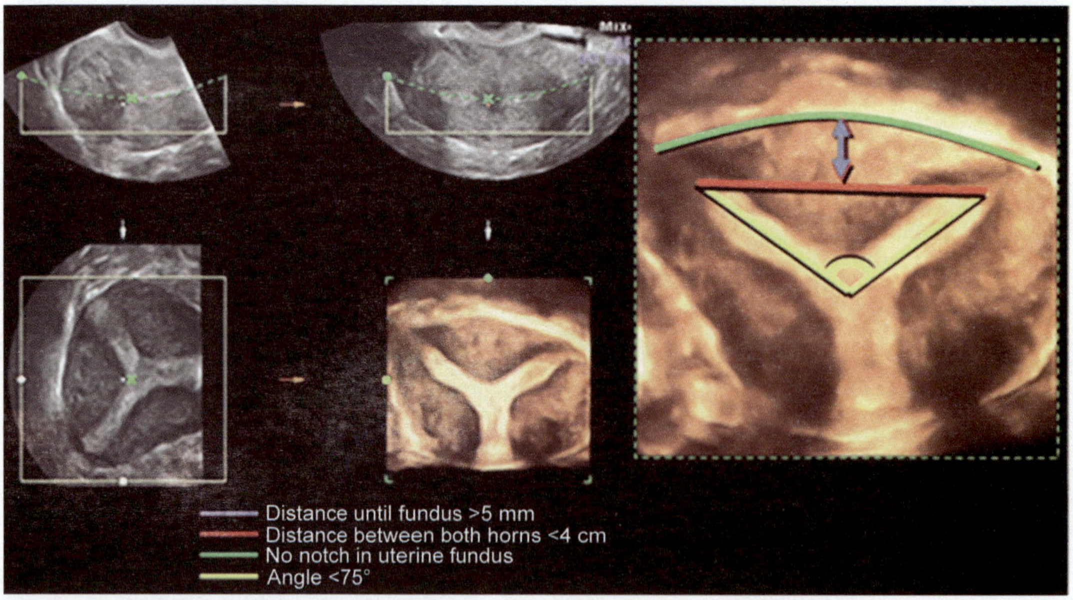

Septate	*Bicornuate*
Angle <75°	Angle >105°
Linear uterine fundus	Fundus with "Notch"
Distance between horns <4 cm	Distance between horns >4 cm
Distance endometrium-fundus >5 mm	Distance endometrium–fundus <5 mm
Vessels in septum	Vessels in septum

Fig. 119: How to make the differential diagnosis with US between septate and bicornuate uterus.

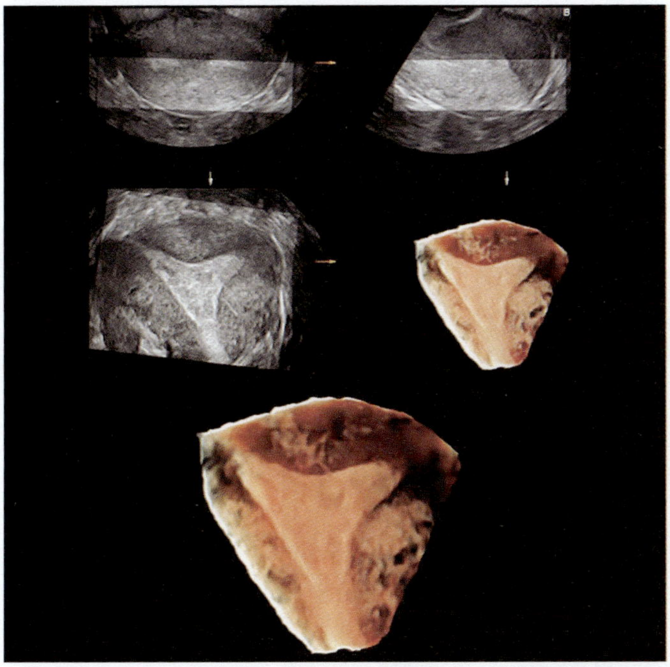

Fig. 120: Arcuate uterus.

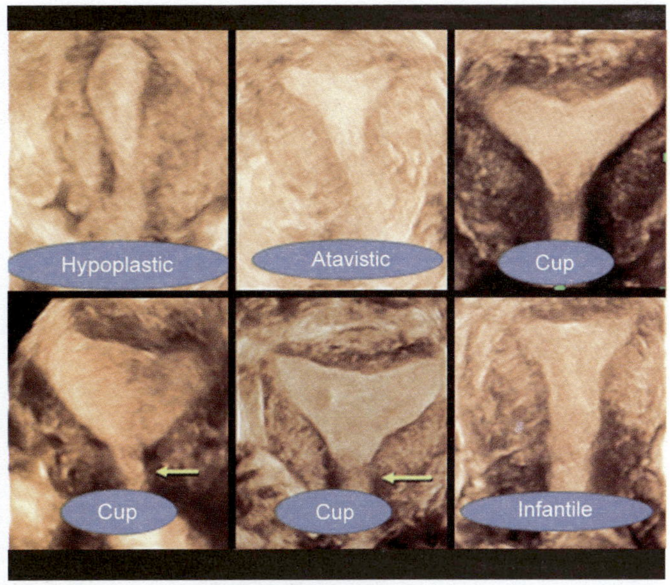

Fig. 121: These groups of minimal malformations are today included the DES group all malformations. Include the so called hypoplastic, atavistic, infantile and cup form uterus.

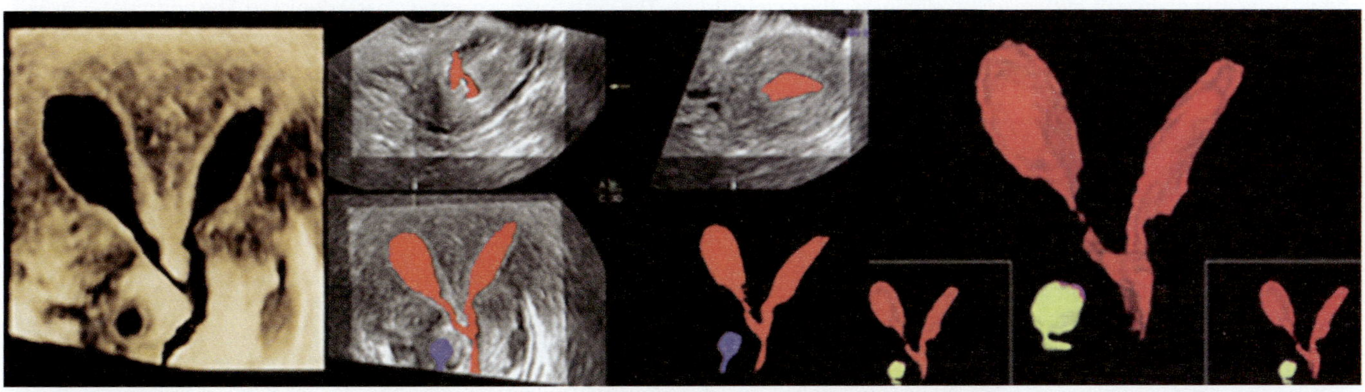

Fig. 122: The American Society classification is very incomplete. We show with 3D and VOCAL a rare case of communicating uterus.

ENDOMETRIAL HYPERPLASIA AND CANCER, FALLOPIAN TUBE PATHOLOGY

Hyperplasias

The ultrasonographic identification of these pathologies is of the outmost interest, especially in postmenopausal patients. It is widely accepted that an endometrial thickness ≤5 mm in asymptomatic postmenopausal patients rules out the presence of a carcinoma with a 97% sensibility. It is important to evaluate not only the endometrial thickness, but also its homogeneity, the delimitation of the outer borders and the presence of intramyometrium vessels.

There are some varieties of endometrial hyperplasia (benign in origin) which should be differentiated from carcinomas.

The atrophic cystic glandular hyperplasia **(Figs. 123 to 126)** is mainly observed in advanced age patients, its endometrial appearance (thickness, irregular delimitation, solid/cystic endometrial findings) is produced by the cystic dilation of the scarce endometrial glands which can be of variable endometrial and glandular size, giving a similar image to cancer.

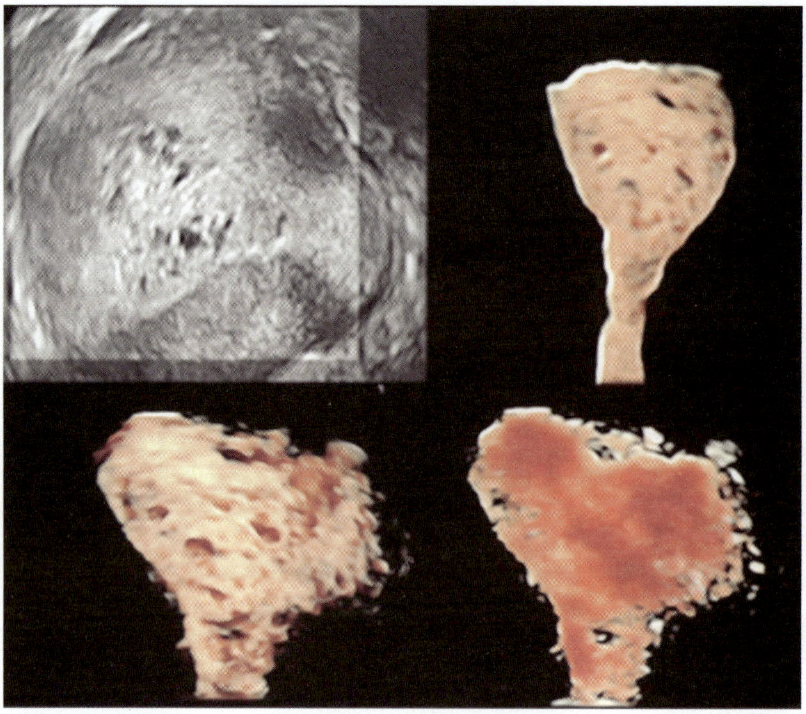

Fig. 123: Atrophic glandular cystic hyperplasia in 72 years old women showed in 2D (above left) and HDlive. The whole endometrium is shown using the magic cut system which eliminates the myometrium. The cystic glands appear clearly depicted. The endometrium with its small cysts is also shown using maximal luminescence (below right). The image can be confused with carcinomas.

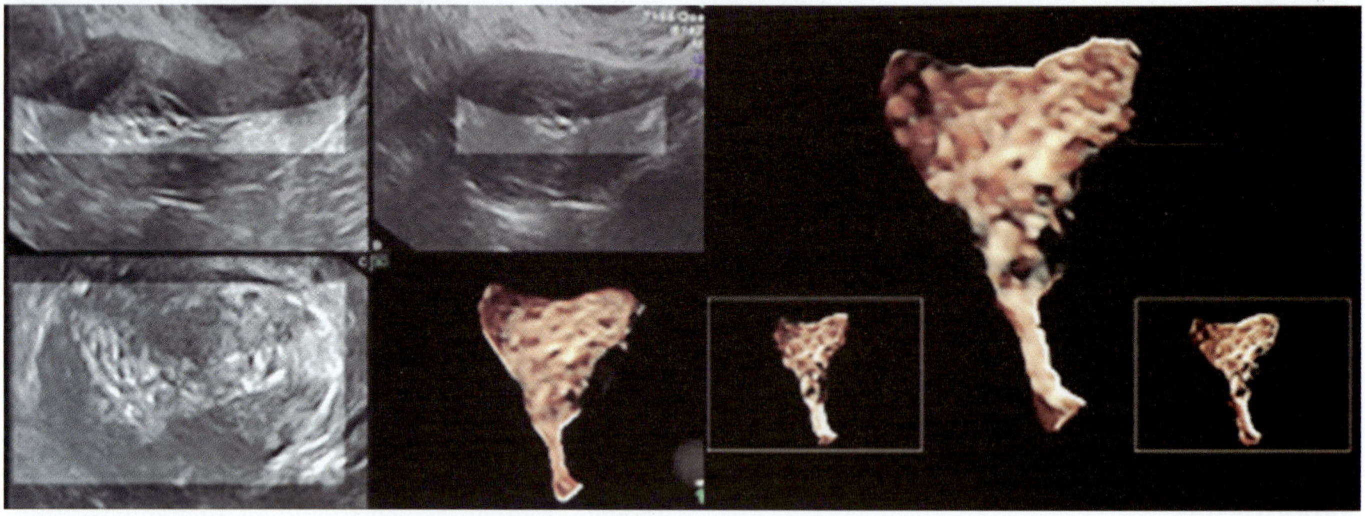

Fig. 124: Atrophic cystic glandular endometrial hyperplasia in an old women showing the whole endometrium fully of small cystic endometrial gland dilatations.

CANCER

In recent years this tumor has changed to be in women of developed countries the most frequent neoplasia.

The ultrasonographic evaluation must take into account:

- An early detection screening in asymptomatic patients (thickness cut-off ≤5 mm)
- Myometrial invasion constitutes the key feature of FIGO endometrial cancer grading system. Unfortunately,

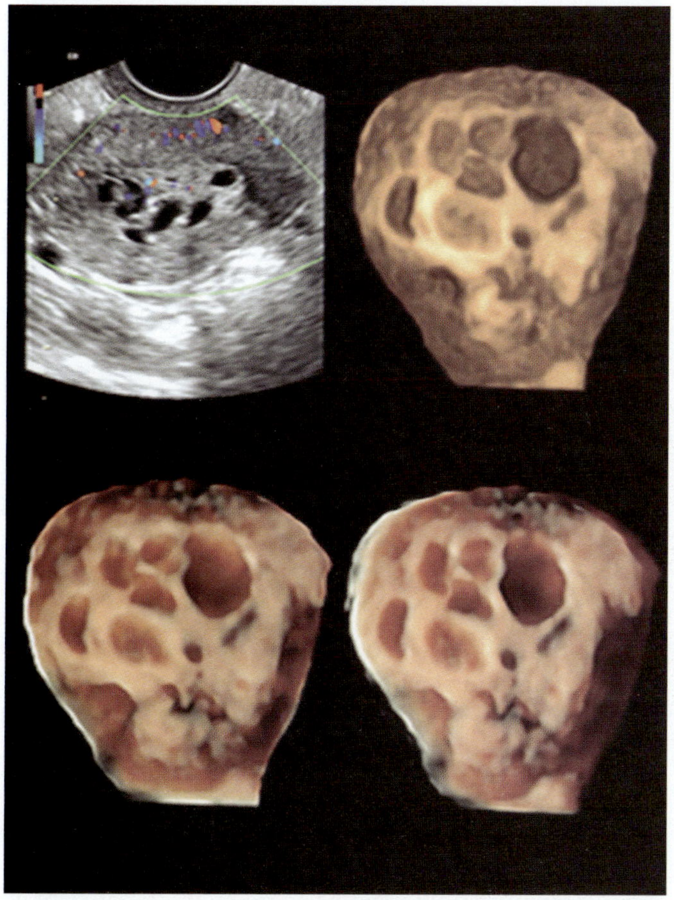

Fig. 125: Atrophic glandular cystic hyperplasia showing multiple cysts. In this case, cysts (dilated endometrial glandule) are of big sizes. This bizarre image is very suggestive of malignancy.

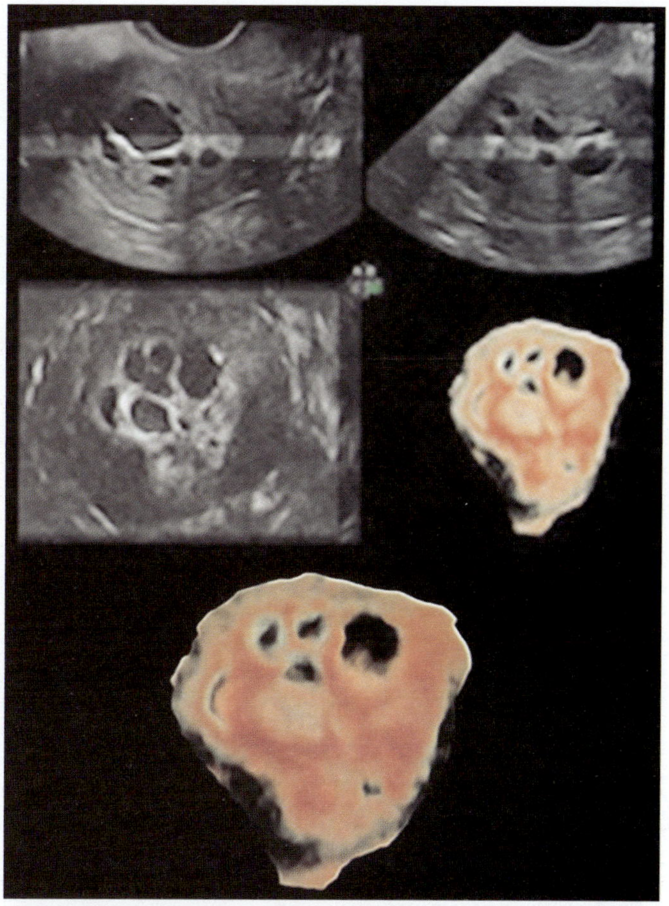

Fig. 126: The same case of **Figure 125** observed with maximum luminescence.

neither 2D nor conventional 3D US had shown any improvement in myometrial invasion evaluation.

Currently this can be evaluated on new 3D softwares such as "shell view" **(Fig. 127)** and HDlive.

Fallopian Tubes

The most frequent pathology is salpingitis and its chronicle consequence: the hydrosalpinx **(Fig. 128)**.

Other tumors and cancer are very infrequent.

Acute salpingitis appears, as an a pelvic inflammatory disease, with numerous irregular cysts of different sizes and forms and containing a gray and relatively homogeneous content.

Chronic adnexitis, sactosalpinx and hydrosalpinx, appears as pure cysts of different forms and sizes always eco negative and located around the ovaries or behind the uterus.

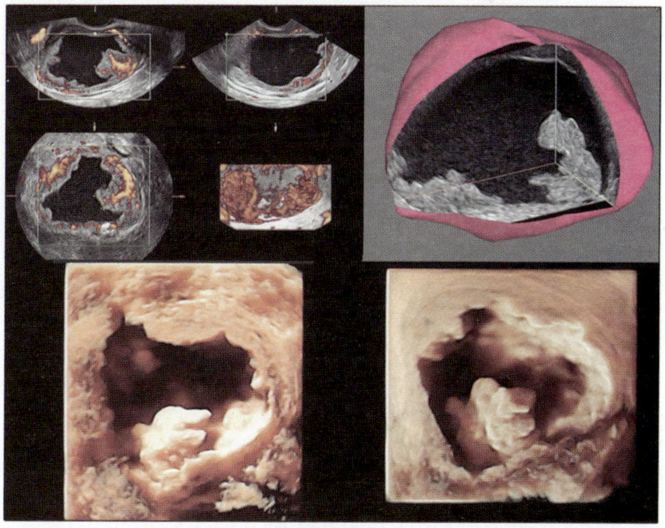

Fig. 127: An adenocarcinoma is show using the orthogonal planes and shell mode (above), and HDlive (below). The myometrium in the uterine fundus is partially invaded by tumor.

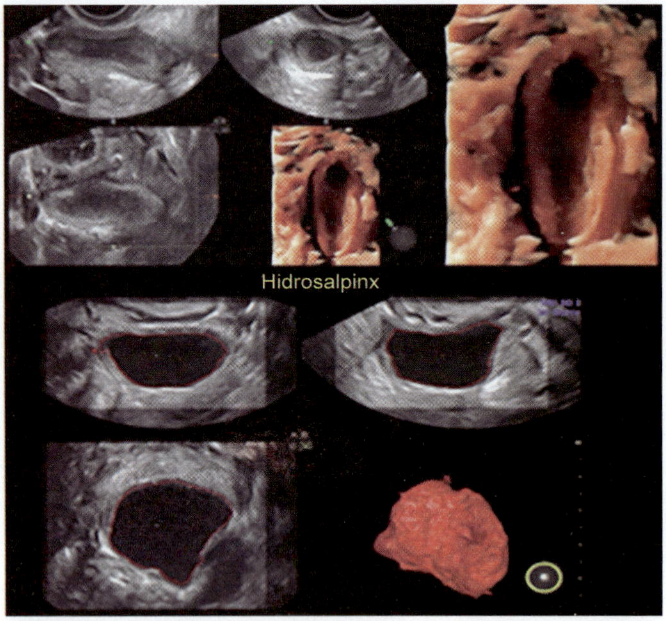

Fig. 128: 2D orthogonal view and HDlive depicting a distended fallopian tube sequelae of a chronic salpingitis. HDlive (above) clearly shows the thickened wall dilated tube and its eco-negative content (also known as sactosalpinx). There is no septums or papillae, but it is not unfrequent to observe them as a consequence of inflammation of the mucosa folds.

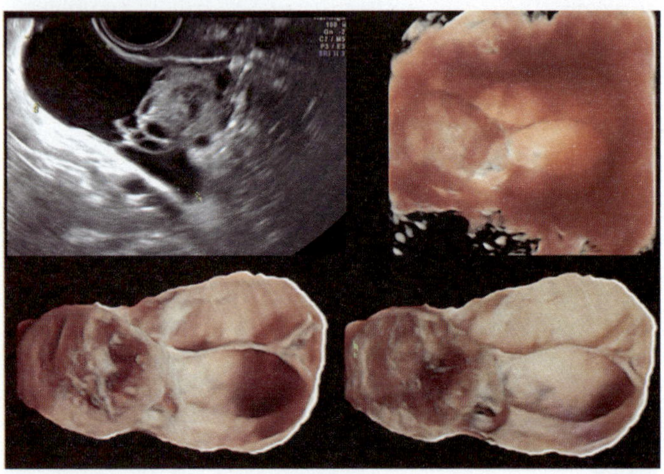

Fig. 129: Chronic salpingitis. From the old inflammatory process remains only the presence of tube dilatations called "sactosalpinx".

In many cases, as in **Figure 129** the tubal walls are thickened.

DIFFERENTIATION OF BENIGN AND MALIGNANT OVARIAN MASSES

Due to its complex embryologic development involving the three embryonic layers, the ovary can be the location of a large list of primary tumors and cancer; only comparable in variety and malignancy to those occurring within the central nervous system.

Albeit its low incidence (only 5% of all types of cancer in women), ovarian cancer is a leading cause of mortality among gynecologic cancers; moreover, from 20 to 30% of all ovarian tumors irrespective of age at diagnosis are malignant.

Many factors contribute to the elevated mortality rate, including:

- Incidence of malignancies of aggressive histologic variety (embryonic tumors)
- Higher lifespan expectancy of women in modern societies which increases the chance of developing age-related diseases and the success in preventing campaigns of other gynecologic cancer, such as cervical and endometrial
- Silent growing into the abdominal cavity also contributes to diagnostic delay.

Given the strong correlation between prognosis and grade of extension of the disease at diagnosis, early diagnosis should be a cornerstone for management protocols; nevertheless, there is a lack of effective screening tests and a paucity of early diagnosis protocols. In clinical practice, the ultrasonographic diagnosis and characteristics of an adnexal mass determine the necessity of complementary diagnostic procedures and management.

Previous studies focused on a systematic gynecologic scanning program for early ovarian cancer detection raised questions about the effectiveness of this screening protocol. Campbell and Andolf performed 6,280 abdominal scans followed by 382 surgeries to detect only 5 carcinomas. Kurjak, van Nagell, and Bourne obtained similar results in 3,905 patients finding 11 carcinomas but requiring 134 laparotomy procedures.

A key issue for an adequate ultrasonographic screening of ovarian masses is the efficacy in the differentiation of benign vs. malignant images. Our group is convinced that an experienced sonographer, on the basis of their skill and own subjective impression, could correctly determine the character of a benign or malignant adnexal mass and, in numerous circumstances, may also refer an approach to the histological nature. However, a high image quality in the evaluation of the ovarian mass has the potential for increasing the diagnostic performance of even young sonographers.

Some recent articles have showed that experienced sonographers achieve sensitivities and specificities regarding malignancy of >95% and of >90%, respectively, and also very high sensitivity in the diagnosis of non-malignant adnexal masses. Nevertheless, serous cystadenomas were misdiagnosed in up to 40,5% of cases.

Use of Scoring Systems

Less experienced sonographers could be helped by scoring systems or mathematical models.

Previous studies described a variety of ultrasonographic scoring systems alone (elegantly described by Finkler, Kurjak, Granberg, Sassone, De Priest, Lerner, Ferrazzi, and Merz) or in combination with vascular Doppler or tumor marker evaluation (essentially CA-125).

None of these descriptions—including the most recent ones, includes the evaluation of optimal sensitivity/specificity values. Finally, international study groups have described ultrasound-based prediction models to evaluate ovarian tumors (International Ovarian Tumor Analysis-IOTA), nevertheless, its clinical worldwide application by general practitioners remains to be fully tested.

Recently, Hata et al. has described a combination of modern three-dimensional (3D) ultrasound and 3D power Doppler (3DPD) ultrasound as well as quantitative 3DPD histogram analysis, for the assessments of the vascularization and further categorization of adnexal masses. The addition of vascular analysis to the standard ultrasonography is not a novel concept; conventional 2D sonographic Doppler was first described by Kurjak et al. in early 80s, this technique paved the way towards new perspectives in the evaluation of vascularity and vascular flow. The 3D sonographic Doppler-introduced 25 years from now and the Angio-power Doppler enhanced image quality, which was nicely illustrated in several publications **(Figs. 130 and 131)**. Doppler scans are nowadays routinely employed in gynecological consultation.

Actually, measuring with APD it is not well known what these indices are really measuring. For these reasons, there is concern about their use in clinical practice.

In this chapter we will explore the state-of-the-art of 3D ultrasound modalities as clinical tools in the differentiation of benign from malignant ovarian masses.

HDlive and Silhouette in the Diagnosis of Ovarian Masses

An important clinical management in order to improve any early diagnosis in ovarian cancer by ultrasonography should begin by differentiating a group of benign tumors and physiologic structures that can be easily confused with ovarian cancer.

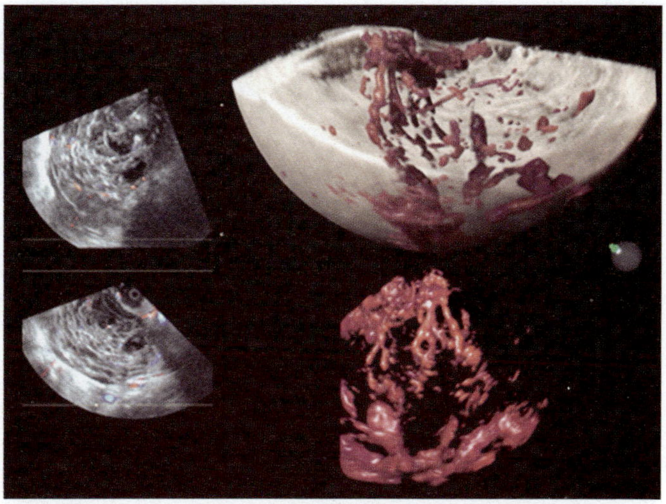

Fig. 130: Two-dimensional angio-Doppler (left) and three-dimensional angio-power Doppler (right) of a solid ovarian cancer with a fantastic view of its tumoral vascular tree.

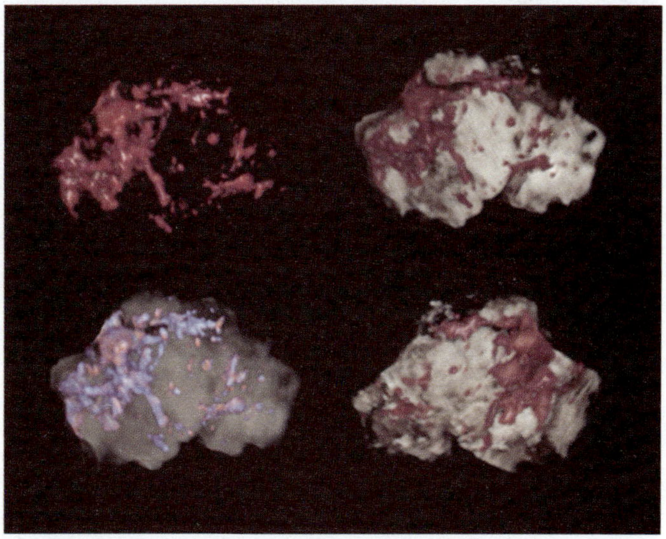

Fig. 131: Three-dimensional angio-power Doppler (3D APD) using color Doppler (red and blue colors, left), Doppler energy (red color, right) and isolated angio-Doppler (red color, upper left). The entire vascular tree is observed cruising the ovarian tumor. The images are of excellent quality; nevertheless, today are well known that the addition of 3D APD does not provide additional information or further improve diagnostic performance.

This includes the followings:

- Endometriomas **(Fig. 132)** which are easily of identify, has typically gray, homogeneous and echoic content

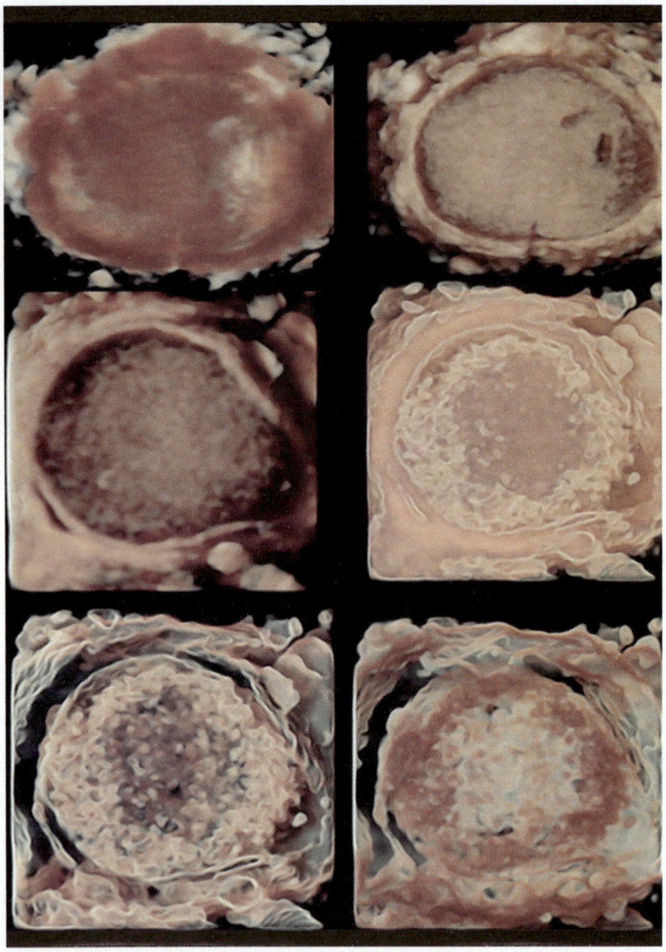

Fig. 132: Typical eco-gray endometrioma depicted with three-dimensional ultrasound (above), HDlive (middle), and silhouette (below) with different illumination ranges.

- Benign teratomas which have a pathognomonic feature known as the Rokitansky papillae (calcic content within the tumor) along with rest of hair, sebaceous material, and importantly a complete absence of vascularization
- Physiologic formations (developing follicles, hemorrhagic follicles, and corpus luteum) show an enhanced vascularization, for this reason they could be mistaken as malignant conditions if the actual scoring systems were applied
- Abscesses from pelvic inflammatory diseases.

Mature Cystic Ovarian Teratomas

Ovarian teratomas comprise a group of tumors containing mature and/or immature tissues of pluripotential germ cells origin, arising from a single of these germ cells after the first meiotic division.

Ovarian teratomas include different histologic type tumors:

- Mature cystic teratoma, also called "Dermoid cyst", which is the most common and contain always tissues arising from, at least, two of the three embryologic layers and showing:
  - Ectodermal—skin derivate, brain, neural tissue (invariably present).
  - Mesodermal—muscle, fat, cartilage, bone (present in over 90% of cases). Teeth are seen in 31% of cases
  - Endodermal: gastrointestinal, bronchial mucinous ciliated epithelium, Thyroid tissue (seen in the majority of cases). Adipose tissue is present in 67–75% of cases.
- Immature teratomas: Very infrequent (<1% of all teratomas). They demonstrate malignant behavior.
- Monodermal teratomas: In these, one type of tissue predominates (e.g., thyroid tissue in struma ovarii, neuro-ectodermal tissue in carcinoid and neural tumors).

Most mature cystic teratomas can be diagnosed at ultrasonography (US) but may have a variety of appearances, characterized by echogenic sebaceous material.

At magnetic resonance (MR) imaging, the sebaceous component is specifically identified with fat-saturation techniques. At computer tomography (CT) fat attenuation within a cyst and calcification is diagnostic.

Mature cystic teratomas are as follows:

- *Cystic tumors generally unilocular* (88%): Filled with sebaceous material, liquid at body temperature and semisolid outside. Cystic dominant lesions may be seen as complex masses. Intracystic fat tissue may be visualized as hyperechogenic and solid when epithelial debris and hair form conglomerates.
- *The wall of the cyst:* A smooth-surfaced lesion is lined by squamous epithelium.
- *Sebaceous material:* Hair follicles, bones, calcifications, skin glands, muscle, and exceptionally thyroid tissue, bronchial mucous membranes are, or can be, within this wall.

Sonographic Appearance

The US appearances of immature teratomas are nonspecific. These tumors are typically heterogeneous. They may be solid or with a prominent solid component with cystic elements usually filled with serous, mucinous or fatty sebaceous material. Scattered calcifications and small fat foci within the solid component are usually recognized.

Monodermal teratomas are composed predominantly or solely of one tissue type. Struma ovarii shows a nonspecific heterogeneous, predominantly solid US feature.

Carcinoid tumors are solid tumors and indistinguishable from other solid malignancies.

Benign cystic teratomas can produce a wide spectrum of sonographic appearances which depends of their major content.

The US imaging of mature teratomas may be predominantly cystic, or a complex mass, or even of solid appearance if the intracystic fat tissue, epithelial debris and hairs are conglomerated filling the entire cyst.

It can also be hyperechogenic view with posterior acoustic shadowing and including diffuse or local shiny echoes or a fluid-fluid/fat-fluid level.

Four manifestations occur most commonly:

1. A cystic lesion with a densely echogenic tubercle (Rokitansky nodule) with sound attenuation owing to sebaceous material and hair within the cystic cavity **(Fig. 133)**. These nodule is also known as "dermoid plug", which represents a protuberance that arises from the tumor wall and contains hair follicles, other solid elements, or both. These nodules are seen as echogenic masses, again with distal acoustic shadowing.
2. A diffuse or partially echogenic mass with the echogenic area usually demonstrating sound attenuation owing to sebaceous material and hair within the cyst cavity **(Figs. 134 and 135)**
3. Two diffuse clearly differentiated partially echogenic masses.

   Figure 136 in two sheets, is absolutely characteristic and pathognomonic.
4. Multiple thin echogenic bands caused by hairs located in the sebum of the cyst cavity **(Figs. 137 and 138)**.

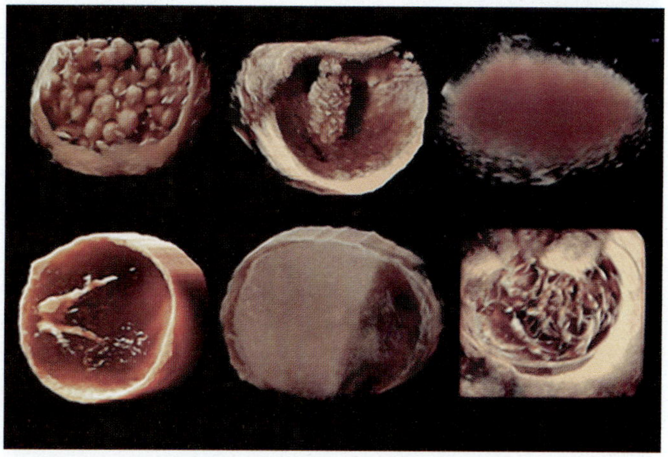

Fig. 133: 2D orthogonal planes and 3D HDlive of a cystic lesion with a densely echogenic tubercle (Rokitansky nodule) located in the inferior part of the cyst. 3D of the Rokitansky nodule showing bones and teeth. Below and right maximal transparency.

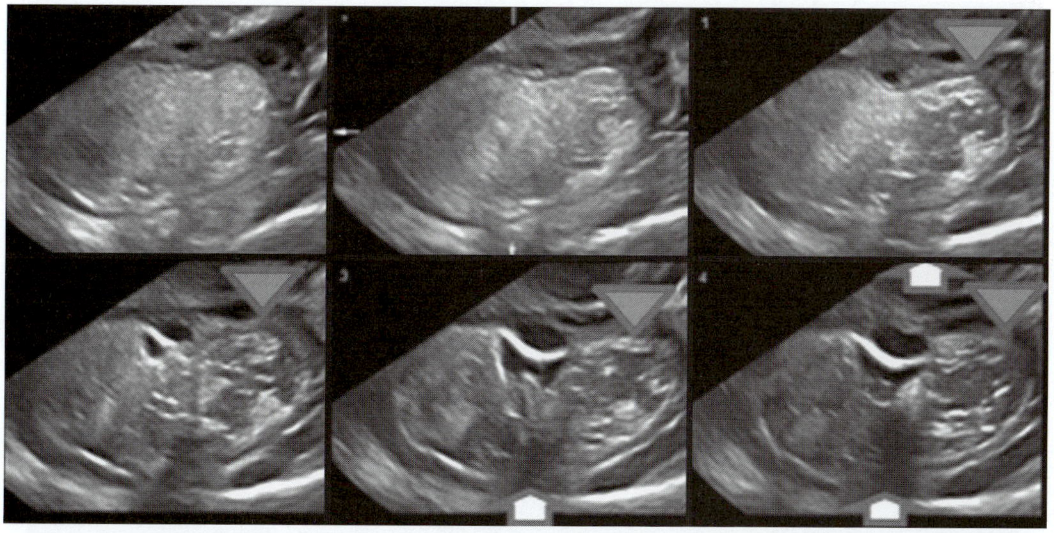

Fig. 134: Tomographic ultrasound image (TUI) of a diffusely echogenic gray mass with the echogenic area showing attenuation owing to sebaceous material and hair within the cyst cavity. To the right (images showed in the second and third TUI lines) the sebaceous and hair material within the cystic cavity produce multiple thin echogenic bands.

The following ultrasonographic "signs" have been also suggested as specific or pathognomonic:

- The cystic lesion with a densely echogenic tubercle (Rokitansky nodule) **(Fig. 139)**.
- The "iceberg" sign. This sign is very similar to the "sound attenuation" sign previously described. The author describes it as "a mass with the amorphous, poorly defined echogenic focus in the near field that causes posterior shadowing and thus obscures the posterior portion of the lesion and any structures behind it". Because these masses are frequently large, the tip of the iceberg sign is readily identified on both transabdominal and transvaginal US scans.

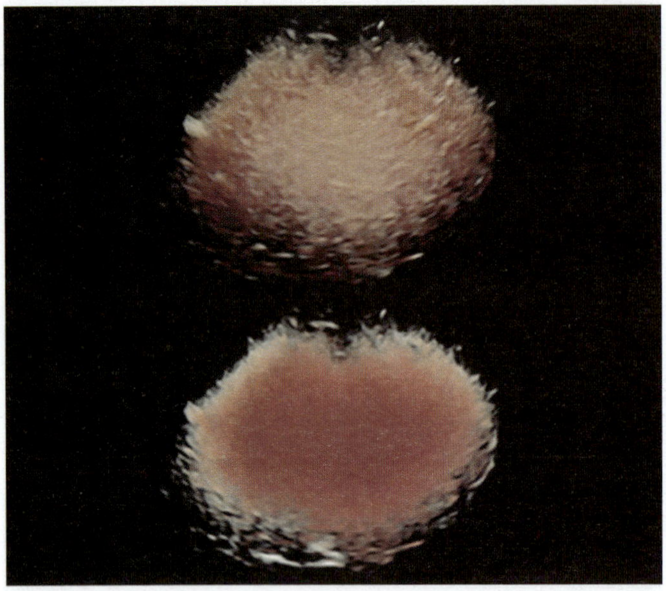

Fig. 135: 2D orthogonal planes a 3D HDlive with and without maximal luminescence of a diffuse echogenic gray mass with the echogenic area showing a small cyst and attenuation owing to sebaceous material. The teratoma has been delimited using the "cut off system" (below).

The echogenic focus at US appears as a solid mass but is actually a cyst that contains a mixture of fatty liquid (i.e., sebum) matted hair, and cellular debris. It is the multiple tissue interfaces within this mixture that are responsible for producing the characteristic acoustic shadowing.

The fat intermixed with the hair strands is echogenic and often attenuates the ultrasound beam. In addition, in vitro scans of surgical specimens have proved that the strongly reflective echo pattern is caused by the multiple tissue interfaces of the hair and sebum within the cyst mass. Acoustic shadowing may totally obscure the back of a large, clinically palpable, mass; hence, the term "tip of the iceberg sign".

- Fluid-fluid/fat-fluid level: This type of levels within a cystic ovarian tumor may strongly suggest cystic teratoma and it has been considered pathognomonic. Pure sebum within the cyst may be hypoechoic or anechoic. Fluid-fluid levels, or fat fluid interface, result from sebum floating above aqueous, which appears more echogenic than the sebum layer.

There is a constant horizontal fluid level within the mass that changes with the patient's position.

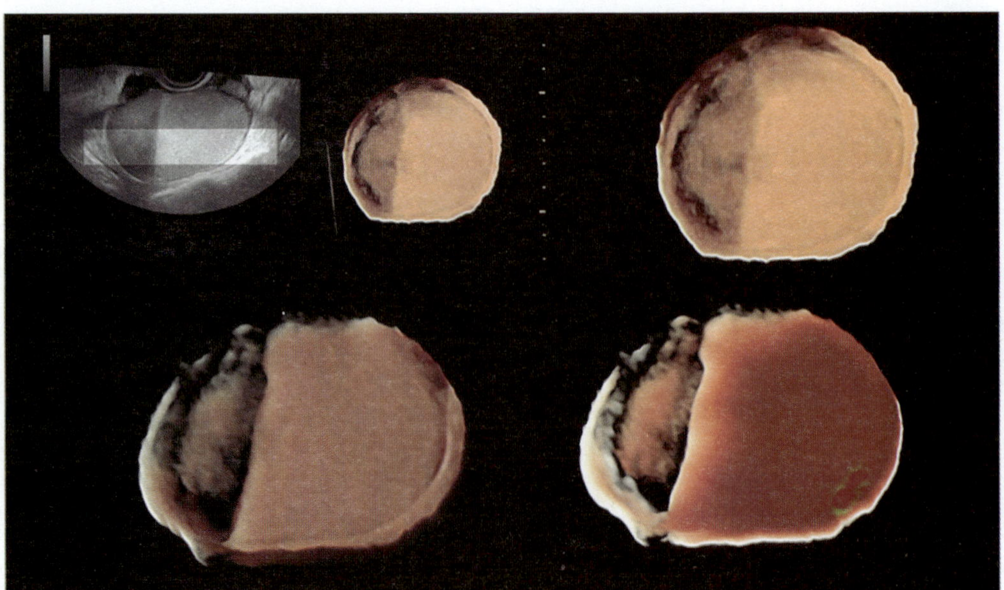

Fig. 136: Two sheets teratoma.

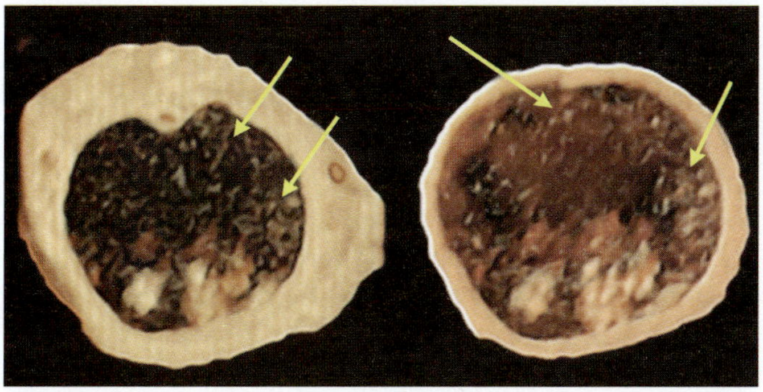

Fig. 137: The use of 3D HDlive allows visualizing multiple very thin echogenic dots and bands caused by hairs in the cystic cavity (arrows).

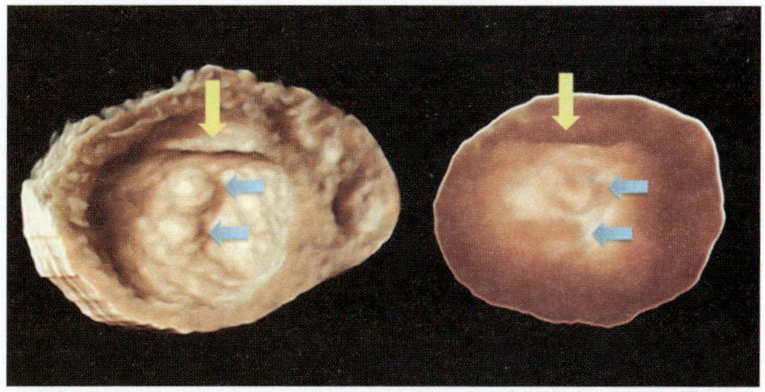

Fig. 139: Fluid-fluid level (yellow arrows) and Rokitansky nodules (blue arrows).

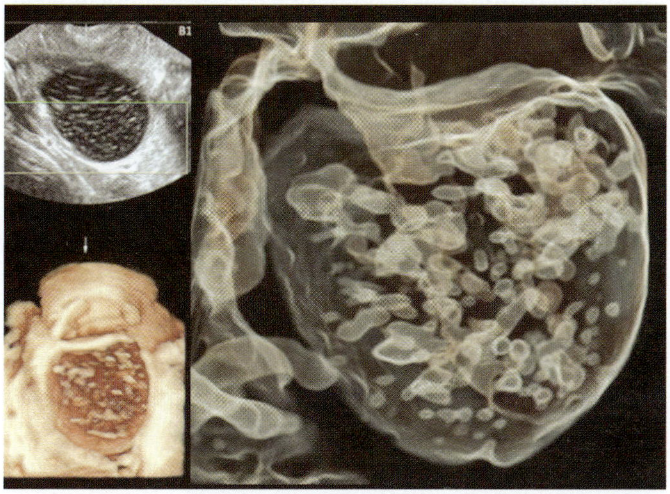

Fig. 138: "Mesh" teratoma containing hairs and sebaceous tissue depicted with 2D (to the left and above) and 3D HDlive and silhouette (to the left and below and to the right). Silhouette allows a perfect delimitation of the internal tumoral dots (hairs).

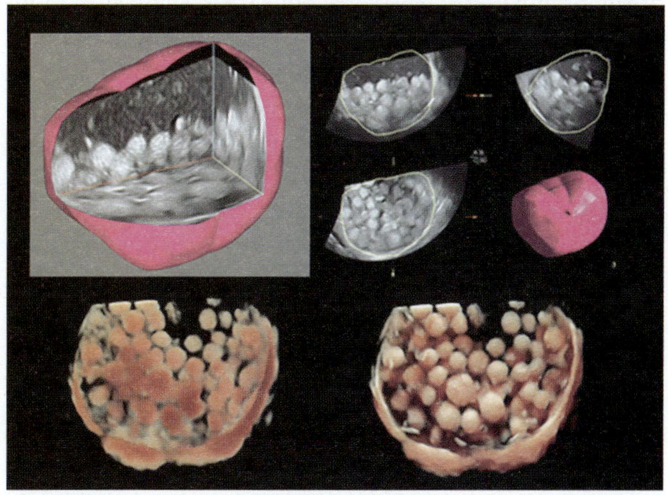

Fig. 140: 2D orthogonal planes, shell mode and HDlive with and without maximal luminescence of fat balls in a mature cystic teratoma.

Associated with the fluid level is, generally, a densely echogenic structure with faint acoustic shadowing behind it **(Fig. 136)**.

- Dermoid mesh. Dermoid mesh with hyperechoic calcifications indicating the presence of bone, teeth, or other ectodermal derivate in a predominantly cystic medium, hyperechoic solid mural components and hair-fluid levels represents multiple echogenic linear interfaces floating within a cyst; this interfaces represent hair fibers.
- The Rokitansky nodule or papillae, a raised protuberance with acoustic shadow, projecting into the cyst cavity. Most of the hair, teeth and bones typically arises from this protuberance **(*see* Figs. 133 and 139)**.
- Dermoid plugs: A broad hyperechogenic area with multiple bright linear echoes and spots

In the literature there is only one 3D US description of these tumors showing wonderful images

- Multiple mobile spherical structures (fat balls) of slightly increased echogenicity floating free in a large cystic mass is one of the most rare patterns **(Fig. 140)**.

In all cases, some degree of mobility was noted when pressure was applied via abdominal probe manipulation.

In some cases, much more exceptional, there were only one big ball between 4 and 7 cm.

Discussion

This type of ovarian tumor was first described more than one century ago. Many references in classic German, English and French medical literature described this entity using curious names, herein mentioned in its original language: Boules de graisse; Butter Kugeln; Caviarlike bodies; Dermoid Kugeln; Epithelial balls; Erbsenartige Köper; Fatty concretions; Fett Kugeln; Floating balls; Inclusions; lipid globules; Pilllike bodies; Rounded balls; Sebum balls; Solid concretions and Spherules.

The last clinical case report was published in 1935; the radiologic and ecographic descriptions start thereafter.

The first case using CT and MR was reported in 1991 (16) and ultrasonographic images were published soon after: three cases and five cases.

The most common denomination in medical literature was "intracystic fat balls" even though fat tissue was a only minimal component of the tumor. The microscopic finding found spherules containing desquamate keratin, fibrin, hemosiderin, and sebaceous debris with squamous skin and fine hair shafts but only a small amount of a fat component. Some spherules had a 2–3 mm thick and an outer sebaceous shell.

The vast majority of authors, including our own group, consider ultrasonographic images as absolutely pathognomonic of this condition. Only echuinococcus involvement of the pelvis—an exceptional condition may be included in the diagnosis differential; moreover, in this condition the vesicles are seen as hypoechogenic images as opposite to the hyperechogenic pattern in teratoma cases.

About its Pathogenesis

The pathogenesis of balls formation is unknown and several theories have been postulated:

1. Predominance of large secretory and absorptive rather than exfoliated surfaces lining the cysts would favor the absorption of most of the contents into the general circulation, leaving the remaining material to solidify and mold into balls.
2. It is speculated that each globule was formed by the aggregation of sebaceous matter around a tiny focus of debris, squames, or a fine hair shaft while moving around the cystic cavity.
3. The spherules appear to have been modeled into discrete masses rather than remaining as an amorphous mass because of the difference in physical and thermal properties of the material being deposited around each nest. Floating balls require space to be remodeled.
4. This type of growth could be related to an unusual pattern of estrogen and progesterone receptor expression in the cystic teratoma, although a definitive agreement has not been reach on this issue.

CRITERIA FOR CATEGORIZING BENIGN VS MALIGNANT OVARIAN MASSES

Since pioneering publications, the criteria have remained unchanged, only the image quality has improved over time

- *Solid and homogeneous tumor component (mainly benign):* It is the typical image of fibroids for instances **(Fig. 141)**.
- *Solid and non-homogeneous tumor component (mainly malignant)* **(Fig. 142)**.

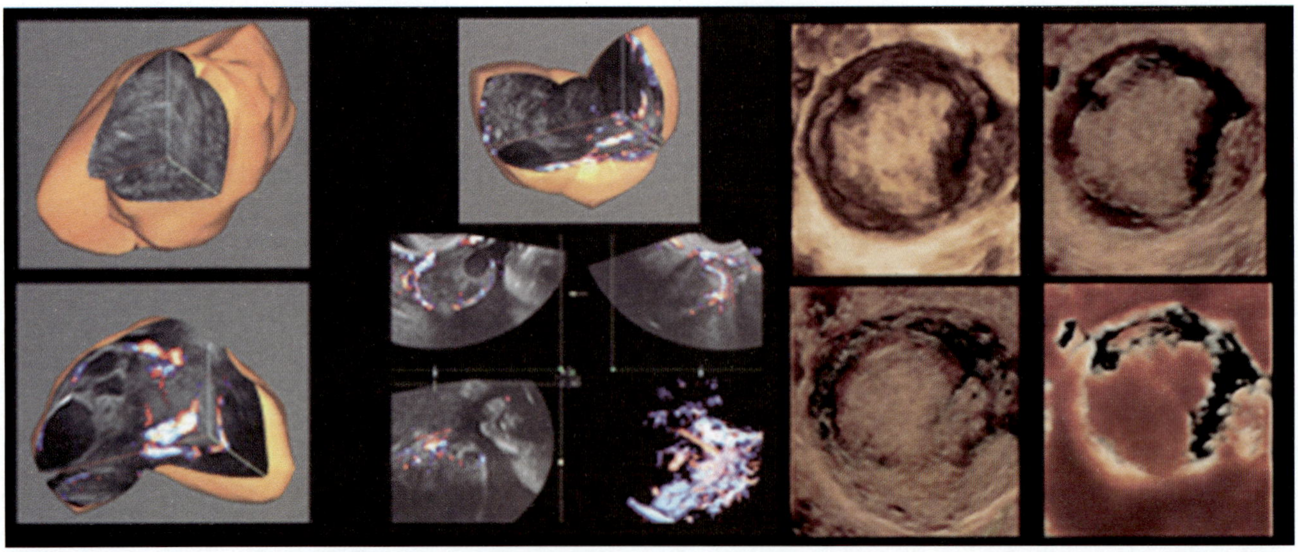

Fig. 141: Three-dimensional "shell" or niche image of a solid ovarian tumor with abnormal vascular component, typical of malignancy (to the left). HDlive visualization of an ovarian mass shows an almost complete solid component. Bottom right: maximum transparency view. The heterogeneous component and the presence of excrescencies in the periphery highly suspicious of malignancy are clearly depicted (to the right).

- *Pure cystic content (always benign)* **(Fig. 143):** Only criteria considered of benignity until 5 cm. and in our opinion until 10 cm. It needs a completely study of it inner cavity using HDlive and silhouette **(Fig. 143)**.
- *Cystic tumor component with small solid components or papillae:* **Figures 144 to 148** provide examples of the evaluation of internal surface of cystic tumors.

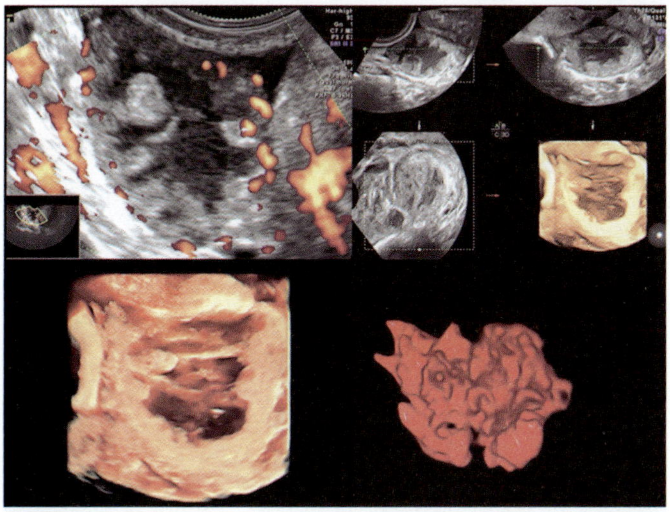

Fig. 142: Two-dimensional Doppler energy (above left), three-dimensional sonographic (above right), HDlive visualizations, and automatic volume calculation (below) of a non-homogeneous mainly solid ovarian mass. The heterogeneous component and the presence of excrescencies in the periphery are highly suspicious of malignancy, and are clearly depicted.

Figures 144 and 145 show small papillary projections, highly suggestive of malignancy if evaluated using 2D sonography. However, under HDlive evaluation although irregular in shape, the surface of this projection is smooth and homogeneous, suggesting a benign finding **(Figs. 145 to 148)**. HDlive and RAS or silhouette, are able to offer a clear evaluation of the internal components tend to rule-out endophytic lesions **(Figs. 145 to 148)**.

- *Cystic multiseptated homogeneous tumor component (mainly benign):* HDlive is shown to be very useful in differentiating this type of masses; when compared to 2D ultrasound, it becomes easier to differentiate between cystoadenomas from cystoadenocarcinomas as shown in **Figures 149 and 150**.
- *Cystic multiseptated non-homogeneous tumor component (mainly malignant)* **(Figs. 151 to 154)**.
- *Cystic multiseptated irregular and heterogeneous tumor component. (mainly malignant)* **(Fig. 155)**: HDlive and silhouette information regarding the shape and components of the intratumoral cystic walls and tumor material (septations, the presence of papillary projections, solid tumoral tissue, etc.).
- *Mixed (solid-cystic) tumor component (mainly malignant):* This typical finding of malignancy is related to an expansive development of a part of the tumor, whereas some other areas develop degeneration or necrosis **(Figs. 155 to 157)**.

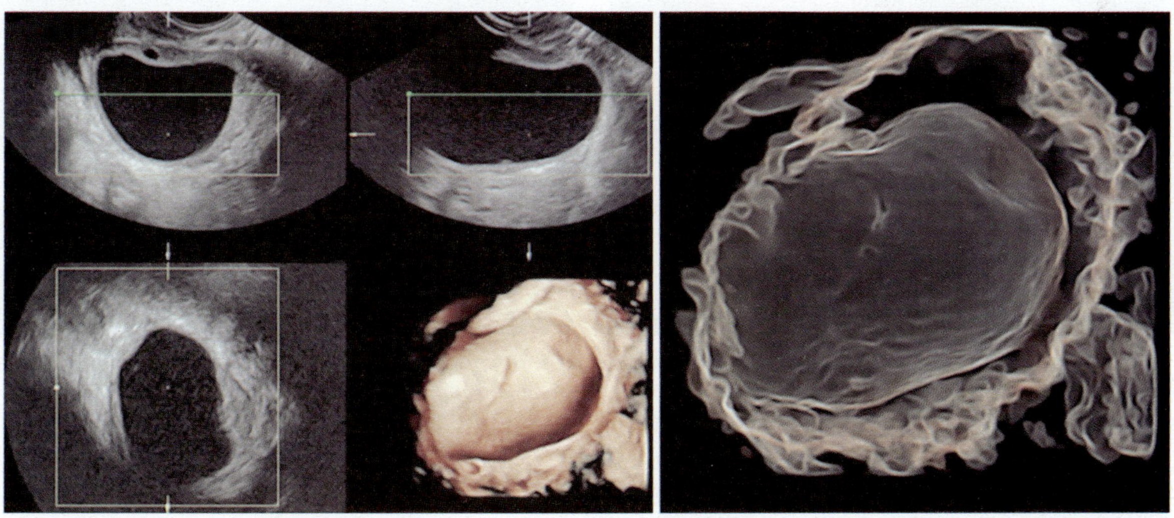

Fig. 143: Left: Orthogonal plane view of a "pure" ovarian cyst. Right: Same structure under Radiance Architecture System view. Notice the external surface (up) showing adhesions to surrounding tissue and the homogeneous and smooth internal surface (down). This finding is considered benign until a maximum diameter of 5 mm, but in our opinion, up to 10 mm can be considered benign providing the absence of papillary projections and septations.

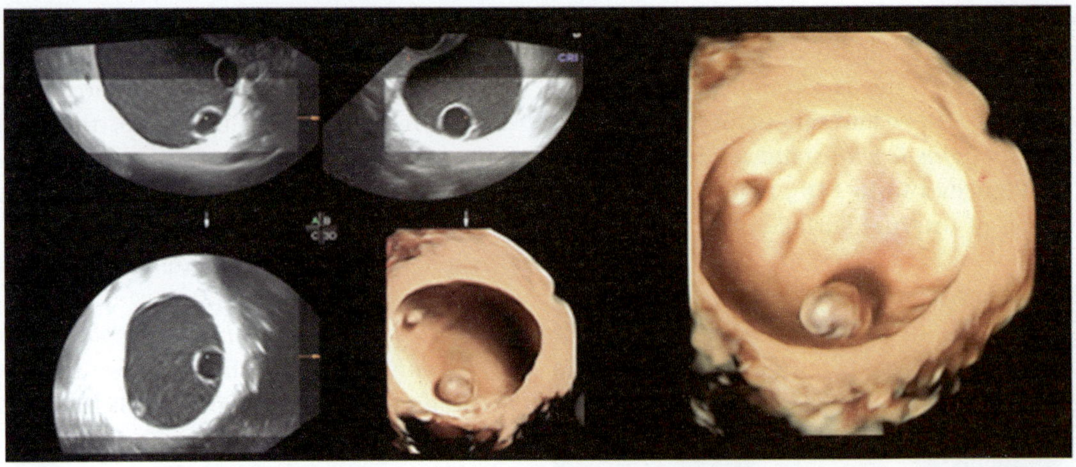

Fig. 144: Cystic formation observed in two-dimensional and HDlive reconstructions. HDlive shows more clearly the inner surface of the cystic mass, which contains two small homogeneous vesicular projections, suggesting a benign pathology.

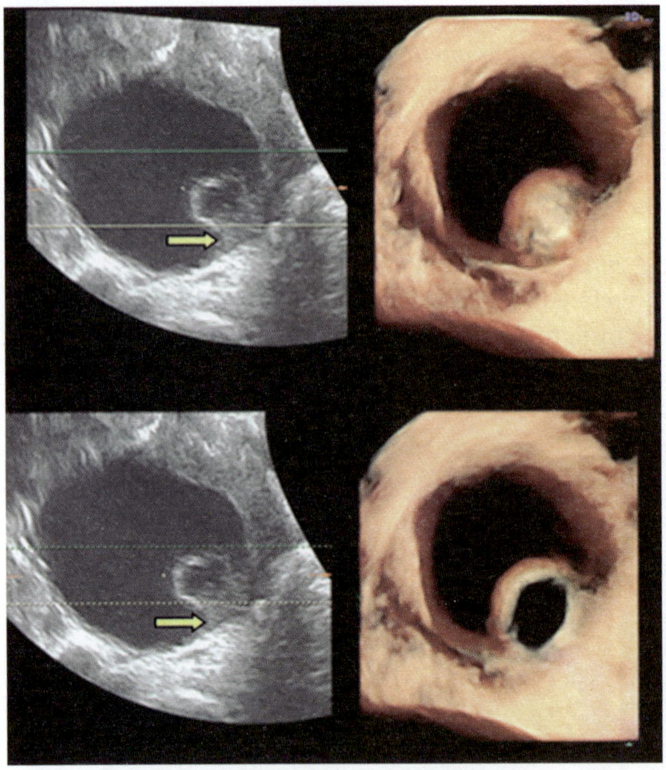

Fig. 145: The 2D US evaluation shows a small vesicle and a solid implantation base (arrows), both showing homogeneous borders, highly suggestive of benignity.

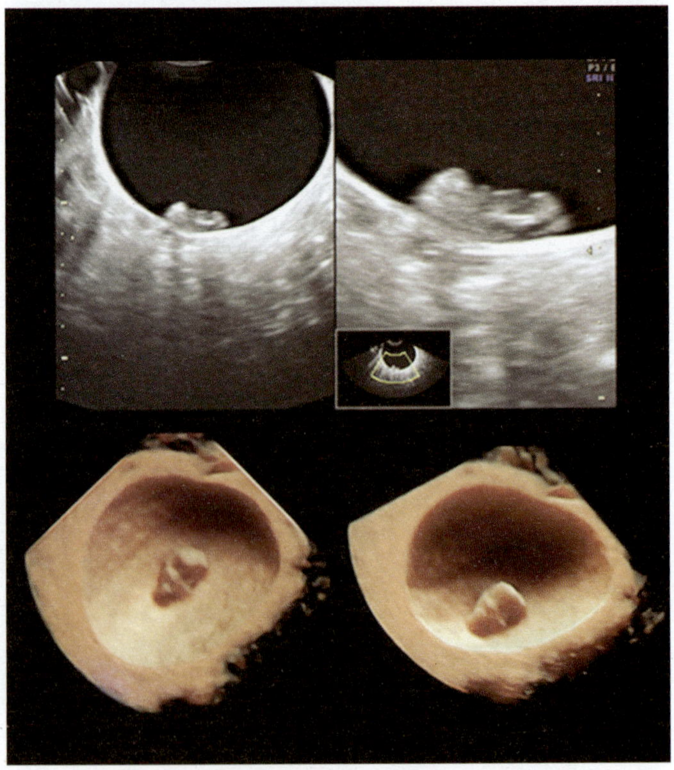

Fig. 146: Above: Two-dimensional image of an ovarian cyst with a small endophytic tumoral component. Bottom: The same ovarian mass under HDlive visualization shows that the endophytic growth has a smooth and uniform surface, thus, benign in nature.

- *The presence of septations and papillae:* They should be clearly observed and described, since they are of enormous help in the differentiation of benign vs. malignant process. Thin and homogeneous septations are always related to benign tumors **(Figs. 158 to 160)**.

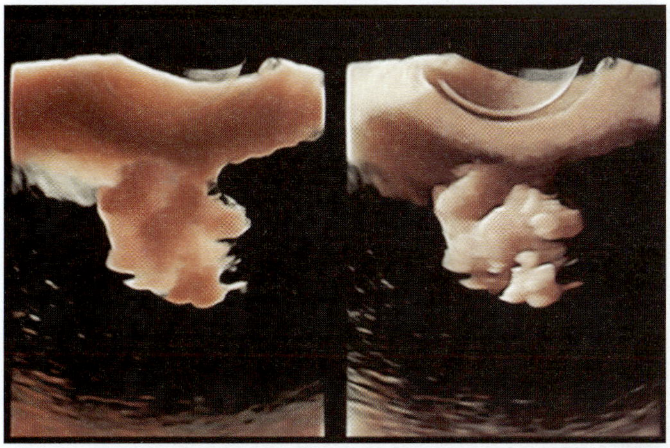

Fig. 147: Close-up view of a small endophytic component within a "pure" ovarian cyst; although small in size, HDlive shows an irregular and heterogeneous surface with small papillary projections. These features are highly suspicious of malignancy. Compare these findings with the ones in **Figures 144 to 146**.

The presence of papillary projections are usually correlated to malignancy when HDlive software is used. Even small and irregular papillae can be clearly studied, and the image obtained is superior to what is usually depicted by 2D sonography. Some other features related with malignancy can be analyzed in-deep by HDlive and silhouette, including increased thickness (more than 3 mm), irregularities of the cyst wall, cyst wall rupture, and the presence of ascites and metastasis **(Figs. 156, 157 and 161)**.

Presence of Papillary Projections (Malignant) (Figs. 156, 157 and 160 to 162)

When studied in HDlive these growths are marked clearly much better than 2D, and papillae and/or endophytic growths are small with very irregular shapes **(Figs. 160 and 161)**.

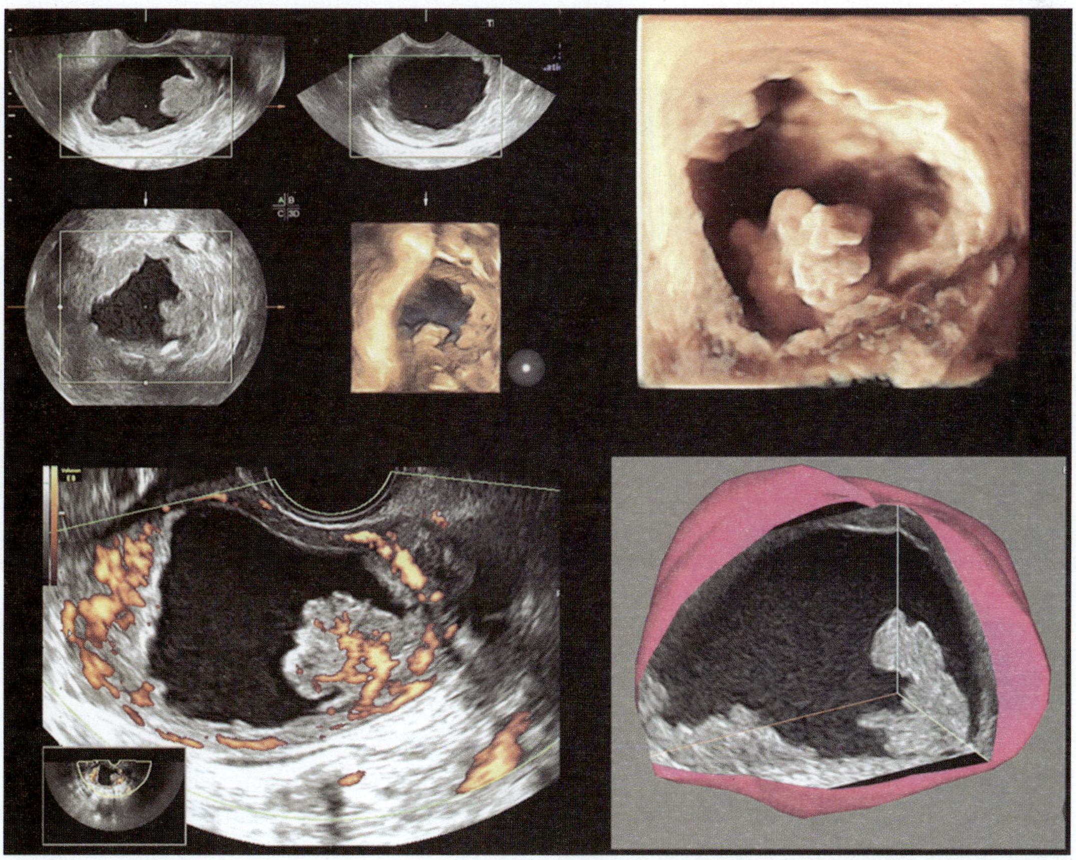

Fig. 148: Cystic ovarian tumor in 2D, 3D and HDlive reconstructions, showing a small papilla (see 2D above left) extremely vascularized (Doppler energy, left and below). Although the capsule is complete (see the "shell" or "niche" image, below right in red color), the whole aspect is of malignancy.

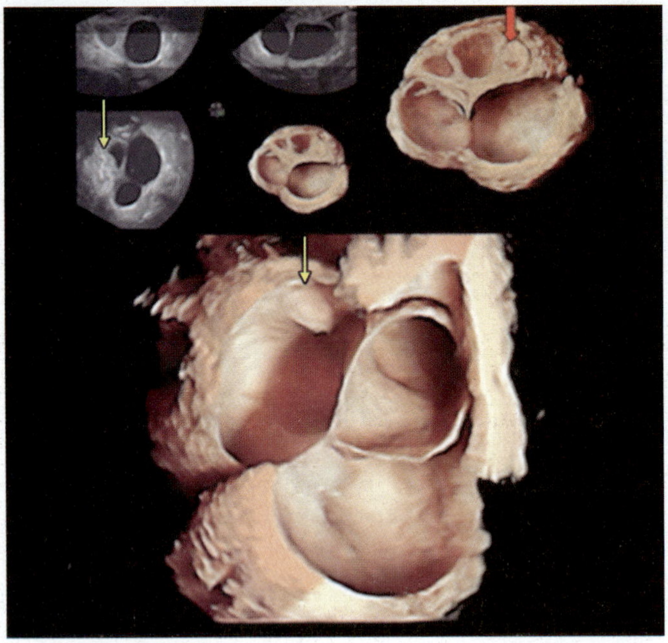

Fig. 149: Multicystic ovarian tumor. Two-dimensional evaluation shows a highly suspicious solid tumoral mass (yellow arrow) adjacent to the cysts. HDlive clearly depicts the inner and external surface of the cysts, showing smooth characteristics of walls and septations compatible with a benign pathology. Moreover, the solid mass seems now more compatible with a corpus luteum under involution. The final pathologic diagnosis was a mucinous ovarian cystoadenoma (Compare with **Figure 148**).

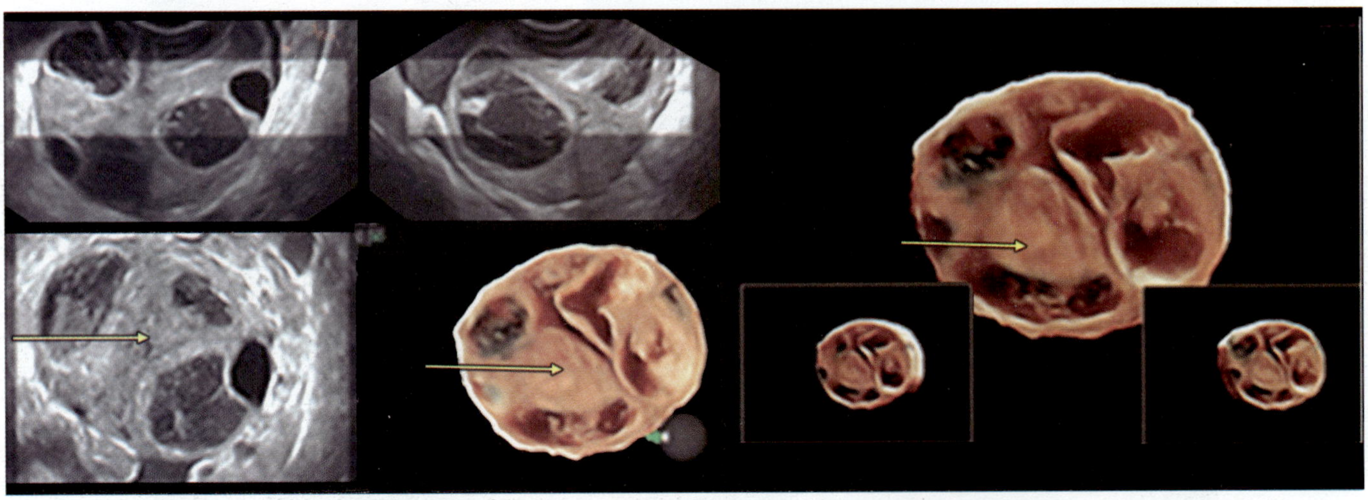

Fig. 150: HDlive image of a mix (cystic-solid) ovarian mass. The yellow arrow shows a solid, irregular part of the mass. The cystic formations have different size, irregular thickness of the walls, and isolated papillae with endophytic growth.

- Tumoral wall thickness bigger >3 mm (malignant) **(Figs. 152, 156 and 161)**
- Irregularities in the tumor wall or irregularities of the proper tumor content (malignant) **(Figs. 153, 157 and 160 to 162)**
- View of the wall rupture (mainly malignant). Although benign ovarían tumors (such as cystoadenomas, etc.) can produce wall rupture, this phenomenon is much frequent and characteristic of malignancy.

It is not easy to visualize with vaginal 2D US. It can be observed with 3D, but we recommend to use the "niche or shell" mode **(Figs. 141 and 161)**.

- View or appearance of ascitis (malignant)
- View of local or lobar metastasis (malignant)

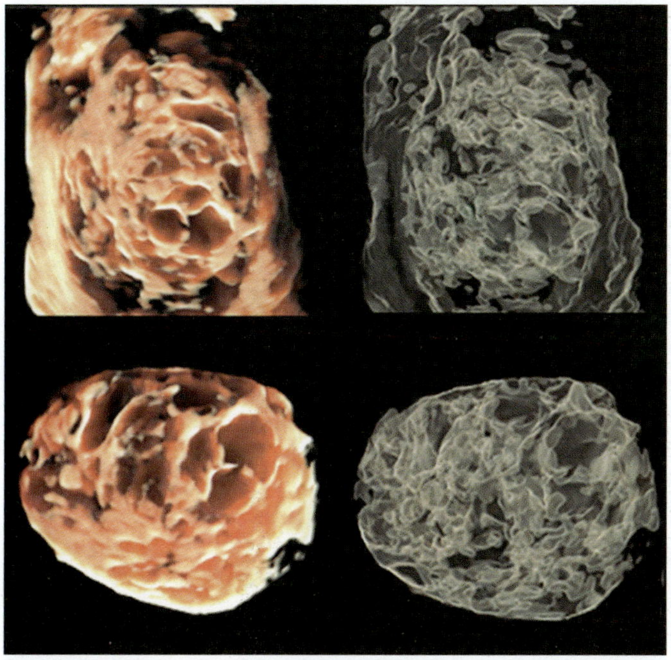

Fig. 151: HDlive and its silhouette mode of an ovarian serous cystoadenocarcinoma. Notice, especially in the silhouette view, the irregular size, shape, and limits of the multiple small cysts. All these findings are strongly suggestive of malignancy.

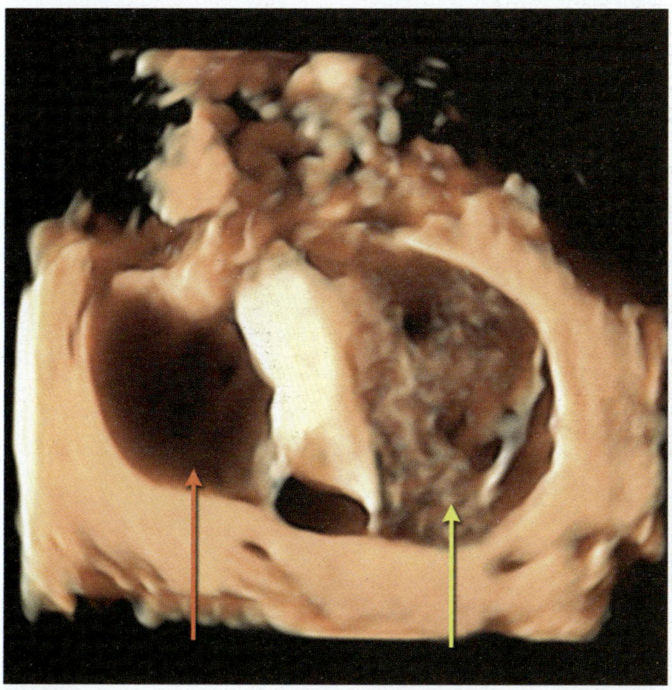

Fig. 152: Cystic multiseptated non-homogeneous tumor. The left cyst (red arrow) is homogeneous and looks benign but the right one (yellow arrow) shows endophytic growth and papillae, very suspicious of malignancy. The septum between the cysts is also thick and amorphous (mainly malignant).

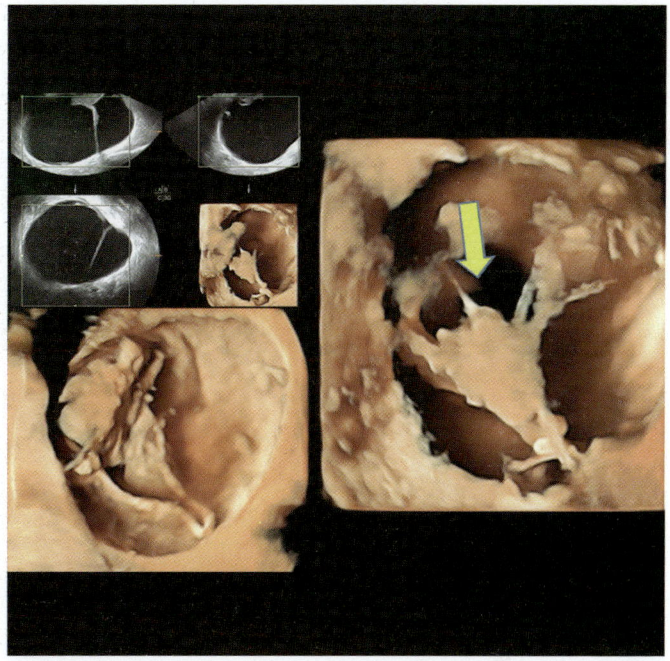

Fig. 153: Ovarian, mainly cystic, malignant tumor. The most interesting tumor part is the one marked with the yellow arrow. It looks like a "malignant star" fool of irregular walls and exophytic papillary projections.

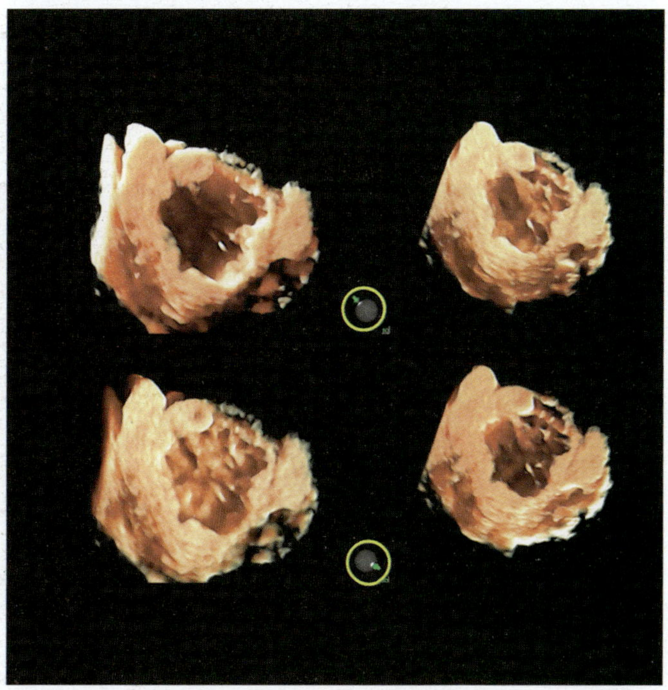

Fig. 154: Cystic, irregular, and nonhomogeneous ovarian tumor. Many necrotic parts and excrescencies are visible. The image is totally compatible with malignancy.

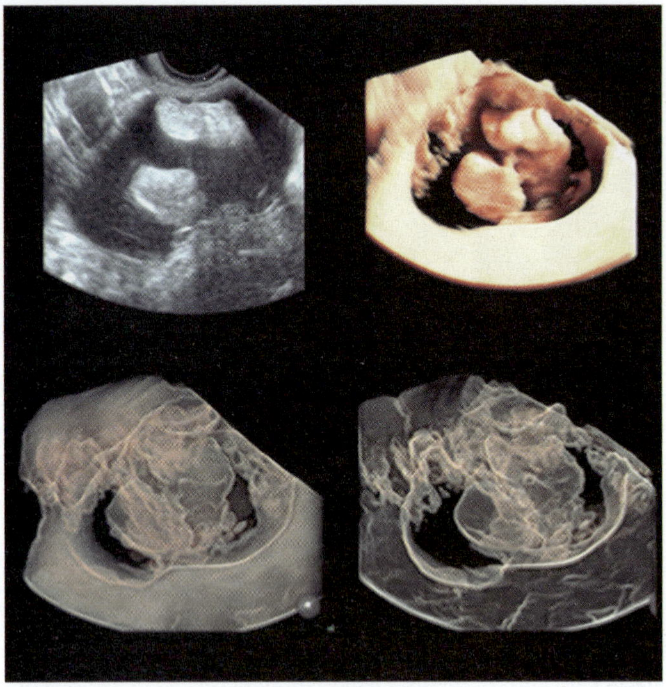

Fig. 155: Comparative images of a heterogeneous solid-cyst ovarian mass. The 3D US mode shows a higher image quality compared with 2D US (above). The mixed component, solid-cystic and fluid, showed in the four-image is completely amorphous, specially the solid component (HDlive view). The silhouette mode shows clearly the internal and external delimitation of the ovarian mass components. These findings are highly suggestive of malignancy.

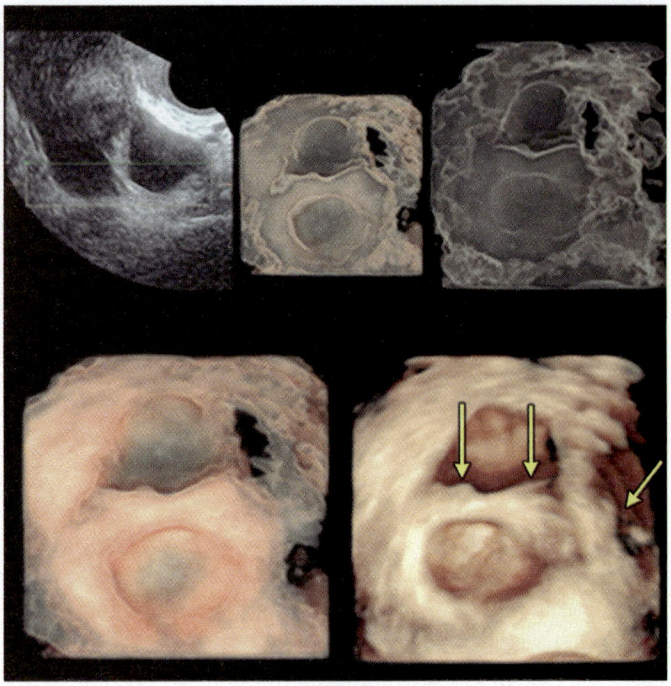

Fig. 156: 2D US (top left), system architecture or radiance silhouette (above center and right) and a characteristic HDlive malignant tumor showing septum (bottom right, arrows) minimum papillary projections not visible in 2D (top left). When RAS is applied, a clear internal and external delimitations and tumor boundaries can be observed.

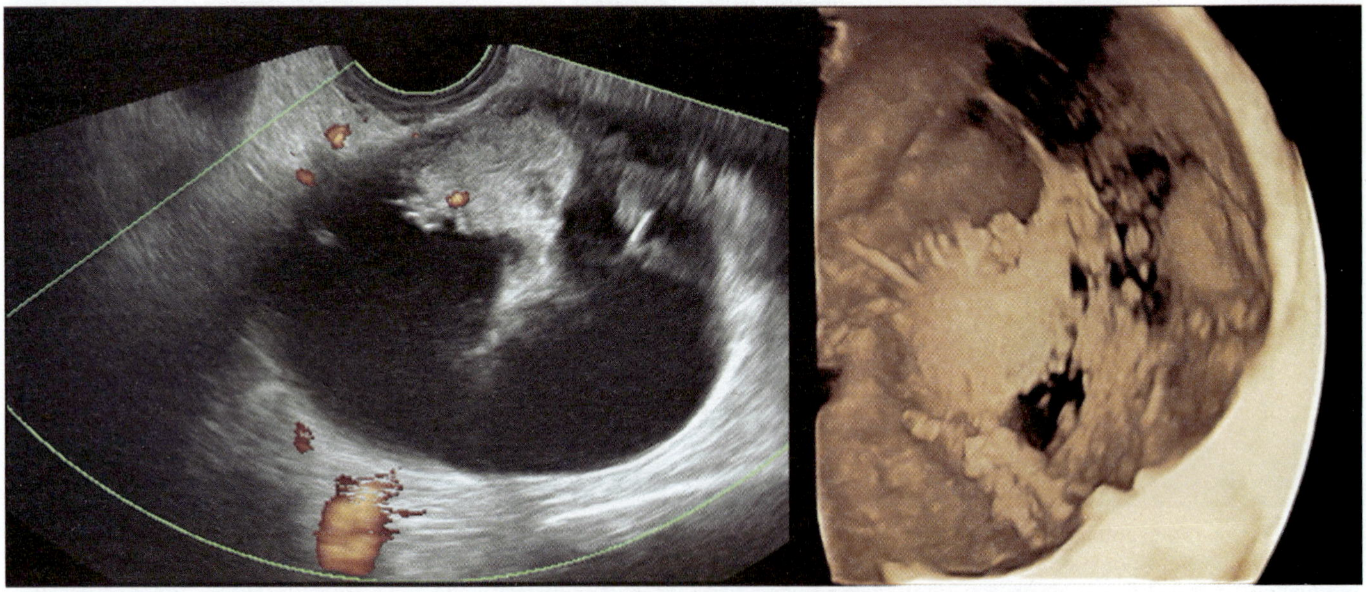

Fig. 157: A solid ovarian tumor area showing numerous septa and irregular, thin and thick walls, larger than 3 mm and/or inhomogeneous. Very suspicious of malignancy.

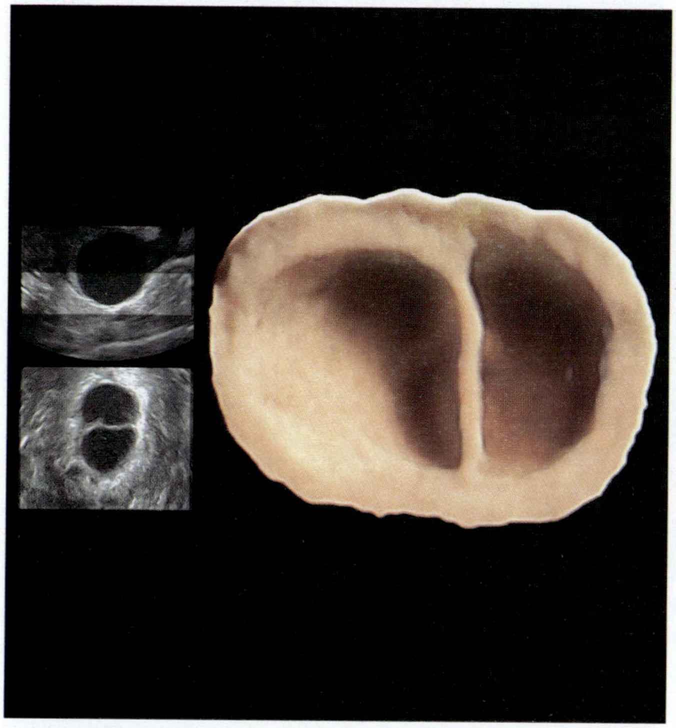

Fig. 158: HDlive view of a pure ovarian cyst. Note the smooth and regular septations, suggesting a benign pathology, whereas the findings of thick (>3 mm) and heterogeneous septations are highly suspicious of malignancy.

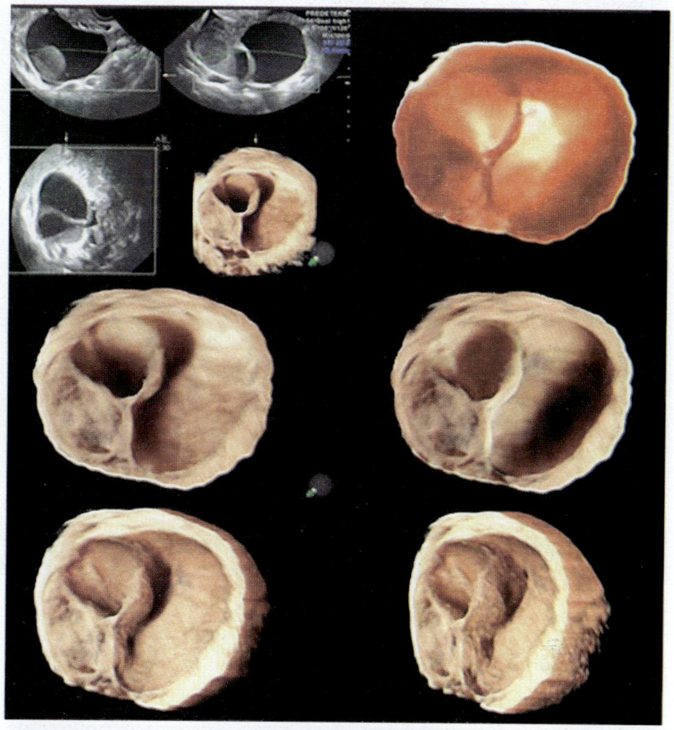

Fig. 159: Ovarian tumor with various cysts of different sizes. All are with fine, homogeneous and septations of same thickness and without endophytic growths. When depicted in different angles and light sources, they are all regular. These tumors are always benign.

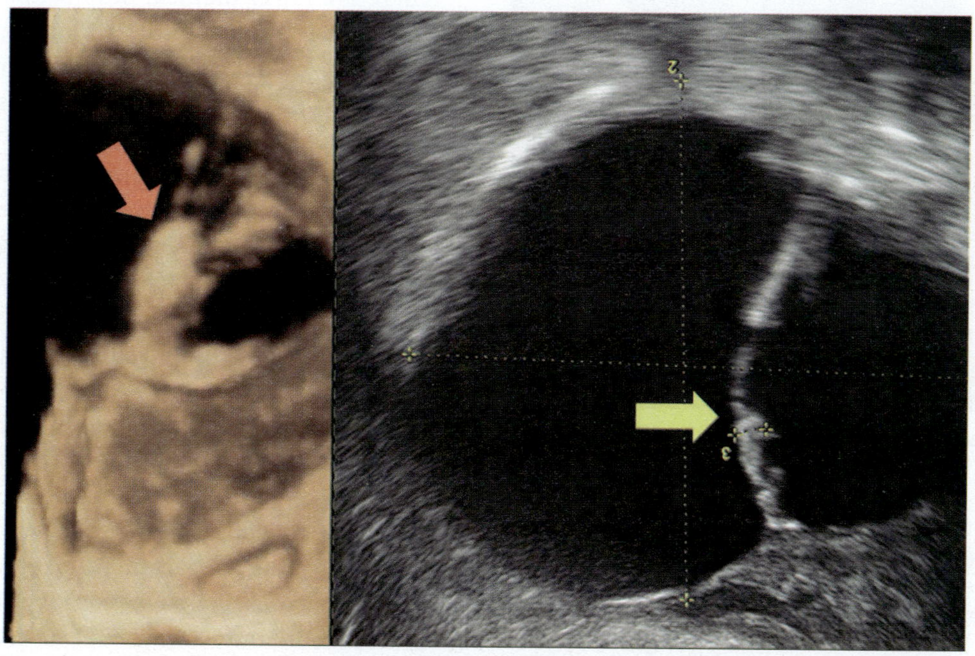

Fig. 160: Septated cyst. The septations are of different thickness (yellow arrows), and 3D shows small papillae and exophytic growths (red arrow). In order to depict the image quality obtained with different ultrasound modes, please compare the two-dimensional orthogonal planes (right) with the 3D picture (left).

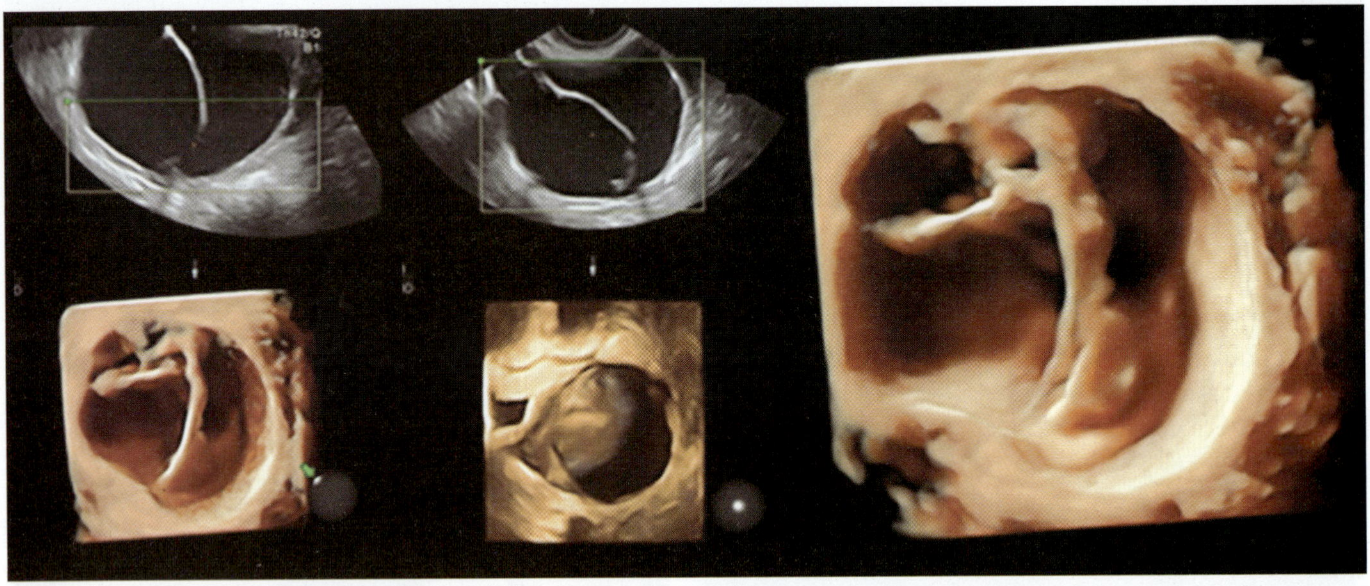

Fig. 161: These fluid-filled cyst with gray color are different from those with low intensity of endometriomas **(Fig. 155)**. This liquid correspond to the serum of a cystoadenocarcinomas. They are always a sign of malignancy as well as appearance of papillae, pathognomonic for malignancy.

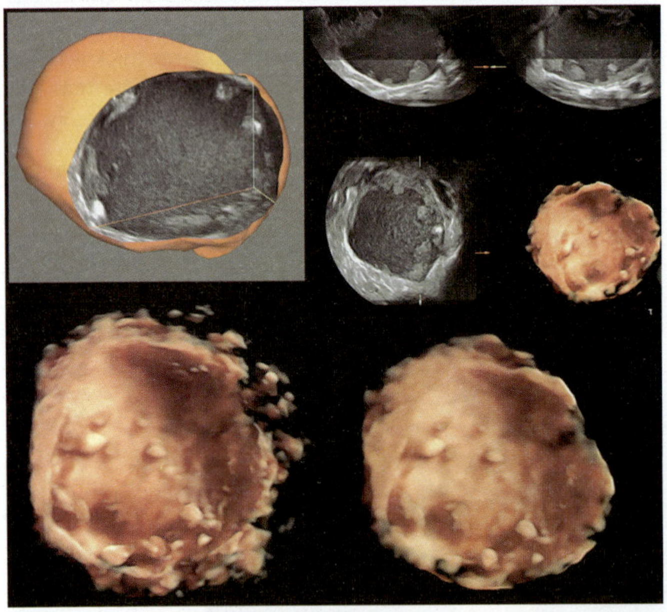

Fig. 162: Small ovarian cancer showing in detail small inner papillary projections typical of malignancy. Above and left "niche" or shell mode showing integral capsule. Below: HDlive showing the inner tumor with small papilae and endophytic growths. Even still, few in number they are specific to tumor malignancy. Means that atypical epithelium is growing. The "niche " mode is used to demonstrate the integrity of the tumor capsule.

CONCLUSION

3D real-time ultrasound has been proved to be better than 2D sonography in the evaluation of adnexal masses. This review adds further on the topic by addressing the role of state-of-the-art 3D ultrasound modalities, namely HDlive and RAS; for the assessing of ovarian masses.

Numerous publications describe the use of 2D sonography in the evaluation of ovarian masses.

There are fewer medical publications describing the study of ovarian tumors by 3D ultrasound with or without Doppler. Nevertheless, it is unquestionable that the image quality and definition of structures are enormously superior with 3D ultrasonography.

HDlive and RAS are innovative tools within 3D ultrasonography; these software provide a more realistic vision and definition of ovarian masses. 3D ultrasound and volumetric reconstruction allow a complete virtual navigation throughout the ovarian tissue in the three spatial planes, facilitating a precise evaluation of intra-tumoral features, such as discrimination of liquid vs solid components, characteristics of papillary projections and septations (if present), and the description of vascular trees (if present); as well as external features, such as tumor diameter, wall thickness, contour, and boundaries. Furthermore, this important information is provided through the reconstruction of realistic 3D images.

The current study shows that HDlive and RAS offer unique ways for assessing women with ovarian masses; anatomically realistic images of the region of interest can be obtained with HDlive; and the spatial relationship and boundaries of intratumoral surface structures can be clearly depicted with RAS. Altogether, this information is extremely important to facilitate the differentiation between benignity and malignancy of ovarian masses, and is in agreement with previous publications on the issue.

Obviously, expertise is a key component for achieving a good diagnostic performance; nevertheless, modern 3D ultrasound modes may facilitate practitioners' diagnostic competence and level on confidence by means of providing high quality and great definition images, moreover, the learning curve in trainee programs could be also significantly reduced as suggested by others.

Our publications and much more specifically the one of Hata et al. have showed that "HDlive facilitated a more precise evaluation of adnexal tumors and accurate characterization of the intratumoral surface structures".

In particular, and what is extremely important to increase image quality and so facilitating the differentiation between benignity and malignancy of adnexal masses, HDlive is more definitely showing particularly, a natural and anatomically more realistic appearance of the smooth thin or irregular thick septum, smooth or irregular papillary projection, and smooth, regular, or irregular inner surface.

Hata et al. finally speaks about a "surgeon's eye" view of unique intratumoral anatomic structures "not easily seen or understood using the conventional 3D sonographic mode".

Summarizing, HDlive, and silhouette mode, provide a much better vision quality of internal tumor structures which facilitate the diagnosis.

In conclusion, state-of-the-art 3D ultrasound tools provide specific and essential information for the differentiation of benign and malignant ovarian masses. Thus, this technique may help to improve diagnostic confidence and accuracy for a correct clinical intervention, and has the potential for reducing the learning curve in trainee programs. However, further studies are needed to validate our findings, and to establish its role in clinical practice.

BIBLIOGRAPHY

Obstetrics

1. AboEllail MAM, Hanaoka U, Numoto A, Hata T. HDlive image of fetal giant hemangioma. J Ultrasound Med; 2015 in press.
2. AboEllail MAM, Kanenishi K, Mori N, Kurobe A, Hata T. HDlive imagen of circumvallate placenta. Ultrasound Obstet Gynecol. 2015;45(4):543-4.
3. AboEllail MAM, Kanenishi K, Tenkumo C, Mori N, Katayama T, Koyano K, et al. 4D power Doppler with HDLive silhouette mode in antenatal diagnosis of right aortic arch with an aberrant left subclavian artery. J Ultrasound Med. 2015. in press
4. AboEllail MAM, Tanaka H, Mori N, Hanaoka U, Hata T. HDLive silhouette mode in antenatal diagnosis of jejunal atresia. Ultrasound Obstet Gynecol. 2015;46: August 2 vol. Doi 10.1002/uog. 1575.
5. AboEllail MAM, Tanaka H, Mori N, Tanaka A, Kubo H, Shimono R, et al. HDlive imaging of meconium peritonitis. Ultrasound Obstet Gynecol. 2015;45(4):494-6.
6. Araujo ED Jr, Machado-Nardozza LM, Fernandes-Moron A. Three-dimensional STIC-HDLive rendering: new technique to assessing of fetal heart. Rev Brasil Cir Cardiovasc. 2013;28(4):5-7.
7. Araujo ED Jr, Martins-Santana EF, Machado-Nardozza LM, Fernandes-Moron A. Assessment of embryo/fetus during pregnancy by three-dimensional ultrasonography using the HDLive software: iconographicessay. Radiol Brasil. 2015;48(1):52-5.
8. Austria BS, Hanaoka U, Sato M, Hata T. Three- and four-dimensional sonographic diagnosis of fetal intra-abdominal umbilical vein varix. J Med Ultrasonics. 2014;41(2):245-6.
9. Bonilla F Jr, Raga F, Caballero-Castillo JC, Machado E, Bonilla-Musoles F. Role of state-of-the-art three-dimensional ultrasound in the differentiation of benign and malignant ovarian masses. DSJUOG. 2015;9(4):446-61.
10. Bonilla-Machado LE, Bailao LA, Osborne NG. Abdominal wall defects. Two versus three-dimensional ultrasonographic diagnosis. J Ultrasound Med. 2001; 20(2):379-89.
11. Bonilla-Musoles F, Bonilla F Jr, Raga F, Caballero O, Cadete C, Machado LE. Second trimester normal fetal scan using 3D/4D ultrasound. DSJUOG. 2015;9(4):372-81.
12. Bonilla-Musoles F, Caballero O, Castillo JC, Bonilla F Jr, Raga F. HDlive and three-dimensional imaging in prenatal diagnosis of sirenomelia in the first trimester: case report and a brief review of the literature. DSJUOG. 2015;9(2):1-4.
13. Bonilla-Musoles F, Caballero O, Castillo JC, Bonilla F Jr, Raga F. HDlive and three-dimensional imaging in prenatal diagnosis of sirenomelia in the first trimester: case report and a brief review of the literature. DSJUOG. 2015;9(2):1-4.
14. Bonilla-Musoles F, Caballero O, Osborne N, Raga F, Bonilla F Jr, Castillo JC. Technical note: HDlive 3D ultrasound and follicular development. J Med Ultrasonics (Japan). 2014;41:401-5.
15. Bonilla-Musoles F, Esquembre MJ, Bonilla F Jr, Raga F, Machado LE, Caballero O. First Trimester. DSJUOG. 2014;8(3):239-49.
16. Bonilla-Musoles F, Esquembre MP, Bonilla F Jr, Raga F, Castillo JC, Machado LE, et al. First trimester. DSJUOG. 2014;8(3):229-33.
17. Bonilla-Musoles F, Machado L, Osborne N, Raga F, Lima-Coury I, Bonilla F Jr, et al. Early diagnosis of

congenital anomalies: 1. Cepahlic pole malformations. In: Controversies in Perinatal Medicine. In: Carreras JM (Ed). Parthenon Publisher. Lancaster; 2003. pp. 1-20.
18. Bonilla-Musoles F, Machado L, Osborne N, Raga F, Lima-Coury I, Bonilla F Jr, et al. Early diagnosis of congenital anomalies: 2. Thoracic and abdominal malformations. In: Carreras JM (Ed). Controversies in Perinatal Medicine. Parthenon Publisher. Lancaster; 2003. pp. 1-20.
19. Bonilla-Musoles F, Machado LE, Osborne N, Blanes J, Bonilla F Jr, Raga F, et al. Two-dimensional and three-dimensional sonography of conjoined twins. J Clin Ultrasound. 2002;30(1):68-75.
20. Bonilla-Musoles F, Machado LE, Osborne N, Muñoz E, Raga F, Blanes Jet al. Two- and three-dimensional ultrasound in malformations of the medullary canal: report of four cases. Prenatal Diagnosis. 2001;21(8):622-6.
21. Bonilla-Musoles F, Machado LE, Osborne N. Multiple congenital contractures (Congenital multiple arthrogryposis). J Perinat Med. 2002;30(1):99-104.
22. Bonilla-Musoles F, Machado LE, Osborne NG, Raga F, Chamusca L, Chagas K, et al. Ultrasound diagnosis of facial and cephalic pole malformations: Comparative study of different three-dimensional modalities and two-dimensional ultrasound. Ultrasound Quaterly. 2000;16(1):97-105.
23. Bonilla-Musoles F, Machado LE, Raga F, Castillo JC, Osborne N, Bonilla F Jr, et al. Three-dimensional/four-dimensional ultrasound. In: Hata T, Kurjak A, Kozuma S (Eds). Fetal Malformations. Part Two: Second Trimester. Cephalic Pole Malformations. In Current Topics on Fetal 3D/4D Ultrasound. Bentham Science Publishers. Busum, Holand; 2009. pp. 56-86. ISSN: 978-1-60805-019-2.
24. Bonilla-Musoles F, Machado LE, Raga F, Castillo JC, Osborne N, Bonilla F Jr, et al. Three-dimensional/four-dimensional ultrasound. In: Hata T, Kurjak A, Kozuma S (Eds). Fetal Malformations. Part Three: Second Trimester. Skeletal Disorders, Thoracic, Abdominal, Kidney and Other Malformations. In Current Topics on Fetal 3D/4D Ultrasound. Bentham Science Publishers. Busum, Holand; 2009. pp- 87-133. ISSN: 978-1-60805-019-2.
25. Bonilla-Musoles F, Machado LE, Raga F. Three- and four-dimensional images of fetal malformations. In: Kurjak A, Jackson D (Eds). An atlas of three- and four-dimensional sonography in obstetrics and gynaecology. Taylor and Francis. London; 2012.
26. Bonilla-Musoles F, Machado LE, Raga F. Three-dimensional ultrasound in the visualization of fetal malformations. In: Kurjak A, Chervenak FK (Eds). Donald School Textbook of Ultrasound in Obstetrics and Gynecology. 2nd Edition. New York. ISBN: 978-81-8448-202-7; 2008, Chapter 42. 625-40.
27. Bonilla-Musoles F, Machado LE, Raga F. Three-dimensional visualization of fetal malformations. Ian Donald School Textbook of Ultrasound in Obstetrics and Gynecology. In: Kurjak A, Chervenak F (Eds). Jaypee Brothers Medical Publishers. New Delhi 38,480-99, 2004. ISBN: 81-8061-198-1.
28. Bonilla-Musoles F, Machado LE. Gastrointestinal tract and internal abdominal wall. In: Kurjark A, Chervenak FA, Carrera JM (Eds). Ian Donald School Atlas of Fetal Malformations. Jaypee Brothers Medical Publishers, New Delhi; 2007. pp. 174-94.
29. Bonilla-Musoles F, Raga F, Bonilla F Jr, Caballero O, Esquembre MJ. HDLive Images in Gynecology and Reproduction. Slide Atlas. In: Pooh RK, Kurjak A (Eds). Donald School Atlas of Advanced Ultrasound in Obstetrics and Gynecology. The Health Science Publisher. Jaypee, New Delhi. 2015. Chapter 10, 787-853. ISBN: 978-93-5152-919-4.
30. Bonilla-Musoles F, Raga F, Bonilla F Jr, Castillo JC, Caballero O. Gynecological tumor images using high definition ultrasound (HDlive US). Donald School Journal of Ultrasound in Obstetric and Gynecology. DSJUOG. 2014;8(1):1-9.
31. Bonilla-Musoles F, Raga F, Bonilla F Jr, Castillo JC, Machado LE, Caballero O. Gynecological tumor images using HDlive US. DSJUOG. 2014;8(2):155-63.
32. Bonilla-Musoles F, Raga F, Bonilla F Jr, Machado L, Cadete C. Second trimester normal fetal scan using 3D/4D ultrasound HDLive and silhouette. IDSJUOG. 2015;9(4):372-81.
33. Bonilla-Musoles F, Raga F, Castillo JC, Bonilla F Jr, Caballero O. Revisión. Alta definición Ecografica en tiempo real (HDlive US) en Obstetricia y Ginecologia. Rev Peru Ginecol Obstet. 2013;59(1):33-41.
34. Bonilla-Musoles F, Raga F, Castillo JC, Bonilla F Jr, Climent MT, Caballero O. High definition real time ultrasound (HDlive) of embryonic and fetal malformations before week 16. DSJUOG. 2012;7(1):1-8.
36. Bonilla-Musoles F, Raga F, Castillo JC, Bonilla F Jr, O Caballero. Revisión. Alta definición Ecográfica en tiempo real (HDlive US) en Obstetricia y Ginecologia. Rev Peru Ginecol Obstet. 2013;59(1):33-41.
37. Bonilla-Musoles F, Raga F, Machado LE, Bonilla F Jr. News on 3D-4D sonographic applications in the diagnosis of fetal malformations. In: Kurjak A, Chervenak (Eds). Donald School Textbook of Ultrasound in Obstetrics and Gynecology. 2nd edition. ISBN: 978-81-8448-202-7; 2008, Chapter 42,640-61.
38. Bonilla-Musoles F, Raga F, Osborne N, Bonilla F Jr, Castillo JC, Caballero O. Pictorial Review. Multimodality 3D volumetric ultrasound in obstetrics and gynaecology with an emphasis in HDlive technique. Ultrasound Quarterly. 2013;29(2):189-201.
39. Bonilla-Musoles F, Raga F, Osborne NG. Three-dimensional ultrasound evaluation of the embryo and the early fetus. In: Kurjak A (Ed). A Textbook of Perinatal Medicine. Parthenon Publish. Lancs. England; 1998. pp. 240-62.
40. Castillo JC, Caballero O, Bonilla F Jr, Raga F, Bonilla-Musoles F. HDlive in Assisted Human Reproduction. DSJUOG. 2014;8(3):229-33.

41. Grigore M, Cojocaru C, Lazar T. The role of HDLive technology in Obstetrics and Gynecology. Present and Future. DSJUOG. 2014;8(3)234-8.
42. Grigore M, Mares A. The role of HDLive technology in improving the quality of obstetrical images. Med Ultrasound. 2013;15(3):209-14.
43. Grigore M, Vulpoi C, Preda C, Martiniuc V, Vasiliu I, Gorduza V. Using HDLive technology to diagnose Turner síndrome in the first trimester of pregnancy. Case Report. Acta Endocrinologica (BUC). 2015;11(1):93-8.
44. Hata T, Hanaoka U, Mashima M, Ishimura M, Marumo G, Kanenishi K. Four-dimensional HDLive rendering image of fetal facial expression: a pictorial essay. J Med Ultrasonics. 2013;40(3):441-8.
45. Hata T, Hanaoka U, Tenkumo CH, Ito M, Uketa E, Mori N, et al. Three-dimensional HDLive rendering image of cystic higroma. J Med Ultrasonics. 2013;40(2):297-9.
46. Hata T, Hanaoka U, Tenkumo CH, Sato M, Tanaka H, Ishimura M. Three- and four-dimensional HDLive rendering images of normal and abnormal fetuses: pictorial essay. Arch Obstet Gynecol. 2012;286(6):1431-5.
47. Hata T, Kanenishi K, Hanaoka U, Marumo G. HDLive and 4D ultrasound in the assessment of fetal facial expressions. DSJOG. 2015;9(1):44-50.
48. Hata T, Kanenishi K, Hanaoka U, Tanaka H. HDlive of the fetal heart. DSJUOG. 2014;8(3):266-72.
49. Hata T, Kanenishi K, Hanaoka U, Uematsu R, Marumo G, Tanaka H. HDlive study of fetal development and behavior. DSJUOG. 2014;8(3):250-65.
50. Hata T, Kanenishi K, Hanaoke U, AboEllai MAM, Marumo G. HDlive and 4D ultrasound in the assessment of twin pregnancy. DSJOG. 2015;9(1):51-60.
51. Hata T, Kurjak A, Kozuma S. Current Topics on Fetal 3D/4D Ultrasound. Bentham Science Publishers. Busum, Holand; 2009. pp. 56-86. ISSN: 978-1-60805-019-2.
52. Hata T, Kurjak A. Current Topics on Fetal 3D/4D Ultrasound. Bentham Science Publishers. Busum, Holand; 2012.
53. Hata T, Mashima M, Ito M, Uketa E, Mori N, Ishimura M. Three-dimensional HDlive rendering images of the fetal heart. Ultrasound Med Biol. 2013;39(8):1513-7.
54. Hata T, Mori N, Tenkumo C, Hanaoka U. Three-dimensional volume-rendered imaging of normal and abnormal fetal fluid-filled structures using inversion mode. J Obstet Gynecol Res. 2011;37(11):1748-54.
55. Hata T, Tenkumo CH, Sato M, Kanenishi K, Ishimura M. Three-dimensional ultrasound HDLive-rendered images of intrauterine abnormalities during pregnancy. J Med Ultrasonics. 2013;40(2):179-80.
56. Hata T, Ukeda E, Tenkumo C, Hanaoka U, Kanenishi K, Tanaka H. Three- and four-dimensional HDlive rendering image of fetal acrania/exencephaly in early pregnancy. J Med Ultrasonics. 2013;40(2):271-3.
57. Hata T. HDlive rendering image at 6 weeks of gestation. J Med Ultrasonics. 2013;40(3):495-6.
58. Kagan KO, Pintoffl K, Hoopmann M. First-trimester ultrasound images using HDlive. Picture of the month. Ultrasound Obstet Gynecol. 2011;38(5):607-9.
59. Kanenishi K, Nitta E, Mashima M, Hanaoka U, Koyano K, Tanaka H, et al. HDlive imaging of intra-amniotic umbilical vein varix with thrombosis. Placenta. 2013;34(4):1110-2.
60. Kurjak A, Chervenak F. Donald School Textbook of Ultrasound in Obstetrics and Gynecology. 2nd Edition. New York. ISBN: 978-81-8448-202-7.
61. Kurjak A, Chervenak F. Ian Donald School Textbook of Ultrasound in Obstetrics and Gynecology. 2008, Jaypee Brothers Medical Publishers, New Delhi, ISBN: 978-81-8061-198-1. Chapter 42.
62. Kurjak A, Jackson D. An atlas of three- and four-dimensional sonography in Obstetrics and Gynecology. Taylor and Francis. London; 2004.
63. Kurjak A. A Textbook of Perinatal Medicine. Parthenon Publish. Lancs. England; 1998.
64. Kurjark A, Chervenak FA, Carrera JM. Ian Donald School Atlas of Fetal Malformations. Jaypee Brothers Medical Publishers, New Delhi; 2007.
65. Kurjark A. Azumendi G. Fetus in three-dimensional imaging, embriology and fetoscopy. Informa Healthcare. Abingdon, England; 2006.
66. Machado LA, Bonilla-Musoles F, Raga F, Bonilla F Jr, Machado LE, Osborne N. Thanatophoric dysplasia, Ultrasound diagnosis. Ultrasound Obstet Gynecol. 2001;18(1):85-6.
67. Machado LE, Bonilla-Musoles F, Osborne N. Skeletal anomalies. In: Kurjark A, Azumendi G (Eds). Fetus in three-dimensional imaging, embryology and fetoscopy. Informa Healthcare. Abingdon, England; 2006. pp. 331-49.
68. Machado LE, Bonilla-Musoles F, Osborne NG. Fetal limb abnormalities. Ultrasound Diagnosis. Ultrasound Quaterly. 2000;16(2):203-19.
69. Merz E, Abramovicz J, Baba K, Blaas HG, Deng J, Glindes L, et al. Three-dimensional imaging of the fetal face-recommendations from the International 3D Focus Group. Ultraschall Med. 2012;33(2):175-82.
70. Merz E. Surface reconstruction of a fetus (28+2 GW) using HDLive technology. Ultraschall Med. 2012;33(2):211.
71. Osborne N, Bonilla-Musoles F, Machado L, Raga F, Bonilla F Jr, Ruiz F, et al. Fetal Megacystic (Prune Belly. Differential Diagnosis). J Ultrasound Med. 2011;30(6):833-41.
72. Pooh RK, Kurjak A. Novel applications of three-dimensional HDLive imaging in prenatal diagnosis from the first trimester. J Perinat Med. 2015;43(2):147-58.
73. POOH RK. Brand new technology of HDLive silhouette and HDLive flow images. In: Pooh RK, Kurjak A (Eds). Donald School Atlas of Ultrasound in Obstetrics and Gynecology. Chapter 1. The Health Science Publishers. New Dehli; 2015. pp. 1-38. ISBN: 978-93-5152-919-4.
74. Raga F, Bonilla F Jr, Castillo JC, Bonilla-Musoles F. HDlive ultrasound images in ART. RBM Online. 2013;26:269-71.

75. Sajapala S, AboEllail MAM, Tanaka T, Nitta E, Kanenishi K, Hata T. New 3D power Doppler (HDlive Flow) with HDLive silhouette mode for diagnosis of malignant ovarian tumor. Ultrasound Obstet Gynecol. 2015;46:August 2 vol. Doi: 10.1002/uog.15730
76. Sanz-Cortés M, Raga F, Bonilla-Musoles F. Three-dimensional sonographic prenatal diagnosis of a lobar holoprosencephaly associated with cebocephaly. Assessment and diagnosis with multiplanar reconstruction. Prenatal Diagnosis. 2007;27(6):585-6.
77. Sanz-Cortes M, Raga F, Leon JL, Sniderman A, Bonilla-Musoles F. MRI and multiplanar 3D ultrasound compared in the prenatal assessment of enlarged posterior fossa. J Perinatal Med. 2007;35(5):422-4.
78. Tenkumo C, Tanaka H, Ito T. Three-dimensional rendering images of the TRP sequence in the first trimester: reverse end-diastolic umbilical artery velocity in a pump twin with an adverse pregnancy outcome. J Med Ultrasonics. 2013;40(2):293-6.
79. Tonni G, Grisolia G. Fetal uvula: navigating and lightening the soft palate using HDLive. Arch Gynecol Obstet. 2013;288(2):239-44.

Reproduction

80. Allemand MC, Tummon IS, Phy JL, Foong SC, Dumesic DA, Session DR. Diagnosis of polycystic ovaries by three-dimensional transvaginal ultrasound. Fertil Steril. 2006;85(1):214-9.
81. Azziz R, Carmina E, Dewailly D, Diamanti-Kandarakis E, Escobar-Morreale HF, Futterweit W, et al. Task Force on the Phenotype of the Polycystic Ovary Syndrome of The Androgen Excess and PCOS Society. The Androgen Excess and PCOS Society criteria for the polycystic ovary syndrome: the complete task force report. Fertil Steril. 2009;91(2):456-88.
82. Ballen AH, Laven JS, Tan SL, Dewailly D. Ultrasound assessment of the polycystic ovary syndrome: International Consensus Definition Human Reprod Update. 2003;9(6): 505-14.
83. Blank SK, Helm KD, McCartney CR, Marshall JC. Polycystic ovary syndrome in adolescence. Ann N Y Acad Sci. 2008;1135:76-84.
84. Bonilla-Musoles F, Ballester MJ, Carrera JM. Doppler color transvaginal Mason-Salvat Medicina. Madrid. 1992. ISBN: 978-84-458-0122-8.
85. Bonilla-Musoles F, Dolz M, Moreno J, Raga F. Reproducción Asistida; Abordaje en la práctica clínica. Panamericana Ed. Madrid; 2008. ISBN: 978-84-9835-156-9.
86. Bonilla-Musoles F. Ecografía vaginal Doppler y Tridimensión. Panamericana Ed. Madrid; 2001. ISBN: 978-84-7903-568-8.
87. Boyle J, Teede HJ. Polycystic ovary syndrome. An update. Australian Family Physician. 2012;41:752-6.
88. Bridges NA, Cooke A, Healy MJ, Hindmarsh PC, Brook CG. Standards for ovarian volume in childhood and puberty. Fertil Steril. 1993;60(3):456-40.
89. Broekmans FJ, De Ziegler D, Howles CM, Gougeon A, Trew G, Olivennes F. The antral follicle count: practical recommendations for better standardization. Fertil Steril. 2010;94(3):96-103.
90. Broekmans FJ, Kwee J, Hendriks DJ, Mol BW, Lambalk CB. A systematic review of tests predicting ovarian reserve and IVF outcome. Human Reprod Update. 2006;12(6): 685-718.
91. Conway G, Dewailly D, Diamanti-Kandarakis D, Escobar Morreala HF, Franks S, Gambineri A, et al. On behalf of the ESE PCOD Special Interest Group Europ. European Survey of diagnosis and management of the polycystic ovary syndrome: results of the ESE PCOS Special Interest Group's Questionnaire. J Endocrinol. 2014;171(4):1-29.
92. Corton M, Botella-Carretero JI, Benguria A, Villuendas G, Zaballos A, San Millan JL, et al. Differential gene expression profile in omental adipose tissue in women with polycystic ovary syndrome. J Clin Endocrinol Metab. 2007;92(1):328-37.
93. Deb S, Campbell BK, Clewes JS, Raine-Fenning NJ. Quantitative analysis of antral follicle number and size: a comparison of two dimensional and automated three-dimensional ultrasound techniques. Ultrasound Obstet Gynecol. 2010;35(3):354-60.
94. Deb S, Jayaprakasan K, Campbell BK, Clewes JS, Johnson IR, Reine-Fenning NJ. Intraobserver and interobserver reliability of automated antral follicle counts made using three-dimensional ultrasound and sono AVC. Ultrasound Obstet Gynecol. 2009;33(4):477-83.
95. Dewailly D, Gronier H, Robin G, Leroy M, Pigny P, Duhamenl A, et al. Diagnosis of polycystic ovary syndrome (PCOS): revisiting the threshold values of follicle count on ultrasound and of the serum AMH level for the definition of polycystic ovaries. Human Reprod. 2011;26(11):3123-9.
96. Dewailly D, Lujan ME, Carmina E, Cedars MI, Laven J, Norman RJ, et al. Definition and significance of polycystic ovarian morphology: a task force report from the Androgen Excess and Polycystic Ovary Syndrome Society. Human Reprod Update. 2014;20(3):334-52.
97. Dolz M, Osborne N, Blanes J, Raga F, Abad de Velasco L, Villalobos A, et al. Polycystic ovarian syndrome: Assessment with color Doppler angiography and three-dimensional ultrasonography. J Ultrasound Med. 1999;18(4):303-13.
98. Fauser BC, Tarlatzis BC, Rebar RW, Legro RS, Balen AH, Lobo R, et al. Consensus on women's health aspects of polycystic ovary syndrome (PCOS): The Amsterdam ESHRE/ASRM-Sonsored 3rd PCOS Consensus Workshop Group. Fertil Steril. 2012;97(1):28-30.
99. Final Report National Institute of Health. Evidence-based Methodology Workshop on Polycystic Ovary Syndrome December 3-5, 2012. http://prevention.nih.gov/workshop/2012/pcos/resourc-es.aspx
100. Franks S. Controversy in clinical endocrinology: diagnosis of polycystic ovarian syndrome: in defense of the Rotterdam criteria. J Clin Endocrinol Metab. 2006;91(3):786-9.

101. Hendriks DJ, Kwee J, Mol BW, TeVelde ER, Broekmans FJ. Ultrasonography as a tool for the prediction of outcome in IVF patients: a comparative meta-analysis of ovarian volume and antral follicle count. Fertil Steril. 2007;87(4):764-75.
102. Hsu Roe A, Dokras A. The Diagnosis of Polycystic Ovary Syndrome in Adolescents. Rev Obstet Gynecol. 2011;4(2):45-51.
103. Jayaprakasan K, Campbell B, Hopkinsson J, Clewes JS, Johnson IR, Reine-Fenning NJ. Establishing the intercycle variability of three-dimensional ultrasonographic predictors of ovarian reserve. Fertil Steril. 2008;90(6):2126-32.
104. Jayaprakasan K, Walker KF, Clewes JS, Johnson IR, Reine-Fenning NJ. The interobserver reliability of off-line antral follicle counts made from stored three-dimensional ultrasound data: a comparative study of different measurement techniques. Ultrasound Obstet Gynecol. 2007;29(3):335-41.
105. Kupesic S, Kurjak A, Bjelos D, Vujisic S. Three-dimensional ultrasonographic ovarian measurements and in vitro fertilization outcome are related to age. Fertil Steril. 2003;79(1):190-7.
106. Lam PM, Johnson IR, Raine-Fenning NJ. Three-dimensional ultrasound features of the polycystic ovary and the effect of different phenotypic expressions on these parameters. Human Reprod. 2007;22(12):3116-23.
107. Lujan ME, Jarrett BY, Brooks ED, Reines JK, Peppin AK, Muhn N, et al. Updated ultrasound criteria for polycystic ovarian syndrome: reliable thresholds for elevated follicle population and ovarian volume. Human Reprod. 2013;28(5)1361-8.
108. Mala YM, Ghosh SB, Tripathi R. Three-dimensional power Doppler imaging in the diagnosis of polycystic ovary syndrome. Int J Gynecol Obstet. 2009;105(1):36-8.
109. March WA, Moore VM, Willson KJ, Phillips DI, Norman RJ, Davies MJ. The prevalence of polycystic ovary syndrome in a community sample assessed under contrasting diagnostic criteria. Hum Reprod. 2010;25(2):544-51.
110. Merce LT, Gomez B, Engels V, Bau S, Bajo JM. Intraobserver and interobserver reproducibility of ovarian volume, antral follicle count, and vascularity indices obtained with transvaginal 3-dimensional ultrasonography, power Doppler angiography, and the virtual-organ computer-aided analysis imaging program. J Ultrasound Med. 2005;24(9):1279-87.
111. Mortensen M, Rosenfield RL, Littlejohn E. Functional significance of polycystic-size ovaries in healthy adolescents. J Clin Endocrinol Metab. 2006;91(10):3786-90.
112. Ng EH, Yeung WS, Fong DY, Ho PC. Effects of age on hormonal and ultrasound markers of ovarian reserve in Chinese women with proven fertility. Human Reprod. 2003;18(10):2169-74.
113. Pascual MA, Graupera P, Hereter L, Tresserra F, Rodriguez I, Alcazar JL. Assessment of ovarian vascularization in the polycystic ovary by three-dimensional power Doppler Sonography. Gynaecol. Endocrinol. 2008;24(11):631-6.
114. Pavlik EJ, De Priest PD, Gallion HH, Ueland FR, Reedy MB, Kryscio RJ. Ovarian volume related to age. Gynecol Oncol. 2000;77:410-2.
115. Pellicer A, Ardiles G, Neuspiller F, Remohi J, Simon C, Bonilla-Musoles F. Evaluation of the ovarian reserve in young low responders with normal basal levels of follicle-stimulating hormone using three-dimensional ultrasonography. Fertil Steril. 1998;70(4):671-5.
116. Raine-Fenning N, Campbell BK, Clewes J, Johnson IR. The interobserver reliability of ovarian volume measurement is improved with three-dimensional ultrasound, but dependent upon technique. Ultrasound Med Biol. 2003;29(12):1685-90.
117. Raine-Fenning N, Jayaprakasan K, Clewes J. Automated follicle tracking facilitates standardization and my improve work flow. Ultrasound Obstet Gynecol. 2007;30(7):1015-8.
118. Ruess ML, Kline J, Santos R, Levin B, Timor-Tritsch I. Age and the ovarian follicle pool assessed with transvaginal ultrasonography. Am J Obstet Gynecol. 1996;174(2):624-7.
119. Scheffer GJ, Broekmans FJ, Bancsi LF, Habbema JD, Looman CW, TeVelde ER. Quantitative transvaginal two- and three-dimensional sonography of the ovaries: reproducibility of Antral Follicles Counts. Ultrasound Obstet Gynecol. 2002;20(3):270-5.
120. Scheffer GJ, Broekmans FJ, Dorland M, Habbema JD, Looman CW, TeVelde TR. Antral follicle counts by transvaginal ultrasonography are related to age in women with proven natural fertility. Fertil Steril. 1999;72(5):845-51.
121. Scheffer GJ, Broekmans FJ, Looman CW, Blankenstein FH, De Jong M, Fauser BC, et al. The number of antral follicles in normal women with proven fertility is the best reflection of reproductive age. Human Reprod. 2003;18(4):700-6.
122. TeVelde ER, Scheffer GJ, Dorland M, Broekmans FJ, Fauser BC. The variability of female reproductive ageing. Developmental and endocrine aspects of normal ovarian ageing. Human Reprod Update. 2002;8(2):141-54.
123. The Rotterdam ESHRE/ASRM-Sponsored PCOS Consensus Workshop Group. Revised 2003 consensus on diagnostic criteria and long-term health risks related to polycystic ovary syndrome (PCOS). Human Reprod. 2004;19(1):41-7.
124. Zawadski JK, Dunaif A. Diagnostic criteria for polycystic ovary syndrome: towards a rational approach. In: Dunaif A, Givens JR, Haseltine FP, Merriam GR (Eds). Polycystic Ovary Syndrome. Boston: Blackwell Scientific Publications; 1992. pp. 377-84.

Gynecology

Benign Ovarian Teratomas

125. Al Hilli E, Ansari N Pathogénesis of balls in mature ovarian teratoma. Report of 3 cases and reviewof literature. Int J Gynecol Pathol. 2006;25:347-53
126. Altinbas SK, Yalvac S, Kandermir O, Altinbas NK, Karcaaltincaba D, Dede H, et al. An unusual growth of

ovarian cystic teratoma with multiple floating balls during pregnancy: a case report. J Clin Ultrasound. 2010;38:325-7.
127. Beller MJ. The "tip of the iceberg" sign. Radiology. 1998;209:395-6.
128. Canda AE, Astarcioglu H, Obuz F, Canda MS. Cystic ovarian teratoma with intracystic floating globules. Abdom Imaging. 2005;30:369-71.
129. Caspi B, Appelman Z, Rabinerson D, Elchalal U, Zalel Y, Katz Z. Pathognomonic echo patterns of bening cystic teratomas of the ovary: classification, incidence and accuracy rate of sonographic diagnosis. Ultrasound Obstet Gynecol. 1996;7:275-9.
130. Chen CP, Chen SR, Wang W, Wang KL, Wang TY. Multiple globules in a cystic ovarian teratoma. Fertil Steril. 2001;75:618-9.
131. Deangelis CE, Yonkers NY. An ovarian dermoid cyst with numerous sebum balls. Am J Obstet Gynecol. 1953;66:443-5.
132. Donnadieu AC, Deffieux X, Le Ray C, Mordefroid M, Frydmn R, Fernandez H. Unusual fast-growing ovarian cyst teratoma during pregnancy presenting with intracystic fat "floating balls" appearance. Fertil Steril. 2006;86:175-8.
133. Fortia ME. Elhajaji E, Elmadani B, Khalil M, Eldergash O. Elhamrouth H. Are they spherules of ovarian cystic teratoma ordoughter cysts of echinococcosis? Ultraschall Der Med. 2006;27:1-3.
134. Gol M, Saygili U, Uslu T, Erten O. Mature cystic teratoma with intracystic fat balls in a postmenopausal women. Eur J Obstet Gynecol Reprod Biol. 2005;119:125-6.
135. Gürel H, Gürel SA. Ovarian cystic teratoma with a pathognomonic appearance of multiple flating balls: a case report and investigation of common characteristics of the cases in the literature. Fertil Steril. 2008;90:17-9.
136. Hutton L, Rankin R. The fat-fluid level: another feature of dermoid tumors of the ovary. J Clin Ultrasound. 1979;7:215-6.
137. Jantarasaengaram S, Siricharo S, Vairojanavong K. Cystic ovarian teratoma with intracystic fat ball. Ultrasound Obstet Gynecol. 2003;22:102-3.
138. Kawamoto S, Sato K, Matsumoto H, et al. Multiple mobile spherules in mature cystic teratoma of the ovary. AJR. 2001;176:1455-7.
139. Kim HC, Kim SH, Lee HJ, Shin SJ, Hwang SJ, Choi YH. Fluid-fluid levels in ovarian teratomas. Abdom Imaging. 2002;27:100-5.
140. Laing FC, Van Dalsem VF, Marks WM, Barton JL, Martinez DA. Dermoid cysts of the ovary: their ultrasonographic appearances. Obstet Gynecol. 1981;57:99-104.
141. Linder D, MaCaw BK, Hecht F. Parthenogenetic origin of benign ovarian teratomas. N Engl J Med. 1975;292:63-6.
142. Malde HM, Kedar RP, Chadha D, Nayak S. Dermoid mesh: a sonographic sign of ovarian teratoma. Am J Roentgenol. 1992;159:1349-50.
143. Muramatsu Y, Moriyama N, Takayasu K, Nawano S, Yamada T. CT and MR imaging of cystic ovarian teratoma with intracystic fat balls. J Comput Assist Tomograph. 1991;15:528-9.
144. Otigbah C, Thompson MO, Lowe DG, Setchell M. Mobile globules in benign cyst teratoma of the ovary. Brit J Obstet Gynaecol. 2000;107:135-8.
145. Outwater EK, Evan S, Siegelman MD, Jennifer L, Hunt MD. Ovarian teratomas: Tumor types and imaging characteristics. Radio Graphics. 2001;21:475-90.
146. Quinn SF, Erickson S, Black WC. Cystic ovarian teratoma: the sonographic appearance of the dermoid plug. Radiology. 1985;155:477-8.
147. Rao JR, Shah Z, Patwardhan V, Hanchate V, Thakkar H, Garg A. Ovarian cystic teratoma: determined phenotypic response of keratocytes and uncommon intracystic floating balls appearance on sonography and computed tomography. J Ultrasound Med. 2002;21:687-91.
148. Rathod K, Kale H, Narlawar R, Hardikar J, Kulkarni V, Joseph J. Unusual "floating balls" appearance of an ovariancystic teratoma: sonographic and CT findings. J Clin Ultrasound. 2001;29:41-3.
149. Sheth S, Fishman EK, Buck JL, Hamper UM, Sanders RC. The variable sonographic appearances of ovarian teratomas: correlation with CT. Am J Roentgenol. 1988;151:331-4.
150. Tampakoudis P, Assimakopoulos E, Zafrakas M, Tzevelekis P, Kostropoulo E, Bontis J. Pelvic echinoccocus mimicking multicystic ovary. Ultrasound Obstet Gynecol. 2003;22:196-8.
151. Tongsong T, Luewen S, Phadungkiatwattana P, et al. Pattern recognition using transabdominal ultrasound for diagnose ovarian mature cysts teratomas. Int J Gynecol Obstet. 2008;103:99-104.
152. Tongsong T, Wanapirak CH, Khunamornpong S, Sukpan K. Numerous intracystic floating balls as a songraphic feature of benign cystic teratoma. J Ultrasound Med. 2006; 25:1587-91.
153. Umesaki N, Nagamatsu A, Yada C, Tanaka T. MR and ultrasound imaging of floating globules in mature ovarian cyst teratoma. Gynecol Oncol Invest. 2004;58:130-2.
154. Yacizi B, Erdogmus B. Floating ball appearance in ovarian cystic teratoma. Diagn Interv Radiol. 2006;12:136-8.

Benign and Malignant Ovarian Tumors

155. Alcázar JL, AubáM Olartecoechea B. Three-dimensional ultrasound in gynecological clinical practice. Reports in Medical Imaging. 2012;5(1):1-13.
156. Alcázar JL, Galán MJ, García-Manero M, Guerriero S. Three-dimensional ultrasound morphologic assessment in complex adnexal masses a preliminary experience. J Ultrasound Med. 2003;22(3):249-54.
157. Alcázar JL, Garcia-Manero M, Galalvan R. Three-dimensional sonographic morphologic assessment of adnexal masses. A reproducibility study. J Ultrasound Med. 2007;26(7):1007-11.

158. Alcázar JL, García-Manero M, Galván R. Three-dimensional sonographic morphologic assessment of adnexal masses: a reproducibility study. J Ultrasound Med. 2007;26(8):1007-11.
159. Alcázar JL, Jurado M. Three-dimensional ultrasound for assessing women with gynecological cancer: a systematic review. Gynecol Oncol. 2011;120(3):340-6.
160. Alcazar JL, Merce L, Laparte C, Jurado M, Lopez-GarciaG. A new scoring system to differentiate benign from malignant adnexal masses. Am J Obstet Gynecol. 2003;188(3):685-62.
161. Alcázar JL. Three-dimensional power Doppler derived vascular indices: what are we measuring and how are we doing it? Ultrasound Obstet Gynecol. 2008;32(4):485-7.
162. Bonilla MF, Ovario El. Tumores malignos in: Ecografia vaginal Doppler y tridimension Panamericana Ed Med. Madrid. 2001;469-559. ISBN: 84-7903-655-8.
163. Bonilla-Musoles F, Ballester MJ, Carrera JM. Doppler color transvaginal. Barcelona. Masson-Salvat Medicina. 1992. ISBN 84-458-0122-8.
164. Bonilla-Musoles F, Cadete C, Raga F, Bonilla F Jr, Osborne NG, Caballero O. HDlive ultrasound images of ovarian dermoid cysts. Diagnostic Accuracy. Clin Exp Obstet Gynecol. 2015;42(4). ref 2073/34 in press.
165. Bonilla-Musoles F, Raga F, Bonilla F Jr, Castillo JC, Machado LE, Caballero O. Gynecological tumor images using HDlive. DSJUOG. 2015;9(2):1-10.
166. Bonilla-Musoles F, Raga F, Osborne N, Bonilla F Jr, Castillo JC, Machado LE, et al. Pictorical review: multimodality 3d volumetric ultrasound in obstetrics and gynecology with emphasis on HDlive technique. Ultrasound Quaterly. 2012;7(1):1-8.
167. Bonilla-Musoles F, Raga F, Osborne NG. Three-dimensional ultrasound evaluation of ovarian masses. Gynecol Oncol. 1995;59(1):129-35.
168. Crade M, Berman M, Chase D. Three-dimensional tissue block ultrasound in ovarian tumors. Ultrasound Obstet Gynecol. 2005;26(6):683-6.
169. Geomini PM, Kluivers KB, Moret E, Bremer GL, Kruitwagen RF, Mol BW. Evaluation of adnexal masses with three-dimensional ultrasonography. Obstet Gynecol. 2006;108(5):1167-75.
170. Hata T, Hata K, Noguchi J, Kanenishi K, Shiota A. Ultrasound for evaluation of adnexal malignancy: from 2D to 3D Ultrasound. JOG. Res. 2011;37(10):1255-68.
171. Hata T, Kanenishi K, Mashima M, Hanaoka U, Tanaka H. HDlive rendering image of adnexal tumors: Preliminary report. J Med Ultrasonics. 2014;41(2):181-6.
172. Hata T, Yanagihara T, Hayashi K, et al. Three-dimensional ultrasonographic evaluation of ovarian tumours: a preliminary study. Human Reprod. 1999;14(3):858-61.
173. Jacobs I, Oram D, Fairbanks J, Turner J, Frost C, Grudzinskas J. A risk of malignancy index incorporating CA-125, ultrasound and menopausal status for the accurate preoperative diagnosis of ovarian cancer. Brit J Obstet Gynaecol. 1990;97(10):922-9.
174. Jokubkiene L, Sladkevicius P, Valentin L. Does three-dimensional power Doppler ultrasound help indiscrimination between benign and malignant ovarian masses? Ultrasound Obstet Gynecol. 2007;29(2):215-25.
175. Jurkovic D. Three-dimensional ultrasound in Gynecology: a critical evaluation. Ultrasound Obstet Gynecol. 2002;19(1):109-17.
176. Kurjak A, Kupesic S, Anic T, Kosuta D. Three-dimensional ultrasound and power Doppler improve the diagnosis of ovarian lesions. Gynecol Oncol. 2000;76(1):28-32.
177. Kurjak A, Kupesic S, Sparac V, Kosuta D. Three-dimensional ultrasonographic and power Doppler characterization of ovarian lesions. Ultrasound Obstet Gynecol. 2000;16(4):365-71.
178. Kurjak A, Kupesić S. Three dimensional ultrasound and power Doppler in assessment of uterine and ovarian angiogenesis: a prospective study. Croat Med J. 1999;40(3):413-20.
179. Laban M, Metawee H, Elyan A, Kamal M, Kamel M, Mansour G. Three-dimensional ultrasound and three-dimensional power Doppler in the assessment of ovarian tumors. Int J Gynaecol Obstet. 2007;99(3):201-5.
180. Martins WP, Raine-Fenning NJ, Ferriani RA, Nastri CO. Quantitative three-dimensional power Doppler angiography: a flow-free phantom experiment to evaluate the relationship between color gain, depth and signal artifact. Ultrasound Obstet Gynecol. 2010;35(3):361-8.
181. Martins WP. Three-dimensional power Doppler: validity and reliability. Ultrasound Obstet Gynecol. 2010;36(4):530-3.
182. Merz E: 25 years of 3D Ultrasound in prenatal diagnosis (1989-2014). Ultraschall Med. 2015;36(1):3-8.
183. Mihaela G. HDlive pictures of a serous ovarian borderline tumor. Ultrasound Obstet Gynecol. 2013;41(5):598-9.
184. Pairleitner H, Steiner H, Hasenoehrl G, Staudach A. Three-dimensional power Doppler sonography: imaging and quantifying blood flow and vascularization. Ultrasound Obstet Gynecol. 1999;14(2):139-43.
185. Raga F, Castillo JC, Bonilla F Jr, Caballero O, Bonilla-Musoles F. HDlive ultrasound images in assisted reproduction treatment. Reprod Biomed Online. 2013;26(3):269-71.
186. Raine-Fenning NJ, Nordin NM, Ramnarine KV, et al. Evaluation of the effect of machine settings on quantitative three-dimensional power Doppler angiography: an in-vitro flow phantom experiment. Ultrasound Obstet Gynecol. 2008;32(4):551-9.
187. Sajapala S, Aboellail MA, Tanaka T, Nitta E, Kanenishi K, Hata T. New 3D power Doppler (HDlive flow) with HDLive silhouette mode for diagnosis of malignant ovarian tumor. Ultrasound Obstet Gynecol. 2015 August 24. doi:10.1002/uog.15730.
188. Sayasneh A, Kaijser J, Preisler J, Smith A, Raslan F, Johnson S, et al. Accuracy of ultrasonography performed by examiners

with varied training and experience in predicting specific pathology of adenexal masses. Ultrasound Obstet Gynecol. 2015;45(4):605-12.

189. Schulten-Wijman MJ, Struijk PC, Brezinka C, De Jong N, Steegers EA. Evaluation of volume vascularization index and flow index: a phantomstudy. Ultrasound Obstet Gynecol. 2008;32(4):560-4.
190. Timmerman D, Testa AC, Bourne T, Ferrazzi E, Ameye L, Konstantinovic ML. International ovarian tumor analysis group. Logistic regression model to distinguish between the benign and malignant adnexal mass before surgery: a multicenter study by the International Ovarian Tumor Analysis Group. J Clin Oncol. 2005;23(34):8794-801.
191. Timmerman D, Valentin L, Bourne TH, Collins WP, Verrelst H, Vergote I. Terms, definitions and measurements to describe the sonographic features of adnexal tumors: a consensus opinion from the International Ovarian Tumor Analysis (IOTA) group. Ultrasound Obstet Gynecol. 2000;16(4):500-5.
192. Utrilla-Layna J, Alcázar JL, Aubá M, Laparte C, Olartecoechea B, Errasti T, et al. Performance of three-dimensional power Doppler angiography as a third-step assessment in differential diagnosis of adnexal masses. Ultrasound Obstet Gynecol. 2015;45(5):613-5.
193. Van Calster B, Van Hoorde K, Valentin L, Testa AC, Fischerova D, Van Holsbeke C, et al. International Ovarian Tumor Analysis Group. Evaluating the risk of ovarian cancer before surgery using the ADNEX model to differentiate between benign, borderline, early and advanced stage invasive, and secondary metastatic tumours: prospective multicentre diagnostic study. Brit Med J. 2014;349:g 5920. doi: 10.1136/bmj.g5920.
194. Van Holsbeke C, Van Calster B, Valentin L, Testa AC, Ferrazzi E, Dimou I, et al. External validation of mathematical models to distinguish between benign and malignant adnexal tumors: A multicenter study by the International Ovarian Tumor Analysis Group. Clin Cancer Res. 2007;13(15 Pt1):4440-7.
195. Vrachnis N, Sifakis S, Samoli E, Kappou D, Pavlakis K, Iliodromiti Z, et al. Three-dimensional ultrasound and three-dimensional power Doppler improve the preoperative evaluation of complex benign ovarian lesions. Clin Exp Obstet Gynecol. 2012;39(4):474-8.
196. Ward GJ. The radiance lighting simulation and rendering system. Proceedings of 94 SIGGRAPH Conference. Computer Graphics; 1994. pp. 459-72.
197. Welsh A. The questionable value of VOCAL indices of perfusion. Ultrasound Obstet Gynecol. 2010;36(1):126-7.

65

CHAPTER

Music and Ultrasound: Origins of our Emotional Connection to Music

Helena Dukić Satinović

INTRODUCTION

In the intricate symphony of prenatal development, the role of external stimuli in shaping the burgeoning human organism has long fascinated researchers and medical professionals alike. Among the multifaceted environmental factors that interact with the developing fetus, music, with its inherent power to evoke emotions and stimulate cognitive processes, stands as a compelling subject of investigation. Music has an extraordinary ability to transcend language barriers and connect individuals on a profound emotional level, serving as a universal form of human communication. This chapter embarks on an exploration of the intricate relationship between music and the human fetus, seeking to unravel the impact of auditory experiences on prenatal development. We delve into the question of how music, as an art form rooted in the expression of human emotions, influences the emotional development of the unborn child. We aim firstly to present a body of relevant research that has been done so far and then to uncover the mechanisms through which music may shape emotional responses, cognitive abilities, and perhaps even the formation of early social bonds. As we journey through this scientific inquiry, we recognize that music's role extends beyond mere auditory stimulation, paving the way for a deeper understanding of how humans communicate and connect, even before birth. We hope to provide valuable insights into the far-reaching implications of music on human experience, from its earliest moments within the womb to its enduring impact on human connection and emotional expression throughout life.

Firstly, this chapter will present the most relevant and current research that explores the effects music has on the life of the fetus. Secondly, it will focus on why this might be the case. Why does music influence a fetus in numerous ways? What is the purpose of children being born with a developed predisposition for emotional responses to music?

DEVELOPMENT OF FETAL HEARING

The development of musical perception in a fetus is a fascinating process that results from the interplay between genetically programmed auditory sensory development and the auditory stimuli experienced by the developing fetus.[1,2] It is intriguing to note that the foundation for this development is laid very early in fetal life, with the formation of ear follicles becoming visible as early as the sixth week of gestation. However, it is during the 10th week of fetal development that the inner ear undergoes intensive growth, leading to the formation of hair cells on the basal membrane within the cochlea. This development, although not yet fully mature, allows the organ of Corti to begin its rudimentary functioning between the 14th and 15th weeks.[3]

Around the 25th week of pregnancy, the emerging auditory system starts to react to external sounds. This response is observable through indicators like an accelerated heart rate and increased fetal movement.[4] As the pregnancy progresses, more milestones in auditory development are achieved. Between the 24th and 28th weeks, both the auditory receptors themselves (the hair cells) and their synaptic connections mature. Additionally, between the 26th and 28th weeks, myelination of the auditory pathways takes place, which plays a crucial role in the speed and synchronization of nerve impulse transmission.

The early responses of the auditory system to sound are specific, typically focusing on a lower frequency range of 250–500 Hz from roughly the 25–27th week. However, as the pregnancy advances to weeks 29–31, the auditory system's capabilities expand to encompass a broader range of frequencies, notably 1,000–3,000 Hz. This expansion leads to increased discrimination between individual frequencies, heightened sensitivity to quieter sounds, and improved temporal processing to rapidly perceive sounds, including those of short duration.[5] It is worth highlighting that the development of fetal auditory sensitivity, particularly the ability to process very quiet sounds, undergoes a period of intensive maturation between weeks 24 and 35.[6]

Interestingly, the type of auditory stimuli experienced by the fetus has observable effects. Loud music, for instance, can lead to an increase in the fetal heart rate and heightened motor activity. Conversely, quiet music has the opposite effect, inducing a calming response.[7]

Notably, the presence of amniotic fluid in the fetal ears acts as a protective barrier, guarding the sense of hearing against potential damage that could be caused by excessively loud sounds.[3]

What Makes Music Music?

If we want to investigate how fetuses respond to music, it is essential to acknowledge that music has a significantly more intricate acoustic composition compared to simple sounds, and it also possesses several distinct emotional and social characteristics that set it apart from them:

- Music is organized and structured with intentional patterns of rhythm, melody, and harmony. These patterns are carefully composed and can evoke emotional responses. In contrast, most everyday sounds lack this intentional organization.
- Music is a form of artistic expression, a medium through which composers, musicians, and performers convey emotions, stories, and ideas. It carries the intention of the creator and often serves as a means of communication or artistic representation.
- Music has a profound ability to evoke emotions and is frequently used to convey or amplify feelings. It can inspire joy, sadness, excitement, nostalgia, and many other feelings that we cannot experience in everyday life.
- Music is deeply embedded in various cultures and plays a significant role in defining and expressing cultural identities. Different cultures have their own unique musical traditions and styles that reflect their history, values, and beliefs.
- Music can tell a story or convey a narrative, either through lyrics in the case of songs or through purely instrumental compositions. This storytelling aspect distinguishes it from most other sounds.
- Music's interpretation is highly subjective. What one person finds beautiful or moving, another may not. This subjectivity makes music a deeply personal and individualized experience.
- Music has been associated with cognitive benefits, such as improved memory and attention, and it is used in therapeutic contexts to aid in physical and mental health. It has a unique ability to stimulate the brain and impact overall well-being.

In contrast, everyday sounds in our environment, like traffic noise, footsteps, or conversations, lack the intentional artistic, emotional, and cultural dimensions that characterize music. While these sounds serve practical purposes, such as communication or warning signals, they typically lack the structured composition and aesthetic qualities that define music. Fetuses will be exposed to different types of sounds while in utero and will through time learn to react emotionally to some of them by associating certain sounds with certain environmental changes that affect them. This forms the basis of our emotional relationship with music. Once we are born, the already formed potential for the emotional processing of sounds will lend itself to more structured and organized forms of sound (music) and will enable us to enjoy it in numerous ways.

FETAL MUSIC PERCEPTION

Maturation of Fetal Responses to Music

Numerous research studies provide evidence of fetal responses to music through a range of manifestations. In this chapter, we will delve into studies that investigate fetal physiological responses to music, such as changes in heart rate and heart rate variability, as well as their behavioral reactions, including body movements and facial expressions. Our exploration will begin with an examination of studies that explore how fetal reactions evolve during various stages of gestation. Next, we will explore research examining how fetuses respond to music when it is played to their mothers and when it is directly presented to them. Finally, we will consider studies focused on fetal memory in relation to music.

So, how does a fetus react to music during its development? Do the reactions of fetuses change in different gestational ages (GAs)? A remarkable study conducted by Kisilevsky et al.[8] delved into the intricacies of fetal responses to music, assessing the maturation of these responses by monitoring fetal heart rate and movement.

Their findings suggested that a notable shift in processing complex sounds, such as Brahms' lullaby, might take place at approximately 33 weeks of gestation.

Collaborating across international borders, research teams in Canada and Paris jointly embarked on this intriguing investigation. Their choice of Brahms' lullaby was deliberate, as its tempo is renowned for its calming effects. The lullaby was delivered to the developing fetuses through a 5-minute recorded piano rendition. To differentiate the fetal reactions from those of the mothers, the mothers wore earphones playing different music, either country or guitar tunes. During the musical exposure, the researchers meticulously measured fetal heart rates and body movements, with particular attention given to the 30 seconds before and after the onset of the music and the 30 seconds before and after the music's conclusion.

The researchers categorized 114 fetuses based on their GA. The first group fell into the 28–32 weeks GA bracket, indicating that their auditory systems were not yet fully developed. The second group comprised fetuses aged 33–34 weeks GA, an age range where prior research had suggested that the auditory system reaches full development. The third group was comprised of fetuses aged 35–36 weeks GA at the time of the study, and the last group was aptly named "term fetuses," as they had reached or surpassed 37 weeks GA and would no longer be considered premature if born.

When the music commenced, all age groups exhibited discernible changes in their heart rates. Robust statistical analysis strongly indicated that these changes were not mere chance occurrences. In the youngest fetuses, the heart rates typically accelerated at the onset of loud music, signifying a state of arousal. However, when the same music was played softly, heart rates generally decelerated at the start, suggesting a state of heightened attention. This deceleration effect became more pronounced in older fetuses. Interestingly, term fetuses exhibited heart rate deceleration, regardless of whether the music was played loudly or softly. This implied that the most mature fetuses might have been displaying a form of rudimentary attention to the music.

The Paris research team introduced a new variable into the study by presenting the lullaby twice to each fetus. In one set, the lullaby was played first at its standard tempo, 69 beats per minute (BPM), and then at a faster tempo of 118 BPM. The other set experienced a faster tempo before the standard-tempo version. Over the course of the 5-minute musical exposure, the term fetuses demonstrated an increase in heart rate in response to the faster tempo but did not exhibit a similar change when exposed to the lullaby at its regular tempo.

Comprehending this study hinges on grasping the technical terms "arousal" and "attention." In the case of the youngest fetuses, the introduction of music into their environment might have evoked excitement or even a sense of alarm. Conversely, more mature fetuses, potentially capable of a rudimentary form of musical attention, could exhibit distinct responses to variations in tempo, whether faster or slower. If tempo and timbre are significant aspects of music for fetuses, it prompts speculation about the extent to which they can differentiate from other musical features, such as pitch, melodic patterns, and even rhythmic structures, Priest[9] points out. Furthermore, it raises questions about whether they can retain memories of the music they encountered in the womb after they are born, which we will discuss later in this chapter.

Fetal Reactions to Mother's Music Listening

As we have seen, fetuses of different ages react to music stimuli differently. Besides fetal age, there are numerous other factors that influence how a fetus perceives musical stimuli. One of the most important factors to consider is whether the music is played to the fetus only, to the fetus and the mother at the same time, or to the mother only. The importance of separating the effects of music listening on mothers and fetuses is crucial because music can induce different emotional states in mothers and thus affect the behavior of the fetus through the mother's responses. Several studies prove that fetuses respond to mothers listening to music even though they does not hear the music directly.

The study by Araki et al. in 2010[10] sought to investigate whether fetal arm movements change in response to music when it is played either to the mother or directly to the fetus via the mother's lower abdomen. Additionally, the study aimed to explore whether the mother's mood has an impact on alterations in fetal arm movements, which were specifically considered indicators of the fetal response to the mother's emotions.

To conduct the study, diagnostic ultrasound equipment was used to measure fetal arm movements in a group of 47 pregnant women during the 35–36th week of pregnancy. The participants were divided into two categories: (1) The maternal presentation group, where mothers listened to music through headphones, and (2) the fetal presentation group, in which music was delivered directly to the fetus through headphones placed on the mother's abdomen. Fetal arm movements were monitored and recorded via ultrasound for a total of 10 minutes, comprising 5 minutes without music followed by 5 minutes with music. The music used for this purpose was Mozart's Sonata for Two Pianos in D Major, K. 448. The researchers also utilized the Profile of Mood States (POMS)—a brief form to examine the influence of maternal mood on fetal arm movements.

The study's findings revealed that in the maternal presentation group, there were no significant variations in fetal arm movement based on the different moods of the mothers. In contrast, in the fetal presentation group, fetal arm movements increased when the mother displayed higher levels of energy and decreased when the mother exhibited lower energy levels. Furthermore, fetal arm movements decreased when the mother experienced elevated fatigue levels and increased when the mother had lower fatigue levels.

They concluded that the direct presentation of music to the fetus while the mother is in a relaxed state holds the potential to enhance the fetal response to the music, potentially contributing to the well-being of the fetus.

The absence of a fetal reaction to the mother's induced emotion could be attributed to the unfamiliarity of the music for the mothers, which may have hindered the elicitation of a significant emotional response. Research indicates that when participants select their own music, referred to as idiographic music, it receives the highest ratings in terms of personal relevance.[11] This suggests that it prompts, thoughts, memories, or images associated with current or past experiences and that participants believe they can personally connect with the emotions conveyed by the music.

It is crucial to note that music is not the sole method for evoking maternal emotions. A research study preceding this one by the same first author (Araki et al.),[12] induced mother's emotions by presenting different film clips and received different results.

This study explored the connection between fetal movements and the immediate emotional changes experienced by expectant mothers during pregnancy. To elicit specific emotional states, the researchers utilized two well-established feature film clips representing happiness and sadness, which were both subjectively and visibly characterized. While these film clips were being shown, the researchers simultaneously monitored fetal arm, leg, and trunk movements using two ultrasound devices. The results revealed that when pregnant women were exposed to the happy film, there was an increase in the number (but not the duration) of fetal arm movements. Conversely, both the number and duration of fetal arm movements decreased when the sad film was presented. It is worth noting that neither the display of happiness nor sadness had any discernible impact on fetal leg or trunk movements. These findings imply that induced emotions in pregnant women primarily influence the arm movements of their fetuses, with positive and negative emotions producing contrasting effects on fetal motion.

Thus, we can see that the mother's emotions, regardless of how they were induced, affect the fetal behavior. What are the possible consequences of this emotional connection and how it affects fetal life and learning will be discussed in the second part of this chapter. Before that, we will look at the effects music has on fetuses when they listen to it directly, without the mother's participation, as well as the fetal musical memory that extends even beyond birth.

Fetal Reactions to Direct Music Listening

A study conducted by López-Teijón et al.[13] compared how fetuses responded to musical stimuli delivered in two ways: (1) Through the vaginal route [intravaginal music (IVM)] and (2) through emitters placed on the mother's abdomen [abdominal music (ABM)]. The researchers used three-dimensional (3D)/four-dimensional (4D) ultrasound to record and measure facial movements of 106 normal pregnancies ranging from 14 to 39 weeks of gestation. The musical stimuli for ABM were standard headphones playing a flute monody at a volume of 98.6 decibels (dB), while IVM used a specially designed device to emit the same monody at a lower volume of 53.7 dB. Additionally, intravaginal vibration (IVV) at a frequency of 125 Hz and a volume of 68 dB was applied with the same device. Facial movements were assessed at three points: (1) Before stimulation, (2) during stimulation, and for (3) 5 minutes after the stimulation ended.

The results showed that in fetuses older than 16 weeks GA, IVM caused mouthing (MT) in 86.7% of the fetuses and tongue expulsion (TE) in 46.6% of the fetuses. These percentages were significantly higher than those observed with ABM and IVV. No significant changes from the baseline were noted in the ABM and IVV groups. Furthermore, TE occurred >5 times in 5 minutes in 13.3% of the fetuses exposed to IVM. The study found a strong association between IVM and a higher occurrence of both MT and TE. The frequency of TE with IVM increased significantly as GA advanced.

In summary, fetuses between 16 and 39 weeks of gestation displayed repetitive mouth and tongue movements in response to intravaginal music (IVM), which were not observed with ABM or IVV. These findings suggest that neural pathways involved in the auditory-motor system develop as early as the 16th week of gestation. Furthermore, several studies in existing literature propose that the MT and TE movements, seemingly triggered by musical stimuli, might be associated with preparations for vocalization. In line with these observations, music has been noted to provoke TE in infants as young as 4 weeks old, possibly linked to this fetal behavior.[14-16] Besides having implications for prenatal hearing screening methods and the study of fetal neurological stimulation, the results of this study suggest that there might be a relationship between music and language processing. There are numerous other studies that confirm this relationship.[17] Recent studies have revealed that music and speech share several common elements, and certain neural processes are involved in both speech and music, as indicated by Tallal and Gaab in 2006.[18] Moreover, there is emerging evidence suggesting that speech and music functions can mutually benefit each other. Two research papers have shown that phonological awareness, a crucial skill for reading and writing, is closely linked to pitch awareness and musical expertise, as demonstrated by Dege and Schwarzer in 2011[19] and Loui et al.[20] in the same year.

Additionally, Giuliano et al. in 2011[21] found that Mandarin speakers display a high sensitivity to small pitch variations and interval distances, a sensitivity that was not observed in the control group. Thus, the very early TEs and MT that were induced by the heard music in López-Teijón study might shed some light on the role of music as a communication tool.

A follow-up study, conducted 4 years later by the same group of researchers (López-Teijón et al.),[13] explored whether different types of sounds could trigger distinct response patterns in fetuses. They investigated the impact of various qualities of music on fetal facial reactions, using an intravaginal sound emitter designed for this purpose.

In a prospective comparative study carried out by a single operator, they evaluated MT and TE movements in fetuses between 18 and 38 weeks of gestation in response to 15 different songs representing three musical styles. A total of 300 participants were randomly assigned to study groups and exposed to classical music (CM), traditional music (TM) from different cultures, or pop-rock music (PR) using a commercially available intravaginal sound emitter designed for this purpose. After a 5-minute baseline observation, each stimulation lasted for 5 minutes, and the fetal movements (MT and TE) were assessed via abdominal ultrasound.

There were no differences in the frequency of movements observed at the baseline between the study groups. However, during stimulation, a higher percentage of fetuses in all study groups displayed MT and TE movements compared to the baseline. Among the stimulation groups, CM (84%) and TM (79%) led to significantly higher percentages of MT compared to the PR group (59%). Similarly, a significantly higher percentage of TE was observed in the CM group (35%) compared to the TM (20%) and PR groups (15%).

Intravaginal sound stimulation using different types of music directly affected fetal facial movements, including MT and TE, which are not typically observed spontaneously during pregnancy. This finding supports the idea that early neurological stimulation can occur during pregnancy through IVM exposure, activating brainstem pathways related to speech. Classical music, in particular, showed a significantly higher rate of complete speech movements (MT + TE), warranting further investigation.

So far, from the studies discussed above, we have learned the following:

- Younger fetuses, particularly those between 28 and 32 weeks of gestation, appear to react to music with a mix of enthusiasm and potential alarm, indicating a form of auditory sensitivity. On the other hand, older fetuses seem to have a more nuanced response to musical tempo changes, suggesting a rudimentary form of musical awareness and attention.
- Furthermore, maternal emotions deliberately induced in pregnant women have a noticeable impact on fetal movements, specifically in the arms. Positive and negative emotions elicit contrasting effects on fetal motion, underscoring the interplay between maternal emotional states and fetal behavior.
- Additionally, the observation of repetitive mouth and tongue movements in fetuses aged 16–39 weeks when exposed to intravaginally emitted music suggests a fascinating connection between musical stimuli and fetal preparations for vocalization. This finding highlights the potential influence of prenatal auditory

experiences on the early development of vocalization skills.

- The ways in which fetuses perceive music, such as their increasing attention to musical stimuli as they mature, their response to music through repetitive mouth and tongue movements indicating readiness for vocalization, and their "attunement" to the mother's emotions, all suggest that fetal music perception likely serves a purpose. It may serve to "train" or prepare fetuses for improved communication with their mothers after birth, or it could establish a solid foundation for language acquisition. In either scenario, it appears that there is a form of early learning and memorization happening in these initial interactions between sound and fetuses, which equips them for their later lives. Thus, in the next paragraph, we will look at the ways in which a fetus memorizes musical content.

FETAL MUSIC MEMORY

Fetal Memory before Birth

The ability of fetuses to memorize music has been tested in several studies.

Brillo et al. conducted a study[22] to examine fetal music memory. They evaluated and compared the cardiac parameters of fetuses under three different conditions, including those who listened to music before and during nonstress tests, those who listened only during the tests, and those who never listened to music.

They randomly assigned 30 healthy mother-fetus pairs to one of three groups: (1) Group A involved fetuses exposed to a "prelistening" phase (between the 33rd and 36th week of gestation) and music during four nonstress tests, (2) group B included fetuses exposed to music during the four nonstress tests, and (3) group C received four nonstress tests without any music exposure. The researchers measured parameters such as the mean fetal heart rate, fetal heart rate accelerations, fetal heart rate decelerations, fetal movements, and uterine contractions.

In Group A, where fetuses had prior exposure to a specific piece of music during previous sessions, they showed a significant increase in heart rate accelerations and fetal movements during the music-listening session of the last nonstress test. However, there were no notable changes in the number of uterine contractions.

The study's findings indicate that fetuses exhibit a mild response to music they are familiar with, but they do not show significant responses to unfamiliar music, which suggests a form of fetal musical memory.

Several other studies have investigated the impact of repeated exposure to complex auditory stimuli during fetal development.[23] Some research has shown that musical stimuli can lead to increased fetal movements,[24] as well as higher average heart rate and heart rate variability in fetuses familiarized with the music compared to control fetuses.[25]

On the other hand, different studies have explored the fetus's ability to remember its mother's voice during the prenatal period. Studies examining prenatal auditory memory, where mothers recited a specific speech passage daily, either between 35 and 38 weeks GA[26] or from 28 to 34 weeks GA,[27] revealed that the targeted story prompted a brief slowing of the fetal heart rate (cardiac deceleration); whereas, the control story did not, also suggesting that a form of memorization occurred.

Fetal Memory after Birth

Other studies demonstrate the ability of the fetus to remember certain musical elements even after birth. Granier–Deferre et al. (2011)[28] conducted a study in which they proved that fatal memory could last more than just a few days after birth: even up to 6 weeks. Experimental fetuses were subjected to carefully regulated exposure to a descending piano melody twice daily during the 35th, 36th, and 37th weeks of gestation. For about 6 weeks later, they examined the cardiac responses of 25 infants who had been exposed to the melody and 25 infants who had not (control group). This assessment took place while the infants were in a state of quiet sleep. The infants were exposed to both the descending melody and an ascending control piano melody. These melodies had inverse shapes but were similar in terms of their sound characteristics, duration, tempo, rhythm, and nearly identical loudness patterns. All infants exhibited noticeable changes in their heart rate. In the exposed infants, the descending melody led to a more significant heart rate decrease, twice as large as the deceleration observed with the ascending melody and both melodies in the control infants.

This suggests that exposure to a specific melodic pattern over a 3-week period during prenatal development impacts infants' auditory processing or perception, influencing their autonomic nervous system responses even when they are 1 month old. Their findings expand the period during which a memory of a particular sound pattern acquired before birth can be observed, from 3 to 4 days to as long as 6 weeks. This long-term memory for the descending melody is interpreted in terms of persistent neurophysiological adjustments and discussed in the context of its significance for the developmental psychobiology of attention and perception, including early speech perception.

PRENATAL ORIGIN OF MUSIC

One of the most widely spread theories about the origin of music includes Dissanayake's theory about motherse.[29] The definition of motherese is that it is a simple form of language mothers often use when talking to their babies, repetitive in its nature, with exaggerated intonation and rhythm. In Dissanayake's paper: *Antecedents of the temporal arts in early mother-infant interaction*, she proposes a different approach to the usual in explaining the origin of music: instead of assuming that music, similarly to other social behaviors, evolved from a competition affecting reproductive success, she suggests that music originated from "perceptual, behavioral, cognitive and emotional competencies and sensitivities that developed from primate precursors in survival enhancing affiliative interactions between mothers and infants under 6 months of age." This would align with the results discussed earlier in this chapter from López-Teijón et al. study,[13] which found that fetuses exposed to music emitted intravaginally displayed MT and TEs. This indicates an intriguing link between musical stimuli and fetal preparations for vocalization. In essence, it suggests that prenatal auditory experiences may have a potential impact on the early development of vocalization skills. When fetuses are exposed to music (or motherese, which closely resembles a melodic line), they respond by demonstrating early attempts of vocalization through MT and tongue movements.

So, the origin of music is seen by Dissanayake as a multifaceted form of expression that involves the presentation and processing of vocal, physical, and even facial movements, occurring over time or in different spaces. This perspective suggests that due to the increasing need for infant care and nurturing during human evolution, the primates' inclination for establishing emotional connections, beyond just being sociable, became highly essential. To ensure and enhance these emotional bonds, specific mechanisms developed, which, in turn, evolved into various forms of temporal arts, including music. These arts played a role in strengthening affiliative bonds among adults in a species where close cooperation became vital for individual survival. It is acknowledged that musical ability can be employed competitively in certain situations. Nevertheless, the hypothesis presented here can account for music's distinctive and widely observed capacity to unite and synchronize individuals both physically and mentally.

Parncutt and Churkrow's Theory

Richard Parncutt also outlines the similarities between music and motherese by pointing out that Dissanayake's theory can explain many of music's basic properties or universals.[30] He defines music as "an acoustic signal that evokes recognizable patterns (segments, structures, etc.) of sound, involves or implies bodily movement, involves social interaction, is created intentionally, and is accepted and valued by most members of a given cultural group."[31]

Furthermore, he emphasizes that music differs from language in that it conveys its meaning or messages without the use of words. This characterization of music could also serve as a definition for "motherese," as Parncutt highlights. Therefore, the striking similarity between "motherese" and music is likely not a mere coincidence.

However, Parncutt delves deeper and poses the question: If the emotional musical vocabulary of music is built upon that of "motherese," what serves as the foundation for "motherese"? He observes that specific melodic patterns in infant-directed speech can trigger particular emotional responses, such as excitement, capturing attention, prompting a response, or providing comfort. Furthermore, he suggests that this emotional vocabulary is probably primarily acquired from the pitch patterns in everyday speech, and this learning process might occur both before and after birth. The research cited in the initial section of this paper strongly suggests the possibility of vocabulary acquisition before birth.

But how does this learning before birth exactly occur? Parncutt has a theory, based on earlier independent work of Churkrow.

As discussed in Dukic and Jakovljevic's paper,[32] Parncutt and Chuckrow[33] put forth the notion that the intricate interconnections between patterns of sound, movement, and emotion, which are characteristic of music, may ultimately have their origins in the prenatal period. They argue that the fetus could acquire knowledge about these relationships through passive exposure.

The consistent patterns of sound and movement to which the fetus is regularly exposed, such as the mother's voice, breathing, heartbeat, digestion, and bodily movements, are influenced by her physical and emotional state. Patterns of sound and movement that are largely tied to the mother's emotional state can also become associated with hormonal changes through classical conditioning. Because the fetus perceives the behavioral aspects of maternal emotional changes (sound and movement patterns) before the physiological changes (hormonal alterations), the behavioral aspects may predict the physiological ones. After numerous repetitions of such patterns in a specific context, the fetus may begin to emotionally respond to variations in sound and movement patterns that occur in a similar context, essentially anticipating the corresponding hormonal changes.

Music-like sequences might emerge after birth when the patterns of sound and movement produced in "motherese" resemble the patterns of sound and movement that the fetus had heard before birth, Parncutt suggests.

But how do the sounds experienced by the fetus in the womb resemble music? Both Chuckrow and Parncutt[34] independently and systematically examined the structural similarities between musical elements and the internal sound patterns of the human body as perceived by the fetus.

Origin of Musical Beat

One of the most important differences between music and speech is that music is by its nature, isochronic. It moves at regular, evenly-spaced intervals. This music feature is referred to as musical beat and is organized in units called measures that can consist of different numbers of beats. What is the origin of this particular music feature?

In his paper titled *Churkrow's theory of the prenatal origin of music*,[33] Parncutt examined how both maternal footsteps and maternal heartbeat might impact the fetus and its subsequent perception of rhythm. While Chuckrow initially mentioned maternal walking as a stimulus, he did not initially identify its specific musical counterpart. Later, he associated the maternal footsteps that the fetus hears before birth with the beat in music, particularly popular music.[35,36]

In musical rhythm, one or more evenly spaced pulse sequences come together to create either a meter or polyrhythm. Since the fetal heart rate is approximately double that of the adult (maternal) heart rate, with the slower maternal heartbeat being louder, Chuckrow proposed that the combination of these two heartbeats could account for both meter and polyrhythm. While the 2:1 ratio is only an approximation, this concept aligns with meters like 3/4 or polyrhythms like 2 against 3. Chuckrow illustrated this by presenting combined maternal and fetal electrocardiograms from a study by Larks and Dasgupta,[37] which displayed the three main types of maternal/fetal rhythms according to the sources available at the time, namely, 1:1, 1:2, and 1:3.

Chuckrow's approach can explain why the slower of the two pulses in a duple pattern typically has a period of around 600 milliseconds, which roughly corresponds to the maternal heartbeat. The faster pulse corresponds to the fetal heartbeat. Of course, the tempo and duration of musical notes are also influenced by the tempo and duration patterns of other bodily movements.

Chuckrow speculated about a potential connection between the changes in combined heartbeat rhythms, resulting from the maternal emotions repeatedly experienced by the fetus, and the heightened excitement or arousal that one experiences when listening to music as the tempo increases or as relationships between rhythmic layers develop.

Additionally, Parncutt linked the slowing down of music, which enhances a sense of conclusion, to the way footsteps decelerate as a destination is approached. Chuckrow considered sinus arrhythmia, or variations in heart rate with inhalation and exhalation, if musical phrases align with maternal breathing, this could explain why musical phrases often speed up at the beginning and slow down towards the end, as observed in the work of Penel and Drake (1998).

Origin of Melodic Lines

But what about the melodic lines that so often prompt our emotions when listening to music? Parncutt[33] drew a connection between the ascending and descending pitch in a musical tune and the way the maternal spoken voice is perceived by the fetus. While not explicitly using the terms "melody" or "phrasing," Chuckrow talked about the similarity between rising and falling inflections in speech and the articulation of syllables in human speech, which he referred to as "tonal patterns in music." Parncutt linked the boundaries of musical phrases to the pauses during a mother's inhalations, whereas Chuckrow discussed the influence of maternal speech and breathing as stimuli without explicitly addressing their musical counterpart, such as phrasing.

Origin of Musical Harmony

There is one more element of music that often goes unnoticed by nonmusicians, but nonetheless greatly influences our emotions, and that is harmony.

Parncutt[33] associated musical harmony with the harmonics present in the mother's vocalizations that are audible to the fetus during pregnancy. A harmonic series (also overtone series) is defined as the sequence of harmonics, musical tones, or pure tones whose frequency is an integer multiple of a *fundamental frequency*. In addition, Chuckrow suggested that because both sides of the fetal eardrum are immersed in amniotic fluid, this could result in greater distortion of the harmonics in the mother's voice. This distortion would lead to the emergence of audible harmonics when exposed to a pure tone, such as the fundamental frequency of the maternal voice when the higher partials are masked. The human ear has evolved to function optimally in an environment with air, not liquid (like amniotic fluid) on both sides of the eardrum. The ideal auditory function involves several factors, including harmonic distortion (as outlined by Petit, El-Amraoui, and Avan).[38] The presence of a different medium, such as amniotic fluid, would increase harmonic distortion compared to postnatal perception. Consequently, louder maternal speech, often indicative of stronger emotions, would generate disproportionately more harmonic distortion in the fetal inner ear, increasing the likelihood of perceiving higher harmonics. Chuckrow argued that this effect aligns with the concept that increased emotional intensity in music is associated with greater harmonic complexity.

Finally, Chuckrow compared the idea of counterpoint, a compositional technique in which multiple melodic lines (or "voices") complement each other while maintaining their independence, with the independent fluctuations in the pitch of maternal formants. In natural human speech, two to four formants are typically identifiable.

Biological and Behavioral Basis of Parncutt's Theory

Assuming that the aforementioned sounds are what the fetus actually hears while in the uterus, we need to look at how it might associate them with the emotional content.

Parncutt[30] examined the time delay between maternal behavioral shifts, such as changes in movement, vocalization, and heartbeat in response to surprises, and the associated hormonal changes that might also impact the fetus. He suggested a classical conditioning model where a predictive conditioned stimulus is paired with a subsequent unconditioned stimulus.

Similarly, Chuckrow considered the time gap between a cause and its effect as hormones linked to changing maternal emotions move from the mother's body into the fetal bloodstream. When there's a change in the mother's emotional state, her heart rate may immediately respond, but the fetal heart rate would not change at once because the hormones related to maternal emotions cannot instantly cross the placenta. Chuckrow also recognized that a change solely on the mother's part would influence the rhythm created by the combination of both heartbeats. This change could potentially alert the fetus to impending maternal hormonal changes, providing an opportunity for preparation or adaptation. After birth, alterations in musical rhythm might similarly trigger corresponding hormonal or emotional patterns.

In summary, the theory proposed by Parncutt and Churkrow offers a compelling hypothesis concerning the source of our musical inclinations. This theory places significant emphasis on the events that occur during gestation, particularly the fetus's capacity to perceive and respond to various sounds, as well as its synchronization with the mother's emotional states.

In the following section, I will explore an equally intriguing theory concerning the emergence of emotion in music, one that also delves into our prenatal development: Narmour's theory of implications and realizations.

Narmour's Theory of Implications and Realizations

As previously discussed, it is believed that a fetus learns emotional responses through a process of conditioning, a hormonal release that triggers an emotional reaction is preceded by a particular sound pattern, and with repeated exposure, a connection is established. At this stage, the fetal emotional responses are likely quite basic, characterized by what we could label as content or calm states and distressed or anxious states.

As mentioned by Dukic,[39] Stern's[40] explanation underscores the early interactions between a mother and her baby as a form of emotional exchange, characterized by the tension of waiting for food and the relaxation experienced when being fed. Stern referred to these brief interactions as "tiny narratives" or "proto-narrative envelopes" and proposed that they serve as fundamental units or building blocks for constructing the child's representational world.

Narmour's[41] implication-realization model of music utilized the concept of a musical plot, involving alternating tension and relaxation, to develop a musical grammar that generates expectations and their subsequent resolutions, mirroring Stern's idea of proto-narrative exchange. Narmour's theory is intriguing because it suggests that when listeners hear a melody, they typically form expectations about its continuation. These expectations are believed to result from a combination of innate and learned factors, encompassing both the bottom-up and top-down systems of melodic implication. While the principles of the former are considered hardwired, innate, and universal, the principles of the latter are viewed as learned and dependent on musical experience.

The top-down influences on expectancy encompass both extrinsic knowledge regarding style-specific norms, such as diatonic interpretations, tonal and metrical hierarchies, and harmonic progressions, and intrinsic knowledge about specific compositional elements, such as distinctive motifs and rhythmic patterns within a particular piece. Since the top-down system operates largely independently of the bottom-up system, it can generate implications that may conflict with those generated by the bottom-up system.

Narmour applies the bottom-up Gestalt principles (innate) to three aspects of melody: The direction of pitch change, the motion between intervals, and the specific pitches involved. The fundamental hypothesis is that small intervals, defined as unison up to and including the major third, imply similarity in both intervallic motion and pitch direction. In contrast, intervals of a minor sixth or larger imply a reversal of pitch direction and intervallic motion. In essence, the innate, bottom-up system is based on two key principles: (1) The implication of continuation and (2) the implication of reversal. If these implications are realized in the way that we expected (small intervals are followed by other small intervals in the same melodic direction, and large intervals are followed by a small interval in the opposite melodic direction), the feeling of tension induced by the melodic implication will be followed by a feeling of relaxation (fulfillment of expectation). This will create a similar "proto-narrative envelope" as proposed by Stern. A "tiny narrative" that is present in our earliest life experience (waiting for food and feeding), as well as presumably before birth where we learn to expect (hearing a certain sound coupled with a delayed hormonal response).

The inclusion and specification of innate factors in this model represent one of its most significant contributions to the field of music psychology. These factors have demonstrated their influence on melodic expectancies across listeners from diverse musical cultures, even when tested in various musical and nonmusical contexts. This universality aligns with their proposed universality. In essence, Narmour's theory, although centered on different aspects of musical emotion compared to Parncutt and Chuckrow's theory, independently suggests a similar hypothesis: We possess preexisting emotional processing for certain aspects of music from birth, implying that these aspects are learned before birth. In this regard, Parncutt and Chuckrow's theory may complement or provide an explanation for specific aspects of Narmour's theory.

CONCLUSION

In this chapter, we initially focused on exploring significant medical research regarding fetal music perception. Our investigation encompassed how fetuses exhibit a growing interest in musical stimuli as they develop, their responses to music, characterized by repetitive mouth and tongue movements that imply readiness for vocalization, and their sensitivity to maternal emotions. Furthermore, we delved into studies that probed fetal musical memory, revealing that fetuses can remember and recognize a melodic line they have encountered, with this memory potentially persisting beyond birth. These findings collectively suggest that fetal music perception has a biologically meaningful purpose.

Subsequently, our attention turned to the prominent psychological and musicological theories that offer insights into why fetuses respond to music as they do. Parncutt and Churkrow's theory proposed a mechanism through which fetuses might acquire musicality before birth, associating intrauterine sounds with the mother's emotional responses and linking it to our need to comprehend our mother's communication postnatally, as seen in motherese. This theory implied a connection between music and language, as mentioned earlier.

Similarly, we explored Narmour's theory of implication and realization, which, although focused on different aspects of musical emotion compared to Parncutt and

Churkrow's theory, independently posited a similar hypothesis: That we possess inherent emotional processing for specific aspects of music from birth, indicating that these aspects are learned before birth. These innate forms of musical processing form the core of emotional music processing, where musical implications create emotional tension and musical realizations generate emotional relaxation.

In conclusion, we have observed that music seems to play a fundamental role in the process of language acquisition. To fully grasp this connection, it is crucial to deepen our understanding of the intricate relationship between the fetus and the mother's emotions. The evidence suggests that prenatal exposure to musical stimuli may not only influence fetal behavior but also lay the foundation for early vocalization skills and, potentially, language development. Recognizing the extent to which the fetus is attuned to the mother's emotional cues and how these cues intersect with musical experiences is vital for unraveling the mysteries of this crucial link between music and language acquisition.

Beyond its role in language acquisition, the connection between the mother and the fetus could also explain various universal features of music. These include shared emotions during group music-making, a preference for rhythmic entrainment and synchronicity, the effects of music on pain perception, its influence on sports performance, and its role in sustaining prolonged repetitive tasks. Additionally, it could account for the transcendental emotions associated with music and the ties between music and religion, as well as its role in religious and spiritual practices.

REFERENCES

1. Barrett MS. Singing and invented song-making in infants' and young children's early learning and development: from shared to independent song-making. In: Welch GF, Howard DM, Nix J (Eds). The Oxford handbook of singing. Oxford, UK: Oxford University Press; 2019. pp. 471-87.
2. Houde M, Narendran N. A literature review of the influence of early childhood mucus education and music therapy on child development. Can J Music Ther. 2018;24:27-39.
3. Pocwierz-Marciniak I, Harciarek M. The effect of musical stimulation and mother's voice on the early development of musical abilities: A neuropsychological perspective. Int J Environ Res Public Health. 2021;18(16):8467.
4. Hepper PG, Shahidullah BS. The development of fetal hearing. Fetal Matern Med Rev. 1994;6:167-79.
5. Parncutt R. Prenatal development. In: McPherson G (Ed). The Child as Musician: The Handbook of Musical Development. Oxford, UK: Oxford University Press; 2016. pp. 3-30.
6. Polin RA, Abman SH, Rowitch DH, Benitz W. In: Fox WW (Ed). Fetal and Neonatal Physiology, 6th edition. Philadelphia: Saunders Co.; 2011.
7. Lecaunet JP. Prenatal auditory experiences. In: Deliege I, Sloboda JA (Eds). Musical Beginnings: Origins and Development of Musical Competence. Oxford University Press; Oxford, UK: 1996. pp. 3-34.
8. Kisilevsky BS, Hains SMJ, Jacquet A-Y, Granier-Deferre C, Lecanuet JP. Maturation of fetal responses to music. 2004;7(5):550-9.
9. Priest J. Research Review: Fetal Responses to Music. Perspectives. 2010;5(2)Spring:20-4.
10. Araki M, Nishitani S, Miyamura T, Masuzaki H, Oishi K, Shinohara K. Fetal Response to Mozart's Music. Acta Medica Nagasakiensia. 2010;55(1):7-13.
11. Ellard KK, Farchione TJ, Barlow DH. Relative effectiveness of emotion induction procedures and the role of personal relevance in a clinical sample: A comparison of film, images, and music. J Psychopathol Behav Assess. 2012;34(2):232-43.
12. Araki M, Nishitani S, Ushimaru K, Masuzaki H, Oishi K, Shinohara K. Fetal response to induced maternal emotions. J Physiol Sci. 2010;60(3):213-20.
13. López-Teijón M, Garcia-Faura A, Prats-Galino A. Fetal facial expression in response to intravaginal music emission. Ultrasound. 2015;23(4):216-23.
14. Jones SS. Exploration or imitation? The effect of music on 4-week-old infants' tongue protrusions. Infant Behav Dev. 2006;29(1):126-30.
15. Kurjak A, Stanojevic M, Andonotopo W, Salihagic-Kadic A, Carrera JM, Azumendi G. Behavioral pattern continuity from prenatal to postnatal life--a study by four-dimensional (4D) ultrasonography. J Perinat Med. 2004;32(4):346-53.
16. Stanojevic M, Kurjak A, Salihagić-Kadić A, Vasilj O, Miskovic B, Shaddad AN, et al. Neurobehavioral continuity from fetus to neonate. J Perinat Med. 2011;39(2):171-7.
17. Jäncke L. The relationship between music and language. Front Psychol. 2012;3:123.
18. Tallal P, Gaab N. Dynamic auditory processing, musical experience and language development. Trends Neurosci. 2006;29(7):382-90.
19. Dege F, Schwarzer G. The effect of a music program on phonological awareness in preschoolers. Front Psychol. 2011;2:124.
20. Loui P, Kroog K, Zuk J, Winner E, Schlaug G. Relating pitch awareness to phonemic awareness in children: implications for tone-deafness and dyslexia. Front Psychol. 2011;2:111.
21. Giuliano RJ, Pfordresher PQ, Stanley EM, Narayana S, Wicha NY. Native experience with a tone language enhances pitch discrimination and the timing of neural responses to pitch change. Front Psychol. 2011;2:146.
22. Brillo E, Tosto V, Ceccagnoli A, Nikolova N, Pinzaglia V, Bordoni F, et al. The effect of prenatal exposure to music on

fetal movements and fetal heart rate: a pilot study. J Matern Fetal Neonatal Med. 2021;34(14):2274-82.
23. Pino O. Fetal memory: The effects of prenatal auditory experience on human development. BAOJ Med Nursing. 2016;2(4):2.
24. Hepper PG. Fetal memory: does it exist? What does it do? Acta Paediatr Suppl. 1996;416:16-20.
25. James DK, Spencer CJ, Stepsis BW. Fetal learning: a prospective randomized controlled study. Ultrasound in Obst Gynecol. Ultrasound Obstet Gynecol. 2002;20(5):431-8.
26. DeCasper AJ, Lecanuet JP, Busnel MC, Granier-Deferre C, Maugeais R. Fetal reactions to recurrent maternal speech. Infant behavior and development. 1994;17(2):159-64.
27. Krueger C, Holditch-Davis D, Quint S, DeCasper A. Recurring auditory experience in the 28-to 34-week-old fetus. Infant Behav Dev. 2004;27(4):537-43.
28. Granier-Deferre C, Bassereau S, Ribeiro A, Jacquet AY, DeCasper AJ. A melodic contour repeatedly experienced by human near-term fetuses elicits a profound cardiac reaction one month after birth. PLoS One. 2011;6(2):e17304.
29. Dissanayake E. Antecedents of the Temporal Arts in Early Mother-Infant Interaction. The origins of music. 2001;27:389.
30. Parncutt R. Prenatal and infant conditioning, the mother schema, and the origins of music and religion. Musicae Scientiae. 2009;13(2_suppl):119-50.
31. Papousek M. Intuitive Parenting: A Hidden Source of Musical Stimulation in Infancy. In Deliage I, Sloboda J (Eds). Musical Beginnings: Origins and Development of Musical Competence. New York: Oxford University Press; 1996. pp. 88-12.
32. Dukic H, Jakovljevic M. Music, religion and health; a scientific perspective on the origin of our relationship to music. Psychiatria Danubina. 2021;33(Suppl 3):143-9.
33. Parncutt R, Chuckrow R. Chuckrow's theory of the prenatal origin of music. Musicae Scientiae. 2019;23(4):403-25.
34. Parncutt R. Prenatal experience and the origins of music. In Blum T (Ed). Prenatal perception, learning, and bonding. Berlin: Leonardo; 1993. pp. 253-77.
35. Chuckrow R. T'ai-chi ch'uan: Embracing the pearl. Briarcliff Manor, NY: Rising Mist Publications; 1995.
36. Chuckrow R. The Tai Chi Book: Refining and Enjoying a Lifetime of Practice, Revised edition. Roslindale, MA: YMAA Publication Center; 1998.
37. Larks SD, Dasgupta K. Fetal electrocardiography, with special reference to early pregnancy. Am Heart J. 1958;56(5):701-14.
38. Petit C, El-Amraoui A, Avan P. Audition: hearing and deafness. In: Neuroscience in the 21st Century: From Basic to Clinical. Cham: Springer International Publishing; 2022. pp. 1075-142.
39. Dukić H. Music, Ultrasound, and Artificial Intelligence: Recent Advances and Future Challenges, Donald School Journal of Ultrasound in Obstetrics & Gynecology. 2022;16(3):187-91.
40. Stern DN. The 'pre-narrative envelope': An alternative view of 'unconscious phantasy' in infancy. Bul Anna Freud Centre. 1992;15(4):291-318.
41. Narmour E. The analysis and cognition of melodic complexity: The implication realization model. Chicago: University of Chicago Press; 1992.

Index

Page numbers followed by *b* refer to box, *f* refer to figure, *fc* refer to flowchart, and *t* refer to table.

A

C

D

E

F

I

M

N

O

P

U

V